5 REASONS

you should

KEEP CALM AND CARRY

Taber's®

5. No need to guess which of the thousands of online search results are accurate, reliable, and objective.

4. Your personal team of nursing, medical, and health sciences experts is at your side.

3. You'll always know how to say it correctly with audio pronunciation for 33,000 terms.

2. On your phone or tablet, Taber's Online, powered by Unbound Medicine, is waiting for you.

#1. TABER'S IS FOR NURSES!

Buy yours today!

www.Tabers.com

F.A. DAVIS COMPANY

D0164193

Learn to

THINK LIKE A NURSE FROM THE VERY FIRST DAY.

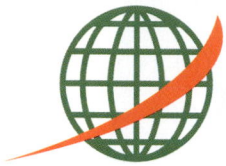

Your nursing education goes well beyond the textbook.

Davis*Plus*.com is your online home for a wealth of learning activities, study tools, and resources that make learning easier. Build your confidence as you prepare for class and clinical.

Your Davis*Plus* Resources are waiting for you.

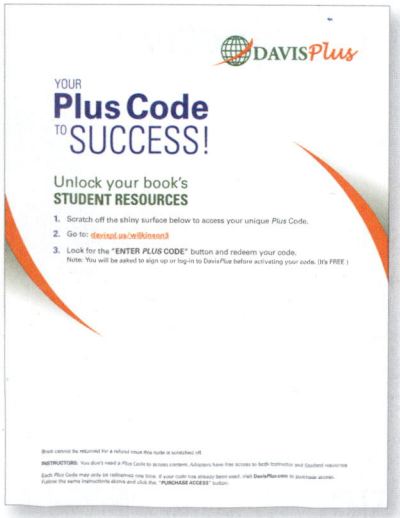

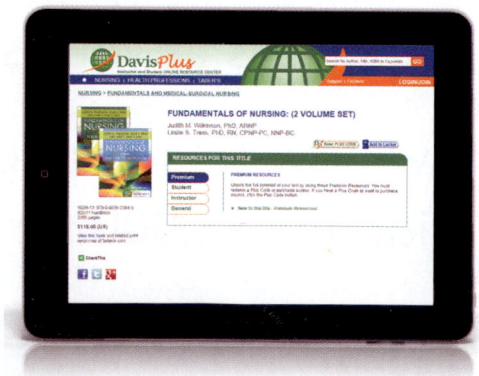

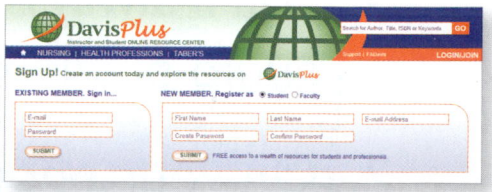

1

Scratch off the shiny surface to reveal your *Plus* Code.*

2

Go to **davispl.us/wilkinson3.** Log in or create your Davis*Plus* account. It's easy and it's FREE.

3

Look for the "Enter *Plus* Code" button to redeem your code and access your resources.

The next time you visit, look for the locker icon. You'll find all of your resources in your locker, making it easy to access the materials you need to study for class, lab, and clinical.

*Each *Plus* Code may only be redeemed one time. If your code has already been used, visit Davis*Plus*.com to purchase access. Follow the same instructions above and click the, "Purchase Access" button.

Everything you need to prepare for class, lab, and clinical.

The Electronic Study Guide Chapter Resources help you master the textbook material chapter by chapter. For each chapter in the book you'll find…

- NCLEX-Style Chapter Review Questions
- Learning Outcomes
- Responses to all Critical-Thinking Questions and Exercises in the text
- Care Plans
- Care Maps
- Knowledge Maps
- Documentation Exercises
- Supplemental Materials such as tables, boxes, figures
- Resources for Caregivers & Health Professionals

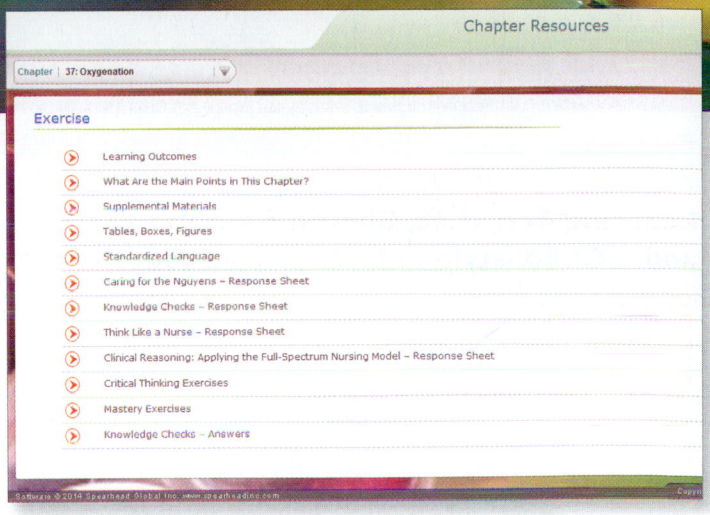

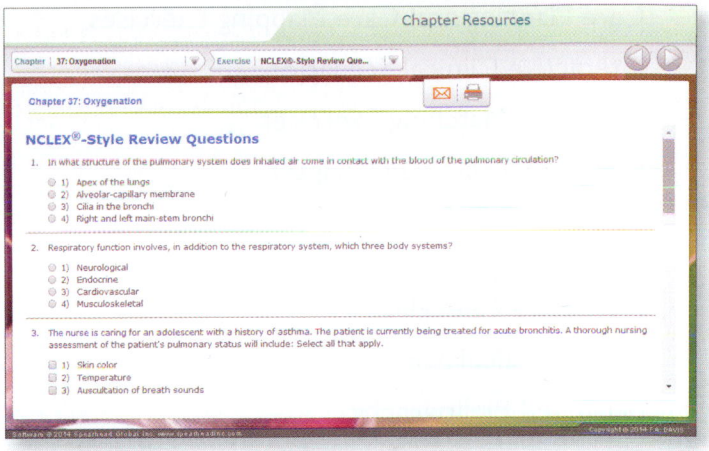

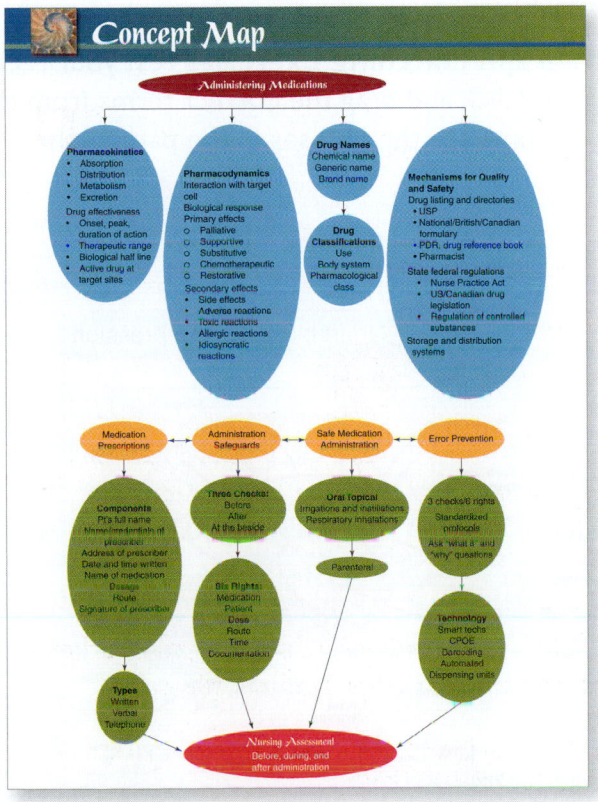

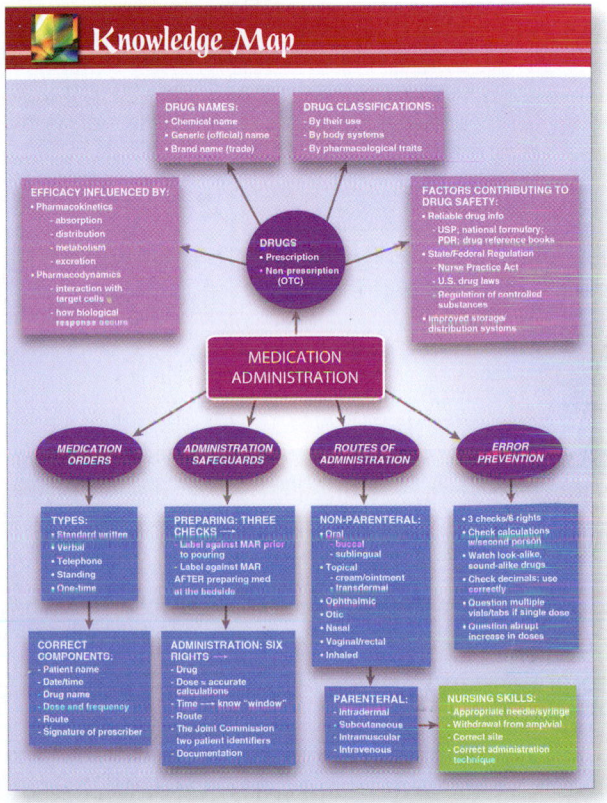

Learning Activities, Clinical Resources, and NCLEX-style quizzes prepare you for class and clinical.

- Davis Digital Version
- Student Question Bank
- Animations
- Concept Care Map Generator
- Care Planning and Care Mapping Exercises
- Interactive Clinical Scenarios
- Paragraph Matching Exercises
- Bonus Microbiology Chapter: *The Human Biome*
- Alphabetical List of NANDA Diagnoses
- Procedure Checklists
- Dosage Calculator
- Expanded Bibliography

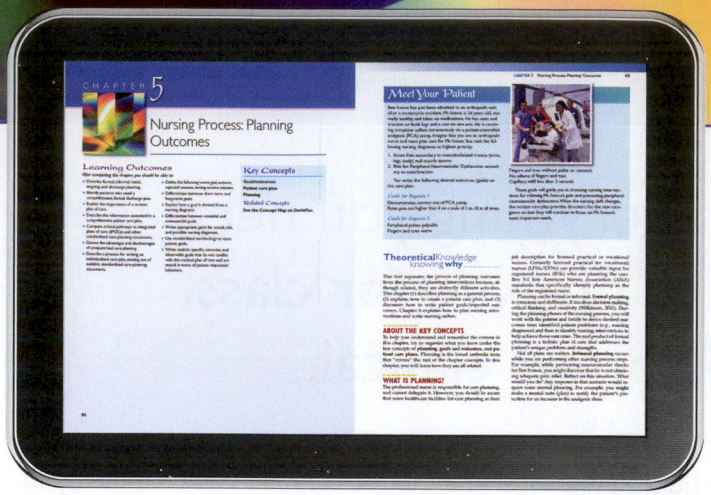

Davis Digital Version is your complete text online. Quickly search for the content you need. Add notes, highlights, and bookmarks.

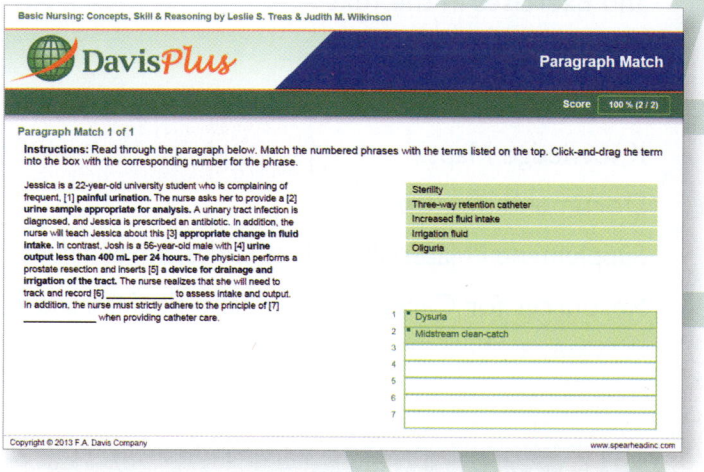

Paragraph Matching Exercises test your recall of facts. Click and drag the correct terms from the list to complete the phrases in the paragraph.

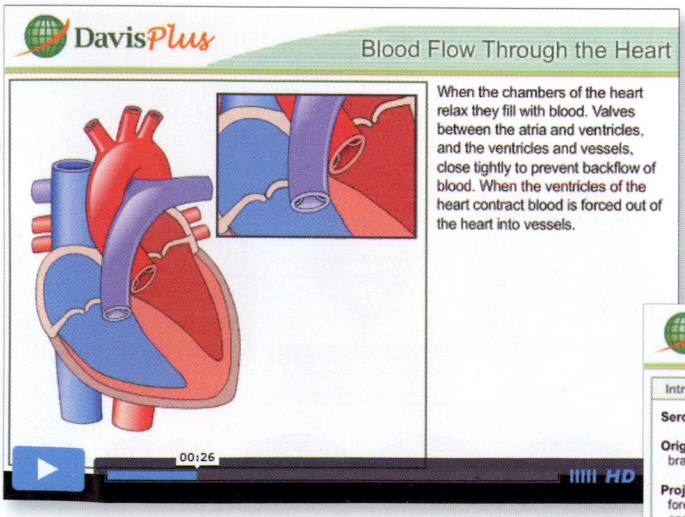

Full-Color Animations make often complex physiological processes easy to understand.

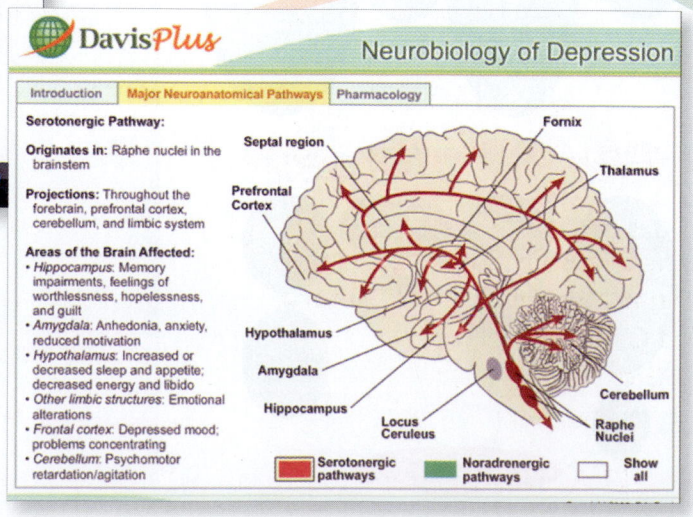

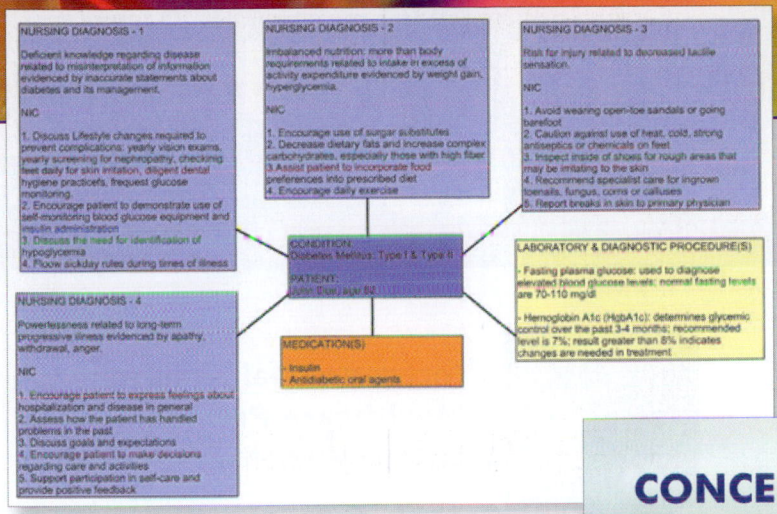

Concept Care Map Generator makes care planning easier. Use it to organize your assessment data, identify patient problems, determine the appropriate nursing diagnoses and interventions, and assess outcomes.

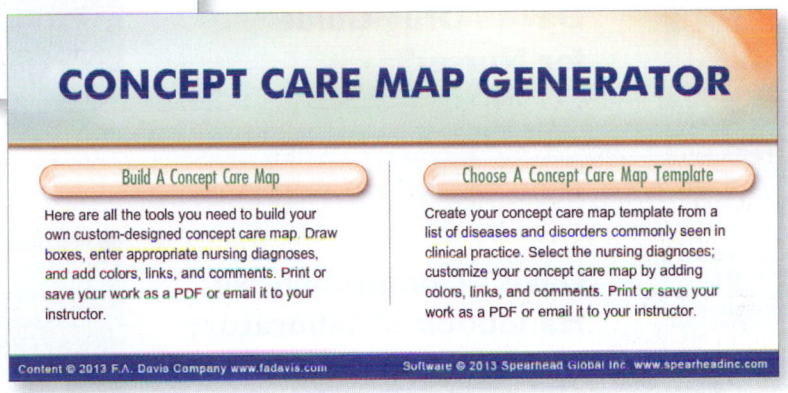

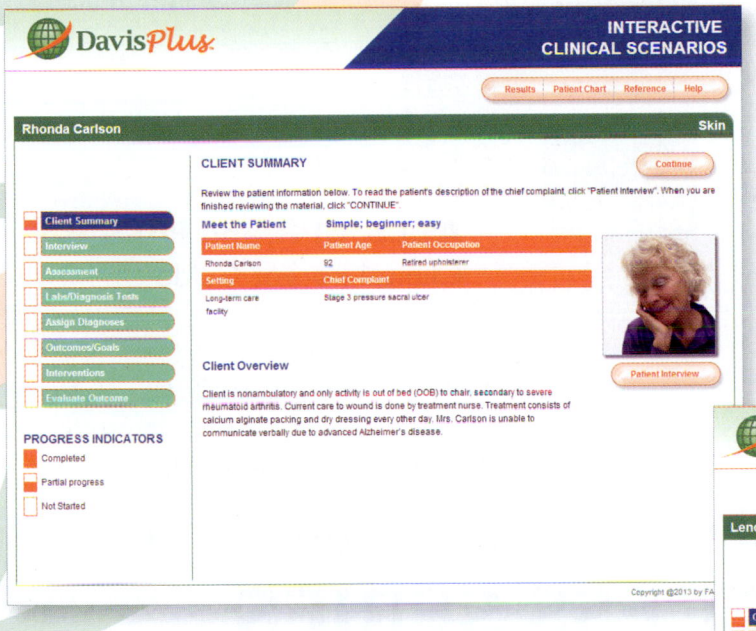

Interactive Clinical Scenarios let you apply your knowledge to virtual patient scenarios to help develop your critical-thinking skills and prepare for common clinical challenges.

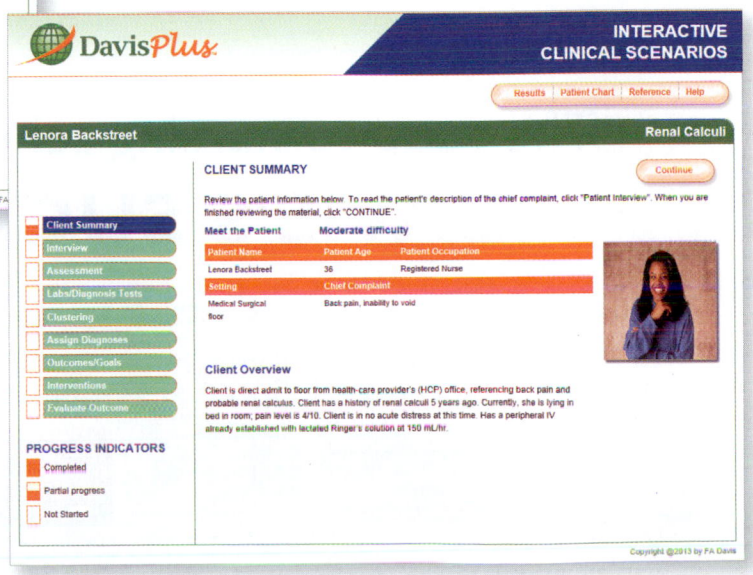

Don't miss these Davis*Plus* Resources

- Chapter Overviews
- Podcasts and Body Sounds Library
- Preventing Medication Errors Tutorial
- Wound Care Tutorial
- Audio Glossary
- And so much more!

Visit **www.Davis*Plus*.com** today!

ESSENTIAL NURSING REFERENCES

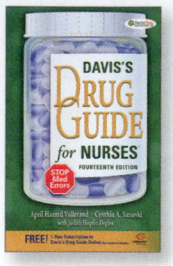

Davis's Drug Guide for Nurses®

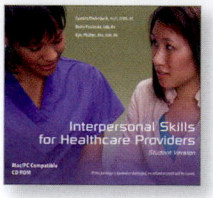

Interpersonal Skills for Healthcare Providers
Student Version

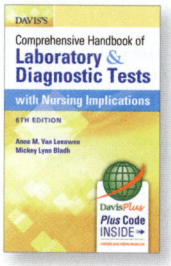

Davis's Comprehensive Handbook of Laboratory and Diagnostic Tests With Nursing Implications

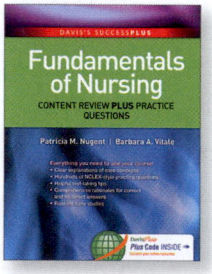

Fundamentals of Nursing
Content Review *Plus* Practice Questions

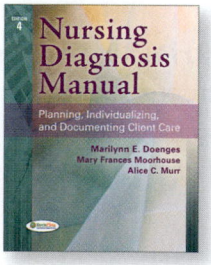

Nursing Diagnosis Manual
Planning, Individualizing, and Documenting Client Care

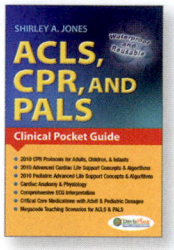

ACLS, CPR, and PALS
Clinical Pocket Guide

The road to nursing school success begins with

DAVIS'S SUCCESS SERIES

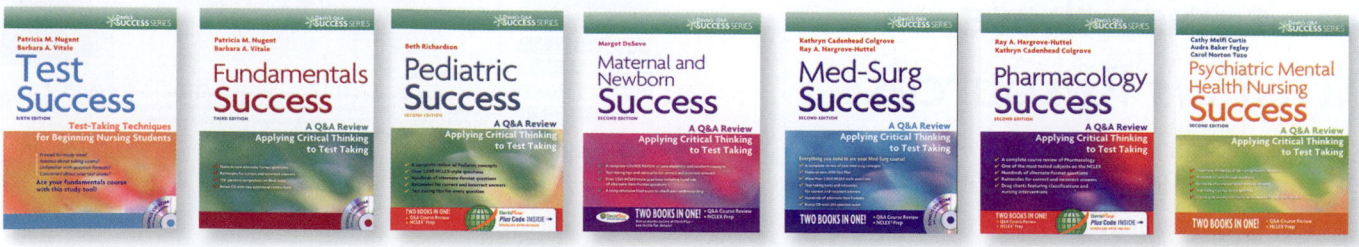

Buy today!

www.FADavis.com

FOR CLASSROOM AND CLINICAL SUCCESS

Watch. Do. Learn.

Davis's Nursing Skills Videos

Real nurses demonstrate essential nursing skills step by step.

All of the skills and procedures you need to master are here! Each video demonstrates a procedure, while a narrator explains clearly what to do. Procedure variations include instructions for what to do in special situations.

Watch each video from beginning to end without interruption, or watch individual sections as many times as you wish.

Select the format you need.

- DVD
- Unlimited Online Streaming Access
- 1-Year Online Streaming Access

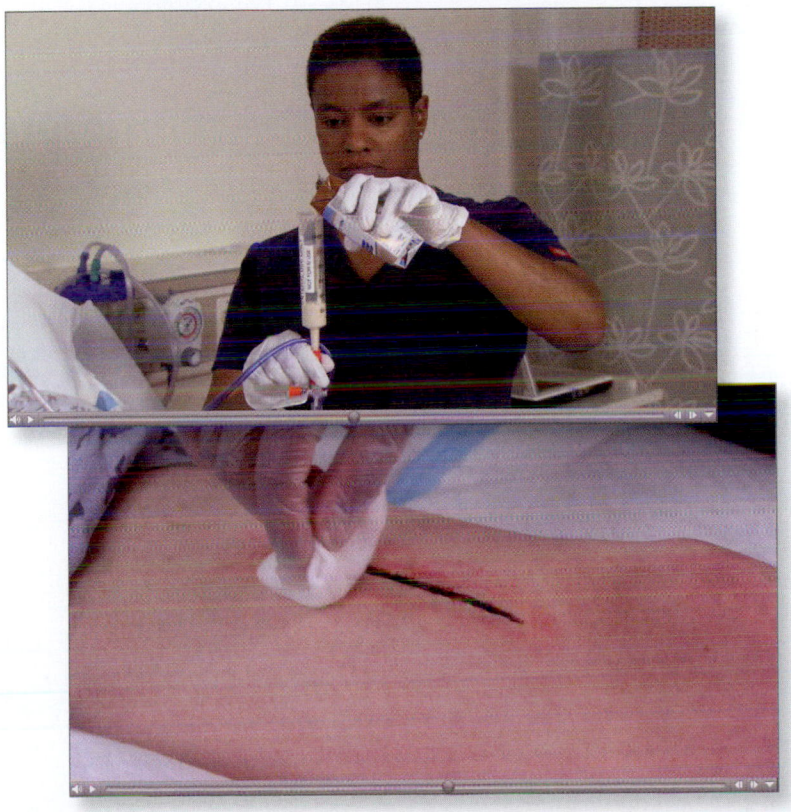

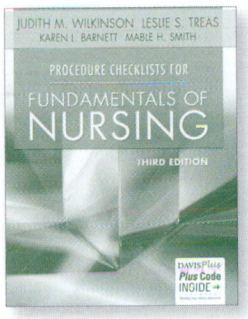

Quick access to every step

Procedure Checklists, 3rd Edition

Quickly reference all of the steps for common nursing procedures.

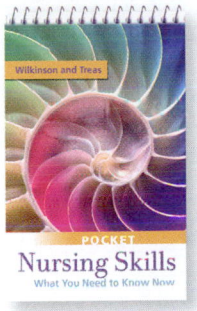

Pocket-perfect guidance

Pocket Nursing Skills, What You Need to Know Now

Put the whats, whys, and hows for fundamentals skills and procedures right at your fingertips.

Buy today!

www.FADavis.com

THIRD EDITION

FUNDAMENTALS OF NURSING

VOLUME 2

THINKING, DOING, AND CARING

Judith M. Wilkinson, PhD, CNS, APRN

Leslie S. Treas, PhD, RN, CPNP-PC, NNP-BC

Karen L. Barnett, DNP, RN

Mable H. Smith, BSN, MN, JD, PhD

F.A. Davis Company • Philadelphia

F. A. Davis Company
1915 Arch Street
Philadelphia, PA 19103
www.fadavis.com

Copyright © 2016 by F. A. Davis Company

Copyright © 2016 by F. A. Davis Company. All rights reserved. This book is protected by copyright. No part of it may be reproduced, stored in a retrieval system, or transmitted in any form or by any means, electronic, mechanical, photocopying, recording, or otherwise, without written permission from the publisher.

Printed in the United States of America

Last digit indicates print number: 10 9 8 7 6 5 4 3 2 1

Publisher, Nursing: Lisa B. Houck
Director of Content Development: Darlene D. Pedersen
Senior Content Project Manager: Adrienne D. Simon
Content Project Manager: Christina L. Snyder
Special Projects Editor: Shirley A. Kuhn
Electronic Project Manager: Katherine E. Crowley
Design and Illustrations Manager: Carolyn O'Brien

As new scientific information becomes available through basic and clinical research, recommended treatments and drug therapies undergo changes. The author(s) and publisher have done everything possible to make this book accurate, up to date, and in accord with accepted standards at the time of publication. The author(s), editors, and publisher are not responsible for errors or omissions or for consequences from application of the book, and make no warranty, expressed or implied, in regard to the contents of the book. Any practice described in this book should be applied by the reader in accordance with professional standards of care used in regard to the unique circumstances that may apply in each situation. The reader is advised always to check product information (package inserts) for changes and new information regarding dose and contraindications before administering any drug. Caution is especially urged when using new or infrequently ordered drugs.

Library of Congress Cataloging-in-Publication Data

Wilkinson, Judith M., 1946- , author.
Fundamentals of nursing / Judith M. Wilkinson, Leslie S. Treas, Karen L. Barnett, Mable H. Smith. — Third edition.
p. ; cm.
Includes bibliographical references and index.
ISBN 978-0-8036-4076-4
I. Treas, Leslie S., author. II. Barnett, Karen L., author. III. Smith, Mable H., author. IV. Title.
[DNLM: 1. Nursing Process. 2. Nursing Care. 3. Nursing Theory. WY 100]

RT41
610.73—dc23

2014025775

Authorization to photocopy items for internal or personal use, or the internal or personal use of specific clients, is granted by F. A. Davis Company for users registered with the Copyright Clearance Center (CCC) Transactional Reporting Service, provided that the fee of $.25 per copy is paid directly to CCC, 222 Rosewood Drive, Danvers, MA 01923. For those organizations that have been granted a photocopy license by CCC, a separate system of payment has been arranged. The fee code for users of the Transactional Reporting Service is: 8036-1169-2/04 0 + $.25.

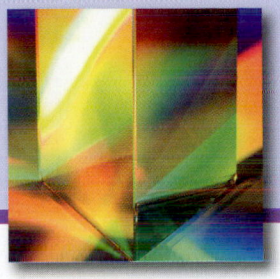

Preface

We chose our book title carefully. We have used the words *theory, concepts, application, thinking, doing,* and *caring* because we believe that excellent nursing requires an equal mix of knowledge, thought, and action. Nurses use all of these to express caring. It is knowledge and its application—not just the tasks nurses do—that delineate the various levels of nursing. Even so, skillful performance of tasks is essential to full attainment of the nursing role.

We present our material in two volumes to enable students to focus on material suitable for use in specific venues. Volume 2 was designed to be a compact, easy-to-carry reference to use in the skills lab and in clinical. This volume contains practical, "how to" information for safely performing nursing actions and interacting with real patients. Rationales for each action explain the "why behind the what" to help you practice nursing based on concepts rather than cookbook-style steps. Volume 2 offers practice-based forms, assessment questionnaires, and other clinical tips, but it is not limited to skills and procedures. It includes both thinking and doing, the same as does Volume 1; however, the emphasis is different in each volume. Volume 2 works seamlessly with Volume 1, the Skills Videos, and Davis*Plus* to provide a user-friendly learning experience that will surely stimulate new enthusiasm for learning. For example, throughout Volume 2, students have access to a simulated experience, known as Caring for the Nguyens, through which they apply our full-spectrum model of nursing to learn about the nursing role, the healthcare system, and the real-world application of the content in Volume 1.

Other features in each chapter of this volume include critical-thinking activities (Critical Thinking and Clinical Reasoning), step-by-step procedures and clinical insights (with rationales); exercises to tie the procedures to the skills videos; assessment guidelines and tools; a summary of the main points that were covered in Volume 1; and a knowledge map of the concepts discussed in the chapter. All of these features will be useful during a student's clinical day.

This volume, like Volume 1, will appeal to nontraditional students of the technological generation, encourage independent learning, promote critical thinking, support a variety of learning styles, and assure students that it is possible to achieve excellent nursing despite today's challenges.

We hope you will read the Preface and other introductory material in the front of Volume 1. It explains the philosophical underpinnings for this text and describes in more detail how to use the various pieces of this highly integrated learning package, which is flexible enough to accommodate a variety of teaching styles and curriculums.

Contents

Unit 1

How Nurses Think 5

CHAPTER 1

Evolution of Nursing Thought & Action 7

Caring for the Nguyens 7
Critical Thinking and Clinical Reasoning 7

Knowledge Map 9

CHAPTER 2

Critical Thinking & Nursing Process 10

Caring for the Nguyens 10

Clinical Reasoning 11
Applying the Full-Spectrum Nursing Model 11
Critical Thinking and Clinical Reasoning 11

Knowledge Map 14

CHAPTER 3

Nursing Process: Assessment 15

Caring for the Nguyens 15

Practical Knowledge: Knowing How 16

Clinical Insights 16

Clinical Insight 3-1: Preparing for a Patient Interview 16

Clinical Insight 3-2: Conducting a Patient Interview 17

Clinical Insight 3-3: Closing a Patient Interview 18

Assessment Guidelines and Tools 18
Patient Assessment Tool—Lawton Instrumental Activities of Daily Living (IADL) 18
Nursing Admission Data Form 19

Clinical Reasoning 22
Applying the Full-Spectrum Nursing Model 22
Critical Thinking and Clinical Reasoning 23

Knowledge Map 25

CHAPTER 4

Nursing Process: Diagnosis 26

Caring for the Nguyens 26

Practical Knowledge: Knowing How 27

Standardized Language 27
Descriptors for NANDA-I Nursing Diagnoses 27

Clinical Reasoning 28
Applying the Full-Spectrum Nursing Model 28
Critical Thinking and Clinical Reasoning 29

Knowledge Map 32

CHAPTER 5

Nursing Process: Planning Outcomes 33

Caring for the Nguyens 33

Practical Knowledge: Knowing How 34

Assessment Guidelines & Tools 34
Discharge Planning Form 34

Standardized Language 35

Clinical Reasoning 36
Applying the Full-Spectrum Nursing Model 36
Critical Thinking and Clinical Reasoning 37

Knowledge Map 39

CHAPTER 6

Nursing Process: Planning Interventions 40

Caring for the Nguyens 40

Clinical Reasoning 41
Applying the Full-Spectrum Nursing Model 41
Critical Thinking and Clinical Reasoning 41

Knowledge Map 44

CHAPTER 7

Nursing Process: Implementation & Evaluation 45

Caring for the Nguyens 45

Practical Knowledge: Knowing How 46

Implementation and Evaluation Tools 46

The Five Rights of Delegation—Checklist 46
NCSBN Delegation Grid 47
Evaluation Checklist 48

Clinical Reasoning 50

Applying the Full-Spectrum Nursing Model 50
Critical Thinking and Clinical Reasoning 51

Knowledge Map 53

CHAPTER 8

Evidence-Based Practice: Theory & Research 54

Caring for the Nguyens 54

Clinical Reasoning 55

Applying the Full-Spectrum Nursing Model 55
Critical Thinking and Clinical Reasoning 55

Knowledge Map 58

Unit 2

Factors Affecting Health 59

CHAPTER 9

Life Span: Infancy Through Middle Adulthood 61

Caring for the Nguyens 61

Practical Knowledge: Knowing How 62

Procedures 62

Procedure 9-1: Assessing for Abuse 63

Assessment Guidelines & Tools 67

Clinical Reasoning 68

Applying the Full-Spectrum Nursing Model 68
Critical Thinking and Clinical Reasoning 69

Knowledge Map 71

CHAPTER 10

Life Span: Older Adults 72

Caring for the Nguyens 72

Clinical Reasoning 73

Applying the Full-Spectrum Nursing Model 73
Critical Thinking and Clinical Reasoning 74

Knowledge Map 75

CHAPTER 11

Experiencing Health & Illness 76

Caring for the Nguyens 76

Practical Knowledge: Knowing How 77

Procedures 77

Procedure 11-1: Admitting a Patient to a Nursing Unit 77
Procedure 11-2: Transferring a Patient to Another Unit in the Agency 80
Procedure 11-3: Transferring a Patient to a Long-Term Care Facility 81
Procedure 11-4: Discharging a Patient From the Healthcare Facility 83

Clinical Insights 86

Clinical Insight 10-1: Preparing the Room for a Newly Admitted Patient 86

Forms 87

Discharge Assessment/Instructions 87
Patient Education Form 88

Clinical Reasoning 89

Applying the Full-Spectrum Nursing Model 89
Critical Thinking and Clinical Reasoning 89

Knowledge Map 91

CHAPTER 12

Stress & Adaptation 92

Caring for the Nguyens 93

Practical Knowledge: Knowing How 93

Clinical Insights 93

Clinical Insight 12-1: Dealing With Angry Patients 93
Clinical Insight 12-2: Crisis Intervention Guidelines 94

Assessment Guidelines and Tools 95

Standardized Language 97

Clinical Reasoning 98

Applying the Full-Spectrum Nursing Model 98
Critical Thinking and Clinical Reasoning 99

Knowledge Map 101

CHAPTER 13

Psychosocial Health & Illness 102

Caring for the Nguyens 102

Practical Knowledge: Knowing How 103

Clinical Insights 103

Clinical Insight 13-1: Assessing Self-Concept Problems 103

Clinical Insight 13-2: Performing a Self-Esteem Inventory 104

Clinical Insight 13-3: Identifying Depressed Patients Who Should Be Referred for Evaluation 105

Assessment Guidelines and Tools 106

Anxiety Assessment Guide 106

Depression Assessment Guide: Patient Health Questionnaire (PHQ-9) 107

Differentiating Depression and Dementia 108

Standardized Nursing Language 108

Anxiety-Related Diagnoses: Selected NOC Outcomes and NIC Interventions 109

Depression-Related Nursing Diagnoses: Selected NOC Outcomes and NIC Interventions 111

Clinical Reasoning 113

Applying the Full-Spectrum Nursing Model 113

Critical Thinking and Clinical Reasoning 113

Knowledge Map 117

CHAPTER 14

The Family 118

Caring for the Nguyens 119

Practical Knowledge: Knowing How 119

Clinical Insights 119

Clinical Insight 14-1: Conducting a Family Assessment 119

Assessment Guidelines and Tools 120

Assessing Family Developmental Tasks 120

Standardized Language 121

NOC Outcomes and NIC Interventions for Caregiver Role Strain 121

Clinical Reasoning 122

Applying the Full-Spectrum Nursing Model 122

Critical Thinking and Clinical Reasoning 122

Knowledge Map 124

CHAPTER 15

Culture & Ethnicity 125

Caring for the Nguyens 125

Practical Knowledge: Knowing How 126

Clinical Insights 126

Clinical Insight 15-1: Assessing for Biological Variations 126

Clinical Insight 15-2: Pain Perception in Selected Cultural Groups 127

Clinical Insight 15-3: Communicating With Clients Who Speak a Different Language 128

Assessment Guidelines and Tools 129

Obtaining Minimum Cultural Information 129

Cultural Assessment Using the Transcultural Assessment Model 130

Clinical Reasoning 131

Applying the Full-Spectrum Nursing Model 131

Critical Thinking and Clinical Reasoning 131

Knowledge Map 135

CHAPTER 16

Spirituality 136

Caring for the Nguyens 137

Practical Knowledge: Knowing How 137

Clinical Insights 137

Clinical Insight 16-1: Praying With Patients 137

S-P-I-R-I-T Assessment 139

Assessment Guidelines and Tools 140

The HOPE Approach to Spiritual Assessment: Examples of Questions 140

Standardized Nursing Language 140

Using Selected NIC Interventions and Activities to Support Spirituality 140

Clinical Reasoning 142

Applying the Full-Spectrum Nursing Model 142

Critical Thinking and Clinical Reasoning 143

Knowledge Map 144

CHAPTER 17

Loss, Grief, & Dying 145

Caring for the Nguyens 146

Practical Knowledge: Knowing How 146

Clinical Insights 146
Clinical Insight 17-1: Communicating With People Who Are Grieving 146
Clinical Insight 17-2: Helping Families of Dying Patients 147
Clinical Insight 17-3: Caring for the Dying Person: Meeting Physiological Needs 148
Clinical Insight 17-4: Caring for the Dying Person: Meeting Psychological Needs 149
Clinical Insight 17-5: Providing Postmortem Care 150
Forms 152
Do Not Resuscitate Orders 152
Assessment Guidelines 153
Assessing Grief and Loss 153
Clinical Reasoning 155
Applying the Full-Spectrum Nursing Model 155
Critical Thinking and Clinical Reasoning 155
Knowledge Map 158

Unit 3
Essential Nursing Interventions 159

CHAPTER 18
Documenting & Reporting 161
Caring for the Nguyens 162
Practical Knowledge: Knowing How 163
Clinical Insights 163
Clinical Insight 18-1: Giving Oral Reports 163
Clinical Insight 18-2: Receiving Telephone and Verbal Orders 164
Clinical Insight 18-3: Guidelines for Documentation 164
Tables 269
Abbreviations Commonly Used in Healthcare 169
Charting Forms 171
Adult Admission History Electronic Screen 171
Intake and Output Sheet 172
Nursing Assessment Flowsheets Are Comprehensive Charting Documents 173
Clinical Reasoning 174
Applying the Full-Spectrum Nursing Model 174
Critical Thinking and Clinical Reasoning 174
Knowledge Map 176

CHAPTER 19
Teaching & Learning 177
Caring for the Nguyens 178
Practical Knowledge: Knowing How 179
Assessment Guidelines and Tools 179
Learning Assessment Guidelines 179
Clinical Reasoning 180
Applying the Full-Spectrum Nursing Model 180
Critical Thinking and Clinical Reasoning 180
Knowledge Map 183

CHAPTER 20
Measuring Vital Signs 184
Caring for the Nguyens 184
Practical Knowledge: Knowing How 185
Procedures 185
Procedure 20-1: Assessing Body Temperature 185
Procedure 20-1A: Taking an Axillary Temperature 186
Procedure 20-1B: Taking an Oral Temperature 186
Procedure 20-1C: Taking a Rectal Temperature 187
Procedure 20-1D: Taking a Temporal Artery Temperature 188
Procedure 20-1E: Taking a Tympanic Membrane Temperature 188
Procedure 20-1F: Taking a Skin Temperature Using a Chemical Strip Thermometer 189
Procedure 20-2: Assessing Peripheral Pulses 191
Procedure 20-2A: Assessing the Radial Pulse 191
Procedure 20-2B: Assessing the Brachial Pulse 192
Procedure 20-2C: Assessing the Carotid Pulse 192
Procedure 20-2D: Assessing the Dorsalis Pedis Pulse 192
Procedure 20-2E: Assessing the Femoral Pulse 193
Procedure 20-2F: Assessing the Posterior Tibial Pulse 193
Procedure 20-2G: Assessing the Popliteal Pulse 193
Procedure 20-2H: Assessing the Temporal Pulse 194
Procedure 20-3: Assessing the Apical Pulse 195
Procedure 20-4: Assessing for an Apical-Radial Pulse Deficit 197
Procedure 20-5: Assessing Respirations 198
Procedure 20-6: Measuring Blood Pressure 200
Procedure Variation A. Measuring Blood Pressure in the Forearm 202
Procedure Variation B. Measuring Blood Pressure in the Thigh 202
Procedure Variation C. Measuring Blood Pressure in the Calf 203
Procedure Variation D. Palpating the Blood Pressure 203

Clinical Insights 204
Clinical Insight 20-1: Choosing a Blood Pressure Cuff Size 204
Clinical Insight 20-2: Taking an Accurate Blood Pressure 204
Forms 205
Graphic Flowsheet 205
Tables 206
Centigrade–Fahrenheit Conversion Chart 206
Clinical Reasoning 206
Applying the Full-Spectrum Nursing Model 206
Critical Thinking and Clinical Reasoning 207
Knowledge Map 209

CHAPTER 21
Communication & Therapeutic Relationships 210
Caring for the Nguyens 210
Practical Knowledge: Knowing How 211
Clinical Insights 211
Clinical Insight 21-1: Enhancing Communication Through Nonverbal Behaviors 211
Clinical Insight 21-2: Technique for Assertive Communication 212
Clinical Insight 21-3: Communicating With SBAR 212
Clinical Insight 21-4: Communicating With Clients From Another Culture 212
Clinical Insight 21-5: Communicating With Clients Who Have Impaired Speech 213
Clinical Insight 21-6: Communicating With Clients Who Have Impaired Cognition or Consciousness 213
Assessment Guidelines and Tools 215
Communication 215
Clinical Reasoning 216
Applying the Full-Spectrum Nursing Model 216
Critical Thinking and Clinical Reasoning 216
Knowledge Map 218

CHAPTER 22
Health Assessment 219
Caring for the Nguyens 219
Practical Knowledge: Knowing How 220
Procedures 220
Procedure 22-1: Performing the General Survey 221
Procedure 22-2: Assessing the Skin 226
Procedure 22-3: Assessing the Hair 234
Procedure 22-4: Assessing the Nails 235
Procedure 22-5: Assessing the Head and Face 236
Procedure 22-6: Assessing the Eyes 238
Procedure 22-7: Assessing the Ears and Hearing 245
Procedure 22-8: Assessing the Nose and Sinuses 249
Procedure 22-9: Assessing the Mouth and Oropharynx 251
Procedure 22-10: Assessing the Neck 255
Procedure 22-11: Assessing the Breasts and Axillae 257
Procedure 22-12: Assessing the Chest and Lungs 260
Procedure 22-13: Assessing the Heart and Vascular System 265
Procedure 22-14: Assessing the Abdomen 271
Procedure 22-15: Assessing the Musculoskeletal System 277
Procedure 22-16: Assessing the Sensory-Neurological System 284
Procedure 22-17: Assessing the Male Genitourinary System 297
Procedure 22-18: Assessing the Female Genitourinary System 301
Procedure 22-19: Assessing the Anus and Rectum 305
Procedure 22-20: Brief Bedside Assessment 306
Clinical Insights 308
Clinical Insight 22-1: Performing Percussion 308
Clinical Insight 22-2: Performing Auscultation 309
Clinical Insight 22-3: Assisting With a Speculum Exam 309
Abnormal Atlas 312
Knowledge Map 316

CHAPTER 23
Promoting Asepsis & Preventing Infection 317
Caring for the Nguyens 317
Practical Knowledge: Knowing How 318
Procedures 318
Procedure 23-1: Hand Hygiene 318
Procedure 23-1A: Using Soap and Water 318
Procedure 23-1B: Using Alcohol-Based Handrubs 319
Procedure 23-2: Donning Personal Protective Equipment (PPE) 320
Procedure 23-3: Removing Personal Protective Equipment (PPE) 322
Procedure 23-4: Surgical Handwashing: Traditional Method 324

Procedure 23-5: Surgical Handwashing: Brushless System 326
Procedure 23-6: Sterile Gown and Gloves (Closed Method) 328
Procedure 23-7: Sterile Gloves (Open Method) 331
Procedure 23-8: Sterile Fields 332
Procedure 23-8A: Setting Up a Sterile Field 332
Procedure 23-8B: Adding Supplies to a Sterile Field 333
Procedure 23-8C: Adding Sterile Solutions to a Sterile Field 334
Clinical Insights 335
Clinical Insight 23-1: Guidelines for Hand Hygiene 335
Clinical Insight 23-2: Providing a Clean Patient Environment 336
Clinical Insight 23-3: Following CDC Standard Precautions 337
Clinical Insight 23-4: Following Transmission-Based Precautions 339
Clinical Insight 23-5: Preventing the Transmission of Multidrug-Resistant Organisms (MDROs) 341
Clinical Insight 23-6: Maintaining a Protective Environment in Special Situations 342
Clinical Insight 23-7: Guidelines for Preparing and Maintaining Sterile Fields 343
Diagnostic Testing 344
Common Tests for Evaluating the Presence of or Risk for Infection 344
Clinical Reasoning 345
Applying the Full-Spectrum Nursing Model 345
Critical Thinking and Clinical Reasoning 345
Knowledge Map 347

CHAPTER 24

Promoting Safety 348

Caring for the Nguyens 349
Practical Knowledge: Knowing How 349
Procedures 350
Procedure 24-1: Using a Bed Monitoring Device 350
Procedure 24-2: Using Restraints 352
Clinical Insights 355
Clinical Insight 24-1: Preventing Needlestick Injury 355
Clinical Insight 24-2: What You Should Know About Using Restraints 356
Assessment Guidelines and Tools 357
Get Up and Go Test 357
The Timed Up & Go Test for Fall Risk Assessment 357
S.A.S. Safety Assessment Scale 358
Clinical Reasoning 359
Applying the Full-Spectrum Nursing Model 359
Critical Thinking and Clinical Reasoning 358
Knowledge Map 362

CHAPTER 25

Facilitating Hygiene 363

Caring for the Nguyens 363
Practical Knowledge: Knowing How 364
Procedures 364
Procedure 25-1: Bathing: Providing a Complete Bed Bath Using a Prepackaged Bathing Product 364
Procedure 25-2: Bathing: Providing a Towel Bath 369
Procedure 25-3: Bathing: Using a Basin and Water 370
Procedure 25-4: Providing Perineal Care 371
Procedure 25-5: Providing Foot Care 374
Procedure 25-6: Brushing and Flossing the Teeth 377
Procedure 25-7: Providing Denture Care 380
Procedure 25-8: Providing Oral Care for an Unconscious Patient 382
Procedure 25-9: Shampooing the Hair 384
Procedure 25-9A: Shampooing the Hair for a Patient on Bedrest—Using Rinse-Free Shampoo 385
Procedure 25-9B: Shampooing the Hair Using Rinse-Free Shampoo Cap 385
Procedure 25-9C: Shampooing the Hair Using a Basin and Water 385
Procedure 25-10: Providing Beard and Mustache Care 387
Procedure 25-11: Shaving a Patient 389
Procedure 25-12: Removing and Caring for Contact Lenses 390
Procedure 25-13: Making an Unoccupied Bed 392
Procedure 25-14: Making an Occupied Bed 394
Procedure 25-15: Caring for Artificial Eyes 397
Procedure 25-16: Caring for Hearing Aids 398
Clinical Insights 401
Clinical Insight 25-1: Assisting With a Shower or Tub Bath 401
Clinical Insight 25-2: Bathing a Patient With Dementia 402
Assessment Guidelines and Tools 402
Guidelines for Assessing Hygiene 402
Clinical Reasoning 404
Applying the Full-Spectrum Nursing Model 404
Critical Thinking and Clinical Reasoning 404
Knowledge Map 408

CHAPTER 26

Administering Medications 409

Caring for the Nguyens 410

Practical Knowledge: Knowing How 410

Procedures 410

Medication Guidelines: Steps to Follow for All Medications (Regardless of Type or Route) 410

Procedure 26-1: Administering Oral Medication 414

Procedure 26-1A: Administering Medication Through an Enteral Tube 416

Procedure 26-2: Administering Ophthalmic Medication 419

Procedure 26-2A: Irrigating the Eyes 421

Procedure 26-3: Administering Otic Medication 422

Procedure 26-4: Administering Nasal Medication 424

Procedure 26-5: Administering Vaginal Medication 426

Procedure 26-6: Inserting a Rectal Suppository 428

Procedure 26-7: Applying Medication to Skin 430

Procedure 26-7A: Applying Topical Lotion, Cream, and Ointment 430

Procedure 26-7B: Applying Topical Aerosol Spray 430

Procedure 26-7C: Applying Prescribed Powder 430

Procedure 26-7D: Applying Transdermal Medication 431

Procedure 26-8: Administering Metered-Dose Inhaler (MDI) Medication 432

Procedure 26-9: Preparing, Drawing Up, and Mixing Medication 435

Procedure 26-9A: Drawing Up Medication From Ampules 435

Procedure 26-9B: Drawing Up Medication From Vials 437

Procedure 26-9C: Mixing Medication From Two Vials 439

Procedure 26-9D: Mixing Medication From One Ampule and One Vial 441

Procedure 26-9E: Using a Prefilled Cartridge and Single-Dose Vial—For Intravenous Administration 442

Procedure 26-10: Recapping Needles Using a One-Handed Technique 443

Procedure 26-10A: Recapping Contaminated Needles 444

Procedure 26-10B: Recapping Sterile Needles 444

Procedure 26-11: Administering Intradermal Medication 445

Procedure 26-12: Administering Subcutaneous Medication 448

Procedure 26-13: Locating Intramuscular Injection Sites 451

Procedure 26-13A: Locating the Ventrogluteal Site 451

Procedure 26-13B: Locating the Deltoid Site 451

Procedure 26-13C: Locating the Vastus Lateralis Site 452

Procedure 26-13D: Locating the Rectus Femoris Site 453

Procedure 26-14: Administering an Intramuscular Injection 453

Procedure 26-14A: Intramuscular Injection: Traditional Method 454

Procedure 26-14B: Intramuscular Injection: Z-Track Method 455

Procedure 26-15: Adding Medications to Intravenous Fluid 457

Procedure 26-15A: Adding Medication to a New IV Bag or Bottle 457

Procedure 26-15B: Adding Medication to an Infusing IV 458

Procedure 26-16: Administering IV Push Medication 459

Procedure 26-16A: Administering IV Push Medications Through a Primary IV Line 459

Procedure 26-16B: Administering IV Push Medications Through an Intermittent Device (IV Lock) When No Extension Tubing Is Attached to the Venous Access Device 460

Procedure 26-16C: Administering IV Push Medications Through an Intermittent Device with IV Extension Tubing 461

Procedure 26-17: Administering Medications by Intermittent Infusion 463

Procedure 26-17A: Using a Volume-Control Administration Set 464

Procedure 26-17B: Using a Piggyback Administration Set With a Gravity Infusion 465

Procedure 26-17C: Using a Piggyback Administration Set With an Infusion Pump 466

Procedure 26-18: Administering Medication Through a Central Venous Access Device (CVAD) 467

Clinical Insights 471

Clinical Insight 26-1: Reusing Needles and Syringes: Home Care 471

Clinical Insight 26-2: Using Prefilled Unit-Dose Systems 472

Clinical Insight 26-3: Reconstituting Medication 473

Clinical Insight 26-4: Measuring Dosage When Changing Needles 474

Clinical Insight 26-5: Mixing Two Kinds of Insulin in One Syringe 475

Clinical Insight 26-6: Administering Anticoagulant Medication Subcutaneously 476

Clinical Insight 26-7: Taking Action After a Medication Error 477

Tables: Abbreviations 477

Common Medication-Related Abbreviations 477

Institute for Safe Medication Practices (ISMP) List of Error-Prone Abbreviations, Symbols, and Dose Designations 478

Measuring and Calculating Dosage 481

Medication Measurement Systems 481
Calculating Dosages 482
Clinical Reasoning 484
Applying the Full-Spectrum Nursing Model 484
Critical Thinking and Clinical Reasoning 485
Knowledge Map 489

Unit 4
Supporting Physiological Functioning 491

CHAPTER 27

Nutrition 493
Caring for the Nguyens 494
Practical Knowledge: Knowing How 494
Procedures 494
Procedure 27-1: Checking Fingerstick (Capillary) Blood Glucose Levels 494
Procedure 27-2: Inserting Nasogastric and Nasoenteric Tubes 498
Procedure 27-3: Administering Feedings Through Gastric and Enteric Tubes 502
Procedure 27-3A: Administering Feedings Through Gastric and Enteric Tubes Using an Open System: Syringe 504
Procedure 27-4: Removing a Nasogastric or Nasoenteric Tube 506
Procedure 27-5: Administering Parenteral Nutrition 508
Procedure 27-6: Administering Lipids 511
Clinical Insights 513
Clinical Insight 27-1: 10 Tips for Building Healthy Meals 513
Clinical Insight 27-2: Skinfold Measurement 514
Clinical Insight 27-3: Measuring Circumferences to Evaluate Body Composition 515
Clinical Insight 27-4: Interventions for Patients With Impaired Swallowing 515
Clinical Insight 27-5: Interventions for Patients Who Have Nausea 516
Clinical Insight 27-6: Assisting Patients With Meals 516
Clinical Insight 27-7: Checking Feeding Tube Placement 517
Clinical Insight 27-8: Monitoring Patients Receiving Enteral Nutrition 519
Clinical Insight 27-9: Preventing Infection in Patients Receiving Enteral Feedings 519
Clinical Insight 27-10: Monitoring and Other Interventions for Patients Receiving Parenteral Nutrition 520
Screening for Nutritional Problems 521
Subjective Global Assessment 521
Nutrition Screening Initiative (NSI), for Older Adults: Indications of Impaired Nutritional Status 521
Mini Nutritional Assessment 522
Focused Nutritional Assessment 522
Focused Nutritional Assessment 522
Diagnostic Testing 525
Tests Reflecting Nutritional Status: Norms 525
Clinical Reasoning 526
Applying the Full-Spectrum Nursing Model 526
Critical Thinking and Clinical Reasoning 526
Knowledge Map 529

CHAPTER 28

Urinary Elimination 530
Caring for the Nguyens 531
Practical Knowledge: Knowing How 531
Procedures 531
Procedure 28-1: Measuring Urine 531
Procedure 28-1A: Measuring Urine Output From a Bedpan or Urinal 532
Procedure 28-1B: Measuring Urine From an Indwelling Catheter 532
Procedure 28-1C: Measuring Post-Void Residual Urine Volume With a Portable Bladder Scanner 533
Procedure 28-2: Obtaining a Urine Specimen for Testing 534
Procedure 28-2A: Collecting a Clean-Catch Urine Specimen 535
Procedure 28-2B: Obtaining a Sterile Urine Specimen From a Catheter 536
Procedure 28-2C: Collecting a 24-Hour Urine Specimen 536
Procedure 28-3: Testing Urine at the Bedside 538
Procedure 28-3A: Dipstick Testing of Urine 538
Procedure 28-3B: Measuring Specific Gravity of Urine 538
Procedure 28-4: Inserting a Urinary Catheter 539
Procedure 28-4A: Intermittent Urinary Catheterization 540
Procedure 28-4B: Indwelling Urinary Catheterization 544
Procedure 28-5: Applying an External (Condom) Catheter 548
Procedure 28-6: Removing an Indwelling Catheter 551
Procedure 28-7: Irrigating the Bladder or Catheter 553
Procedure 28-7A: Intermittent Bladder or Catheter Irrigation 553
Procedure 28-7B: Continuous Bladder Irrigation 554

Clinical Insights 556
Clinical Insight 28-1: Caring for a Patient With an Indwelling Catheter 556
Clinical Insight 28-2: Caring for Patients With Urinary Incontinence 558
Clinical Insight 28-3: Caring for Patients With Urinary Diversions 559
Clinical Insight 28-4: Teaching Clients About Clean, Intermittent
Self-Catheterization 560
Assessment Guidelines and Tools 561
Urinary Elimination History Questions 561
Guidelines for Physical Assessment for Urinary Elimination 561
Diagnostic Testing 562
Urinalysis 562
Blood Studies: BUN and Creatinine 563
Studies of the Urinary System 564
Clinical Reasoning 565
Applying the Full-Spectrum Nursing Model 565
Critical Thinking and Clinical Reasoning 566
Knowledge Map 568

CHAPTER 29
Bowel Elimination 569
Caring for the Nguyens 569
Practical Knowledge: Knowing How 570
Procedures 570
Procedure 29-1: Testing Stool for Occult Blood 570
Procedure 29-2: Placing and Removing a Bedpan 572
Procedure 29-2A: Placing a Bedpan 573
Procedure 29-2B: Removing a Bedpan 574
Procedure 29-3: Administering an Enema 575
Procedure 29-3A: Administering a Cleansing Enema 575
Procedure 29-3B: Administering a Prepackaged Enema 577
Procedure 29-3C: Administering an Oil-Retention Enema 577
Procedure 29-3D: Administering a Return-Flow Enema 578
Procedure 29-4: Removing Stool Digitally 579
Procedure 29-5: Inserting a Rectal Tube 581
Procedure 29-6: Changing an Ostomy Appliance 582
Procedure 29-7: Irrigating a Colostomy 586
Procedure 29-8: Placing Fecal Drainage Devices 588
Procedure 29-8A: Applying an External Fecal Collection System 589
Procedure 29-8B: Inserting an Indwelling Fecal Drainage Device 590
Clinical Insights 592
Clinical Insight 29-1: Caring for a Patient With an Indwelling Fecal Drainage Device 592
Clinical Insight 29-2: Guidelines for Ostomy Care 593
Assessment Guidelines and Tools 594
Bowel Elimination 594
Diagnostic Testing 594
Direct Visualization Studies of the Gastrointestinal Tract 594
Indirect Visualization Studies of the Gastrointestinal Tract 595
Clinical Reasoning 596
Applying the Full-Spectrum Nursing Model 596
Critical Thinking and Clinical Reasoning 596
Knowledge Map 598

CHAPTER 30
Sensation, Perception, & Cognition 599
Caring for the Nguyens 599
Practical Knowledge: Knowing How 600
Procedures 600
Procedure 30-1: Performing Otic Irrigation 600
Clinical Insights 602
Clinical Insight 30-1: Seizure Precautions 602
Clinical Insight 30-2: Communicating With Visually Impaired Clients 604
Clinical Insight 30-3: Communicating With Hearing-Impaired Clients 604
Assessment Guidelines and Tools 605
Hearing Screening in Older Adults 605
Other Sensory Assessment Tools 605
Nursing History: Sensory Perceptual Status 605
Bedside Assessment of Sensory Function 606
Clinical Reasoning 607
Applying the Full-Spectrum Nursing Model 607
Critical Thinking and Clinical Reasoning 607
Knowledge Map 609

CHAPTER 31
Pain 610
Caring for the Nguyens 611
Practical Knowledge: Knowing How 611
Procedures 611
Procedure 30-1: Setting Up and Managing Patient-Controlled Analgesia by Pump 611
Clinical Insights 614
Clinical Insight 31-1: Caring for the Patient With an Epidural Catheter 614
Clinical Insight 31-2: Guidelines for Assessing Pain 615
Assessment Guidelines and Tools 616

Pain Assessment 616
Pain Relief Diary 618
Richmond Agitation-Sedation Rating Scale 618
Clinical Reasoning 619
Applying the Full-Spectrum Nursing Model 619
Critical Thinking and Clinical Reasoning 619
Knowledge Map 621

CHAPTER 32
Physical Activity & Mobility 622
Caring for the Nguyens 623
Practical Knowledge: Knowing How 623
Procedures 623
Procedure 32-1: Moving and Turning Patients in Bed 623
Procedure 32-1A: Moving a Patient Up in Bed 624
Procedure 32-1B: Turning a Patient in Bed 625
Procedure 32-1C: Logrolling a Patient 626
Procedure 32-2: Transferring Patients 628
Procedure 32-2A: Transferring a Patient From Bed to Stretcher 628
Procedure 32-2B: Dangling a Patient at the Side of the Bed 629
Procedure 32-2C: Transferring a Patient From Bed to Chair 630
Procedure 32-3: Assisting With Ambulation 632
Procedure 32-3A: Assisting With Ambulation (One Nurse) 632
Procedure 32-3B: Assisting With Ambulation (Two Nurses) 633
Clinical Insights 635
Clinical Insight 32-1: Applying Principles of Body Mechanics 635
Clinical Insight 32-2: Using Common Positioning Devices 636
Clinical Insight 32-3: Tips for Performing Passive Range-of-Motion Exercises 638
Clinical Insight 32-4: Assisting With Physical Conditioning Exercises to Prepare for Ambulation 638
Clinical Insight 32-5: Sizing Walking Aids 639
Clinical Insight 32-6: Teaching Patients to Use Canes, Walkers, and Crutches 639
Assessment Guidelines and Tools 641
Assessing Activity and Exercise 641
Tables 643
Range of Motion at the Joints 643
Clinical Reasoning 648
Applying the Full-Spectrum Nursing Model 648
Critical Thinking and Clinical Reasoning 648
Knowledge Map 650

CHAPTER 33
Sexual Health 651
Caring for the Nguyens 652
Practical Knowledge: Knowing How 652
Clinical Insights 652
Clinical Insight 33-1: Providing Care After Sexual Assault 652
Clinical Insight 33-2: Guidelines for Taking a Sexual History 653
Clinical Insight 33-3: Teaching Your Patient to Use a Condom 654
Tables 654
Fertility Control Methods 654
Assessment Guidelines and Tools 656
Guidelines and Questions for Taking a Sexual History 656
Clinical Reasoning 658
Applying the Full-Spectrum Nursing Model 658
Critical Thinking and Clinical Reasoning 658
Knowledge Map 661

CHAPTER 34
Sleep & Rest 662
Caring for the Nguyens 662
Practical Knowledge: Knowing How 664
Procedures 664
Procedure 34-1: Giving a Back Massage 664
Assessment Guidelines and Tools 666
Questions for a Sleep History 666
Clinical Reasoning 667
Applying the Full-Spectrum Nursing Model 667
Critical Thinking and Clinical Reasoning 668
Knowledge Map 670

CHAPTER 35
Skin Integrity & Wound Healing 671
Caring for the Nguyens 672
Practical Knowledge: Knowing How 672
Procedures 672
Procedure 35-1: Obtaining a Wound Culture by Swab 673
Procedure 35-2: Performing a Sterile Wound Irrigation 675

Procedure 35-3: Taping a Dressing 678
Procedure 35-4: Removing and Applying Dry Dressings 680
Procedure 35-5: Removing and Applying Wet-to-Damp Dressings 682
Procedure 35-6: Applying a Negative Pressure Wound Therapy (NPWT) Device 685
Procedure 35-6A: Open-Pore Reticulated Polyurethane Foam Therapy (i.e., Vacuum-Assisted Closure [V.A.C.]) 687
Procedure 35-6B: Gauze Dressing Application (i.e., Chariker–Jeter Method) 688
Procedure 35-7: Applying and Removing a Transparent Film Dressing 690
Procedure 35-8: Applying a Hydrating Dressing (Hydrocolloid or Hydrogel) 693
Procedure 35-9: Placing Skin Closures 695
Procedure 35-10: Applying Binders 697
Procedure 35-11: Applying Bandages 699
Procedure 35-12: Removing Sutures and Staples 703
Procedure 35-12A: Removing Sutures 703
Procedure 35-12B: Removing Staples 704
Procedure 35-13: Shortening a Wound Drain 705
Procedure 35-14: Emptying a Closed-Wound Drainage System 706
Clinical Insights 708
Clinical Insight 35-1: Applying Local Heat Therapy 708
Clinical Insight 35-2: Applying Local Cold Therapy 709
Assessment Guidelines and Tools 709
History Questions for Skin and Wound Assessment 709
Physical Examination: Wound Assessment 710
The Braden Scale for Predicting Pressure Sore Risk 711
The Norton Scale for Assessing Risk of Pressure Ulcers 712
The PUSH Tool for Evaluation of Pressure Ulcers 713
Diagnostic Testing 715
Tests for Assessing Wounds 715
Standardized Language 716
Selected Standardized Outcomes and Interventions for Skin and Wound Diagnoses 716
Clinical Reasoning 717
Applying the Full-Spectrum Nursing Model 717
Critical Thinking and Clinical Reasoning 718
Knowledge Map 721

CHAPTER 36

Oxygenation 722
Caring for the Nguyens 722
Practical Knowledge: Knowing How 723
Procedures 723
Procedure 36-1: Collecting a Sputum Specimen 723
Procedure 36-1A: Collecting an Expectorated Sputum Specimen 724
Procedure 36-1B: Collecting a Suctioned Sputum Specimen 725
Procedure 36-2: Monitoring Pulse Oximetry (Arterial Oxygen Saturation) 726
Procedure 36-3: Performing Percussion, Vibration, and Postural Drainage 728
Procedure 36-4: Administering Oxygen 731
Procedure 36-5: Performing Tracheostomy Care Using Sterile Technique 736
Procedure 36-6: Performing Tracheostomy Suctioning (Open System) 741
Procedure 36-7: Performing Tracheostomy or Endotracheal Suctioning (Inline Closed System) 744
Procedure 36-8: Performing Orotracheal and Nasotracheal Suctioning (Open System) 745
Procedure 36-9: Performing Upper Airway Suctioning 749
Procedure 36-10: Caring for Patients Requiring Mechanical Ventilation 752
Procedure 36-11: Setting Up Disposable Chest Drainage Systems 755
Procedure 36-12: Inserting an Oropharyngeal Airway 759
Procedure 36-13: Inserting a Nasopharyngeal Airway 760
Clinical Insights 762
Clinical Insight 36-1: Tips for Obtaining Accurate Pulse Oximetry Readings 762
Clinical Insight 36-2: Guidelines for Preventing Aspiration 762
Clinical Insight 36-3: Oxygen Therapy Safety Precautions 763
Clinical Insight 36-4: Caring for Patients With Endotracheal Airways 763
Clinical Insight 36-5: Managing Chest Tubes 764
Assessment Guidelines and Tools 765
Oxygenation 765
Diagnostic Testing 766
Lung Volumes and Capacities 766
Tests Related to Oxygenation 767
Reading a Tuberculin Skin Test Result 768
Clinical Reasoning 768
Applying the Full-Spectrum Nursing Model 768
Critical Thinking and Clinical Reasoning 769
Knowledge Map 771

CHAPTER 37

Circulation 772

Caring for the Nguyens 773

Practical Knowledge: Knowing How 773

Procedures 773

Procedure 37-1: Performing Cardiac Monitoring 774

Assessment Guidelines and Tools 776

Assessing Circulation 776

Diagnostic Testing 777

Tests Related to Circulation 777

Clinical Reasoning 777

Applying the Full-Spectrum Nursing Model 777

Critical Thinking and Clinical Reasoning 778

Knowledge Map 780

CHAPTER 38

Fluids, Electrolytes, & Acid–Base Balance 781

Caring for the Nguyens 782

Practical Knowledge: Knowing Why 782

Procedures 783

Procedure 38-1: Initiating a Peripheral Intravenous Infusion 783

Procedure 38-2: Regulating the IV Flow Rate 788

Procedure 38-3: Setting Up and Using Volume-Control Pumps 790

Procedure 38-4: Changing IV Solutions and Tubing 793

Procedure 38-4A: Changing the IV Solution 793

Procedure 38-4B: Changing the IV Administration Tubing and Solution 794

Procedure 38-5: Changing IV Dressings 796

Procedure 38-5A: Peripheral IV Dressings 796

Procedure 38-5B: Central Line Dressings 797

Procedure 38-5C: PICC Line Dressings 798

Procedure 38-6: Converting a Primary Line to a Peripheral IV Lock 800

Procedure 38-7: Discontinuing a Peripheral IV 803

Procedure 38-8: Administering a Blood Transfusion 804

Procedure 38-8A: Administering Blood and Blood Products 805

Procedure 38-8B: Managing a Transfusion Reaction 807

Procedure 38-9: Assisting With Percutaneous Central Venous Catheter Placement 808

Clinical Insights 810

Clinical Insight 38-1: Assessing for Trousseau's and Chvostek's Signs 810

Clinical Insight 38-2: Guidelines for Measuring Intake and Output (I&O) 810

Clinical Insight 38-3: Guidelines for Selecting a Peripheral Venipuncture Site 812

Clinical Insight 38-4: Caring for Patients With a Central Venous Access Device (CVAD): CVC and PICC 813

Clinical Insight 38-5: Managing Infiltration and Extravasation 814

Assessment Guidelines and Tools 815

Assessing Fluids, Electrolytes, and Acid–Base Balance 815

Diagnostic Testing 817

Assessing Fluid, Electrolyte, and Acid–Base Balance 817

Clinical Reasoning 817

Applying the Full-Spectrum Nursing Model 817

Critical Thinking and Clinical Reasoning 818

Knowledge Map 821

Unit 5

Nursing Functions 823

CHAPTER 39

Perioperative Care 825

Caring for the Nguyens 825

Practical Knowledge: Knowing How 826

Procedures 826

Procedure 39-1: Teaching a Patient to Deep-Breathe, Cough, Move in Bed, and Perform Leg Exercises 826

Procedure 39-1A: Teaching a Patient to Deep-Breathe and Cough 827

Procedure 39-1B: Teaching a Patient to Move in Bed 827

Procedure 39-1C: Teaching Leg Exercises 828

Procedure 39-2: Applying Antiembolism Stockings 829

Procedure 39-3: Applying Sequential Compression Devices 832

Procedure 39-4: Managing Gastric Suction 834

Procedure 39-4A: Initial Equipment Setup 835

Procedure 39-4B: Emptying the Suction Container 835

Procedure 39-4C: Irrigating the Nasogastric Tubing 836

Procedure 39-4D: Providing Comfort Measures 836

Clinical Insights 839

Clinical Insight 39-1: Preoperative Teaching 839

Clinical Insight 39-2: Preparing a Room for a Patient's Return From Surgery 840

Clinical Insight 39-3: Creating an Operative Field 840

Assessment Guidelines and Tools 841

Preoperative Assessment Topics 841
Example of a Preoperative Checklist 842
Example of a Surgical Safety Checklist 844
Intraoperative Care Questionnaire 844
Postanesthesia Assessment: Essential Elements 845

Diagnostic Testing 845
Common Preoperative Screening Tests 845

Standardized Language 846
Preoperative Patients: Selected Standardized Nursing Diagnoses, Outcomes, and Interventions 846
Intraoperative Patients: Selected Standardized Nursing Diagnoses, Outcomes, and Interventions 848
Postoperative Patients: Selected Standardized Nursing Diagnoses, Outcomes, and Interventions 851

Clinical Reasoning 855
Applying the Full-Spectrum Nursing Model 855
Critical Thinking and Clinical Reasoning 856

Knowledge Map 858

CHAPTER 40

Leading & Managing 859

Caring for the Nguyens 859

Clinical Reasoning 860
Applying the Full-Spectrum Nursing Model 860
Critical Thinking and Clinical Reasoning 860

Knowledge Map 863

CHAPTER 41

Nursing Informatics 864

Caring for the Nguyens 865

Practical Knowledge: Knowing How 865

Standardized Language 865
American Nurses Association Recognized Languages for Nursing 865

Clinical Reasoning 866
Applying the Full-Spectrum Nursing Model 866
Critical Thinking and Clinical Reasoning 867

Knowledge Map 870

CHAPTER 42

Promoting Health 871

Caring for the Nguyens 871

Assessment Guidelines and Tools 872
Health Promotion: Physical Fitness Assessment 872
Lifestyle and Risk Assessment 873
Life Stress Review 875
Selected Health Screening Activities 876

Standardized Language 877
Examples of NANDA-I Health Promotion Diagnoses 877
Selected NIC Health Promotion Interventions 877

Clinical Reasoning 879
Applying the Full-Spectrum Nursing Model 879
Critical Thinking and Clinical Reasoning 879

Knowledge Map 881

Unit 6

The Context for Nurses' Work 883

CHAPTER 43

Community & Home Health Nursing 885

Caring for the Nguyens 886

Practical Knowledge: Knowing How 886

Clinical Insights 887

Clinical Insight 43-1: Safety Considerations in Home Care 887

Clinical Insight 43-2: Infection Control in the Home 888

Standardized Language 888
The Omaha System 888
Omaha System: Domains and Examples of Problem Labels 889
Omaha Problem Rating Scale for Outcomes 889
NIC Community Health Classes and Interventions 890
Omaha Intervention Categories and Examples of Targets 891
Clinical Care Classification System for Home Health Care 891
An Example of CCC Nursing Diagnoses and Interventions 892

Clinical Reasoning 892
Applying the Full-Spectrum Nursing Model 892
Critical Thinking and Clinical Reasoning 892

Knowledge Map 896

CHAPTER 44

Ethics & Values 897

Caring for the Nguyens 898

Practical Knowledge: Knowing How 898

Clinical Insights 899

Clinical Insight 44-1: Using the MORAL Model for Ethical Decision Making 899
Clinical Insight 44-2: Guidelines for Advocacy 899
Clinical Reasoning 900
Applying the Full-Spectrum Nursing Model 900
Critical Thinking and Clinical Reasoning 900
Knowledge Map 904

CHAPTER 45
Legal Accountability 905
Caring for the Nguyens 906
Practical Knowledge: Knowing How 906
Clinical Insights 906
Clinical Insight 45-1: Using Equipment Safely 906
Clinical Insight 45-2: Tips for Avoiding Malpractice 907
Clinical Insight 45-3: Guidelines for Documenting Care 907
Clinical Reasoning 908
Applying the Full-Spectrum Nursing Model 908
Critical Thinking and Clinical Reasoning 908
Knowledge Map 911

CHAPTER 46
Holistic Healing (on Davis*Plus*)

Credits 912
References Cited 914
Index 1000

Meet the Nguyens

Throughout this text, you will be applying what you have learned as you care for the Nguyen family. In Chapter 1, you will meet Nam Nguyen, a construction work supervisor, who arrives at the Family Medicine Center for his first physical exam in 10 years. It is Nam's knee pain that causes him to seek help because it affects his work. But as you will see, Nam will discover that he has other serious health problems that require him to be more vigilant about his health. As you read and work through the exercises in Caring for the Nguyens, you will also get to know Nam's wife, Yen Nguyen, his grandchild, Kim Phan, other members of his extended family, and his friends as they deal with health issues and life changes.

Your experience in caring for the Nguyens will show you that patients come to you with symptoms but each person brings unique values, lifestyle, and relationships to the encounter. From the Nguyens, you will learn what it means to care for the whole person and how to be a full-spectrum nurse.

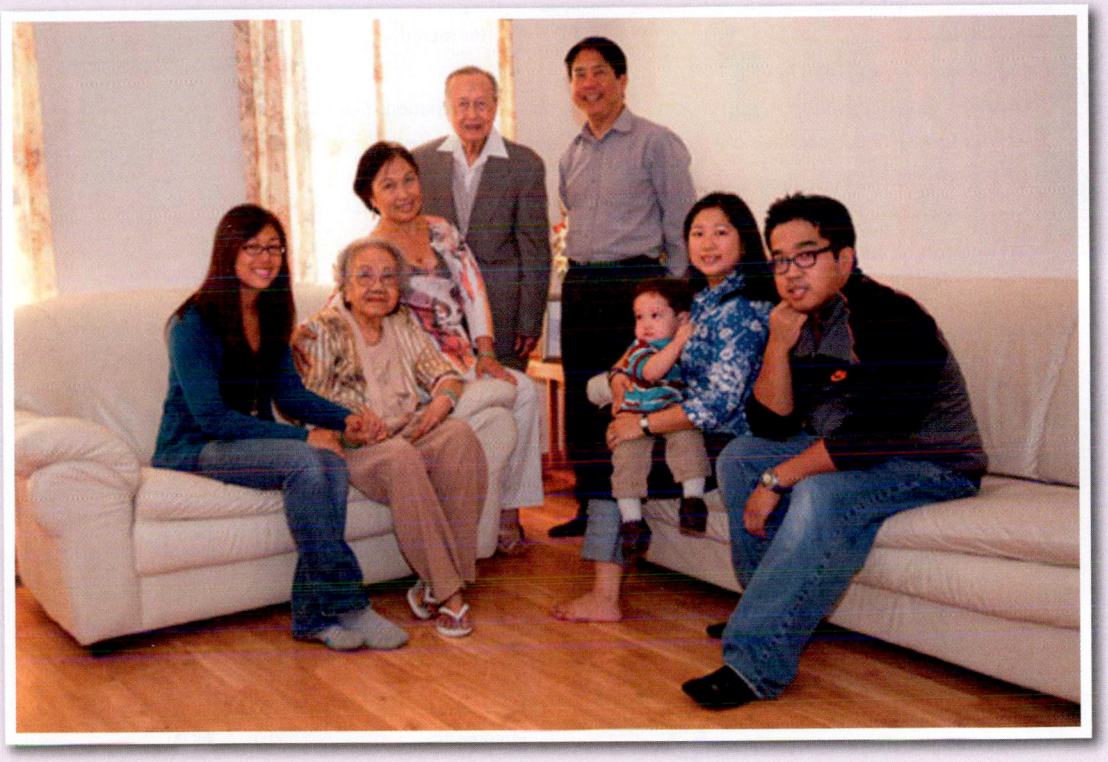

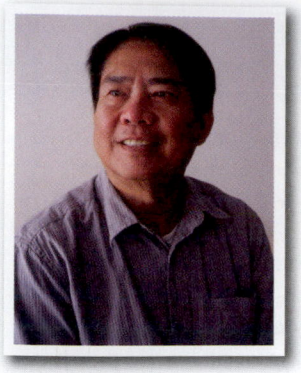

Mr. Nam Nguyen is a new patient at the Family Medicine Center. He arrives at the Center for an appointment for a physical exam and completes the following admission questionnaire.

Name: *Nam Nguyen* DOB: *7 / 12 / 50*

Marital Status S (M) W D Partnered

If applicable, spouse/partner name: *Yen*

Occupation: *Construction supervisor* Spouse/partner occupation: *Daycare teacher*

Does your spouse or partner have any health care problems? If so, please list:

High blood pressure

Do you have children? *Yes* Ages? *30, 27, 22*

Please circle yes or no if you have had the following:

AIDS/HIV +	YES	(NO)	Headaches	YES	(NO)
Allergies	(YES)	NO	Heart Disease	YES	(NO)
Anemia	YES	(NO)	Hernia	(YES)	NO
Anorexia	YES	(NO)	Herpes	YES	(NO)
Anxiety	YES	(NO)	High Cholesterol	YES	(NO)
Arthritis	YES	(NO)	High Blood Pressure	YES	(NO)
Bleeding Disorder	YES	(NO)	Kidney Problems	YES	(NO)
Breast Problems	YES	(NO)	Liver Problems	YES	(NO)
Cancer	YES	(NO)	Abnormal Mammogram (N/A)	YES	NO
Chicken Pox	(YES)	NO	Menopause (N/A)	YES	NO
Colon Disorder	YES	(NO)	Mononucleosis	YES	(NO)
COPD/Emphysema	YES	(NO)	Multiple Sclerosis	YES	(NO)
Depression	YES	(NO)	Osteoporosis	YES	(NO)
Diabetes	YES	(NO)	Pneumonia	YES	(NO)
Epilepsy/Seizures	YES	(NO)	Polio	YES	(NO)
Eye Problems	(YES)	NO	Prostate Problems	YES	(NO)
Gallbladder Disorder	YES	(NO)	Skin Problems	YES	(NO)
Stomach Problems/Ulcer	YES	(NO)	Stroke	YES	(NO)
Gout	YES	(NO)	Suicide Attempt	YES	(NO)
Gynecological Problems	YES	(NO)	Thyroid Problems	YES	(NO)
Sexually Transmitted Disease	YES	(NO)	Other	YES	(NO)

Please list your current medications and dosages. Also list over-the-counter and herbal products you use regularly.

Ibuprofen
MultiVitamin 1 per day
Acetaminophen

Ben-Gay Balm on knees

The Diagnosis

During the visit, the clinic nurse records the following information in Nam's chart.

Height	5 ft 4 in.
Weight	165 lb
BP	162/94 mm Hg
Pulse	84 beats/min
RR	20 breaths/min
Temp	98.2°F oral

Presenting Complaint: Patient states he is here to become established as a patient at the Center and that he has not had a physical exam in more than 10 years. Wife accompanies. He is currently experiencing bilateral knee pain that is affecting his work performance. "I supervise construction workers. To check on things, I have to climb up and down ladders, lift things, and crawl around a lot." Has not missed any work but has been using increasing amounts of acetaminophen and ibuprofen "to get through the day." The medications provide only limited relief. States pain occurs daily even if not at work. Describes the pain as achy and dull. Feels best when he is off his feet. Desires pain relief and checkup. Explains that both parents had heart disease. Wife expresses worry that he may be developing heart problems "because he's so tired after work and he gets short of breath easy."

The nurse explains to Nam that he will be seen by the nurse practitioner shortly. She asks Mr. Nguyen if he would like his wife to be present for the exam. Mr. Nguyen requests that his wife remain in the room.

Zach Jackson, MSN, FNP-BC, is on duty at the Center today. Zach worked as a registered nurse (RN) for more than 10 years in the local emergency department and urgent care clinic. He has been a family nurse practitioner (FNP-BC) for more than 5 years. Zach enters the room and introduces himself to the Nguyen couple. To begin the exam, Zach reviews the information Mr. Nguyen supplied on the admission form, and then asks Nam about his family history.

Zach: Are your parents still living?

Nam: Yes, they're both alive. My father is 80 years old and my mother is 76.

Zach: I'd like to hear a little more about your family history. Tell me about your father's cancer. How old was he when he was first diagnosed? Has he had treatment?

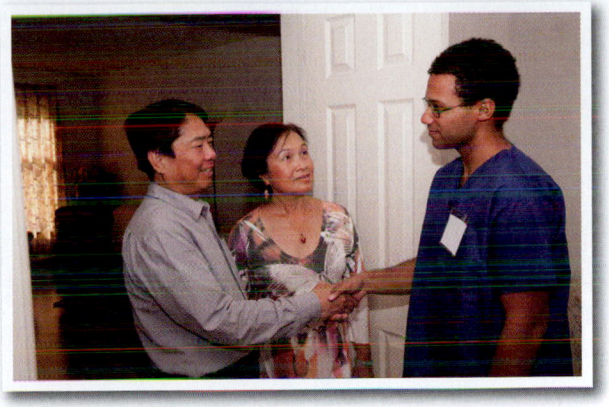

Nam: He was probably about 60 when he first found out about it. I know he had some kind of surgery and takes medicines but I don't know the details. He seems all right though.

Zach: Your father also has high blood pressure and heart disease. Please tell me a little more about that.

Nam: My father and mother both have high blood pressure and heart disease. They both take medicines for their blood pressure. My father had a small heart attack about 10 years ago. My mother has never had a heart attack that I know of, but she sometimes has chest pain.

Zach: Your mother also has diabetes?

Nam: She's had that for a long time. A lot of people in my family have diabetes, especially on my father's side—but nobody in my mother's family. Yet my mother is the one with the diabetes!

Yen: A lot of people in my family have diabetes too. But so far I'm okay, I think.

Zach: Have you had a health exam lately, Mrs. Nguyen?

Yen: Not in about a year, but I'm going to schedule an appointment here.

The Nguyen couple and Zach continue to review the health information. After reviewing the history and discussing current complaints, Zach performs a complete physical exam.

unit 1

How Nurses Think

1 Evolution of Nursing Thought & Action

2 Critical Thinking & Nursing Process

3 Nursing Process: Assessment

4 Nursing Process: Diagnosis

5 Nursing Process: Planning Outcomes

6 Nursing Process: Planning Interventions

7 Nursing Process: Implementation & Evaluation

8 Evidence-Based Practice: Theory & Research

CHAPTER 1

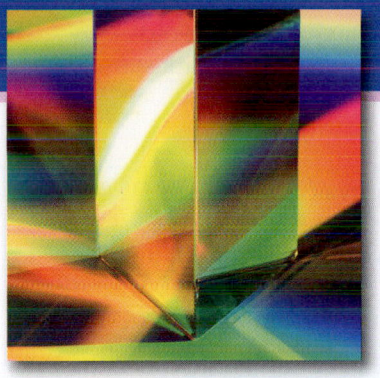

Evolution of Nursing Thought & Action

STUDENT RESOURCES

*The questions and exercises in Volume 2 allow you to practice the kind of thinking you will use as a full-spectrum nurse. Critical-thinking questions usually have more than one correct answer, so we do not provide "answers" for these features. It is more important to develop your nursing judgment than to just cover content. You will learn by discussing the questions with your peers. If you are still unsure, consult your instructor. You will find Response Sheets (for writing your responses to the questions) on Davis*Plus.

To explore learning resources for this chapter,

Go to Davis*Plus* at DavisPl.us/Wilkinson3.

Chapter Resources for Chapter 1:

- **Response sheets for all learning exercises**
- **Resources for Caregivers and Health Professionals**
- **Reading More About Evolution of Nursing Thought & Action (suggested readings)**
- **Concept Map of chapter content**

Interactive Case Studies

NCLEX-Style and Chapter Review Questions

CHAPTER OVERVIEW

For a podcast of an overview of this chapter,

Go to Student Resources: Chapter 1, **Podcast—Chapter Overview,** on Davis*Plus*.

Caring for the Nguyens

Review the opening scenario in the front of the book. On Nam Nguyen's preliminary visit to the Family Medicine Center, he is examined by Zach Miller, MSN, FNP-BC.

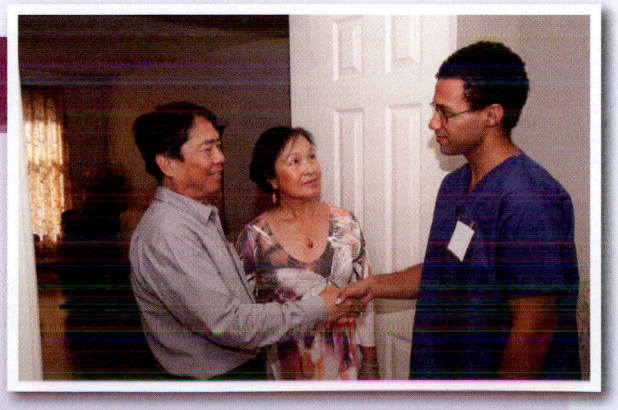

A. How would you respond to Mr. Nguyen's concerns that he was examined by someone who is "just a nurse"?

B. What factors might be causing Mr. Nguyen to question care by "a male nurse"?

Critical Thinking and Clinical Reasoning

1. At a holiday family gathering, you are at the dinner table with your 60-year-old aunt, your 85-year-old grandmother, and your 15-year-old sister-in-law. Your aunt and grandmother are retired RNs. Your sister-in-law aspires to be a nurse, and you are in school studying to be a nurse.
   a. What factors will influence how each of you views nursing?
   b. Your sister-in-law asks you to define nursing. What would you say?
   c. How could you explain to her how a nurse is different from a nurse's aide or a physician?
2. Review the information on educational pathways into nursing.
   a. What do you believe is the minimum level of education that should be required in order to practice nursing?
   b. What reasons can you give to support your opinion?
3. Review the description of the National Student Nurses Association (NSNA). If your program has a local chapter of the NSNA, consider attending a meeting or consulting the association's Web site for more information. Identify at least three potential benefits of joining this organization.
4. For each of the following concepts, use critical thinking to describe how or why it is important to nursing, patient care, or the evolution of nursing thought and action. Note that these are *not* to be merely definitions.

Healthcare delivery system	Nursing organizations
The Nightingale era	The national economy
ICN and ANA definitions of nursing	Better-informed healthcare consumers
Regulation of nursing practice	Use of nursing assistive personnel
Benner's stages of nursing skill	Use of life-extending, high-technology equipment

What Are the Main Points in This Chapter?

- Religious organizations and the military have played a major role in the development of nursing and healthcare organizations.
- Initially the role of the nurse was limited to bathing, feeding, and supporting the patient; keeping the patient environment clean and orderly; and providing support for the physician.
- Contemporary nursing care includes activities that are performed in collaboration with other members of the healthcare team and also independently.
- Licensed practical nurses (LPNs or LVNs) are nurses who have successfully completed a practical nursing program and have passed a licensure exam (NCLEX-PN). They are prepared to give direct patient care.
- Registered nurses (RNs) are nurses who have successfully completed a registered nurse education program and have passed a licensure exam (NCLEX-RN). There are several types of RN education programs.
- Graduate nursing education is designed to prepare the RN for advanced practice, expanded roles, nursing education, or research.
- Benner has identified a five-step progression of skill acquisition in nurses: novice, advanced beginner, competence, proficiency, and expert.
- Nurse practice acts are laws that regulate nursing practice at the state level.
- Nurses engage in health promotion, illness prevention, health restoration, and care of the dying.
- Nurses work in a variety of inpatient and outpatient settings, including hospitals, extended care facilities, ambulatory care, and community or home health settings.
- Nurses provide care using either the case method, functional, team, primary, or differentiated model.
- The economy, technology, an aging population, increased consumer involvement in healthcare, the women's movement, and the change in nursing role are all forces that have strongly affected nursing.
- The healthcare delivery system is complex and involves a multitude of players.
- Managed care models of insurances (HMOs, PPOs, POS, IDNs) reduce cost by reimbursing providers at discounted, predetermined rates and limiting the consumers' choice of providers.
- Government funded programs, such as Medicare, Medicaid, and CHIP, provide health insurance for persons with disabilities, are 65 years of age or older, or have a low income.
- Nurses care for sicker inpatients due to changes in reimbursement rates to hospitals.
- Nurses are essential members of the interdisciplinary healthcare team.
- Nurses must engage in lifelong learning activities to remain knowledgeable of and competent in professional practice.

Knowledge Map

Factors Affecting the Evolution of Nursing

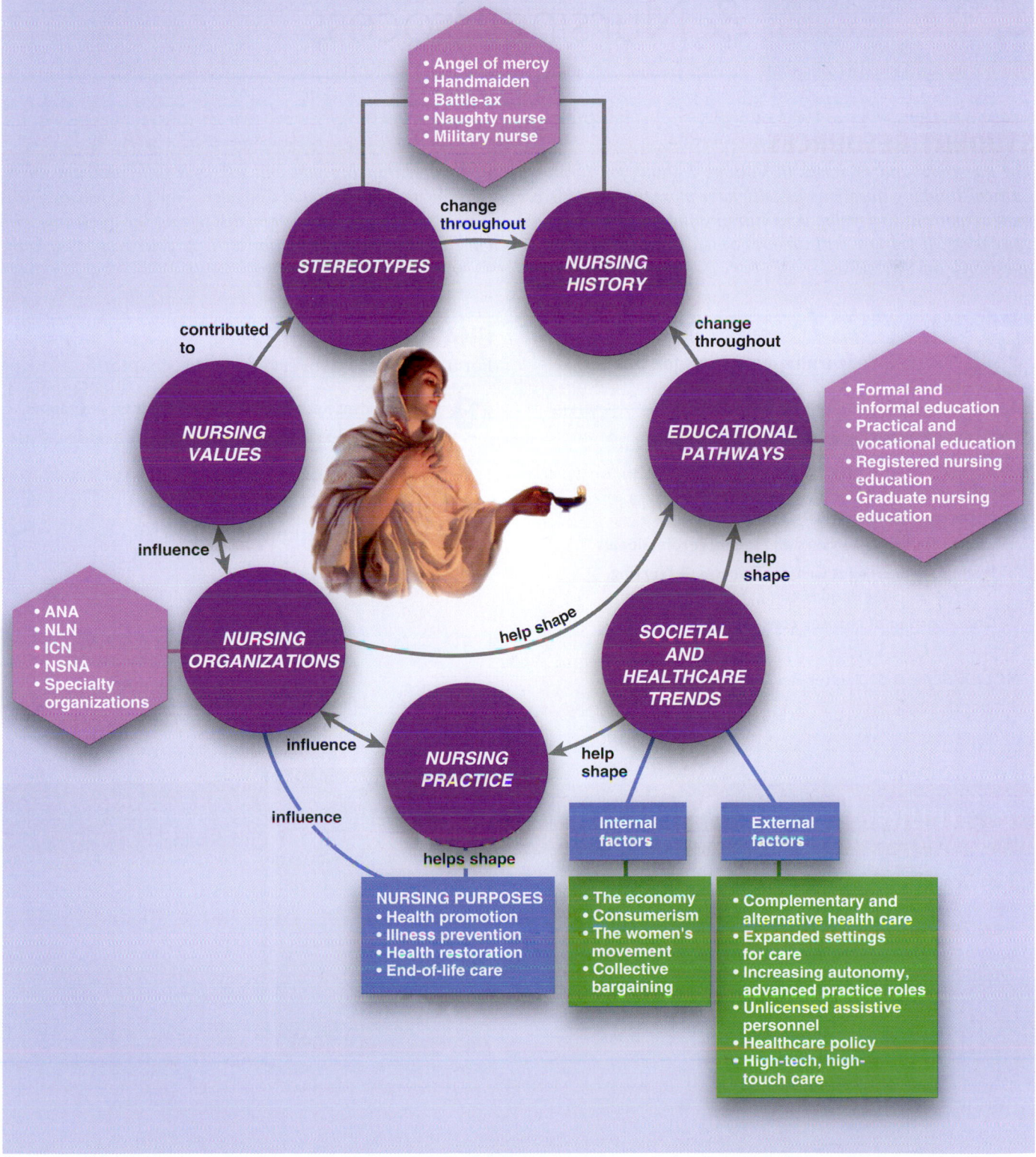

CHAPTER 2

Critical Thinking & Nursing Process

STUDENT RESOURCES

*The questions and exercises in Volume 2 allow you to practice the kind of thinking you will use as a full-spectrum nurse. Critical-thinking questions usually have more than one correct answer, so we do not provide "answers" for these features. It is more important to develop your nursing judgment than to just cover content. You will learn by discussing the questions with your peers. If you are still unsure, consult your instructor. You will find Response Sheets (for writing your responses to the questions) on Davis*Plus.

To explore learning resources for this chapter,

Go to Davis*Plus*, at DavisPl.us/Wilkinson3.

Chapter Resources for Chapter 2:

- **Response Sheets for all learning exercises**
- **Resources for Caregivers and Health Professionals**
- **Reading More About Critical Thinking & Nursing Process (suggested readings)**
- **Concept Map of chapter content**

Interactive Case Studies

NCLEX-Style and Chapter Review Questions

CHAPTER OVERVIEW

For a podcast of an overview of this chapter,

Go to Student Resources: Chapter 2, **Podcast— Chapter Overview,** on Davis*Plus*.

Caring for the Nguyens

Review the opening scenario of Nam Nguyen in the front of this book. Imagine that you are the clinic nurse at the Family Medicine Center. Based on the information presented in the scenario, work through the following questions:

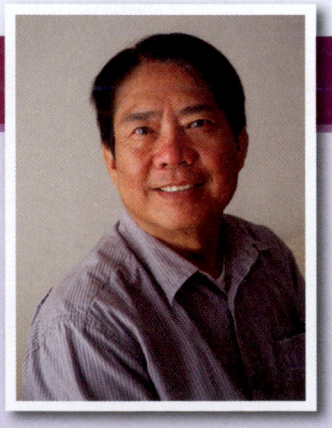

Caring for the Nguyens (continued)

A. Patient Situation

- Why is Mr. Nguyen at the clinic?
- What are his wife's concerns?
- Are his wife's concerns similar to or different from his?

B. Critical Thinking

- How do I go about getting the data I need? What sources should I use?
- Are my data congruent?
- What is one possible explanation for what is happening in this situation?

C. Nursing Knowledge

What type of nursing knowledge (theoretical, practical, ethical, or self-knowledge) is needed to answer the following questions?

- What health concerns does Mr. Nguyen have that should be addressed by the healthcare team?
- What is the role of Zach Jackson on the healthcare team?
- What role will you play in the care of Mr. Nguyen?

D. Nursing Process

- In what phase of the nursing process are you engaged when you are asking Mr. Nguyen about the reason for his visit?
- What activities are involved in the diagnosis phase? In planning outcomes? In planning interventions?
- Why would you not, at this point, be using the evaluation phase?

CLINICALREASONING

Applying the Full-Spectrum Nursing Model

PATIENT SITUATION

Mrs. Castillo has late-stage cancer and is not expected to live more than a few months. With chemotherapy, she could live perhaps a year or two more. She cannot decide what to do. She knows the chemotherapy will have unpleasant side effects and will be very expensive, and she wants to protect her family from the emotional and financial hardships of a lingering illness. She is showing physical signs of anxiety and distress (e.g., increased heart rate, restlessness, tearfulness). You want to provide support for her decision, whatever it may be.

THINKING

1. *Theoretical Knowledge*: What theoretical knowledge do you need to help Mrs. Castillo?
2. *Critical Thinking (Contextual Awareness)*: What details in the scenario represent *patient situation* or *context*?

DOING

3. *Practical Knowledge*:
   a. What practical knowledge do you need to help Mrs. Castillo?
   b. Which skills are you already competent in, and which ones would you need to learn or review before caring for this patient?

CARING

4. *Ethical Knowledge*: Depending on Mrs. Castillo's decision, can you think of one ethical issue that might arise for you or members of her family later on?

Critical Thinking and Clinical Reasoning

1. At the end of your first nursing class, your instructor gives an overview of a long-term assignment. She informs you that each semester of the program the class is required to complete a project that provides some

type of service to the college community or the local community, and that demonstrates the role or importance of nursing. The instructor asks you to begin discussing potential projects and come to class next week prepared to discuss several proposals for your community and the potential benefits of each option. You and several friends gather to talk about the class. "What an odd assignment!" you tell your friends. "How can we possibly do this now? We aren't nurses. We don't have any skills. What could we possibly do?" Your friends echo similar views.

This exercise is designed to help you actually work through the imaginary assignment you have just read. Use the *critical-thinking model* shown in Figure 2-1 and the sample questions in Table 2-1 of Volume 1 to complete the assignment.

Go to Volume 1, **Chapter 2: Critical Thinking & Nursing Process.**

a. *Contextual awareness* is one concept in the critical-thinking model. Consider the context in which the assignment was given.
- What exactly is this assignment?
- Your instructor is perfectly aware of your knowledge and skill levels. Why do you think she would ask students to complete such an assignment so early in their nursing studies?

To complete this assignment you would need to gather information to find ways to answer the following questions. You would also need to use credible sources (another task of critical thinking) to address these questions.

b. What sources might you use to answer the following two questions?
- What will I learn this semester?
- What skills will I have by the time this assignment is due?

c. What are some ways in which you could answer the following two questions?
- What do nurses do?
- How do nurses interact with the community?

d. What are some ways in which you could obtain information to answer this question: What does my community need?

e. If you had actually gathered the preceding information, you would then need to consider possible solutions. One way would be to develop a list of community needs, a list of activities nurses engage in, and a list of skills and knowledge you will have at the end of the term. Then look at the overlap between the lists. This should help you to get some ideas for projects. Imagine now that you have a list of possible projects similar to the following:
- Take blood pressures at a neighborhood grocery store for a day.
- Hold a health fair at a neighborhood shopping center.
- Create some materials for teaching about a healthy diet; distribute them at a community event.

Now think critically about this list of projects (this involves *reflective skepticism and exploring and imagining alternatives*). What questions could you ask about each project to help you decide which to actually do?

2. Review the following scenarios. Is critical thinking occurring? If so, which part of the critical-thinking model is the student using, or which critical-thinking skill or attitude from Chapter 2 in Volume 1? If there is no evidence of critical thinking, revise the scenario to include it.

a. Juan is a first-year nursing student. His clinical rotation is at a skilled nursing facility (SNF). He arrives at the unit at 0700 for the start of the day shift. After hearing the shift change report, he prepares to give his client a bedbath per unit policy.

b. Lily is teaching her patient, Mr. Johannsen, about the medications he will be taking when he is discharged from the hospital. When Lily reviews the list with him, he says, "That's too many medicines. It's too confusing." Lily devises a schedule and information sheet about the medicines that she gives to her client. She reviews the medications and their schedules with Mr. Johannsen and his wife before discharge.

c. Erin is caring for a young man who has had orthopedic surgery after a skiing accident. She is unable to hear his blood pressure when she attempts to take his vital signs. He is alert and able to converse with her. Since she is unable to hear the blood pressure, she records "0" in the client record.

d. As you are walking down the hall on the hospital unit, you hear a patient call out, "Nurse!" When you enter the room, you notice that the bedside is crowded with equipment. The patient is receiving several fluids intravenously, and a unit of blood is hanging from the IV pole. Since you have limited clinical experience you say to the patient, "I'll get you some help."

3. For each of the following concepts, use critical thinking to describe how or why it is important to nursing, patient care, or critical thinking in the nursing process. Note that these are *not* to be merely definitions.

Caring
Critical-thinking skills
Critical-thinking attitudes
Exploring alternatives
The nursing process
Assessment phase
Planning outcomes phase
Planning interventions phase
Implementation phase
Evaluation phase
Theoretical knowledge

What Are the Main Points in This Chapter?

- Nursing involves thinking, doing, and caring; and all are equally important.
- Critical thinking is a combination of reasoned thinking, openness to alternatives, an ability to reflect, and a desire to seek the truth.
- Critical thinking involves both attitudes and cognitive skills.
- Critical thinking attitudes include independent thinking, intellectual curiosity, intellectual humility, intellectual empathy, intellectual courage, intellectual perseverance, and fair-mindedness.
- Nurses use critical thinking in all aspects of their practice.
- Practical knowledge (knowing what to do and how to do it) and theoretical knowledge (knowing why) are equally important in nursing.
- The nursing process is a systematic problem-solving process that guides all nursing actions.
- The nursing process consists of six overlapping and interdependent phases: assessment, diagnosis, planning outcomes, planning interventions, implementation, and evaluation.
- Critical thinking is used in each phase of the nursing process; it is related to, but not the same as, the nursing process.
- Your ability to think critically depends on your theoretical knowledge about critical thinking, your motivation to practice it, and your fund of nursing knowledge.
- In full-spectrum nursing the nurse applies thinking, doing, and caring to the patient situation to help effect positive patient outcomes.

Knowledge Map

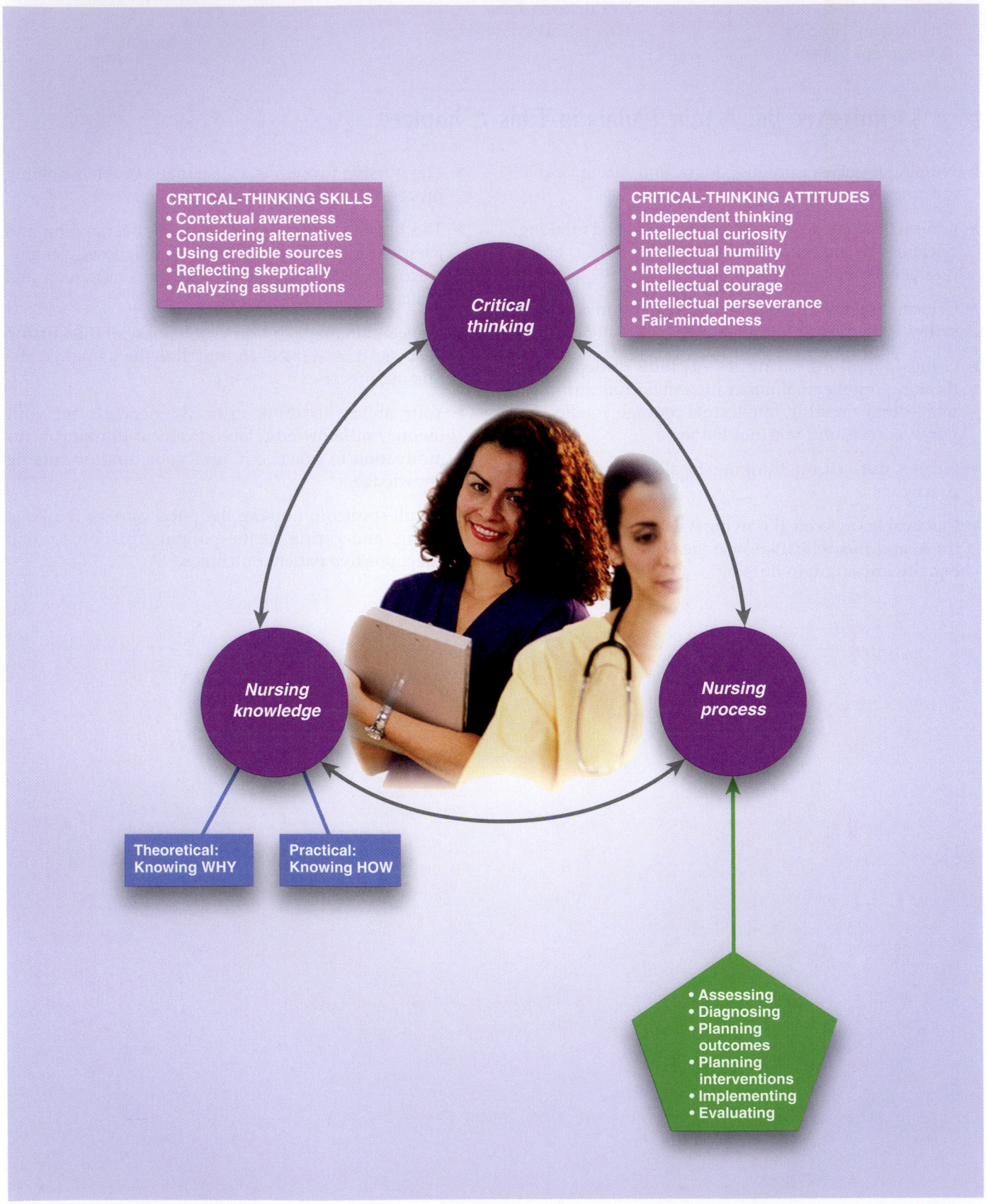

CHAPTER 3

Nursing Process: Assessment

STUDENT RESOURCES

*The questions and exercises in Volume 2 allow you to practice the kind of thinking you will use as a full-spectrum nurse. Critical-thinking questions usually have more than one correct answer, so we do not provide "answers" for these features. It is more important to develop your nursing judgment than to just cover content. You will learn by discussing the questions with your peers. If you are still unsure, consult your instructor. You will find Response Sheets (for writing your responses to the questions) on the Electronic Study Guide or Davis*Plus.

To explore learning resources for this chapter,

Go to Davis*Plus* at DavisPl.us/Wilkinson3.

Chapter Resources for Chapter 3:

- **Response Sheets for all learning activities**
- **Resources for Caregivers and Health Professionals**
- **Reading More About Nursing Process: Assessment (suggested readings)**
- **Concept Map of chapter content**

Interactive Case Studies

NCLEX-Style and Chapter Review Questions

CHAPTER OVERVIEW

For a podcast of an overview of this chapter,

Go to Student Resources, Chapter 3, **Podcast—Chapter Overview,** on Davis*Plus*.

Caring for the Nguyens

Review the opening scenario of Nam Nguyen in the front of Volume 2. Imagine that you are the clinic nurse at the Family Medicine Center. Using the information presented in the scenario, work through the following questions:

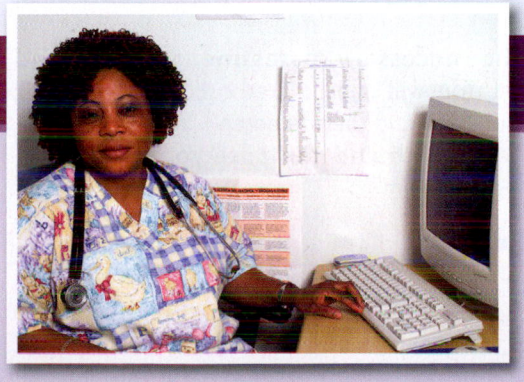

A. What type of assessment, comprehensive or focused, is being performed at this clinic visit? Explain your thinking.

B. Identify the types of data (e.g., subjective/objective, primary/secondary) that have been gathered so far. Give an example of each type.

(Continued)

Caring for the Nguyens (continued)

C. How might you verify data that Mr. Nguyen provided on the intake sheet?

D. Based on what you know about Mr. Nguyen, what follow-up assessments would provide useful data to help with the care of Mr. Nguyen? Why would you make these assessments?

Practical Knowledge knowing how

In this chapter, practical knowledge pertains to your skill in applying the concepts of assessment and data, for example, by using structured and unstructured methods of data collection.

CLINICAL INSIGHTS

Clinical Insight 3-1 ➤ Preparing for a Patient Interview

Prepare Yourself

- **Know your purpose.** Be sure you know why you are conducting the interview and how the data will be used. As a student, this may simply mean preparing thoroughly for your clinical assignment.
- **Read the patient's chart.** This will give you an idea of where to start with the interview and keep you from covering topics already assessed by other caregivers. Be careful to keep an open mind, though. If you approach an interview with preconceived ideas, you may overlook important data.
- **Form some goals** for the interview.
- **Think of some opening questions.**
- **Schedule some uninterrupted time** for the interview. Giving the patient your undivided attention builds rapport and helps her to feel freer to share information with you.
- **Gather the necessary assessment forms and equipment.** You will need a stethoscope, pen, pencil, blood pressure cuff, and thermometer.
- **Take a deep breath and compose yourself** just before entering the room.

Prepare the Space

- **Provide privacy** (e.g., ask visitors to wait outside, shut the door). Unless you need information from the visitor (e.g., when the client cannot communicate clearly) you may wish to postpone the interview until it can be done in private. The presence of even a close family member may inhibit the client in some situations. For example, a wife may not want her husband to know that she had a miscarriage before they were married.
- **Keep the focus on the client** as much as possible. If others must be present, sometimes the client's spouse, family, or partner will offer information that may or may not be pertinent. Focus on the client, but do not ignore the information provided by others.
- **Remove distractions** (e.g., turn off the television, arrange for someone to watch the children for a while, if they are present).
- **Sit down. Do not hover over the bed.** Position yourself at the same level as your client, even if the client is in bed.

Prepare the Patient

- **Introduce yourself** to the patient and others in the room.
- **Call the patient by name.** First ask what name the patient prefers. Don't use endearing terms like "grandma," "dear," and "sweetie." You may think you are being friendly or expressing caring, but many people feel belittled by these terms.
- **Tell the patient what you will be doing and why.** Explain that you will be taking notes and that you will keep all information confidential.
- **Assess and provide comfort** (e.g., assess and medicate for pain, offer the bedpan, offer a drink of water).
- **Assess for anxiety.** Be sure the patient is comfortable emotionally as well as physically. A very anxious person cannot provide good information, so you may need to intervene to relieve anxiety before proceeding.
- **Assess readiness to discuss health issues.** If the patient indicates that now is not a good time, reschedule (e.g., if the patient has just received some bad news about his condition, or in his personal life, he may need some time to process that information before he can concentrate on interview questions).
- **Interviews** are recorded only when done during research projects. The researcher must be sure to obtain institutional review board approval and written permission from the patient, using an approved consent form.

Clinical Insight 3-2 ➤ Conducting a Patient Interview

- **Individualize your approach.** Ask yourself, for example, "What approach is best considering the client's age and developmental level?" Respect the generational differences of a person older or younger than you are.
- **Be sensitive to cultural differences** (e.g., comfort with eye contact, the need for space).
- **Begin with neutral topics**, such as the biographical data (e.g., address, contact person, occupation). Ask more personal or sensitive questions after you and the client are more comfortable with each other.
- **Key Point:** *Use active listening. This is the most important interviewing technique. Focus intently on trying to understand what the client is saying, rather than thinking ahead to what your response to the statement will be.*
- **Use the mnemonic FOLK** to remember other active listening behaviors:

  Face the patient (either sitting or standing).
  Open, relaxed posture (arms and legs uncrossed).
  Lean toward the patient.
  Keep eye contact.
- **Do not get caught up in note taking.** Excessive writing interferes with eye contact and may inhibit the client's responses, especially when you are discussing personal issues such as sexuality or drug and alcohol use.
- **Pay attention to nonverbal communication.** Body language may signal that the person is tired or in pain but is too polite to say so. If the person is fatigued, you may need to end the interview and finish it at another time.
- **Use open-ended questions** as much as possible to encourage the client to talk.
- **Avoid asking too many questions.** Asking too many questions may make you seem merely curious instead of genuinely interested in the client.
- **Use neutral statements instead of questions** (e.g., instead of asking, "How many children do you have?" say, "Tell me about your family").
- **Avoid asking "why"** (e.g., "Why have you stopped taking your pills?"). For some people, "why" suggests disapproval and causes them to become defensive. (This may be because parents frequently ask their children, "Why did you do that?")
- **Do not use healthcare jargon** (e.g., say, "I want to take your temperature and blood pressure" instead of "I want to take your vital signs").
- **Do not "talk down" to the client** (e.g., Don't say, "How often do you go potty?" when interviewing an adult).
- **Be sure your client understands what he says.** Confirm that clients actually understand the terminology they use. If a client says, "It's the inflammation that causes me the trouble, you know," you might say, "Tell me where the inflammation is and what happens when you have it." People may repeat words they hear from care providers without really knowing what the words mean.
- **Refocus and redirect the client as needed** (e.g., when a response becomes scattered or does not produce useful information). Encourage the client to talk about the topics of importance to her, but direct her to topics that need to be covered (e.g., "We haven't talked about your surgery. What do you expect to happen?").
- **Curb your curiosity.** Do not get caught up in the details of the client's story. Focus on the information you need to plan care.
- **Do not give advice or voice approval or disapproval.** Even if the advice is good (e.g., "It is good that you take your pills on time"), it may cause the client to be less open because he feels you are judging him. This can interfere with your ability to gather data.

Clinical Insight 3-3 ➤ Closing a Patient Interview

- Prepare the patient for closure. Begin by informing her that the interview is nearly finished.
- Summarize the key points of the interview.
- Be sure you have recorded all the important data. Ask the patient, "Is there anything else you would like to tell me?" or "Is there anything else we should talk about?"
- Thank the patient for answering the questions.
- Encourage the patient to keep you informed. For example, you might say, "Please let us know if you think of anything else we should know."
- Tell the patient what to expect next. Let the patient know when you will be leaving, when you will see him again, and what he can expect for the rest of the day (e.g., tests, treatments).
- And finally, ask, "Is there anything I can do for you before I leave?"

ASSESSMENT GUIDELINES AND TOOLS

You can use the forms in this section to perform a focused assessment of activities of daily living and to perform a comprehensive patient assessment. If you want to use an interactive assessment tool to create your own assessment form,

Go to **Davis's Care Planning & Nursing Diagnosis Resource Center, Interactive Assessment Tool,** at **http://davisplus.fadavis.com/daviscareplans/assessment tool.cfm.**

Patient Assessment Tool—Lawton Instrumental Activities of Daily Living (IADL)

Date:_____ Name:_____

Please check the box that most applies for each activity:

Activity	Needs no help (2 pts. each)	Needs some help (1 pt. each)	Unable to do at all (0 pts. each)
1. Using the telephone	___	___	___
2. Getting to places beyond walking distance	___	___	___
3. Grocery shopping	___	___	___
4. Preparing meals	___	___	___
5. Doing housework or handyman work	___	___	___
6. Doing laundry	___	___	___
7. Taking medications	___	___	___
8. Managing money	___	___	___
Total score:___ =	(___ × 2 =) ___ +	(___ × 1 =) ___ +	0

A patient is awarded 2 points for each area in which he/she can function totally without help, 1 point in those areas that they need some help, and 0 points for those activities that somebody else must do completely for them. The maximum score is 16, minimum score is 0.

Like other evaluations, the IADL scale provides a baseline of data that can be compared with the results of future evaluations. (Note that some activities may be gender specific. Omit these items if the patient does not usually perform those tasks.)

Permission obtained from M. Powell Lawton, Ph.D., Philadelphia Geriatric Center, Philadelphia, PA. May be used freely for patient assessment. Formatted and posted May 25, 1996, to www.acsu.buffalo.edu/~drstall/assessmenttools.html by Robert S. Stall, M.D.

NURSING ADMISSION DATA FORM

Nursing Admission Data Form

Name: Ben J. Ivanos Age: 24 Phone #: 618-445-2300 Date: mm/dd/yyyy Time: 10:30
Primary Physician: Charles Katz Phone #: 618-446-8160
Chief Complaints/Procedure: ORIF fx (L) leg, Fx (R) femur + (R) ulna Height: 5' 10" Weight (lbs.): 155
Historian: Patient Temp: 100 Pulse: 90 Resp: 16 BP: 140/82
Religious Affiliation: Catholic Hospitalized within 30 days: Yes [X] No [ ]

UNABLE TO OBTAIN HISTORY [ ]
Reason:

NEUROLOGICAL/SENSORY PERCEPTION
- Glaucoma [ ]
- Hearing Loss/Deaf ... Right [ ] Left [ ]
- Motion Sickness [ ]
- Paresthesia ... Right [ ] Left [ ]
- Fibromyalgia/Migraine [ ]
- Spina Bifida [ ]
- Stroke/CVA/TIA [ ]
- Altered Mental Status [ ]
- Other:

CARDIOVASCULAR/HEMATOLOGY
- Bleeding Problems [ ]
- Blood transfusion in the past 3 months [ ]
- Chest Pain/Angina [ ]
- Heart Attack/Date: [ ]
- Heart Disease [ ]
- High Blood Pressure [ ]
- Irregular Beats/Pacemaker/AICD [ ]
- Mitral Valve Prolapse [ ]
- Murmur [ ]
- Peripheral Vascular Disease [ ]
- Sickle Cell Disease [ ]
- Venous Access Device/Type [ ]
- Other:

RESPIRATORY
- Asthma [ ]
- Bronchitis ... 6 months ago [X]
- COPD/Emphysema [ ]
- Post Nasal Drip/Rhinitis/Sinusitis [X]
- Pneumonia [ ]
- Tracheostomy [ ]
- Other:

GASTROINTESTINAL
- Dysphagia [ ]
- Hiatal Hernia [ ]
- Liver Disease/Jaundice [ ]
- Pancreatitis [ ]
- Gall Stones [ ]
- Ostomy [ ]
- Last Bowel Movement: 5/19/2013
- Other:

GENITOURINARY/RENAL
- Kidney Disease/Urogenital [ ]
- Prostate Problems [ ]
- Voiding Problems [ ]
- Other:

MUSCULOSKELETAL
- Arthritis [ ]
- Back/Disc Problem [ ]
- Fractures ... present admission [X]
- Other:

ENDOCRINE
- Diabetes/type: [ ]
- Thyroid Disease [ ]
- Other:

INFECTIOUS DISEASE
- Fevers [ ]
- Hepatitis/type/active [ ]
- HIV/AIDS [ ]
- Recent Cold [ ]
- Sexually Transmitted Disease/type [ ]
- Tuberculosis/Active: [ ]
- Other:

- Pregnant [ ]
- Lactating [ ]
- LMP/Date:

VACCINATION/DATE
- Flu: Hepatitis B:
- Pneumonia:

BEHAVIORAL HEALTH
- Anxiety Disorder [ ]
- Depression [ ]
- Suicide (thoughts/attempts) [ ]
- Patient is a Baker Act [ ]
- Other:

CANCER
- Type [ ]
- Radioactive Seeds/Implant [ ]
- Date:
- Other:

SOCIAL HISTORY
- Tobacco [X]
  - Number of years: 3
  - # of packs per day: 1/2
  - Year Quit: 2003
- Would you like smoking cessation info? [X] No [ ] Yes [ ] information provided
- Alcohol [X]
  - Drinks per day: 1
  - Amount:
  - Type:
- Recreational Drug [ ]
  - Amount:
  - Type:
  - Year Quit:
- Detoxification Protocol Initiated [ ]

ALLERGIES & REACTION None Known [X] Allergy Bracelet on [ ]

Medications: none
Symptoms:

Blood Reaction: [ ]
Latex: [ ]
Latex Allergy Protocol Initiated: [ ]

Food/Shellfish/other allergies: No
Contrast/Dye: No

PAST HOSPITAL/PROCEDURE (Surgical/Medical/Behavioral Health)
None

CURRENT MEDICATIONS (include ASA/Anticoagulant, over the counter medications, ointments, patches, eye drops, herbal, vitamins and nutritional supplements)

Medication	Dose	Frequency	Last Dose
ASA	"2"	occasionally for HA	

Food/Drug Interaction information provided [ ]
Initiate Social Service Consult
(Note: Additional medication can be listed on last page)

ADDRESSOGRAPH

Nursing Admission Data Form *(continued)*

PAIN HISTORY

Have you been experiencing pain? ☒ Yes
If yes, when *Now* Intensity (0-10): *10* Goal (0-10): *2*
Location: *Legs and arm, muscles in back*
Radiation: *No*
Duration: *Constant*
Quality: *Sharp, aching*
Aggravating factors *Movement*

What medications/interventions are effective in relieving your pain?
Taking PCA Demerol

Acute Pain Management - It is Your Right brochure provided ☒

PSYCHOSOCIAL ASSESSMENT

☒ Lives alone ☐ Lives with spouse/SO ☐ Nursing Home/ALF
☐ Homeless ☐ Rehab Facility ☐ Other:
Marital Status ☒ Single ☐ Married ☐ Divorced ☐ Widowed ☐ Separated
Next of Kin: *Mother, Clara Ivanos* **Phone #:** *618-446-3816*
Supportive Adult: - **Phone #:** -
Has anybody threatened/hit/abused you within the last year?
☐ Yes **(refer to policy RA 004015 mauve manual)** ☒ No

EDUCATIONAL LEARNING ASSESSMENT

Learner ☒ Patient ☐ Family ☐ Significant Other
Readiness to learn ☐ Eager to learn ☒ Asks questions
☐ Extremely anxious ☐ Denies need for Education
Knowledge of current health status ☐ No knowledge
☒ Partial understanding ☐ Full understanding
Barriers to learning ☒ Physical ☐ Emotional
☐ Language ☐ Religious ☐ Cultural
☐ Reading Ability ☐ Changes in Short Memory
☐ None
Preferred Learning Method ☒ Reading ☐ Lecture
☒ Video ☒ Demo/Practice
Communication ☒ English ☐ Spanish ☐ Creole
☐ Sign Language ☐ Other:
Do you have any religious/cultural practices that are important to you or may alter your care or education? ☒ No ☐ Yes

☒ **Patient Handbook provided** ☒ **Patient safety information provided**
☒ **Patient's Bill of Rights and Responsibilities information provided**
Other Educational Materials:

PERSONAL EFFECTS: Do you use the following:

	YES	WITH PT.	FAMILY/SO
Wheelchair	☐	☐	☐
Braces	☐	☐	☐
Cane/Crutches	☐	☐	☐
Walker	☐	☐	☐
Prothesis	☐	☐	☐
Medications	☐	☐	☐
Dentures: (Full)	☐	☐	☐
Upper	☐	☐	☐
Lower	☐	☐	☐
Glasses	☐	☐	☐
Contacts	☒	☒	☐
Hearing Aids	☐	☐	☐

Other:

Initiate Social Service Consult

ADVANCE DIRECTIVES

Do you have an Advance Directive?
(must check one)
☒ **No** Information provided to patient
☐ **No** Patient elects not to receive information
☐ **Yes** (check advance directive patient states he/she has)
☐ **Living Will** ☐ **Health Care Surrogate** ☐ **State DNAR form**
☐ **Durable Power of Attorney** ☐ **Organ Donation**
(If patient has an Advance Directive, inform patient to provide copy within 24 hours or they may complete a new advance directive or verbalize their wishes)
Do you have a guardian? ☐ **Yes name**
(Inform patient to provide guardianship form within 24 hours)
☐ **Patient unable to respond/family not available**

FALL SCREEN: *If any of the following are checked, initiate* ***Safety/Protective Intervention Protocol***

Inability to understand or follow instructions		☐
Impaired mobility, visual impairment, drug therapy, surgical procedure, unsteady gait, incontinence	*Casts, Traction*	☒
Unable to use call light		☐
Altered mental status	*Taking Demerol PCA*	☒
Nocturnal/urgency/frequency in elimination		☐
Dizziness		☐
History of falls		☐
No Criteria Met		☐

NUTRITIONAL SCREEN: *If any of the following are checked, enter in the computer request for* ***Nutritional Consult***

Nausea/vomiting > 5 days	☐
No food/drink for 3 days	☐
Recent unexplained weight loss > 10 lbs.	☐
Difficulty swallowing/dysphagia	☐
Evidence of Stage III - IV pressure ulcer	☐
Feeding tube	☐
New onset diabetes	☐
TPN	☐
Pregnant/lactating	☐
Surgical patients > 70 years of age	☐
Ethnic diet/special needs **(include in diet order and order for Preference consult)**	☐
Difficulty chewing **(include in diet order and order for Preference consult)**	☐
No Criteria Met	☒

FUNCTIONAL SCREEN: *If any of the following are checked, please request physician order for physical therapy consult.*

New onset of paralysis		☐
New onset stroke/CVA		☐
New amputation		☐
Unsteady gait		☐
Decreased mobility	*Casts, Tx for Fx*	☒
Dysphagia		☐
No Criteria Met		☐

Nursing Admission Data Form *(continued)*

MARK LOCATION

Anterior View | Posterior View | Right Lateral | Left Lateral | Left Foot | Right Foot

* Label Wound Type

WOUND TYPE

P = Pressure ulcer
ST = Skin tear
S = Surgical
L = Laceration
B = Burns
A = Abrasions
LU = Leg/Foot ulcers
BR = Bruising
M = Maceration
O = Other

STAGE

Pressure ulcer only

I: Reddened area, does not resolve with pressure relief.
II: Blister or superficial break in skin.
III: Full thickness wound into subcutaneous tissue.
IV: Full thickness with muscle, bone or tendon tissue exposed.
U = Unable to stage: Necrotic

COLOR WOUND BED

R = Red (new tissue)
P = Pink
Y = Yellow (slough)
B = Black (eschar)

EXUDATE

O = None
S = Serous
SS = Serosanguinous
P = Purulent

ODOR

N = None
S = Slight
F = Foul

SURROUNDING SKIN

OK = Clean & Intact
C = Cellulitis (red & tender)
R = Raw & denuded
M = Maceration
I = Induration
Ra = Rash

Skin Breakdown Present ☐ Consent Obtained ☐ Photograph Taken ☐ Acute/Chronic Wound Flow Sheet Initiated ☐ Swat Consult Initiated ☐

BRADEN SCALE - PRESSURE ULCER RISK ASSESSMENT

SENSORY PERCEPTION Ability to respond meaningfully to pressure-related discomfort	1. Completely Limited:	2. Very Limited:	3. Slightly Limited:	4. No Impairment:	4
MOISTURE Degree to which skin is exposed to moisture	1. Constantly Moist:	2. Very Moist:	3. Occasionally Moist:	4. Rarely Moist:	4
ACTIVITY degree of physical activity	1. Bedfast:	2. Chairfast:	3. Walks Occasionally:	4. Walks Frequently:	1
MOBILITY ability to change and control body position	1. Completely Immobile:	2. Very Limited:	3. Slightly Limited:	4. No Limitations:	3
NUTRITION usual food intake pattern	1. Very Poor:	2. Probably Inadequate:	3. Adequate:	4. Excellent:	4
FRICTION AND SHEAR	1. Problem:	2. Potential Problem:	3. No Apparent Problem:		2

RN Signature: [signature] Date: mm/dd/yyyy **TOTAL SCORE:** 18

NOTE: Patients with a total score of 16 or less are considered to be at risk of developing pressure ulcers. Implement Skin Care Protocol. Refer to Surface Bed Decision Tree. (12 or less = high risk)

ATICIPATED DISHARGE NEEDS

☒ Transportation ☐ Placement needed

Medical Equipment: ☐ Oxygen ☐ CPAP ☐ Nebulizer ☐ Blood Glucose Meter Other: Crutches, Wheelchair

Community Services: (Home Health, Reach to Recovery, Meals On Wheels, etc.): Home Health for f/u on cast care and pain medication. Transportation to physicians office for return visit.

Nurse Signature: [signature] Unit: 3E Date: mm/dd/yyyy Time: 10:45

Nurse Signature: _____ Unit: _____ Date: _____ Time: _____

Nursing Admission Data Form *(continued)*

DATE & TIME	INTERDISCIPLINARY NOTES/ADVANCE DIRECTIVES INFORMATION
mm/dd/yyyy, 11:00	Healthy young adult, on no meds, admitted via E.D. p̄ motorcycle accident, and reduction and casting of
	multiple fx (L tibia + fibula, R femur, and R elbow and ulna). Experiencing severe pain r/t fx, bruises
	and muscle spasms. Plan:
	1 Traction per Rx; check weights q̄ 4th
	2 Control pain w/PCA Demerol. Assess + instruct prn
	3 Neurovascular + circulatory checks, all extremities, q̄ 2h -
	4 Monitor adema of extremities; re-cast after 3 days if edema has subsided.

Nurse Signature: Jon Rhodes RN Unit: 3E Date: mm/dd/yyyy Time: 11:00

Nurse Signature: _____ Unit: _____ Date: _____ Time: _____

Current Medications: (Continued)

Medication	Dose	Frequency	Last Dose

Page 4 of 4 WHITE - INPATIENT/OUTPATIENT LITE GREEN - OUTPATIENT ONLY DARK GREEN - ANESTHESIA LITE BLUE - INPATIENT ONLY

CLINICALREASONING

Applying the Full-Spectrum Nursing Model

PATIENT SITUATION

As the intake nurse in a community-based clinic, your role is to complete a comprehensive nursing assessment and initiate a plan of care for the clients. Your first client is a 27-year-old single woman, Sami, who is requesting clinic services for her general healthcare needs. Sami is Cuban American and lives alone in a one-bedroom apartment. She works as a fitness trainer at the local fitness club while attending college part-time. Her family lives in another city about 200 miles away. Sami's earnings place her at the poverty level, but she realizes that she must have healthcare to prevent illness and to detect and receive treatment of illnesses should they arise.

THINKING

1. *Theoretical Knowledge:* To care for Sami, what knowledge would you need that you do not already have? List the URL for at least one reputable online source for this information.
2. *Critical Thinking:* The nurse asks Sami, "If you can't afford healthcare, couldn't you get a roommate to save some money on rent?" What are some critical-thinking questions you should ask yourself when reflecting on this question later?

DOING

3. *Practical Knowledge:* What practical knowledge will you, as the nurse, use in this scenario?
4. *Nursing Process:* What kind of assessment will you perform for Sami (e.g., comprehensive, focused, special needs, discharge, etc.)?

CARING

5. *Self-Knowledge:* In what ways are you similar to Sami? In what ways are you different?

Critical Thinking and Clinical Reasoning

1. Recall the definition of subjective data. Make a list of the kinds of patients from whom you might not be able to get subjective data or who might give unreliable data. One example is a baby who cannot talk yet. How many others can you think of?
2. What are some factors that might make it difficult, but not impossible, for a patient to provide you with subjective data? One example is when the person is severely anxious.
3. For each of the factors in question 2, state what you could do to facilitate collection of reliable subjective data from that person.
4. List your present assessment skills and indicate your comfort level using each skill. Include observation, physical assessment, and interviewing skills. Use a scale of 1–5, with 1 = slightly comfortable; 2 = somewhat comfortable; 3 = moderately comfortable; 4 = fairly comfortable; and 5 = very comfortable.
5. For any skill that you score as 3 or lower, write a plan describing what you need to do to move to the higher comfort level.
6. The following are excerpts from criteria in the American Nurses Association (ANA) (2010) professional practice Standard 1. For each of the criteria, write an example of what would constitute evidence (proof) that the standard is being followed in a healthcare agency. The first one is done for you.
   a. "Collects data . . . in a systematic and ongoing process."
      I would look in the care plan for nursing orders that call for some kind of assessment on a scheduled basis. For example, an order might read, "Temperature q4hr" or "Check dressing for drainage once per shift." I would also look at the nursing notes, especially for flow sheets (e.g., vital sign flow sheets, input and output records, neurological checks) to see whether assessment findings were recorded at regular intervals. I would look for nursing diagnoses or other conclusions they have charted in the nurses' notes (e.g., stating that the medication has effectively relieved pain). Other evidence would be to observe the nurses doing systematic and ongoing data collection.
   b. "Involves the healthcare consumer, family, and other healthcare providers, as appropriate, in holistic data collection."
   c. "Prioritizes data-collection activities based on the healthcare consumer's immediate condition, or the anticipated needs . . ."
   d. "Uses appropriate evidence-based assessment techniques, instruments, and tools."
   e. "Synthesizes available data, information, and knowledge relevant to the situation to identify patterns and variances."
   f. "Documents relevant data in a retrievable format."
7. Your client, Sami (Meet Your Patient, in Volume 1), was born in Cuba. Having worked with many clients of Cuban heritage and being familiar with nursing literature regarding various cultural patterns, you are aware of the following:
   - Many Hispanic people who live in Sami's city are bilingual.
   - When communicating, especially with strangers, it is not unusual for Hispanic women not to maintain eye contact. (During the interview, Sami speaks rapidly and does not maintain eye contact with you.)
   - Many people of Cuban descent are Catholic and consider birth control to be taboo.
   - Many Cuban American women do not obtain annual physical examinations (Purnell & Paulanka, 2008).

   a. Looking at the four points from the literature, how is Sami's cultural background similar to or different from your own? Remember that you are looking at cultural patterns, not Sami's individual and personal values and behaviors.
   b. On the basis of your understanding of your own and Sami's culture, what questions might you want to ask Sami to support her reproductive health?
8. What physical examination techniques would you use to:
   a. Assess for a distended bladder?
   b. Get information about a patient's headache?
   c. Obtain data about a patient's ankle edema?
   d. What subjective data could you obtain by using one of the four physical assessment techniques?

9. For each of the following concepts, use critical thinking to describe how or why it is important to nursing, patient care, or assessment. Note that these are *not* to be merely definitions.

Active listening
Agency policies
ANA standards of practice
Assessment
Comprehensive assessments
Focused assessments
Nursing frameworks/models
Pain assessment
Recording data
Reflecting critically about your assessment
Special needs assessments
Spiritual health assessment
The Joint Commission
The nursing health history
Validating data
Wellness assessment

What Are the Main Points in This Chapter?

- Assessment is a systematic, ongoing process of collecting, categorizing, and recording holistic data about client health status.
- Accurate, complete data are essential to effective nursing diagnosis and care planning.
- Nursing assessments focus on client responses to illness and stressors rather than on identifying disease processes.
- ANA standards of practice state that professional nurses are responsible for assessing clients.
- A comprehensive assessment provides information about the client's overall health, whereas a focused assessment provides data about a particular topic, body part, or functional ability.
- Special needs assessments provide in-depth information about a particular area of client functioning (e.g., nutrition, pain, lifestyle).
- Subjective data can be perceived only by the client; objective data are measurable or observable by the nurse or other healthcare providers.
- Nurses obtain data by observing and interviewing patients, and by performing physical assessment.
- The formats and frameworks for the nursing health history vary among agencies; however, all have essentially the same components (e.g., chief complaint, family history, review of body systems).
- Effective interviews require preparation by the nurse and use of both closed and open-ended questions.
- Active listening is one of the most important interviewing techniques.
- Validating data helps to ensure that they are accurate, complete, and factual.
- Documentation of assessment findings is of critical importance and has professional and legal implications.
- When documenting assessments, the nurse should record cues (observations), not inferences (conclusions).

Knowledge Map

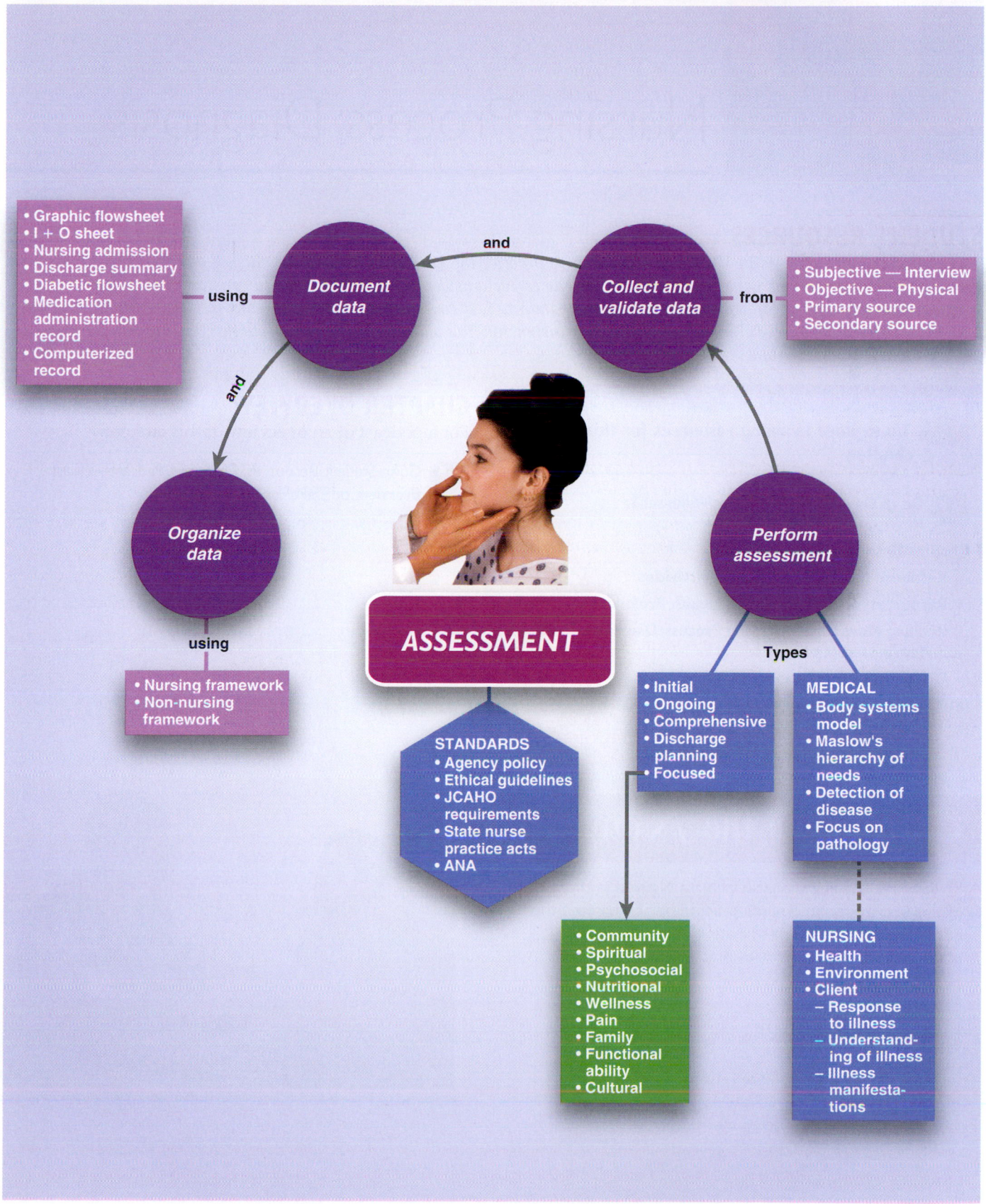

CHAPTER 4

Nursing Process: Diagnosis

STUDENT RESOURCES

*The questions and exercises in Volume 2 allow you to practice the kind of thinking you will use as a full-spectrum nurse. Critical-thinking questions usually have more than one correct answer, so we do not provide "answers" for these features. It is more important to develop your nursing judgment than to just cover content. You will learn by discussing the questions with your peers. If you are still unsure, consult your instructor. You will find Response Sheets (for writing your responses to the questions) on Davis*Plus.

To explore learning resources for this chapter,

Go to Davis*Plus* at DavisPl.us/Wilkinson3.

Chapter Resources for Chapter 4:

- **Response sheets for all learning activities**
- **Resources for Caregivers and Health Professionals**
- **Reading More About Nursing Process: Diagnosis (suggested readings)**
- **Concept Map of chapter content**

Interactive Case Studies

NCLEX-Style and Chapter Review Questions

CHAPTER OVERVIEW

For a podcast of an overview of this chapter,

Go to Student Resources: Chapter 4, **Podcast—Chapter Overview,** on Davis*Plus*.

Caring for the Nguyens

Review the opening scenario of Nam Nguyen in the front of this book. After the nurse practitioner completed the interview and physical examination of Mr. Nguyen, he listed the following diagnoses on the problem list:

- Hypertension
- Obesity
- Musculoskeletal pain
- Tobacco abuse
- Family history of prostate cancer
- Family history of cardiovascular disease
- Family history of diabetes mellitus (DM)

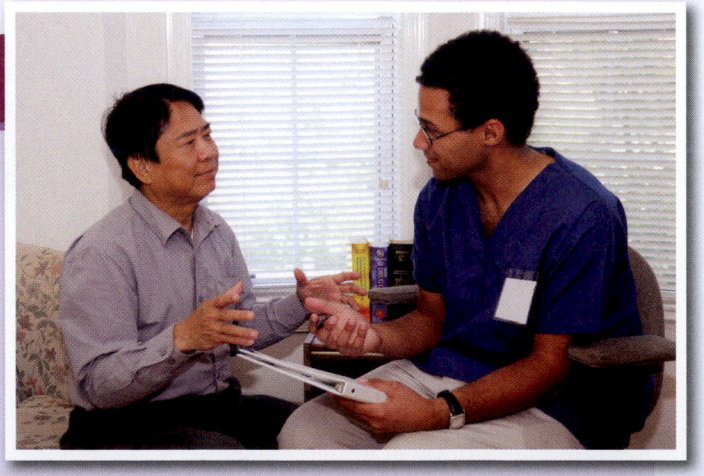

Caring for the Nguyens (continued)

A. What type of problem list does this represent? How is it similar to or different from a problem list that you might generate?

B. Based on the data in the scenario, identify at least one actual, one potential, and one wellness diagnosis for Mr. Nguyen. Identify the NANDA-I labels, and describe the cues that support your choices.

C. The nurse has identified a problem of Imbalanced Nutrition: More Than Body Requirements for Mr. Nguyen.
- What information do you need in order to determine the etiology of this problem?
- Because you do not have that information, write a two-part diagnostic statement describing Mr. Nguyen's nutritional status.

D. Now rewrite the nutrition statement as a three-part statement, including the phrase *"as evidenced by."*

E. The nurse has identified Acute Pain (knees) for Mr. Nguyen. If the pain were caused by a medical condition, osteoarthritis, how would you write a two-part diagnostic statement to describe this health status?

PracticalKnowledge knowing how

In this section, you will find a list of descriptors for NANDA-I nursing diagnoses. To see an alphabetical list of NANDA-I nursing diagnoses,

Go to Additional Resources, **NANDA-I Nursing Diagnoses, 2012-2014 Alphabetical List,** on Davis*Plus*.

To see NANDA-I labels organized into taxonomy categories,

Go to Student Resources: Chapter 4, **Standardized Language, NANDA-International Taxonomy II: Domains, Classes, and Diagnoses (Labels),** on Davis*Plus*.

Refer to these lists as you develop nursing diagnoses for your patients.

STANDARDIZED LANGUAGE

Descriptors for NANDA-I Nursing Diagnoses

Axis 1. The Diagnostic Focus This describes the "human response or experience" that is the core of the diagnosis. Examples are activity tolerance, airway clearance, anxiety, and pain

Axis 2. Subject of the Diagnosis This is defined as the person(s) for whom a nursing diagnosis is determined. The values (descriptors) in Axis 2 are:

Descriptor	Definition
Individual	A single human being distinct from others, a person
Family	Two or more people having continuous or sustained relationships, perceiving reciprocal obligations, sensing common meaning, and sharing certain obligations toward others; related by blood or choice
Group	A number of people with shared characteristics
Community	A group of people living in the same locale under the same governance (e.g., neighborhoods, cities)

Axis 3. Judgment A descriptor or modifier that limits or specifies the meaning of the diagnostic focus (or concept). The values (descriptors) in Axis 3 are:

Descriptor	Definition
Complicated	Intricately involved, complex
Compromised	Damaged, made vulnerable
Decreased	Lessened (in size, amount, or degree)
Defensive	Used or intended to defend or protect
Deficient	Insufficient, inadequate
Delayed	Late, slow, or postponed
Disabled	Limited, handicapped
Disorganized	Not properly arranged or controlled

(Continued)

Descriptors for NANDA-I Nursing Diagnoses—cont'd

Disproportionate	Too large or too small in comparison with norm
Disturbed	Agitated; interrupted, interfered with
Dysfunction	Not operating normally
Effective	Producing the intended or desired effect
Enhanced	Improved in quality, value, or extent
Excess	Greater than necessary or desirable
Failure	Cessation of proper functioning or performance
Imbalanced	Out of proportion or balance
Impaired	Damaged, weakened
Ineffective	Not producing the intended or desired effect
Insufficient	Quantity or quality that is not able to fulfill a need or requirement
Interrupted	Having its continuity broken
Low	Below the norm
Organized	Properly arranged or controlled
Perceived	Observed through the senses
Readiness for	In a suitable state for an activity or situation
Situational	Related to a particular circumstance

Axis 4. Location The parts/regions of the body and/or their related functions. The values (descriptors) in Axis 4 are:

Descriptor	Definition
Auditory	Neurovascular
Bladder	Olfactory
Body	Oral
Bowel	Peripheral
Breast	Peripheral neurovascular
Cardiac	Peripheral vascular
Cardiopulmonary	Renal
Cerebral	Skin
Gastrointestinal	Tactile
Gustatory	Tissue
Intracranial	Vascular
Kinesthetic	Verbal
Liver	Visual
Mucous membranes	Urinary

Axis 5. Age Refers to the age of the person who is the subject of the diagnosis. The values (descriptors) in Axis 5 are:

Fetus	School-age child
Neonate	Adolescent
Infant	Adult
Toddler	Older adult
Preschool child	

Axis 6. Time The duration of the diagnostic concept (Axis 1). The values (descriptors) in Axis 6 are:

Descriptor	Definition
Acute	Lasting less than 6 months
Chronic	Lasting more than 6 months
Intermittent	Stopping or starting again at intervals, periodic, cyclic
Continuous	Uninterrupted, going on without stopping

Axis 7. Status of the Diagnosis Refers to the actuality or potentiality of the problem or to its categorization as a wellness/health promotion diagnosis. The values (descriptors) in Axis 7 are:

Descriptor	Definition
Actual	Existing in fact or reality, existing at the present time
Health Promotion	Behavior motivated by the desire to increase well-being and actualize human health potential (Pender, Murdaugh, & Parsons, 2006, cited in *NANDA-I Nursing Diagnoses: Definitions & Classification 2012–2014*)
Risk	Vulnerability, especially as a result of exposure to factors that increase the chance of injury or loss
Syndrome	Clinical judgment describing a specific cluster of nursing diagnoses that occur together, and are best addressed together and through similar interventions

Source: From NANDA International. (2012). *NANDA international nursing diagnoses: Definitions and classification 2012–2014.* Ames, IA: Wiley-Blackwell.

CLINICALREASONING

Applying the Full-Spectrum Nursing Model

PATIENT SITUATION

Recall Todd from Volume 1, Meet Your Patient. You have admitted him from the emergency department (ED). His admitting medical diagnosis is chronic renal failure, and that he has a medical history of type 2 diabetes mellitus. Todd is married, 58 years old, and employed. In the past 3 days, he has developed decreased sensation in his bilateral lower extremities with slight mobility impairment.

You will need to ask Todd about his medication regimen, his compliance with his diabetes treatment plan, and the extent to which his family is involved. You will also need to find out what laboratory tests have been completed and how severe his renal dysfunction has become. Your initial impressions about possible problems are the following:

- Because he has chronic renal failure, you can anticipate a problem with fluid balance.
- He has been admitted to the hospital and is acutely ill, so he may be anxious and fearful.
- He has decreased sensation in his lower extremities, so he may have a mobility or a safety problem.
- He has diabetes, so he is at risk for impaired skin and tissue integrity.
- Because diabetes and renal failure require complex regimens and patient self-care, it is possible that Todd may not be managing his therapy effectively, either because he is not motivated to do so or because he lacks the knowledge to do so.

When Todd and his family arrive on your unit, you begin gathering additional data. Armed with comprehensive data, you then make a list of Todd's health problems, in priority order. These actions illustrate the diagnosis phase of the nursing process phase. The purpose of diagnosing is to identify the client's health status, from which you will create your plan of care.

THINKING

1. *Theoretical Knowledge:* What theoretical knowledge will you need to identify the collaborative problems and nursing diagnoses for Todd?
2. *Critical Thinking (Inquiry Based on Credible Sources):*
   a. What resources would you use to find out more about the pathophysiology of renal failure? How do you know the source is credible?
   b. One of your first impressions was that Todd seemed anxious and fearful. What data do you need in order to decide whether to write an Anxiety nursing diagnosis? How will you obtain the data?
   c. When you are making your assessments of Todd, who is your best source of data? Why?

DOING

3. *Nursing Process (Diagnosis):*
   a. Write one collaborative problem for Todd. If you do not know the potential complications of chronic renal failure, look them up in a medical–surgical or pathophysiology textbook. Also explain why you would not use a nursing diagnosis to describe the problem.
   b. After further assessment, you observe that Todd's skin is intact and without redness or lesions. Write a nursing diagnosis (problem and etiology) to describe your concerns about his skin.
   c. Based on Maslow's Hierarchy of Needs, which problem has the highest priority?

CARING

4. *Ethical Knowledge:* The scenario doesn't provide enough information for you to identify the ethical dimensions of Todd's care. However, based on what you already know about him, speculate about some things that might create ethical questions for you.

PATIENT SITUATION

5. *Patient Preferences:* Think critically about the patient's preferences and concerns. Suppose that Todd's main concern is not the same as the high-priority problem you identified. Speculate about some other concerns he might have. What other things might he want to have resolved that could—for him—be more important than his chronic renal failure? Aside from his physical condition, what life concerns do you think Todd might have right now?

Critical Thinking and Clinical Reasoning

1. Sally Jones, a 45-year-old woman, was admitted to your surgical unit directly from the surgical suite. She was in a motorcycle accident this evening. In the emergency department, her blood pressure was falling, and she was bleeding profusely from many sites. She was sent directly to the operating room for a splenectomy, internal fixation of a compound fracture of bilateral femurs, and traumatic amputation of

the right hand. During surgery she lost 2,000 mL of blood and received three units of packed red blood cells (volume = 750 mL) along with 1,000 mL of fluid administered intravenously.

You receive the report on the client at 1900. Sally is receiving IV fluid through several peripheral lines and through a central line (a catheter inserted into a major vein leading to the heart). She has a Foley catheter, which is draining 30 mL of concentrated urine each hour. Sally's vital signs are as follows: temperature, 102.8°F (39.3°C) (rectal); heart rate, 120 beats/min; respirations, 28 breaths/min; and blood pressure, 160/86 mm Hg. Her skin is flushed, dry, and warm to the touch. On assessment, you find the following: skin turgor > 3 seconds, dry mucous membranes, and bloodstained dressing on right upper extremity.

She is complaining of thirst, weakness, and pain at a level of 10 on a scale of 1 to 10 (10 highest). Sally is receiving a continuous infusion of morphine. She refuses to deep-breathe, cough, or attempt to turn. She lies very still and is rigid. Sally drifts in and out of sleep but remains asleep for less than 30 minutes each time. She is irritable and restless. She communicates with one-word answers only. Frequently, she displays facial grimaces and becomes increasingly stiff. Her eyes appear dull. She complains of severe pain with any passive or active movements. In answering the following questions, use a nursing diagnosis handbook to look up the NANDA-I defining characteristics, definitions, and so forth, as needed.

a. Based on the data provided, which of the following NANDA-I labels would you use for Sally? Explain your reasoning.
   Deficient Fluid Volume or Risk for Deficient Fluid Volume
b. For Sally, what cues are present for a diagnosis of Deficient Fluid Volume? What related factors are present?
c. Using your responses to (a) and (b), write a diagnostic statement that includes problem, etiology, defining characteristics (cues), and the medical condition that the problem is "secondary to."
d. Think of other explanations for these cues: temperature, 102.8°F (39.3°C); heart rate, 120 beats/min; respirations, 28 breaths/min; blood pressure, 160/86 mm Hg.
e. Sally certainly has the defining characteristics for the nursing diagnosis Impaired Physical Mobility. If you use this problem label, what would the etiological factors be?
f. Which of those etiological factors could you treat with independent nursing interventions?
g. Sally has the nursing diagnoses (problem labels only are listed) and collaborative problems listed below. Answer the two following questions about that list:
   - From Sally's perspective, which is probably the highest priority problem?
   - Using an urgency (or threat to life) criterion, name Sally's three most important problems and why you consider them most important.

   Problems:
   Deficient Fluid Volume
   Acute Pain (abdominal incision, amputation site, fractures)
   Risk for Disturbed Body Image
   Potential Complication of trauma, surgery, and IV lines: infection
   Risk for Ineffective Airway Clearance
h. Examine your theoretical knowledge. To care for Sally, what additional theoretical knowledge do you need?
i. What practical knowledge will you need to use in her care?

2. You have a homebound client with diabetes who has the beginning of a ressure ulcer. You have been treating the client for Impaired Skin Integrity related to decreased circulation and mobility. However, the client's skin continues to break down.
   a. Your client has diabetes mellitus type 2. What type of problem is that (medical, nursing, or collaborative)?
   b. What is the client's nursing diagnosis?
   c. The client has Impaired Skin Integrity. The break in the body's first line of defense (intact skin) increases the risk for infection. Write a problem statement reflecting that risk nursing diagnosis.
3. For each of the following concepts, use critical thinking to describe how or why it is important to nursing, patient care, or nursing diagnosis. Note that these are *not* to be merely definitions.

The diagnosis step of the nursing process	Wellness nursing diagnosis
NANDA International	Cues
Patient strengths	Diagnostic label definition
Maslow's hierarchy	Defining characteristics
Documenting priorities	Risk factors
Nursing diagnoses	Etiological factors
Possible nursing diagnoses	Theoretical knowledge
Collaborative problems	Standardized nursing languages

What Are the Main Points in This Chapter?

- Nursing diagnosis is the unique obligation of the professional nurse; it cannot be delegated.
- An accurate nursing diagnosis is the foundation for the plan of care because it directs the choice of client-centered goals and nursing interventions.
- A nursing diagnosis is a statement of health status that nurses can identify, prevent, or treat independently.
- A medical diagnosis describes a disease, illness, or injury. A nursing diagnosis, in contrast, more holistically describes human responses to disease, illness, or injury.
- Collaborative problems are potential physiological complications of diseases, treatments, or diagnostic studies that nurses monitor and help to prevent but that cannot be treated primarily by independent nursing interventions.
- You must determine the "status" of each nursing diagnosis—that is, actual, potential, or possible problem; wellness diagnosis; or syndrome—because each status requires (1) different wording and (2) different nursing interventions.
- Diagnostic reasoning involves analyzing and interpreting data, verifying problems with the patient, and prioritizing the problems.
- You can never be certain that an inference is accurate, but you can have more confidence in an inference that is well supported by data.
- A problem etiology consists of the factors causing or contributing to the problem.
- You should involve patients in verifying and prioritizing their problems.
- Sound diagnostic reasoning is based on critical thinking and good theoretical and self-knowledge.
- A NANDA-I nursing diagnosis consists of a diagnostic label, a definition, defining characteristics, and related or risk factors.
- To choose the correct NANDA-I problem label, match the patient's cue clusters to the NANDA-I definition and defining characteristics.
- A diagnostic statement consists basically of "problem + etiology"; however, a variety of formats is needed to describe client health status.
- In general, the problem side of the diagnostic statement directs the choice of goals; the etiology directs the choice of nursing interventions.
- Diagnostic statements should be descriptive, accurate, clear, concise, and nonjudgmental.
- One criticism of standardized diagnostic language is that it represents a threat to creative, holistic thinking.

Knowledge Map

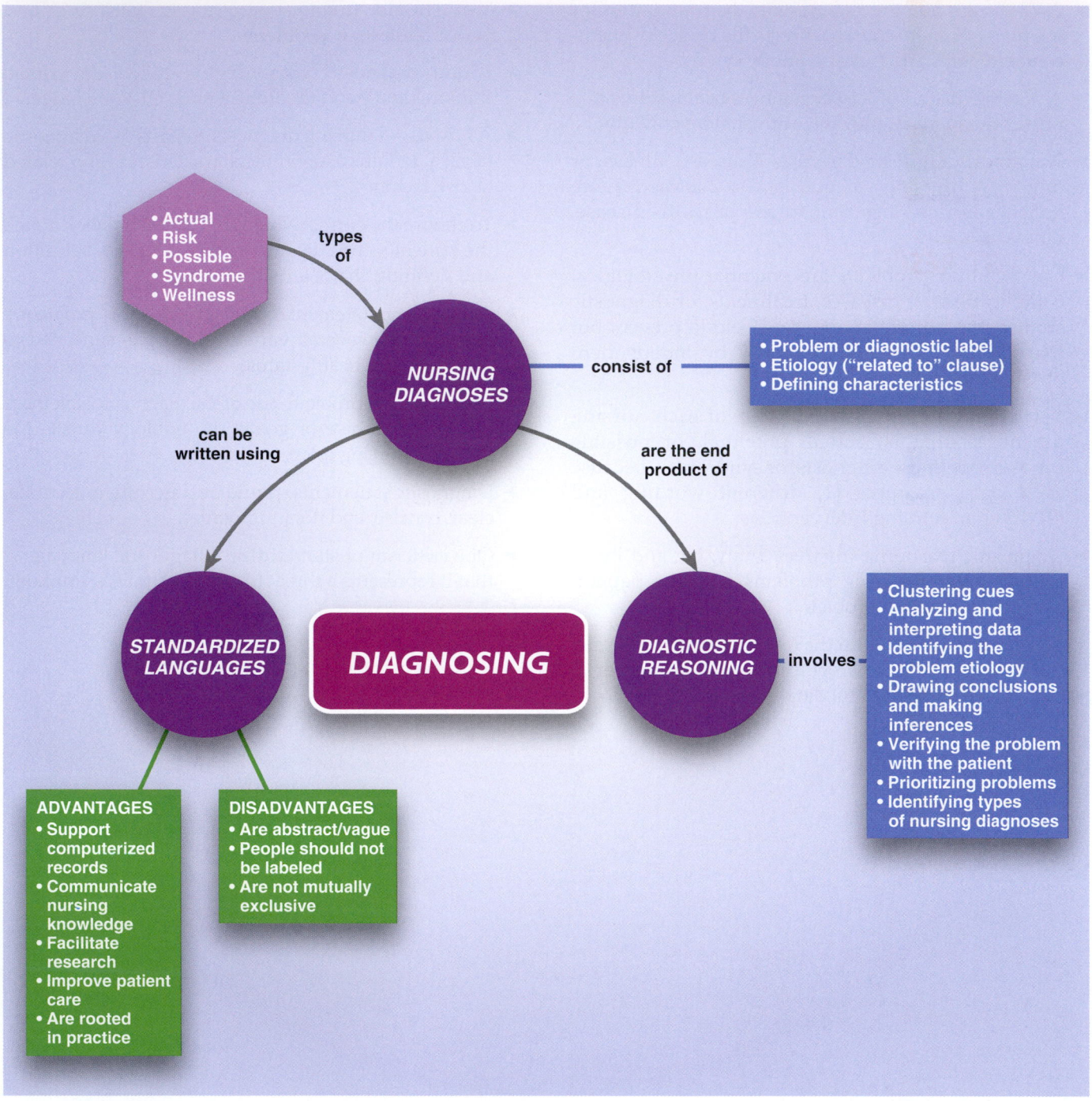

CHAPTER 5

Nursing Process: Planning Outcomes

STUDENT RESOURCES

The questions and exercises in Volume 2 allow you to practice the kind of thinking you will use as a full-spectrum nurse. Critical-thinking questions usually have more than one correct answer, so we do not provide "answers" for these features. It is more important to develop your nursing judgment than to just cover content. You will learn by discussing the questions with your peers. If you are still unsure, consult your instructor. You will find Response Sheets (for writing your responses to the questions) on DavisPlus.

To explore learning resources for this chapter,

Go to Davis*Plus* at DavisPl.us/Wilkinson3.

Chapter Resources for Chapter 5:

- **Response Sheets for all learning activities**
- **Resources for Caregivers and Health Professionals**
- **Reading More About Nursing Process: Planning Outcomes (suggested readings)**
- **Concept Map of chapter content**

Interactive Case Studies

NCLEX-Style and Chapter Review Questions

CHAPTER OVERVIEW

For a podcast of an overview of this chapter,

Go to Student Resources: Chapter 5, **Podcast—Chapter Overview,** on Davis*Plus*.

Caring for the Nguyens

Review the opening scenario of Nam Nguyen in the first pages of this volume. As the clinic nurse, you have written the following nursing diagnostic statement: Imbalanced Nutrition: More Than Body Requirements related to inappropriate food choices and serving size as evidenced by body mass index (BMI) of 28.5.

Write at least two short-term and two long-term goals for Mr. Nguyen based on this diagnostic statement. Remember that your goals must be realistic and take into account Mr. Nguyen's other health problems.

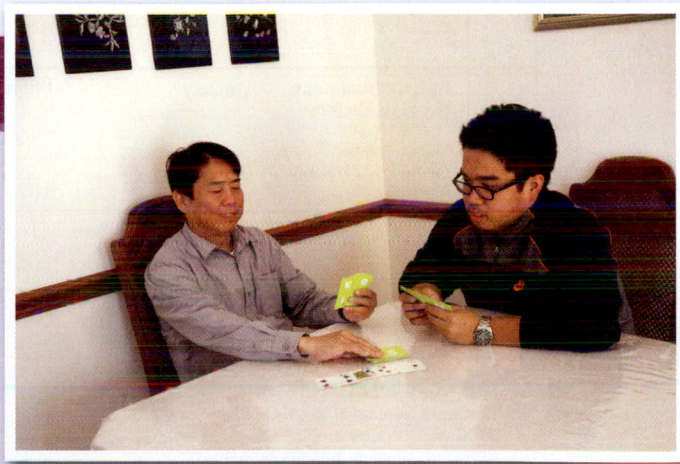

Practical Knowledge knowing how

Practical knowledge in the planning phase of the nursing process requires you to use a variety of care planning forms and, in some organizations, standardized language. This section includes a discharge planning form, as well as a table of Nursing Outcomes Classification (NOC) measurement scales. The remainder of the chapter consists of activities to help you apply critical thinking and clinical reasoning to the concepts you learned in Volume 1.

ASSESSMENT GUIDELINES & TOOLS

Discharge Planning Form

FOLLOW-UP CARE

When to call the doctor; symptom management (pain, nausea); plan for meeting outcomes not met during hospitalization:

Call your primary physician to find out if an insurance referral form is needed for follow-up appointments.
After discharge, you need to call for an appointment to see physician.

Clinic/Physician	Phone #	Date	Time			
_____	_____	_____	_____	or	____days	____weeks ____months
_____	_____	_____	_____	or	____days	____weeks ____months
_____	_____	_____	_____	or	____days	____weeks ____months

Plans for follow-up Labs/Tests/Treatments

Date	Time	Test/Treatment	Location	Ordered by
_____	_____	_____	_____	_____
_____	_____	_____	_____	_____
_____	_____	_____	_____	_____

PERSONAL CARE

Bathing: ❑ No restrictions ❑ Other:

Treatment/Therapy/Wound or Skin Care/ Supplies Needed 2-Day Supply Sent Home ? ❑ Yes

ACTIVITY/ REHAB

❑ No restrictions ❑ Do not climb stairs ❑ Drive_____ ❑ Return to Work _____
❑ Do not lift ❑ May lift up to _____lbs ❑ Weight Bearing _____# ❑ Other

DIET

❑ No restrictions ❑ Other:

Food/Drug Interactions: ❑ Coumadin ❑ MAO Inhibitors ❑ Other:

MEDICAL EQUIPMENT

❑ 2nd pair of TED hose given

COMMUNITY RESOURCES

Referral Resource	Agency	Phone #
Home IV Therapy	_____	_____
Home Health	_____	_____
Home Oxygen	_____	_____
Home PT/OT/Speech	_____	_____
Ask-A-Nurse	_____	816-932-0000

Transportation Arrangements for discharge: ___
_____

Education/Community Resources:_____
_____

Preprinted Discharge Instruction Sheet given to patient ❑ NA ❑ Yes
List Instruction Sheets:

I understand these instructions and agree with this plan of care _____
Patient/SO Signature

MULTIDISCIPLINARY DISCHARGE INSTRUCTIONS
Shawnee Mission Medical Center
9100 W. 74th Street
Shawnee Mission, Kansas 66204

Form # 60869 Revised: 4/01 PILOT Page 1 of 2

Source: Courtesy of Shawnee Mission Health System, Shawnee Mission, KS

STANDARDIZED LANGUAGE

By combining the following scale with NOC labels and indicators, you can write observable, concrete patient goals to use in evaluating a patient's response to care.

NOC Measurement Scales

SCALE NUMBER	1	2	3	4	5*
01	Severely compromised	Substantially compromised	Moderately compromised	Mildly compromised	Not compromised
02	Severe deviation from normal range	Substantial deviation from normal range	Moderate deviation from normal range	Mild deviation from normal range	No deviation from normal range
06	Not adequate	Slightly adequate	Moderately adequate	Substantially adequate	Totally adequate
07	10 and over	7–9	4–6	1–3	None
09	None	Limited	Moderate	Substantial	Extensive
11	Never positive	Rarely positive	Sometimes positive	Often positive	Consistently positive
12	Very weak	Weak	Moderate	Strong	Very strong
13	Never demonstrated	Rarely demonstrated	Sometimes demonstrated	Often demonstrated	Consistently demonstrated
14	Severe	Substantial	Moderate	Mild	None
17	Poor	Fair	Good	Very good	Excellent
18	Not at all satisfied	Somewhat satisfied	Moderately satisfied	Very satisfied	Completely satisfied
19	Consistently demonstrated	Often demonstrated	Sometimes demonstrated	Rarely demonstrated	Never demonstrated
20	No knowledge	Limited knowledge	Moderate knowledge	Substantial knowledge	Extensive knowledge

Source: Moorhead, S., Johnson, M., Maas, M., & Swanson, E. (2013). *Nursing outcomes classification (NOC)* (5th ed.). St. Louis, MO: C.V. Mosby, pp. 12–17. Used with permission.

*The scores (1 through 5) are constructed so that 5 is usually the most desirable and 1 is the least desirable condition relative to the outcome.

CLINICALREASONING
Applying the Full-Spectrum Nursing Model

PATIENT SITUATION

Ivan Benjamin has just been admitted to an orthopedic unit after an automobile accident. He was driving. Mr. Benjamin is 80 years old and has been living at home. His preexisting comorbidities are type 2 diabetes and osteoarthritis. He has casts and traction on both legs and a cast on one arm. He is receiving morphine sulfate intravenously via PCA pump. Imagine that you are an orthopedic nurse and must plan care for Mr. Benjamin. The admitting nurse wrote the following diagnoses and goals on the plan of care:

NURSING DIAGNOSES	GOALS/EXPECTED OUTCOMES
1. Acute Pain secondary to musculoskeletal trauma (arms, legs, body) and muscle spasms	▪ Demonstrates correct use of PCA pump ▪ Rates pain not higher than 4 on a scale of 1 to 10 at all times
2. Risk for Peripheral Neurovascular Dysfunction secondary to casts/traction	▪ Peripheral pulses palpable ▪ Fingers and toes warm ▪ Fingers and toes without pallor or cyanosis ▪ No edema of fingers and toes ▪ Capillary refill less than 3 seconds

THINKING

1. *Theoretical Knowledge:* What general *theoretical knowledge* will you need to care for this patient? Identify just the topics; limit the answer to about 150 words.
2. *Critical Thinking (Considering Alternatives):* Older adults are especially sensitive to certain medications, including morphine sulfate. What is one thing you could do to ensure Mr. Benjamin's safety while managing his acute pain? (There are several; think of just one.)
3. *Critical Thinking (Inquiry):* List at least two more things you need to know about Mr. Benjamin in order to begin his discharge planning.

DOING

4. *Practical Knowledge:* What general practical knowledge will you need? What would you do to obtain this knowledge?
5. *Nursing Process:*
   a. *Diagnosis:* What is another nursing diagnosis you might want to assess for Mr. Benjamin?
   b. *Planning Goals:* On the care plan rewrite the goals/expected outcomes for Acute Pain so that they will have all the required components. Assume that today's date is January 4.

CARING

6. *Self-Knowledge:* What beliefs, values, biases, or emotional responses might interfere with your ability to provide the best care to Mr. Benjamin?

CONTEXT

7. Think critically about the context. Is there anything in this situation that you have seen before? Identify any familiar elements. For example, you may have an elderly male relative, even if you have never cared for an 80-year-old patient before.

Critical Thinking and Clinical Reasoning

1. Merle Quinn is visiting a family planning clinic where she has just been informed that she is 6 weeks pregnant. She looks worried and makes the following statements: "This is a shock. I've just started a new business, and I need to work 7 days a week to make it go. . . . I don't know if I am ready to be a mother. . . ." Her husband agrees: "I just don't see how we can afford this. We don't even have any insurance now."

   "Still," Mrs. Quinn says, "I don't see how I could deal with having an abortion. My parents would be devastated. I'm sure they'd never speak to me again." Her husband says, "Not to speak of the fact that the Church forbids it. It would be a sin."

   A week later Mrs. Quinn calls the clinic in tears. She says she has not been able to eat or sleep and that she doesn't know what to do about her pregnancy. "I don't want this baby, but I can't bring myself to have an abortion." The nurse diagnoses Decisional Conflict related to unexpected/unwanted pregnancy and possibly assuming that abortion is her only alternative, as evidenced by statements of indecision, tearfulness, and inability to sleep. She makes an appointment to see Mr. and Mrs. Quinn that same day. Imagine that you are the nurse writing the care plan for the Quinns.

   a. Analyze your assumptions. What values and beliefs do you have that may influence the goals you write for the Quinns? Specifically, how could your values affect the goals you write?
   b. Develop a short-term goal to address the problem clause of this nursing diagnosis. The goal should be one you expect the Quinns to be able to achieve during their appointment that same day.
   c. You also write a goal stating: "By the end of this visit, clients will verbalize and demonstrate decreased anxiety and stress." Which part of the nursing diagnosis does this goal address?
   d. The NOC standardized outcomes linked to the NANDA-I diagnosis of Decisional Conflict are the following (definitions are given):
      Decision Making: Ability to choose between two or more alternatives
      Information Processing: Ability to acquire, organize, and use information
      Participation: Health Care Decisions: Personal involvement in selecting and evaluating health care options
      Which of those outcomes is most important for the Quinns to achieve *today*? Why?
   e. Now imagine that you have written the following individualized goals/outcomes for today's visit with the Quinns:
      By the end of this visit, clients will:
      1. Verbalize and demonstrate decreased anxiety and stress.
      2. Verbalize awareness that they have options for coping with whatever decision they make about the pregnancy.
      3. Discuss with the nurse options for continuing or terminating the pregnancy.
      4. Verbalize intent to discuss their feelings with family (i.e., their parents).
      5. Verbalize intent to discuss feelings with a member of the clergy.
      6. Decide whether to continue the pregnancy.
         - Why is outcome 2 so important?
         - What would you have had to assume in order to write outcome 4?
         - What would you have had to assume in order to write outcome 5?
         - Which of the outcomes is/are probably *not* appropriate for today's visit? Why?

2. For each of the following concepts, use critical thinking to describe how or why it is important to nursing, patient care, or the process of planning care. Note that these are *not* to be merely definitions.

   Discharge planning
   A written, individualized nursing care plan
   Standardized care-planning documents (e.g., protocols)
   Critical pathways
   Computerized care planning
   Goals (expected outcomes)
   Short-term goals
   Long-term goals
   Action verbs (in goals)
   Essential patient goals
   The Nursing Outcomes Classification (NOC)
   Aggregate goals
   Wellness goals
   Concrete, specific goal/outcome statements (as opposed to vague statements)

What Are the Main Points in This Chapter?

- During the planning outcomes phase, you will derive goals/expected outcomes from identified nursing diagnoses.
- Goals/expected outcomes (1) suggest nursing interventions, (2) serve as criteria for use in the evaluation step of the nursing process, and (3) provide motivation for patients and nurses.
- To ensure continuity of care, you should begin discharge planning with the initial patient assessment.
- Discharge planning is especially important for older adults and patients with complex needs.
- A holistic, individualized patient care plan contains information needed to address (1) basic needs and ADLs, (2) medical and collaborative therapies, (3) nursing diagnoses and collaborative problems, and (4) special teaching and/or discharge needs.
- Ideally, a care plan consists of a combination of standardized and individualized goals and interventions.
- Standardized approaches to care planning include institutional policies and procedures, protocols, unit standards of care, standardized care plans, critical pathways, and integrated plans of care (IPOCs).
- Computer-assisted care planning helps ensure that the nurse considers a variety of interventions and does not overlook common and important interventions; it reduces the time spent on paperwork.
- Nursing-sensitive goals (expected outcomes, predicted outcomes, desired outcomes) describe the changes in patient health status that are intended to result from and can be influenced by nursing interventions.
- Goals for collaborative problems are usually not nursing sensitive, and should not be included on a nursing care plan.
- A goal statement should include a subject, an action verb, a performance criterion, a target time, and special conditions if needed.
- For every nursing diagnosis, you must state one "essential" goal—one that, if achieved, would demonstrate problem resolution or improvement.
- Among the ANA-recognized standardized vocabularies/taxonomies for describing patient outcomes are NOC, the Omaha System, and the Clinical Care Classification System.
- Goals should be concrete, specific, and observable; they should be valued by the patient/family; and they should not conflict with the medical treatment plan.

Knowledge Map

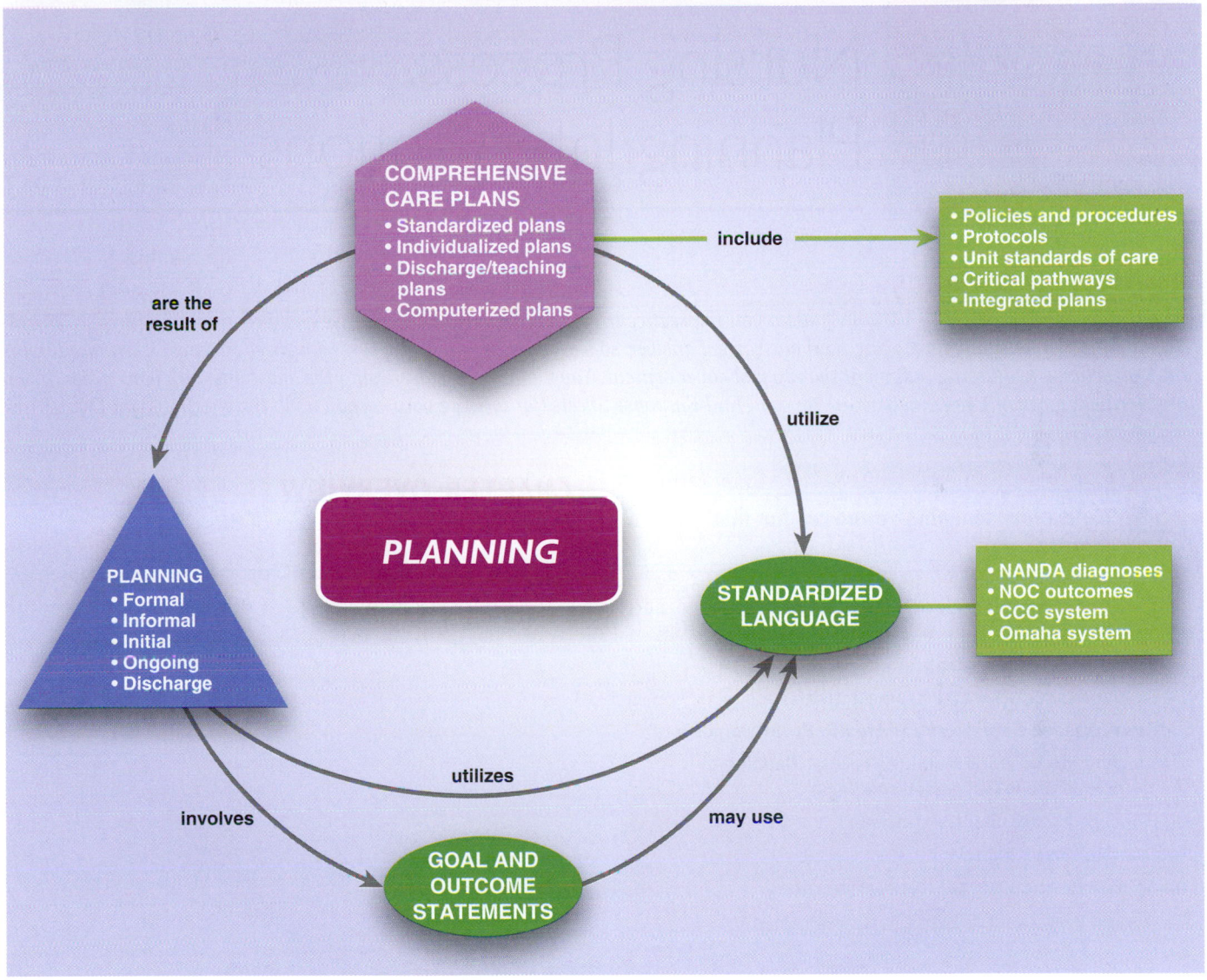

CHAPTER 6

Nursing Process: Planning Interventions

STUDENT RESOURCES

*The questions and exercises in Volume 2 allow you to practice the kind of thinking you will use as a full-spectrum nurse. Critical-thinking questions usually have more than one correct answer, so we do not provide "answers" for these features. It is more important to develop your nursing judgment than to just cover content. You will learn by discussing the questions with your peers. If you are still unsure, consult your instructor. You will find Response Sheets (for writing your responses to the questions) on Davis*Plus.

To explore learning resources for this chapter,

Go to Davis*Plus* at DavisPl.us/Wilkinson3.

Chapter Resources for Chapter 6:

- **Response sheets for all learning activities**
- **Resources for Caregivers and Health Professionals**
- **Reading More About Nursing Process: Planning Interventions (suggested readings)**
- **Concept Map of chapter content**

Interactive Case Studies

NCLEX-Style and Chapter Review Questions

CHAPTER OVERVIEW

For a podcast of an overview of this chapter,

Go to Student Resources: Chapter 6, **Podcast—Chapter Overview,** on Davis*Plus*.

Caring for the Nguyens

Recall that you have written the following nursing diagnosis for Mr. Nguyen: Imbalanced Nutrition: More Than Body Requirements related to inappropriate food choices and serving size, as evidenced by body mass index (BMI) of 28.5.

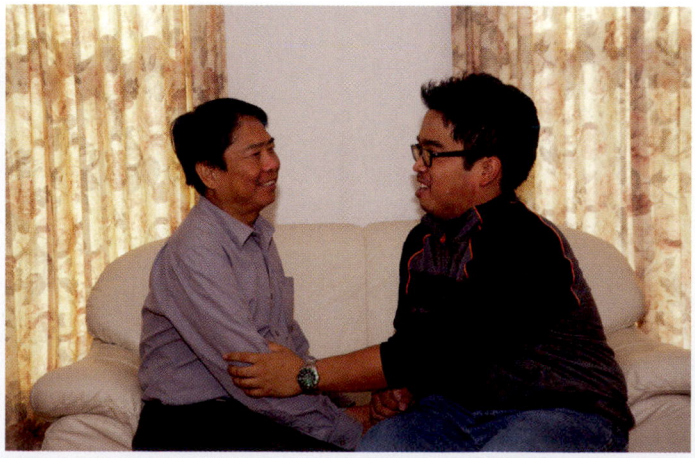

Caring for the Nguyens (continued)

A. Based on the outcomes you wrote in Chapter 5, Nursing Process: Planning Outcomes, identify four possible interventions to address the diagnosis and outcomes.

B. Review the interventions, and identify two that would be most appropriate for Mr. Nguyen given all of the information you have about his health status.

C. Write a nursing order for each of the two interventions you identified above.

CLINICALREASONING

Applying the Full-Spectrum Nursing Model

PATIENT SITUATION

Mr. Sanborn is a 65-year-old man who has come to the clinic for a complete physical checkup. He has no health complaints and his physical examination is negative except for a few minor changes associated with aging. During the interview, he tells you that he is gay, and that he has had the same partner for 5 years. On further questioning, he reveals that he has had numerous sex partners during his lifetime. He says, "I was wondering if I should be tested for HIV" and "Mike, that's my partner, says I ought to get a flu shot and maybe a hepatitis shot. What do you think?"

THINKING

1. *Theoretical Knowledge:* What principles and concepts do you need to know in order to help Mr. Sanborn today?
2. *Inquiry:* Which of those do you already know enough about, and which ones will you have to study further?

DOING

3. *Practical Knowledge:* What psychomotor and communication skills will you need in order to help Mr. Sanborn?
4. *Nursing Process (Assessment):* What further data do you need about Mr. Sanborn's sexual activity?
5. *Nursing Process (Planning Interventions):* What is one important nursing intervention for today?

CARING

6. *Self-Knowledge:* How do you feel about same-sex relationships? Would you be able to care for Mr. Sanborn effectively?
7. *Ethical Knowledge:* What does the American Nurses Association (ANA) *Nursing Code of Ethics* say about relationships to patients and the nature of patient health problems? To see the *Nursing Code of Ethics,*

Go to http://www.nursingworld.org/MainMenuCategories/EthicsStandards/CodeofEthicsforNurses/Code-of-Ethics.aspx

Critical Thinking and Clinical Reasoning

1. Recall the Quinns from Chapter 5. Merle Quinn is visiting a family planning clinic, where she has just been informed that she is 6 weeks pregnant. She looks worried and makes the following statements: "This is a shock. I've just started a new business and I need to work 7 days a week to make it go. . . . I don't know if I am ready to be a mother. . . ." Her husband agrees: "I just don't see how we can afford this. We don't have any insurance now."

   "Still," Mrs. Quinn says, "I don't see how I could deal with having an abortion. My parents would be devastated. I'm sure they'd never speak to me again." Her husband says, "Not to speak of the fact that the Church forbids it. It would be a mortal sin."

   A week later, Mrs. Quinn calls the clinic in tears. She says she has not been able to eat or sleep and that she doesn't know what to do about her pregnancy. "I don't want this baby, but I can't bring myself to have an abortion." The nurse diagnoses Decisional Conflict related to this unplanned/unwanted pregnancy and inability to accept the only perceived alternative (abortion), as evidenced by statements of indecision, tearfulness, and inability to sleep. The nurse makes an appointment to see Mr. and Mrs. Quinn that same day. Imagine that you are the nurse writing the care plan for the Quinns.

a. *Critical Thinking and Self-Knowledge (Analyzing Assumptions):* To set aside your assumptions and care for the Quinns, you will need to focus on the Quinns' immediate problem, Decisional Conflict, rather than thinking about what they "ought" to do. Remember, the nurse's role is not to make decisions for clients, but to provide information, clarification, and support.
   - What questions must you ask in this case to analyze your assumptions?
   - What are the answers to those questions?

b. *Critical Thinking (Contextual Awareness) and Knowledge of Patient Situation (Context):*
   - What is going on in the Quinns' lives that may affect your choice of interventions?
   - What is going on with Mrs. Quinn's health status that may affect your choice of interventions?

Now imagine that the nurse has written the following care plan for today's visit with the Quinns:

OUTCOMES	INTERVENTIONS
NOC Outcomes Decision Making Participation: Health Care Decisions	**NIC Interventions** Decision-Making Support Family Planning: Contraception Family Planning: Unplanned Pregnancy
Individualized Goals By the end of this visit, clients will: 1. Verbalize and demonstrate decreased anxiety and stress. 2. Verbalize awareness that they have options for coping with whatever decision they make about the pregnancy. 3. Discuss with the nurse options for continuing or terminating the pregnancy. 4. Verbalize intent to discuss their feelings with family (i.e., their parents). 5. Verbalize intent to discuss feelings with a member of the clergy.	**Computer-Generated Nursing Activities** 1. Offer emotional support. 2. Inform client(s) of alternative views or solutions. 3. Help to identify advantages and disadvantages of each alternative. 4. Encourage client(s) to explore options, including termination, keeping the infant, or adoption. 5. Provide information as requested by client(s). 6. Serve as liaison between patient and family. 7. Assist in identifying support system. 8. Refer to community agency for counseling, if needed (e.g., family-planning clinic). 9. Discuss factors related to unplanned pregnancy (e.g., no use or misuse of contraceptives). 10. Teach and clarify misinformation about contraceptive use. 11. Teach regarding preparation and procedures. 12. Monitor for complications of procedure.

c. *Nursing Process:* Which NIC intervention, based on its label alone, does *not* appear to be relevant to producing the stated goals. (Note that it also does not appear that it would relieve the problem, reduce the etiology, or relieve Mrs. Quinn's symptoms of anxiety and distress.)

d. *Nursing Process:* Which of the computer-generated activities is/are *not* appropriate for today's visit with the Quinns?

e. *Nursing Process:* For which individualized outcome is there apparently *not* a computer-generated nursing activity?

f. *Critical Thinking:* Look at intervention 6 ("Serve as liaison between patient and family"). What critical-thinking questions should you ask about that intervention with regard to:
   - Contextual awareness?
   - Credible sources?
   - Reflecting skeptically?

g. *Critical Thinking (Prioritizing):* Which of the computer-generated interventions will you probably need to do first today?
h. *Critical Thinking (Prioritizing):* Look at computer-generated interventions 2, 3, and 4. Which of these is most important to do today? Which one could you encourage the Quinns to do during the next week or so? Why?
i. *Nursing Process (Planning Interventions):* What would you need to do to nursing activity 1 to turn it into a nursing order that another nurse could use to care for the Quinns?
j. *Nursing Process (Assessment):* What questions would you need to ask to individualize activity 1 for the Quinns' care plan?

2. For each of the following concepts, use critical thinking to describe how or why it is important to nursing, patient care, or the process of planning interventions. Note that these are *not* to be merely definitions.

Nursing interventions/strategies/activities/actions
Individualized interventions
Independent interventions
Collaborative interventions
Dependent interventions
Theories
Research
Evidence-based practice
The patient's problem status
The nursing diagnosis etiology
Client outcomes
Critical thinking (e.g., contextual awareness, reflecting skeptically)
Computerized care planning program
Standardized intervention vocabularies
Nursing Interventions Classification (NIC)
Wellness interventions
Spiritual care interventions
Nursing orders

What Are the Main Points in This Chapter?

- Nursing interventions are treatments that nurses perform (1) in response to nursing diagnoses and (2) for the purpose of achieving client outcomes.
- Nursing interventions include such activities as teaching, counseling and emotional support, referral, physical care, and environmental management.
- Independent interventions are nurse-initiated treatments—those that nurses perform or delegate based on their knowledge and skills.
- Nursing interventions are performed for the purpose of assessing health status, preventing and treating disease/illness, and promoting health.
- The RN is responsible for choosing interventions and writing nursing orders; however, the RN can delegate actual performance of some interventions to nursing assistive personnel (NAPs) and LPN/LVNs.
- Theories influence your perspective: What you notice and identify as a problem, as well as how you define a problem, more or less determines your choice of interventions.
- Ideally, a nursing intervention should have a sound basis in research.
- When generating interventions, nurses use critical-thinking skills such as making interdisciplinary connections, predicting, generalizing, explaining, and making therapeutic judgments.
- The American Nurses Association has approved the following three standardized vocabularies for nursing interventions: (1) the Nursing Interventions Classification (NIC), (2) the Omaha System (developed for community health nursing), and (3) the Clinical Care Classification (CCC).
- Standardized vocabularies are especially useful in agencies that have computerized care planning systems.
- Standardized vocabularies include terminology for describing wellness interventions and spiritual interventions.
- Nursing orders, written on the nursing care plan, consist of the detailed instructions for performing nursing interventions.

Knowledge Map

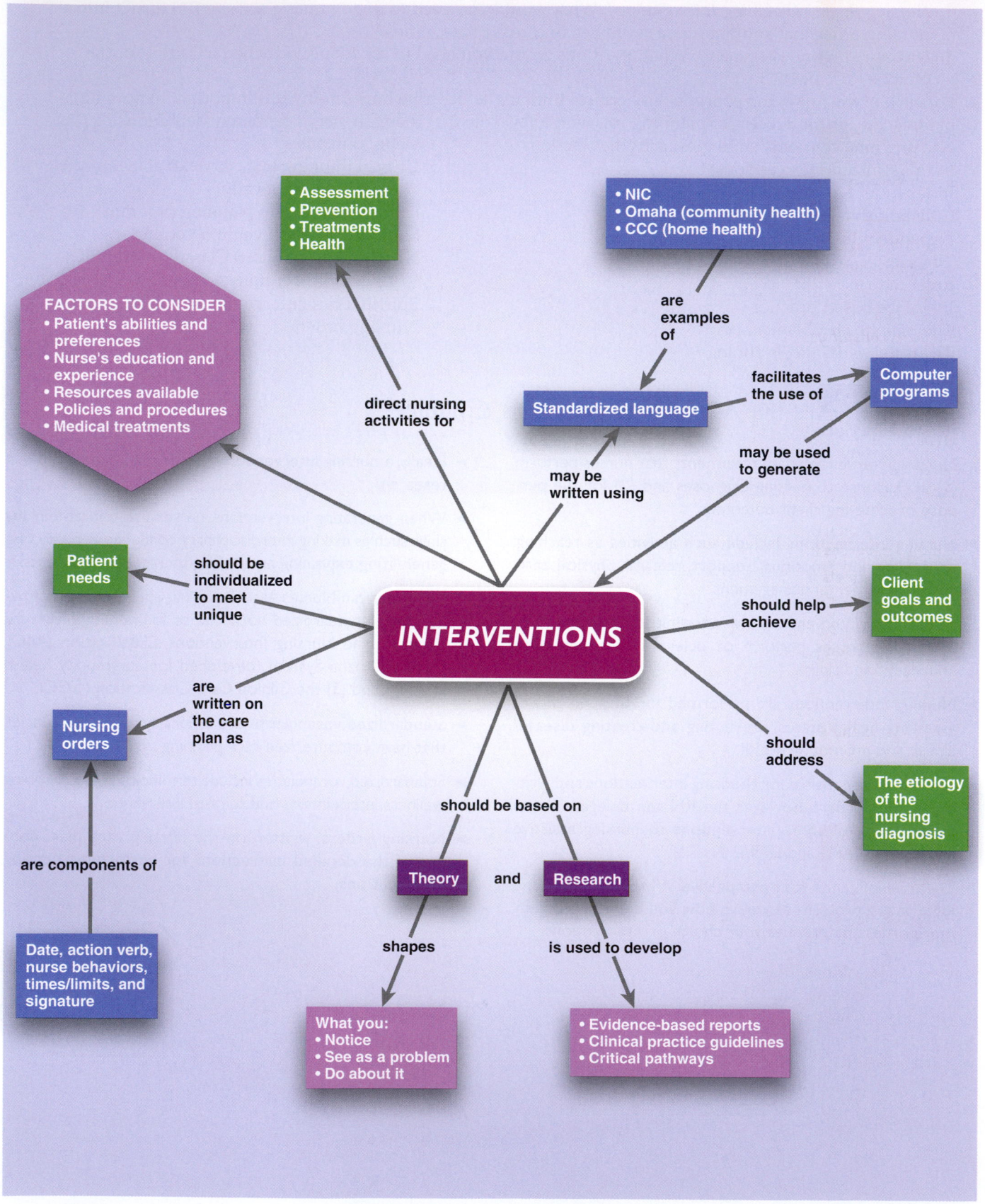

CHAPTER 7

Nursing Process: Implementation & Evaluation

STUDENT RESOURCES

*The questions and exercises in Volume 2 allow you to practice the kind of thinking you will use as a full-spectrum nurse. Critical-thinking questions usually have more than one correct answer, so we do not provide "answers" for these features. It is more important to develop your nursing judgment than to just cover content. You will learn by discussing the questions with your peers. If you are still unsure, consult your instructor. You will find Response Sheets (for writing your responses to the questions) on Davis*Plus.

To explore learning resources for this chapter,

Go to Davis*Plus*, at DavisPl.us/Wilkinson3.

Chapter Resources for Chapter 7:

- **Response sheets for all learning activities**
- **Resources for Caregivers and Health Professionals**
- **Reading More About Nursing Process: Implementation & Evaluation (suggested readings)**
- **Concept Map of chapter content**

Interactive Case Studies

NCLEX-Style and Chapter Review Questions

CHAPTER OVERVIEW

For a podcast of an overview of this chapter,

Go to Student Resources: Chapter 7, **Podcast—Chapter Overview,** on Davis*Plus*.

Caring for the Nguyens

The following information is recorded on Mr. Nguyen's clinic health record:

9/1/16 Imbalanced Nutrition: More Than Body Requirements related to inappropriate food choices and serving size, as evidenced by BMI of 28.5

Outcome: Will lose 5 lb by 10/15/2016

Interventions:

- Collect 3-day nutrition history 9/2/2016 through 9/4/2016.

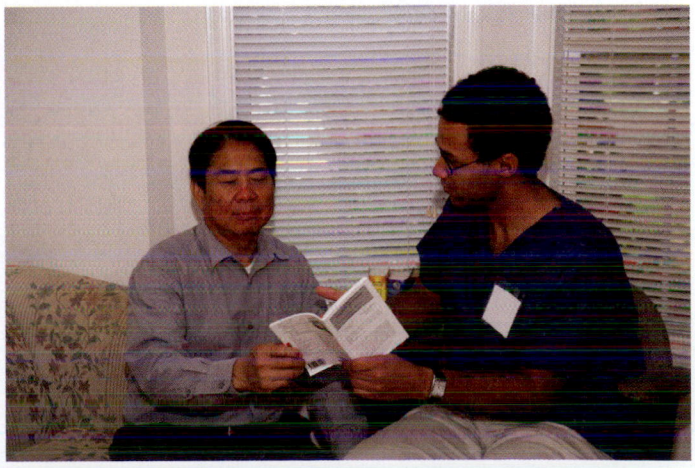

(Continued)

Caring for the Nguyens (continued)

- Have patient meet with clinic nurse for diet review and nutrition instruction 9/8/2016.
- Provide sample meal plans at 9/8/2016 instruction.
- Phone patient 9/22/2016 to discuss nutrition questions and review progress.
- Have patient return to clinic 10/15/2016 for follow-up visit.

A. What must you do before implementing each nursing intervention?

B. Identify at least two strategies that will help promote Mr. Nguyen's participation in and adherence to the plan.

C. How will you determine whether Mr. Nguyen has met his goal?

PracticalKnowledge knowing how

When implementing and evaluating care, you will need to make good decisions about administering and delegating care. In this section, you will find forms to help you delegate, implement, and evaluate patient care.

IMPLEMENTATION AND EVALUATION TOOLS

The first tool is a small checklist, followed by a delegation grid (to help you make wise delegation decisions). The final tool is an Evaluation Checklist.

For a worksheet for organizing nursing care that you can print and use in clinical,

Go to Student Resources: Chapter 7, Tables, Boxes, Figures: **ESG Figure 7-1, Worksheet for Organizing Nursing Care,** on Davis*Plus*.

That worksheet allows you to see at a glance the total work you need to accomplish for all your patients. Write on it, in priority order, only the most important things you must accomplish during this one day. Room numbers take up less space than names, but remember to refer to your patients by name, not by number or diagnosis. At first, you may also need to make a time-sequenced list, the size of a 3 × 5 card, to help you organize your day. For example, it might read in part:

0700 – Assessments, all patients, begin with Room 310
0730 – Ambulation: 315, 318
0800 – Change IV, meds 310; check intake
0815 – Meds 315, 318, 319; check intake
0845 – Toilet and bath, 310

and so on for the rest of the day.

The Five Rights of Delegation—Checklist

Right Task *(Can I delegate it?)*

The task is:

—Delegable for a specific patient.

—Within the nurse's scope of practice.

—Permitted by the state's nurse practice act.

—Permitted by the agency's policies.

Right Circumstance *(Should I delegate it?)*

Consider patient safety:

—Is the patient setting appropriate?

—Are adequate resources available?

—Other factors to maintain safety?

Right Person *(Who is best prepared to do it?)*

The right person:

—Is delegating the task (the nurse must be competent to delegate).

—Will be performing the task (the NAP must be competent to do the task).

—Will receive the care (i.e., the severity of the patient's illness is considered).

Right Direction/Communication *(What does the NAP need to know?)*

—The task is described clearly, including its objective, limits, and expectations.

—The delegatee (NAP) understands the communication.

Right Supervision *(How will I follow up?)*

—The nurse monitors, evaluates, and intervenes as needed.

—The nurse obtains feedback from the patient.

—The nurse obtains feedback from the delegatee.

Source: National Council of State Boards of Nursing. (1995). *Delegation: Concepts and decision-making process.* National Council Position Paper. Chicago: Author.

NCSBN Delegation Grid

Elements for review		Client A	Client B	Client C	Client D
Activity/Task Level of client stability	Describe activity/task: Score the client's level of stability: **Client condition:** 0 – Is chronic/stable/predictable 1 – Has minimal potential for change 2 – Has moderate potential for change 3 – Has unstable/acute/strong potential for change				
Level of NAP competence	Score the NAP competence in completing delegated nursing care activities in the defined client population: **NAP is:** 0 – Expert in activities to be delegated, in defined population 1 – Experienced in activities to be delegated, in defined population 2 – Experienced in activities but not in defined population 3 – Novice in performing activities and in defined population				
Level of licensed nurse competence	Score the licensed nurse's competence in relation to both knowledge of providing nursing care to a defined population and competence in implementation of the delegation process: 0 – Expert in the knowledge of nursing needs/activities of defined client population *and* expert in the delegation process 1 – Either expert in knowledge of needs/activities of defined client population and competent in delegation *or* experienced in the needs/activities of defined client population and expert in the delegation process 2 – Experienced in knowledge of needs/activities of defined client population *and* competent in the delegation process 3 – Either experienced in knowledge of needs/activities of defined client population *or* competent in the delegation process 4 – Novice in knowledge of defined population *and* novice in delegation				
Potential for harm	Score the potential level of risk the nursing care activity has for the client *(risk is probability of [the client] suffering harm):* 0 – None 1 – Low 2 – Medium 3 – High				
Frequency	Score based on how often the NAP has performed the specific nursing care activity: 0 – Performed at least daily 1 – Performed at least weekly 2 – Performed at least monthly 3 – Performed less than monthly 4 – Never performed				
Level of decision making	Score the decision-making needed, related to the specific nursing care activity, client (both cognitive and physical status) and client situation: 0 – Does not require decision making 1 – Minimal level of decision making 2 – Moderate level of decision making 3 – High level of decision making				
Ability for self care	Score the client's level of assistance needed for self-care activities: 0 – No assistance 1 – Limited assistance 2 – Extensive assistance 3 – Total care or constant attendance				
	Total Score				

Scoring: A low score on the grid suggests that an activity can be safely delegated. For example if a client's stability is ranked 3 (unstable) and the level of NAP competence is also 3 (novice in the activity), then you probably should *not* delegate to that NAP. Each agency should establish a policy regarding the individual and/or total scores to be considered acceptable for delegating.

Source: Used by permission from the National Council of State Boards of Nursing (NCSBN), Chicago, IL (1997). Retrieved February 1, 2008, from the NCSBN web site (www.ncsbn.org)

Evaluation Checklist

Evaluation Checklist

Instructions: Check the appropriate response and follow the associated instructions

Assessment Review

1. Were the assessment data complete and accurate?
   - ___ YES. No action.
   - ___ NO. Reassess client. Record the new data. Change care plan as indicated
2. Have all data been validated, as needed?
   - ___ YES. No action.
   - ___ NO. Validate with client (by interview and physical examination), significant others, or other professionals. Record validation (or failure to validate). Change care plan as indicated.
3. Have new data become available that require changes in the plan (e.g., a different problem etiology, new goals/ outcomes, new medical orders)?
   - ___ NO. No action.
   - ___ YES. Record the new data in the progress notes; redefine problem, goals, nursing orders, as needed.
4. Has the patient's condition changed?
   - ___ NO. No action.
   - ___ YES. Record data about present health status. Change care plan as indicated.

Move to a review of the diagnosis step.

Diagnosis Review

1. Is the diagnosis relevant and related to the data?
   - ___ YES. No action.
   - ___ NO. Revise the diagnosis.
2. Is the diagnosis well supported by the data?
   - ___ YES. No action.
   - ___ NO. Collect more data. Support or revise diagnosis.
3. Has the problem status changed (actual, potential, possible)?
   - ___ NO. No action.
   - ___ YES. Restate the problem.
4. Is the diagnosis stated clearly?
   - ___ YES. No action.
   - ___ NO. Revise the diagnostic statement.
5. Does the etiology correctly reflect the factors contributing to the problem?
   - ___ YES. No action.
   - ___ NO. Revise the etiology.
6. Is the problem one that can be treated primarily by nursing actions?
   - ___ YES. No action.
   - ___ NO. Label as collaborative and consult appropriate health professional.
7. Is the diagnosis specific and individualized to the patient?
   - ___ YES. No action.
   - ___ NO. Revise diagnosis. Revise outcomes and nursing orders as suggested by the new nursing diagnosis.
8. Does the problem (diagnosis) still exist?
   - ___ YES. No action.
   - ___ NO. Delete diagnosis and related outcomes and nursing orders.

Proceed to a review of client goals.

Planning Review: Outcomes

1. Have nursing diagnoses been added or revised?
   - ___ NO. No action.
   - ___ YES. Write new outcomes.
2. Are the outcomes realistic in terms of patient abilities and agency resources?
   - ___ YES. No action.
   - ___ NO. Revise outcomes.
3. Was sufficient time allowed for outcome achievement?
   - ___ YES. No action.
   - ___ NO. Revise time frame.
4. Do the outcomes address all aspects of the client's problem?
   - ___ YES. No action.
   - ___ NO. Write additional outcomes.

Evaluation Checklist *(continued)*

5. Do the expected outcomes, as written, demonstrate resolution of the problem specified in the nursing diagnosis?
   __ YES. No action. __ NO. Revise outcomes.
6. Have client priorities changed, or has the focus of care changed?
   __ NO. No action. __ YES. Revise outcomes.
7. Is the client in agreement with the goals?
   __ YES. No action. __ NO. Get client input. Write outcomes valued by the client.

→ ***Proceed to a review of nursing orders.*** ←

Planning Review: Nursing Orders

1. Have nursing diagnoses or outcomes been added or revised in previous review steps?
   __ NO. No action. __ YES. Write new nursing orders.
2. Are the nursing orders clearly related to the stated patient outcomes?
   __ YES. No action. __ NO. Revise or develop new nursing orders.
3. Is the rationale sufficient to justify the use of the nursing order?
   __ YES. No action. __ NO. Revise or develop new nursing orders.
4. Are the nursing orders unclear or vague, so that other staff may have had questions about how to implement them?
   __ NO. No action. __ YES. Revise nursing orders. Add details to make more specific or individualized to the patient.
5. Do the nursing orders include instructions for timing of the activities?
   __ YES. No action. __ NO. Revise nursing orders: add times, schedules.
6. Was an order clearly and obviously ineffective?
   __ NO. No action. __ YES. Delete it.
7. Are the orders realistic in terms of staff and other resources?
   __ YES. No action. __ NO. Revise orders or obtain resources.
8. Have new resources become available that might enable you to change the goals or nursing orders?
   __ NO. No action. __ YES. Write new goals or nursing orders reflecting the new capabilities.
9. Do the nursing orders address all aspects of the client's health goals?
   __ NO. No action. __ NO. Add new nursing orders.

→ ***Proceed to a review of implementation step*** ←

Implementation Review

1. Did the nurse [or NAP] get client input at each step in developing and implementing the plan?
   __ YES. No action. __ NO. Obtain client input, revise plan and implementation as needed. [Coach NAP or role model, as needed.]
2. Were the nursing interventions acceptable to the patient?
   __ YES. No action. __ NO. Consult patient; change nursing orders or implementation approach.
3. Did the nurse [NAP] prepare the patient for implementation of the nursing order (e.g., explain what the patient should expect or do)?
   __ YES. No action. __ NO. Continue same plan, but prepare patient before implementing. Reevaluate.
4. Did the nurse [NAP] have adequate knowledge and skills to perform techniques and procedures correctly?
   __ YES. No action. __ NO. Continue same plan. Have someone else implement or help the nurse [or NAP] to acquire the needed knowledge or skills. If neither of these is possible, delete nursing order.

(continued)

5. Did client or family comply with the therapeutic regimen? Were self-care activities performed correctly?
   __ YES. No action.
   __ NO. Reassess motivation, knowledge, and resources. Add outcomes and nursing orders aimed at teaching, motivating, and supporting, patient in carrying out the regimen. Set time for reevaluation.
6. Did other staff members follow the nursing orders?
   __ YES. No action.
   __ NO. Implement the omitted nursing orders or ensure that others will do so. Set time for reevaluation. Find out why order was not carried out.
7. Was the plan of care implemented in a manner that communicated caring?
   __ YES. No action.
   __ NO. This is a problem that must be addressed by personal and staff development.

After making the necessary revisions to the care plan, implement the new plan and begin the nursing cycle again.

Source: Wilkinson, J. (2011). *Nursing process and critical thinking* (5th ed.). Upper Saddle River, NJ: Prentice Hall, pp. 325–327.

CLINICALREASONING
Applying the Full-Spectrum Nursing Model

PATIENT SITUATION

Recall Jeannette Wu from Volume 1. Jeannette Wu is a frail 80-year-old woman who is in the hospital after fracturing her hip. Her hip was surgically repaired 4 days ago, but because of her overall fragile health and some postsurgery confusion, her recovery is slower than usual. One of her nursing diagnoses is Self-Care Deficit (Bathing, Dressing, and Toileting) related to weakness, pain, confusion, and decreased mobility. Her nursing orders (NIC) include Bathing and Self-Care: Activities of Daily Living (ADLs). As the nurse is helping a nursing assistive personnel (NAP) with Mrs. Wu's bath, she notices a reddened area on Mrs. Wu's sacrum. Realizing that this may be the beginning of a pressure ulcer, the nurse observes carefully and notes a small skin excoriation (abrasion) in the reddened area. She repositions Mrs. Wu to prevent further pressure on her sacrum. After finishing the bath, the nurse records her findings and enters on Mrs. Wu's care plan a nursing diagnosis of Impaired Skin Integrity related to impaired bed mobility and minimal subcutaneous tissue. She writes nursing orders, including an order to observe skin over bony prominences every 4 hours, and then delegates to the NAP the task of turning and repositioning Mrs. Wu every 2 hours. The nurse also sends a consultation request to a wound care nurse specialist.

THINKING

1. *Theoretical Knowledge:*
   a. What facts and principles do you already know about the causes of pressure ulcers?
   b. Do you have enough information to provide interventions for Mrs. Wu's actual Impaired Skin Integrity? If not, what do you still need to find out?
2. *Critical Thinking (Inquiry):* What resource would be best to use to find out exactly what is meant by Mrs. Wu's diagnosis of Self-Care Deficit? Why?

DOING

3. *Practical Knowledge:* What do you know about positioning patients? How would you explain to the NAP about how to position Mrs. Wu "to prevent further pressure on her sacrum"?
4. *Nursing Process (Evaluation):*
   a. To evaluate Mrs. Wu's Impaired Skin Integrity problem, what reassessments would you make?
   b. To evaluate Mrs. Wu's Self-Care Deficit problem, what reassessments would you make? Who can or should make them? How often, or when, would you reassess?

CARING

5. *Self-Knowledge:* How comfortable would you be in caring for Mrs. Wu, who is a frail older adult? What is one problem that might arise that is not described in the scenario?

Critical Thinking and Clinical Reasoning

1. You are working a 12-hour shift (1900 to 0700) on a medical unit at a local hospital. You will be caring for six adult patients. Make a list of the theoretical and practical knowledge you need about the patients to begin organizing your work for the shift. You may not yet have enough experience to make a complete list, but speculate about the kinds of information you think you might need. For example, to organize your work, you will need to know whether you have an NAP or LVN/LPN to assist you or whether you are providing total care for the patients.
2. Create a form for organizing your work. You will need to use a separate sheet of paper for this. Be sure it has space for at least six patients. You might begin by making a column for each patient's name and age, for example. Be sure to leave enough room to write the necessary information. For example, you will need more room to write the patients' tests and treatments than for writing in age and gender.
3. Alma Newport, who is 80 years old, has diabetes, severe arthritis, and mild dementia secondary to Alzheimer's disease. She lives alone. She refuses to consider an assisted living facility or nursing home, although her primary provider and children, who live out of town, believe it would be safer for her to do so. On more than one occasion, she has forgotten to turn off a stove burner while cooking, burning the contents of the pan and smoking up the house.

   A home health nurse visits Mrs. Newport once a week. The physician wants Mrs. Newport to check and record her blood sugar levels before each meal. When the nurse asks, she says her blood sugar level is "OK" and shows the nurse the record she has kept, on which she has recorded many extremely low readings (e.g., 17, 20, 80, 24, 17 mg/dL). When the nurse checks Mrs. Newport's blood sugar, she obtains a reading of 210 mg/dL. After calibrating the glucose meter, the nurse writes the following care plan:

   Nursing Diagnosis:
   Deficient Knowledge related to cognitive deficits secondary to dementia
   Desired Outcomes:
   Mrs. Newport will demonstrate correct method for checking her blood sugar by next visit.
   Mrs. Newport will obtain correct readings.
   Nursing Orders:
   Teach correct method of fingerstick and checking blood glucose.
   Evaluate patient's technique at each visit.

   Over the next few weeks, the home health nurse checks Mrs. Newport's log and fingerstick method at each visit. The logs continue to show low readings, and Mrs. Newport remains unable to perform a fingerstick blood glucose test correctly in spite of repeated demonstrations.

   a. Evaluate Mrs. Newport's progress. Has she met, partially met, or not met the desired outcome?
   b. What possible reasons may account for your evaluation (of Mrs. Newport's outcome status)? Hints:
      (1) Use your theoretical knowledge and personal experience with physical changes that occur with aging.
      (2) Use the data you have about Mrs. Newport.
      (3) Use your practical knowledge about nursing diagnoses.
4. A NAP is helping a patient with a shower when her pager goes off. After ensuring the patient's safety, the NAP goes into the hallway and answers her page. You observe that the NAP is still wearing her gloves. How would you handle this situation?
5. For each of the following concepts, use critical thinking to describe how or why it is important to nursing, patient care, or the processes of implementing and evaluating. Note that these are *not* to be merely definitions.

   Overlapping (of implementation and other nursing process steps)
   Preparing for implementation
   Client participation and adherence
   Coordination of care
   Delegation of care
   The "five rights" of delegation
   Supervision
   Reflecting critically about implementation
   Evaluation
   Outcomes evaluation
   Evaluative statements
   Quality assurance programs

What Are the Main Points in This Chapter?

- Implementation is the nursing process phase in which you perform or delegate the nursing activities that were planned in preceding steps.
- Before performing interventions, you should organize supplies and equipment and ensure the client's readiness.
- While implementing care, you will continue to make assessments and evaluate client responses.
- Collaboration and coordination of care are important nursing functions.
- Delegation is the transfer of responsibility for an action while retaining the accountability for the outcome—this implies that you must supervise those to whom you delegate care.
- The "five rights" of delegation are right task, right circumstance, right person, right direction/communication, and right supervision.
- The final activity in the implementation step is documentation of the care provided. Documenting client responses is actually a part of the evaluation phase; however, you will document both at the same time, often in the same note.
- Evaluation is the final step of the nursing process; it is a planned, ongoing, systematic activity in which you use predetermined standards and criteria to make judgments about: (1) patient progress toward health goals; (2) the effectiveness of the nursing care plan; and (3) the overall quality of care on a unit, in an organization, or in a geographical area.
- When evaluating client health status, you will compare the client's present data/responses to the desired outcomes (goals) set in the planning outcomes phase.
- When evaluating the effectiveness of the nursing care plan, remember that you cannot control all of the variables that influence the success of a nursing activity.
- Quality improvement programs are specially designed to promote excellence in nursing; they include structure, process, and outcomes evaluation.

Knowledge Map

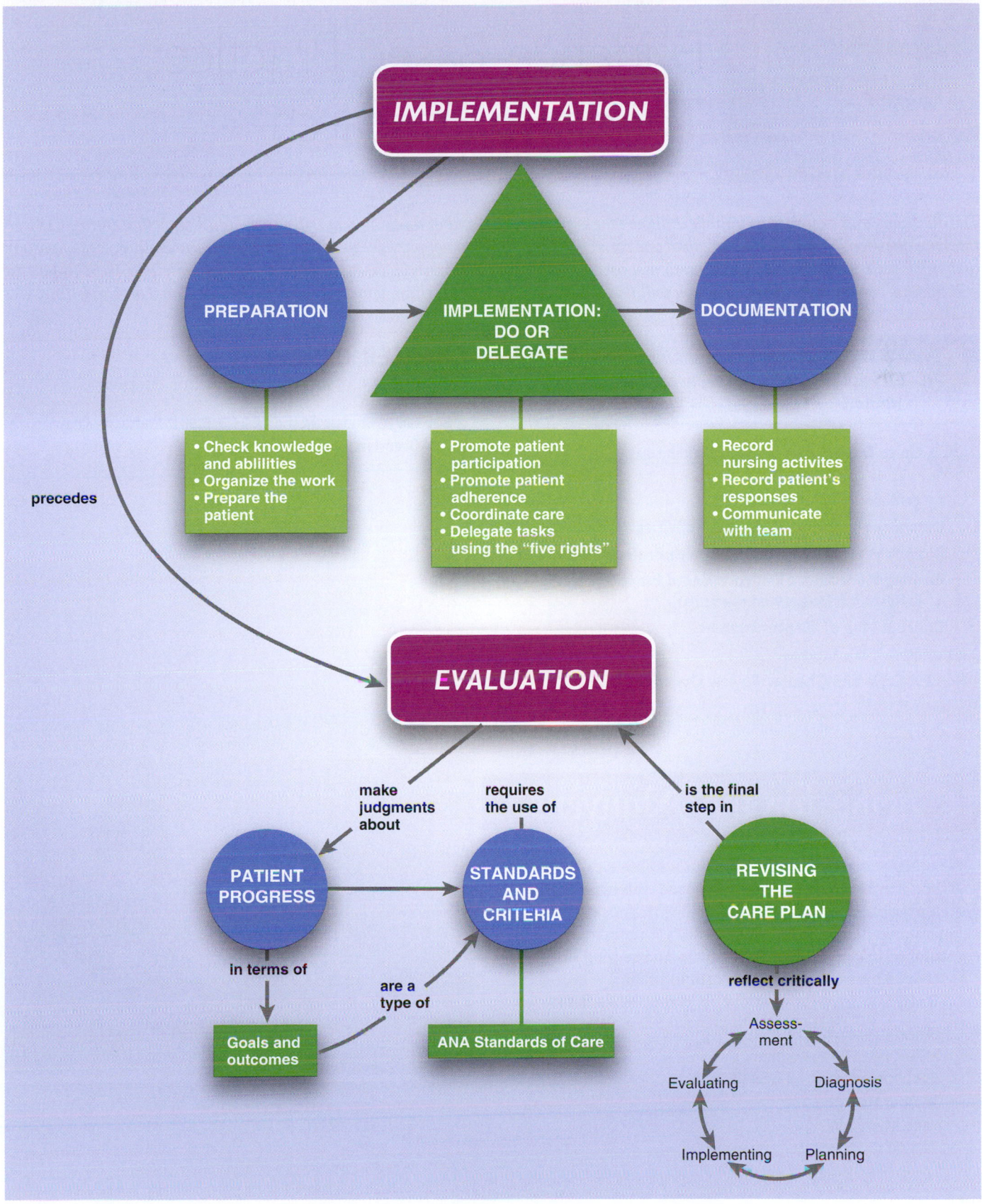

CHAPTER 8

Evidence-Based Practice: Theory & Research

*The questions and exercises in Volume 2 allow you to practice the kind of thinking you will use as a full-spectrum nurse. Critical-thinking questions usually have more than one correct answer, so we do not provide "answers" for these features. It is more important to develop your nursing judgment than to just cover content. You will learn by discussing the questions with your peers. If you are still unsure, consult your instructor. You will find Response Sheets (for writing your responses to the questions) on Davis*Plus.

To explore learning resources for this chapter,

Go to Davis*Plus* at DavisPl.us/Wilkinson3.

Chapter Resources for Chapter 8:

- **Response sheets for all learning activities**
- **Resources for Caregivers and Health Professionals**
- **Reading More About Evidence-Based Practice: Theory & Research (suggested readings)**
- **Concept Map of chapter content**

Interactive Case Studies

NCLEX-Style and Chapter Review Questions

CHAPTER OVERVIEW

For a podcast of an overview of this chapter,

Go to Student Resources: Chapter 8, **Podcast—Chapter Overview,** on Davis*Plus*.

Caring for the Nguyens

Nam Nguyen arrives at the clinic for a follow-up visit. As you may recall, he has been diagnosed with hypertension. At a previous visit, you wrote a nursing diagnosis of Imbalanced Nutrition: More Than Body Requirements related to inappropriate food choices and serving size, as evidenced by a body mass index (BMI) of 28.5.

Today you have gathered the following intake data:

Blood pressure: 174/96 mm Hg
Heart rate: 88 beats/min
Respiratory rate: 18 breaths/min
Temperature: 98.5°F
Weight: 175 lb

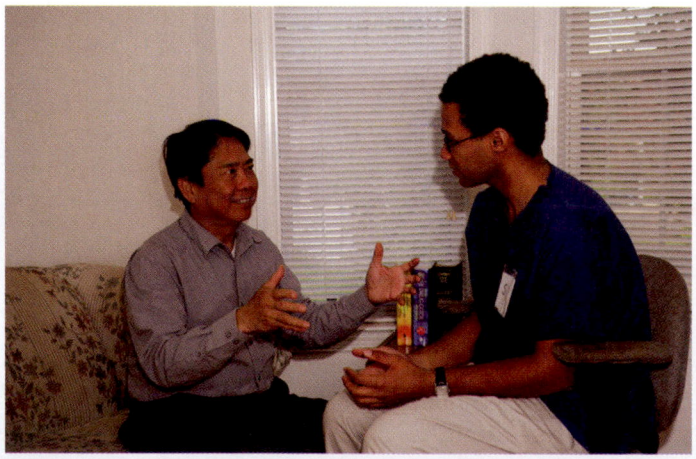

Caring for the Nguyens (continued)

A. What observations can you make about today's data in comparison with his initial visit?

B. As part of the treatment plan for Nam Nguyen, you have been asked to educate him about a diet to assist with weight loss and hypertension management. How would you determine the most appropriate diet to include in your treatment plan?

C. A number of sources recommend the DASH (Dietary Approaches to Stop Hypertension) eating plan. Go to the Internet and search for "Dietary Approaches to Stop Hypertension." Is there sufficient research to support incorporating this information into Mr. Nam's treatment plan? If so, describe the research, and summarize the DASH eating plan.

CLINICALREASONING

Applying the Full-Spectrum Nursing Model

PATIENT SITUATION

You are caring for a 90-year-old patient in a long-term care facility. He is completely dependent for activities of daily living (ADLs). In addition, he has been unresponsive, cannot swallow safely, and for many months has been receiving fluids and nutrition through a feeding tube. His adult grandson has recently discovered a living will, in which the patient had stated that he does not wish to be kept alive by "artificial means, including being tube fed." The grandson, John, insists that the patient's wishes be honored, but the patient's son (Mr. Lee) threatens a lawsuit if the caregivers discontinue the feedings. They argue loudly, and Mr. Lee yells to his son, "You just want him gone because you're in a hurry to get his money! You know you're getting the major part of it."

THINKING

1. *Theoretical Knowledge:* What facts are important to know in order to decide whether or not to stop the feedings?
2. *Critical Thinking (Analyzing Assumptions):* Without thinking too carefully about it, what is your first thought about what is causing the disagreement between Mr. Lee and his son, John? Examine your assumption. How certain are you it is true? What else might be going on in their lives to cause father and son to disagree on this issue?

DOING

3. *Nursing Process (Assessment):* In order to provide some information about the patient that might be helpful in restoring peace between Mr. Lee and John, what patient assessments should you make?

CARING

4. *Ethical Knowledge:* State one ethical issue involved in this case—or one moral problem that it would be present for you if you were involved in it.

Critical Thinking and Clinical Reasoning

1. Recall the scenario about Mr. Wilkey (Meet Your Patient) in Volume 1. Imagine you are the charge nurse on the night shift at a long-term care facility. You hear the certified nursing assistant (CNA) and another person talking loudly down the hall. You immediately go to see what has happened. You are surprised and shocked by what you see. An older patient, Mr. Wilkey, is sitting on the bed of another patient, Mrs. Fredrickson, who is crying and shouting, "Get out! Get out!" Mr. Wilkey is tearful and looks frightened. He keeps repeating, "Where is Momma? Where is Momma?" The CNA is visibly upset and is grabbing at Mr. Wilkey in an effort to get him off the bed. Use any nursing theory you wish, or your own idea, and describe each of the following concepts as they apply in this scenario:
   a. Patient (Who is the patient? How do you know?)
   b. Nurse (Who is the nurse? What is she doing that is "nursing"?)
   c. Health (Is the patient healthy? What is the patient's state of health?)
   d. Environment (Where is the nurse–patient encounter occurring?)

2. Recall Maslow's Hierarchy of Needs. Give one example of a specific nursing intervention a nurse could do to meet each of those needs. If you think the nurse cannot address a need, explain.
   a. Physiological
   b. Safety and security (mental and physical protection)
   c. Love and belonging
   d. Self-esteem (achievement, reputation)
   e. Cognitive needs (knowledge, self-awareness)
   f. Aesthetic needs (beauty, balance, form)
   g. Self-actualization (personal growth, fulfillment)
   h. Transcendence (helping others to self-actualize)
3. You are an emergency department nurse taking care of a 4-year-old child who has had a bike accident. The child has an open abrasion and a few cuts that will require some minor care. However, he is frightened and crying.
   a. Using Nightingale's theory, what interventions might you use?
   b. Using Watson's theory, what might you do?
   c. Using Henderson's theory, what would be the focus of your interventions?
   d. Choose one of the following theories: Neuman, Orem, or Rogers. Look it up on the URL listed in Volume 1 or on Davis*Plus*. Describe how that theory would direct you in this case.
4. You are working the night shift, and while making your 0200 rounds, you are surprised. As you look into the room of 22-year-old Angela Kindred, you see her mother sitting at her bedside sobbing. Visits are not encouraged at that time of night, and you didn't know Mrs. Kindred was on the unit. Even though Angela's leukemia prognosis is terminal, you understood from the day nurse that the family, as well as Angela, had accepted the inevitable outcome. Explain how you can demonstrate caring to this mother who will soon lose her beloved daughter. Look at Watson's (1988) 10 caring processes, repeated below from your textbook. How can you use them to demonstrate caring to this mother and daughter? Be specific in your answers.

Watson's Ten Caring Processes:

1. Forming a humanistic–altruistic system of values
2. Instilling faith and hope
3. Cultivating sensitivity to self and others
4. Forming helping and trusting relationships
5. Conveying and accepting the expression of positive and negative feelings
6. Systematic use of the scientific problem-solving method that involves caring process
7. Promoting transpersonal teaching–learning
8. Providing for supportive, protective, and corrective mental, physical, sociocultural, and spiritual environment
9. Assisting with gratification of human needs
10. Sensitivity to existential–phenomenological forces

5. You are an emergency department nurse taking care of a 4-year-old child who has had a bike accident. The child has an open abrasion and a few cuts that will require some minor care. However, he is frightened and crying, even though his mother is sitting in the treatment room with him. You ask the mother to hold the child while he is being treated and restrain him, if necessary. In reflecting on this intervention afterward, you decide to find the best evidence for your intervention to be certain you will want to use it in similar situations in the future. Write a PICO question to guide your literature search. Write each part, then write the full statement. Note that you do not need to add the "Time" element to this statement.
   P—
   I—
   C—
   O—
   Full statement of the question.
6. Read analytically an article in a research journal. Answer the following questions about the article:
   a. What is the article about as a whole? Answer using one sentence.
   b. What are the author's main conclusions?
   c. Do you think these conclusions are true? If not, why not?
   d. Is this article of any significance in nursing? That is, how could it be used to improve patient care or nursing education?

7. For each of the following concepts, use critical thinking to describe how or why it is important to nursing, patient care, or nursing theory and research. Note that these are *not* to be merely definitions.

Nursing theory	Nursing research
The science of human caring	Institutional review board
From novice to expert	Informed consent
Culturally competent care	Research utilization
Evidence-based practice	Analytical reading

What Are the Main Points in This Chapter?

- According to Florence Nightingale, nursing theories describe "what is" and "what is not" nursing.
- The four basic components of a nursing theory are person, nurse, environment, and health.
- A theory is developed by recognizing a need in nursing or by having an idea, using research to determine whether the idea is effective, and then using the research results to define a theory.
- Theories help nurses (1) find meaning in their experiences of nursing; (2) organize their thinking around pertinent ideas; and (3) develop new, evidence-based ideas and insights into the work they do.
- Nurses use theories as an evidence-based framework for their nursing practice.
- Three leaders in nursing caring theories are Dr. Jean Watson, Dr. Patricia Benner, and Dr. Madeleine Leininger.
- Nursing research is a systematic, objective process of analyzing phenomena of importance in nursing.
- Quantitative research may be generalized to populations similar to the one studied. It has tight controls and large numbers of participants, and the data are statistically analyzed.
- Qualitative research tells the lived experience of a person or group of people. It is analyzed by examining the words and actions of a small number of participants.
- The research process is a systematic way of organizing, preparing, and presenting research.
- Research participants (people in a research study) are protected from harm by specific laws and regulations.
- Research reports are critiqued by reading analytically and using preselected criteria.
- Nursing research evolved slowly. The advanced education currently available to nurses is speeding up the evolution of research.
- Evidence-based nursing requires evaluating research to find the best evidence, and then applying it in practice.
- The process of finding best evidence consists of: identifying a clinical nursing problem, formulating a searchable question, searching the literature, evaluating the quality of the research, and integrating the research into practice.
- The parts of a PICOT question are: **P**atient problem, **I**ntervention, **C**omparison intervention, **O**utcome, and **T**ime.

Knowledge Map

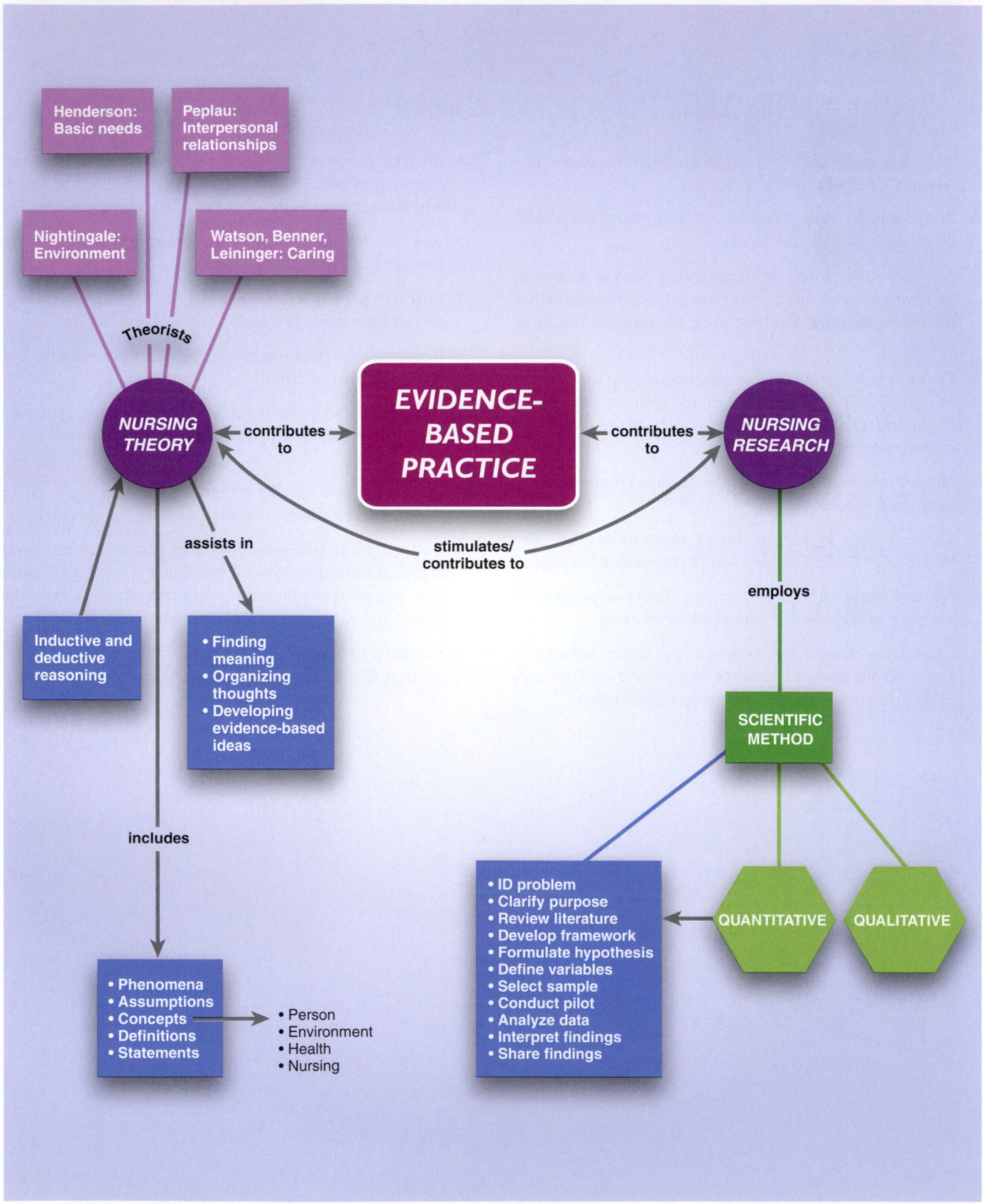

unit 2

Factors Affecting Health

9 Life Span: Infancy Through Middle Adulthood

10 Life Span: Older Adults

11 Experiencing Health & Illness

12 Stress & Adaptation

13 Psychosocial Health & Illness

14 The Family

15 Culture & Ethnicity

16 Spirituality

17 Loss, Grief, & Dying

CHAPTER 9

Life Span: Infancy Through Middle Adulthood

STUDENT RESOURCES

The questions and exercises in Volume 2 allow you to practice the kind of thinking you will use as a full-spectrum nurse. Critical-thinking questions usually have more than one correct answer, so we do not provide "answers" for these features. It is more important to develop your nursing judgment than to cover content. You will learn by discussing the questions with your peers. If you are still unsure, consult your instructor. You will find response sheets (for writing your responses to the questions) on DavisPlus.

To explore learning resources for this chapter,

Go to Davis*Plus* at DavisPl.us/Wilkinson3.

Chapter Resources for Chapter 9:

- **Response Sheets for all activities**
- **Resources for Caregivers and Health Professionals**
- **Reading More About Life Span: Infancy Through Middle Age (Suggested Readings)**
- **Concept Map of chapter content**

Interactive Case Studies

NCLEX-Style and Chapter Review Questions

CHAPTER OVERVIEW

For a podcast of an overview of this chapter,

Go to Student Resources: Chapter 9, **Podcast—Chapter Overview,** on Davis*Plus*.

Caring for the Nguyens

Review the scenario of Nam Nguyen, in the Meet the Nguyens section before Chapter 1 in the front of this book. Answer the following questions based on that scenario:

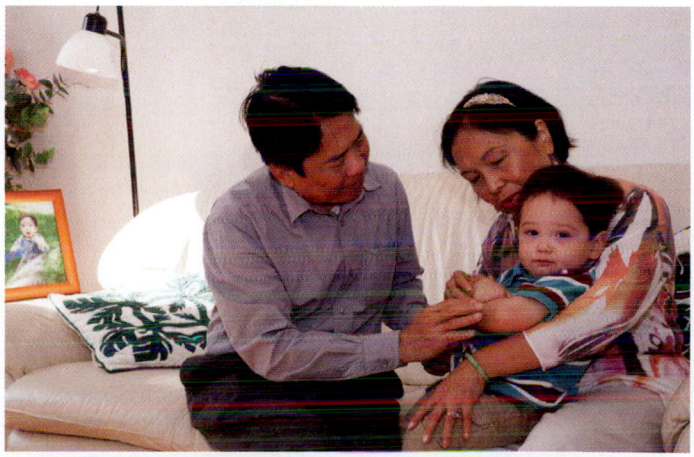

(Continued)

Caring for the Nguyens (continued)

A. Evaluate Mr. Nguyen's physical health status in comparison with what is expected for someone in his age group.

B. Mr. Nguyen and his wife are raising their 3-year-old grandson. What effect might this have on Mr. Nguyen's ability to accomplish his developmental tasks?

Practical Knowledge knowing how

One important aspect of developmental care across the life span is to identify abuse and intervene with patients who are being abused.

PROCEDURES

You will find information on elder abuse in Chapter 10; however, the following procedure can be used for patients of all ages.

Keep in mind that if there is an injury, there is the possibility that it was inflicted. The following flow chart and Procedure 9-1 will aid you in identifying cases of abuse.

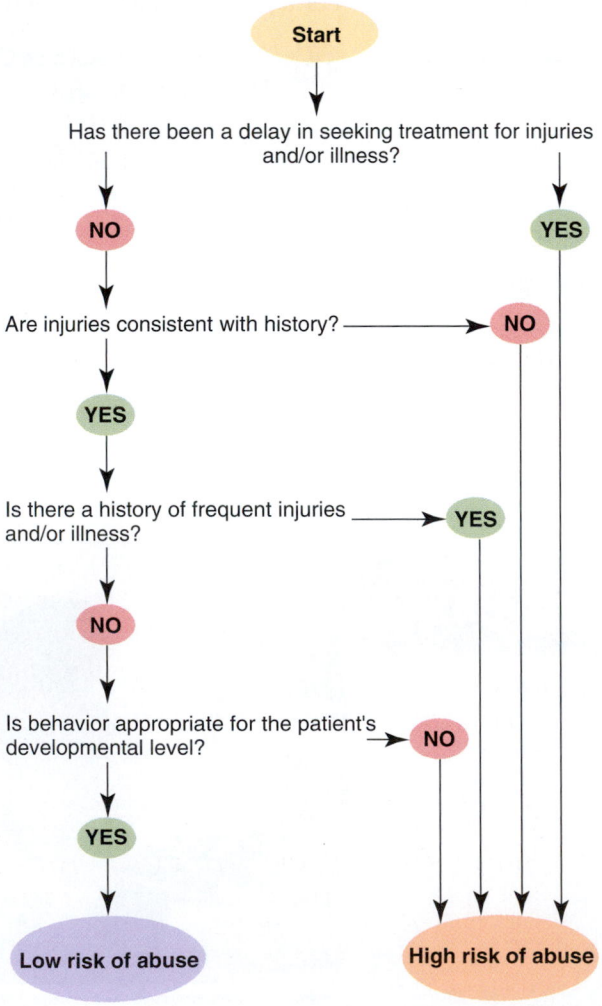

Procedure 9-1 ■ Assessing for Abuse

➤ For steps to follow in *all* procedures, refer to the Universal Steps for All Procedures found on the inside back cover of Volume 2.

Delegation

Key Point: ***Assessment is a nursing responsibility and cannot be delegated.***

Pre-Procedure Assessment

- If you suspect sexual abuse, request a forensic nurse or sexual assault nurse examiner (SANE) be present.
  A forensic nurse and SANE are specially trained to identify findings that indicate abuse, to support the patient, and to handle the evidence to ensure validity in a court of law.
- Assess for abuse routinely in elderly or vulnerable adults and women of childbearing age, and any time a child, dependent person, or spouse has an injury.
  Although there is not a strong base of evidence to support screening, The Joint Commission requires that all patients be screened for abuse and domestic violence.

➤ When performing the procedure, always identify your patient according to agency policy and be attentive to standard precautions, hand hygiene, patient safety and privacy, body mechanics, and documentation.

➤ Privacy and confidentiality are extremely important for this procedure.

Procedure Steps

Obtain a Focused Health History.

1. **Interview the patient and family** members or caregivers separately. If more than one caregiver is present, separate them for the interview, as well.
   Allows the patient more freedom to express his concerns. An abused person may be afraid to talk with the abuser present. Victims have often been intimidated and will usually support the abuser's version of events. If two adults accompany a child, it may be that one of them is abusing both the partner and the child. To help rule that out, separate the caregivers to be certain that they tell the same story.

2. **Approach the subject in a nonthreatening and caring manner.** For example, you might say: "The law requires us to ask about certain injuries. We are not accusing you of anything. I know you care about your child/parent/spouse and want to do everything possible for her health."

3. **Consider the patient's developmental and cognitive level** in assessing whether the story of how the injury occurred is consistent with the injuries.
   The patient must be developmentally capable of performing an activity in a situation in which an injury occurred. For example, an infant is not likely to have opened a medication bottle and taken pills; if a child cannot yet walk, it is not likely that he reached up to pull a hot pan off the stove.

4. **Observe the patient's behavior.** Is it inconsistent with his developmental level?
   In the presence of the abuser, it is common for the abuse victim to appear passive and withdrawn and avoid eye contact. The victim may exhibit anxious or fearful behavior; may look to the parent or caregiver before answering questions; may be overly compliant; or may let the abuser answer the questions for him.

5. **Ask about the injury or incident.** Ask detailed questions about how and when the injury occurred or the illness began: "When did this injury happen or when did you first begin to feel ill?" "How did you get this injury?" "What happened to you?" "What have you been doing to treat your symptoms since you first became ill?"
   A delay of treatment of 12 to 18 hours may indicate abuse. If the details of the history of an injury change during the interview, the likelihood of abuse increases.

6. **Ask about past injuries or incidents:** "Have you ever had similar injuries?" "Have you ever required emergency care in the past?"
   Abusive behavior typically occurs over and over. If an injury is due to abuse, the patient would most likely have experienced abuse in the past and would have evidence of old injuries.

7. **Ask about the patient's usual diet:** "What do you usually eat for breakfast? Lunch? Dinner? What kind of snacks do you have during the day?"
   Neglect and/or abuse may be exhibited by an inadequate or inappropriate diet.

Assess for Sexual Abuse.

8. **Ask directly whether the patient has been touched** inappropriately or forced to have sexual relations.
   Whenever possible, question the patient directly so your question will not be misunderstood.

9. **Ask whether the patient has genitourinary symptoms:** "Have you had any burning or itching when you urinate? How about any vaginal discharge?"
   In a child, genitourinary symptoms may indicate sexual abuse or neglect.

10. **Does the child display knowledge or interest in sexual acts** inappropriate to his or her age, or even seductive behavior?

11. **Does the child appear to avoid another person,** or display unusual behavior—either very aggressive or very passive?

12. **Does the victim display destructive behaviors,** such as alcohol or drug abuse, self-mutilation, or suicide attempts?

(continued on next page)

13. **Is the victim pregnant,** particularly if no intimate relationship is known or the victim is very young?

Assess for Psychological Abuse.

14. **Ask parents or caregivers,** "Are there family members or friends who help you with problems?"
Isolation is a risk factor for abuse. Parents or caregivers may not have the support they need.

15. **Ask the patient, "Whom do you talk to** when you are having problems?"
An abuser will try to isolate the victim from family and friends over time. Ask questions to determine what the relationship is between the victim and family and friends.

16. **Ask, "Tell me how you feel about yourself."**
An abuser demeans and degrades the victim so that the victim has a low self-worth and feels the "punishment" is deserved; conversely, the victim may desire the attention.

17. **Observe if the child acts fearful,** shies away from touch, or appears to be afraid to go home.

18. **Ask, "Who manages the family finances,** and how are decisions made regarding spending?"
An abuser frequently controls all the finances, and restricts the resources of the victim. Abusers typically seek control of victims by fostering dependency and powerlessness.

Perform a Focused Physical Assessment.

19. **If sexual abuse is suspected** from the interview, have a forensic nurse or SANE present if possible.
For any sexual examination, always have a witness in the room to protect the patient and the examiner.

20. **Assess the current injury** and look for evidence of previous injuries. Look for the following cues:
    a. Bruises that form an outline of a hand, cord loop, buckle, or belt
Injuries of different ages and multiple injuries may show a pattern of abuse. Be careful to assess the bruise accurately. Some home treatments may cause what looks like bruising. For example, ***moxibustion*** *(includes such things as firmly rubbing a warm spoon down the affected area) is used in some Asian cultures.*
    b. Injuries that are of varying ages (e.g., bruises of different colors, cuts in various stages of healing)
    c. Obvious nonaccidental burns, such as burns to both feet and lower legs from immersion in hot water
One method of abuse is to immerse the victim's hands or feet into scalding water. The resulting injury has a well-defined border and usually occurs on both extremities.
    d. Circular burns, possibly from cigarettes
Burns at several locations on the body are signs of abuse.
    e. Bite marks
    f. Oral ecchymosis or injury from forced oral sex
Forced oral sex will cause injuries to the mouth.
    g. Bruising at the crease above the eyelids, tense fontanel if the victim is an infant, hyphema, subconjunctival hemorrhage or retinal bleeding, detached retina, ruptured tympanic membrane
Key Point: ***Injuries to the head are common in abuse. Abusive head trauma (AHT, previously referred to as shaken-baby syndrome) is one of the most common and most serious injuries for a young child.***
    h. Bleeding or bruising of genitalia, poor sphincter tone, encopresis (poor bowel control) and bruises on inner thighs
    i. Positive culture for sexually transmitted infection (STI) or positive pregnancy test
STI, particularly in a child, can indicate sexual abuse.
    j. Bruises on wrists and ankles from being restrained
Abused individuals may be tied or locked in a closet or other small space.
    k. Refer to the figure for typical features of injuries that may be nonaccidental:
        Injuries to both sides of the body
        Injuries to soft tissue
        Injuries in the "triangle of safety" (ears, side of face, neck, and top of the shoulders)
Accidental injuries are usually over bony prominences. One suspicious pattern is the "swimsuit zone" on the trunk, breast, abdomen, genitalia, and buttocks. ▼

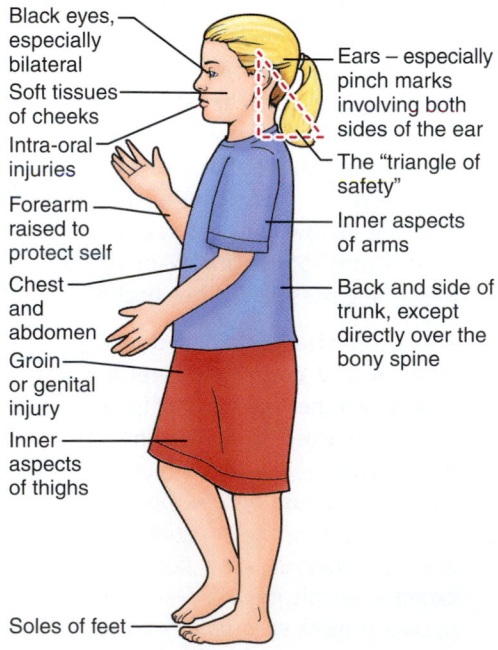

21. **Assess whether injuries are consistent with the history.**
If injuries are not consistent with the history, you must assume abuse.

22. **Observe for signs of neglect:**
- Malnutrition, such as a distended abdomen, or weight markedly below ideal body weight
- Excess body weight for height and age
- Poor hygiene, including oral hygiene
- Ingrown nails
- Untreated sores or pressure sores or other medical conditions
- Matted hair
- Dehydration
- Confusion
- Clothing that is inappropriate for the weather, such as heavy, long-sleeved pants and shirts on hot days
- Periods of time a young child or frail, older adult is left alone without care or supervision

Signs of neglect occur because of long-term starvation or underfeeding, poor personal care, untreated sores or injuries, and inadequate fluid intake. Neglect can also result in childhood obesity as a result of food of poor quality, erratic eating patterns, and poor supervision of the diet.

After The Examination.

23. **If the forensic nurse or primary care provider determines** that abuse has occurred, follow legal procedures to ensure that all evidence is secured. If possible, have a forensic nurse and social worker work with the patient.
In situations in which violation of the law has occurred, strict procedures are essential to ensure that your findings can be used in a court of law and to protect yourself against legal liability.

24. **Provide referrals, if appropriate,** for the abused person, partner, family member, or caregiver to obtain assistance in escaping the abusive situation and/or stopping the abuse.
Resources are available to assist the abused individual and to assist the parent or caregiver to stop the abuse. Be aware of local and national resources.

25. **Report concerns regarding abuse** according to agency and state guidelines.

Key Point: ***Suspected child and elder abuse must be reported to the appropriate agency, according to federal and state laws. Spousal abuse may be mandatory to report, depending on state law. The Joint Commission requires that all cases of possible abuse or neglect are immediately reported in the hospital.***

26. **Treat physical injuries** or refer to the primary care provider for medical care, as needed.
Detection and prevention of abuse require collaborative efforts of the health-care team.

? What if. . .

- **My patient is a child? Are there any special assessments I should make or actions I should take?**

Follow steps 1 through 25 above, with these modifications:

➤ *Note: The interview is important in ruling out sexual abuse in children. Physical findings are often absent, even when the perpetrator admits to penetration of the child's genitalia. Most expert interviewers do not interview children younger than 3 years.*

a. To assess for sexual abuse, ask whether the patient has been touched inappropriately:
- *Child older than 2:* Ask about being touched in "private parts."
- *Older child:* Ask a question such as, "Sometimes people you know may touch or kiss you in a way that you feel is strange or wrong. Has this ever happened to you?"
- *Adolescent:* Ask, "Sometimes people touch you in ways you feel are wrong. This can be frightening, and it is wrong for people to do that to you. Has this ever happened to you?"

b. Ask the parent or caregiver:
- "Has the child started wetting the bed or soiling himself?"
- "Does the child have fears that seem unreasonable?"

Abuse may result in regression to former behaviors. Symptoms of sexual abuse in children may be general and nonspecific, such as sleep disturbances, bed-wetting, or excessive fears.

- "Has the child been masturbating or sexually acting out with other children?"

A child who is sexually abused may exhibit inappropriate sexual behavior.

- "Has the child ever run away? If she leaves, does she go to somewhere safe?" "Is the child/adolescent sexually active?"

An abused child may have feelings of low self-worth and may demonstrate risk-taking behavior, such as running away to places that are unsafe.

c. To assess for psychological abuse, ask the parent or caregiver:
- "Was the child a result of a planned pregnancy? What were the pregnancy, birth, and postpartum period like?"

Risk factors for abuse include an unplanned pregnancy, complications during pregnancy, stressors (e.g., moving, illness, loss of job, divorce), a difficult pregnancy or birth, and lengthy stay in the neonatal intensive care unit.

- "How would you describe the child now?"

An abusive parent may describe the child as a "problem child" who is always doing something wrong. The opposite is sometimes seen, when the child is "perfect."

- "How does the child's behavior compare with that of others in the family?"

Determine whether the parent sees the child differently from siblings. This is a risk factor for abuse.

- "Has the child experienced physical or emotional problems in the past?"
- "What are your expectations of the child's behavior [e.g., school performance, following instructions]?"

The expectations of parents or caregivers who are more at risk to abuse a child may be that the child will "always be a problem" or will be a "perfect" son or daughter.

- "What form of discipline works best with the child?"

(continued on next page)

Determine whether the parents or caregivers use physical or emotional punishment that may be abusive or disproportionate for the act or situation.

- "Do you have any history of depression, anxiety, difficulty coping with situations or everyday life, or other history of mental health problems?"

Mental health disorders interfere with a person's ability to perceive others and situations in a realistic and appropriate way. When coping is compromised, the risk for abuse escalates.

d. Perform a physical assessment. Signs of physical abuse and neglect in children include the following:
   - Bruises on head, face, ears, buttocks, and lower back that are inconsistent with the history of the injury and are of varying stages of healing (different colors)
   - Hemorrhage of the eye, detached retina, ruptured ear drum

Bruising may occur in different patterns. One pattern is the "swimsuit zone" on the trunk, breast, abdomen, genitalia, and buttocks. Children often have accidental bruises over bony areas, but usually not on the abdomen. Injuries to the head are common in abuse. The abusive head trauma (AHT) syndrome may cause detached retina(s), hemorrhages, and subdural hematomas.

   - Abdominal pain

Abdominal pain may be a symptom of sexual abuse in children. Signs of sexual abuse may be general and nonspecific in children.

? What if. . .

- **My patient is an older adult? Are there any special assessments I should make or actions I should take?**

a. Ask the patient and caregiver:
   - "Describe the patient's personal support network. Who visits the patient? How often does the patient have visitors?"

As in spousal abuse, people who victimize older people often isolate the person from any support network.

   - "Who is the patient's primary healthcare provider?"

Multiple healthcare providers, or lack of a provider, can be an indication of abuse. The caregiver may bring the patient to a different physician with each injury or illness to avoid discovery.

   - "Has the patient ever received the wrong dose of medication?"

Getting the wrong medication or dosage of medication (especially oversedation) may indicate abuse or inability to provide safe care.

   - "Who manages the patient's finances?"

Financial abuse is a fairly common form of abuse in this population. Determine who has control of the older person's finances and makes the decisions regarding spending.

b. Ask the patient:
   - "Do you feel safe in your home?"

The patient who is being abused does not feel safe. Keep in mind that abandonment is a form of abuse.

   - "Tell me about your usual day." "Are you able to take care of yourself?" "Who helps you shower and dress?" or "Do you require help with showering or dressing?" "Who is responsible for grocery shopping and cooking in your home?" "How do you get to your appointments or other places you want or need to go?"

To determine the patient's usual level of self-care

c. Observe for signs of self-neglect.

? What if . . .

- **You feel that you are or the patient is in immediate danger?**

If the patient's or your safety is at risk, immediate intervention is required. You may need to secure the area (e.g., by closing the door), notify the in-house security officer, and then call the police.

Evaluation

- Determine whether abuse may have occurred.
- Ensure that appropriate agencies have been notified of the possible abuse.
- Evaluate whether it is safe to let the patient leave the facility.

Patient Teaching

- Inform the patient, parent, partner, and/or caregiver of local resources for prevention or intervention in situations of child, spousal, or elder abuse.
- Inform the patient that abuse is suspected. Ask for her perceptions of the situation.
- Emphasize to the patient that her safety is the primary concern.

Home Care

- If potential abuse is identified in the home, follow agency and state legal guidelines.
- If the patient's safety is at risk, immediate intervention is required. You may need to notify the police or call an ambulance. Be sure to carry a fully charged cell phone with you.
- If you believe that you are at risk for harm (common in abusive situations), leave the setting before notifying the police.

Documentation

- Chart all findings factually—do not add any interpretations. For example:

Do Chart:

4-year-old boy admitted with second-degree burns to both feet extending to midpoint of shins. Father says, "I put him in the bathtub and didn't realize how hot the water was."

Do Not Chart:

4-year-old boy admitted with immersion burns to both feet extending to midpoint of shins, such as those found in abuse.

- Follow legal requirements for documenting possible abuse, including disposition of potential evidence.

- If possible, include pictures of the injuries in the charting, using a digital camera. Place a ruler or other common object next to the injury for reference by a third party viewer. *Photos must be saved and stored in-house because of the requirement to protect confidentiality.*

Practice Resources

Smith & Segal, 2012; The Joint Commission, 2012; National Guideline Clearinghouse 2004, 2007; U.S. Preventive Services Task Force, 2012a.

ASSESSMENT GUIDELINES & TOOLS

Apgar Scoring

CATEGORY	0	1	2
Breathing effort	Not breathing	Respirations slow (less than 30 breaths/min) or irregular	Infant cries well
Heart rate (by stethoscope)	None	Less than 100 beats/min	Greater than 100 beats/min
Muscle tone	Loose and floppy	Some muscle tone, weak flexion	Active motion, full flexion
Grimace response or Reflex irritability (re-sponse to stimulation such as mild pinch)	No reaction	Grimacing	Grimacing and cough, sneeze, or vigorous cry
Skin color	Pale blue	Pink with blue extremities	Entire body is pink

Source: Medline Plus, U. S. National Library of Medicine, National Institutes of Health. APGAR. (Last updated August 27, 2012). Retrieved August 30,2012 from http://www.nlm.nih.gov/medlineplus/ency/article/003402.htm#top

Focused Assessment

Breast Self-Examination (BSE)

The best time to examine your breasts is when they are not tender or swollen. Have your technique reviewed periodically by your healthcare professional. It is acceptable to choose not to do BSE or to do BSE once in a while. Report any changes to your healthcare provider right away.

1. Lie down. Place a pillow under your right shoulder and place your right arm behind your head. (Lying down spreads the breast tissue evenly over the chest wall, making it easier to feel all the tissue.)
2. Using the finger pads (not the tips) of the three middle fingers of your left hand, feel for lumps in the right breast. Use overlapping dime-sized circular motions of the fingers to feel the breast tissue. Move in an up-and-down pattern (see step 4).

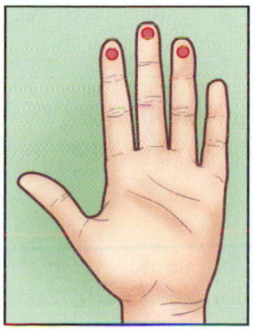

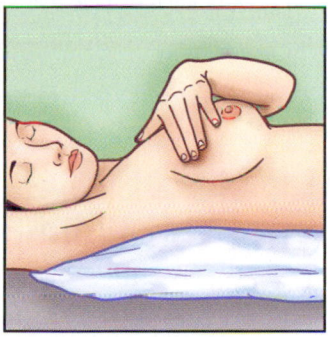

3. Use three different levels of pressure to feel all the breast tissue:
   - Light pressure to feel the tissue closest to the skin
   - Medium pressure to feel a little deeper
   - Firm pressure to feel the tissue closest to the chest and ribs

   Use each pressure level to feel the breast tissue before moving on to the next spot.
4. Start at an imaginary line drawn straight down your side from the underarm. Move across the breast to the middle of the chest bone (sternum), moving in an up-and-down pattern. Check the entire breast area, moving down until

continued

Focused Assessment

Breast Self-Examination (BSE)—cont'd

you feel only ribs, and moving up to the neck or collar bone (clavicle). Evidence suggests that this vertical (up-and-down) pattern is the most effective way to avoid missing any breast tissue.

5. After completely examining your right breast, put the pillow under your left shoulder and examine your left breast using the same methods.
6. Next stand in front of a mirror, arms at your sides, and look at each breast. Note the size, shape, contour, and direction of your breasts and nipples.
7. Press your hands firmly on your hips and look at your breasts for any changes in size, shape, contour, or dimpling, or redness or scaliness of the nipple or skin.
8. While standing (or sitting) with your arm raised slightly, examine each underarm. If you raise your arm straight up, it tightens the tissue and makes it harder to examine.

Source: Adapted from the American Cancer Society (December 31, 2013). How to perform a breast self-exam. Retrieved August 30, 2012, from http://www.cancer.org/docroot/CRI/content/CRI_2_6x_How_to_perform_a_breast_self_exam_5.asp

Focused Assessment

Testicular Self-Examination

Note: The U.S. Preventive Services Task Force (USPSTF) (2011b) recommends against routine screening with testicular self-examination (TSE). However, from the point of view of the individual patient, because there is no harm in self-examination, and because that is the way most testicular cancers are discovered, we see no reason to discourage it. If a patient chooses to perform TSE, you can teach him to use the following method monthly after a warm bath or shower when the scrotal skin is relaxed.

1. Stand in front of the mirror and look for swelling on the skin or scrotum.
2. Using both hands, with the fingers under the scrotum and thumbs on top, gently roll each testicle, feeling for lumps.
3. Palpate the epididymis, a normal cord-like structure on the top and back of each testicle that carries the sperm.

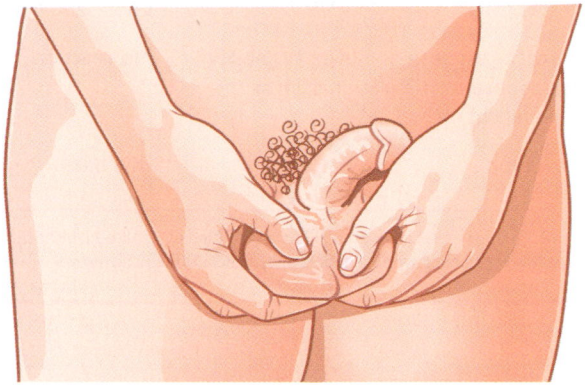

4. Contact your healthcare provider as soon as possible if you palpate a lump or if the area is painful or swollen.

CLINICALREASONING
Applying the Full-Spectrum Nursing Model

PATIENT SITUATION

Lani Ettinger is a 30-year-old woman, married, with three school-age children. She has just had a mastectomy (removal of a breast) because her biopsy was positive for cancer. The surgery was uncomplicated, the cancer was removed at an early stage, and she is expected to recover completely. As you are helping her prepare to leave the hospital, she begins crying.

THINKING

1. *Theoretical Knowledge:* What are Havighurst's developmental tasks of young adulthood?
2. *Critical Thinking (Contextual Awareness):* Which of those developmental tasks is/are most likely to be affected by Lani's mastectomy and her emotional reaction to it?

DOING

3. *Nursing Process (Assessment):* When you see that Lani is crying, what do you need to do?

CARING

4. *Self-Knowledge:* Suppose Lani tells you, "My husband has gone to get the car, but when he was here, he didn't want to hug me or kiss me. I asked him if he will still love me and he didn't say anything. He was crying when he left." What would your feelings be about the husband? You do not need to speculate on exactly what he meant; just imagine what your initial feelings would be.

Critical Thinking and Clinical Reasoning

1. Now that you have an understanding of the stages of growth and development, let us return to the three pediatric patients you met in Meet Your Patients, in Volume 1. All three children are diagnosed with pneumonia. You have introduced yourself to Miguel's and Tamika's caregiver and spoken by phone to Carrie's mother. Each is asking you how this hospitalization will affect their child or grandchild.
   - Tamika, a 3-year-old, lives with her grandparents. Her elderly grandmother is present only during afternoon visiting hours because she must care for her husband, who suffers from numerous health problems.
   - Miguel, a 2-month-old, lives with his mother. Since his admission yesterday, his mother has stayed at his bedside and provided most of her son's care. Miguel's mother is 17 years old and is very concerned about her son's condition.
   - Carrie, a 13-year-old, lives with her parents. Both parents are able to visit only during evening visiting hours, when they leave work.
     a. Based on Erikson's stages of development, contrast the developmental stages of Miguel, Tamika, and Carrie.
     b. How will nursing care differ for each child?
     c. Analyze each caregiver's developmental stage, and discuss the impact it may have on health teaching.
     d. Would it be a good idea to have the children's caregivers meet for a group teaching session to provide information about pneumonia? Explain.
2. For each of the following concepts, use critical thinking to describe how or why it is important to nursing, patient care, or growth and development. Note these are *not* to be merely definitions.

Ego defense mechanisms	Preschooler development
Cognitive development	School-age development
Psychosocial development	Puberty
Fetal development	Adolescent development
Infant development	Young adult development
Reflexes	Middle adult development
Toddler development	Older adult development

What Are the Main Points in This Chapter?

- Growth and development occur across the life span in a predictable pattern.
- Developmental theories help nurses identify what to expect behaviorally, cognitively, socially, and morally from patients at various ages.
- Fetal growth begins at the time of conception and continues for 10 lunar months until birth.
- Critical adaptations at birth include the establishment of respirations and independent circulation, thermoregulation, and the production of urine.
- Between birth and 1 year, infants develop a sense of trust when the caregiver provides the child with love, warmth, and food.
- The toddler period (12 to 36 months) is the time when the child explores the environment and attempts to become autonomous.
- In the preschool period (4 to 5 years) children are able to separate from their parents, communicate needs through language, and control bodily functions.
- The school-age child (6 to 12 years) begins to develop relationships outside the home. This leads to increasing confidence and independence.
- In the adolescent period (12 to 18 years) children establish their own identities and begin to make decisions that will affect their future.
- The young adult (20 to 40 years) leaves home and begins to function as an independent person.
- Middle adulthood (40 to 65 years) is a time when people balance aspirations with reality. It is often a time when the needs of children diminish whereas the needs of aging parents increase.

- Growth and developmental differences result in each age group's having specific health problems requiring specific assessment techniques. Data from these assessments are used to plan and provide care and anticipatory guidance that are developmentally appropriate.
- Abuse of both children and adults is common. Assess all patients for signs of abuse.

Knowledge Map

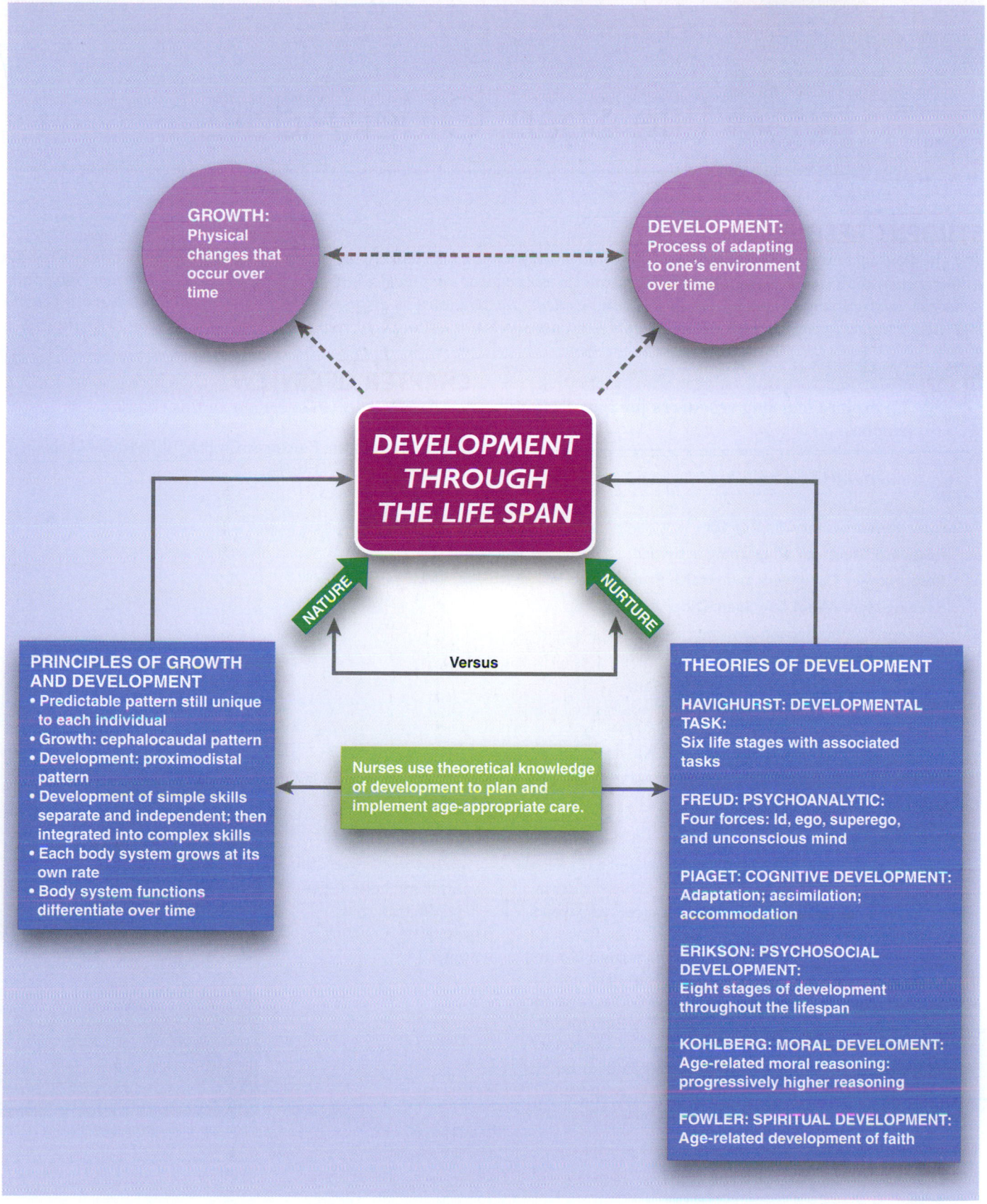

CHAPTER 10

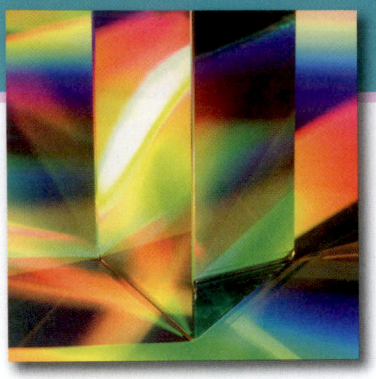

Life Span: Older Adults

STUDENT RESOURCES

*The questions and exercises in Volume 2 allow you to practice the kind of thinking you will use as a full-spectrum nurse. Critical-thinking questions usually have more than one correct answer, so we do not provide "answers" for these features. It is more important to develop your nursing judgment than to just cover content. You will learn by discussing the questions with your peers. If you are still unsure, consult your instructor. You will find Response Sheets (for writing your responses to the questions) on Davis*Plus.

To explore learning resources for this chapter,

Go to DavisPlus, at DavisPl.us/Wilkinson3.

Chapter Resources for Chapter 10:
- **Response Sheets for all learning activities**
- **Resources for Caregivers and Health Professionals**
- **Reading More About Life Span: Older Adults**
- **Concept Map of chapter content**

Interactive Case Studies

NCLEX-Style and Chapter Review Questions

CHAPTER OVERVIEW

For a podcast of an overview of this chapter,

Go to Student Resources: Chapter 10, **Podcast—Chapter Overview,** on Davis*Plus*.

Caring for the Nguyens

Nam Nguyen's father, Binh, is 80 years old and has multiple health problems. He has hypertension and heart disease. Although he had surgery for prostate cancer many years ago, the cancer has now metastasized. Because Binh's health was declining rapidly, Nam and Yen moved him and his wife, Mai, into their home last year. Both Nam and his wife work outside the home, so the elderly Mai cares for her husband as best she can during the day. Binh is too weak to get out of bed without help, and his wife is not strong enough to support him. She cooks for him, but he eats only a few bites, then pushes the plate away. Nam telephones today to say, "We can't take care of him safely at home any longer. Can you tell me how to get him admitted to a hospital or a nursing home?"

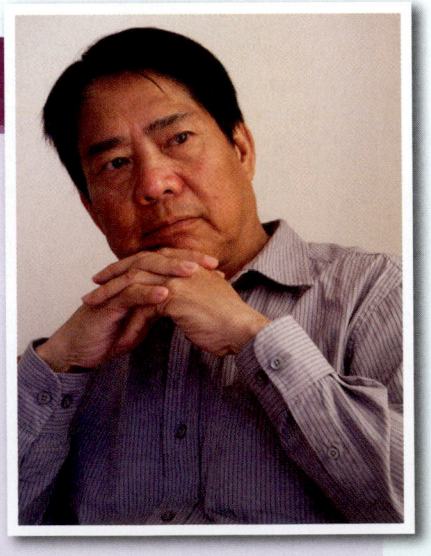

Caring for the Nguyens (continued)

A. What other ideas do you have for helping the Nguyens to care or to find care for Binh other than placing him in a hospital or nursing home?

B. Nam's first concern seems to be about getting help for his father. What do you think his next concern will be?

C. What actual data do you have about Binh Nguyen's nutritional status?

D. What else do you need to know to fully assess Binh's nutritional status? If you do not know the answer to this, you will find some information in the Assessment sections of this chapter in Volume 1. For more complete information, refer to Screening for Nutritional Problems and in Focused Nutritional Assessment, in Chapter 27 of this volume. Also

Go to **Assessment,** in Chapter 27 of Volume 1.

E. Would you consider Binh Nguyen to be a frail elderly person? Why or why not?

CLINICALREASONING

Applying the Full-Spectrum Nursing Model

PATIENT SITUATION

Alvin Bell, 82 years old, was just discharged from the hospital following a myocardial infarction (heart attack). On your first home visit to supervise his medication regimen, you notice that the house looks as though it has not been cleaned in weeks. Piled on every flat surface, including the floor, is what appears to be months' accumulations of newspapers, magazines, and other clutter. Dishes are piled in the sink, apparently from before his hospitalization. There is hardly any food in the cupboard. When you weigh Mr. Bell, you see that he has lost 3 lb in the 3 days he has been home. He admits he has not been eating: "I'm not hungry, and it's too much trouble." As you talk with him, you learn that his wife died of cancer 7 months ago. He says, "I don't know what to do without her. I hate living alone. I don't have much reason for going on." Mr. Bell is alert and oriented, but talks and moves very slowly.

THINKING

1. *Theoretical Knowledge:*
   a. What do you know about depression in older adults? Do you have enough knowledge of that topic to be able to assess whether Mr. Bell is depressed? If not, what resources would you use to find out (list specific resources; that is, give the URL, don't just say "the Internet"; give the name or author of the book, not just "my psych-nursing book").
   b. You will also need to know whether it is normal for appetite to decrease in older adults, and what their calorie needs are compared with other age groups. Where can you go to find this information?
2. *Critical Thinking (Considering Alternatives):*
   a. As you survey Mr. Bell's overall situation, what is your first impulse to improve his situation? What questions come to you?
   b. What community services might be helpful for Mr. Bell?
   c. How would you handle referrals? Would you leave a list of telephone numbers? Would you call the agencies yourself? Explain your thinking.

DOING

3. *Practical Knowledge:* In your physical examination of Mr. Bell, you find no old or recent bruises or other injuries. However, because he is depressed and losing weight, you wonder if he is suffering neglect or financial abuse. What questions could you ask to find out?

CARING

4. *Self-Knowledge:* Think of one patient you have cared for who has something in common with Mr. Bell. Describe the way(s) in which they are alike.

Critical Thinking and Clinical Reasoning

1. Margaret O'Malley, age 67, tells you that even though she has new reading glasses, she still cannot see as well as she would like to for reading or sewing. She says, "My eyes often feel dry and scratchy. I wonder if something is wrong."
   a. What would you advise her to do that might improve her reading ability?
   b. What age-related change do you think may be causing Mrs. O'Malley's eyes to feel dry and scratchy?
2. Tony King, age 78, is having difficulty controlling his diabetes. As he leads a sedentary life, his physician has advised him to take daily walks to help regulate his blood sugar. Mr. King says, "Doc, I can't do that. With the arthritis in my back and hips, every step is agony. I walk just enough to take care of myself, get to the store, come here, and do whatever I have to. I'm already taking a lot of drugs for the pain; I can't take more when I walk." What kind of program could the physician recommend to Mr. King?
3. For each of the following concepts, use critical thinking to describe how or why it is important to nursing, patient care, or growth and development. Note that these are *not* to be merely definitions.
   a. Gender disparities in life expectancy
   b. Age distribution in the population (population pyramid)
   c. Aging in place

What Are the Main Points In This Chapter?

- The number of older adults (age 65 and older) has risen significantly because of increasing life expectancy.
- Older adulthood is a time of transition. Most health problems experienced by older adults are chronic in nature and often affect the person's ability to live independently.
- Most older adults live independently.
- Aging can be examined from a life expectancy, percentage of total population, or life-span perspective.
- Aging in place means that as they age, persons live in their own elder-friendly residences and receive supportive services for their changing needs, rather than moving to another location or alternative type of housing.
- Retirement communities are planned and built specifically to provide elder-friendly dwellings and environments for independent living and allow older adults to "downsize" their dwelling.
- Continuing care retirement communities (CCRC) offer a wide range of living accommodations, including residential living, assisted living, skilled nursing care, rehabilitation, and dementia care on a large campus-like setting.
- Assisted-living facilities (ALFs) are congregate residential settings that provide or coordinate personal services, 24-hour supervision and assistance, activities, and health-related services.
- Nursing care facilities, or nursing homes, provide skilled and unskilled nursing care for older adults and adults with disabilities.
- The stages of older adulthood are typically referred to as the *young-old* (age 65 to 74), *middle-old* (age 75 to 84), and *oldest-old* (age 85+).
- The fastest growing segment of older adults is the oldest-old, some of whom are the frail elderly and *centenarians* (people over 100 years old).
- Older adults learn new material more slowly. However, there is no loss of intelligence as a person ages.
- Disengagement theory and activity theory attempt to explain the psychosocial development of older adults.
- **Dementia**, a loss of cognitive ability, is not a normal result of aging. It is important to differentiate dementia from depression, acute confusion, or delirium that may be precipitated by dehydration, infection, or a medication side effect or overdose.
- Developmental differences result in each age group's having specific health problems requiring specific assessment techniques. Data from these assessments are used to plan and provide care and anticipatory guidance that are developmentally appropriate.
- Older adults should have an annual physical examination, including a focused assessment of functional status.
- Frailty is set of characteristics that describe a heightened state of vulnerability for developing adverse health outcomes.
- Abuse of adults is common. Assess all patients for signs of abuse.
- Suspicion of elder abuse must be reported to adult protection services and/or the authority designated by law in each state.

Knowledge Map

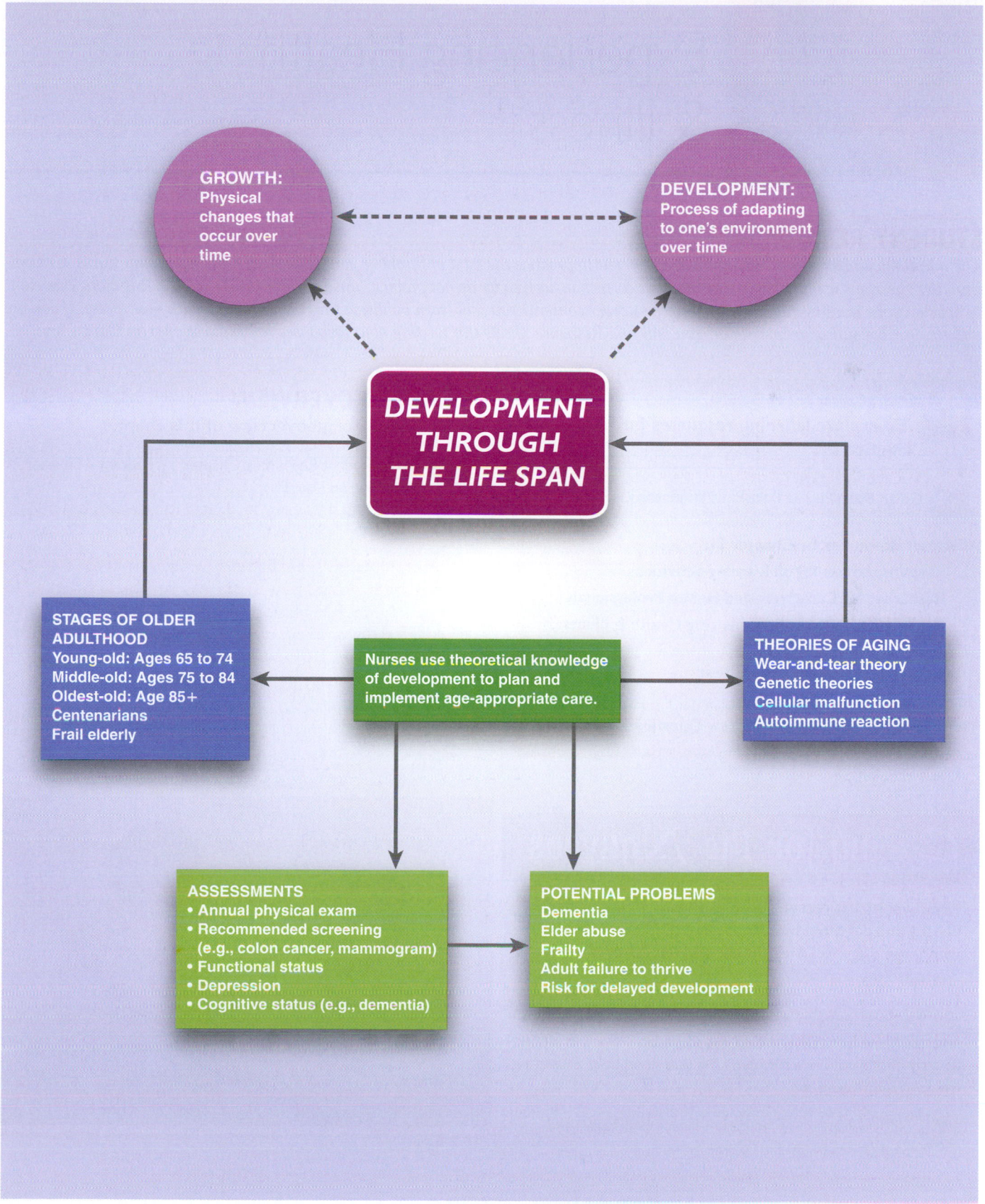

CHAPTER 11

Experiencing Health & Illness

STUDENT RESOURCES

*The questions and exercises in Volume 2 allow you to practice the kind of thinking you will use as a full-spectrum nurse. Critical-thinking questions usually have more than one correct answer, so we do not provide "answers" for these features. It is more important to develop your nursing judgment than to just cover content. You will learn by discussing the questions with your peers. If you are still unsure, consult your instructor. You will find Response Sheets (for writing your responses to the questions) on Davis*Plus.

To explore learning resources for this chapter,

Go to Davis*Plus* at DavisPl.us/Wilkinson3.

Chapter Resources for Chapter 11:

- **Response sheets for all learning activities**
- **Resources for Caregivers and Health Professionals**
- **Reading More About Experiencing Health & Illness (suggested readings)**
- **Concept Map of chapter content**

Interactive Case Studies

NCLEX-Style and Chapter Review Questions

CHAPTER OVERVIEW

For a podcast of an overview of this chapter,

Go to Student Resources: Chapter 11, **Podcast—Chapter Overview,** on Davis*Plus*.

Caring for the Nguyens

Nam Nguyen has recently been diagnosed with hypertension, obesity, and degenerative joint disease (DJD). He is struggling with these diagnoses. He tells his wife, Yen, "I feel so old now. These are the kind of things my parents are dealing with." At a clinic visit Nam tells you, "It's hard to think of myself as sick. I've been depressed ever since Zach told me about his findings. Now he's asked me to get some lab work. I'm afraid he may find even more problems." If you need help answering the following questions,

Go to Chapter 11, The Health-Illness Continuum and Dunn's Health Grid in Volume 1.

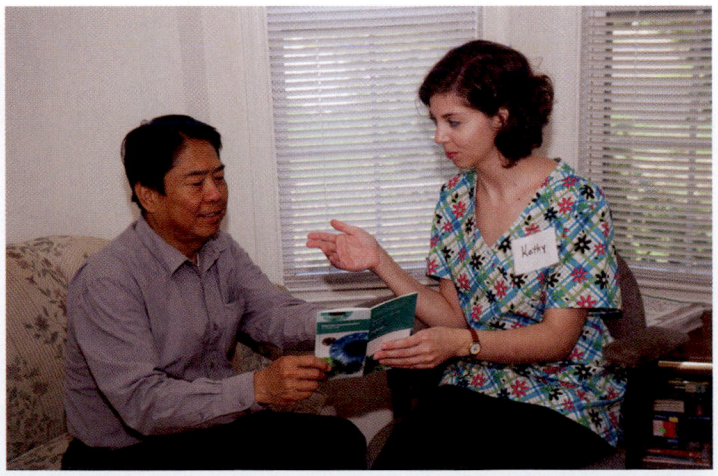

Caring for the Nguyens (continued)

A. Identify the disruptions that Mr. Nguyen must deal with based on these diagnoses. Explain your reasons for choosing these disruptions.

B. How would you evaluate Mr. Nguyen health status? To review the concepts of health status,

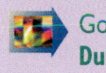
Go to Chapter 11, **The Health-Illness Continuum and Dunn's Health Grid** in Volume 1.

C. What kinds of activities could you suggest to Nam to improve his health status?

D. What stage of illness behavior is Mr. Nguyen exhibiting in regard to his recent medical diagnoses?

Practical Knowledge knowing how

Practical knowledge in this chapter means using the nursing process to apply what you have learned about how people experience health, wellness, and illness.

PROCEDURES

The procedures in this chapter are designed to help you admit, transfer, and discharge patients in such a way that you can begin to establish trust at the first patient contact.

Procedure 11-1 ■ Admitting a Patient to a Nursing Unit

➤ For steps to follow in *all* procedures, refer to the Universal Steps for All Procedures found on the inside back cover.

Equipment

- Identifying armband (if this has not been supplied by the admissions department)
- Patient's chart, including physician's orders and nursing admission record
- Thermometer, blood pressure cuff, and stethoscope
- Scales for height and weight
- Gown
- Admission pack (e.g., water pitcher, soap, comb, toothbrush, mouthwash, and facial tissues)
- Nursing care plan or clinical pathway, if one has already been made
- Hospital brochures, Patient Care Partnership, and other forms
- Admission assessment form

Delegation

A registered nurse is responsible for managing medical orders and assessing the patient's need for nursing care in all settings, although this may vary in some specifics according to hospital policy, the law, and regulations. Most other admission activities can be delegated to nursing assistive personnel (NAP) if the patient is stable.

Pre-Procedure Assessments

- Assess for signs of emotional and/or physical distress.
- Assess ability to ambulate and/or move.
- Assess ability to communicate and understand what is occurring.

➤ When performing the procedure, always identify your patient according to agency policy and be attentive to standard precautions, hand hygiene, patient safety and privacy, body mechanics, and documentation.

Procedure Steps

1. **Ensure placement of patient labels** (e.g., on the chart, at the bedside, outside the door).
2. **Introduce yourself to the patient and family.** Explain who you are. Don't be afraid to tell a client that you are a nursing student.
   Many clients are aware that students have more time to spend with them. Talking to the patient and family reassures them and provides information about the patient's level of consciousness and awareness, social relationships, and so on.
3. **Assist the patient into a hospital gown.**
   If the patient is able to stand, assist her into a gown before weighing her to obtain the most accurate weight.

(continued on next page)

Procedure 11-1 ■ Admitting a Patient to a Nursing Unit (continued)

4. **Measure height and weight** while the patient stands on a scale, if possible. If she is unable to stand, transfer her into the bed and measure her weight using a bed scale.
   Weigh in the same manner each time to ensure accuracy.

5. **Assist the patient into the bed.**
   Get the patient comfortable before continuing the admission to prevent overtiring her.

6. **Check the patient's identification band** to ensure the information, including allergies, is correct. Verify this information with the patient or family.
   Questioning the patient about allergies and verifying with the family will ensure that the information is accurate and documented on the wristband and the chart.

7. **Measure vital signs.**
   Measuring the vital signs before completing the rest of the admission ensures that you will be aware of the patient's status. If the vital signs are abnormal, further assess the patient's condition before continuing. Report your findings to the admitting care provider.

8. **Complete the nursing admission assessment**, including health history and physical assessment. Be sure to include the patient's expectations and concerns. For inpatients, this must be completed within 24 hours after admission. All patients should be screened on admission for risk for pressure ulcers. (Chapter 22 provides a step-by-step approach to physical assessment.)
   An admission assessment is needed to identify problems and establish a baseline. The Joint Commission requires that each patient have an admission assessment performed by a registered nurse.

9. **Check the list of the patient's current medications** (created in the admitting department) to be sure it is complete and accurate. Usually the patient's own medications are sent home with the family, or they may be sent to pharmacy for storage.
   It is important to know what medications the patient has been taking. The pharmacy will identify medicines from home when necessary. When medications are ordered and given during the patient's stay, they are compared with those on the list so any discrepancies can be resolved.

10. **Orient the client to the room.**
    These actions ensure that the patient and family will be able to call for assistance if needed and increase the patient's and family's level of comfort and ability to function in the hospital setting. Remember that one of the disruptions associated with illness is anxiety about the unknown. If you tell your client what to expect, you help to minimize his anxiety.
    a. Make sure the client knows how to use the bed, the call light, and any equipment that you expect him to use.
    b. Point out the location of personal care items.
    c. Show the client the location of the restroom.
    d. If you will be measuring the client's intake and output, tell him so during your orientation.

    If the client is alert, he may be able to assist you with these measures.

11. **Explain hospital routines**, including use of side rails, meal times, and so on. Answer the patient's and family's questions.
    Hospitalization takes away control of basic decisions. Knowing the routines and available choices increases patient and family comfort.

12. **Verify with the patient all other admission data** on the chart for completeness and accuracy.
    Basic data such as name, address, marital status, name of admitting physician, admitting diagnosis, consent to treatment, and so on, will usually be obtained in the admitting office. However, you will need to be sure all the admitting information is complete, and complete it if it is not.

13. **Ask if the patient has an advance directive** (e.g., power of attorney or living will). If so, place a copy in the hospital record. If not, explain the purpose of the document and give the patient a form to fill out if he wishes to do so. (See Chapters 17 and 45, Volume 1, if you need more information about advance directives.)
    Advance directives enable patients to indicate their preferences about treatments and prolonging life.

14. **Advise the patient of his privacy rights under HIPAA.** See that he has a written explanation of his privacy rights (see Chapter 45 as needed).

15. **Inventory the patient's belongings.** Encourage the family to take home valuable items and money. If that is not possible, arrange to have valuables placed in the hospital safe. Most agencies require money in excess of $5.00 to be sent home or to the cashier's office.
    Patient belongings, including valuables, are frequently lost during hospitalization. Documenting the disposition of everything ensures being able to return the belongings to the patient upon discharge.

16. **Complete all admission orders** or ensure that they have been completed (e.g., laboratory tests, medications, diet and fluid orders).
    Unless it is an unscheduled admission, diagnostic tests are usually completed on an outpatient basis before admission to the hospital. However, there may still be some orders that need to be done immediately, while others can be delayed. Make sure the orders are completed in the most appropriate time frame.

17. **Ensure patient comfort** (e.g., positioning, pain, water at bedside).

18. **Make one last safety check** (i.e., call light within reach, bed in low position, siderails up as appropriate, equipment functioning properly).

19. **Before leaving, ask if you can do anything else** for the patient and family.

20. Initiate the care plan or clinical pathway.
Identifying the patient's priority problems enables the nurse to develop the most appropriate nursing orders.

? What if. . .

- **The patient may be at risk for falls?**

  Perform falls risk assessment as appropriate to the patient, and according to agency policy.
  Falls are common in inpatient facilities, especially among older adults. If a patient has falls risk factors, risk reduction measures can be instituted.

- **The patient has special care needs?**

  When the patient has special needs, such as allergies, a "nothing by mouth" order or an "intake and output" order, post patient care reminders at the head of the bed or at the door to remind other care providers.

- **The patient needs a more in-depth assessment in some areas?**

  Perform special needs assessments as relevant to the care and condition of the patient (social situation, nutrition and hydration status, functional abilities, spiritual and cultural variables). If these are warranted, they must be completed within 24 hours after admission or prior to surgery.
  In-depth assessment of these topics is not a part of all admission assessments, but should be done if the patient's condition warrants.

- **The patient has a learning disability?**

  If possible, preadmissions should be arranged for the patient and main caregiver. This allows more time to discuss issues of consent, alleviate anxiety, and set up links with a learning disability specialist or social worker. Whether or not this is possible: Allow more time for the admission process.

  Use short sentences, with one idea at a time.

  Include the caregiver in the admission process, but encourage the patient to participate as much as possible.

  Document the main caregiver and contact numbers.

  Expect the patient to be anxious.

  Include special communication and personal needs in the plan of care.

  Give the patient hospital information with pictures, such as those given to children, if appropriate for her developmental level.

- **The patient is an older adult?**

  Ask all older adults if they have had any falls in the past year. If they report a fall, observe them as they stand up from a chair without using their arms, walk several paces, and return ("get up and go"). If they are steady, no further assessment is required. If there is unsteadiness or if the person reports more than one fall, further assessment is required.
  The incidence and severity of fall-related complications rise steadily after age 60. Fall rates in nursing homes and hospitals are almost three times the rate for those living at home.

- **The patient is a child?**

  Use a friendly approach.
  The first priority is to establish a trusting relationship with the child and parents to help relieve fears and anxiety. Children younger than 3 years may fear being separated from parents. Older children usually worry more about what is going to happen to them.

  Explain the visiting and rooming-in policies to the parents.

  Ask about the child's usual routine (e.g., toileting, bedtime rituals, favorite foods).

  Speak to the child directly if she is old enough to understand.

  Direct the family to the bathroom, playroom, television, and snack room, if those are available.

  Encourage the parents to bring toys and other favorite items from home.
  It helps the child feel more comfortable in the unfamiliar surroundings.

Documentation

- Document all assessment findings on the admission database provided by the institution. If you need an example, see Chapter 3, Tables, Boxes, Figures, Nursing Admission Data Form, Assessment Forms: Nursing Admission Data Form, in this volume.
- Document an admission note and any teaching or other interventions in the nursing notes or flowsheet (according to agency policy).
- Recall that a discharge plan is created on admission. You will find forms for discharge assessment and teaching under Forms, after the Procedures in this chapter. For another example of a discharge plan, see Chapter 5, Discharge Planning Form, in Volume 2.

Practice Resources

The American Geriatrics Society (n.d.); The Joint Commission (2008, 2012b); Michael, Y., Lin, J., Whitlock, E., et al. (December 2010).

Procedure 11-2 ■ Transferring a Patient to Another Unit in the Agency

➤ For steps to follow in *all* procedures, refer to the Universal Steps for All Procedures found on the inside back cover.

Equipment

- Medical record or chart
- Care plan
- Patient's medications
- Supplies for any ongoing treatments
- Patient's belongings, clothes, and personal care articles
- Standardized handoff form, if available
- A utility cart, if belongings are numerous
- Wheelchair or transfer cart, if bed is not being moved

Delegation

If the patient's condition allows, you can delegate the physical transfer of the patient and have the nursing assistive personnel (NAP) move the patient's belongings to the other room. However, as the nurse, you are responsible for obtaining and completing the necessary records, making the final assessment, and gathering and checking the medications. You must also give the handoff report to another nurse.

Pre-Procedure Assessment

- Make a final, brief focused physical assessment.
- Assess the patient's mobility and ability to assist.
- Assess for emotional and/or physical distress (administer medications, as needed).
- Assess the patient's ability to communicate and understand what is occurring.

➤ When performing the procedure, always identify your patient according to agency policy and be attentive to standard precautions, hand hygiene, patient safety and privacy, body mechanics, and documentation.

Procedure Steps

1. **Obtain the number of personnel needed** to make a safe transfer.
   For efficiency and patient and staff safety.

2. **Gather the patient's medications and label them** correctly for the new room.
   Ensures availability of medications when the patient arrives at the new unit; helps prevent medication administration errors.

3. **Notify the receiving unit of the time to expect the transfer**; notify other departments (e.g., dietary, pharmacy, admitting), primary care provider, and family of the transfer.
   You need to schedule the transfer with the receiving nurse so he can plan his work and so you can arrange the transfer time to limit the number of interruptions during the handoff. Limiting interruptions minimizes the possibility of failing to communicate or forgetting information. Other departments must have the transfer data so that services such as meals and physical therapy treatments will not be interrupted. The primary care provider and family, of course, need to know where to find the patient.

4. **Gather the patient's personal belongings and supplies**, including: treatment-related supplies and equipment (e.g., isolation supplies, clean dressings), chart, Kardex, and care plan. Place in a container (e.g., the patient's bath basin) or on a utility cart if necessary.
   Having the supplies and equipment "ready to go" makes the transfer more efficient for you and less stressful for the patient.

5. **Bring the wheelchair or transfer cart to the bedside** and assist the patient to the chair or cart. If using a wheelchair, the patient can hold the pan of supplies; if using a bed or cart, place supplies on the bed.

6. **Take the patient to the new room and give the handoff report.** Follow agency procedure for handoff reports. However, the method chosen should allow both the giver and receiver of patient information the opportunity for questioning.
   a. If you need to review content of an oral handoff report, see Chapter 18. In general, the report should include name, age, sex, physicians, surgical procedures, medical diagnoses, medications, allergies, laboratory data, special equipment (e.g., oxygen, suction), the patient's current health status, and whether there are advance directives and resuscitation status. Identify the nursing diagnoses and priorities for nursing care.
   b. Consistently use a structured framework or memory aid to guide the handoff process and the oral report.
   The objective of a handoff is to provide accurate information about the patient. The information communicated must be accurate in order to ensure patient safety.
   c. **Be sure to point out to the nurse if patient is taking corticosteroids, anticoagulants, diabetic medications, antibiotics, or narcotic analgesics.**
   These medications can have serious side effects and need careful monitoring.

? What if. . .

- **The patient has intravenous (IV) lines and other equipment that cannot be turned off?**

  It is common to transfer patients with IV lines. Some wheelchairs are equipped with an IV pole; for others, you may need to obtain a rolling pole from the unit supply room. The patient may be able to maneuver the rolling pole. Most beds and transfer carts also have portable IV poles, sometimes stored along the underside. Portable oxygen and suction are also available for patients who must have them even during transfer. Be sure to obtain these, set them up, and check their functioning prior to moving the patient from his bed.

- **The patient has too many personal belongings for one person to carry?**

  If the patient's condition requires two staff members to transfer, one person can manage the utility cart while the other manages the patient. If only one person can make the actual move, load a utility cart and move all the supplies and belongings to the new room before transferring the patient.

- **The patient is being transferred to the intensive care unit (ICU)?**

  If this is an urgent transfer, you may need to notify the receiving nurse and move the patient with his records and medications. Later you can make the other notifications, finish the charting, and move belongings and other supplies. In some ICUs, the family may need to take the patient's personal belongings home.

Evaluation

With the receiving nurse, evaluate the patient's response to the move. The receiving nurse will take vital signs and make a preliminary admission assessment.

Documentation

- Just before moving, document as much information as you can, including the patient's status at that time.
- After handoff, document the information reported in the handoff, the name and title of the person who received the patient, and your report.
- Sign the note. Some agencies have a standardized form for the transfer note.

Example documentation

3/13/15, 1615. Client transferred to room 501 by stretcher, with both siderails up, with assistance of one. Temperature 104.8°F, pulse 100 beats/min, BP 138/88, respirations 20 breaths/min and shallow. Drowsy upon arrival. Responds to verbal stimuli with moaning. Last pain medication given at 1515. Denies pain when asked. No urine noted since 12:00 pm; will encourage voiding by offering urinal every 2 hr. #22 IV in RAC and #18 IV in R hand flushed with 3 mL of normal saline; flushes without redness, edema, or induration. Receiving 3 L/min of oxygen during transfer. Placed on 3 L/min in room; will wean oxygen as tolerated. Handoff report given to Linda Hamm, RN.——————— Sarah Fields, RN

Practice Resources

The Joint Commission (2012a); McFetridge, B., Gillespie, M., Goode, D., et al. (2007); Riesenberg, L. A., Leisch, J., & Cunningham, J. M. (2010).

Procedure 11-3 ■ Transferring a Patient to a Long-Term Care Facility

➤ For steps to follow in *all* procedures, refer to the Universal Steps for All Procedures found on the inside back cover.

Equipment

- Medical record or chart
- Care plan
- Patient's medications
- Supplies for any ongoing treatments
- Patient's belongings, clothes, and personal care articles
- Standardized transfer form, if available
- A utility cart, if belongings are numerous
- Wheelchair or transfer cart

Delegation

If the patient's condition allows, you can delegate the physical transfer of the patient and have the NAP move the patient's supplies and belongings. However, as the nurse, you are responsible for obtaining and completing the necessary records, making the final assessment, and gathering and checking the medications. You must also give the handoff report to another nurse.

Pre-Procedure Assessment

- Make a final, brief focused physical assessment.
- Assess the patient's mobility and ability to assist.
- Assess for emotional and/or physical distress (administer medications, as needed).
- Assess the patient's ability to communicate and understand what is occurring.

(continued on next page)

Procedure 11-3 ■ Transferring a Patient to a Long-Term Care Facility (continued)

➤ When performing the procedure, always identify your patient according to agency policy and be attentive to standard precautions, hand hygiene, patient safety and privacy, body mechanics, and documentation.

Procedure Steps

1. **Notify the patient and family well in advance** of the upcoming transfer to another facility. Include information about the reasons the patient is being transferred, as well as any alternatives to transfer. You will also need to determine which agency is to arrange transportation for the patient.
   Allows them time to adjust emotionally and to make any necessary plans.

2. **Prepare the patient's records.** You may need to send a copy of the patient's chart to the receiving facility. The original remains with the hospital. You will usually also send a copy of the comprehensive nursing assessment and a detailed nursing care plan, as well as prescriptions and cards for future appointments (e.g., with physicians or social workers).
   Ensures continuity of care, thus minimizing patient stress.

3. **Gather and pack the patient's personal items** and treatment supplies to send to the long-term care facility with the patient.
   Having the supplies and equipment "ready to go" makes the transfer more efficient for you.

4. ✚ Be certain the medications are labeled correctly.
   Ensures availability and correct administration of medications when the patient arrives at the new facility.

5. **Coordinate the transfer.** Notify the receiving facility of the time to expect the transfer and of any special equipment the patient will need (e.g., IV pole, portable oxygen); notify other hospital departments (e.g., dietary, pharmacy, admitting), primary care provider, and family of the transfer.
   You need to schedule the transfer with the receiving agency so they can plan their work and so you can arrange the transfer at a time that will limit the number of interruptions during the transfer. Other in-house departments must have the transfer data so that services such as meals and physical therapy treatments will be discontinued. The primary care provider and family, of course, need to know where to find the patient.

6. **Just before transfer, make your final quick assessment and sign off your charting** (usually there is a preprinted, standardized discharge form for this purpose).
   It is important to complete documentation in a timely manner, but it is also important to provide the most recent assessment data to the long-term care facility.

7. **Take the patient off the unit and out of the hospital after you are notified** that transportation has arrived (or delegate this task). Alternatively, a transporter may come to your unit to get the patient. (Note: Some agencies ask you to remove the patient's identification band at time of transfer.)
   Keeping the patient on the unit as long as practical helps to minimize his anxiety and fatigue that may occur from a long wait in the hospital lobby.

8. **Give an oral report** to the nurse at the long-term care facility. You will usually give a telephone report unless a nurse comes to your hospital to accompany the patient. The report should include, as appropriate for the care, treatment, and services provided, the following:
   a. The reason the patient is being transferred
   b. The patient's physical and psychosocial status
   c. A summary of care, treatment, and services provided and progress toward outcomes
   d. Referrals, community resources provided to the patient

   A report helps ensure continuity of care and provide a baseline for later changes in the patient's health status.

- ✚ It is best to consistently use a structured framework or memory aid to guide the handoff process and the oral report.
  The objective of a handoff report is to provide accurate information about the patient. The information communicated must be accurate in order to ensure patient safety.

- ✚ Notify the long-term care agency if the patient is colonized or infected with methicillin-resistant *Staphylococcus aureus* (MRSA) or other contagious microorganisms.
  So they can arrange for and communicate any special isolation or care activities to their staff. MRSA is a serious problem for long-term care residents.

- ✚ If the patient is taking corticosteroids, anticoagulants, diabetic medications, antibiotics, and/or narcotic analgesics, be sure to point out to the nurse
  These medications confer particularly high risk of adverse postdischarge drug events, and the long-term-care nurses will need to continue careful monitoring.

What if. . .

- **The patient has intravenous (IV) lines and other equipment that cannot be turned off?**

  It is common to transfer patients with IV lines. Some wheelchairs are equipped with an IV pole, or you may need to hold the IV bag while taking the patient to the transporting vehicle. If so, always hold the bag well above the patient's chest and arm so that blood does not back up in the tubing. Also, you should notify the long-term care facility so they will have the necessary equipment in the transport vehicle. Portable oxygen and suction are also available for patients who must have them. Usually the receiving facility will bring these, but you need to coordinate that in advance.

- ✚ **When you are ready to transfer the patient, her condition worsens and she becomes unstable?**

  Perform interventions to stabilize the patient, call for help if needed, and notify the medical provider. Notify the transporter and the long-term care center of the change and postpone the transfer until further medical assessment is done.

Evaluation

The receiving nurse at the long-term care facility will evaluate the patient's response to the move.

Documentation

- Just before the transfer, document your final assessment and complete the agency's discharge summary.
- You will probably put your final nursing note on a transfer or discharge summary, similar to the ones shown in the Forms section in this chapter of Volume 2.

Practice Resources

The Joint Commission (2012a); McFetridge, B., Gillespie, M., Goode, D., et al. (2007); Riesenberg, L. A., Leisch, J., & Cunningham, J. M. (2010).

Procedure 11-4 ■ Discharging a Patient From the Healthcare Facility

➤ For steps to follow in *all* procedures, refer to the Universal Steps for All Procedures found on the inside back cover.

Equipment

- Medical record or chart
- Patient's medications
- Supplies for any ongoing treatments
- Patient's belongings, clothes, and personal care articles
- Standardized discharge form, if available, with instructions for patient
- A utility cart, if belongings are numerous
- Wheelchair

Delegation

If the patient's condition allows, you can delegate to the NAP such tasks as packing belongings, helping the patient dress, and taking the patient out of the facility. However, as the nurse, you are responsible for obtaining and completing the necessary records, making the final assessment, gathering and checking the medications, and coordinating care.

Pre-Procedure Assessment

- Make a final, brief focused physical assessment.
- Assess the patient's mobility.
- Assess for emotional and/or physical distress.
- Assess the patient's ability to communicate and understand what is occurring.

➤ When performing the procedure, always identify your patient according to agency policy and be attentive to standard precautions, hand hygiene, patient safety and privacy, body mechanics, and documentation.

Procedure Steps

1. **Notify the patient and family** as much in advance of the discharge as possible. This is often done early in the hospital stay.
   Allows them time to adjust emotionally and to make any necessary plans.

A Day or Two Before Discharge (Steps 2 and 3)

2. **Make or confirm necessary arrangements.**
   a. Arrange for or help the family arrange for services (e.g., home healthcare, physical therapy, intravenous therapy, social worker) that will be needed at home.
   NOTE: To reimburse for home care, insurers require a physician's order for all services, and the patient must meet certain eligibility criteria.
   b. Confirm or arrange for equipment needed in the home (e.g., portable oxygen).
   c. Confirm or arrange for transportation.
   d. Make necessary referrals (e.g., medical specialists, physical therapists); book appointments, if necessary and if in line with agency policy.
   Hospital stays are short, and many patients are still ill enough to require complex treatments and care by family members when they go home.
3. Communicate and provide teaching to the patient and caregivers.
   Patients who have a clear understanding of their after-hospital care (e.g., medications, follow-up visits) are 30% less likely to visit the emergency department or be readmitted than patients who lack this information (Agency for Healthcare Research and Quality [AHRQ], 2009).
   a. Discuss the patient's diagnosis, care needs, and functional abilities with the family/caregiver.
   b. Train the patient and caregiver in the use of equipment. Arrange for follow-up evaluation at home to check that equipment is working and being used correctly, and that further training is given if needed.
   In the stress of illness and the disruption of transition home, patients may not retain what they are taught in the hospital. Therapies will be ineffective if equipment

(continued on next page)

Procedure 11-4 ■ Discharging a Patient From the Healthcare Facility (continued)

is used incorrectly, so follow-up is essential to help avoid further illness and hospital readmission.

c. Educate about medication use and side effects.

Medication errors at home are a frequent cause of adverse events and readmissions to the hospital.

d. Ask relatives or the caregiver to bring clothing for the patient to wear home, if needed.

If this was an unplanned admission, the patient may have come in nightwear and a robe.

Day of Discharge (Steps 4 Through 16)

4. **Make and document final assessments.**
   a. Assess that the patient's condition remains as expected.
   b. Confirm that the patient has house keys, heating is turned on, and food is available.
   c. Follow up on diagnostic and laboratory test results.

5. **Bring a wheelchair or other transport** device to the bedside.

6. **Make final notifications.**
   a. Contact the family or guardian; confirm transportation.
   b. Notify community service agencies and home health nursing of the discharge, as needed.

7. **Gather prescriptions and instruction sheets**, including a list of current medications and appointment cards; give to the patient along with the discharge instructions at discharge. **Key Point:** ***Be certain that either the patient or caregiver can read the instructions. Inadequate literacy has been shown to be a risk factor for readmission.***

8. **Gather and pack the patient's personal items** and treatment supplies.

   Having the supplies and equipment ready to go makes the transfer more efficient for you and less stressful for the patient and family.

9. **Prepare the patient's medications.** Be certain the medications are labeled correctly; pack them; and record which medications he is taking home.

   Ensures availability and correct administration of medications when the patient arrives home. Provides a legal record that the patient left with the medications.

10. **Review discharge instructions** with patient and caregiver (and provide a written copy to take home): Review:
    a. Medication instructions
    b. Symptom management and treatments
    c. When and with which care provider the follow-up appointment(s) takes place
    d. How to obtain further care, treatment, and services, as needed
    e. How and when to call the physician or primary care provider, including signs of a change in condition
    f. Whom to contact in an emergency
    g. Diet restrictions
    h. Maintenance of hydration
    i. Activities of daily living, focusing on safety and mobility

    Teaching should occur throughout the hospital stay. However, it is important to reinforce with a last-minute summary and written instructions to take home. With the stress of illness and anticipation of discharge, patients may not retain what they are taught.

11. **Address any questions or concerns** of the patient and caregiver.

    To ensure the ability to safely transition to home.

12. **Give new prescriptions and reminder cards** (e.g., for appointments with physicians, social services) to the patient.

    Ensures continuity of care, thus minimizing patient stress.

13. **Document your final nursing note and complete the discharge summary** (the patient often receives a copy of the summary). The patient needs a copy of (1) his instructions for care at home, which may be called a discharge plan, and (2) his discharge summary, a summary of the progress of his illness and treatment from admission through discharge. Some agencies combine these into one form.

    It is important to document the patient's condition at the time he leaves the unit. This provides a baseline for comparison if his condition should deteriorate after discharge.

14. **Accompany the patient off the unit** and out of the hospital (or delegate this task) when you are notified that transportation has arrived.

    Keeping the patient on the unit as long as practical helps to minimize the anxiety and fatigue that may occur from a long wait in the hospital lobby while a family member brings a car to the door.

15. **Notify the admissions department** of the discharge. Depending on agency policy, notify the primary care or admitting physician.

    This will stop all scheduled services, such as meals, and notify the housekeeping department that the room needs to be cleaned.

16. **Ensure the patient's records are sent** to the medical records department.

    Whether paper or electronic, the chart is a legal document and remains permanently in storage in the medical records department.

What if. . .

■ **Near the time of discharge, the patient's condition worsens and he becomes unstable?**

Perform interventions to stabilize the patient, call for help if needed, and notify the provider. Notify the family that discharge will be delayed.

Communicate with other hospital departments and community agencies as necessary.

- **The patient is an older adult?**
  - Allow for more time to dress and leave the hospital.
  - Allow for more time to communicate, teach, and answer questions.
  - Obtain feedback to be certain the caregivers have heard and understood instructions.
  - Consider having a geriatric nurse specialist make follow-up home visits.

  Hearing, visual, and mobility deficits become more common with advanced age.

- **The patient is taking "high-risk" drugs postdischarge?**

  Medications with a high risk of postdischarge adverse events include corticosteroids, anticoagulants, diabetic medications, antibiotics, antianxiety agents, sedatives, and narcotic analgesics.
  - Provide teaching for patient, family, and other caregivers throughout the hospital stay. A day or two before discharge, review teaching with patient and family; evaluate their understanding.
  - On discharge, summarize medication precautions and provide clear written instructions. Be sure the patient and family can read them.

Evaluation

A few weeks after discharge, the facility will contact the patient to evaluate the quality and appropriateness of the discharge process. This may be done by making a home visit, telephoning, or sending a questionnaire. As a nurse, you may or may not be involved in this evaluation. The best evaluation of the multidisciplinary care will be whether the patient must be readmitted to the acute care facility.

Documentation

- For the medical record, the primary provider will write a discharge progress note that contains the following information:

  Reason for hospitalization

  Significant findings during the stay, including significant changes in status since admission

  Procedures performed; care, treatment, and services provided during the stay

  Status of goals for the stay

  Condition at discharge
- Agency policy determines the format and content of nursing documentation. This is often a combination of a structured discharge form or checklist and a narrative progress note. Regardless of format, you should document the following information:
  - Your final assessment of the patient's health status
  - Information and teaching provided to the patient and caregivers
  - Referrals, medications
  - How patient left the unit (e.g., in wheelchair) and who accompanied him (e.g., wife, name of staff member)

The Joint Commission recommends standardized formats for documentation (2008, p. 367).

To see examples of discharge summaries,

Go to Forms, later in this chapter.

Practice Resources

AHRQ (2009); Closson, B., Mattingly, L., Finne, K., et al. (2012).; Greenwald, J. L., Denham, C. R., & Jack, B. W. (2007); The Joint Commission (2008, 2012a); Lim, F., Foust, J., & VanCleave, J. (2011); Naylor, M., Brooten, D., Jones, B., et al. (1994); Phillips, C. O., Wright, W. M., Kern, D. E., et al. (2004); U.S. Department of Health and Human Services (2007).

CLINICAL INSIGHTS

Clinical Insight 11-1 ➤ Preparing the Room for a Newly Admitted Patient

Delegation

As a general rule, these tasks can be delegated to NAPs. The nurse is responsible for evaluating and supervising, as well as for setting up special equipment (although the NAP may obtain it from storage).

Clean the Room

Agencies differ; however, it is common for the housekeeping department to clean the room and change the bed linens when a patient is discharged, so you should find the room ready for your preparations. The rest of these guidelines assume that fact.

Prepare the Bed

- Position the bed according to patient status. If the patient is ambulatory, put the bed in the lowest position and lock the wheels. If the patient will arrive on a stretcher, place the bed at stretcher height.
- If necessary, rearrange the furniture to allow easy access to the bed.
- Fold back the top linens to "open" the bed (see the figure).
- The patient may need to go to bed immediately, so it should be ready when she arrives.

Prepare Routine Supplies

- Most agencies have an admission pack containing a bath basin, soap, lotion, tissues, water pitcher, and drinking glass. Open it and put it in the room.
- Place a hospital gown on the bed and nonslip footware by the bedside. Patients may choose to wear their own sleep clothing, though.

Prepare Equipment

You will need:

- A stethoscope, thermometer, and blood pressure cuff in the room for taking vital signs
- A scale for measuring and weighing the patient
- Bedpan and urinal if the patient is not ambulatory; possibly a bedside commode
- A clean-catch urine specimen container if laboratory work has not already been done
- Set up and check special equipment (e.g., oxygen, suction, cardiac monitor, pulse oximeter, IV pump).

Prepare the Environment

Turn on the lights, adjust the room temperature. Open or close curtains, as needed.

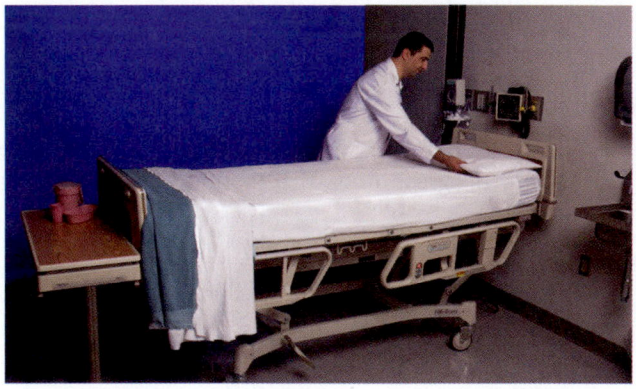

FORMS

The forms in this section are copies that are put into the patient's permanent record in paper form. Many agencies have computer-based discharge processes, however.

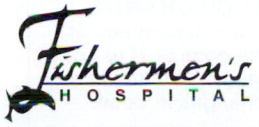

Discharge Assessment/Instructions

Date of Discharge	Time of Discharge	Mode of Discharge ☐ Ambulatory ☐ Wheelchair ☐ Stretcher ☐ Ambulance	Accompanied by:
Belongings sent with patient/family ☐ Yes ☐ No		Personal Medications sent with patient family ☐ Yes ☐ No	
Temp	P	Discharge Destination	Transfer Information Sent
R	BP	☐ Home ☐ AMA ☐ Facility_____ ☐ Home Health	☐ Yes ☐ No
Special Instructions			

Patient Assessment and Health Status

	Yes	No		Yes	No		Yes	No
Afebrile	☐	☐	Skin Intact	☐	☐	Hygiene	☐	☐
Able to live independently	☐	☐	Eating Well	☐	☐	Self-Care	☐	☐
Pain Controlled	☐	☐	Adequate Hydration	☐	☐	Assist	☐	☐
Oriented	☐	☐				Total Care	☐	☐
Appropriate Behavior	☐	☐				Adequate Elimination	☐	☐
Functions Independently	☐	☐						

Additional Comments:

Weight monitoring daily **Avoid all tobacco products**

Instructions

Diet
☐ No Restrictions

Activity
☐ No Restrictions

Special Equipment/Treatment
☐ No Restrictions

Discharge Medications (Name, Amount, Special Instructions)
☐ No Meds See Patient Education

Special Instructions/Discharge Summary
Call MD or go to the ER if symptoms worsen

☐ Pt or Caregiver given instructions about and counseled on potential for drug-food interactions

Physician Follow-up Appointment	Outpatient Visit

Referral
☐ None Required

I have received all personal belongings.
I have received a copy and understand the above Instructions.
I have received a copy of the Patient Education form.

Patient Identification

Signature/Responsible Party

Physician/Nurse Signature **Date**

0916065

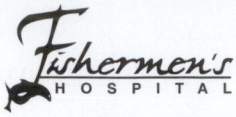

3301 Overseas Highway, Marathon, FL 33050 • Ph 305-743-5533 • Fax 305-743-3962

Allergies/Reactions	No known drug allergies ❑	IN-PATIENT Circle Y to continue or N to not continue and sign below to authenticate order.	AT DISCHARGE Circle Y to continue at same dose or N to not continue or document any changes in dose.

MEDICATION NAME (Include Herbal, OTC, Vitamins)	Dose / Route / Freq	Reason Taken	LAST DOSE DATE/TIME	Continue on Admission		Continue at home on same dose		Continue with the following changes:
Patient takes no medication ❑								
				Y	N	Y	N	
				Y	N	Y	N	
				Y	N	Y	N	
				Y	N	Y	N	
				Y	N	Y	N	
				Y	N	Y	N	
				Y	N	Y	N	
				Y	N	Y	N	
				Y	N	Y	N	
				Y	N	Y	N	
				Y	N	Y	N	
				Y	N	Y	N	
				Y	N	Y	N	
				Y	N	Y	N	

Source-of-Medication list *(check all used)*:

___ Bottles/List
___ Patient/Family
___ Retail pharmacy_____
_____
___ MD office records
___ Previous discharge medical record
___ Medication Administration Record from_____
_____
___ Med Reconciliation Form

Meds:
___ Sent home with_____
___ Removed
Sent to Pharmacy for approval

New medications prescribed for patient discharge:

Meds	Dose / Route / Freq	Reason

ADMITTING NURSE SIGNATURE DATE

DISCHARGE NURSE SIGNATURE DATE

Patient Education Form

Page ____ of ____

FORM N-100, Rev. 12-07 White: Chart Yellow: Patient

CLINICALREASONING

Applying the Full-Spectrum Nursing Model

PATIENT SITUATION

Recall Evelyn (Meet Your Patient). She is 87 years old and has lived in a nursing home for the past 5 years. She suffers from congestive heart failure (CHF), hypertension, diabetes, macular degeneration resulting in near blindness, a severe hearing deficit, urinary incontinence, and immobility resulting from a hip fracture. Despite these limitations, she keeps current in the lives of all of her family members and friends. At the nursing home, staff members confide in Evelyn and she knows about their children, their romances, and the gossip around the nursing home. Whenever there is an election, she makes sure that she gets to vote. She "reads" every audio book she can get her hands on.

Recently Evelyn was admitted to the hospital in severe CHF. When leaving the nursing home, she told her pastor, "I don't want to die yet. I'm having too much fun!" You notice that the papers from the nursing home do not contain an advance directive, and it was not mentioned in their report to you.

THINKING

1. *Critical Thinking (Considering Alternatives):*
   a. What are some possible reasons that there is no advance directive?
   b. Which of those seems most likely to you?
   c. How might you find out about the status of Evelyn's advance directive?

DOING

2. *Nursing Process (Nursing Diagnosis):* On the care plan from the nursing home, there were two nursing diagnoses:
   - Urge Urinary Incontinence related to difficulty ambulating to bathroom
   - Impaired Skin Integrity related to immobility and incontinence

   Which of these can you remove from the care plan for now? Explain your decision.

CARING

3. *Self-Knowledge:* The next day, despite aggressive treatment, Evelyn's condition worsens. She is not responding to verbal stimuli and her oxygen level is decreasing. There is discussion about putting her on a ventilator.
   a. What would you be feeling?
   b. If Evelyn has an advance directive that says "no ventilator," how would that change your feelings?
   c. If there is an advance directive that says "do everything possible to keep me alive," how would that change your feelings?

   Note: We are not asking you what you would do; rather, you should consider how you would feel.

Critical Thinking and Clinical Reasoning

1. Describe your personal view of health.
2. Identify an individual in your life, personally or professionally, who personifies health. What characteristics do you identify in this individual that represent health? What factors do you think contribute to this individual's health status?
3. Use the nursing process to develop a plan to improve your personal health.
4. What attributes, resources, or life experiences do you have as an individual to offer in your role as a nurse?
5. For each of the following concepts, use critical thinking to describe how or why it is important to nursing, patient care, or experiencing health and illness. Note that these are *not* to be merely definitions.

Health	Hardiness
Wellness	Responses to illness
Illness	Health–illness continuum
Disruptions	

What Are the Main Points in This Chapter?

- Health is a complex phenomenon that involves physical, mental, and spiritual aspects. Having good health is an almost universal desire.
- Wellness is a way of life oriented toward optimal health and well-being.
- Life and wellness require nourishment. Nourishment comes in the form of food, exercise, sleep, relationships, meaningful work, the environment, and memories.
- The person with an illness rarely perceives the experience as a medical diagnosis. Instead, illness is usually described in terms of how it makes the person feel, such as pain, sadness, loss, fatigue, or being overwhelmed.
- People dealing with life-threatening illness have to figure out how to live and still be dying. Dealing with death is one of the most difficult experiences you will face as a nurse.
- One aspect of persevering in illness and life disruption is maintaining as much normalcy as possible. Normalcy helps clients cope with illness.
- Nurses deal with people who have been thrust into new life situations, situations they did not ask for and for which they were not prepared.
- People who are suffering experience loneliness. Part of aloneness can be related to the actual physical separation, part of it from a sense of the world going on without them, and part of it from a sense of no one really being in their world.
- Several factors influence a person's responses to disruptions. These factors include age; family patterns; culture; hardiness; support; access to healthcare resources; the stage and nature of the illness; and the intensity, duration, and multiplicity of the disruption.
- Chronic illnesses are a large and growing healthcare concern, especially among older adults.
- The top three risks for functional decline are cognitive impairment, depression, and disease burden.
- You can ease patients' disruptions experienced during admission, transfers, and discharge from a healthcare setting by discharge planning, communication, coordination, and teaching.
- As a nurse, you will need to cultivate a healing presence. Listening, being attentive, being willing to learn from those in your care, and recognizing and respecting others' ways of coping are behaviors associated with a healing presence.
- Most people experience health, illness, and wellness as an ever-changing continuum on which they move.
- Communicating genuine care, concern, and sensitivity comes from who you are as a person, not from assuming a professional persona that you "put on" to fulfill a role.
- Patients and families may not recognize the strengths and creative abilities that they bring to a situation. Part of the art of nursing is to envision strengths and potential in patients and families who may be too overwhelmed to identify them on their own.
- Your healing presence may be the most memorable aspect of nursing care that you have to offer.

Knowledge Map

EXPERIENCING HEALTH & ILLNESS

WELLNESS
- A state of optimal health
- Well-being
- Integration of body, mind, and spirit
- Influenced by attitude and lifestyle choices

HEALTH
- Perfect body
- Absence of illness/disease
- Something one can buy
- Ideal state of physical and mental well-being
- Power of the soul to cope with varying body conditions

ILLNESS
- To some, a disease
- Response to a disruption in health
- A lived experience
- Unique to each individual
- Not a medical diagnosis

CONCEPTUAL MODELS:
- Health–illness Continuum
- Dunn's Health Grid
- Neuman's Continuum

FACTORS THAT INFLUENCE HEALTH
- Genetics; gender; age; developmental stage
- Nutrition
- Activity level
- Quantity/quality of sleep/rest
- Meaningful work
- Lifestyle choices
- Family relationships
- Culture
- Spirituality
- Environment
- Finances
- Hardiness

FACTORS THAT DISRUPT HEALTH
- Physical disease
- Injury
- Mental illness
- Pain
- Loss
- Impending death
- Competing demands
- The unknown
- Imbalance
- Isolation

STAGES OF ILLNESS BEHAVIOR
- Experiencing symptoms
- Sick role behavior
- Seeking professional care
- Dependence on others
- Recovery

NATURE OF ILLNESS
- Acute
- Chronic
  - Exacerbation
  - Remission

CHAPTER 12

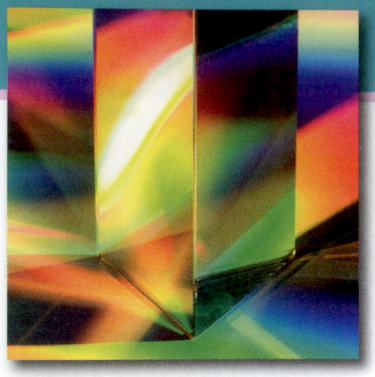

Stress & Adaptation

STUDENT RESOURCES

*The questions and exercises in Volume 2 allow you to practice the kind of thinking you will use as a full-spectrum nurse. Critical-thinking questions usually have more than one correct answer, so we do not provide "answers" for these features. It is more important to develop your nursing judgment than to just cover content. You will learn by discussing the questions with your peers. If you are still unsure, consult your instructor. You will find Response Sheets (for writing your responses to the questions) on Davis*Plus.

To explore learning resources for this chapter,

Go to Davis*Plus* at DavisPl.us/Wilkinson3.

Chapter Resources for Chapter 12:

- **Response sheets for all learning activities**
- **Resources for Caregivers and Health Professionals**
- **Reading More About Stress & Adaptation (suggested readings)**
- **Concept Map of chapter content**

Interactive Case Studies

NCLEX-Style and Chapter Review Questions

CHAPTER OVERVIEW

For a podcast of an overview of this chapter,

Go to Student Resources: Chapter 12, **Podcast—Chapter Overview,** on Davis*Plus*.

Caring for the Nguyens

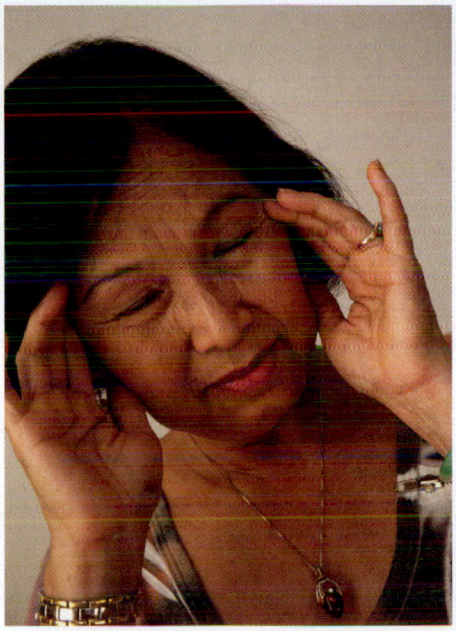

After having a comprehensive physical exam at the family health center, Yen Nguyen has been scheduled to have a mammogram and screening laboratory work. When she arrives at the clinic for her mammogram, she tells you she is very nervous. "I have a good friend who just found out she has breast cancer. She's very depressed now. Do I really have to do this test?"

A. What kind of stress is Yen experiencing?

B. Three days later, the radiologist contacts Yen requesting that she return to the family health center for additional films of the upper outer quadrant of the right breast. "There are some calcifications I want to check out," explains the radiologist.

- What factors might affect Yen's adaptation to this stress?
- Evaluate what you know about Yen's perception of her stress, her overall health status, her support system, and her coping methods. What more do you need to know about these topics to fully answer this question?

C. Later, Yen calls the office frantically explaining that she is very upset about this recent event. She says, "Not knowing is killing me. I'm so nervous I can't stand it. I can't sleep. I can't eat." She asks how she can handle the stress until she comes in for the additional tests next week. What strategies would you recommend to help Yen deal with the stress?

Practical Knowledge knowing how

CLINICAL INSIGHTS

Clinical Insight 12-1 ➤ Dealing With Angry Patients

- ***Be aware of how you are responding to angry patients.*** Are you relieving your own stress, or are you relieving the client's stress? If you respond angrily to relieve your own stress, you may provoke further anger in the patient and even escalate the situation to the point of violence.
- ***Keep reminding yourself not to take anger personally;*** remind family members of this as well.
- ***Recognize that anger and anxiety are normal feelings*** when facing adversity, such as a life-threatening or debilitating illness. Do not discount feelings by saying something like, "Please, don't be so angry," or "You shouldn't talk like that." Or, "Everything will be OK. Don't worry."
- ***Encourage the client and family to express feelings*** verbally and appropriately.
- ***Listen instead of defending.*** If the patient yells, "Everything about this place stinks," don't respond with something like, "This hospital is highly rated by The Joint Commission," or, "We really are all trying to do the best we can for you." Instead, say something to encourage the person to express his feelings or give you more information: "You seem really angry; what's going on?" or "Maybe I can help. Tell me a little more about what stinks."
- ***Do not take responsibility for the patient's anger.*** It is not your fault, so don't apologize (unless you really *do* have

(Continued)

Clinical Insight 12-1 ➤ Dealing With Angry Patients *(continued)*

something to apologize for). In the preceding example, for instance, it is not your fault that "the place stinks" or that the patient feels that way. So do *not* say, "I'm sorry we haven't been meeting your expectations."

- ***Remain calm;*** this reassures the patient.
- ***Help the patient identify what is causing the anger*** and try to meet those needs.
- ***Be alert to your own and to the patient's safety needs.***
  - If the person seems violent, do not allow him to get between you and the door.
  - Be sure you know how to call for help from staff or security personnel if you think you or someone else is in danger.
  - Do not wear a stethoscope around your neck, dangling jewelry, or anything a patient might use to hurt you.
  - Do not go into a room alone with an angry patient who seems to have a potential for violence.
  - Remain at least an arm's length away from an angry and potentially violent patient.
  - Do not turn your back on an angry patient.
- ***If you believe the patient's anger may escalate to violence, your priority is your own safety and the safety of others in the area.***

In addition to the above, if you want more information,

Go to Chapter 24, **Box 24-8,** in Volume 1.

Also refer to the NIC intervention, Anger Control Assistance (Bulechek, Butcher, & Dochterman, 2013, pp. 81—82).

Clinical Insight 12-2 ➤ Crisis Intervention Guidelines

For nurses who are at an entry level of practice, the goals of crisis intervention include the following (Brammer & MacDonald, 2003; Neeb, 2006):

1. Assess the situation.

What is the nature of the patient's condition and the severity of the crisis?

2. Ensure safety.

- Call for help if you or the patient is in physical danger.
- Do not leave the patient unless you think you are in imminent danger.
- First ensure your own safety; then provide for the patient's safety.

3. Defuse the situation.

- Keep in mind that a person in crisis may not be in control of his actions.
- Try to calm the person verbally.
- Attempt physical restraint only as a last resort and only when there is enough help to do it safely for both the staff and the patient.

4. Decrease the person's anxiety.

- Reassure the person that he is in a safe place and that you are concerned and want to help.
- Explain gently but firmly that you need his help and cooperation.
- Help the person to vent feelings of fear, guilt, and anger.
- Use physical contact very cautiously. The person in turmoil may interpret touch as aggression or a sexual approach.

5. Determine the problem.

- Find out what the patient believes to be the cause of the crisis.
- Remain calm, and do not pressure the patient to give reasons. Any tension on your part will create further panic in the patient.

6. Decide on the type of help needed.

- You may be able to calm the person enough for him to understand what just happened, or you may not. Evaluate your ability to calm the patient based on your assessment of his coping skills and resources.
- Put in place the help needed to restore the person to a minimal level of functioning. This may require long-term treatment. In that case, make the referrals.

7. Return the person to his precrisis level of functioning. This may involve crisis counseling and/or home crisis visits.

- The goal of crisis counseling is to provide immediate relief, solve the most urgent problems, and give long-term counseling if needed. Crisis centers often rely on telephone counseling ("hotlines").
- If telephone counseling is not adequate or if observations of the home environment are needed, home visits may be necessary.

ASSESSMENT GUIDELINES AND TOOLS

Focused Assessment

The Holmes–Rahe Social Readjustment Scale

This is a way to check your stress level, measured in "life change units." Of course it is not possible to score the exact "amount" of stress. However, this will give you a general idea of your stress level and should provide some insight about the sources of your stress. The following are based on the number of life change units over a 1- to 2-year period:

Over 300 points (Major amount of change): 80% chance of major illness

200–299 (Moderate amount of change): 50% chance of major illness

150–199 (Mild amount of change): 33% chance of major illness

0–149 (Insignificant amount of change): Minimal chance of major illness

Of course, your personality and your ability to cope also determine the likelihood of your becoming ill.

Life Event	Life Change Units	Life Event	Life Change Units
Death of spouse	100	Son or daughter leaving home	29
Divorce	73	Trouble with in-laws	29
Marital separation	65	Outstanding personal achievement	28
Imprisonment	63	Spouse begins or stops work	26
Death of a close family member	63	Begin or end school	26
Personal injury or illness	53	Change in living conditions	25
Marriage	50	Revision of personal habits	24
Dismissal from work	47	Trouble with boss	23
Marital reconciliation	45	Change in work hours or conditions	20
Retirement	45	Change in residence	20
Change in health of family member	44	Change in schools	20
Pregnancy	40	Change in recreation	19
Sexual difficulties	39	Change in church activities	19
Gain of new family member	39	Change in social activities	18
Business readjustment	39	Minor mortgage or loan	17
Change in financial state	38	Change in sleeping habits	16
Change in number of arguments with spouse	35	Change in number of family reunions	15
Major mortgage	32	Change in eating habits	15
Foreclosure of mortgage or loan	30	Vacation	13
Change in responsibilities at work	29		

Source: Reprinted from Holmes, T., & Rahe, R. (1967). Social readjustment rating scale. *Journal of Psychosomatic Research, 11*(2), 213–218. Reprinted with permission from Elsevier.

Focused Assessment

Assessing for Stress: Questions to Ask

1. **Assess stressors and risk factors.** Ask the client to complete a stress inventory, such as the preceding Holmes-Rahe Social Readjustment Scale. Then ask the client the following questions:
   - What is causing the most stress in your life?
   - On a scale of 1 to 10 (where 1 is "not much" and 10 is "extreme"), rate the stress you are experiencing in each of these areas: work or school, finances, community responsibilities, your health, health of a family member, family relationships, family responsibilities, relationships with friends.
   - How long have you been dealing with the stressful situation(s)?
   - Can you track the accumulation of stress in your life?
   - How long have you been under this stress?
   - Note the client's developmental stage, and determine whether he is functioning as expected for this stage. Review Chapter 9 if you need help to identify developmental milestones. To help you assess for stressors that can be predicted to occur in each stage, you might ask questions such as:

     What challenges do you face as a result of your life and your age?

     Have you had recent life changes?

     Do you anticipate any life changes?

To review developmental stage changes,

Go to **Chapters 9 and 10,** in Volume 1. Also see Chapter 12, **Box 12-1: Stressors Throughout the Life Span,** in Volume 1.

2. **Assess coping methods and adaptation.**
   - What coping strategies have you used previously? What was successful, and what was not successful?
   - Tell me about previous experiences you have had with stressful situations in your life.
   - What do you usually do to handle stressful situations? (If the client needs prompting, you can ask, "Do you cry, get angry, avoid people, talk to family or friends, do physical exercise, pray? Some people laugh or joke, others meditate, others try to control everything, others just work hard and look for a solution. What is your usual response?")
   - How well do these methods usually work for you?
   - What have you been doing to cope with the present situation?
   - How well is that working?
   - During the interview, you should also observe for the use of psychological defense mechanisms.

To review psychological defense mechanisms,

Go to Chapter 12, **Table 12-1: Psychological Defense Mechanisms,** in Volume 1.

   - If the patient has not exhibited any defense mechanisms, you could ask about the common ones. For example, "Do you ever cope with a situation by denying it exists or just by trying to put it out of your mind?"
   - Also ask the client about physiological changes and diseases caused by ongoing stress. Check the client's records for a history of somatoform disorders. Ask the client:

     What physical illnesses do you have? How long have you had them?

     What, if any, physical changes have you noticed?

     Do you have other physical conditions, for example, hypertension, cardiac disease, diabetes, arthritis, joint pains, cancer?

To review findings that might indicate maladaption to stress,

Go to Chapter 12, **Table 12-2, Organic Disorders Brought About by Failure of Adaptive Mechanisms,** in Volume 1.

3. **Assess physiological responses to stress.**

   The following are examples of questions you should ask:
   - What do you do to stay healthy?
   - Tell me about your health habits.
   - How often do you have a checkup?
   - What are your health concerns?
4. **Assess emotional and behavioral responses to stress.**

Emotional Responses

Observe for:

- Anger
- Anxiety
- Depression
- Fear
- Feelings of inadequacy
- Low self-esteem
- Irritability
- Lack of motivation
- Lethargy

Behavioral Responses

Observe for:

- Crying, emotional outbursts
- Dependence
- Poor job performance
- Substance use and abuse
- Sleeplessness (or sleeping too much)
- Change in eating habits (e.g., loss of appetite, overeating)
- Decrease in quality of job performance
- Preoccupation (i.e., daydreaming)
- Illnesses
- Increased absenteeism from work or school
- Increased number of accidents
- Avoiding social situations or relationships
- Rebellion, acting out

Examples of Assessment Questions

- Do you smoke?
- How much alcohol do you drink every day?
- What do you eat? What is your typical eating pattern?
- How much fluid do you drink daily?
- How many hours do you sleep at night? Do you feel rested when you wake up?

Focused Assessment

Assessing for Stress: Questions to Ask—cont'd

- Do you often wake up very early in the morning and have difficulty getting back to sleep?
- What prescribed medications, vitamins, over-the-counter medications, or herbs do you take?
- What regular physical activity or exercise do you engage in?
- How much time do you spend at work versus at leisure and play?
- Do you constantly take work home with you? Or think about work almost all the time?
- How do you relax?
- Have you given up activities and relationships you previously enjoyed because you "don't have enough time" or are too tired?
- How do you express anger?
- Do you try to be perfect?
- Would you describe yourself as having the stress-filled lifestyle of a type A personality?
- How often do you find yourself feeling hopeless? Sad?

5. **Assess cognitive responses to stress.**

   Observe for the following responses when you assess other functional areas:

   - Difficulty concentrating
   - Poor judgment
   - Decrease in accuracy (e.g., in counting money)
   - Forgetfulness
   - Decreased problem-solving ability
   - Decreased attention to detail
   - Difficulty learning
   - Narrowing of focus
   - Preoccupation, daydreaming

6. **Assess support systems.**

   Ask the following questions:

   - Tell me about your home. Describe your living environment. (Make a home visit if possible, or contact the case manager or social worker to arrange a home evaluation.)
   - Who are the persons who provide the most support for you? In what ways do they support you?
   - What support is available from family, friends, significant others, community agencies, and clergy that you may not have required until now?
   - Do you have or do you seek spiritual support?
   - How has your stress affected the family?
   - What are your financial resources? What are your financial obligations?

STANDARDIZED LANGUAGE

NANDA-I Nursing Diagnoses Associated With Stress

Physical

Constipation
Deficient Fluid Volume
Delayed Growth and Development
Diarrhea
Disturbed Energy Field
Disturbed Sleep Pattern
Fatigue
Imbalanced Nutrition (can be More Than or Less Than Body Requirements)
Nausea
Pain (e.g., backache)
Risk for Injury
Sleep Deprivation

Behavioral

Decisional Conflict
Impaired Home Maintenance
Impaired Verbal Communication
Ineffective Coping
Ineffective Health Maintenance
Ineffective Self-Health Management
Ineffective Therapeutic Regimen Management
Risk-Prone Health Behavior
Self-Neglect

Cognitive

Acute Confusion
Disturbed Thought Processes
Impaired Memory

Emotional

Anxiety
Defensive Coping
Disturbed Body Image
Disturbed Personal Identity
Fear
Grieving, Complicated
Ineffective Coping
Ineffective Denial
Low Self-Esteem (Chronic or Situational)

Interpersonal Relationships

Caregiver Role Strain
Compromised or Disabled Family Coping
Dysfunctional Family Processes
Impaired Parenting
Impaired Social Interaction
Ineffective Community Coping

(Continued)

NANDA-I Nursing Diagnoses Associated With Stress—cont'd

- Interrupted Family Processes
- Post-Trauma Syndrome
- Relocation Stress Syndrome
- Risk for Compromised Resilience
- Risk for Other-Directed Violence
- Risk for Self-Directed Violence
- Risk for Suicide
- Social Isolation
- Stress Overload

Spiritual Domain

- Hopelessness
- Spiritual Distress
- Impaired Religiosity

Source: Adapted from NANDA International. (2012). *Nursing diagnoses: Definitions & classification 2012–2014.* Ames, IA: Wiley-Blackwell. Used with permission.

Standardized Outcomes and Interventions for Stress-Related Nursing Diagnoses

Examples of NOC Outcomes

- Anxiety Level
- Caregiver Stressors
- Coping
- Decision-Making
- Family Coping
- Family Resiliency
- Nutritional Status
- Psychosocial Adjustment: Life Change
- Rest
- Sleep

NIC Interventions Listed Under "Stress" in the NIC Index

- Anxiety Reduction
- Art Therapy
- Caregiver Support
- Case Management
- Cognitive Restructuring
- Coping Enhancement
- Counseling
- Dementia Management
- Emotional Support
- Relocation Stress Reduction
- Resiliency Promotion
- Sleep Enhancement

Source: Adapted from Bulechek, G. M., Butcher, H. K., & Dochterman, J. M. (2013). *Nursing interventions classification (NIC)* (6th ed.). St. Louis, MO: C.V. Mosby; Moorhead, S., Johnson, M., Maas, M. L., et al. (Eds.). (2013). *Nursing outcomes classification (NOC)* (5th ed.). St. Louis, MO: C.V. Mosby. Used with permission.

CLINICALREASONING

Applying the Full-Spectrum Nursing Model

PATIENT SITUATION

Mrs. Williams is a 76-year-old Indian American woman who was admitted yesterday after suffering a stroke that paralyzed her right side. She has had diabetes and high blood pressure for many years. Since the stroke, she has been unable to speak clearly and becomes frustrated as she attempts to communicate her needs. Her daughter says Mrs. Williams is a proud, independent, and tidy woman who has been living alone since her husband's death last year. Until her stroke, she had been driving her car, cleaning the house, doing her grocery shopping, and maintaining the yard and garden. She wears eyeglasses for reading and driving and has a hearing aid, although she rarely uses it.

THINKING

1. *Theoretical Knowledge:*
   a. What stroke risk factors probably functioned as stressors for Mrs. Williams? (*Hint:* Look up stroke risk factors in a medical-surgical nursing or pathophysiology text, or online.)
   b. What are common stressors for patients who must be hospitalized?
2. *Critical Thinking (Contextual Awareness):*
   c. Now that Mrs. Williams is in the hospital, what new stressors might she have?

DOING

3. *Practical Knowledge:* What might you advise Mrs. Williams's daughter to do to help her mother adapt more comfortably to the stressors in the hospital?
4. *Nursing Process (Diagnosis):* Based on only the data in the scenario, write one actual nursing diagnosis for Mrs. Williams. Do not use potential diagnoses. Remember, the defining characteristics must be present in the scenario. State the data you would need in order to make the diagnosis more descriptive.

CARING

5. *Self-Knowledge:* Imagine yourself in Mrs. Williams's situation.
   a. What is the one thing that would cause you the most stress? Why would that be the most stressful thing?
   b. What is the single most important thing you would want your nurse to do for you?

Go To Chapter 12, **Applying the Full-Spectrum Nursing Model Response Sheet,** on Davis*Plus*.

Critical Thinking and Clinical Reasoning

1. Gloria and her husband, John, (Meet Your Patient, in Volume 1) live in a residential community from which John commutes to work in a nearby city. Gloria runs an accounting business from their home. They have two teenage boys who are active in sports, church activities, Boy Scouts, and the school band. The boys need transportation to activities. Gloria and John teach Sunday school and are Boy Scout leaders. Gloria's mother needs knee replacement surgery and so cannot take care of Gloria's father, who is in the early stage of Alzheimer's disease. In addition to her own home responsibilities, Gloria must go to her parents to prepare meals and to provide care for her parents during the day. Gloria's sister comes at 8:00 p.m. to sleep in the parents' home during the night.
   a. What resources may be available to help Gloria?
   b. What stress-reducing techniques can you suggest to help Gloria?
   c. What may reduce John's stress?
   d. On a scale of 1 to 10 (1 being low and 10 being high), what number will you give to Gloria's stress level?
2. Look again at Gloria and John's situation. Using the following defense mechanisms, create a possible scenario for each. That is, what might Gloria (or John) say and/or do if they use the defense mechanism in this situation? If you need to review ego defense mechanisms,

Go to **Table 12-1,** in Volume 1.

   a. **Avoidance**—unconsciously staying away from events or situations that might open feelings of aggression or anxiety.
   b. **Conversion**—changing emotional conflict into physical symptoms that have no physical basis.
   c. **Denial**—transforming reality by refusing to acknowledge thoughts, feelings, desires, or impulses. This is unconscious; the person is *not* consciously lying.
   d. **Displacement**—"kicking the dog." Transferring emotions, ideas, or wishes from one original object or situation to a substitute inappropriate person or object that is perceived to be less powerful or threatening.
   e. **Reaction formation**—similar to compensation, except the person develops the exact opposite trait. The person is aware of her feelings but acts in ways opposite to what she is really feeling.
3. Mary is a nursing student. She works part-time to maintain health insurance coverage for herself and her children and to earn tuition money for school. She has to do her studying after the children are in bed, so she gets little sleep herself. Her grades are low and do not reflect Mary's true knowledge level. Nursing faculty suggest that Mary seek counseling for exam anxiety and test-taking strategies. Mary realizes she may fail out of nursing school without this counseling, but she does not know how she will fit weekly sessions into her already full schedule.
   a. List Mary's stressors.
   b. *Self-Knowledge*:
      - What life experiences do you have that may help you to understand Mary's situation?
      - How could these same life experiences interfere with your empathy for and understanding of Mary?
      - How much of Mary's story can you identify with as being part of your own experience now?
   c. Which type of intervention do you think would be most helpful to Mary: (1) helping her to change her perception of her stressors, or (2) the health promotion activities discussed in Volume 1? Explain your reasoning.
   d. Before deciding specifically how to help Mary, what data do you still need?
   e. Based on the information you have, what do you think Mary's two most important goals are?
   f. If you discover that Mary's most important goals actually are to (1) provide for her children and (2) succeed in nursing school, how might you use this information to help her?
4. *Self-Knowledge:* In Volume 1, you listed your stressors. Let's assess further.
   a. What are your two (or three) *most* important goals? List them in order of importance.
   b. What support do you have that can help you to achieve each of these goals?

5. *Self-Knowledge and Theoretical Knowledge:* Use the Script for Visualization to lead a partner through a visualization exercise; then reverse roles, and have your partner lead you through it. To see the script,

Go to Chapter 12, **Tables, Boxes, Figures: ESG Box 12-2,** on Davis*Plus*.

   a. Before beginning, what were your thoughts and feelings about the exercise?
   b. After doing the visualization exercise, how did you feel? Did you feel more relaxed?
   c. How do you think your attitudes and perceptions prior to the exercise affected how you felt *after* the exercise?

6. For each of the following concepts, use critical thinking to describe how or why it is important to nursing, patient care, or stress and adaptation. Note that these are *not* to be merely definitions.

Stress
Developmental stressors
Coping strategies
Ego defense mechanisms
Inflammatory response
Somatoform disorders
Relaxation techniques for stress reduction

What Are the Main Points in This Chapter?

- Stress is a disturbance in normal homeostasis caused by internal or external stimuli called stressors.
- Adaptive coping techniques are those that offer healthy choices to the person and reduce the negative effects of stress.
- Approaches to coping include altering the stressor, adapting to the stressor, and avoiding the stressor.
- Whether the outcome of stress is positive (adaptation) or negative (disease) depends on the balance between the strength and duration of the stressors and the effectiveness of the person's coping methods.
- The three stages of Selye's general adaptation syndrome (GAS) are alarm, resistance, and exhaustion. Each stage in the GAS produces different physical or psychological responses.
- In the alarm stage of the GAS, responses are produced primarily by adrenal hormones, epinephrine, mineralocorticoids, and the sympathetic nervous system.
- The exhaustion stage can lead to stress-induced illness, burnout, or death.
- The two most common responses of the local adaptation syndrome (LAS) are the reflex pain response and the inflammatory response.
- Examples of psychological responses are anxiety, fear, anger, and ego defense mechanisms.
- Ego defense mechanisms are unconscious mental mechanisms that help to decrease the inner tension associated with stressors; when overused, they are maladaptive.
- Unsuccessful adaptation can lead to crisis, organic disease (e.g., stomach ulcers), somatoform disorders (e.g., hypochondriasis), and psychological disorders (e.g., mental illness).
- Crisis exists when (1) an event in a person's life drastically changes his or her routine and is perceived as a threat to self, and (2) the person's usual coping methods are ineffective, resulting in high anxiety and reduced ability to function.
- Burnout occurs when nurses or other professionals cannot cope effectively with the demands of the workplace.
- You should assess for data about the patient's stressors, risk factors, coping and adaptation, support systems, and psychosocial and physiological responses to stress.
- Interventions for stress must be individualized to the patient. They include (1) health promotion activities for preventing and improving the ability to cope with stressors; (2) managing anxiety, fear, and anger; (3) stress management techniques that focus on discharging tension or producing relaxation; (4) techniques to alter perception (i.e., cognitive restructuring and positive self-talk); (5) identifying and using support systems; (6) reducing the stress of hospitalization; (7) providing spiritual support; (8) crisis intervention; (9) stress management in the workplace; and (10) making referrals.

Knowledge Map

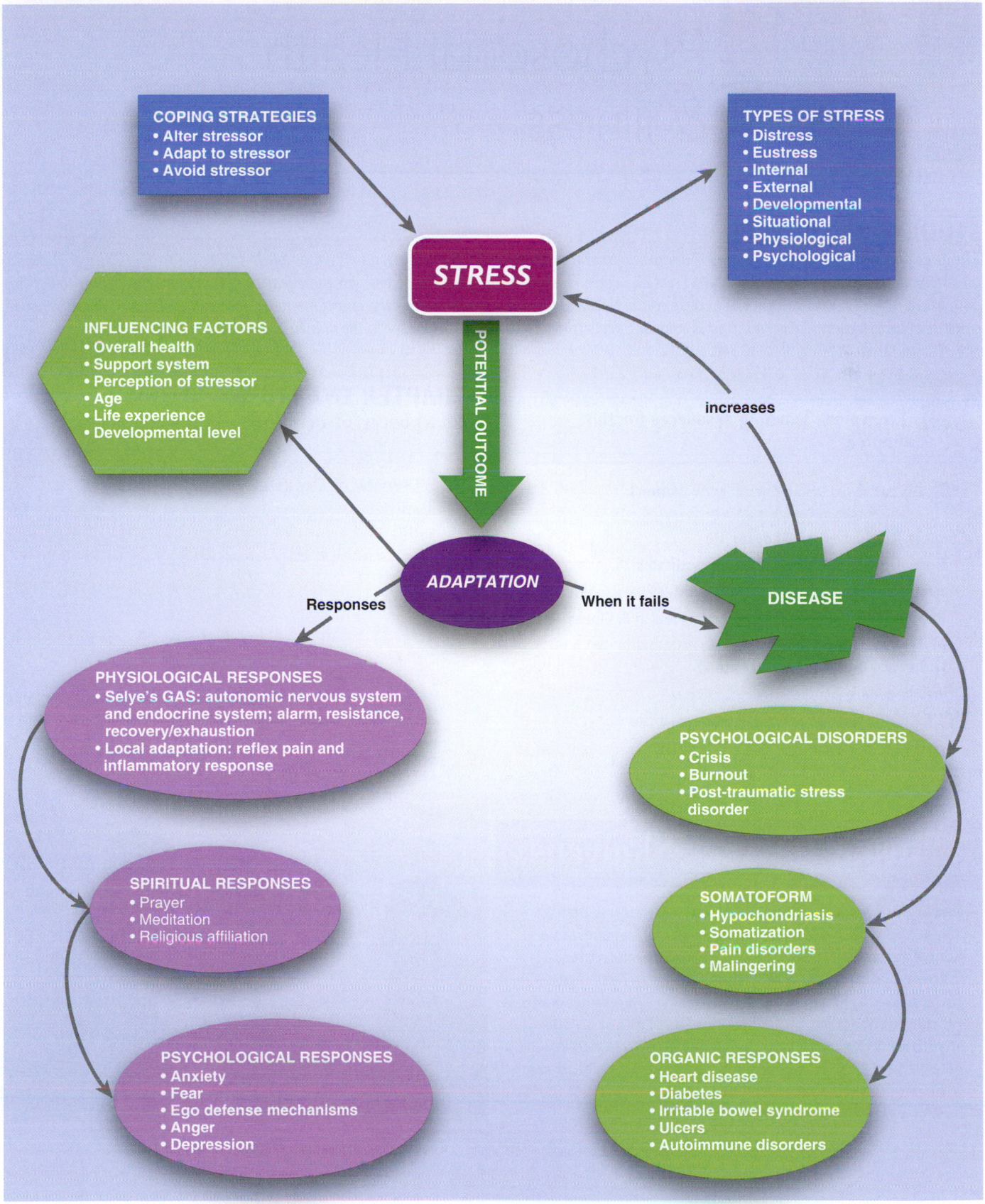

CHAPTER 13

Psychosocial Health & Illness

STUDENT RESOURCES

The questions and exercises in Volume 2 allow you to practice the kind of thinking you will use as a full-spectrum nurse. Critical-thinking questions usually have more than one correct answer, so we do not provide "answers" for these features. It is more important to develop your nursing judgment than to just cover content. You will learn by discussing the questions with your peers. If you are still unsure, consult your instructor. You will find Response Sheets (for writing your responses to the questions) on DavisPlus.

To explore learning resources for this chapter,

Go to Davis*Plus* at DavisPl.us/Wilkinson3.

Chapter Resources for Chapter 13:

- **Response sheets for all learning activities**
- **Resources for Caregivers and Health Professionals**
- **Reading More About Psychosocial Health & Illness (suggested readings)**
- **Concept Map of chapter content**

Interactive Case Studies

NCLEX-Style and Chapter Review Questions

CHAPTER OVERVIEW

For a podcast of an overview of this chapter,

Go to Student Resources: Chapter 13, **Podcast—Chapter Overview,** on Davis*Plus*.

Caring for the Nguyens

Recall the case of Nam Nguyen. Mr. Nguyen has been diagnosed with hypertension, obesity, and degenerative joint disease (DJD). At clinic visits he has made the following comments: "Every time I come in here, I get some new diagnosis. I guess it's amazing I'm not dead yet. I thought I had a lot more time left, but I'm not so sure anymore." When you ask him what his main concerns are, he tells you, "Just take a look at me! I'm a mess. Nothing is turning out the way I planned. I might as well just die now. It would save my family a lot of grief."

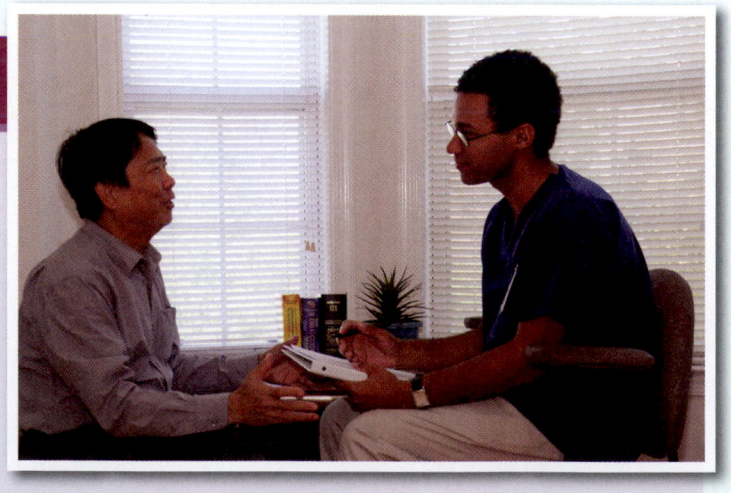

Caring for the Nguyens (continued)

A. What information do you need in order to respond to Mr. Nguyen?

B. How should you respond to Mr. Nguyen?

C. What actions should you take?

D. What conclusions can you make about Mr. Nguyen's self-concept (body image, role performance, personal identity, and self-esteem)? What additional information do you need about his self-concept?

Practical Knowledge knowing how

This section provides guidelines and forms for assessing self-concept, self-esteem, anxiety, and depression, which are basic to psychosocial health and illness. In addition, you will find tables of selected standardized outcomes and interventions to consider when planning care for patients with problems related to anxiety and depression.

CLINICAL INSIGHTS

Clinical Insight 13-1 ➤ Assessing Self-Concept Problems

Assessment Category	Examples of Assessment Questions
Body image	■ When you look in the mirror, what do you see? ■ How do you think others see you? ■ How does your current ability to engage in work and leisure activities compare with how you would like to be?
Role performance	■ What are your three or four major roles (e.g., daughter, student)? ■ How successful are you in each of these roles? ■ How important is it to you to be successful in each of these roles? ■ What is interfering with your ability to perform any of these roles? What can you do about it?
Personal identity	■ How did you see yourself before your illness/injury/loss? ■ How do you see yourself now? ■ How would you describe yourself to others? ■ What special abilities do you have? ■ How do you think others see you?
Self-esteem (also refer to the Assessment Box, Performing a Self-Esteem Inventory)	■ How do you feel about yourself? ■ What do you like about yourself? ■ To what extent do you feel you are in control of your life? ■ If you could change one thing about yourself, what would it be? ■ Where would you like to be 5 years from now? ■ How realistic are your expectations of yourself? ■ How do you see your illness/injury/loss in relation to yourself?

Clinical Insight 13-2 ➤ Performing a Self-Esteem Inventory

Place a check mark in the column that most closely describes the client's answer to each statement. Each check is worth the number of points listed.

	3 Often or a great deal	2 Some-times	1 Seldom or occasionally	0 Never or not at all
1. I become angry or hurt when criticized.				
2. I am afraid to try new things.				
3. I feel stupid when I make a mistake.				
4. I have difficulty looking people in the eye.				
5. I have difficulty making small talk.				
6. I feel uncomfortable in the presence of strangers.				
7. I am embarrassed when people compliment me.				
8. I am dissatisfied with the way I look.				
9. I am afraid to express my opinions in a group.				
10. I prefer staying home alone rather than participating in group social situations.				
11. I have trouble accepting teasing.				
12. I feel guilty when I say no to people.				
13. I am afraid to make a commitment to a relationship for fear of rejection.				
14. I believe that most people are more competent than I am.				
15. I feel resentment toward people who are attractive and successful.				
16. I have trouble thinking of any positive aspects about my life.				
17. I feel inadequate in the presence of authority figures.				
18. I have trouble making decisions.				
19. I fear the disapproval of others.				
20. I feel tense, stressed out, or "uptight."				

Problems with low self-esteem are indicated by items scored with a 3 or by a total score higher than 46.

Source: Townsend, M. C. (2010). *Psychiatric mental health nursing: Concepts of care* (5th ed.). Philadelphia: F.A. Davis, p. 248.

Clinical Insight 13-3 ➤ Identifying Depressed Patients Who Should Be Referred for Evaluation

One way to identify depression that is more than simple, situational depression is to ask the following two questions. A Yes answer merits a referral.

1. "Over the past 2 weeks, have you felt down, depressed, or hopeless?"
2. "Over the past 2 weeks, have you felt little interest or pleasure in doing things?"

Source: U.S. Preventive Services Task Force (USPSTF). (2009). Screening for depression in adults. Retrieved January 18, 2013, from http://www.uspreventiveservicestaskforce.org/uspstf/uspsaddepr.htm

SIGECAPS

Another method is to use the mnemonic SIGECAPS, a concise version of the *DSM-5* diagnostic criteria. Ask the patient if he has experienced, for 2 or more weeks:

Sleep increase/decrease
Interest in formerly compelling or pleasurable activities diminished
Guilt, low self-esteem
Energy poor
Concentration poor
Appetite increase/decrease
Psychomotor agitation or retardation
Suicidal ideation

Both of the following require referral for evaluation and treatment:

Major depression = depressed mood or interest *plus* 4 SIGECAPS for 2 or more weeks
Mild depression (mood disorder) = depressed mood or interest plus 3 SIGECAPS most days for 2 or more years

Source: Breggin, P. (2009). *Medication madness: The role of psychiatric drugs in cases of violence, suicide, and crime.* New York: St. Martin's Press.

IN SAD CAGES

Some people prefer a mnemonic from an older source, IN SAD CAGES, which you would use in essentially the same way. Ask the patient whether he has experienced, for 2 or more weeks:

Interest reduced
Negative thoughts

Sleep disturbance
Appetite change
Decreased confidence or self-esteem

Concentration reduced
Affect blunt or flat
Guilt
Energy reduced
Suicidal ideas

The original reference does not include a suggested total that requires referral. However, you can assume that the more symptoms there are, the more severe the depression will be. We would suggest the following:

IN (reduced interest and negative thoughts or depressed mood) plus 4 of the other SAD CAGES requires referral.

Do not try to differentiate mild and major depression with this method.

Adapted from Leng, L. B. (2011). Overview of major depressive disorder. *The Singapore Family Physician, 37*(4), 18–21.

ASSESSMENT GUIDELINES AND TOOLS

Focused Assessment

Anxiety Assessment Guide

Rating Scale: None = 0, Mild = 1, Moderate = 2, Severe = 3, Disabling (Panic) = 4

PHYSIOLOGICAL EFFECTS	Rating	PSYCHOLOGICAL EFFECTS	Rating
Shortness of breath (dyspnea)	____	Depersonalization (unreal)	____
Choking sensation	____	Feeling "on edge"	____
Dry mouth	____	Poor concentration	____
Pounding heart, increased heart rate	____	Poor memory	____
Chest pain	____	Depressed mood	____
Increased sweating and clamminess	____	Loss of interest	____
Feeling faint, dizzy, unsteady	____	Restlessness	____
Nausea and abdominal upsets	____	Sense of panic	____
Numbness (pins and needles)	____	Worry, anticipation of the worst	____
Hot/cold flashes	____	Irritability	____
Trembling, shaking	____	Nightmares	____
Muscle tension and aches	____	Feeling of fear and foreboding	____
Exaggerated startle response	____	Excessive apprehension	____
Difficulties in falling asleep and staying asleep	____	Feeling lack of control	____

Assessing Overall Scores

0–28	Mild anxiety
29–56	Moderate anxiety
57–84	Severe anxiety
85–112	Disabling anxiety

Creating a total score from this table can help you assess whether overall anxiety is mild, moderate, severe, or disabling. However, individual physiological or psychological symptoms that are rated as severe (3) or disabling (4) may be more important and relevant to your nursing assessment. For example, your patient's overall or total assessment may be 26 (in the mild range, 0–27) but she has rated "Excessive apprehension" as 4 (disabling).

Focused Assessment

Depression Assessment Guide: Patient Health Questionnaire (PHQ-9)

This is a valid and reliable measure of depression developed in 1999 by Pfizer, Inc. It can be self-administered (Kroenke, Spitzer, & Williams, 2001). It may be useful across cultures (Arthurs, Steele, Hudson, et al., 2012; Chen, Huang, Chang, et al., 2006).

Over the past 2 weeks, how often have you been bothered by any of the following problems? (Check or circle your answers.)

	NOT AT ALL	SEVERAL DAYS	MORE THAN HALF THE DAYS	NEARLY EVERY DAY
1. Little interest or pleasure in doing things	0	1	2	2
2. Feeling down, depressed, or hopeless	0	1	2	3
3. Trouble falling or staying asleep, or sleeping too much	0	1	2	3
4. Feeling tired or having little energy	0	1	2	3
5. Poor appetite or overeating	0	1	2	3
6. Feeling bad about yourself—or that you are a failure or have let yourself or your family down	0	1	2	3
7. Trouble concentrating on things, such as reading the newspaper or watching television	0	1	2	3
8. Moving or speaking so slowly that other people could have noticed. Or the opposite—being so fidgety or restless that you have been moving around a lot more than usual	0	1	2	3
9. Thoughts that you would be better off dead or of hurting yourself in some way	0	1	2	3
ADD COLUMNS		☐ +	☐ +	☐

TOTAL: ☐

10. If you checked off any problems, how difficult have these problems made it for you to do your work, take care of things at home, or get along with other people?

Not difficult at all _____

Somewhat difficult _____

Very difficult _____

Extremely difficult _____

(Healthcare professional: For interpretation of TOTAL, please refer to the accompanying score card. *[Note to students: Interpretation requires training. You should report the patient's score to your instructor or your immediate supervising nurse.])*

Source: Pfizer, Inc. Retrieved January 23, 2013, from http://www.phqscreeners.com/. Used by permission.

Focused Assessment

Differentiating Depression and Dementia

This table may help you to identify older adults who should be referred for further evaluation to determine whether symptoms are related to depression or dementia. To screen for depression,

Go to Chapter 13, **Tables, Boxes, Figures: Geriatric Depression Rating Scale (Short Form),** on Davis*Plus*.

To determine whether the patient should be referred to a mental health professional, refer to Clinical Insight 13-3.

CHARACTERISTIC	DEPRESSION	DEMENTIA
Cause/triggers	Loss (e.g., of spouse, of independence); stress	Physiological causes (e.g., Alzheimer's disease, brain infarcts)
Onset	Acute or chronic; can be related to specific events	Chronic, gradual, and insidious
Course	Varies, depending on cause	Progressive, over a long period of time
Alertness	Usually reduced	Usually normal
Memory	Memory loss and forgetfulness	Recent and remote memory impaired; loss of recent memory is first sign; some loss of common knowledge
Thinking	Inability to concentrate	Difficulty with abstraction and word finding, especially nouns; difficulty with calculations; decreased judgment
Response to questions	Often says, "I don't know."	Answers inappropriately or with "near misses"
Language	Speaks slowly; slow to respond to verbal stimuli	Disoriented, rambling, incoherent; difficulty using nouns
Sleep	Difficulty falling asleep, early morning awakening, much day sleeping	Sleep fragmented; awakens often during night
Reversibility	Potential	Irreversible, progressive

Source: Adapted from Edwards, N. (2003). Differentiating the three D's: Delirium, dementia, and depression. *MedSurg Nursing: Official Journal of the Academy of Medical-Surgical Nurses, 12*(6), 347.

STANDARDIZED NURSING LANGUAGE

You can use the tables in this section when planning care for patients with problems of anxiety, depression. The tables provide standardized wording for nursing diagnoses, outcomes, and interventions. You can use the NOC indicators with the outcomes to write goals. Non-NOC outcomes are also suggested. In addition to the broad NIC interventions, the tables provide specific nursing activities suggested by NIC.

Anxiety-Related Diagnoses: Selected NOC Outcomes and NIC Interventions

CUE CLUSTER	NANDA-I DIAGNOSIS*	NOC OUTCOMES†	SELECTED INDICATORS	NIC INTERVENTIONS AND SPECIFIC ACTIVITIES‡
Susan is pacing the floor and does not make eye contact when she speaks to you. Her hands are shaking. Her BP is 140/88 mm Hg, P is 100 beats/min, and R is 24 breaths/min. She says she is worried.	Anxiety	Anxiety Self-Control ***Other Outcomes*** Anxiety Level Concentration Coping	(Often demonstrated) ▪ Monitors intensity of anxiety. ▪ Maintains concentration.	Anxiety Reduction ▪ Use a calm, reassuring approach. ▪ Explain all procedures, including sensations the patient is likely to experience during the procedure. ▪ Help the patient identify situations that precipitate anxiety. ***Other Interventions*** Anger Control Assistance Anticipatory Guidance Calming Technique Coping Enhancement Emotional Support
Martin has a terminal illness. He looks very sad. He states that he is worried that his dying will be prolonged and difficult for his family and that he is afraid of dying.	Death Anxiety	Acceptance: Health Status ***Other Outcomes*** Anxiety Self-Control Comfortable Death Depression Level Dignified Life Closure Fear Self-Control Hope Spiritual Health	(Often demonstrated) ▪ Appears peaceful. ▪ Reports positive self regard. ▪ Clarifies personal values.	Emotional Support ▪ Listen to and encourage expressions of feelings and beliefs. ▪ Provide support during denial, anger, bargaining, and acceptance phases of grieving. ***Other Interventions*** Anxiety Reduction Coping Enhancement Decision-Making Support Dying Care Hope Instillation Pain Management Presence Religious Ritual Enhancement Spiritual Support
Ms. Eng says, "I just don't know whether to have this chemotherapy or not. I know I could live a little longer, but the side effects . . ." She has decided twice to do it and each time has changed her mind. She says, "I just can't focus on anything else."	Decisional Conflict	Decision Making ***Other Outcomes*** Information Processing Participation: Health Care Decisions Personal Autonomy	(Not compromised) ▪ Identifies alternatives. ▪ Identifies needed resources to support each alternative.	Decision-Making Support ▪ Determine whether there are differences between the patient's view of own condition and the views of healthcare providers. ▪ Serve as a liaison between the patient and family. ▪ Serve as a liaison between patient and other healthcare providers. ***Other Interventions*** Assertiveness Training Health System Guidance Learning Facilitation Mutual Goal Setting

(Continued)

Anxiety-Related Diagnoses: Selected NOC Outcomes and NIC Interventions—cont'd

CUE CLUSTER	NANDA-I DIAGNOSIS*	NOC OUTCOMES†	SELECTED INDICATORS	NIC INTERVENTIONS AND SPECIFIC ACTIVITIES‡
Bryan is to have his burns debrided today. He is crying. He says, "I wish my mom was here. It hurts so bad when they do that. I'm so scared."	Fear	Fear Self-Control ***Other Outcomes*** Fear Level Fear Level: Child	(Often demonstrated) ▪ Uses relaxation techniques to reduce fear. ▪ Maintains concentration. ▪ Controls fear response.	Security Enhancement ▪ Spend time with the patient. ▪ Answer questions about health status in an honest manner. ▪ Hold a young child or infant, as appropriate. ***Other Interventions*** Anxiety Reduction Calming Technique Coping Enhancement Presence
Mr. Paul's blood pressure remains dangerously high, yet he does not make the changes in diet and exercise that are needed, and he often fails to take his pills. "I feel OK. This is a bunch of mumbo jumbo. My folks ate fried foods, and they lived to be over 80."	Ineffective Denial	Health Beliefs: Perceived Threat ***Other Outcomes*** Acceptance: Health Status Anxiety Self-Control Fear Self-Control Symptom Control	(Strong) ▪ Perceived threat to health ▪ Perceived vulnerability to progressive health problems ▪ Perceived impact on functional status	Self-Awareness Enhancement ▪ Assist the patient to identify the values that contribute to self-concept. ▪ Assist patient to identify the impact of illness on self-concept. ▪ Verbalize the patient's denial of reality, as appropriate. ***Other Interventions*** Anxiety Reduction Calming Technique Coping Enhancement Counseling Emotional Support Health Education Security Enhancement Self-Awareness Enhancement Self-Modification Assistance Self-Responsibility Facilitation Teaching: Disease Process

*NANDA International. (2012). *Nursing diagnoses: Definitions and classification 2012–2014*. Philadelphia: Author. Used with permission.

†Johnson, M., Bulechek, G., Butcher, H., et al. (2011). *NANDA, NOC, and NIC linkages: Nursing diagnoses, outcomes, and interventions* (3rd ed.). St. Louis, MO: C.V. Mosby; and Moorhead, S., Johnson, M., Maas, M. L., et al. (Eds.). (2013). *Nursing outcomes classification (NOC)* (5th ed.). St. Louis, MO: C.V. Mosby. Used with permission.

‡Johnson, M., Bulechek, G., Butcher, H., et al. (2011). *NANDA, NOC, and NIC linkages: Nursing diagnoses, outcomes, and interventions* (3rd ed.). St. Louis, MO: C.V. Mosby; and Bulechek, G. M., Butcher, H. K., & Dochterman, J. M. (Eds.). (2012). *Nursing interventions classification (NIC)* (6th ed.). St. Louis, MO: C.V. Mosby. Used with permission.

Depression-Related Nursing Diagnoses: Selected NOC Outcomes and NIC Interventions

CUE CLUSTER	NANDA-I DIAGNOSIS*	NOC OUTCOMES†	SELECTED INDICATORS	NIC INTERVENTIONS AND SPECIFIC ACTIVITIES‡
John is dying of AIDS. He sleeps most of the time. During care activities (e.g., bath), he closes his eyes and remains passive. When asked to move or participate, he sighs and says, "I can't." When friends visit, he turns away from them; when they talk to him, he just shrugs. He has quit eating. He says, "It doesn't matter what I do. Nothing can change the way this turns out."	Hopelessness	Hope ***Other Outcomes*** Depression Level Depression Self-Control Mood Equilibrium Psychomotor Energy Quality of Life Will to Live	(Often demonstrated) Expresses meaning in life. Expresses inner peace. Expresses belief in self. Expresses belief in others. Expresses sense of self-control.	Hope Inspiration ▪ Demonstrate hope by recognizing the patient's intrinsic worth and viewing the patient's illness as only one facet of the individual. ▪ Help the patient expand spiritual self. ▪ Create an environment that facilitates patient practicing religion, as appropriate. ▪ Facilitate the patient's or family's reliving and savoring past achievements and experiences. ▪ Teach the family about the positive aspects of hope (e.g., develop meaningful conversational themes that reflect love and need for the patient). ▪ Avoid masking the truth. ***Other Interventions*** Coping Enhancement Counseling Mood Management Resiliency Promotion Self-Modification Assistance Spiritual Growth Facilitation Values Clarification
Jennifer is 16 and pregnant. She does not follow good health practices. She angrily says, "It's my body, and I don't want this baby. But my parents say abortion is a sin. I should honor my parents, but I hate them. I hate having to depend on them, and I hate being pregnant."	Powerlessness	Health Beliefs: Perceived Control ***Other Outcomes*** Depression Self-Control Family Participation in Professional Care Health Beliefs Health Beliefs: Perceived Ability to Perform Health Beliefs: Perceived Resources Hope Participation in Health Care Decisions	(Strong) Requested involvement in health decisions. Efforts at gathering information. Belief that own actions control health outcomes. Willingness to designate surrogate decision maker.	Self-Responsibility Facilitation ▪ Discuss with the patient the extent of responsibility for present health status. ▪ Determine whether the patient has adequate knowledge about healthcare condition. ▪ Encourage verbalizations of feelings, perceptions, and fears about assuming responsibility. ▪ Discuss consequences of not dealing with own responsibilities. ▪ Encourage patient to take as much responsibility for own self-care, as possible. ▪ Provide positive feedback for accepting additional responsibility and/or behavior change. ***Other Interventions*** Cognitive Restructuring Decision-Making Support Emotional Support Family Involvement Promotion

(Continued)

Depression-Related Nursing Diagnoses: Selected NOC Outcomes and NIC Interventions—cont'd

CUE CLUSTER	NANDA-I DIAGNOSIS*	NOC OUTCOMES†	SELECTED INDICATORS	NIC INTERVENTIONS AND SPECIFIC ACTIVITIES‡
		Personal Autonomy		Financial Resource Assistance Health Education Health System Guidance Hope Inspiration Mood Management Mutual Goal Setting Patient Rights Protection Self-Esteem Enhancement Values Clarification
Tim has attempted suicide twice. He now says, "I will get it right this time. I know where I can get a gun."	Risk for Suicide	Suicide Self-Restraint ***Other Outcomes*** Mood Equilibrium Will to Live	(Often demonstrated) Obtains assistance as needed. Controls impulses. Refrains from gathering means for suicide. Refrains from giving away possessions. Upholds suicide contract. Expresses feelings.	Suicide Prevention ▪ Refer patient to mental healthcare provider . . . for evaluation and treatment. . . . ▪ Administer medications to decrease anxiety, agitation, or psychosis and to stabilize mood, as appropriate. ▪ Conduct mouth checks after medication administration to ensure that patient is not "cheeking" the medications for later overdose attempt. ▪ Initiate suicide precautions (e.g., ongoing observation and monitoring of the patient, provision of a protective environment) . . . ▪ Limit access to windows, unless locked and shatterproof, as appropriate. ▪ Monitor patient during use of potential weapons (e.g., razor). ▪ Assist patient to identify network of supportive persons and resources (e.g., clergy, family, providers). ***Other Interventions*** Behavior Management: Self-Harm Hope Inspiration Mood Management Spiritual Support

*NANDA International. (2012). *Nursing diagnoses: Definitions and classification 2012–2014.* Philadelphia: Author. Used with permission.

†Johnson, M., Bulechek, G., Butcher, H., et al. (2011). *NANDA, NOC, and NIC linkages: Nursing diagnoses, outcomes, and interventions* (3rd ed.). St. Louis, MO: C.V. Mosby; and Moorhead, S., Johnson, M., Maas, M., et al. (Eds.). (2013). *Nursing outcomes classification (NOC)* (5th ed.). St. Louis, MO: C.V. Mosby. Used with permission.

‡Johnson, M., Bulechek, G., Butcher, H., et al. (2011). *NANDA, NOC, and NIC linkages: Nursing diagnoses, outcomes, and interventions* (3rd ed.). St. Louis, MO: C.V. Mosby; and Bulechek, G. M., Butcher, H. K., & Dochterman, J. M. (Eds.). (2012). *Nursing interventions classification (NIC)* (6th ed.). St. Louis, MO: C.V. Mosby. Used with permission.

CLINICALREASONING

Applying the Full-Spectrum Nursing Model

PATIENT SITUATION

Matthew has been admitted to the emergency department with extensive wounds to both forearms, including tendon and vascular damage, from a suicide attempt. Matthew seems very quiet, almost withdrawn, and answers most of your questions in monosyllables.

Matthew reports the following: He is the third child in a family of five. Matthew's middle-class parents are now retired, and his brothers and sisters are scattered across the country in various large cities. Although Matthew claims his schooling years were unremarkable, he reminisces about several occasions when he was bullied and physically beaten by gangs of older adolescents.

Matthew further states that he graduated from Harvard Law School and became vice president of an influential law firm. Despite his apparent success in life, he has continued to question his self-worth since childhood. Plagued by worries and depression that have increased over the past few years, he says he wrote a note indicating that he now realizes what a failure he is and proceeded to slash both of his forearms with a sharp razor.

Matthew reports that he has not been eating much, feels tired all the time, and has no interest in going outside the house. He says, "I just don't feel like doing anything; I just want to sleep all the time."

THINKING

1. *Theoretical Knowledge:* Using just the information you have in the Patient Situation, use the SIGECAPS method outlined in Clinical Insight 13-3 to assess Matthew's level of depression. You will need to assume that he is reporting what he has experienced in the past 2 weeks (unless he is obviously referring to the past).
2. *Critical Thinking (Inquiry):* What items of the SIGECAPS cannot be completed with the information in the Patient Situation? What do you need to ask Matthew to complete them?

DOING

3. *Nursing Process (Interventions):* Based on your SIGECAPS data, what do you need to do right away (or be certain it was done in the emergency department)?

CARING

4. *Self-Knowledge:* What do you have in common with Matthew that might help you to empathize with him?
5. *Ethical Knowledge:* Try to put aside your own beliefs now, and answer the following questions from the perspective of (a) Matthew and (b) one of your nursing colleagues on the unit:
   a. Give one reason to support Matthew's claim that he has a right to commit suicide if his despair is too deep to bear.
   b. Give one reason to support a colleague's claim that Matthew does not have a right to commit suicide, no matter how he feels.

Critical Thinking and Clinical Reasoning

1. Review the scenario about Karli (Meet Your Patient from Volume 1):

   You are caring for a 16-year-old patient named Karli who is suffering from fractures to both arms and several ribs, as well as extensive first- and second-degree burns to 30% of her body after a motor vehicle accident. Karli was driving her parents' car home from her part-time job when she lost control of the car and crashed into a wall. The car exploded in flames. A passerby quickly reported the accident, and fast action by the emergency response team saved Karli's life.

   Karli is suffering from a moderate amount of shock and pain. She alternates among outbursts of anger, self-directed sarcasm, and despondence. She tells you that she cannot understand how the accident happened, that one moment she was adjusting the car radio, and the next moment she awoke in the hospital. Then suddenly she explodes. "It's not fair! I just took my eyes off the road for a second; that's all!" She bursts into tears. Picking at her bandages, she sobs, "No one will ever love me the way I'm going to look. My life is over. I hate myself!" You take her hand. "I used to be pretty," she says, "but now I'll look like a freak! What did I do to deserve this? I know plenty of kids who drive drunk or high all the time. I wasn't doing anything wrong! Why did this happen to me?"

a. Now that you have completed Chapter 13 in Volume 1, make a list of the multiple physical, psychological, and social issues that you would need to consider in developing a comprehensive care plan for Karli.
b. Compare your list with the one you made when you first began reading the chapter. How is it different? Or is it the same?

2. In the Meet Your Patient scenario, Karli perceives herself as unlovable "looking this way." Which of the following nursing activities do you think might be helpful in *exploring and changing her perception*? For those you *do not* choose, explain why.

Role Enhancement

- Help the patient distinguish ideal and actual self. Help her describe realistic roles and expectations tailored to specific health changes.
- Compare realistic roles with previous and less functional roles.

Conflict Mediation

- Provide a quiet, private, neutral setting for mediation to take place.
- Maintain your own neutrality in the process; do not "take sides."

Promoting Family Integrity

- Encourage and facilitate communication among family members.
- Encourage family members to care for the patient as much as possible.

Family Mobilization

- Help the family to identify strengths they can use to support the patient.
- Teach family members how to provide home care for the patient.
- Help the family identify community resources and/or support groups.
- With the patient's permission, keep the family informed about the patient's progress.

Enhancing Socialization

- Explore and reinforce the individual's established relationships.
- Provide opportunities to rehearse relationship-building skills.
- Investigate, assist, and promote any developing relationships with persons of similar interests and goals.
- Provide information and links to community activities that relate to the person's past, current, and future interests.
- Promote access to education in social skills development.
- Encourage the patient to communicate and engage in interpersonal relationship activities by providing ongoing positive feedback.
- Organize small, cohesive group activities.
- Provide or act as a role model where appropriate.

3. Mrs. King is being admitted into the orthopedics unit for a scheduled total knee replacement. Even though she appears to be in good health for a 72-year-old woman, you are concerned about her excessive weight, which can be described as moderate to severe obesity. You are troubled by how the obesity may negatively affect postsurgical recovery, wound healing, and mobility.

a. What theoretical knowledge will you draw on to plan care to meet her biopsychosocial needs?
b. What assumptions are you making? What stereotypes do you have that might affect your understanding of Mrs. King's situation?
c. What do you think might be contributing to Mrs. King's obesity?
d. What facts do you have to support those ideas?
e. How could you find out for sure what is contributing to Mrs. King's obesity?

4. Day by day, you notice that your patient is eating less and complaining about constipation and tiredness. You carefully review her nutritional requirements against the food menu, as well as check nursing records for bowel movements. You have exhausted your initial search for obvious reasons your patient's appetite has changed. After sitting down next to your patient, you cannot help noticing how tired she looks.

a. What psychosocial problem do you suspect (low self-esteem, depression, anxiety, or disturbed personal identity)?

b. What data do you have to support your inference in (a)?
c. Objective data in her chart indicate that the patient has been eating very little and that she has been having bowel movements only every 3 or 4 days—and even then only with a laxative or enema. What other symptom do you need to investigate further?
d. How could you obtain more information about that symptom?
e. Think of depressed people you have known or depressed patients you have cared for. What have you found to be difficult about dealing with them?

5. Edna Jackson is 42 years old. She has had a hysterectomy (removal of her uterus). Her surgery was uncomplicated, her overall health is good, and she is expected to make a full and rapid physical recovery. Her husband was not present when she was admitted and has not been to see her since the surgery. He did not want her to have the surgery. He told Edna that he doesn't know whether he will want to have sex with her when she is no longer "a whole woman." He has had casual affairs during their marriage, which Edna has tolerated because she feels that difficulty is balanced by the many positive benefits of their relationship, which include a "good sex life."

Edna has seven brothers and sisters, and she has five children of her own, ages 23, 21, 18, 6, and 4. She comes from a culture and a religion that value children and motherhood. She believes she is a good mother, although she must work full-time outside the home. Edna is an office manager—respected by her boss and by those who work for her. She has an internal locus of control and evaluates her job performance as "better than most people would do."

a. Look at the context. What aspects of this situation may negatively impact Mrs. Jackson's recovery?
b. Based on your answers in (a), what nursing diagnoses might be useful in describing the psychosocial aspects of Mrs. Jackson's health? (State both the problem and the etiology.)
c. What strengths does Mrs. Jackson have that may help her to avoid and/or overcome those problems?

6. Matthew has been admitted to the emergency department with extensive wounds to both forearms, including tendon and vascular damage, from an attempted suicide. Matthew seems very quiet, almost withdrawn, and answers most of your questions in monosyllables.

Matthew reports that he is the third child in a family of five. Matthew's middle-class parents are now retired, and his brothers and sisters are scattered across the country in various large cities. Although Matthew claims his schooling years were unremarkable, he reminisces about several occasions when he was bullied and physically beaten by gangs of older adolescents.

Matthew graduated from Harvard Law School and became vice president of an influential law firm. Despite his apparent success in life, he has continued to question his self-worth from early childhood. Plagued by worries and depression that have increased over the past few years Matthew wrote a note indicating that he now realized what a failure he is and proceeded to slash both his forearms with a sharp razor.

During the nursing assessment, Matthew reports that he has not been eating much, feels tired all the time, and has no interest in getting outside the house. He says, "I just don't feel like doing anything; I just want to sleep all the time."

a. After Matthew's tendon and vascular repair, he is admitted to your medical-surgical unit. What, broadly speaking, are your first two priorities for Matthew's care?
b. Which of these nursing diagnoses— Risk for Suicide or Risk for Self-Mutilation—would you use, and why? (Consult a NANDA-I handbook, if necessary)
c. Prioritize the following interventions for Matthew. Rank them (1 = highest rank, 4 = lowest rank). Explain your thinking.
   ____ Refer to a mental health professional for help with his depression.
   ____ Examine Matthew's belongings and the room for anything he might use to harm himself.
   ____ Encourage Matthew to tell you if he begins having thoughts of suicide.
   ____ Begin establishing a therapeutic relationship and gaining his trust.
d. Evaluate your self-knowledge. To plan comprehensive care for Matthew, in what areas do you need to increase your theoretical and practical knowledge? How will you do that?

7. For each of the following concepts, use critical thinking to describe how or why it is important to nursing, patient care, or psychosocial health and illness. Note that these are *not* to be merely definitions.

Self-concept
Self-esteem
Body image
Biopsychosocial well-being
Anxiety
Defense mechanisms
Depression
Therapeutic relationships
Hopelessness

What Are the Main Points in This Chapter?

- Health and well-being are influenced by psychological, social, and spiritual development.
- Psychosocial theory provides a way to understand people as interactions of psychological and social events.
- Self-concept is one's overall view of oneself; it answers the question, "Who do you think you are?"
- Self-concept is developed throughout the life span and is influenced by multiple factors. Four dimensions contribute to self-concept: body image, role performance, personal identity, and self-esteem.
- Body image is a person's mental image of his physical self.
- Role performance consists of the actions a person takes and the behaviors she demonstrates in fulfilling a role, such as the role of a student.
- Personal identity is a person's view of himself as a unique human being, different and separate from all others.
- Self-esteem evaluations arise from the differences between the ideal and the actual self.
- Communication skills are important because psychosocial information is personal and sometimes sensitive.
- When you formulate psychosocial diagnoses it is difficult, but important, to determine what is cause and what is effect.
- Many of the NOC standardized psychosocial outcomes are found in the domains of Psychosocial Health and Family Health.
- Many of the NIC standardized psychosocial interventions are found in the Behavioral and Family domains.
- Anxiety is a common emotional response to a (usually unknown) stressor; it results from psychological conflicts, and it is accompanied by physical symptoms (e.g., trembling).
- Assessment should identify the presence, level, and cause of anxiety.
- Interventions for anxiety should help the patient become aware that he is anxious, identify the source of anxiety, and deal with the symptoms it produces.
- Depression is characterized by diminished interest or pleasure in previously enjoyed activities, sadness, emptiness, a flat or hollow feeling (absence of feeling), tearfulness, difficulty concentrating, feelings of worthlessness, and some physical symptoms (e.g., constipation).
- Assessment of depression includes a comprehensive history of mood, thoughts, behavior, and physical status.
- If you suspect severe depression, you should refer the patient to a mental health specialist; if there is a risk of suicide, referral should be immediate.
- In communicating with depressed persons, it is important not to be overly cheerful and to avoid phrases such as "Cheer up."

Knowledge Map

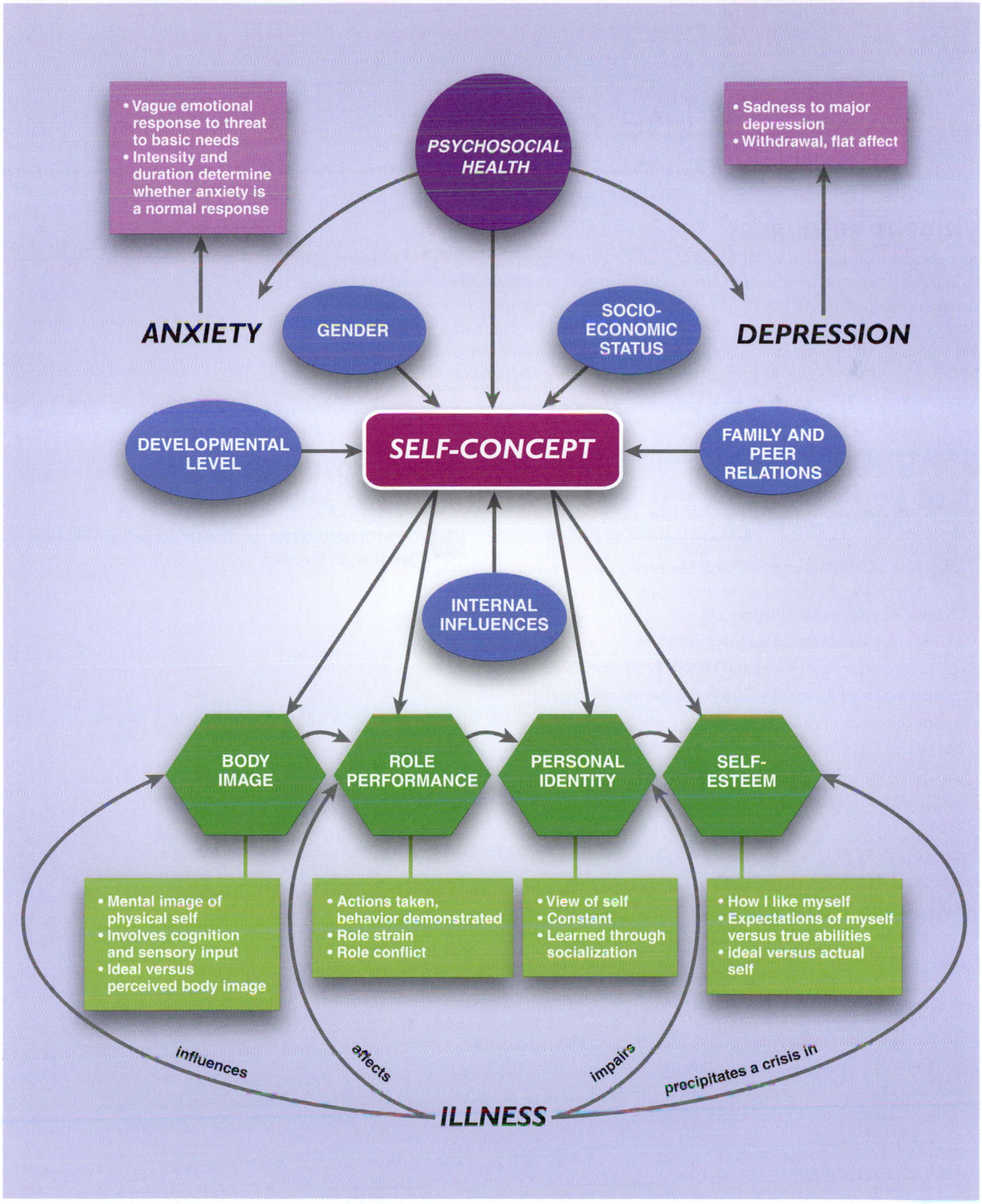

CHAPTER 14

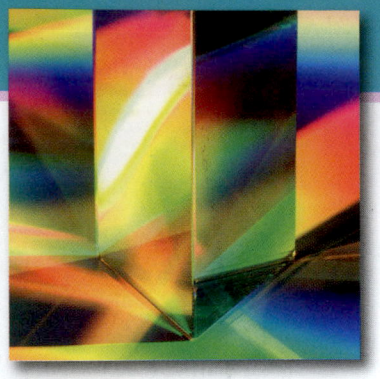

The Family

STUDENT RESOURCES

*The questions and exercises in Volume 2 allow you to practice the kind of thinking you will use as a full-spectrum nurse. Critical-thinking questions usually have more than one correct answer, so we do not provide "answers" for these features. It is more important to develop your nursing judgment than to just cover content. You will learn by discussing the questions with your peers. If you are still unsure, consult your instructor. You will find Response Sheets (for writing your responses to the questions) on Davis*Plus.

To explore learning resources for this chapter,

Go to Davis*Plus* at DavisPl.us/Wilkinson3.

Chapter Resources for Chapter 14:
- **Response sheets for all learning activities**
- **Resources for Caregivers and Health Professionals**
- **Reading More About the Family (suggested readings)**
- **Concept Map of chapter content**

Interactive Case Studies

NCLEX-Style and Chapter Review Questions

CHAPTER OVERVIEW

For a podcast of an overview of this chapter,

Go to Student Resources: Chapter 14, **Podcast—Chapter Overview,** on Davis*Plus*.

Caring for the Nyugens

Kim Phan, 3 years old, is the first grandchild for Nam and Yen Nguyen. Until recently, Kim lived with his mother, Trinh Phan, the Nguyen's daughter. Trinh was diagnosed with schizophrenia at age 18, and initially was functioning adequately on her medications. However, her condition has been worsening and for the past year she has not been taking her medications. When Trinh became unable to care for Kim, Nam and Yen assumed the child's care. Trinh rarely visits Kim. Nam and Yen convinced Trinh to obtain residential care at a mental health facility. Nam tells you at a clinic visit that he wishes his family were "normal."

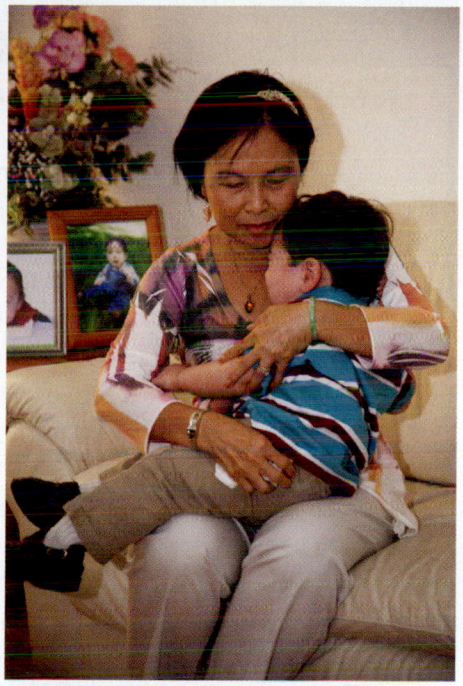

A. What do you need to clarify about Nam's statement about his family?

B. What do *you* think Nam means by a "normal" family?

C. How would you respond to Nam's comments?

D. What effect might this new family structure have on Nam's and Yen's health?

E. How might you promote family functioning for the Nguyens? What assessments should you make? What interventions should you consider?

F. What personal values or biases do you have that may affect your ability to care for the Nguyens?

Practical Knowledge knowing how

Material in this section will help you to assess and plan care for families.

CLINICAL INSIGHTS

Clinical Insight 14-1 ➤ Conducting a Family Assessment

In general, a family assessment should include the following:

Identifying data	Include such information as name, address, phone number, cultural/ethnic background, religious identification, social affiliation.
Family composition	For each member of the family, include gender, age, relationship, date and place of birth, occupation, and education.
Family history and developmental stage	This refers to the stages and developmental tasks in the table Assessing Family Development Tasks.
Environmental data	Include a description of the home, neighborhood, larger community, family's social supports, and their transactions with the community.

(Continued)

Clinical Insight 14-1 ➤ Conducting a Family Assessment—*(continued)*

Family structure	In addition to identifying the structural type (e.g., traditional nuclear, single-parent, etc.), assess: ■ Communication patterns: Functional and dysfunctional patterns; the manner in which emotions are expressed, and contextual variables that affect communication ■ Power and role structures (e.g., How are family decisions made? What are the roles of each member? Have there been changes in these?) ■ Family values (e.g., What are their values? What are their priorities? How do they compare with the values of their cultural group? Are there value conflicts in the family?)
Family functions	Assess the effectiveness of the family's: ■ Nurturing (e.g., Are the members close? Are they separate or connected?) ■ Socialization and child rearing (e.g., Who is the socializing agent(s) for the children? What are their child-rearing practices? Are needs for play being met?)
Health beliefs, values, and behaviors	How do they define health and illness? What are their dietary, sleep, physical, and drug habits? What are their dental and medical health practices, including physicals, eye exams, immunizations, etc.? Do they have access to health services?
Family stressors and coping	What are their stressors (e.g., financial, family communication or relationships, neighbors, holidays, children's behavior)? What successful coping strategies have they used? What dysfunctional strategies?
Abuse and violence within the family	Because of the prevalence of abuse and because families are likely to be ashamed to discuss it, you should assess every family to see if any abuse or neglect is occurring. For detailed guidelines, go to Procedure 9-1, Assessing for Abuse.

ASSESSMENT GUIDELINES AND TOOLS

Focused Assessment

Assessing Family Developmental Tasks

STAGES	TASKS	CHILDREN'S AGES (IF ANY) (APPROXIMATE)
Beginning family	■ Relinquishing the family of origin as the major emotional and economic resource ■ Gaining a sense of autonomy and independence ■ Making the relationship/marriage work; investment in spouse as the major emotional resource ■ Finding a place in the kin network of each partner ■ Exploring options for career development ■ Deciding whether to have children	None
Childbearing family	■ Achieving pregnancy and birth ■ Adjusting to life changes after birth and to the infant's needs ■ Determining ways to meet all members' needs ■ Renegotiating marriage ■ Increasing contact with extended family	Newborn to 2 years
"No longer newlyweds" (with no children)	■ Establishing a sense of the permanence of the relationship ■ Establishing long-term residency ■ Being involved in the community/promoting the well-being of the community	Not applicable
Family with preschool children	■ Adjusting to increased costs associated with family life ■ Socializing the preschoolers ■ Coping with loss of parental energy and privacy	3–5 years

Focused Assessment

Assessing Family Developmental Tasks—cont'd

STAGES	TASKS	CHILDREN'S AGES (IF ANY) (APPROXIMATE)
Mature family (with no children)	■ Renegotiating relationship on basis of more maturity ■ Adjusting to changing levels of responsibility in work and community ■ If not done already, achieving financial security	Not applicable
Family with school-age children	■ Adjusting to the needs and demands of growing children ■ Promoting joint decision making among parents and children ■ Encouraging and supporting educational and school-related activities	6–12 years
Family with teenagers and young adults	■ Maintaining open communication among family members ■ Reinforcing ethical and moral values ■ For teens, balancing independence with parental rules	13–20 years
Family launching young adults	■ Maintaining support to young adults as they leave the security of family ■ Rediscovering marriage	18–30 years
Postparental family	■ Preparing for retirement ■ Adjusting to children's moving into new phases of adulthood, marriage or other relationship, and childbearing and to becoming a grandparent	Adult
Middle-aged couple (with no children)	■ Accepting that it may be too late to reconsider childbearing or child rearing ■ Reaching the peak of a career or realizing that the peak may not occur ■ Planning for retirement	*None*
Aging family (applies to family with no children)	■ Adjusting to retirement and changes associated with aging ■ Adjusting to the loss of a spouse and friendships	Adult *(or none)*

Source: Adapted from Friedman, M. M., Bowden, V. R., & Jones, E. G. (2003). *Family nursing: Research, theory, and practice* (5th ed.). Upper Saddle River, NJ: Prentice Hall; Hanson, S., Gedaly-Duff, V., & Kaakinen, J. (Eds.). (2005). *Family health care nursing: Theory, practice, and research* (3rd ed.). Philadelphia: F.A. Davis; McGoldrick, M., & Carter, E. (1985). The family life cycle: Its stages and dislocations. In J. Henslin (Ed.), *Marriage and family in a changing society* (4th ed.). New York: Free Press, pp. 372–389.

STANDARDIZED LANGUAGE

NOC Outcomes and NIC Interventions for Caregiver Role Strain

NOC OUTCOMES	NIC MAJOR INTERVENTIONS
Caregiver Emotional Health	Caregiver Support, Coping Enhancement
Caregiver Lifestyle Disruption	Caregiver Support, Respite Care
Caregiver-Patient Relationship	Coping Enhancement, Role Enhancement
Caregiver Performance: Direct Care	Teaching: Disease Process; Teaching: Prescribed Diet; Teaching: Prescribed Medication
Caregiver Performance: Indirect Care	Decision-Making Support, Health System Guidance
Caregiver Physical Health	Energy Management, Nutrition Management
Caregiver Well-Being	Caregiver Support, Respite Care

Source: Johnson, M., Bulechek, G., Butcher, H., et al. (2012). *NANDA, NOC, and NIC linkages* (3rd ed.). St. Louis, MO: C.V. Mosby. Used with permission.

CLINICALREASONING

Applying the Full-Spectrum Nursing Model

PATIENT SITUATION

Sandra Jackson is the 22-year-old single mother of an 18-month-old child. She has type 1 diabetes mellitus. Sugar control has been unstable at times, primarily during times of stress and illness. Sandra lives with her mother, two younger sisters, and a brother. At times her boyfriend will stay in the home, depending on the status of their relationship. Sandra works part-time at a retail chain, struggling to meet the financial responsibilities of rearing a child. She is showing physical signs of depression and distress (e.g., apathy, anorexia, excessive sleeping, and episodes of crying). Sandra says to you during your home visit, "Something is really wrong with me. I can't snap out of this feeling of darkness. Life is too hard for me and is nothing but pain. I can't take it anymore and want it to be over." You believe she needs immediate mental health support.

THINKING

1. *Theoretical Knowledge:*
   a. What facts and principles do you already know about stress and depression?
   b. How does the emotional well-being of one family member affect others living in the home and the family as a whole?
2. *Critical Thinking (Inquiry):*
   a. What factors in Sandra's life are possibly contributing to her feelings of hopelessness and thoughts of self-harm?
   b. Name at least three nursing diagnoses that would best suit Sandra's health needs.

DOING

3. *Practical Knowledge:* Based on the knowledge you have about stress and depression, (see #1 above) how would you explain to the family about how best to support Sandra?
4. *Nursing Process (Evaluation):* What measures would you identify to determine whether your nursing plan of care was effective?

CARING

5. *Self-Knowledge:*
   a. How comfortable would you be caring for a patient who is at risk for self- injury?
   b. What is one problem with Sandra and her family, not described in the scenario, that could possibly arise?
6. *Ethical Knowledge:* What ethical concerns might you have for a woman with a young child who is at risk for self-injury, but has no financial resources to cover the expenses of mental health care?

Critical Thinking and Clinical Reasoning

1. You are caring for a 58-year-old woman who was admitted for surgery of the foot. Today is the second day you have cared for the patient. You notice that the family seems quiet and subdued. You ask the client whether something is wrong. She says that her 29-year-old niece just lost her job as a TV programming assistant because her employer found out she is HIV positive. Apparently the diagnosis was revealed on her health insurance claim forms when they were processed.
   a. Name two things in this scenario that you, as a nurse, *cannot* change.
   b. Do the client and family have a problem that you *can* help them with? How could you find out?
   c. Imagine you were your client (the aunt). What concerns would you have?
   d. Try to depict this situation by using systems theory. Draw circles for each system involved and show where they interact.
   e. Use your self-knowledge. What biases or values do you have that might affect your thinking in this case, either positively or negatively?
2. You are the nurse in the intensive care unit (ICU) who is caring for a 45-year-old man who was involved in a serious car accident. He suffered severe head trauma and, if he lives, probably will have serious deficits. He was admitted 24 hours ago and has not made significant improvements. The family is aware of his status and likely outcome.
   a. What are some concerns this family might have?
   b. Using structural-functional theory, describe how this family might be affected.
   c. How could you help this family?

3. You are the nurse in the emergency department caring for a 3-year-old child who experienced a fall. The child will be fine and is being discharged. As you are reviewing the discharge instructions, the mother reveals that she and the child spent the previous night in a hotel because of violence in the home. She tells you that her husband (the child's stepfather) drinks excessively and at times has become violent, hitting her but not the child. She did not call him when they went to the emergency room, and is afraid to go home.
   a. What do you think this woman's main concerns might be?
   b. Do you think this is a common or an unusual problem?
   c. What is the developmental stage of this family?
   d. What theoretical knowledge do you need to help this family?
   e. What kinds of help do you think this woman might need if she decides to escape from her husband?
   f. How could you help her at this moment?
4. For each of the following concepts, use critical thinking to describe how or why it is important to nursing, patient care, or the family. Note that these are *not* to be merely definitions.

Family relationships
Blended families
Communication
Systems theory
Structural–functional theories
Developmental theory
Family interactional theory
Family as the unit of care
Family health risk factors
The national economy
Health beliefs
Family coping mechanisms
Unexpected illness

What Are the Main Points in This Chapter?

- *Family* is not limited to the traditional definition of husband, wife, and their children; defined more broadly, it is a group of individuals who provide physical, emotional, economic, and/or spiritual support while maintaining involvement in each other's lives.
- Families are structured in a variety of ways. Three examples are the traditional nuclear family, dual-earner families, and single-parent families.
- Family nursing views the family from three perspectives: as the context for care of an individual, as the unit of care, and as a system.
- Wellness of each member is critical to the health of the family unit.
- Under general systems theory, the family is viewed as a system in interaction with other systems (e.g., other families, groups, communities, and individuals).
- Under structural–functional theories, families are viewed as social systems with a focus on outcomes.
- Developmental theories focus on family stages: beginning family, childbearing family, family with preschool children, family with school-age children, family with teenagers and young adults, family launching young adults, postparental family, and aging family.
- Family interactional theory views the family as a unit of interacting personalities with a major emphasis on family roles.
- The family teaches health beliefs, values, and behaviors to its individual members.
- Assessment of family communication patterns consists of interviewing the family and the individual seeking care, as well as astute observation by the nurse.
- How families cope with everyday life situations and hospitalization can influence the effectiveness of care rendered.
- Nurses can promote family wellness by addressing both individual and family concerns.
- The family can be a source of support or a source of difficulties for the ill person.

Knowledge Map

FAMILY RISK FACTORS
- Adapting to new roles
- Financial needs
- Adolescent's risk-taking behaviors
- Children leaving home
- Illness
- Sandwich generation

CHALLENGES TO HEALTH
- Poverty
- Disease
- Homelessness
- Violence
- HIV/AIDS
- Developmental changes

interrelated

FAMILY STRUCTURES
- Single parent
- Without children
- Extended
- Single individuals
- Gay and lesbian couples
- Families with adopted and foster children

occur in response to; and modify

FAMILY COPING PATTERNS

affect

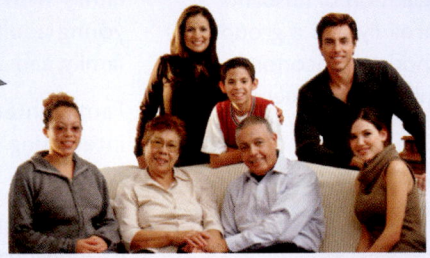

guide thinking about

FAMILY THEORIES
- General systems theory
- Structural–functional theories
- Developmental theories
- Family interactional theory

influence and reflect

FAMILY COMMUNICATION PATTERNS

FAMILY HEALTH

INDICATORS OF FAMILY HEALTH
- State of family well-being
- Sense of belonging and connectedness
- Shared responsibility
- Trust and respect
- Spending time together, sharing rituals and traditions
- Flexibility
- Commitment: working together to maintain the family
- Spiritual well-being
- Respect for privacy of individual members
- Positive, effective communication
- Ability to compromise and disagree
- Appreciation and affection for each other
- Responding to the needs and interests of all members
- Egalitarian distribution of power
- Health-promoting lifestyle of individual members

HOLISTIC FAMILY NURSING

CHAPTER 15

Culture & Ethnicity

STUDENT RESOURCES

The questions and exercises in Volume 2 allow you to practice the kind of thinking you will use as a full-spectrum nurse. Critical-thinking questions usually have more than one correct answer, so we do not provide "answers" for these features. It is more important to develop your nursing judgment than to just cover content. You will learn by discussing the questions with your peers. If you are still unsure, consult your instructor. You will find Response Sheets (for writing your responses to the questions) on DavisPlus.

To explore learning resources for this chapter,

Go to Davis*Plus* at DavisPl.us/Wilkinson3.

Chapter Resources for Chapter 15:

- **Response sheets for all learning activities**
- **Resources for Caregivers and Health Professionals**
- **Reading More About Culture & Ethnicity (suggested readings)**
- **Concept Map of chapter content**

Interactive Case Studies

NCLEX-Style and Chapter Review Questions

CHAPTER OVERVIEW

For a podcast of an overview of this chapter,

Go to Student Resources: Chapter 15, **Podcast—Chapter Overview,** on Davis*Plus*.

Caring for the Nguyens

Review the initial assessment of Nam Nguyen, found just before Chapter 1.

A. How might the Nguyens' cultural heritage affect their health beliefs?

B. What factors would you want to consider when performing a cultural assessment of the Nguyen family?

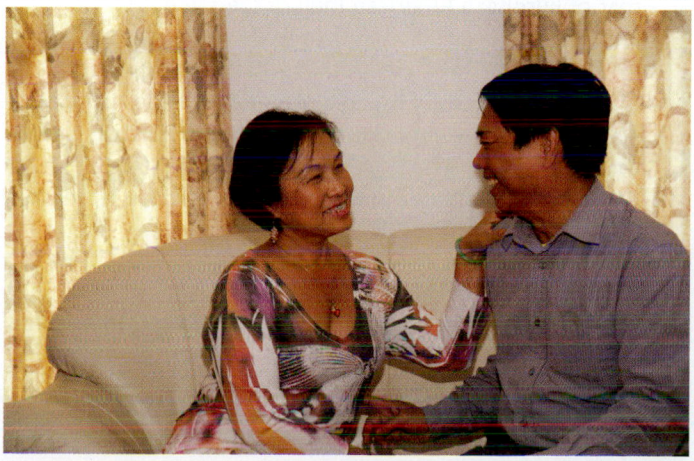

Practical Knowledge knowing how

Information in this section may be useful for assessing and communicating with clients of cultures different from your own.

CLINICAL INSIGHTS

Clinical Insight 15-1 ➤ Assessing for Biological Variations

People differ genetically and physiologically. Some biological variations create susceptibility to certain diseases and injuries. The following are examples:

Body Build and Structure

- 12% of Native Americans have 25 vertebrae instead of 24, which relates to an increased number of back problems.
- The lower a person's socioeconomic status, the more likely he is to be obese.
- Black and white men are on average about 3.5 inches taller than Asian American men and 2 inches taller than Mexican American men.

Skin Color

- Darker skin challenges the nurse to be more observant when assessing skin color changes (e.g., when assessing oxygenation or skin rashes). Obtain a baseline skin color by asking a family member or someone who knows the patient well.
- To assess for oxygenation and cyanosis in dark-skinned people, examine the sclera, buccal mucosa, tongue, lips, nailbeds, palms of the hands, and soles of the feet.
- To assess for jaundice in Asians, examine the sclera.

Vital Signs

- The average systolic blood pressure of black men between the ages of 35 and 65 is 5 mm Hg higher than that of European American men of the same age.

Laboratory Tests

- Native Americans, Hispanic Americans, and Japanese Americans, on average, have higher blood glucose levels than do whites.
- Bone density is greater in whites than in Chinese, Japanese, and Eskimos.

Susceptibility to Disease

- Blacks have a higher incidence of hypertension and sickle cell anemia than do other groups.
- Asian Americans have a higher incidence of tuberculosis compared with the white population.
- Blacks, Native Americans, and Mexican Americans are more likely to have diabetes mellitus than their white counterparts.

Nutritional Variations

- All groups demonstrate food preferences.
- Soy sauce, used in many Asian foods, is high in sodium.
- There is a high incidence of diabetes mellitus in areas where sugar cane is a major crop.

Enzymatic and Genetic Variations and Body Secretions

- Lactose intolerance, caused by a deficiency of the enzyme lactase, is more commonly seen in blacks, Native Americans, and Asians.

Drug Metabolism

- Native Americans and Asians are more likely to experience facial flushing and palpitations after ingesting alcohol.
- Blacks metabolize alcohol, nicotine, antihypertensives, and beta blockers differently from European Americans; they are more susceptible to side effects of haloperidol and tricyclic antidepressants; and they respond better to diuretic therapy than do whites.
- Asian Americans tend to experience more gastrointestinal side effects from opiates, even though the analgesic effect is less.
- Chinese Americans are more sensitive to the cardiovascular effects of propranolol; they have increased absorption of antipsychotics, antihypertensives, and some narcotics.
- Recall that most drug studies in the past were normed on European Americans, so "variations" refer to differences from those norms.

Practice Resources

Andrews, M. M., & Boyle, J. S. (2011); Purnell, L. D., & Paulanka, B. J. (2008); Spector, R. E. (2013); Suzuki, L. A., & Ponterotto, J. G. (2007).

Clinical Insight 15-2 ➤ Pain Perception in Selected Cultural Groups

The following are some general cultural beliefs about and responses to pain. Remember that these are only a starting point (archetypes) and that you must never stereotype a person on the basis of culture. Assess each person individually.

Cultural Group	Pain Perception and Responses
Black heritage	Depending on the religion, may believe that pain is inevitable and must be endured; therefore, may tolerate a great deal of pain. Depending on the religion, may seek prayers and the laying on of hands for pain relief. May see pain as a test of faith. May see pain as the only sign of illness or disease, so may not follow medical therapies (e.g., for hypertension) if pain is absent.
European American heritage, New England subculture	(These are chronic pain responses.) Copes by working and keeping busy. Stoicism; lack of expressiveness and behavioral pain response, including little wincing and groaning. Pain is viewed as a biological abnormality that can be treated and lived with; may be angry with care providers if treatment is ineffective. *Polish American subgroup*: Strong tendency for nonexpressiveness.
Arab heritage	View pain as unpleasant and something to be controlled. Expect medical science to be able to relieve their suffering. Express pain openly with family members, less so with health professionals. This may cause the nurse to evaluate pain relief as adequate even though the family may be demanding more medication for the patient.
Chinese heritage	Pain expression is similar to traditional U.S. culture, but description of pain may be different (i.e., described more often as "dull" and "diffuse"). Use external pain relief methods, such as massage, oils, warmth, and relaxation.
Filipino heritage	View pain as a part of living an honorable life or as an opportunity to atone for sins. Commonly tolerate severe pain, with stoic acceptance. May not complain of pain or ask for interventions.
Irish heritage	Value stoic response to pain. Ignore, deny, or minimize pain. Delay seeking treatment.
Italian heritage	Verbalization of pain is common and acceptable, even with chronic pain. Women are especially likely to report and express pain. Expect immediate treatment for pain.
Japanese heritage	It is a virtue, and a matter of family honor, to bear pain without expressing it. There may be taboos against use of narcotics for pain relief. May be more accepting of analgesics if reassured that pain control enhances healing.
Jewish heritage	Verbalization of pain is common and acceptable. Knowing the reason for pain is as important as obtaining relief.
Mexican heritage	View pain as the will of God or a part of life. May view pain as punishment for immoral behavior. May view enduring pain as a sign of strength. May endure pain longer and report it less frequently than other groups, or may express vocally with groaning and crying out. May delay seeking help for pain, hoping it will go away. May interpret pain as a loss of manhood or provider role.

(Continued)

Clinical Insight 15-2 ➤ Pain Perception in Selected Cultural Groups—cont'd

Navajo Indian heritage	View pain as a part of life. Do not express pain openly. May hide the intensity of their pain. May not request pain medication. May prefer herbal medications for pain.
Puerto Rican heritage	Loud and outspoken expression of pain is not an exaggeration, but a socially learned coping mechanism. May experience low self-esteem because of pain. Older or rural people may not be able to interpret pain-rating scales. Most prefer oral or intravenous analgesics to intramuscular or rectal routes. Many use herbal teas, heat, and prayer to manage pain.

Practice Resources

Andrews, M. M., & Boyle, J. S. (2011); Bates (1996); Giger, J. N., & Davidhizar, R. (2008); Purnell, L. (2012); Spector, R. E. (2013); Todd, K. (1996); Zborowski, M. (1952).

Clinical Insight 15-3 ➤ Communicating With Clients Who Speak a Different Language

When possible, use a qualified interpreter or a translator.

An **interpreter** is specially trained to provide the meaning behind spoken words from one language to another, whereas a **translator** merely restates into the targeted language. An interpreter can serve as a cultural broker by conveying the client's responses to questions, and by providing general information about the client's culture (Munoz & Luckmann, 2005).

When using any type of interpreter, it is important to do the following:

- Because of confidentiality issues, avoid asking a family member, especially a child or spouse, to act as an interpreter.
- Avoid using an interpreter who is socially or politically incompatible with the client (e.g., you would not ask an Israeli to interpret for a Palestinian).
- Be aware of gender and age differences. (It usually is preferable to have an interpreter of the same gender as the client.)
- Have the interpreter spend some time alone with the patient.
- Ask the interpreter to interpret the words used by the healthcare provider as closely as possible, except where literal translation might be offensive or misunderstood. In such cases, an interpreter (as compared with a translator) would provide the meaning of your words in terms acceptable to the client.
- Do not use metaphors ("happy as a clam") or medical jargon.
- Observe nonverbal communication (e.g., body language) when the client is listening and talking to the interpreter.
- Address your questions to the client, not the interpreter.
- Maintain eye contact with both the client and interpreter.
- Speak slowly and distinctly, facing the client; do not speak loudly.
- Ask one question at a time; allow time for interpretation and response from the client before asking another question.
- Use active rather than passive voice (e.g., say, "The doctor will see you tomorrow." rather than "You will be seen by the doctor tomorrow.")
- Be aware that many clients can understand more English words than they can express.
- Have health education materials translated into the client's language, or have an interpreter audiotape or videotape instructions.

If there is no one available to interpret for you:

In addition to the strategies listed above, Munoz and Luckmann (2005) suggest the following:

- Greet the client with respect. Greet the person formally, using Mr., Ms., and so forth, until given permission to do otherwise. People in some groups consider it disrespectful to use a person's first name.
- Identify the client's primary language, and use any words that you are familiar with in her language to show that you are trying to communicate.
- Use the Internet or computer software to translate words into the client's native language.
- If appropriate, use a third language that both of you speak. For example, some Vietnamese and some Cambodians speak French.
- Speak slowly and clearly, using simple sentences to talk about one question or need at a time.
- Use gestures to help convey meaning.
- Restate in different words, if needed.
- Use pictures or diagrams.
- Be aware that some clients may answer yes even if they don't understand what you have said.

Practice Resources

Munoz, C., & Luckmann, J. (2005); Purnell, L. D. (2012).

ASSESSMENT GUIDELINES AND TOOLS

Focused Assessment

Obtaining Minimum Cultural Information

You should obtain at least this much cultural information from every client. For some, you may need a more in-depth assessment.

- Begin the interview with open-ended questions, such as the following:

  I would like to know more about your family.

  Who will be able to help you when you go home?

  What do you do to help keep yourself well?

- When you and the client are comfortable, be sure to ask a question such as, "What concerns you the most about your illness and treatment?" This allows you to focus on the individual rather than just on his culture.
- You will not need to perform an in-depth cultural assessment on every patient, but you will need to recognize situations in which this is needed. Lipson and Meleis (1985) suggest that the following minimum information is important:

Language(s) spoken; proficiency in the language of the host country	➤ What language(s) do you speak? ➤ Are you comfortable speaking [English], or would you like to have an interpreter?
Length of time client has been here; where client was raised	➤ Where were you raised? ➤ How long have you lived here?
Ethnic affiliation and identity	➤ With what racial and ethnic group(s) do you identify? ➤ How closely do you identify with the values of those groups?
Usual religious practices	➤ What religion do you practice, if any? ➤ Are there any special beliefs, rituals or practices you want us to be aware of?
Nonverbal communication style	➤ You will need to observe the patient and draw on your theoretical knowledge of the patient's cultural group for this information.
Family roles, primary decision maker	➤ Who is in your family? ➤ What is your role in your family? ➤ Who makes most of the decisions? ➤ How are decisions made in your family? ➤ Who should I talk to for decisions about your healthcare?
Social support in the new country	➤ Do you have family and friends here? ➤ Who can you go to when you need help? ➤ Where do you work? ➤ Will you need any help with your healthcare expenses?

Practice Resources

Giger, J. N., & Davidhizar, R. (2008); Giger, J. (2012); Lipson, J., & Meleis, A. (1985); Spector, R. E. (2013); Suzuki, L. A., & Ponterotto, J. G. (2007).

Focused Assessment

Cultural Assessment Using the Transcultural Assessment Model

Assess information listed in the following categories.

Cultural Uniqueness

- Cultural and ethnic identification
- Place of birth
- Time in country

Communication

- Voice quality
- Pronunciation and enunciation
- Use of silence
- Use of nonverbal communication
- Touch
- Spoken language

Space

- Degree of comfort
- Distance in conversations
- Definition of space
- Body movement

Social Organization

- Normal state of health
- Marital status
- Number of children
- Parents living or deceased
- Friends
- Work
- Leisure

Time

- Orientation to time
- View of time
- Physiochemical reaction to time

Environmental Control

- Locus of control
- Value orientation
- Health and illness beliefs

Biological Variations

- Physical assessment (including body structure, skin color, skin discoloration, hair color and distribution, other visible physical characteristics, weight, height, lab variances)
- Susceptibility to illness
- Nutritional preferences
- Psychological characteristics

Other

In addition to the Giger and Davidhizar categories, obtain information about the following:

- Educational experiences (formal and informal)
- Family patterns of healthcare
- Family role and function
- Healthcare beliefs and practices (folk and professional)
- Religious practices and beliefs
- Social networks
- Values orientation

Source: Adapted from Giger, J. N., & Davidhizar, R. E. (2008). *Transcultural nursing: Assessment and intervention* (5th ed.). St. Louis, MO: C.V. Mosby.

CLINICALREASONING

Applying the Full-Spectrum Nursing Model

PATIENT SITUATION

Mrs. Vasquez, a 70-year-old Mexican American woman, has diabetes mellitus and has come to the hospital because of a sore on her lower leg that will not heal. Mrs. Vasquez, a widow, cares for herself at home. She speaks only broken English and has some difficulty understanding your questions. After great effort on your part, you determine that she has missed her last appointment with her diabetes specialist because she has no transportation, so she has just been putting a dressing on the sore. Mrs. Vasquez tells you that she loves to see her grandchildren, who visit often, and that she enjoys cooking and eating Mexican food. She also says that she believes she is sick because she has not pleased God. However, God is a source of comfort and assurance to her. She prays a lot and has rosary beads in her hand.

THINKING

1. *Theoretical Knowledge (Recall of Facts and Principles):* List six important culture specifics.
2. *Critical Thinking (Application of Knowledge):* Based on your theoretical knowledge, what are your expectations about communicating with Mrs. Vasquez?
3. *Critical Thinking (Compare and Contrast):* Compare your expectations to the actual data you have about her ability to communicate.

DOING

4. *Nursing Process (Assessment):* What are some pertinent cultural data that you should assess for Mrs. Vasquez?
5. *Nursing Process (Analysis/Diagnosis):* Which nursing diagnosis do you think would be best for planning Mrs. Vasquez's care? (Recall that the etiology should suggest your nursing interventions, and the diagnostic label should suggest the expected patient outcomes.) Explain your reasoning.
   - Noncompliance (with clinic appointments) r/t lack of transportation
   - Impaired Skin Integrity r/t self-treatment of ulcer
   - Noncompliance (with clinic appointments) r/t beliefs about God and illness

CARING

6. *Self-Knowledge:* What areas of commonality do you have with Mrs. Vasquez, around which you might form a caring relationship?
7. *Self-Knowledge:* Do you agree with Mrs. Vasquez that illness may be caused by displeasing God?
8. *Ethical Knowledge:* Suppose you do not agree with Mrs. Vasquez that she is ill because she has displeased God. Discuss whether you would explain to her that this is most likely not true and then teach her about the cause of diabetic ulcers.

Critical Thinking and Clinical Reasoning

1. Mrs. Vasquez, a 70-year-old Mexican American woman, has diabetes mellitus and has come to the hospital because of a sore on her lower leg that will not heal. Review the details of Mrs. Vasquez's case in the Full Spectrum Nursing Model Situation, preceding.
   a. Identify Mrs. Vasquez's cultural data and group it under the following culture specifics:

      Communication

      Space

      Time orientation

      Social organization

      Environmental control

      Biological variations

b. What does your theoretical knowledge lead you to expect about Mrs. Vasquez's personal space? What, if any, actual patient data do you have about that?
c. What does your theoretical knowledge lead you to expect about her time orientation, social organization, and environmental control? Compare your expectations with the actual patient data that you have.
d. What theoretical knowledge do you have regarding biological variations among Hispanic people? How does this compare to the actual data, if any, that you have for Mrs. Vasquez?
e. You have learned that cultural data can have implications for nursing care. Answer each of the following:
   - What additional information should you assess for in this situation?
   - What biases do you have that affect your thinking in this situation?

2. An Asian woman comes to your clinic for assessment of her blood pressure. In casual conversation, she tells you that her oldest daughter is about to be married. She reveals that her daughter has some type of anemia for which she needs medication. She tells you that she has recently heard terrible stories about sickle-cell anemia and is afraid that this is what her daughter has.
   a. What additional data do you need to collect in order to answer this client's questions?
   b. What are the biological variations that normally affect this cultural group?
   c. What assurances, if any, can you give this client about her daughter?
3. At times we must care for clients who do not speak our language. This poses a challenge to the nurse who strives to provide culturally competent care to all clients. Even with the assistance of interpreters, this can be difficult because of such barriers as differing dialects, street talk, and jargon. Keeping these facts in mind, answer the following questions:
   a. What options do you have when you encounter a person who cannot speak English?
   b. How do you communicate with such a client if no interpreter is available?
   c. What biases do you have about such a situation? Why?
4. Alma is of European descent; she is Caucasian. She is a Roman Catholic and believes abortion is wrong. She believes that it should be illegal to own a gun. She is a nursing student.

   Violetta's parents came to the United States from Europe. They were born in France. Before that, her great-grandparents lived in Africa. Violetta is an African American. She is Roman Catholic, and she believes that abortion is wrong. She believes that it should be illegal to own a gun. She is a nursing student.

   Darcy is of European descent. She is Caucasian. She laughs at the idea of religion, saying, "Nobody's 'up there' looking out for me; and when you're dead, you're dead." Darcy is a gang member and carries a gun in her purse or her pocket at all times. She did not finish high school, and by the age of 19 she had had two abortions.

   All of the women live in the United States. Which two women do you think share the most cultural commonalities? Explain your thinking.
5. Helen is a 52-year-old divorced African American. Her only child, Tamika, is incarcerated for prostitution and possession of narcotics. Helen is now raising her two grandchildren, Calvin, age 13 years, and Jevetta, age 2. Helen is a nursing assistant at the local hospital. It's hard for her to make ends meet because she has hypertension and diabetes, for which she takes a number of medications, including insulin—that is, when she can afford them. Helen has not applied for medical assistance because she believes she should be able to take care of herself, but she does receive assistance for Jevetta's day-care costs. In addition to her grandchildren, Helen has a large group of friends, many of whom attend her church. She has little time to spend with her friends since she took custody of the children. Jevetta has been admitted to the hospital for asthma. You are Jevetta's student nurse.
   a. Using your data collection skills, identify NANDA-I diagnostic labels that you could apply to Jevetta and to Helen as Jevetta's caregiver.
   b. What resources may be helpful to Helen?
6. Examine the following nursing diagnosis labels. For this set of labels, write an etiology that might be caused by cultural differences. The first one is completed for you as an example.
   - Imbalanced Nutrition: Less than (or More Than) Body Requirements *r/t patient's lack of knowledge about how to adapt his preferred ethnic foods to her prescribed low-fat diet.*
   - Ineffective Health Maintenance
   - Ineffective Role Performance
   - Anxiety
   - Powerlessness
   - Deficient Knowledge

7. For the following set of labels, explain or give an example of how the nurse might misdiagnose or misperceive the data because of cultural differences. The first one is done for you.

- Decisional Conflict

The nurse might ask a woman to make some decision about her care. The woman may seem very indecisive and unable to reach a conclusion. The reason may be that the husband is the decision maker in the family. When the husband arrives, the Decisional Conflict ("problem") may disappear.

- Confusion
- Readiness for Enhanced Breastfeeding or Ineffective Breastfeeding
- Impaired Social Interaction
- Social Isolation
- Noncompliance
- Pain (Acute or Chronic)

8. For each of the following concepts, use critical thinking to describe how or why it is important to nursing, patient care, or cultural competence. Note that these are *not* to be merely definitions.

Culture
Subculture
Ethnicity
Race
Religion
Acculturation
Health and illness belief
Health and illness practice
Phenomena of culture
Ethnocentric
Folk medicine
Cultural competence
Transcultural nursing
Giger and Davidhizar assessment model
Biological variations among cultures
Prejudice and racism
Professional (e.g., nursing) subculture
Cultural sensitivity
Cultural awareness
Culture universals
Culture specifics

What Are the Main Points in This Chapter?

- The cultural and ethnic composition of North America has changed dramatically over the past several decades, making it essential that nurses understand the healthcare beliefs and practices of diverse populations.
- Culture includes shared values, beliefs, norms, and practices that guide a particular group's thinking, decision making, and actions in a patterned way.
- Through acculturation, most ethnic and cultural groups modify some of their traditional cultural characteristics, values, beliefs, and practices.
- You should be familiar with the common characteristics of different cultural groups in your community.
- The U.S. Census Bureau has identified the following racial categories on the 2010 Census questionnaire:

  White
  Black, African American, or Negro
  American Indian or Alaska Native
  Asian Indian
  Chinese
  Filipino
  Japanese
  Korean
  Vietnamese
  Other Asian
  Native Hawaiian
  Guamanian or Chamorro
  Samoan
  Other Pacific Islander (specify, e.g., Tongan)

- The Census Bureau (2010) categories for ethnicity (or "origin") are (1) Hispanic, Latino, or Spanish and (2) Not Hispanic, Latino, or Spanish. Subcategories under Hispanic origin are Mexican, Mexican American, Chicano; Puerto Rican; Cuban; and Another Hispanic, Latino, or Spanish origin.
- **Culture universals** (commonalities) are the values, beliefs, and practices that people from *all* cultures share. **Culture specifics** (diversities) are those values, beliefs, and practices that are unique to a culture.
- A **cultural archetype**, similar to a model, is an example of something that is recurrent and has its basis in facts. A **cultural stereotype** is a widely held but oversimplified and unsubstantiated belief that all people of a certain racial or ethnic group are alike in certain respects.
- Six organizing phenomena of culture that influence health include communication patterns, space, social organization, time, environmental control, and biological variations.

- Healthcare providers cannot understand the health beliefs and practices of diverse populations if they view them through the lens of the conventional (Western, U.S.) culture of healthcare.
- A variety of "alternative" healing systems exists. Remedies have been passed down from generation to generation and include the use of herbs, customs, and rituals.
- An understanding of cultural concepts, theories, and models can help you develop cultural competence.
- Ethnocentrism, stereotyping, prejudice, and racism are barriers to culturally competent care.
- When assessing a client and making nursing diagnoses, you must consider the client's cultural values, beliefs, and practices related to health and healthcare.
- Culturally competent care requires a nonjudgmental attitude, self-awareness, sensitivity, respect for differences, theoretical knowledge, and the desire to be culturally competent.

Knowledge Map

Culture & Ethnicity Concepts

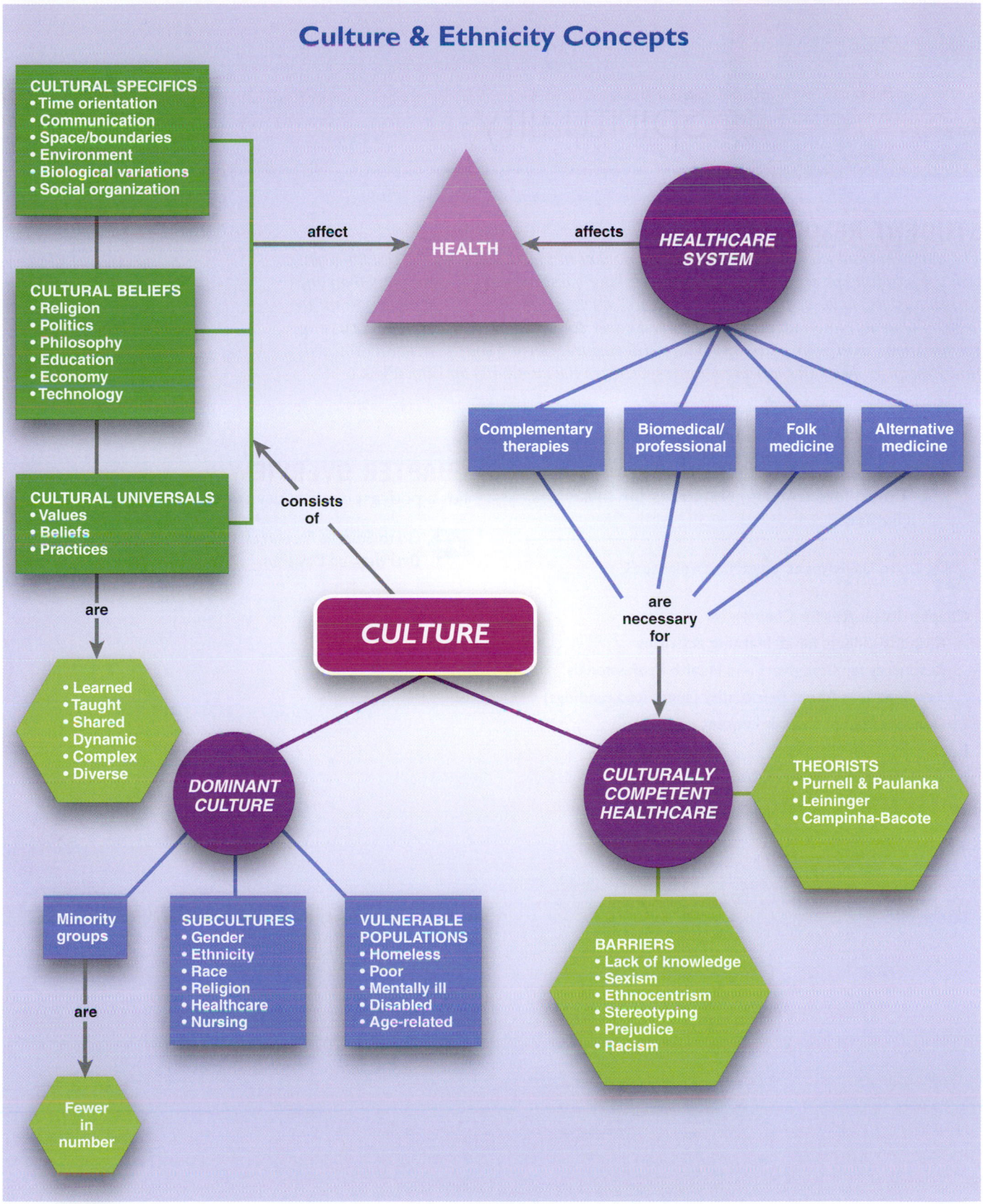

CHAPTER 16

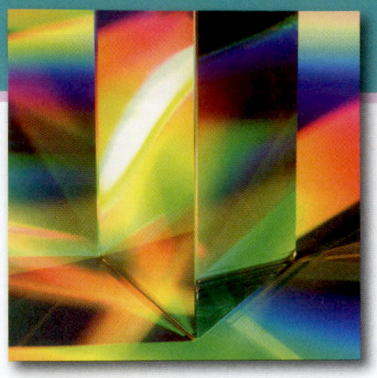

Spirituality

STUDENT RESOURCES

*The questions and exercises in Volume 2 allow you to practice the kind of thinking you will use as a full-spectrum nurse. Critical-thinking questions usually have more than one correct answer, so we do not provide "answers" for these features. It is more important to develop your nursing judgment than to just cover content. You will learn by discussing the questions with your peers. If you are still unsure, consult your instructor. You will find Response Sheets (for writing your responses to the questions) on Davis*Plus.

To explore learning resources for this chapter,

Go to Davis*Plus* at DavisPl.us/Wilkinson3.

Chapter Resources for Chapter 16:

- **Response sheets for all learning activities**
- **Resources for Caregivers and Health Professionals**
- **Reading More About Spirituality (suggested readings)**
- **Concept Map of chapter content**

Interactive Case Studies

NCLEX-Style and Chapter Review Questions

CHAPTER OVERVIEW

For a podcast of an overview of this chapter,

Go to Student Resources: Chapter 16, **Podcast—Chapter Overview,** on Davis*Plus*.

Caring for the Nguyens

Kim Phan is the 3-year-old grandson of Nam and Yen Nguyen. The Nguyens are both practicing Catholics. Kim's mother, Trinh, is the Nguyens' daughter. Trinh feels that Catholicism is "a waste of time" and does not attend church. Kim has had no formal religious experiences or training.

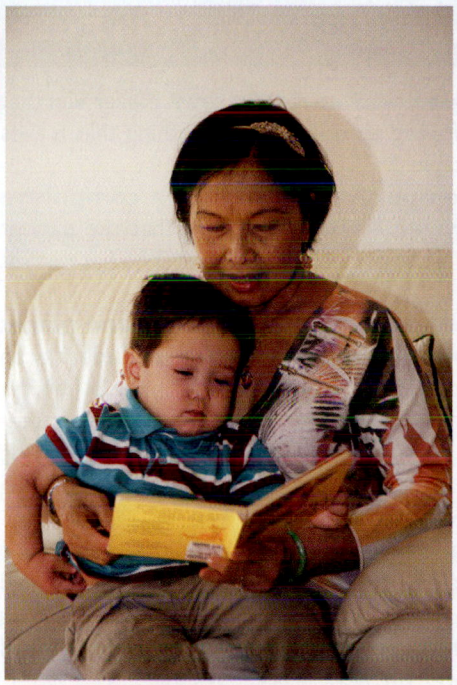

A. At a clinic visit, Nam asks you what you think about keeping religion away from a child. How would you respond?

B. Mr. Nguyen explains his views on the situation: "If anything were to happen to him, he would go to hell. I think we should take him to church and get him baptized right away. I don't know how anyone can live like that. He has no connection to God." Do you agree with this statement? Explain your views.

C. Nam asks you to pray for Kim and his mother. How would you feel about this situation? What would you say to Nam?

Practical Knowledge knowing how

In this section, you will find guidelines for performing spiritual interventions and for performing focused spiritual assessments.

CLINICAL INSIGHTS

Clinical Insight 16-1 ➤ Praying With Patients

Because there is a rich diversity in religious expression, keep the following guidelines in mind when you pray for or with patients:

Ask how the patient prefers to address the divine. Some people prefer the use of parental language in their prayers, for example, *Father God* or *Divine Mother*. Some use the word *Jehovah*, *Yahweh*, or *Allah*. Hindus may address one or more of multiple Gods, each of whom has several names. So don't be afraid to seek direction from the patient in these matters: Most people are honored to be able to explain their beliefs and practices to someone who is open to the experience.

Before the prayer begins, ask the patient whether any rituals or religious items are necessary. Muslims may want water to wash the mouth, nostrils, and hands before beginning prayer. Roman Catholics may want to hold their rosary beads while praying, and some Buddhists and Hindus meditate with a set of beads called a mala. Others may have a prayer cloth or other item that needs to be accessible.

(Continued)

Clinical Insight 16-1 ➤ Praying With Patients *(continued)*

Always feel free to pray or not to pray. Never feel that you are being forced to do or say something that makes you uncomfortable.

Do not be a compulsive "prayer" or a compulsive avoider of prayer. Always make sure that the patient (and/or family) is comfortable with prayer if he has not yet requested it.

Know that there are appropriate times and places for the offering of prayer. Prayer at the bedside may be most appropriate, although it may make people uncomfortable in a crowded waiting room. Perhaps the statement "I will be praying for you and your family" might be more appropriate for some patients than actually praying aloud at that moment.

When a patient asks for prayer, consider using this reply: "I would be honored to offer prayer. What would you like me to *especially* address in the prayer?" Knowing what the patient hopes for in prayer gives you an idea of the type of prayer the person is requesting.

When the patient tells you what he wants you to pray for, be sure to focus your prayer around the request.

- It is always good to summarize the results of previous conversations with the patient and his needs in the course of your prayer. For example, imagine that a patient with cancer who has been treated with chemotherapy now finds his blood counts are coming back to normal levels. The chemotherapy treatment seems successful at this point, but the patient is afraid of a relapse and asks you to pray for the cancer to be cured.
- Analyze the situation in terms of what has happened in the past, what is happening now, and what the patient is requesting. This will help you organize your thoughts and then put them into the form of a prayer.

Perhaps you would want to take the patient's hand in yours (if appropriate, based on your intuition and the nature of your nurse–patient relationship) and compose a prayer in the following manner:

Dear [Lord], I give you thanks that [John] has done so well with his treatments. Please continue to help him be strong and open to your healing presence. We pray for his family, doctors, and nurses that all may be a part of [John's] continued healing and sense of comfort. I pray that the treatments that he is receiving, together with the prayers that we are offering, may all be effective in his care and in the treatment of his cancer. Watch over [John], and visit us all at this time with your healing presence. [Amen.]

When a terminally ill patient requests a prayer for a cure, total healing, or a miracle, you may be challenged. Knowing how to offer prayers that are "realistic" allows for the occurrence of miracles and healings of all types while also keeping in perspective the physical realities of the nature of disease and the reality of death.

If composing a prayer is difficult for you, you may want to explore the use of the Psalms in the Hebrew Bible (Old Testament) or some New Testament scriptures, if appropriate for the patient. (See especially Psalms 43, 51, 67, 121). In terms of larger themes, the following sources for patients who profess Christianity may be helpful:

Forgiveness and guilt: Psalm 51, Isaiah 55:7, and Matthew 6:9–15
Comfort: Psalm 23, John 14
Hope: Psalm 42, Romans 15:4
Love and acceptance: Matthew 5:11
Caring: 1 Corinthians 12

For exact quotations of these passages,

Go to Chapter 16, **Psalms for Prayers,** on Davis*Plus*.

For patients of religions other than your own, ask whether they have examples of their sacred writings from which you might be allowed to read. Perhaps the patient has a favorite prayer or a text from an authoritative source that brings comfort and hope.

It is always good to include in the course of your prayer a request for God's help and direction with the patient's healthcare team. This expresses the reality that we are all working together for a common good and purpose and that we depend on God and others for our welfare and place in life.

Once the prayer is over, thank the patient for asking you to participate. In that way you can ask whether you can be of any further assistance.

Focused Assessment

S-P-I-R-I-T Assessment

- Obtain information from the patient when possible.
- For an emergency admission or if the patient cannot give information, consult the next of kin or a designated power of attorney (DPOA) as soon as possible for information.

S—Spiritual/religious belief system

Religion, tradition, sect, or denominational affiliation

Text/writing(s) that provide source of authority and codes for behavior

Name and phone number of supporting or affiliated church, synagogue, temple, or other place of worship

Past experience with a belief system (positive or negative)

Beliefs related to health, illness, healthcare, healthcare providers, Western medicine, adjuvant therapies, herbal or natural healing methods or techniques

Beliefs about suffering, terminal or chronic illness, advance directives, autopsy, organ donation

Stigmas related to illness, if applicable

P—Personal spirituality

Individual beliefs and practices of affiliation that the patient or family accepts and attempts to follow (may be directly or indirectly related to above assessment areas)

Individual beliefs that may differ or even be contrary to affiliation beliefs

Whether spirituality is a part of personal experience of religion or a separate entity

Level of comfort discussing spirituality

Whether personal spirituality is viewed positively or negatively at the present time

I—Integration within a spiritual community

Name and title of religious or spiritual leader or authority figure(s)

Names and titles of religious groups that may need to be contacted: Stephen Ministry, prayer group leader, prayer chain support person, shaman, medicine man or woman, men's or women's group within denomination

Role of patient or individual in any of above named groups

R—Ritualized practices and restrictions

Activities that patient's or family's faith encourages or forbids

Needs for modesty and covering of body parts or appendages

Any special beliefs or needs in relation to drawing blood or to laboratory tests or procedures

Dietary needs and restrictions: food preferences, preparation of foods, and location of food preparation areas

Gender-specific roles and responsibilities of care providers

Prayer needs and restrictions: Who delivers and offers such practices?

Articles or other materials needed for worship, devotion, or prayer (rosaries, prayer beads, prayer books, religious tracts, Bibles, crosses, prayer shawls or cloths)

I—Implications for medical care

Beliefs and practices that healthcare providers should remember while providing care

Specific medications that may not be administered and withheld; implications for pain control

Specific medical procedures or products that may not be administered (abortion, blood products)

Communication patterns and needs for effective care delivery: Who makes decisions? What is the role of parents or guardians when children or other vulnerable populations are the recipients of care? Does the guardian reflect the beliefs of patient, if these are known?

T—Terminal events planning

Wishes for advance directives (cardiopulmonary resuscitation, intubation, ventilator assist, feeding tubes)

Wishes for transplantation or organ donation

Need for religious services (last rites, ministries of healing, baptism, initiation, confession, communion)

Clergy or ministry groups to be contacted and when

Ideas of an afterlife

Treatment of the body at the time of death

Funeral planning

Source: Adapted from Highfield, M. E. F. (2000). Providing spiritual care to patients with cancer. *Clinical Journal of Oncology Nursing, 4*(3), 115–120.

ASSESSMENT GUIDELINES AND TOOLS

Focused Assessment

The HOPE Approach to Spiritual Assessment: Examples of Questions

Mnemonic	Examples of Questions
H—Sources of **hope**, meaning, comfort, strength, peace, love and connection	What are your sources of internal support? What do you hold onto to get you through difficult times? For some people, religious or spiritual beliefs are a source of comfort in dealing with life's ups and downs. Is this true for you?
O—Organized religion	Do you belong to a religious or spiritual community? Does it help you? How important is this to you? What aspects of your religion are helpful to you?
P—Personal spirituality/ Practices	Do you believe in God? What is your relationship with God? Do you have personal spiritual beliefs that are not a part of organized religion? If so, what are they? What aspects of your spirituality are most helpful to you (e.g., meditation, prayer, reading scripture, listening to music, nature)?
E—Effects on medical care and end-of-life issues	Has your illness affected your relationship with God? Or to do the things that usually help you spiritually? Are you concerned about conflicts between your beliefs and your healthcare treatment plan? Do you have any dietary restrictions or other practices I should know about in planning your care? Would you like to speak to a clinical chaplain (or community spiritual leader)?

Source: Based on Gowri, A., & Hight, E. (2001). Spirituality and medical practice: Using the HOPE questions as a practical tool for spiritual assessment. *American Family Physician, 63*, 36–41.

STANDARDIZED NURSING LANGUAGE

Using Selected NIC Interventions and Activities to Support Spirituality

Nursing Diagnoses	
Moral Distress	Impaired Religiosity
Spiritual Distress	Risk for Impaired Religiosity
Risk for Spiritual Distress	Readiness for Enhanced Religiosity
Readiness for Enhanced Spiritual Well-Being	

NURSING INTERVENTIONS	NURSING ACTIVITIES
Dying Care	Facilitate obtaining spiritual support for patient and family. Support the patient and family through stages of grief (see Chapter 17). Facilitate discussion of funeral arrangements.
Emotional Support	Explore with the patient what has triggered emotions. Embrace or touch the patient supportively. Make supportive or empathetic statements. Encourage the patient to express feelings of anger, anxiety or sadness.
Forgiveness Facilitation	Listen empathetically without moralizing or offering platitudes. Explore forgiveness as a process.

Using Selected NIC Interventions and Activities to Support Spirituality—cont'd

NURSING INTERVENTIONS	NURSING ACTIVITIES
	Assist client to seek out an arbitrator (objective party) to facilitate the process of individual or group concern.
	Explore possibilities of making amends and reconciliation with self, others, and/or higher power.
Hope Inspiration	Assist the patient/family to identify areas of hope in life.
	Help the patient expand his spiritual self.
	Facilitate the patient/family's reliving and savoring past achievements and experiences.
	Create an environment that facilitates patient's practicing religion, as appropriate.
Presence	Be physically available as a helper.
	Remain physically present without expecting interactional responses.
	Offer to remain with the patient during the initial interaction with others in the unit.
	Listen to the patient's concerns.
	Stay with the patient to promote safety and reduce fear.
Religious Ritual Enhancement	Coordinate or provide healing services, communion, meditation, or prayer in the place of residence or other setting.
	Encourage the use of and participation in usual religious rituals or practices that are not detrimental to health.
	Assist with modifications of the ritual to meet the needs of the disabled or ill.
	Treat the individual with dignity and respect.
Self-Awareness Enhancement	Assist the patient to realize that everyone is unique.
	Assist the patient to identify life priorities.
	Assist the patient to identify guilty feelings.
	Assist the patient to identify his source of motivation.
Self-Esteem Enhancement	Encourage the patient to identify strengths.
	Provide experiences that increase the patient's autonomy, as appropriate.
	Explore previous achievements of success.
	Assist the patient to identify the significance of culture, religion, race, gender, and age on self-esteem.
	Monitor the frequency of self-negating verbalizations. Reinforce the personal strengths that the patient identifies.
Spiritual Growth Facilitation	Encourage conversation that assists the patient in sorting out spiritual concerns.
	Assist the patient with identifying barriers and attitudes that hinder growth or self-discovery.
	Offer individual and group prayer support, as appropriate.
	Encourage participation in devotional services, retreats, and special prayer/study programs.
	Assist the patient to explore beliefs as related to healing of body, mind, and spirit.
	Refer for pastoral care or primary spiritual caregiver as issues warrant.
Spiritual Support	Be open to the patient's expressions of loneliness and powerlessness.
	Encourage chapel service attendance, if desired.
	Provide desired spiritual articles, according to individual preferences.
	Be available to listen to the individual's feelings.
	Listen carefully to the individual's communication, and develop a sense of timing for prayer or spiritual rituals.
	Be open to the individual's feelings about illness and death.

continued

Using Selected NIC Interventions and Activities to Support Spirituality—cont'd

NURSING INTERVENTIONS	NURSING ACTIVITIES
Values Clarification	Consider the ethical and legal aspects of free choice, given the particular situation, before beginning the intervention. Pose reflective, clarifying questions that give the patient something to think about. Encourage the patient to make a list of what is important and not important in life and the time spent on each. Encourage the patient to list values that guide behavior in various settings and types of situations. Avoid use of the [preceding] intervention with persons with serious emotional problems.

Other NIC Spiritual Care Interventions

Active Listening	Crisis Intervention	Meditation Facilitation	Resiliency Promotion
Anticipatory Guidance	Decision-Making Support	Mood Management	Self-Esteem Enhancement
Anxiety Reduction	Emotional Support	Music Therapy	Self-Modification Assistance
Bibliotherapy	Grief Work Facilitation	Referral	Self-Responsibility Facilitation
Coping Enhancement	Guilt Work Facilitation	Role Enhancement	Support Group
Counseling	Humor	Religious Ritual Enhancement	Touch

Sources: Bulechek, G. M., Butcher, H. K., & Dochterman, J. M., et al. (Eds.). (2012). *Nursing interventions classification (NIC)* (6th ed.). St. Louis, MO: C.V. Mosby; and Gaskamp, C., Sutter, R., Meraviglia, M., et al. (2006). Evidence-based guideline: Promoting spirituality in the older adult. *Journal of Gerontological Nursing, 32*(11), 8–13.

CLINICALREASONING: Applying the Full-Spectrum Nursing Model

PATIENT SITUATION

Review the Meet Your Patient scenario to answer the questions below about Charles Johnson, a 75-year-old black man with newly diagnosed cancer of the lung. His physicians want to start chemotherapy to try to increase his life span. He is unsure whether he wants to have chemotherapy.

Go to Chapter 16, **Meet Your Patient,** in Volume 1.

THINKING

1. *Theoretical Knowledge (Recall of Facts and Principles):* Define *forgiveness,* and explain the benefits of forgiving self and others.
2. *Critical Thinking (Application of Knowledge)*: Based on your theoretical knowledge about forgiveness, with whom might Mr. Johnson need to reconcile? Why do you think so?

DOING

3. *Practical Knowledge (HOPE Assessment):* Use the Focused Assessment box, The HOPE Approach to Spiritual Assessment: Examples of Questions, and enter Mr. Johnson's data. Identify sections for which you need additional data.

CARING

4. *Self-Knowledge:* How is your religious background similar to or different from Mr. Johnson's?
5. *Self-Knowledge:* (a) How would you feel if Mr. Johnson said to you, "Church folk are all a bunch of hypocrites, if you ask me. I choose not to be a part of any of that"? (b) How would you respond?
6. *Ethical Knowledge:* Imagine that Mr. Johnson's sister comes to visit and leaves some religious pamphlets on a chair, where he will not see them before she leaves. What would you do?

Critical Thinking and Clinical Reasoning

1. A 5-year-old boy was admitted to the hospital last night with a fever of 103°F (39.4°C). He was diagnosed with a serious infection that is easily treated with intravenous (IV) antibiotics. However, his parents are Christian Scientists, and they do not want the boy to be given antibiotics. They have called their Christian Science practitioner to visit as soon as possible.
   a. What practical knowledge do you have that will give you some insight into this situation?
   b. What essential piece of knowledge do you need that is *not* given in this scenario?
   c. If the parents do not agree to accept IV antibiotics for their child, what can you do to (1) ensure that the child receives treatment and (2) support their spiritual needs?
2. A woman is admitted to the emergency department and gives birth to a premature baby boy who is in severe respiratory distress. The woman is a devout Roman Catholic. What interventions could you use to ensure holistic spiritual care in such an emergency situation?
3. Interview nurses in the area where you have your clinical experiences. Discuss the interviews with classmates.
   a. Ask them to describe spiritual problems their patients have had.
   b. Ask them to tell you of any spiritual interventions they have used with patients, and to evaluate their effectiveness.
   c. Ask them how comfortable they are in using spiritual interventions, especially prayer.
4. For each of the following concepts, use critical thinking to describe how or why it is important to nursing, patient care, or spirituality. Note that these are *not* to be merely definitions.
   Spirituality and religion
   Nursing research in religion and healthcare
   Major religions and healthcare
   The nurse and spirituality
   Assessment of the spiritual domain of care
   Spiritual care nursing interventions
   Spiritual well-being

What Are the Main Points in This Chapter?

- Spirituality is a powerful force in the lives of many patients.
- Nursing has historical roots in religion and spirituality.
- Religion is a sort of "map" that outlines and integrates essential beliefs, values, and codes of conduct into a manner of living.
- Spirituality, like a journey, takes place over time and involves the accumulation of life experiences and understandings.
- Religion and spirituality affect health and well-being; in turn, health and well-being affect a person's religion and spirituality.
- Research suggests that patients' beliefs in religion and spirituality are important to healthcare outcomes; however, it does not explain *how* or *why* this is so.
- The more you know about the world's major religions, the more you will be able to offer comprehensive, compassionate care to patients.
- People vary greatly in the degree to which they follow the rituals and practices of their own religion.
- Barriers to spiritual care include (1) lack of awareness of spirituality and your own spiritual belief system, (2) differences in spirituality between you (the nurse) and the patient, (3) fear that your spiritual knowledge is insufficient, and (4) fear of where spiritual discussions might lead.
- Nursing interventions related to spiritual care require you to be self-aware, fully present, supportive, empathetic, and nonjudgmental and to have a desire to benefit the patient.
- When a patient asks you to pray, determine whether he wishes you to pray *for* or *with* him, and ask what he would like you to *especially* address in the prayer.
- A miracle does not necessarily involve the notion of a cure; miracles are more often events that proceed according to natural law but still have a powerful impact on the person's expectations.

Knowledge Map

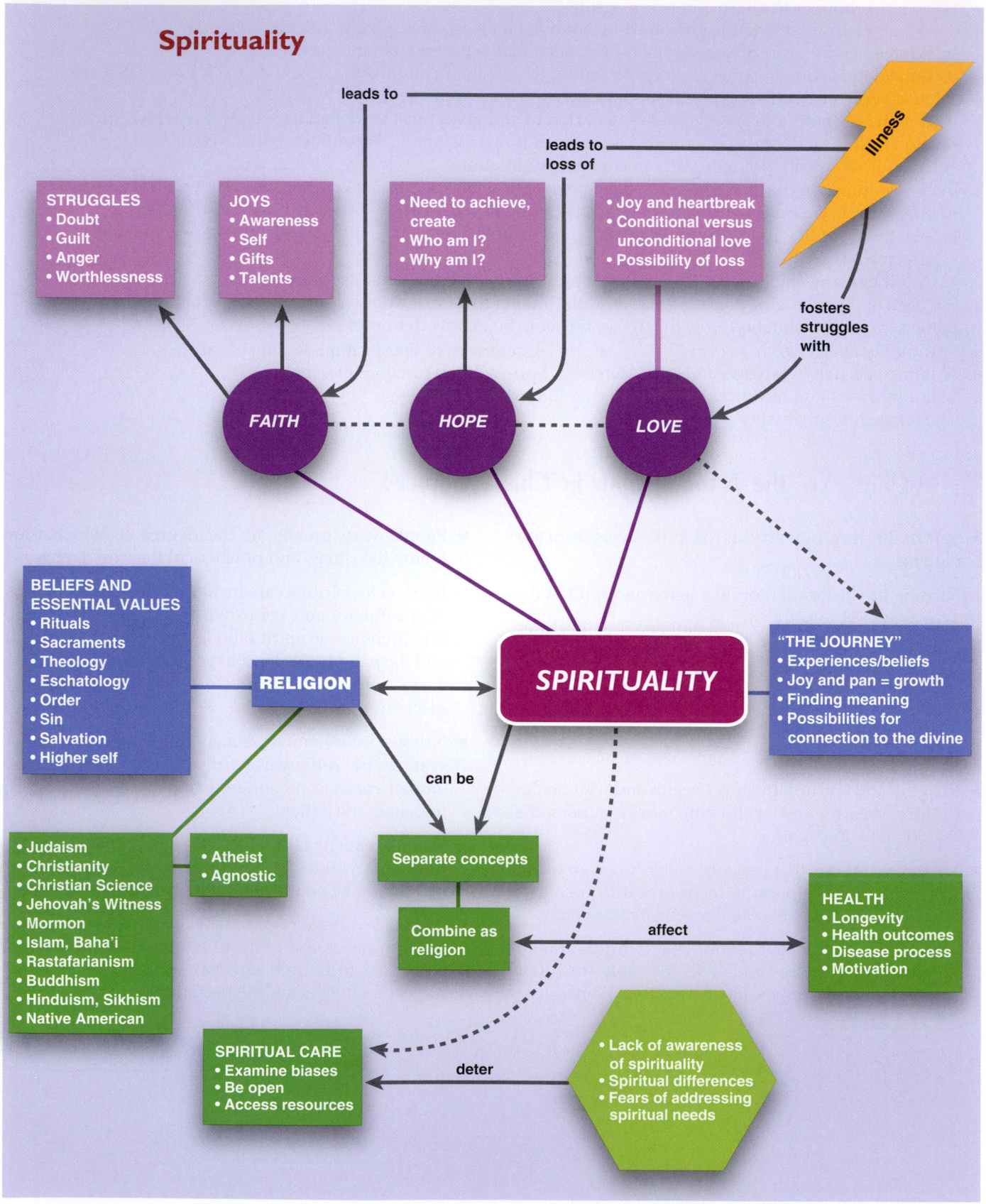

CHAPTER 17

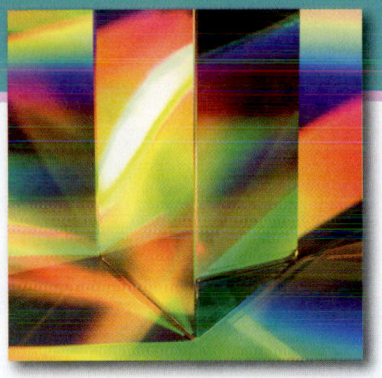

Loss, Grief, & Dying

STUDENT RESOURCES

*The questions and exercises in Volume 2 allow you to practice the kind of thinking you will use as a full-spectrum nurse. Critical-thinking questions usually have more than one correct answer, so we do not provide "answers" for these features. It is more important to develop your nursing judgment than to just cover content. You will learn by discussing the questions with your peers. If you are still unsure, consult your instructor. You will find Response Sheets (for writing your responses to the questions) on Davis*Plus.

To explore learning resources for this chapter,

Go to Davis*Plus* at DavisPl.us/Wilkinson3.

Chapter Resources for Chapter 17:

- **Response sheets for all learning activities**
- **Resources for Caregivers and Health Professionals**
- **Reading More About Loss, Grief, & Dying (suggested readings)**

Concept Map of chapter content

Interactive Case Studies

NCLEX-Style and Chapter Review Questions

CHAPTER OVERVIEW

For a podcast of an overview of this chapter,

Go to Student Resources: Chapter 17, **Podcast—Chapter Overview,** on Davis*Plus*.

Caring for the Nguyens

At a clinic visit, Nam Nguyen tells you that his father's health is declining rapidly. Mr. Nguyen tells you, "I thought he was doing okay. I knew he had surgery for his prostate, so I thought it was all over. Lately he's been having lots of low back and hip pain. So my mom begged him to go to the doctor, and he told him he has cancer all over." Mr. Nguyen shakes his head and looks away from you. You notice tears in his eyes.

Mr. Nguyen tells you that his family has avoided discussions about serious illness and death. "It just never got discussed. The whole idea made my parents uncomfortable. When my father got sick the first time, he refused to discuss it. 'I'm going to get better. Don't even think about it,' he would say." Now Mr. Nguyen feels the need to discuss this situation with his parents but doesn't know how to bring up the topic. He asks for your advice.

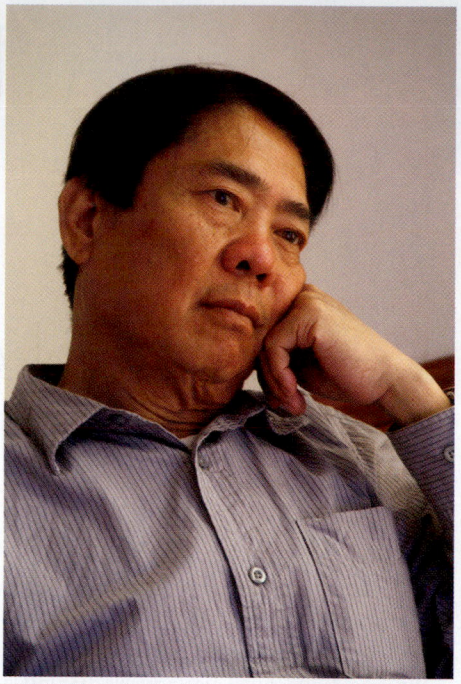

A. What would you think and feel when you see Nam's tears and when Mr. Nguyen asks for this advice?

B. What would you advise Mr. Nguyen?

C. What type of grief is Mr. Nguyen experiencing?

D. Examine the factors that affect grief. Apply these factors to Mr. Nguyen's situation. You will need to review the family history included in the introduction to the Nguyens (in the front of this book) to fully answer this question. Indicate whether the information for any of the factors to be evaluated is insufficient.

Practical Knowledge knowing how

This section provides guidelines for communicating with people who are grieving, caring for dying patients and their families, and providing postmortem care.

CLINICAL INSIGHTS

Clinical Insight 17-1 ➤ Communicating With People Who Are Grieving

Perfect your listening skills. Listen for what is *not* said as well as what is said.

Be alert for and respond to nonverbal cues with appropriate touch and eye contact. A smile, a gentle touch, sitting with a patient, and eye contact all relay a message of genuine care and concern. You may not need to say very much at all.

Encourage and accept expressions of feelings.

- Receiving expressions of intense feelings (e.g., anger and guilt) may be painful for you. It may help to remember that it is therapeutic for people to express their feelings.
- You don't need to change the person's feelings or "make them better." As much as we would like to do this, it is not possible.
- You do need to validate the person's feelings (e.g., "It is normal to feel that way; it is okay").

Reassure the person that it is not "wrong" to feel anger, guilt, relief, or other feelings she may believe to be unacceptable. A dying patient might say, "I know it's awful, but I feel so angry with God for giving me this disease." Or a bereaved spouse might admit, "I shouldn't feel this way, but I'm relieved that it's finally over." Patients need

Clinical Insight 17-1 ➤ Communicating With People Who Are Grieving *(continued)*

to hear you say their feelings are not "wrong" or "bad" and that they are going through a normal process.

Increase your self-awareness. Become more conscious of your own attitudes and feelings regarding death and dying. *If you are comfortable with your perspective, you will be able to hear patients' expressions of anger, guilt, frustration, fear, and loneliness more comfortably.*

Continue to communicate with dying patients even if they are in a coma. Encourage family members to do so as well.

- Talk to the patient. Tell him what is going on around him, what care you are providing, and when you or others enter or are about to leave the room.
- Avoid discussing the dying person as though he were not present. *Research indicates that patients continue to hear even though they cannot respond, sometimes up to the moment of death.*

Practice Resources

Eisenhandler, S. (2004); Emanuel, L., Ferris, F., von Gunten, C., et al. (2008); The Joint Commission (2010, 2013); Kruse, B. (2004); Traylor, E., Hayslip, B., Kaminski, P. L., et al. (2003); Wittenberg-Lyles, Goldsmith, Oliver, et al. (2012).

Clinical Insight 17-2 ➤ Helping Families of Dying Patients

- **View the family as your unit of care.** *Family members often rate communication with clinicians as one of their most important needs.*
- **Provide information, support, and a listening ear.** Include specific facts about the patient's condition and prognosis and whom to call about changes in condition.
- **Communicate medical updates daily.** *Information can relieve anxiety and is useful to the family when making decisions.*
- **Encourage family members to help with care if they are able.** Instruct and supervise as appropriate. If family members are not physically or emotionally able to provide care, accept that. *This helps meet their need to be useful, promotes family ties, and makes the patient more comfortable.*
- **Encourage family members to ask questions.** *They may hesitate to do so for various reasons (e.g., they may not want to interrupt busy care providers).*
- **Listen actively to the patient's and family's concerns.** Make eye content; clarify when you don't understand. *This helps you avoid misinterpreting the family's concerns and needs.*
- **Help the family to understand the goals of care and solve problems when needed.**
- **Follow up with other healthcare team members promptly** if the family has questions that are outside your scope of practice.
- **Arrange for a formal multidisciplinary meeting with the family** soon after the patient's admission, if possible. Discussions should cover personal, cultural, and religious traditions (e.g., how prayers are to be conducted, how the body is to be handled after death, and so on).
- **Encourage the family to visit the hospital chapel and to speak with a chaplain** or with their own spiritual adviser.
- **Provide anticipatory guidance regarding the stages of loss and grief,** so that they will know what to expect after their loved one dies.
- **Acknowledge the family's feelings** and the loss they are experiencing. *Many times family members begin the grieving process before the loved one dies.*
- **Help the family members explore past coping mechanisms;** reinforce successful past coping mechanisms.
- **Refer for ethics consultation** if decision making may become a problem.
- **Remind family members and significant others to take care of themselves.** *Watching a loved one die is a very difficult experience. A sensitive, caring nurse can make it a little easier.*
  - Many times they need "permission" to go to eat or to go home and rest.
  - If the patient is near death and family and friends do not want to leave the patient's side, make them as comfortable as possible.
  - Provide comfortable chairs, coffee, and snacks (according to organizational policy), and be alert for other needs they may have.
- **Teach the family what to expect with regard to medications, treatments, and signs of approaching death.** *If family members know what is normal, they will be less likely to panic or fear the inevitable.*
- **As physical signs of death become apparent, keep the family informed.** You may say something like, "Her blood pressure is becoming difficult to hear. That is one of the signs that she is closer to death." Help the family to understand what the patient is experiencing, as this may be very different from what they are seeing.
- **Reassure families of patients who become withdrawn near the time of death** that this does not mean the patient is rejecting them, but only that his body

(Continued)

Clinical Insight 17-2 ➤ Helping Families of Dying Patients *(continued)*

is conserving energy and that he has come to terms with dying and letting go of his connections with life.

- **When approaching death is apparent, ask family members directly, "Do you want to be present while he is dying?"** Tell them what to expect, if they do not know.
- **When an expected death occurs, shift the focus of your care** to the family and those who were caregivers. *Death does not end the relationship; family and caregivers need support during bereavement.*

Practice Resources

Ahrens, T., Yancey, V., & Kollef, M. (2003); Boyle, D. K., Miller, P. A., & Forbes-Thompson, S. A. (2005); Emanuel, L., Ferris, F., von Gunten, C., et al. (2008); Hospice Foundation of America (2005); Hudson, P. (2006); The Joint Commission (2010, 2013); von Gunten C., Ferris, F., & Emanuel, L. (2000).

Clinical Insight 17-3 ➤ Caring for the Dying Person: Meeting Physiological Needs

Active dying usually occurs over a period of 10 to 14 days (although it can take as little as 24 hours). The "final hours" refer to the last 4 to 48 hours of life, in which failure of body systems results in death (Brennan, 2011; Pitorak, 2003).

Encourage the patient to be as independent as possible. *This helps the patient to maintain a sense of control.*

Provide adequate pain control. *This can be a major issue for patients and caregivers. In fact, dying patients are often more concerned about pain and loss of control than about dying itself. Pain is difficult to assess in semiconscious or unconscious patients. See Chapter 31 if you need more information about pain management.*

- Dispel the myths about pain medication (e.g., addiction, overdose). Effective pain control medications exist and can be administered by various routes. Assure the patient and family that analgesics will not be addictive in this situation.
- Respect the patient's informed decision to refuse pain medications. For example, a patient may prefer to endure pain in order to be awake and alert when his family is at the bedside.
- Follow the prescribed pain protocols to ensure that pain is controlled.
- Administer pain medication on a regular schedule instead of waiting until the patient asks (prn), to ensure pain control.
- Teach and perform nonpharmacological pain-relief measures when you judge these may be helpful (e.g., meditation, heat/cold therapies, massage, distraction, imagery, deep breathing, and herbal-scented lotions). It may be soothing to play soft music, add "white noise," or turn off the television.
- Patients who are near death may moan or grunt as they breathe; this does not necessarily indicate pain. Be sure that families understand this. When accompanied by agitation and restlessness, these symptoms may indicate terminal delirium, which may require medications for control.

Monitor the patient's energy level. *Fatigue is a normal part of the dying process. Most dying patients sleep much of the time.*

- Perform hygiene and other care, if the patient tires easily or lacks the energy for self-care (i.e., activities of daily living).
- Remove environmental stressors that interfere with sleep (e.g., noise, too much light, a room that is too hot or too cold).
- Identify psychosocial stressors (e.g., depression, anxiety, fear) that may keep the patient awake (see Clinical Insight 17-4).

Maintain skin integrity. *During the final hours of life, the goal changes from preserving skin integrity to providing comfort. Realize that during this time even excellent care may not prevent skin breakdown.*

- Turn the patient frequently unless contraindicated. Refer to the pain control interventions in the preceding list.
- Assess for increased diaphoresis and/or incontinence.
- Maintain adequate nutrition.

If the patient is comatose or unconscious, provide special care for the eyes so they do not become too dry. Many agencies use a form of artificial tears for this purpose.

If the patient is not able to take fluids, wet the lips and mouth frequently with cool water or with a prepared product to prevent dryness and cracking of lips and mucous membranes of the nose, mouth, and eyes.

There is some evidence that glycerin swabs dry the mucous membranes and should not be used.

Provide artificial hydration (unless the patient has an advance directive requesting no artificial hydration) per nasogastric (NG) or IV route. *IV fluids can cause edema, nausea, and even pain in a patient who is actively dying. Dehydration is thought not to cause distress during the last hours, and may even be protective (Campbell, 2010; Emanuel, Ferris, von Gunten, et al., 2008).*

Take the vital signs often, unless contraindicated; observe for decreased level of consciousness and pallor.

Assess and provide interventions for constipation, urinary retention, and incontinence. *Constipation may be associated with decreased fluid intake, inactivity, weakness, hypercalcemia, hyperkalemia, and lack of privacy. It can contribute to pain, nausea, vomiting, and anorexia, so intervention is an important comfort measure. Incontinence may occur because of fatigue and loss of sphincter control. It can be distressing to patients and family members.*

Clinical Insight 17-3 ➤ Caring for the Dying Person: Meeting Physiological Needs *(continued)*

- Administer laxatives, stool softeners, and lubricants for constipation.
- Catheterize the patient if he is unable to void and the bladder becomes distended.
- Use pads for incontinence, but change them frequently to prevent skin breakdown and, near the end, to promote comfort.
- Use a rectal tube if diarrhea is severe.

Intervene for "death rattle" if it occurs and if it is distressing to the family.

- Turn the patient on his side, and elevate the head of the bed.
- Administer antispasmodic and anticholinergic medications if necessary.

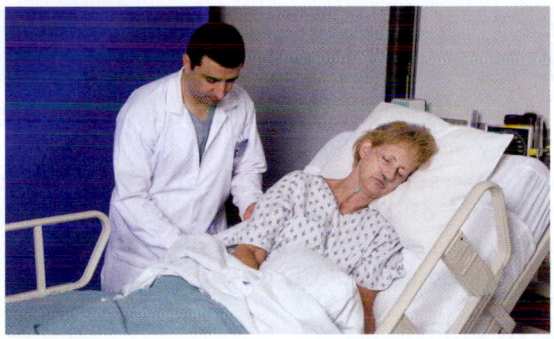

Provide medication for other symptoms, such as nausea and breathlessness.

Continue to speak to the patient as if he can hear.

Do not talk about the patient to others in his presence. *The patient is usually able to hear even after he can no longer respond to sounds and other stimuli. Assume the unconscious patient hears everything.*

Document changes in vital signs and level of consciousness. Record intake and output, noting changes. Document the times of cardiac arrest and cessation of respirations.

Practice Resources

American Nurses Association (2010); Covington (2013); Emanuel, L., Ferris, F., von Gunten C., et al. (2005); Harvey, J. (2001); The Joint Commission (2010, 2013); Qaseem, A., Snow, V., Shekelle, P., et al. (2008).

Clinical Insight 17-4 ➤ Caring for the Dying Person: Meeting Psychological Needs

Patients experience many emotions at end of life, including anger, sadness, depression, fear, relief, loneliness, and grief. At this time, communication and support are most helpful. Discussing concerns and issues is a viable means of coping.

If there is an advance directive or living will, locate the documents. Review the documents to be certain you understand the patent's wishes. If you have not already done so, notify all relevant health professionals of the existence of these documents.

Answer all questions honestly.

Explain all care and treatments even if the patient is unconscious. *He may still be able to hear.*

Realize that the patient may feel he is losing control.

- Help the person recognize what he does have control over.
- Include the patient in care decisions as much as he is able.

Attend to social needs. *Relationships are a priority at this time. Some patients may simply need to keep the bonds with family members and friends intact. For other patients, this may be a time to reestablish or mend relationships.*

- Notify family members when the patient wishes to see them.
- Allow the patient and family to discuss death at their own pace.
- Offer to contact a chaplain or other spiritual leader if the patient chooses.
- Pray with the patient if he requests it and you are comfortable doing so.

Encourage the patient to express feelings. Be prepared to accept a wide range of feelings, including anger, hopelessness, loneliness, and depression.

Early in the dying process, assess the sources of financial support for the patient and family. *Finances may be a concern and may place an additional burden on the family; or the patient may feel he is a burden to care for.*

Be aware of sexual needs. Provide realistic information about these issues. For example, suggest ways a couple can be close and affectionate at this time. Be aware that expressions of sexuality may change as a person becomes closer to death. *Some people may feel it is not right to have sexual feelings when the person they love is dying. Others may be afraid of harming the patient if they are sexually intimate.*

When the patient is very near death, focus on relieving symptoms (e.g., pain, nausea) and emotional distress.

(Continued)

Clinical Insight 17-3 ➤ Caring for the Dying Person: Meeting Physiological Needs *(continued)*

If the person can communicate, ask about immediate concerns:

- "Are you in pain?" "Are you comfortable?"
- "What are you afraid of now?"
- "What can we do to help you go peacefully?"
- "Who do you want in the room with you right now?"

If the patient asks whether he is dying, be honest.

If the patient cannot communicate, ask a significant other what the patient would want. Ask the family member or person who is most likely to know.

When the patient is very near death, it may be helpful to say something like, "Your family will be fine" rather than, "It is okay for you to go now." *Be aware that some people seem to wait to die until after a significant date (birthday, anniversary, and so on) has passed. Others wait for family to gather; whereas, others wait until loved ones leave so they will not upset the family by dying in their presence.*

Practice Resources

Brennan, C., Prince-Paul, M., & Wiencek, C. (2011); Duffy, S., Jackson, F., Schim, S., et al. (2006); Emanuel, L., Ferris, F., von Gunten, C., et al. (2008); Hancock, K., Clayton, J., Parker, S., et al. (2007); Law, R. (2009); The Joint Commission (2010, 2013); Pitorak, E. (2003).

Clinical Insight 17-5 ➤ Providing Postmortem Care

Supporting the Family

- **At the moment of death, do not interrupt or intrude on the family.** Wait quietly and observe, or if they would feel more comfortable being alone with the patient, leave the room. Give them as much time as they need. When they move away from the body, or have expressed their last good-byes, then it is time to assess the patient and report the lack of vital signs.
- **Immediately after death, express sympathy to the family.** This is very important. Make a simple statement, such as, "I am sorry for your loss." Avoid statements that interpret the situation for the family, such as, "It's God's will." Also avoid attempts to mitigate the family member's grief, for example, "It will get better in time," or "You still have your son."
- **If the family wishes to be alone with the body,** straighten the bedcovers and make the patient look as natural as possible. Remove any tubes, IV lines, and so on, according to the institution's policy, and have the patient positioned in a way that appears comforting (e.g., bedcovers pulled up, hands at the side).
- **Be accepting of family members' behavior at this time,** no matter how strange it may seem to you. A family might want to take a picture, or the spouse may lie down beside the deceased person.
- **If no family members are present, identify the next of kin** and be sure the family is informed of the patient's death.
- **If family members arrive after the death, offer to take them to the bedside.**
- **If family members wish to be involved in postmortem care,** encourage them to do so. This can facilitate their grieving process.
- **Ask whether each family member wishes to spend time alone with the deceased person,** and arrange for them to do so. Never remove the body until the family is ready. Viewing the body is useful to many individuals.
- **Ask, "How can I help?" "What do you need?" "What would you like for me to do?"**
- **Locate personal effects and give them to the family/next of kin.** If you can't remove a ring, wrap it with gauze, tape it in place, and tie the gauze to the wrist to prevent subsequent loss.

Legal Responsibilities

- **Notify the primary provider of the death.** Usually the physician must pronounce death; however, in some areas a coroner or a nurse may also perform this task.
- **The person who pronounces death must sign the death certificate.** In some agencies, the nurse is responsible for checking to see that it has been signed.
- **If the patient is donating organs,** review and make any necessary arrangements.
- **If an autopsy is to be performed,** as a rule, the physician (or other person designated by the institution) is responsible for obtaining signed permission from the next of kin.

Care of the Body

- **Follow agency policies, and respect cultural and spiritual preferences.**
- **Wash the body if there has been any incontinence or drainage.** Place absorbent (ABD) pads between the buttocks to absorb rectal drainage. Ask the family before washing the body. *In some cultures, the body is not washed, or family members arrange to have someone special do it.*
- **Dress the body in a clean gown, comb the hair, and straighten the bed linens.**
- **Place the body supine in a natural position.**
  - Place the dentures in the mouth before rigor mortis occurs.
  - Close the eyes and mouth before rigor mortis occurs. Close the eyes by gently pressing on the lids with your fingertips. If they do not stay closed, place a moist

Clinical Insight 17-5 ➤ Providing Postmortem Care *(continued)*

compress on the eyelids for a few minutes and then try to close them again.
  - Tie a strip of soft gauze (e.g., Kling) under the chin and around the head if your institution requires it (not all do). Alternatively, you can place a folded towel under the chin to keep the jaw closed. *This keeps the mouth set in a natural position in case there is a viewing later.*
  - Place a pillow under the head and shoulders. *This prevents blood from settling there and causing discoloration.*
- **Be sure that dressings are clean, and unless an autopsy is to be done, remove all tubes and drains.** Be careful when removing tape or dressings. Apply small adhesive bandages to puncture sites. *After death, the skin loses its elasticity and can be torn easily.*
- **If the family asks about the coldness and color of the body, explain to them about algor mortis and livor mortis.**
- **After the family has spent time with the body, arrange to have it sent to the morgue,** where either an autopsy will be performed, or, if not, the funeral home in charge of arrangements will arrive to transport the body.
  - Pad the wrists and ankles to prevent bruising; tie them together with gauze.
  - Wrap the body in a shroud or body wrap for transfer to the morgue.
  - If no relatives were present to receive patient belongings, bag them, label the bag, and send with the patient to the morgue.
  - If possible, close doors to adjoining rooms before transport.
- **Make sure there are identification tags on the body, on the shroud or body bag, and on the patient's possessions; and if necessary, hazard labels.** Follow agency policy for number and location of tags. They will usually include the patient's name, room and bed numbers, date and time of death, and the physician's name. Misidentification can create legal problems, for example, if the body is prepared incorrectly for a funeral.
- **Follow institutional policy if the patient has died of a communicable disease.** By law, there are special preparations to perform in such cases.
- **Handle the body with dignity.**

Documentation

Documentation varies among healthcare facilities. However, you will almost always document the time that you noted absence of heartbeat and respirations, any auxiliary equipment still present (e.g., mechanical ventilator), the disposition of the patient's possessions (especially money and jewelry), and the date and time the body is transported to the morgue or funeral home.

Practice Resources

College of American Pathologists (2007); Harvey, J. (2001); Smith-Stoner, M., & Hand, M. (2012); The Joint Commission (2010, 2013).

FORMS

DO NOT RESUSCITATE ORDERS

Physician: Complete Part I & II to initiate order. Part III is to be completed every seven days.

☐ **DNR forms completed on previous admission. Verified by:** _____.
Date of original order: _____. **Signature** **Date**

NOTE: Words that appear in the directions in all capital letters are listed in the DNR definitions.

PART I: ☐ If this patient suffers a cardiac or respiratory arrest, a Cart is not to be called and no resuscitation measures are to be carried out.

PART II: ☐ This order is to be transcribed and instituted immediately. All required documentation is complete.

or

☐ This order is to be transcribed and instituted only after the CONCURRING PHYSICIAN'S statements have been completed. I have requested Dr. _____ to be the CONCURRING PHYSICIAN.

_____, M.D. _____, R.N.
Signature of ATTENDING PHYSICIAN Signature of Transcribing Nurse

_____ _____ _____ _____
Date Time Date Time

PART III: Review of DNR ORDER

This is to verify that review and determination of continued appropriateness of the DNR ORDER and the conditions under which it was obtained was done: (to be documented at least every 7 days)

Date	By	Date	By
			Continued on reverse side

PART IV: Wavier to DNR ORDER

I, the undersigned, have previously consented to a DO NOT RESUSCITATE ORDER. During the procedure and until I am returned to my room, I hereby waive my consent to the DO NOT RESUSCITATE ORDER and authorize my ATTENDING PHYSICIAN to write such an order.

_____ _____ _____ _____
Signature of patient or SURROGATE or PROXY (or parent or legal guardian for minor) Date Signature of WITNESS Date

☐ DNR ORDER suspended during the peri-operative period, as noted above.

_____, M.D. _____, R.N.
Signature of ATTENDING PHYSICIAN Signature of Transcribing Nurse

_____ _____ _____ _____
Date Time Date Time

PART V: Revocation of DNR ORDER

I, the undersigned, hereby revoke the DO NOT RESUSCITATE ORDER previously consented to by me.

_____ _____ _____ _____
Signature of patient or SURROGATE or PROXY (or parent or legal guardian for minor) Date Signature of WITNESS Date

☐ DNR ORDER revoked.

_____, M.D. _____, R.N.
Signature of ATTENDING PHYSICIAN Signature of Transcribing Nurse

_____ _____ _____ _____
Date Time Date Time

13610 3/01 side 1 of 2

ASSESSMENT GUIDELINES

You can use these guidelines for assessing dying patients as well as for other types of loss.

Focused Assessment

Assessing Grief and Loss

1. Assess the patient and significant others for common grief reactions.

Physical	Emotional	Behaviors	Cognition
Loss of appetite	Sadness	Forgetfulness	Decreased concentration
Weight loss/gain	Guilt	Withdrawal	Forgetfulness
Fatigue	Relief	Insomnia or too much sleep	Impaired judgment
Decreased libido	Shock	Dreaming of deceased	Obsessive thoughts of the deceased or lost object
Decrease in immune system	Numbness	Verbalizing the loss	Preoccupation
Decreased energy	Loneliness	Crying	Confusion
Possibly physical symptoms, such as headache or stomach pain	Fear	Loss of productivity at work or school	Questioning spiritual beliefs
	Anxiety		Searching to understand
	Powerlessness		Searching for purpose and meaning
	Helplessness		
	Depression		

2. Assess knowledge base of patient and significant others.

a. Can they make informed decisions about healthcare choices? You might ask the following questions:

- "Tell me what you understand about your illness."
- "Are there any questions about your illness that you'd like me to answer?"
- "What are your options for treatment?"
- "Do you know how to reach your provider if you have questions about your care?"

b. What and how much do the patient and family want to know? *Some people wish to have all the details of their condition and care. For others, the details cause anxiety.*

3. Assess the history of loss. Determine whether the patient or family has sustained recent losses or major changes (e.g., death, moving, divorce, retirement). Ask such questions as:

- "Have you had any recent changes in your life?"
- "Tell me about your family."
- "Are your parents still living?" (as appropriate)
- "What previous experiences have you had with the loss of someone you loved (or with this condition)?"

4. Assess coping abilities and support systems. Questions to assess coping include the following:

- "What do you do to reduce stress?"
- "Which family/friends can you talk with?"
- "What would you say is your greatest support when going through difficult times?"
- "Tell me about a previous loss and what you did to cope with it."
- "Are you using any community resources to help you get through this? Do you know what they are?"

The way individuals have coped in the past will affect how they cope with dying or with their current loss. It may also be therapeutic for them to identify their resources and supports.

5. Assess the meaning of the loss or illness. Be alert for statements that may indicate the patient or family is struggling to find meaning, such as:

- "I'm being punished."
- "She doesn't deserve this."
- "Why is this happening to me?"

In trying to "make sense" of their loss or their dying, people try to attach a meaning to their suffering.

6. Differentiate between grief and depressive disorder.

a. Symptoms common to both grief and depressive disorder: sadness, insomnia, poor appetite and weight loss. Feelings of sadness and depression are a normal part of grief, provided the depression does not linger too long.

b. Symptoms that indicate grief. For example, the person may feel relatively better in certain situations, such as when she is with friends and family. However, triggers, such as the deceased person's birthday, an anniversary, or holidays, cause the feelings to resurface more strongly.

c. Symptoms that indicate depressive disorder:

- The depression is more pervasive. That is, the person rarely gets any relief from the symptoms.
- Feelings of guilt not related to the loved one's death
- Thoughts about own death or of suicide (other than feelings the person would be better off dead now that the loved one is gone)

(Continued)

Focused Assessment

Assessing Grief and Loss—cont'd

- Preoccupation with own "worthlessness"
- Sluggishness
- Hesitant and confused speech
- Prolonged and marked difficulty in carrying out activities of daily living
- Hallucinations, other than thinking he hears the voice of or sees the deceased person

7. Perform a physical assessment. Look for signs of increased stress, such as tension, forgetfulness, distraction, increased or decreased appetite and sleep, weight gain or loss, fatigue, and decreased self-care (e.g., deficient hygiene). *A thorough physical examination adds data to help you determine how well the patient is coping with the loss or illness.*

8. Perform a cultural and spiritual assessment.

a. Assess the patient's and family's religious beliefs, any spiritual needs they may have (e.g., forgiveness, hope, meaning, love), and cultural influences that may affect the way they cope.

b. Do not assume that a person adheres closely to the dominant values of his religious or cultural group. Always assess. For example, ask: "To what religious and ethnic groups do you belong?" and "How closely do you identify with those groups?"

See Chapters 15 and 16 for details of cultural and spiritual assessment, if you need them.

9. Perform these specific assessments for dying patients. For dying patients, in addition to the other assessments in this guideline, you should also assess the following:

a. When the patient and family are ready, encourage them to talk about what the patient might want for burial or cremation or whether there are tasks that the person would like taken care of (e.g., giving away valuables, calling family members).

b. Determine whether the dying person has a living will or advance directives.

c. Discuss with the patient and family the possibility of organ donation if appropriate for the patient's circumstances.

d. Observe for physical changes indicating the approach of death:

1 to 3 months before death: Beginning withdrawal from others, increased sleep, decreased appetite, difficulty digesting food (especially meats), prefers liquids. *Anorexia may be protective, as the resulting ketosis can diminish pain and increase the person's sense of well-being.*

1 to 2 weeks before death: Cardiovascular deterioration brings decreased blood pressure, pulse and respiration changes (decreased or increased), a yellowish pallor to the skin, extreme pallor of extremities. Observe for temperature fluctuations, increased perspiration, brief periods of apnea during sleep, rattling breathing sounds caused by congestion, nonproductive cough

Days to hours before death: A brief surge of energy and mental clarity, with a desire to eat and talk with family members

- Dehydration, difficulty swallowing, decreasing blood pressure, weak pulse
- Mucous membranes dry and tacky; cracked lips. *Dehydration during the last hours of dying is thought to not cause distress, and perhaps to stimulate endorphin release.*
- Sagging of tongue and soft palate, diminished gag reflex, secretions accumulating in the oropharynx and/or bronchi
- Shallow, rapid, or irregular breathing; respiratory congestion; Cheyne-Stokes respirations; apnea of 10 to 30 seconds; "death rattle." *Cheyne-Stokes breathing is a cyclic pattern consisting of a 10- to 60-second period of apnea and then a gradual increase in depth and rate of respirations. Respirations gradually become slow and shallow, and then the cycle begins again with apnea.*
- Decreased peripheral circulation, increased perspiration, "clammy" skin; extremities cool and mottled; dependent body parts darker than the rest of the body
- Decreased urinary output, concentrated and foul-smelling urine, secondary to decreased kidney function
- Slack facial muscles ("drooping")
- Retained feces; bowel and bladder incontinence *due to decreased peristalsis and relaxation of sphincters*
- Blurred vision; eyes open but unseeing
- Restlessness or agitation (check for impacted stool, distended bladder, pain, medications, cerebral hypoxia, unresolved emotional or spiritual issues)
- Decreased communication, quiet, withdrawal. Some become more coherent and energized for a time.
- Fatigue

Moments before death: Does not respond to touch or sound; cannot be awakened. There may be a short series of long-spaced breaths before breathing stops entirely and the heart stops beating. Auscultate to determine whether apical pulse and respirations are absent.

Sources: Emanuel, L., Ferris, F., von Gunten, C., et al. (2008); Ferszt, G. G., & Leveillee, M. (2006); Pitorak, E. (2003); Widera, E., & Block, S. (2012).

CLINICALREASONING

Applying the Full-Spectrum Nursing Model

PATIENT SITUATION

Marie is 84 years old and has had a right-sided cerebrovascular accident (CVA, stroke, or brain attack). Doctors say she is unlikely to regain much physical function, if she even awakens from the coma. She was alert and active before her stroke and was able to maintain her independence with the help of a home health aide, who assisted her with ADLs and meal preparation three times a week. Kelly and Dan, her children, have met with the physician, who tells them that Marie's chance of survival is slim. He wants to put a feeding tube into Marie and has asked whether they want Marie to be resuscitated in case of cardiac or respiratory arrest. Kelly wants to do what is best for her mother, but she feels that Marie would not want to be kept alive in this condition. She is also concerned about putting her through uncomfortable procedures if there is no chance of recovery. Her brother, Dan, thinks Marie should have the feeding tube. Kelly asks to speak with you and wants to know the best thing to do for her mother.

THINKING

1. *Theoretical Knowledge (Recall of Facts and Principles):* If Marie and Dan agree that they do not want Marie to be resuscitated, the physician will complete a DNAR (AND) order. What do the letters *DNAR* and *AND* represent?
2. *Critical Thinking (Problem-Solving):* At this stage of your education, you probably need more information about CVAs and tube feedings. Write a PICO question you could use to search the literature for information about these two topics and how they are related. See Chapter 8 if you need to review PICO questions.

DOING

3. *Practical Knowledge (Nursing Diagnosis):* Write a possible nursing diagnosis to describe Kelly's situation.
4. *Practical Knowledge (Basic Skills):* If Marie and Dan agree to tube feedings for Marie, as her nurse, what basic nursing skills will you need to perform? How will you learn to perform these skills, if you do not already know how to do them?

CARING

5. *Ethical Knowledge:* How do you think the situation came to this? What might Kelly, Dan, and Marie have done before the stroke to prevent this confusion and indecision?
6. *Self-Knowledge:* What are your responsibilities in this situation? What could you do to help Kelly and Dan?

Critical Thinking and Clinical Reasoning

1. Jessie McCarthy is a 69-year-old woman who is terminally ill with multiple myeloma. She is currently hospitalized for a week of chemotherapy. Her husband of 49 years is recuperating from recent hip surgery and has difficulty getting around. Her daughter and son-in-law are very close to them, and her granddaughter, 14 years old, has a very special relationship with her "Gammie." The side effects of Mrs. McCarthy's chemotherapy include nausea and headaches. She doesn't like to have people around when she feels this way. Jessie's pastor comes to visit every other day and seems to bring her comfort. Her 50th wedding anniversary will occur when she is in the hospital. She verbalizes fear of "not making it home this time." You are her nurse in a hospital where palliative care is provided. Initiate a holistic plan of care for Mrs. McCarthy, addressing the main issues noted.
   a. What immediate physical problems does Mrs. McCarthy have? Do not use her medical diagnosis as an answer.
   b. What might you do to meet her physical needs?
   c. What psychological needs does Mrs. McCarthy have: (1) What are her fears? (2) What social and emotional issues is she facing? (3) How might you help meet her needs?
2. You are caring for Jack Wirtz, a 37-year-old man who was admitted to the hospital for a lumbar laminectomy (surgery of his lower spine). As you are doing Jack's preoperative assessment, he tells you that his 12-year-old son died 6 months ago in an automobile accident in which Jack was the driver. He is a builder and has been out of work since the accident. His wife now works to help support them. Jack's affect is flat, and he talks in a monotone.
   a. What losses has Jack experienced?
   b. What further assessments need to be made for Jack, and why?

3. A patient requests your participation in a plan for assisted suicide or passive euthanasia. What are your options as a nurse? Use the Internet to get information about this.
   a. List the URLs for the pages you found to be helpful in answering the question. Beside each URL, state the name of the organization, person, or agency to which the Web site belongs.
   b. For each URL, state what you believe to be the *purpose* of the Web site.
4. Find a partner. Take 5 minutes to describe to her a personal loss you have had (e.g., a person, a pet, an object, an aspect of health). The partner must listen silently and not speak at all during these 5 minutes. When you have finished, answer the following questions:
   a. What did you feel when describing your loss?
   b. Did you feel that the listener was really listening to you?
   c. How did the listener respond to you?
5. Now reverse the process; you become the listener. When you have finished, answer the following questions:
   a. What did you feel while you were listening?
   b. Did the time go quickly or seem long?
   c. What did you learn from this listening experience?
6. John is 17 years old and volunteers at the hospital. He has just moved from another state because of his father's work, so he is a new senior in high school. As you chat with him, he reveals that his mother is getting radiation and chemotherapy treatments for breast cancer and has been very ill. What are some loss issues this young man is facing?
7. Sharon is your 48-year-old patient who is in the hospital for a hysterectomy (removal of her uterus) because of fibroids and heavy bleeding. With teary eyes, she shares with you that she is feeling "down" and doesn't want any visitors this evening. She says, "I really thought I would feel better after having this surgery done."
   a. Why do you think Sharon is teary and feeling "down"?
   b. What should you do to begin helping Sharon cope with her loss?
8. You are having lunch with a nursing colleague, who reveals to you that her mother has Alzheimer's disease. Her mother has been placed in a nursing home because she is losing her memory and is not safe at home. Your friend describes feeling distracted, angry for no reason, and unable to shake her feelings of sadness.
   a. What might be causing your colleague to feel distracted and angry?
   b. How would you respond to her?
9. You are caring for Mr. Bishop, a 57-year-old man who is terminally ill with metastatic bone cancer. He wants to donate his organs for research after his death, but his wife is totally against this.
   a. What could you do or say to him to help resolve this issue? Go to the following URL, and download the Organ Donation and Transplantation page for information to use in this situation: http://organdonor.gov/about/index.html
   b. Now go to the top of the Web page and look at the logo and other information. Who do you think provides and maintains the content for this Web site? What else would give you a clue about the source of the site?
   c. Look at the bottom of the Web page. What department of the U.S. government "owns" this page?
10. For each of the following concepts, use critical thinking to describe how or why it is important to nursing, patient care, or loss, grief, and dying. Note that these are *not* to be merely definitions.

Physical loss	Stages of grief
Actual loss	Advance directives
Complicated grief	Assisted suicide
Disenfranchised grief	Palliative care
Significance of the loss	

What Are the Main Points in This Chapter?

- How people cope with loss directly affects their healing and well-being.
- Loss may be actual or perceived, physical or psychological, external or internal.
- Grief is the physical, psychological, and spiritual response to loss.
- People do not move neatly from one stage of grief or dying to the next; there is constant movement and overlap between and among them.
- Factors that affect the grieving process include the significance and circumstance of the loss, the timeliness of the death, the bereaved support system, spiritual beliefs, cultural values, the person's developmental stage, and conflicts existing at the time of death.
- Patients experience loss of independence, body image, self-esteem, and so on, when they are ill and/or hospitalized. Recognizing these as losses, you can assist the patient with the grieving process, thus promoting physical, emotional, and spiritual healing.
- The Uniform Determination of Death Act states that death has occurred when "an individual . . . has sustained either (1) irreversible cessation of circulatory and respiratory functions, or (2) irreversible cessation of all functions of the entire brain, including the brainstem. . . ."
- Palliative care focuses on providing comfort care and symptom relief, without further efforts to stop the disease process or prevent death.
- Hospice care is a movement and an approach to allow terminally ill persons to face death with dignity and surrounded by the comfort of their home and family.
- Healthcare providers are responsible for educating staff and patients about advance directives.
- A do not attempt resuscitation (DNAR) or allow natural death (AND) order is a specific order to *not* perform cardiopulmonary resuscitation.
- Nurses should be aware of what is involved with assisted suicide and euthanasia. You should think ahead about what your response might be if a patient wants to discuss these topics. You may find the American Nurses Association (ANA) position statement on the nurses' roles and responsibilities in end-of-life care helpful.
- An autopsy is a medical examination of the body to determine the cause of death.
- When a patient is dying or has experienced a loss, you should perform a thorough, holistic assessment.
- Most grief is normal, not dysfunctional; you should not diagnose Complicated Grieving for every person who is grieving a loss.
- You can facilitate grief work by validating feelings ("It's normal to feel that way") and providing an opportunity and encouragement to talk about the lost person or object.
- Active dying usually occurs over a 10- to 14-day period, although it can take as little as 24 hours. During the final 4 to 48 hours, failure of body systems results in death.
- When the patient is very near death, focus on relieving physical symptoms and emotional distress. If he can communicate, ask about immediate concerns, such as, "Who do you want in the room right now?"
- At the moment of death, do not interrupt or intrude upon the family; give them as much time as they need to say good-bye to their loved one. Express your sympathy.
- Care of the body includes making it presentable for the family, carefully placing identification tags, and arranging to have the body sent to the morgue.
- The death certificate must be signed by the person who legally pronounced the death (usually a physician).
- It is normal for the nurse to feel grief when a patient dies.

Knowledge Map

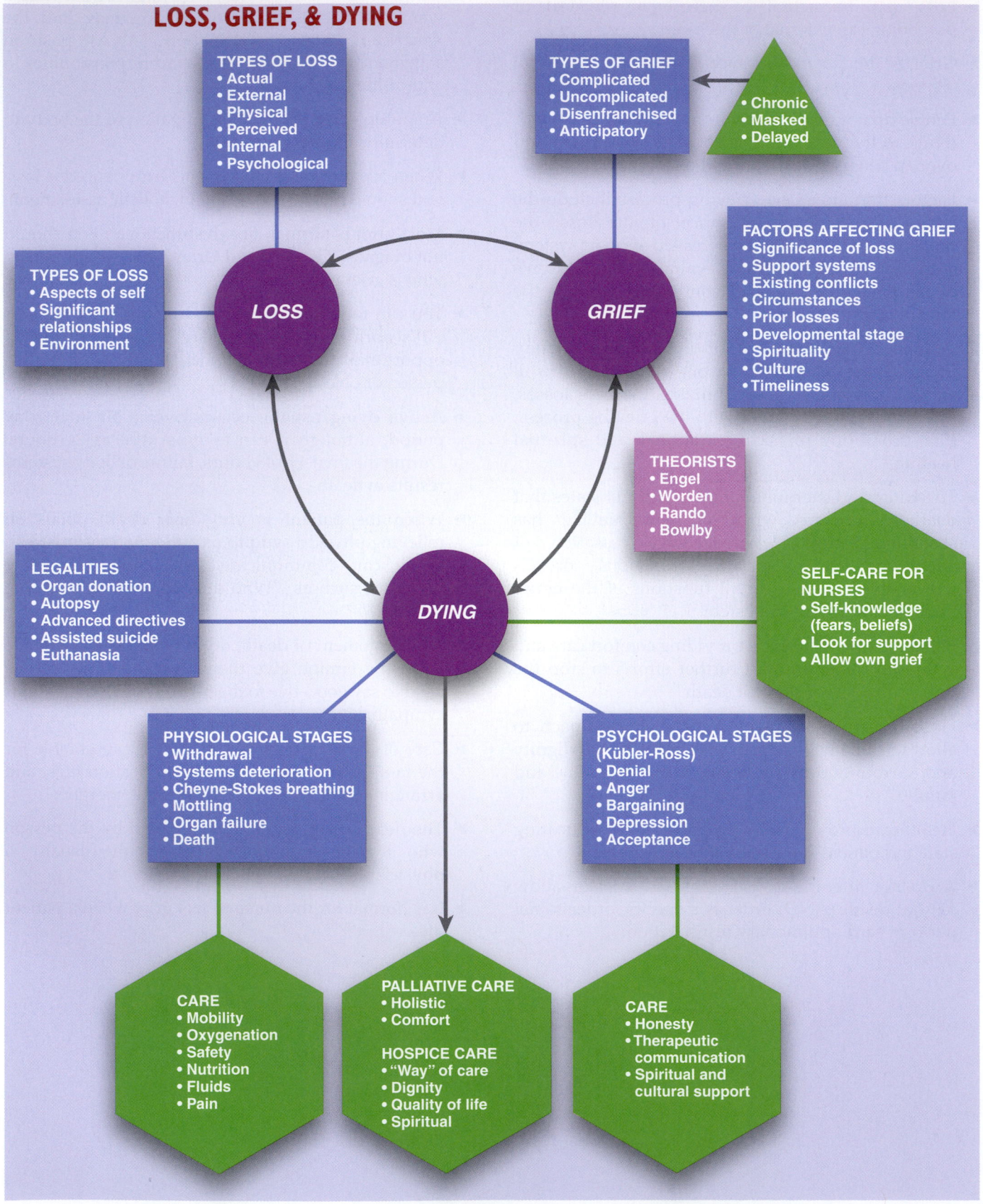

unit 3

Essential Nursing Interventions

18 Documenting & Reporting

19 Teaching & Learning

20 Measuring Vital Signs

21 Communication & Therapeutic Relationships

22 Health Assessment

23 Promoting Asepsis & Preventing Infection

24 Promoting Safety

25 Facilitating Hygiene

26 Administering Medications

CHAPTER 18

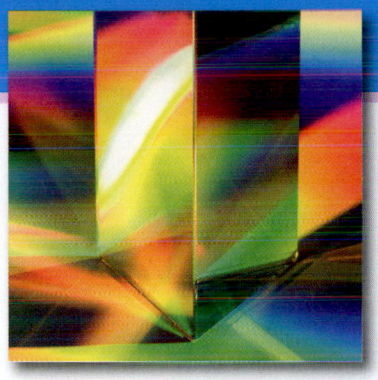

Documenting & Reporting

STUDENT RESOURCES

*The questions and exercises in Volume 2 allow you to practice the kind of thinking you will use as a full-spectrum nurse. Critical-thinking questions usually have more than one correct answer, so we do not provide "answers" for these features. It is more important to develop your nursing judgment than to just cover content. You will learn by discussing the questions with your peers. If you are still unsure, consult your instructor. You will find Response Sheets (for writing your responses to the questions) on Davis*Plus.

To explore learning resources for this chapter,

Go to Davis*Plus* at DavisPl.us/Wilkinson3.

Chapter Resources for Chapter 18:

- **Response sheets for all learning activities**
- **Resources for Caregivers and Health Professionals**
- **Reading More About Documenting & Reporting (suggested readings)**
- **Concept Map of chapter content**

Interactive Case Studies

NCLEX-Style Review Questions

CHAPTER OVERVIEW

For a podcast of an overview of this chapter,

Go to Student Resources: Chapter 18, **Podcast—Chapter Overview,** on Davis*Plus*.

Caring for the Nguyens

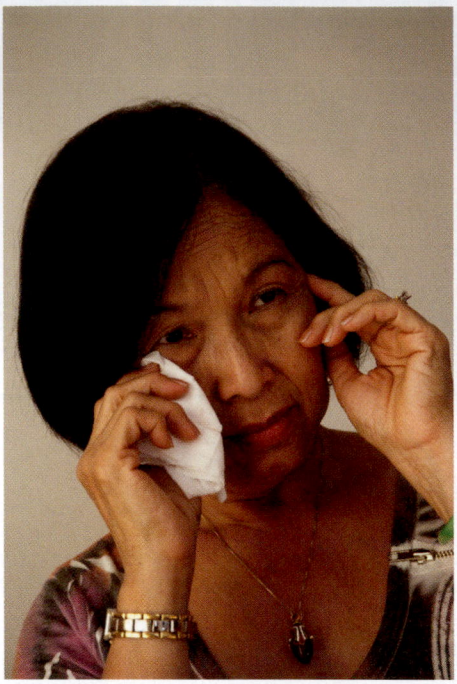

Yen Nguyen arrives at the Family Medicine Clinic complaining of pain and drainage from her right eye. She requests an appointment. As part of your clinical experience working as a triage nurse at the clinic, you must evaluate the patient's status and determine whether she needs to be seen today. Below is your conversation with Mrs. Nguyen.

Mrs. Nguyen: I don't have an appointment, but I need to see someone today. My husband is a patient here. I have an appointment in 2 weeks for a physical, but I've never been here before. I just can't wait 2 weeks.

You: What seems to be the problem?

Mrs. Nguyen: My eye is killing me. My right one. It burns and stings, and there's all this nasty gunk coming out. I think I need some medicine for it.

You: Tell me a little more about this problem. When did this start?

Mrs. Nguyen: I woke up yesterday with a painful, itchy eye. I used some saline drops, but the eye seems to be worse. I work at a preschool, and they won't let me work unless I take care of this. I also think I need to be checked for other things. I haven't had an appointment in a long time. I suppose I just need some tests. My husband just found out he has high blood pressure, but I don't think I do. I guess I'm not old enough. I'm 55, but my mother got high blood pressure when she was 70.

As she is talking, you notice a large amount of thick, yellow-green drainage in the corner of her right eye and the eye is reddened. She is rubbing this eye vigorously and dabbing at it with a tissue. The skin is puffy around the eye as well. Her left eye is slightly red, but there is no drainage.

Her vital signs are as follows: blood pressure, 132/76 mm Hg; heart rate, 88 beats/min; respirations, 18 breaths/min; and temperature 98.9°F (37.2°C). Based on your brief assessment, you ask the receptionist to give Mrs. Nguyen an urgent appointment.

A. Make two charting entries to describe the above events. First make a brief narrative note.

B. Next, construct a SOAPIER note. Be sure to follow charting guidelines when you prepare your note.

Practical Knowledge knowing **how**

CLINICAL INSIGHTS

Clinical Insight 18-1 ➤ Giving Oral Reports

For all types of report formats

Remember the acronym CUBAN (Currie, 2002):
Confidential, **U**ninterrupted, **B**rief, **A**ccurate, **N**amed nurse

Use a Standardized Format Such as the Following:

PACE

Patient/Problem—Include patient's name, room number, diagnosis, reason for admission, and recent procedures. State the present problem. Briefly summarize medical history relevant to the current problem.

Assessment/Actions—Nursing assessments and interventions directed to the problem.

Continuing/Changes—Continuing needs and potential changes include:

- Patient care and treatments that must be monitored on other shifts (e.g., dressing changes)
- Changes in the patient's condition or the care plan, recent or anticipated (e.g., new orders, changes in discharge date)

Evaluation—Evaluation of responses to nursing and medical interventions, progress toward goals, and effectiveness of the plan

SBAR/SBAR-R

Identify yourself, the patient, and the agency.
S*ituation*—"Here's the situation . . ."
B*ackground*—"The supporting background information is . . ."
A*ssessment*—"My assessment of the situation is that . . ."
R*ecommendation*—"I recommend that you . . ."
R*ead back*—"To repeat the information and . . ."
For additional information about SBAR, see Clinical Insight 21-3.

Include the Following Content:

In a handoff report:

- Patient's name, age, and room number
- Patient's admitting diagnosis—one or several may exist.
- Patient's relevant past medical history
- Treatments the patient has received during this admission, such as surgery, line placements, breathing treatments
- Upcoming diagnostic tests, surgeries, or treatments
- Patient restrictions, such as diet, bed rest, isolation, activity limits
- Plan of care, such as IV therapy, pain management, current medications, wound care, and patient or family concerns
- Significant assessment findings from the previous shifts

In a transfer report:

- Your name, facility, and phone number
- Patient's name, age, gender, and admitting and current diagnoses
- Patient's physician(s), if still following patient
- Procedures or surgeries performed
- Current medications and last date/time each was taken/time next dose is due
- Patient status at present as well as progression since admission
- Last set of vital signs, plus any pertinent trends since admission
- Tubes in the patient, such as IVs, catheters, drainage tubes, along with the intake and output of each tube or drain
- Presence of wounds or open areas of the skin plus current interventions for each
- Names and contact numbers for family and significant others
- Special directives, such as code status, presence of advanced directives, preferred intensity of care, or isolation required
- Reason the patient is being transferred
- Location of above information (on transfer form, in medical records, etc.)

When Your Report Is Finished:

- Ask the receiving nurse whether he has any questions.
- Get the nurse's full name, and then record it plus the transfer date and time in your transfer documentation.

Practice Resources

Children's Hospital of Wisconsin (n.d.); Grbach, W., Vincent, L., & Struth, D. (2008); Haig, K., Sutton, S., & Whittington, J. (2006); Kaiser Permanente of Colorado (updated 2011); Schroeder, M. (2011); Schroeder, S. (2006).

Clinical Insight 18-2 ➤ Receiving Telephone and Verbal Orders

You should accept verbal and telephone orders only in specific situations when the primary care provider is not able to write or enter the orders personally.

- **Have a second nurse listen to the order**, if possible, to verify its accuracy.
- **Write or enter the order electronically only if you heard it yourself**; no third-party involvement is acceptable.
- **Repeat the written order** even if you believe you have clearly understood it.
- **Spell unfamiliar names** when repeating to be sure the spelling is correct.
- **Pronounce digits of numbers separately.** For example, instead of "seventeen," say "one, seven." Mishearing a number can lead to a serious error in medication dosage.
- **Make sure the order makes sense** given the patient's current status.
- **Transcribe the order directly into the chart as quickly as possible.** Writing it on a piece of paper, then copying it again onto a paper order sheet introduces an additional chance of error. If entering the order electronically, it's best to have the EHR's order entry area open and begin entering the order as the prescriber is dictating it to you.
- **Write the order while the prescriber remains on the telephone or in the building** so that you can ask any necessary questions immediately without the need for a return call.
- **When writing the order on a paper order sheet, first document the date and time.** Next write the text of the order. Following the text of the order, depending on how you received the order, write "TO" (telephone order) or "VO" (verbal order) followed by the ordering provider's name and then your name. The following is an example of a telephone order:

  12/17/16 0815 Morphine 2 mg IV push 1 for pain now. _____
  TO Dr. Clayton Kent/Sarah Hogan, RN; order read back for verification and validated. _____

- **Sign electronically to activate the order.** If entering the order electronically, indicate during order entry that the order was given verbally or over the telephone, the date and time the order was given, and then search for and select the ordering provider's name. Click "sign" or whatever option in your EHR indicates the order is signed and is now active.
- **Be sure you have the provider's phone number** so that you can reach her if future questions arise.
- **All verbal and telephone orders must be countersigned** by the physician, physician assistant, or nurse practitioner within 24 hours.

Practice Resources

The Joint Commission (2008).

Clinical Insight 18-3 ➤ Guidelines for Documentation

When to Document

Guideline	*How to Apply*	*Rationale or Example*
Documentation begins at the start of your shift.	▪ *Hospital or long-term care facility*—start of shift ▪ *Home visit or outpatient facility*—when you first encounter the client ▪ Document the condition of your patient when you first observed him. Was he awake? Was he in bed? Did he have any complaints? What did you do?	
Document immediately.	Discipline yourself to document as soon as possible after making an observation or providing care.	The longer you wait, the more likely you will forget important details.
Never chart ahead.	Never chart before performing an intervention.	It is impossible to see into the future and be sure that what you expect to happen will actually happen. To do this threatens the record's credibility.

Clinical Insight 18-3 ➤ Guidelines for Documentation *(continued)*

Guideline	How to Apply	Rationale or Example
Avoid "block" charting.	Each entry needs to be made individually; record the time each was done	Do not chart an entry time as "From 1300 to 1500."
Chart chronologically.	■ *On paper:* Document times in chronological order. ■ *EHRs:* Most automatically insert the current date and time when forms are opened. Follow the documentation system's guidelines for changing those dates and times before signing.	Chronological charting communicates the changing status of the patient.
Designate late entries (paper).	■ If you forget to make an important entry while charting, you will later need to add "late entry" to the first available line. ■ Record the time and date you are making the addition; clearly designate it is a late entry. ■ If you know legal action is pending, do not place a late note in the health record without notifying the nurse manager or risk management officer first.	■ Late entry example: 5/11/16, 1400; late entry for 5/11/16, 1200 ■ It is a criminal offense to alter a patient record after the organization's approved time limit for doing so has passed.
Designate late entries (EHR).	■ Open the appropriate form and change the automatically generated current date/time to the date/time your care was actually done; then sign. ■ Follow the agency policy regarding the time period for making a late entry.	
	What to Document	
Questions to aid your recall.	As your shift or visit progresses, you will perform assessments and nursing interventions. To remind yourself what to record, ask yourself these example questions.	■ What were your assessment findings? ■ Did any abnormalities exist? ■ What was the patient's response to your intervention? Did any changes occur from the initial assessment?
Interventions, patient responses, and evaluation of progress toward goals.	■ These are often recorded on an IPOC. ■ Clearly describe what your patient is experiencing. ■ **Key Point:** *Do not chart a symptom without also documenting what you did about it and how the patient responded.*	(Symptom) Pt complained of pain, rated 6 on a 0–10 scale. (Intervention) Administered Tylenol 1,000 mg, by mouth, at 0900. At 1030, pt rated pain as 3.
Significant events or changes in condition.	When possible, quote the patient's interpretation of the event or change.	Quoting the patient directly gives all healthcare providers objective data.
Informed consent.	■ If you are asked to obtain informed consent for a procedure, document your actions. ■ In most states, your signature (paper or electronic) confirms only that the patient signed the consent. ■ For further discussion of informed consent, see Chapters 44 and 45.	The primary provider conducting the procedure is legally responsible for discussing the procedure and its risks and benefits.

(Continued)

Clinical Insight 18-3 ➤ Guidelines for Documentation *(continued)*

Guideline	*How to Apply*	*Rationale or Example*
Patient teaching.	■ Include instruction about medications and patient diagnoses. ■ Include discharge teaching. ■ If the patient's physical or cognitive condition prevents teaching, explain that in your documentation.	Documenting patient teaching can positively affect insurance and other payments to the institution.
Spiritual or other concerns expressed by the patient and/or family.	Document your interventions.	Addressing spiritual concerns ensures that the patient receives holistic healthcare.
Attempts made to contact the primary care provider.	■ Contacts may, for example, be to notify the provider of the patient's condition, or to clarify orders. ■ If you are unable to contact the primary provider, document your contacts with your charge nurse, nurse manager, supervisor, medical director, and hospital administrator.	You must indicate that you made every effort to communicate your concerns.
Patient leaving the facility against medical advice. (AMA)	■ Chart the patient's condition, any explanations of risks and consequences given to the patient, the patient's destination (if known), and your notification of the patient's care providers. ■ If your facility has specific forms for AMA departures, use the designated form. ■ If the form is hard-copy paper, have the patient sign the form before leaving. ■ If the patient refuses to sign, note this in your chart.	Your actions and responsibilities in the situation must be made clear in the record.
Patient's refusal of treatment.	■ Try to determine the reason for refusal. ■ Quote the exact language the patient used in this situation whenever possible.	Helps ensure charting facts instead of inferences.
Use of restraints.	■ Most facilities have a separate form that allows you to document the reason for restraint use, the type of restraint, and frequent checks of the patient. ■ You must have contacted the primary care provider.	■ The primary care provider must place a signed order for restraints in the chart or in the EHR. ■ Restraint orders must be reordered inside a specific time frame set by the organization or the restraints are discontinued (see Chapter 24).
"Occurrences."	■ Chart your findings accurately and objectively. ■ Fill out a separate occurrence form and send to the risk manager (paper forms). ■ Do not make reference to the occurrence form anywhere in your charting.	■ Examples of occurrences: falls and medication errors. ■ Occurrence forms are not part of the client's health record. See **Occurrence Reports** in Volume 1.

Clinical Insight 18-3 ➤ Guidelines for Documentation *(continued)*

Guideline	How to Apply	Rationale or Example
Complete data about medications.	■ *Paper MAR*—Include the date, time, and medication given, and your initials. ■ *Electronic MAR*—Ensure your entry is accurate, then sign electronically that administration was accomplished successfully.	Accurate documentation is an essential component of the nurse's role.
prn, unscheduled, IV infusions,and STAT medications.	■ Record on the MAR. ■ Include comments regarding the medication in your narrative charting or insert a comment in your electronic charting. ■ Chart a timely evaluation of patient's response to the medication.	Certain prn medications require a follow-up response be documented within a specific period of time set by the organization, usually 15 to 30 minutes after the medication is given.
Medications not administered.	■ Document omission on the MAR. ■ If the patient states a reason for refusing the medication: *Paper notes*—Quote the patient in your narrative notes. *Electronic MAR*—Use pull-down or other menu.	■ *Examples:* Patient refuses medication; dose accidentally omitted. ■ Most electronic MARs include an explain with a selection from a drop-down list such as "Patient refused" or "Patient not available." ■ Some MARs also contain a narrative section to type a comment about why a medication was not given.

How to Document

Know your organization's requirements for reimbursement.

- Requirements typically specify frequency of charting and the type of data that must be recorded.
- Fulfilling documentation requirements helps to ensure appropriate reimbursement.
- Home care, hospitals, clinics, office settings and long-term care facilities have specific guidelines for documentation necessary for payment.

Date and time all your documentation.

- Most organizations use a 24-hour clock or military time to avoid confusion between a.m. and p.m.
- For detailed guidelines for converting a 12-hour clock to military time (24-hour clock),

Go to **Tables, Boxes, Figures: ESG Box 18-1,** on Davis*Plus*.

- The day begins at 0001 (1 minute past midnight) and ends at 2400 (12 midnight).
- *Morning hours*—Most people have little difficulty with early morning hours. Example: 9:00 a.m. is 0900.
- *Hours after 12 noon*—To convert to military time after 12 noon, simply add 12 to the clock time. Example: 7:30 p.m. + 12 = 1930 in military time.

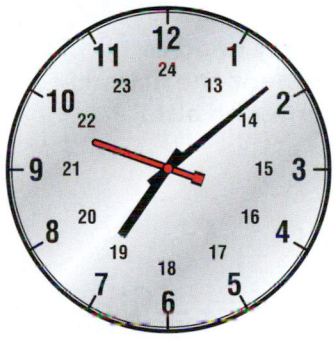

Many healthcare facilities use the 24-hour clock.

(Continued)

Clinical Insight 18-3 ➤ Guidelines for Documentation *(continued)*

Guideline	*How to Apply*	*Rationale or Example*
Document accurately and objectively, using nonjudgmental language.	■ Avoid labeling patients or team members. ■ Do not chart judgments about decisions made by members of the care team. ■ Document objective facts, so the reader can draw an informed conclusion. ■ Quote the patient in his own words, when possible.	■ *Chart:* "Pt says, 'I'm not taking that medicine. Take it away." ■ *Do not chart:* "Patient obnoxious and refuses prescribed medication."
Avoid vague, subjective words.	■ When possible, give specific examples.	■ Terms such as *good*, *average*, or *normal* do not clearly define the status of the client. ■ Descriptive details allow caregivers to better understand your patient's individual needs.
Use only the abbreviations authorized by your organization.	See Tables, Abbreviations Commonly Used in Health Care, following.	
Use correct spelling and grammar.	Incorrect spelling may raise questions about what you are attempting to communicate. Incorrect grammar implies carelessness on your part and creates a question of your competence if your chart is reviewed.	
Chart your own nursing actions.	Do not allow anyone to chart for you; do not document the actions of others as though you had performed them.	Each nurse is responsible for documenting his assessments, interventions, and evaluations. A deviation from this principle can imply coverup, carelessness, or a blatant disregard of policy and standards of practice.
You may need to document the actions of someone else.	■ Try to avoid this, but if you must do it, be sure to designate clearly whose actions they are. ■ *EHRs*—You can indicate another person performed the action in an added comment, or by searching for and selecting the other care provider in the appropriate field, then signing.	For example, if the NAP (nursing assistive personnel) helps the patient ambulate: *Do not chart:* "Patient assisted to bathroom." *Do chart:* "J. Scott, NAP, assisted patient to bathroom."
Avoid charting what someone else said, heard, felt, or smelled.	■ If the information is critical and you *must* chart it, use quotations and attribute the remarks to the person who made them.	*Example:* "Wife stated, 'My husband told me that he is in a lot of pain, but does not want to bother the nurses.'"

TABLES

Abbreviations Commonly Used in Healthcare

ABBREVIATION	MEANING	ABBREVIATION	MEANING
ADL	Activities of daily living	GI	Gastrointestinal
ad lib	As desired, if the patient desires	gtt(s)	Drop(s)
AKA	Above-knee amputation	GU	Genitourinary
amb	Ambulation, ambulatory	GYN	Gynecology
amt	Amount	HA	Headache
ASAP	As soon as possible	HMO	Health maintenance organization
bid	Twice a day	h/o	History of
BM	Bowel movement	hob or HOB	Head of bed
BR	Bedrest	HOH	Hard of hearing
BRP	Bathroom privileges	H&P	History and physical
BSC	Bedside commode	hr	Hour
$\bar{c}$	With	ht	Height
cal	Calories	HTN	Hypertension
Cath	Catheter	hyper	Above or high
CBC	Complete blood count	hypo	Below or low
CCU	Critical care unit or coronary care unit	ICU	Intensive care unit
c/o	Complaint of	I&O	Intake and output
CO_2	Carbon dioxide	isol	Isolation
CPR	Cardiopulmonary resuscitation	IV	Intravenous
CVA	Cerebrovascular accident (stroke)	IVP	Intravenous push (caution: do not use to mean "IV piggyback")
D&C	Dilation and curettage	L	Liter
DM	Diabetes mellitus	lb	Pound
dsg or drsg	Dressing	LPN	Licensed practical nurse
DX or Dx	Diagnosis	LMP	Last menstrual period
EBL	Estimated blood loss	LVN	Licensed vocational nurse
EKG/ECG	Electrocardiogram	mcg	Microgram
ED/ER	Emergency department, emergency room	MD	Medical doctor
EEG	Electroencephalogram	med	Medication
EENT	Eyes, ears, nose, throat	mg	Milligram
ETOH	Alcohol	mL	Milliliter
F	Female	MN	Midnight
FBS	Fasting blood sugar	NAS	No added salt
Ft	Foot	N/V/D	Nausea, vomiting, diarrhea
Fx	Fracture		

continued

Abbreviations Commonly Used in Healthcare—cont'd

ABBREVIATION	MEANING	ABBREVIATION	MEANING
NKA or NKDA	No known allergies or no known drug allergies	qam	Every morning
NG	Nasogastric	qh	Every hour
NGT	Nasogastric tube	qid	Four times a day
noc	At night	RN	Registered nurse
NPO	Nothing by mouth	R/O	Rule out
O_2	Oxygen	RX or Rx	Treatment or prescription
OB	Obstetrics	$\bar{s}$	Without
OOB	Out of bed	SCD	Sequential compression device
OPD	Outpatient department	SOB	Short of breath
ortho	Orthopedics	$\bar{ss}$	One-half
OR	Operating room	SSE	Soapsuds enema
os	Mouth, opening	Stat	Immediately
OT	Occupational therapy	STI or STD	Sexually transmitted infection or sexually transmitted disease
oz	Ounce	TB	Tuberculosis
pc	After meals	TO	Telephone order
PCA	Patient-controlled analgesia	TPR	Temperature, pulse, respirations
PO	By mouth	tid	Three times a day
P, $\bar{p}$	After	VO	Verbal order
PPBS	Postprandial blood sugar	VS	Vital signs
prn	As needed	WBC	White blood count
Pt	Patient	w/c	Wheelchair
PT	Physical therapy	WNL	Within normal limits
q	Every	wt	Weight

Caveat: Abbreviations vary among healthcare agencies. Furthermore, they change rather often because of regulating agency guidelines (e.g., The Joint Commission). Therefore, you will need to be familiar with the abbreviations in the agency in which you work.

CHARTING FORMS

Adult admission history electronic screen.

Hill, Richard - BWMC 006-829 Opened by Simms RN, Chris

Task Edit View Patient Chart Links Notifications Documentation Options Documentation Orders Help

PAL PMLaunch New Sticky Note View Sticky Notes Tear Off Attach Change Suspend Charges Charge Entry Exit Calculator AdHoc Medication Administration

Hill, Richard | Browne, Cindy

Hill, Richard — Age:52 years DOB:7/27/1956 — Sex:Male MRN:BWMC 006-829 — Location: BW5E; 5E01; 02 Fin Number: 013504 — Allergies: No Known Allergies Inpatient [mm/dd/yy 3:10 PM – <No - Discharg...

Menu - All: Overview, 24 Hr Summary, Results, Orders (Add), Flowsheet, MAR, Activities, Allergies (Add), Browser, Chart Review, Clinical Trials, Demographics, Documentation (Add), Dx/Problems, Growth Chart, Health Maintenance, Histories, Immunizations, MAR Summary, Medications (Add), Med Profile, Notes, Reference, Schedule, Condition Summary

Flowsheet — Print — 0 minutes ago

Nursing Assessment: Vital Signs, Primary Pain Assessment, Measurements, IV Drips, Cardiovascular, Respiratory, Breath Sounds Assessment, O_2 Therapy/Titration, Neurological, Neurovascular Check, Gastrointestinal, Genitourinary, Urinary Catheter, Glycemic Control, Notes, Miscellaneous, Phone Messages/Calls, Urine Dipstick, Diagnostic Radiology, Routine Chemistry, Routine Urinalysis, Office/Clinic Notes, Progress Notes

Med Surg Assessment; Graphs; Intake and Output; Ongoing Pediatric Assessment; Summary Report

mm/dd/yy 10:28 PM - mm/dd/yy 10:59 PM — MORE

Find Item — Critical High Low Abnormal Flag New

Vital Signs		mm/dd/yy 10:28 PM	6:00 AM	2:00 PM	mm/dd/yy 10:00 PM	6:00 AM	mm/dd/yy 2:00 PM	10:00 PM
Temperature Axillary	DegC							
Temperature Oral	DegC							
Temperature Tympanic	DegC				37.7			
Peripheral Pulse Rate	bpm				104 ↑			
Respiratory Rate	br/min				24 ↑			
SBP/DBP Cuff	mmHg				104/68			

USPRES NURSE October 06, 2011 10:33 PM

(Courtesy of Cerner Corporation.)

Nurses use intake and output (I&O) records to record data about the patient's fluid status.

INTAKE AND OUTPUT SHEET

DATE	Time	INTAKE						OUTPUT						SIGNATURE OF NURSE
		ORAL	IV	IV MED	BLOOD PRODUCT	OTHER	TOTAL	URINE	EMESIS	STOOL	SUCTION	OTHER	TOTAL	
	6 A.M.-2 P.M.													
	2 P.M.-10 P.M.													
	10 P.M.-6 A.M.													
	TOTAL													
	6 A.M.-2 P.M.													
	2 P.M.-10 P.M.													
	10 P.M.-6 A.M.													
	TOTAL													

Nursing assessment flowsheets are comprehensive charting documents.

DATE / /

VS	TIME							
	BP							
	P R							
	TEMPERATURE							
ASSESSMENTS / INTERVENTIONS	ACTIVITY							
	PAIN LEVEL:							
	INTERVENTION							
	RESPONSE							
	DR. VISIT							
LAB								
INTAKE	DIET / APPETITE							
	PO							
	IV							
	IV TUBE / SITE CONDITION							
OUTPUT	URINE							
	BM							
	SAFETY							
	PERSONAL CARES							
RESPIRATORY	❑ HEATED / ❑ COOL MIST / ❑ CROUP TENT — F102 / ✓ LIST							
	O2 — LPM / ADJ							
	O2 SAT — RA / O2							
	INC SPIRO							
	INITIAL							

TIME	PULSE Before	PULSE After	BREATH SOUNDS LU LL RU RL
			❑ ❑ CLEAR ❑ ❑
			❑ ❑ CRACKLES ❑ ❑
			❑ ❑ RHONCHI ❑ ❑
			❑ ❑ WHEEZING ❑ ❑
			❑ ❑ DIMINISHED ❑ ❑
			❑ ❑ ABSENT ❑ ❑

After Treatment Eval: ❑ NO CHANGE ❑ IMPROVED ❑ ADVERSE

DRUG | ❑ P&PD | INITIAL

TIME	PULSE Before	PULSE After	BREATH SOUNDS LU LL RU RL
			❑ ❑ CLEAR ❑ ❑
			❑ ❑ CRACKLES ❑ ❑
			❑ ❑ RHONCHI ❑ ❑
			❑ ❑ WHEEZING ❑ ❑
			❑ ❑ DIMINISHED ❑ ❑
			❑ ❑ ABSENT ❑ ❑

After Treatment Eval: ❑ NO CHANGE ❑ IMPROVED ❑ ADVERSE

DRUG | ❑ P&PD | INITIAL

TIME	PULSE Before	PULSE After	BREATH SOUNDS LU LL RU RL
			❑ ❑ CLEAR
			❑ ❑ CRACKLES
			❑ ❑ RHONCHI
			❑ ❑ WHEEZING
			❑ ❑ DIMINISHED
			❑ ❑ ABSENT

After Treatment Eval: ❑ NO CHANGE ❑ IMPROVED ❑ ADVER

DRUG | ❑ P&PD | INITIAL

PATIENT CARE FLOW SHEET

PUPIL SIZE

1 mm 2 mm 3 mm 4 mm 5 mm 6 mm 7 mm 8 mm

GLASGOW COMA SCALE

Child		Adult	
Eye Opening		**Eye Opening**	
Spontaneous	4	Spontaneous	4
To sounds	3	To speech	3
To painful stimulation	2	To pain	2
None	1	Nil	1
Motor Responses		**Motor Responses**	
Spontaneous Movement	6	Obeys commands	6
Localizes to pain	5	Localizes pain	5
Withdraws	4	Withdrawal	4
Reflex flexion	3	Abnormal flexion	3
Reflex extension (decerebrate)	2	Extensor rigidity	2
None (flaccid)	1	Nil	1
Verbal Responses		**Verbal Responses**	
Appropriate words or social smile; fixes and follows	5	Oriented	5
Cries, but consolable	4	Confused	4
Persistently irritable	3	Inappropriate	3
Restless, agitated	2	Incomprehensible	2
None	1	Nil	1

NEUROVASCULAR RATING SCALE

EXTREMITY: RA, LA, RL, LL CAP REFILL: NOR = <3 SEC * = >3 SEC
COLOR: NOR = NORMAL DU = DUSTY RED = RED PALE = PALE
SENSATION: NOR = INTACT NUMB = NUMBNESS TIN = TINGLING Ø = ABSENT
MOTION: FULL = FULL LTD = LIMITED Ø = NONE PAIN: RATE (0-10)
PULSES: NOR = NORMAL ↓ = DIMINISHED Ø = NOT PALPABLE DOP = DOPPLER

STRENGTH (DESIGNATE EXTREMITY)

5 = NORMAL STRENGTH
4 = LIFTS AGAINST RESISTANCE
3 = LIFTS AGAINST GRAVITY
2 = LIFTS, FALLS BACK
1 = MUSCLE CONTRACTION, NO MOVEMENT
0 = NO MUSCLE CONTRACTION, NO MOVEMENT

ADJUCANTS FOR 02 ADMINISTRATION

NC Nasal Cannula M Mask NRB Non Rebreather
TT Trans Trach ET Endotrachial Tube

Activity
AMB - Ambulating
ARMS - Being held
BR - Bed rest
CH - Chair
L - Lavatory
ROM - Range of motion
SLP - Sleeping
T/P - Turned/Positioned
↑ c̄ - Up with assist
↑ s̄ - Up without assist
DA - Dangle
CO - Commode

IV Site/Condition
✔- No redness, swelling, leakage
DC - Discontinued
INF - Infiltrated
SWL - Swelling
D△ - Dressing change
T△ - Tubing change

Personal Cares/Safety
AM - AM Care
PA - PM/HS Care
CLWR - Call Light Within Reach
OR - Oral Care
SH - Shower
SP - Sponge
SK - Skin Care
SR↑ - Side rails up
SR↓ - Side rails down
L△ - Linen changed
PE - Peri care
FO - Foley care
SN - Snack
BA - Backrub

Lab Values
✔- Physician notified

Diet
R - Regular
S - Soft
NA - Low Sodium
LF - Low Fat
MS - Mechanical Soft
ADA - Diabetic Diet
CL - Clear Liquids
FL - Full Liquids
ICE - Ice Chips
ø - Refused

Wound Interventions
DDI - Dressing dry, intact
DRNG - Drainage
D△ - Dressing change
SSG - Serosanguinous
SWL - Swelling
O - Odor

PAIN ASSESSMENT IN ADULTS

0 (NO PAIN) 1 2 3 4 5 6 7 8 9 10 (WORST PAIN)

INIT.	SIGNATURE / TITLE	INIT.	SIGNATURE / TITLE

PATIENT NAME

(Courtesy of Teton Valley Hospital, Driggs, ID.)

CLINICAL REASONING

Applying the Full-Spectrum Nursing Model

PATIENT SITUATION

Ellen is 85 years old and has sustained a right-sided cerebrovascular accident (CVA, stroke, or brain attack). Doctors say she is unlikely to regain much physical function, if she even awakens from the coma. Her children, Mary and Dale, have met with the physician, who tells them that Ellen is not likely to survive. The physician wants to insert a feeding tube and has asked whether they want Ellen to be resuscitated in case of cardiac or respiratory arrest. Mary tells you she wants to do what is best for her mother, but she feels that Ellen would not want to be kept alive in the condition she is in. She is also concerned about putting her through uncomfortable procedures if there is no chance of recovery. Her brother, Dale, says, "Mom needs the feeding tube. I can't sit and watch her starve to death. As long as she's alive, there's hope."

THINKING

1. *Theoretical Knowledge (Recall of Facts and Principles):* You plan to use the Focus Charting® format to document this interaction.
   a. Write the focus for this note.
   b. What does the acronym DAR stand for?
2. *Critical Thinking (Contextual Awareness):*
   a. What aspects of this situation have you experienced or observed before in your role as a caregiver?
   b. How might those past experiences affect your perception in this situation?

DOING

3. *Practical Knowledge (Handoff Report):* Ellen's last name is Smith; assume her children are also named Smith. Ellen is in room 820. Using the PACE format, what would you say to the oncoming nurse during handoff report? You will be able to address only a small amount of physiological information because the scenario does not provide it.

CARING

4. *Self-Knowledge:* In what way(s) can you identify with any of the people involved?

Critical Thinking and Clinical Reasoning

1. You are caring for a 96-year-old patient, James Wilson. Mr. Wilson has been admitted to the hospital for pneumonia. He is normally alert and oriented to place, time, and person. However, during this admission he has become confused and agitated. He frequently yells at staff and resists care by kicking and hitting. While you are providing morning care, Mr. Wilson becomes very agitated and yells and curses at you. When you attempt to provide oral hygiene, he throws his dentures at you. The dentures break when they hit the floor.
   a. Construct a nurse's note about this situation using the paper charting format you prefer.
   b. You will need to complete an occurrence report regarding the broken dentures. The report asks you to identify actions that you might have taken to prevent this incident. Brainstorm this question with your peers. Identify one or two actions that might have prevented this incident.
2. The primary care provider has written an order on your patient's paper chart that you find illegible. A veteran nurse states that she can read it, and she translates it for you. What factors should you consider before determining how to proceed?
3. For each of the following concepts, use critical thinking to describe how or why it is important to nursing, patient care, or documenting and reporting. Consider both paper and electronic documentation in each. Note that these are *not* to be merely definitions.

Narrative charting	Flowsheets
SOAP(IER) charting	Charting by exception
Nursing admission form	Signing documentation forms
Medication administration record	Handoff report
Occurrence report	Late entry

What Are the Main Points in This Chapter?

- The client record is a collection of documents that form a legal record of the client's healthcare experience.
- The client record is used by health professionals to communicate about the client's care, to legally document the care delivered to the client and the client's responses to that delivered care, to document care for reimbursement, to educate students, to determine whether care is adequate, as a data source for health research, and as the basis for determining the cost of care.
- In source-oriented records, members of each discipline record findings in a separately labeled section.
- In problem-oriented records, members of each discipline chart on shared notes, and the record is organized around a problem list.
- In electronic health records (EHRs), members of each discipline all chart inside the same EHR. The EHR can be organized as source-oriented, problem-oriented, or a combination of the two.
- The EHR can be accessed by many members of the healthcare team at the same time.
- In narrative charting, the writer tells the story of what has occurred in a chronological format.
- SOAP(IER) is an acronym for Subjective data, Objective data, Assessment, Plan (and Intervention, Evaluation, and Revision). This format may be used to address a single problem or to document summative notes on a patient.
- In Focus Charting®, data is entered in a Data–Action–Response (DAR) format.
- Charting by Exception (CBE) utilizes pre-printed or electronic flowsheets to document most aspects of care. CBE assumes that unless a separate entry is made—an exception—all standards have been met and the patient has responded as expected.
- Paper and electronic flowsheets and graphic records are used to record recurring assessments, such as vital signs, intake and output, weight, hygiene, and ADLs.
- Paper progress notes are used to document the patient's responses to care. They may be in the form of narrative, SOAP(IER), PIE, or Focus-style notes.
- A discharge summary should be completed when the patient is discharged from the organization. A transfer form should be completed when the patient is transferred within the organization.
- An occurrence report, or incident report, is a formal record of an unusual occurrence or accident that is not part of the patient's chart.
- The most commonly used paper and electronic home health documentation form is OASIS, a federally required form that includes history, assessment, demographics, and information about the client's and caregiver's abilities.
- Federal law requires that a resident in long-term care be evaluated using the Minimum Data Set for Resident Assessment and Care Screening (MDS) within 4 days of admission. The MDS must be updated every 3 months and with any significant change in client condition.
- The handoff report is designed to alert the next nurse about the client's status, changes in the client condition, planned activities, tests or procedures, or concerns that require follow-up.
- A consistent, structured (standardized) format should be used in handoff reports that contain critical key items to minimize miscommunication and other errors.
- Nurses should not take verbal and telephone orders unless the ordering provider is in a situation in which the order can't be written or entered or the patient is in a life-threatening situation.
- Telephone orders offer more room for error because of unfamiliar terminology and differences in background noise.
- Charting should be accurate and nonjudgmental.
- You should document as soon as possible after you make an observation or provide care.
- You should never share your electronic username or password with someone else.
- Document any significant events or changes in condition, teaching performed, use of restraints, and patient refusal of treatment or medications.
- You are responsible for documenting the care you provided. Never chart the actions of others as though you had performed them.
- If you believe a provider's order is inappropriate or unsafe, you are legally and ethically required to question the order.

Knowledge Map

Documenting & Reporting

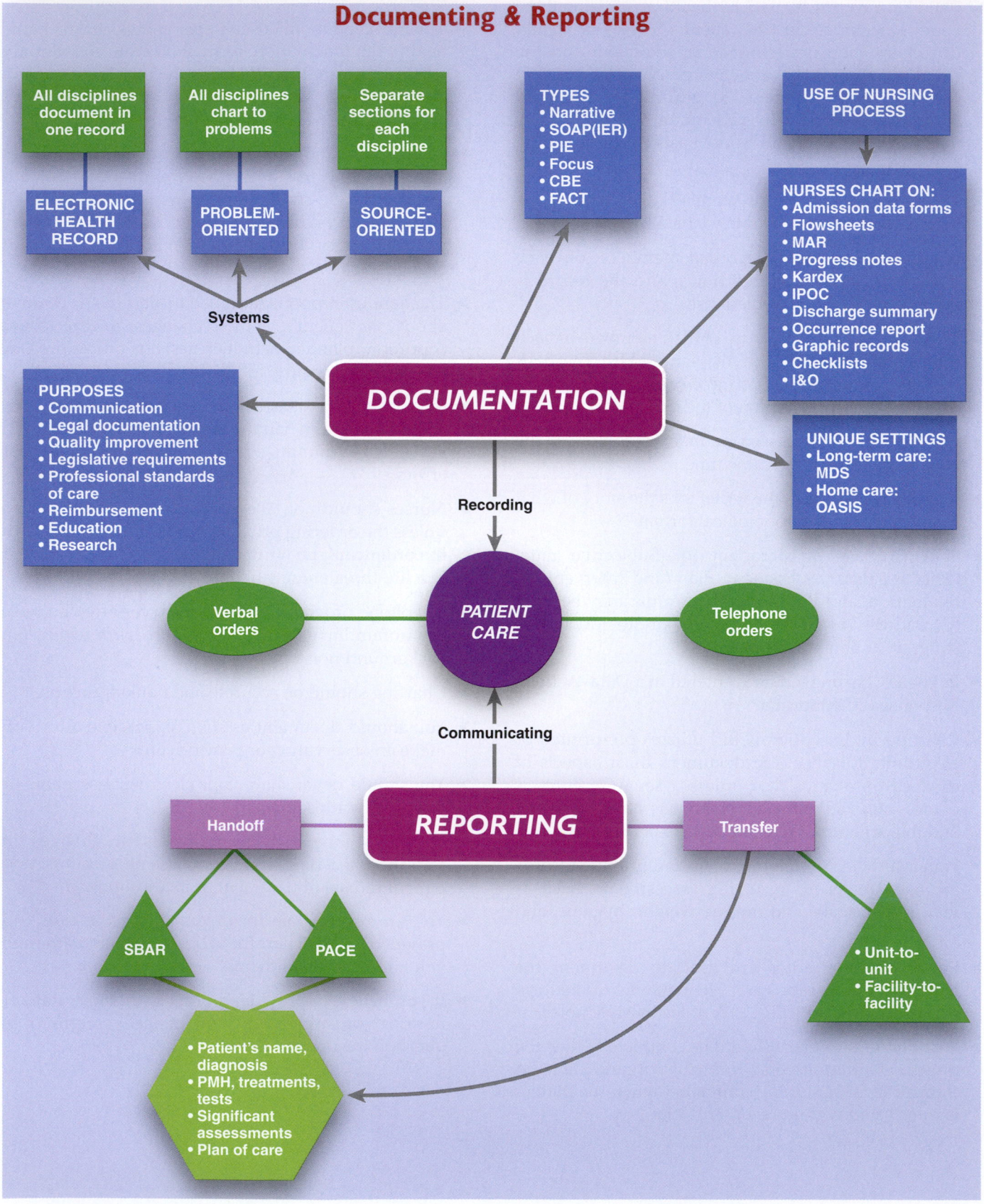

CHAPTER 19

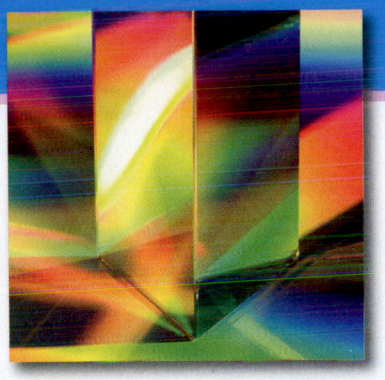

Teaching & Learning

STUDENT RESOURCES

*The questions and exercises in Volume 2 allow you to practice the kind of thinking you will use as a full-spectrum nurse. Critical-thinking questions usually have more than one correct answer, so we do not provide "answers" for these features. It is more important to develop your nursing judgment than to just cover content. You will learn by discussing the questions with your peers. If you are still unsure, consult your instructor. You will find Response Sheets (for writing your responses to the questions) on Davis*Plus.

To explore learning resources for this chapter,

Go to Davis*Plus* at DavisPl.us/Wilkinson3.

Chapter Resources for Chapter 19:

- **Response sheets for all learning activities**
- **Resources for Caregivers and Health Professionals**
- **Reading More About Teaching & Learning (suggested readings)**
- **Content Map of chapter content**

Interactive Case Studies

NCLEX-Style and Chapter Review Questions

CHAPTER OVERVIEW

For a podcast of an overview of this chapter,

Go to Student Resources: Chapter 19, **Podcast—Chapter Overview,** on Davis*Plus*

Caring for the Nguyens

Nam Nguyen has medical diagnoses including hypertension, type 2 diabetes mellitus, obesity, and osteoarthritis. There is a positive history of tobacco abuse. Based on the information you know about Nam and his family, consider the following questions.

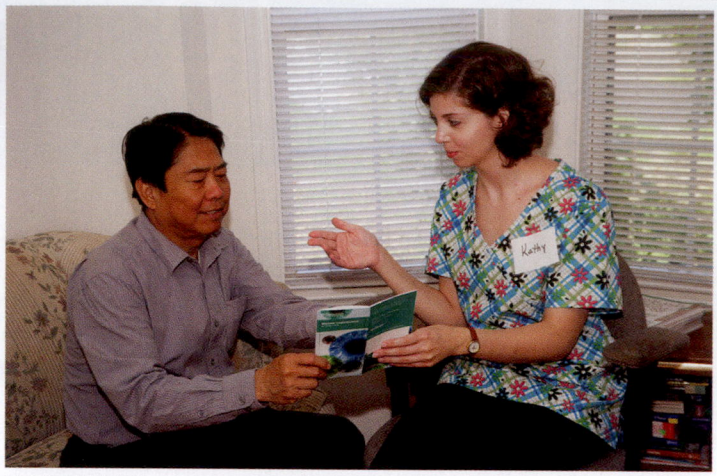

A. What kinds of information does Nam probably need?

B. What would be the best approach to teach Nam about his healthcare conditions?

C. You have been asked to teach Nam about weight loss. What theoretical knowledge must you have, and where can you obtain it?

D. What patient information do you need to know before planning your teaching?

E. Nam tells you that he feels overwhelmed with his recent diagnoses. He does not believe he can begin a weight-loss program or attend any teaching sessions. How might you handle this concern?

F. Nam has been prescribed the following medicines. Devise one or more teaching sessions focused on these medications. You will need to use your pharmacology reference books to devise this plan. As you plan your teaching, recall that Nam is overwhelmed by his recent diagnoses.

Lisinopril 20 mg PO daily
Hydrochlorothiazide 25 mg PO daily
Metformin 500 mg PO bid

Practical Knowledge knowing **how**

ASSESSMENT GUIDELINES AND TOOLS

Focused Assessment

Learning Assessment Guidelines

Pre-assessment

Before assessing the learner, think about the following:

- ***Time constraints.*** How much information do you need to present? How much time do you have to do it?
- ***Available resources.*** What equipment and supplies do you have to work with? Do you have access to the Internet? Audiovisual and projection equipment? A whiteboard? A scanner? Books? Do learners have mobile devices with downloaded applications for interactive classroom learning?

Assessing the Learner

You can assess the learner in several ways: through informal conversations, structured interviews, interviews, questionnaires, tests, observations, and information obtained from the client's chart. You will pick up many cues in your initial comprehensive assessment of the client. A teaching/learning assessment should include the following:

- ***Intended audience.*** Who are you teaching? What is the person's age, occupation, developmental level, and cultural affiliation? Will you be teaching a person or a group?
- ***Learning needs.*** The client's need for information is based on actual or anticipated healthcare or developmental needs. What is the client's health (or other) problem? What behavioral changes are needed? What self-care knowledge and skills does the client need?
- ***Client's knowledge level.*** Determine what the client already knows so that you can reinforce accurate information, correct misinformation, and adapt the teaching plan to the client's learning needs. Ask questions such as: "What do you think caused or worsened your health problem? What are your concerns about it? How has the problem affected your usual activities? What are your concerns about treatment (tests, surgery, and so on)?"
- ***Health beliefs and practices.*** Teaching will not be effective unless it falls into the range of beliefs and practices that are acceptable to the client. People are unlikely to incorporate changes that do not fit into their value system. Ask the client to give a general description of her health. Ask: "What do you usually do to stay healthy? What problems do you think you are at risk for? What lifestyle changes would you be willing to make in order to improve your health?"
- ***Physical readiness.*** The client must have adequate concentration, manual dexterity skills, and minimal pain to be able to listen and learn.
- ***Emotional readiness.*** Find out whether the client is experiencing anxiety or emotional distress that will interfere with the learning process. Also ask the client whether she would like a family member or friend to be present during the learning.
- ***Ability to learn.*** What are the learner's cognitive and psychomotor developmental level and ability? How does the client learn best (e.g., by memorization or recall, or by problem-solving or applying information)? How well does the client recall previously presented material?
- ***Health literacy level.*** Does the patient have the ability to understand basic health information and services needed to make appropriate healthcare decisions? Is the information the healthcare provider offers in the patient's primary language? Is the health teaching provided in a format the patient can understand? Is medical jargon or unnecessary technical information used? Can the person read and write?

  Adults who have low health literacy may react to learning situations by withdrawal, avoidance, or repeated noncompliance. They may claim that they were too tired, were too busy, or just didn't feel like reading. They may also ask you to read to them with the excuse that their eyes are tired, they are not interested, or they have no energy. They may fail to ask questions or ask for clarification.
- ***Neurosensory factors.*** What is the client's ability to feel, see, hear, and grasp? Does the client have a medical condition that causes neurosensory compromise?
- ***Learning styles.*** Ask the person: "How do you prefer to learn new things? For example, do you prefer to read about them, talk about them, watch a video, be shown how to do it, listen to the teacher, or use a computer? Do you like to read? Where do you get information about your health—online, from books, magazines, your family, your healthcare provider? Do you learn best alone or with other people?"

CLINICAL REASONING

Applying the Full-Spectrum Nursing Model

PATIENT SITUATION

Katrina Peplowsi is a 22-year-old college student from Ukraine who is transported to the emergency department of a local hospital after passing out in her dorm room. Katrina had been sick with a viral illness and she had a fever for 5 days with nausea, vomiting, and diarrhea. She had been drinking large amounts of Gatorade because of her insatiable thirst, thought to be related to the fever and vomiting. Before the illness, Katrina's friends and family had been commenting about her remarkable weight loss since she started school 2 months earlier in spite of her increased appetite. On arrival to the emergency department, Katrina's blood sugar is 585 mg/dL. She is diagnosed with diabetes mellitus, type 1. After her blood sugar is stabilized with fluid therapy and insulin infusion, Katrina regains consciousness. Although Katrina speaks some English, her proficiency is somewhat limited.

THINKING

1. *Theoretical Knowledge (Recall of Facts and Principles):* As your patient is newly diagnosed with diabetes mellitus, type 1, there are many areas in which Katrina will need healthcare education. List at least six important topics that are relevant to her care.
2. *Critical Thinking (Application of Knowledge):* What considerations do you make as you are devising a teaching plan for Katrina?
3. *Critical Thinking (Synthesis of Knowledge):* What factors would you consider important for customizing her teaching plan, considering the extent of her ability to communicate?

DOING

4. *Nursing Process (Assessment):* What are some pertinent personal factors that you should assess for Katrina when devising a teaching plan that is best suited to her learning needs?
5. *Nursing Process (Planning):* When setting up a teaching plan involving other members of the healthcare team, how would you plan to optimize Katrina's motivation to learn how to best manage her diabetes after discharge?

CARING

6. *Self-Knowledge:* What areas of commonality do you have with Katrina, around which you might form a caring relationship?
7. *Ethical Knowledge:* Suppose Katrina refuses to receive information from you about diabetes mellitus. She states she is not interested in knowing how to give herself insulin because she doesn't want to give herself injections at home. How should you best respond to Katrina's requests?

Critical Thinking and Clinical Reasoning

1. For the following Nursing Outcomes Classification (NOC) standardized outcomes (Moorhead, Johnson, & Maas, 2013), try to figure out which NANDA-I diagnoses might be linked to each outcome. Consult the NANDA-I handbook as necessary.

   Knowledge: Breastfeeding
   Knowledge: Child Physical Safety
   Knowledge: Diabetes Management
   Knowledge: Infant Care
   Knowledge: Disease Process
   Knowledge: Energy Conservation
   Knowledge: Health Behavior
   Knowledge: Healthy Diet
   Knowledge: Prescribed Activity
   Knowledge: Infection Management

2. Recall that Heather (Meet Your Patient in Volume 1) is a 20-year-old mother of a 4-year-old preschooler. They have come to a family practice clinic for a well-child checkup. You notice that the child speaks only in one- or two-word phrases. Heather is impatient with her and repeatedly tells her to "stop using that baby talk." Your nursing instructor tells you that you need to assess for teaching needs and provide anticipatory guidance to the mother regarding safety, nutrition, and normal preschooler growth and development.
   a. Heather says, "I don't know what I'm doing wrong. All her little friends are taller and talking more. She was even small when she was born, so I suppose it's my fault." How do you assess Heather's learning needs without reinforcing her feelings of self-blame?

b. Your assessment shows that although the child is below the 5th percentile for height and weight, she has grown appropriately since her last clinic visit. What teaching could you provide that might help address her mother's learning needs related to childhood growth and development?
c. In addition to information on growth and development, your anticipatory guidance should include safety measures and nutrition for a 4-year-old. How can you evaluate whether your teaching has been effective and further promote Heather's retention of all of this new information?

3. As a student, you have learned about discharge planning. Your instructor tells you that you need to begin teaching for discharge as soon as the client is admitted. You hear the nurses complaining that they just don't have time for any teaching. So where do you begin? You will need to use the teaching process for your assigned client.

   Your client is a 9-year-old girl who is being admitted to the outpatient procedures unit for testing because of chronic recurrent urinary tract infections. Daily, she receives an antibiotic, methylphenidate (Ritalin) for attention deficit-hyperactivity disorder (ADHD), and an asthma inhaler for sports activities. She is accompanied by her mother and father, a younger sister, and her big, pink teddy bear. She is scheduled for x-ray studies and blood work. Depending on the results of her tests, she may require surgery or dilation of her ureters. The parents appear very anxious and tell you that their daughter "has a hard time understanding things and needs a lot of repetition." You have an hour to prepare her for the procedures and testing.

   a. Assessment
      (1) What information do you already have that will be significant for your teaching plan?
      (2) What other information will you need to gather?
   b. Diagnosis
      (1) What possible diagnoses are involved in this situation? Consider a diagnosis for your client and another one for at least one of her family members.
   c. Planning
      (1) What information will you present first?
      (2) What teaching techniques would you use for this situation?
      (3) Who would you include in the teaching?
      (4) Where would you complete the teaching?
   d. Goals and interventions
      (1) Write an appropriate goal for your client (the child). Remember to make the goal client-centered, timed, and realistic. You have only an hour to complete this teaching.
      (2) What content and methods would you include in your teaching plan?
      (3) How can you incorporate a stuffed teddy bear in your teaching?
   e. Evaluation
      (1) How would you determine whether your teaching was effective?
      (2) What further teaching do you need to continue to prepare your client for discharge?

4. For each of the following situations, determine which teaching techniques would be most effective.
   a. A group of adolescents with diabetes needs to plan for their prom. The after-prom party lasts until 6:00 a.m. and will interfere with their usual schedule for insulin administration. You need to help them decide how to manage this problem. They are all busy with after-school activities and attend three different schools.
   b. An 80-year-old man has experienced a cerebrovascular accident (CVA) (stroke) with right-sided weakness. He will need mobility training and assessment of his home situation for safety hazards. Currently he lives alone.
   c. A new mother must learn how to feed her infant, who has a cleft palate. She is in considerable pain after an emergency cesarean section and unexpected blood loss.

5. You are assigned to a client with a diagnosis that you are unfamiliar with. You are expected to prepare a teaching session for this client and family as well as for your classmates. How should you prepare for this assignment?

6. Give an example of teaching content you might need to present to a 58-year-old patient who has been diagnosed with hypertension. What chapters in this text (Volume 1) might be useful if you need theoretical knowledge about hypertension to answer this question? Where would you look to verify where this information is located?

7. Do you think it is appropriate for a nurse to offer personal experiences in the teaching process? Explain your thinking.

8. A client refuses to make eye contact during a teaching session. This makes it difficult for you to determine whether she is actually paying attention to what you are saying. How can you assess whether she is focused on the teaching session?

9. For each of the following concepts, use critical thinking to describe how or why it is important to nursing, patient care, or teaching clients. Note that these are *not* to be merely definitions.

Role of teaching in nursing practice
Principles of teaching and learning
Factors that affect the learning process
Factors that affect the teaching process
Timing
Choice of techniques
Relevance
Learning styles
Amount of information to be presented

What Are the Main Points in This Chapter?

- Teaching is an essential component of professional nursing.
- Nurses do formal and informal teaching for individuals and groups.
- To be effective, teaching requires cooperation between the learner and the teacher.
- Learning is a change in behavior, knowledge, skills, or attitudes that occurs as a result of exposure to environmental stimuli.
- Bloom and Krathwohl (1956) identified three domains of learning: cognitive, psychomotor, and affective.
- Teaching includes motivating the learner.
- Teaching is interactive and requires communication.
- Readiness means that the learner is both motivated and able to learn at a specific time.
- Other factors that affect learning include emotions, timing, active involvement, feedback, repetition, environment, amount and complexity of the content, communication, developmental stage, culture, and literacy.
- Common barriers to teaching in the hospital setting include failure to see teaching as a priority and lack of time, preparation, space, privacy, poor coordination, and third-party reimbursement for teaching.
- Barriers to learning include illness, physical discomfort and fatigue, anxiety, low health literacy, environmental distraction, overwhelming amount of behavioral change needed, not enough time, lack of positive reinforcement, and feelings of discouragement.
- The teaching process is similar to the nursing process.
- The nursing diagnosis Deficient Knowledge may be the primary problem or the etiology of other problems; this diagnosis is often overused or used incorrectly.
- A teaching plan is similar to a nursing care plan, except that (1) interventions are actually teaching strategies and (2) the plan includes the content of the teaching, the sequencing of the content, and the materials to be used.
- Demonstration and return demonstration are the most effective strategies for teaching psychomotor skills.
- A certain amount of forgetting is normal. You can aid learner retention by using strategies that require learner participation and by providing printed materials to use at a later time.
- It is important to document specifically what teaching you did as well as your evaluation of the learning that occurred.

Knowledge Map

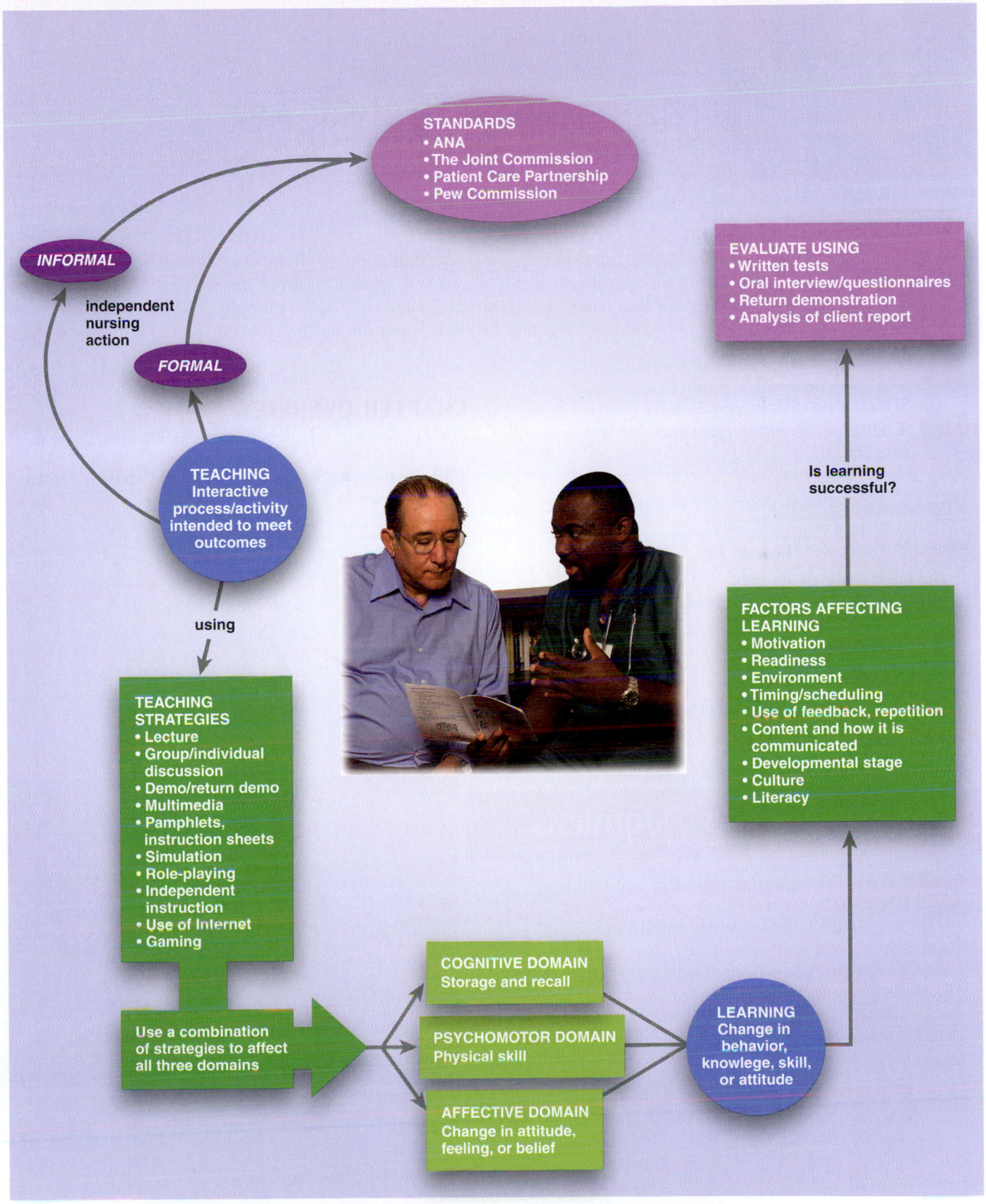

CHAPTER 20

Measuring Vital Signs

STUDENT RESOURCES

*The questions and exercises in Volume 2 allow you to practice the kind of thinking you will use as a full-spectrum nurse. Critical-thinking questions usually have more than one correct answer, so we do not provide "answers" for these features. It is more important to develop your nursing judgment than to just cover content. You will learn by discussing the questions with your peers. If you are still unsure, consult your instructor. You will find Response Sheets (for writing your responses to the questions) on Davis*Plus.

To explore learning resources for this chapter,

Go to Davis*Plus* at DavisPl.us/Wilkinson3.

Chapter Resources for Chapter 20:
- **Response sheets for all learning activities**
- **Resources for Caregivers and Health Professionals**
- **Reading More About Vital Signs (suggested readings)**
- **Concept Map of chapter content**

Interactive Case Studies

NCLEX-Style and Chapter Review Questions

CHAPTER OVERVIEW

For a podcast of an overview of this chapter,

Go to Student Resources, Chapter 20, **Podcast—Chapter Overview,** on Davis*Plus*.

Caring for the Nguyens

Recall that on Nam Nguyen's preliminary visit to the Family Medicine Center, his blood pressure (BP) was 162/94 mm Hg. On subsequent visits, his BP was 168/100 and 174/96 and he was continuing to gain weight. Mr. Nguyen was diagnosed with hypertension and prescribed an antihypertension medication to be taken each morning. This morning Mr. Nguyen has come to the clinic for follow-up. The following information is gathered as he checks in for his visit.

VS: BP, 168/92; pulse, 80 beats/min; respirations, 20 breaths/min; temperature, 98.4°F (36.9°C)
Weight: 180 lb (82 kg)

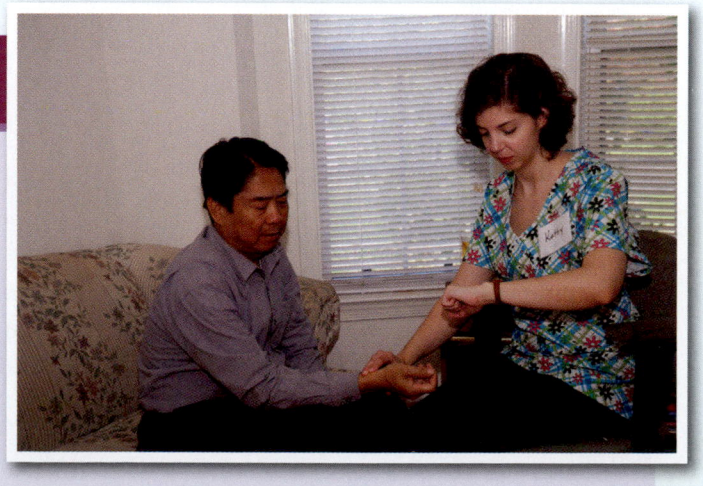

Caring for the Nguyens (continued)

Review the preliminary data and the preceding information to answer the following questions:

A. What patterns do you see in the data?

B. Do you have enough information to draw any conclusions? If not, what other information should you gather?

C. Identify three alternatives that may explain what is happening with Mr. Nguyen's vital signs.

D. How could you determine which of these alternatives provides the best explanation of what is happening?

E. Why is it important to intervene in this situation?

Practical Knowledge knowing how

Use the Procedures, Clinical Insights, and tables in this section when assessing your patients' vital signs.

PROCEDURES

Procedure 20-1 ■ Assessing Body Temperature

➤ For steps to follow in *all* procedures, refer to the Universal Steps for All Procedures found on the inside back cover.

Equipment

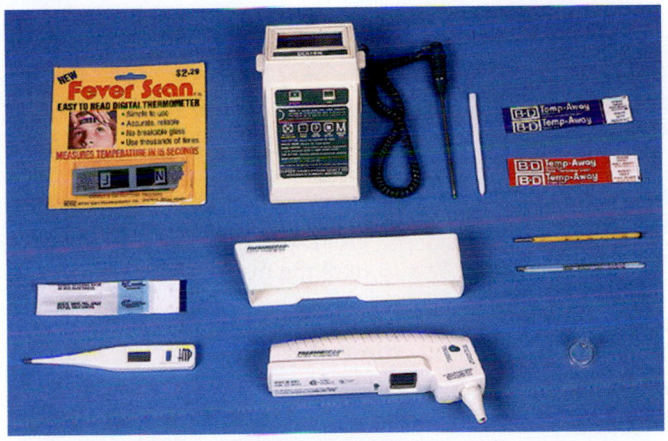

- Thermometer (An oral thermometer generally has a blue tip. A rectal thermometer generally has a red tip.)
- ✚ Glass-and-mercury thermometers should not be used in any healthcare setting, but because some people still use them at home, we include them in this procedure. They should be used with disposable covers, and cleaned and sterilized regularly according to the manufacturer's instructions.
- Thermometer cover, if needed
- Procedure gloves, if taking a rectal temperature or if there is risk of contact with body fluids (e.g., saliva)
- Water-soluble lubricant, if taking a rectal temperature
- Towel, if needed, for taking an axillary temperature (*to dry the axillae*)
- Tissues

Delegation

You can delegate temperature measurement to nursing assistive personnel (NAP) if you conclude that the patient's condition and the NAP's skills allow. Perform the pre-procedure assessments that follow, and inform the NAP of the route and type of thermometer used. Explain any special considerations (e.g., tell the NAP if the patient had food or oral fluids in the last 20 to 30 minutes; inform the NAP if the patient is confused). Ask the NAP to record and report the temperature to you, and to report immediately if the temperature is elevated (e.g., greater than 100°F [37.8°C]).

(continued on next page)

Procedure 20-1 ■ Assessing Body Temperature (continued)

Pre-Procedure Assessments

- Determine the site that is most appropriate for the patient. Consider patient comfort, safety, and accuracy. For example, do not use the oral route for patients who are unable to hold the thermometer properly, for children or others who cannot follow instructions (e.g., unconscious patients), or for patients who use "mouth breathing."
- For an oral temperature: Determine how long it has been since the patient smoked, had anything to eat or drink, or chewed gum.
  Smoking, eating, drinking, and chewing gum can all affect an oral reading. If any of these have occurred, wait 20 to 30 minutes before taking an oral temperature.
- Assess for any contraindications to using the site you have chosen. For example:
  Tympanic: Assess for impacted earwax or hearing aid.
  Rectal: Check the client record for diarrhea or impacted stool.
  Axillary: Check the client record for presence of fever or hypothermia.
  Skin: Assess for the presence of conditions that require a very precise, reliable reading (e.g., fever, hypothermia).
  Some conditions increase the risk for patient injury; others contribute to inaccurate, unreliable temperature measurement.
- What were the previous recordings, if any?
  Noting changes over time is important in all patient assessments.
- Assess for clinical signs and symptoms of temperature alterations.

Procedure 20-1A ■ Taking an Axillary Temperature

➤ When performing the procedure, always identify your patient according to agency policy, using two identifiers, and be attentive to standard precautions, hand hygiene, patient safety and privacy, body mechanics, and documentation.

Procedure Steps

1. **Slide the thermometer into a** protective sheath (depending on type of thermometer).
   A protective sheath provides a barrier to prevent transmission of organisms.
2. **Dry the patient's axilla,** as needed.
   Moisture from perspiration alters the temperature reading.
3. **Position the patient** and the thermometer.
   a. Assist the patient to a supine or sitting position.
   b. Place the thermometer tip in the middle of the axilla.
   c. Position the patient's upper arm down, with the lower arm across the chest.
   Puts the thermometer in close proximity to the axillary blood vessels, allowing it to better reflect the core temperature. ▼

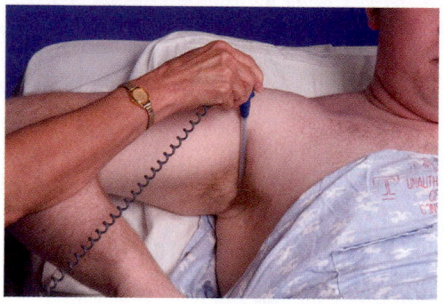

4. **Hold the thermometer in place** for the recommended time.
   a. Leave an electronic probe in place until it beeps.
   b. Leave a glass or plastic thermometer in place for 8 minutes, or according to agency policy (usually 5 minutes for children).
   Study findings differ for accuracy of temperature measurements at the axillary site. Follow agency policy.
5. **Remove the thermometer** and discard the thermometer cover. If there is no cover, wipe the thermometer with a tissue.
   Removes any moisture that may have accumulated in 8 minutes' time.
6. **Read the temperature.**
   a. Electronic thermometer: Read the digital display.
   b. Glass or plastic thermometer: Hold at eye level, and rotate it until the markings are clear.
7. **Clean and replace the thermometer** in the storage base, following agency policy.
   Prevents microbial growth on thermometers and recharges the battery.

Procedure 20-1B ■ Taking an Oral Temperature

➤ When performing the procedure, always identify your patient according to agency policy, using two identifiers, and be attentive to standard precautions, hand hygiene, patient safety and privacy, body mechanics, and documentation.

Procedure Steps

1. **For a glass or plastic thermometer,** shake down the liquid if necessary. Use a glass thermometer only if you must.
   a. Stand in an open area away from tables and other objects.
   Prevents thermometer breakage.
   b. Hold the end opposite the bulb between your thumb and forefinger, and snap your wrist downward.
   c. Shake the thermometer until the reading is less than 96°F (36°C).
   The reading must be lower than the anticipated temperature measurement.
2. **Slide the thermometer into** a protective sheath.
   Provides a barrier to prevent transmission of microorganisms.

3. **Place the thermometer tip** under the tongue in the posterior sublingual pocket (right or left of frenulum).
Puts the tip in close proximity to the major blood vessels under the tongue, allowing the thermometer to reflect the core temperature. ▼

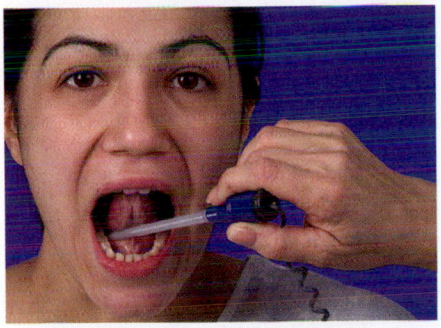

4. **Have the patient close her lips** around the thermometer, cautioning her not to bite down on it.
Protects the thermometer from exposure to the air, which could alter the reading. Biting may break a glass thermometer, injuring the mouth.

5. **Leave the thermometer in place** for the recommended time.
   a. Glass or plastic thermometer: 5 to 8 minutes
   b. Electronic (digital) thermometer: Until it beeps
   c. According to agency policy
   Research findings differ on the optimal time for measuring an oral temperature, so follow agency policy.

6. **Remove the thermometer;** discard the cover. If there is no cover, wipe the thermometer with a tissue.
Wiping removes mucus that can make the markings on a glass or plastic thermometer difficult to read.

7. **Read the temperature.**
   a. Glass or plastic thermometer: Position the thermometer at eye level, and rotate it until the markings are clear. ▼

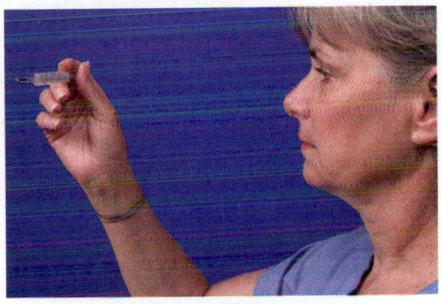

   b. Electronic thermometer: Read the digital display.

8. **Clean and replace the thermometer.** Follow agency policy.
Prevents microbial growth on thermometers and recharges battery of electronic thermometers.

Procedure 20-1C ■ Taking a Rectal Temperature

➤ When performing the procedure, always identify your patient according to agency policy, using two identifiers, and be attentive to standard precautions, hand hygiene, patient safety and privacy, body mechanics, and documentation.

➤ *Note:* This procedure primarily describes use of an electronic (digital) thermometer.

Procedure Steps

1. **Slide the thermometer into** a protective sheath.
A protective sheath provides a barrier to prevent transmission of microorganisms.

2. **Position an adult patient** in Sims' position (on the side with the knees flexed); place a child in the prone position. Drape the patient so that only the anal area is exposed. ▼

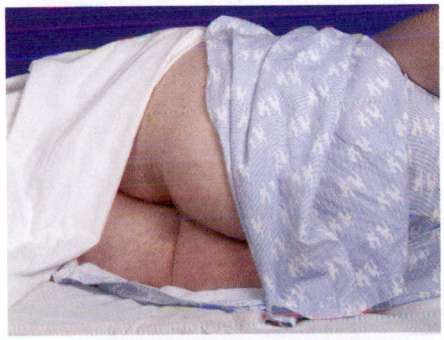

Procedure Variation for a Small Child
You can lay the child face down across your lap or a parent's lap.
Flexing the knees helps relax the muscles to ease insertion and aid in visualization. Draping provides privacy and decreases embarrassment.

3. **Lubricate the tip** of the thermometer by squeezing water-soluble lubricant onto a tissue and then applying it to the thermometer.
Prevents injury to the rectal mucosa and eases insertion. Inserting the thermometer into the lubricant container would contaminate contents of the container.

4. **Don a procedure glove** on your dominant hand, or on both hands if necessary.

5. **With your nondominant hand,** separate the patient's buttocks to visualize the anus.

6. **Gently insert** the thermometer approximately:
   Adult: 1 to 1.5 in. (2.5 to 3.7 cm)
   Child: 0.9 in. (2.5 cm)
   Infant: 0.5 in. (1.5 cm)
   The thermometer must be placed past the rectal sphincter.
   a. Have the patient take a deep breath. Insert the thermometer as he exhales.
   Taking a deep breath helps relax the anal sphincter.
   b. If you feel resistance, do not use force.
   Inserting the thermometer too far or forcing against resistance may injure the rectal mucosa. ▼

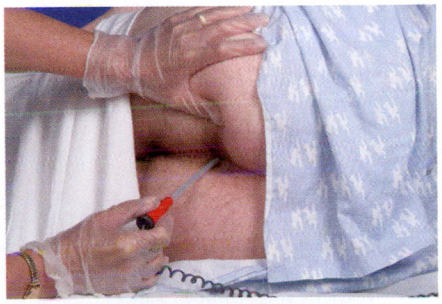

7. **Hold the thermometer in place** until it beeps. (For a glass thermometer, hold the thermometer 3 to 5 minutes. Avoid using a glass thermometer when at all possible.)
The thermometer must be held in place to prevent inadvertent injury to the patient. An electronic thermometer will beep when a constant temperature is reached. Research differs on the optimal time for measuring a rectal temperature, so follow agency policy.

(continued on next page)

Procedure 20-1 ■ Assessing Body Temperature (continued)

8. **Remove the thermometer**, discard the cover, and read the digital display.

9. **Remove the procedure glove(s)** and discard in a biohazards container.

10. **Follow agency policy** for cleaning and storing thermometers.

Prevents microbial growth on thermometers and recharges electronic thermometer battery.

Procedure 20-1D ■ Taking a Temporal Artery Temperature

➤ When performing the procedure, always identify your patient according to agency policy, using two identifiers, and be attentive to standard precautions, hand hygiene, patient safety and privacy, body mechanics, and documentation.

Procedure Steps

NOTE: If the patient has been lying down, do not measure the temperature on the side that was lying on the pillow. Do not measure if a cap or hair has been covering the area over the temporal artery.
These can prevent heat dissipation and produce a falsely high reading.

1. **Remove the protective cap** from the instrument; clean the lens/probe according to the manufacturer's instructions.

2. **Place the probe flat** on the center of the forehead, midway between the eyebrow and the hairline. ▼

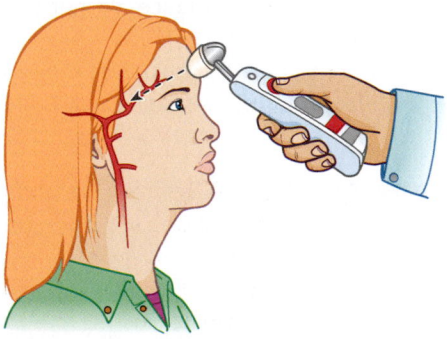

3. **Press and hold the button** while you stroke the thermometer medially to laterally across the forehead; keep the lens/probe flat and in contact with the skin, and slide in a reasonably straight line until you reach the hairline. ▼

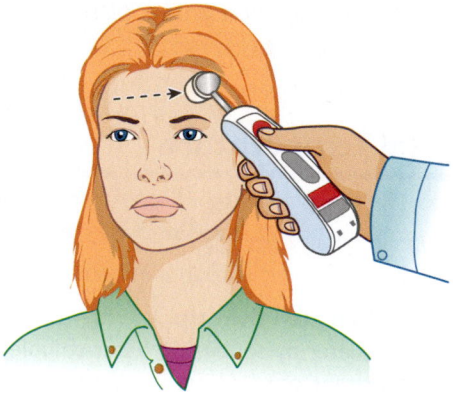

4. **Still holding the button,** touch the thermometer lens/probe behind the ear lobe, in the soft depression below the mastoid.
This step is necessary for an accurate reading if there is any moisture at all on the patient's forehead. ➤

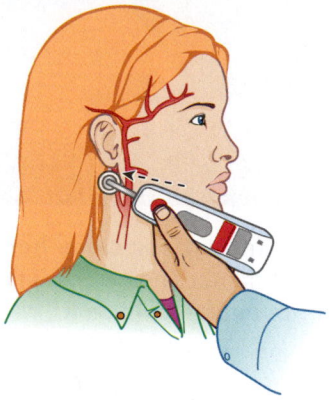

5. **Release the button for** the temperature reading. ▼

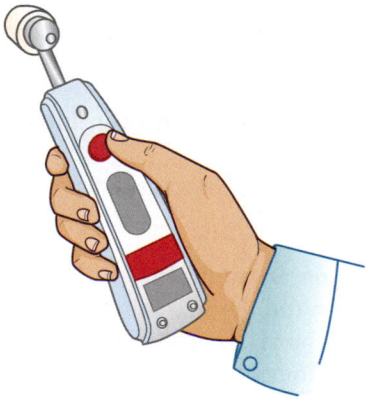

Procedure 20-1E ■ Taking a Tympanic Membrane Temperature

➤ When performing the procedure, always identify your patient according to agency policy, using two identifiers, and be attentive to standard precautions, hand hygiene, patient safety and privacy, body mechanics, and documentation.

Procedure Steps

1. **Make sure the thermometer** lens is intact and clean.
Ensures an accurate reading.

2. **Place a disposable cover tightly** over the lens, making sure the clear film is smooth across the lens.
Ensures an accurate reading and prevents cross-contamination.

3. **Position the patient's head** to one side. If you are right-handed try to use the right ear; if you are left-handed, use the left ear.
This allows you to better visualize the ear canal.

4. **Straighten the ear canal,** or follow the manufacturer's instructions. As a rule: ➤

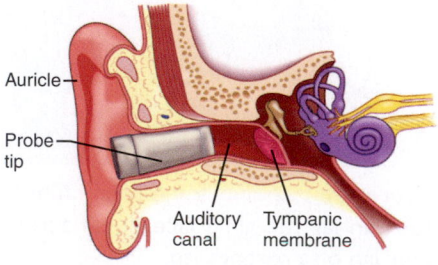

a. For an adult, pull the pinna up and back.

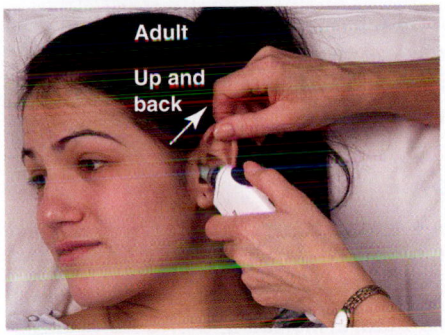

b. For a child, pull the pinna down and back.

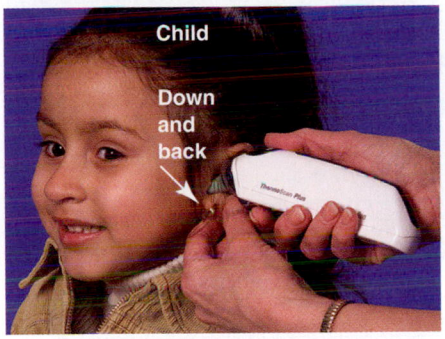

Some tympanic thermometers require you to straighten the ear canal; others do not. Some instruct, for adults, to pull the ear up, backward, and slightly away from the head. Some models instruct, for a child, to pull the pinna straight back instead of down and back. The external auditory canal is curved upward in children younger than 3 years of age. In an adult, it is a slightly S-shaped structure.

5. **Insert the probe into the ear** canal gently and firmly, directing it toward the tympanic membrane and inserting far enough to seal the opening.
   Creates a seal to obtain an accurate reading without causing trauma to the ear canal.

6. **Rotate the probe handle** towards the jaw (for some thermometer models). Follow the manufacturer's instructions; not all models require this.
   Aims the lens toward the tympanic membrane.

7. **Take the measurement.**
   a. Press and release the button to obtain the reading.
   b. Follow the instructions for the specific tympanic thermometer being used.
   Some tympanic thermometers record the reading immediately; for some you must wait for about 3 seconds.

8. **Remove the thermometer** when you hear a beep and the display flashes. Note the reading in the display window.

9. **Repeat the measurement** in the other ear.
   A study of 132 adults found significant differences in temperature in the left compared with the right ear. In addition, the left ear tended to register a lower temperature than the right ear at temperatures below 36.7°C (98.1°F) and a higher temperature above 36.7°C (Heusch & McCarthy, 2005) or when taken by a female (Helton & Carter, 2011).

10. **Discard the probe cover** (usually you will press an "eject" button to do this), and replace the thermometer in its charging base.
    Recharges the battery and protects the instrument.

Procedure 20-1F ■ Taking a Skin Temperature Using a Chemical Strip Thermometer

➤ When performing the procedure, always identify your patient according to agency policy, using two identifiers, and be attentive to standard precautions, hand hygiene, patient safety and privacy, body mechanics, and documentation.

Procedure Steps

1. **Place the thermometer strip** (paper or tape) on the patient's skin, generally on the forehead or abdomen.
   The thermometer strip must be in contact with the skin to work properly.

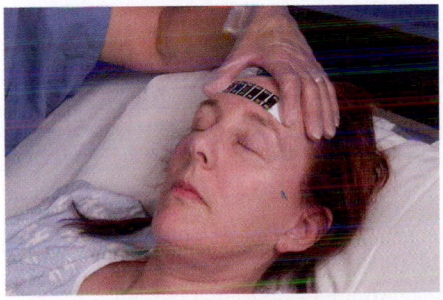

2. **Leave the thermometer strip** in place 15 to 60 seconds (or as the manufacturer directs).

3. **Observe for color changes.**
   Chemical strips have indicators that change colors to indicate temperature changes.

4. **Read the temperature before** removing the strip from the patient's skin.
   Ensures the most accurate reading.

5. **Remove and discard** the thermometer strip.

? What if . . .

- **The patient's temperature is not within normal range?**
  Identify whether the temperature reading indicates hypothermia, fever, or hyperthermia (e.g., heat stroke). Perform other assessments to determine the cause or severity of the findings.
  Assess for clinical signs to confirm an abnormal temperature reading.
  Institute interventions to raise or lower temperature, as appropriate.
  Provide comfort measures (e.g., change linens if they are wet from diaphoresis).
- **You are must use a glass thermometer?**
  Be sure the thermometer does not contain mercury.

- **Before and after using, shake down the thermometer as needed.**
- **Clean the thermometer** before and after using with soap and water or approved solution; rinse.
- **Use disposable covers, if available.**
- **When reading the thermometer,** hold it at eye level and rotate it until the markings are clear and easy to read.
  Handle carefully and store in an appropriate container to avoid breakage.

(continued on next page)

Procedure 20-1 ■ Assessing Body Temperature (continued)

Evaluation

- Compare to normal range for developmental stage, site used, and client's baseline data.
- Look for trends to identify potential concerns.
- Notify the appropriate healthcare provider of abnormal findings.

Patient Teaching

- Inform the patient of the temperature reading.
- Explain the significance of the temperature reading and any interventions that may be needed.

Home Care

- Clients commonly use chemical strip (disposable), glass, or tympanic membrane thermometers at home. Teach the following points:
- Do not use an oral thermometer to take a rectal temperature. Use a specially shaped, more rounded, rectal thermometer *to avoid injury to the rectum.*
- Do not use glass-and-mercury thermometers. If you discover a glass-and-mercury thermometer, or any kind of glass thermometer, urge the client to replace it with a safer instrument (e.g., a plastic thermometer). Arrange for an exchange if there is a procedure for this in your agency or community.

  Glass-and-mercury thermometers carry the risk of breakage, cuts, and exposure to toxic mercury.
- If you obtain a high or low reading using a chemical strip or a tympanic thermometer, retake the temperature using a plastic or digital thermometer.
- Teach the same procedures you have learned for measuring temperature. Observe as the client takes a temperature to ensure correct technique.
- Clients often use the oral site. Remind them to not drink, eat, or smoke for 30 minutes before taking the temperature.
- Reinforce the following points about care of reusable thermometers:
  - If you use the same thermometer for more than one person, use disposable covers, if possible; clean the thermometer well between uses.
  - If the person has an infection or communicable illness, soak the thermometer in 70% isopropyl alcohol between uses.
  - Clean the thermometer after each use, even if it is used for only one person. Wash with soap and water, rinse with cold water, dry well, and store in a clean, dry container.
  - If you store a thermometer in alcohol, rinse it with cold water before taking the temperature.
  - Do not use the same thermometer for both oral and rectal temperatures.

Documentation

You will usually record temperature on a graphic flowsheet (see Forms section). In some situations (e.g., a fever), you may need to write a nurse's note. If so, follow these suggestions:

- Document the temperature, indicating the route of measurement, according to agency policy.
- Notify the appropriate provider of abnormal findings.
- Document supporting findings, such as "Skin is hot and dry" and state whether the temperature reading is consistent with the client's condition.

Sample documentation

mm/dd/yyyy 1230 Oral temperature 105°F: it has risen steadily since the first elevation at 0630, when it was 100°F. Skin hot and dry. Patient is voiding only small amounts, but states no burning. Urine dark but clear. No chills. I & O begun. Gave Tylenol 650 mg by mouth and notified Dr. Anderson of patient's condition and medication. — Mary Clinton, RN

Practice Resources

Amoore, D. (2010); Heusch, A., & McCarthy, P. (2005); Lockwood, C., Conroy-Hiller, T., & Page, T. (2004); Quatrara, B., Coffman, J., Jenkins, T., et al. (2007); Rabinowitz, R., Cookson, S., Wasserman, S., et al. (1996); Robinson, J., Jou, H., & Spady, D. (2005); Therapeutic Research Center (2007); Vital Signs (1999).

Thinking About the Procedure

To practice applying clinical reasoning to these procedures,

Go to the *Davis's Nursing Skills Videos*, **Taking an Axillary Temperature, Taking an Oral Temperature, Taking a Rectal Temperature, Taking a Temporal Artery Temperature,** and **Taking a Tympanic Membrane Temperature.**

For questions and suggested responses,

Go to Chapter 20, **Thinking About the Procedure Questions and Suggested Responses** on Davis*Plus*.

Procedure 20-2 ■ Assessing Peripheral Pulses

➤ For steps to follow in *all* procedures, refer to the Universal Steps for All Procedures found on the inside back cover.

Equipment

- Watch with a second hand or digital readout
- Pen, pencil, and flowsheet or personal digital assistant (PDA)

Delegation

You can delegate measurement of pulses to the nursing assistive personnel (NAP) if you conclude that the patient's condition and the NAP's skills allow. For example, if pedal circulation is critical and you suspect it may be difficult to palpate, you should not delegate assessment of the pedal pulse. If you do delegate, perform the pre-procedure assessments and tell the NAP which site (e.g., radial, brachial) to use. Inform the NAP of any special considerations (e.g., to note what the patient's activity has been just before taking the pulse). Ask the NAP to record and report the pulse to you and to report immediately if it is outside normal limits (you must specify what is "normal" for each patient).

Pre-Procedure Assessments

- Determine why assessment of pulses is indicated.
  Conditions requiring an assessment of pulses include blood loss, cardiac or respiratory disease, diabetes mellitus, and other conditions that affect oxygenation.
- Assess factors that may alter the pulse, such as activity and medications. If the client has been active recently, wait 5 to 10 minutes before measuring.
  Activity increases the pulse rate; increased intracranial pressure decreases the rate; medications such as digoxin decrease the rate; other medications, such as albuterol, increase the pulse rate.

Procedure 20-2A ■ Assessing the Radial Pulse

➤ When performing the procedure, always identify your patient according to agency policy, using two identifiers, and be attentive to standard precautions, hand hygiene, patient safety and privacy, body mechanics, and documentation.

Procedure Steps

1. **With the patient sitting or supine,** flex the patient's arm, and place the patient's forearm across his chest.

2. **Palpate the radial artery.**
   The radial site is the most frequently used to calculate the patient's heart rate because it is generally the easiest site to use.
   a. Place the pads of your index or middle fingers (or both) in the groove on the thumb side of the patient's wrist, over the radial artery.
   b. Press lightly but firmly until you are able to feel the radial pulse. Start with light pressure to prevent occluding the pulse, and gradually increase the pressure until you feel the pulse.
   The fingertips are the most sensitive parts of the hand to palpate arterial pulsations. Avoid using the thumb, because it has its own pulsation and may interfere with the accuracy of your count. ➤

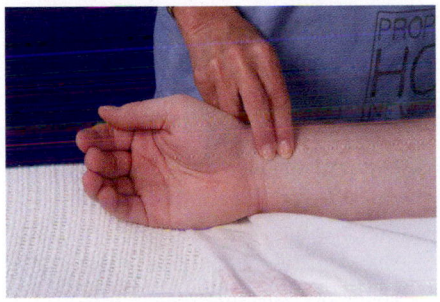

3. **Note the rhythm and quality** of the pulse. Note whether the thrust of the pulse against your fingertips is bounding, strong, weak, or thready.
   The rhythm and quality of the pulse are a reflection of the patient's cardiac output. The strength of the pulse reflects the volume of the blood that is ejected against the arterial wall with each contraction of the heart. An irregular or weak pulse indicates decreased cardiac output. A bounding pulse indicates increased cardiac output.

4. **Count the pulse:**
   a. Count for 60 seconds the first time you take a patient's pulse. After that, you can count a pulse with a regular rhythm for 15 seconds and multiply by 4, or count for 30 seconds and multiply by 2 to get the beats per minute. If you do not know the patient well, count for a full minute to be certain to detect irregularities. See Step 4c rationale.
   b. Begin timing with the count of 1—starting with the first beat that you feel.
   c. Count an irregular pulse for 1 full minute (60 seconds).
   Research is conflicting. Some studies indicate that a 60-second count is most accurate; others say that accuracy is not affected by a 30-second, or even a 15-second, count if the pulse is regular. You must count an irregular pulse for 1 full minute to be accurate.

5. **For an admission assessment** or peripheral vascular check, palpate the radial pulses on both wrists simultaneously. Note any difference in the quality of the pulse between arms. Is the pulse on one side weaker than that on the other?
   Palpating simultaneously enables the recognition of small differences in the peripheral circulation.

(continued on next page)

Procedure 20-2 ■ Assessing Peripheral Pulses (continued)

Procedure 20-2B ■ Assessing the Brachial Pulse

➤ When performing the procedure, always identify your patient according to agency policy, using two identifiers, and be attentive to standard precautions, hand hygiene, patient safety and privacy, body mechanics, and documentation.

Procedure Steps

1. **Palpate the brachial artery.**
   a. Using firm pressure, press in the inner aspect of the antecubital fossa until you palpate the brachial artery.
   b. If you have difficulty palpating the pulse, ask the patient to pronate the forearm (i.e., turn the palm of the hand downward).

   This brings the brachial artery over a bony prominence and makes the pulse easier to feel. ▼

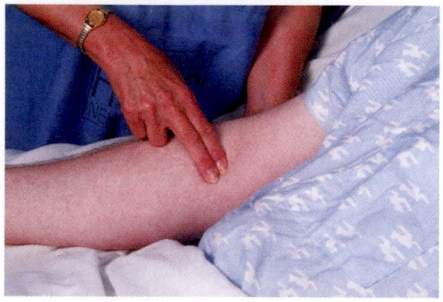

2. **Assess pulse rate, rhythm, and quality, and assess bilaterally (see Procedure 20-2A).**
   The brachial pulse is used most frequently to assess blood pressure and to identify the presence of a pulse during cardiopulmonary resuscitation (CPR) in an infant.

Procedure 20-2C ■ Assessing the Carotid Pulse

➤ When performing the procedure, always identify your patient according to agency policy, using two identifiers, and be attentive to standard precautions, hand hygiene, patient safety and privacy, body mechanics, and documentation.

Caution! Do not palpate the carotid pulse except during cardiopulmonary resuscitation in an adult, and in certain situations to assess for circulation to the head.
Pressure on the carotid (especially in older adults) can stimulate the vagus nerve, causing the pulse and blood pressure to drop suddenly, and perhaps fainting or circulatory arrest. It can also decrease circulation to the brain.

Procedure Steps

1. **Palpate the carotid artery lightly.** Place your fingers on the patient's trachea, and slide them to the side into the groove between the trachea and the sternocleidomastoid muscle.
   Compressing the carotid arteries can stimulate the carotid bodies and significantly decrease the patient's heart rate and blood pressure.

   NEVER compress the carotid artery on both sides of the neck at the same time. ➤

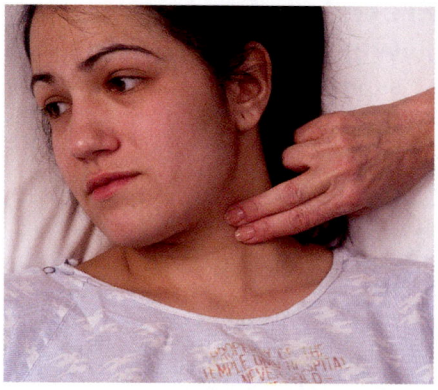

2. **Assess the rate, rhythm, and quality, and compare bilaterally.**

Procedure 20-2D ■ Assessing the Dorsalis Pedis Pulse

➤ When performing the procedure, always identify your patient according to agency policy, using two identifiers, and be attentive to standard precautions, hand hygiene, patient safety and privacy, body mechanics, and documentation.

Procedure Steps

1. **Palpate the dorsalis pedis pulse.**
   a. Run your fingers up the groove between the great and first toes to the top of the foot.
   b. Palpate very lightly.
   The dorsalis pedis pulse is easily obliterated, so use very light pressure.

   The dorsalis pedis pulse is used to access circulation of the foot.

   Owing to atherosclerosis or hardening of the arteries, the dorsalis pedis may be difficult to palpate in older adults.

2. **Assess pulse rate, rhythm, and quality, and assess bilaterally.** ➤

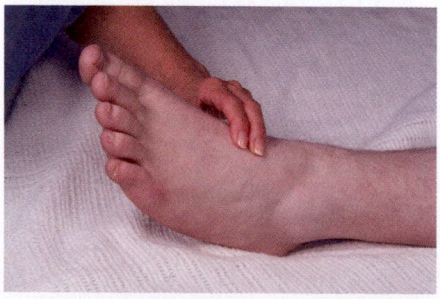

3. **If you are unable to palpate the dorsalis pedis pulse,** use a Doppler ultrasound device to assess the pulse and circulation to the lower extremity.

Procedure 20-2E ■ Assessing the Femoral Pulse

➤ When performing the procedure, always identify your patient according to agency policy, using two identifiers, and be attentive to standard precautions, hand hygiene, patient safety and privacy, body mechanics, and documentation.

Procedure Steps

1. **Palpate the femoral pulse** by pressing deeply in the groin midway between the anterosuperior iliac spine and the symphysis pubis.
   The femoral artery lies very deep and requires significant pressure to palpate. You may need to use both hands to feel the pulse on an adult. ➤

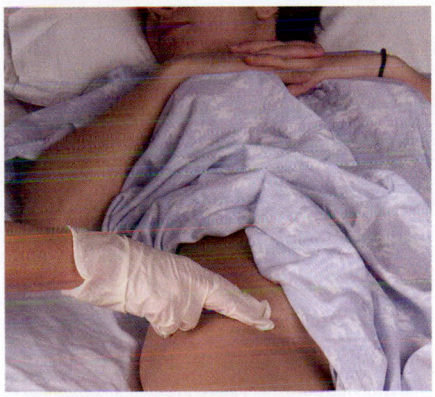

2. **Assess pulse rate, rhythm, and quality, and assess bilaterally.**
   The femoral pulse is used to determine the presence of a pulse during CPR and to assess circulation to the leg.

Procedure 20-2F ■ Assessing the Posterior Tibial Pulse

➤ When performing the procedure, always identify your patient according to agency policy, using two identifiers, and be attentive to standard precautions, hand hygiene, patient safety and privacy, body mechanics, and documentation.

Procedure Steps

1. **Palpate the posterior tibial pulse** by pressing on the inner (medial) side of the ankle below the medial malleolus.
   The posterior tibial pulse is usually palpated easily, but it may be deeper in some people. So, press down moderately and then increase pressure until you feel the pulse. It is relatively easy to obliterate. ➤

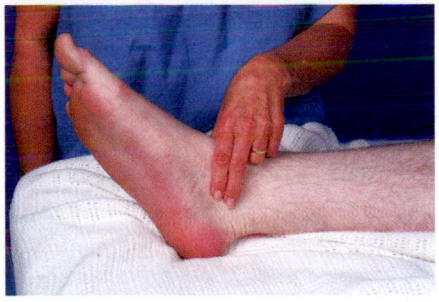

2. **Assess pulse rate, rhythm, and quality, and assess bilaterally.**
   The posterior tibial pulse is used to assess circulation to the lower extremity; it is assessed along with the dorsalis pedis pulse.

Procedure 20-2G ■ Assessing the Popliteal Pulse

➤ When performing the procedure, always identify your patient according to agency policy, using two identifiers, and be attentive to standard precautions, hand hygiene, patient safety and privacy, body mechanics, and documentation.

Procedure Steps

1. **Palpate the popliteal pulse** by pressing behind the knee in the middle of the popliteal fossa.
   The popliteal pulse can be difficult to feel. It is used only when specifically indicated because of absence of pedal pulses or for taking a thigh blood pressure. ➤

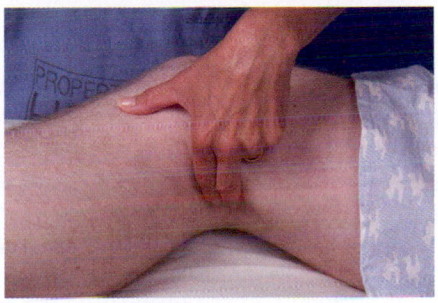

2. **Assess pulse rate, rhythm, and quality, and assess bilaterally.**
   The popliteal pulse is used to assess circulation of the lower leg and auscultate a thigh blood pressure.

(continued on next page)

Procedure 20-2 ■ Assessing Peripheral Pulses (continued)

Procedure 20-2H ■ Assessing the Temporal Pulse

➤ When performing the procedure, always identify your patient according to agency policy, using two identifiers, and be attentive to standard precautions, hand hygiene, patient safety and privacy, body mechanics, and documentation.

Procedure Steps

1. **Palpate the temporal pulse** by pressing lightly lateral (outside area) and superior to (above) the eye. ▼

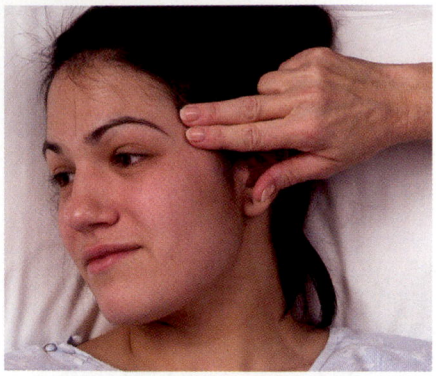

2. **Assess pulse rate, rhythm, and** quality, and assess bilaterally as for the radial pulse (see Procedure 20-2A).
The temporal pulse is easily accessible and is used frequently in infants.

? What if . . .

- **The patient is an infant or a child younger than age 3 years?**
Auscultate an apical pulse rate. Rates are faster and small arteries more difficult to feel in a child or infant.
If a parent is present, encourage the parent to hold the child to reduce anxiety.
Fear increases the pulse rate.

- **The patient is an older adult?**
Have the patient at rest for 15 to 20 minutes after activity and before assessing the pulse.
The pulse tends to return to baseline more slowly in older adults.
If the pulse is fast, take repeated measures; if a pattern of fast rate emerges, note this for the primary care provider for further evaluation.
An elevated heart rate is related to increased mortality in older adult women, so it is a simple index of general health status.

- **The pulse is faint or weak?**
Use a Doppler ultrasound device to detect blood flow.
Lack of pulses indicates inadequate circulation to the lower extremities. If you cannot feel the pulse, you must determine whether the pulse is absent or whether you are having difficulty feeling. To draw the conclusion that the pulse is "absent," you must use a Doppler.

Apply transmission gel to the end of the probe. Do not use water-soluble lubricant as a substitute for transmission gel.
Place the probe lightly on the skin over the artery you are using.
Turn on the instrument and set the volume control to the lowest setting.
Tilting the probe to a 45° angle to the artery, move the probe slowly in a circular motion to locate the signal (a rhythmic hissing noise). Count for 60 seconds.
Move the probe slowly to avoid distorting the signal.
When you are finished, wipe the gel off the patient's skin. Clean the probe with soapy water or an antiseptic solution. Do not immerse the probe or bump it against anything hard.
Clean the probe to prevent cross-contamination to other patients. Probes are fragile and may malfunction if bumped against a hard surface.

Evaluation

Especially if pedal pulses are decreased, observe for other indications of inadequate circulation, such as cool skin, decreased capillary refill, and bluish or ashen skin tone. You must provide supporting evidence if you chart that pedal pulses are decreased or absent. The complete absence of a pulse requires immediate intervention.

Patient Teaching

- Teach the patient about the significance of any abnormalities in pulse rate or rhythm.
- Explain any interventions that may be needed.

Home Care

Assess the skill level of the person who will be assessing the client's peripheral pulses in the home, and provide instruction if necessary.

Documentation

Usually you will document routine vital signs (VS), including pulse, on a flowsheet or graphic. If you record it in a nurse's note, document the pulse rate, rhythm, quality, and site (e.g., "radial pulse 64 beats/min, regular, and strong bilaterally").

Practice Resources

Alexis, O. (2010); *Best Practices* (2007); Lockwood, C., Conroy-Hiller, T., & Page, T. (2004); Perk, G., Stessman, J., Ginsberg, G., et al. (2003); Trim, J. (2005); Vital Signs (1999).

Thinking About the Procedure

To practice applying clinical reasoning to this procedure,

Go to the *Davis's Nursing Skills Videos*, **Assessing Peripheral Pulses.**

For questions and suggested responses,

Go to Chapter 20, **Thinking About the Procedure Questions and Suggested Responses** on Davis*Plus*.

Procedure 20-3 ■ Assessing the Apical Pulse

➤ For steps to follow in *all* procedures, refer to the Universal Steps for All Procedures found on the inside back cover.

Equipment

- Watch with a second hand or second readout
- Stethoscope
- Alcohol wipes (to clean stethoscope)

Delegation

You can delegate measurement of the apical pulse to the nursing assistive personnel (NAP) if you conclude that the patient's condition and the NAP's skills allow. First perform the pre-procedure assessments. Then inform the NAP of any special considerations (e.g., to note what the patient's activity has been just before taking the pulse, or to mark the time exactly so you can compare it to the patient's ECG). Ask the NAP to record and report the pulse to you, and to report immediately if it is outside normal limits (you must specify what is "normal" for each patient).

Pre-Procedure Assessments

- Determine why assessment of the apical pulse is indicated.
  Conditions that require assessment of the apical pulse include digitalis therapy, blood loss, cardiac or respiratory disease, or other conditions that affect oxygenation status.
- Assess factors that may alter the pulse, such as activity and medications. If the client has been recently active, wait 10 to 15 minutes before obtaining a measurement.
  The apical pulse is generally best heard at the point of maximum impulse (PMI) in the 5th intercostal space at the midclavicular line. The PMI is located over the apex of the heart.

➤ When performing the procedure, always identify your patient according to agency policy, using two identifiers, and be attentive to standard precautions, hand hygiene, patient safety and privacy, body mechanics, and documentation.

Procedure Steps

1. **With the client supine or sitting,** expose the left side of the chest, but only as much as necessary.
   Prevents distortion of sound from the patient's gown rubbing on the stethoscope, while also protecting the patient's privacy. ▼

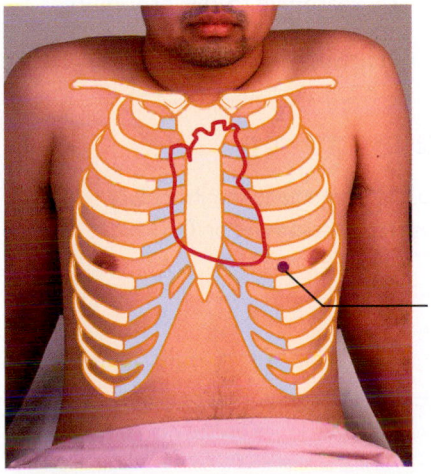

2. **Wipe the stethoscope with** a 70% alcohol or benzalkonium chloride wipe before and after examining the patient.
   Cleaning can reduce the bacterial count by up to 100%.

3. **Palpate the 5th intercostal space** at the midclavicular line for the apical pulse.
   The left ventricle of the heart and the point of maximum impulse lie in this area. The apical pulse is generally best heard at the PMI, over the apex of the heart.
   a. To locate the 5th intercostal space, slide your finger down from the sternal notch to the angle of Louis (the bump where the manubrium and sternum meet).
   b. Slide your finger over to the left sternal border to the 2nd intercostal space.
   c. Now place your index or ring finger (depending on which hand you use) in the 2nd intercostal space, and count down to the 5th intercostal space by placing a finger in each of the spaces.
   d. Slide over to the midclavicular line, keeping your finger in the 5th intercostal space.

4. **Palpate the apical pulse.**
   a. The palpated apical pulse is also called the point of maximal impulse (PMI).
   b. The pulse area should be about the size of a quarter, without lifts or heaves.
   A larger than normal pulsation may indicate ventricular hypertrophy.

5. **Warm the stethoscope** in your hand for 10 seconds. Then place the diaphragm over the PMI, and listen to the normal S_1 and S_2 heart sounds (lub dub).
   A cold stethoscope placed on the skin may startle the patient and increase the heart rate. Heart sounds result when blood moves through the valves of the heart. The first heart sound is louder at the apical area and should be audible when the pulse is auscultated.

Go to Student Resources, **Sound files, Heart Sounds,** on Davis*Plus*.

6. **Count the apical heart rate** for 1 full minute.
   Ensures accuracy. Because the apical heart rate is needed as an assessment measure for the administration of some medications (e.g., digoxin), accuracy is essential. Some cardiac conditions cause either slow or irregular rates, both of which must be counted for a full minute to ensure accuracy.

(continued on next page)

Procedure 20-3 ■ Assessing the Apical Pulse (continued)

? What if . . .

- **The apical rate is less than 60 beats/min?**

  (**Note:** You may also see "bpm" as an abbreviation for "beats per minute" or for "beats/min.")
  If the patient is taking cardiac medications, withhold them and consult with a physician about whether to adjust dosage.
  Certain cardiac medications (e.g., digoxin) are given to slow the heart rate; bradycardia may indicate that blood levels are too high.
  Assess for chest pain, dizziness, dyspnea.
  May indicate decreased cardiac output

- **The apical rate is greater than 100 beats/min?**

  Obtain a complete set of vital signs. Assess for pain, anxiety, fever, dehydration, decreased oxygenation, hypotension, and decreased exercise.
  These factors may increase pulse rate.

Evaluation

- Are the findings within normal limits?
- Are there other factors supporting the findings?
- What are the trends over time?
- Is the skin pink, warm, and dry?
- Is there any cyanosis?

Patient Teaching

- Teach the patient about the significance of any abnormalities in the pulse rate or rhythm.
- Explain any interventions that may be necessary.

Home Care

- Assess the skill level of the person who will be assessing the client's apical pulse in the home, and provide instruction if necessary.
- Teach the home caregiver when to hold medications and/or to call primary care provider (e.g., to hold the digitalis if the rate is <60).
- Before leaving the home, clean the stethoscope with detergent or disinfectant, when possible; or place it in a plastic bag for transporting to the reprocessing location.
- If the patient has a multidrug-resistant organism infection, reusable equipment such as stethoscopes should remain in the home. If the stethoscope cannot remain in the home, clean and disinfect it before leaving the home, using a low to intermediate level disinfectant. If this is not practical, place the stethoscope in a plastic bag and transport it to another site for cleaning and disinfection.

Documentation

Document the pulse rate, rhythm, and site.

Sample documentation

mm/dd/yyyy 0800 Apical pulse regular rhythm, and strong, rate of 64.
Janice Jonas, RN

Practice Resources

Alexis, O. (2010); *Best Practices* (2007); Centers for Disease Control and Prevention (CDC) (2008); Lockwood, C., Conroy-Hiller, T., & Page, T. (2004); Vital Signs (1999); Wall, R. (2009).

Thinking About the Procedure

To practice applying clinical reasoning to this procedure,

Go to the *Davis's Nursing Skills Videos*, **Assessing the Apical Pulse.**

For questions and suggested responses,

Go to Chapter 20, **Thinking About the Procedure Questions and Suggested Responses** on Davis*Plus*.

Procedure 20-4 ■ Assessing for an Apical-Radial Pulse Deficit

➤ For steps to follow in *all* procedures, refer to the Universal Steps for All Procedures found on the inside back cover.

Equipment

- Watch or clock with a second hand or second readout
- Procedure gloves, if indicated
- Stethoscope
- Alcohol wipes to clean the stethoscope

Delegation

Instead of delegating measurement of an apical-radial pulse to a NAP, you would most likely ask the NAP to assist you in this procedure because it is best performed by two persons working together.

Pre-Procedure Assessments

- Determine why assessment of pulse deficit is indicated.
  Conditions that require assessment of pulse deficit include digitalis therapy, blood loss, cardiac or respiratory disease, and other conditions that affect oxygenation status.
- Assess factors that may alter the pulse, such as activity and medications.

➤ When performing the procedure, always identify your patient according to agency policy, using two identifiers, and be attentive to standard precautions, hand hygiene, patient safety and privacy, body mechanics, and documentation.

Procedure Steps

1. **Wipe the stethoscope with** a 70% alcohol or benzalkonium chloride wipe before and after examining the patient.
   Cleaning can reduce the bacterial count by up to 100% and prevent the transmission of microbes.

2. **Expose the left side** of the patient's chest, minimizing patient exposure.
   Prevents distortion of sound from the patient's gown rubbing on the stethoscope and protects privacy.

3. **Place the watch so that the** second hand is visible to both nurses (if two nurses are performing the procedure).
   Using one watch increases accuracy of counts.

4. **Nurse 1 palpates the** 5th intercostal space at the midclavicular line for the apical pulse, and holds the diaphragm of the stethoscope in place, using firm pressure.
   Aids in hearing high-pitched sounds and ensures good contact between the diaphragm of the stethoscope and the skin. ➤

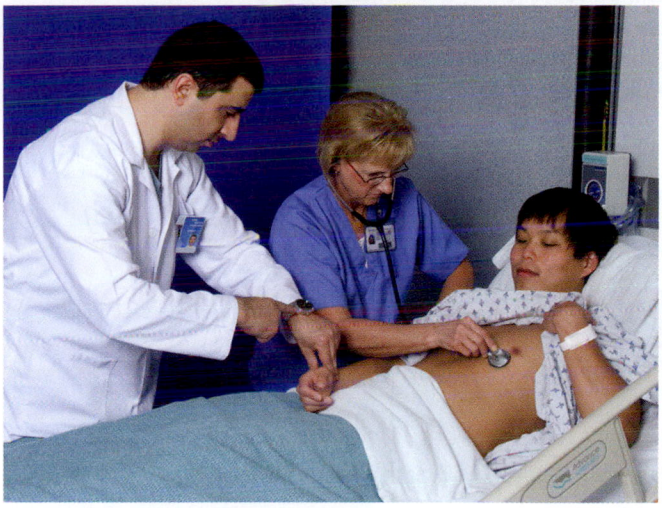

5. **Nurse 2 palpates the radial pulse** and assesses rate, rhythm, and quality.

6. **Nurse 2 says "Start"** when ready to begin and "Stop" when finished. Both nurses count the pulse simultaneously for 1 full minute.
   Count simultaneously to ensure accuracy. Counting for 1 full minute is necessary for an accurate assessment of any discrepancies that may exist between the two sites.

7. **To obtain pulse deficit, subtract** the radial rate from the apical rate.

   Apical Rate – Radial Rate = Pulse Deficit

   Atrial and ventricular dysrhythmias may cause beats that do not perfuse, so although you hear an apical heart beat, you do not feel a peripheral pulse. The pulse deficit is the number of heartbeats that do not perfuse.

? What if . . .

- **There is not another nurse available to assist?**
  Hold the stethoscope in place with the one hand while palpating the radial pulse with the hand wearing the watch.
  Even if you cannot manage to count both rates, you should be able to feel any differences between the apical and radial pulses.

- **There has been an increase in pulse deficit since the last measurement?**
  An increase in pulse deficit means that the patient's cardiac output has decreased.

(continued on next page)

Procedure 20-4 ■ Assessing the Apical Pulse (continued)

Evaluation

- Identify the presence of an apical-pulse deficit, and compare to previous findings.
- Assess other measures of cardiopulmonary status to identify a decline in the patient's condition.
- Look for trends.

The presence of any apical-radial pulse deficit is abnormal.

Patient Teaching

- Teach the patient about the significance of an apical-radial pulse deficit.
- Explain any necessary interventions.

Home Care

- Assess the skill level of the person(s) who will be measuring the client's apical-radial pulse deficit in the home, and provide instruction if necessary.
- Before leaving the home, clean the stethoscope as described in the Home Care section of Procedure 20-3.

Documentation

Document the apical-radial pulse deficit.

Sample documentation

01/15/15 0900 Apical-radial pulse deficit is 4 beats/min. ——— Jon Albertson, RN

Practice Resources

Alexis, O. (2010); *Best Practices* (2007); CDC (2008); Lockwood, C., Conroy-Hiller, T., & Page, T. (2004); Siegel, J., Rhinehart, E., Jackson, M., et al. (2006); U.S. Department of Health and Human Services, Agency of Healthcare Research and Quality (AHRQ) (2008); Vital Signs (1999).

Thinking About the Procedure

To practice applying clinical reasoning to this procedure,

Go to the *Davis's Nursing Skills Videos*, Assessing for an Apical-Radial Pulse Deficit.

For questions and suggested responses,

Go to Chapter 20, **Thinking About the Procedure Questions and Suggested Responses** on Davis*Plus*.

Procedure 20-5 ■ Assessing Respirations

➤ For steps to follow in *all* procedures, refer to the Universal Steps for All Procedures found on the inside back cover.

➤ NOTE: To listen to breath sounds,

Go to **Student Resources, Sound Files: Breath Sounds,** on Davis*Plus*.

Equipment

- A watch with a second hand (or a wall clock)

Delegation

You can delegate the counting of respirations to the nursing assistive personnel (NAP) if you conclude that the patient's condition and the NAP's skills allow. Perform the pre-procedure assessments, and inform the NAP of any special considerations (e.g., the need to keep the patient in a certain position). Ask the NAP to record and report the respirations to you, and to report immediately if they are not within the normal range for this patient (specify the range).

Pre-Procedure Assessments

- Observe for signs of respiratory distress—breathing faster or slower than normal, gasping breaths, confusion, circumoral (around the month) cyanosis.

  Signs of hypoxemia may indicate that the patient is not adequately oxygenated.
- Determine the baseline respiratory rate and character of respirations.
- Assess for factors that may affect the respiratory rate (e.g., pain, activity, fever, respiratory disorders).

➤ When performing the procedure, always identify your patient according to agency policy, using two identifiers, and be attentive to standard precautions, hand hygiene, patient safety and privacy, body mechanics, and documentation.

Procedure Steps

1. **Position the patient.** With the patient in a sitting position (preferably), flex the patient's arm, and place her forearm across her chest.
   Aids in counting the patient's pulse rate by making the rise and fall of the chest more discernible and by making the patient less aware that you are measuring the respiratory rate. The patient's awareness might alter the respiratory rate and/or pattern because respirations are partially under voluntary control.

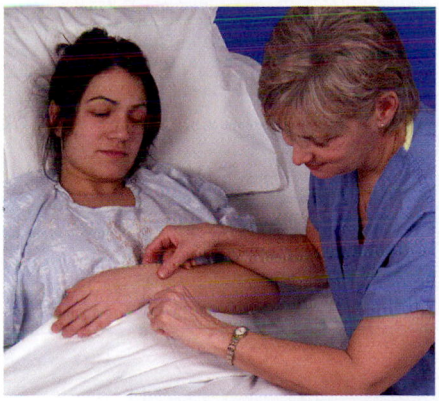

2. **Palpate and count the radial** pulse; remember that number.
3. **Then, keeping your hand** on the patient's wrist, count the respirations.
   Allows you to count the respirations unobtrusively.
4. **Observe the respiratory rate,** rhythm, and depth.
   - *Rate*: Normal for patient's age, fast (tachypnea), or slow (bradypnea)
   - *Rhythm*: Regular or irregular
   - *Depth*: Normal, shallow, or deep (e.g., Kussmaul's)

   All of these characteristics are necessary to evaluate respiratory status. Different pathologies affect each of these characteristics differently.
5. **Count the number of breaths** per minute. Begin timing the respirations with a count of 1, not 0 (the same as with pulse measurement).
   a. If the respiratory rhythm is regular, count the rate (one inhalation and one exhalation is one respiration) for 30 seconds, and multiply by 2.
   b. If the rhythm is irregular, count the rate for 1 full minute (60 seconds).
   Variations in rhythm may cause an inaccurate rate when counted for less than 1 minute.

? What if . . .

- **The patient is an infant?**
  Place your hand on the abdomen to assess the respiratory rate. Auscultate breath sounds with a stethoscope.
  Infants and young children breathe rapidly and are abdominal breathers, so it is difficult to see each and every rise and fall of the abdomen. Using a stethoscope increases the accuracy of the count, as well as providing information about the breath sounds.

  For infants and very young children, count for 1 full minute.
  Infants and young children have irregular respirations. Counting for a full minute provides a more accurate rate for irregular respirations.
- **The patient is receiving oxygen therapy, or requires careful assessment of respiratory status?**
  Apply a pulse oximeter (see Procedure 36-2, Monitoring Pulse Oximetry).
  Evidence suggests that pulse oximetry is useful for detecting deterioration of physiological function that might otherwise be missed (e.g., during the perioperative period or in seriously ill patients).

Evaluation

- Compare the respiratory rate and rhythm with previous readings.
- Note other vital signs, especially temperature.
- Look for trends, and note whether the respiratory rate and rhythm are changing in conjunction with changes in the other vital signs.
  If the patient has an elevated temperature, the respiratory rate will increase. Corresponding elevation in pulse with respiratory rate may indicate hypoxemia. If respirations are not within normal parameters, assess oxygenation with a pulse oximeter.

Patient Teaching

Teach the patient about factors that affect respiratory status, such as smoking and activity.

Home Care

Assess the skill level of the person(s) who will be measuring the client's respiratory rate in the home, and provide instruction as needed.

Documentation

You will document routine VS (including respirations) on a graphic or flowsheet. When a nurse's note is needed, follow these guidelines.

- Document the respiratory rate and rhythm.

Document that respirations are either labored or unlabored; if labored, describe in what way (e.g., intercostal retractions, use of accessory muscles, nasal flaring).

(continued on next page)

Procedure 20-5 ■ Assessing the Apical Pulse (continued)

Example of Electronic Health Record

Flowsheet

Print 4 minutes ago

Nursing Assessment
Med Surg Assessment
Graphs
Intake and Output
Intake
Oral
Enteral
Gastric
Transfusions
Parenteral
Other Intake Sources
Output
Urine Output
Emesis Output
Gastric Tube Output
Stool Output
Other Output Sources
Drains and Chest Tubes
Ongoing Pediatric Assessm...
Summary Report

mm/dd/yyyy 10:28 PM - mm/dd/yyyy 10:59 PM MORE

Find Item Critical High Low Abnormal Flag New Unauth

		mm/dd/yyyy 10:28 PM	6:00 AM	mm/dd/yyyy 2:00 PM	10:00 PM	mm/dd/yyyy 6:00 AM	2:00 PM	10:00 PM
Vital Signs								
Temperature Axillary	DegC							
Temperature Oral	DegC							
Temperature Tympanic	DegC				37.7			
Peripheral Pulse Rate	bpm				104 ↑			
Respiratory Rate	br/min				24 ↑			
SBP/DBP Cuff	mmHg				104/68			

mm/dd/yyyy 7:00 AM - mm/dd/yyyy 6:59 AM MORE

Today's Intake: 0 Output: 250 Balance: -250 Yesterday's Intake: Output: Balance:

		Clinical	24 Hour	Night Shift	mm/dd/yyyy 3:00 AM	mm/dd/yyyy 11:00 PM	Evening Shift	mm/dd/yyyy 7:00 PM	3:00 PM	Day Shift	10/E 11:0
Intake Total		0	0				0	0			
Oral		0	0				0	0			
Oral Intake	mL	0	0				0	0			
Transfusions											
Output Total		250	250				250	250			
Urine Output		250	250				250	250			
Urine Voided	mL										
Urine Catheter	mL	250	250				250	250			
Emesis Output											
Balance		-250	-250				-250	-250			

Practice Resources

CDC (2008); Lockwood, C., Conroy-Hiller, T., & Page, T. (2004); Parkes, R. (2011); Vital Signs (1999).

Thinking About the Procedure

To practice applying clinical reasoning to this procedure,

Go to the *Davis's Nursing Skills Videos*, Assessing Respirations.

For questions and suggested responses,

Go to Chapter 20, **Thinking About the Procedure Questions and Suggested Responses** on Davis*Plus*.

Procedure 20-6 ■ Measuring Blood Pressure

➤ For steps to follow in *all* procedures, refer to the Universal Steps for All Procedures found on the inside back cover.

Equipment

- Stethoscope

NOTE: Do not wear a stethoscope around your neck. There is a slight risk that you can entangle it in intravenous and other lines. There is also a risk that a psychotic or delirious patient could use it to harm you. Also, wearing a stethoscope can be a source of cross-contamination.

- 70% alcohol or benzalkonium chloride wipes.
  For cleaning stethoscope before and after use. Clean all parts.
- Sphygmomanometer with a cuff of the appropriate size. Refer to Clinical Insight 20-1.
  Using a cuff that is too small will result in a false-high reading; using a cuff that is too large will result in a false-low reading.
- *Note:* This procedure describes the use of an aneroid manometer or an electronic measuring device.

Delegation

You can delegate measurement of BP to the NAP if you conclude that the patient's condition and the NAP's skills allow. Perform the pre-procedure assessments, and inform the NAP of the site (e.g., radial, brachial) to use. Inform the NAP of any special considerations (e.g., not to place a BP cuff on the same side as the site of a mastectomy). Ask the NAP to record and report the BP to you, and to report immediately if it is outside normal limits (you must specify what is "normal" for each patient). Tell the NAP that if BP is elevated, to note which arm, the patient's position during measurement, and activity immediately preceding the measurement.

Pre-Procedure Assessments

- Check for factors or activities that may alter the readings.
  Caffeine, smoking, exercise, and stress can all elevate the BP. Be certain the patient has been lying or sitting for at least 5 minutes (30 minutes after strenuous exercise) and is relaxed.
- Check the previous recording, if any.
  Noting changes over time is important with all patient assessments. Because BP changes constantly and because so many factors affect it, you cannot draw conclusions from a single measurement.

➤ When performing the procedure, always identify your patient using two identifiers according to agency policy, using two identifiers, and be attentive to standard precautions, hand hygiene, patient safety and privacy, body mechanics, and documentation.

➤ *Note:* To improve the accuracy of your readings, also refer to Clinical Insights 20-1 and 20-2.

Procedure Steps

1. **Clean the stethoscope before** and after the procedure.
   Although only a small percentage of microorganisms are pathogenic, cleaning can reduce the bacterial count by 94% to 100%.

2. **Position the patient** comfortably, ensuring that:
   a. The legs are uncrossed, the back is supported, and the feet are resting on the floor (if the patient is sitting in a chair); or that the patient is supine.
   This position allows for the most accurate reading. Crossing the legs may elevate the BP reading.
   b. The measurement arm is supported at heart level, slightly flexed, with the palm facing upward.
   The blood pressure will decrease if the arm is above the heart and increase if the arm is below the heart or not supported.

3. **Fully expose the arm**, being careful that clothing is not tight. Remove clothing rather than rolling up a sleeve. *Note:* There is some evidence to suggest that readings taken over sleeves do not affect blood pressure results, and that it may actually be preferable because of concerns about hygiene, privacy and religious beliefs (Pinar, Ataalkin, & Watson, 2010). While you are learning, and until there is evidence, we advise that you will find it easier to hear the BP sounds on a bare arm.
   Clothing that is tight enough to restrict blood flow will alter the reading.

4. **Place the cuff** on the upper arm. ➤

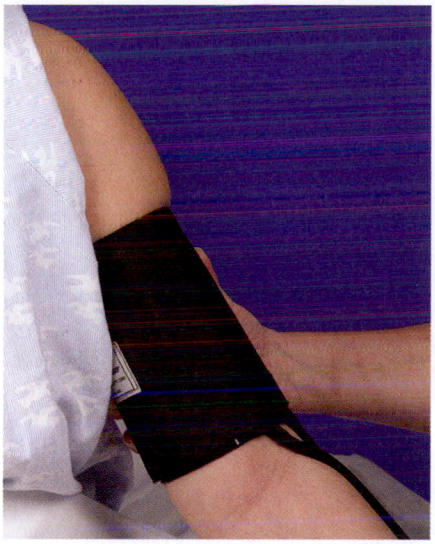

   a. Wrap the cuff snugly.
   b. Ensure that the cuff is totally deflated, and palpate the brachial artery.
   c. Place the bottom edge of the cuff approximately 1 in. (2.5 cm) above the antecubital space.
   d. Place the center of the cuff bladder directly over the brachial artery (the center is often indicated with an arrow on the BP cuff).
   The center of the cuff bladder needs to be directly over the brachial artery to obtain an accurate reading. Loose application of the cuff results in overestimation of the pressure.

5. **Place the stethoscope ear pieces** in your ears, pointing slightly forward.
   When the earpieces point slightly forward, they direct sound into the ear canal, making the sounds more audible.

6. **Palpate the brachial artery** on the arm with the cuff. (Use the radial artery for this step if you prefer.)
   For correct stethoscope placement

7. **Inflate the cuff, as follows:**
   a. Close the sphygmomanometer valve and inflate the cuff rapidly to about 80 mm Hg.
   b. Then palpate the pulse while you continue inflating in 10 mm Hg increments until you no longer feel the pulse.
   c. Note the pressure at which the pulse disappears.
   d. Go to step 8 or the variation, as you prefer.
   Palpating the artery while inflating the cuff ensures that the cuff is inflated higher than the systolic BP. If the patient has an auscultatory gap, the systolic pressure can be mistakenly identified as lower than it actually is. Palpation is particularly important if the baseline systolic BP is unknown or if the patient is hypertensive.

8. Continue inflating the cuff to a pressure that is 20 to 30 mm Hg above the level at which the pulse disappeared. Move to Step 9.
   Helps ensure you will not miss an auscultatory gap or a faint first sound.

Variation in Cuff Inflation Technique

- Do not continue palpating after the pulse disappears; instead, deflate the cuff rapidly.
- Wait 2 minutes, then place the stethoscope over the brachial artery and inflate the cuff to a pressure that is 20 to 30 mm Hg above the palpated level.
- Continue with steps 9 and 10.

9. **Place the stethoscope over** the brachial artery as follows: ▼

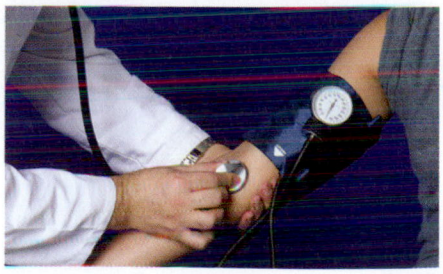

(continued on next page)

Procedure 20-6 ■ Measuring Blood Pressure (continued)

a. Be certain that the stethoscope tubing is not touching anything and that the diaphragm is not tucked under the edge of the cuff.
When the tubing rubs against clothing, for example, it produces artifact sounds that make it difficult to hear the BP sounds. Placing the bell or diaphragm under the cuff can partially occlude the brachial artery, delaying the appearance of the Korotkoff sounds.

b. Using the bell will enable you to hear BP sounds more accurately, especially at diastolic pressures. However, most people use the diaphragm because it is easily placed and because some stethoscopes do not have a bell.

10. Deflate the cuff slowly (2 to 3 mm Hg per second or per beat), listening for the Korotkoff sounds as you deflate.
Deflating the cuff slowly increases patient discomfort and may alter the reading. Deflating the cuff faster may cause errors in hearing the Korotkoff sounds.

a. Note the point on the manometer at which you hear the first sound. This is the systolic BP. (If you are using an electronic BP device, read the digital screen when the numbers appear. Follow the manufacturer's instructions.)
The 1st Korotkoff sound is the systolic pressure.

b. Continue deflating the cuff, and note the level at which the sounds become muffled and disappear. The diastolic pressure is the point at which the sound disappears.
The 5th Korotkoff sound (the disappearance of sound) is the diastolic BP in adults. The 4th Korotkoff sound (the muffling of sounds) is the diastolic BP in children. The AHA recommends recording the first sound, muffling, and last sound in children younger than 13 years, pregnant women, and people with high cardiac output or peripheral vasoconstriction.

11. If you need to repeat the measurement, deflate the cuff completely, and wait 2 minutes before reinflating it.
Prevents venous congestion and false high readings.

? What if . . .

- **You cannot feel the brachial pulse?**
  While supporting the arm at the elbow, have the patient pronate her forearm.
  This moves the brachial artery more over a bony prominence, making the pulsation easier to feel.

- **You have difficulty hearing BP sounds for many patients?**
  You may need a stethoscope with a built-in amplifier.

- **You are not certain of the systolic reading when you begin to deflate the cuff?**
  Do not stop cuff deflation to recheck the systolic reading. Deflate the cuff completely and wait 2 to 3 minutes before taking another measurement.
  Stopping deflation and retaking the BP too soon can lead to a muffling of the Korotkoff sounds and inaccurate results.

- **You must use a mercury manometer?**
  Because mercury is a health hazard, mercury manometers should not be found in healthcare agencies. Use an aneroid manometer or an electronic BP device if one is available. If you must use a mercury manometer, be certain the meniscus of the mercury is at eye level when taking the reading. Take care not to bump equipment against the glass cover over the column of mercury.

- **You are using an automatic blood pressure device?**
  Follow the same guidelines as for a manual BP (e.g., cuff size and placement, patient position).
  Turn on the machine; be sure the cuff is deflated.
  Apply the cuff.
  Press the button to start the measurement.
  At the tone, read the digital measurement.

- **You do not have a cuff size to fit the upper arm?**
  Use the forearm, thigh, or calf. See procedure Variations A, B, and C, respectively.

- **The patient requires contact or isolation precautions?**
  Follow agency guidelines for equipment (e.g., stethoscope, BP cuff). Generally the equipment remains in the room with the patient; otherwise it must be disinfected before leaving the room. For information about contact precautions and protective isolation, see Chapter 23, Clinical Insights 2, 3, and 4.

Procedure Variation A. Measuring Blood Pressure in the Forearm

- Place a properly sized cuff on the forearm, midway between the elbow and the wrist. Auscultate over the radial artery.
- Note that a forearm reading is not interchangeable with an upper arm reading.

Procedure Variation B. Measuring Blood Pressure in the Thigh

- Use the thigh or the calf if the cuff will not fit either the upper or lower arm.

  Note: The thigh systolic measure may be 20 to 30 mm Hg higher than an arm BP reading. The diastolic reading is generally comparable.

- Place the patient in a prone position. If patient cannot be prone, place supine with knee slightly bent.
- Choose the correct cuff size. Wrap the cuff snugly around the thigh so that the lower edge of the cuff is approximately 1 in. (2.5 cm) above the popliteal fossa and the center of the cuff bladder is

positioned directly over the popliteal artery (often indicated with an arrow on the blood pressure cuff).

- Palpate and auscultate over the popliteal artery. ▼

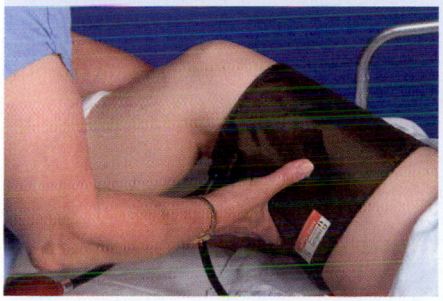

Procedure Variation C. Measuring Blood Pressure in the Calf

- Use the thigh or the calf if the cuff will not fit either the upper or lower arm.
- Place the patient supine.
- Choose the correct size cuff. Wrap the cuff snugly around the calf so that the lower edge of the cuff is approximately 2.5 cm above the malleoli or ankle.
- Place the stethoscope over either the dorsalis pedis or the posterior tibial artery.

Note: Calf BP measurements are not equivalent to upper arm measurements in adults; they tend to produce a higher systolic BP.

Procedure Variation D. Palpating the Blood Pressure

- Apply the cuff, and palpate for the radial or brachial pulse.
- Begin to inflate the cuff. When you can no longer feel the pulse, inflate the cuff about 30 mm Hg more.
- As you release the valve and slowly deflate the cuff, note the reading on the manometer at which you once again feel the pulse.
- Record the palpated blood pressure according to the way it was assessed (e.g., "Palpated, low Fowler's, left arm 86/——" [or "86 systolic"]).

Evaluation

- Compare the BP reading with previous readings.
- Look for trends. Is the BP slowly decreasing (e.g., impending shock) or slowly increasing (e.g., hypervolemia)?
- Look for a corresponding change in pulse rate, indicating potential hypoxemia.
- If this is the first BP measurement for the client, check readings in both arms.
  A difference of 10 mm Hg or less is normal.
- Report any significant changes in the BP reading.

Patient Teaching

Teach the patient about:

- Normal BP values (keep in mind that prehypertension is diagnosed at a lower level when using self-monitored readings).
- Significance of the BP reading.
- Further follow-up that may be necessary.

Home Care

- The American Heart Association (AHA) and other guidelines recommend self-monitoring of BP at home. It is thought that self-measurement of BP provides more reliable data than office BP because of the availability of multiple readings. It is also thought to improve adherence to treatment regimens.
- If possible, use the same equipment each time to prevent false changes in measurement.
- Explain the need for frequent recalibration of the home-monitoring device.
- Assess the skill level of the person(s) who will be measuring the patient's BP in the home, and provide instruction if necessary.
- Assess whether self-monitoring is causing the client to be anxious.

  Some clients do become overly anxious when they know they must monitor their BP, or when they obtain a high reading. Self-monitoring should not be used if it produces too much anxiety; this raises the BP even more.
- Teach clients not to change their medication dosage without consulting their primary provider when their BP goes up or down.
- ✚ Before leaving the home, clean the stethoscope and sphygmomanometer with detergent or disinfectant, when possible; or place them in a plastic bag for transporting to the reprocessing location.
- ✚ If the client has an infection with a multidrug-resistant organism, reusable equipment such as stethoscopes should remain in the home. If the stethoscope and sphygmomanometer cannot remain in the home, clean and disinfect them before leaving the home, using a low to intermediate level disinfectant. If this is not practical, place them in a plastic bag and transport them to another site for cleaning and disinfection.

Documentation

- You will usually document BP on a flowsheet (such as in Procedure 20-5, Documentation).
- Document the blood pressure systolic/diastolic readings (e.g., 130/80).
- If you hear the 4th Korotkoff sound or muffling, document systolic/muffling/diastolic (e.g., 130/80/70). If you hear an auscultatory gap, document "systolic/diastolic with an auscultatory gap from ..." For example, "170/90 with an auscultatory gap from 170 to 140."
- Follow agency policy regarding the recording of muffled sounds.
- If you chose an alternate site, document the site used and the reason for not using the upper arm.

(continued on next page)

Procedure 20-6 ■ Measuring Blood Pressure (continued)

Practice Resources

Alexis, O. (2010); American Association of Critical-Care Nurses (2010); American Heart Association (n.d.a); American Heart Association (2012); British Hypertension Society, Hypertension Influence Team (2006); CDC (2011); Joint National Committee on Prevention, Detection, Evaluation, and Treatment of High Blood Pressure (2004); Lockwood, C., Conroy-Hiller, T., & Page, T. (2004); Pinar, R., Ataalkin, S., & Watson, R. (2010); Rhinehart, E. (2001); Siegel, J. D., Rhinehart, E., Jackson, M., et al. (2007); Vital Signs (1999).

Thinking About the Procedure

To practice applying clinical reasoning to this procedure,

Go to the *Davis's Nursing Skills Videos*, **Measuring Blood Pressure.**

For questions and suggested responses,

Go to Chapter 20, **Thinking About the Procedure Questions and Suggested Responses** on Davis*Plus*.

CLINICAL INSIGHTS

Clinical Insight 20-1 ➤ Choosing a Blood Pressure Cuff Size

- The *width* of the bladder should cover approximately two-thirds of the *length* of the upper arm (or other extremity) for an adult, and the entire upper arm for a child.
- Another method for sizing: (1) The cuff width should be 40% of the arm circumference, and (2) the *length* of the bladder should encircle 80% of the arm.
- Perhaps the easiest sizing method is to measure *arm circumference* and follow the chart in columns 2 and 3. →

For arm circumference	Cuff should be
22–26 cm (8½ × 10¼ in.)	"small adult" size: 12 × 22 cm (4¾ × 8¾ in.)
27–34 cm (10½ × 13½ in.)	"adult" size: 16 × 30 cm (6¼ × 11¾ in.)
35–44 cm (13¾ × 171/4 in.)	"large adult" size: 16 × 36 cm (6¼ × 14¼ in.)
45–52 cm (17¾ × 101/2 in.)	"adult thigh" size: 16 × 42 cm (6¼ × 16⅝ in.)

Source: Pickering, Hall, & Appel (2005).

Clinical Insight 20-2 ➤ Taking an Accurate Blood Pressure

To improve your technique and accuracy of measurement, use the following tips in addition to Procedure 20-6.

- Explain the procedure, particularly on admission or when changing the routine.

Reduces patient anxiety

- Wait 30 minutes before assessing BP after client has ingested caffeine or smoked.
- Do not assess BP while the client is in pain.
- Apply the cuff over bare skin, if possible. Controversy surrounds this issue, so follow the manufacturer's instructions and agency policy. Advise clients who are home monitoring to apply the cuff over bare skin.
- Instruct the client not to talk during BP measurement. You should not talk either.
- Keep environmental noise and client movement to a minimum.
- Hold the stethoscope lightly but completely against the skin; do not put your thumb on top of the bell or diaphragm. Try not to allow the tubing to brush against your clothing or the bed.
- Do not be influenced by the client's previous BP measurements.
- Use the same limb for each measurement, unless you are comparing arms or averaging readings from both arms.
- For the initial reading, measure the BP in both arms and use the arm with the higher reading for subsequent measurements.
- If you obtain an elevated reading, confirm in the other arm.
- Do not draw conclusions based on one reading. Take two or more readings, at least 2 to 5 minutes apart, and average them. If the readings differ by more than 5 mm Hg, obtain and average additional readings.

Practice Resources

Joint National Committee on Prevention, Detection, Evaluation, and Treatment of High Blood Pressure (2004); Ma, G., Sabin, N., & Dawes, M. (2008); McKay, D. (2008); Tomlinson, B. (2010).

FORMS

Graphic Flowsheet

VITAL SIGNS
24 HOUR FLOW SHEET

ACCOUNT NO. 37681A
MED. REC. NO. 00005674321
NAME Fred D Abbott
BIRTHDATE 1-25-39

DATE mm/dd/yy WEIGHT 285 lb.

ISOLATION Standard Precautions

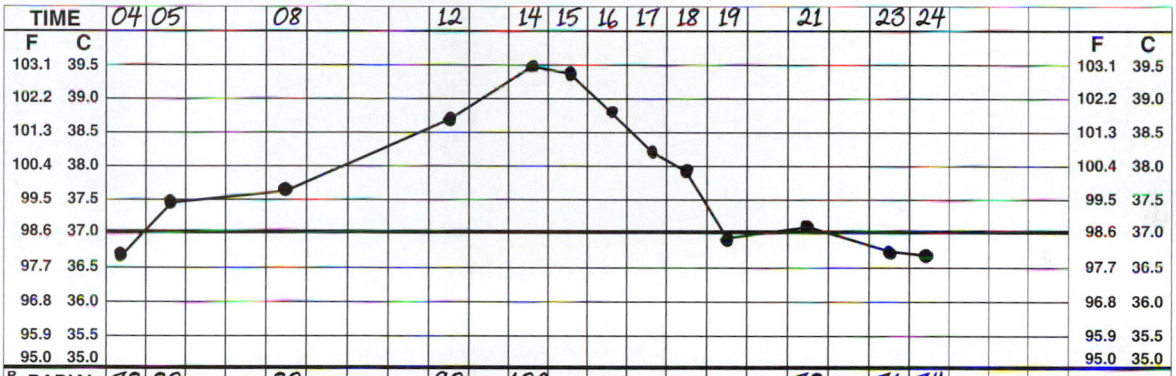

TIME	04	05			08				12		14	15	16	17	18	19		21		23	24			
PULSE RADIAL	78	80			80				90		102							78		76	74			
PULSE APICAL											100	98	92	90	82	80								
RESP.	12	14			16				20		21	22	20	18	16	16		14		12	12			
B/P	118				120				138		144	146	140	138	130	124		118			118			
	84				86				90		90	90	86	84	84	82		80			78			
PAIN																								
SAO_2	96%				96%				94%		94%		92%	96%	98%	99%		99%			98%			

PAIN LEVEL
0–NONE
10–SEVERE

TABLES

Centigrade–Fahrenheit Conversion Chart

°CENTIGRADE	°FAHRENHEIT	°CENTIGRADE	°FAHRENHEIT
34.0	93.2	38.8	101.8
34.2	93.6	39.0	102.2
34.4	93.9	39.2	102.5
34.6	94.3	39.4	102.9
34.8	94.6	39.6	103.2
35.0	95.0	39.8	103.6
35.2	95.4	40.0	104.0
35.4	95.7	40.2	104.3
35.6	96.1	40.4	104.7
35.8	96.4	40.6	105.1
36.0	96.8	40.8	105.4
36.2	97.1	41.0	105.8
36.4	97.5	41.2	106.1
36.6	97.8	41.4	106.5
36.8	98.2	41.6	106.8
37.0	98.6	41.8	107.2
37.2	98.9	42.0	107.6
37.4	99.3	42.2	108.0
37.6	99.6	42.4	108.3
37.8	100.0	42.6	108.7
38.0	100.4	42.8	109.0
38.2	100.7	43.0	109.4
38.4	101.1	44.0	111.2
38.6	101.4		

CLINICALREASONING: Applying the Full-Spectrum Nursing Model

PATIENT SITUATION

A patient in the critical care unit had a stable pulse and BP for the first few days. He has become more ill and now his pulse and BP are weak and difficult to palpate. His last BP reading was abnormally low, so it must be monitored frequently. He is receiving intravenous fluids in both arms.

THINKING

1. *Critical Thinking (Reflecting and Deciding What to Do):* Which of the patient's vital signs (TPR and BP) might you delegate to a NAP?

DOING

2. *Practical Knowledge:* How would you take the patient's blood pressure? Be specific: (a) What site would you use? (b) What equipment would you use?
3. *Nursing Process (Assessment):*
   a. Will you need to validate any of the vital signs you obtain? If so, why?
   b. How could you validate those vital signs?

CARING

4. Assume that you are very busy. How would you demonstrate caring to this patient while you are assessing his vital signs (the ones you did not delegate to a NAP)?

Critical Thinking and Clinical Reasoning

1. Recall the clients in the Meet Your Patients scenario (in Volume 1 of your textbook). Two-year-old Jason's oral temperature was 102°F (38.9°C) and his skin was warm, dry, and flushed. His mother told you that he had been eating poorly and was very irritable. What cues alert you that something is wrong?
2. You have already established (in Think Like a Nurse 20-3, Vol. 1) what, if any, additional information you need to determine the meaning of Jason's temperature elevation.
   a. What theoretical knowledge may account for Jason's temperature?
   b. Are there any actions you should take while meeting with Jason and his mother? If so, what?
   c. What biases do you have that affect your thinking about this situation? (This requires self-knowledge.)
3. Suppose you have the following data: In a long-term care center, where most patients are older, the average normal oral temperature of the patients is 97.1°F (36.2°C). In a local well-baby nursery, the average skin temperature of the newborns ranges from 97.7°F to 98.6°F (36.5°C to 37.0°C), but it fluctuates during the first 24 hours after birth. At a walk-in surgery center, the average oral temperature of the healthy clients is 98°F (36.7°C).
   a. What conclusion might you draw about what is causing the differences in average body temperature among these three groups? (*Clue:* First list the average temperatures in order, from highest to lowest.)
   b. What theoretical knowledge did you use to answer that question?
4. Suppose you have the following data about patients' temperatures:
   Patient A, 58 years old: 0600, 97.7°F (36.5°C); 1200, 98.8°F (37.1°C); 2100, 99°F (37.2°C)
   Patient B, 14 years old: 0600, 97.5°F (36.4°C); 1200, 97.9°F (36°C); 2100, 98.4°F (36.9°C)
   Patient C, 80 years old: 0600, 96.4°F (35.8°C); 1200, 96.8°F (37.1°C); 2100, 97.2°F (36.2°C)
   What conclusion can you draw about what is probably affecting the patients' temperatures? (*Clue:* Look at the pattern for each patient. How are the patterns similar?)
5. Organize a small group of classmates. Obtain several different sizes of blood pressure cuffs for each member of the group. Practice checking blood pressures on each other. Vary the size of the cuffs used, and note the variation generated by the change in cuff size. List your findings here (for at least three different people and at least two cuff sizes).

	Cuff Size		
BP READING	**LARGE**	**MEDIUM**	**SMALL**
Person A			
Person B			
Person C			

6. Analyze the following scenario. A 46-year-old man is hospitalized for multiple trauma after a mountain bike accident.
   Vital signs on admission: BP, 138/90; pulse, 108 beats/min; respirations, 24 breaths/min; temperature, 37.2°C (98.9°F)
   8 hours later: BP, 162/100; pulse, 122 beats/min; respirations, 26 breaths/min; temperature, 37.9°C (100.2°F)
   He is restless, agitated, and in pain.
   a. What is going on in this situation that may be influencing the VS?
   b. Do you have enough patient information to determine what is happening?
   c. What nursing actions should you consider?
   d. Should you involve others in your discussion of possible actions? If so, who?
   e. What can you delegate in this situation?
   f. Should you report this change in vital signs to the primary care provider? Why or why not?
7. Ms. Alvin is an 80-year-old patient in a long-term care facility. Her blood pressures have been in the range of 120/70 to 130/80 mm Hg for the past month. When she is newly assigned to your care, you see that according to her medical records, she has a history of hypertension. She is taking an antihypertensive medication. You observe that she is very thin, especially her extremities. She weighs only 90 lb (40.8 kg), although she is of average height.
   a. Do you think the charted BPs are probably accurate? Why or why not?
   b. How could you make sure that the recorded BP readings are accurate?
   c. After looking for a small BP cuff, you discover that there is only one size available in the agency: a standard adult size. What should you do?
8. For each of the following concepts, use critical thinking to describe how or why it is important to nursing, patient care, and measuring vital signs. Note that these are not to be merely definitions.

Vital signs	Radial artery
Circadian rhythm	Brachial artery
Metabolism	Apical pulse
Shivering	Diaphragm
Fever	Oxygen saturation and pulse oximetry
Pulse	Blood pressure
Stethoscope	Peripheral resistance

What Are the Main Points in This Chapter?

- Vital signs (temperature, pulse, respirations, and blood pressure) are indicators of a person's state of health and functioning of the body systems.
- Many factors, such as age, activity, smoking, and gender, cause normal variations in vital signs.
- Body temperature is the balance between heat production and heat loss.
- Fever is a symptom, but it is also beneficial to the immune response.
- A normal pulse rate varies widely according to age, from an average of 120 beats/min for newborns to 80 beats/min for adults.
- Assess the pulse for quality, bilateral equality, volume, and rate.
- Respiration is the process of supplying the body with oxygen and disposing of carbon dioxide.
- Assess respirations for rate, depth, rhythm, and associated clinical signs (e.g., breath sounds, chest movement, cough, pallor, and cyanosis).
- Blood pressure is the pressure of the blood as it is forced against arterial walls during cardiac contraction.
- Prehypertension is blood pressure ranging between 120 and 139 systolic or between 80 and 89 mm Hg diastolic obtained with two readings taken 6 minutes apart.
- Hypertension is persistent elevated BP (> 140 systolic or > 90 mm Hg diastolic) on more than two separate occasions.
- Clients can prevent or modify hypertension through certain lifestyle changes (e.g., exercise, weight control, and stress management).
- Nurses can delegate the activity of taking vital signs, but the nurse is responsible for evaluating the meaning of the data.

Knowledge Map

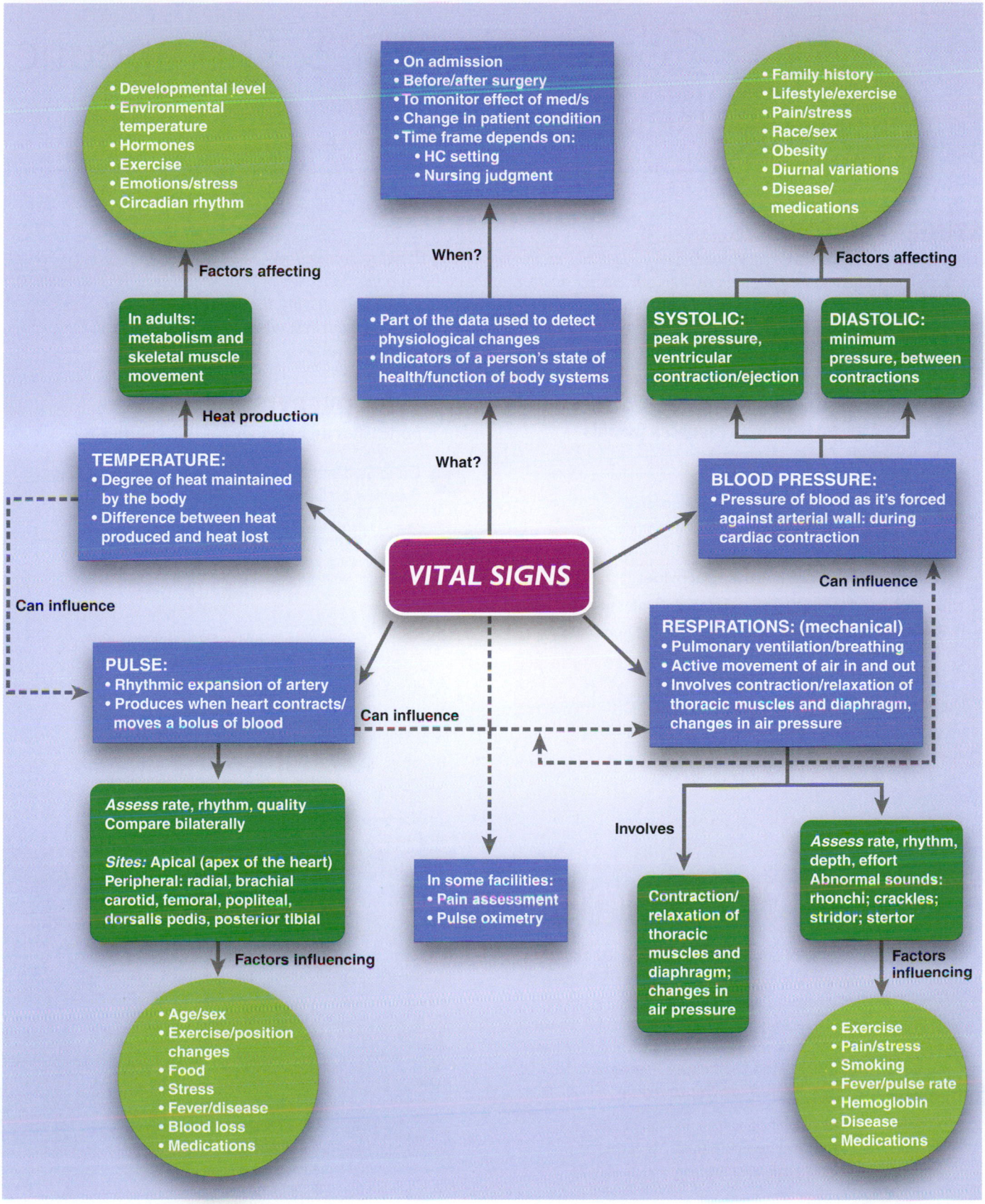

CHAPTER 21

Communication & Therapeutic Relationships

STUDENT RESOURCES

*The questions and exercises in Volume 2 allow you to practice the kind of thinking you will use as a full-spectrum nurse. Critical-thinking questions usually have more than one correct answer, so we do not provide "answers" for these features. It is more important to develop your nursing judgment than to just cover content. You will learn by discussing the questions with your peers. If you are still unsure, consult your instructor. You will find Response Sheets (for writing your responses to the questions) on Davis*Plus.

To explore learning resources for this chapter,

Go to Davis*Plus* at DavisPl.us/Wilkinson3.

Chapter Resources for Chapter 21:

- **Response sheets for all learning activities**
- **Resources for Caregivers and Health Professionals**
- **Reading More About Communication & Therapeutic Relationships**
- **Concept Map of chapter content**

Interactive Case Studies

NCLEX-Style and Chapter Review Questions

CHAPTER OVERVIEW

For a podcast of an overview of this chapter,

Go to Student Resources, Chapter 21, **Podcast—Chapter Overview,** on Davis*Plus*.

Caring for the Nguyens

Below is a transcript of an interaction that occurred during Nam Nguyen's first visit to the family healthcare clinic. As you may recall, Zach Jackson is a family nurse practitioner who is examining Nam Nguyen. Analyze the interaction. Identify open-ended and closed questions and therapeutic communication techniques. Comment on responses that Zach might have improved on.

Zach: "Are your parents still living?"
Nam: "Yes, they're both alive. My father is 80 years old and my mother is 76."

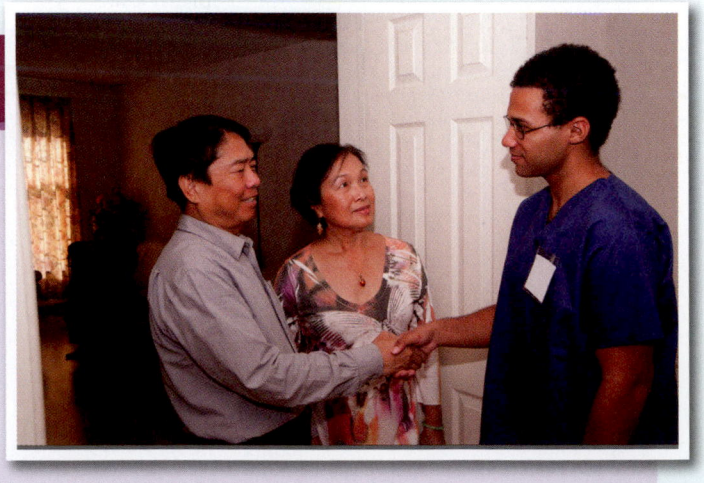

Caring for the Nguyens (continued)

Zach: "I'd like to hear a little more about your family history. Tell me about your father's cancer. How old was he when he was first diagnosed? Has he had treatment?"

Nam: "He was probably about 60 when he first found out about it. I know he had some kind of surgery and takes medicines, but I don't know the details. He seems all right though."

Zach: "Your father also has high blood pressure and heart disease. Please tell me a little more about that."

Nam: "My father and mother both have high blood pressure and heart disease. They both take medication for their blood pressure. My father had a small heart attack about 10 years ago. My mother has never had a heart attack that I know of, but she sometimes has chest pain."

Zach: "Your mother also has diabetes?"

Nam: "She's had that for a long time. A lot of people in my family, especially on my father's side, have diabetes but nobody in my mother's family. Yet my mother is the one with the diabetes!"

Yen: "A lot of people in my family have diabetes too. But so far I'm okay, I think.

Zach: "Have you had a health exam lately, Mrs. Nguyen?"

Yen: "Not in about a year, but I'm going to schedule an appointment here."

Practical Knowledge knowing how

This section provides clinical insights and assessments for communicating with patients.

CLINICAL INSIGHTS

Clinical Insight 21-1 ➤ Enhancing Communication Through Nonverbal Behaviors

Nonverbal Behaviors	*Interpretation*
Direct eye contact	Demonstrates interest and attention. Consider the client's cultural heritage when determining how much eye contact is appropriate.
Concerned facial expression	Lends credibility, if congruent with conversation.
Leaning forward	Shows interest in the conversation.
Personal space	Maintaining a distance of 18 inches to 4 feet allows most clients to feel comfortable during the interaction. Adjust the distance within that range based on the client's preference.
Professional appearance	Gives people an impression of how you may act in your role as a healthcare provider.
Sitting down to talk	Communicates willingness to listen and a sense of not wanting to rush the interaction with the client.
Touch	Conveys caring and concern when used appropriately.

Clinical Insight 21-2 ➤ Techniques for Assertive Communication

- Maintain eye contact, as culturally appropriate.
- Speak clearly and firmly.
- Project a clear tone of voice.
- Communicate self-confidently.
- Maintain professional composure.
- Communicate in a positive manner.
- Refrain from sarcasm.
- Ensure congruence between verbal and nonverbal messages.
- Guide the direction of the discussion.
- Use "I" statements.
- Focus on the issues.
- Do not invite negative responses.
- Avoid overly modest or timid statements.

Clinical Insight 21-3 ➤ Communicating With SBAR*

Situation — In 10 seconds, identify yourself and the patient and describe the present situation that prompted you to call. State:
your name
your unit
the patient's name and room number
the problem

Background — Give other information pertinent to the situation—not the patient's entire history since admission, but circumstances leading up to the situation (e.g., medications, lab results, current symptoms).

Assessment — State the problem and what you think is causing it. This is an inference rather than traditional data collection.

Recommendation — State what you think will correct the problem, or what you need from the physician.

*If you need other information about SBAR, see Clinical Insight 18-1, Giving Oral Report. Also,

Go to to **Chapter 18,** in Volume 1.

Practice Resources

De Meester, K., Verspuy, M., Monsiers, K. G., et al. (2013); Institute for Healthcare Improvement (2011, updated 2013); Military Health System, U.S. Department of Defense. (n.d.).

Clinical Insight 21-4 ➤ Communicating With Clients From Another Culture

General Guidelines

- Most important: Be aware of your own cultural beliefs and attitudes.
- Learn about other cultures, especially those in your area.
- Convey empathy and show respect.
- Be certain the communication strategies you usually use are culturally appropriate for the individual.
  - Is direct eye contact viewed as aggressive or impolite? Or is it perceived as engaged and caring?
  - How much space should you keep between yourself and the patient?
- Use touch cautiously. In some cultures, it is inappropriate to touch certain parts of the body.
- Proceed slowly. Rushing may cause the patient to be more anxious, and is offensive to some.
- Smile and be polite, but not overfriendly or casual. Use the patient's title and last name when introducing yourself.
- Use short words and sentences. Don't give too much information in one sentence.
- Present one idea at a time.
- Provide written teaching materials.

If There Is a Language Barrier

- Written information provided must be appropriate to the population served and the language of the patient (The Joint Commission, 2011).
- Use a trained medical interpreter, if possible.
- To review guidelines for communicating with clients who speak a different language, see Clinical Insight 15-3 in Chapter 15 of this book.
- Some medical dictionaries or Web-based resources have a comprehensive list of English–Spanish phrases.

Clinical Insight 21-4 ➤ Communicating With Clients From Another Culture *(continued)*

- The following are some useful Spanish words and phrases.

English	*Spanish*	*English*	*Spanish*
How do you feel?	¿Como se siente?	Cough	Tosa
Good	Bien	Open your mouth	Abra la boca
Bad	Mal	Take a deep breath	Respire profundamente
Have you any difficulty breathing?	¿Tiene dificultad al respirar?	You may eat	Puede comer
		Tea	Té
Are you thirsty?	¿Tiene sed?	Coffee	Café
Have you any pain?	¿Tiene dolor?	I will give you something for	Le dare algo para eso
Show me where	Enséñeme dónde	A pill	Una píldora
Is it worse now?	¿Está peor ahora?		

Spanish Patient-Education Materials

Several U.S. government Web sites offer free, reliable patient education materials in Spanish. For links to these and other online resources:

Go to Chapter 21, **Resources for Caregivers & Health Professionals,** on Davis*Plus*.

Clinical Insight 21-5 ➤ Communicating With Clients Who Have Impaired Speech

Healthcare agencies should address the communication needs of those with vision, speech, hearing, language, and cognitive impairments. .

- Nonverbal communication is the key to communication with clients with impaired speech.
- Ask the client to use hand gestures and a picture board, as appropriate.
- Solicit family assistance in understanding the client's speech.
- Provide a comfortable environment for the client to practice speaking.
- Be positive and patient.
- Although the client may have difficulty speaking, you should continue to speak and explain all procedures.
- A referral to a speech pathologist may be necessary.

Practice Resources

The Joint Commission (2010a, 2010b).

Clinical Insight 21-6 ➤ Communicating With Clients Who Have Impaired Cognition or Consciousness

Clients Who Are Cognitively Impaired

Always try to communicate.	Make every effort to communicate, even if you think that the client cannot understand you.
Do not use the in-room intercom to speak with the patient.	A voice sounding from the intercom on the bedside call system might frighten the patient and cause confusion, delirium, or other cognitive impairments. It is better to talk face-to-face.
Don't rush the client.	Provide adequate time to allow the client to communicate. He needs time to respond to your questions or commands.
Reduce environmental distractions.	Extraneous noises, lights, and even smells can compete for attention when talking with or providing instructions to the patient. For example, you might turn off the TV or close the door if you want to reduce distractions.
Approach the patient directly.	To avoid frightening the patient, approach the patient from the front, make eye contact, address the person by name, smile, and speak in a calm, friendly voice.

(Continued)

Clinical Insight 21-6 ➤ Communicating With Clients Who Have Impaired Cognition or Consciousness *(continued)*

Talk first and touch second.	Touching a patient before establishing a basic trust might frighten the confused or cognitively impaired patient.
Do not argue or insist the patient agree with you.	The patient with altered perception or cognition might not have the capacity to understand or accept reality. Pushing him to agree with you simply can create anxiety or hostility.
Use multiple communication modalities.	Provide verbal and written discharge instructions. Review the instructions several times with the client before discharge, and include family members in the teaching.
Provide reminders.	Use memory aids, schedules, and reminder notices to reinforce information.
Orient the client.	Verbally orient to time, person, and place, and provide visual orientation materials, such as a calendar or schedule.
Stimulate memory.	If the client loses his place in the conversation, stimulate memory by repeating his last expressed thought (e.g., "We were talking about your back pain. Tell me more about your back pain").
Use short sentences.	Use short sentences containing a single thought (e.g., "Are you hungry?"). Avoid complex statements (e.g., "You look hungry. Would you like a sandwich or a milk shake, or can you hold off until dinner?")
Ask yes or no questions.	Ask direct questions that require only a yes or no answer (e.g., "Are you hungry?").
Limit choices.	Limit choices to avoid confusing or frustrating the patient.
Be concrete and specific.	Do not use vague comments to indicate that you are listening. The client may be unable to interpret comments such as, "I see." Instead, repeat the client's words and directly state your response (e.g., "You are cold. I will bring you a blanket").
Avoid slang and jargon.	The client may not understand, and may become anxious.
Use gestures.	Model desired behaviors. You might say "Brush your teeth now" and then pantomime brushing your teeth.
Don't assume.	Bear in mind that the client cannot behave differently and that he may be confused about reality. When the person is talking about superficial, routine matters, he may seem more competent than he is.
For clients with expressive difficulties:	■ If you are sure of the word the person is trying to say, repeat it. Don't guess, though. ■ Pay close attention to nonverbal communication. ■ Assess for and anticipate unmet needs, such as hunger, thirst, and pain. ■ Respond to the emotion, not the words. ■ Do not reprimand the patient if she curses or is aggressive.

Patients Who Are Unconscious

- Touch and speak to unconscious or sedated patients, and advise them of the care you are providing. Although the patient may not be able to respond, she may be able to hear your comments. The patient may also benefit physiologically when hearing your voice or that of his loved ones.
- Consult with previous caregivers or the family to determine what the patient responds to.
- Begin each interaction by identifying yourself and calling the patient by name.
- Speak calmly and slowly, even if the patient doesn't seem to be alert and oriented.
- Explain all healthcare procedures as you are doing them.
- Provide soothing music and periods of rest.

Patients Who Have Suffered a Stroke

- Remember that many stroke survivors may have trouble communicating their thoughts. They also commonly experience emotional ups and downs. Do not take these moods personally.
- With aphasia, speak slowly, not louder. Be careful not to use patronizing tone.
- **Augmentive and alternative communication** (AAC) might be helpful to patients experiencing expressive aphasia. AAC includes all forms of communication other than speech to express thoughts, needs, wants, and ideas, such as communication boards and electronic devices.
- Be a good listener and allow time for the patient to express his thoughts.

Practice Resources

Alzheimer's Society (2012); American Heart Association (2012); American Speech-Language-Hearing Association (n.d.); Miller, C. A. (2008); Simoes, J., Jesus, L. M. T., & Voegeli, D. (2009); Zembrzuski, C. (2013, revised).

ASSESSMENT GUIDELINES AND TOOLS

Focused Assessment

Communication

A focused assessment should identify factors that alter a patient's ability to receive, understand, and transmit verbal and nonverbal messages.

Medications

Is the patient taking medications that might interfere with speech, cognition, or level of consciousness?

Language Barriers

- What is the patient's primary language?
- Does the patient have sufficient command of the dominant language?
- Is an interpreter (foreign language or sign language) required?
- Can the patient read and write? At what level and in what language?

Cognitive Function

- What is the patient's level of consciousness?
- Is there short-term or long-term memory loss, or both?
- Is intellectual function at, below, or above expectations for age?
- Can the patient read simple instructions?
- Can the patient follow simple spoken instructions?
- Can the patient understand a yes or no choice?
- Are there symptoms or a diagnosis of mental illness or dementia?
- If the patient is unconscious, are there nonverbal responses that indicate he can hear you (e.g., blinking, moving the head, squeezing your hand)?

Hearing

- Ask the patient, and observe, whether there are hearing problems.
- Is the patient wearing a hearing aid? If so, is it working properly? Does the patient appear to be reading your lips?
- Is the patient trying to use sign language to communicate?
- Refer to Chapter 19 for tests of hearing (e.g., ticking watch).

Vision

- Is the patient wearing glasses or contact lenses?
- Is the patient able to see adequately?
- Refer to Chapter 22 for vision tests.

Also see Procedure 22-20, **Brief Bedside Assessment,** in this volume.

Aphasia

- Is there a history of stroke, or a diagnosis of aphasia?
- Is there receptive aphasia (inability to receive or interpret verbal or nonverbal messages)?
- Is there expressive aphasia (inability to express verbal or nonverbal messages)?

Physiological Barriers

Does the patient have conditions that cause difficulty speaking, such as:

- Dyspnea?
- Artificial airway?
- Oral problems, such as poorly fitted dentures?
- Cleft palate or other structural problems?

Communication Style

- Is it difficult to understand what the patient says (e.g., slurring words, stuttering, inability to pronounce certain sounds)?
- Does the patient speak readily, or refuse to speak?
- Does the patient speak slowly or rapidly; spontaneously or hesitantly?
- Is the vocabulary adequate for the purpose needed?
- Has the vocabulary changed from the person's normal vocabulary?

Other

- Are verbal communication and nonverbal communication congruent?

CLINICALREASONING: Applying the Full-Spectrum Nursing Model

Choose *two* of the following communication techniques and plan to consciously use them with your next patient. Use the following thinking, doing, and caring questions to reflect on your interaction.

- Active listening
- Communicating assertively by making "I" statements
- Restating a message
- Clarifying messages
- Validating messages
- Sharing observations about body language
- Asking open-ended questions
- Using silence
- Summarizing the conversation

THINKING

1. *Critical Thinking (Contextual Awareness):* Before you have the conversation, make a note of what is going on in the situation (e.g., values, environment, culture) that might influence the effectiveness of the two techniques you will be using.

DOING

2. *Nursing Process (Assessment):* Before using the two techniques, assess for factors that might affect the patient's ability to communicate. Make a note of them.
3. *Nursing Process (Implementation):* As soon as possible after using the techniques, record the conversations. Try to remember the exact words.
4. *Nursing Process (Evaluation):* Evaluate your ability to use the two techniques you chose.
   a. Did you use them at appropriate times in the conversations: as an appropriate response to something the patient said?
   b. What effect did what you said have on the interaction? How did the patient respond to what you said?
   c. Do you think your communication was therapeutic for the patient?

CARING

5. *Self-Knowledge:*
   a. What were your thoughts and feelings before, during, and after the interaction?
   b. In what way has your comfort level with these two techniques changed?
   c. Describe the type of patient or situation in which you would be the least confident in your ability to communicate therapeutically.

Critical Thinking and Clinical Reasoning

1. Mrs. Washington arrives at the clinic complaining of a painful lump in her left breast. She is 40 years old and appears very nervous. She tells you, "I was afraid to come in, but I guess I have to find out what this is."
   a. How might you acknowledge Mrs. Washington's feelings? Give examples.
   b. What might you say to clarify and validate her messages?
   c. Write a hypothetical conversation with Mrs. Washington that:
      - What will I learn this semester?
      - Acknowledges her feelings
      - Establishes trust
      - Explores the issue
      - Clarifies and validates the client's messages
      - Uses silence
      - Summarizes the conversation
2. Paramedics bring a 35-year-old man and his 14-year-old son to the emergency department (ED). Both have been involved in a recreational vehicle gas explosion and have suffered burns. The son is placed in one of the trauma rooms adjacent to his father. He has partial and full-thickness burns over his face, neck, chest, arms, and hands, and he is unresponsive. The father has partial-thickness burns on his right hand and

forearm. He appears to be in a lot of pain and is screaming for his son in Spanish. He speaks limited English. Thirty minutes later, his wife (who is also the boy's mother) arrives at the ED. She is crying and asking whether her husband and son will be okay. Her English is fluent.

a. Identify at least two interventions to help you communicate with the father.
b. What kind of body language would you expect from the father?
c. How could you show acceptance of and establish trust with the father?
d. Identify at least two factors that will influence communication with the son.
e. Identify at least two communication strategies to use with the son.
f. Explain or give an example of how to use the following techniques as you communicate with the anxious wife and mother:
   - Establishing trust
   - Using silence
   - Offering nonverbal support

3. For each of the following concepts, use critical thinking to describe how or why it is important to nursing, patient care, or communication. Note that these are *not* to be merely definitions.

Verbal communication	Therapeutic communication
Nonverbal communication	Therapeutic relationship
Intrapersonal communication	Barriers to therapeutic communication
Interpersonal communication	Distance between sender and receiver
Group communication	Communication strategies

What Are the Main Points in This Chapter?

- Communication is a dynamic, reciprocal process of sending and receiving messages.
- Communication occurs on three levels: intrapersonal, or self-talk; interpersonal (between two or more people); and group communication.
- The sender delivers a message to the receiver via verbal and/or nonverbal communication. The receiver provides feedback to the sender.
- Verbal communication is the use of spoken and written words.
- Nonverbal communication, sometimes called body language, communicates how someone is feeling and gives a more accurate account of an individual's true sentiment.
- Physical development, maturity, language skills, intellectual abilities, culture, gender, roles, and relationships influence the communication process
- Collaborative professional communication is assertive without being aggressive.
- Communication is most successful in a comfortable environment. A favorable environment is quiet, private, free of noxious smells, and at a comfortable temperature.
- The distance between individuals engaged in communication is affected by the relationship of the individuals, the nature of the conversation, the setting, and cultural influences.
- Relationships affect the choice of vocabulary, tone of voice, use of gestures, and distance associated with the communication.
- Therapeutic communication is the use of communication skills that results in a positive effect on client care; it is the foundation of professional nursing practice.
- Therapeutic communication occurs in the context of a helping relationship. The helping relationship has four phases: pre-interaction, orientation, working phase, and termination.
- Group communication occurs when you are interacting with a family, a community, or a committee. Groups may be focused on a task, self-improvement, coping skills, or work-related issues.
- To enhance communication, listen actively, establish trust, be assertive, restate messages, clarify and validate messages, interpret body language, share observations, explore issues, use silence, summarize the conversation, and make use of process recordings while you are learning.
- Barriers to communication include asking too many questions; asking why; fire-hosing information; changing the subject inappropriately; failing to listen; failing to probe; expressing approval or disapproval; offering advice; providing false reassurance; stereotyping; and using patronizing language.
- Language barriers, sensory perceptual alterations, impaired cognitive skills, and physiological barriers make therapeutic communication challenging, but nursing activities can enhance communication with these clients.

Knowledge Map

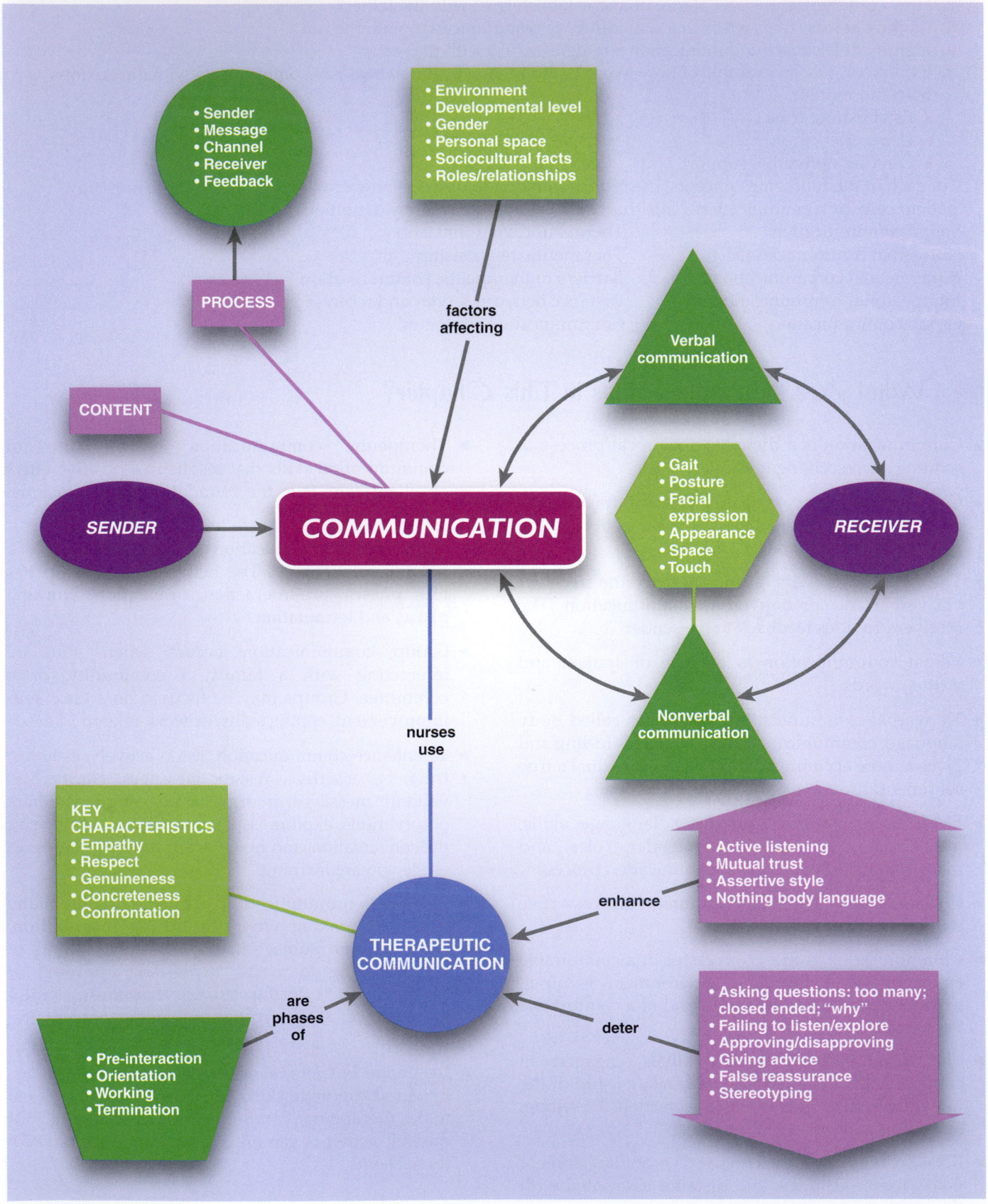

CHAPTER 22

Health Assessment

STUDENT RESOURCES

*The questions and exercises in Volume 2 allow you to practice the kind of thinking you will use as a full-spectrum nurse. Critical-thinking questions usually have more than one correct answer, so we do not provide "answers" for these features. It is more important to develop your nursing judgment than to just cover content. You will learn by discussing the questions with your peers. If you are still unsure, consult your instructor. You will find Response Sheets (for writing your responses to the questions) on Davis*Plus.

To explore learning resources for this chapter,

Go to Davis*Plus* at DavisPl.us/Wilkinson3.

Chapter Resources for Chapter 22:

- **Response sheets for all learning activities**
- **Resources for Caregivers and Health Professionals**
- **Reading More About Health Assessment (suggested readings)**
- **Concept Map of chapter content**

Interactive Case Studies

NCLEX-Style and Chapter Review Questions

CHAPTER OVERVIEW

For a podcast of an overview of this chapter,

Go to Student Resources: **Chapter 22, Podcast—Chapter Overview** on Davis*Plus*.

Caring for the Nguyens

Nam Nguyen has had a comprehensive physical examination with Zach Jackson, the nurse practitioner at the clinic. To review the note written by Zach,

Go to Chapter 22, **Documenting Physical Assessment Findings,** in Volume 1.

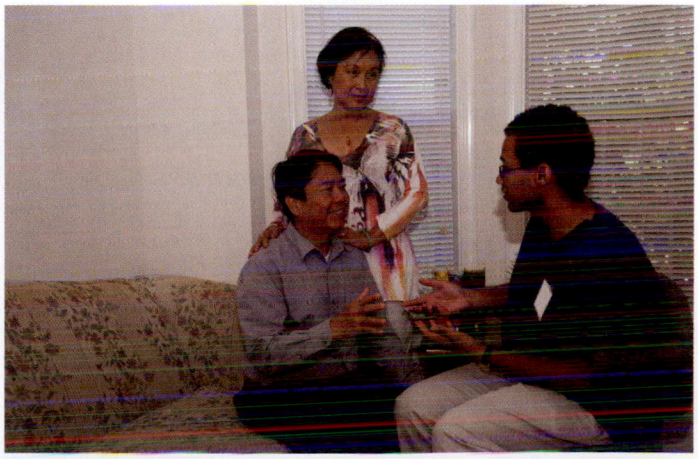

(Continued)

Caring for the Nguyens (continued)

A. Discuss how each of the following would differ from the examination Zach Jackson conducted and what would be expected if:
- A registered nurse conducted the exam.
- A nursing student performed the exam.

B. Review Zach's documentation of the exam. Identify the abnormal findings.

C. Review the laboratory work. Identify the abnormal findings.

D. What conclusions, if any, can you draw from these findings? What actions should you consider based on these conclusions?

E. Identify at least two nursing diagnoses based on these findings.

F. Zach Jackson has identified a problem of Imbalanced Nutrition: More Than Body Requirements for Mr. Nguyen.
- What information do you need to determine the etiology of this problem?
- Because you do not have that information, write a two-part diagnostic statement describing Mr. Nguyen's nutritional status.

G. Now rewrite the nutrition statement as a three-part statement, using "as evidenced by."

H. Zach Jackson has identified the diagnosis Acute Pain (knees) for Mr. Nguyen. If the pain is caused by a medical condition, osteoarthritis, how would you write a two-part diagnostic statement to describe this health status?

I. How would the examination of Yen Nguyen differ from the exam Nam experienced?

J. How would the examination of Kim Phan, Nam's 3-year-old grandson, differ?

K. If you were responsible for examining Nam Nguyen, what aspects of the exam would you find most challenging? Explain why.

Practical Knowledge knowing how

The registered nurse is responsible for patient assessment. As the RN, you should (1) perform the initial assessment to establish a baseline and (2) perform follow-up assessments for any changes. You can instruct nursing assistive personnel (NAPs) to report any changes to you. You can delegate measurement of height, weight, and vital signs to the NAP. However, you may want to obtain the first set of vital signs yourself, because they will serve as a baseline.

In the remainder of this chapter, you will find all the procedures and assessment guidelines necessary for a complete physical examination (Procedures 22-1 through 22-19). Procedure 22-20 describes a brief bedside assessment. In addition, you will find Clinical Insights and an Abnormal Atlas at the end of the chapter.

PROCEDURES

When examining each body system be sure to compare findings on both sides of the body. The following procedures are described mainly for adult patients, but modifications for children and older adults are also included. If you want to further review ways in which to adapt your examination to people of different ages,

Go to **How Do I Modify Assessment for Different Age Groups?,** in Volume 1.

Procedure 22-1 ■ Performing the General Survey

➤ For steps to follow in *all* procedures, refer to the Universal Steps for All Procedures found on the inside back cover.

Equipment

See Equipment Needed for Physical Examination, below.

Equipment Needed for Physical Examination

Usual Equipment for Ongoing Assessment

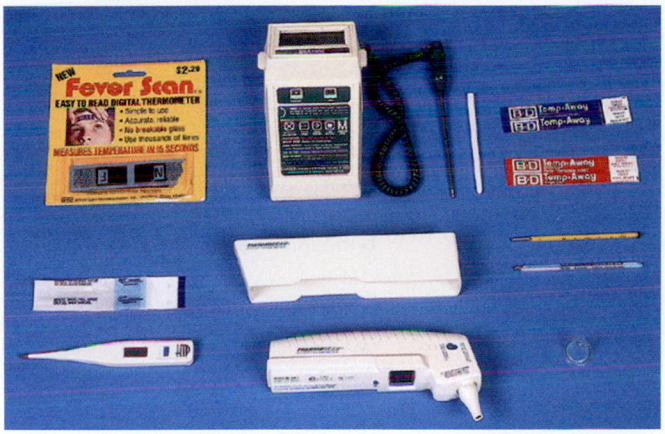

Thermometer (for measuring temperature)

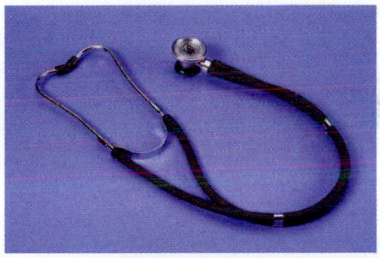

Stethoscope (for measuring blood pressure and listening to heart, lung, and bowel sounds)

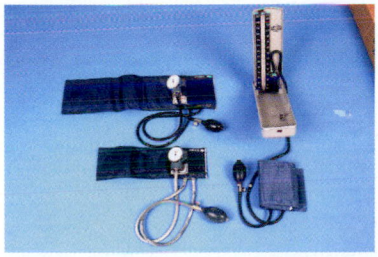

Sphygmomanometer (for measuring blood pressure)

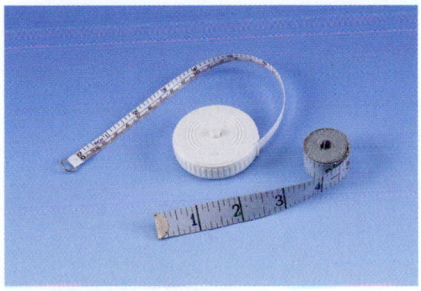

Tape measure (to measure circumference and length)

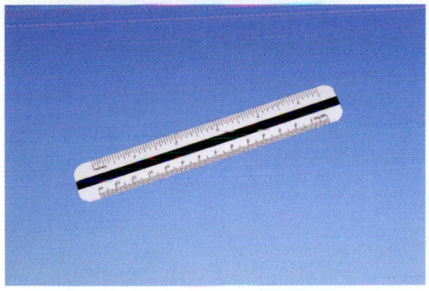

Pocket ruler (to measure size or distance)

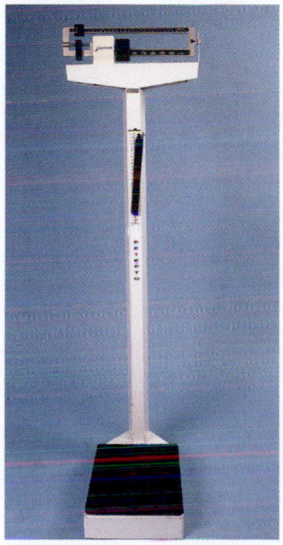

Scale (to measure weight and height)

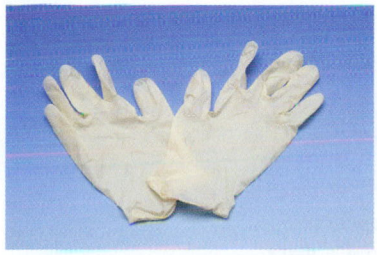

Gloves (to wear if there is any possible exposure to blood or body fluids)

(continued on next page)

Procedure 22-1 ■ Performing the General Survey (continued)

Equipment Needed for Physical Examination—cont'd

Additional Equipment for a Comprehensive Assessment

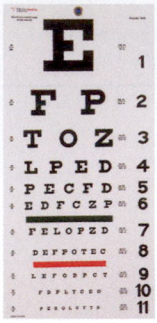

Snellen acuity chart (for screening vision)

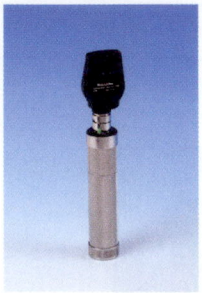

Ophthalmoscope (for inspection of the internal structures of the eye)

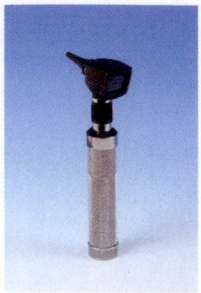

Otoscope (for examining the external auditory canal and tympanic membrane)

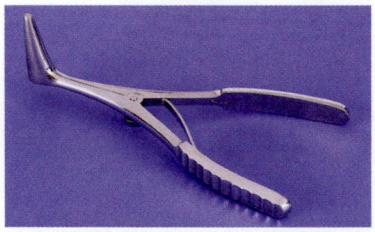

Nasal speculum (for examining the nasal turbinates)

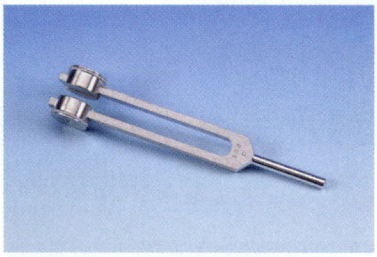

Tuning fork (for auditory screening and assessment of vibratory sensation during the neurological exam)

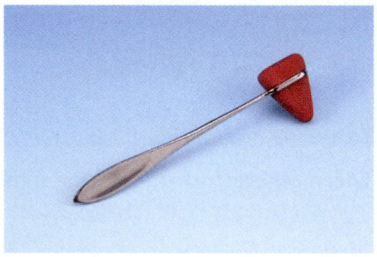

Percussion hammer (for eliciting deep tendon reflexes)

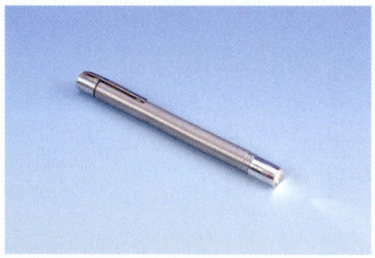

Penlight (for visualizing the eyes and inside of mouth, or highlighting a skin lesion)

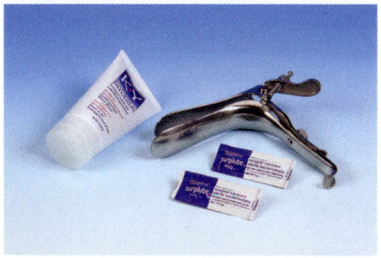

Vaginal speculum and lubricant (for examining the female pelvis; lubricant is also used for rectal exams)

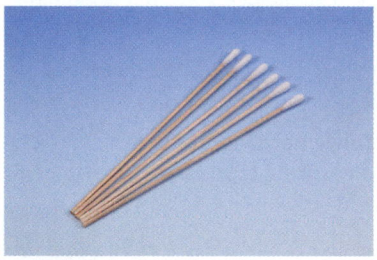

Cotton-tipped applicators (for obtaining specimens)

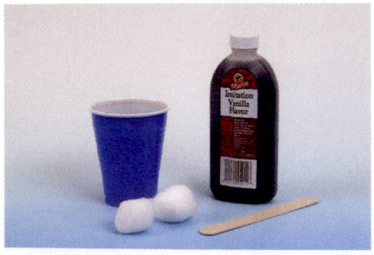

Cotton balls, tongue depressor, strong-smelling substance, a glass of water (for testing various cranial nerves)

Positioning

- Have the client seated as you begin the examination (on an exam table or on the side of the bed).
- If the client is unable to sit, use Fowler's or semi-Fowler's position.

Focused History Questions

- How are you feeling today?
- (If the client is an outpatient) What brings you to the clinic today?
- Are you in any discomfort or pain?
- Have you had any hospitalizations or surgeries?
- What medicines do you take? That means prescribed as well as over-the-counter drugs.
- How much alcohol do you drink per day? Do you smoke cigarettes? If so, how many per day? Do you use drugs for non-medical purposes?
- Do you use any herbal products or natural remedies?
- Do you have any difficulty falling asleep or staying asleep?

Developmental Modifications for Infants and Children

- Encourage the parents to be present for the examination. Position an infant on a padded examination table or held against the parent's chest.
  Infants and toddlers usually feel most secure if a parent is present.
- Offer toddlers choices. Involve the parent in the exam. Praise the toddler for cooperation.
- Allow the preschool child to sit in the parent's lap if she wishes. Let the child help with the exam. Give reassurance as you proceed. Compliment the child on her cooperation.
  Preschoolers often are fearful of body injury and invasive procedures.
- Support the school-age child's independence. Develop rapport by asking the child about his teacher or favorite school and play activities. Allow the child to undress himself and get up and down from the exam table. Demonstrate and let the child touch your equipment before you use it.
  Equipment will seem less threatening to the child if she touches it. It is unlikely that the child would break the equipment.
- Adolescents should be examined without parents or siblings present unless they request otherwise. Provide privacy.
  Adolescents are self-conscious and introspective.

Developmental Modifications for Older Adults

- Observe the older adult's energy level during the physical examination, and provide rest periods if needed. If the client tires easily, arrange the exam sequence to limit position changes.
- Allow extra time to interview and examine older adults.
- Be aware that stiff muscles and arthritic joints may make it impossible for older adults to assume certain positions.
- Be alert for hearing and vision deficits in older adults, and adapt your interview techniques accordingly (e.g., elicit feedback to be sure the client has heard you correctly).
- Assess the older adult's functional status. You can use the Lawton Instrumental Activities of Daily Living (IADL), found in the section Assessment Guidelines and Tools in Chapter 3 of this volume.
- Work the SPICES assessment into the examination of various body systems: **S**leep disorders, **P**roblems eating or feeding, **I**ncontinence, **C**onfusion, **E**vidence of falls, **S**kin breakdown.

➤ When performing the procedure, always identify your patient according to agency policy, using two identifiers, and be attentive to standard precautions, hand hygiene, patient safety and privacy, body mechanics, and documentation

Procedure Steps	Expected and Abnormal Findings
1. **Identify signs of distress** (e.g., pain, fear, or anxiety). If signs of distress are present, perform a focused assessment, and address the immediate problem.	**Expected findings:** The client is in no apparent distress. Appears relaxed, with no evidence of pain, fear, or anxiety. **Abnormal findings:** Pain, grimacing, breathing problems, skin color changes
2. **Observe apparent age, sex, and race.** Ask the patient, "What racial or ethnic group do you identify with?" Ask yourself, ▪ Is apparent age consistent with biological age? ▪ Are there cultural or gender-related factors that influence the exam or findings?	**Expected findings:** Client appears his stated age. Makes eye contact consistent with his cultural norms. Is reasonably comfortable with being examined.
3. **Note facial characteristics**, including facial expression, symmetry of facial features, and the condition and color of the skin. Ask yourself, ▪ What is the client's face telling me? ▪ Is the facial expression appropriate to the situation?	**Expected findings:** Face is symmetrical; visible skin is intact without excessive wrinkling, discoloration, or deformity.

(continued on next page)

Procedure 22-1 ■ Performing the General Survey (continued)

- Are facial features symmetrical (palpebral fissure and nasolabial folds)?
- Are there any changes in condition or color of skin?
- Does the client maintain eye contact?

---

4. Note body type and posture. Greet the client with a handshake. Be aware that shaking hands is not acceptable in all cultures.

Allows you to assess muscle strength and surface skin characteristics while at the same time conveying that you care.

Ask yourself,

- Is the body build stocky, slender, average, obese, or **cachectic** (very thin, wasted appearance)?
- Are the body parts proportional to the client's overall size?
- Does the client have abnormal fat distribution?
- Does the client assume a specific position for comfort (e.g., sitting versus supine)?

Expected findings: Posture is upright, and body appears proportionate. Grip is strong.

---

5. Observe gait, and note any abnormal movements. If the client has Impaired Bed Mobility, determine ability to move and amount of assistance needed. Ask yourself,

- Does the client move in a coordinated manner?
- Are there any obvious gait problems?
- Does the client walk with a wide base of support or short stride length?
- Does the client use assistive devices?
- Are there any abnormal or spastic movements?

Expected findings: Movements are coordinated; gait is steady; does not use assistive devices.

Abnormal findings: Unstable or shuffling gait; spastic movements, stiff movements

---

6. Listen to your client's speech pattern, pace, quality, tone, vocabulary, and sentence structure. Ask yourself,

- Are the responses appropriate?
- Is there any difficulty with speech?
- Does the client's tone of voice match her statements?

Expected findings: Client responds appropriately to questions. Tone of voice matches responses. Speech is clear, evenly paced, and rises and falls based on content.

Abnormal findings: Rapid speech, slow speech, slurred speech

---

7. Assess mental state and affect.

a. Determine level of consciousness.

b. Determine orientation to time, place, and person.

Ask yourself,

- If the client is disoriented, does he reorient easily?
- What is the client's mood? Is it appropriate for the situation?

Many medical conditions and medications can affect mental status. If you note any abnormal findings: During the general survey, be sure to focus on them when you assess mental status during the sensorineurological examination.

Expected findings: Awake, alert, and oriented to time, place, person, and self. Mood is appropriate for the situation.

Abnormal findings: Confusion and irritability, inability to recall information or provide history, lethargy and somnolence, bizarre responses

---

8. Observe dress, grooming, and hygiene. Ask yourself,

- Is the client appropriately and neatly dressed?
- Is the client well groomed?
- Are there any unusual odors?

Expected findings: Client is dressed appropriately for the climate. Skin is clean, and clothing is in good repair. No noticeable odor.

Abnormal findings: Poor hygiene, dirty skin or nails, uncombed hair, visible soiling of clothing, mismatched or wrinkled clothing, objectionable odor

9. **Measure vital signs**: blood pressure, temperature, radial pulse, respiratory rate. If your initial observations and interview indicate that the client is in pain, perform a pain assessment, as well. See Chapter 31.

Expected findings: BP: < 120/80 mm Hg
Temperature: 97.3°F–98.6°F (36.3°C–37°C) oral
Pulse: 60–100 beats/min, regular, and easily palpated
Respiratory rate: 12–20, regular and even

Abnormal findings: See Chapter 20.

10. **Measure height and weight.**
    a. For adults: Calculate BMI, or use the accompanying table.

$$\frac{\text{Wt (lb)} \times 703}{\text{Ht (in.)}^2} = \text{BMI}$$

    b. For children: Plot height and weight on growth chart.

Expected findings: For adults: BMI is 18.5–24.9.
For children: Height and weight are consistent with previous trend on growth chart.

Abnormal findings: BMI < 18.5 = underweight
BMI 25–29.9 = overweight
BMI > 30 = obese
BMI 30–34.9 = Level I Moderate obesity
BMI 35–39.9 = Level II Severe obesity
BMI > 40 = Level III Morbid obesity

Developmental Modifications

Infants and children
- Weigh infants without clothing; weigh older children in their underwear.
- For infants and children younger than 2 years, position supine to measure height; be sure knees are extended.
- For infants and children younger than age 2, also measure head circumference.

? What if . . .

- **There is an apparent language barrier?**
  Obtain an interpreter; and refer to Clinical Insight 21-4, in Chapter 21 of this volume.

Use this table to find body mass index, based on height and weight, or use a BMI calculator such as the ones found at, http://www.nhlbi.nih.gov/health/educational/lose_wt/BMI/bmi_tbl.htm

Weight (lb)

Height (ft/in)	120	130	140	150	160	170	180	190	200	210	220	230	240	250	260	270	280	290	300	310	320	330
4'5"	30	33	35	38	40	43	45	48	50	53	55	58	60	63	65	68	70	73	75	78	80	83
4'6"	29	31	34	36	39	41	43	46	48	51	53	56	58	60	63	65	68	70	72	75	77	80
4'7"	28	30	33	35	37	40	42	44	47	49	51	54	56	58	61	63	65	68	70	72	75	77
4'8"	27	29	31	34	36	38	40	43	45	47	49	52	54	56	58	61	63	65	67	70	72	74
4'9"	26	28	30	33	35	37	39	41	43	46	48	50	52	54	56	59	61	63	65	67	69	72
4'10"	25	27	29	31	34	36	38	40	42	44	46	48	50	52	54	57	59	61	63	65	67	69
4'11"	24	26	28	30	32	34	36	38	40	43	45	47	49	51	53	55	57	59	61	63	65	67
5'0"	23	25	27	29	31	33	35	37	39	41	43	45	47	49	51	53	55	57	59	61	63	65
5'1"	23	25	27	28	30	32	34	36	38	40	42	44	45	47	49	51	53	55	57	59	61	62
5'2"	22	24	26	27	29	31	33	35	37	38	40	42	44	46	48	49	51	53	55	57	59	60
5'3"	21	23	25	27	28	30	32	34	36	37	39	41	43	44	46	48	50	51	53	55	57	59
5'4"	21	22	24	26	28	29	31	33	34	36	38	40	41	43	45	46	48	50	52	53	55	57
5'5"	20	22	23	25	27	28	30	32	33	35	38	38	40	42	43	45	47	48	50	52	53	55
5'6"	19	21	23	24	26	27	29	31	32	34	36	37	39	40	42	44	45	47	49	50	52	53
5'7"	19	20	22	24	25	27	28	30	31	33	35	36	38	39	41	42	44	46	47	49	50	52
5'8"	18	20	21	23	24	26	27	29	30	32	34	35	37	38	40	41	43	44	46	47	49	50
5'9"	18	10	21	22	24	25	27	28	30	31	33	34	36	37	38	40	41	43	44	46	47	49
5'10"	17	19	20	22	23	24	26	27	29	30	32	33	35	36	37	39	40	42	43	45	46	47
5'11"	17	18	20	21	22	24	25	27	28	29	31	32	34	35	36	38	39	41	42	43	45	46
6'	16	18	19	20	22	23	24	26	27	29	30	31	33	34	35	37	38	39	41	42	43	45
6'1"	16	17	19	20	21	22	24	25	26	28	29	30	32	33	34	36	37	38	40	41	42	44
6'2"	15	17	18	19	21	22	23	24	26	27	28	30	31	32	33	35	36	37	39	40	41	42
6'3"	15	16	18	19	20	21	23	24	25	26	28	29	30	31	33	34	35	36	38	39	40	41
6'4"	15	16	17	18	20	21	22	23	24	26	27	28	29	30	32	33	34	35	37	38	39	40
6'5"	14	15	17	18	19	20	21	23	24	25	26	27	29	30	31	32	33	34	36	37	38	39
6'6"	14	15	16	17	19	20	21	22	23	24	25	27	28	29	30	31	32	34	35	36	37	38
6'7"	14	15	16	17	18	19	20	21	23	24	25	26	27	28	29	30	32	33	34	35	36	37
6'8"	13	14	15	17	18	19	20	21	22	23	24	25	26	28	29	30	31	32	33	34	35	36
6'9"	13	14	15	16	17	18	19	20	21	23	24	25	26	27	28	29	30	31	32	33	34	35
6'10"	13	14	15	16	17	18	19	20	21	22	23	24	25	26	27	28	29	30	31	32	34	35

Less risk — More risk

(continued on next page)

Procedure 22-1 ■ Performing the General Survey (continued)

Documentation

- Document BP as right or left arm, and note the patient's position: sitting, standing, or lying.
- Document temperature measurement route: oral, rectal, or tympanic membrane.
- For children, document height and weight on a growth chart.

Go to Chapter 22, **Supplemental Materials: Growth Charts,** on Davis*Plus*.

- If you need more information about documenting, see the form, Graphic Flowsheet, in the Forms section of Chapter 20. Also,

Go to Chapter 18, **Documenting and Reporting,** in Volume 1.

Practice Resources

Centers for Disease Control and Prevention (CDC) (last updated September 13, 2011); CDC (last updated April 27, 2012); National Guideline Clearinghouse (NGC) (2005, revised January 2013); National Heart, Lung, and Blood Institute (n.d.).

Procedure 22-2 ■ Assessing the Skin

➤ For steps to follow in *all* procedures, refer to the Universal Steps for All Procedures found on the inside back cover.

Equipment

- Nonlatex gloves (if exposure to body fluids is a possibility)
- Flexible transparent ruler
- Penlight
- Magnifier
- Pen and record form

Focused History Questions

Ask the patient about the history or presence of any:

- Rashes
- History of allergies
- Areas of skin that have changed color
- Skin lesions
- Skin with rough or unusual texture
- Skin that is always warm or cool, regardless of room temperature

Developmental Modifications for Older Adults

- Assess the level of risk for pressure ulcers. For assessment tools (Braden scale, Norton scale), go to Chapter 35 in this volume.
  As adults age, the subcutaneous tissue layer thins. The dermal layer loses elasticity as a result of changes in collagen fibers; and the strong bond between the epidermal and dermal layers decreases. These changes make the skin prone to breakdown.

➤ When performing the procedure, always identify your patient according to agency policy, using two identifiers, and be attentive to standard precautions, hand hygiene, patient safety and privacy, body mechanics, and documentation.

Procedure Steps

1. **Inspect skin color**, including mucous membranes, tongue, and conjunctiva.
   To assess color changes of exposed and unexposed areas. Color changes and odors may indicate underlying disease and should be fully investigated.
   a. Provide good lighting.
   b. In dark-skinned clients, look for color changes in the conjunctiva or oral mucosa, tongue, lips, nailbeds, palms of the hands, and soles of the feet.
   Skin color varies widely among individuals by age and ethnicity, but in each individual skin color is fairly uniform over his body.▼

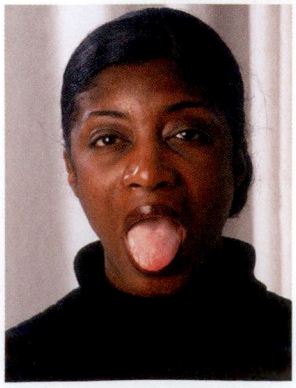

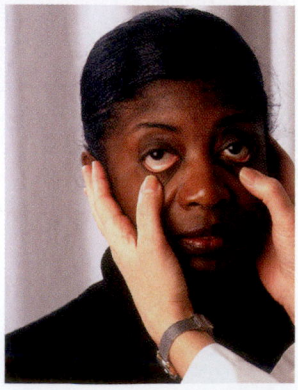

Step 1

Expected and Abnormal Findings

Expected findings: Skin color is uniform, with darker exposed areas. Mucous membranes and conjunctiva are pink and moist. No unusual odors.

Developmental Variations

Newborns—May be jaundiced for a few weeks. Blue-black Mongolian spots and pink-red capillary hemangiomas are common and fade with time.

Older adults—May have thin, translucent skin and wrinkles due to loss of elasticity. Fragile skin is not uncommon among lighter skinned, older adults.

Abnormal findings: Pallor, jaundice, cyanosis, erythema, hyperpigmentation, hypopigmentation. If there are abnormal findings, ask the patient (or someone who knows him well) about the baseline skin color. See the Abnormal Atlas: Skin Color Changes at the end of this chapter for examples of color changes.

c. Note any unusual odors.
d. To assess for cyanosis, be sure to examine the tongue.
Exposure to cold causes the lips to turn blue, but not the tongue. Cyanosis affects the color of the skin, mucous membranes, and tongue.

---

2. Palpate skin for temperature.
a. Wear procedure gloves and discard after examining any open areas of the skin.
b. Use dorsal aspect of hand or fingers.
c. Compare bilaterally.
The dorsa of the hands and the fingers are most sensitive to temperature variations.

Expected findings: Skin is warm; temperature is the same bilaterally.

Abnormal findings: Local area(s) that are warmer or cooler than the rest of the skin; generalized temperature increase or decrease. If the skin is excessively warm, assess for fever. Localized warmth with erythema can indicate an infection. Cool skin might be a sign of compromised circulation or dehydration, particularly in the older adult.

---

3. Palpate skin for turgor. Test an unexposed area, such as the area below the clavicle, inner thigh, sternum, or forehead, by gently pinching up the skin, noting its return when you release it.

Developmental Modifications

Infants—Check skin turgor on the abdomen.

Older adults—Check skin turgor over the sternum or clavicle.▼

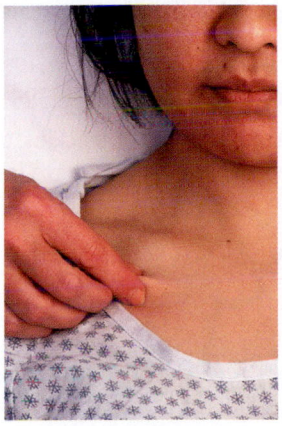

Skin turgor

Expected findings: Skin returns immediately to its original position.

Developmental Variations

Older adults have decreased skin turgor due to decreased elasticity.

Abnormal findings: Decreased or increased turgor. Tenting (decreased turgor): Skin takes several seconds to return to original position.

Decreased turgor or tenting is seen with dehydration or normal aging. It predisposes the patient to skin breakdown.

Increased turgor: Skin tension does not allow the skin to be pinched up.

---

4. Palpate the skin for texture.
Texture varies, depending on the area being assessed and the age of the client.

Expected findings: Skin is smooth and soft. Exposed areas and extensor surfaces (e.g., elbows and knees) are drier and coarser than other areas.

Developmental Variations

Infants and young children—Have smooth skin.

Abnormal findings: Coarse, thick, rough, or dry skin; very smooth, thin, fine-textured, shiny skin

---

(continued on next page)

Procedure 22-2 ■ Assessing the Skin (continued)

5. Palpate skin for moisture/hydration. Use the dorsum of your hand.

Expected findings: Skin is warm and dry.

Developmental Variations

Older adults—Skin may be dry and flaky because of decreased activity of sebaceous and sweat glands.

Adolescents—May have skin that is oilier than normal.

Abnormal findings: Increased moisture (skin feels damp, visible diaphoresis); decreased moisture (skin feels dry)

6. Inspect for edema.

a. Press firmly with your fingertip for 5 seconds over a bony area, such as the tibia.
b. Release your finger, and observe the skin for the reaction.
c. If edema is present, note the location, degree, and type of swelling. For example, if you observe edema in the lower leg, how far up the leg does it extend?

Expected findings: No edema. Normally there will be no evidence of the pressure once you release your finger. If pitting edema is present, you will see a depression in the skin.

Grading System

Trace: Minimal depression with pressure.

+1: 2 mm depression; rapid return of skin to position.

+2: 4 mm depression that disappears in 10–15 seconds.

+3: 6 mm depression that lasts 1–2 minutes. Area appears swollen.

+4: 8 mm depression that persists for 2–3 minutes. Area is grossly edematous.

Abnormal findings: Edema is an abnormal finding.

7. Identify any skin lesions.

a. Inspect and palpate lesions.
b. When you notice bruises, be alert for signs of abuse (see Chapter 9).
c. Ask the client: "Do you have any new moles or other lesions? Has there been any change in existing moles/lesions?"
d. Assess for malignant lesions using ABCDE:
   A (asymmetry)
   B (irregular borders)
   C (color variations)
   D (diameter: 0.5 cm)
   E (elevation).

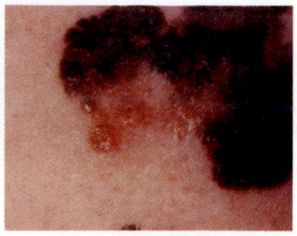

Malignant melanoma

Expected Finding: No lesions are present.

Normal variations include moles, freckles, birthmarks, striae (in pregnant women or clients who have lost much weight), and wrinkles.

Developmental Variations

Newborns—**Milia** (tiny collections of sebum, usually on the face) are common.

Adults—**Acrochordons** (skin tags) may be seen around the neck, axillae, skinfolds, or areas where clothing rubs.

Older adults—Flat beige or brown macules are common on exposed skin areas.

Abnormal findings: See the Abnormal Atlas: Skin Lesions at the end of this chapter. Also see the table Describing Skin Lesions following this procedure.

Adolescents—Acne is a common abnormal finding among adolescents.

Describing Lesions

When you observe a lesion, evaluate and describe the following:

- **Size.** Measure the length, width, and depth of the lesion.
- **Shape and pattern.** Describe the *shape* of individual lesions. If there are clusters or groups, describe the *pattern*. Is it linear or circular? Are the *borders* distinct, or do they run together? Is the border smooth or irregular?
- **Color.** Describe the color of the lesion, and determine whether there is any variation of color within the lesion.
- **Distribution.** Are the lesions distributed over the entire body? Are they confined to a specific region? What parts of the body are affected?
- **Texture.** The texture (e.g., smooth, rough, scaly) of a lesion helps with classification.
- **Surface relationship.** To assess surface relationship, you will need to palpate the lesion. Is it flat, raised, or depressed? Is it firmly attached to the surrounding skin or mobile?
- **Exudate.** Examine the lesion(s) for signs of drainage. Describe the color, appearance, amount, and odor of drainage, if present.
- **Tenderness, pain, or itching.** Press on the lesion, and determine the patient's reaction. Does touching the lesion cause pain or discomfort?

Patient Teaching

Teach the patient the signs and symptoms of skin cancer, the importance of the skin exam, and preventive measures.

Home Care

- Assess the skill level of the caregiver. Instruct the caregiver in the importance of skin assessment and measures to prevent skin breakdown.
- Be alert for lesions (e.g., burns, bruises) that may signal physical abuse. For more signs of abuse, refer to Procedure 9-1.

Documentation

- If lesions are present, describe the history: onset, duration, associated or aggravating factors (e.g., itching), factors that relieve symptoms, treatments that have been used, and responses to treatment.
- Sketch the location of skin lesions on body diagrams, if available (see example below); or sketch a body if necessary. ➤

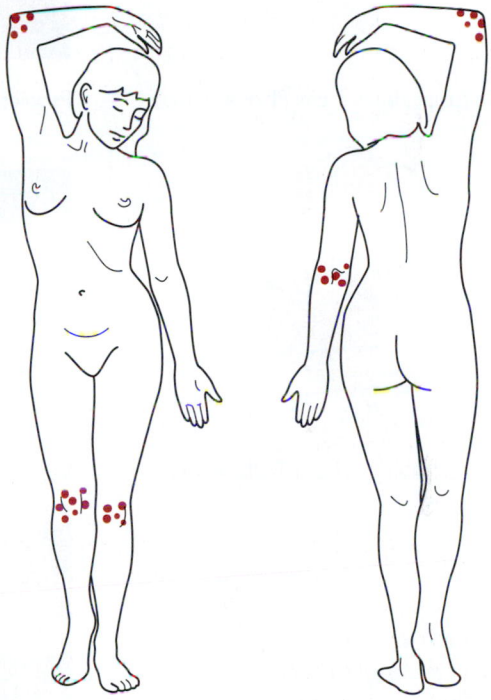

If you need more information about documenting, review Caring for the Nguyens, and

Go to Chapter 22, **Documenting Physical Assessment Findings,** in Volume 1.

(continued on next page)

Procedure 22-2 ■ Assessing the Skin (continued)

Describing Skin Lesions

TYPES		DESCRIPTION
Primary Lesions Macule (nonpalpable, < 1 cm) 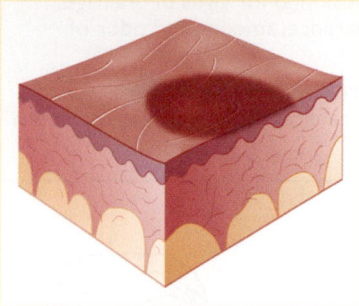	Macule (nonpalpable, < 1 cm) 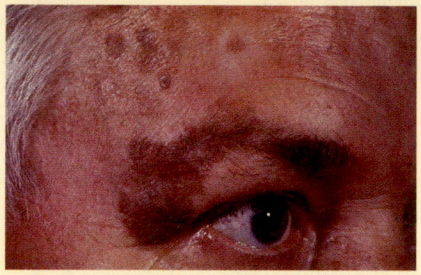	Flat and colored. Examples: freckle, petechiae, birthmark, Mongolian spot
Papule (palpable) < 1 cm; Plaque > 1 cm 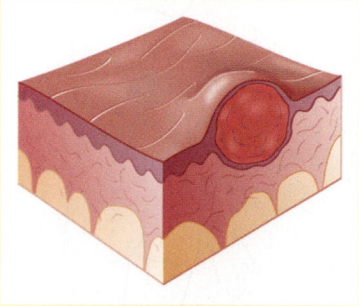	Papules (seborrheic keratosis) 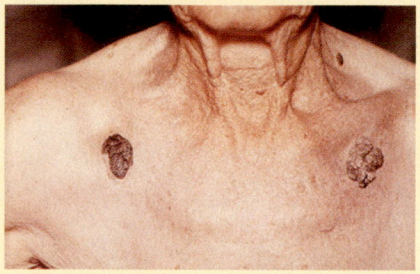	Elevated and raised, but superficial Examples: mole, psoriasis
Vesicle (palpable), < 1 cm; Bulla, > 1 cm 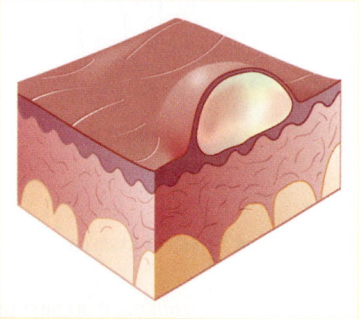	Vesicles (blisters) 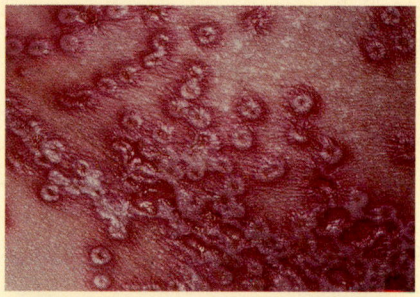 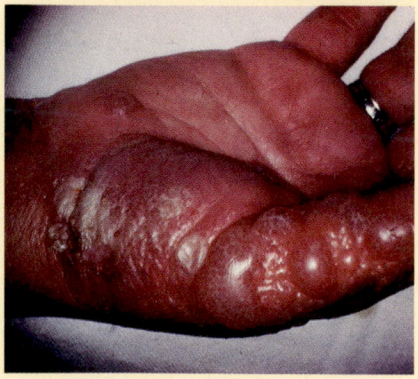	Elevated and filled with serous fluid. Examples: blister, herpes simplex

Describing Skin Lesions—cont'd

TYPES		DESCRIPTION
Cyst (palpable), < 2 cm 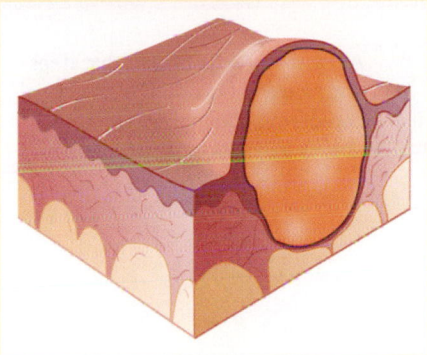	Keratogenous cyst 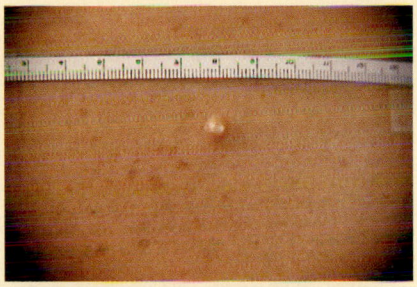	Palpable, fluid-filled, and encapsulated. If not fluid-filled, called a nodule
Pustule (palpable) 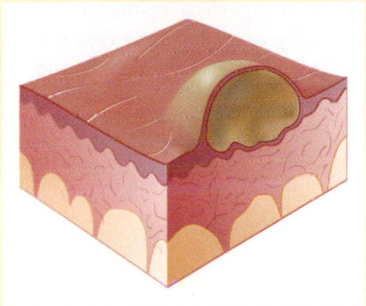	Pustules (acne) 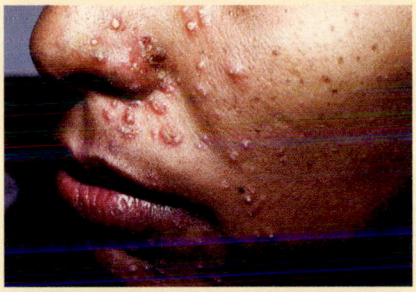	Elevated and filled with pus. Examples: acne, folliculitis, impetigo
	Nodule (palpable) 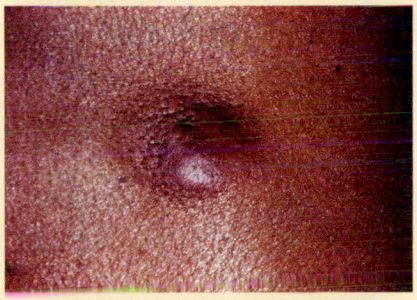	Elevated, solid, and firm, with depth into dermis. Examples: wart, lipoma (fatty cyst)
Wheal 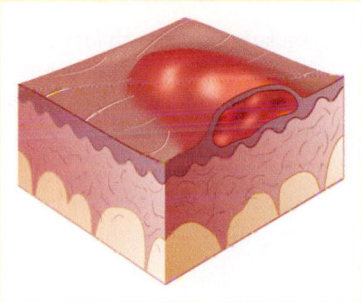	Hive 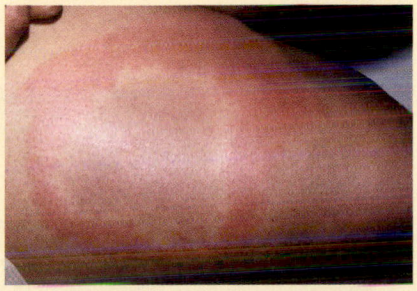	Elevated, superficial, with localized edema. Examples: insect bites, hives

(continued on next page)

Procedure 22-2 ■ Assessing the Skin (continued)

Describing Skin Lesions—cont'd		
TYPES		**DESCRIPTION**
Secondary Lesions Excoriation	Excoriation from pruritus	Abrasion or loss of skin that does not extend beyond the superficial epidermis. Examples: scratches, stasis dermatitis, atopic dermatitis
Erosion	Erosions	Loss of superficial epidermis, usually secondary to rupture of a blister. Examples: abrasions and impetigo
Fissure	Cheilitis	Linear break in the skin ("crack"); may extend to the dermis. Examples: athlete's foot, cheilitis
Ulcer	Stasis ulcer	Irregularly shaped with loss of tissue. Graded based on depth and tissue involvement. Examples: pressure ulcers, stasis ulcers

Describing Skin Lesions—cont'd

TYPES		DESCRIPTION
Crust 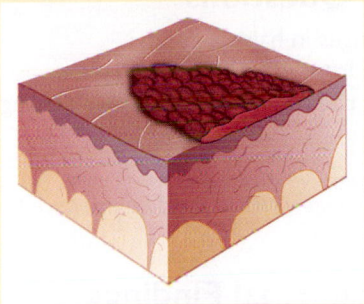	Crust 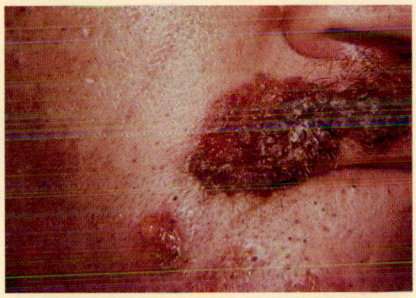	Elevated, rough texture with dried exudate. Examples: impetigo, herpes simplex
Scales 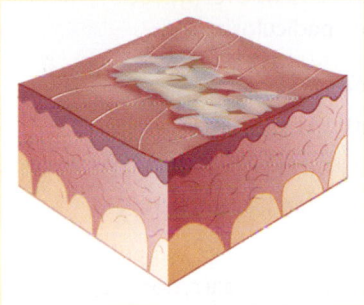	Psoriasis 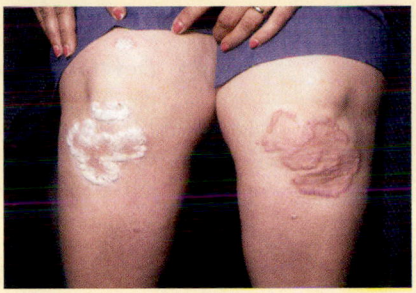	White to tan flaking, dead skin cells; may be adherent or loose. Examples: psoriasis and dandruff
Scar 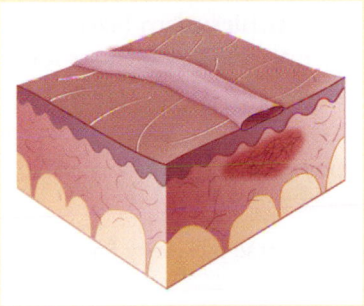		Fibrous tissue at site of injury, trauma, or surgery. Examples: surgical site, trauma site
Keloid 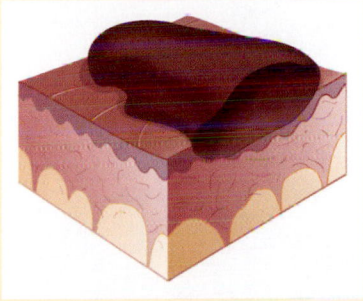	Keloids 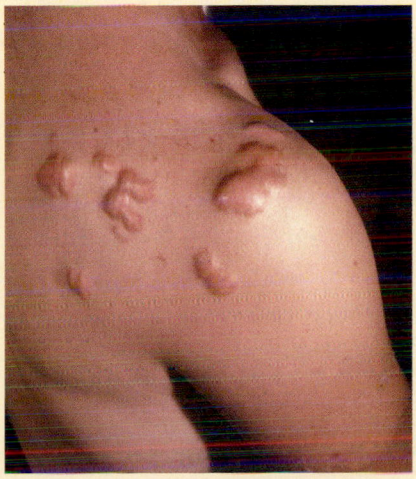	Raised and irregular scar due to excess collagen formation. Examples: surgical scars, ear piercing

Practice Resources

Linton, C. P. (2011); Reddy, M. (2008).

Procedure 22-3 ■ Assessing the Hair

➤ For steps to follow in *all* procedures, refer to the Universal Steps for All Procedures found on the inside back cover.

Equipment

- Nonlatex procedure gloves (if exposure to body fluids is a possibility)
- Pen and record form

Focused History Questions

- Have you had any changes in hair texture?
- Have you had any hair loss?
- Do you use dyes or chemical treatments for curling or straightening?

➤ When performing the procedure, always identify your patient according to agency policy, using two identifiers, and be attentive to standard precautions, hand hygiene, patient safety and privacy, body mechanics, and documentation.

Procedure Steps

Expected and Abnormal Findings

1. **Inspect the hair and scalp.** Check the color, quantity, and distribution of the hair and the condition of the scalp. Note the presence of lesions or pediculosis.
   Sex, genetics, and age affect hair distribution on the head, legs extremities, pubis, and axillae. With aging, melanocyte function declines and sebaceous gland function decreases.

Expected findings: The hair is evenly distributed on the scalp, and fine body hair is present over the body. The hair is clean and free of debris or pediculosis.

Developmental Variations

Infants—May have very little scalp hair.

Adolescents—May have oily hair. Puberty marks the onset of pubic hair growth and increased hair growth.

Older adults—Scalp, axillary, leg, and pubic hair may be dry and thin; hair of the ears, nostrils, and eyebrows may become coarse.

Abnormal findings: Generalized hair loss not attributed to genetics or aging; patchy hair loss; **hirsutism** (excess facial or trunk hair). See the Abnormal Atlas at the end of this chapter.

2. **Palpate the texture of the hair.**

Expected findings: Hair texture varies (fine, medium, coarse) depending on genetics and treatments.

Abnormal findings: Very dry, coarse hair; very fine, silky hair

3. **Palpate the scalp for mobility and tenderness.**

Expected findings: Scalp is smooth, firm, symmetrical, nontender, and without lesions.

Abnormal findings: Tenderness, lesions.

Patient Teaching

If indicated, teach the patient to check for head lice, and provide preventive measures.

Go to Chapter 22, **Documenting Physical Assessment Findings,** in Volume 1.

Documentation

If you need more information about documenting, review Documentation of Physical Assessment Findings for Nam Nguyen, in Volume 1.

Procedure 22-4 ■ Assessing the Nails

➤ For steps to follow in *all* procedures, refer to the Universal Steps for All Procedures found on the inside back cover.

Equipment

- Nonlatex gloves (if exposure to body fluids is a possibility)
- Pen and record form

Focused History Questions

- Have you had any recent changes in the way your nails grow or look?
- Have you had any recent trauma to your nails?
- Do you use acrylic nails?
- Do you have any medical problems, such as peripheral vascular disease or diabetes?

➤ When performing the procedure, always identify your patient according to agency policy, using two identifiers, and be attentive to standard precautions, hand hygiene, patient safety and privacy, body mechanics, and documentation.

Procedure Steps

1. **Inspect nails.**
   - Check nails for color, condition, texture, and shape.
   - Examine nails on both hands and feet. However, for efficiency you may defer examination of the toenails until the assessment of peripheral circulation. ▼

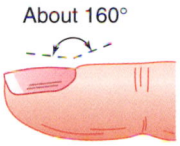

Expected and Abnormal Findings

Expected findings: Healthy nailbeds are level, firm, and similar to the color of the skin. The shape is convex, with a nail plate angle of about 160°.

Developmental Variations

Newborns—Have very thin nails.

Children—May bite their nails. Most children outgrow this habit.

Older adults—Nails grow more slowly, become thicker, and tend to split.

Abnormal findings: Yellow, blue, or black discoloration. White spots may indicate zinc deficiency. Spoon-shaped (concave) nails are associated with iron deficiency. See the Abnormal Atlas: Nail Appearance at the end of this chapter.

2. **Inspect and palpate for texture.**
   Grooves or lines in the nails provide information about nutrition and health problems.

Expected findings: Nails are smooth and uniform in texture.

Abnormal findings: Thickened, brittle, or soft nails; nails with deep vertical grooves

(continued on next page)

Procedure 22-4 ■ Assessing the Nails (continued)

3. **Assess capillary refill.** Briefly press the tip of the nail with firm, steady pressure; then release and observe for changes in color.
   This test assesses circulatory adequacy rather than the nails themselves. However, circulatory insufficiency affects the nails and nailbeds. It is convenient to perform the assessment at this point in the exam.

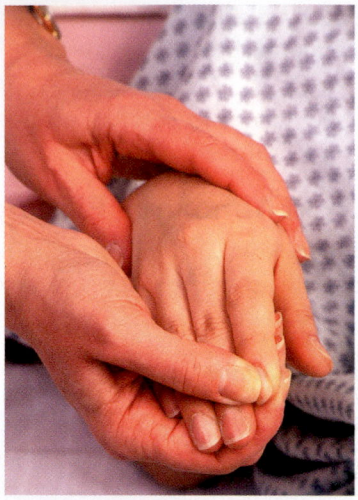

Step 3

Expected findings: Normal capillary refill is < 2 to 3 seconds.

Developmental Variations

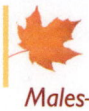

Older adults—Capillary refill time (CRT) is slower.

Males—CRT faster than in women

Environment—CRT is slower in a cool environment.

Abnormal findings: Delayed capillary refill.

Documentation

If you need more information about documenting

Go to Chapter 22, **Documenting Physical Assessment Findings,** in Volume 1.

Practice Resources

Anderson, B., Kelly, A. M., Kerr, D., et al. (2008); Linton, C. P. (2012).

Procedure 22-5 ■ Assessing the Head and Face

➤ For steps to follow in *all* procedures, refer to the Universal Steps for All Procedures found on the inside back cover.

Equipment

- Nonlatex gloves (if exposure to body fluids is a possibility)
- Penlight (to transilluminate the sinuses)
- Pen and record form

Positioning

The client should be sitting, if possible.

Focused History Questions

- Have you had any recent headaches?
- Have you ever had a head injury or loss of consciousness?
- Have you ever had a seizure?
- Do you have jaw or facial pain?

➤ When performing the procedure, always identify your patient according to agency policy, using two identifiers, and be attentive to standard precautions, hand hygiene, patient safety and privacy, body mechanics, and documentation.

Procedure Steps

1. **Inspect the head.** Check for size, shape, symmetry, and position.

Developmental Modifications

- *Newborns and infants*—Assess and transilluminate fontanels, and measure head circumference.

Expected and Abnormal Findings

Expected findings: There is wide variation in head size and shape, although the shape should be symmetrical and rounded. The head should be erect, midline, and proportional to the body size based on age.

Developmental Variations

Newborns and infants—Cranial bones are not fused at birth, and head shape may reflect normal pressure or trauma during vaginal birth for several weeks. The anterior fontanel ("soft spot") fuses at about 18 months; the posterior, at about 8 weeks. Infants normally cannot hold their head up until about 6 months of age.

Abnormal findings: Larger or smaller than expected size for age, asymmetry of skull

---

2. **Inspect the face.** Note the client's facial expression. Ask yourself,
   - Are the facial features symmetrical?
   - Are there any abnormal facial movements?
   - Are there any visible lesions of abnormal hair distribution?

Helpful hint: Look for symmetry in the palpebral fissures and the nasolabial folds. ▼

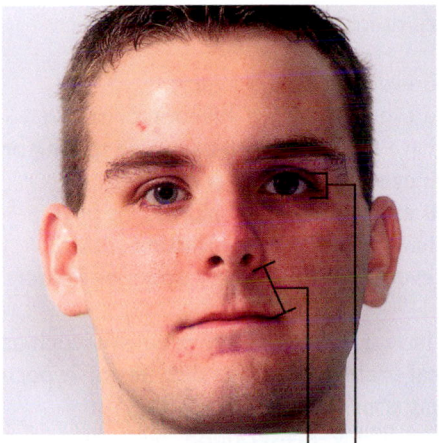

Step 2

Expected findings: Facial expression is appropriate for the situation. No visible lesions. Facial features and movement are symmetrical.

Abnormal findings: Facial appearance inconsistent with sex, age, or racial/ethnic group; asymmetry of facial features or facial movement. ▼

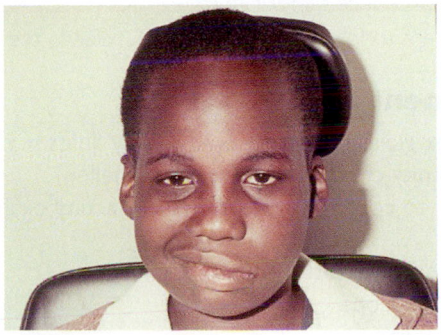

Bell's Palsy

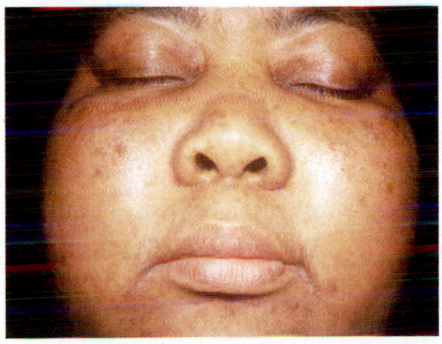

Cushing's Syndrome

---

3. **Palpate the head.** Check for masses, tenderness, and scalp mobility.

Developmental Modifications

Newborns and infants—Palpate anterior and posterior fontanels.

Expected findings: The head should be relatively smooth, with no tenderness or lesions.

Abnormal findings: Contour abnormalities (e.g., indentations, "bumps")

(continued on next page)

Procedure 22-5 ■ Assessing the Head and Face (continued)

4. **Palpate the face for symmetry, tenderness,** muscle tone, and temporomandibular joint function. ▼

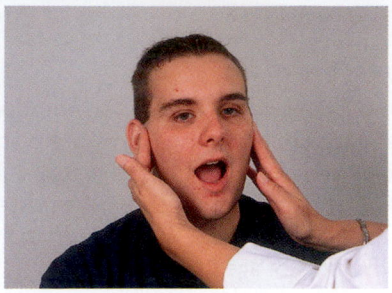

Palpating the TMJ

Expected findings: Smooth, symmetrical movement with no pain, crepitus, or clicking of the jaw

Abnormal findings: Irregular or uneven movement of the jaw; pain or popping with movement

Documentation

- If you need more information about documenting, review Documentation of Physical Assessment Findings for Nam Nguyen,

Go to Chapter 22, **Documenting Physical Assessment Findings,** in Volume 1.

Procedure 22-6 ■ Assessing the Eyes

➤ For steps to follow in *all* procedures, refer to the Universal Steps for All Procedures found on the inside back cover.

Equipment

- Nonlatex gloves—if exposure to body fluids is a possibility
- Visual acuity chart with color bars (Snellen)
- A card—to cover one eye during the acuity exam
- Penlight
- Cotton ball and cotton-tipped applicator
- Ophthalmoscope
- Pen and form

Positioning

The client should be sitting, if possible.

Focused History Questions

- Have you noticed any changes in your vision?
- Do you wear glasses or contact lenses?
- Have you ever had an eye injury?
- Have you ever had an eye infection or stye?
- Do you have problems with excessive tearing or dry eyes?
- Have you ever had eye surgery?
- Have you ever experienced blurred vision?
- Do you have difficulty with nighttime vision?
- Do you ever see halos of light, spots or floaters, or flashes of light?
- Do you have a history of eye problems, such as glaucoma, or medical problems, such as diabetes or hypertension?
- When was your last eye exam?
- Do you use any prescription or over-the-counter eye medications?

➤ When performing the procedure, always identify your patient according to agency policy, using two identifiers, and be attentive to standard precautions, hand hygiene, patient safety and privacy, body mechanics, and documentation.

Procedure Steps

1. **Test distance vision.**
   - Depending on patient's age and literacy level, use the Snellen standard eye chart or Snellen E chart (for those who cannot read). Picture charts are available for preschoolers.
   - If the client wears corrective lenses, they should be worn during a test.
     a. Have the patient sit or stand 6 m (20 ft.) from the chart. With a card, cover the eye not being tested;

Expected and Abnormal Findings

Expected findings: Expect 20/20 vision in the right eye, left eye, and both eyes. The top number of the fraction indicates the distance the person was standing from the chart; the bottom number is the distance from which a person with normal vision would be able to read the chart.

Developmental Variations

Children—Distance vision does not reach 20/20 until around 6 or 7 years of age.

ask the patient to read the smallest line of print that he can distinguish. Consider a line to be read correctly if the client makes no more than two mistakes in that line.

b. Test the opposite eye.
c. Test both eyes together.
d. At the end of each line of the Snellen chart is a fraction—the top line is 20/200. After each test, record the resulting fraction: the number at the end of the smallest line the patient could read with no more than two errors.

Middle adults—At about middle age, the lens of the eye begins to lose some ability to accommodate to near objects.

Abnormal findings: A smaller fraction (e.g., 20/100) indicates diminished distant vision or myopia. A larger fraction (e.g., 20/15) indicates diminished near vision, called hyperopia.

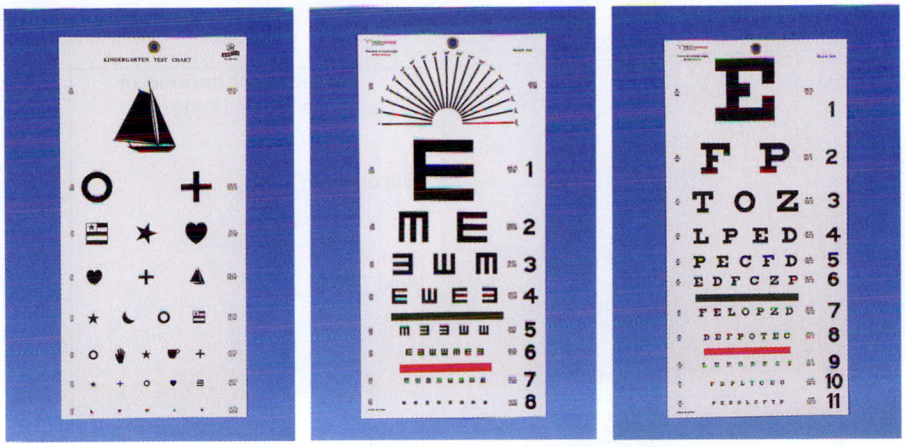

Preliterate chart Snellen E chart Snellen standard chart

2. Test near vision. Test the client's ability to read newsprint at a distance of 35.5 cm (14 in.) from the eyes. Use print-sized pictures if the patient is unable to read.

Expected findings: The client reads newsprint at a distance of 35.5 cm (14 in.).

Abnormal findings: The need to hold the print at a greater distance indicates hyperopia or presbyopia.

3. Test color vision.

a. Have the patient differentiate patterns of colors on color cards or identify the color bars on the Snellen eye chart.
b. Inability to distinguish colors requires a thorough evaluation using the Ishihara cards to determine the scope of the color deficit.

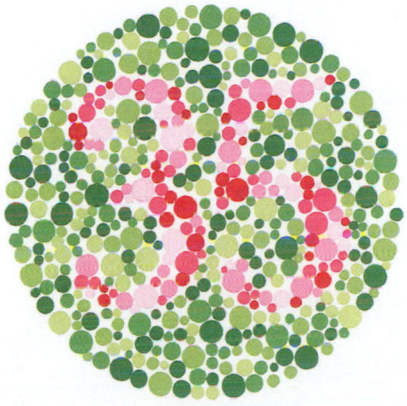

Ishihara card

Expected findings: Color vision is intact.

Developmental Variations

Older adults—Experience some decline in color vision, especially in the ability to see purples and pastels.

Abnormal findings: Inability to distinguish colors

(continued on next page)

Procedure 22-6 ■ Assessing the Eyes (continued)

4. Test peripheral vision.

a. Seat the client 60–90 cm (2–3 ft) from you.

b. Have client cover one eye and fix the gaze straight ahead while you bring an object in from the periphery to the center of the visual fields. Be sure to begin by holding the object well outside the range of normal peripheral vision. Instruct the client to identify when the object becomes visible.

c. Repeat this in each of the four visual fields, moving clockwise.

Expected findings: Expect no deficits in the visual fields.

Abnormal findings: Loss of peripheral vision. Report gross deficits to an ophthalmologist for further assessment.

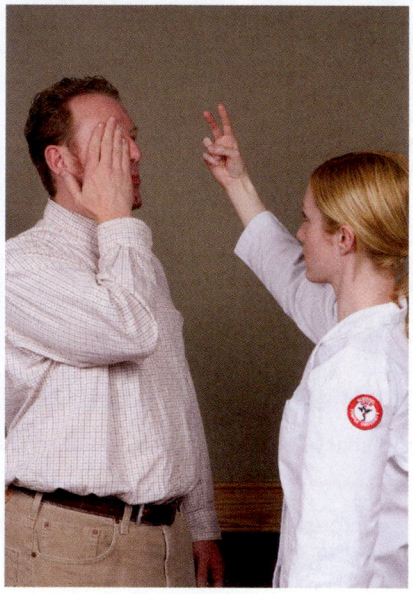

Step 4

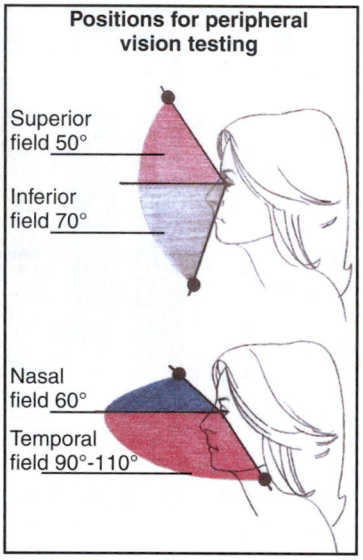

Testing peripheral vision.

5. Assess extraocular movements.

a. Inspect the eyes for parallel alignment.

b. Test the corneal light reflex by shining a penlight at the bridge of the nose. Note where the light reflects on the cornea of each eye.

a. **Expected findings:** The eyes should be in parallel alignment.

b. **Expected findings:** Corneal light reflex appears at the same position in each eye.

Abnormal findings: An asymmetrical corneal light reflex may indicate weak extraocular muscles or strabismus.

c. Test the six cardinal fields of gaze. Stand in front of the patient, and have the patient follow an object through the six cardinal fields without moving his head.

c. **Expected findings:** The eyes move through all six gaze positions.

Abnormal findings: Inability to move through all gaze positions

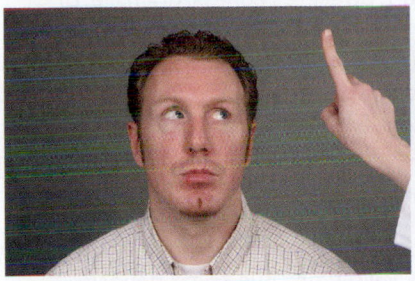

Up left

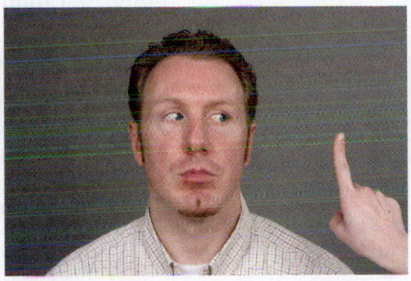

Side left

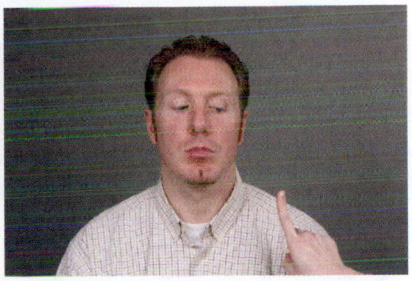

Down left

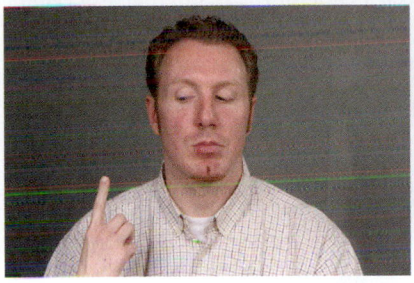

Down right

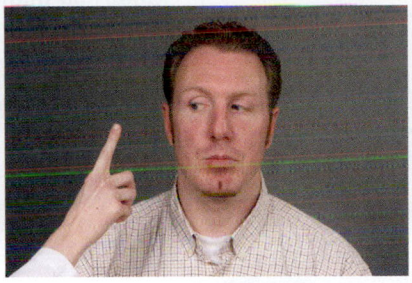

Side right

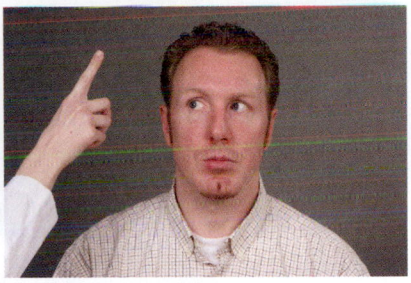

Up right

d. Perform the cover/uncover test. Cover one eye and have the patient gaze at a distant object. Uncover the eye. Repeat on the opposite side.

d. **Expected findings:** The gaze should be steady when the eye is covered and uncovered.

Abnormal findings: A shift in gaze indicates weak eye muscles.

---

6. Inspect the external structures.

a. **General appearance.** Check the color and alignment of the eyes.

a. **Expected findings:** Eyes clear, bright, and in parallel alignment.

Developmental Variations

Older adults—A decrease in periorbital fat may give the eyeballs a sunken appearance.

Abnormal findings: Glazed eyes may indicate a febrile state.

b. **Inspect the eyelids.** Note the presence of any lesions, edema, or lid lag. Refer to Eyes: Abnormal Lesions, at the end of this chapter.

b. **Expected findings:** No lesions present; lids move freely. Upper eyelid covers half of the upper iris.

Developmental Variations

Older adults—The lower lids may sag; skinfolds are prominent in the upper lids.

Abnormal findings: Asymmetry of lids may result from CN III damage or from a stroke. Lesions may be benign (e.g., a stye) or pathological (e.g., basal cell carcinoma).

c. **Inspect the eyelashes.** Note symmetry and distribution.

c. **Expected findings:** Eyelashes are evenly distributed and curve outward. No crustations or infestations are present.

Abnormal findings: Inflammation of the eyelids, which may be caused by infection; inverted eyelashes (entropion); everted eyelashes (ectropion); visible sclera between the iris and upper lid

(continued on next page)

Procedure 22-6 ■ Assessing the Eyes (continued)

d. **Inspect the lacrimal ducts and glands.** Note any edema, excessive tearing, or drainage.

d. **Expected findings:** No periorbital edema or lesions are present. No drainage.

Abnormal findings: Swelling, redness, drainage, or tenderness.

e. **Inspect the conjunctivae.** Note the color, moisture, and contour of the conjunctivae.
   (1) The palpebral conjunctivae cover the lids. To assess, have the patient look up as you place a cotton-tipped applicator on the upper lid, gently grasp the upper lid and lashes, and evert the lid over the cotton-tipped applicator.
   (2) The bulbar conjunctiva covers the eyeball. To assess, pull the lower lid down. ▼

e. **Expected findings:** The palpebral conjunctivae are smooth, glistening, and peach in color. Minimal blood vessels are present. The bulbar conjunctivae are clear with few underlying blood vessels and white sclera visible.

Developmental Variations

Older adults—The conjunctivae may be pale or have a slightly yellow tint due to fat deposits.

Abnormal findings: Pallor, dryness, edema; pterygium; subconjunctival hemorrhage

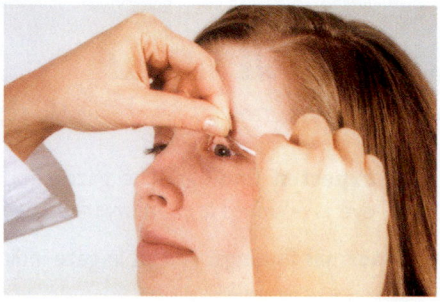

Examining the palpebral conjunctiva

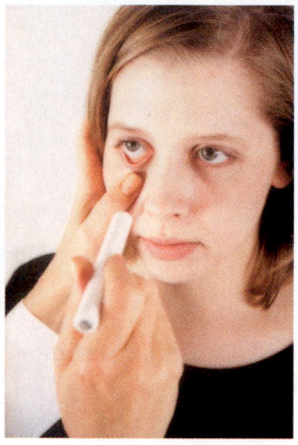

Examining the bulbar conjunctiva

f. **Inspect the sclera.** Note the color of the sclera and whether lesions are present.

f. **Expected findings:** The sclera should be smooth, white, and glistening. Dark-skinned patients may have a yellowish cast to the peripheral sclera or small brown spots more centrally.

Abnormal findings: Yellow (icteric) sclera

g. **Inspect the cornea and lens.** As the client looks straight ahead, shine a penlight at an angle to the eye, and move it across the corneal surface. Note the color and whether any lesions are present.

g. **Expected findings:** The cornea and lens are clear, smooth, and glistening.

Developmental Variations

Older adults—**Arcus senilis** (white, gray, or blue opaque ring in the corneal margin) is a normal variant.

Abnormal findings: Lens opacities (cataracts); roughness or irregularity of the cornea

h. **Test the corneal reflex.** Touch the cornea with a wisp of sterile cotton, or use a needleless syringe to shoot a small amount of air over the cornea.

Note: This is not routinely performed on conscious patients. A conscious person can blink intentionally, so there is no need. In addition, there is a slight risk of corneal abrasion from cotton.

h. **Expected findings:** Blink reflex is prompt.

Abnormal findings: Failure to blink may result from neurosensory deficits.

i. **Inspect the iris and pupils.** Note the color, size, shape, and symmetry.

i. **Expected findings:** The iris is blue, green, brown, or a combination of these colors; its shape is circular. The pupils are round and of equal size. Unequal pupils (anisocoria) can be a normal variation if the difference is less than 0.5 mm.

Developmental Variations

Older adults—Pigment degeneration may cause the iris to be pale with brownish discolorations.

Abnormal findings: Damage to one eye may cause the iris to be a different color. Absence of part or all of the iris is a congenital problem. Unequal pupils may result from CN III damage, brain herniation, or increased intracranial pressure.

j. **Test pupillary reaction.** In a dimly lighted room, have the patient look straight ahead. Bring a penlight in from the side, and shine the light onto one eye. Note the reaction, equality, and speed of response of both eyes. For example, when you shine a light onto the right eye, the right pupil reaction is direct; the left eye is consensual. Repeat the test on the opposite eye.

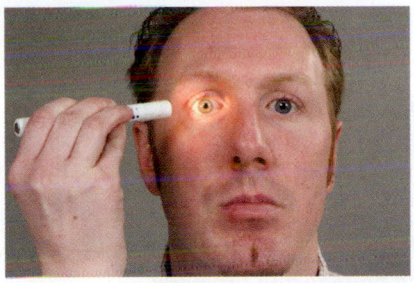

Testing pupillary reaction to light

j. **Expected findings:** Normal direct and consensual response to light is brisk, with equal constriction of both pupils.

Developmental Variations

Older adults—Pupil reaction may be slower but should be symmetrical.

Abnormal findings: Sluggish or fixed pupils may result from CN II damage or brain injury. Absence of consensual response may result from nerve compression or anoxia.

k. **Test pupil accommodation.** Have the patient look straight ahead and focus on an object about 30 cm (12 in.) from his face. Slowly bring the object in toward the patient's eyes. Note pupil size and location.

k. **Expected findings:** The pupils constrict and the eyes cross as a person attempts to focus on a near object.

Developmental Variations

Older adults—Accommodation may be slow.

Abnormal findings: One or both pupils fail to accommodate, or they accommodate slowly.

l. **Inspect the anterior chamber.** Shine a penlight across the eye from the side as the patient looks straight ahead. Observe color, size, shape, and symmetry.

l. **Expected findings:** The chamber should be clear and symmetrically curved.

Abnormal findings: Blood or pus in the chamber. Also see the Abnormal Atlas: Eyes at the end of this chapter.

(continued on next page)

Procedure 22-6 ■ Assessing the Eyes (continued)

7. Palpate the external structures.

a. Gently palpate the globe (eyeball) with your fingertips on the upper lids over the sclera. Note the consistency and any tenderness.

b. Palpate the lacrimal glands and ducts by palpating below the eyebrow and below the inner canthus of the eye. Note tenderness and excessive tearing or discharge.

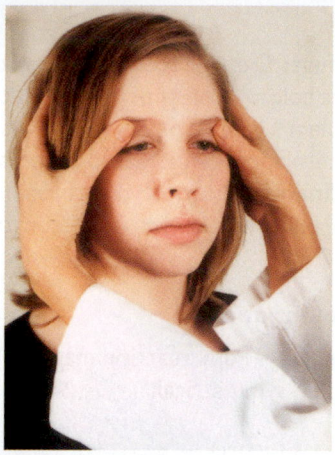

7. Expected findings: The globe is firm and nontender. Lacrimal glands are nonpalpable; no tenderness is present.

Abnormal findings: Firm or tender globe; swelling and tenderness over the lacrimal glands. Also,

Go to the Abnormal Atlas at the end of this chapter.

8. Assess the internal structures via ophthalmoscopy. This is an advanced physical assessment technique.

a. Darken the room.

b. Stand about 1 foot from the patient at a 15° lateral angle.

c. Dial the lens wheel to zero with your index finger. Hold the ophthalmoscope to your brow.

d. Have the patient look straight ahead while you shine the light on one pupil and identify the red light reflex.

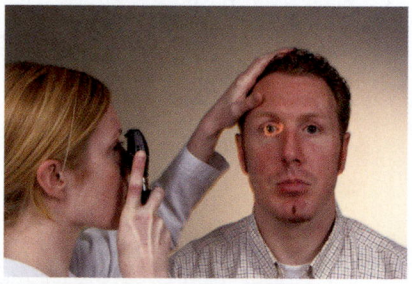

Checking red reflex

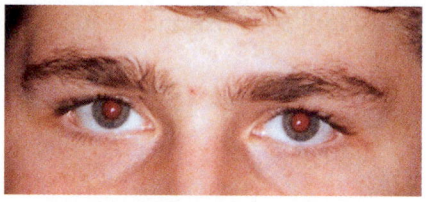

Red reflex over pupil area

Expected findings: A positive red light reflex. On internal examination, the optic disk is round with sharp margins. There are no opacities and the cup to disk ratio is 1:2. The disk is yellow with a white cup.

Abnormal findings: Any findings not consistent with the above should be reported promptly.

e. Once you identify the red light reflex, move in closer to within a few inches of the eye and observe the internal structures of the eye. Adjust the lens wheel to focus as needed. Use your right eye to examine the patient's right eye, and your left eye to examine the patient's left eye.

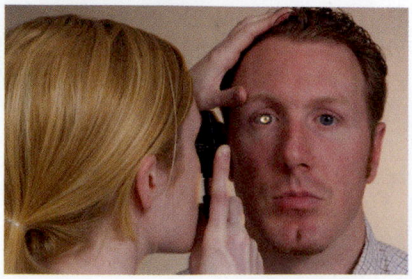

Examining internal structures of the eye

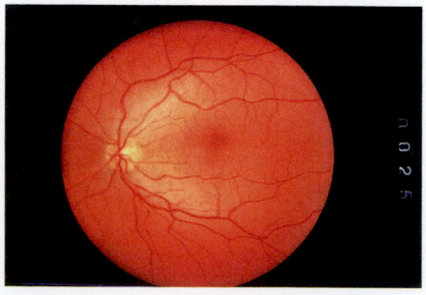

Normal fundus

f. Repeat for the opposite eye.

Patient Teaching

Teach the patient the importance of routine eye examinations.

Documentation

If you need more information about documenting, review

Documenting Physical Assessment Findings, in Volume 1.

Procedure 22-7 ■ Assessing the Ears and Hearing

➤ For steps to follow in *all* procedures, refer to the Universal Steps for All Procedures found on the inside back cover.

Equipment

- Nonlatex gloves (if exposure to body fluids is a possibility)
- Tuning fork
- Watch
- Otoscope with pneumatic tube
- Pen and record form

Positioning

Have the patient seated, if possible.

Focused History Questions

- Do you have any hearing problems?
- Have you ever had ringing in your ears?
- Have you had any changes in your hearing?
- Do you have any ear drainage? If yes, how much and what color?
- Do you have any ear pain?
- Do you have any balance problems, dizziness, or vertigo?
- Do you have a history of head trauma?
- Are you exposed to noise pollution at work or in your home environment?

➤ When performing the procedure, always identify your patient according to agency policy, using two identifiers, and be attentive to standard precautions, hand hygiene, patient safety and privacy, body mechanics, and documentation.

Procedure Steps

1. **Inspect the external ear.**
   a. Check the placement and angle of attachment of the ear. ▼

Expected and Abnormal Findings

a. **Expected Findings:** The normal angle of attachment is 10°.

Abnormal findings: High or low placement of the ear may be a sign of hearing deficit or genetic problems.

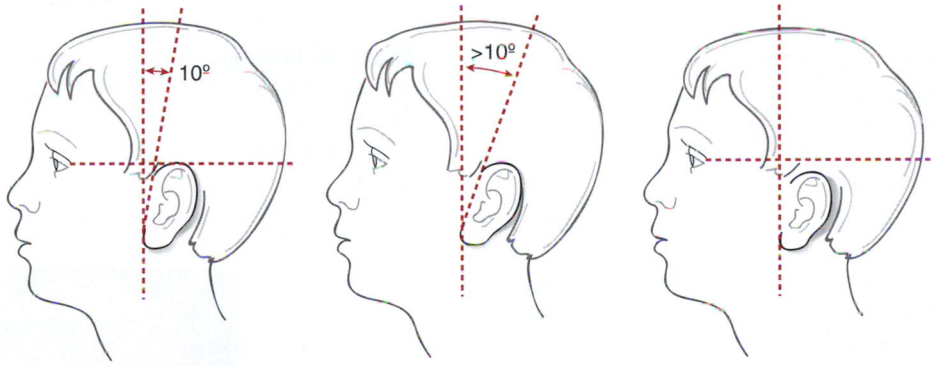

Normal ear attachment — Deviated alignment — Low-set ear attachment

(continued on next page)

Procedure 22-7 ■ Assessing the Ears and Hearing (continued)

b. Note the shape, size, and symmetry of the ears.

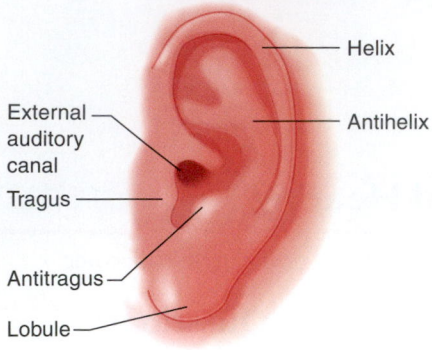

b. **Expected findings:** The helix, antihelix, antitragus, tragus, and lobule are present. The ears are 4–10 cm in length and symmetrical in size and shape.

Developmental Variations

Older adults—The ear changes shape as the lobe elongates.

Abnormal findings: Absence of any of the landmarks may indicate a hearing deficit. Ears that are <4 cm long or >10 cm long may indicate a genetic disorder.

c. Observe the color of the ear.

c. **Expected findings:** Color is consistent with skin color.

Abnormal findings: Redness may indicate inflammation or infection.

d. Observe the condition of the skin; observe for drainage and visible lesions.

d. **Expected findings:** Skin is intact with no drainage or lesions. Piercings may be present.

Developmental Variations

Older adults—May have coarse hair on the helix, antihelix, and tragus; skin may be dry.

Abnormal findings: Bloody or purulent drainage; lesions. The ears are a common location for skin cancer.

---

2. Palpate the external structures of the ear. Note the consistency of the skin, the presence of lesions, and any signs of tenderness.

Expected findings: Skin is soft, pliable, and nontender. No nodules or lesions are present.

Abnormal findings: Tenderness is often associated with infection.

---

3. Perform an otoscopic exam.

a. This is an advanced physical assessment technique.
b. Use a speculum with the largest diameter and shortest length that the ear canal can accommodate. 4 mm is a common size for adults.
c. Have the patient tilt his head to the side not being examined.
d. For adults, grasp the pinna and gently pull upward and back. For a child, position the pinna down and back. *Positions the ear canal with more direct alignment, allowing for improved visualization.*

Expected findings: The ear canal is light in color and patent, with a small amount of yellow cerumen (color may vary). TM is shiny and pearly gray with a cone of reflective light on the nasal aspect that would be 7 o'clock in the left ear and 5 o'clock in the right ear. Bony landmarks are visible. The TM is mobile. No bulging or retraction of the TM. ▼

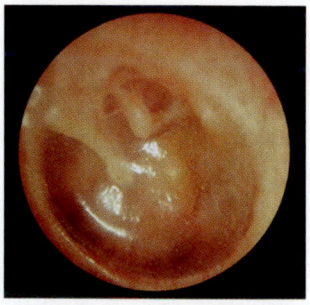

Normal fundus

e. Insert the speculum no further than halfway into the ear canal. As you advance the speculum, examine the canal for redness, open areas, drainage, foreign objects, and so on.

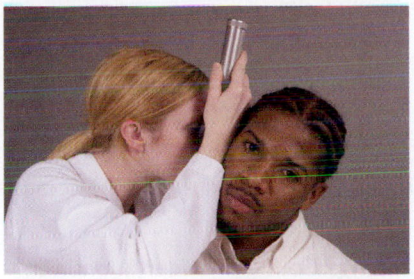

Otoscope insertion with handle up

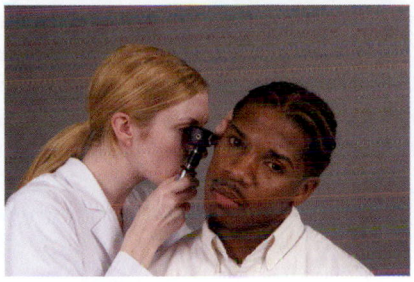

Otoscope insertion with handle down

f. Look through the magnifying lens.
   (1) Observe the ear canal.
   (2) Observe the tympanic membrane.

g. Test the mobility of the tympanic membrane by using the otoscope's pneumatic tube to gently "puff" air into the external ear canal while observing movement of the cone of light.

NOTE: The ears are mirror images, with the cone of light at 7 o'clock in the left ear and 5 o'clock in the right ear.

Developmental Modifications

Children—Many young children fear the otoscopic examination. Demonstrating the procedure on a parent or a doll may relieve their anxiety.

h. Carefully remove the otoscope from the ear canal, being careful not to traumatize the delicate tissue.

Developmental Variations

Older adults—May have dry ear wax. The TM is translucent, and the light reflex may be diminished.

Abnormal findings: Excessive wax may occlude the canal. TM that is red, with a distorted light reflex, suggests otitis media. A change in the position or shape of the cone of light reflex indicates an imbalance in middle ear pressure.

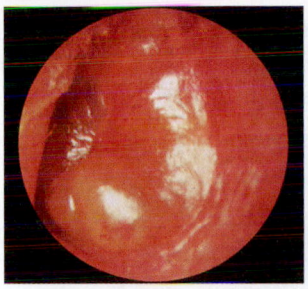

Otitis media

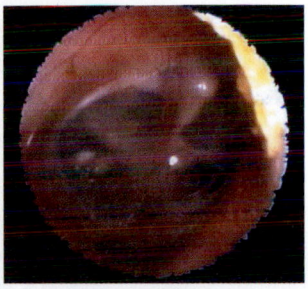

Perforated TM

4. Test gross hearing.

a. Stand 1–2 ft behind the patient. Have the patient cover one ear as you whisper some words. Repeat on the other side. Have the patient repeat the words she heard. *A test of hearing also indicates cranial nerve XIII is intact.*

b. Have the patient occlude one ear. Hold a ticking watch next to the patient's unobstructed ear. Slowly move it away until the patient says she can no longer hear the sound. Repeat for the opposite ear.

Expected Findings: The patient is able to hear you whisper on both sides. The patient hears the watch at a distance of about 12 to 13 cm (5 in.).

Developmental Variations

Older adults—Often have a generalized loss of hearing. It first occurs in the high-frequency sounds (*f, s, sh,* and *ph*) and then progresses to include all frequencies.

(continued on next page)

Procedure 22-7 ■ Assessing the Ears and Hearing (continued)

Developmental Modifications

Infants—For infants younger than 3 months of age, loudly clap your hands behind the infant and observe whether he startles. After 3 months of age, the infant should turn his head or eyes toward a sound, for example, when the parent stands behind the infant and calls his name.

Abnormal findings: Problems with the whisper test indicate low-tone hearing loss. Problems with the watch-tick test indicate a high-pitch deficit.

5. **Perform the Weber test.** Place a vibrating tuning fork on top of the patient's head. Ask the patient whether the sound is the same in both ears or louder in one ear. ▼

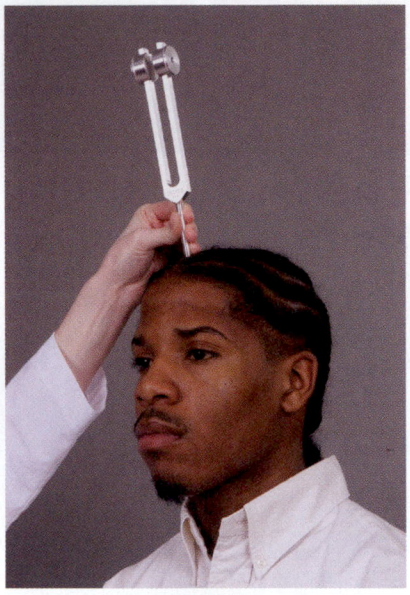

Weber test

Expected findings: The patient hears the sound equally in both ears.

Abnormal findings: Sound is louder in one ear.

- If there is a conductive hearing loss, the vibration will be louder in the impaired ear. Conductive hearing loss may be caused by external or middle ear problems, such as infection, blockage of the canal by cerumen, or trauma to the TM.
- If there is a sensorineural hearing loss, the sound will be louder in the unaffected ear. Sensorineural loss may result from inner ear problems or from some medications.

6. **If the Weber test is positive: Perform the Rinne test.**
   a. Strike a tuning fork on the table. While it is still vibrating, place it on the patient's mastoid process.
   Tests bone conduction of sound.
   b. Measure the elapsed time in seconds that the patient hears the vibration.
   c. Move the tuning fork to 2.5 cm (1 in.) in front of the ear, and measure the elapsed time until the patient can no longer hear the vibration.
   Tests air conduction of sound.

Expected findings: Normally, sound transmission through air (step 6c) is twice as long as transmission through bone (step 6b); that is, AC = 2 × BC.

The ratio of AC to BC is similar in both ears.

Abnormal findings:

- Conductive loss: AC is less than 2 × BC.
- Sensorineural loss: AC is greater than BC but not 2 × longer; or the patient is unable to hear the tuning fork through BC.
- A difference between ears indicates unilateral hearing loss.
- Inability to hear the tuning fork through BC indicates sensorineural hearing loss.

d. Repeat for the opposite ear.

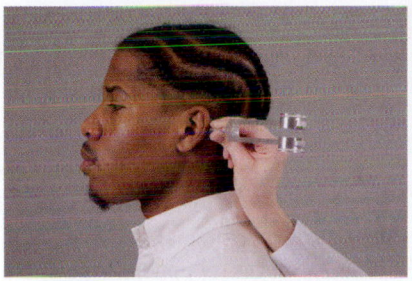

Rinne test

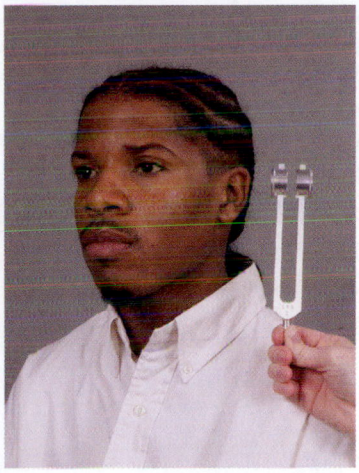

Step 6c

7. **Perform the Romberg test.** Have the patient stand with feet together, hands at side, with eyes opened and then with eyes closed. Note the patient's ability to maintain balance.

- Stand nearby in case the client loses his balance.

Tests for balance. Strictly speaking, it does not assess the ears, but the vestibular nerve and other parts of the central nervous system. Therefore, you may prefer to perform the test during the neurological exam.

Expected findings: The patient maintains balance with minimal sway.

Abnormal findings: Positive Romberg (swaying) is seen with vestibular and cerebellar disorders.

Patient Teaching

Teach the patient the importance of routine hearing examinations.

Documentation

- If you need more information about documenting,

Go to Chapter 22, **Documenting Physical Assessment Findings,** in Volume 1.

Procedure 22-8 ■ Assessing the Nose and Sinuses

➤ For steps to follow in *all* procedures, refer to the Universal Steps for All Procedures found on the inside back cover.

Equipment

- Nonlatex procedure gloves (if exposure to body fluids is a possibility)
- Penlight
- Nasal speculum or otoscope with a wide-tipped speculum
- Pen and record form

Positioning

Have the patient seated, if possible.

Focused History Questions

- Do you have any nasal congestion?
- Do you have a history of nose or sinus problems?
- Do you have problems with seasonal or environmental allergies?
- Do you have a history of sinus headaches?
- Do you experience nose bleeds (*epistaxis*)?
- Have you ever broken your nose?
- Have you had any changes in your sense of smell?
- Do you use any nasal sprays or allergy medications?

(continued on next page)

Procedure 22-8 ■ Assessing the Nose and Sinuses (continued)

➤ When performing the procedure, always identify your patient according to agency policy, using two identifiers, and be attentive to standard precautions, hand hygiene, patient safety and privacy, body mechanics, and documentation.

Procedure Steps	Expected and Abnormal Findings
1. Position the client for the exam.	
2. Inspect the external nose. Note the position, shape, and size. Observe for discharge and flaring.	**Expected findings:** The nose is midline and symmetrical. No discharge or flaring **Abnormal findings:** Asymmetry suggests congenital deformity or trauma. Flaring suggests respiratory distress (especially in infants, who cannot breathe through the mouth). Clear drainage suggests allergy; yellow or green drainage suggests upper respiratory infection; bloody drainage may result from trauma, hypertension, or a bleeding disorder.
3. Check for patency of the nasal passages. Ask the patient to close his mouth, hold one naris closed, and breathe through the other naris. Repeat with the opposite naris.	**Expected findings:** The client breathes freely through both nares.
4. Inspect the internal structures. a. Use a nasal speculum or an otoscope with a large speculum (or a penlight with a speculum) to assess the internal structures. b. Tilt the patient's head back to facilitate speculum insertion and visualization. c. Brace your index finger against the patient's nose as you insert the speculum. d. Insert the speculum about 1 cm into the nares. Use the other hand to position the client's head and to hold the penlight if you do not have a lighted scope. ➤ e. Observe the nasal mucosa for color, edema, lesions, erosion or ulceration, blood, and discharge. Inspect the septum for position and intactness. f. Check for sense of smell using commonly recognized objects, such as a lemon or vanilla. Do not use a noxious odor. You can defer this test until the sensorineurological part of the exam if you choose, but keep the same order for every exam. *Cranial nerve I is intact when the patient shows an ability to detect odor.* ***Developmental Modifications*** *Infants and children*—You will not need a speculum to examine internal structures. Push the tip of the nose upward with your thumb, and direct a penlight into the nares.	**Expected findings:** Nasal mucosa is pink and moist. Septum is intact and midline. No lesions **Abnormal findings:** Deviated septum; polyps. Pale boggy mucosa is seen with allergies; bright red mucosa is associated with rhinitis, sinusitis, and cocaine use. Clustered vesicles suggest herpes infection. Erosion of nasal mucosa should signal you to investigate further for other signs or history of crack/cocaine use. Blood in the nasal passage indicates trauma, nose bleeds, or polyps. 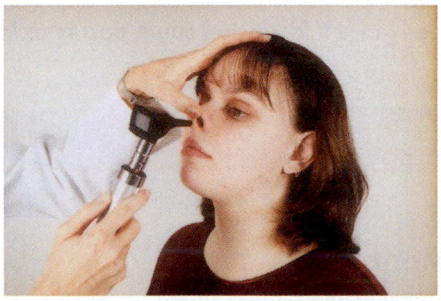 Step 4d

5. Transilluminate the frontal and maxillary sinuses.
First, darken the room.

a. *Frontal sinuses:* Shine a penlight or the otoscope with speculum below the eyebrow on each side.

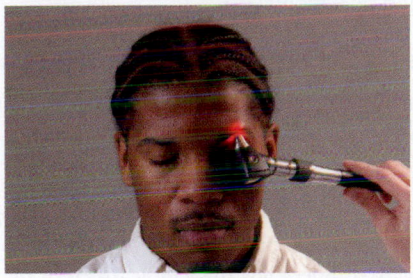

Step 5a

a. **Expected findings:** A red glow is seen above the eyebrow, indicating that the frontal sinus is patent.

b. *Maxillary sinuses:* Place the light source below the eyes and above the cheeks. Look for a glow of red light at the roof of the mouth through the client's open mouth.

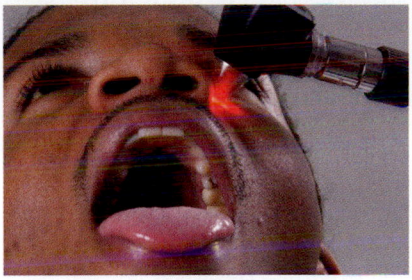

Step 5b

b. A red glow may be (but is not always) seen in the roof of the mouth, indicating that the maxillary sinus is patent.

Abnormal findings: Absence of transillumination may result from mucosal thickening or sinusitis.

6. Palpate the external structures.

Expected Findings: No tenderness, lesions, or deformity

7. Palpate the frontal and maxillary sinuses.

Expected findings: No tenderness

Abnormal findings: Tenderness may indicate infectious or allergic sinusitis.

Documentation

- If you need more information about documenting,

Go to Chapter 22, **Documenting Physical Assessment Findings,** in Volume 1.

Procedure 22-9 ■ Assessing the Mouth and Oropharynx

➤ For steps to follow in *all* procedures, refer to the Universal Steps for All Procedures found on the inside back cover.

Equipment

- Nonlatex procedure gloves
- Penlight
- Tongue blade
- Small gauze pad
- Pen and record form

Positioning

Have the patient seated, if possible.

Focused History Questions

- Do you have any problems with your mouth or teeth?
- When was your last dental exam?
- Do you have any discomfort in your mouth or throat?
- Have you had any recent changes in your mouth or teeth?
- How often do you brush your teeth? Floss?
- Do you smoke or chew tobacco?
- Do you have any sores or irritation in your mouth? If so, when did you first notice this?

(continued on next page)

Procedure 22-9 ■ Assessing the Mouth and Oropharynx (continued)

➤ When performing the procedure, always identify your patient according to agency policy, using two identifiers, and be attentive to standard precautions, hand hygiene, patient safety and privacy, body mechanics, and documentation.

Procedure Steps

1. **Inspect the mouth externally.** Locate the placement of the lips and their color and condition. Ask the client to purse his lips.

Expected and Abnormal Outcomes

Expected findings: The lips are midline, symmetrical, moist, and intact with no lesions. Coloring is consistent with ethnic group/race. The client can purse his lips.

Abnormal findings: Asymmetry (may be due to congenital deformity, trauma, paralysis, or surgical alteration); pallor; cyanosis; redness; inability to purse lips (may indicate facial nerve damage); lesions (may be caused by bacteria, viruses, or trauma)

2. **Note the color and condition of the oral mucosa and gums.**
   a. Don procedure gloves.
   b. Inspect and palpate the lower lip. Pull the lower lip away from the teeth, and inspect the inner side of the lip. Palpate any lesions for size, mobility, and tenderness. ▼

Expected findings: Oral mucosa is pink, moist, and intact; no lesions. Gingiva is consistent in color with the other mucosae and is intact, with no bleeding. Buccal mucosa is pink and moist, with no lesions. Mucosa is darker in dark-skinned clients.

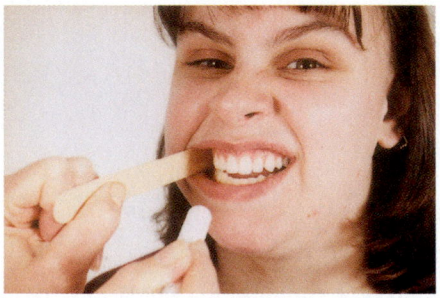

Step 2b

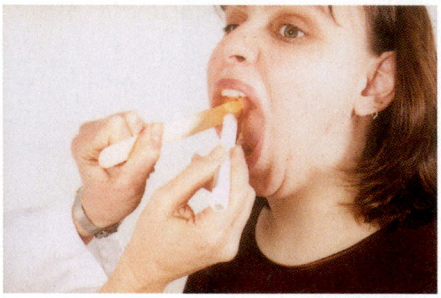

Step 2b

   c. Inspect the buccal mucosa, top to bottom and back to front.
      - Ask the client to open his mouth. Use a tongue depressor to retract the cheek, then shine a penlight onto the mucosa.
      - Using a tongue blade and penlight, inspect the Stensen's duct openings to the parotid glands.
   d. Finally, palpate inside each cheek by placing a finger inside and thumb outside. Grasping the cheek between them, move the finger about. Repeat on both sides.
   e. As you are inspecting the buccal mucosa, also examine the gums. Check for color, bleeding, edema, retraction, and lesions. Press gum tissue gently with gloved finger or tongue blade to assess firmness.

Developmental Variations

Older adults—Mucosa is drier than in young adults because of decreased salivary gland activity; brownish pigmentation of gums may be seen, especially in dark-skinned people.

Abnormal findings: Receding gums, sponginess, bleeding, inflammatory changes, gingival hyperplasia, ulcerations, or other lesions ▼

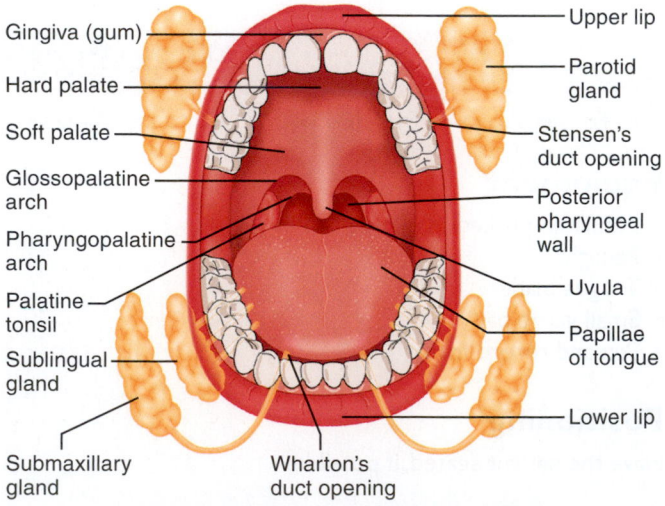

Structures of the mouth and oropharynx

3. **Inspect the teeth.** You can do this while you are inspecting the oral mucosa and gums, in step 2.
   a. Observe the number, color, and condition of the teeth. Note the occlusion ("bite") and any loose teeth.
   b. If the client wears dentures, ask her to remove them. Inspect for cracked or worn areas; assess the fit. ▼

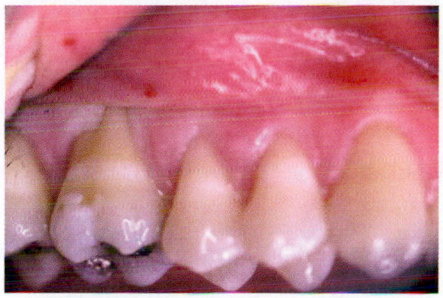

Gingival recession

Expected findings: Most adults have 28 teeth, or 32 if the wisdom teeth have erupted. Children have 20 teeth. The teeth should be white, in good repair, with no caries and good occlusion. The top front teeth should slightly override the lower ones.

Developmental Variations

Older adults—May have receding gums, so teeth appear longer. Teeth may be chipped, eroded, or stained.

Abnormal findings: Missing or poorly anchored teeth, misalignment, and brown or black enamel (indicative of dental caries or staining, e.g., from taking tetracycline). White spots may indicate excessive fluoride intake.

4. **Inspect the tongue and the floor of the mouth.**
   a. Ask the client to "stick out" his tongue. Examine the upper surface for its color, texture, position, and mobility.
   b. Ask the client to roll his tongue upward and move it side to side.
   c. Have the client place the tip of his tongue on the roof of his mouth, as far back as possible. Using the penlight, inspect the underside of the tongue, the frenulum (which fastens the tongue to the floor of the mouth, in the center), and the floor of the mouth.
   d. Inspect the two Wharton's duct openings to the submaxillary glands, on either side of the frenulum.
   e. Use a tongue blade or gloved finger to move the tongue aside and examine the lateral aspects of the tongue and the floor of the mouth bilaterally. Use caution when placing your finger into the mouth of a noncompliant client. ▼

Expected findings: Tongue is moist, and the coloring is consistent with the client's race. Mucosa has no lesions or discoloration. Papillae are intact. Tongue is midline with full mobility. The base of the tongue is smooth with prominent veins. No tenderness; no palpable nodules. A geographic tongue is a common normal variant.

Developmental Variations

Older adults—May have varicosities under the tongue.

Abnormal findings: Red, smooth, or painful tongue; inflamed mucosa or ducts; tongue that is not midline or has restricted mobility; ulcerations of the tongue or the floor of the mouth (e.g., from trauma, viral infection, or cancerous changes); white plaque or black, hairy tongue (fungal infection).

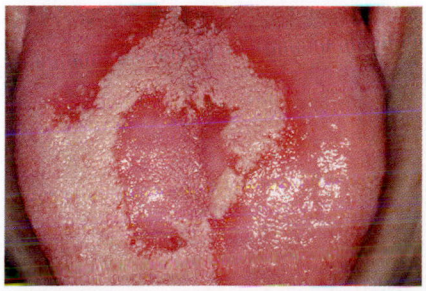

Geographic tongue

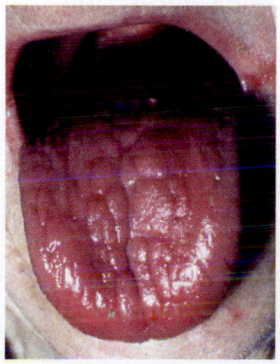

Red, beefy tongue

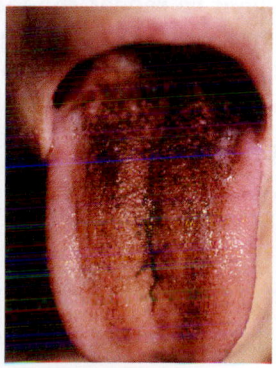

Black, hairy tongue

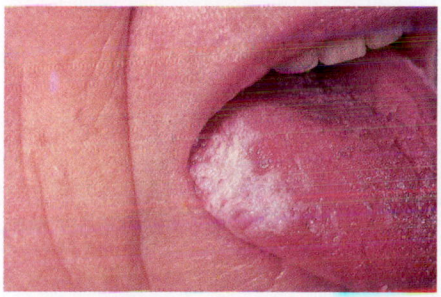

Leukoplakia

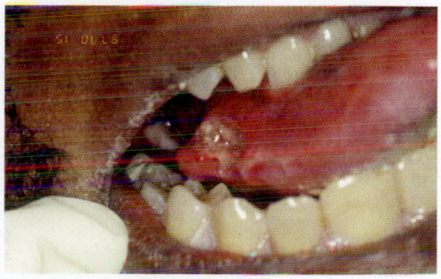

Cancer of the tongue

(continued on next page)

Procedure 22-9 ■ Assessing the Mouth and Oropharynx (continued)

5. **Palpate the tongue and floor of the mouth.** Stabilize the tongue by grasping it with a gauze pad. Palpate top, bottom, and sides with your other index finger.

6. **Inspect the oropharynx (hard/soft palate, tonsils, and uvula).** Note the color, shape, texture, and condition.
   a. Have the client tilt his head back and open his mouth as widely as possible. Depress the tongue with a tongue blade, and shine a penlight on the areas to be inspected.
   b. To inspect the uvula, ask the client to say "ah," and watch the uvula as the soft palate rises.
   c. Inspect the oropharynx by depressing one side of the tongue at a time, about halfway back on the tongue.
   d. Note the size and color of the tonsils; note any discharge, redness, swelling, or lesions.
   e. Look and palpate for cleft palate, especially in infants.

Expected findings: Hard and soft palates are pink and smooth. Uvula is midline and rises symmetrically. Tonsils are pink, symmetrical, and without lesions or exudate.

Developmental Variations

Children—Until about age 12, the tonsils may extend beyond the palatine arch.

Abnormal findings: Redness, edema, lesions, plaques, drainage; yellow or greenish streaks on the posterior wall of pharynx (indicate postnasal drainage); tonsils that are red, edematous, or enlarged or have white or pale patches of exudates. Asymmetrical rise of the uvula may indicate a problem with CN IX or X.

7. **Test the gag reflex** by touching the back of the soft palate with a tongue blade.

Expected findings: Positive gag reflex is present.

Developmental Variations

Older adults—May have a slightly slower gag response.

Abnormal findings: Absence of a gag reflex is seen with extreme sedation, head injury, or damage to CN IX and X. Also see the Abnormal Atlas: Mouth and Oropharynx, at the end of this chapter. Inability to articulate the specified words indicates CN XII is not intact.

8. **Ask the client to repeat the following words:** Light, tight, dynamite. Again, you may defer this test to the sensorineurological portion of the exam if you choose.

Patient Teaching

Instruct the patient in the importance of dental care and the need for regular checkups.

Go to Chapter 22, **Documenting Physical Assessment Findings,** in Volume 1.

Documentation

- If you need more information about documenting,

Procedure 22-10 ■ Assessing the Neck

➤ For steps to follow in *all* procedures, refer to the Universal Steps for All Procedures found on the inside back cover.

Equipment

- Stethoscope and antiseptic wipe
- Pen and record form

Positioning

- Have the client seated, if possible.
- For infants and children, position supine.

Focused History Questions

- Do you have any difficulty swallowing?
- Do you have any neck pain or stiffness?
- Do you have any neck masses or lumps?
- Do you have any history of thyroid disease?
- Do you have any difficulty swallowing?

➤ When performing the procedure, always identify your patient according to agency policy, using two identifiers, and be attentive to standard precautions, hand hygiene, patient safety and privacy, body mechanics, and documentation.

Procedure Steps

1. **Inspect the neck**. Note symmetry, range of motion (ROM), and the condition of the skin.
   - Inspect the neck in a neutral position.
   - Inspect the neck when it is hyperextended.
   - Inspect the neck when the patient swallows water.

Expected and Abnormal Findings

Expected findings: Neck is erect, midline, and symmetrical with full ROM. No masses are present; skin is intact. Larynx and trachea rise with swallowing. Thyroid is not visible.

Abnormal findings: Swollen lymph nodes may be visible. An enlarged thyroid may be visible in the lower half of the neck.

2. **Palpate the cervical lymph nodes**. Note the size, shape, symmetry, consistency, mobility, tenderness, and temperature of any palpable nodes.
   a. Use light palpation with one or two fingerpads in a circular movement.
   b. Palpate the cervical nodes in the following order:
      (1) *Preauricular*—in front of the ear
      (2) *Posterior auricular*—behind the ear
      (3) *Tonsilar*—at the angle of the jaw
      (4) *Submandibular*—halfway up the lower jaw
      (5) *Submental*—under the tip of the chin
      (6) *Occipital*—at the base of the skull in the occipital area
      (7) *Superficial cervical*—below the tonsilar node over the sternocleidomastoid muscle
      (8) *Deep cervical*—under the sternocleidomastoid muscle
      (9) *Posterior cervical*—in posterior triangle along trapezius muscle
      (10) *Supraclavicular*—above the clavicle
   c. Use the same sequence every time so that the steps will become automatic and you will not omit any area.

Expected findings: Lymph nodes are supple and nontender; no masses are palpable. ▼

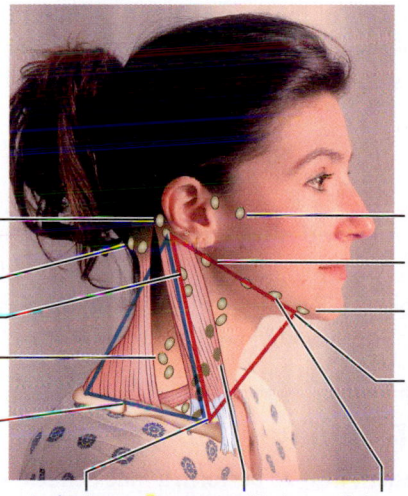

Abnormal findings: Lymphadenopathy (palpable nodes 1 cm or greater). Immobile nodes may indicate malignancy, inflammation, or infection in the area they drain.

(continued on next page)

Procedure 22-10 ■ Assessing the Neck (continued)

3. Palpate the thyroid.

To use the posterior approach:

a. Stand behind the client, and ask her to flex her neck slightly forward and to the left.
b. Position your thumbs on the nape of the client's neck.
c. Using the fingers of your left hand, locate the cricoid cartilage, which is located below the thyroid cartilage. Push the trachea slightly to the left with your right hand as you palpate just below the cricoid cartilage and between the trachea and sternocleidomastoid muscle.
d. Ask your client to swallow (give her small sips of water if necessary), and feel for the thyroid gland as it rises up.
e. Reverse and repeat the same steps to palpate the right thyroid lobe (use the fingers of your left hand to displace the trachea to the right, while using the fingers of your right hand to palpate the thyroid to the right of the trachea).

To use the anterior approach:

f. Stand in front of the client, and ask her to flex her neck slightly forward and in the direction you intend to palpate.
g. Place your hands on the neck, and apply gentle pressure to one side of the trachea while palpating the opposite side of the neck for the thyroid as the client swallows.
h. Reverse and repeat the same steps on the opposite side.

? What if . . .

■ **The thyroid gland is enlarged or there is a mass?**

Auscultate the thyroid for bruits using the bell portion of the stethoscope. Ask the client to hold her breath as you auscultate. There should be no bruits.

Expected findings: The thyroid is generally nonpalpable. If some tissue is palpable, the consistency is firm and smooth. There is no nodularity, enlargement, or tenderness.

Abnormal findings: An enlarged thyroid may signify a tumor or goiter. A tender thyroid is associated with inflammation.▼

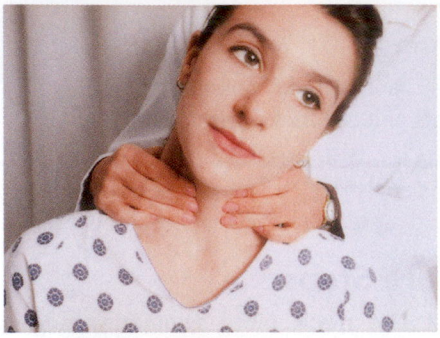

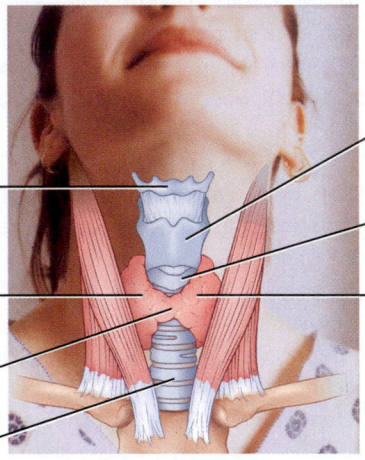

Steps 3a–d

Patient Teaching

Teach the patient how to perform a "neck check"—self-check the thyroid with a glass of water and a handheld mirror. Tell the patient: "Hold the mirror in your hand and focus on your neck just below the Adam's apple and above your collarbone. Tip your head back, take a drink of water, and swallow. As you swallow look at your neck. Check for any bulges in this area as you swallow." To download Neck Check instructions, and for more information about thyroid health,

Go to **http://www.thyroidawareness.com.**

Documentation

■ If you need more information about documenting,

Go to Chapter 22, **Documenting Physical Assessment Findings,** in Volume 1.

Procedure 22-11 ■ Assessing the Breasts and Axillae

➤ For steps to follow in *all* procedures, refer to the Universal Steps for All Procedures found on the the inside back cover.

Equipment

- Nonlatex procedure gloves, if exposure to body fluids is possible
- Glass slide
- Culturette
- Pen and record form

Positioning

The patient must assume several positions during breast examination (see step 1).

Focused History Questions

- Do you have a lump or thickening in your underarm or breasts that persists throughout your menstrual cycle?
- Do you have any breast pain or discharge?
- Have you noticed any changes in the skin on your breasts, nipples, or underarms?
- Have you had any changes in your nipples?
- Have your breasts changed in size, shape, or contour?
- Do you perform breast self-examination (BSE)?
- Are you taking any medications or hormones?
- If you are premenopausal, when was your last period?

➤ When performing the procedure, always identify your patient according to agency policy, using two identifiers, and be attentive to standard precautions, hand hygiene, patient safety and privacy, body mechanics, and documentation.

Procedure Steps

1. **Inspect the breasts.** Note size, shape, symmetry, and color. Inspect with the client in each of the following positions:
   a. Sitting or standing with arms at her side
   b. Sitting or standing with arms raised slightly but not over her head
   Aids in detecting dimpling or retraction of breast tissue
   c. Seated or standing with her hands pressed on her hips
   Aids in detecting dimpling or retraction of breast tissue
   d. With the client leaning forward
   Helpful when examining large, pendulous breasts
   e. With the client supine with a pillow under the shoulder of the breast being examined
   Helps spread the breast tissue over the chest wall

Expected and Abnormal Findings

Expected findings: The breasts are symmetrical; however, the dominant side may be more developed, resulting in a slightly asymmetrical appearance. Skin color is lighter than exposed areas, and there are no lesions, redness, or edema. Texture is smooth, with no dimpling or retraction. Striae are a normal variation.

Developmental Variations

Newborns—You may see breast enlargement and watery, white discharge from the nipples during the first 2 weeks of life.

Children—Breasts typically begin to develop at about 13 years of age; the breasts may not develop at equal rates.

Pregnancy—Breast size increases; areolae and nipples darken; superficial veins become prominent; stretch marks may be present; colostrum (a thick, yellow precursor to breast milk) can sometimes be expressed as early as the second trimester.

Older adults—Breasts lose firmness and become flaccid and pendulous.

Abnormal findings:

- Asymmetry warrants further investigation.
- Swelling or erythema may be seen in infection (mastitis).
- **Peau d'orange** (dimpled skin texture) skin changes may be seen with lymphatic obstruction that is present in some forms of breast cancer.
- Puckering, lesions, and retraction may also be seen with breast cancer.
- **Gynecomastia** (enlargement of breasts in males) may indicate hormone imbalance.

(continued on next page)

Procedure 22-11 ■ Assessing the Breasts and Axillae (continued)

2. **Inspect the nipples and areolae.** Note color, shape, and symmetry. Observe for any discharge.

Expected findings: The areolae and nipples are darker in color than breast tissue. Nipples are everted and point in the same direction. No discharge is present, except in newborns and during pregnancy and lactation. No lesions or erosion is present.

Abnormal findings:
- Nipple discoloration that is not associated with pregnancy
- Nipples pointing in different directions. Such findings warrant follow-up as a potential sign of an underlying mass.
- Flat or inverted nipples, which are caused by shortening of the mammary ducts. May make breastfeeding difficult.
- Any nipple discharge not associated with newborns, pregnancy, or breastfeeding requires a thorough evaluation
- Cracks and nipple redness, which may occur with breastfeeding

3. **Inspect the axillae.** Note the color, condition of the skin, and hair distribution.

Expected findings: Skin is intact with no lesions or rashes. Presence of hair depends on the age of the client and personal preference. Axillary hair develops with puberty. Some women may choose to shave the hair, whereas others will allow it to grow.

Abnormal findings: Rashes, redness, or unusual pigmentation may indicate infection or allergy to deodorants. Dark-pigmented, velvety skin may be seen with ***acanthous nigricans,*** a condition associated with obesity and type 2 diabetes mellitus.

4. **Palpate the breasts,** wearing procedure gloves if necessary. Using the fingerpads of your three middle fingers, make small circles with light, medium, and deep pressure. Begin at an imaginary line drawn straight down the side from the underarm; move across the breast to the middle of the sternum. Check the entire breast area, moving down until you feel only ribs and up to the clavicle.

   Follow one of the following three patterns (evidence suggests the vertical strip method is best).

   a. ***Vertical strip method:*** Start at the sternal edge, and palpate the breast in parallel lines until you reach the midaxillary line. Go up one area and down the adjacent strip (like "mowing the grass").
   b. ***Pie wedge method:*** This method examines the breast in wedges. Move from one wedge to the next.
   c. ***Concentric circles method:*** Start at the outermost area of the breast at the 12 o'clock position. Move clockwise in concentric, ever smaller, circles.

Expected findings: Breasts are soft and nontender with no lesions or masses. Consistency depends on age; premenopausal women have firm and elastic tissue, whereas postmenopausal women have softer tissue that may be stringy or cord-like.

Abnormal findings: Breast lumps or masses may be benign or malignant and require follow-up.

Technique Hints

- Do not remove your fingers from the skin surface once you have begun palpating. Move from area to area by sliding the fingers along the skin.
- Most breast lesions in women are found in the upper outer quadrant.
- Most breast cancer in men occurs in the areola.

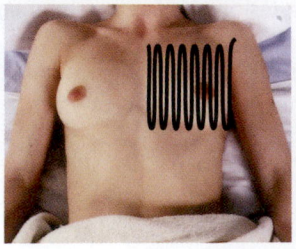

Vertical strip method

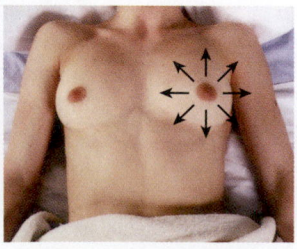

Pie wedge method

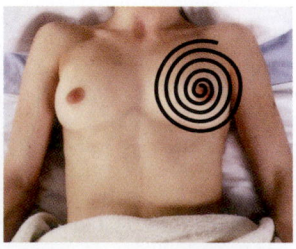

Concentric circle method

5. **Palpate the nipples and areolae.**
   a. If the woman is supine, place a small pillow or folded towel under the shoulder of the breast you are examining.
   b. Squeeze the nipple gently between your thumb and finger to check for discharge.
   c. Note tissue elasticity and tenderness.

Expected findings: Nipples are elastic and nontender. No discharge is present.

Abnormal findings: Loss of elasticity may indicate underlying malignancy. Bloody, purulent discharge may indicate infection. Other forms of drainage may indicate malignancy. Nipple tenderness is normal when establishing breastfeeding.

6. **Palpate the axillae and clavicular lymph nodes.**
   a. Have the woman sitting with her arms at her sides or supine.
   b. Using your fingerpads, move your fingers in circular fashion.
      - *Central nodes:* located high in the midaxillary region
      - *Anterior pectoral nodes:* located on the lower border of the pectoralis major in the anterior axillary fold
      - *Lateral brachial nodes:* located high in the axilla on the inner aspect of the humerus
      - *Posterior subscapular nodes:* located high in the axilla on the lateral scapular border
      - *Epitrochlear nodes:* located above the elbow
      - *Infraclavicular nodes:* located below the clavicle
      - *Supraclavicular nodes:* located above the clavicle

Expected Findings: Nodes are nonpalpable.

Abnormal findings: Palpable nodes may be seen with infection or malignancy. Enlarged lymph nodes caused by infection are tender.

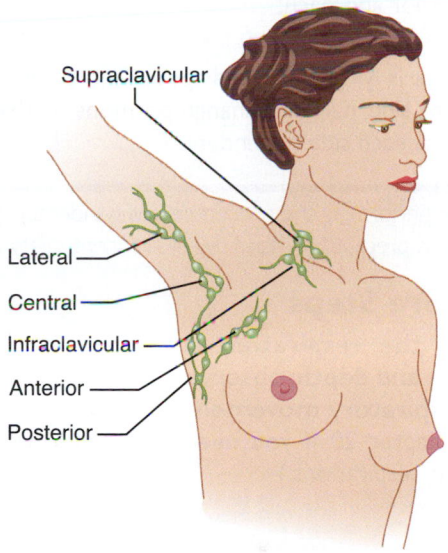

Location of normal lymph nodes

? What if . . .

- **There is a nipple discharge?**

  If there is nipple discharge in a woman who is not pregnant or breastfeeding, obtain a specimen by placing a glass slide up to the breast to capture a drop of discharge. Transport the slide to the laboratory as soon as possible. If there is ample discharge, obtain a swab of the discharge with a culturette.

Patient Teaching

You should demonstrate BSE procedure as part of client teaching for self-care, if the patient chooses to perform BSE. Instruct clients that clinical breast exams should be done annually for women aged 40 and older, and every 1 to 3 years for women aged 20 to 39 (ACOG, 2011). Guidelines vary as to the age at which women should start having clinical breast exams (CBE) and mammograms to screen for breast cancer. Annual or biennial mammograms or breast thermography most commonly begin after age 40, or at a younger age and more often for those at high risk (American Cancer Society, n.d., revised 2013a, n.d., revised 2013b). Evidence at present does not support the need for a CBE if a mammogram is done (AHRQ, 2005 October, revised March 2013).

Documentation

- If you palpate a mass or lump, document its size, shape, symmetry, mobility, tenderness, and skin color changes. To document the location, divide the breast into four quadrants by intersecting vertical and horizontal lines. With the nipple as the center, locate the mass or lump as though the breast were a clock; state the distance in cm from the nipple (e.g., 4 o'clock, 2.5 cm from nipple).
- If you need more information about documenting,

Go to Chapter 22, **Documenting Physical Assessment Findings,** in Volume 1.

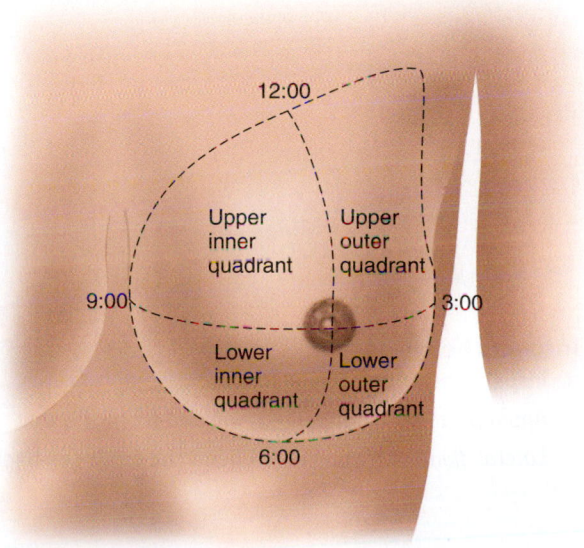

Practice Resources

Agency for Healthcare Research and Quality (AHRQ) (2005 October, revised March 2013); American Congress of Obstetricians and Gynecologists (ACOG) (2009, 2011); American Cancer Society (n.d., last revised 2013b); Maurice, A. Evans, D.G. Affen, J. et al. (2012); Smith, R. A., Duffy, S. W., & Tabár, L. (2012).

Procedure 22-12 ■ Assessing the Chest and Lungs

➤ For steps to follow in *all* procedures, refer to the Universal Steps for All Procedures found on the inside back cover.

Equipment

- Stethoscope and antiseptic wipe
- Felt-tipped marker and ruler
- Pen and record form

Positioning

- Have the client sitting, if possible, and leaning forward for the posterior approach.
  If the client is unable to sit up, findings will be distorted.
- If the client is lying down, findings are more evident on the dependent side; help her change positions so that you can assess with each side dependent.

Focused History Questions

- Do you have fatigue or activity intolerance?
- Do you have any current respiratory problems?
- Have you had any recent respiratory problems?
- Do you have a cough?
- Do you have any difficulty breathing?
- What, if anything, causes you to be short of breath?
- Have you had any chest pain?
- Do you have a history of allergies or asthma?
- Do you smoke? If so, how much and for how long?
- If you smoke, have you tried to quit? Would you like to quit?
- Are you exposed to air pollutants at home or at work?

➤ When performing the procedure, always identify your patient according to agency policy, using two identifiers, and be attentive to standard precautions, hand hygiene, patient safety and privacy, body mechanics, and documentation.

Procedure Steps

1. **Count the respiratory rate, and observe the rhythm and depth; observe the symmetry of chest and respiratory movements.**
   (See Chapter 20 if you need more information about counting respirations.)

Expected and Abnormal Findings

Expected findings:

- Respirations are quiet with a regular rhythm and depth; rate 12–20 breaths/min for adults. Chest movement is symmetrical.

Developmental Variations

Infants and children—The normal respiratory rate varies by age. A newborn may have a respiratory rate of 40–90. The rate gradually declines as the child matures. Newborns breathe abdominally, so you will see little chest movement.

Older adults—Rate changes very little; however, respirations decrease in depth as muscles become weakened.

Abnormal findings:

- Chest asymmetry may be seen with musculoskeletal disorders of the spine, such as kyphosis or scoliosis.
- Asymmetrical movement during breathing is seen in rib fractures, pneumothorax, and atelectasis; affected chest area may not move at all with respiration.
- Sternal and intercostal retractions are seen with hypoxia, respiratory distress, and airway obstruction.
- Respiratory rate may be increased with activity, smoking, fever, pain, or anemia.

2. **Inspect the chest.**
   a. Inspect the anteroposterior (AP):lateral ratio.
   Anteroposterior diameter—as viewed from the side
   Lateral diameter—as viewed from the front (or back)

a. **Expected findings:** The normal adult AP:lateral ratio is 1:2.

Developmental Variations

Infants—AP is equal to the lateral diameter

Older adults—Kyphosis and osteoporosis change the size and shape of the chest; weakening thoracic and diaphragm muscles allow the chest to widen and become more barrel-shaped, as does COPD.

Abnormal findings: AP:lateral ratio is increased in COPD (barrel chest).

b. Inspect the costal angle.

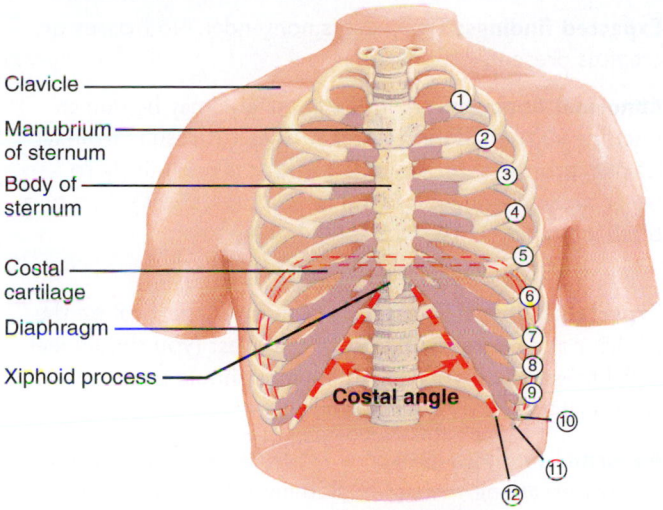

b. **Expected findings:** The costal angle is < 90°.

Abnormal findings: Costal angle is > 90° in COPD.

c. Identify any spinal deformities.

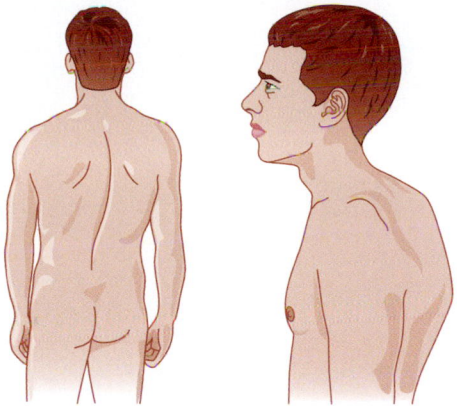

Scoliosis Kyphosis

c. **Expected findings:** The spine is straight without lateral curvatures or deformity.

Abnormal findings: Scoliosis is a lateral curvature of the spine. Kyphosis is excessive thoracic curvature.

d. Observe the effort required to breathe.

d. **Expected findings:** Respirations appear effortless. No retraction or use of accessory muscles.

Abnormal findings: Sternal and intercostal retractions are seen in severe hypoxia or respiratory distress.

e. Note the color and condition of skin.

e. **Expected findings:** Skin color and hair distribution are consistent with the client's gender, ethnicity, and exposure to the sun. The skin is intact with no scars.

Abnormal findings: Cyanosis of the chest wall (due to extreme hypoxia or cold temperature).

---

3. **Palpate the trachea.** Place your fingers and thumb on either side of the trachea and note its position. (In a comprehensive exam, you may have already done this with the neck examination.)

Developmental Modifications

Infants—Neck is short, so it may not be possible to palpate the trachea.

Expected findings: Trachea is in the midline.

Abnormal findings: Tracheal deviation may occur from a mass in the neck (e.g., thyroid enlargement) or from excess pressure in the lungs (e.g., tension pneumothorax).

(continued on next page)

Procedure 22-12 ■ Assessing the Chest and Lungs (continued)

4. Palpate the chest.

- Observe for tenderness, masses, or **crepitus** (crackling skin due to air in the subcutaneous tissue).
- Palpate the anterior, posterior, and lateral chest by placing your hands on the chest wall.

Expected findings: The chest is nontender. No masses or crepitus present.

Abnormal findings: Pain in the chest wall may be due to fracture, inflammation, or trauma. Crepitus results from air leaking into the subcutaneous tissue. It is most likely to occur around wounds, central IV line sites, chest tubes, or a tracheostomy.

5. Palpate chest excursion (expandability).

a. Place your hands at the base of the client's chest with fingers spread and thumbs about 5 cm (2 in.) apart (at the costal margin anteriorly and at the 8th to 10th rib posteriorly).
b. Press your thumbs toward the client's spine to create a small skinfold between them.
c. Have the client take a deep breath, and feel for chest expansion. This may be performed on the anterior or posterior portion of the chest, or both.

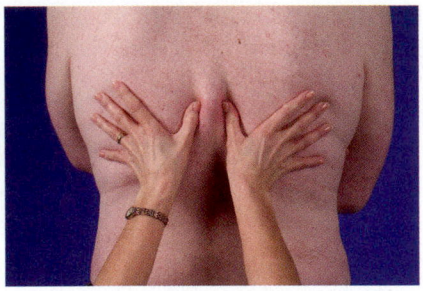

Expected findings: Chest excursion is symmetrical on the anterior and posterior aspect of the chest (you should feel equal pressure on your hands; thumbs should move apart equal distances).

Abnormal findings: Limited chest excursion may occur with shallow breathing, restrictive clothing, or restrictive airway disease. Asymmetrical excursion may result from airway obstruction, pleural effusion, or pneumothorax.

6. Follow the same pattern and sequence for palpating fremitus, percussing, and auscultating the chest. See the accompanying diagram.

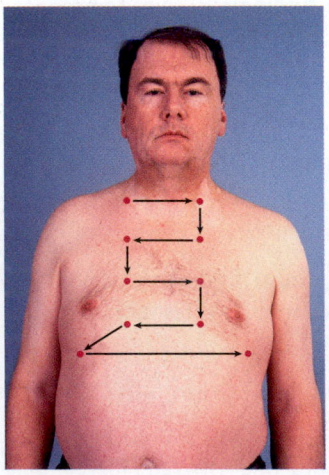

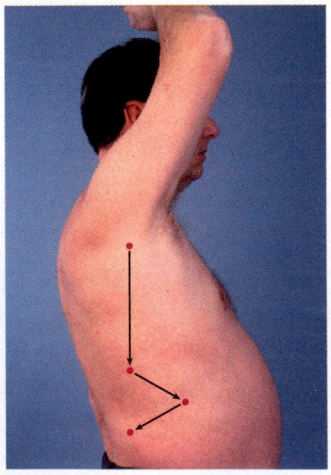

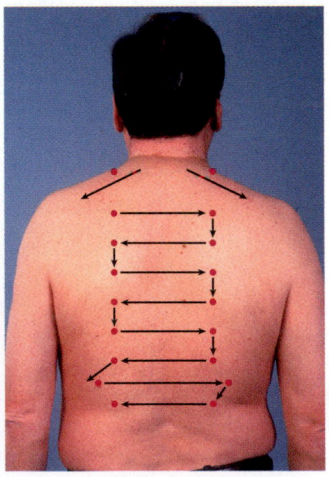

7. Palpate the chest for tactile fremitus.

a. Use the palmar surface of your hands, but raise the fingers off the client's chest so that you palpate with the bony metacarpophalangeal joints of your hands.

Bony prominences are best for detecting vibrations.

Expected Findings: Tactile fremitus is equal bilaterally on the anterior and posterior chest; it is diminished at midthorax. Fremitus is normally diminished if the chest wall is very thick or the voice very soft.

b. Palpate for vibrations as the client says "99."

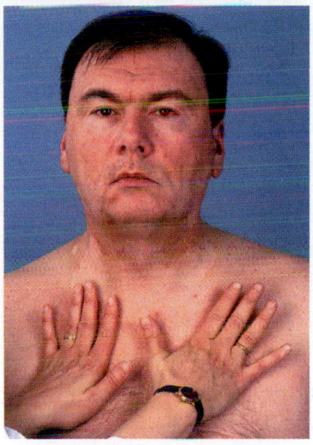

Developmental Modifications

Infants—Place your hand over the chest while the infant is crying.

Developmental Variations

Children and thin adults—May have increased fremitus.

Abnormal findings: Increased fremitus occurs with conditions that cause fluid in the lungs (e.g., pulmonary edema). Decreased or absent fremitus occurs when there is decreased air movement or tissue consolidation (e.g., emphysema, asthma).

---

8. Percuss the chest.

- Percuss over the intercostal spaces rather than over the ribs.

  Percussion over bone produces less resonance.
- Use the indirect percussion method on the anterior, posterior, and lateral chest, following the diagram in step 6. Compare the right side to the left side.

Expected findings:

- The anterior chest is resonant to the 2nd ICS on the left and to the 4th ICS on the right.
- The lateral chest is resonant to the 8th ICS.
- The posterior chest is resonant to T12.

Abnormal findings: Dullness is heard with fluid or masses in the lungs. Hyperresonance is heard with air trapping that occurs with emphysema.

---

9. Percuss the posterior chest for diaphragmatic excursion.

a. Percuss the level of the diaphragm on full expiration. Have the client exhale completely and hold his breath while you percuss (beginning just below the scapula) from resonance over the lung downward toward the diaphragm. The sound will become dull at the diaphragm. Mark the area with a pen.

b. Percuss the diaphragm level on full inspiration. Have the client take a deep breath and hold it as you percuss again. Mark the location.

c. Measure the distance between the two marks.

Expected findings: Diaphragmatic excursion (the distance between the two marks) is normally 3–6 cm.

Abnormal findings: Decreased excursion may indicate paralysis, atelectasis, or COPD with overinflated lungs.

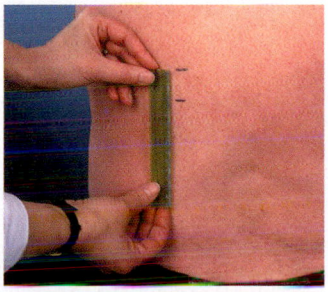

---

10. Auscultate the chest.

a. Follow the pattern in Step 6.

b. Use the diaphragm of the stethoscope.

c. Have the client take slow, deep breaths through his mouth as you listen at each site through one full respiratory cycle.

For lung sounds, refer to the tables at the end of this procedure. To listen to some lung sounds,

Go to the sound file, **Breath Sounds,** on Davis*Plus*.

Expected findings: No abnormal or adventitious sounds are heard. Lung fields are clear to auscultation. *Bronchial* breath sounds are heard over the trachea. *Bronchovesicular* breath sounds are heard over the sternum anteriorly and between the scapulae posteriorly. *Vesicular* breath sounds are heard over most of the lung fields.

Developmental Variations

Infants—Breath sounds are louder than in adults.

Abnormal findings: Crackles or rales, rhonchi, wheezing, stridor, friction rub, grunting

(continued on next page)

Procedure 22-12 ■ Assessing the Chest and Lungs (continued)

11. **Auscultate for abnormal voice sounds if there is evidence of lung congestion.** Follow the pattern in Step 6.
    a. Assess for *bronchophony* by having the client say "1, 2, 3" as you listen over the lung fields.
    b. Assess for *egophony* by having your client say "eee" as you listen over the lung fields.
    c. Assess for *whispered pectoriloquy* by having your client whisper "1, 2, 3" as you listen over the lung fields.

Expected findings: No abnormal voice sounds are heard.

Abnormal findings:

a. **Bronchophony** is present if the words are clearly heard over the lungs.
b. **Egophony** is present if the sound you hear is "ay."
c. **Whispered pectoriloquy** is present if you hear, "One, two, three" clearly.

Patient Teaching

Instruct the patient about the dangers of tobacco use, especially smoking; exposure to air pollutants and environmental pollutants, such as radon or asbestos; and the signs and symptoms of lung cancer.

Home Care

- Instruct clients or caregivers to identify any pollutant within the home that may cause respiratory problems, such as radon, dirty heating/air-conditioning systems, or mold.
- Instruct caregivers or patients with allergies and/or asthma to eliminate potential allergens, such as cigarette smoke, dust, feathers, and pet dander.

Documentation

If you need information about documenting your findings,

Go to Chapter 22, **Documenting Physical Assessment Findings,** in Volume 1.

Normal Lung Sounds

NORMAL LUNG SOUNDS	LOCATION	DESCRIPTION	ILLUSTRATION
Bronchial or tubular	Heard over the trachea	Blowing, hollow sounds; inspiration is shorter than expiration and lower-pitched.	Inspiration / Expiration
Bronchovesicular	Heard over the 1st and 2nd ICS anteriorly and over the scapula posteriorly	Medium-pitched, medium intensity, blowing sounds; inspiration and expiration are equal length and similar pitch	Inspiration / Expiration
Vesicular	Heard over the lung periphery	Soft, low-pitched sounds; inspiration is longer, louder, and higher-pitched than expiration	Inspiration / Expiration

Abnormal Lung Sounds

ABNORMAL LUNG SOUNDS	CAUSE	CHARACTERISTICS	EXAMPLES
Crackles (sometimes called rales)	Air bubbling through moisture in the alveoli	Bubbling, crackling, popping. Soft, high-pitched, and very brief sounds, usually heard during inspiration	Pneumonia Congestive heart failure (CHF) Bronchitis Emphysema
Rhonchi	Mucous secretions in the large airways	Coarse, snoring, continuous low-pitched sounds heard during inspiration and expiration. May clear with coughing.	Bronchitis Emphysema Narrowed airways Fibrotic lungs
Wheezes	Narrowing of small airways by spasm, inflammation, mucus, or tumor	High-pitched musical or squeaking sounds heard during inspiration or expiration	Acute asthma Emphysema
Stridor*	Partial upper airway obstruction or tracheal or laryngeal spasm	High-pitched, continuous honking sounds heard throughout the respiratory cycle but most prominent on inspiration	Acute respiratory distress Foreign body in airway Epiglottitis
Friction Rub	Rubbing together of inflamed pleural layers	A high-pitched grating or rubbing sound that may be heard throughout the respiratory cycle. Loudest over lower lateral anterior surface.	Pleuritis
Grunting	Retention of air in the lungs	A high-pitched tubular sound heard on expiration	Emphysema

*Patients with stridor need immediate medical evaluation.

Procedure 22-13 ■ Assessing the Heart and Vascular System

➤ For steps to follow in *all* procedures, refer to the Universal Steps for All Procedures found on the inside back cover.

Equipment

- Combination stethoscope with bell and diaphragm
- Alcohol or other antiseptic wipes
- Two rulers
- Pen and record form

Clean stethoscope and rulers before and after use unless they are only used for one patient.

Positioning

Place the client in three positions: sitting, supine, and left lateral (to facilitate hearing specific sounds).

Focused History Questions

- Have you experienced any fatigue or activity intolerance?
- Do you have a history of high blood pressure or stroke?
- Have you ever passed out or felt light-headed?
- Do you have any problems with your heart or circulation?
- Do you ever experience chest pain? If so, describe the circumstances that triggered the pain.
- What was the pain like? What did you do to relieve it?
- Do you ever experience palpitations or a rapid heart beat?
- Do you ever feel short of breath?
- Do you ever get swelling in your feet?
- What medications are you taking?

(continued on next page)

Procedure 22-13 ■ Assessing the Heart and Vascular System (continued)

➤ When performing the procedure, always identify your patient according to agency policy, using two identifiers, and be attentive to standard precautions, hand hygiene, patient safety and privacy, body mechanics, and documentation.

Procedure Steps

1. **Inspect the neck.**
   a. With the patient supine, inspect the carotid and jugular venous system in the neck for pulsations.

   b. Assess jugular flow: Compress the jugular vein below the jaw. The vein collapses, and the jugular wave is more prominent at the supraclavicular area. ▼

   The jugular venous pulse is easily obliterated with gentle pressure.

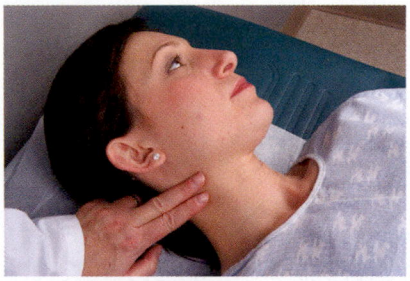

Assessing jugular flow

   c. Assess jugular filling: Compress the jugular above the clavicle. The vein distends and the jugular wave disappears. ▼

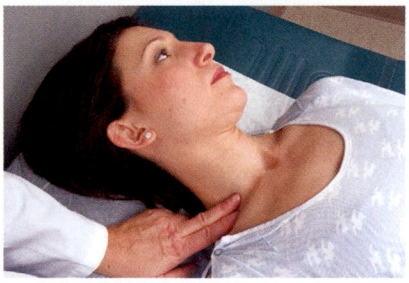

Assessing jugular filling

Expected and Abnormal Findings

Expected Findings: Carotid pulsation is easily visible. A slight pulsation in the supraclavicular area or suprasternal notch indicates jugular venous pressure. The pulsation should be easily obliterated when you apply pressure to the area.

Abnormal findings: Significant jugular vein distention suggests right-sided heart failure.

2. **Measure jugular venous pressure (JVP).**
   a. Elevate the head of the bed to a 45° angle.
   b. Identify the highest point of visible internal jugular filling.
   c. Place a ruler vertically at the sternal angle (where the clavicles meet).
   d. Place another ruler horizontally at the highest point of the venous wave.
   e. Measure the distance in centimeters vertically from the chest wall. ▼

Expected findings: Normal jugular venous pressure is <3 cm.

Abnormal findings: Elevated JVP (in CHF or constricted flow into the right side of the heart); low JVP (in hypovolemia)

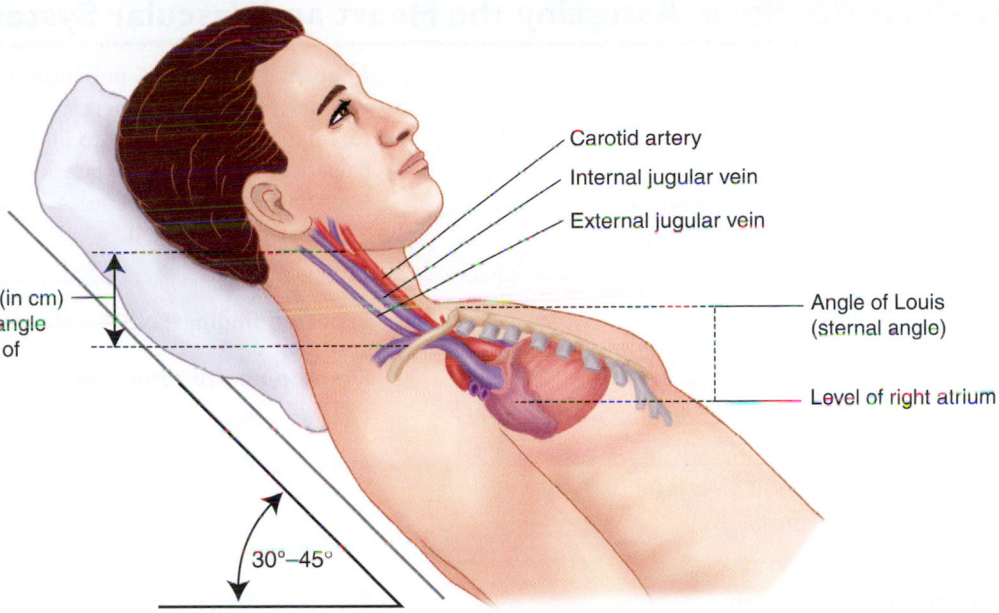

Measuring Jugular Venous Pressure

3. Inspect the precordium for pulsations. (Have the patient supine with tangential lighting.)

Developmental Modifications

Children—Look for the PMI more medially and at about the 4th ICS in children younger than age 8.

Expected findings: Visible pulsation at the point of maximal impulse (PMI, the 5th ICS in the midclavicular line)

Developmental Variations

In thin adults and children, a pulsation may also be visible over the base of the heart.

Abnormal findings: A pulsation (a heave or lift) displaced toward the axillary line indicates left ventricular hypertrophy. Pulsations to the right of the sternum may indicate an aortic aneurysm.

4. Very gently palpate the carotid arteries. **NOTE:** that this step is not done for all patients. It is a part of a thorough cardiovascular assessment and is done only when indicated.

a. Palpate each side separately.
Bilateral pressure may impair cerebral blood flow.

b. Avoid massaging the carotid artery as you palpate.
Increased pressure on the carotid will lead to a drop in the heart rate and blood pressure.

c. Note the rate, rhythm, amplitude, and symmetry of the pulse.

d. Note the contour, symmetry, and elasticity of the arteries.

e. Note any thrills.

Expected findings:
- Rhythm is regular with +2 amplitude.
- Contour: There should be a smooth upstroke with less acute descent.
- Symmetry: Pulses are equal bilaterally.
- Elasticity: Carotids are soft and pliable.

Developmental Variations

Pulse rate is age dependent.

Older adults—The carotids may be stiff and cord-like.

Abnormal findings: A thrill indicates turbulent flow.

5. Palpate the precordium.

a. For this part of the examination, have the patient sit up and lean forward. If lying down, have him turn to the left side.

b. Palpate in all five areas: apex, left lateral sternal border, epigastric area, base left, and base right.

Expected Findings: PMI is palpable at the apex over a 1–2 cm area. Slight pulsation from the abdominal aorta may be felt at the epigastric area. No pulsations, lifts, heaves, or thrills are palpable.

(continued on next page)

Procedure 22-13 ■ Assessing the Heart and Vascular System (continued)

c. Feel for pulsations, lifts, heaves, and thrills.
Brings the apex of the heart closer to the chest wall.

Helpful Hint: ***Perform cardiac palpation and auscultation from the patient's right side, whenever possible.***
This allows you to stretch the stethoscope during auscultation so that you minimize interference and "static."

Abnormal findings: A pulsation, lift, or heave may be seen with left ventricular hypertrophy. A ***lift*** is a pulsation that is forceful enough to seem to lift the examiner's fingers with palpation. A **heave** is a pulsation that feels rolling under your fingers. A **thrill** indicates turbulent flow and feels like a vibration over the PMI.

---

6. Auscultate the carotids.

b. Place the bell portion of the stethoscope over the carotid artery to listen for bruits.
Bruits are low-pitched sounds, best heard by the bell portion.

c. Have the patient hold his breath as you listen.
Breath sounds over the trachea are loud and could interfere with the ability to hear a bruit.

Expected findings: No audible bruit is present.

Developmental Variations

Children—Bruit may be heard because of a high-output state.

Abnormal findings: In adults, a bruit suggests carotid stenosis.

---

7. Auscultate the jugular veins.

a. Place the bell portion of the stethoscope lightly over the jugular veins to listen for a low-pitched venous hum.

b. Have the patient hold his breath as you listen.

Expected findings: No venous hum is audible.

Developmental Variations

Children—A venous hum may be heard. This is a benign condition whereby, blood travels to the brain and back down again to the heart, causing the vein walls to vibrate.

---

8. Auscultate the precordium. To review heart sounds,

Go to the Sound File, **Heart Sounds,** on Davis*Plus*.

- Ask the patient to sit upright and lean forward a bit.
  This will position the heart closer to the chest wall for clearer auscultation.
- Listen for the S_1, S_2, S_3, and S_4 sounds.
- Listen for murmurs.
- Listen with both the bell and the diaphragm at the sites in the following figure:
  These sites are located along the pathway the blood takes as it flows through the atria, ventricles, and valves of the heart.

Expected findings: No extra sounds are heard. No murmurs, clicks, or rubs are present.

Developmental Variations

Infants—You may hear a split S_2 when the child takes a deep breath.

Children—The chest wall is thinner, so heart sounds are louder than in adults.

Older adults—An S_4 sound is considered normal; extra systoles per minute are considered normal. ▼

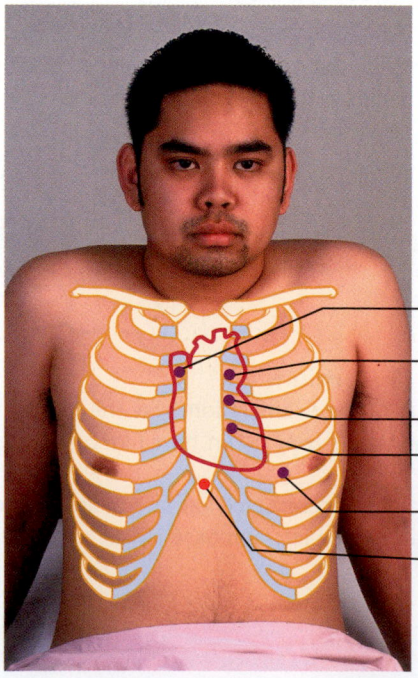

Cardiac auscultation sites

a. *Base right (aortic valve).* Locate the angle of Louis. (It is the prominence on the sternum, two to three finger-breadths below the suprasternal notch.) Slide your fingers laterally until you feel the 2nd ICS.

The right 2nd ICS is the best place to auscultate the aortic valve.

a. **Expected Findings:** $S_1 < S_{2t}$

b. *Base left (pulmonic valve).* Locate the angle of Louis (the prominence on the sternum, two to three finger-breadths below the clavicular notch). Slide your fingers laterally until you feel the 2nd ICS.

The left 2nd ICS is the best place to auscultate the pulmonic valve.

b. **Expected findings:** $S_1 < S_2$

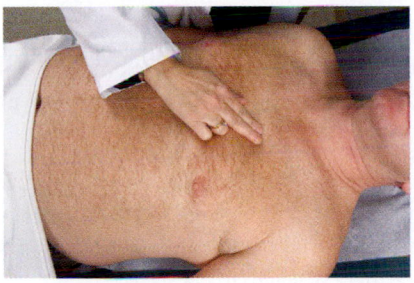

Palpating base left

c. *Apex (mitral valve).* You may be able to locate the apex by observing the pulsation at the PMI. It is at the 5th ICS in the midclavicular line.

c. **Expected findings:** $S_1 > S_2$

Developmental Variations

Children—You will hear S_3 at the apex in about 30% of children.

d. *Left lateral sternal border (LLSB) (tricuspid valve).* From the apex, *slide* your finger up to the 4th ICS, then move close to the sternum.

d. **Expected findings:** $S_1 \geq S_2$. You may hear a split S_1.

Abnormal findings: Extra sounds (S_3 or S_4), murmurs, clicks, or rubs. NOTE: A diastolic murmur or a murmur greater than grade ⅙ is never innocent. Also, *in infants,* a split S_2 sound during normal respirations may indicate an atrial-septal defect.

Assessing Murmurs

Auscultating murmurs is an advanced technique that requires practice and experience. However, if you hear a murmur, assess its:

- Location
- Quality
- Frequency (high, medium, or low pitch)
- Intensity (loudness)
- Timing (in relation to S_1 and S_2)
- Duration
- Configuration (constant or crescendo/decrescendo)
- Radiation (can you hear this in other locations?)
- Respiratory variation (does it change with breathing?)

Classifying Murmurs

Grade

1/6 Very faint, comes and goes

2/6 Quiet, but heard immediately

3/6 Moderately loud

4/6 Loud, associated with a thrill

5/6 Heard with stethoscope half off the chest wall; thrill present

6/6 Heard with stethoscope entirely off the chest wall; thrill present

For a description of murmurs,

Go to Chapter 22, **Tables, Boxes, Figures: ESG Table 22-1,** on Davis*Plus*.

(continued on next page)

Procedure 22-13 ■ Assessing the Heart and Vascular System (continued)

9. Inspect the periphery for color, temperature, and edema. (You will probably already have done this when examining the integumentary system.)

Expected findings: Skin is warm. No edema is present. Color is appropriate for race.

Abnormal findings: Pallor, cyanosis, coolness, shininess, sparse hair growth, and clubbing of the nails (may indicate pulmonary oxygenation problems or impaired central or peripheral circulation)

10. Palpate the peripheral pulses: radial, brachial, femoral, popliteal, dorsalis pedis, and posterior tibial.

- Using the distal pads of your second and third fingers, firmly palpate pulses.
- Palpate firmly but not so hard that you occlude the artery.
- If you have trouble finding a pulse, vary your pressure, feeling carefully at the correct anatomical location.
- Assess pulses for rate, rhythm, equality, amplitude, and elasticity.
- Describe pulse amplitude on a scale of 0–4:
  0 = absent, not palpable
  1 = weak, barely palpable, easily obliterated by the finger
  2 = normal, obliterated by strong finger pressure
  3 = full, increased, not easily obliterated
  4 = bounding, forceful, obliterated only by strong finger pressure

Expected findings: All pulses are regular, strong, and equal bilaterally. Pulse amplitude is +2.

Developmental Variations

Older adults—Arterial pulses may be difficult to palpate because of decreased arterial perfusion.

Abnormal findings: Weak, absent, or asymmetrical pulses may indicate partial or complete occlusion of the artery. Other signs of arterial occlusion include pain, pallor, cool temperature, paresthesia, or paralysis.

11. Inspect the venous system. If a client has varicosities, assess for valve competence with the manual compression test, following:

a. With the client standing, compress the distal portion of the vein.
b. Still holding the distal portion, compress the proximal portion.

Expected Findings: Veins are not distended. Superficial spider-like veins, especially on the lower extremities, may occur with normal aging.

If the valves are competent, you will not feel backflow. If the valves are incompetent, you will feel a wave pulsation with your lower hand as a result of backflow when you press on the proximal segment of the veins.

Developmental Variations

Older adults—Often have peripheral edema as a result of chronic venous insufficiency.

Abnormal findings: Rope-like, distended, tortuous, or painful veins **(varicosities)**

? What if . . .

- **The patient is obese and heart sounds are difficult to hear?**

  The larger the body mass over the heart, the more difficult it is to hear heart sounds clearly. However, it may help to have the patient sit upright and lean forward as you auscultate.

- **Findings from inspecting and palpating peripheral pulses are abnormal?**

  If inspection or palpation findings are abnormal, perform the tests in the table, More Extensive Tests for Abnormal Findings, at the end of this procedure.

Patient Teaching

Instruct the patient in the risk factors of heart disease and stroke and in the signs and symptoms of heart disease.

Documentation

If you need information about documenting your findings,

Go to Chapter 19, **Documenting Physical Assessment Findings,** in Volume 1.

If you need more information about assessing apical and peripheral pulses and measuring blood pressure,

Go to *Davis's Nursing Skills Videos,* **Vital Signs.**

More Extensive Tests for Abnormal Findings	
TESTS	**EXPECTED FINDINGS**
1. *Perform the capillary refill test* anywhere you note signs of diminished blood flow. a. Press the skin with sufficient pressure to produce blanching. b. Release the pressure and observe the return of color.	1. Color returns in <3 seconds.
2. *Perform Allen's test* to assess abnormal pulse findings and arterial flow in the hands. a. Have the client form a tight fist with one hand. b. With her fist still clenched, compress her radial and ulnar arteries. c. Ask the client to open her hand; observe for pallor. d. Release the ulnar artery and watch for natural color to return. e. Then repeat the process, but release the radial artery.	2. In a healthy individual skin color returns rapidly with each maneuver. Failure to return to normal color indicates impaired flow through the open artery. Normally pallor resolves in 3–5 seconds.
3. *Check the ankle–brachial index (ABI)* to assess circulatory impairment of the feet. a. Use a Doppler (handheld ultrasonic device) to measure blood pressure at the posterior tibialis or dorsalis pedis pulse sites. b. Compare that pressure with blood pressure obtained over the brachial artery. c. To calculate the ABI, divide the systolic pressure at the ankle by the systolic pressure at the brachial site.	3. Normally ankle pressure is higher than brachial pressure. The following is a summary of ABI findings. Normal: 1 or greater Minimal disease: 0.8–0.95 Moderate disease: 0.79–0.4 Severe disease: 0.39–0 *Example:* If the systolic pressure at the ankle is 75 and at the brachial artery is 100, the ABI is 75/100, or 0.75. This indicates moderate peripheral vascular disease.
4. *Perform the color change test* to assess arterial circulation in the legs. a. While the client is lying supine, elevate the legs to increase venous return. b. Have the client quickly move to a sitting position with the feet dangling.	4. Normal color should return to the feet in less than 10 seconds. Pallor with the legs elevated and dependent rubor (reddish-purple color) are signs of arterial insufficiency.

Procedure 22-14 ■ Assessing the Abdomen

➤ For steps to follow in *all* procedures, refer to the Universal Steps for All Procedures found on the inside back cover.

Equipment

- Stethoscope and antiseptic wipe
- Felt-tipped marker
- Tape measure and ruler
- Penlight or examination light
- Pen and record form

Clean stethoscope and other equipment before and after using unless they are only used for one patient.

Positioning

Begin with the client supine, arms at sides, with small pillows under the head and knees.

Relaxes the abdominal muscles.

Focused History Questions

- What types of foods do you typically eat?
- Are there any foods that you cannot eat? If so, why?

(continued on next page)

Procedure 22-14 ■ Assessing the Abdomen (continued)

- How many cups of coffee, tea, cola, or caffeinated beverages do you drink per day?
- Do you smoke? If so, how much and at what age did you start?
- Do you drink alcohol? If so, how many drinks per day? Per week?
- Do you use any drug for non-medical purposes?
- Do you have any abdominal pain?
- How often do you have a bowel movement (BM)?
- Have you noticed any changes in your BMs?
- Are you having any problems with constipation, diarrhea, or getting to the bathroom in time to use the toilet?
- Have you ever seen blood in your stool or noticed blood when you wipe after a BM?
- Have you ever had black, tarry stools?
- How often do you use antacids, laxatives, enemas, aspirin, or anti-inflammatory medicines such as Anaprox or Motrin?
- What home remedy, herbal, or over-the-counter medicines do you use?
- What prescription medicines do you use?
- Have you ever been immunized for hepatitis?
- Have you ever had a blood transfusion?
- What is your occupation?
- Have you ever been diagnosed with an ulcer, hemorrhoids, hernia, bowel problem, cancer, hepatitis, liver problems, cirrhosis, or appendicitis?
- Have you ever had abdominal surgery? If so, when, what type, and what if any follow-up was done for the problem?
- Do you have any family history of abdominal problems, such as ulcers, gallbladder disease, bowel disease, or cancer?
- Do you ever have trouble with: swallowing, heartburn, nausea, vomiting, diarrhea, bloating, excess gas, yellowing of the skin?

Developmental Modifications

For older adults, recall that "Problems with eating" is a part of the SPICES assessment. Ask clients, for example:

- Do you have difficulty chewing or swallowing your food?
- How is your appetite?
- Are you able to shop for and prepare your food?

➤ When performing the procedure, always identify your patient according to agency policy, using two identifiers, and be attentive to standard precautions, hand hygiene, patient safety and privacy, body mechanics, and documentation.

Procedure Steps

Expected and Abnormal Findings

1. Have the client void before the exam.
Empties the bladder so that you do not mistake a full bladder for a mass.

2. Position the client supine with the knees slightly flexed.
Relaxes the abdominal muscles.

3. Inspect the abdomen.

a. Observe the size, symmetry, and contour of the abdomen.
   (1) Stand at the client's side and view across the abdomen.
   (2) If distention is present, use a tape measure to measure girth at the level of the umbilicus.
   (3) Have the client raise his head and check for bulges.
   Accentuates hernia, if present.

a. **Expected Findings:** Abdomen is flat, slightly rounded, scaphoid (concave), or slightly protuberant; sides are symmetrical. No visible masses or distention are present.

Developmental Variations

Infants and toddlers—Protuberant abdomen is normal.

Abnormal findings: Tumors, cysts, bowel obstruction, or scoliosis may cause asymmetry.

b. Observe the condition of skin and skin color. Look for lesions, scars, striae, superficial veins, and hair distribution (if you have not already done this in your examination of the integumentary system).

b. **Expected findings:** Skin color is consistent with ethnicity but is usually lighter in color than exposed areas. No lesions are present. Hair distribution is appropriate for age and gender. Striae, superficial veins, and scars are common variations.

Abnormal findings:
- Skin color changes may be associated with bruising, internal bleeding, or jaundice.
- Striae occur after periods of rapid growth or weight gain. Pink striae are new. Older striae are silver-white in color.
- Dilated veins are associated with liver disease and obstruction of the vena cava.

c. Note abdominal movements.

c. **Expected findings:** On a thin client, peristalsis and aortic pulsations may be visible. Men tend to use their abdominal muscles for breathing.

Developmental Variations

Infants and children—Peristaltic waves are often visible. Abdominal breathing is common in infants and young children.

Older adults—Abdomen may be more rounded because of decreased muscle tone.

Abnormal findings:

- Peristaltic waves may be seen if there is intestinal obstruction.
- Abnormal respiratory movements may be seen with respiratory distress.
- Pulsations (in other than a thin client) may indicate an aortic aneurysm.

d. Note the position, contour, and color of the umbilicus.

d. **Expected findings:** Umbilicus is inverted and in the midline. No discoloration or discharge is present.

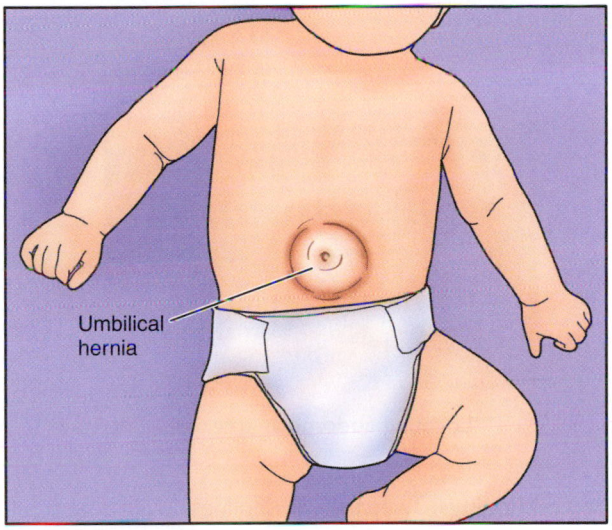

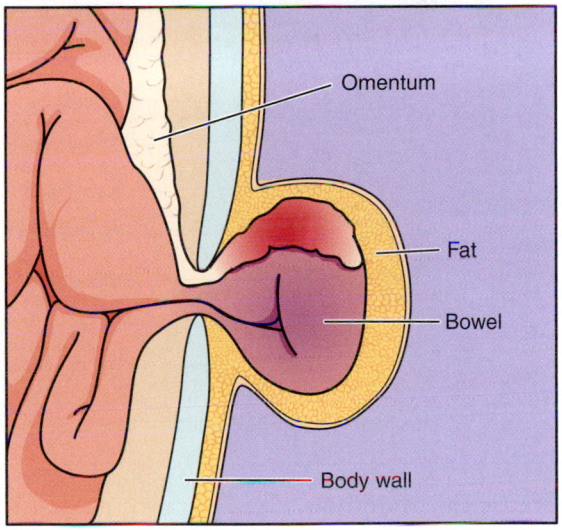

Abnormal findings: Protrusion of the umbilicus may result from a hernia or underlying mass.

---

4. Auscultate the abdomen. To hear a sample of bowel sounds,

Go to **Sound Files: Bowel Sounds,** on Davis*Plus*.

a. Ask the client when he last ate.

Bowel sounds are loudest 5 or 6 hours after the person eats, when the small intestine contents empty through the ileocecal valve into the large intestine. They also increase immediately after eating.

(continued on next page)

Procedure 22-14 ■ Assessing the Abdomen (continued)

b. Listen for bowel sounds.
   (1) Using the stethoscope diaphragm, listen in several areas in all four quadrants (see the figure).

The diaphragm of the stethoscope is used because bowel sounds are high-pitched.

   (2) If bowel sounds are infrequent or difficult to hear, listen to the right of the umbilicus over the ileocecal valve.
   (3) Listen for up to 5 minutes before concluding that bowel sounds are absent.

c. Use the stethoscope bell to listen for bruits over the aorta and the renal, femoral, and iliac arteries. ▼

b. **Expected findings:** Audible bowel sounds, occurring every 5–15 sec or 5–30 times per min.

Abnormal findings:
- ***Hyperperistalsis*** (hyperactive): >2 or 3 sounds per sec or >30 sounds per min
- ***Hypoperistalsis*** (hypoactive): <5 sounds per min
- ***Absent*** bowel sounds: none after listening for 5 min

c. **Expected Findings:** No audible bruits are present.

Abnormal findings: A bruit is abnormal and may indicate an aneurysm or altered blood flow.

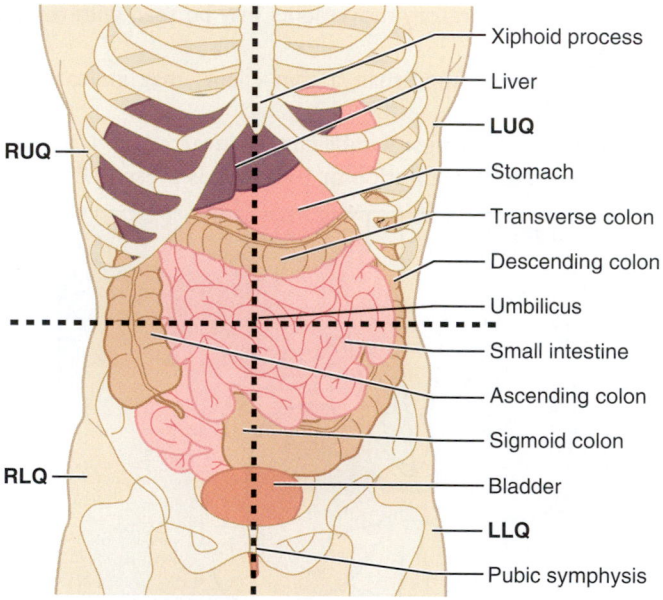

The four abdominal quadrants

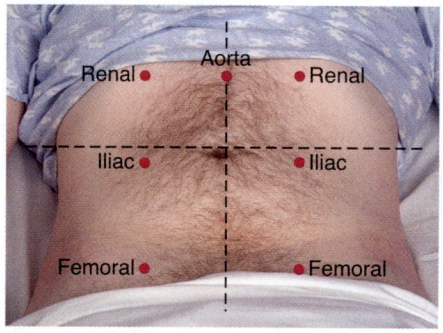

Locating abdominal arteries

5. Percuss the abdomen. (See Clinical Insight 22-1.)
   a. Use indirect percussion to assess at multiple sites in all four quadrants.
   b. Estimate organ size by noting the change in sounds as you percuss over the liver, spleen, and bladder. ▼

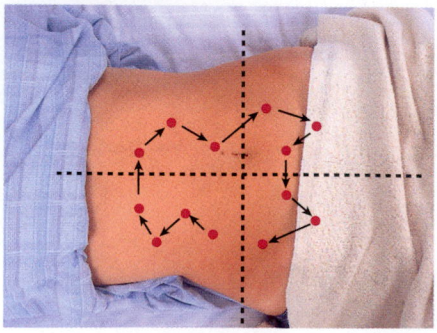

Expected findings: Tympany, with dullness over organs or fluid, is present. No tenderness

Abnormal findings: Extremely high-pitched tympanic sounds are heard with distention. Extensive dullness indicates organ enlargement or underlying mass.

6. **Using fist or blunt percussion, percuss the costovertebral angle** (where the end of the rib cage meets the spine) bilaterally to assess for kidney tenderness.

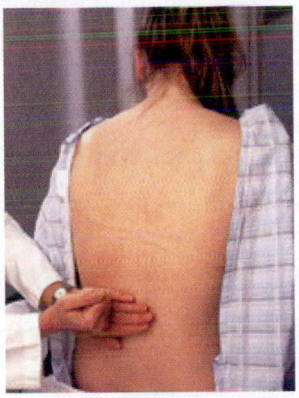

Expected findings: No costovertebral angle tenderness is present.

Abnormal findings: Pain or tenderness is associated with kidney infection or musculoskeletal problems.

7. **Palpate the abdomen.**
   a. **Begin with light palpation** throughout the abdomen. Identify surface characteristics, tenderness, muscular resistance, and turgor.
      (1) If the client is having pain in one area of the abdomen, palpate that area last.

   A guarding response to pain from palpation can interfere with your assessment of the other areas.

      (2) Using your fingertips, press down 1–2 cm in a rotating motion.
      (3) Lift your fingers and move to the next site.
      (4) Palpate the entire abdomen if possible.
      (5) Proceed in an organized fashion through all quadrants, using the same sequence in every examination.
      (6) Observe for grimacing, guarding, or verbal statements of tenderness or pain.

Developmental Modifications

Encourage a child to place her hand lightly over yours as you palpate.

Caution: Do not palpate the abdomen if the client has a Wilms' tumor, a large diffuse pulsation, or a history of organ transplant.

a. **Expected findings:** The abdomen is soft and nontender, with no masses. Muscles are easily palpated; no guarding is present.

Abnormal findings: Guarding and rigidity may indicate peritonitis. Tenderness on light palpation indicates the need for further evaluation.

   b. **Use deep palpation** to palpate organs and masses. See the table Deep Palpation Techniques at the end of this procedure.

b. **Expected Findings:** Tenderness may be noted in a normal adult near the xiphoid process and over the cecum and sigmoid colon.

Developmental Variations

Older adults—May have a higher pain threshold, so they may not react to palpation even if there is an abnormality in the abdomen.

Abnormal findings: A mass indicates the need for further evaluation.

(continued on next page)

Procedure 22-14 ■ Assessing the Abdomen (continued)

c. **Palpate the liver.**
   (1) Stand at the client's right side.
   (2) Place your right hand at the client's right midclavicular line under the costal margin, parallel to the right costal.
   (3) Place your left hand under the client's back at the lower (11th to 12th) ribs, and press upward. This elevates the liver toward the abdominal wall.
   (4) Ask the client to inhale and deeply exhale while you press in and up, gently but deeply, with your right fingers.

Alternative approach: Hooking technique. Place your hands over the right costal margin, and hook your fingers over the edge. Have the client take a deep breath, and feel for the liver's edge as the liver drops down on inspiration and then rises up over your fingers during expiration. ➤

c. **Expected findings:** The liver is not normally palpable unless the client is very thin. If it is palpable, the edge should be smooth and nontender.

Developmental Variations

Children—Liver is relatively large and can be palpated 1–2 cm (0.5–1 in.) below the right costal margin.

Abnormal findings: Palpation below the costal margin indicates enlargement.

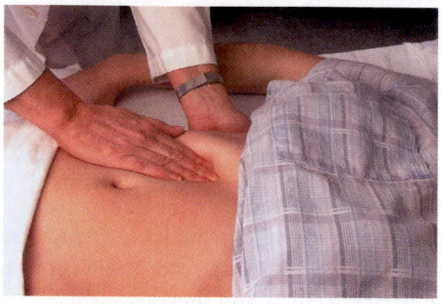

d. **Palpate the Spleen**
   (1) Stand at the client's right side.
   (2) Reach across the client to place your left hand under the costovertebral angle, and pull upward to move the spleen anteriorly.
   (3) Place your right hand under the left anterior costal margin, and have the client take a deep breath.
   (4) During exhalation, press your hands together (inward) to try to palpate the spleen. ➤

d. **Expected Findings:** The spleen is not normally palpable.

Abnormal findings: Splenic enlargement or tenderness may result from infection, trauma, or cancer.

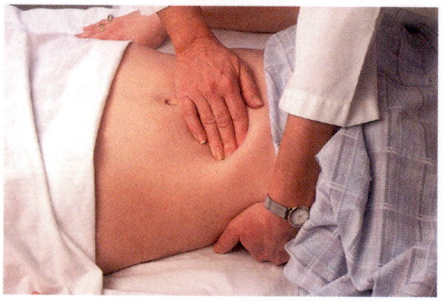

? What if . . .

■ **The patient is ticklish or guarding when you palpate the abdomen?**

Distract the person by giving her a task, such as "Count aloud to 10" or "Count backward from 100." Alternatively, have the client place her hand on her abdomen; place your hand on hers and begin light palpation. When she begins to feel more relaxed, slip your hand underneath hers and continue.

■ **The patient complains of abdominal pain?**

Check for rebound tenderness: Place your hand perpendicular to the abdomen. Press firmly and slowly then release quickly.

If pain increases when you remove your hand, this indicates peritoneal irritation. Rebound tenderness in the right lower quadrant may be a sign of appendicitis.

Patient Teaching

Instruct the patient in the importance of proper diet, the signs and symptoms of colorectal cancer, and the importance of screening colonoscopy.

Documentation

If you need more information about documenting your findings,

Go to Chapter 22, **Documenting Physical Assessment Findings,** in Volume 1.

Deep Palpation Techniques

DEEP PALPATION: ONE-HANDED TECHNIQUE

- Using your fingertips, press down 4 to 6 cm in a dipping motion.
- Proceed in an organized fashion through all four quadrants.

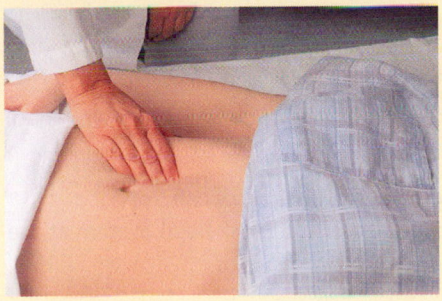

DEEP PALPATION: BIMANUAL TECHNIQUE

- This technique is useful when palpating a large abdomen.
- Place your nondominant hand on your dominant hand.
- Depress your hands 4 to 6 cm (1.5 to 2 in.) in a dipping motion.
- Proceed in an organized fashion through all four quadrants.

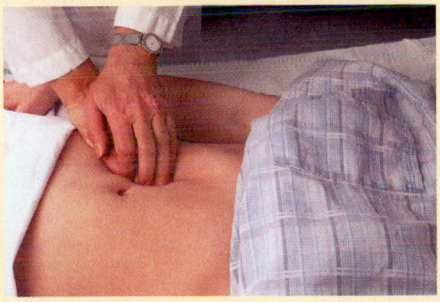

? What if . . .

- **You palpate a mass?**

  Have the client tighten her abdominal muscles.
  If the mass is in the abdominal wall, it will become easier to palpate. If it is deep in the abdomen, it will be difficult to palpate.

Procedure 22-15 ■ Assessing the Musculoskeletal System

➤ For steps to follow in *all* procedures, refer to the Universal Steps for All Procedures found on the inside back cover.

Equipment

- Tape measure
- Goniometer
- Pen and record form

Developmental Modifications

For older adults, recall that "Problems with falls" is a part of the SPICES assessment. If your facility has a falls assessment tool, perform that focused assessment.

Focused History Questions

- Do you have any difficulty with coordination (e.g., folding clothes, brushing your teeth)?
- Do you now have, or have you ever had, musculoskeletal problems, pain, or disease? If so, what medications or treatments are you using?
- Have you ever injured your bones or joints?
- Do your joints, muscles, or bones limit your activities?
- Do you lose your balance or fall?
- Do you have any occupational hazards that could affect your muscles and joints?

➤ When performing the procedure, always identify your patient according to agency policy, using two identifiers, and be attentive to standard precautions, hand hygiene, patient safety and privacy, body mechanics, and documentation.

Procedure Steps

1. **Assess posture.**
   a. Note the body and head position.

   b. Check the alignment and symmetry of the shoulders, scapula, and iliac crests. Inspect from the front, back, and side.

Expected and Abnormal Findings

a. **Expected findings:** Posture is erect, with the head in the midline.
b. **Expected findings:** The shoulders, scapula, and iliac crests are symmetrical.

(continued on next page)

Procedure 22-15 ■ Assessing the Musculoskeletal System (continued)

Developmental Modifications

Newborns—Palpate clavicles for fractures that may have occurred at birth. Check for congenital hip dysplasia (dislocation) by examining for asymmetry of the gluteal folds or shortening of the femur.

c. Assess the spinal curvature by:
   (1) Observing the client's profile while he is standing erect.
   (2) Having the client bend forward at the waist with arms hanging free at the sides.▼

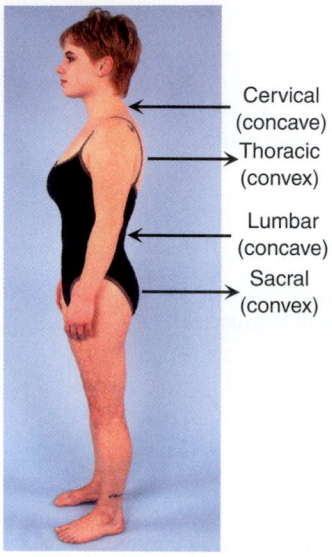

Assessing for normal curves

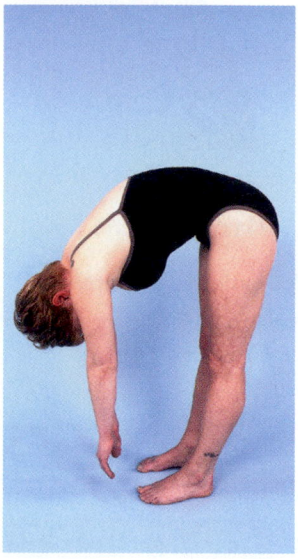

Assessing for kyphosis and scoliosis

c. **Expected findings:** Cervical and lumbar curves are concave; thoracic and sacral curves are convex.

Developmental Variations

Children—**Lordosis** (exaggerated lumbar curve) is normal before age 5.

Abnormal findings: Kyphosis, scoliosis, lordosis
See the Abnormal Atlas: Musculoskeletal System at the end of this chapter.

d. Have the client stand upright with the feet together. Note the position of the knees.▼

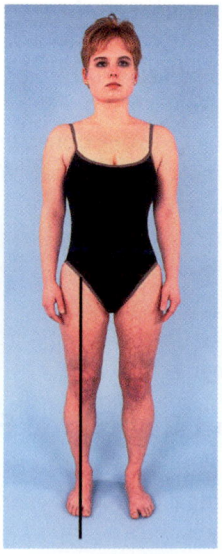

d. **Expected findings:** Patella is in the midline on an imaginary line drawn from the anterior superior iliac crest to the feet.

Developmental Variations

Children—**Genu varum** (bowlegs) is normal for 1 year after a child begins to walk.

2. Assess gait by observing the client walking.

Developmental Modifications

Children—Observe them at play.

a. Pay attention to the base of support (distance between the feet) and stride length (distance between each step).

a. **Expected findings:** Average base of support for an adult is 5–10 cm (2–4 in.). Average stride length is 30–35 cm (12–14 in.); the longer the legs, the longer the stride length.

Abnormal findings: Abnormal gait can be caused by muscle weakness, joint stiffness, pain, deformities, and central nervous system dysfunction. A wide base of support and shortened stride length reflect a balance problem, placing the client at risk for falls.

b. Observe the phases of the gait.

b. **Expected findings:** Movements are smooth and coordinated, weight is evenly distributed, arms swing in opposition, and toes point forward.

Abnormal findings: Toeing in or out, jerky or shuffling movements, touching the floor first with the toe rather than the heel, arms held out to the side or front.

Also refer to the Abnormal Atlas: Abnormal Gaits at the end of this chapter.

Stance Phase

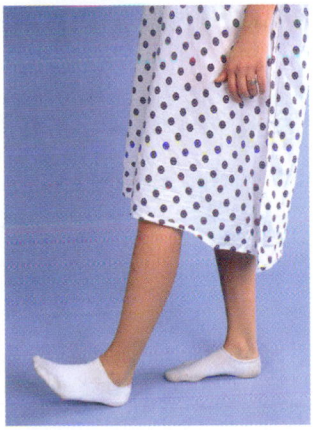

Heel strike

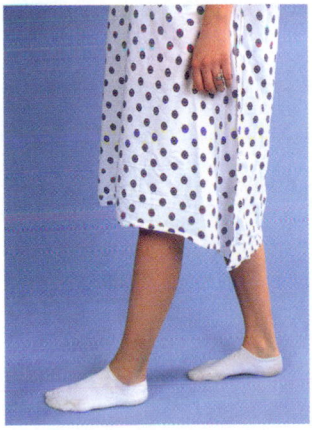

Foot flat

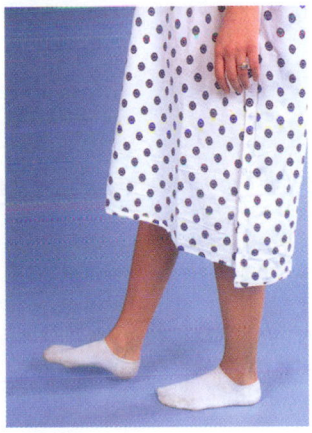

Midstance

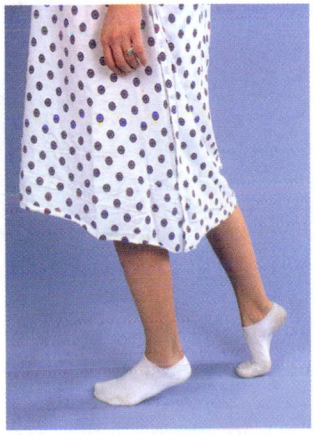

Push-off

Swing Phase

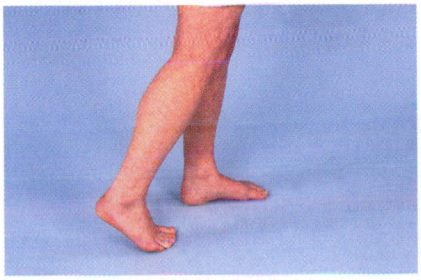

Accelerate

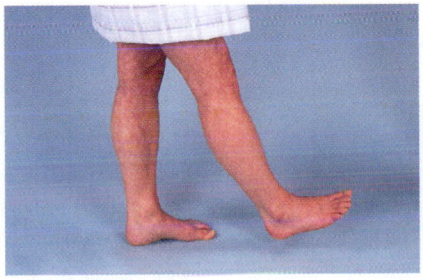

Swing-thru

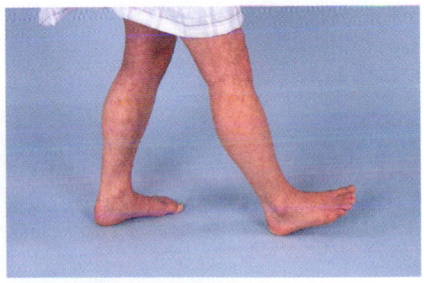

Decelerate

(continued on next page)

Procedure 22-15 ■ Assessing the Musculoskeletal System (continued)

3. Assess balance.

If the client was unsteady when walking, do not complete this portion of the exam. Proceed only if the gait is steady; stand nearby in case the client loses his balance.

a. Have the client tandem walk heel-to-toe.
b. Have the client walk alternately on heels and toes.
c. Ask the client to do a deep knee bend.
d. Ask the client to hop in place on each foot several times.
e. Perform the Romberg test (if you did not already do so when examining the ears): Have the client stand with feet together and eyes open. Then have him close his eyes and stand still.

Expected Findings: The client is able to perform each of these maneuvers smoothly. The Romberg test (see Procedure 22-7) is negative—the client is able to maintain balance with minimal sway with eyes open and closed.

Developmental Variations

Infants—Should be able to sit alone by age 8 months.

Abnormal findings: Balance problems may indicate a cerebellar disorder, an inner ear problem, or muscle weakness.

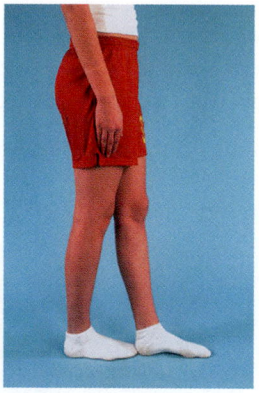

Step 3a. Walking heel-to-toe

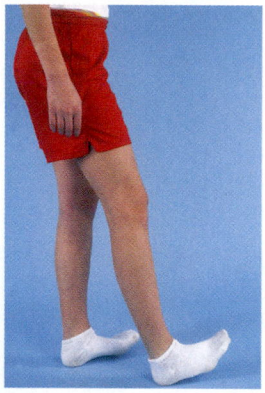

Step 3b. Walking on heels

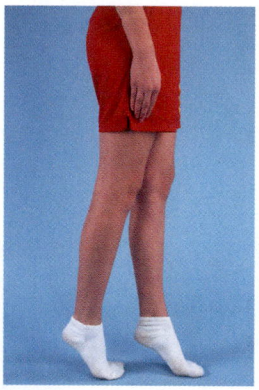

Step 3b. Walking on toes

Developmental Modifications

Infants—Observe sucking, swallowing, and kicking movements.
Children—To assess a child's movement, coordination, ROM, and so on, watch the child at normal play. Cerebellar function cannot be tested on infants and toddlers because of their immature neuromuscular system.

4. Assess coordination while the client is seated.

a. Test upper extremity coordination by having the client perform finger–thumb opposition. Test one side and then the other.

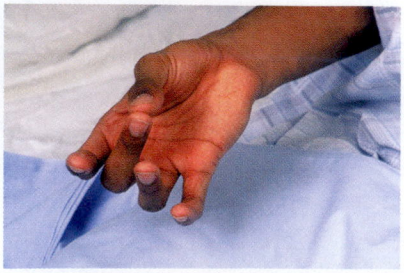

b. Test rapid alternating movements by having the client alternate between supinating and pronating her hands.
c. Assess lower extremity coordination by having the client perform rhythmic toe-tapping, one side at a time.
d. Have the client run the heel of one foot down the shin of the other leg. Repeat on the opposite side.

Expected findings: The client is able to perform these movements smoothly and in a coordinated fashion. The dominant side (usually the right) may be slightly more coordinated.

Developmental Variations

Older adults—Decreased coordination and reaction time may result from slower nerve conduction and loss of muscle tone.

Abnormal findings: Slowness or awkwardness with movement may indicate a cerebellar disorder or muscle weakness.

5. Test accuracy of movements. Have the client touch his finger to his nose with his eyes open. Repeat with his eyes closed.

Expected findings: The movement is accurate with eyes open and closed.

Abnormal findings: Inaccurate movements indicate cerebellar dysfunction.

6. Measure the limbs.

a. Measure arm length from the acromion process to the tip of the middle finger.

b. *Apparent leg length*—Measure from the umbilicus (a nonfixed point) to the medial malleolus.

c. *True leg length*—Measure from the anterior superior iliac crest, crossing over the knee to the medial malleolus ▼

a., b., c. **Expected findings:** The differences in length between the right and left arm and leg are 1 cm or less.

Abnormal findings: Leg length discrepancies may cause back and hip pain and gait problems. A *true leg length* discrepancy results from unequal bone length; an *apparent leg length* discrepancy may result from a pelvic tilt or flexion deformity of the hip.

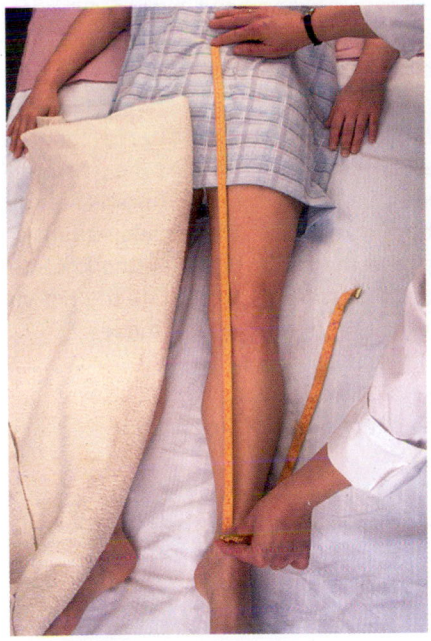

Apparent leg length

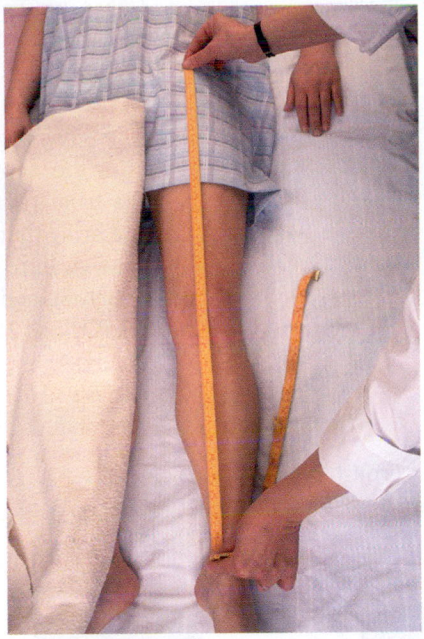

True leg length

d. Measure the circumference of the forearms, upper arms, thighs, and calves.

d. **Expected findings:** The differences in circumference between the right and left arm and leg are 1 cm or less.

Abnormal findings: Circumference differences >1 cm may reflect atrophy or hypertrophy.

7. Inspect muscles and joints bilaterally for symmetry and shape.

Developmental Modifications

Older adults—Observe for surgical scars indicating joint replacement or joint surgeries.

Expected findings: Size and shape are symmetrical. Muscles and joints are smooth, nontender, and similar in color and temperature to surrounding tissue.

Developmental Variations

Older adults—Muscle mass and tone decrease.

Abnormal findings:

- Hot, red, swollen, stiff, or painful joints may indicate injuries, arthritis, gout, bursitis, or other inflammatory diseases.
- ***Heberden's nodes*** are hard, painless nodules over the distal interphalangeal joints—usually seen with degenerative joint disease (DJD), but they may be seen with rheumatoid arthritis (RA).
- Severe misalignment and deformity are more often a result of DJD than of RA.
- Crepitus may be heard in DJD.

(continued on next page)

Procedure 22-15 ■ Assessing the Musculoskeletal System (continued)

8. Test active ROM by asking the client to move the following joints through ROM:

a. Temporomandibular joint (TMJ)

b. Neck

c. Thoracic and lumbar spine

d. Shoulder

e. Upper arm and elbow

f. Wrist

g. Hands and fingers

h. Hip

i. Knee

j. Ankles and feet

Expected findings:

a. *TMJ*—Able to flex, extend, move side to side, protrude, and retract the jaw.

b. *Neck*—Flexes, extends, hyperextends, bends laterally, and rotates side to side.

c. *Spine*—Able to bend at the waist, stand upright, hyperextend (bend backward), bend laterally, and rotate side to side.

d. *Shoulder*—Able to move the arm forward and backward, abduct, adduct, and rotate internally and externally.

e. *Upper arm and elbow*—Able to bend, extend, supinate, and pronate the elbow.

f. *Wrist*—Flexes, extends, hyperextends, and moves side to side.

g. *Hands and fingers*—Able to spread the fingers (abduct), bring them together (adduct), make a fist (flex), extend the hand (extend), bend fingers back (hyperextend), and bring thumb to index finger (palmar adduction).

h. *Hip*—Able to extend the leg straight, flex the knee to the chest, abduct and adduct the leg, rotate the hip internally and externally, and hyperextend the leg.

i. *Knee*—Able to flex and extend the knee.

j. *Ankles and feet*—Able to dorsiflex, plantar flex, evert, invert, abduct, and adduct the feet and ankles.

If a patient cannot move the limb, put the joint through passive ROM. Never force a joint against resistance or if it causes discomfort.

Joint movements

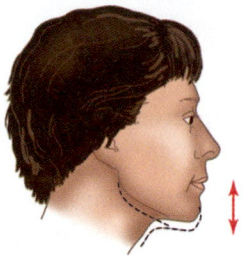

Depression: lowering a body part
Elevation: raising a body part

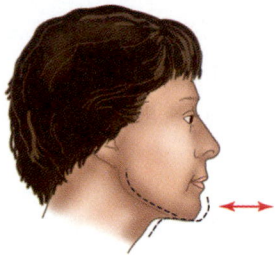

Retraction: moving backward
Protraction: moving forward

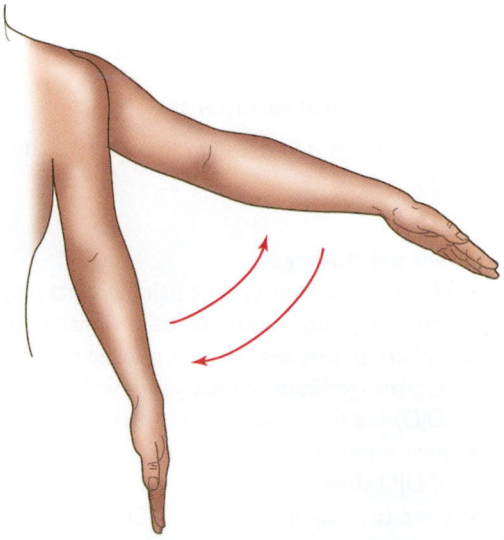

Abduction: moving away from midline
Adduction: moving toward midline

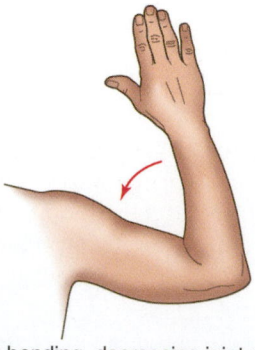

Flexion: bending, decreasing joint angle

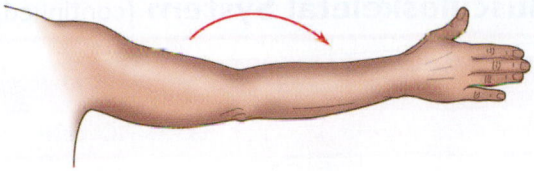

Extension: straightening, increasing joint angle

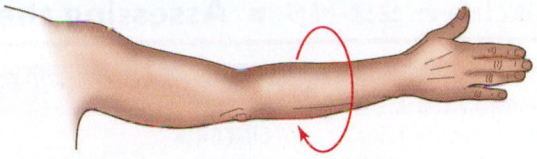

Circumduction: moving in a circular fashion

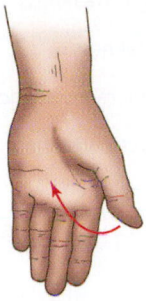

Reposition

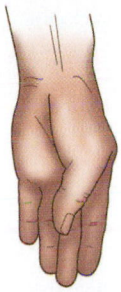

Opposition

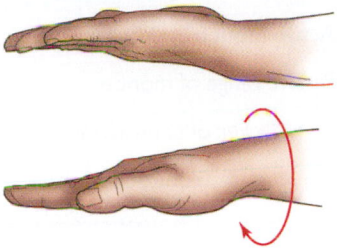

Supination: turning upward

Pronation: turning downward

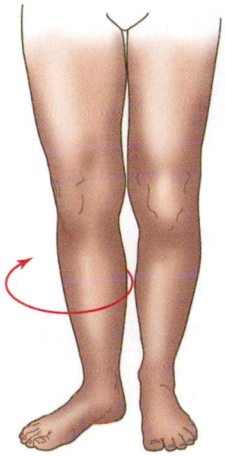

External rotation: turning away from midline

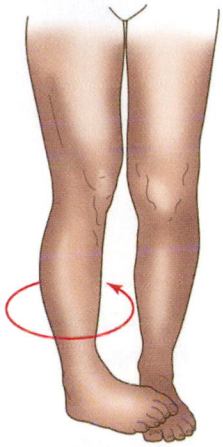

Internal rotation: turning toward midline

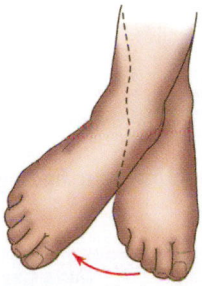

Eversion: turning outward

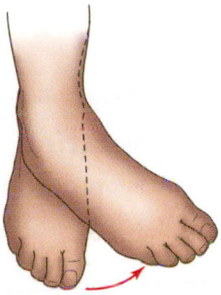

Inversion: turning inward

9. **Test muscle strength by repeating ROM against resistance.** Use the rating scale at the end of this step.
   a. **Test hand grip** by crossing your middle and index fingers and asking the patient to squeeze. (*Tip: If you are wearing rings, a strong hand grip on those fingers can be painful.*)
   b. **Test biceps strength.** Place one hand on the client's biceps and have the patient raise the forearm (flex the elbow) as you apply resistance at the wrist.
   c. **Test triceps strength** by having the client straighten the arm at the elbow (extend the elbow) as you apply resistance at the wrist.
   d. **Test leg strength** by having patient raise leg (straighten the knee) against your hand as you apply resistance.
   e. **Test ankle strength** by asking the patient to point the toes downward (plantar flexion) at the ankle while you apply resistance to the plantar surface of the foot.
   f. **Test ankle strength** by having the client point the toes toward the knee (dorsiflexion) as you apply resistance to the top of the foot.

Expected findings: Expect active motion against full resistance. There should be no crepitus (clicking) or pain with joint movement. ▼

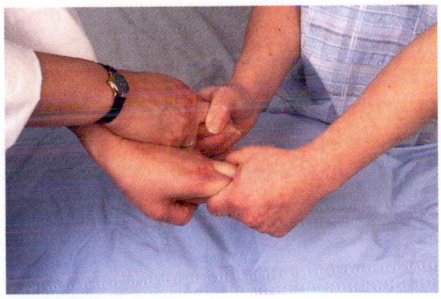

Step 9a

(continued on next page)

Procedure 22-15 ■ Assessing the Musculoskeletal System (continued)

Muscle Strength Rating Scale

RATING	CRITERIA	CLASSIFICATION
5	Active motion against full resistance	Normal
4	Active motion against some resistance	Slight weakness
3	Active motion against gravity	Weakness
2	Passive range of motion	Poor range of motion
1	Slight flicker of contraction	Severe weakness
0	No muscular contraction	Paralysis

? What if . . .

- **There is limited range of motion in a joint?**

  Use a goniometer to measure the limited motion in degrees. Place the goniometer over the joint, matching the angle of the joint.

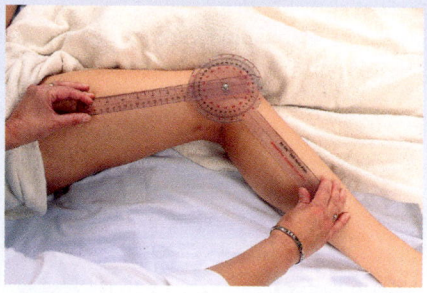

Using a goniometer

Documentation

If you need information about documenting your findings,

Go to Chapter 22, **Documenting Physical Assessment Findings,** in Volume 1.

Procedure 22-16 ■ Assessing the Sensory-Neurological System

➤ For steps to follow in *all* procedures, refer to the Universal Steps for All Procedures found on the inside back cover.

➤ *Note:* This procedure provides guidelines for performing a comprehensive neurological exam. Steps 1–10 assess cognitive status, and the box at the end of the procedure contains questions that are useful for screening cognitive status.

Equipment

- Pen and record form
- Wisp of cotton
- Sharp object, such as a toothpick or sterile needle
- Objects to touch, such as a coin, button, or key
- Something fragrant, such as coffee or rubbing alcohol
- Something to taste, such as sugar, salt, or lemon
- Tongue blade
- Two test tubes
- Reflex hammer
- Ophthalmoscope

Developmental Modifications for Children

- For children younger than age 5 years, use the Denver Developmental Screening Test II to assess neurological and motor function.
- Check the child's ability to understand and follow instructions.

Developmental Modifications for Older Adults

You may need to perform the sensorineurological exam over several sessions. The full exam is lengthy, and older adults fatigue easily. If the client seems to be getting tired, stop the test and finish at a later time.

Focused History Questions

- Do you have any neurological ("nerve") problems?
- Have you ever had head trauma, loss of consciousness, dizziness, headaches, or seizures?
- Do you have memory problems, forgetfulness, or inability to concentrate?
- Have you noticed any changes in your ability to see, smell, taste, hear, feel, or maintain balance?
- Do you have any weakness, numbness, or paralysis?
- Do you have any problems performing activities of daily living (ADLs)?

- Do you have any problems walking?
- Do you have mood problems or depression?
- Do you use alcohol or drugs for non-medical purposes? If so, how much and how often?
- Have you ever been treated for neurological or psychiatric problems?
- Do you have a history of hypertension, diabetes, stroke, or circulation problems?

➤ When performing the procedure, always identify your patient according to agency policy, using two identifiers, and be attentive to standard precautions, hand hygiene, patient safety and privacy, body mechanics, and documentation.

Procedure Steps

1. **Assess behavior**. Note the client's facial expression, posture, affect, and grooming.

Expected and Abnormal Findings

Expected findings: The client is well groomed, with an erect posture, pleasant facial expression, and appropriate affect.

Abnormal findings: Inappropriate behavior may result from neurological or psychological problems, as well as from a variety of medications, alcohol, and street drugs.

2. **Determine level of arousal (LOA):**
   a. Note the client's response to verbal stimuli.
   b. If the client does not respond to verbal stimuli, try **tactile stimulation**: Gently shake the client's shoulder.
   c. If the client does not respond to tactile stimuli, try **painful stimuli**: Squeeze the trapezius muscle, rub the sternum, apply pressure on the mandible at the angle of the jaw, or apply pressure over the "moon" of the nail.

The Glasgow Coma Scale and the FOUR Scale at the end of this procedure provide standard references for assessing LOA for a patient with head injury.

Expected findings: The patient is awake and alert and readily responds to verbal stimuli.

Abnormal findings: Lethargy, stupor, or coma may result from trauma, neurological disorder, hypoxia, or chemical substances

A changing level of arousal (along with forgetfulness, restlessness, or sudden quietness) is one of the earliest indicators of increased intracranial pressure, which can be life threatening.

3. **Determine the level of orientation.**
   a. *Orientation to time:* Ask the client to state the year, date, and time of day.
   b. *Orientation to place:* Ask the client to state where he is (i.e., city, state, where he lives).
   c. *Orientation to person:* Ask the names of family members. Ask, "Do you know who I am?" If the client cannot answer these questions, ask him to state his name.

Self-identity remains intact the longest.

Expected findings: The client is awake, alert (see Step 2), and oriented to time, place, and person (AAO × 3).
a. Hospitalized patients commonly lose track of date and time of day, but they easily reorient. As a rule, they should at least know the year.
b. Interpret data carefully. In some situations (e.g., after an automobile accident away from home), the patient may know he is in the hospital but not know which hospital or which city.
c. Patient should know you are a healthcare worker, but not necessarily your name.

Developmental Variations

Older adults—The stress of an unfamiliar situation can create confusion in an older adult.

Abnormal findings: Disorientation may result from physical or psychological problems. Bizarre responses are usually associated with psychiatric problems.

4. **Assess memory.**
   a. *Assess immediate memory* by asking the client to repeat a series of three numbers that you speak slowly (e.g., 1, 5, 8). Gradually increase the length of the series until the client cannot repeat the series correctly. Record the length of the last correct series (e.g., "Successfully repeats a series of 7 numbers correctly.")

Expected findings: Immediate, recent, and remote memory are intact. Average series recall is 5–8 numbers in sequence and 4–6 numbers in reverse order.

Developmental Variations

Children—Number of objects recalled is usually fewer than the child's age in years.

(continued on next page)

Procedure 22-16 ■ Assessing the Sensory-Neurological System (continued)

b. *Repeat the test,* beginning with a series of three numbers, but ask the client to repeat them back to you in reverse order.
c. *Assess recent memory* by naming three items (e.g., "mirror, truck," and "the letter *X*") and asking the client to recall them later during the exam. Alternatively, you can ask questions such as, "How did you get to the hospital? What did you have for breakfast?" However, you will need to verify the patient's answers.
d. *Assess remote memory* by asking the client his birth date or the date of a major historical event.

Developmental Modifications

Children—Assess memory by using names of toys (e.g., truck, ball, puzzle), names of people in his family, or names of familiar cartoon characters.

Older adults—Loss of immediate and recent memory is common; long-term memory is usually not impaired.

Abnormal findings: Memory problems may be benign or may signal underlying neurological problems. Temporary memory loss may occur after trauma.

---

5. Assess mathematical and calculation skills.

a. Have the client solve a simple mathematical problem, such as 3 + 3.
b. If he is able to solve that problem, present a more complex example, yet simple enough that regardless of math skills the client could still determine the appropriate response, such as, "If you have $3 and you buy an item for $2, how much money will you have left?"
c. To assess both calculation skills and attention span, ask the client to count backwards from 100.
d. A more difficult test is to have the client perform serial threes or serial sevens. Ask him to begin at 100 and keep subtracting 3 (or 7).

Consider the person's language, education, and culture in deciding whether this test is appropriate for him.

Expected findings: Mathematical and calculation ability is appropriate for the patient's age, education level, and language ability. The average adult can solve simple mathematical problems and can complete serial sevens in about 90 seconds with 3 or fewer errors.

Abnormal findings: Inability to calculate at a level appropriate for age and educational level may indicate neurological impairment or developmental delay.

---

6. Assess general knowledge.

You can ask questions directly or work this into the overall interaction with the client.

Ask the client how many days in the week or months in the year.

Expected findings: Vocabulary and general knowledge are intact.

---

7. Evaluate thought processes. Assess throughout the exam. Notice attention span, logic of speech, ability to stay focused, and appropriateness of responses.

Expected findings: Thought processes are clear, client responds appropriately, and speech is coherent and logical.

Abnormal findings: Alteration in thought processes may be due to physical disorders, such as dementia; psychiatric disorders, such as psychosis; or alcohol and drugs.

---

8. Assess abstract thinking. Ask the client to interpret a maxim (or saying), such as "A penny saved is a penny earned" or "A rolling stone gathers no moss."

Expected findings: Abstract thinking is intact.

Abnormal findings: Inability to think abstractly is associated with dementia, delirium, mental retardation, and psychoses.

Developmental Modifications

Children—The ability to think abstractly does not develop until the late school-age years or adolescence. To assess a child under the age of 12, ask her to describe things that are like and unlike a named object (e.g., "Tell me something that is like a cup").

9. Assess judgment.
Ask the client to respond to a hypothetical situation, such as, "If you were walking down the street and saw smoke and flame coming from a house, what would you do?"

Expected findings: Judgment is intact.

Abnormal findings: Impaired judgment may be associated with dementia, psychosis, or substance abuse.

10. Assess communication ability.

a. **Listen to the client's speech.** Note the rate, flow, choice of vocabulary, and enunciation.

a. **Expected findings:** Speech flows easily, and patient enunciates clearly. Vocabulary is consistent with the client's age, education, and language fluency.

Abnormal findings: Problems with flow (e.g., halting speech, stuttering, very rapid speech, slurred words) may be due to language problems, nervousness, anxiety, or neurological problems.

b. **Test spontaneous speech:** Show the client a picture, and have him describe it.

b. **Expected findings:** Spontaneous speech is intact.

Abnormal findings: Impaired spontaneous speech is associated with cognitive impairment.

c. **Test motor speech** by having the client say "Do, re, mi, fa, so, la, ti, do." Assess ability to swallow. Observe for clarity of speech, facial mobility, drooling, and oral hypotonia. Ask the client to repeat a short phrase 2 or 3 times and observe for lack of coordination.

c. **Expected findings:** Motor speech is intact.

Abnormal findings: Impaired motor speech is associated with problems with CN XII or with coordination of speech muscles.

d. **Test automatic speech** by having the client recite the days of the week.

d. **Expected findings:** Automatic speech is intact.

Abnormal findings: Cognitive impairment or memory problems cause difficulty with automatic speech.

e. **Test sound recognition** by having the client identify a familiar sound, such as clapping hands.

e. **Expected findings:** Sound recognition is intact.

Abnormal findings: Temporal lobe problems may be the cause of impaired sound recognition.

f. **Test auditory–verbal comprehension** by asking the client to follow simple directions (e.g., "Point to your nose; rub your left elbow").

f. **Expected findings:** Auditory–verbal comprehension is intact.

Abnormal findings: Temporal lobe problems affect reception. Frontal lobe problems affect expression.

g. **Test visual recognition** by pointing to objects and asking the client to identify them.

g. **Expected findings:** Visual recognition is intact.

Abnormal findings: Impaired visual recognition indicates parieto–occipital lobe problems.

h. **Test visual-verbal comprehension** by having the client read a sentence and explain its meaning.

h. **Expected findings:** Visual–verbal comprehension is intact.

Abnormal findings: Impaired visual–verbal comprehension indicates cognitive impairment.

i. **Test writing** by having the client write her name and address.

i. **Expected findings:** Writing ability is intact.

j. **Test ability to copy figures** by having the client copy a circle, letter *X*, square, triangle, and star.

j. **Expected findings:** The client is able to copy figures.

(continued on next page)

Procedure 22-16 ■ Assessing the Sensory-Neurological System (continued)

11. Test cranial nerve I—olfactory nerve.

NOTE: You can assess CN I with your examination of the nose and sinuses (see Procedure 22-8).

a. Before testing, check the patency of the nostrils by gently occluding each nostril and having the client sniff.

b. Have the client occlude one nostril and hold an aromatic substance (e.g., lemon, coffee, vanilla, alcohol) under the nostril.

c. Repeat with a different substance under the other nostril.▼

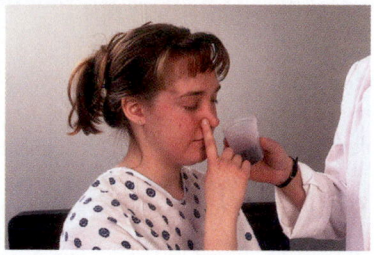

Developmental Modifications

Children—Select a substance that you are certain the child is familiar with (e.g., bananas or apples).

Expected findings: The client can identify the substances.

Developmental Variations

Older adults—May have a decreased sense of smell.

Abnormal findings: Anosmia is the loss of the sense of smell. It may be genetic, related to chronic nose or sinus problems, heavy tobacco use, snorting cocaine, or zinc deficiency.

12. Test cranial nerve II—optic nerve.

NOTE: You can assess CN II with your examination of the eyes (see Procedure 22-6).

a. Test visual acuity by asking the client to identify the smallest print readable on the Snellen chart.

Developmental Modifications

Use picture chart for small children, Snellen E for school-age children.

b. Identify visual field by having the client describe the boundaries of the visual field while her eye is in a fixed position.

c. Perform a fundoscopic exam. (See Procedure 22-6.)

a. **Expected findings:** Visual acuity is 20/20 in the right eye, left eye, and both eyes.

Abnormal findings: Many visual deficits are correctable with eyeglasses or contact lenses. They are not necessarily caused by optic nerve damage.

b. **Expected findings:** Peripheral vision range is approximately 50° in the superior field, 70° in the inferior field, 60° in the nasal field, and 90°–110° in the temporal field.

c. **Expected findings:** Disc margins are sharply demarcated. The cup is half the size of the disc or less.

Abnormal findings: CN II deficits may be due to tumor or CVA.

13. Test cranial nerves III, IV, and VI—oculomotor, trochlear, and abducens nerves.

a. Test EOMs by having the client move the eyes through the six cardinal fields of gaze while holding her head steady.▼

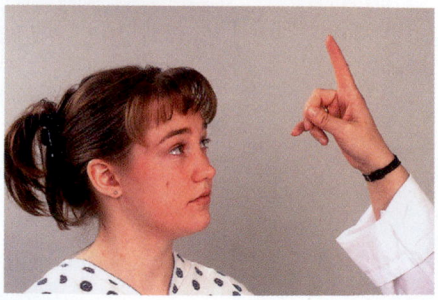

b. Test pupillary reaction to light and accommodation.

NOTE: See Procedure 22-6 for further details on each of these tests.

Expected findings: Client can move her eyes through the six cardinal fields of gaze. Pupils are equal in size and react to light and accommodation.

Abnormal findings: Changes in intracranial pressure (ICP) may affect EOMs and pupillary reaction.

14. Test cranial nerve V—trigeminal nerve.

a. Test motor function by having the client move his jaw from side to side, clenching his jaw, and biting down on a tongue blade.

NOTE: You can assess this function in your examination of the mouth and oropharynx (see Procedure 22-9).

b. Test sensory function by having the client close her eyes and identify when you are touching her face at the forehead, cheeks, and chin bilaterally—first with your finger and then repeat with a toothpick.

c. Test the corneal reflex by touching the cornea with a wisp of cotton or puffing air from a syringe over the cornea.

The corneal reflex is not usually tested on a conscious person because the procedure is unpleasant and a corneal abrasion can occur. A conscious person can blink intentionally, so there is no need to stimulate the blink.

NOTE: You can assess the corneal reflex in your examination of the eyes (see Procedure 22-6).

Expected findings: The client is able to perform all motor functions and can perceive light touch and superficial pain bilaterally; corneal reflex is intact.

Abnormal findings: Inability to perceive light touch and superficial pain may indicate peripheral nerve damage. An absent corneal reflex is an ominous neurological sign.

---

15. Test cranial nerve VII—facial nerve.

a. Test motor function by having the client make faces, such as smile, frown, or whistle.

Note: You can assess this function in your examination of the head and face (see Procedure 22-5).

b. Test taste on the anterior portion of the tongue by placing sweet (sugar), salty (salt), or sour (lemon) substance on the tip of the tongue. Do not test taste by using pungent, bitter, or markedly unpleasant flavors.

Note: You can assess this function in your examination of the mouth and oropharynx (see Procedure 22-9).

Expected findings: The client is able to perform all movements and can distinguish sweet, salty, and sour tastes.

Developmental Variations

Older adults—Have decreased taste sensation, especially sweet and salty, due to taste bud atrophy and diminished sense of smell.

Abnormal findings: Asymmetrical movement may be seen with nerve damage from a CVA or Bell's palsy. Impaired taste may be associated with nerve damage, chemotherapy, or radiation to the face or neck.

---

16. Test cranial nerve VIII—acoustic nerve.

Note: You can assess this function in your examination of the ears (see Procedure 22-7).

a. Perform watch-tick test for hearing by holding a watch close to the client's ear.

b. Perform Weber and Rinne tests to assess air and bone conduction.

c. Test balance with the Romberg test, if it has not already been performed.

See Procedures 22-7 and 22-15 for further details on these tests.

Developmental Modifications

Children—Romberg test is appropriate only after age 3.

Expected findings: Hearing is intact. Romberg test is negative.

Abnormal findings: Hearing loss, loss of balance, or vertigo may result from acoustic nerve damage.

(continued on next page)

Procedure 22-16 ■ Assessing the Sensory-Neurological System (continued)

17. Test cranial nerves IX and X—glossopharyngeal and vagus nerves.

a. Observe ability to talk, swallow, and cough.
b. Test motor function by asking the client to say "ah" while you depress a tongue blade and observe the soft palate and uvula.
c. Test sensory function by taking a tongue blade and gently touching the back of the pharynx to induce a gag reflex.
d. Test taste (sweet, salty, and sour) on the posterior portion of the tongue. Avoid bitter or repulsive tasting substances.

Expected findings: Swallow and cough reflex are intact. Speech is clear. The uvula and soft palate rise symmetrically, and the gag reflex is intact. Taste on the posterior tongue is intact.

Developmental Variations

Older adults—Have decreased taste sensation, especially sweet and salty, due to atrophy of the taste buds and a diminished sense of smell.

Abnormal findings: Damage to CN IX and X impairs swallowing. Damage to CN X changes voice quality.

18. Test cranial nerve XI—accessory nerve.

NOTE: You can assess this motor nerve function with your examination of the musculoskeletal system (see Procedure 22-5).

a. Place your hands on the client's shoulder, and have the client shrug his shoulders against resistance.
b. Have the client turn his head from side to side against resistance. ▼

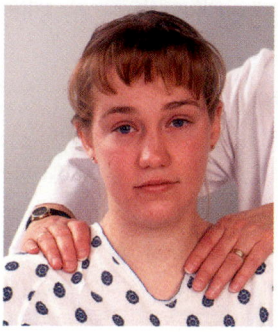

Expected findings: Movement is symmetrical and pain-free. Full ROM of the neck with +5 strength.

Abnormal findings: Asymmetrical movement, pain, or absent movement indicates CN XI disorders.

19. Test cranial nerve XII—hypoglossal nerve.

a. Ask the client to say "d, l, n, t."
b. Have the client protrude the tongue and move it from side to side.

Expected findings: The client can articulate the sounds and move the tongue easily.

Abnormal findings: Tongue paralysis

20. Test superficial sensations.

- Begin with the most peripheral part when testing the limbs (e.g., test the foot before the leg). ➤

If the client can feel sensation in the most peripheral part, you can assume the sensory nerve is intact to that point.

- If the client does not perceive the touch in an area, determine the boundaries of the dysfunction by testing at about every inch (2.5 cm). Sketch the area of sensory loss.
- Wait about 2 seconds before moving to each site.

Wait so that you can be sure that the patient is perceiving each stimulus separately.

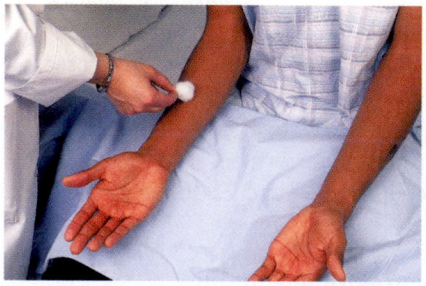

Testing light touch

a. *Light touch:* With the patient's eyes closed, brush a cotton wisp on various areas of the body, comparing sides. Ask the client to say, "Now," when he feels your touch and to point to the spot you are touching.

b. *Pain:* With the patient's eyes closed, use a toothpick (or sterile needle) with dull and sharp ends. Touch various areas of the body (except the face), and have the patient identify whether the sensation is dull or sharp. Alternate the dull and sharp ends as you move from spot to spot. Compare sides of the body.

c. *Temperature sensation:* Test only if the patient's perception of pain is abnormal. Use test tubes filled with hot and cold water. Touch the tube to various areas of the body, comparing sides; have the client say "Hot," "Cold," or "Don't know."

If pain sensation is intact, temperature will be, too, because sensations for pain and temperature are transmitted along the same tracts.

a. **Expected findings:** Able to identify areas of light touch.

Abnormal findings: Diminished sensation or areas of absent perception

b. **Expected findings:** The client is able to identify the areas stimulated and the type of sensation.

Abnormal findings:
- **Hyperalgia:** increased pain sensation
- **Analgesia:** no pain sensation
- **Paresthesia:** numbness and tingling

Developmental Variations

Older adults—May have a decreased perception of temperature and deep pain.

21. Test deep sensations.

a. *Assess vibratory sensation* by placing a vibrating tuning fork on a metatarsal joint and distal interphalangeal joint. Have the patient identify when she feels the vibration and when it stops.

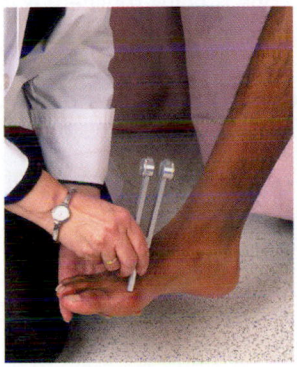

a. **Expected findings:** Vibratory sense is intact bilaterally in the upper and lower extremities.

Abnormal findings: Diminished or absent vibration sense is seen with peripheral nerve damage from vascular disease, diabetes, alcoholism, or damage to the posterior column of the spinal cord.

22. Test kinesthetic sensation (position sense).

By holding the client's finger or toe on the sides and moving it up or down. Keeping her eyes closed, have the client identify the direction of the movement.

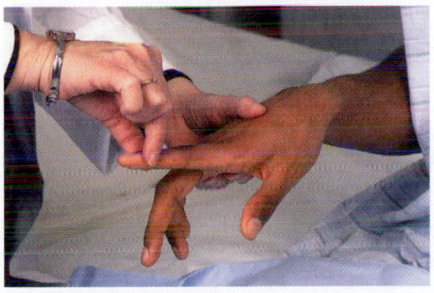

Expected Findings: Position sense is intact bilaterally in the upper and lower extremities.

Developmental Variations

Older adults—May lose position sense in the great toes.

Abnormal findings: Diminished or absent position sense indicates nerve or spinal cord damage.

(continued on next page)

Procedure 22-16 ■ Assessing the Sensory-Neurological System (continued)

23. Test discriminatory sensations.

a. *Assess stereognosis* by placing a familiar object (e.g., a coin or a button) in the palm of the client's hand and having her identify it.

b. *Assess graphesthesia* by drawing a number or letter in the palm of your patient's hand and having the patient identify what was drawn.

c. *Test two-point discrimination* with toothpicks. Have the patient close her eyes. Touch her on the finger with two toothpicks simultaneously. Gradually move the points together, and have the patient say, "One," or "Two," each time you move the toothpicks. Document distance and location at which she can no longer feel two separate points. ➤

a. **Expected findings: Stereognosis** (the ability to recognize the form of solid objects by touch) is intact bilaterally.

b. **Expected findings: Graphesthesia** (the ability to recognize outlines, numbers, or symbols written on the skin) is intact bilaterally.

c. **Expected findings: Point discrimination** (recognizing whether 1 or 2 areas of the skin are being touched). Discriminates between two points on fingertips no more than 0.5 cm apart.

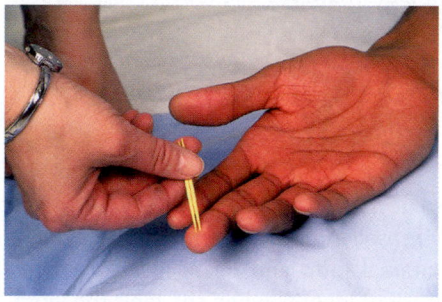

d. *Test point localization* by having the patient close her eyes while you touch her. Have her point to the area you touched. Repeat on both sides and the upper and lower extremities.

e. *Test sensory extinction* by simultaneously touching the patient on both sides (e.g., on both hands, both knees, both arms). Have the patient identify where he was touched.

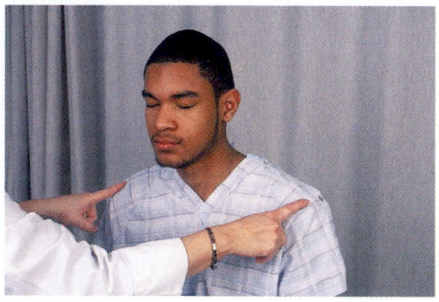

d. **Expected findings: Point localization** (the ability to identify where one is being touched) is intact bilaterally in the upper and lower extremities.

e. **Expected findings:** Extinction is intact: Client should feel the sensation on both sides of his body.

Abnormal findings: Abnormalities in any of the discriminatory sensation tests may indicate a lesion or disorder of the sensory cortex or disorder of the posterior column of the spinal cord.

Developmental Modifications

Older adults—May need more time to respond to a stimulus, as reaction time may be slower.

24. Test deep tendon reflexes.
(See the accompanying scale to grade responses.)

Deep Tendon Reflex Grading Scale

0 No response detected
+1 Diminished response
+2 Response normal
+3 Response somewhat stronger than normal
+4 Response hyperactive with **clonus** (involuntary contractions that continue after the first contraction is elicited by the hammer)

Developmental Variations

Older adults—Reflex responses may not be as strong as in young adults. Reaction time is slower as well.

a. *Biceps reflex* (spinal cord level C5 and C6). Rest the patient's elbow in your nondominant hand, with your thumb over the biceps tendon. Strike the percussion hammer to your thumb.

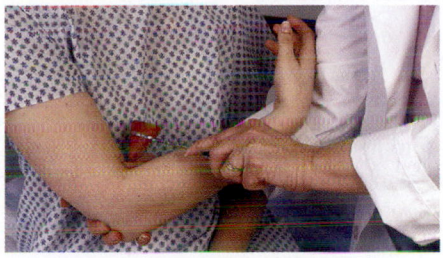

a. **Expected findings:** +2 response: You can feel the biceps contract with your thumb; slight flexion of the elbow.

b. *Triceps reflex* (spinal cord level C7 and C8). Abduct the patient's arm at the shoulder, and flex it at the elbow. Support the upper arm with your nondominant hand, letting the forearm hang loosely. Strike the triceps tendon about 2.5–5 cm (1–2 in.) above the olecranon process.

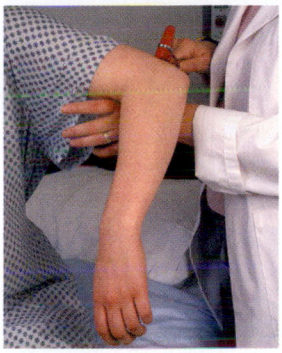

b. **Expected findings:** +2 response: Contraction of triceps with slight extension at elbow.

c. *Brachioradialis reflex* (spinal cord level C3 and C6). Rest the client's arm on her leg. Strike with the percussion hammer 2.5–5 cm (1–2 in.) above the bony prominence of the wrist on the thumb side.

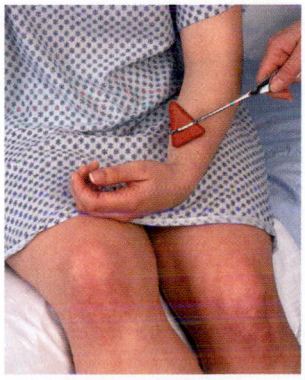

c. **Expected findings:** +2 response: Flexion at elbow and supination of forearm

d. *Patellar reflex* (spinal cord level L2, L3, and L4). Have the client sit with her legs dangling. Strike the tendon directly below the patella.

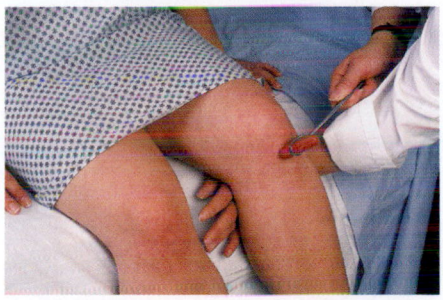

d. **Expected findings:** +2 response: Contraction of quadriceps with extension of leg

(continued on next page)

Procedure 22-16 ■ Assessing the Sensory-Neurological System (continued)

e. *Achilles reflex* (spinal cord level S1, S2). Have the patient lie supine or sit with her legs dangling. Hold the patient's foot slightly dorsiflexed, and strike the Achilles tendon about 5 cm (2 in.) above the heel with the percussion hammer.

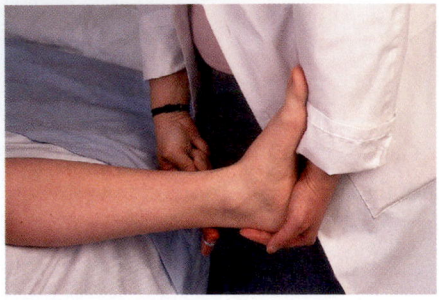

Developmental Modifications

Newborns—test the following reflexes:

- **Rooting reflex**—Stroke the cheek; the head should turn to the side you touched.
- **Palmar grasp**—Place one finger in the baby's hand; his fingers should curl around your finger.
- **Tonic neck reflex**—Position the baby supine; turn his head to one side. The arm and leg on that side should extend, and those on the other side will flex.

e. **Expected findings:** +2 response: Plantar flexion of foot.

Developmental Variations

Older adults—May lose this reflex.

Abnormal findings:

- Absent or diminished responses are seen with degenerative disease, nerve damage, or lower motor neuron disease.
- Hyperactive reflexes are seen with spinal cord injuries and upper motor neuron disease.
- Rooting, palmar grasp, and tonic neck reflexes present after 6 months of age.

25. Test superficial reflexes.

- Plantar reflex (Babinski response): With your thumbnail or pointed object, stroke the sole of the client's foot in an arc from the lateral heel to medially across the ball of the foot. Record response as negative (normal) or positive (abnormal).

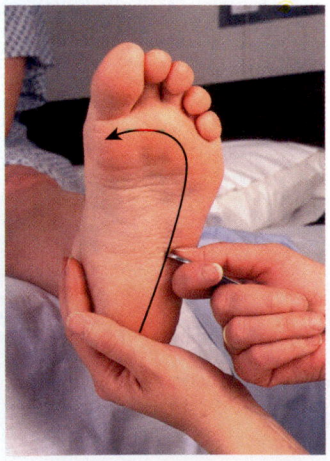

Developmental Modifications

Older adults—This reflex may be difficult to elicit.

Expected findings: Babinski response is negative. All the toes curl downward or there is no response.

Infants and children—Positive Babinski is normal until age 2 or until the child begins walking.

Abnormal findings: A positive Babinski response: dorsiflexion of the great toe and fanning of the other toes. Seen with drug or alcohol intoxication or upper motor neuron disease.

26. Mental status screening.
The following questions may be used for a rapid evaluation of cognitive status. You may have already assessed for some aspects of mental status (e.g., orientation to time).

Questions for Evaluating Cognitive Status

This complete set of questions is included so you can use them for a mental status exam that is not part of a comprehensive assessment. In a comprehensive assessment, do not repeat questions you have already covered in other portions of the assessment.

QUESTION	FUNCTION ASSESSED
What is today's date?	Orientation to time
What time is it?	Orientation to time
Where are you?	Orientation to place
What is the reason for your visit? (If the patient is hospitalized, modify the question as: Why are you in the hospital?)	Communication, vocabulary, thought processes, recent memory
Ask the patient to count backward from 100.	Word comprehension, abstract reasoning
Ask the patient to name several objects that you point to. Be sure to use common objects such as a pen, shoe, or window.	Vocabulary, general knowledge, and word comprehension
Write a brief command, such as "Clap your hands," on a slip of paper. Hand the paper to the patient and ask him to follow the instructions.	Reading comprehension
Ask the patient to write the names of his family members, along with their relationship to him.	Writing, thought processes, memory, sound recognition
Ask the patient to name three things that begin with the letter *D*.	Auditory comprehension, thought processes
Ask the patient to draw a circle, square, and triangle next to each other on a sheet of paper.	Word comprehension, mathematical and calculation skills, communication (naming
Difficulty with any of these questions requires further evaluation.	

? What if . . .

- **The patient is an older adult?**

For a mental-status exam for older adults,

Go to the link to the Mini-Cog exam in **Chapter 22, Resources for Caregivers & Health Professionals,** on Davis*Plus*.

You should also assess older adults for dementia, which is characterized by these four features:

- Mental status change of sudden onset, or fluctuating course
- Difficulty focusing attention, distractible
- Disorganized, illogical thinking
- Increased or decreased level of consciousness (e.g., hyperalert, lethargic)

Delirium occurs in 15% to 60% of older hospitalized patients. You should assess them frequently to facilitate prompt identification and management of delirium.

For a reliable tool for assessing confusion and dementia in older adults,

Go to the link for the Confusion Assessment Method Instrument In **Chapter 22, Resources for Caregivers & Health Professionals,** on Davis*Plus*.

Home Care

Instruct caregivers in home safety if the client has cerebral function deficits or sensory or motor deficits.

Go to Chapter 22, Documenting Physical Assessment Findings, in Volume 1.

Documentation

If you need more information about documenting,

(continued on next page)

Procedure 22-16 ■ Assessing the Sensory-Neurological System (continued)

Glasgow Coma Scale

EYE RESPONSE	SCORE	MOTOR RESPONSE	SCORE	VERBAL RESPONSE	SCORE
Opens spontaneously	4	Obeys verbal commands for movement	6	Oriented and converses	5
Opens to verbal commands	3	Reacts purposefully to localized pain	5	Disoriented but converses	4
Opens to pain	2	Withdraws in response to pain (generalized body response)	4	Uses inappropriate words	3
No response	1	Assumes flexor posture (decorticate posturing—arms flexed to chest, hands clenched and internally rotated) in response to pain. *Indicates problem is at or above the brainstem*	3	Makes incomprehensible sounds	2
				No response	1
		Assumes extensor posture (decerebrate posturing—arms extended, hands clenched and hyperpronated); *Indicates problem at the brainstem level*	2		
		No response	1		
Totals					

Full Outline of UnResponsiveness (FOUR)

Eye Response

4—Eyelids open or opened, tracing, or blinking on command
3—Eyelids open but not tracking
2—Eyelids closed but open to loud voice
1—Eyelids closed but open to pain
0—Eyelids remain closed with pain

Motor Response

4—Thumbs-up, fist, or peace sign
3—Localizing to pain
2—Flexion response to pain
1—Extension response to pain
0—No response to pain or generalized myoclonus status

Brainstem Reflexes

4—Pupil and corneal reflexes present
3—One pupil wide and fixed
2—Pupil or corneal reflexes absent
1—Pupil and corneal reflexes absent
0—Absent pupil, corneal, and cough reflexes

Respirations

4—Not intubated, regular breathing pattern
3—Not intubated, Cheyne-Stokes breathing pattern
2—Not intubated, irregular breathing
1—Respirations greater than ventilator rate
0—respirations at ventilator rate or apnea

***Note:* Education is necessary to use this scale properly.**

To see how to use it,

Go to Iyer, V., Mandrekar, J., Danielson, R., et al. (2009). Validity of the FOUR score coma scale in the medical intensive care unit. *Mayo Clinic Proceedings, 84*(8), 694–701, at http://www.ncbi.nlm.nih.gov/pmc/articles/PMC2719522/

Sources: NGC (2008); Rauen, A., Chylay, M., Bridges, E., et al. (2008); Wijdicks, E. F. M., Bamlet, W. R., Maramattom, B. V., et al. (2005).

Procedure 22-17 ■ Assessing the Male Genitourinary System

➤ For steps to follow in *all* procedures, refer to the Universal Steps for All Procedures found on the inside back cover.

Equipment

- Nonlatex procedure gloves
- Penlight
- Pen and record form

Developmental Modifications for Children

- Obtain the parent's permission to perform this assessment.
- Explain to the child what you are going to do, and expect some resistance or embarrassment.

Children are taught to not let strangers touch their genitals, and many children are modest.

Developmental Modifications for Older Adults

- Assess for incontinence.

Incontinence is one of the elements of the SPICES assessment model for older adults.

Focused History Questions

- Have you noticed any redness, swelling, discharge, or odor in your genital area?
- Have you noticed asymmetry, lumps, or masses in your genitals? If so, describe them, and show me where they are.
- Have you ever been told you have a hernia?
- Have you ever had trauma to your genitals?
- Are you having any problems urinating?
- Are you sexually active? If not, have you ever been?
- Do you have sex with men, women, or both?
- What types of sexual activity do you engage in? Oral, anal, genital?
- Do you have more than one partner? How many partners have you had in the past 6 months?
- Do you use birth control? If so, what type and how often?
- Have you ever been treated for a sexually transmitted infection (STI)? If so, what type?
- Are you concerned about STIs or HIV?
- Do you take any precautions to avoid infections?
- Do you have any concerns about your sexual function?
- Do you have any difficulty achieving or maintaining an erection?
- Have you been taught to examine your testicles?

  In spite of the low prevalence of testicular cancer, men should be aware that a lump in the testicle and/or a feeling of heaviness or swelling in the scrotum could be a sign of testicular cancer and should report these findings to his healthcare provider immediately (American Cancer Society, n.d., last revised 2013a).
- How often do you do testicular self-examination?
- Have you had any surgery of your reproductive tract?

➤ When performing the procedure, always identify your patient according to agency policy, using two identifiers, and be attentive to standard precautions, hand hygiene, patient safety and privacy, body mechanics, and documentation.

Procedure Steps

1. **Instruct the client to empty his bladder and undress** to expose the groin area.

2. **Have the patient stand while you sit at eye level to the genitalia;** alternatively, the patient can lie supine on the exam table with his legs slightly apart.

3. **Inspect the external genitalia.**
   a. *Hair.* Note the hair distribution pattern and condition of pubic hair. See the table discussing Tanner staging, at the end of this procedure.

   The appearance of the external genitalia depends on the client's developmental stage.

Expected and Abnormal Findings

a. **Expected findings:** Hair distribution is triangular and appropriate for age. No pediculosis is present.

Abnormal findings: Sparse or absent hair may result from genetic factors, aging, or local or systemic disease.

(continued on next page)

Procedure 22-17 ■ Assessing the Male Genitourinary System (continued)

b. *Skin:* Inspect the condition of the skin of the penis. Observe for the presence or absence of the foreskin. Note the position of the urethral meatus and any lesions or discharge.

b. **Expected findings:** Skin is intact with no lesions or discharge. Color is consistent with ethnicity. The urethral meatus is midline. The foreskin may be absent (circumcised); if present, it covers the glans and easily retracts.

Developmental Variations:

Infants—Foreskin is difficult to retract in the uncircumcised male until about age 3 months.

Older adults—Penis and testes decrease in size.

Abnormal findings: Ulcerations or lesions (may be seen with a number of STIs, such as genital warts and genital herpes); **phimosis** (foreskin cannot be retracted and becomes swollen).

c. *Scrotum:* Observe the condition, size, position, and symmetry of the scrotal sacs.

c. **Expected findings:** The skin should be free of lesions, nodules, swelling, rash, and erythema. The skin is rugated and deeper in color than the rest of the body. Size and shape vary greatly. The left scrotal sac is usually lower than the right.

Abnormal findings: A rash may be caused by **tinea cruris,** a fungal infection often called "jock itch." Swelling may indicate hernia, tumor, or infection.

d. *Inguinal area:* Note the condition of the inguinal areas. Look for swelling or bulges. The best way to do this is to have the client bear down while you palpate the inguinal canal.

d. **Expected findings:** The inguinal area should be free of swelling or bulges.

Abnormal findings: A bulge may indicate a hernia or enlarged lymph node.

---

4. Palpate the penis.

a. With a gloved hand, use your thumb and fingers to palpate the shaft of the penis. Note consistency, tenderness, masses, or nodules.

b. Retract the foreskin if present.

Expected findings: The penis is nontender with no masses or nodules. Pulsations are present on the dorsal side. The foreskin, if present, easily retracts.

Abnormal findings: Inability to palpate a pulse may indicate vascular insufficiency; difficulty retracting the foreskin or problems with its return to position need further evaluation.

---

5. Palpate the scrotum, testes, and epididymis.

a. Don a procedure glove and use your thumb and fingers to palpate. ▼

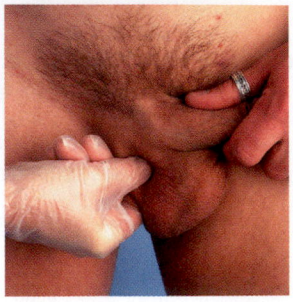

Expected findings: The scrotal skin is rough but without lesions. Each testicular sac contains a testicle and epididymis. The testes are rubbery, round, movable, and smooth. They are sensitive to pressure but nontender. The epididymis is comma shaped. The spermatic cord is smooth and round. There is no swelling or nodules. The left scrotal sac is usually lower than the right.

Abnormal findings:

- A unilateral mass
- Painless intratesticular masses may represent testicular cancer.
- A testicle that is swollen or tender may indicate infection or torsion.

b. Note size, shape, consistency, mobility, masses, nodules, or tenderness.
c. Transilluminate any lumps, nodules, or edematous areas by shining a penlight over the area in a darkened room.

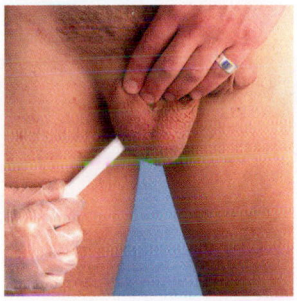

6. Palpate the inguinal and femoral area for hernias.

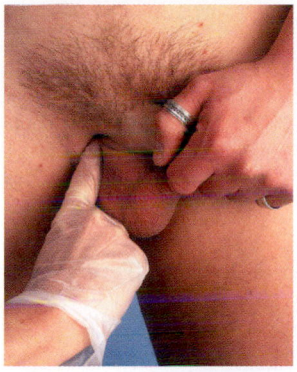

a. Assess for inguinal hernias with a gloved hand. Have the patient hold his penis to one side. Place your index finger in the client's scrotal sac above the testicle, and invaginate the skin. Follow the spermatic cord until you reach a slit-like opening (Hesselbach's triangle). Ask the client to cough or bear down as you feel for bulges.
b. Palpate for femoral hernias by palpating below the femoral artery while having the client cough or bear down.

Expected findings: No bulges or palpable masses are present in the inguinal or femoral area.

Abnormal findings: A bulge or mass often represents a hernia. Refer to the Abnormal Atlas at the end of this chapter.

Direct hernia: protrusion through the abdominal wall.

Indirect hernia: protrusion into the inguinal canal or into the scrotum.

7. Palpate the lymph nodes in the groin area and the vertical chain over the inner aspect of the thigh.

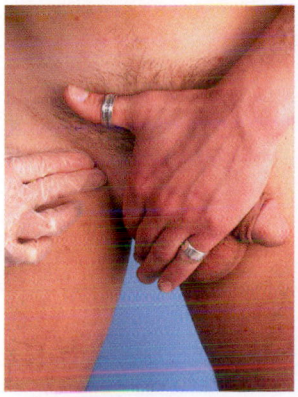

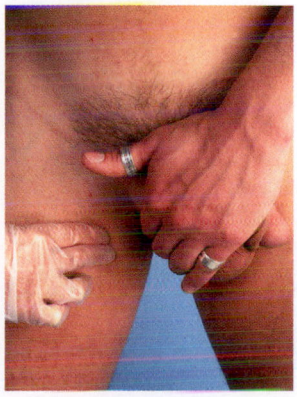

Expected findings: Nodes should be <1 cm in size and freely mobile.

Abnormal findings: Enlarged or tender lymph nodes may indicate local or systemic disease. Also see the Abnormal Atlas: Male Genitourinary System.

(continued on next page)

Procedure 22-17 ■ Assessing the Male Genitourinary System (continued)

Documentation

If you need more information about documenting,

Go to Chapter 22, **Documenting Physical Assessment Findings,** in Volume 1.

Tanner Staging

STAGE	PUBIC HAIR	PENIS	TESTES AND SCROTUM
Stage 1: Preadolescent	No pubic hair except for fine body hair similar to that on abdomen	Same size and proportions as in childhood	Same size and proportions as in childhood
Stage 2	Sparse growth of long, slightly pigmented, downy hair, straight or only slightly curled, chiefly at base of penis	Slight or no enlargement	Testes larger, scrotum larger, somewhat reddened and altered in texture
Stage 3	Darker, coarser, curlier hair spreading sparsely over pubic symphysis	Larger, especially in length	Further enlarged
Stage 4	Coarse and curly hair, as in adult; area covered greater than in stage 3 but not as great as in adult	Further enlarged in length and breadth, with development of glans	Further enlarged; scrotal skin darkened
Stage 5 Adult	Hair same as adult in quantity and quality, spreading to medial surfaces of thighs but not up over abdomen	Adult in size and shape	Adult in size and shape

Adapted from: Tanner, J. (1962). *Growth at adolescence* (2nd ed.). Oxford: Blackwell Scientific

Procedure 22-18 ■ Assessing the Female Genitourinary System

➤ For steps to follow in *all* procedures, refer to the Universal Steps for All Procedures found on the inside back cover.

Equipment

- Patient drape
- Additional light source
- Nonlatex procedure gloves (if exposure to body fluids is a possibility)
- Pen and record form

Positioning

Lithotomy position, if possible.

Developmental Modifications for Older Adults

- Assess for incontinence.

Incontinence is one of the elements of the SPICES assessment model for older adults.

- Older women may have arthritis, which, along with muscle weakness, may make it difficult for them to assume the lithotomy position. You may need to use Sims' position and/or provide support for them to maintain a position.

Developmental Modifications for Children

- Obtain parental permission for this examination.
- Explain to the child what you are going to do, and expect some resistance or embarrassment.

Children are taught to not let strangers touch their genitals, and many children are modest.

Key Point: ***Do not perform internal assessment of an adolescent unless the girl is sexually active.***

Focused History Questions

- Are you having any problems urinating?
- Have you noticed any redness, swelling, discharge, or odor in your genital area?
- Have you ever been told you have a hernia?
- Have you ever had trauma to your genitals?
- Are you sexually active? If not, have you ever been?
- Do you have sex with men, women, or both?
- What types of sexual activity do you engage in? Oral, anal, or genital?
- How many partners do you currently have?
- How many partners have you had in the past 6 months?
- Do you use birth control? If so, what kind and how often?
- Have you ever been treated for a sexually transmitted infection (STI)? If so, what type?
- Are you concerned about STIs or HIV?
- Do you take any precautions to avoid infection?
- Do you have any concerns about your sexual function?
- Have you had any surgery of your reproductive tract?
- When was your last menstrual period?
- How often are your periods?
- Do you have any problems with your periods, such as cramping, breast pain, or heavy flow?
- How often do you have a gynecological health exam?
- When was your last Pap smear?
- Have you ever had an abnormal Pap smear? If so, how was it treated?
- How many times have you been pregnant?
- How many children do you have?
- Have you ever had a miscarriage? An abortion?

➤ When performing the procedure, always identify your patient according to agency policy, using two identifiers, and be attentive to standard precautions, hand hygiene, patient safety and privacy, body mechanics, and documentation.

Procedure Steps

1. Inspect the external genitalia.
   a. Note the hair distribution pattern and the condition of pubic hair. See the table Maturation Status in Females at the end of this procedure.

   The appearance of the external genitalia depends on the developmental stage of the client.

   b. Inspect the condition of the skin of the mons pubis and labia. Observe for color, condition, lesions, and discharge.

Expected and Abnormal Findings

a. **Expected findings:** Hair distribution in the pubic region is inverse triangular. Some hair may extend onto her abdomen and upper thighs. Hair distribution is appropriate for age. No **pediculosis pubis** (pubic lice).

Abnormal findings: Sparse or absent hair (may result from genetic factors, aging, or local or systemic disease); lice, **nits** (white lice eggs), or flecks of dried blood on the skin.

b. **Expected findings:** Skin is intact with no lesions or discharge. Labia majora and minora are symmetrical, with smooth to moderate wrinkling. Skin color is consistent with ethnicity. No ecchymosis, excoriation, nodules, edema, rash, or lesions are present.

(continued on next page)

Procedure 22-18 ■ Assessing the Female Genitourinary System (continued)

Developmental Variations

Older adults—Labia and vulva are atrophied.

Abnormal findings: Ulcerations or lesions may occur with a number of STIs.

2. Inspect the clitoris, urethral meatus, and vaginal introitus.

a. Wearing gloves, use your thumb and index finger to separate the labia and expose the clitoris. Observe the clitoris for size and position.

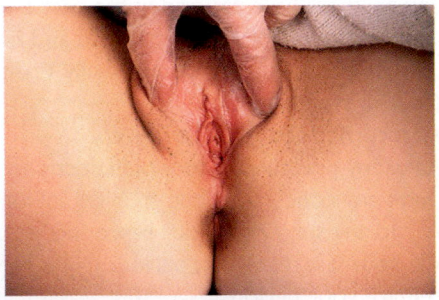

a. **Expected findings:** The clitoris is about 2 cm long and 0.5 cm in diameter. No redness or lesions are present.

Abnormal findings: Enlargement of the clitoris may result from androgen excess or swelling related to trauma. Absence of the clitoris, along with parts of the labia, is seen with female circumcision.

b. With the labia separated, observe the urethral meatus and vaginal introitus. Observe for color, size, and presence of discharge or lesions.

c. Have the client bear down while you observe the introitus.

b. **Expected findings:** The urethral meatus is slit-like, midline, and free of discharge, lesions, swelling, or erythema. The mucosa of the introitus is pink and moist. Some clear to white discharge may be present and is odor-free.

c. **Expected findings:** The introitus is patent, and there is no bulging or discomfort with bearing down.

Abnormal findings: Discharge, redness, or swelling may result from infection. Pale and dry mucosa may result from aging or use of topical steroids. Bulging may indicate prolapse of the uterus, bladder, or rectum.

3. Palpate Bartholin's glands, the urethral glands, and Skene's ducts.

a. Lubricate the index and middle fingers of your dominant hand with water-soluble lubricant.

b. To palpate Bartholin's glands, insert your lubricated fingers into the vaginal introitus, and palpate the lower portion of the labia bilaterally between your thumb and fingers.

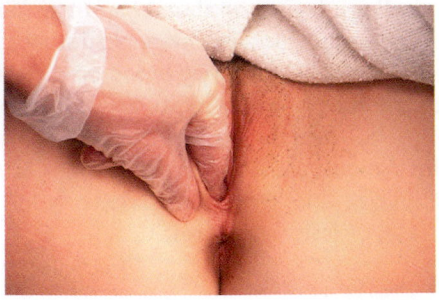

Expected findings: No swelling, masses, or tenderness of the glands is present. There is no urethral discharge. The labia are uniform in texture, and there is no discharge or pain with palpation. The perineum is smooth and firm in **nulliparous** women (women who have had no children), thinner in **parous** women (women who have had children).

Abnormal findings: Pain or discharge from the glands may indicate infection. Fissures or tears in the perineum are painful and require treatment.

c. To palpate Skene's ducts, rotate your internal fingers upward, and palpate the labium bilaterally. ➤

d. To milk the urethra, apply pressure with your index finger on the anterior vaginal wall, and observe for urethral discharge. Culture any discharge you see.

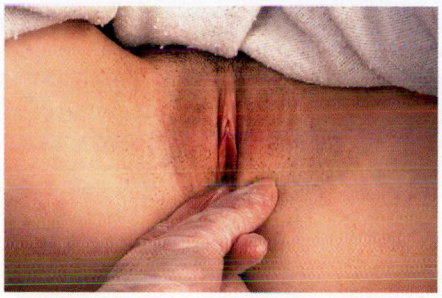

4. Assess vaginal muscle tone and pelvic musculature.

a. Insert two gloved fingers into the vagina.

b. Ask the woman to constrict her vaginal muscles and then to bear down as though she were having a bowel movement.

Expected findings: Muscle tone should be strong in women who have never given birth. With increasing **parity** (number of births), pelvic muscle tone diminishes. Diminished tone may also result from injury, age, or medication. No bulges should be noted.

5. Palpate the inguinal and femoral area for hernias.

Expected findings: No bulges or palpable masses are present in the inguinal or femoral area.

6. Palpate the lymph nodes **in the groin area and the vertical chain over the inner aspect of the thigh.**

Expected findings: Nodes should be <1 cm in size and freely mobile.

Abnormal findings: Enlarged or tender lymph nodes may indicate local or systemic disease. Also see the Abnormal Atlas: Female Genitourinary System at the end of this chapter.

Documentation

If you need more information about documenting,

Go to Chapter 22, **Documenting Physical Assessment Findings,** in Volume 1.

Maturation Status in Females

STAGE OF DEVELOPMENT	BREASTS	PUBIC HAIR
Stage 1. Prepuberty	Elevation of papilla. 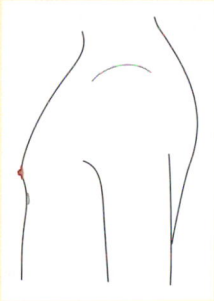	No pubic hair except for fine body hair similar to hair on abdomen. 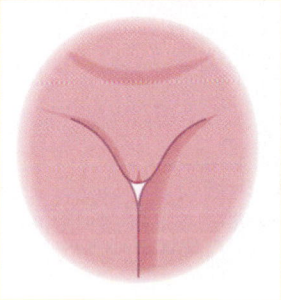
Stage 2	Breast bud. Elevation of breast and nipple and increased diameter of areola. 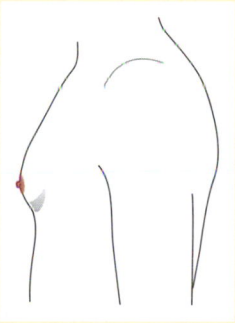	Sparse growth of long, slightly pigmented, downy hair, straight or only slightly curled, mostly along labia. 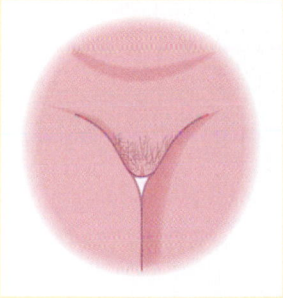

(continued on next page)

Procedure 22-18 ■ Assessing the Female Genitourinary System (continued)

Maturation Status in Females—cont'd

STAGE OF DEVELOPMENT	BREASTS	PUBIC HAIR
Stage 3	Areola deepens in color and enlarges further. Glandular tissue begins to develop beneath areola. 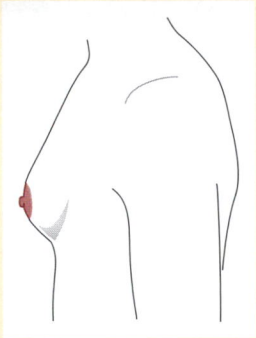	Hair becomes darker, coarser, and curlier and spreads sparsely over pubic symphysis. 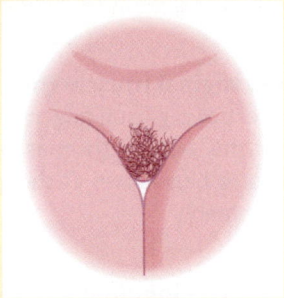
Stage 4	Areola appears as a mound; breast appears as a mound; papilla and areola form a secondary mound. 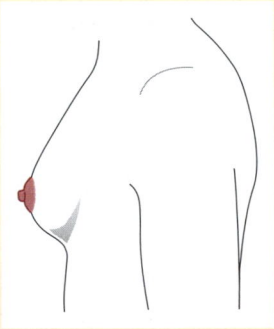	Pubic hair is coarse and curly as in adults. It covers more area than in stage 3, but does not extend to the medial thighs. 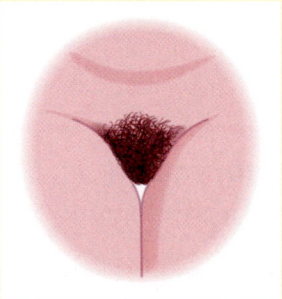
Stage 5. Adult	Mature breast. Areola recesses to general contour of breast; nipple projects forward. 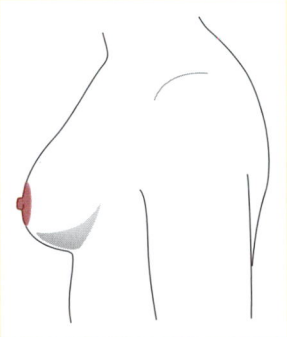	Quality and quantity are consistent with adult pubic hair distribution and spread over medial surfaces of thighs but not over abdomen. 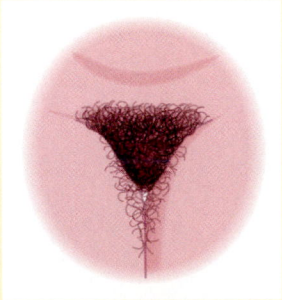

Adapted from: Tanner, J. (1962). *Growth at adolescence* (2nd ed.). Oxford: Blackwell Scientific.

Procedure 22-19 ■ Assessing the Anus and Rectum

➤ For steps to follow in *all* procedures, refer to the Universal Steps for All Procedures found on the inside back cover.

Equipment

- Water-soluble lubricant
- Hemoccult test
- Nonlatex procedure gloves
- Pen and record form

Developmental Modification for Infants and Children

You will not usually perform a rectal exam on infants and children.

Focused History Questions

- Do you have any pain or discomfort around your anus?
- Do you ever have difficulty passing stool?
- Have you ever noticed blood on your stool or when you wipe?
- Do you have or have you ever been told you have hemorrhoids?
- For men, have you ever had a prostate exam or a prostate-specific antigen (PSA) blood test? If so, what were the results?

➤ When performing the procedure, always identify your patient according to agency policy, using two identifiers, and be attentive to standard precautions, hand hygiene, patient safety and privacy, and body mechanics.

Procedure Steps

1. **Inspect the anus.** Note the condition of the skin and the presence of any lesions.

Expected and Abnormal Findings

Expected findings: Anal area is intact, with no inflammation or lesions. Anus is a darker color than surrounding tissue.

Abnormal findings:
- A fissure or tear may be due to trauma, severe constipation, or an abscess.
- External hemorrhoids or skin tags may be visible.

2. **Palpate the anus and rectum.**
   a. *For women,* change gloves to prevent cross-contamination. Insert a lubricated index finger gently into the rectum. Palpate the rectal wall, noting masses or tenderness.
   b. *For men,* have the client bend over the exam table or turn on his left side to recumbent. Insert a lubricated index finger gently into the rectum. Palpate the rectal wall, noting masses or evidence of tenderness. ▼

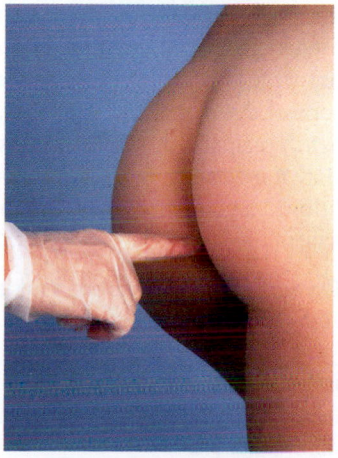

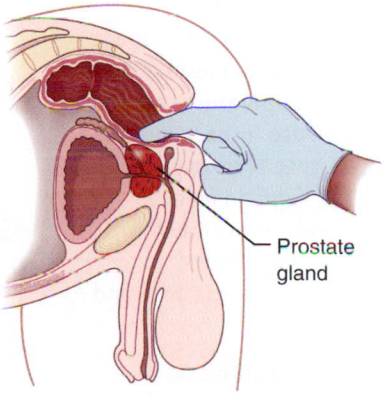

Step 2b

Test any stool on the gloved finger for occult blood. See Procedure 29-1.

Expected findings: Good sphincter tone. Rectum is nontender. No palpable masses or hard stool. The stool is brown and negative for occult blood.

Abnormal findings:
- Hard stool in the rectum indicates impaction.
- Positive occult blood indicates bleeding in the GI tract.
- A palpable mass or enlarged prostate gland requires further evaluation.
- Internal hemorrhoids may be present.

(continued on next page)

Procedure 22-19 ■ Assessing the Anus and Rectum (continued)

Patient Teaching

Instruct the client in the importance of colonoscopy and prostate exam.

Documentation

If you need more information about documenting,

Go to Chapter 22, Documenting Physical Assessment Findings, in Volume 1.

Procedure 22-20 ■ Brief Bedside Assessment

Note: This assessment is not as detailed as in Procedures 22-1 through 22-19. You might perform such an assessment when admitting a patient to a hospital unit. You can also use it for ongoing assessments. For daily patient assessments, you will modify the procedure to fit the patient's health status. You may be able to omit some portions, and you may need to add in-depth, focused assessments of some body systems. The entire assessment should take no more than 15 minutes after you become skilled.

➤ For steps to follow in *all* procedures, refer to the Universal Steps for All Procedures found on the inside back cover.

Equipment

- Thermometer, stethoscope, sphygmomanometer
- Procedure gloves

Focused History Questions

- Ask about any health problems, allergies, or medications.
- Ask your patient how she feels currently and during the previous month and year.
- Ask other questions as you assess each body system.

➤ When performing the procedure, always identify your patient according to agency policy, using two identifiers, and be attentive to standard precautions, hand hygiene, patient safety and privacy, body mechanics, and documentation.

Procedure Steps

1. **Greet the patient and explain what you need to do.** Ask the patient her name and confirm by checking her identity band.
   Assures that you have the correct patient and also allows you to assess mental status and communication.

2. **Observe the environment** (e.g., IV lines, oxygen, urinary catheter) and patient's general appearance (including signs of distress).
   This allows you to identify any immediate actions you may need to take before performing the assessment.

3. **Begin by measuring the vital signs (patient supine or sitting):**
   a. temperature, pulse, respirations, blood pressure
   b. pain status
   c. pulse oximetry

4. **Now assess each body system.**
   a. Use a systematic approach such as head-to-toe.
   b. As you assess each system, observe for mobility, range of motion (ROM), balance, and coordination.
   c. As you talk with the patient, observe her thought processes and level of consciousness.

5. **Assess the integument.**
   a. Ask about any hair, nail, or skin changes, including rashes.
   b. With each body system, inspect skin color, rashes, and lesions; and palpate for temperature, turgor, and texture. Also inspect the hair and nails in that area (e.g., when assessing the legs and feet).
   c. Assess wounds: appearance, size, drainage, dressings, drains.
   d. Inspect and palpate the hair and scalp.

6. **Assess the head and neck.**
   a. Ask the patient about any problems with the head and neck.
   b. **Key Point:** ***Remember to continue assessing mental status and orientation to time, place, and person.***
   c. Inspect the external ears; observe for apparent hearing deficit.
   d. Check the eyes for pupil reaction and cardinal fields of gaze. Ask about and observe for any problems with vision.
   e. Inspect the color of the lips, mucous membranes, and conjunctiva.
   f. Inspect the tongue and oropharynx.
   g. Inspect for hydration, color, and lesions of the mucous membranes.
   h. Lightly palpate the carotid pulse (only if indicated by patient's condition) and listen for carotid bruits.

Do not palpate both carotid arteries at the same time. See Procedure 22-16.

7. **Assess the heart.**
   a. Have the patient sit up and lean forward a bit.
   b. Ask about any cardiovascular problems.
   c. Auscultate heart sounds. Note rate, rhythm, S_1, S_2, and extra sounds.

8. **Assess the back while patient is in the sitting position.**
   a. Inspect skin.
   b. Auscultate breath sounds; compare side to side and apex to base.
   c. Assess respiratory rate, rhythm, and effort.
   d. Note cough, secretions, how many pillows used to sleep on, and whether head of bed is elevated for breathing.
   e. Check oxygen order, SaO_2, ability to use incentive spirometer.

9. **Assess the anterior chest.**
   a. Ask about any respiratory problems.
   b. Palpate skin turgor, temperature, and point of maximal impulse (PMI).
   c. Auscultate breath sounds.

10. **Assess the abdomen, with the patient supine.**
   a. Inspect the size, shape, symmetry, and condition of the abdominal skin.
   b. Observe abdominal movements including respirations, pulsations, and peristalsis.
   c. Auscultate bowel sounds in all four quadrants, and the aorta for bruits.
   d. Palpate all four quadrants for tenderness, guarding, and masses; and inspect for rebound tenderness.
   e. Ask the patient about any weight changes, gastrointestinal (GI) complaints, a change in appetite or diet.
   f. Review the pattern for bowel movements, and when examining a woman, ask of her last menstrual period.

11. **Assess urinary status.**
   a. Review voiding pattern with the patient (including frequency and dysuria).
   b. If there is an indwelling catheter, observe for patency, kinks in the tubing, and color of urine; monitor intake and output.
   c. Palpate for bladder distention.

12. **Assess the upper extremities.**
   a. Ask about any problems with the hands and arms, such as weakness, arthritis, change in sensation, temperature or color.
   b. Inspect the condition of the skin and nails.
   c. Palpate skin temperature and bilateral brachial and radial pulses.
   d. Check capillary refill.
   e. Note any stiffness or limited range of motion of the hands and arms.
   f. Test muscle strength by having the patient grip your hands or two fingers.
   g. Note whether the patient has any casts, traction, splints, or slings.
   h. Observe for edema.

13. **Assess the lower extremities.**
   a. Ask about any problems with the legs, such as weakness, numbness, tingling, arthritis, edema, change in sensation, and temperature or color.
   b. Observe ROM and ability to ambulate or move about in bed.
   c. Inspect the condition of the skin and nails.
   d. Palpate skin temperature and pedal pulses; check capillary refill.
   e. Test for leg strength by asking the patient to raise the leg against your counterpressure. (This is more easily done with the patient sitting.)
   f. Check sensation through light touch, proceeding to pain as needed.
   g. Observe for problems such as paralysis.
   h. Observe for edema.

14. **Ask the patient to stand, and inspect for:**
   a. Gross spinal deformities
   b. Balance and coordination of movements
   c. ROM and gait

15. **With the patient seated in bed, legs extended, check for:**
   a. Babinski reflex
   b. Homans' sign

Documentation

- Document your findings and report any significant changes or findings to the primary care provider. As a student, report your findings to the instructor and the patient's assigned RN for validation and action.
- To print out a form to use as a documentation worksheet when performing a brief physical exam,

Go to Chapter 22, ESG Figure 22-2, Documentation Worksheet for Bedside Assessment, on DavisPlus.

- If you need more information about documenting,

Go to Chapter 22, Documenting Physical Assessment Findings, in Volume 1.

Thinking About the Procedure

To practice applying clinical reasoning to this procedure,

Go to *Davis's Nursing Skills Videos*. For questions and suggested responses, go to Chapter 22, **Thinking About the Procedure Questions and Suggested Responses** on Davis*Plus*.

CLINICAL INSIGHTS

Clinical Insight 22-1 ➤ Performing Percussion

Direct Percussion

Tap lightly with the pads of the fingers directly on the skin.

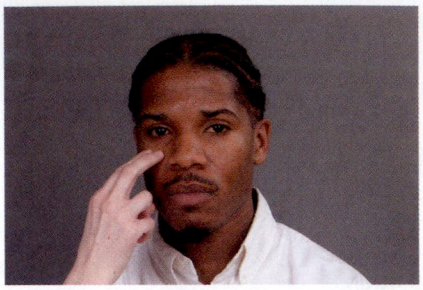

Direct percussion over the sinuses

Indirect Percussion

- Keep your fingernails short.
- Strive for a quiet environment: Turn off all entertainment media and music, shut the door, and so on. This allows you to better perceive the subtle differences in percussion notes.
- One hand is considered the stationary hand; the other is the striking hand.
- Hyperextend the middle finger of your stationary hand, and place its distal portion firmly against the client's skin over the area you wish to percuss.
- Lift the rest of your fingers off the patient's skin. Prevents dampening the sounds produced.
- Be sure both of your hands are relaxed to best perform the technique. Stiff hands will not effectively produce the percussion sounds for assessment.
- Use the middle finger of your dominant hand as the striking finger (**plexor**), and tap the distal portion of the middle finger of the stationary hand using a quick motion from your wrist.

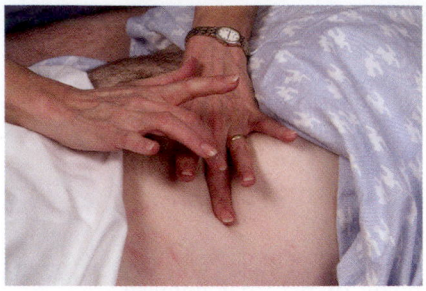

Indirect percussion.

- Use enough force to elicit a clear sound.
- Percuss two times over each location, then move to a new body location and repeat.

Describing Sounds

Use the terms in the following list to describe the sounds you hear. The terms are based on the components of the sounds produced by percussion:

Amplitude—The loudness or softness of a sound

Pitch—The number of vibrations per second; either high or low in nature

Quality—A distinctiveness about the sound produced

Duration—How long the sound lingers

Percussion Notes

SOUND	AMPLITUDE	PITCH	QUALITY	DURATION	EXAMPLE
Resonant	Medium-loud	Low	Hollow	Medium	Normal lung
Hyperresonant	Louder	Lower	Booming	Longer	Hyperinflated lung (as in emphysema)
Dull	Soft	High	Muffled thud	Short	Liver/spleen
Flat	Very soft	High	Absolute dullness	Very short	Thigh or tumor
Tympany	Loud	High	Musical	Longest	Gastric air bubble, intestinal air

Clinical Insight 22-2 ➤ Performing Auscultation

- Provide a quiet environment to facilitate auscultation.

  Clean your stethoscope with a 70% alcohol or benzalkonium chloride wipe before and after using it to examine a patient. Most stethoscopes are colonized by bacteria, although only a small percentage are pathogenic. Cleaning can reduce the bacterial count by 94% to 100%.

- Use the diaphragm to listen to high-pitched sounds that normally occur in the heart, lungs, and abdomen. Press the diaphragm hard enough to produce an obvious ring on the patient's skin.
- Use the bell to hear low-pitched sounds, such as extra heart sounds (murmurs) or turbulent blood flow (bruits). Apply the bell lightly with just enough pressure to produce an air seal with its full rim.
- Place the earpieces facing forward. Seals the ear canal and improves detection of sounds.
- Warm the stethoscope before you place it on the client's skin.
- Place the stethoscope directly on the client's skin. Do not listen through clothing. Clothing can create artifact or reduce the quality of auscultation.
- If body hair prevents good contact with the skin, dampen the hair before you listen.
- Close your eyes as you listen through the stethoscope. This helps improve your focus.
- Concentrate on one sound at a time. Do not try to evaluate breath and heart sounds at the same time. Improves the quality of the data.

Practice Resources

CDC (2009); Muniz, J., Sethi, R. K., Zaghi, J., et al. (2012); Russell, A., Secrest, J., & Schreeder, C. (2012).

Clinical Insight 22-3 ➤ Assisting With a Speculum Exam

Equipment

- Patient drape
- Nonsterile gloves
- Vaginal speculum (see accompanying figure)
  The speculum may be plastic or metal.
  The size of the speculum depends on the patient's history. Use a small speculum for a woman who has never been sexually active or an older woman who is not sexually active.
  If a culture or a Pap smear is to be obtained, lubricate the speculum with warm water. Otherwise, use a water-soluble lubricant.
- Lubricant
- Pap smear slide, spatula, brush, or specimen broom and container with solution
- Fixative, if the smear technique is used
- Genital culture supplies
- Additional light source

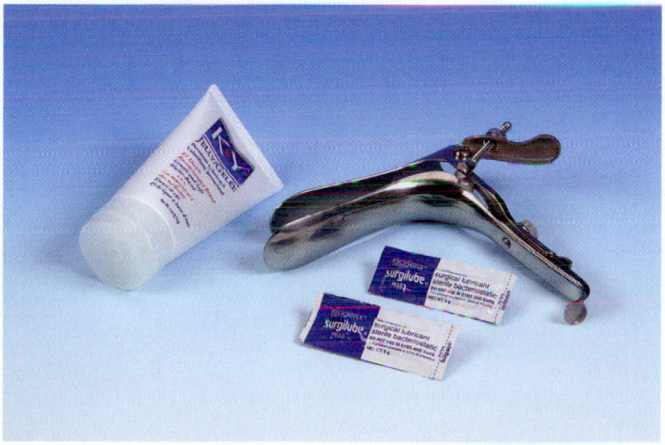

Equipment. A vaginal speculum

Preparing the Patient

- Explain to the patient that an internal examination of her vagina and pelvic organs will be performed. The examination usually takes only a few minutes, and although it might not be comfortable it should not be painful.
- Have the woman urinate before the examination if needed. Emptying the bladder helps the patient to feel more comfortable during the exam.
- Provide privacy and keep the patient warm during the procedure.
- Assist the woman to the lithotomy position, and cover her with a drape.

Inserting the Speculum

The speculum is inserted into the vagina to visualize the cervix (see accompanying figure). Once the speculum is inserted, you may need to adjust the light source for the examiner.

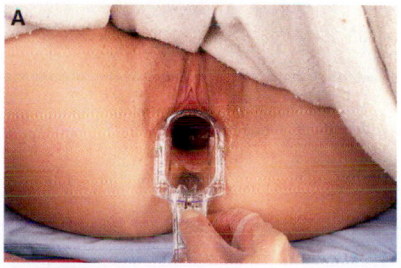

A. A vaginal speculum examination. Placement of the speculum in the vagina.

(Continued)

Clinical Insight 22-3 ➤ Assisting With a Speculum Exam—cont'd

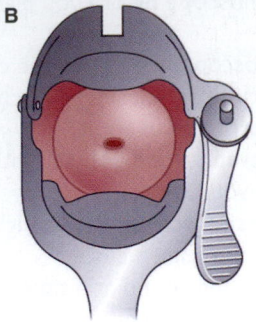

B, View through the speculum

Collecting Specimens

If a routine screening for cervical and uterine cancer is being done, a specimen will be collected. Additional cultures or screens may be required if there is unusual discharge or risk of sexually transmitted infection (STI). Genital cultures are endocervical smears.

Pap Smear Procedure

Most commonly, the examiner inserts a small brush through the cervical os and rotates it to obtain cells from within the cervical canal (endocervical smear). The brush is then rolled onto the slide.

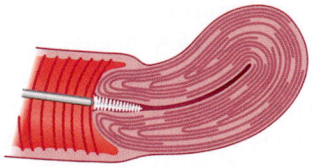

Using a specimen broom to obtain endocervical cells

A second specimen may be obtained by lightly scraping the cervix with a wooden spatula to obtain cells from the ectocervix (the lowest portion of the cervix that protrudes into the vagina).

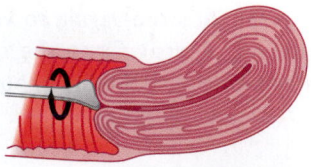

Using a spatula to obtain ectocervical cells.

The spatula is then smeared on the slide. Some examiners use both specimen sources and then apply a fixative, usually a spray or liquid, on top of the specimen to preserve it for examination. After the samples are obtained, the speculum is removed.

Pap Smear, Alternative Method

The examiner inserts a specimen broom into the cervical os and rotates it. The broom is then inserted into a fixative solution and rotated to disperse cells into the solution. This technique is gaining popularity because it is considered more sensitive for detection of cervical changes. After the samples are obtained, the speculum is removed.

Bimanual Exam

After removing the speculum, the examiner inserts lubricated gloved fingers into the vagina while pressing down on the lower abdomen and suprapubic area. This is known as a **bimanual exam.** It is used to assess the consistency of the cervix and the size of the uterus, and to detect tenderness over the ovaries, fallopian tubes, or with movement of the cervix.

Post-Procedure

- Assist the woman to a sitting position at the end of the exam.
- You may need to assist the woman with perineal care.
- If there is any bleeding or discharge, provide a perineal pad.
- Document the date and time of the procedure, the name of the examiner, the patient's tolerance of the procedure, and any nursing assessments or interventions performed.

Practice Resources

ACOG (2010a, 2010b); Bates, C. K., Carroll, N., & Potter, J. (2011).

What Are the Main Points in This Chapter?

- A physical examination may be conducted to obtain data about the patient, to further investigate an identified health problem, to monitor a client's health status, or to screen for health problems.
- A comprehensive physical assessment includes a complete head-to-toe examination of every body system. Data from a comprehensive physical assessment provide guidance for care and determine the need for further assessment.
- A focused physical assessment is performed to obtain data about an actual, potential, or possible problem that has been identified. A focused exam adds to the database created from the comprehensive assessment.
- An ongoing assessment is appropriate for periodic reassessment of the client and reflects the dynamic state of the client. This is a less detailed examination than a comprehensive assessment.
- Before a physical assessment, you will need to gather equipment, prepare the environment, review the skills you will use, familiarize yourself with the patient situation, review the nursing plan of care, and assist the patient to relax by taking the time to develop a rapport.
- *Inspection* is the use of sight to gather data. Inspection begins the moment you meet the client.
- *Palpation* is the use of touch to gather data. Use palpation to assess temperature, skin texture, moisture, anatomical landmarks, and abnormalities such as edema, masses, or areas of tenderness.
- *Percussion*, tapping on the skin with short strokes from your fingers, produces vibrations that allow you to determine the location, size, and density of underlying structures.
- *Auscultation* is the use of hearing to gather data. Direct auscultation is unassisted listening. Indirect auscultation is listening to the sounds produced by the body with the help of a stethoscope.

Abnormal Atlas

Skin Color Changes

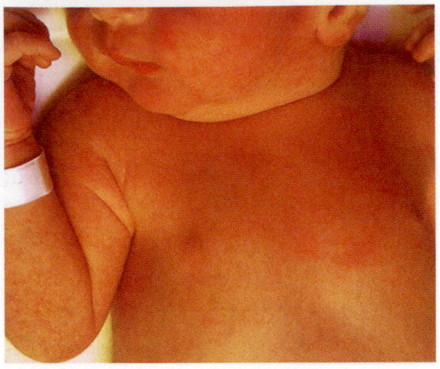

Jaundice

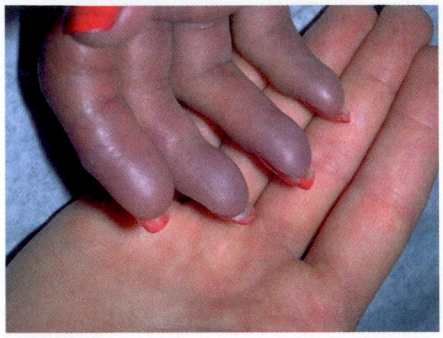

Cyanosis

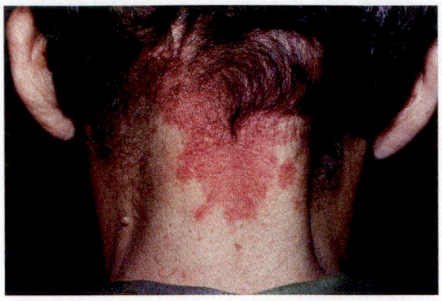

Port-wine stain (nevus flammeus)

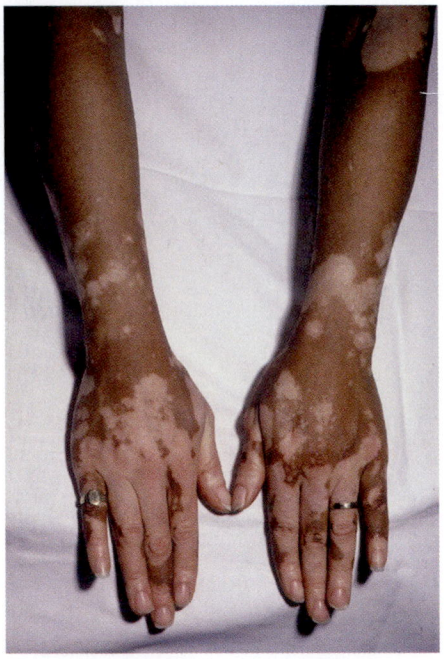

Vitiligo

Skin Lesions

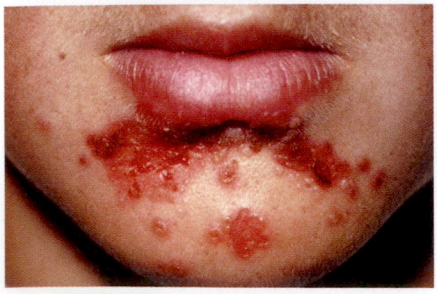

Herpes simplex

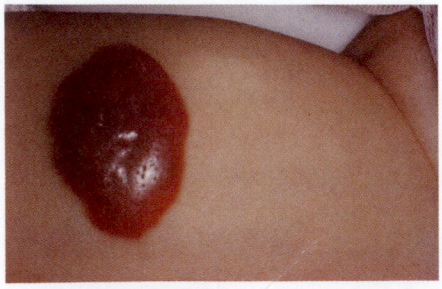

Capillary hemangioma

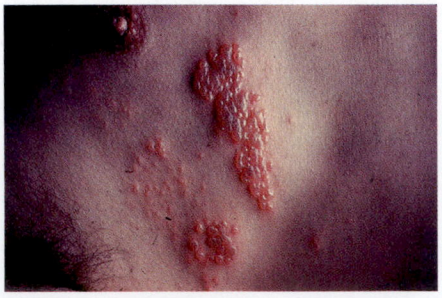

Vesicles (blisters)

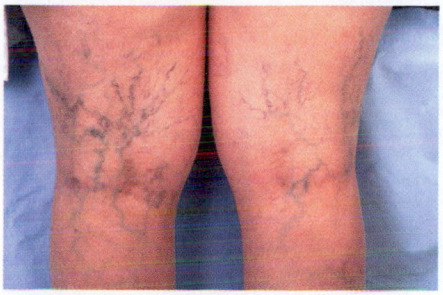

Venous star

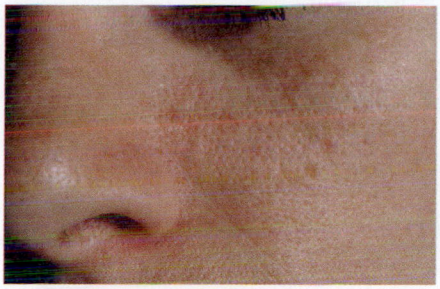

Petechiae

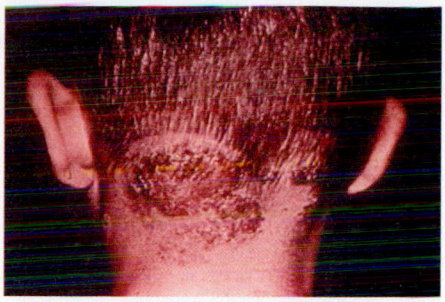

Ringworm

Hair

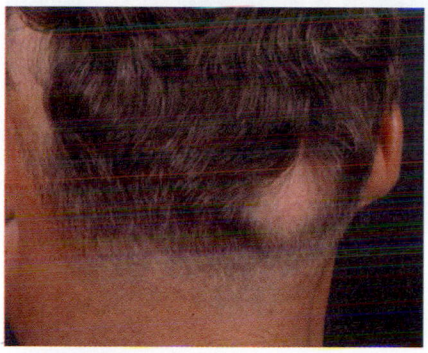

Alopecia areata

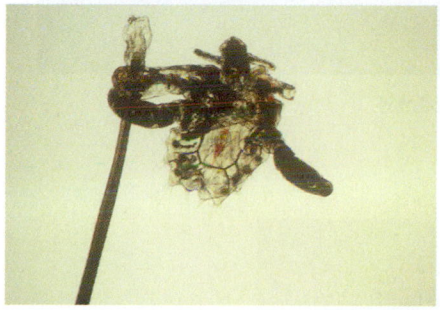

Pediculosis (lice)

Nail Appearance

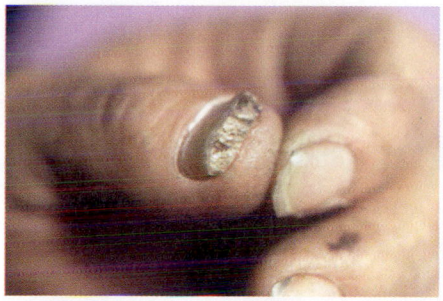

Fungal infection

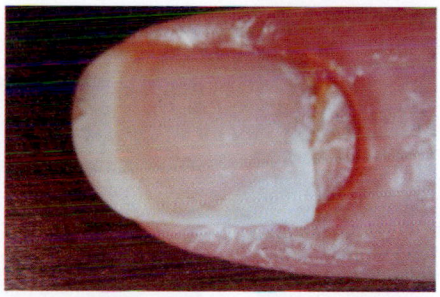

Paronychia

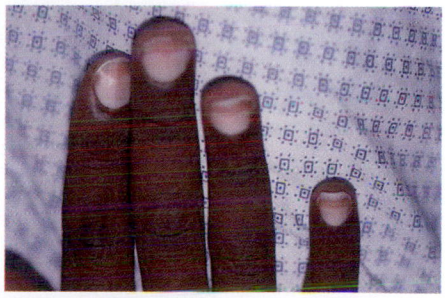

Half-and-half nails

Eyes

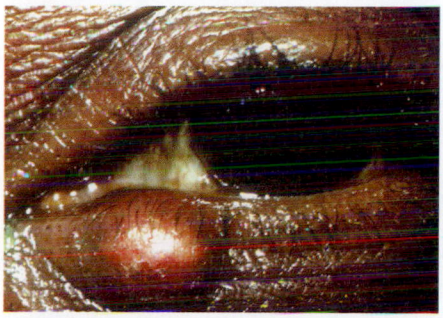

Hordeolum (stye)

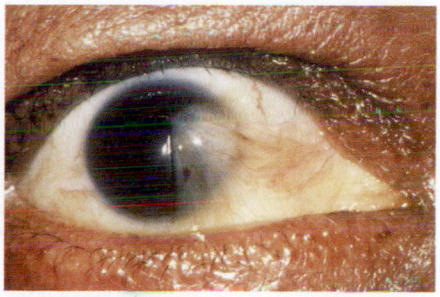

Pterygium

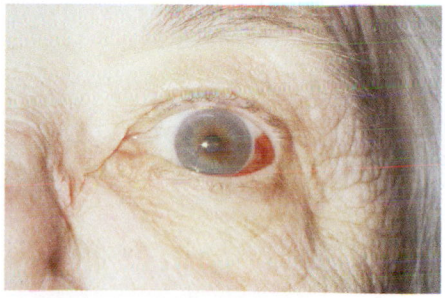

Subconjunctival hemorrhage

Musculoskeletal System

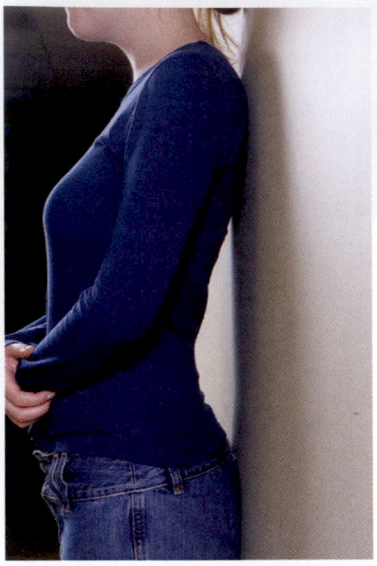

Lordosis

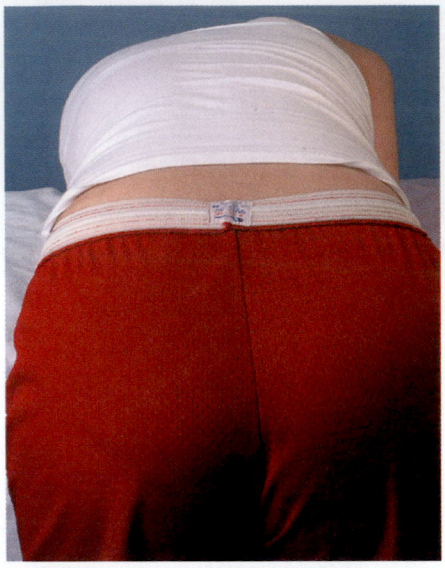

Scoliosis

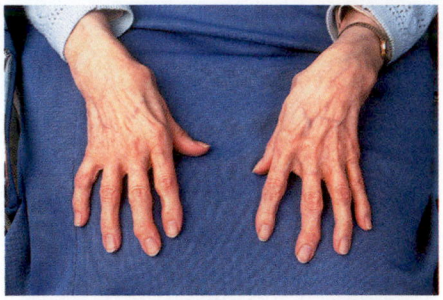

Degenerative joint disease (Heberden's nodes)

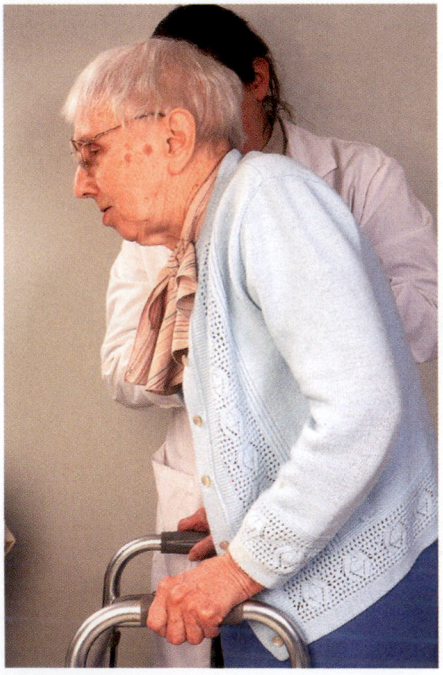

Kyphosis

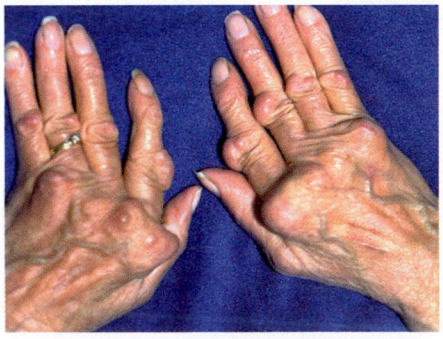

Rheumatoid arthritis

Abnormal Gaits

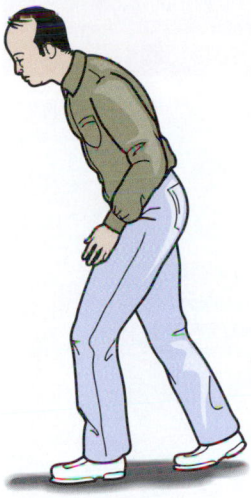

Propulsive gait

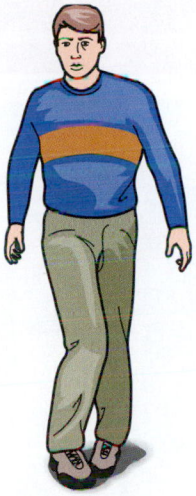

Scissors gait

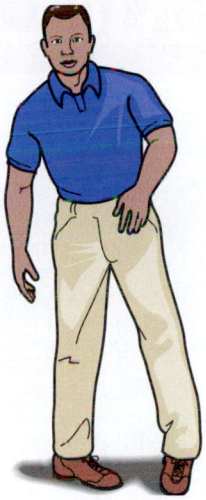

Spastic gait

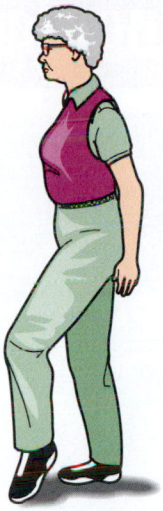

Steppage gait

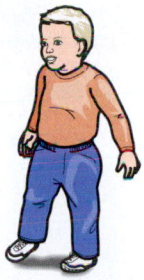

Waddling gait

Male Genitourinary System

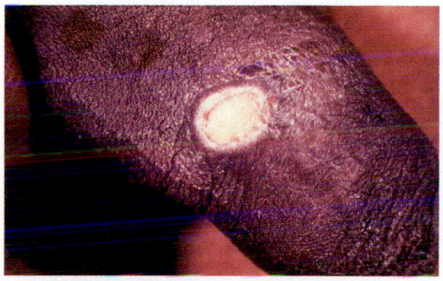

Syphilitic chancre

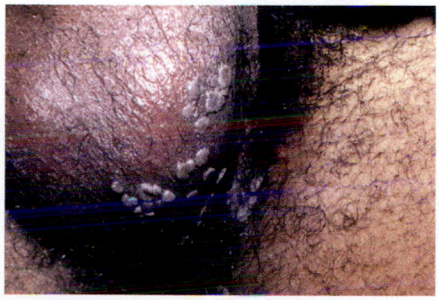

Genital warts

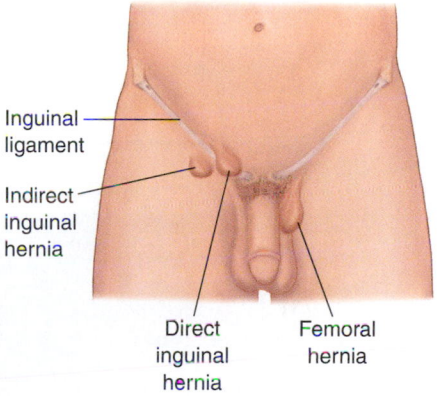

Locations of direct and indirect hernias

Female Genitourinary System

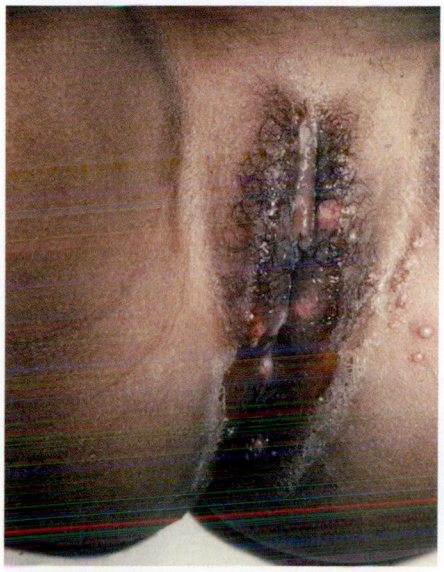

Herpes vulvovaginitis

Knowledge Map

PHYSICAL EXAMINATION

Health Assessment
- Physical Assessment

PURPOSE:
- Obtain baseline data
- Identify nursing diagnoses, PCs, Wellness dx
- Monitor status of identified problems
- Screening

TYPES:
- Comprehensive:
  - interview
  - head-to-toe
- Focused:
  - data gathered on particular topic, body part/functional ability
- Ongoing:
  - prn with every pt. contact

APPROACHES:
ways to gather data
- Head to toe
- Body systems

PREPARATION

SELF
- Know A&P
- What is purpose of exam
- Know pt. situation & plan of care
- Be familiar with equipment
- Exam technique
- Therapeutic communication
- How to document

ENVIRONMENT
- Provide privacy
- Decrease extraneous noise
- Adequate lighting
- Comfortable temperature

PATIENT
- Promote relaxation
- Develop a rapport
- Position patient properly
- Have patient void prior
- Alert patient to touch
- Attend to cultural preferences

AGE MODIFICATIONS:

Infant: have parent hold

Toddler:
- allow to sit on parent lap
- allow choices; use praise
- invasive assessments last

Preschooler:
- demo assessment on doll
- let child help
- give reassurance

School-age Child:
- develop rapport
- allow independence
- demo equipment

Adolescent:
- no parent/sibling present
- respect privacy during exam
- emphasize healthy lifestyle habits
- assess for suicide potential

Young/Middle-Aged Adult:
- no specific modifications unless acute/chronic disease

Older Adult:
- tailor exam to energy and mobility levels
- adapt techniques for vision & hearing changes

ASSESSMENT SKILLS:

Inspection:
- use of sight/observation

Palpation:
- use of touch: fingertips, dorsum/palm of hand, finger/thumb grasp

Percussion:
- vibrations elicited through tapping
- sound indicates location, size, density of underlying structure

Auscultation:
- use of hearing
- direct via stethoscope

Olfaction: not a formal skill
- use of sense of smell

GENERAL SURVEY:
- Appearance/behavior
- Body type; posture
- Dress; grooming; hygiene
- Mental status
- Vital signs/height/weight assessment

Proceeding to:

Assessment of all body systems

CHAPTER 23

Promoting Asepsis & Preventing Infection

STUDENT RESOURCES

The questions and exercises in Volume 2 allow you to practice the kind of thinking you will use as a full-spectrum nurse. Critical-thinking questions usually have more than one correct answer, so we do not provide "answers" for these features. It is more important to develop your nursing judgment than to just cover content. You will learn by discussing the questions with your peers. If you are still unsure, consult your instructor. You will find Response Sheets (for writing your responses to the questions) on DavisPlus.

To explore learning resources for this chapter,

Go to Davis*Plus* at DavisPl.us/Wilkinson3.

Chapter Resources for Chapter 23:

- **Response sheets for all learning activities**
- **Resources for Caregivers and Health Professionals**
- **Reading More About Promoting Asepsis & Preventing Infection (suggested readings)**
- **Concept Map of chapter content**

Interactive Case Studies

NCLEX-Style and Chapter Review Questions

CHAPTER OVERVIEW

For a podcast of an overview of this chapter,

Go to Student Resources, Chapter 23, **Podcast—Chapter Overview,** on Davis*Plus*.

Caring for the Nguyens

Mrs. Nguyen works as a preschool teacher in her community. Kim, her grandchild, has been attending the preschool since he came to live with his grandparents. Mrs. Nguyen tells you at a recent visit to the clinic that Kim has had "a lot of problems with colds and a runny nose since he started preschool."

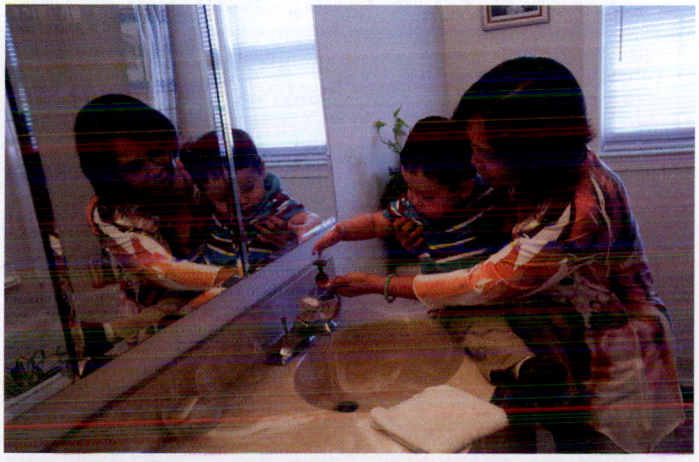

(Continued)

Caring for the Nguyens (continued)

A. Based on your theoretical knowledge of asepsis and immunity, what is the most likely explanation for Kim's symptoms?

B. Do you have enough patient data to make any conclusions? If not, what other information should you gather?

C. Identify three alternatives that may explain what is happening.

D. What strategies could you recommend that Mrs. Nguyen implement at the preschool to help limit the number of infections? Identify at least two strategies.

Practical Knowledge knowing how

As a nurse, you play a vital role in preventing the transmission of infection. Most infection control measures are independent nursing activities that require theoretical knowledge and scrupulous medical and surgical asepsis technique. The procedures and clinical insights in this volume provide the guidance you will need to implement your theoretical knowledge about infection and infection-control concepts.

PROCEDURES

Procedure 23-1 ■ Hand Hygiene

➤ For steps to follow in *all* procedures, refer to the Universal Steps for All Procedures found on the page facing inside back cover. For this procedure, also refer to Clinical Insight 23-1.

Equipment

- Liquid soap
- Paper towels
- Warm, running water
- Hand moisturizer (recommended)

Assessments

- Check your hands for breaks in the skin.
  Breaks in the skin provide a route for microbial entry.
- Inspect the condition of your nails.
  —Nails should be no longer than 1/4 inch from the fingertips.
  —Do not wear artificial nails or extensions.
  —Preferably, do not use nail polish.
  Research indicates the area under the nails, artificial nails/extensions, and chipped polish act as reservoirs for microorganisms.

Procedure 23-1A ■ Using Soap and Water

➤ When performing the procedure, always identify your patient according to agency policy, using two identifiers, and be attentive to standard precautions, hand hygiene, patient safety and privacy, body mechanics, and documentation.

Procedure Steps

1. **Bare your hands and forearms.** Push your sleeves above your wrists, and remove your wristwatch and rings.
   Moist clothing facilitates transfer of microorganisms; jewelry harbors bacteria and creates a moist area on the skin, which facilitates bacterial growth.
2. **Turn on the water.** Adjust the water temperature to warm.
   Warm running water opens pores to aid in removing microorganisms without removing excess skin oils. It also reduces chapping.
3. **Wet your hands and wrists.** Keep your hands below your wrists and forearms.
   The hands are considered more contaminated than the wrists and arms, so prevent water from running from your hands onto your wrists and forearms.
   a. Avoid splashing water onto clothing.
   b. Avoid touching the inside of the sink.
   Microorganisms travel in moisture. The inside of the sink is considered contaminated. ▼

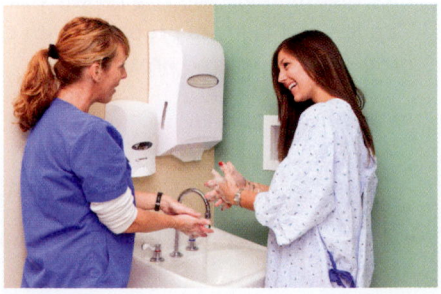

4. **Apply 3 to 5 mL of liquid soap,** which is typically 3 to 4 pumps using a soap dispenser. Rub the soap over all surfaces of your hands.
Three to 5 mL of liquid soap provides adequate amounts to completely cover the hands for maximum effectiveness to remove transient microorganisms.

5. **Vigorously rub your hands together** for at least 15 seconds, lathering all surfaces, interlacing fingers, rubbing around each finger and thumb, rubbing the backs and palms of the hands in a circular motion.
Washing for at least 15 seconds is required for mechanical removal of microorganisms and to give antimicrobial products adequate contact with the skin surfaces to be effective. Attention to all areas of the hands is necessary; research indicates areas of the hands most often missed are the thumb, the wrist, and areas between the fingers.

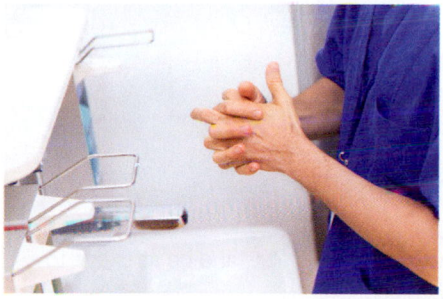

6. **Clean under your fingernails,** if needed, using a disposable nail cleaner.
Areas under the nails harbor high concentrations of microorganisms. Chipped nail polish and artificial nails/extenders support growth of microorganisms, especially gram-negative bacteria.

7. **Rinse your hands thoroughly.** Keep your hands below your wrists and forearms.
Rinsing hands from wrist to fingertips mechanically washes away debris and microorganisms to flow into the sink and not back up the hand and arm.

8. **Dry your hands thoroughly,** moving from your fingers up to your forearms and blotting with paper towel.
Move from the area you wish to keep cleanest (hands). Blotting decreases skin irritation.

9. **Turn off the faucet with** a dry paper towel if it is not automatic. Do not handle the paper towel with the opposite hand.
Prevents contamination of hands from the faucet. The paper towel has had contact with the contaminated faucet and may transfer microorganisms to your freshly washed hand. Many pathogens can live on environmental surfaces, such as faucets and countertops.

10. **Apply a hand moisturizer** at least twice daily; use hand care products recommended by infection preventionists.
Hand moisturizer is recommended to prevent skin from drying and chaffing, which may lead to transmission of infection. Petroleum-based products compromise latex gloves, resulting in permeability. Anionic-based moisturizers can neutralize the residual effects of chlorhexidine gluconate and chloroxylenol. In most agencies, you will use the moisturizer recommended by the infection preventionist. Many facilities use soaps that contain moisturizer.

Procedure 23-1B ■ Using Alcohol-Based Handrubs

➤ When performing the procedure, always identify your patient according to agency policy, using two identifiers, and be attentive to standard precautions, hand hygiene, patient safety and privacy, body mechanics, and documentation.

Procedure Steps

1. **Use alcohol-based handrubs** when hands are not visibly soiled and when certain pathogens are suspected.
Antiseptic solutions are not effective when organic material or dirt from hands is present. Alcohol handrubs cannot remove spores, and therefore should not be used for hand hygiene when Clostridium difficile *or* Bacillus anthracis *is suspected of being present.*

2. **Bare your hands and forearms.** Push your sleeves above your wrists. Remove your jewelry and wristwatch.

3. **Apply antiseptic solution** in a quantity sufficient (at least 3 mL) to cover the hands and wrists.
All surfaces must be covered with sufficient product to effectively remove microorganisms.

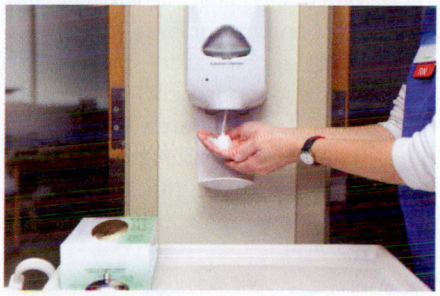

4. **Vigorously rub antiseptic solution** into your hands for 15 to 30 seconds (or as long as it takes to sing "Happy Birthday" if no clock is available), interlacing fingers, rubbing around each finger and thumb, and rubbing the backs and palms of the hands in a circular motion including under the nails until the solution is completely dry.
Fifteen to 30 seconds is recommended by the Centers for Disease Control and Prevention (CDC) for effective disinfection by alcohol handrubs.

(continued on next page)

Procedure 23-1 ■ Hand Hygiene (continued)

Procedure 23-1B ■ Using Alcohol-Based Handrubs

Evaluation

Hands are free of handrub and dry.

Documentation

Hand hygiene is a responsibility of all healthcare providers. It does not require documentation.

Practice Resources

Association of periOperative Registered Nurses (AORN) (2010); Boyce, J., & Pittet, D. (2002); Siegel, J., Rhinehart, E., Jackson, M., et al. (2007).

Thinking About the Procedure

To practice applying clinical reasoning to this procedure,

Go to *Davis's Nursing Skills Videos*, **Asepsis: Hand Hygiene.**

For questions and suggested responses,

Go to Chapter 23, **Thinking About the Procedure Questions and Suggested Responses,** on Davis*Plus*.

Procedure 23-2 ■ Donning Personal Protective Equipment (PPE)

➤ For steps to follow in *all* procedures, refer to the Universal Steps for All Procedures found on the page facing the inside back cover.

Equipment

Following CDC recommendations, you will usually use some combination of gloves, gown, mask, and eye protection, depending on the organism and level of precaution. In certain situations, you may need hair covers and shoe covers (e.g., when full barrier precautions are needed).

- Disposable gloves of the proper size
- Disposable isolation gown
- Face mask (or N-95 respirator mask, as indicated)
- Face shield or goggles
- Hair cover
- Shoe covers

➤ When performing the procedure, always identify your patient according to agency policy, using two identifiers, and be attentive to standard precautions, hand hygiene, patient safety and privacy, body mechanics, and documentation.

Procedure Steps

1. **Assess the need for PPE.** If you need more information about choosing PPE, refer to Clinical Insights 23-3, 23-4, and 23-5.
   a. **Gloves:** When you may be exposed to any body secretions directly or indirectly
   Gloves provide a barrier against body fluids. All patients are considered potentially infected per Standard Precautions (see Clinical Insight 23-3).
   b. **Gowns:** When your uniform (e.g., scrubs) may become exposed to potentially infective secretions
   Examples of such situations include excessive wound drainage, fecal incontinence, or other discharges from the body, or when fluids may be splashed (as in eye irrigation).
   c. **Face mask:** When splashing may occur during close contact (3 ft or less) and potentially contaminate your mouth or nose
   Surgical masks provide a barrier to large-particle droplets (>5 microns in diameter), helping prevent transmission of pathogens to the nurse's mucous membranes.
   d. **Face shield or eye goggles:** When splashing might occur and fluids enter your eyes (e.g., blood splashes, respiratory droplets, or wound debridement). To protect the entire facial area, wear a face shield (for maximum protection, it should protect the crown and chin and wrap around the face to the ear).
   Helps prevent pathogens from entering the conjunctiva directly or indirectly.
   e. **N-95 respirator:** When caring for clients infected with airborne organisms (<5 microns) such as the tuberculosis bacillus.
   This device prevents the airborne transmission of the tuberculosis bacterium. The respirator mask shown is disposable; some are reusable. ▼

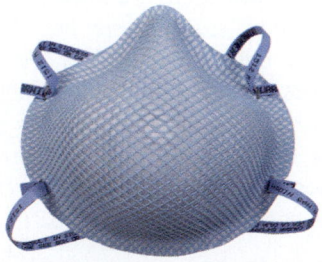

   f. **Hair covers:** When there is a potential for spraying or splashing of body fluids
   Although this is not in the CDC report (Siegel, Rhinehart, Jackson, et al.,

2007), agency policy may advise hair covers in certain situations.

g. **Shoe covers:** When there is a potential for contamination of shoes with body fluids
Although this is not in the CDC report (Siegel, Rhinehart, Jackson, et al., 2007), agency policy may require shoe covers in certain situations. The floor (and anything in contact with it) is considered contaminated. However, certain categories of pathogens require full protective gear, and in those circumstances shoe covers are necessary.

2. Determine the availability of appropriate PPE.
A patient gown is not a substitute for a disposable isolation gown. Isolation gowns must be made of moisture-repelling materials to prevent contamination of underlying clothing and skin.

3. Don the isolation gown.
While donning PPE, the goal is to not contaminate the PPE.

a. Pick up the gown by the shoulders, allowing the gown to fall open without touching the floor or other surfaces.
Touching the floor or other surfaces will contaminate the gown with environmental pathogens.

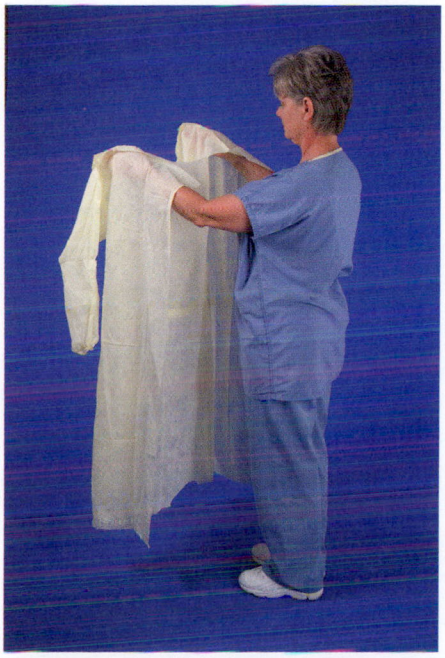

b. Slip your arms into the sleeves.

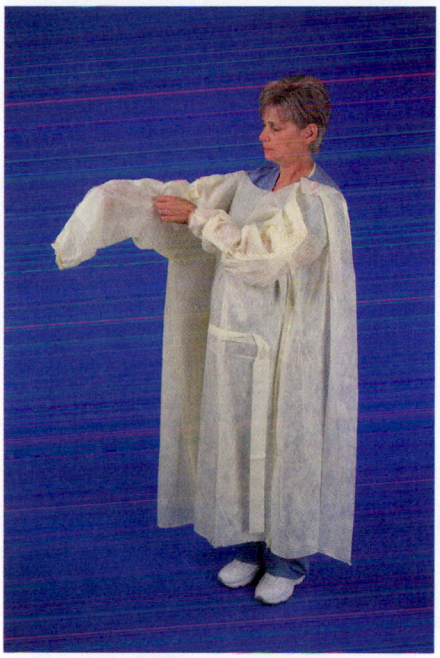

c. Fasten ties at the neck.

d. Position the gown so that it covers the back, and fasten the ties at the waist. Do not bring ties around to the front of the gown.
The front of the gown is considered contaminated after you enter the patient's room. If the ties are at the front of the gown, they will be contaminated, making it difficult to remove the gown safely.

e. If the gown does not completely cover your clothing in the back, wear two gowns. Don the first gown so that the opening is in the front, and then place the second gown over the first, so that the opening is in the back.

4. Don the face mask or N-95 respirator.

a. Determine how the mask is secured. Identify the top edge of the mask by locating the thin metal strip (nosepiece) that goes over the bridge of the nose.
Surgical masks may be secured by ties at the back of the head and neck, loops around the ears, or elastic bands.

b. Pick up the mask with the top ties or ear loops. Place the mask over your nose, mouth, and chin. Press the flexible metal strip so that it conforms to the bridge of your nose.
The mask must fit snugly to the face for maximum barrier protection. Correct positioning will also keep your glasses or goggles from fogging.

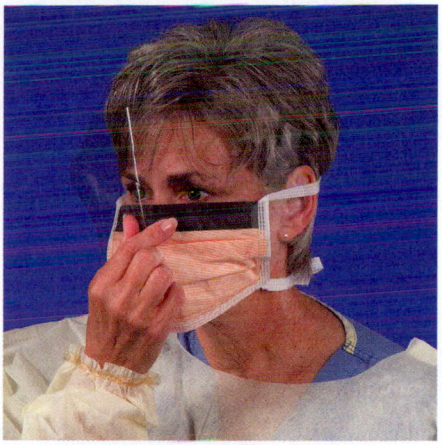

c. Tie the upper ties to the back of your head and the lower ties to the back of your neck or slip the loops around your ears or place the elastic bands as with the ties.

d. Place the lower edge of the mask below your chin, and tie the lower ties.
Covering the nose and mouth creates a barrier to prevent droplet pathogens from entering through the nasal and oral mucous membranes or the respiratory system.

5. Don the face shield or goggles.

a. *Face shield:* Place the shield over your eyes, adjust the metal strip over the bridge of your nose, and tuck the lower edge below your chin. Secure the straps behind your head.

b. *Safety glasses or goggles:* Set them over the top edge of the mask. See Step 1c, d, e for rationale.

6. Don hair cover, if indicated.
Hair covers can be worn to protect from contamination when you anticipate sprays or airborne exposure.

7. Don shoe covers, if indicated.
Shoe covers protect against exposure to airborne organisms or contact with a contaminated environment and as a part of full barrier precautions (e.g., active bleeding).

(continued on next page)

Procedure 23-2 ■ Donning Personal Protective Equipment (PPE) (continued)

8. Don gloves.

a. Select nonsterile disposable gloves of the appropriate size. See Clinical Insight 23-3.
The correct size will prevent gloves from falling off or ripping while you are working with the client.

b. If you are wearing a gown, make sure that the glove cuff extends over the cuff of the gown. If skin is visible between the gown and the glove, tape the glove cuff to the gown cuff, covering all visible skin.
To provide complete protection of hands and wrists, no skin should be visible between the glove and gown.

Patient Teaching

Answer questions the patient may have and educate about the need for PPE, his disease process, and the purpose of isolation.

Home Care

- Identify the type of PPE needed, and ensure that the necessary supplies are available.
- Develop a plan with the client and family for using and disposing of personal protective equipment and contaminated items.
- Teach family members to don PPE as needed.
- Obtain referral for a home health agency to provide support.

Documentation

The use of personal protective equipment is generally assumed and does not require documentation.

Practice Resources

AORN (2013a); Minnesota Dept. of Health (n.d.); Siegel, J. D., Rhinehart, E., Jackson, M., et al. (2007).

Thinking About the Procedure

To practice applying clinical reasoning to this procedure,

Go to *Davis's Nursing Skills Videos*, **Asepsis: Donning Personal Protective Equipment.**

For questions and suggested responses,

Go to Chapter 23, **Thinking About the Procedure Questions and Suggested Responses,** on Davis*Plus*.

Procedure 23-3 ■ Removing Personal Protective Equipment (PPE)

➤ For steps to follow in *all* procedures, refer to the Universal Steps for All Procedures found on the inside back cover. For this procedure, also refer to Clinical Insights 23-2 and 23-3 if you need more information.

Key Point: ***Considered contaminated: front areas, sleeves, mask, and gloves of the PPE (as well as head and shoe covers if you are wearing them).***

Key Point: ***Considered clean: the inside of the gown, gloves, the ties on the mask, and ties at the back of the gown (as well as the inside of the head and shoe covers if you are wearing them).***

➤ When performing the procedure, always identify your patient according to agency policy, using two identifiers, and be attentive to standard precautions, hand hygiene, patient safety and privacy, body mechanics, and documentation.

Procedure Steps

1. Remove gloves first (unless the gown ties in front; in that case, see the section What If . . . ?).
Gloves are the most contaminated PPE and must be removed first to avoid contamination of clean areas of the PPE during their removal.

a. Remove the first glove by grasping the outside cuff of the glove with the opposite gloved hand and pulling downward so that the glove turns inside out. Do not touch the skin of your wrist or hand with your gloved hand.
The outside of both gloves are contaminated. To prevent contamination, touch only the outside (contaminated) surface of first glove to outside (contaminated) surface of second glove. "Dirty touches dirty" and "clean touches clean." ➤

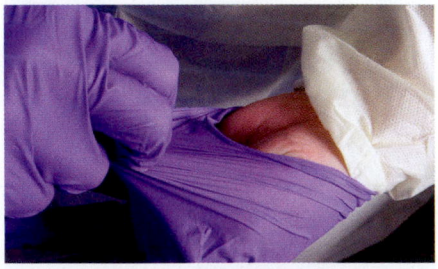

b. Hold the removed glove in the palm of your gloved hand. Slip two ungloved fingers inside the cuff of the remaining glove. Pull the glove off, inside out, over the glove that hand is holding. Do not touch the outside of the soiled glove with your ungloved fingers.

The inside of gloves are considered "clean" because they have not been in contact with client or contaminated surfaces. Therefore, you can touch the insides with your bare hands.

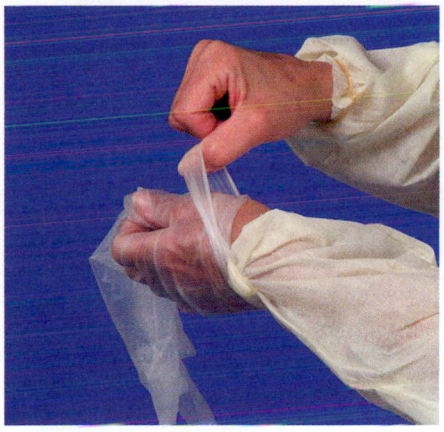

c. Dispose of the gloves in a designated waste receptacle.

2. **Remove the gown**:
   a. Release the waist ties and the neck ties of the gown, bending slightly forward to allow the gown to fall forward.
   The ties and the inside area of the gown are considered clean areas. Gown front and sleeves are contaminated. Allowing the gown to fall forward exposes the clean area for the hands to grasp more readily.
   b. Slip your hands inside the neck and peel the gown away from the shoulders. Reach inside to pull off the cuff and remove your arm from the sleeve. Repeat the maneuver to remove the second sleeve. Do not touch the front of the gown, even if it is not visibly soiled.
   The inside of the gown is clean and will not contaminate your hands. The front of the gown and the sleeves are considered contaminated.

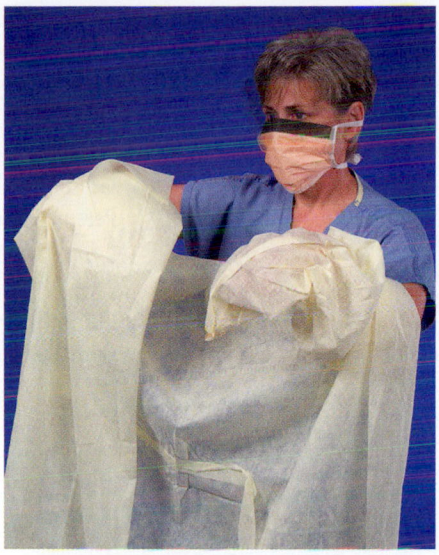

3. **Fold the gown so the inside of the gown is to the outside.** Holding the gown away from your uniform, roll it up with the contaminated front and sleeves in the center, and place in the designated waste receptacle.
   The inside of the gown is considered clean. Folding the gown prevents contamination of your hands, clothing, and the environment.

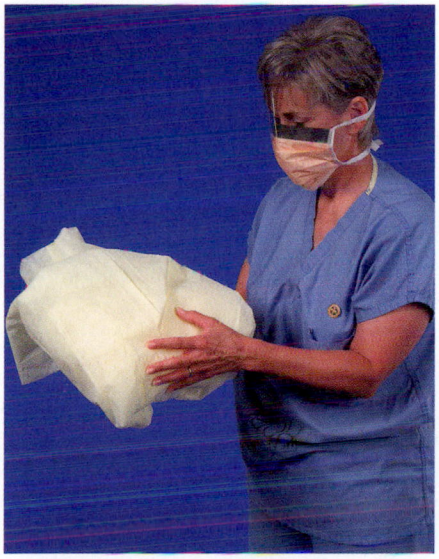

4. **Remove goggles** (if wearing them). Grasp only the earpieces (or head band) of the goggles and pull off the face. Place in the receptacle provided for disinfection if the goggles are not disposable.
   Earpieces are considered clean. Some goggles are cleaned and reused.
5. **Remove your mask or face shield** (if wearing one). Untie the lower ties first. Untie the upper ties next, being careful not to let go of the ties. Touch only the ties; do not touch the front of the mask. Dispose of the mask by holding on to the ties and placing it in a designated waste receptacle.
   Ties are considered clean. The front of the mask is potentially contaminated; do not touch it with your bare hands.
6. **Remove your hair covering**, if you are wearing one. Slip your bare fingers under the edge of the hair cover, being careful not to touch the outside of it. Lift it up and away from your hair. Touching only the inside of it, place it in a designated waste receptacle.
   The inside of the hair covering is considered clean, so you may touch it with your bare hands.
7. **Remove shoe covers**, if wearing them. Be careful to touch only the insides of the covers.
8. **Perform hand hygiene** before leaving the room. Wash your hands after all patient contact even if gloves are worn to prevent contamination.
9. **Close the door.**
   Keeping the door closed contains contaminants and makes signage more visible.

What if . . .

- **The gown is tied in front?**
  This would be an unusual circumstance, but if that occurs, you must untie the front gown ties before removing your gloves; then remove the gloves and untie any back ties (e.g., at the neck).
  Because the front of the gown (including a front tie) is considered contaminated, once you remove your gloves, you could not use your bare hands to untie a front tie.
- **You are wearing two gowns (top one tied in back, inner one tied in front)?**
  Remove gloves; untie waist ties of outer gown, remove the gown and fold it inside out. Remove the inner gown by untying it in front. Fold inner gown inside out. Take off goggles and face mask or shield.

(continued on next page)

Procedure 23-3 ■ Removing Personal Protective Equipment (PPE) (continued)

Patient Teaching

See Procedure 23-2.

Home Care

See Procedure 23-2.

Documentation

The removal of personal protective equipment is generally assumed and does not require documentation.

Practice Resources

AORN (2013a, 2013c); Siegel, J., Rhinehart, E., Jackson, M., et al. (2007); U.S. Department of Labor (n.d.a); U.S. Department of Labor (n.d.b).

Thinking About the Procedure

To practice applying clinical reasoning to this procedure,

Go to *Davis's Nursing Skills Videos*, **Asepsis: Removing Personal Protective Equipment.**

For questions and suggested responses,

Go to Chapter 23, **Thinking About the Procedure Questions and Suggested Responses,** on Davis*Plus*.

Procedure 23-4 ■ Surgical Handwashing: Traditional Method

➤ For steps to follow in *all* procedures, refer to the Universal Steps for All Procedures found on the inside back cover. For this procedure, also refer to Clinical Insights 23-2, 23-3, and 23-7 if you need more information.

Equipment

- Antimicrobial soap (FDA-approved for surgical hand asepsis)
- Soft, nonabrasive scrub sponge
- Disposable single-use nail cleaner
- Deep sink with foot or knee controls
- Surgical shoe covers, cap, and face mask
- Sterile gloves of the correct size
- Surgical pack containing a sterile towel

➤ When performing the procedure, always identify your patient according to agency policy, using two identifiers, and be attentive to standard precautions, hand hygiene, patient safety and privacy, body mechanics, and documentation.

Procedure Steps

1. **Determine that sterile gloves,** gown, and towel are set up for use after the scrub.
   To maintain sterility, the sterile towel, gown, and gloves must be ready for use immediately after you scrub. If you need to gather supplies after the scrub, you will need to start the scrub procedure over again.

2. **Determine the agency policy for** the duration of the surgical scrub and the type of cleansing agent used. This is typically 2 to 5 minutes.
   The type of cleansing agent determines how long to scrub. Typically, an alcohol-based antimicrobial soap requires 2 to 6 minutes.

3. **Avoid nail polish** and artificial nails. Trim so nails do not extend beyond fingertips. Remove rings, watches, and bracelets.
   Rings are a substantial risk factor for harboring moisture and gram-negative bacilli and Staphylococcus aureus; artificial nails and chipped polish are more likely to carry gram-negative pathogens, including pseudomonas, because water collects between the artificial and real nails.

4. **Don surgical shoe covers, cap,** and face mask before the surgical scrub.

5. **Perform a prewash** before the surgical scrub (see Procedure 23-1).
   The prewash removes any visible soil, reduces the number of microorganisms on your skin, and allows you to begin the surgical scrub with clean hands.

6. **Remove debris from under your nails** using a single-use nail file under running water.
   Decreases the number of microorganisms. ➤

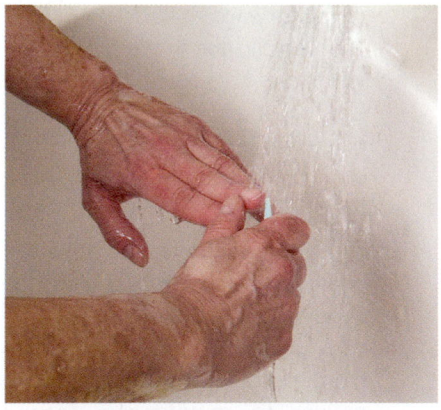

7. **To begin the surgical scrub,** turn on the water, using the knee or foot controls or motion sensors. Adjust the temperature so that the water is warm.
   Hot water removes too many of the skin's protective oils. Knee and foot controls help to prevent contamination of the hands. You cannot touch any unsterile surfaces once you begin the surgical handwash. ➤

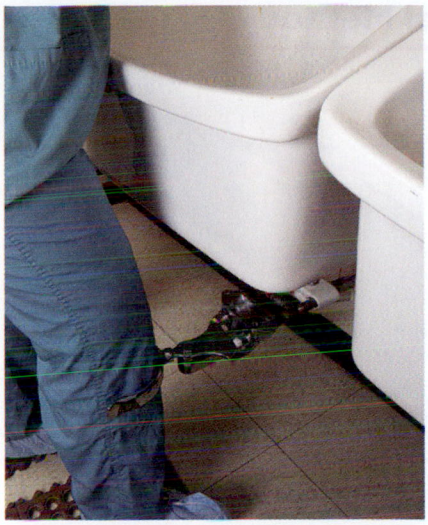

8. **Wet your hands and forearms** from elbows to fingertips, keeping hands above elbows and away from your body. If using a scrub sponge, wet the sponge.
Prevents water running down from your elbows and forearm over rinsed hands.

9. **Apply soap** onto your hands and the sponge. Use a liberal amount of antimicrobial; lather well to 2 inches above the elbow. Do not touch the inside of the sink with your fingers, hands, or elbows. Avoid splashing your surgical attire.
Scrub brushes are harsh on the skin. Soft, nonabrasive sponges are recommended instead. Antimicrobial soap reduces the number of microorganisms.

10. **Scrub all the surfaces** of one hand and arm, all surfaces, using a circular motion. Start at the fingers. Scrub at least 10 strokes each on nail, all four sides of each finger, hands, and arms. When scrubbing the arm, use 10 strokes each for the lower, middle, and upper areas of the forearm. Keep your hands higher than your elbows.
All surfaces of the skin must be scrubbed effectively.

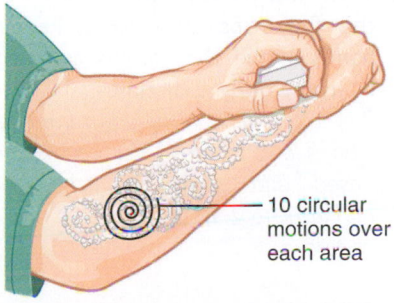

11. **Rinse the brush, and reapply soap.** Repeat the scrub on the second hand and arm. Normally the scrub takes at least 2 to 6 minutes.
The purpose of the scrub is to decrease the number of microorganisms on the hands. The length of the scrub depends on the time needed for the particular scrub agent to be effective.

12. **Rinse your hands and arms,** keeping your fingertips higher than your elbows.
Prevents contamination of hands from water running from the upper arm down onto hands.

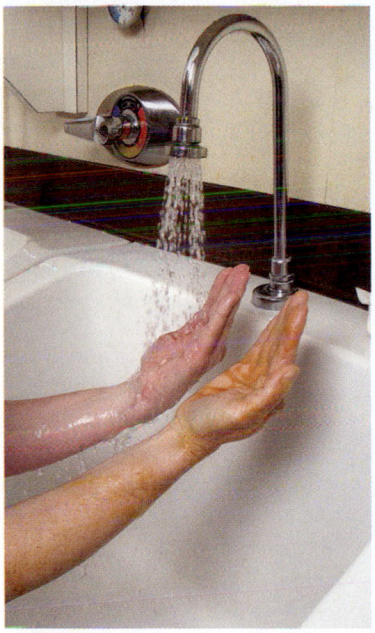

13. **Repeat Steps 8 through 12** if directed to do so by the soap manufacturer or agency policy.

14. **With arms flexed and your hands** held higher than your elbows, move to the area with the sterile towel and gown.
Avoids contamination of hands from water runoff.

15. **Grasp the sterile towel,** and move away from sterile field.
Moving away keeps the sterile field dry and prevents you from inadvertently brushing against the table, which would contaminate the field.

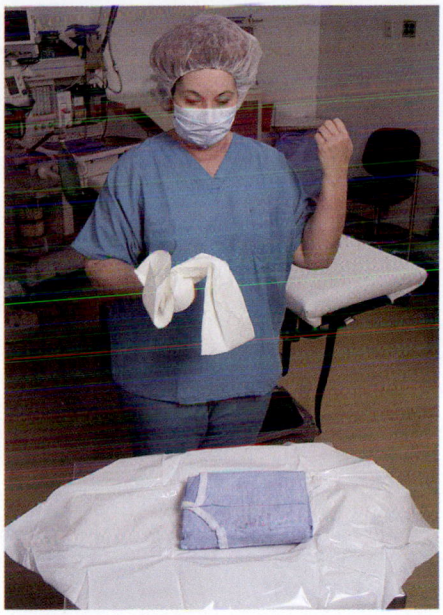

16. **Lean forward slightly,** and allow the towel to fall open, being careful not to let it touch your clothing.
The towel would be contaminated if it brushed against your uniform.

17. **Use one end of the towel** to dry one hand and arm. Use the opposite end to dry the other hand and arm. Be certain your skin is thoroughly dry before donning sterile gloves.
Dry skin prevents maceration and allows gloves to go on much more easily. Use a separate section of the towel to prevent rewetting the skin.

? What if . . .

- **The agency uses an alcohol-based surgical hand-scrub product?**
  a. Perform Steps 1 through 6. Omit Steps 7 through 17.
  b. Using the indicated amount of handrub, rub all surfaces of the hands, including the nails and up the arm to 2 inches above the elbow, according to the manufacturer's recommendations and agency policy.
  Many different products are on the market. Be careful to follow the manufacturer's guidelines for use for maximum effectiveness.
  c. Allow the handrub to dry completely before you don sterile gloves.

(continued on next page)

Procedure 23-4 ■ Surgical Handwashing: Traditional Method (continued)

Patient Teaching

If the patient is able to observe the procedure, explain the purpose of the surgical scrub and sterility.

Documentation

A surgical hand scrub does not require documentation. Instead, chart the procedure (or surgery) and how the patient tolerated it.

Practice Resources

AORN (2010b); Boyce, J., & Pittet, D. (2002); Siegel, J., Rhinehart, E., Jackson, M., et al. (2007).

Procedure 23-5 ■ Surgical Handwashing: Brushless System

➤ For steps to follow in *all* procedures, refer to the Universal Steps for All Procedures found on the inside back cover. For this procedure, also refer to Clinical Insights 23-2, 23-3, and 23-7 if you need more information.

Equipment

- Antimicrobial soap (60% to 95% alcohol, or other FDA-approved product for surgical hand asepsis)
- Disposable single-use nail cleaner
- Deep sink with foot or knee controls
- Surgical shoe covers, cap, and face mask
- Sterile gloves of the correct size
- Surgical pack containing a sterile towel

➤ When performing the procedure, always identify your patient according to agency policy, using two identifiers, and be attentive to standard precautions, hand hygiene, patient safety and privacy, body mechanics, and documentation.

Procedure Steps

1. **Determine agency policy** for duration of the surgical scrub and the type of cleansing product to be used. This is typically 2 to 5 minutes.
   Policies vary from institution to institution, although all should be based on sound principles for infection control designed in accordance with CDC and the Association of periOperative Registered Nurses (AORN) guidelines and follow manufacturer's directions for product use. The type of cleansing agent determines how long to scrub. Typically, alcohol-based handrub is rubbed onto hands and arms until dry.

2. **Before starting the scrub,** gather supplies and set up sterile gloves, gown, and towel for use after the scrub.
   To maintain sterility of the hands after the scrub, the sterile gloves, gown, and towel must be ready before washing.

3. **Observe recommended hygiene.**
   a. Do not wear artificial nails and extendors and chipped polish: Nails should be free of polish and not extend beyond the end of the fingers (¼ inch or less).
   The AORN and CDC recommend avoiding these when in direct contact with patients or in high-risk situations, such as the perioperative setting or among those receiving immunosuppressant therapy. Individuals wearing artificial nails have been shown to harbor more pathogenic organisms in the subungual area than those with natural nails, particularly gram-negative bacilli, especially pseudomonas, and various strains of yeast. Long nails can tear gloves.
   b. Remove rings, watches, and bracelets before starting the scrub.
   Hand jewelry can prevent the handrub from reaching all skin areas and increase the spread of potential pathogens. Risk of infection from microorganisms increases exponentially in relation to the number of rings worn.

4. **Don shoe covers, a cap, and** a mask. Tuck hair completely under the cap.
   Masks filter out possible airborne pathogens carried in the nose or mouth, preventing contamination of sterile areas. Covering the hair reduces the transmission of pathogenic organisms that adhere to the hair shaft or scalp, which is a warm, moist environment for organisms.

5. **Perform a prewash** before the surgical scrub. Use a pick to remove dirt and debris from under the nails; discard.
   Prewash removes any visible soil, reduces the number of microorganisms on your skin, and allows you to begin the surgical scrub with clean hands. The nailbed harbors dirt and debris in which microorganisms live.

6. **To begin the surgical scrub,** turn on the water, using the knee or foot controls or motion controls. The temperature usually adjusts automatically in a surgical scrub sink.
   Water temperature that is too hot can cause injury to the skin, making it prone to disruption in the skin integrity. In addition, it can remove the skin's normal flora and natural oil, which has a protective effect.

7. **Wet hands and forearms** from the fingertips to elbows, keeping hands above the elbows and away from the body at all times.
   Prevents water running down from your elbows and forearm over washed and rinsed hands. a. First scrub the hands and arms to 2 inches above the elbows, as follows:

8. **Dispense a palm full of** antibacterial cleansing solution into your dominant hand. Insert the fingertips of your nondominant hand into the cleansing solution using a twisting motion to apply the product to the fingertips and nails. Then dispense soap into your nondominant hand and repeat.

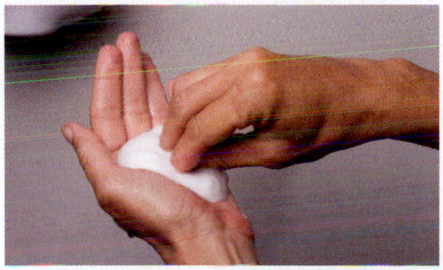

9. **Vigorously rub all surfaces** of your nondominant hand and fingers, adding water as needed. Be sure to rub each digit on all sides. Do not touch the inside of the sink during the cleansing procedure.
Complete contact and friction are necessary for removal of microorganisms adherent to the skin's surface. The inside of the sink is considered contaminated with microbes and should be avoided. Incidental contact necessitates repeating the cleansing procedure.

10. **Rub the hands together** palm to palm.
    a. Bend the fingers of both hands and "hook" the curved fingers together at the ends. Using your right palm, clean the back of your left hand. Then rub your left palm over your right hand.
    b. Then rub your palms together with your fingers interlaced.
    c. Rub the back of your fingers on your closed right hand and rub them back and forth across your left palm, again with your curved fingers "hooked" together. Do the same with your other hand.
    d. Using a rotational movement, clasp your right thumb with your left hand. Repeat on the other hand.
    e. Hold your fingers together on the right hand and move them back and forth and in a circular pattern against your other palm, and vice versa.
    Although the palmar surface carries more organisms than the back side of the hands and arms, this area nonetheless should be cleansed thoroughly to reduce microbial colonization.

11. **Rinse using deep basin sink** with knee-, foot-, or motion-operated controls.
Improved adherence to sterile technique commonly results from use of motion- or foot/knee-operated or motion controls for faucets.

12. **Next cleanse the remaining 2/3** of the arms, beginning at the wrist, to 2 inches above the elbow. Cover every aspect of the middle and upper third of the forearm.

13. **Dispense cleansing solution** into the hands each time you cleanse a new area. Be sure the dispenser is not blocked.
A blocked dispenser can interfere with obtaining the amount of product needed for reducing bacterial colonization.

14. **First, scrub the nondominant arm** wrist-to-elbow. Then repeat the wrist-to-elbow scrub on the dominant arm. Rinse each arm thoroughly and independently on the dominant arm.

15. **This completes 1 washing cycle.** Using the same motions, beginning with Step 8, perform a 2nd cycle. Then finish with a 3rd cycle in which you scrub only the hands (Steps 8–11). The scrub is complete after cleansing every aspect of the hands and forearms for 3 full minutes.
The AORN promotes a 2- to 3-minute scrub time using an antiseptic detergent in order to achieve maximal microbicidal activity while avoiding irritant contact dermatitis associated with use of an abrasive sponge. Reduced time required to perform the surgical scrub often results in increased compliance with the prescribed technique.

16. **With arms flexed and hands** held higher than the elbows away from the body, move to the area with the sterile towel and gown.
This position prevents water running down from your elbows and forearm over rinsed hands.

17. **Grasp the sterile towel,** and back away from the sterile field. Lean forward slightly, and allow the towel to fall open, being careful not to let it touch clothing or gown.
This motion is performed to maintain a dry sterile field and prevent inadvertent brushing against the table and contaminating the field.

18. **Use one end of the towel** to dry one hand and arm using a dabbing motion. Dry the other hand and arm with the opposite end of the towel.
Use of a separate section of the towel guards against inadvertently rewetting the skin or contaminating an already clean area.

19. **Allow time for the skin to dry** thoroughly before donning sterile gloves.
Dry skin prevents maceration and allows the gloves to go on more easily. Moisture left on the skin can be a source of further microbial contamination.

20. **Once the brushless scrub is** complete, prevent contamination of the hands and forearms when moving from the scrub sink to the sterile table by keeping the hands in front of the body and above the waist. It may be necessary to enter backwards through the door of the surgical suite to prevent contamination of the scrubbed hands.

(continued on next page)

Procedure 23-5 ■ Surgical Handwashing: Brushless System (continued)

Documentation

A brushless surgical hand scrub does not require documentation in the patient's medical record. However, you must adhere to the institution's policy for performing the technique.

Patient Teaching

If the patient is able to observe the procedure, explain the purpose of a diligent approach to surgical scrub for promoting a low-risk environment for infection.

Home Care Adaptations

Sinks in the home environment typically do not have knee- or foot-operated controls or motion-sensor on/off devices. Therefore, when scrubbing for a sterile procedure in the home, contact with the faucet handles is performed with barrier objects (e.g., a paper towel) between the clean hands and the environmental surface.

Practice Resources

AORN (2013a, b); Association for Surgical Technologists (2008); CDC (2002); George, D., & Bhabra, M. A. (2010).

Thinking About the Procedure

To practice applying clinical reasoning to this procedure,

Go to *Davis's Nursing Skills Videos*, **Asepsis: Surgical Handwashing: Brushless System.**

For suggested questions and responses,

Go to Chapter 23, **Thinking About the Procedure Questions and Suggested Responses,** on Davis*Plus*.

Procedure 23-6 ■ Sterile Gown and Gloves (Closed Method)

➤ For steps to follow in *all* procedures, refer to the Universal Steps for All Procedures found on the inside back cover. For this procedure, also refer to Clinical Insights 23-2, 23-3, and 23-7 if you need more information.

Equipment

- Sterile gloves of the right size
- Sterile gown

(These should be lying on a sterile field. If they are not, you will need to create a sterile field to place them on.)

➤ When performing the procedure always identify your patient according to agency policy, using two identifiers, and be attentive to standard precautions, hand hygiene, patient safety and privacy, body mechanics, and documentation.

Procedure Steps

1. **Grasp the gown at the neckline.** Hold the gown up and allow it to fall open as you step back from the table. Be careful not to allow the gown to come into contact with nonsterile areas while you are lifting it off the table and opening it.
   The gown will be contaminated if it touches unsterile objects. ▼

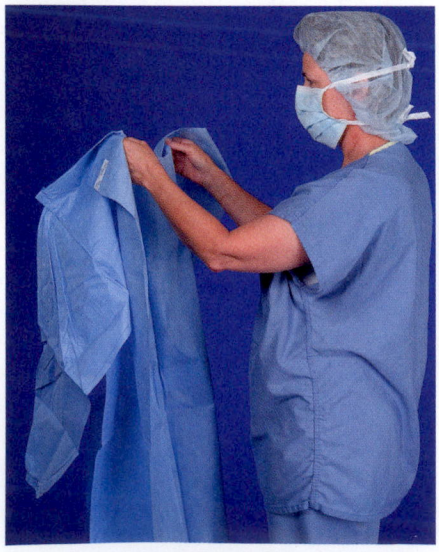

2. **Slide both arms into** the sleeves, but do not extend your hands through the cuffs. ▼

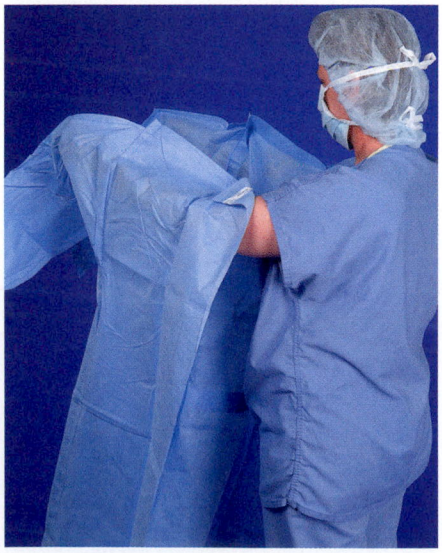

3. **Keep the sleeves of the gown** above waist level.
   Hands will contaminate the sleeve edge if allowed to pass through the cuff.
4. **Have a coworker (or the circulating** nurse, if you are in the operating room) stand behind you and pull the shoulders of the gown up and tie the neck tie. The coworker touches only the inside of the gown while pulling it up.
   Touching only the inside prevents contamination of the gown with the nurse's hands.
5. **Don sterile gloves** using the closed method.
   a. Open the sterile glove wrapper, keeping your fingers inside the sleeve of the gown. The outer wrapper has already been discarded.
   b. Glove the dominant hand first:
      (1) With your nondominant hand, keeping your hands inside the gown sleeves, grasp the cuff of the glove for your dominant hand. Turn your dominant hand palm up.

Keeping the hand inside the cuff ensures that you are making contact with the sterile gown; sterile is touching sterile.

(2) Lay the glove on the dominant gown cuff, thumb side down with the glove opening pointed toward the fingers, and thumb of glove positioned over the thumb-side of the hand.

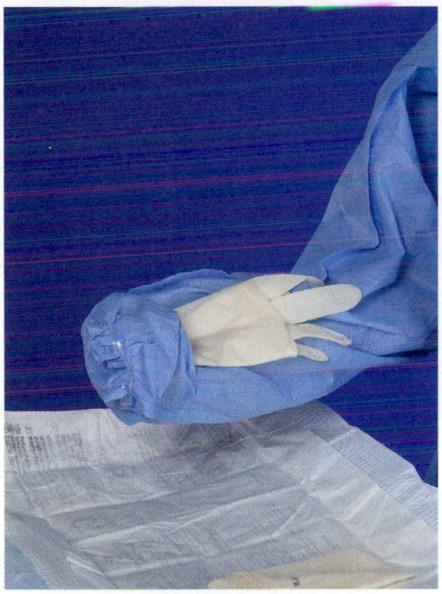

(3) Keeping your dominant hand inside the sleeve, grasp the inside of the glove cuff.

(4) With your other hand (inside its sleeve), grasp the upper side of the glove cuff and stretch it over the gown cuff.

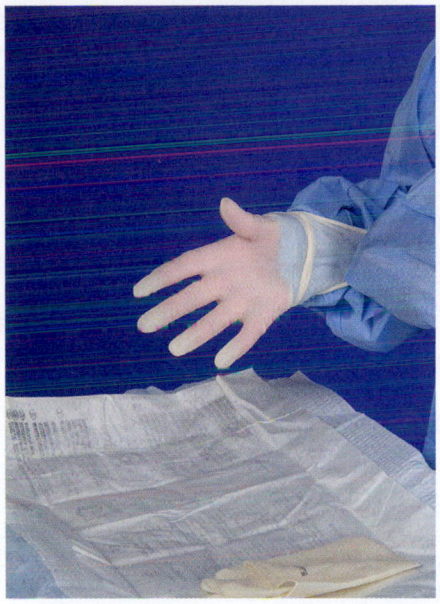

(5) Pull the sleeve of your gown up to pull the glove cuff over your wrist as you move your fingers into the glove fingers.

c. **Glove the nondominant hand.**

(1) Place the fingers of your gloved hand under the cuff of the second glove. Lay the glove on the forearm of your nondominant hand. Grasp and anchor the inside glove cuff with your nondominant (ungloved) hand through the gown, being careful to keep fingers inside the gown.

(2) With your dominant (gloved) hand, pull the glove cuff over the cuff of the gown as you move your fingers into the glove.

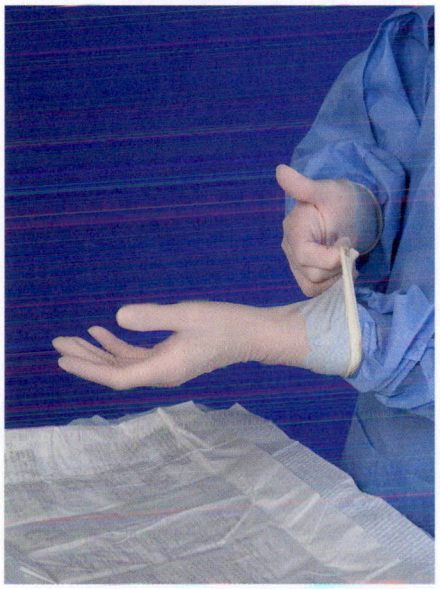

d. **Adjust the fingers in both gloves so the excess glove is pulled over the fingertips.**

Maintains sterility of the gown and gloves by maintaining a closed system. The final adjustment of the gloves is done when both gloves are in place to prevent contaminating the gloves. Taut gloves, especially over the fingertips, allow better feel and dexterity.

6. **Grasp the waist tie on the gown,** and hand the tie to the circulating nurse or a coworker who is wearing a hair cover and mask. Your coworker will grab the tie with sterile forceps.

The tie is considered sterile. You will need help pulling it around you. A coworker can help you. Using sterile forceps keeps the tie sterile.

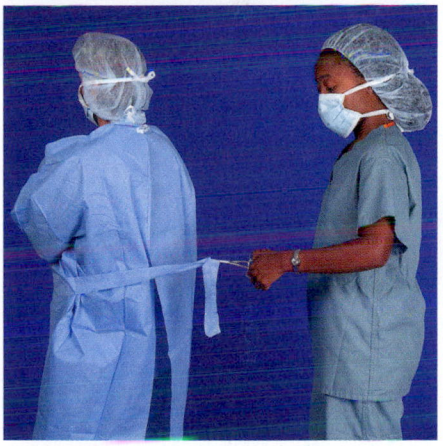

7. **Make a three-quarter turn,** and receive the tie from your coworker.

Because only areas within your field of vision are considered sterile, a coworker must pull the waist tie around you.

8. **Secure the waist tie.**

Ensures that the gown is secured and will not expose clothing to a sterile field.

(continued on next page)

Procedure 23-6 ■ Sterile Gown and Gloves (Closed Method) (continued)

Patient Teaching

If the patient is alert during the procedure, explain:

- The need for the sterile procedure
- Why he must not touch the drapes
- Why he must not move or talk once the drapes are in place
- Explain any special precautions during the procedure

Documentation

- Donning sterile gown and gloves does not require documentation.
- You will need to chart the procedure performed and how the patient tolerated it.
- In the operating room, the circulating nurse charts about the surgery and the patient's response.

? What if . . .

- **Your hand inadvertently comes through the cuff opening when putting on the gown?**

  Change gowns. The cuff would have been contaminated and would then contaminate your glove.

Practice Resources

AORN (2010a, 2013a, 2013b); CDC (2002).

Thinking About the Procedure

To practice applying clinical reasoning to this procedure,

Go to *Davis's Nursing Skills Videos*, **Asepsis: Sterile Gown and Gloves (Closed Method).**

For questions and suggested responses,

Go to Chapter 23, **Thinking About the Procedure Questions and Suggested Responses,** on Davis*Plus*.

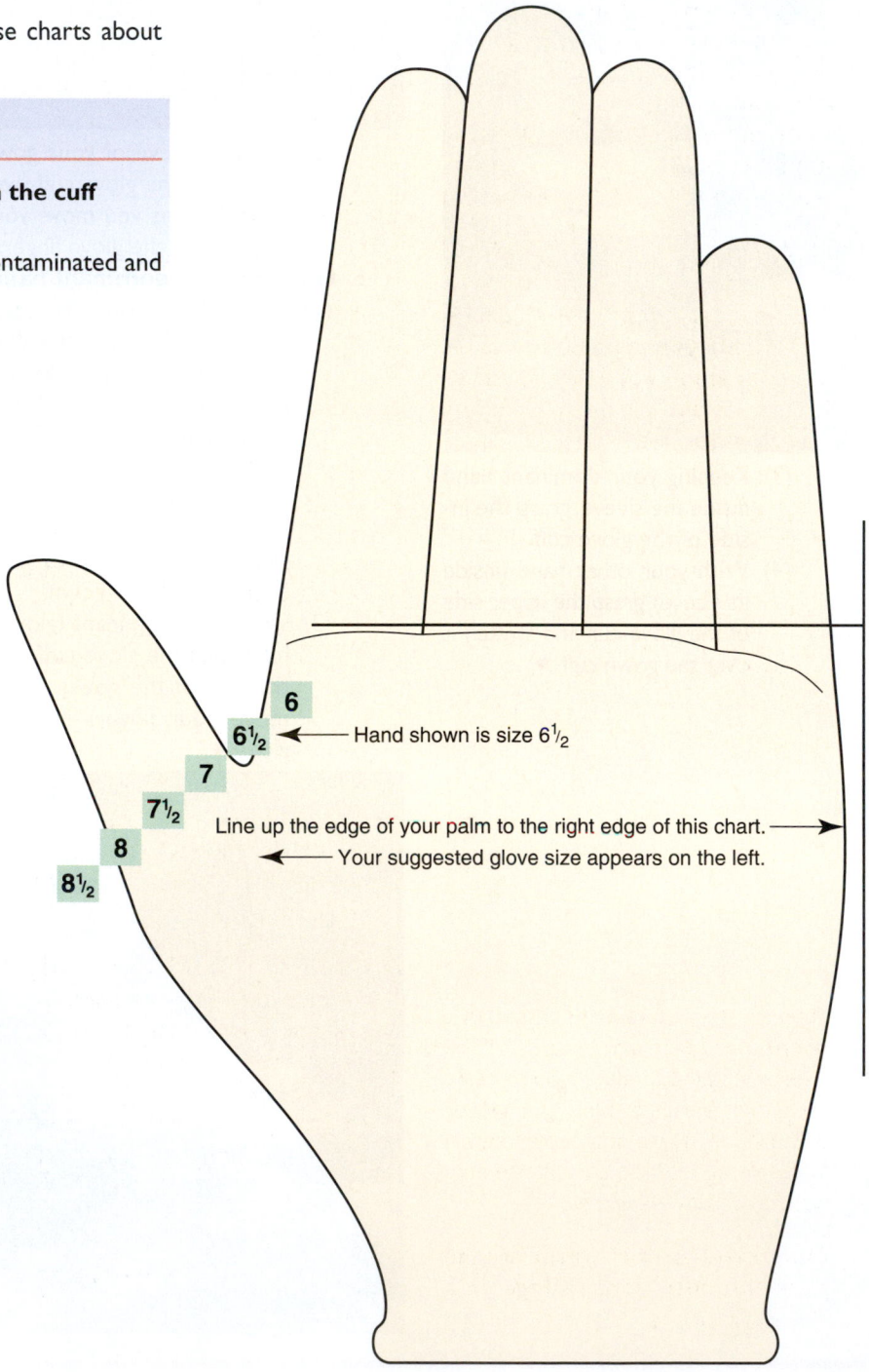

Sterile glove sizes. This can help you determine the proper size glove you need for your hand.

Procedure 23-7 ■ Sterile Gloves (Open Method)

➤ For steps to follow in *all* procedures, refer to the Universal Steps for All Procedures found on the inside back cover 2. For this procedure, also refer to Clinical Insights 23-2, 23-3, and 23-7 if you need more information.

Equipment

- Sterile gloves of the correct size

➤ When performing the procedure, always identify your patient according to agency policy, using two identifiers, and be attentive to standard precautions, hand hygiene, patient safety and privacy, body mechanics, and documentation.

Procedure Steps

1. **Determine the correct size** of sterile gloves (see the drawing of glove sizes accompanying Procedure 23-6). The gloves should be snug, but not tight.
   Gloves that are too loose are more easily contaminated and make handling equipment or supplies difficult. Gloves that are too tight are uncomfortable and may tear during use.

2. **Assess the glove package** for intactness and expiration date. Do not use the gloves if the package is torn, has become moist, or is past the expiration date.
   Torn packaging may allow the gloves to become contaminated. Moisture allows wicking and may cause contamination. Expired gloves are not considered sterile.▼

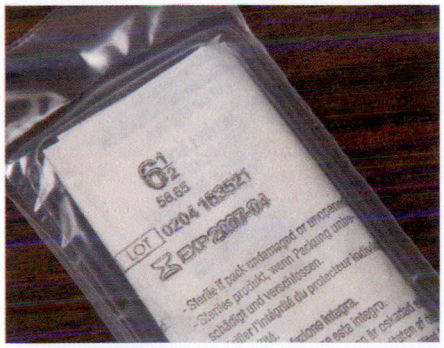

3. **Assess the patient's environment** for a space that is clean and has adequate space to allow you to open the glove package. Don the gloves without touching a nonsterile item.
   Inadvertently touching a nonsterile item will contaminate the gloves.

4. **Open the outer wrapper** and place the inner glove package on a clean, dry surface.

5. **Open the inner glove package** so that the glove cuffs are closest to you. Be careful to fully open the flaps of the package so that they do not fold back over and contaminate the gloves.
   The outer 1-inch border of the glove package is considered contaminated.▼

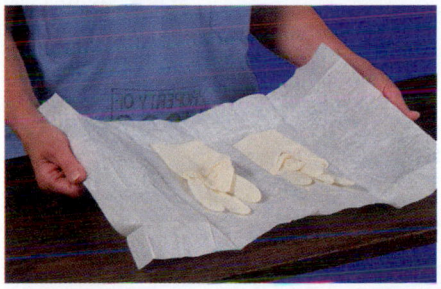

6. **With your nondominant hand** grasp the inner surface of the glove for the dominant hand. Lift the glove up and away from the table, keeping it away from your body. Take care to not touch anything else on the sterile field
   The inside of the glove is not considered sterile because it is in contact with your skin. Lifting the glove up and away from the table prevents you from accidentally touching the table or your clothing while donning the glove and thereby contaminating the glove.

7. **Slide your dominant hand into** the glove, keeping your hand and fingers above your waist and away from your body.
   The area below the waistline is considered contaminated. Keeping gloves away from your body prevents accidental contamination.➤

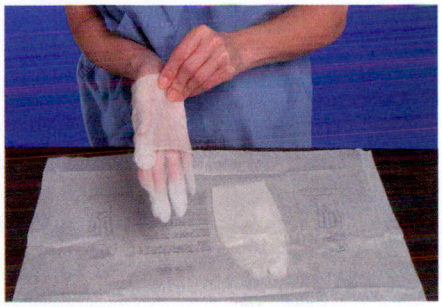

8. **Slide your gloved fingers under** the cuff of the glove for the nondominant hand, keeping your gloved thumb well away from your ungloved hand. Lift the glove up and away from the table and away from your body.
   The outside of the glove is sterile and may be touched with your sterile gloved hand.▼

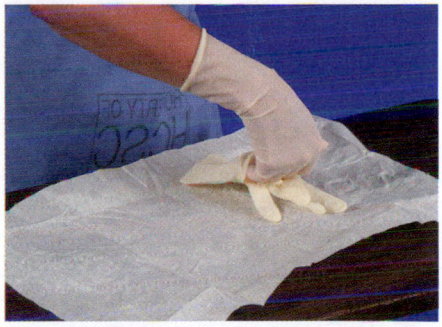

9. **With gloved fingers still under** the cuff, slide your nondominant hand into the glove and pull it on, being careful to avoid contact with your gloved hand, especially the thumb.▼

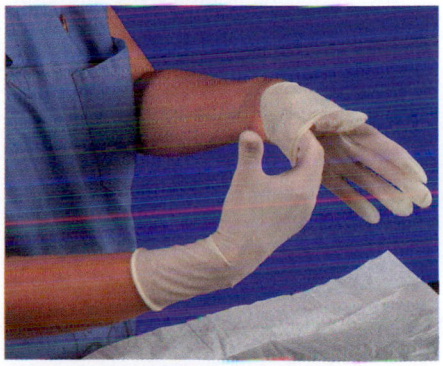

(continued on next page)

Procedure 23-7 ■ Sterile Gloves (Open Method) (continued)

10. **Adjust both gloves to fit your** fingers. If necessary, pull the fingers of the gloves down so that no excess is at the fingertips.
Adjusting your gloves after both have been donned decreases the risk of contamination and allows for greater dexterity during the procedure.

11. **Keep your hands between** shoulder and waist level in front of you.
Keeps the gloves within your field of vision to avoid contamination.

NOTE: To remove soiled gloves after the procedure, refer to Procedure 23-3.

Patient Teaching

Explain the reason sterile gloves are needed for the procedure.

Home Care

- Many home care procedures are clean rather than sterile. The client is in his own environment and not surrounded by other patients, who may serve as hosts for infection.
- You may need to teach caregivers how to apply sterile gloves for some procedures. No modifications are required. Demonstrate the procedure, and have the caregiver do a return demonstration.

Documentation

- No special documentation is needed for sterile gloving.
- Chart the procedure you performed and the patient's response to the procedure.

Practice Resources
AORN (2010a, 2013a, 2013b).

Thinking About the Procedure

To practice applying clinical reasoning to this procedure,

Go to *Davis's Nursing Skills Videos*, **Asepsis: Sterile Gloves (Open Method).**

For questions and suggested responses,

Go to Chapter 23, **Thinking About the Procedure Questions and Suggested Responses,** on Davis*Plus*.

Procedure 23-8 ■ Sterile Fields

➤ For steps to follow in *all* procedures, refer to the Universal Steps for All Procedures found on the inside back cover. For this procedure, also refer to Clinical Insights 23-2, 23-3, and 23-7 if you need more information.

Equipment

- Package of sterile supplies required for the procedure
- Sterile gloves of the correct size

Procedure 23-8A ■ Setting Up a Sterile Field

➤ When performing the procedure, always identify your patient according to agency policy, using two identifiers, and be attentive to standard precautions, hand hygiene, patient safety and privacy, body mechanics, and documentation.

Procedure Steps

1. **Assess the sterility of all** packages and equipment. Check to make sure the packaging is intact and the expiration dates have not passed.
Only sterile items should enter a sterile field. Any compromise in packaging means that the item is assumed not to be sterile.

2. **Arrange the environment** for performing the sterile procedure.
   a. Remove all items from the surface you will use to set up the sterile field.
   Inadequate space causes inadvertent contamination during sterile procedures.
   b. Position the patient as needed for the procedure.
   Allows you to immediately proceed with the planned procedure. Once the sterile field is established, air movement can create contamination of the sterile items.

Procedure Variation. Using Sterile Packaged Equipment

3. **Place the sterile package on a** clean, dry surface.
Prevents contamination of the sterile item. If a surface is damp, strike-through may occur, making the item unsterile. ▼

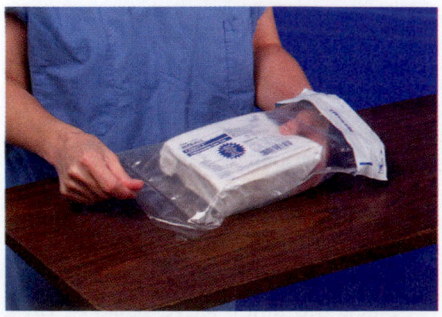

4. **Open the flap away from you** first to prevent passing an unsterile arm over the sterile items.
If you move an unsterile item over a sterile field, the field is no longer considered to be sterile. ▼

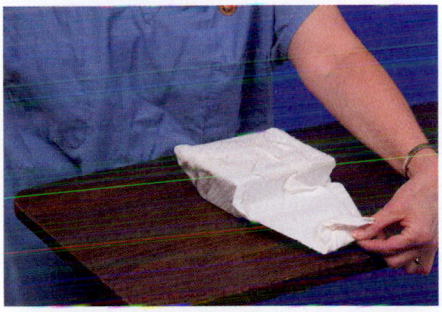

5. **Open the side flaps.** ▼

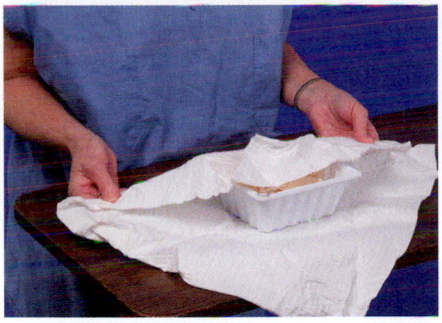

6. **Pull the final flap toward you.** The wrapper is now the sterile field. The area 1 inch from the edge of the wrapper and 1 inch from the table edge is considered unsterile. Do not readjust the sterile area after the package has been opened.
Only the horizontal surface of the draped area is considered sterile. Any part of the sterile wrapper that falls below the level of the sterile area (e.g., top of the table) is considered unsterile. If you move the field after opening, the field shifts and places unsterile areas of the wrapper on the surface. ▼

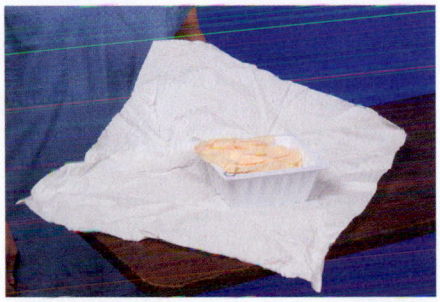

Procedure Variation. Opening a Fabric- or Paper-Wrapped Sterile Package

7. **Check and remove** the chemical indicator strip.
The indicator tape per manufacturer or institution confirms that the package was sterilized. The pack usually is also dated.

8. **Remove the outer wrapper** and place the inner wrapped package on a clean, dry surface.
The outer wrapper is not considered sterile and is discarded.

9. **Open the inner wrapper** following the same technique described in Steps 3 through 6.

Procedure Variation. Using a Sterile Drape

Omit Steps 3 through 9.

10. **Place the package on a clean,** dry surface. Hold the edge of the package flap down toward the table, grasp the top edge of the package, and peel back.
The sterile drape is inside the outer wrapper. This maneuver opens the package without contaminating the sterile drape. ▼

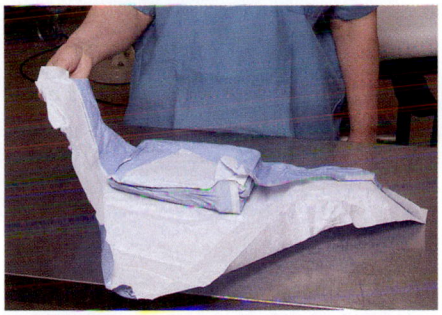

11. **Pick up the sterile drape by the corner.** Allow the drape to fall open, away from your body and away from unsterile surfaces. Place it on a clean, dry surface by touching only the edge of the drape. Avoid fanning the drape.
A 1-inch border around the sterile drape is considered unsterile.

Procedure 23-8B ■ Adding Supplies to a Sterile Field

➤ When performing the procedure, always identify your patient according to agency policy, using two identifiers, and be attentive to standard precautions, hand hygiene, patient safety and privacy, body mechanics, and documentation.

Procedure Steps

1. **Hold the sterile package in your** dominant hand. Grasping the corner of the wrapper, peel each corner back with your nondominant hand.
The inside of the wrapper is sterile and will be used as a barrier when placing the sterile item onto a sterile field.

2. **Holding the contents several** inches above the field, allow the supplies to drop onto the field inside the 1-inch border of the sterile field. Do not let your arms pass over the sterile field.
By holding the package upside down, you ensure that the sterile part of the package is facing the sterile field and that you deposit the item onto the sterile field. ▼

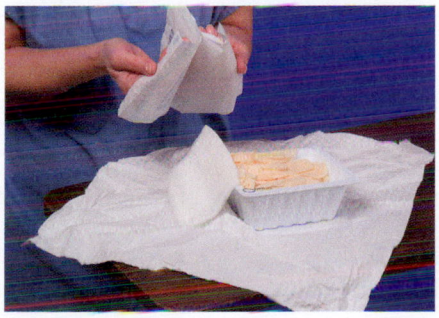

3. **Dispose of the wrapper**, and continue opening any needed supplies for the procedure.
Key Point: *Once sterile gloves are on, you will not be able to add items without contaminating the gloves.*

(continued on next page)

Procedure 23-8 ■ Sterile Fields (continued)

Procedure 23-8C ■ Adding Sterile Solutions to a Sterile Field

Procedure Steps

1. **Use a sterile bowl or receptacle** if the sterile field is fabric or at risk for soaking through. You may add a sterile bowl to the field by unwrapping (as discussed above) and holding the bowl through the sterile wrapper as you place it near the edge of the sterile field. The sterile bowl may also be placed next to the sterile field.
   If you place the sterile bowl on the field, place it near the edge so that you can pour the sterile solution from the back of the sterile field. This prevents you from reaching over and thereby contaminating the field.

2. **Check that the sterile solution** and concentration are correct, and confirm that the expiration date has not passed.

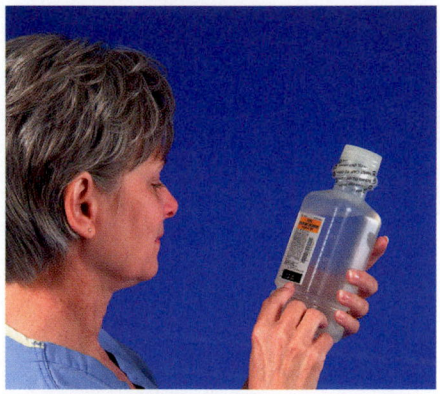

3. **Remove the cap off the solution** bottle by lifting it directly up and throw it away.
   The edge of the container is considered contaminated after the contents have been poured and the sterility of the contents cannot be ensured if the cap is replaced.

4. **Hold the bottle 4 to 6 inches** above the bowl and pour the needed amount of the solution into the bowl.
   Prevents you from inadvertently touching the sterile bowl with the bottle and thereby contaminating the bowl. Limited height reduces the risk of splashing, which strikes through and contaminates a cloth or permeable sterile field. A disposable sterile drape generally has a plastic membrane in the middle to prevent strike-through.

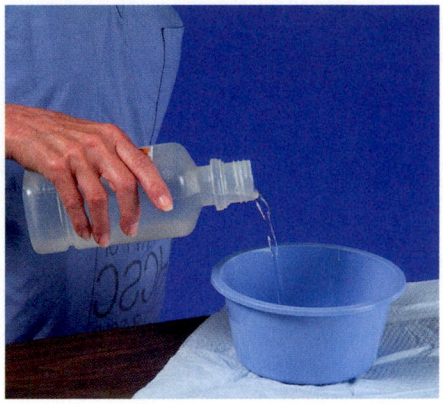

5. **Discard the remaining solution.**
   Reusing open containers may cause contamination due to drops contacting the unsterile areas and running back over the container opening.

6. **Before donning sterile gloves** to perform the procedure, double-check that all supplies have been added to the field using sterile technique. Do not leave the sterile field unattended. Do not turn your back to the sterile field.
   If a sterile item is out of your field of vision, it is no longer considered sterile because airborne particles, insects, or liquids could contaminate the field.

Home Care

- Most sterile procedures in the home are done by visiting nurses.
- Procedures performed by clients or family members are usually clean rather than sterile.

Documentation

- You will not document the actual setting up of the sterile field.
- Document the procedure, your assessment of the patient's tolerance for the procedure, and your assessment of the area being treated by the procedure.

? What if . . .

- **The nurse observes a breach in sterility by the surgeon?**

  The nurse's duty is to protect the patient above all else, even when fearing an uncomfortable confrontation with the healthcare provider. The nurse is obligated to follow the institution's policy and advocate for patient safety.

Practice Resources

AORN (2010a; 2013b); Simko (2012).

Thinking About the Procedure

To practice applying clinical reasoning to this procedure,

Go to *Davis's Nursing Skills Videos*, **Asepsis: Sterile Fields.**

For questions and suggested responses,

Go to Chapter 23, **Thinking About the Procedure Questions and Suggested Responses,** on Davis*Plus*.

CLINICAL INSIGHTS

Clinical Insight 23-1 ➤ Guidelines for Hand Hygiene

Handwashing

When to Wash

- When hands are visibly dirty or soiled with blood or body fluids
- When arriving on and leaving the patient care unit
- Before direct contact with a patient, even if you intend to wear procedure gloves
- Before donning gloves (either procedure or sterile)
- When gloves are changed during a procedure
- After removing gloves
- After contact with a patient's intact skin (e.g., when lifting a patient or taking a blood pressure)
- After contact with body fluids, mucous membranes, non-intact skin, and wound dressings even if hands are not visibly soiled
- When moving from a contaminated body site to a clean body site during patient care
- Before and after contact with objects and equipment in the patient's immediate vicinity
- Before eating and after using a restroom. Use soap and water.
- Before and after touching any area on your face and hair

What to Use

- Use alcohol-based handrub (at least 60% alcohol) for routine hand hygiene and if hands are not visibly soiled.
- Use soap and water when hands are dirty or visibly soiled.
- Use soap and water after using a restroom.
- Use soap and water if there is potential for exposure to *Bacillus anthracis* (or other spore-producing bacteria such a *C. difficile*). *Alcohol-based solutions are not effective against spores.*
- Use warm, not hot, water.
- Use disposable paper towels.

If you are interested in a comparison of the effectiveness of various hand-hygiene antiseptic agents,

Go to Chapter 23, **ESG Table 22-2, Antimicrobial Spectrum and Characteristics of Hand-Hygiene Antiseptic Agents,** on Davis*Plus*.

How to Wash

Refer to Procedure 23-1 and also the *Nursing Fundamentals Skills*, **Asepsis: Hand Hygiene.**

Fingernails

- Do not wear artificial nails or extenders when caring for patients at high risk (e.g., in intensive care and oncology units).
- The 2007 epic2 guidelines in the United Kingdom recommend artificial nails and extenders not be worn at all (Pratt, Pellowe, Wilson, et al., 2007). The CDC's position is that although studies provide evidence that wearing artificial nails poses an infection hazard, additional studies are warranted.
- It is best to not wear nail polish because it chips easily and can harbor microorganisms.
  The area under the nails, artificial nails/extensions, and chipped polish act as reservoirs for microorganisms.
- Keep nail tips less than ¼ inch long from the fingertips (CDC).
  Longer nails are associated with increased microbial carriage on the hands.

Jewelry

- We recommend that you not wear a watch or rings in the clinical setting, especially rings with stones.
  The CDC has stated jewelry is still an unresolved issue. They noted that hand contamination with pathogens increased when nurses wear rings, but that no studies have related that practice to the transmission of pathogens to patients. However, the epic2 guidelines advise against wearing wrist and hand jewelry.
- If your agency permits you to wear jewelry, clean it thoroughly and often.

Practice Resources

AORN (2013b, 2013c); Boyce, J., & Pittet, D. (2002); Pratt, R., Pellowe, C., Wilson, J., et al. (2007); Rupp, M., Fitzgerald, T., Puumala, S., et al. (2008); Siegel, J., Rhinehart, E., Jackson, M., et al. (2007).

Clinical Insight 23-2 ➤ Providing a Clean Patient Environment

The following guidelines are used along with standard precautions for all patients. A clean environment includes the surfaces in a patient's room, as well as supplies, equipment, and other objects brought into the room.

Supplies and Equipment

- Do not stock rooms with unnecessary supplies.
- Consider supplies that are brought into a patient's room contaminated. Do not return them to the linen or supply cart; instead, handle them according to agency policy.
- Consider contaminated any items brought from the patient's home, gifts from visitors, and so forth.
- Mobile computing devices should be cleaned (e.g., pagers, smart phones, point-of-care keyboards, and medication administration devices). However, most hospitals lack infection prevention policies for mobile devices. Be sure to wash your hands after using such a device.
  Often, electronic devices cannot be decontaminated without damage; in that case, only hand hygiene can protect you and the patient from these vectors.
- Clean stethoscopes with alcohol before use on a patient. Disposable stethoscopes are commercially available, but not commonly seen in healthcare agencies (some hospitals do have disposable stethoscopes for patients in isolation or on transmission-based precautions).
  Stethoscopes are often contaminated with Staphylococcus aureus because care providers do not clean them adequately between patients.
- Clean reusable equipment that is soiled with blood or body fluids according to agency policy—typically, autoclaving, ethylene oxide gas, or dry heat.
- Do not reuse equipment for the care of another patient until it has been cleaned and reprocessed appropriately.
- Dispose of single-use equipment that is soiled with blood or body fluids in appropriate biohazard containers.
- Wear gloves when handling equipment that is visibly contaminated. Perform hand hygiene.

Linens

- Carefully handle contaminated linens to prevent skin and mucous membrane exposures, contamination of clothing, and transfer of microorganisms to other patients or the environment.
  Linens may harbor microorganisms that may transfer to your clothing, open skin, or mucous membranes, to then be carried to other clients or environment.
- Bag and remove soiled linens from the room immediately.

Uniforms and Lab Coats

- Do not wear a uniform (e.g., scrubs) or a lab coat for more than one day without laundering.
  Care provider clothing is often contaminated as care providers move from patient to patient. The traditional white lab coats are being banned in some hospitals because they are vehicles for dangerous pathogens. Although contaminated clothing has not been implicated directly, the potential exists for it to transfer pathogens to patients (CDC, 2008).
- If you wash your uniforms at home, they require only washing with warm or hot water and detergent (except in the case of possible exposure to multidrug-resistant organisms, for which you should add bleach).

Spills and Waste

- Empty and clean bedpans, urinals, and emesis basins immediately after use.
- Place soiled dressings, drains, and so forth, in appropriate waterproof bags for disposal. Do not leave such used supplies in an open trashcan.
- Wipe up small spills from tabletops and floors. Notify the housekeeping or environmental services department for large spills.

Needles and Sharps

Do not recap, bend, break, or hand-manipulate used needles. If recapping is necessary, use a one-handed "scoop" technique. Place used sharps in puncture-resistant containers.

For Home Care

- Teach patients and caregivers to keep the home environment clean.
- To disinfect the home environment, use and teach caregivers to create, a dilute bleach solution. Mix 1 part regular-strength bleach to 50 parts water. The mixture may be stored for a month in an opaque container. NEVER mix the solution with other household cleaners. *Note:* Be careful not to splash the bleach because it removes color from fabric and other objects, and keep it out of reach of children.
- Washing dishware and eating utensils in a dishwasher with hot water and detergents is sufficient decontamination.
- Healthcare workers in the home are a potential source of pathogens and should use caution to avoid infecting the patient.

Practice Resources

Carling, P., Parry, M., & Von Beheren, S. (2008); CDC(2008); Siegel, J., Rhinehart, E., Jackson, M., et al. (2007).

Clinical Insight 23-3 ➤ Following CDC Standard Precautions

Standard precautions (Tier 1) apply to all clients and should be used whenever there is a possibility of coming in contact with blood, body fluids (except sweat), excretions and secretions, mucous membranes, and breaks in the skin.

These precautions are designed to protect you from exposure to potential pathogens, to decrease the likelihood that you will transmit pathogens among patients, and to protect the patient from microorganisms that you may carry.

Assume that every person may be infected or colonized with an organism that could be transmitted to others.

TIER 1 COMPONENT	RECOMMENDATIONS
Hand Hygiene	▪ Perform hand hygiene after touching blood, body fluids, secretions, excretions, contaminated items; immediately after removing gloves; between patient contacts. Refer to Clinical Insight 23-1 for details.
Respiratory Hygiene/Cough Etiquette for Patients	▪ Instruct symptomatic persons to cover mouth/nose when sneezing/coughing. ▪ Provide and use tissues and dispose in a no-touch receptacle. ▪ Perform hand hygiene after soiling hands with respiratory secretions or after using a tissue or covering the mouth/nose. ▪ Wear a surgical mask if tolerated (some patients may not be able to tolerate the decreased oxygen that is available when breathing room air through a mask), or do not come within 3 feet of another person if possible.
Masks and Eye Protection (for the Nurse)	▪ Wear a mask and eye protection or a face shield to protect mucous membranes of the eyes, nose, and mouth during patient care activities that are likely to generate splashes or sprays of blood, body fluids, secretions, and excretions. *Barrier protection helps keep microorganisms from accidentally entering your mucous membranes, eyes, nose, or mouth.*
Patient Placement	▪ Place in a single-patient room if the patient is at increased risk of transmitting or acquiring infection, does not maintain appropriate hygiene, is likely to contaminate the environment, or is at increased risk of developing adverse outcome following infection.
Gowns	▪ Wear a clean, nonsterile, nonpermeable gown during procedures and activities when you anticipate contact of clothing or exposed skin with blood or body fluids, secretions, and excretions (e.g., when there is a risk of spray or splash onto clothing). ▪ Promptly remove the gown once it is soiled. Avoid contaminating clothing when removing the gown. ▪ Wash hands after removing the gown. ▪ See Procedures 23-2 and 23-3, Donning PPE and Removing PPE.
Needles and Sharps	▪ Never recap, bend, or break used needles, or otherwise manipulate them using both hands, or use any other technique that involves directing the point of a needle toward any part of the body. Instead, use either a one-handed "scoop" technique or a mechanical device designed for holding the needle sheath (see Procedure 25-10, Recapping needles...). ▪ Use safety features when available. ▪ Place "sharps" (e.g., scalpels, needles, and so on) in puncture-resistant containers for disposal.
Patient Resuscitation	▪ Use one-way valve mouthpieces, resuscitation bags, or other ventilation devices as an alternative to mouth-to-mouth resuscitation methods in situations when the need for resuscitation is predictable. *To prevent contact between rescuer's and client's mucous membranes and airflow, preventing transmission of microorganisms.*
Soiled Patient Care Equipment, Environment, Textiles & Laundry	▪ See Clinical Insight 23-2 for details. ▪ Wear gloves if the equipment or laundry is visibly contaminated. ▪ Handle equipment, textiles, and laundry in a manner to prevent transfer of microorganisms to others and the environment.

(Continued)

Clinical Insight 23-3 ➤ Following CDC Standard Precautions—cont'd

TIER I COMPONENT	RECOMMENDATIONS
	▪ Perform hand hygiene. ▪ Develop procedures for routine care, cleaning, and disinfection of environmental surfaces, especially frequently touched surfaces in patient care areas.
Gloves	***When to Wear*** ▪ If you have an area of irritation or a break in the skin, wear gloves or apply an occlusive dressing during patient contact. ▪ Wear gloves when contact with blood or other potentially infectious materials, mucous membranes, and nonintact skin could occur.
	When to Remove or Change ▪ Remove gloves immediately after caring for a patient. Avoid touching clean items, environmental surfaces, or another patient. ▪ Do not wear the same gloves for care of more than one patient; do not wash gloves and reuse gloves between patient contact. *Research shows that washing and reusing gloves between patient contacts results in increased bacterial counts on the hands.* ▪ Change gloves during patient care if moving from a contaminated body site to a clean site. ▪ Change gloves between tasks or procedures on the same patient if you have made contact with material that may contain a high concentration of microorganisms.
	Use and Storage ▪ When preparing for a procedure, first collect equipment and place at the bedside ready for use; then wash your hands and don gloves just before performing the procedure. Donning gloves ahead of time allows them to become contaminated before the procedure. ▪ Do not carry gloves in your pocket. Keep them in their original box and remove them when and where required. ▪ Do not store gloves on top of trash containers or on windowsills. ▪ Handwashing or disinfection is required regardless of whether gloves are used or changed. Gloves are not completely impermeable to microorganisms; furthermore, they may leak or tear. Hands can be easily contaminated when removing gloves, as well.

For a comparison of glove materials (latex, nitrile, vinyl, and polyethylene),

Go to Chapter 23, **DP Table 23-4, Comparison of Glove Materials,** on Davis*Plus*.

Practice Resources

Boyce, J., & Pittet, D. (2002); Occupational Safety & Health Administration, U.S. Department of Labor (n.d.); Pratt, R., Pellowe, C., Wilson, J., et al. (2007); Siegel, J., Rhinehart, E., Jackson, M., et al. (2007); U.S. Department of Labor (n.d.a).

Clinical Insight 23-4 ➤ Following Transmission-Based Precautions

Note: Refer to Clinical Insight 23-3 if you need to review standard precautions.

When to Use: Use transmission-based (Tier 2) precautions when the routes of transmission are not completely interrupted using Standard Precautions alone. Pathogens may be transmitted by contact, droplet, or air. Each mode of transmission requires a different approach to prevent infection, and has a different set of precautions. For some diseases, you may need to use more than one of the categories.

Contact Precautions

Follow all standard precautions.

When to Use: Use contact precautions when direct contact with the patient or the patient's environment can lead to spread of the pathogen. This is the most common form of transmission. Draining wounds, dressings, patient supplies, and secretions are sources of infection. Indirect contact, or contact with fomites, can also transmit pathogens that spread by this method.

Patient Placement and Transport

- Always choose a private room if one is available. When there is no private room, and when you have no choice but to place the patient with one who has a different infection, ensure that the patients are physically separated by more than 3 feet. Keep the privacy curtain closed. This minimizes contact between patients. Ideally, consult with an infection preventionist for patient placement. A private room provides the most effective protection.
- Limit transport outside the room to medically necessary purposes; if transport is necessary, the patient should wear a mask. The transporter is not required to mask.
- Ideally, consult with an infection preventionist for patient placement.
- Place in a private room, if available. Private room provides the most effective protection.
- If no private room is available, place patient in a room with a patient with an active infection caused by the same organism and no other infections.
- When transporting the patient, ensure that infected or colonized areas of the body are contained and covered.
- *Ambulatory care:* Place the patient in an exam room or cubicle as soon as possible.

Personal Protective Equipment

- Wear clean nonsterile gloves when touching the patient's intact skin. Don gloves on entry to the room.
- Wear a clean gown if you anticipate your clothing may contact the patient or any contaminated items in the room.
- Remove PPE and observe hand hygiene before leaving the room. Take care that your skin and clothing do not contact environmental surfaces on the way out of the room.

Equipment, Supplies, and Environment

- Keep contact precaution supplies just outside the patient's room on a cart.
- Double bag all linen and trash (or use a single waterproof bag), and clearly mark them contaminated.
- Use disposable equipment (e.g., blood pressure cuffs) if possible; otherwise, clean and disinfect the equipment per institutional policy before removing them from the room and before use on another patient.
- Ensure that the patient room is cleaned and disinfected at least daily.
- *Home care:* Limit the amount of nondisposable equipment brought into the home. If possible, leave the equipment in the home until discharge from home care.
- *Home care:* If equipment cannot remain in the home, clean and disinfect items before taking them from the home, or place them in a plastic bag for transport to a reprocessing area.

Other

- Follow any additional precautions specific to the microorganism.
- Discontinue contact precautions after signs and symptoms have resolved or according to pathogen-specific recommendations.

(Continued)

Clinical Insight 23-4 ➤ Following Transmission-Based Precautions—cont'd

Droplet Precautions

Follow all standard precautions.
Follow all contact precautions.

When to Use: Use droplet precautions when the pathogen can be spread via moist, large droplets (e.g., sneezing, coughing, talking). Droplets can spread infection by direct contact with mucous membranes or through indirect contact, for example, suctioning or touching a bedside table that was contaminated with moist droplets and then rubbing your eyes.

Patient Placement and Transport

- Always choose a private room if one is available. If there is no private room, and when you have no choice but to place the patient with one who has a different infection, ensure that the patients are physically separated by more than 3 feet. Keep the privacy curtain closed. This minimizes contact between patients. Ideally, consult with an infection preventionist for patient placement. A private room provides the most effective protection.
- Limit transport outside the room to medically necessary purposes; if transport is necessary, the patient should wear a mask. The transporter is not required to mask.

Personal Protective Equipment

- Keep droplet precaution supplies just outside the patient's room on a cart.
- Wear a mask when working within 3 feet of the patient. Don the mask on entry into the room. Whether to wear goggles is an unresolved issue. Follow agency policy.
- Change PPE and perform hand hygiene between contact with patients in the same room, regardless of whether one or both patients are on droplet precautions.

Other

- Instruct patients to observe respiratory hygiene/cough etiquette.
- Discontinue droplet precautions after signs and symptoms have resolved or according to pathogen-specific recommendations.

Airborne Precautions

Follow all standard precautions.
Follow all contact precautions.

When to Use: Use airborne precautions to control the spread of infections that are transmitted person-to-person on air currents. These include tuberculosis, varicella (chickenpox), severe acute respiratory syndrome (SARS), and rubeola (measles). Pathogens spread by this method are very small and can be easily transmitted through ventilating systems as well as by any activities that stir the air, such as fanning sheets, shaking out towels, or sweeping the floor.

Patient Placement and Transport

- Place the patient in an airborne infection isolation room (AIIR)—one with negative pressure that discharges and exchanges the air outside or through a high-efficiency particulate air (HEPA) filtration system. Monitor air pressure daily (usually this is via an electronic device with an alarm).
- If such a room is not available, transfer the patient to a facility where one is available.
- Keep the room door closed when not required for entry and exit. To maintain the negative pressure and contain the airborne organisms.
- In the event of an outbreak involving large numbers of patients who require airborne precautions, consult with infection preventionists for patient placement.
- Limit transport of the patient outside the room to medically necessary purposes. If transport is necessary, cover any infectious skin lesions and have the patient wear a mask. The transporter is not required to mask if the patient is wearing a mask and infectious skin lesions are covered. Notify the receiving department. So the receiving department can take airborne precautions.
- *Ambulatory care:* Triage and identify patients with suspected airborne precautions upon entry to the agency. Place the patient in an AIIR as soon as possible. If one is not available, place a mask on the patient and place him in an exam room. Do not reuse the room for at least an hour after the patient leaves it.

Clinical Insight 23-4 ➤ Following Transmission-Based Precautions—cont'd

Personal Protective Equipment

- Keep airborne isolation supplies just outside the patient's room on a cart.
- Don a mask on entering the room. Wear a special, fit-tested, approved mask (e.g., N-95 respirator) if the patient is suspected of having pulmonary tuberculosis or smallpox.
- Remove your respirator/mask outside the room after closing the door. If the respirator is not disposable, clean and store according to the manufacturer's instructions.
- When using a respirator mask, check the seal. Hold your hands over the respirator and exhale. If you feel air around your nose, adjust the nosepiece; if you feel air at the edges, adjust the straps.
- When the patient has rubeola, chickenpox, or disseminated zoster, CDC makes no recommendation about use of PPE if, based on your history of vaccination or disease, you think you are presumed immune to the disease.
- If the patient has or is suspected of having measles (rubeola) or varicella (chickenpox), only immune caregivers should provide care. Immune caregivers do not need to wear masks.

Other

- Discontinue airborne precautions according to pathogen-specific recommendations of the CDC.
- Tape a waterproof bag to the bedside. To facilitate proper disposal of tissues.

Practice Resources

Pratt, R. J., Pellowe, C. M., Wilson, J. A., et al. (2007); Siegel, J. D., Rhinehart, E., Jackson, M., et al. (2007); U.S. Department of Labor (n.d.a).

Clinical Insight 23-5 ➤ Preventing the Transmission of Multidrug-Resistant Organisms (MDROs)

Note: Refer to Clinical Insights 23-1, 23-2, 23-3, and 23-4, which are also followed in preventing the transmission of MDROs.

Preventing the transmission of MDROs requires some measures over and above the other precautions, but does not replace them.

Note: The CDC recommends that hospitals try to reduce infection rates by improving hygiene and standard precautions; and resorting to special measures, such as screening all high-risk patients, only if other methods fail.

General Recommendations

- **Perform meticulous hand hygiene, for *all* patient care.**
- **Observe standard precautions for *all* patients.** See Clinical Insight 23-2.
  Standard precautions, including hand hygiene, are absolutely essential in preventing spread of infection. There is some evidence that standard precautions alone may be as effective as isolating methicillin-resistant Staphylococcus aureus (MRSA) patients in private rooms and wearing PPE (Halcomb, Griffiths, & Fernandez, 2008a). However, most studies reporting successful MDRO control used a combination of several control measures.
- **Observe (or modify) contact precautions** routinely for patients infected or colonized with target MDROs. Usually this continues until the patient has a negative culture for the organism.
  The type of organism and extent of disease it causes vary by population and institution. Approaches to prevention and control must be tailored to the needs of individual institutions and populations.
  - ***MRSA:*** Prevention is a national priority. The organism can survive on hands, clothing, environmental surfaces, and equipment, so healthcare institutions are targeting it with staff education, aggressive handwashing, increased use of protective gloves and gowns, and targeted screening (Klevens, Morrison, Nadle, et al., 2007).
  - ***C. difficile:*** Prevention focuses on the following:
    Contact precautions for patients with diarrhea
    Accurate patient identification
    Consistent hand hygiene, using soap and water rather than alcohol-based handrubs (for mechanical removal of spores)

(Continued)

Clinical Insight 23-5 ➤ Preventing the Transmission of Multidrug-Resistant Organisms (MDROs)—cont'd

Patient Placement and Transport

- Assign the patient to a single room, if available. Give highest priority to those having conditions that may lead to transmission of infection (e.g., uncontained secretions or excretions, inability to follow cough hygiene).
- If no single room is available, place with a patient with the same MDRO.

Personal Protective Equipment

- Use masks according to standard precautions when performing splash-generating procedures (e.g., wound irrigation). Masks are not recommended for routine care (e.g., upon room entry).
- Use gloves and gowns according to standard precautions.
- *Home care and ambulatory care:* Follow standard precautions for PPE.

Equipment, Supplies, and Environment

- Ensure that patient rooms are cleaned well and often. Disinfect high-touch surfaces (e.g., bedrails, door knobs, bedside commodes) in the room.
- Dedicate noncritical equipment (e.g., stethoscope, blood pressure cuff) to use on individual patients colonized or infected with MDROs.
- Follow standard precautions for handling linens and eating utensils.
- For *C. difficile:* Use a bleach-containing disinfectant for environmental disinfection.
- *Home care:* Limit the amount of patient care equipment brought into the homes of patients infected or colonized with MDROs. See Contact Precautions in Clinical Insight 20-4 to review this.

Other

- Actively observe for symptoms of infections, such as MRSA. Some institutions require screening cultures at admission, or on admission to certain units (e.g., intensive care).
- Be aware of and practice preventive measures, such as:
  - Use intravenous and urinary catheters only when essential, and with scrupulous sterile technique.
  - Special measures to prevent lower respiratory tract infection in intubated patients
  - Judiciously select and use antimicrobials.
- *For C. difficile:* Use a bleach-containing disinfectant for environmental disinfection.

If Further Measures Are Needed

Note: If MDROs continue to be a problem in spite of diligent infection control measures, your agency might consider intensifying infection control practices. For example:

- Donning gowns and gloves before or upon entry to the patient's room
- Assigning the same personnel to the care of MDRO patients only
- Stopping new admissions to the unit or facility
- Obtaining environmental cultures
- Screening high-risk patients on admission

Practice Resources

AORN (2013a); Association for Professionals in Infection Control and Epidemiology (APIC) (2010); CDC (n.d.f, last modified February 5, 2013); Halcomb, E., Griffiths, R., & Fernandez, R. (2008); Institute for Healthcare Improvement (n.d.a, n.d.b); Siegel, J., Rhinehart, E., Jackson, M., et al. (2006).

Clinical Insight 23-6 ➤ Maintaining a Protective Environment in Special Situations

The CDC recommends a protective environment (isolation) for a special class of stem cell transplant patients, who are neutropenic (and therefore immunocompromised) secondary to chemotherapy. You may, in some facilities, encounter protective isolation for other types of patients, as well. However, in most instances, standard and transmission-based precautions are adequate protection for those patients.

In special situations:

- **Follow standard precautions** meticulously, including hand hygiene before and after patient contact.
- **Follow transmission-based precautions** as indicated by a suspected or proven infection.

Patient Room

- Maintain a protective environment (PE) room.
- Avoid a standing collection of water in the room (e.g., with fresh flowers or humidifiers) to prevent fungi and bacteria typically found in this water.

Personal Protective Equipment

- PPE is not required for care providers or visitors for routine entry into the room, unless approaching the patient.
- If the patient must have diagnostic or other procedures that cannot be performed in the PE room, provide respiratory protection (e.g., an N-95 respirator, minimal contact with others).
- Gown, gloves, and mask are used for visitors and care providers according to standard precautions and as indicated for suspected or proven infections for which they are recommended.

Clinical Insight 23-6 ➤ Maintaining a Protective Environment in Special Situations—cont'd

- Refer to Clinical Insight 23-2 and Procedure 23-5 to review donning and removing PPE.

Care Providers, Visitors

- Only healthy caregivers should provide care. Do not care for such a patient if you have an upper respiratory infection, for example.
- Healthcare workers caring for patients in protective isolation should not also be providing care for other patients with active infections.
- Restrict visitors who have a cold or contagious illness.

Housekeeping/Environmental Services

- Carpeting in patient rooms or halls traps soil and can wick moisture, creating an environment for growth of microbes.
- Upholstered furniture and furnishings tend to harbor microbes.
- Avoid dusting methods that scatter particles in the air.
- If vacuum cleaning is necessary, use a vacuum cleaner equipped with a HEPA filter.
- Wet-dust horizontal surfaces daily with EPA-registered disinfectant or detergent.

Engineering

- Use of 99.7% efficiency particulate air (HEPA) filters to remove particles for incoming air at a specified flow rate of air
- Well-sealed rooms—no air leaks
- Ventilation as for airborne precautions
- Directed air flow within the room
- Positive room air pressure in relation to the corridor
- Back-up ventilation equipment (e.g., portable fans or filters)
- For patients who require both protected environment and airborne isolation, use an anteroom to control air in and out of the room.

Practice Resources

AORN (2013a); American Society of Healthcare Engineering (n.d.); Bartley, J. M., Olmsted, R. M., & Haas, J. (2010); Siegel, J. M., Rhinehart, E., Jackson, M., et al. (2007).

Clinical Insight 23-7 ➤ Guidelines for Preparing and Maintaining Sterile Fields

For steps in setting up a sterile field and adding supplies and solutions, see Procedure 23-7.

Key Point: *Sterile touches sterile. Unsterile touches unsterile.*

Setting Up the Field

- Close doors and limit foot traffic when setting up a sterile field.
  Air currents can carry dust and microorganisms.
- Prepare a sterile field as close as possible to the time of use.
  To minimize the opportunity for contamination via air currents.
- You may establish a sterile field by using a sterile drape or by using the inner side of a sterile package wrapping. Touch the inside of the wrapper only after you don sterile gloves.
- When you are placing a sterile drape, protect your gloved hands by cuffing the drape over your hands.

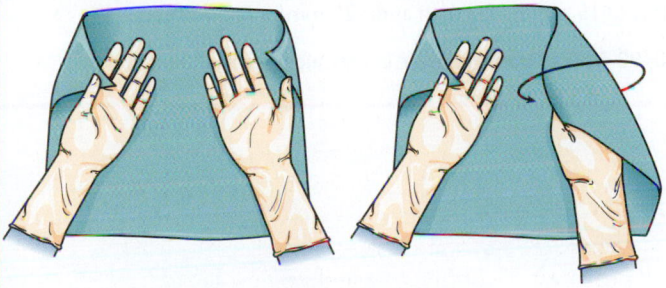

Protecting gloved hands.

What Areas Are Considered Sterile?

- A sterile field is sterile only on the horizontal plane. Consider nonsterile any material that drapes over the horizontal plane.
- Consider a 1-inch margin around the drape unsterile, even if it remains on a horizontal surface.
  Because it is in contact with contaminated surfaces.
- If you are wearing sterile attire, only in the front of your body from the chest to the level of the sterile field is considered sterile.
- Sleeve cuffs are considered unsterile when your hands pass beyond the cuff (they are sterile if you don gloves using the closed method).

Keeping the Field Sterile

- No one in unsterile garb should come near a sterile field.

Remain at least 1 foot away from nonsterile areas if you are wearing sterile garb. Never turn your back to a sterile field. A sterile field or open sterile items must be kept in constant view. *You are responsible for monitoring and maintaining the sterility. If you cannot see the field, you do not know if it has become contaminated.*

- Keep conversation to a minimum around the sterile field.
  To reduce the spread of droplets.

(Continued)

Clinical Insight 23-7 ➤ Guidelines for Preparing and Maintaining Sterile Fields

- Avoid reaching over a sterile field even if you are in sterile garb.
- Handle sterile equipment only if you are wearing sterile gloves.
- Limit the amount of time a sterile field remains set up in advance of a procedure.
- Liquid can act as a wick and contaminate a field. Sterile liquids must be contained in sterile bowls on the field or the sterile drape must be nonpermeable in order to avoid wicking.

Adding Sterile Items

- Only sterile items can be placed on a sterile field.
- Before adding items to a sterile field, inspect them immediately for proper packaging, integrity, and inclusion of a sterilization indicator.
- Never assume an item is sterile. If there is any doubt about its sterility, consider it contaminated.
- All items applied to a sterile field must be sterilized in an approved manner.

Practice Resources

AORN (2010a, 2013a, 2013b); Association for Surgical Technologists (2008); Siegel, J., Rhinehart, E., Jackson, M., et al. (2006).

DIAGNOSTIC TESTING

Common Tests for Evaluating the Presence of or Risk for Infection

TEST	DESCRIPTION
White blood cell (WBC) count with differential	A breakdown of the number and types of WBCs; normal WBC count is 5,000–10,000/mm^3.
Blood cultures	A sample of blood placed on culture media and evaluated for growth of pathogens. Normally, should show no growth of infectious microorganisms.
Urine cultures	Urine is normally sterile with no microorganism growth.
Throat cultures, wound cultures	Presence of microorganisms is normal, but there should be no growth of infectious microorganisms. To yield the most reliable results, blood cultures should be obtained from peripheral sites, using venipuncture by trained phlebotomists, unless a culture is specifically ordered from a central catheter or peripherally inserted central catheter.
Disease titers	Blood tests for specific disease immunity (e.g., to rubella)
Panels to evaluate specific disease exposure	Blood tests to evaluate exposure to specific diseases (e.g., HIV, hepatitis)
Immunoglobulin (IgG, IgM) levels	Blood tests to evaluate humoral immunity status
C-reactive protein (CRP)	A blood test to measure inflammatory change or bacterial infection
Agglutinins, warm or cold	Used to diagnose atypical infections by detecting antigens in the blood
Erythrocyte (red blood cell) sedimentation rate (ESR or sed rate)	A measure of inflammatory changes. Sed rate increases with inflammation. Normally it is @15 mm/hr for men and <20 mm/hr for women.
Iron level	Normally 60–90 grams/100 mg. Lower in chronic infection.

CLINICALREASONING

Applying the Full-Spectrum Nursing Model

PATIENT SITUATION

Mr. Long, a frail elderly man, is in the hospital because he has become dehydrated and needs intravenous fluids and other supportive care. The nurse administered intravenous fluids. Mr. Long also has a fairly large decubitus ulcer (bedsore), which was cultured recently and found to be infected with *Staphylococcus aureus*. The nurse wore gloves to treat the ulcer. While doing so, she noticed that the IV was infusing too fast and, without thinking, regulated the IV without removing her soiled gloves. The next nurse to regulate the IV did so with her bare hands, and then, without realizing it, rubbed her neck. Later, the nurse developed a boil on her neck, which was infected with *S. aureus*.

THINKING

1. *Theoretical Knowledge:*
   a. What are the six links in the chain of infection?
   b. Why do you think the *S. aureus* was able to thrive in Mr. Long's decubitus ulcer?
   c. What are the three modes of transmission of microorganisms? Which one is the most frequent mode of transmission?
2. *Critical Thinking (Reflecting):*
   a. What was the reservoir for the *S. aureus*?
   b. What was the exit from Mr. Long?
   c. What was (were) the fomite(s) for transmission to the nurse?
   d. What was the portal of entry into the nurse?

DOING

3. *Nursing Process (Implementation):* In addition to wearing gloves, what other PPE (if any) does the nurse need if she is performing decubitus care and changing Mr. Long's bed linens?

CARING

4. *Self-Knowledge and Ethical Knowledge:* Think of one instance in the clinical setting in which you did *not* follow standard precautions? Why do you think that happened?

Critical Thinking and Clinical Reasoning

1. You notice that your clinical instructor is not washing his hands between patients. What should you do?
2. As you are gowning and gloving for your first experience in the operating room, you become nervous and forget the proper procedure for applying sterile surgical garb. How should you handle this situation?
3. What action should you take if you contaminate yourself while gowning and gloving?
4. Refer to Procedure 23-7, the open method for donning sterile gloves. In the photograph at Step 7, you can see that the nurse has a sterile glove on her right hand and is touching the glove with her bare left hand. Is the nurse breaking the "sterile-touches-sterile" principle? Explain your thinking.
5. Refer to Procedure 23-6, the closed method of donning a sterile gown and gloves. Examine the very last photograph, in which one nurse is preparing to turn and receive her gown tie from a coworker. The gowned nurse has already donned sterile gloves, using the closed method. When the gowned nurse turns to receive the tie, what must she take care to not touch? What can she touch?
6. For each of the following concepts, use critical thinking to describe how or why it is important to nursing, patient care, or promoting asepsis and preventing infection. Note that these are *not* to be merely definitions.

Chain of infection	Standard precautions
Pathogens	Transmission-based precautions
Asepsis	Protective isolation
Healthcare-related infections	Sterile
Multidrug-resistant organisms (MDROs)	Medical asepsis
Contamination	Surgical asepsis

What Are the Main Points in This Chapter?

- Healthcare-related infections (infections that are acquired in healthcare facilities) are a major health problem worldwide.
- The chain of infection consists of six links that must all be present for infection to be transmitted from one individual to another: infectious agent, reservoir, portal of exit, mode of transmission, portal of entry, and susceptible host.
- Pathogens are strains of bacteria, viruses, fungi, protozoa, helminths, and prions that cause disease.
- Drug-resistant and multidrug-resistant organisms (MDROs) have mutated to develop resistance to one or more classes of antimicrobial drugs. They are a serious problem because: (1) options for treating MDRO infections are limited; (2) they are associated with increased hospital lengths of stay and hospital charges; and (3) they are associated with serious illness and increased mortality.
- Many emerging pathogens are airborne and widely spread by air travel before the carrier shows any symptoms. They have the potential for causing epidemics and pandemics.
- Infectious illnesses typically follow five predictable stages: incubation, prodromal stage, illness, decline, and convalescence.
- Primary body defenses, such as intact skin and mucous membranes, block entry of pathogens into the body.
- Invading microorganisms trigger the body's secondary defenses, which include phagocytosis, the complement cascade, the inflammatory response, and fever.
- The humoral immune response results in the production of antibodies that neutralize pathogens or trigger their destruction.
- The cell-mediated immune response results in the production of T cells that destroy infected body cells.
- Nutrition, hygiene, rest, exercise, stress reduction, and immunization protect the body against infection.
- Anything that weakens the body's defenses or increases the person's exposure to pathogens makes the person more susceptible to infection. Such factors include illness, injury, medical treatment, infancy or old age, frequent public contact, and various lifestyle habits.
- Medical asepsis requires that objects and surfaces in the healthcare environment be disinfected.
- Scrupulous handwashing markedly decreases the transmission of infection and is the most important aspect of medical asepsis.
- Standard precautions are used with all clients whenever there is a possibility of coming in contact with blood, body fluids (except sweat), excretions and secretions, mucous membranes, and any break in the skin.
- Transmission-based precautions are added to standard precautions when there is concern about transmission of infection via contact, droplets, or air currents.
- Isolation precautions are designed to prevent the spread of disease, not to isolate the person who has the disease.
- Surgical asepsis is an attempt to prevent the patient from coming in contact with *any* microorganisms.
- Sterile technique is required in many patient activities, such as administering an injection, starting an intravenous line, or performing a sterile dressing change.
- Exposure to blood, body secretions, or body tissues containing blood or secretions requires immediate action. Minimize the exposure by washing hands or flushing the area thoroughly. Contact the infection preventionist or employee health nurse as soon after the exposure as possible, complete an injury report, and seek medical care.
- The task of the infection preventionist is to minimize the number of infections in the healthcare facility.
- A key factor in minimizing infectious outbreaks is recognizing unusual disease patterns.

Knowledge Map

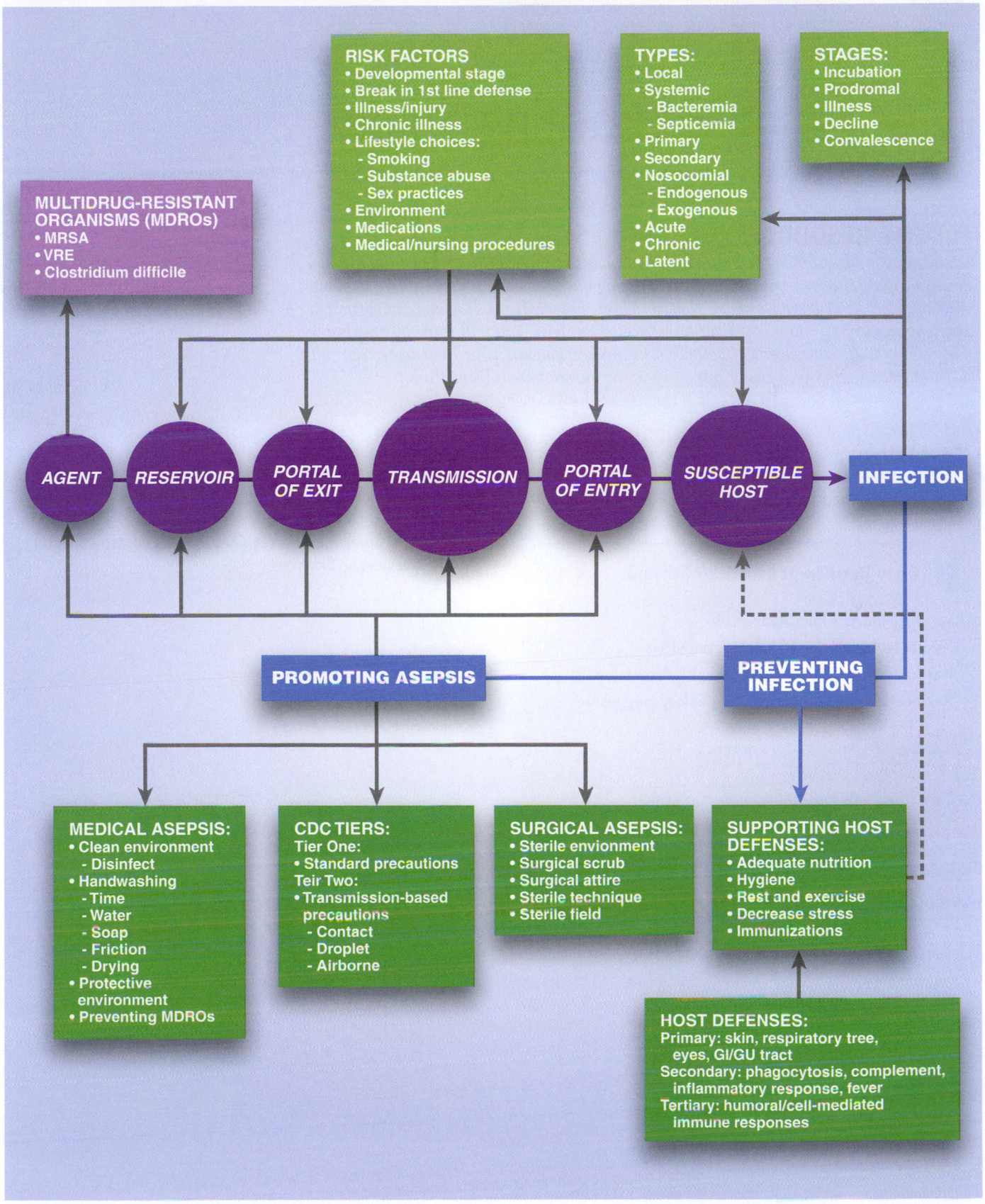

CHAPTER 24

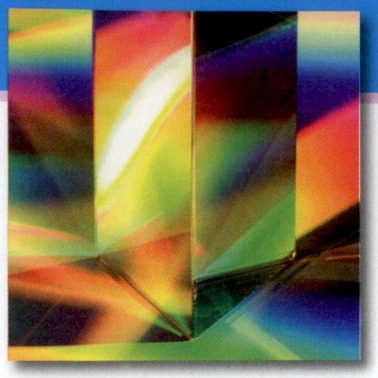

Promoting Safety

STUDENT RESOURCES

*The questions and exercises in Volume 2 allow you to practice the kind of thinking you will use as a full-spectrum nurse. Critical-thinking questions usually have more than one correct answer, so we do not provide "answers" for these features. It is more important to develop your nursing judgment than to just cover content. You will learn by discussing the questions with your peers. If you are still unsure, consult your instructor. You will find Response Sheets (for writing responses to the questions) on Davis*Plus.

To explore learning resources for this chapter

Go to Davis*Plus* at DavisPl.us/Wilkinson3.

Chapter Resources for Chapter 24:

- **Response sheets for all learning activities**
- **Resources for Caregivers and Health Professionals**
- **Reading More About Promoting Safety (suggested readings)**
- **Concept Map of chapter content**

Interactive Case Studies

NCLEX-style and Chapter Review Questions

CHAPTER OVERVIEW

For a podcast of an overview of this chapter,

Go to Student Resources, **Chapter 24, Podcast—Chapter Overview,** on Davis*Plus*.

Caring for the Nguyens

Refer to the database for Nam Nguyen in the front of this book. Use full-spectrum thinking to identify safety hazards for Mr. Nguyen, his 3-year-old grandchild (Kim Phan, who lives with him), and his widowed mother, Mai Nguyen, who lives alone.

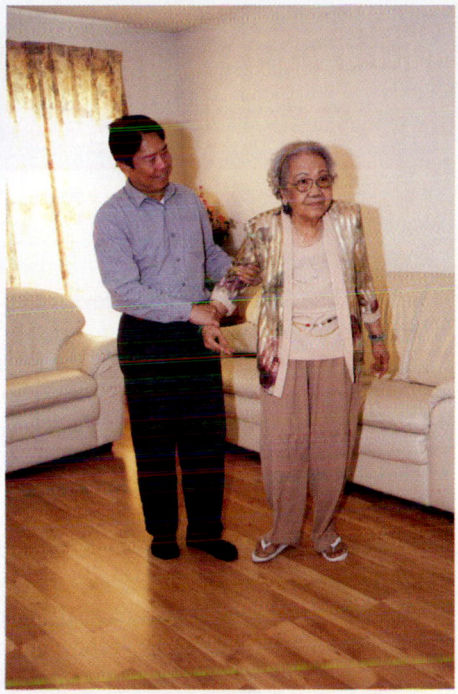

A. Without even using any patient data from the database (except ages), what theoretical knowledge do you have that will help you to identify risks that commonly occur in the developmental stages represented by these three clients?
Mr. Nguyen
Mr. Nguyen's 3-year-old grandchild, Kim
Mr. Nguyen's widowed mother, Mai

B. From Mr. Nguyen's database, what data can you put with your theoretical knowledge to identify the most likely safety risks for him? What are those risks?

C. From the risks and possible risks you have identified, for which one do you definitely need more data before deciding whether it increases his risk for accidents? That is, which piece of data is especially vague? What do you need to find out?

D. You know the theoretical (or possible) risks for Mr. Nguyen's mother. What data do you need in order to determine her *actual* safety risks?

E. What, if any, data do you have that would help you to identify any *actual* safety risks for Mr. Nguyen's grandchild? What, if any, are those risks?

F. What would you want to assess at the child's preschool to be sure that safety measures exist for preventing falls?

Practical Knowledge knowing how

Nursing interventions to promote safety in the home focus mainly on patient teaching. In hospitals and long-term care facilities, however, you will take a more proactive role in preventing injury to patients. In addition to patient advocacy activities, you will need practical knowledge of measures other than restraints (e.g., bed and chair monitors) you can use to prevent falls. You must also know how to apply and manage restraints safely.

PROCEDURES

Procedure 24-1 ■ Using a Bed Monitoring Device

➤ For steps to follow in *all* procedures, refer to the Universal Steps for All Procedures found on the inside back cover.

Equipment

Bed or chair exit monitoring device

There are at least four types of staff notification systems that may be utilized to warn caregivers that a patient is leaving a bed or chair: (1) pressure sensitive, (2) posture indicators, (3) motion sensors, and (4) pull-cord and combination alarms.

Delegation

As the nurse, you must determine whether a monitoring device is needed. You must also select the appropriate device and provide ongoing evaluation of its effectiveness. You may delegate to a nursing assistive personnel (NAP) the installation of the device, after verifying the NAP has the necessary knowledge and skill.

Pre-Procedure Assessments

- Assess for intrinsic factors that increase the risk for falls:
  - Older than age 75
  - History of a recent fall or fear of falling
  - Bowel and bladder incontinence (particularly urge bladder incontinence)
  - Cognitive impairment
  - Mood changes, lability
  - Dizziness
  - Functional impairment
  - Medications (especially new medications or changes in regimen)
  - Comorbidities (diseases such as dementia, hip fracture, type 2 diabetes, Parkinson's disease, arthritis, and depression)
- Assess for environmental factors that increase the risk for falls:
  - Use of an assistive device
  - Equipment in the room
  - Wet or uneven floors
  - The use of physical restraints
  - Inappropriate footwear
  - Poor lighting
  - Lack of grab rails and bars in the bathroom
  - Furniture and adaptive aids that are in disrepair or unstable (e.g., bed rails, IV poles)
  - Clothing that may cause tripping
- Identify factors that increase risk for more severe injury in the case of a fall. These include use of anticoagulants (e.g., Coumadin, Plavix, or aspirin) and osteoporosis.
- Check the alarm on the monitoring device to ensure that it is working properly.

➤ When performing the procedure, always identify your patient according to agency policy, using two identifiers, and be attentive to standard precautions, hand hygiene, patient safety and privacy, body mechanics, and documentation.

Procedure Steps

1. Apply the device.

Bed or Chair Monitor

Place sensor pads under the patient's buttocks.

The sensor will alarm when the patient attempts to get out of the bed or chair; it alarms when there is no weight on it for more than a few seconds. Many electronic beds have bed exit and patient position monitors for which you must select the desired alarm sensitivity. For example, you may set the system to alarm when the patient exits the bed, when the patient attempts to exit the bed, or even when the patient moves in the bed.▼

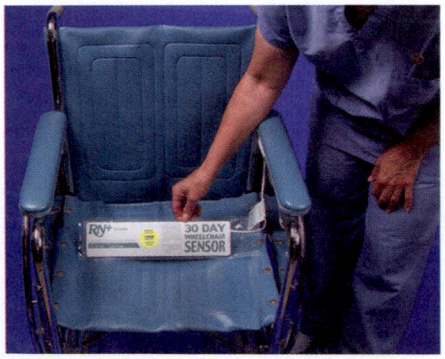

Leg Sensors

Place sensors on the patient's thigh.

The alarm will sound when the leg assumes a near-vertical position.▼

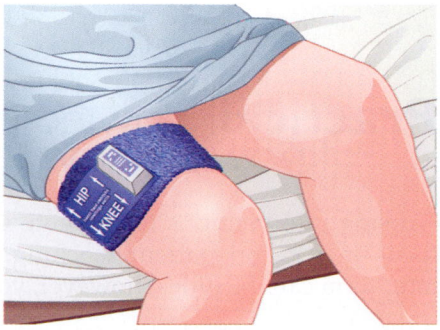

Infrared Beam Detector
Attach next to the bed or on the wall.

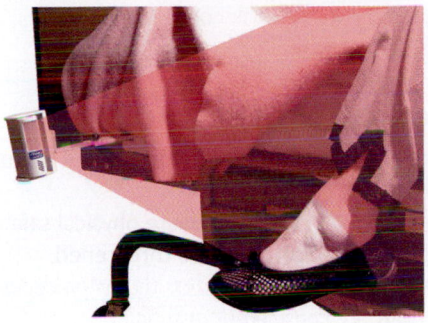

Cord-Activated Sensor
Attach one end of the cord (clip) to the patient's garment. Attach the other end to the control unit. The cord should be long enough to allow moderate movements, but short enough to prevent false alarms. Be sure the cord is free to pull straight out from the monitor and is not blocked by pillows, bedding, or bedrails.
The alarm is activated when the patient's movement causes the cord to be detached from the control unit. Some patients will deactivate the alarms, including removing the alarms clipped to their garments.

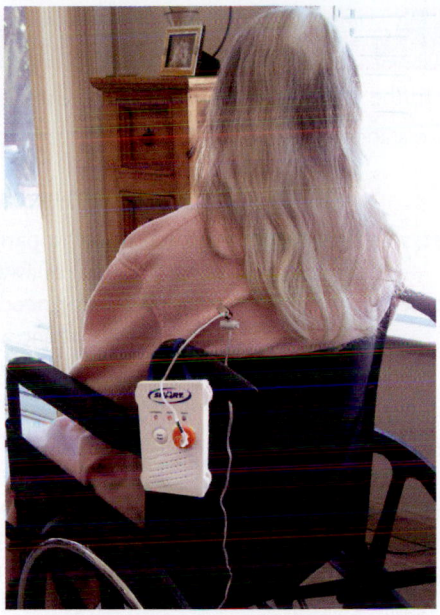

2. **Connect the control unit to the sensor pad.**

Bed or Chair Monitor
Mount the control unit on the bed or chair.

Leg Sensor
Mount the control unit directly on the leg sensor.

Infrared System
Mount the control unit next to the bed or on the wall.

Cord-Activated System
Mount the control unit next to the bed or on the wall.

3. **Connect the control unit to the nurse call system,** if possible.
Allows for a quicker response; however, not all call systems will accommodate this.

4. **Disconnect or turn off the alarm** before assisting the patient out of the bed or chair.
Prevents false alarms. Some systems have a standby setting to allow the alarm to be temporarily suspended.

5. **Reactivate the alarm** after assisting the patient back to the bed or chair.
Helps improve the timeliness of staff response, which may prevent patient falls.

6. **Be sure the patient can access** to the nurse call light easily.

Evaluation

- Assess the sensitivity of the monitoring device, and adjust as needed to ensure that the alarm is activated if the patient tries to get out of the bed or chair.
- Continue to assess fall risk per agency policy and as indicated by the patient's physical and/or mental status.
- In the event of a fall, perform a post-fall assessment to identify possible causes. Monitor patients closely for 48 hours after a fall.

Patient Teaching

- Explain to the patient and family that a bed or chair exit monitoring device alerts the staff when the patient tries to get out of the chair or bed.
- Explain that the purpose of the device is to help prevent falls using the least restrictive method possible will reassure the patient and family.
- Explain to the patient that she will need to call for assistance when she wants to get up.
Calling for assistance will prevent the alarm from sounding. Summoning for help can prevent the patient from falling.

Documentation

Document the initial sensor placement, including type of sensor used and the location of placement.

- After documenting initial placement, follow agency policy for documenting the use of bed exit monitor. Usually, the minimum documentation for exit monitors is every 8 hours.
- Place the patient on fall risk precautions according to agency policy.
- Document on the fall risk assessment sheet, restraint flowsheet, and nursing notes according to agency policy.

Sample documentation

9/14/16 1230. Client becomes easily disoriented while sitting in wheelchair and attempts to rise to a standing position. Safe standing and walking with assistance x1. Reminded to ask for assistance when standing or walking and placed next to nurse's station.

Mary Clinton, RN

Practice Resources

Gray-Micelli, D., & Quigley, P. (2011); National Guideline Clearinghouse (2003, updated 2008); Park, K., & Tang, J. (2007).).

Thinking About the Procedure

To practice applying clinical reasoning to this procedure,

Go to the *Davis's Nursing Skills Videos*, **Using Bed and Chair Monitoring Devices.**

For questions and suggested responses,

Go to Chapter 24, **Thinking About the Procedure Questions and Suggested Responses,** on DavisPlus.

Procedure 24-2 ■ Using Restraints

➤ For steps to follow in *all* procedures, refer to the Universal Steps for All Procedures found on the inside back cover.

➤ **Caution:** This procedure describes Medicare standards, but state and agency policies may be more restrictive.

Equipment

- Restraint of the appropriate size: belt, vest, wrist or ankle, or mitt
- Soft gauze or cotton padding for bony prominences

Delegation

As the nurse, you must determine whether restraints are needed in each specific situation. You must also select the least restrictive type of restraints, evaluate their effectiveness, and continue to assess for complications that may occur. You may delegate to NAPs the application and periodic removal of ordered restraints, after verifying that the NAP has the knowledge and skill to do so.

Pre-Procedure Assessments

- Assess the patient's risk for falls, including mobility status and level of awareness.
- Assess for need for restraints: The immediate physical safety of the patient, a staff member, or others is threatened.
  If a patient must be temporarily restrained so that a procedure may be performed, this is not considered "restraint."
- Determine that all less restrictive interventions have been tried unsuccessfully.
- Identify the appropriate restraint:
  - The least restrictive possible
  - Does not interfere with care or exacerbate patient's medical condition.
  - Does not pose a safety risk to the patient.
  - Can be changed easily to keep it clean.

➤ When performing the procedure, always identify your patient according to agency policy, using two identifiers, and be attentive to standard precautions, hand hygiene, patient safety and privacy, body mechanics, and documentation.

Procedure Steps

1. **Determine whether dangerous** behaviors continue despite attempts to eliminate causal factors using less restrictive interventions.

2. **Obtain a physician's prescription** for restraint, including type of restraint, indications for use, site of restraint application, and duration. Determine if the restraint is being used for medical–surgical or behavioral reasons.
   Federal and state regulations and laws permit healthcare facilities to use restraints only when they are medically needed. Restraints can be used only with a physician's or advanced registered nurse practitioner's (ARNP) order for a specified and limited time. When you apply restraint in an emergency, obtain the order as the restraint is being applied, or as quickly as possible afterward. When the restraint prescription expires (maximum 24 hr), physician assessment and a new prescription are needed.

3. **Notify the family of the change in patient status and the need for restraints.** Obtain patient and family consent when clinically feasible.
   Patients have the right to refuse treatment. Consent may not be necessary if there is an immediate threat to patient safety; however, as a rule, the family must be notified of the use of restraints if the patient has cognitive impairment. Many times family members prefer to sit with the patient as an alternative to restraint.

4. **Pad bony prominences** and apply the appropriately sized restraint, using appropriate knotting techniques. ➤

   ✚ Use a quick-release knot, such as the half-bow, when tying restraints to the bed frame or wheelchair. Do not tie restraints to the siderails.

   A quick-release knot is used to prevent patient injury and for ease of caring for the patient. Tie the knot on an immovable part of the bed to prevent injuring the patient if the siderails or head of bed is lowered. A quick-release knot will not tighten or slip when the patient moves about, but unties quickly when you pull on the loose end.

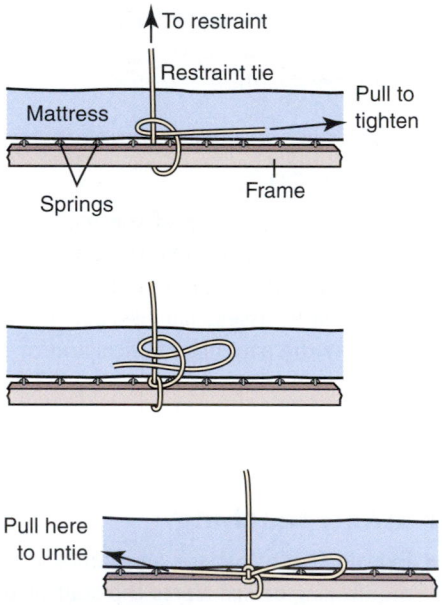

Belt Restraint

a. Place the belt restraint at the patient's waist, removing any wrinkles.
b. Make sure that the belt is snug but does not constrict the patient's waist.
c. Some belts have a key-locked buckle to prevent slipping.

A belt restraint is used mainly to prevent a patient from falling when getting up from a chair or wheelchair and may be used to remind a patient not to get out of bed unassisted.▼

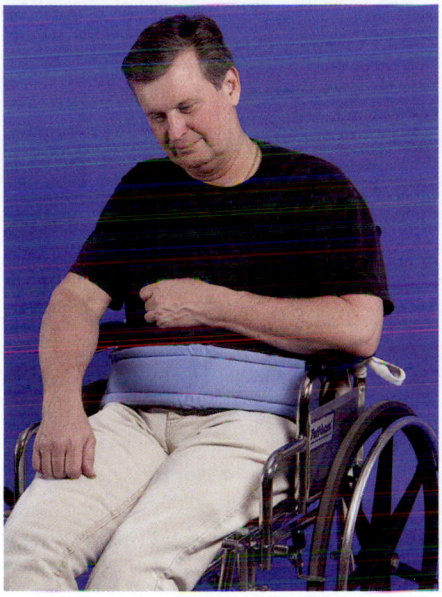

Vest or Jacket Restraint

a. Place the patient in the vest restraint. A zipper-style vest is preferred.
A vest restraint with a rear zipper is less likely to accidentally strangle the patient.

b. Attach the vest straps to the bed or wheelchair.
A vest restraint is used mainly to prevent a patient from falling out of a chair or wheelchair and sometimes to prevent a patient from getting out of bed unassisted.▼

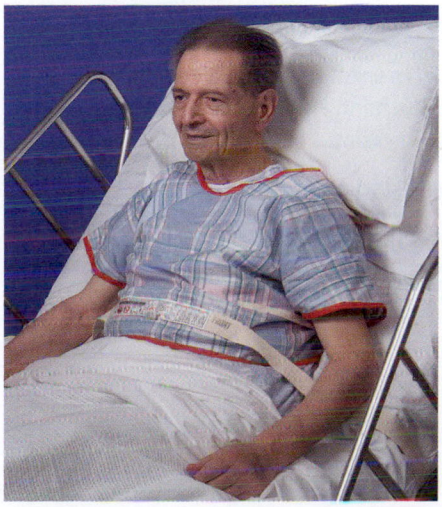

Wrist or Ankle Restraint

a. Apply the padded portion of the wrist or ankle restraint around the patient's wrist or ankle.

b. Make the restraint snug enough to prevent the patient from being able to slip it off, but not tight enough to impair circulation.

c. Attach the restraint strap to the bed frame. Do not attach to bed rails.
A wrist restraint is used mainly to prevent an agitated patient from pulling at tubes, such as IV sites and nasogastric tubes.▼

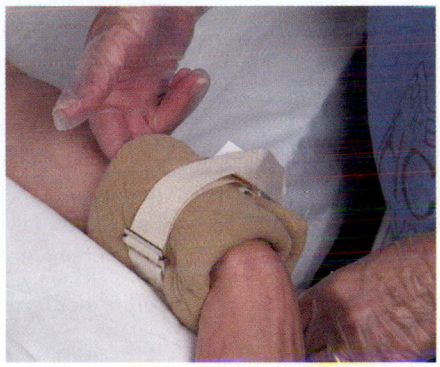

Mitt Restraint

a. Place patient's hand in the mitt restraint, ensuring that fingers are slightly flexed in the mitt.

b. Attach restraint strap to the bed frame if necessary.
A mitt restraint is used mainly to prevent a patient from pulling at tubes, such as IV sites and nasogastric tubes. Mitt restraints limit the use of the fingers, which may be enough to prevent the patient from grasping the tube. If this is the case, mitts that are not tied to the bed frame are the least restrictive restraint.▼

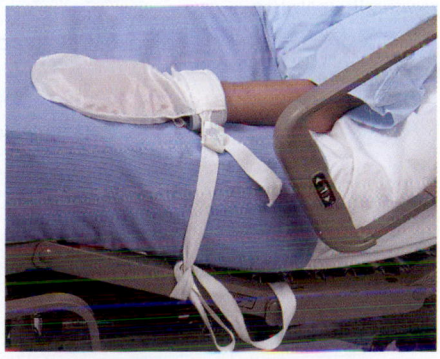

Enclosed Bed

a. Place patient in the bed and zip all sides. Be sure zippers are completely closed and zipper tabs are positioned in the upper aspects of the net panels out of the patient's reach.

b. Adhere to the manufacturer's minimum height and weight recommendations.

c. Never leave the bed in the high position with the patient unattended.
An enclosed bed is a canopy-like padded bed that is used mainly to keep a patient from wandering or from falling out of bed. The bed has nylon netting on all four sides, with zippered panels that can be opened to provide care. The patient has full freedom of movement and access to all parts of his body. Patients in enclosed beds have a higher risk of becoming entrapped between the bed rails and the mattress, risking suffocation. The dangers are greater for smaller patients and when the bed is left in a high position.

5. **Adjust the restraint** to maintain good body alignment, comfort, and safety. You should be able to slide two fingers under a wrist or ankle restraint.
The restraint should be snug enough to prevent it from slipping off, but not tight enough to impair circulation.

6. **Release restraints at least** every 2 hr to provide skin care, passive and active range of motion (ROM), ambulation, toileting, hydration, and nutrition at least every 2 hr. Assess for the continued need for restraint.

Prevents impaired circulation and injury. Medicare- and Medicaid-certified healthcare agencies must ensure that a patient's abilities do not decline unless the decline cannot be avoided because of the patient's medical condition. Patients often lose the ability to bathe, dress, walk, toilet, eat, and communicate when they are regularly restrained. If restraints are necessary, they must be used in a way that does not cause these losses.

(continued on next page)

Procedure 24-2 ■ Using Restraints (continued)

7. **Place the patient on fall risk** precautions according to agency policy.
   Patients who are restrained have a higher incidence of falls.

? What if . . .

- **I must apply a restraint in an emergency, for the safety of the patient or others?**

In such an emergency, an RN may initiate a restraint. When you apply restraint in an emergency, obtain the order as the restraint is being applied, or as quickly as possible afterward.

Evaluation

- Assess the initial restraint placement, circulation, and skin integrity. Observe for pallor, cyanosis, and coolness of extremities when extremities are restrained.
- Check the restraint every 30 minutes (more often for a behavioral restraint).
- Reassess the restraint, circulation, the patient's response to the intervention, and the need for continuing the use of the restraint every 2 hours; remove it when it is no longer needed.
  Ensures that the restraint is still functioning as intended. Monitoring and reassessment are critical components of caring for patients in physical restraints. Frequency of monitoring is determined by the type of restraint (behavioral vs. medical-surgical). Patients in behavioral restraints require more frequent monitoring and in some circumstances require continual observation.
  - Check every 24 hours to see that the restraint prescription has been renewed.
  - Remove the restraint as soon as possible.
  - Modify the plan of care to reflect the application of restraints and the plan for monitoring.

Patient Teaching

- Explain to the patient and family the need for the restraints.
- Explain that the restraints will be removed as soon as possible.

Home Care

- The same guidelines apply to clients in the home.
- Evaluate caregivers' knowledge and skill in using restraints, and provide teaching as needed (e.g., regarding padding bony prominences and the need to periodically release restraints).
- If an enclosed bed is used in the home, instruct the caregiver in safe use.

Documentation

Document the following:

- All nursing interventions that were done to eliminate the need for the restraint (e.g., moving patient closer to the nurses' station, asking a family member to remain with the patient, reorienting the patient)
- Reasons for placing the restraint (e.g., patient behaviors)
- The initial restraint placement, location, circulation, and skin integrity
- The teaching session with the patient and family members
- Circulation checks, ROM, and restraint removal per agency protocol
- Entries on fall risk assessment sheet, restraint flowsheet, and nursing notes according to agency policy

Sample documentation

12/24/16 1230. Continues to be confused, pulling at IV lines. Physician notified and evaluated patient. Mitt restraints ordered and placed on bilateral hands. Fall risk precautions initiated. Mitt restraints explained to patient and wife. Wife agreed that mitt restraints would help keep her husband from removing IV line.
Mary Clinton, RN

Practice Resources

American Nurses Association (ANA) (2001); Centers for Medicare & Medicaid Services (2006b).

Thinking About the Procedure

To practice applying clinical reasoning to this procedure,

Go to the *Davis's Nursing Skills Videos*, **Safety, Using Restraints: Belt Restraint, Mitt Restraint, Vest Restraint, and Wrist/Ankle Restraint.**

For questions and suggested responses,

Go to Chapter 24, **Thinking About the Procedure Questions and Suggested Responses,** on Davis*Plus*.

CLINICAL INSIGHTS

Clinical Insight 24-1 ➤ Preventing Needlestick Injury

Use needleless systems (e.g., retractable needles) when possible. More than 80% of needlestick injuries can be prevented with the use of safe needle devices (ANA, 2002).

Before beginning a procedure:

- Provide adequate lighting and space to perform the procedure.
- Place the sharps container near the work area, if it is moveable.
- Obtain assistance if there is a risk the patient may be uncooperative, combative, or confused.
- Inform the patient about the procedure and explain the importance of avoiding any sudden movement.

During the procedure:

- Be sure you can see the sharps container at all times.
- When handling a sharp, be aware of other persons in the immediate area.
- Do not hand-pass exposed sharps from one person to another.
- When using a safety needle, observe for audio or visual cues that the feature has engaged.

Handling needles:

- Do not shear or break contaminated needles
- Avoid recapping, bending, or removing contaminated needles and other sharps unless there is no feasible alternative.
- When you must recap a sterile needle, use a mechanical recapping device or a modified "scoop" technique (see Procedure 26-10).
- Never carry syringes in your uniform pocket.

Sharps containers:

- Keep puncture-proof needle disposal containers in every room.
- Place sharps containers at eye level; do not overfill the container.
- Make sure the container is large enough to hold the entire sharp device.
- Dispose of sharps immediately. Do not wait until you have finished the procedure.
- Inspect sharps and waste containers for protruding sharps. If found, notify safety personnel for removal of the hazard.

If your agency does not use needleless systems or protective devices you should do the following:

- Explain the OSHA Bloodborne Pathogens Standard (BPS) to your employer, including the need to provide needleless systems or protective devices for blood products and parenteral medication administration.

Refer your employer to the OSHA Web site at www.osha.gov/needlesticks/needlefaq.html

- OSHA requires worker involvement in evaluating, selecting, and implementing the use of safer needle products; volunteer to serve on that committee.
- Ask your agency for a copy of their exposure control plan, which is required by the BPS for monitoring compliance with the new law.
- Keep a record of needlestick injuries on your unit and of "near-misses" (e.g., overfilled sharps containers, sharps left on bed or overbed table).
- Submit written concerns to your employer.
- If your employer refuses to purchase safety devices, you may want to file an OSHA complaint. If you do so, refer to Chapter 44's Whistleblowing section. Complaints can be filed anonymously.
- For complaint filing,

http://www.osha.gov/as/opa/worker/complain.html

Practice Resources

Adapted from: ANA (2002); Centers for Disease Control and Prevention (CDC) (2011b.); National Institute for Occupational Safety and Health (NIOSH) (n.d., updated 2010.); U.S. Department of Labor, Occupational Safety and Health Administration (OSHA) (n.d.); Wilburn, S. (2004).

Clinical Insight 24-2 ➤ What You Should Know About Using Restraints

- ***Restraints are a last resort.*** The current standard of care is restraint-free. Restraints should be a last-resort intervention.
- ***Individualize care.*** Before using restraints, try to understand the message in the patient's behavior. The best way to achieve restraint-free care is to individualize care to avoid the risky behavior.
- ***Try less restrictive interventions*** before resorting to restraints. For example, request family involvement as an alternative to restraint. Family members may be able to interpret a patient's gestures or understand what is bothering him. For other suggestions,

Go to Volume 1, **Preventing the Need for Restraints.**

- ***Follow agency policy,*** professional guidelines, and state laws for using restraints.
- ***Use restraints only for safety*** to ensure the immediate physical safety of the patient or others.
- ***No standing orders*** or "as needed" orders for physical restraint are allowed.
- ***You must obtain a medical prescription*** from a physician or other licensed care provider.
- ***Guidelines are more restrictive when restraints are used for behavior management.***
- ***You must renew restraint prescriptions every 24 hours*** (more often for behavioral restraints).
- ***You must modify the plan of care*** to reflect the application of restraints and the plan for monitoring.
- ***Explain the need for the restraints*** if you must use them.
- ***Obtain consent*** from the patient and family when feasible.
- ***Always use the least restrictive restraint that ensures safety.***
- ***Remove the restraint as soon as possible.***
- ***Monitor and reassess.*** These are critical components of caring for patients in physical restraints. Assess restraints every 30 minutes (more frequently for patients with behavioral restraints, who may need continuous monitoring).
- ***Remove restraints for assessment, feeding, toileting, and skin care every 2 hours.*** Patients in medical-surgical restraints should be evaluated by an RN at least every 2 hours. Those in behavioral restraints require more frequent monitoring.
- ***Medications are considered a restraint*** when they are used to restrict the patient's freedom of movement or to manage behavior.
- ***Physical holding of a patient is not always considered restraint.*** Sometimes it is necessary to use devices or methods that involve the physical holding of a patient for routine physical examinations or tests.

ASSESSMENT GUIDELINES AND TOOLS

Focused Assessment

Get Up and Go Test

Conduct the Get Up and Go Test as part of a routine assessment when dealing with older persons. Its purpose is to detect "fallers" and to identify those who need evaluation. The staff should be trained to perform the Get Up and Go Test at check-in and query those with gait or balance problems for falls.

Initial Check

All older persons who report a single fall should be observed as they "get up and go":

- Move from a sitting position and stand without using their arms to help them rise and stand.
- Walk several paces, turn, and return to the chair.
- Sit back in the chair without using their arms for support.

Those who have difficulty or demonstrate unsteadiness performing this test require the following follow-up assessment.

Follow-Up Assessment

In the follow-up assessment, ask the person to:

- Sit.
- Stand without using their arms for support.
- Close his eyes for a few seconds, while standing in place.
- Stand with eyes closed, while you push gently on his sternum.
- Walk a short distance and come to a complete stop.
- Turn around and return to the chair.
- Sit in the chair without using his arms for support.

If the client has difficulty performing those tests, refer for a comprehensive evaluation.

Referring for Comprehensive Evaluation

A comprehensive evaluation should be performed by a practitioner with advanced skills and experience (AHI of Indiana, n.d.; American Academy of Neurology, 2008a, 2008b; Hendrich, 2007; Kenny, Rubenstein, & Tinetti, et al., 2011). In any of the following situations, you should refer the patient for a comprehensive fall evaluation.

- The patient is seeking care because of a fall.
- The patient or family reports recurrent falls in the past year.
- The patient's gait or balance is abnormal.

Focused Assessment

The Timed Up & Go Test for Fall Risk Assessment

Physicians are asked to assess annually all patients who are 65 years or older using the **Timed Up & Go Test.**

Timed Up & Go Test

1. Have the patient in a seated position.
2. Place a visible object 8 feet away from the patient.
3. Ask the patient to get up and walk around the object, and then sit back down.
   - Allow the patient to practice once.
   - Then time the patient three times as he performs these steps.
   - Scores greater than 8.5 seconds are associated with high fall risk in community-dwelling older adults.

Practice Resources

American Academy of Neurology (2008a, 2008b); Hendrich, A. (2007); Kenny, R., Rubenstein, L., Tinetti, F., et al. (2011); Podsiadlo, D., & Richardson, S. (1991).

FOCUSED ASSESSMENT: S.A.S. SAFETY ASSESSMENT SCALE

Name _____

CLSC CÔTE-DES-NEIGES

S.A.S. SAFETY ASSESSMENT SCALE

CAREGIVER AND LIVING ENVIRONMENT (1)

a) This person lives on her own. Yes [1] No [0] _____

b) This person is alone at home.
Always [4] Most of the time [3] Occasionally [2] Never [1] _____

SMOKING (2)

This person leaves cigarette bum marks on the floor, furniture, or clothing.
Yes [1] No [0] _____

FIRE AND BURNS (3)

a) The stove on/off buttons are located...
on the front of the stove [1] on the top of the stove [2]
behind the hotplates [3] _____

b) This person is capable of turning on the stove him/herself
Yes [1] No [0] Doesn't know [1] _____

c) This person cooks his/her own food.
Always [4] Most of the time [3] Occasionally [2] Never [1] _____

d) This person forgets a pan on the stove.
Very often [4] Often [3] Sometimes [2] Never [1] _____

e) The heating system uses...
electricity [1] natural gas [2] wood [3] _____

NUTRITION (4)

a) This person receives meals-on-wheels or other prepared meals.
More than once a day [1] Once a day [2]
A few times a week (2 to 6 times a week) [3] Once a week or less [4] _____

b) This person's meals contain foods from different food groups (dairy products, meat or fish, cereals, fruit and vegetables).
Always [1] Most of the time [2] Occasionally [3] Never [4] _____

FOOD POISONING AND TOXIC SUBSTANCES (5)

This person can tell the difference between food that is fresh and food that is spoiled. Yes [0] No [1] _____

MEDICATION AND HEALTH PROBLEMS (6)

a) This person takes, on a regular basis...*
1 to 3 medications [2] 4 to 6 medications [3]
7 medications or more [4] Does not take any medication [1]
*prescribed medications only _____

b) This person takes medication to help him/her sleep or relax.
Yes [1] No [0] _____

c) Does this person suffer from any physical health problem?
None [1] Minor [2] Moderate [3] Severe [4] _____

d) This person accepts treatment for his/her physical health problems.
Yes [0] No [1] Does not apply [0] _____

WANDERING AND ADAPTATION TO CHANGING TEMPERATURE (7)

a) This person gets lost in familiar surroundings.
Very often [4] Often [3] Sometimes [2] Never [1] _____

b) Has this person ever gotten lost? Yes [1] No [0] _____

c) Can this person find his/her way home? Yes [0] No [1] _____

d) Does this person dress appropriately according to the changing temperature, both indoors and outdoors?
Yes [0] No [1] _____

An Affiliated University Centre
Affiliated with McGill University

Assessed by _____

SCORE _____ / 47

Source: Dr. Louise Poulin de Courval ©CLSC Côte-des-Neiges. Used with permission.

CLINICALREASONING

Applying the Full-Spectrum Nursing Model

PATIENT SITUATION

Recall your patient, Alvin Lin, from Meet Your Patient in Volume 1. Mr. Lin is a 79-year-old man who was just transferred from a long-term care facility to your medical unit. His admitting diagnosis is dehydration and pneumonia. In the handoff report you were told he had rested well during the night and was alert and oriented. When you enter his room, he is confused and does not know where he is. He is becoming combative and is trying to get out of bed.

THINKING

1. *Theoretical Knowledge:*
   a. What is the pathophysiology of pneumonia?
   b. When the oxygen level of the blood falls, what is the effect on the central nervous system? If you don't know the answer to this question, consult a reliable reference.
   c. What are the defining characteristics for the NANDA-I diagnosis, Deficient Fluid Volume?
2. *Critical Thinking (Considering Alternatives):*
   a. Which of the three defining characteristics (in 1c) may increase Mr. Lin's risk for falls? Why?
   b. What else may be increasing his confusion and his risk for falls?

DOING

3. *Practical Knowledge:* Suppose you have tried all the less restrictive restraints, but Mr. Lin still attempts to get out of bed. He has even pulled out his intravenous line. You decide you must apply restraints to keep him safely in bed. You have called the physician, but he has not returned your call. You cannot wait any longer because you have other patients who need you, and yet you must stay with Mr. Lin to keep him from falling. What should you do right now?
4. *Nursing Process (Diagnosis):* Which nursing diagnosis seems more useful to you in planning care for Mr. Lin?
   Confusion related to disease process
   Risk for Falls related to confusion and possibly r/t weakness

CARING

5. *Self-Knowledge:*
   a. Do you think having a restraint-free facility is a valuable goal, or not? Explain your thinking.
   b. How did you come to believe that?
6. *Ethical Knowledge:* Suppose Mr. Lin is too confused to give consent for restraints, and you cannot reach his family by telephone. How can you justify applying restraints, and what must you do later to follow up?

Critical Thinking and Clinical Reasoning

1. Recall from Meet Your Patient in Volume 1 the clients you encountered in the community setting. Teresa was caring for her 2-year-old daughter and her elderly grandmother. The grandmother has a fear of falling. In Volume 1, we addressed some of the issues related to child-proofing the home. You would like to suggest ways for Teresa to make the home safe for her frail grandmother.
   a. Refer to the critical-thinking model and questions in Table 2-1 of Volume 1. What questions in the Inquiry section should you ask before making suggestions to Teresa?

Go to Table 2-1, **Critical Thinking Model,** in Volume 1.

   b. What specific information do you need about the grandmother? About the home?
   c. Once you have the necessary information, what suggestions could you make about home safety measures?
   d. Consider alternatives. What types of assistive devices might be helpful in preventing falls?
   e. Explore the alternatives. For example, are they practical? What do you need to know about this family to determine whether it is practical for them to obtain such devices?
   f. Think now about Teresa. Given the situation, what might create a safety risk for her?

2. Recall Alvin Lin (Meet Your Patients, in Volume 1), the 79-year-old man you were assigned to care for on your first day on the medical unit. The initial report you received was that he was alert and oriented, but you find that he is now confused and is becoming combative.
   a. What should be your first two priorities in this situation?
   b. What specific patient data do you need to determine what might have caused this change in behavior? How could you get that data?
   c. What alternatives to restraints might you consider?
3. A friend calls to tell you she thinks her 18-month-old daughter swallowed some of her sleeping pills. The child is very sleepy, and your friend is having difficulty arousing her. Your friend has ipecac in her medicine cabinet and wonders whether she should try to get her awake enough to take it.
   a. What is the first thing that you would recommend that the mother do?
   b. What is a major concern with inducing vomiting, given that you must assume from the mother that the child is very drowsy? What could go wrong if the child vomits?
   c. If the mother decides to take the daughter to the hospital instead of taking time to call the poison control center (PCC), what should you remind her to take with her?
4. An older couple has health problems and both are taking several medications. The husband has assumed care for himself and his wife, Ethyl, because Ethyl has been exhibiting confusion at times. He says he sometimes becomes overwhelmed with everything he has to do, and he is not sure that he always gives the medicine at the right times.
   a. What information do you need to know to be able to help with this situation? About the medications? About resources? How would you obtain the information?
   b. What suggestions can you make to help the husband organize the medications?
5. You are caring for a patient 12 hours after surgery following an abdominal hysterectomy for cancer. She asks you to help her to walk to a chair. You note that she has IV fluids infusing and is receiving opioids via a patient-controlled analgesia (PCA) pump. She states that she has not been out of bed since surgery and that she has just administered some medication and would like to get up while she has pain relief. You also notice that there is a Foley (indwelling urinary) catheter connected to a bedside drainage.
   a. What environmental factors could be safety hazards when this patient gets out of bed?
   b. What assessments and other interventions would help to ensure safe ambulation despite those obstacles?
6. For each of the following concepts, use critical thinking to describe how or why it is important to nursing, patient care, or promoting safety. Note that these are *not* to be merely definitions.

Environmental hazard	Choking rescue maneuver
Pathogens	Refrigeration
Poisoning	Mosquito control
Scald injuries	Rodent control
Falls	Reduce, reuse, recycle, respond
Teaching firearm safety to children	Back injuries
Pollution	Needlestick injuries
Radiation	Time, distance, and shielding
Restraint	Gang culture
Ambularm	Morse Fall Scale

What Are the Main Points in This Chapter?

- Safety is a basic human need.
- Unintentional injuries are the fifth leading cause of death in the United States.
- Major causes of unintentional deaths in the United States are motor vehicle accidents, poisoning, and falls.
- The environment includes the physical and psychosocial factors that contribute to the life and well-being of each person. It may be identified as any setting where the nurse and client interact.
- A person's safety is influenced by developmental factors as well as individual factors, such as lifestyle, cognitive awareness, sensoriperceptual status, ability to communicate, mobility status, and sensory losses, particularly hearing and vision losses.
- The main safety hazards in the home are poisoning, carbon monoxide poisoning, scalds and burns, fires, falls, firearm injuries, suffocation and drowning, and take-home toxins.
- Most fatal home fires occur while people are asleep, and most deaths result from smoke inhalation.
- More than half of all falls occur in the home; about 80% involve people older than age 65.
- Community hazards include motor vehicle accidents, pathogens, improper sanitation, pollution (air, water, noise, and soil), and electrical storms.
- Safety hazards in the healthcare agency include falls, equipment-related accidents, fires and electrical hazards, restraints, mercury exposure, and biological hazards.
- When possible, nurses should use alternative interventions instead of restraints.
- Medical prescriptions for restraints must be renewed at least every 24 hours.
- Workplace hazards to nurses include back injuries, needlestick injuries, radiation injury, and violence.
- All inpatients should be assessed for their risk for falls.
- Identifying anxiety may allow the nurse to intervene before a patient becomes aggressive.
- The Heimlich maneuver differs from the American Red Cross choking rescue maneuver in that the Heimlich does not include back blows.
- Nursing interventions for promoting safety in the home focus on client teaching.
- Nursing interventions for promoting safety in the healthcare facility focus on assessing for risk and creating a safe environment.

Knowledge Map

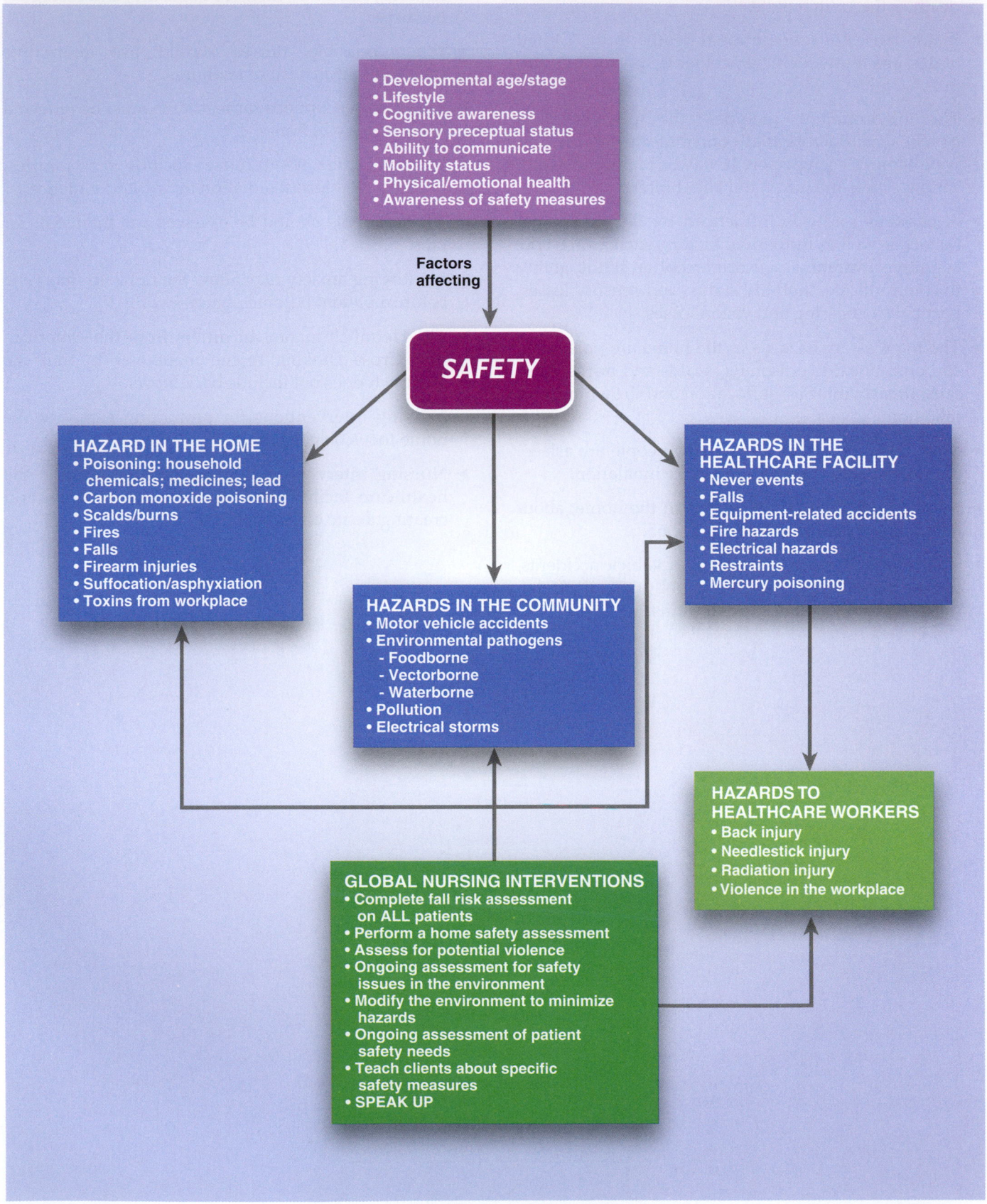

CHAPTER 25

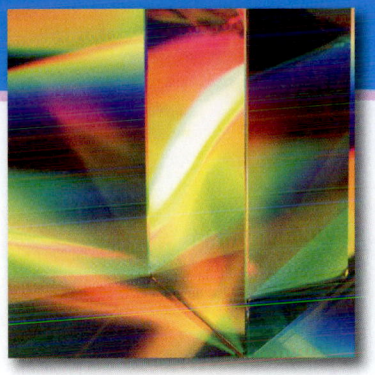

Facilitating Hygiene

STUDENT RESOURCES

*The questions and exercises in Volume 2 allow you to practice the kind of thinking you will use as a full-spectrum nurse. Critical-thinking questions usually have more than one correct answer, so we do not provide "answers" for these features. It is more important to develop your nursing judgment than to just cover content. You will learn by discussing the questions with your peers. If you are still unsure, consult your instructor. You will find Response Sheets (for writing your responses to the questions) on Davis*Plus.

To explore learning resources for this chapter,

Go to Davis*Plus* at DavisPl.us/Wilkinson3.

Chapter Resources for Chapter 25:

- **Response sheets for all learning exercises**
- **Resources for Caregivers and Health Professionals**
- **Reading More About Facilitating Hygiene (suggested readings)**
- **Concept Map of chapter content**

Interactive Case Studies

NCLEX-Style and Chapter Review Questions

CHAPTER OVERVIEW

For a podcast of an overview of this chapter,

Go to Student Resources, **Chapter 25, Podcast—Chapter Overview,** on Davis *Plus*.

Caring for the Nguyens

Yen Nguyen works as a preschool teacher. She schedules a clinic visit to discuss a variety of concerns. For each of the concerns she mentions, answer the following four questions:

1. What theoretical knowledge do you need?
2. Where could you find it?
3. What, if any, additional patient information do you need?
4. How would you respond to Mrs. Nguyen's concerns?

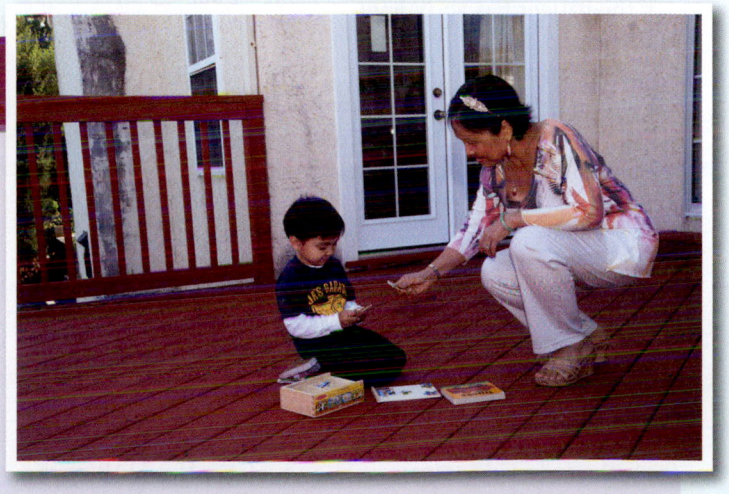

(Continued)

Caring for the Nguyens (continued)

A. Yen tells you that her skin is very dry and irritated.

B. Yen tells you that several of the children at the preschool have recently been diagnosed with head lice. She would like to know how to assess for pediculosis.

C. Yen tells you that her 3-year-old grandson, Kim, frequently refuses to bathe. She asks for advice on how to handle this.

Practical Knowledge knowing how

The following procedures and techniques provide the practical knowledge you will need to assist patients with personal cleanliness and grooming. As a nurse you are responsible for providing the necessary assistance and, at the same time, promoting as much self-care as possible. Self-care in activities of daily living (ADLs) promotes increased activity, independence, and self-esteem.

This Practical Knowledge section also contains clinical insights for providing hygiene care and a guideline for assessing hygiene needs. For standardized language tables for Self-Care Deficits and other nursing diagnoses related to hygiene,

Go to Chapter 25, **Standardized Language,** on Davis *Plus*.

PROCEDURES

Procedure 25-1 ■ Bathing: Providing a Complete Bed Bath Using a Prepackaged Bathing Product

➤ For steps to follow in *all* procedures, refer to the Universal Steps for All Procedures found on the inside back cover.

Equipment

- Prepackaged bathing product with disposable wipes (e.g., Comfort Bath)
- Bath blanket
- Clean patient gown (with shoulder snaps or Velcro closures if the patient has an IV line)
- Clean bed linen
- Orangewood stick
- Deodorant, lotion, and/or powder as needed
- Emollient (if not included in prepackaged bathing product)
- Procedure gloves (for anal and perineal care)
- Bedpan or urinal
- Laundry bag
- Plastic trash bag for used wipes and other disposable soiled items

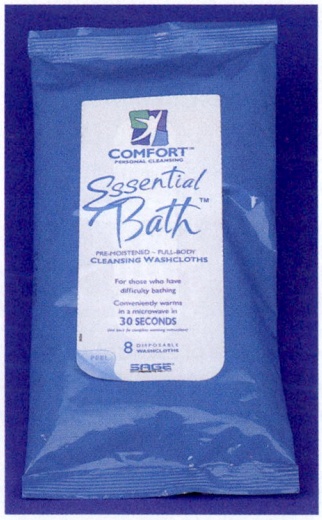

Delegation

You can delegate this procedure to the NAP if you conclude that the patient's condition and the NAP's skills allow. Perform the following assessments, and inform the NAP of the specific type of bath (e.g., packaged bath, bag bath) and the amount of help the patient needs. Inform the NAP of any special considerations, such as IV lines, drains, and so on. Ask the NAP to report the condition of the patient's skin, level of self-care, and ability to tolerate the procedure.

Pre-Procedure Assessments

- Assess mobility, activity tolerance, type of bath needed, and level of ability to perform bathing self-care.

A patient who has decreased activity tolerance or mobility (e.g., chest pain or shortness of breath with exertion) may have limited ability to assist with the bath. Having the patient assist as much as possible increases mobility and sense of control and comfort.

- **Check for positioning or activity restrictions (e.g., maintaining hip abduction following a total hip replacement).**
  Prevents injuring the patient during the procedure.
- **Determine the number of people you need to safely bathe and reposition the patient.**
  Helps prevent injury to the patient or the nurse.
- **Assess for personal and cultural issues that may be of concern to the patient regarding the bath.**
  Bathing may conflict with the patient's sense of privacy or modesty. Cultural norms and individual preferences must be considered.
- **Assess for specific patient needs and preferences during a bath, such as lotions and extra wipes or towels.**
  Advanced age, certain skin conditions, or skin breakdown may require special soaps and/or lotions. Incontinence or drainage may require additional wipes, towels, and precautions. Meeting patient preferences helps prevent depersonalization and promotes patient cooperation with the procedure.

➤ When performing the procedure, always identify your patient according to agency policy, using two identifiers, and be attentive to standard precautions, hand hygiene, patient safety and privacy, body mechanics, and documentation.

➤ *Note:* You may find that you need to adapt the bathing order and other steps to meet individual needs.

Procedure Steps

1. **Provide for patient privacy** and comfort.
   a. Close the door or privacy curtains, adjust room temperature, and assist the patient with elimination as needed.
   b. Ask the patient and family if they wish family members to assist with the bath.
   Assisting the patient with elimination before beginning the bath helps prevent interruptions during the procedure. Bathing practices differ among cultures and individuals, but are often private. The patient or family may wish to have a family member assist with the bath, or the patient may prefer that they leave the room.

2. **Peel open the label on the commercial bath** without completely removing it.
   Allows for steam to escape as contents heat without spilling the contents.

3. **Heat the package** in the microwave for no longer than 1 minute. The temperature of the contents should be approximately 105°F (41°C). This is controversial. Some references suggest, for safety, using the commercial bag bath at room temperature.
   Heating to 105°F (41°C) brings contents to a safe and comfortable temperature. This must be done with caution to prevent burning, especially in patients who have fragile skin.

If Using a Warmer Unit

You do not need Step 3 because the bags are always warm.

4. **Adjust the bed** to working height, lower the siderail nearest you, and position the patient supine close to the side of bed you will be working on.

   Raise the siderail before you leave that side of the bed.

   Prevents patient falls and keeps you from having to lean over the patient or reach across the siderail, which can cause back strain or injury.

5. **Remove the bedspread,** and spread the bath blanket over the top sheet; then ask the patient to hold the bath blanket in place while you remove the top sheet.
   Protects modesty and prevents chilling. If no bath blanket is available, you can use the top sheet in its place. However, if the sheet becomes damp, it may chill the patient.

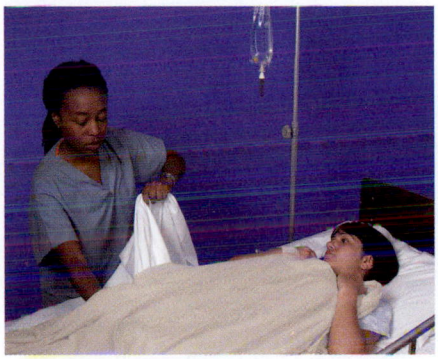

Note: Before proceeding, assist the patient with oral hygiene as needed. See Procedures 25-6 and 25-7.

6. **Remove the patient's gown,** keeping the patient covered with the bath blanket. During the bath, expose just the part of the body you are bathing.
   Maintains the patient's modesty and prevents chilling.

Patient With an IV Line

The patient may be wearing a gown that has snap-open sleeves.

a. Some tubing systems include a needlefree 2-way connector that maintains a closed line even when you disconnect the tubing. In that case, you simply open the connection, remove the gown, and then reconnect the tubing. After the bath, follow the same procedure to place the clean gown on the patient.
b. If there is no 2-way, needlefree connector on the tubing, remove the gown first from the arm without the IV. Lower the IV container, and pass the gown over the tubing and the container, taking care to keep the container above the level of the patient's arm.
   Keeps blood from backing up into the IV line.

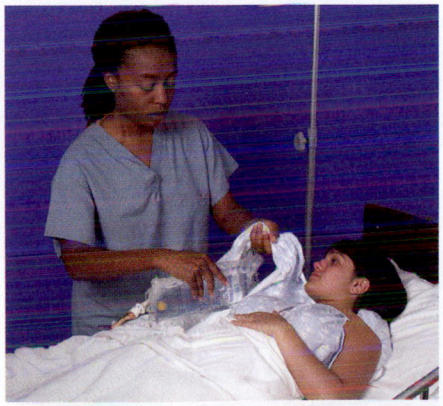

c. Never disconnect this type of IV tubing connection; this breaks the sterile system and provides a portal of entry for pathogens.

(continued on next page)

Procedure 25-1 ■ Bathing: Providing a Complete Bed Bath Using a Prepackaged Bathing Product (continued)

d. Rehang the container; check the flow rate.
Manipulating the IV equipment may change the flow rate; flow rate must be maintained as prescribed.

e. After the bath, replace the gown by threading the IV equipment from inside the arm of the gown and onto the affected arm. Then place the unaffected arm through the other gown sleeve.

7. **Don clean procedure gloves** if exposure to body fluids is likely or if either you or the patient has any breaks in the skin.
Follows universal precautions; helps prevent transfer of microorganisms.

8. **Wash the patient's face, neck, and ears.**
a. Fold the wipe around the hand to make a mitt, tucking in loose corners.
Keeps loose ends from dragging across the skin. This is uncomfortable because loose ends cool quickly.
b. Wash the face using one wipe.
c. Use a different corner of the wipe to gently wipe each eyelid outward from the inner canthus.
Some wipes contain chlorhexidine gluconate (CHG) an antimicrobial, which can be irritating to the eyes and mucous membranes. Use pH-balanced prepackaged wipes for the face, or use gauze squares moistened with agency-approved water or normal saline. A major principle is cleaning from "clean to dirty" to prevent contamination of a cleaner area. The inner canthus is considered the cleanest area. Prevents moving debris toward the nasolacrimal duct, which is located near the inner canthus.

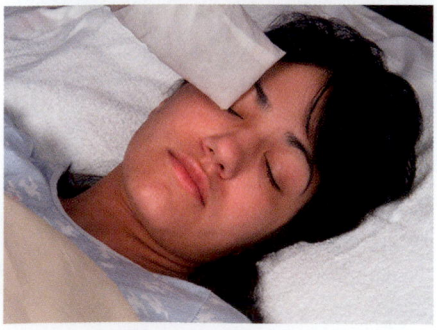

d. Wash the rest of the patient's face, neck, and ears.
Move sequentially through the bath to make it less tiring for the patient and more efficient for the nurse.
e. Allow areas to air dry. Do not rinse.
Prevents the emollient and surfactant skin protectants from being removed.

9. **Discard each wipe after use.**
Ensures following the "clean to dirty" principle.

10. **Wash the patient's arms**, using a new, clean wipe.
a. Fold the bath blanket off one arm at a time, and place a folded bath towel under the arm. Beginning with the patient's far arm, support the arm, and wash the arm from the hands upward using long strokes.
Long strokes increase circulation in the extremity. Washing from distal to proximal increases venous return from the periphery. Lifting the arm provides range of motion (ROM) to preserve joint mobility.
b. Continue to support the arm while washing the axilla.
Prevents potential injury to the joints. A sprain, subluxation, or dislocation of the joint can occur when an extremity is not properly supported, especially in older adults.
c. Allow the areas to air dry; do not rinse.
Prevents the emollient and surfactant skin protectants from being removed.
d. Apply deodorant and/or powder if desired.
Follow patient preferences whenever possible to increase feelings of comfort.
e. Clean under the nails with an orangewood stick as needed.
f. Repeat the preceding Steps 8a–d for the arm nearest you.

11. **Wash the patient's chest**, using a new clean wipe.
a. Cover the patient's chest with a bath towel, and lower the bath blanket to the patient's waist.
Maintains patient comfort and modesty.
b. For women, gently lift each breast to wash the skinfold if needed. Keep the chest covered between the wash and rinse.
Skinfolds are a source of odor and can become reddened and irritated because of skin-to-skin irritation and dampness from perspiration.
c. Cover to maintain privacy and warmth.
d. Allow the areas to air dry; do not rinse.
Prevents the emollient and surfactant skin protectants from being removed

12. **Wash the abdomen,** using a new, clean wipe.
a. Fold the bath blanket down to the perineal area, and cover the chest with a bath towel.
b. Wash the abdomen, including the umbilical area; allow to air dry. Pay special attention to skinfolds.
Perspiration and moisture do not evaporate well from skinfolds, predisposing them to maceration.
c. Cover the abdomen and chest with the bath blanket.
Prevents chilling.

13. **Wash the legs and feet**, using a new, clean wipe for each leg.
a. Uncover one leg at a time, beginning with the leg farthest from you. Place the bath towel under the leg.
Keeps the sheet dry; prevents chilling.
b. Wash the leg from distal to proximal with long, gentle strokes. Allow the leg to air dry.

Do not massage the calves of the legs.

Washing from distal to proximal may help to promote venous return. If a venous thrombus is present, massaging might dislodge the clot and cause an embolus.

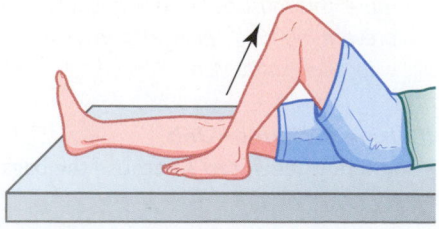

c. Thoroughly wash the foot and toes. Allow the foot to air dry. Apply lotion if the prepackaged bath product does not include emollient and as needed, but not between the toes.
Disease processes frequently decrease circulation to the feet and lower legs, increasing the likelihood that minor skin irritations may become more severe. Applying emollient between the toes can lead to skin breakdown.

d. Repeat the procedure on the other leg and foot.

14. Wash the back and buttocks, using a new, clean wipe.

a. Position the patient on his side with his back facing you, or in the prone position. Make sure the siderail on the far side of the bed, facing the patient, is still up.
Provides for clear visualization of back and access to the area.

b. Exposing only the back and buttocks, place the bath towel under the back and buttocks. Wash the back first and then the buttocks. Observe for redness and skin breakdown in the sacral area.
Maintains the principle of "clean to dirty." The sacral area is a common site of pressure sores.▼

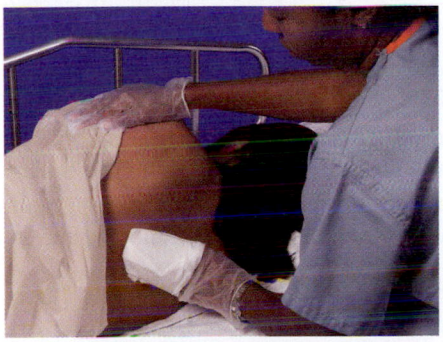

c. Unless contraindicated, give the patient a back rub, applying lotion to the back and buttocks (see Chapter 34, Procedure 34-1: Giving a Back Rub).
Stimulates circulation and maintains the health of the skin. Because the patient is in bed, he is at risk for skin irritation and breakdown from immobility and friction. A back rub may be contraindicated for patients with musculoskeletal injuries or cardiovascular disease.

d. Don procedure gloves if you have not already done so, and wash the rectal area, removing any fecal matter with tissues before washing with the wipe. Wash from front to back.
Washing the rectal area at this time removes the need for the patient to turn to his side again and helps prevent soiling clean linen when changing the linen in an occupied bed. Fecal matter usually contains microorganisms. Washing from front to back helps prevent transferring bacteria from the rectum to the vagina and urethra.▼

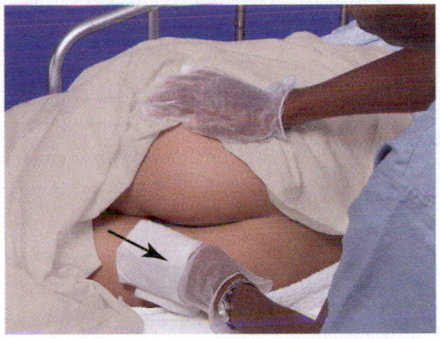

e. Discard the soiled wipe. If linens are soiled, cover them with a clean sheet before repositioning the patient.

f. Remove soiled gloves and wash hands or use an alcohol-based handrub. Don new procedure gloves before providing perineal care.
Prevents transferring microorganisms from anal to genital area—cleansing the gluteal and anal areas contaminates the wipe. Maintains standard precautions during the bath and prevents soiling of clean linens during bed change and cross-contamination to other body sites.

15. Cleanse the perineal area. See Procedure 25-4: Providing Perineal Care.

16. After providing perineal care, reposition and cover the patient with the bath blanket. Remove soiled gloves and wash hands or use alcohol-based handrub. Help the patient put on a clean gown, and attend to other hygiene needs (e.g., hair grooming).
Prevents contaminating clean linen with soiled gloves. Ensures proper body position and warmth.

17. Change the bed linen as needed, including soiled linen or linen that became damp during the bath. See Procedure 25-14: Making an Occupied Bed.
Ensures patient safety, comfort, and privacy.

? What if . . .

- **You are bathing the patient without assistance, or you are not tall enough to comfortably reach across the patient?**

  These situations put you at risk for back strain. Thus, you may want to bathe one side of the body—that is, the right arm, trunk, right leg—and then move to the other side of the bed to bathe the opposite side of the body (instead of the order given in Steps 8 and 9). Move the patient close to you before beginning the bath.

- **You are bathing a patient in leg traction?**

  You may decide to bathe the arms and trunk first. Then have the patient sit forward so that you can cleanse his back. Then have the patient lift up slightly so that you can wash his buttocks. Finally, wash the lower extremities.

- **You are bathing a patient with dementia?**

  Use your knowledge of the person's bathing practices and preferences to determine a time of day and a routine the person will accept. Keep stimulation to a minimum. Turn on some calming music, speak softly and reassuringly, and don't rush. Keep the patient warm. If the patient becomes agitated and you cannot calm him, do not force him to bathe. You may wish to consider a towel bath (Procedure 25-2) for patients with dementia. Also refer to Clinical Insight 25-2.
  Many steps in the bathing process may be misinterpreted or stressful for the person with dementia and may present with disruptive or agitated behaviors. If forced to bathe, the patient may be upset for hours. Towel baths are effective hygiene measures.

(continued on next page)

Procedure 25-1 ■ Bathing: Providing a Complete Bed Bath Using a Prepackaged Bathing Product (continued)

- **Your patient becomes agitated and uncooperative during the bath?**

  Speak calmly and softly. Give the patient a few minutes to calm down. Discontinue the bath if the patient remains upset.

- **Your patient is an older adult?**

  a. Some clinicians recommend bathing older adults every other day instead of daily, and it is generally agreed that they should not bathe more than once a day unless soiling occurs.
  These help prevent skin dryness.

  b. Assure that the wipes are warm prior to use, but not hot.
  Prevents burns (older adults may have decreased sensation in their extremities).

  c. If you are not using a commercial packaged bath, use antibacterial soap or a mild soap substitute. If you must use soap, it should be non-perfumed and rich in moisture. If you use soap, rinse the skin well.
  To avoid skin irritation.

  d. Pat the skin dry or air dry; do not rub.

  e. Apply a moisturizer immediately after drying, while there is still moisture in the skin. Wash your hands before applying the moisturizer.

  f. Cleanse the skin immediately after every incident of soiling (e.g., when the patient has a bowel movement).
  Prevents maceration and irritation from enzyme activity.

Evaluation

- Assess how well the patient tolerated the procedure. Was there any discomfort, shortness of breath, and so on?
- Observe the patient's mobility, both ROM and ease of movement.
- Note the condition of the patient's skin, including redness and other abnormal findings, especially in skinfolds.
- Ask the patient whether he is comfortable and satisfied.
- If someone other than the nurse performs the procedure, the nurse must still evaluate the care to be certain that it was done and performed satisfactorily.

Patient Teaching

- Discuss the need for activity (e.g., moving about in bed) and the hazards of immobility.
- Discuss usual skin care and how to increase the health of the skin.
- Demonstrate bathing procedure to family or other caregivers.

Home Care

Note: Many of the following apply to older adults and others with self-care deficits.

- Evaluate the home for bathing safety considerations (not limited to bed bath), such as the following:

  Safety bars in the bathroom?
  To facilitate transfers and provide support while washing.

  A safe water supply for bathing?

  Bathing supplies that are available and accessible?

  Nonskid mat or abrasive strips for shower or tub?

  Stool for shower; transfer bench or stool for getting into the tub?

  Handheld shower spray?

  Long-handled brush or sponge?

- Assess the client's ability to help with the bath or to bathe independently.
- Ask how the client usually bathes (e.g., shower, at the sink). Follow the client's preference as much as possible.
- Ask what supplies the client usually uses for the bath, and ask where they are stored. You will need to adapt the procedure depending on the available equipment and supplies.
- Suggest the use of large plastic trash bags or a shower curtain to protect the mattress during a bed bath.
- Instruct caregivers to wear gloves when handling linens that are soiled with blood or other body fluids. Linens should be washed in cold water, separately from other household laundry, and then washed again, using hot water, detergent, and bleach.
  Hot water coagulates proteins in the blood and makes it more difficult to remove. Detergent and bleach are used to destroy pathogens.

Documentation

Chart the type of bath given, how much patient was able to help with the bath, how well the patient tolerated the procedure, the patient's mobility, and any abnormal findings. Hygiene care is charted on checklists and flowsheets in most agencies.

Sample electronic documentation

0630 complete bed bath given, pt. unable to assist in care. Patient tolerated procedure well, VSS, denied pain. Patient turned side to side with assist of one. Skin warm, dry and intact. Emollient applied to dry areas. Encouraged patient to shift weight while in bed to prevent injury to skin.
K. Barnett, RN

Practice Resources

American Association of Critical-Care Nurses (AACN); (2013); D'Hondt, A., Kaasalainen, S., Prentice, D., et al. (2012); Downey, L., & Lloyd, H. (2008); Flori, L. (2007); Haas, J., & Larson, E. (2008); Johnson, Lineweaver, & Maze (2009); O'Flynn, J. (2007); Powers, J., Peed, J., Burns, L., et al. (2012); Siegel, J., Rhinehart, E., Jackson, M., et al. (2007); Sievert, D., Armola, R., & Halm, M. (2011).

Thinking About the Procedure

To practice applying clinical reasoning to this procedure,

Go to *Davis's Nursing Skills Videos*, **Bathing: Providing a Complete Bed Bath Using a Prepackaged Bathing Product. Also go to Providing Perineal Care, Brushing and Flossing the Teeth, and Providing Foot Care.**

For questions and suggested responses,

Go to Chapter 25, **Thinking About the Procedure Questions and Suggested Responses,** on Davis *Plus*

Procedure 25-2 ■ Bathing: Providing a Towel Bath

➤ For steps to follow in *all* procedures, refer to the Universal Steps for All Procedures found on the inside back cover.

➤ *Note:* Because the towel bath is a variation of the bed bath, only the steps differing from a bed bath are listed.

Equipment

- Large plastic bag containing a bath blanket (or a very large towel, about 3 ft × 6 ft), one standard bath towel, and two or three washcloths
- Dry bath blankets (two or more) and dry bath towels.
- Pitcher and approximately 2 qt (2,000 mL) of warm distilled, sterile or filtered water (105°F [41°C]), according to agency policy
- 30 mL of no-rinse liquid soap or commercial solution of soap, moisturizer, and disinfectant (preferably a CHG and water solution)
- Other supplies for a bed bath; see Procedure 25-1.

Delegation

You can delegate this procedure to the NAP if you conclude that the patient's condition and the NAP's skills allow. Perform the pre-procedure assessments and inform the NAP of the amount of help the patient needs and any special considerations, such as IV lines and drains. Ask the NAP to report the condition of the patient's skin, level of self-care, and ability to tolerate the procedure.

Pre-Procedure Assessments

- Assess the patient's mobility and activity tolerance to determine whether she will be able to assist with the bath, whether a towel bath is appropriate, and the amount of help you will need.
  A patient with decreased activity tolerance or mobility (e.g., because of chest pain or shortness of breath with exertion) may have a limited ability to assist with the bath, making a towel bath the most appropriate choice. For severely compromised patients, having two nurses give the bath will make the procedure much quicker and less demanding on the patient.

➤ When performing the procedure, always identify your patient according to agency policy, using two identifiers, and be attentive to standard precautions, hand hygiene, patient safety and privacy, body mechanics, and documentation.

Procedure Steps

1. **Prepare the towel bag.**
   a. Prefold the bath blanket.
   Allows for organized application and ease of handling the blanket.
   b. Fill a large pitcher with 2,000 mL warm water (approximately 105°F [41°C]). Distilled, sterile, or filtered water is recommended (follow agency policy).
   Using tap water for bathing exposes patients to waterborne pathogens if biofilm is present in the water lines or faucets. This differs among agencies. The amount of water varies depending on the size of the bath blanket and bath towel. Use enough water to saturate them. Hot water can injure the patient and removes more of the skin's protective oils, but if the water is too cool, the patient may become chilled.
   c. Add 30 mL of no-rinse soap or commercial solution to the water according to the manufacturer's instructions.
   Adding a prescribed amount of soap to the water before pouring into the bag prevents excessive sudsing.
   d. Pour the about 2,000 mL of the solution into the bag, over the bath blanket, bath towel, and wash cloths. Ensure even distribution.
2. **If you do not plan to change** the linen, work one dry bath blanket under the patient.
   Protects the linen and provides warmth.
3. **Spread a dry bath blanket** over the patient; remove the patient's clothing, working underneath the blanket.
   Protects privacy and prevents chilling.
4. **Replace the dry blanket with** the wet blanket:
   a. Take the wet bath blanket or towel out of the bag, squeezing out excess water so that it does not drip.
   b. Push the dry bath blanket down to the patient's waist, and place the wet bath blanket on the patient's chest.
   c. Continue to unfold the wet bath blanket until it covers the patient, pushing the dry bath blanket out of the way as you do so.
   The wet bath blanket will feel warm and relaxing. You will use the dry bath blanket to dry the patient.
   d. If necessary, place yet another dry blanket on top of the wet one.
   This helps hold in the warmth if the patient is chilling or the room is cool.
5. **Bathe the patient**, beginning at the feet and working toward the head.

(continued on next page)

Procedure 25-2 ■ Bathing: Providing a Towel Bath (continued)

a. Keeping the patient covered, use the wet bath blanket to wash the legs, abdomen, and chest.

b. As you work, replace the wet bath blanket with the dry one.
Keeps the patient from chilling.

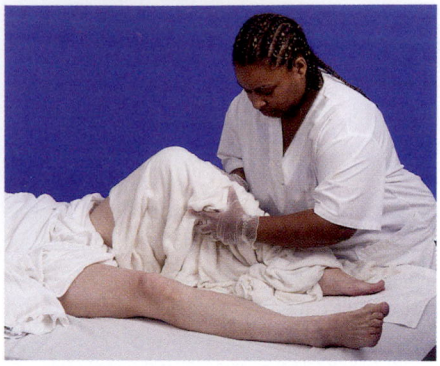

c. Fold the wet bath blanket as each area is bathed, allowing only clean surfaces to contact clean surfaces.
Prevents contamination of the clean side of the wet bath blanket.

d. Use one of the wet washcloths to wash the patient's face, neck, and ears.
Notice that this varies from the order of most baths, which proceed from head to toe. However, this is the most efficient way to accomplish a towel bath. It does not really compromise the "clean to dirty" principle because the legs, abdomen, and chest are usually equally "clean," and you are washing those before the back, buttocks, and perineum.

6. **Don procedure gloves.** Roll the client to one side, unfold the wet bath towel so the clean surface covers the patient, and use the wet bath towel to wash the back and then the buttocks.

7. **Remove procedure gloves,** wash your hands. Wash the perineal area with a washcloth. See Procedure 25-4: Providing Perineal Care.

8. **Finish the bath** as in Procedure 25-1. Follow patient preferences whenever possible to increase feelings of comfort.

9. **Change linen as needed,** including soiled linen or linen that became damp during the bath. You will almost certainly need to change the linen if you have not padded the bottom sheet well before the bath.
Ensures patient safety and comfort. Because the bath is finished rapidly, there is no real need to pad the bottom sheet if you know that you will have time to change the linens after the bath.

? What if . . .

- **Your patient becomes agitated and uncooperative during the bath?**
  Speak calmly and softly. Give the patient a few minutes to calm down. Discontinue the bath if the patient remains upset.

Practice Resources

AACN (2013); Downey, L., & Lloyd, H. (2008); Flori, L. (2007); Joanna Briggs Institute (2007); Larkin, C. (2011); Warchol, K. (2013).

Procedure 25-3 ■ Bathing: Using a Basin and Water

Key Point: ***The potential exists (1) that bath basins can become a reservoir for microorganisms and for cross-contamination of the immediate environment and healthcare personnel and (2) biofilm is commonly present in hospital water lines and faucets. Use this method only when a patient is grossly contaminated or a patient refuses other types of bath.***

➤ For steps to follow in *all* procedures, refer to the Universal Steps for All Procedures found on the inside back cover of Volume 2.

Equipment

- Disposable water basin for single-patient use
- Tap, distilled, filtered, or sterile water (depending on facility policy)
- CHG and water solution (for bathing the patient and cleaning the basin)
- Lotion, deodorant, and/or powder as needed
- Bath blanket
- Clean patient gown (gown with shoulder snaps or Velcro closures if the patient has an IV line)
- Clean linen
- Procedure gloves

Delegation

You can delegate this procedure to the NAP if you conclude that the patient's condition and the NAP's skills allow. Perform the pre-procedure assessments, and inform the NAP of the amount of help the patient needs and of any special considerations, such as IV lines and drains. Ask the NAP to report the condition of the patient's skin, level of self-care, and ability to tolerate the procedure.

Pre-Procedure Assessments

Assessments are the same as in Procedure 25-1: Bathing: Providing a Complete Bed Bath Using a Prepackaged Bathing Product.

➤ When performing the procedure, always identify your patient according to agency policy, using two identifiers, and be attentive to standard precautions, hand hygiene, patient safety and privacy, body mechanics, and documentation.

Procedure Steps

1. **Fill the disposable basin** with warm water (approximately 105°F [41°C]). Check the temperature with a thermometer or your hand. If possible, ask the patient to test the water temperature.

   Using tap water for bathing exposes patients to waterborne pathogens; use distilled, filtered, or sterile water if available. This differs among institutions, so follow agency requirements. Use water that is comfortable for the patient. Hot water removes protective skin oils and can injure the patient. If the water is too cool, the patient may become chilled.

2. **Prepare a solution** of 60 mL CHG solution diluted in 3 qt (2.85 L) of water for bathing the patient (Powers, Peed, Burns, et al., 2012).

   Evidence indicates that use of CHG is effective in preventing the bath basin from becoming a reservoir for microorganisms and in helping to prevent HAIs.

3. **Prepare the patient for the bath** as described in Procedure 25-1.
4. **Using one washcloth for each body area**, wash the patient following the sequence in Procedure 25-1. Rinse and wring water from the washcloth as you move from each body area.
5. **Rinse body areas as needed**, if you use soap, and pat dry.

   Preserves skin integrity by preventing the drying effect of the soap on the skin.

6. **Apply emollients** after the bath.

   Aids in preventing dry skin.

7. **Put used washcloths in the laundry** for future use.
8. **Help patient don a clean gown.**
9. **Provide a back rub**, if not contraindicated.
10. **Reposition patient**, as needed.
11. **Change linens**, as needed.
12. Clean and dry the basin.
    a. Wipe the basin with a paper towel and place upside down on a table to air dry.
    b. Label the basin for bathing only. Discard it if it becomes contaminated with vomit or other body fluids.
    c. Designate an additional basin for storage of bath supplies.

For Evaluation, Documentation, and Patient Teaching, see Procedure 25-1: Bathing: Providing a Complete Bed Bath Using a Prepackaged Bathing Product.

Practice Resources

Doughty, D., Junkin, J., Kurz, P., et al. (2012); Joanna Briggs Institute (2007); Larson, E., Ciliberti T., Chantler, C., et al. (2004); Ritz, J., Pashnik, B., Padula, C., et al. (2012); Rönner, A. C., Berland, C. R., Runeman, B., et al. (2010).

Procedure 25-4 ■ Providing Perineal Care

➤ For steps to follow in *all* procedures, refer to the Universal Steps for All Procedures found on the inside back cover.

Equipment

- Procedure gloves
- Prepackaged bathing product (i.e., Comfort Care)
- Bedpan or portable sitz tub (optional)
- Bath towel
- Toilet paper
- Plastic trash bag for used wipes and other disposable soiled items
- Perineal ointment or lotion if needed

If prepackaged bathing product is not available:

- Sterile, filtered, distilled, or tap water according to agency policy
- Disposable basin or perineal wash bottle, if needed
- Perineal cleansing solution or no-rinse soap
- Wash cloths

Delegation

You can delegate perineal care to the NAP if the patient's condition and the NAP's skills allow. Perform the pre-procedure assessments, and inform the NAP of the amount of help the patient needs and any special considerations (e.g., presence of a urinary catheter, vaginal drainage). Ask the NAP to report the condition of the patient's perineum (skin, drainage), level of self-care, and ability to tolerate the procedure.

Pre-Procedure Assessments

- Assess the patient's mobility and activity tolerance.

  Determine whether the patient will be able to assist with the perineal care. Doing as much self-care as possible increases the patient's sense of independence and maintains modesty .

- Check for positioning or activity restrictions, such as maintaining hip abduction following a total hip replacement.

  Prevents injuring the patient during the procedure.

- Assess for psychosocial issues that may concern the patient regarding perineal care.

  You must consider cultural norms to ensure that the perineal care is appropriate for the patient. For example, in some cultures a woman would find it completely unacceptable for a male nurse to perform her perineal care (pericare).

- Assess for any specific patient needs for perineal care.

  For example, if there are lesions or skin breakdown, you may need to use special soaps and/or lotions. Incontinence or drainage requires assessment and follow-up to prevent Impaired Skin Integrity.

- Assess for the presence of a urinary drainage catheter, perineal surgery, or lesions.

  You may need to adapt the procedure to clean around an indwelling urinary catheter or surgical incisions.

(continued on next page)

Procedure 25-4 ■ Providing Perineal Care (continued)

➤ When performing the procedure, always identify your patient according to agency policy, using two identifiers, and be attentive to standard precautions, hand hygiene, patient safety and privacy, body mechanics, and documentation.

Procedure Steps

1. **Adjust the room temperature,** and assist with elimination as needed.
   Assisting the patient with elimination before perineal care helps prevent interruptions during the procedure and allows for thorough cleansing. Adjusting room temperature prevents chilling.

2. **Warm the perineal bathing** product.

If Using a Microwave

Heat the package in the microwave for no longer than 1 minute. The temperature of the contents should be approximately 105°F (41°C). This step is controversial. Some references suggest, for safety, using the commercial bag bath at room temperature.

If Using a Warmer Unit

You do not need Step 2 because the bags are always warm.

3. **Prepare the patient.**
   a. Position the patient on her back (supine). Place waterproof pads under the patient if they are not already in place. You may wish to place the patient on a bedpan or portable sitz tub, especially if the perineum is grossly soiled. Place a waterproof bag within reach to discard wipes.
   Placing the patient on a bedpan raises the hips to increase visualization and allows for more thorough cleansing. A bedpan also allows for using water when needed.
   b. Wear procedure gloves (and other protective wear as needed) when providing perineal care. If you are using a basin and water you may wear a procedure gown and goggles if you are concerned about splashing (e.g., if the patient is confused and may be unable to follow instructions).
   When providing perineal care there is a possibility of coming in contact with urine, vaginal secretions, or fecal material.
   c. Drape the patient to protect privacy.

For Female Patients

- Drape the bath blanket so that one point faces the patient's head (drape it in the shape of a diamond).
- Take one of the side points of the diamond, and wrap it around the patient's leg. Anchor the end of the blanket under the patient's foot.
- Repeat on the other leg with other point of the diamond.▼

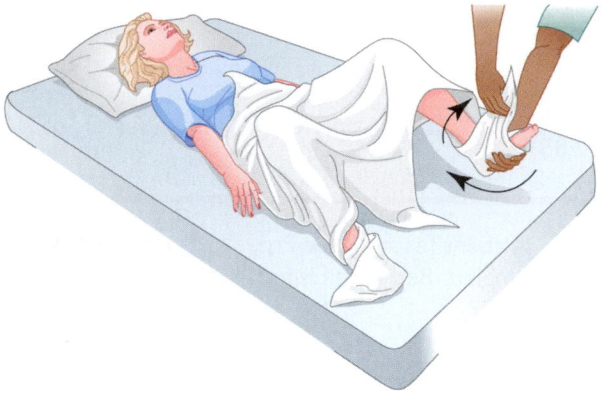

- Fold the center lower point of the diamond up to expose the patient's perineum.▼

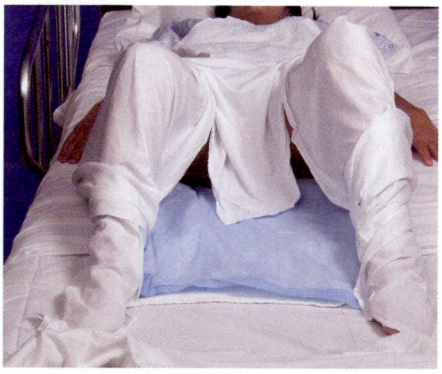

This draping technique covers the patient as much as possible, which helps maintain privacy and prevents chilling during the procedure. The patient can also relax her legs against the bath blanket.

For Male Patients

- Place the bath blanket over the patient's chest.
- Fold the bed linens down to expose only the patient's groin.
   d. Remove any fecal material with toilet paper.
   Prevents contamination of the perineum with feces, which can lead to bladder or incisional infections. If you are providing perineal care as part of giving a bed bath, you will have cleaned the anal area when the patient was in the lateral position.

4. **Wash the perineum,** using a warm wipe. In both males and females, cleanse the skinfolds of the groin area thoroughly. Examine the skin creases for redness or excoriation.

For Female Patients

Wash the perineum from front to back, using a clean portion of the wipe for each stroke. Cleanse the labial folds and around the urinary catheter, if one is in place.
Prevents contaminating the urethra with fecal material. Any fecal particles that are left can cause skin breakdown due to enzyme activity, and may increase the risk of a urinary tract infection because of the presence of Escherichia coli in the feces.▼

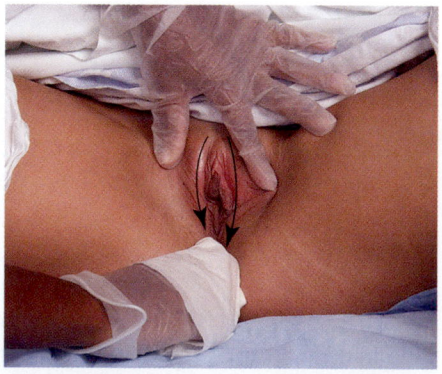

Male Patient

Retract the foreskin, if present, and gently cleanse the head of the penis using a circular motion. Replace the foreskin, and finish washing the shaft of the penis, using firm strokes. Then wash the scrotum, using a clean portion of the wipe with each stroke. Handle the scrotum with care, because the area is sensitive.

To adequately clean the head of the penis in an uncircumcised male, you must retract the foreskin. After cleaning, replace the foreskin to prevent constriction and edema of the penis. Firm strokes may help to prevent an erection. Using a clean portion of the wipe for each stroke prevents fecal contamination of the urethra and perineum.

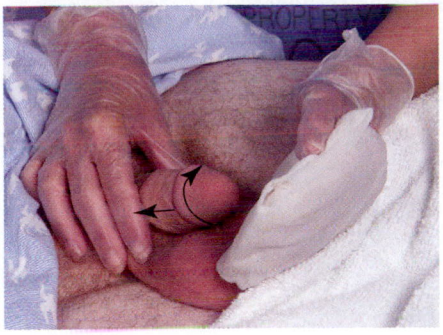

Detects and prevents excoriation in skinfold areas, where moisture accumulates.

5. **Allow body areas to air dry**; do not rinse.
   Prevents the emollient and surfactant skin protectants from being removed.

6. **Discard each wipe after use**, or place on the waterproof pad to discard when finished.
   Ensures following the "clean to dirty" principle.

7. **If perineal care is not being** done as part of the bath, also clean the anal area. Ask the patient to turn to the side, wipe the buttocks and anal area as needed.
   Fecal contamination of the perineum can lead to urinary tract infections and skin irritation. Therefore, the anal area is cleansed last.

8. **Apply skin protectants** as needed. Powder only if the patient requests it.
   If urinary or fecal incontinence is present, skin barriers may be used to prevent urine, feces, or other drainage from contacting the skin. This helps prevent skin breakdown. For female patients, powder is a medium for bacterial growth. In the presence of moisture, it also creates a paste, which irritates the skin.

9. **If the patient has an indwelling** catheter and if agency policy requires special catheter care, you will usually provide the care at this point. Don clean gloves before providing catheter care, and follow the agency's procedure. For more information about catheter care, see Clinical Insight 28-1: Caring for a Patient With an Indwelling Catheter.

10. **Reposition and cover the patient** with the bath blanket. Remove soiled gloves, discarding in a waterproof bag.
    Prevents contaminating clean linen with soiled gloves.

11. **Change linen as needed**, including soiled linen or linen that became damp during perineal care.
    Ensures patient safety, comfort, and privacy.

? What if . . .

- **The patient is unable to control bowel and/or bladder?**

  Gently cleanse the perineal/perigenital area after each incontinence/soiling and apply a moisture barrier according to agency protocols.
  Minimizing contact with irritants such as moisture, urine, and stool can decrease the development of incontinence-associated dermatitis.

  Use a spray, no-rinse cleanser and soft wipes.
  These aid in preventing irritation from friction, and reducing drying effects on the skin.

  Follow agency policy and use skin assessment tools (some geared particularly to perineal skin).

  Assess for signs of secondary infection in addition to irritation and report as needed.

  Consider bowel and bladder retraining and scheduling to reduce frequency of incontinence.

- **Your patient is postpartum?**

  Educate the patient about perineal care. Include the importance of handwashing before and after cleansing the perineum, measures to keep the perineum clean, frequent changing of sanitary pads, and checking for signs and symptoms of abnormal lochia. If the patient had an episiotomy, laceration, or tear, teaching should also include management of discomfort and signs of wound infection.

Evaluation

- Assess the patient's responses to the procedure. Was there any discomfort?
- Observe for difficulty with movement or ROM during the procedure.
- Note the condition of the skin, including redness and other abnormal findings.
- Ask the patient whether she feels comfortable now.

Patient Teaching

- Discuss adaptations to perineal care. For example, if the area is tender, (1) wash the area with warm moistened wipe after going to the bathroom, instead of using toilet paper; or (2) use a skin protectant on the area.
- Review the importance of handwashing after elimination.
- If appropriate, teach the caregiver how to provide perineal care, including the major concept of cleaning front to back ("clean to dirty"). Stress the importance of wearing gloves and washing hands.
- Advise women not to douche because it disturbs the balance of normal vaginal flora and can irritate or injure mucosal cells.
- Explain that scented and deodorant feminine hygiene products are not necessary for cleanliness and may even be harmful. Daily cleansing is the most effective means of odor control.

Home Care

- Evaluate the ability of the client or caregiver to provide perineal care.

(continued on next page)

Procedure 25-4 ■ Providing Perineal Care (continued)

- Determine the availability of supplies needed for perineal care.
- You will need to adapt the procedure depending on the available equipment and supplies. Major issues involved in perineal care in the home are the lack of clean water and/or linens. In some instances, you may need to use bottled water or boil water for the procedure. One option is to use prepackaged moistened towelettes to provide the care (e.g., Comfort Bath towelettes).

Documentation

Usually perineal care is part of routine hygiene care and is charted on a flowsheet. If you need to write a narrative note, chart that perineal care was given, any patient responses to the procedure, and the condition of the perineal area.

Sample documentation

8/16/16 1430 Perineal care given. Patient had no complaint of discomfort. No redness or discharge noted. ——— *Nora Noyes, RN*

Practice Resources

AACN (2013); Bliss, D., Zehrer, C., Savik, K., et al. (2006); Gray, M., Bliss, D., Doughty, D., et al. (2007); National Guideline Clearinghouse (NGC) (2006, revised 2011); Siegel, J., Rhinehart, E., Jackson, M., et al. (2007).

Thinking About the Procedure

To practice applying clinical reasoning to this procedure,

Go to *Davis's Nursing Skills Videos*, **Providing Perineal Care.**

For questions and suggested responses,

Go to Chapter 25, **Thinking About the Procedure Questions and Suggested Responses,** on Davis *Plus*.

Procedure 25-5 ■ Providing Foot Care

➤ For steps to follow in *all* procedures, refer to the Universal Steps for All Procedures found on the inside back cover.

➤ *Note:* This procedure describes foot care using a basin and water. It may also be done with prepackaged wipes, along with the bath.

Equipment

- Procedure gloves (if there are open lesions)
- Pillow (if procedure is done with the patient in bed)
- Disposable basin for water (distilled, sterile or filtered tap water, per agency requirement)
- Liquid no-rinse soap
- Bath towel and washcloth
- Waterproof pad
- Orangewood stick
- Toenail clippers and nail file
- Lotion or prescribed ointment or cream

Delegation

You can delegate foot care to the NAP if the patient's condition and the NAP's skills allow. For example, as a rule you should not delegate care if the patient has impaired peripheral circulation or foot ulcers. Perform the following pre-procedure assessments, and inform the NAP of the amount of help the patient needs and any special considerations (e.g., ability to sit in a chair). Ask the NAP to report the condition of the patient's skin and nails, level of self-care, and ability to tolerate the procedure.

Pre-Procedure Assessments

- As you assess the feet and toenails, compare findings for both feet.
- Assess bilateral dorsalis pedis pulses, capillary refill, skin color, and warmth. Compare right and left feet. Palpate pulses at the same time bilaterally to determine whether one side is weaker than the other.

  Decreased circulation to the feet increases the risk for tissue injury and infection. A variety of diseases can cause poor circulation. For example, cardiac or renal disease may cause pedal edema, which impairs circulation to the skin, and diabetes causes vascular changes leading to poor circulation to the lower extremities.
- Assess for diseases (e.g., diabetes mellitus and peripheral vascular disease) that create risks for foot problems.
- Thoroughly assess all areas of the feet for skin integrity, edema, condition of toenails, and any abnormalities. Check carefully between the toes.

  Decreased circulation in the feet commonly causes such problems as thickened toenails, dry skin, and increased risk of infection. Changes in vision and mobility can increase the risk for injuries to the feet. Patients with diabetes also may have neuropathy, which prevents them from knowing when they have injured their feet. Identifying abnormalities enables you to provide interventions to help prevent potential problems.

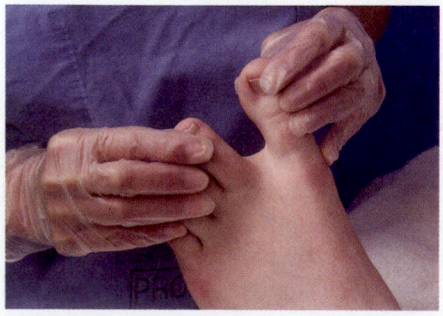

- Check institutional policy to verify whether a nurse is allowed to trim nails. Obtain a primary provider's prescription for trimming the patient's nails, if necessary.
  Patients who have diabetes or impaired circulation to the lower extremities require a prescription for trimming their nails. Refer the patient to a podiatrist if the circulation is severely compromised or if edema would make the procedure difficult.
- Assess the patient's usual footwear.
  Improperly fitting shoes, especially if they are too tight, are a common cause of foot problems (e.g., bunions, ingrown toenails).
- Assess the patient's self-care ability to provide foot care. Evaluate the need for a referral. Determine whether the patient has the necessary vision and mobility to be able provide his own foot care.
- Assess the patient's knowledge about foot care, including usual foot care practices.

  Identify potential deficits in understanding that may require additional teaching or referral to a podiatrist, general practice physician, or advanced practice nurse.
  Many home remedies for foot problems can damage the tissue. For example, corn pads can increase pressure on the tissue, compromising circulation and causing local tissue ischemia. Cutting the sides of the toenails can lead to ingrown toenails.

➤ When performing the procedure, always identify your patient according to agency policy, using two identifiers, and be attentive to standard precautions, hand hygiene, patient safety and privacy, body mechanics, and documentation.

Procedure Steps

1. **Wear procedure gloves** and other protective wear as needed when providing foot care.
   Follows standard precautions. The heel is a common place for skin breakdown, so use gloves if you are unable to see the area without lifting the foot. If the patient has significant drainage to the area, such as a draining wound, you may need to wear a protective gown.

2. **Ask the patient to sit in a chair** with a waterproof pad or bath towel under the feet, if possible. If the patient is unable to sit in a chair, place him in semi-Fowler's position in bed; place a pillow under his knees.
   It is easier to perform the procedure with the patient in a chair. The pillow supports the knee joints and prevents muscle fatigue.

3. **Fill the basin halfway** with warm water (approximately 105°F to 110°F [40°C to 43°C]).
   Recent research recommends the use of filtered, distilled or sterile water. Using tap water for bathing exposes patients to waterborne pathogens that may be contained in biofilm in water lines and faucets. Hot water can injure the skin. Warm water promotes circulation. Filling the basin halfway prevents spilling when the patient places his foot in the water.

4. **Help the patient place one foot** in the water, first checking with the patient that the temperature is comfortable.
   a. If the patient is in a chair, place the basin on the floor (on the waterproof pad).
   b. If the patient is in bed, place the basin near the foot of the bed on the waterproof pad; pad the basin with a towel.
   The waterproof pad keeps the bed dry. Padding the basin prevents pressure on the back of the leg, which could cause discomfort and interfere with circulation.

5. **Allow the foot to soak** for 5 to 20 minutes, depending on the patient's tolerance and the condition of his feet.
   Soaking is not recommended for patients with diabetes or peripheral vascular disease (PVD).
   Soaking softens the skin and helps relax the patient. For patients who have diabetes or PVD, soaking is not recommended because it may remove natural oils, cause cracking of the skin, and may cause burns even if the water is at the recommended temperature.

6. **Cleanse the foot** with mild or no-rinse soap.
   Removes loose debris. No-rinse soaps do not dry the skin.

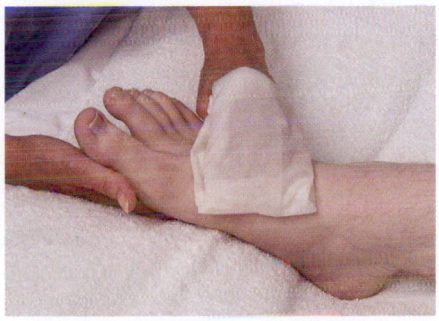

7. **Clean under the nails** with the orangewood stick while the foot is still in the water.
   Water softens the nails and makes cleaning easier.

8. **Remove the foot from** the water, and dry it gently and thoroughly.
   Remaining moisture, especially between the toes, can cause maceration and promotes development of fungal infections.

9. **Change the water.**
   Ensures proper temperature and prevents cross-contamination.

10. **Soak the opposite foot** while performing Steps 11 through 14 for the first (clean) foot.
    Saves time.

11. **Gently push the cuticles back** with the orangewood stick or towel.
    Increases cuticle health. Do not damage the cuticle; doing so can increase the risk of infection.

12. **Trim the nails straight across** with toenail clippers, if not contraindicated by the patient's condition and if permitted by agency policy. Note whether the nail has cut into the skin of the toe being trimmed or the adjacent toes. If the nails are brittle or thick, allow the foot to soak for 10 to 20 minutes before trimming.
    Trimming straight across prevents ingrown toenails. Early recognition

(continued on next page)

Procedure 25-5 ■ Providing Foot Care (continued)

and treatment of problems will prevent further complications, such as infection.

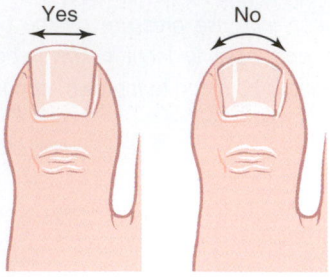

13. File the nails with an emery board.
Smooths the edges to prevent scratching the skin with the toenails.

14. Apply cream, lotion, or foot powder lightly to the feet and toes.
Cream hydrates the skin; however, excess cream can cause maceration. Foot powder absorbs moisture and functions as a nonirritating deodorant for patients whose feet perspire heavily.

15. Repeat Steps 11 through 14 with the second foot.

16. Check the patient's footwear for rough edges that may injure feet.

What if . . .

- **My patient has Impaired Bed Mobility?**

  Apply protective devices (e.g., lamb's wool) as needed.

- **My patient has an injury, lesions, or pain?**

  You may need to use a bed cradle to keep the pressure of the bedding off the patient's feet. Refer to Chapter 35 for other measures to preserve skin integrity.

- **My patient has diabetes mellitus?**

  In addition to controlling blood glucose levels, adhering to a specific foot care plan is essential for people with diabetes. Include the following in your teaching:
  - The importance of inspecting the feet daily
  - Ways to protect the feet (e.g., by wearing shoes when out of bed)
  - Potential complications involving the feet
  - Management of symptoms
  - When to seek advice from a healthcare professional
  - What to include in the foot care regimen (apply moisturizing lotion on tops and bottoms of feet but not between toes)—and what not to do (cut corns and calluses, use topical corn removers, or soak the feet)

Elderly patients with diabetes are especially at risk for development of foot-related complications. Visual changes and loss of flexibility could make it challenging to bend and visualize the feet. Plastic mirrors may be helpful in this regard.

Early detection and treatment of problems can minimize foot-related complications.

Evaluation

- Observe that feet are clean, smooth, and intact; nails are trimmed and smooth; skin is pink and warm.
- Be sure that foot problems are identified and interventions provided.
- Ask the patient to demonstrate or describe correct foot care.

Patient Teaching

For patient teaching,

Go to the **Self-Care box, Teaching Your Client About Foot Care,** in Volume 1.

Home Care

The procedure does not vary in the home. The nurse must:

- Work with the client and care provider to determine the availability of supplies needed for foot care (clean water and so on).
- Identify home care practices, and teach the client and/or caregiver proper foot care techniques. Influencing older adults can be especially difficult if they have usual routines, such as walking barefoot, that put them at risk for injury. For clients with diabetes, the biggest risk to foot health is inadequate regulation of their blood glucose levels.

Documentation

In most agencies you will not document routine foot care (except, perhaps, on a checklist) unless there are problems. If you do document, chart that foot care was given, and chart assessment findings.

Sample documentation

09/25/16 0900. Foot care given. 2 cm circular reddened area on right heel. Skin abrasion outer lateral aspect of 5th toe, left foot —bioocclusive dressing applied.
—Ann Hopkins, RN

Practice Resources

AACN (2013); NGC (2008); Plummer, E., & Albert, S. (2008); Powers, J., Peed, L., et al. (2012); Siegel, J., Rhinehart, E., Jackson, M., et al. (2007).

Thinking About the Procedure

To practice applying clinical reasoning to this procedure,

Go to *Davis's Nursing Skills Videos,* **Providing Foot Care.**

For questions and suggested responses,

Go to Chapter 25, **Thinking About the Procedure Questions and Suggested Responses, on DavisPlus.**

Procedure 25-6 ■ Brushing and Flossing the Teeth

➤ For steps to follow in *all* procedures, refer to the Universal Steps for All Procedures found on the inside back cover.

Equipment

- Toothbrush or sponge toothettes
- Toothpaste
- Dental floss (two pieces, each about 10 in. long) and floss holder (optional)
- Tonsil-tip suction connected to suction source (if aspiration is a concern)
- Emesis basin
- Towel
- Glass of water (distilled, sterile or filtered water, according to agency requirements)
- Mouthwash and/or lip moisturizer, if desired
- Procedure gloves; mask and goggles if splashing may occur

Delegation

You can delegate oral hygiene to the NAP if the patient's condition and the NAP's skills allow. Perform the following assessments, and inform the NAP of the specific type of oral care and the amount of help the patient needs. Ask the NAP to report the condition of the patient's mouth, level of self-care, and ability to tolerate the procedure.

Pre-Procedure Assessments

- Assess the patient's ability to assist with oral care.
  Having the patient assist whenever possible promotes independence and supports a positive self-image.
- Determine whether the patient has dentures, bridgework, or partial plates.
  Determines how you will provide oral care.
- Assess general oral health, including gag reflex and the condition of the teeth, gums, and mucous membranes. If a patient has dentures, examine the mouth with and without the dentures.
  If the patient has a hypoactive or absent gag reflex, you will need a suction setup to prevent aspiration. Inflammation or lesions in the mouth increase the patient's risk of infection and may make eating difficult or painful, leading to malnutrition. Poorly fitting dentures can cause irritation of the gums.
- Assess the patient's usual oral care, including cultural practices.
  Helps determine the type of oral care you will provide and identifies areas of patient teaching needed.

➤ When performing the procedure, always identify your patient according to agency policy, using two identifiers, and be attentive to standard precautions, hand hygiene, patient safety and privacy, body mechanics, and documentation.

Procedure Steps

1. **Position the patient** in a high-Fowler's position or in a chair, if possible. Position the patient on her side if the head of bed cannot be elevated.
   Prevents aspiration and makes the procedure easier.

2. **Set up suction**, if needed. Attach suction tubing and tonsil-tip suction; check suction.
   Suctioning equipment may be needed to prevent aspiration of secretions during the procedure, especially if the gag reflex is decreased.

3. **If the patient is able to perform self-care:**
   a. Arrange supplies within the patient's reach.
      Promotes the patient's ability to do self-care and therefore independence.
   b. Assist the patient with brushing and flossing as needed.
      Ensures that the teeth are thoroughly cleaned.

For Nurse-administered Brushing and Flossing,
Follow the remaining steps.

4. **Place the towel across** the patient's chest.
   Prevents getting the patient's gown or linen wet during the procedure.

5. **Don procedure gloves** as needed. Wear gown and goggles if splashing might occur, such as with a confused patient.
   Follows standard precautions.

6. **Adjust the bed to working** height; lower the siderail nearest you.
   Prevents you from having to lean over the patient or reach across the siderail, possibly causing back strain or injury.

7. **Moisten a small, soft toothbrush**, and apply a small amount of toothpaste. See Equipment for type of water to use.
   A small toothbrush fits more easily into the mouth and reaches more areas. The soft bristles can be used to brush the tongue and also the gums if the patient is edentulous. Excessive toothpaste does not increase the cleaning, and toothpaste residue has a drying effect on the mucosa. Moistening the toothbrush increases patient comfort because patients frequently have a dry mouth.

8. **Place, hold, or ask the patient** to hold the emesis basin under the chin.
   Collects oral secretions and protects clothing and linens.

9. **Brush the teeth**, holding the bristles at a 45° angle to the gumline.
   a. Using short circular motions, gently brush the inner and outer surfaces of the teeth, from the gumline to the crown of each tooth.
   b. Brush the biting surface of the back teeth by holding the brush bristles straight up and down to the teeth and brushing back and forth.
      This is the most effective technique for removing all food particles and plaque from the teeth and gums. Removing debris and subsequent plaque helps to decrease microbial colonization.

(continued on next page)

Procedure 25-6 ■ Brushing and Flossing the Teeth (continued)

c. If the patient is frail, perform oral suctioning when fluid accumulates in the mouth.
Prevents choking and aspiration.

Brush teeth, holding bristles at a 45° angle to the gumline. Using short circular motions, gently brush the inner and outer surfaces of the teeth, including the gumline.

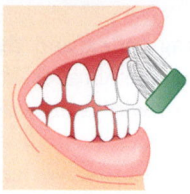

Clean front teeth.

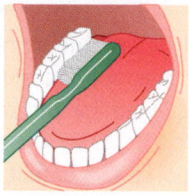

Clean both inner and outer surfaces of the teeth.

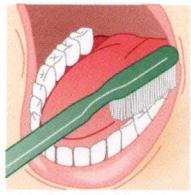

Brush the biting surfaces of the back teeth with the brush bristles straight up and down.

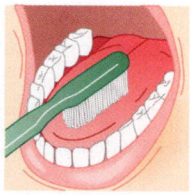

Brush the surface of the tongue.

10. Gently brush the patient's tongue.
Removes coating and accumulated debris that can be a reservoir for bacteria. Brush gently to prevent gagging or vomiting.

11. Floss the teeth. Grasp dental floss in both hands, or use a floss holder.

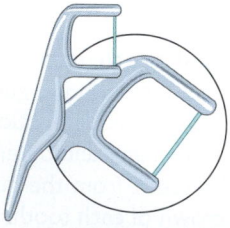

If you are not using a floss holder

a. Wrap one end of the floss around the middle finger of each hand.

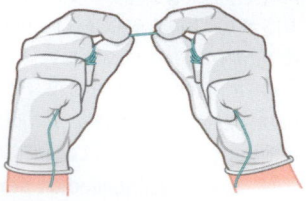

b. Stretch the floss between your thumbs and index fingers, and move the floss up and down against each tooth.

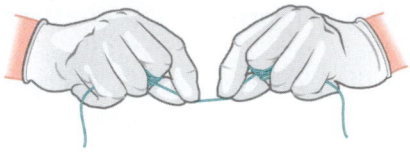

c. Floss between and around all teeth.
Moving the floss up and down instead of back and forth prevents damaging the gums.

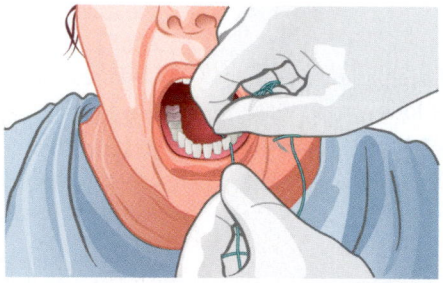

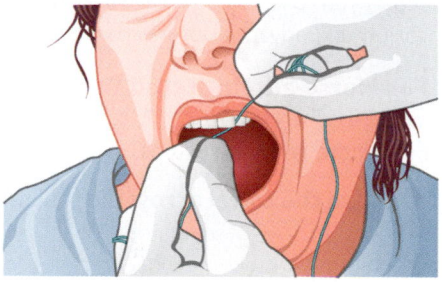

12. Assist the patient in rinsing his mouth, suctioning as needed. Or, ask the patient to rinse vigorously and spit the water into the emesis basin.
Removes food particles from mouth. Suction if the patient has a decreased or absent gag reflex.

Key Point: ***Recent studies recommend that hospitalized patients at high risk for infection avoid exposure to hospital water and use distilled, sterile, or filtered water instead (follow agency policy).***

13. Offer a mild or dilute mouthwash, and apply lip moisturizer, if desired.
Prevents irritation of the mucous membranes. Apply lip moisturizer for dry lips, for unconscious patients, or those on a ventilator, or per patient preference.

14. Reposition the patient as needed and return the bed to the low position.
Ensures patient comfort and safety.

? What if . . .

- **My patient has an excessively dry oral cavity?**

  You may need to use a saliva substitute.
  Aging, adverse medication effects, and illness often lead to decreased salivary production.

- **My patient has viscous (thick) mucus?**

  Use appropriately diluted sodium bicarbonate to dissolve viscous mucus.

- **My patient has a high risk of gum bleeding (e.g., such as associated with thrombocytopenia), has painful mouth lesions, or toothbrushing is otherwise contraindicated?**

  You may use foam or cotton mouth swabs instead of a toothbrush. Do not use glycerin swabs, lemon glycerin swabs, or gauze squares. Use normal saline mouthwash.
  Foam swabs are less effective in removing debris and plaque, so it is best to brush when not contraindicated. Lemon glycerin swabs are drying to the mucosa and may cause decalcification of tooth enamel. Mouthwashes may be painful.

- **My patient has dementia or is uncooperative and agitated for other reasons?**

  Use dementia-focused behavior management strategies:
  Older adults with dementia frequently accumulate greater amounts of plaque and calculus, exhibit a higher incidence of periodontal gingival bleeding, and demonstrate a greater prevalence of denture-related oral mucosal lesions, yet they often resist oral care.

  - Provide oral hygiene at the same time every day, not necessarily at bathing time.
  - Use as many staff members as necessary.

- Give care in a quiet, distraction-free environment. Keep stimulation to a minimum, turn on some calming music.
- Speak softly; give one-step directions in short, simple sentences.
- Use a relaxed, slow approach; be sure your facial expression does not reflect tension.
- Give reassuring body contact and use gentle touch.
  Promotes trust. Quick or forceful touch may frighten the patient.
- Provide diversion.
  Occupies the patient's hands and prevents "grabbing."
- Never place your fingers between the teeth.
- Try placing a spare toothbrush or a rolled facecloth in the patient's hands while you provide oral care.
  Minimizes "grabbing."
- Use the "hand over hand" technique to gently guide the patient's own hand.
- Try starting the task (e.g., brushing), then having the resident help finish it.
- If the procedure is not going well, find another caregiver to come in and attempt the task.
- Use modified equipment and aids, if available (e.g., mouth props, backward-bent and suction toothbrushes).

- **My patient is on a ventilator, is a frail older adult, or has undergone cardiac surgery?**

  Be certain the teeth are brushed twice a day.

  In addition to brushing, use moisturizer on lips and oral mucosa every 2 to 4 hours.

  Apply a 0.12% chlorhexidine gluconate solution twice daily to complement oral care.

- **My patient is receiving chemotherapy?**

  Stress the importance of good oral hygiene, including brushing the teeth after meals and before going to bed.

  Chemotherapy can cause neutropenia (reduced white blood cell count), predisposing the patient to infections. The oral cavity is a common site for infections in patients with neutropenia.

  Routine rinses of mouthwashes with chlorhexidine are not recommended. Instead, use a bland rinse of diluted salt and/or sodium bicarbonate. Patients should swish for a minimum of 30 seconds and then expectorate the residue.

  Chlorhexidine products have not proved superior to bland rinses in preventing or reducing either chemotherapy/radiation-induced mucositis or yeast colonization. In addition, chlorhexidine products may contain alcohol, may cause discomfort, may alter taste sensations, and may stain teeth. Bland rinses containing 1 teaspoon of salt or sodium bicarbonate per pint of water reduce the acidity of oral secretions, lessen mucus accumulation, and discourage yeast colonization.

  An antifungal agent or a multiagent rinse (sometimes labeled "magic" or "miracle" rinse) may be used, followed by a short NPO period of 30 to 60 minutes. If other mouthwashes or rinses are also being used, allow 30 minutes to pass between their use and the use of an antifungal agent.

  Multiagent rinses typically contain lidocaine. The resulting numbing effect may pose risks for a biting injury or aspiration. These rinses can neutralize antifungal agents.

Evaluation

- Inspect the teeth, gums, and mucous membranes to verify that they are free of food particles.
- Inspect for abnormalities, such as bleeding, that may have been stimulated by the brushing or flossing.
- Observe for patient discomfort or gagging during the procedure.
- If the procedure was performed by the NAP, the nurse should still perform an evaluation of the care. This includes a physical assessment of the oral cavity as well as objective and subjective findings related to the patient's tolerance of and satisfaction with the care.

Patient Teaching

- Discuss the importance of daily oral care.
- Review any areas of brushing or flossing that the patient has not been performing adequately.
- Discuss any problems that need further follow-up, such as inflammation, bleeding, dryness, caries, missing teeth, or broken or missing dentures.

Home Care

The procedure does not vary in the home. The nurse must:

- Work with the client and care provider to determine supplies needed for the home.
- Determine whether suction is needed (e.g., if the client is unconscious or has a decreased gag reflex). Explain to the client and/or caregiver how to obtain a portable suction unit.
- Demonstrate how to position the client and perform the procedure if the height of the bed is not adjustable or if both sides of the bed are not accessible.

Documentation

Document that oral care was given, the patient's response, any abnormal findings, and nursing interventions. Oral care is usually charted on a flowsheet.

Sample documentation

mm/dd/yyyy 0815 *Oral care given. Mucous membranes intact, pink, and dry. No choking or complaints of discomfort. Patient encouraged to increase fluid intake.* — Nancy Botha, RN

(continued on next page)

Procedure 25-6 ■ Brushing and Flossing the Teeth (continued)

Practice Resources

AACN (2007); Berry, A. Davidson, P., Nicholson, L., et al. (2012); Coughlan, M., & Healy, C. (2008); Harris D., Eilers J., Harriman, A., et al. (2008); Joanna Briggs Institute (2004); Philip, P., Rogers, C., Kruger, E., et al. (2012); Weening-Verbree, L., Huisman-de Waal, G., van Dusseldorp, L., et al. (2013).

Go to *Davis's Nursing Skills Videos*, **Brushing and Flossing the Teeth.**

Thinking About the Procedure

To practice applying clinical reasoning to this procedure,

For questions and suggested responses,

Go to Chapter 25, **Thinking About the Procedure Questions and Suggested Responses,** on Davis*Plus*.

Procedure 25-7 ■ Providing Denture Care

➤ For steps to follow in *all* procedures, refer to the Universal Steps for All Procedures found on the inside back cover.

Equipment

- See Procedure 25-6: Brushing and Flossing the Teeth.
- Denture cup

Delegation

You can delegate denture care to the NAP if the patient's condition and the NAP's skills allow. Perform the pre-procedure assessments, and inform the NAP of the specific care and the amount of help the patient needs. Ask the NAP to report the condition of the patient's mouth and dentures, level of self-care, and ability to tolerate the procedure.

Pre-Procedure Assessments

See Procedure 25-6: Brushing and Flossing the Teeth.

➤ When performing the procedure, always identify your patient according to agency policy, using two identifiers, and be attentive to standard precautions, hand hygiene, patient safety and privacy, body mechanics, and documentation.

Procedure Steps

1. **Don gloves, and remove** dentures (if the patient cannot do so).
   a. ***Upper denture:*** With a gauze pad, grasp the denture with your thumb and forefinger, and move it gently up and down. Tilt the denture slightly to one side to remove it, without stretching the lips. Place the denture in the denture cup.
   The gauze gives you a better grip. Breaking the seal on the top dentures can be difficult; movement breaks the suction. Always place dentures in a denture cup as soon as you remove them to prevent accidental breakage. ▼

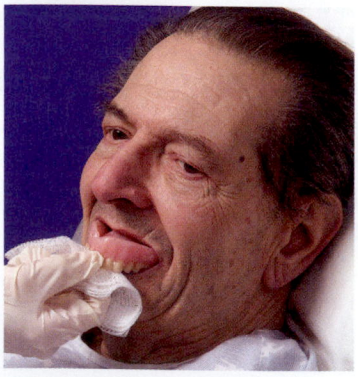

   b. ***Lower denture:*** Use your thumbs to push up gently on the denture at the gumline to release from the lower jaw. Grasp the denture with your thumb and forefinger, and tilt it to remove it from the patient's mouth. Place the denture in the denture cup.
   A gauze pad is not usually needed to grasp the lower dentures; however, you can use one if the dentures are difficult to grasp. Pushing up on the dentures breaks the seal. Rotating the dentures is necessary to remove the dentures from the patient's mouth. ▼

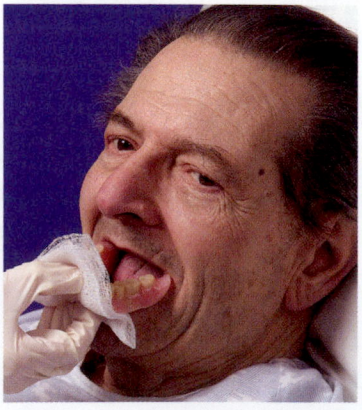

2. **Place the towel in the sink**, and pour cool water over the dentures to cleanse them. Follow agency policy for type of water to use.
   Heat can damage some dentures. The towel helps prevent the dentures from breaking if they are accidentally dropped. Dentures are expensive and usually not reimbursed by insurance. Institutions vary with regard to the existence of biofilm in the water lines.
   c. Apply a small amount of special denture paste to a soft-bristled toothbrush.
   Denture paste assists in cleaning. Toothpaste and stiff-bristled brushes may be too abrasive for dentures. However, follow the patient's preference in use of denture cleaner. Some patients prefer to soak their dentures in a cleanser overnight. If dentures have been soaking, rinse them well before placing them in the patient's mouth.
   d. Brush all surfaces of each denture.
   Loosens all food particles and any old denture adhesive.

e. Rinse thoroughly with cool water.
Removes loosened particles and the cleaning agent. Do not use hot water with dentures, because hot water can react to make the denture material sticky. Hospitalized patients at high risk for infection should avoid exposure to hospital water and use distilled sterile or filtered water instead.

Note: You can soak stained dentures in a commercial cleaner, following the manufacturer's instructions. Do not soak the denture overnight if the appliance has metal parts.
Soaking can cause corrosion of the metal parts.

3. **Inspect dentures** for rough, worn, or sharp edges.
These can irritate the tongue, gums, or mucous membranes of the mouth.

4. **Inspect the mouth** under the dentures for redness, irritation, lesions, or infection.
If present, refer to a dentist to check the fit of the dentures or to make needed repairs.

5. **Apply denture adhesive** as needed (ask the patient whether he uses denture adhesive).
Adhesives are needed to "seal" some dentures and prevent slipping and irritation of the gums.

6. **Moisten the top denture**, if it is dry. Then insert the top denture, at a slight tilt, and press it up against the roof of the mouth.
Moistening the dentures eases insertion. You can tell when you have securely seated the dentures by checking to feel for any slippage or to confirm that the dentures stay in place. Because the top denture is larger, it is removed first and inserted first for ease of insertion.

7. **Moisten the bottom denture**, if it is dry. Then insert bottom denture, rotating it as you put it in the patient's mouth.
Because it is smaller, the bottom denture is inserted after the top one. ▼

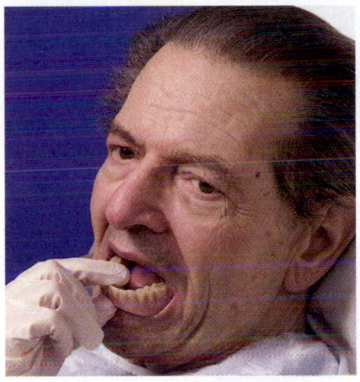

8. **Ask the patient whether** the dentures are comfortable.
Ensures that the dentures are properly placed.

9. **If the patient does not wish to** wear the dentures, cover them with water in a clean denture container with a lid. Label the container with the patient's name and the agency identifying number. Place denture container in bedside drawer rather than on top of bedside table for safekeeping.
Drying can cause dentures to warp. Hospitalized patients at high risk for infection avoid exposure to hospital water and use sterile water instead. Having the denture out of the mouth for several hours a day relieves pressure on the oral tissues, allows saliva to clean the tissues, and helps to minimize gingival irritation.

10. **Offer mouthwash.**

? What if . . .

- **My patient develops Candida-related denture stomatitis?**
Follow agency protocols. Microwave disinfection of complete dentures has been documented as an effective treatment of *Candida*-related denture stomatitis and can reduce the recurrence of infections.
Denture stomatitis ranges in severity. Treatment includes good oral and denture hygiene and administration of antifungal agents. Recurrence of infection after treatment can be due to colonization of Candida on the dentures.

Evaluation

- See Procedure 25-6: Brushing and Flossing the Teeth.
- Check to see that dentures are comfortable and fit properly.

Other

For Documentation, Patient Teaching, and Home Care, see Procedure 25-6: Brushing and Flossing the Teeth.

Practice Resources

Neppelenbroek, K., Pavarina, A., Spolidorio, D., et al. (2008); Pappas, P., Rex, J., Sobel, J., et al. (2009); Siegel, J., Rhinehart, E., Jackson, M., et al. (2007); Silva, M., Mima, E., Colombo, A., et al. (2012).

Thinking About the Procedure

To practice applying clinical reasoning to this procedure,

Go to *Davis's Nursing Skills Videos*, **Providing Denture Care.**

For questions and suggested responses,

Go to Chapter 25, **Thinking About the Procedure Questions and Suggested Responses,** on Davis *Plus*.

Procedure 25-8 ■ Providing Oral Care for an Unconscious Patient

➤ For steps to follow in *all* procedures, refer to the Universal Steps for All Procedures found on the inside back cover.

Equipment

- Toothbrush with soft bristles or sponge oral swabs
- Toothpaste
- Denture cup, if the patient has dentures
- 4 in. × 4 in. gauze pad to remove dentures if present
- Tonsil-tip suction connected to suction source (you may use a product that combines the toothbrush or oral swab with the suction device)
- Tongue blade (padded) or bite-block
- Towel
- Waterproof linen protector
- Disposable emesis basin
- Water-soluble lip moisturizer
- Procedure gloves and goggles

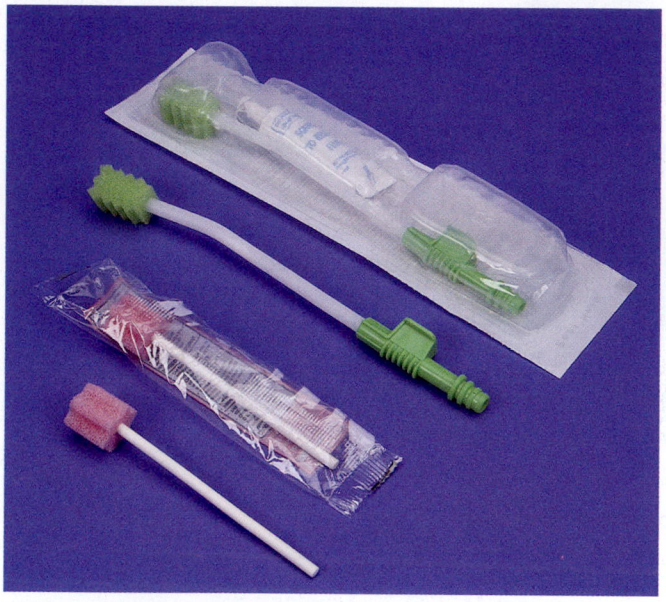

Source: Courtesy of Sage Products, Inc., Cary, IL.

Delegation

As a rule, you probably should not delegate oral hygiene for an unconscious patient to a NAP. However, in some situations it may be acceptable—for example, when the NAP has a great deal of experience caring for unconscious patients and when the NAP's ability to perform oral hygiene safely for them is documented. Perform the pre-procedure assessments, and inform the NAP of any special considerations for care (e.g., if the patient must have the head of the bed elevated to facilitate breathing). Ask the NAP to report the condition of the patient's mouth and the patient's ability to tolerate the procedure (e.g., ask the NAP to take vital signs before and after the procedure, or to note the oxygen saturation if it is being monitored).

Pre-Procedure Assessments

- Determine whether the patient has dentures or partial plates.
  The presence of these appliances determines how you will provide oral care. You may leave dentures out for an unconscious patient to decrease the risk that the dentures will be damaged or block the airway. However, when possible, keep the dentures in place to help ensure they will fit adequately later. Remove partial plates in an unconscious patient to prevent the plate from causing aspiration or damage to the mouth if it becomes loosened.
- Assess the patient's gag reflex.
  If the patient has an intact gag reflex, the risk of aspiration is lower.
- Assess the patient's general oral health, including the condition of the teeth and gums, and hydration of the mucous membranes. If the patient has dentures, examine the mouth with and without the dentures.
  Unconscious patients tend to breathe through the mouth, so oral mucosa are often dry. Because the oral mucosa acts as a barrier against microorganisms, inflammation or lesions in the mouth increase the risk for infection. The lips, gums, and mucous membranes should be pink, moist, and intact. The teeth should be intact and clean. The condition of the mouth determines what you will use to provide oral care. Assess the fit of dentures and the condition of the skin under the dentures to determine whether the fit is proper and whether any irritation is present.

➤ When performing the procedure, always identify your patient according to agency policy, using two identifiers, and be attentive to standard precautions, hand hygiene, patient safety and privacy, body mechanics, and documentation.

Procedure Steps

1. **Position the patient side-lying** with head turned to the side and, if possible, with the head of the bed down.
   Secretions will pool in the dependent side of the mouth. This position helps prevent aspiration and facilitates the removal of secretions by gravity.
2. **Don procedure gloves and eye goggles.**
   Follows standard precautions. Eye protection is needed when suctioning because of the risk of splashing.
3. **Place a waterproof pad** and then a towel under the patient's cheek and chin.
   The towel and pad will absorb water and keep the bed linens dry.
4. **Set up suction.** Attach suction tubing and tonsil-tip suction; check suction.
   Suctioning helps ensure that the patient does not aspirate oral secretions during mouth care.

5. **Brush the patient's teeth.**
   a. Use a padded tongue blade or bite-block, as needed, to hold the patient's mouth open.
   A padded tongue blade or bite block is used to hold the mouth open so you can visualize and reach the different areas of the mouth without injuring the oral mucosa. It also keeps the patient from biting the nurse's fingers.

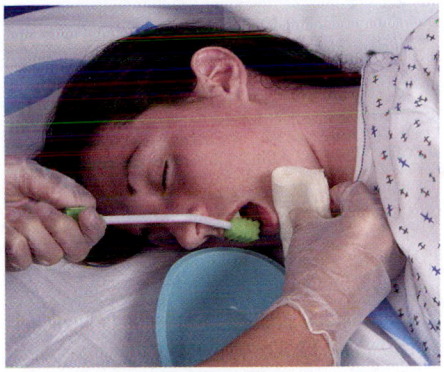

   b. Place an emesis basin under the patient's cheek.
   Catches the secretions draining from the patient's mouth.
   c. Moisten the toothbrush, and apply a small amount of toothpaste. Use hospital-approved water (e.g., sterile, distilled, or filtered tap water).
   Excessive toothpaste does not increase the cleaning. Brushing the teeth with a soft-bristled brush stimulates the mucosa, which increases the health of the gums.
   d. Brush the teeth, holding the bristles at a 45° angle to the gumline.
      (1) Using short, circular motions, gently brush the inner and outer surfaces of the teeth, including the gumline.
      (2) Brush the biting surface of the back teeth by holding the brush bristles vertical to the teeth and brushing back and forth.
      (3) Brush the patient's tongue.
      This is the most effective technique for removing plaque and debris from the teeth and gums. The tongue can be a reservoir for bacteria.
   e. Perform oral suctioning when fluid accumulates in the mouth.
   Removing fluid prevents choking and aspiration.
   f. Draw about 10 mL of distilled, sterile or filtered water or mouthwash (e.g., dilute hydrogen peroxide) into a syringe; eject it gently into the side of the mouth. Allow the fluid to drain out into the basin, or suction as needed.
   Removes any toothpaste residue, which may have a drying effect. Remove all fluid from the mouth to prevent aspiration into the lungs. Use a minimal amount of solution to prevent aspiration.

6. **Provide denture care**, if necessary. See Procedure 25-7: Providing Denture Care.

7. **Clean the tissues in the oral** cavity according to agency policy. Use foam swabs or a moistened gauze square wrapped around a tongue blade. Use a clean swab for each area of the mouth: cheeks, tongue, roof of the mouth, and so on.
   Oral tissues may be dry and sticky from mouth breathing. Using separate swabs prevents transfer of microorganisms from one area to another.

8. **Remove and dispose of the** basin, dry the patient's face and mouth, and apply water-soluble lip moisturizer.
   Petroleum-based lip moisturizers (e.g., mineral oil, petroleum jelly) are not recommended because of the possibility of aspiration, which might cause pneumonia. Never use petroleum-based jelly for patients receiving oxygen therapy; it can cause burns.

9. **Remove the waterproof pad** and towel; turn off suction equipment; discard gloves and used supplies.

10. **Reposition the patient** as needed.
    Maintains good body alignment.

11. **Cleanse and store reusable** oral hygiene tools in clean containers, separate from other articles of personal hygiene.
    Prevents possible contamination from the environment and other personal hygiene tools.

? What if . . .

- **You are providing oral care to a patient receiving mechanical ventilation?**

  Provide oral cleansing, including subglottic suctioning, at least every 2 hours and prn. Brush the teeth at least twice a day.
  Keeping the oral cavity clean and clear of secretions has been proved to decrease the incidence of ventilator-associated pneumonia (VAP). Pooled oral secretions become rapidly colonized with pathogens that contribute to VAP.

  Avoid tap water. Use normal saline or a half-strength solution of saline for oral rinses.
  Studies show hospital plumbing and tap water are often colonized with microbial organisms.

  Apply a 0.12% chlorhexidine gluconate solution twice daily to complement oral care.

- **It is difficult to floss the patient's teeth, or the patient doesn't tolerate flossing?**

  Handheld interdental tools may be used instead of floss. These devices are special small brushes, picks, or sticks.
  Toothbrush bristles can't reach between teeth to dislodge food particles and bacteria. Interdental cleaners can be as effective as floss in keeping these areas clean.

- **Oral tissues are dry and sticky?**

  Use appropriately diluted sodium bicarbonate to dissolve viscous mucus.

(continued on next page)

Procedure 25-8 ■ Providing Oral Care for an Unconscious Patient (continued)

Evaluation

- Inspect the teeth, gums, and mucous membranes for cleanliness.
- Observe the oral mucosa and gums for hydration, inflammation, bleeding, or infection.
- Observe the patient's overall responses to the procedure (e.g., gagging, coughing, vital signs, skin color).

Patient Teaching

- Discuss with family members any problems that need further follow-up.
- Teach oral hygiene measures, as needed.

Home Care

- The procedure steps do not vary in the home.
- Work with the client and caregiver to determine supplies needed for the home.
- Determine whether suction is needed, and explain to caregivers how to obtain a portable suction unit.
- Demonstrate how to position the client and perform the procedure if the height of the bed is not adjustable or if both sides of the bed are not accessible.

Documentation

Document that oral care was given, any abnormal findings, and nursing interventions. Typically, though, oral care is documented on a checklist or flowsheet.

Sample documentation

mm/dd/yyyy 0730 *Oral care given. Mucous membranes pink and moist. White coating on tongue—physician notified. Patient had no coughing during the procedure. Gag reflex is intact. Patient did not aspirate. Respiratory rate 18.* Susan Hiam, RN

Thinking About the Procedure

To practice applying clinical reasoning to this procedure,

Go to *Davis's Nursing Skills Videos*, **Providing Oral Care for an Unconscious Patient.**

For questions and suggested responses,

Go to Chapter 25, **Thinking About the Procedure Questions and Suggested Responses,** on Davis *Plus*.

Practice Resources

AACN (2007); American Dental Association (n.d.); Ames, N., Sulima, P., Yates, J., et al. (2011); Berry, A., Davidson, P., Nicholson, L., et al. (2012); Cason, C., Tyner, T., Saunders, S., et al. (2007); Karki, S., & Cheng, A. C. (2012); NGC (2008); Slot, D., Dörfer, C., & Van der Weijden, G. (2008).

Procedure 25-9 ■ Shampooing the Hair

➤ For steps to follow in *all* procedures, refer to the Universal Steps for All Procedures found on the inside back cover.

Delegation

You can delegate this procedure to the NAP if the patient's condition and the NAP's skills allow. Perform the pre-procedure assessments, and inform the NAP of the specific type of procedure needed (e.g., in bed, at sink, disposable shampoo equipment) and the amount of help the patient needs. Inform the NAP of any special considerations, such as positions the patient cannot assume or presence of scalp lesions. Ask the NAP to report the condition of the patient's scalp and hair, level of self-care, and ability to tolerate the procedure.

Pre-Procedure Assessments

- Assess for contraindications to a shampoo (e.g., scalp sutures or limited head or neck movement). A rinse-free shampoo would be more appropriate in these cases.
- Determine the patient's ability to assist with the procedure.
  Promotes independence and provides active ROM.
- Assess the condition of the patient's hair and scalp. Note any dryness or irritation.
  Dry and brittle hair may indicate hypothyroidism or malnutrition and may require special shampoos or conditioners.
- Determine the need for special hair care products.
  Dandruff, lice, and dry hair are examples of conditions that require medicated shampoos or conditioners.
- Ask the patient how she normally cares for her hair.

Procedure 25-9A ■ Shampooing the Hair for a Patient on Bedrest—Using Rinse-Free Shampoo

Equipment

- Rinse-free shampoo (no water is needed); conditioner is optional
- Bath towel
- Brush or hair pick, and comb
- Procedure gloves (if scalp lesion or infestation present)

➤ When performing the procedure, always identify your patient according to agency policy, using two identifiers, and be attentive to standard precautions, hand hygiene, patient safety and privacy, body mechanics, and documentation.

Procedure Steps

1. **Elevate the head** of the bed, if possible.
   Makes it easier to maintain good body mechanics during the procedure.
2. **Place a protective pad** or bath towel under the patient's shoulders.
   Prevents the linen from getting wet.
3. **Don procedure gloves** if lesions or infestations are present.
   Helps prevent transmission of disease.
4. **Work your fingers through the hair**, or comb the hair to remove tangles before washing. If the patient has her hair in small braids, do not take out the braids to wash the hair.
5. **Apply rinse-free shampoo.** Apply enough shampoo to thoroughly wet the hair. One application is usually sufficient to clean the hair.
6. **Work the shampoo through the hair**, from scalp down to ends.
   Helps prevent pulling on and damaging the hair.
7. **Dry the hair** with a bath towel.
   Removes the shampoo. Leaves the hair feeling clean and soft.
8. **Comb or brush hair** to remove tangles, starting at the ends and working toward the scalp.
   Prevents excessive pulling on the patient's hair, which may cause breakage.
9. **Dry the hair** with a hair dryer at a medium temperature, if desired.
   Use a medium temperature to prevent burning the patient.
10. **When you are finished**, be sure that the patient's clothing and bed linens are dry. Wash and store brushes and combs.

Procedure 25-9B ■ Shampooing the Hair Using Rinse-Free Shampoo Cap

➤ When performing the procedure, always identify your patient according to agency policy, using two identifiers, and be attentive to standard precautions, hand hygiene, patient safety and privacy, body mechanics, and documentation.

Procedure Steps

1. **Warm the shampoo cap** using a water bath or microwave according to package instructions. Be careful to not overheat. Check the temperature before placing on the patient's head to prevent burns.
   A commercial no-rinse shampoo cap is a microwavable cap that contains a no-rinse shampoo and conditioner. Different products are available. Be sure to follow the directions on the package.
2. **Place the cap on the patient's hair**, and gently massage.
3. **Remove the cap**, and towel-dry the patient's hair.
   Removes the shampoo and excess water.
4. **Complete hair care** according to the patient's needs (see Procedure 25-9A, Steps 7–10, preceding).

Procedure 25-9C ■ Shampooing the Hair Using a Basin and Water

Key Point: ***The use of prepackaged shampoo products is recommended. However, some patients prefer the traditional shampooing technique or may have excessive soiling of the hair and scalp requiring the use of water and basin. This traditional method of hair hygiene can result in significant variation from caregiver to caregiver and increase the risk of hospital-associated infection from contaminated basins and/or tap water. Such techniques also take longer so they require more nursing time. They may also be more tiring for the patient.***

Equipment

- Shampoo; conditioner is optional
- Disposable shampoo tray or commercial system, if available
- Disposable washbasin, plastic pail, small easy-to-handle plastic container
- Towels (2), washcloth, bath blanket
- Waterproof pads or plastic trash bag
- Brush and comb
- Procedure gloves, if indicated by the presence of lesions or infestation
- Hair dryer
- For inpatients, filtered tap water, distilled, or sterile water are recommended (see Key Point above). Follow agency policy, as conditions vary among institutions.

(continued on next page)

Procedure 25-9 ■ Shampooing the Hair (continued)

➤ When performing the procedure, always identify your patient according to agency policy, using two identifiers, and be attentive to standard precautions, hand hygiene, patient safety and privacy, body mechanics, and documentation.

Procedure Steps

1. **If lesions or infestation is** present, don procedure gloves.
   Observes standard precautions.

2. **Unless contraindicated** (e.g., by a neck condition), lower the head of the bed, take the pillow from under the patient's neck, and place it under her shoulders.
   Hyperextends the neck and helps keep water from the eyes.

3. **Place the waterproof pad** or plastic trash bag under patient's shoulders, and cover with towels. A commercial system will have a drain hose to use.
   Protects the bed from getting wet.

4. **Collect warm, not hot, water** (see Equipment) in a container and bring to the bedside.

5. **Place the shampoo tray** under the patient's shoulders (or head, depending on the type of tray). If you are using a hard plastic tray, pad the neck area with a towel. An inflatable shampoo tray needs minimal padding, but you will need to inflate it before beginning the procedure, either by mouth or with an air pump.
   Protects the patient from lying on a hard surface and prevents water from leaking out onto the bed.

6. **Ensure that the tray will drain** into the washbasin or plastic pail.
   Prevents water draining onto the bed or floor.

7. **Fold the top linens down** to the patient's waist, and cover her upper body with a bath blanket.
   Keeps the linen dry; keeps the patient warm.

8. **Work your fingers through** the patient's hair, or comb the hair to remove tangles prior to washing.
   It is easier to remove tangles from dry hair. Note that very tangled or matted hair may sometimes indicate a lice infestation.

9. **Wash the hair.**
   a. Wet the hair, pouring warm water from the pitcher. Do not get water in the person's eyes or ears.
   b. Next, apply shampoo and lather well, working from the scalp out and from the front to the back of the head.
   c. Gently lift the patient's head to rub the back of the head.

10. **Rinse thoroughly.**
    Shampoo is drying if left in the hair. ▼

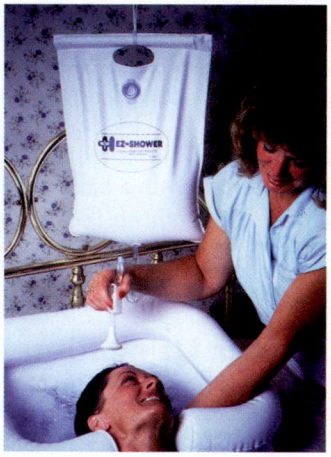

11. **Apply conditioner to the hair**, if desired, especially for patients with hair that tangles easily, such as dry, long, curly, or kinky hair. Rinse if needed. Leave-in conditioner can be used and is recommended for curly hair.

12. **Remove the tray**, and blot-dry the hair with the towel. Do not use circular motions to dry the hair.
    Circular motions will increase tangles.

13. **Comb or brush hair** to remove tangles, starting at the ends and working toward the scalp.
    Prevents excessive pulling on the patient's hair, which may cause breakage.

14. **Dry the hair** with a hair dryer at a medium temperature, if desired.
    Use a medium temperature to prevent burning the patient.

15. **When you are finished**, be sure that the patient's clothing and bed linens are dry. Wash the shampoo tray and the brushes and combs.

Procedure Variation: Shampooing the Hair of African American Patients

16. **If the hair is in cornrows or braids**, do not take out the braids to wash the hair. You may need to apply a cloth or net cap to the head prior to shampooing.

17. **Handle the patient's hair very gently**, being careful not to pull on the hair.
    Many African Americans have fragile hair that breaks easily. Because it is fragile, apply moisturizer, if needed, to untangle the hair.

18. **When shampooing**, thread your fingers through the hair from the scalp out to the ends. Do not massage the hair in circular motions.

19. **Rinse thoroughly**, then apply a conditioner on the hair if the hair is dry and fragile.
    A leave-in conditioner helps minimize tangles and breakage.

20. **Comb through the hair.**
    a. Use a wide-toothed comb or hair pick. Do not use a brush or fine-toothed comb.
    b. Part the hair into four sections and begin combing near the ends of the hair, working through each section.
    c. Use additional moisturizer to help soften and ease combing.
    Never pull on the hair, because it will break easily.

21. **Apply a natural oil to the hair**, if desired. Examples of natural oils are coconut, sweet almond, shea butter, and avocado. Many commercial products use these oils.
    Mineral oil and Vaseline tend to clog pores and damage the hair, so use

them only if the patient still prefers them after receiving this information.

22. **Let the hair air-dry** if possible.
Prevents the hair from becoming frizzy. A high temperature, such as from a hair dryer, will also damage the hair.

? What if . . .

- **You do not have a shampoo tray?**
Improvise by using a new bedpan, and reserve it only for washing the hair. Pad it liberally with towels.
- **You discover head lice or nits as you begin the shampoo?**
Stop the procedure. Discuss your findings with the patient and offer reassurance. Leave the patient in a position of comfort and safety. Perform hand hygiene. Report the findings and obtain an order for a prescriptive shampoo.

Evaluation

- Observe that the hair is clean, dry, and free of tangles.
- Observe for patient discomfort or fatigue during the procedure.
- Ask the patient how the hair and scalp feel.

Patient Teaching

- Educate patients and their families about how bathing technology has changed to improve patient care and reduce risk of infection. Products such as rinse-free shampoos or a shampoo cap can make shampooing easier to accomplish for a bedridden patient.
- Advise patients with coarse hair to wash it less frequently (every 3 to 7 days, depending on dryness). Leave-in conditioners are often recommended for dry, curly, or kinky hair.

Home Care

- In the home care setting, determine how the client usually washes her hair.
- If the client is confined to bed, work with the caregiver to develop an effective plan for washing the client's hair. For example, if a shampoo tray is not available, you can make one by using a plastic garbage bag and pillows or rolled towels.
- The newer rinse-free products or the inflatable shampoo tray may be good choices for the client.
- If the client cannot afford the adaptive equipment needed, refer the caregiver to the local resources, such as senior services.
- If the client is ambulatory, recommend a shower stool. The stool needs to fit into the shower or bathtub securely, without wobbling, to prevent the client from falling.
- If the client has only a bathtub, an adaptor for the faucet can be used to attach a handheld showerhead. Using a shower stool will make the procedure easier.

Documentation

Chart that hair was shampooed, the condition of the hair and scalp, and the patient's responses to the procedure.

Sample documentation

mm/dd/yyyy 2045 *Hair shampooed. Scalp without signs of irritation. Hair dry. Conditioner applied. No c/o discomfort. Pt states, "My hair feels wonderful now, and my head doesn't itch anymore."* Alicia Nelson, RN

Practice Resources

EZ-Shampoo Instructions for Use (2005); Thompson Healthcare, Inc. (2012). (Caveat: These are not research articles; they are manufacturers' recommendations.)

Procedure 25-10 ■ Providing Beard and Mustache Care

➤ For steps to follow in *all* procedures, refer to the Universal Steps for All Procedures found on the inside back cover.

Equipment

- Scissors or beard trimmer
- Wide-toothed comb
- Mild shampoo; conditioner for coarse and/or dry hair
- Basin (single-patient use, disposable)
- Bath towel
- Procedure gloves (if skin nicks occur, contact with blood may occur)

Delegation

You can delegate beard and mustache care to the NAP if the patient's condition and the NAP's skills allow. Perform the pre-procedure assessments, and inform the NAP of the specific type of care needed (e.g., in bed, at sink, safety razor, electric razor). Inform the NAP of any special considerations, such as skin irritation or activity intolerance. Ask the NAP to report the condition of the patient's skin and beard, level of self-care, and ability to tolerate the procedure.

Pre-Procedure Assessments

- Ask the patient or family about preferences for beard and mustache care.
Beards and mustaches may have personal and/or cultural meaning. Men in some cultures never cut or trim their beards. Some patients use a comb and scissors to do a slight trim of their beard and/or mustache, whereas others use a beard trimmer for a closer trim.
- Assess the patient's skin and hair condition.
Determine whether the skin has any reddened or dry areas and whether skin treatments are needed.

(continued on next page)

Procedure 25-10 ■ Providing Beard and Mustache Care (continued)

➤ When performing the procedure, always identify your patient according to agency policy, using two identifiers, and be attentive to standard precautions, hand hygiene, patient safety and privacy, body mechanics, and documentation.

Procedure Steps

1. **Drape the towel around** the patient's shoulders.
   Protects the patient's clothing from falling pieces of hair and water from shampooing the beard or mustache.

2. **Trim the beard and mustache** when they are dry.
   The beard and mustache are often shorter when dry. If they are cut when wet, they may be shorter than desired after they dry.

If Using a Comb and Scissors

a. Comb through the beard, and cut the hair on the outside of the comb. Be conservative; cutting too little is better than cutting too much.
   Trimming too much off the beard can be upsetting for the patient, whereas if you cut too little, you can always trim off more.

b. Trim from the front of the ear to the chin on one side, and repeat on the other.
   Keeps the beard equal on both sides of the face.

If Using a Beard Trimmer

c. Select the trimming guide to the correct length. Adjust the guide to a longer length rather than a shorter length.
   Ensures that you do not cut the beard too short.

d. Trim from the front of the ear to the chin on one side, and repeat on the other.

3. **Trim the mustache.**
   a. Comb the mustache straight down.
   Cuts the length equally so that the mustache is just above the upper lip. ▼

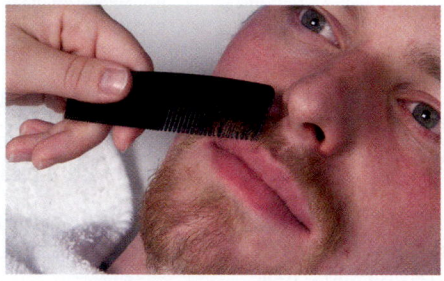

   b. Using either scissors or a beard trimmer, start in the middle, and trim toward one side of the mouth and then toward the other. Do not trim the top of the mustache.
   Trimming from the center out toward each side helps you cut both sides equally.

4. **Define the beard line** by one of the following methods:
   a. Using either the scissors or a beard trimmer, trim the line of the beard so that it is well defined. Trim very little to ensure that you only define the beard and do not change the length. ▼

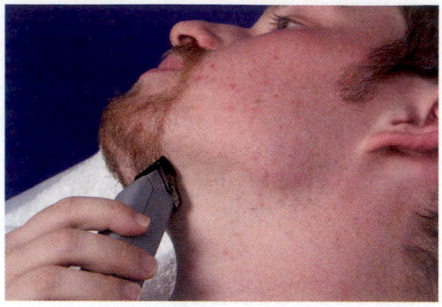

   b. Shave the neck to define the beard line, particularly for short beards.

5. **Apply procedure gloves**, if needed, and shampoo the beard and mustache using warm sterile, distilled, or tap water and a mild shampoo.
   The skin under a beard or mustache can be tender, so treat it gently with a mild shampoo. Follow standard precautions, because it is possible to nick the skin and cause bleeding. Policies about use of tap water vary among institutions.

6. **Rinse well, and pat and wipe** the beard and mustache dry with the towel.
   Any shampoo left can irritate the skin, as can rubbing motions with the towel.

7. **Apply conditioner**, if desired.

8. **Comb the beard and mustache** with a wide-toothed comb or a brush.
   Do not use a fine-toothed comb, because it will pull the hair.

Evaluation

- Make sure that the beard and mustache are trimmed to the desired length and are clean.
- Verify that skin problems are identified and treatment initiated.

Home Care

No adaptations are required in the home. The patient's usual supplies are sufficient, as a rule.

Documentation

Chart that beard and mustache were trimmed and shampooed; chart the condition of the skin.

Practice Resources

Procter & Gamble (2008). (Caveat: This is not an evidence-based practice article. It is a manufacturer's recommendation.)

Procedure 25-11 ■ Shaving a Patient

➤ For steps to follow in *all* procedures, refer to the Universal Steps for All Procedures found on the inside back cover.

Equipment

- Safety razor or electric razor
- Shaving cream or soap; after-shave lotion, if desired
- Shaving brush, if desired
- Warm water (sterile, distilled, or tap water per agency policy)
- Face towel and bath towel
- Procedure gloves

Delegation

You can delegate shaving to the NAP if the patient's condition and the NAP's skills allow. Perform the pre-procedure assessments, and inform the NAP of the amount of help and specific type of care (e.g., safety or electric razor, in bed, or at the sink), the patient needs. Inform the NAP of any special considerations, such as skin irritation or activity intolerance. Ask the NAP to report the condition of the patient's skin, level of self-care, his ability to tolerate the procedure.

Pre-Procedure Assessments

- Determine how much assistance the patient needs.
  Aids you in promoting as much independence as possible.
- Assess the patient's skin and hair condition for redness, skin lesions, or moles.
  Identifies skin problems, and determines whether skin treatments are needed or the procedure must be modified. To prevent abrading the skin, do not shave any areas that have skin lesions or moles.
- Assess the patient's usual shaving method, including use of electric razor or safety razor.
  When possible, follow the patient's routine. The patient may or may not use shaving cream or shaving soap, shaving brush, and after-shave lotion.
- Check for any contraindications to shaving, such as an increased risk of infection or bleeding (e.g., because of neutropenia, thrombocytopenia, or the administration of anticoagulants, such as warfarin or heparin).

➤ When performing the procedure, always identify your patient according to agency policy, using two identifiers, and be attentive to standard precautions, hand hygiene, patient safety and privacy, body mechanics, and documentation.

Procedure Steps

1. **Don procedure gloves.**
   To prevent exposure to blood if skin is nicked or scratched.
2. **Place a warm, damp face towel** on the patient's face for 1 to 3 minutes.
   Opens the pores and softens the beard to prevent pulling. Do not use hot water, because it will dehydrate the skin and can burn sensitive skin.
3. **Apply shaving lotion** to the face with your fingers or a shaving brush. Lather well for 1 to 2 minutes.
   Lathering well helps to further soften the beard. Do not use shaving creams that contain numbing agents, because they close the pores and stiffen the beard.
4. **Shave the patient.**
   a. Pull skin taut with your nondominant hand, and gently pull the razor across the skin. If you are using a safety razor, hold the blade at a 45° angle to the skin.
   b. Shave the face and neck in the same direction of hair growth (the direction is not the same for all people). Using short strokes, start shaving at the sideburns, and work down to the chin on each side and then the neck.
   c. Last, shave the chin and upper lip.
   Usually the hair on the face will grow down toward the chin and on the neck up toward the chin. The hair is generally thickest on the chin and upper lip, so shaving them last allows more time for the shaving cream to soften the hair. Shave in the same direction as the hair is growing to prevent skin irritation. ▼

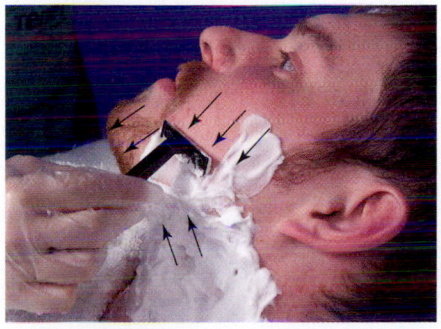

5. **Rinse the razor** frequently while you are shaving.
   Avoids clogging the blade.
6. **When you are finished shaving,** rinse the patient's face with cool water (see Equipment), and gently pat it dry.
   Cool water helps close the pores. Pat dry, do not rub, to prevent irritating the skin.
7. **Apply after-shave lotion,** if desired.
   After-shave lotions that contain alcohol are not recommended, because alcohol stings and dries out the skin. A moisturizer is recommended.
8. **Dispose of the single-use razor** in the sharps container.
   Prevents cutting injury to others.

If Using a Multiuse Razor

Shake the razor to remove excess moisture. Do not bang the razor against objects or dry with a towel. Store the razor in a covered container.

Banging or wiping the razor edge will dull the razor and may damage the holding mechanism. A covered container protects others from a cutting injury.

? What if . . .

- **Your patient has a condition that predisposes him to bleeding (e.g., thrombocytopenia) or infection (e.g., neutropenia)?**

  Such patients must be shaved carefully using an electric razor, if at all.

  A razor scratch or cut causes a break in skin integrity, providing a portal of entry for pathogens. This could be especially serious for a patient whose defenses against infection are compromised. For a patient with a delayed clotting time, a cut could cause excessive blood loss.

(continued on next page)

Procedure 25-11 ■ Shaving a Patient (continued)

Evaluation

- Inspect the patient's face, closeness of the shave, and for nicks or cuts.
- If the procedure was performed by the NAP, ask the patient about his satisfaction with and tolerance of the care.

Patient Teaching

Teach patients about changes that need to be made in their shaving technique as a result of changes in health status. For example, a patient who has begun taking anticoagulants may need to change from a blade to an electric razor because of an increased risk of bleeding.

Home Care

The procedure does not vary in the home. The nurse must:

- Determine the availability of supplies
- Assess the client's or caregiver's ability to perform the procedure.

Documentation

Chart that the patient was shaved and the condition of the skin. There will probably be a flowsheet or checklist for this information.

Practice Resources

Coughlan, M., & Healy, C. (2008); Proctor & Gamble (2008); Men's Health (updated 2011). (Caveat: Except for Coughlan & Healy, the preceding are not evidence-based resources. They are information from manufacturers.)

Procedure 25-12 ■ Removing and Caring for Contact Lenses

➤ For steps to follow in *all* procedures, refer to the Universal Steps for All Procedures found on the inside back cover.

Equipment

- Contact lens wetting solution
- Contact lens soaking solution
- Sterile saline (optional)
- Contact lens case
- Contact lens remover (optional)
- Procedure gloves

Delegation

You can delegate this procedure if the patient's condition and the NAP's skills permit. For example, if the patient is unconscious, you must determine whether contact lenses are present, and you should not delegate their removal.

Pre-Procedure Assessments

- Determine whether the patient is wearing contact lenses. If the patient is unconscious, examine the eyes for the presence of contact lenses by shining a penlight across the eye. You should be able to see the edge of the lens.
- Determine the type of contact lenses in place.
  Hard lenses are smaller than soft lenses. Each type of contact lens has different care requirements. Hard lenses can be worn for only up to 18 hours. Rigid gas-permeable (RGP) lenses may be worn overnight or for about 7 days, depending on the kind. Soft contacts are used for either short or longer periods.
- Ask the patient whether he is able to remove his contact lenses.

➤ When performing the procedure, always identify your patient according to agency policy, using two identifiers, and be attentive to standard precautions, hand hygiene, patient safety and privacy, body mechanics, and documentation.

➤ *Note:* It is difficult to remove a contact lens when wearing procedure gloves. For hard lenses, you can use a suction cup device if one is available.

If you must use ungloved hands (e.g., in an emergency situation), it is extremely important to wash your hands thoroughly before and after the procedure. *Do not* use your fingernails.

➤ *Note:* Lens cases are marked "L" and "R" to indicate left and right lenses. Clean, rinse, and place the lens you remove first into its designated cup before removing the second lens.

Procedure Steps

1. **Perform hand hygiene** and don gloves.
2. **Instill one to two drops** of contact lens wetting solution to moisten the lenses.
   Aids in lens removal.
3. **Remove the lenses.**

For Hard or Gas-Permeable Contact Lens

- *Alternative 1:* If the lens is not centered over the cornea, place your finger on the patient's lower eyelid, and apply gentle pressure to move it into position. Place your index finger at the outer corner of the eye, and gently pull sideways toward the ear; position your other hand below the eye to "catch" the lens. Ask the patient to blink. As the skin tightens, the palpebral fissure narrows, the lids catch on the edge of the lens and pop it out. ▼

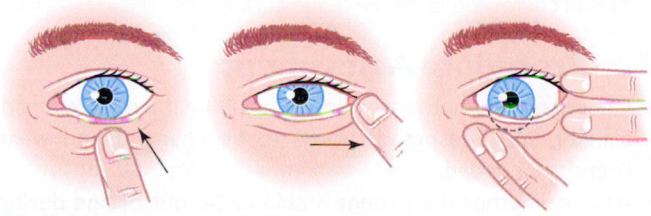

- *Alternative 2:* Use a small suction cup contact lens remover. Gently press the suction cup end of the remover onto the contact lens, and lift straight up off the eye.
- *Alternative 3:* Gently pull the top eyelid up and the lower lid down beyond the top and bottom edges of the lens. Then gently press the lower eyelid up against the bottom of the lens. When the lens is slightly tipped, move the eyelids together. This should cause the lens to slide out. ▼

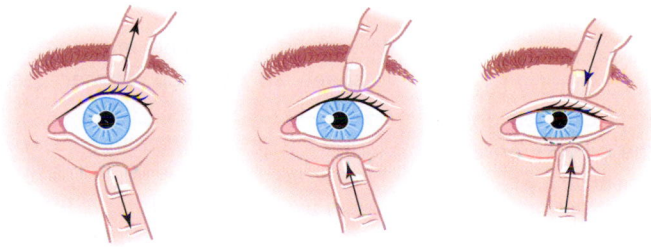

For Soft Contact Lens

a. Hold the eye open with your nondominant hand.
Allows you to visualize the contact lens.

b. Gently place the tip of your index finger on the contact lens, and slide it down off the pupil to the white area of the eye.

To prevent potential damage to the eye, do not pinch a lens directly over the pupil. ▼

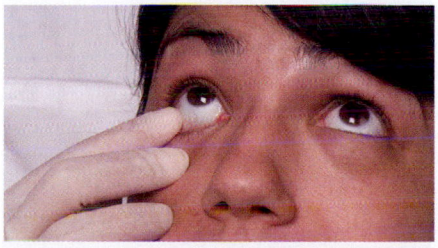

c. Using your thumb and index finger pads, gently pinch the lens, and lift it straight up off the eye. If the edges stick together, moisten with a few drops of wetting solution. Rub gently until edges separate.
A soft contact lens is very flexible and pinches easily. ▼

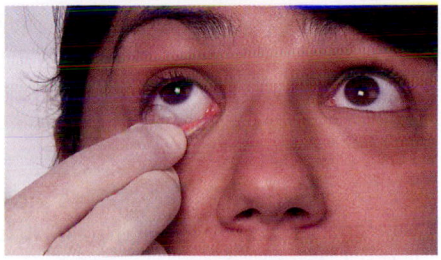

4. **Clean the lens** according to the instructions on the cleaning solution bottle. If there is no lens cleaner, use sterile saline. Be careful not to tear soft lenses.

5. **Rinse the lenses** with contact lens solution or sterile saline.
Removes any particles from the lenses.

6. **Place the lenses in a contact** lens case containing soaking solution or sterile saline (see note above regarding lens cases).
Prevents bacterial growth on the contacts and keeps the lenses from drying out.

Evaluation

Examine the eyes for redness or irritation.

Patient Teaching

- Review with the patient and/or family the importance of keeping the contact lenses clean and moist.
- If hard contact lenses are used, they must be removed at bedtime to prevent hypoxia of the cornea.

Documentation

Chart that contacts were removed, what type of lenses they are, what solution they are stored in, and the condition of patient's eyes.

Practice Resources

Bausch & Lomb (2008, 2009); Holman, C., Roberts, S., & Nicol, M. (2005); Massachusetts Eye and Ear Infirmary (n.d., last updated January 5, 2009).

Procedure 25-13 ■ Making an Unoccupied Bed

➤ For steps to follow in *all* procedures, refer to the Universal Steps for All Procedures found on the inside back cover.

Equipment

- Bottom and top sheets, possibly drawsheet
- Pillowcase for each of the pillows
- Linen bag or hamper
- Procedure gloves (if exposure to body fluids is possible)
- Moisture-proof gown (if heavy soiling of linens with body fluids is possible).

Delegation

You can delegate this procedure to the NAP. You are responsible for supervising to ensure that the procedure is performed correctly.

Pre-Procedure Assessments

- Check to see whether the linen (including the mattress pad, blanket, and bedspread) needs to be changed, and what linens are needed.
- Assess whether the patient is able to be out of bed during the linen change.
- Assess for drainage or incontinence to determine whether personal protective equipment, such as procedure gloves and gown, is needed.

Note: This procedure describes bed making by one person. It is more efficient for two people to work together on opposite sides of the bed.

➤ When performing the procedure, always identify your patient according to agency policy, using two identifiers, and be attentive to standard precautions, hand hygiene, patient safety and privacy, body mechanics, and documentation.

Procedure Steps

1. **Assist the patient to a chair.** Provide a robe and/or blanket if needed.
   Ensures that the patient is comfortable and will be warm enough during the bed change.

2. **Prepare the environment:** Position the bed flat, raise to appropriate working height, put on the brakes, and lower the siderails. Move the overbed table and other furniture, as needed. Place the linen bag or hamper conveniently near the bed.
   Maintains good body mechanics and prevents back strain during the procedure. Remove obstacles to allow easy access to the bed. Place all items so you can work efficiently, saving time and energy.

3. **Don protective gloves** and other gear if necessary. Loosen all the bedding.
   This observes Standard Precautions and reduces the risk of contaminating your clothing.

4. **If the blanket or bedspread is** clean, fold it and place it on a clean area (e.g., on the back of a chair). *Do not* place on another patient's bed or furniture.
   Reuse the blanket and/or bedspread if it is not soiled. Placing the item on a clean area prevents cross-contamination.

5. **Remove the bottom and top sheet**, draw sheet, and pillowcases.
   a. Do not shake the linens.
      Minimizes dispersal of dust, skin cells, and microorganisms into the environment.
   b. Holding the items away from your body, place them in a laundry bag or hamper. Never place linen on the floor. Place the pillows on a clean area (e.g., on a chair).
      Hold dirty linen away from your uniform to prevent contamination. Cross-contamination can occur if you place linens on the floor.▼

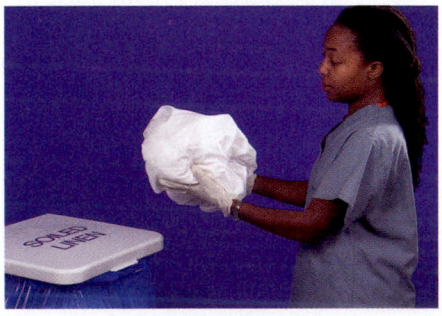

6. **Working from one side of bed,** to save steps:

   For a Contour-Bottom Sheet
   a. Fit the contour-bottom sheet on one side of the bed, and smooth it out over half the mattress.

   For a Flat-Bottom Sheet
   b. Fold the flat-bottom lengthwise with the center crease in the middle of bed and unfold with the rough side facing down.
   c. Position the bottom sheet so that approximately 10 inches hang over at the top and sides. The hem of the bottom sheet should be just even with the bottom edge of the mattress.
   d. Tuck in the sheet, mitering the sheet at the top corner (see Step 11).
      When using a flat bottom sheet, having extra sheet at the top helps keep it in place when the head of the bed is raised and lowered. Unfold the sheet rather than shake or fan to reduce dispersing microorganisms into the air. The sheet will not be long enough to tuck in at the bottom.

7. **Place the drawsheet** with the center fold in the middle of the mattress and unfold. Tuck the side in under the mattress, and smooth out over half of the mattress.
   Ensures that all wrinkles are out of the bottom sheet and drawsheet.▼

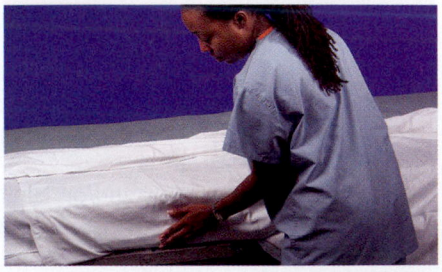

8. **Go to the other side** of the bed, straighten the linen, and finish tucking in the bottom sheet and drawsheet.
   a. Make the drawsheet tight, and smooth any wrinkles in the bottom sheet and drawsheet.

b. If desired, place a waterproof pad on or under the drawsheet.
Pulling the drawsheet tight helps prevent wrinkles from developing under the patient when she moves around in bed.

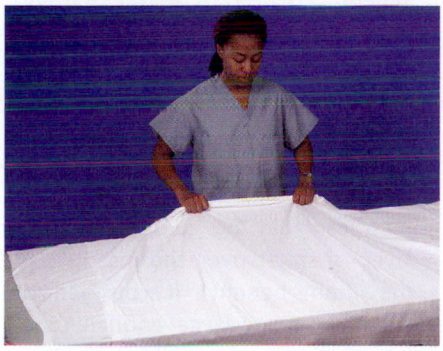

9. **Place the top sheet and** bedspread along one side of the mattress. Center the top sheet and bedspread, so that when you straighten them from the other side of the bed, they fall equally over each side of the bed.
Putting the linen on one side of the bed saves steps.

10. **At the foot of the bed**, make a small pleat in the top sheet and bedspread.
Prevents the top covers from placing pressure on the patient's toes.

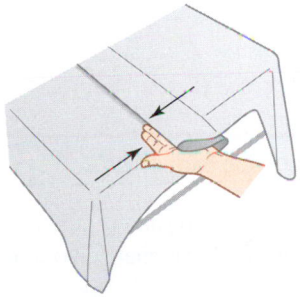

11. **Tuck in the top sheet** and bedspread at the same time, mitering the corners.
   a. Tuck in the sheet and bedspread at the bottom of the mattress.

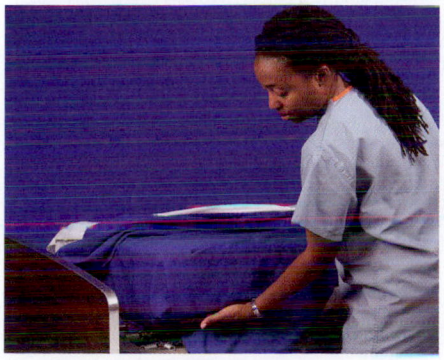

   b. Bring the edge of sheet and the bedspread up to make a right angle.

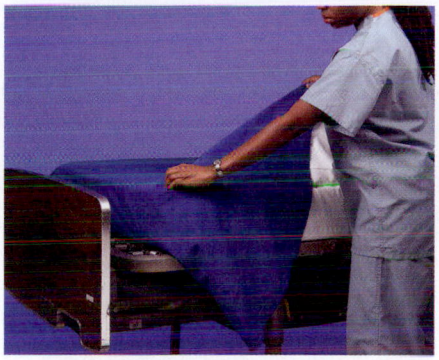

   c. Tuck the lower edge of sheet and bedspread under the mattress.

Mitered corners help secure the linen at the foot of the bed.

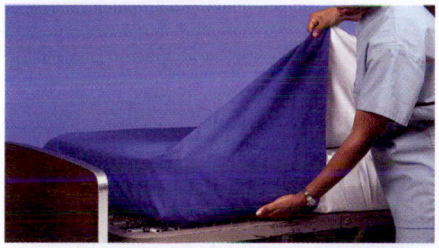

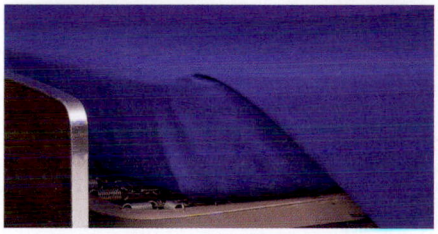

12. **Move to the other side** of the bed, smooth top linens, and repeat Step 11. At the head of the bed, fold the edge of sheet down over the bedspread.
Prevents the bedspread from rubbing against the patient's skin.

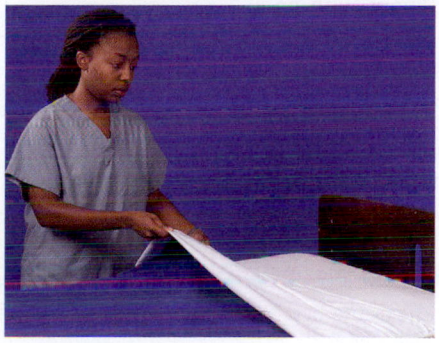

13. **Fanfold the top sheet** and bedspread back to the foot of the bed.
Makes it easier for the patient to get into bed.

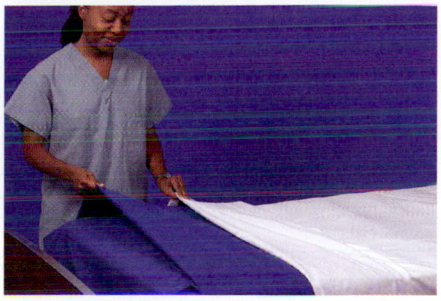

14. **Change pillowcases.**
   a. Turn the pillowcase wrong side out.
   b. Grasp the middle of the closed end of the pillowcase.
   c. Reaching through the pillowcase, grasp the end of the pillow.

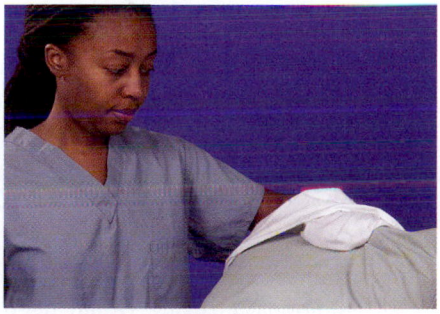

   d. Continuing to grasp the end of the pillow, pull the pillowcase down over the pillow.
Do not hold the pillow under your arm or chin to put on pillowcase because contamination can occur.

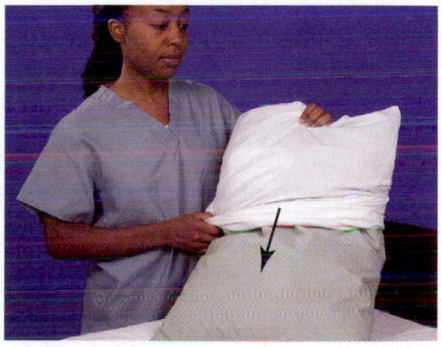

15. **Assist the patient back to bed**, return the bed to the low position, place the call signal within reach, and place the bedside table and overbed table so that they are accessible to the patient.
Provides for patient comfort and safety.

(continued on next page)

Procedure 25-13 ■ Making an Unoccupied Bed (continued)

? What if . . .

- **The linens have been contaminated by body fluids?**

  Follow recommended infection control procedures for laundering of linens (e.g., wear procedure gloves, place linen in moisture-proof bags, and so on).

- **The mattress has become contaminated by body fluids?**

  Follow agency policies for cleaning the mattress before putting on clean linens. This often involves notifying another department, such as housekeeping or environmental services, whose members are trained in this procedure.

- **The mattress cover is damaged or worn?**

  Regularly check each mattress cover for any visible signs of damage or wear such as cuts, tears, cracks, pinholes, snags, or stains. Routinely remove the mattress cover and check its inside surface for wet spots, staining, or signs of damage or wear. Check all sides and the bottom of the mattress. Remove any damaged, worn, or visibly stained medical bed mattress according to the healthcare facility's procedures and immediately replace any damaged mattress cover to reduce the risk of infection to patients.

- **The patient has a specialty bed or specialty mattress?**

  Several products are available with specific criteria to match patients' needs in terms of comfort, prevention, or treatment of pressure ulcers, and movement (e.g., specialty beds designed for bariatric patients). Follow the manufacturer's directions (e.g., a recommendation for a specific mattress may be to use only one layer of sheet over the mattress for maximum benefit). If you find the sheets are not large enough to accommodate a specialized mattress, you may need to use two flat sheets to cover it.

Home Care

The only adaptations at home depend on the type of bed the patient has. If the height of the bed is not adjustable or the bed is not accessible from both sides, the procedure may be more difficult.

Documentation

Linen changes are generally recorded on a checklist, if at all. Additional charting would need to be done only if something abnormal occurred, for example, "The drawsheet had a 20-cm circular area of serosanguineous drainage."

Practice Resources

Bloomfield, J., Pegram, A., & Jones, A. (2008); Mitchell, B., Wilson, F., McGregor, A., et al. (2012); Sergent, A. P., Slekovec, C., Pauchot, J., et al. (2012); Siegel, J., Rhinehart, E., Jackson, M., et al. (2007); U.S. Food and Drug Administration (2013).

Procedure 25-14 ■ Making an Occupied Bed

➤ For steps to follow in *all* procedures, refer to the Universal Steps for All Procedures found on the inside back cover.

Equipment

- Bottom and top sheets; drawsheet
- Pillowcase for each of the pillows
- Bath blanket (as needed)
- Linen bag or hamper
- Procedure gloves (if exposure to body fluids is possible)
- Moisture-proof gown (if heavy soiling of linens with body fluids is possible).

Delegation

You can delegate this procedure if the patient's condition and the NAP's skills permit. For example, if the patient is very ill, in pain, or requires two people for turning and repositioning, you should assist with or perform the linen change yourself.

Pre-Procedure Assessments

- Determine the patient's ability to assist with the procedure and whether additional help or assistive devices are needed.
- Make other assessments listed in Procedure 25-13.

➤ When performing the procedure, always identify your patient according to agency policy, using two identifiers, and be attentive to standard precautions, hand hygiene, patient safety and privacy, body mechanics, and documentation.

➤ *Note:* If linen change is done at the same time as the bed bath, some of these steps will vary.

Procedure Steps

1. **Prepare the environment:** Move the overbed table and other furniture, as needed, to allow access to the bed. Place the linen bag or hamper conveniently near the bed.
   To allow easy access to the bed and enable you to work efficiently, saving time and energy.

2. **Don protective gloves** and other gear if necessary.
   This observes standard precautions and reduces the risk of contaminating your clothing.

3. **Position the bed flat** if possible, and raise it to working height. Lower the siderail nearest you.
   Maintains good body mechanics and prevents back strain during the procedure. Having the head of the bed flat makes it easier to smooth the bottom sheet. To prevent the patient from falling out of bed, lower the siderails only on the side where you are standing.

4. **Disconnect the call device**, and remove the patient's personal items from the bed.
   Prevents items from getting lost.

5. **Check that no tubes** (e.g., IV, nasogastric) are entangled in the bed linens.
   Prevents dislodging tubes accidentally.

6. **If the blanket or bedspread** is clean, fold it and place it on a clean area (e.g., the back of a chair); do not place it on another patient's bed or furniture.
   Reusing the blanket and/or bedspread if it is not soiled conserves resources.

7. **Cover the patient** with a bath blanket, if available, or leave the top sheet over the patient.
   Covering the patient prevents chilling and preserves modesty.

8. **Slide the patient to the far side** of bed and place him in a side-lying position, facing the siderail. Place a pillow under his head. If needed for support, place a pillow between the patient and the siderail.
   Placing the patient close to the side rail will allow you to place the clean linen over a larger area, making it easier to roll the patient back onto the clean linen. Patients who cannot maintain the side-lying position should have a pillow placed between their chest and the siderail to prevent them from accidentally rolling into the siderail.

9. **Roll or tightly fanfold** the soiled linens toward the patient's back. Tuck the roll slightly under the patient. Cover any moist areas with a waterproof pad.
   Cover any moist areas to prevent contact with the clean linen or patient. ▼

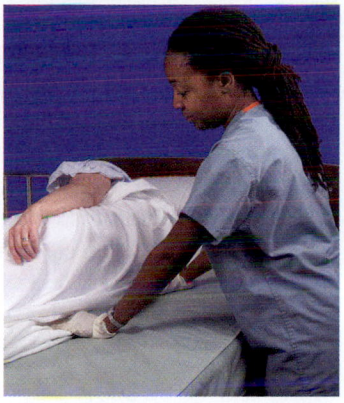

10. **Remove soiled gloves**, perform hand hygiene, and don clean gloves.

11. **Place the clean bottom sheet** and drawsheet (or pad) on the near side of the mattress, with the center vertical fold at the center of the bed. Fanfold the half of the clean linen that is to be used on the far side, folding it as close to the patient as possible and tucking it under the dirty linen. Tuck the lower edges of clean linen under the mattress. Smooth out all wrinkles.
    Wrinkles under the patient can cause skin irritation. ▼

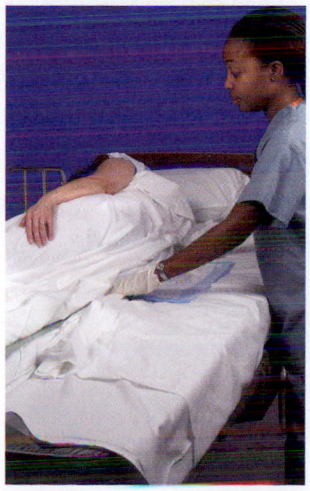

12. **Roll the patient over the clean and dirty linen**, turning him toward you. Explain to him that he will be rolling over a "lump," and then gently pull the patient toward you so that he rolls onto the clean linen. ▼

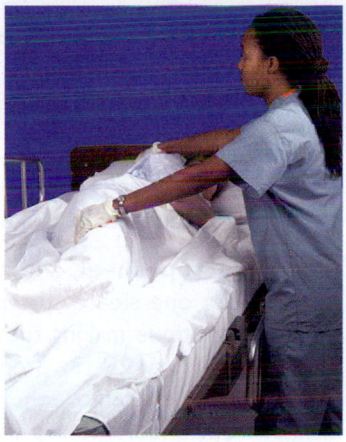

13. **Raise the siderail** on the clean side of the bed.
    Prevents the patient from falling.

14. **Move the pillows** to the clean side. Position the patient comfortably on his side, near the siderail.
    Always ensure patient comfort and safety before going to the other side of the bed.

15. **Go to the opposite side of bed**, and lower the rail. Pull the soiled linen from under the clean linen, and place it in laundry bag or hamper. Never place linen on the floor.
    Prevents cross-contamination. ▼

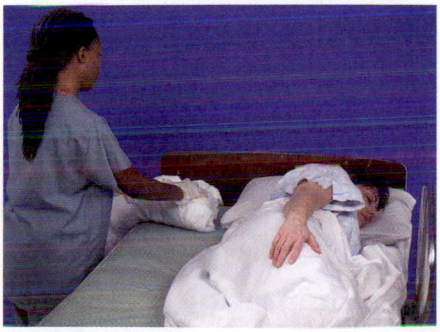

16. **Remove soiled gloves and** don clean gloves. Pull clean linens through, and tuck them in. Pull taut, starting with the middle section.
    Ensures that no wrinkles will be under the patient. ▼

(continued on next page)

Procedure 25-14 ■ Making an Occupied Bed (continued)

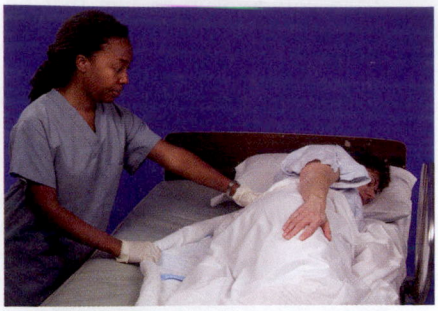

17. **Assist the patient to a supine** position close to center of the mattress.

18. **Place the top sheet** and bedspread along one side of the mattress, and continue making the bed as in Procedure 25-13, Steps 9 through 14, *except* remove the bath blanket from under the top linens before tucking them in.▼

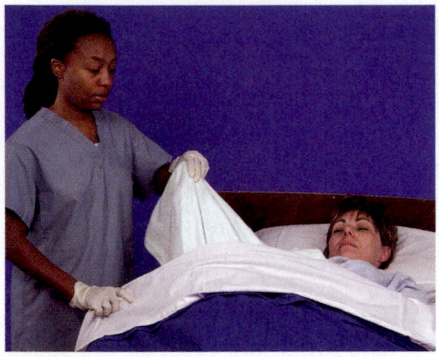

19. **Return the bed to the low** position, raise the siderails, and attach the call light within patient's reach. Position the bedside table and overbed table within patient's reach.

Ensures patient safety and comfort.

What if . . .

- **You are making the bed with a patient in leg traction?**

  It may be easier to make the bed from top to bottom, as follows:
  - Loosen all bed linens and bring the dirty linens from the top of the bed to hip area. Put the clean bottom sheet on the top corners of the mattress, bring down to hip level and tuck under the dirty linen. Cover any moist areas with a waterproof pad.
  - Ask the patient to grasp the trapeze and raise his buttocks. If the patient is unable to raise his buttocks, use an assistive device per agency policy.
  - Bring the dirty bottom sheet along with the clean bottom sheet toward the foot of the bed. Remove dirty linen and place in the laundry bag.
  - Tuck the clean sheet under the mattress. Cover with the top sheet. To accommodate traction equipment, do not tuck in the top sheet.

- **You need to move or reposition a patient in bed who is not able to assist or is obese?**

  Before making the occupied bed, assess the patient's ability to move.

  Use assistive equipment such as friction reducing devices, mechanical lifts, air powered mattresses and or lateral transfer devices.

  These are essential tools in preventing work-related injuries. You should limit the need to use your own strength while lifting, turning, or repositioning the patient in bed, because of the stress placed on the weaker muscles in the arms and shoulders.

  Follow agency policies and use of patient moving devices appropriately. *Many healthcare facilities have adopted safe lifting and patient-handling policies as a means to protect both the patient and the healthcare worker.*

Evaluation

- Assess how well the patient tolerated the procedure. Was there any discomfort, shortness of breath, and so on?
- Ask the patient whether he feels comfortable.

Home Care

The only adaptations at home depend on the type of bed the client has. If the height of the bed is not adjustable or the bed is not accessible from both sides, the procedure may be more difficult.

Documentation

Linen changes are usually recorded on a checklist. Additional charting needs to be done only if something abnormal occurred.

Practice Resources

American Nurses Association (ANA) (2013); Bloomfield, J., Pegram, A., & Jones, A. (2008); Collins, J., Nelson, A., Sublet, V. (2006); Siegel, J., Rhinehart, E., Jackson, M., et al. (2007).

Thinking About the Procedure

To practice applying clinical reasoning to this procedure,

Go to *Davis's Nursing Skills Videos*, **Making an Occupied Bed.**

For questions and suggested responses,

Go to Chapter 25, **Thinking About the Procedure Questions and Suggested Responses,** on Davis *Plus*.

Procedure 25-15 ■ Caring for Artificial Eyes

➤ For steps to follow in *all* procedures, refer to the Universal Steps for All Procedures found on the inside back cover.

Equipment

- Procedure gloves
- Normal saline solution
- Labeled container filled with saline or sterile, distilled, or filtered water
- Cotton balls

Delegation

You can delegate this procedure to the NAP if the patient's condition and the NAP's skills allow. Perform the pre-procedure assessments, and inform the NAP of any special considerations. Ask the NAP to report the patient's ability to tolerate the procedure.

Pre-Procedure Assessments

- Assess the patient's activity tolerance and whether you will need another caregiver to assist.

➤ When performing the procedure, always identify your patient according to agency policy, using two identifiers, and be attentive to standard precautions, hand hygiene, patient safety and privacy, body mechanics, and documentation.

Procedure Steps

1. **Wash hands and don gloves.**
2. **Position the patient lying down.**
   If you accidentally drop the eye when removing it, it will fall onto the bed instead of the floor.
3. **To remove the artificial eye:**
   a. Raise the upper eyelid with your nondominant hand, and depress the lower lid with your dominant hand.
   b. Apply slight pressure below the eye to release the suction holding it in place.
   c. Catch the eye in the palm of your dominant hand.
   d. Alternatively, you can use a small bulb syringe, place it directly on the eye, and squeeze to create suction and lift the eye straight up from the socket.▼

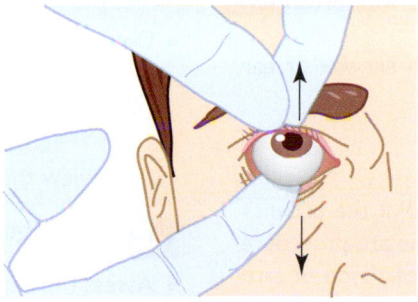

4. **Clean the eye with saline**, and store it in a labeled container filled with saline or sterile, distilled or filtered water. ✚ Do not use solvents, disinfectants, or alcohol. These chemicals may irritate the socket or damage the artificial eye.
5. **Wipe the edge of the patient's** eye socket with a moistened cotton ball, wiping from outer canthus toward the nose.
6. **Inspect the socket** for redness, swelling, or drainage.
   Irritation or infection can occur if debris has entered the socket.
7. **To reinsert the eye:**
   a. Remove the prosthetic eye from the container, but do not dry it.
   b. Hold the eye between your thumb and the index finger of your dominant hand.
   c. With your nondominant hand, pull down on the lower lid while lifting the upper lid and guide the eye into the socket.
   The prosthesis will slide into place more easily when it is wet.

Evaluation

- Observe that the eye has been placed correctly in the socket.
- Ask the patient how the eye area feels.
- Observe the eye area for redness or irritation.

Patient Teaching

- Advise the patient to periodically inspect the eye area.
- Review the importance of hand hygiene and proper handling of the eye.
- If the eye wearer experiences dryness or irritation, a lubricant made for ocular prosthetics can be used.
- If the eye needs to be wiped but not removed, wipe from outer canthus toward the nose.
  Wiping outward may dislodge the prosthesis.
- Encourage the patient to sleep in the prosthesis at night and remove it every 1 to 3 weeks for cleaning (follow prosthesis specialist's advice). Some patients do find that it is necessary to remove and clean the prosthesis every day.
  Frequent removal irritates the lining of the socket and increases the amount of discharge produced by the eye socket.
- The eye should be professionally polished every 6 to 12 months. Symptoms that may indicate the need for a polish are irritated or itchy lids, increased drainage or discomfort, or changes in the appearance of the artificial eye.

(continued on next page)

Procedure 25-15 ■ Caring for Artificial Eyes (continued)

Home Care

- In the home care setting, determine how the client usually performs eye care.
- Discuss ways to promote the safety of the artificial eye.
- Work with the client or caregiver to develop a plan of care for cleaning the eye and care of the area associated with the socket.

Documentation

Chart that the artificial eye was cleansed, the condition of the socket, care given to the area around the socket, and the patient's responses to the procedure.

Practice Resources

Erikson Labs Northwest (n.d.); Hospital Info (2008); Peters, R. (2010).

Procedure 25-16 ■ Caring for Hearing Aids

➤ For steps to follow in *all* procedures, refer to the Universal Steps for All Procedures found on the inside back cover.

Equipment

- Face cloth, dry towel
- Damp cloth
- Cotton applicators
- Wax-loop and wax brush, if available
- Pipe cleaner or toothpick, if wax-loop and wax brush unavailable
- Procedure gloves (to prevent contact with earwax or ear drainage)

Delegation

You can delegate hearing aid care to the NAP if the patient's condition and the NAP's skills allow. Perform the pre-procedure assessments, and inform the NAP of the specific type of care needed (e.g., type of hearing aid), and the amount of help the patient needs. Inform the NAP of any special considerations, such as skin irritation or usual volume setting. Ask the NAP to report the condition of the patient's ear, level of self-care, his ability to tolerate the procedure, and his ability to hear in a normal conversation.

Pre-Procedure Assessments

- Determine how much assistance the patient needs.
  Aids you in promoting independence as much as possible.
- Determine the type of hearing aid in use. The three common types of hearing aids are (1) postaural hearing aid, (2) in-the-canal hearing aid, and (3) in-the-ear hearing aid.
  The cleaning procedure varies according to the type of hearing aid.

  To review the types of hearing aids,

Go to **Figure 25-6,** in Volume 1.

- Assess the patient's ear and outer canal for redness, skin lesions, earwax buildup, or drainage.
  Identify skin problems and determine whether any symptoms of infection exist. Earwax buildup increases with age and doesn't necessarily indicate a health problem.

➤ When performing the procedure, always identify your patient according to agency policy, using two identifiers, and be attentive to standard precautions, hand hygiene, patient safety and privacy, body mechanics, and documentation.

Procedure Steps

1. **Don procedure gloves.**
   The hearing aid may contain earwax buildup or drainage.
2. **Place a towel on a nearby table** or flat surface.
   The towel helps prevent the hearing aid from breaking if it is accidentally dropped. Hearing aids are expensive.
3. **To remove the hearing aid:**
   a. Turn the hearing aid off by applying slight pressure against the volume control wheel and turning it backward (away from the nose).
   Stops the hearing aid from whistling.
   b. Rotate the earmold slightly forward (toward the nose), and gently pull it out. Do not pull on the battery door or the volume wheel.
   Pulling on the battery door or the volume wheel may damage the faceplate.
   c. Place the hearing aid on the towel.
   The towel will prevent the hearing aid from rolling off the table or banging against the table.
4. **Clean the hearing aid.**
   a. Wipe all external surfaces with a damp cloth.
   b. Clean the canal portion of the hearing aid using the wax-loop and wax brush, cotton-tipped applicator, pipe cleaner, or toothpick. Clean the top portion only. Do not insert anything into the hearing aid itself.
   Poking utensils into any part of the hearing aid except for the canal portion may damage the hearing aid.

For a Detachable Earmold

   c. Disconnect the earmold, and soak it in soapy water. Rinse and dry well, and then reattach it. Do not use alcohol. Never immerse a hearing aid in water, only the earmold.

Detaching an earmold that is glued or fastened by a small metal ring will break the hearing aid. Alcohol will damage the earmold material.

d. Check the hearing aid and any tubings for cracks and loose connections.
A damaged hearing aid will be less effective and may cause injury to the ear. Early detection of hearing aid damage may allow for repair rather than replacement of the device.

5. **Cleanse the outer ear** using the corner of a washcloth or a cotton-tipped applicator. Inspect these areas for redness, abrasions, swelling, drainage, or other irregularities.
Poorly fitting or improperly positioned hearing aids may cause trauma to the ear.

6. **Insert the hearing aid.**
   a. Check that the battery is functioning. Hold the hearing aid in your hand. Close the battery compartment door if open. Turn the power on, turn the volume high, and listen for a whistling sound.
   Whistling indicates proper power level and functioning of the battery.
   b. Set the volume control to "Off."
   Prevents whistling during insertion and a sudden, loud noise.
   c. Handle the hearing aid by the edges using your thumb and forefinger.
   Prevents whistling during insertion.
   d. Holding the hearing aid in your dominant hand, use your nondominant hand to gently pull the ear up and back.
   Opens the ear canal slightly for an easier insertion and better fit.
   e. Insert the canal portion of the hearing aid into the ear. Apply slight pressure and gently rotate the hearing aid back and forth until the canal portion rests flat in the ear.
   Allows a better fit and prevents hearing aid from falling out.

When Inserting a Postaural Hearing Aid
Insert the earmold first and then place the earmold over the ear.

When Inserting an In-the-Canal Hearing Aid
Insert with the volume control at the top. The canal should be facing away from your hand.

When Inserting an In-the-Ear Hearing Aid
Insert with the volume control at the bottom.

7. **Turn the hearing aid on** and adjust the volume by turning the volume control wheel toward the nose. Set the volume control as low as possible.
Normal setting requires a one-third to two-thirds turn of the volume control wheel. A noisier environment requires less volume, or one-fourth turn.

8. **Protect the hearing aid** from curling irons, hair dryers, and hair spray and other hair products.
Heat and moist aerosols will damage the hearing aid.

Procedure Variation: Storing the Hearing Aid

9. **Open the battery compartment** and place the hearing aid in a closed container labeled with the patient's name.
Saves battery power and allows any moisture to evaporate. Protects the hearing aid from accidental damage or loss.

10. **If the hearing aid is to be kept stored** and not worn for a week or more, remove the battery completely.
Prevents battery acid from leaking and damaging the hearing aid.

11. **Store the hearing aid** in a cool, dry place, preferably in the bedside drawer. Keep the hearing aid away from children and pets.
Moisture and heat will damage the hearing aid. Hearing aids and containers are easily lost. A child may choke on the hearing aid. Dogs and cats are attracted to the whistling noise and odor of the hearing aid and sometimes attempt to eat the device.

Procedure Variation: Replacing the Battery

12. **Use your finger** to swing the battery door open. Never force the door.

13. **Peel the tab off the new battery.**

14. **Hold the battery with the** positive (+) side up and slide it into the door, not into the hearing aid itself.

15. **Gently close the battery door.** Never force the door.

16. **Dispose of the old battery** in the regular trash.

Guidelines for Care of the Batteries

- Always dispose of old batteries. Do not throw into a fire.
  Minimizes damage from leaking battery acid and prevents mistaking fresh battery from used battery. Heat and fire may cause the battery to explode.
- Store batteries in a cool, dry place. Do not place zinc-air batteries in the refrigerator.
  Heat shortens the life of the battery. Cold batteries warming to room temperature are exposed to condensation and subsequent corrosion.
- Do not store batteries near coins or other metals.
  Contact with other metals can short-circuit the batteries.
- Do not remove the tab from the battery until the battery is ready for use.
  The tab keeps air out of the battery. Once the tab is removed, the battery is activated. Early removal decreases the life of the battery.
- Keep batteries away from children, confused adults, and pets.
  Minimizes accidental swallowing.

? What if . . .

- **The hearing aid becomes wet?**
  If the hearing aid becomes exposed to moisture, dry it as much as possible. Remove the battery and throw it

(continued on next page)

Procedure 25-16 ■ Caring for Hearing Aids (continued)

away. Keep the battery door open. Place the hearing aid in its container and allow it to dry overnight. Do not place a new battery in the hearing aid until the next morning.
Moisture will cause the battery to corrode.

- **The patient wears bilateral hearing aids?**

Be sure to identify which hearing aid is for the left ear and which hearing aid is for the right ear. Most hearing aids have a color marking for easy identification: red = right ear and blue = left ear.
Attempting to force a hearing aid into the wrong ear may cause trauma to the ear.

- **The patient continues to have hearing difficulties despite hearing aids?**

Hearing aids will not restore full hearing. General tips when communicating with a person with a hearing deficit are listed in Chapter 30, Clinical Insight 30-3: Communicating With Hearing-Impaired Clients.
Hearing aids will not block out background noise. A clear, distinct, low-pitched voice helps the client to understand what is being said.

Evaluation

- Assess how well the patient tolerated the procedure. Was there any discomfort, difficulty with insertion, and so on?
- Note the condition of the patient's skin, including pain, redness, and abnormal discharge.
- Note the condition of the hearing aid itself.
- Assess the patient's ability to hear normal speaking voices.
- Ask the patient whether he feels comfortable and hears satisfactorily.

Patient Teaching

- Discuss the importance of daily hearing aid care.
- Review any areas of care that the patient has not been performing adequately.
- Discuss any problems that need further follow-up, such as earwax build up, faulty or broken hearing aid, or ill-fitting hearing aid.

Home Care

The procedure does not vary in the home. The issues are that the nurse must:

- Work with the patient and care provider to determine supplies needed for the home.
- Determine whether further knowledge is required (e.g., if the patient must expose hearing aids to prevailing weather conditions, uses a telephone extensively, must make several adaptations from quiet to noisy environments throughout the day, and so on).
- Provide a list of available resources (e.g., AARP, National Institutes of Health, Better Hearing Institute).

Documentation

Chart that the patient is wearing a hearing aid, the condition of the ear, and the ability to hear. There will probably be a flowsheet or checklist for this information.

Practice Resources

Department of Veteran Affairs (n.d.); National Institute on Deafness and Other Communication Disorders (2007); U.S. Food and Drug Administration (2009).

CLINICAL INSIGHTS

Clinical Insight 25-1 ➤ Assisting With a Shower or Tub Bath

- Assess the patient's self-care abilities: sensorimotor, musculoskeletal, and cognitive function; activity tolerance; level of knowledge.
- Ensure that the patient has the necessary supplies (e.g., soap, washcloth, towel, clean gown, and so forth).
- Check agency policy regarding the safety of the tap water for general use in bathing patients.
- Hang a sign on the door to ensure privacy.
- Help wash and dry any areas that the patient cannot reach (e.g., feet, back).
- Avoid showering and exposure to faucet water in patients who are immunocompromised or at high risk of infection. Use prepackaged wipes instead.
- Assist the patient to the shower or bathroom as needed.
- Prevention of nosocomial infections related to the use of tubs should include stringent maintenance and cleaning according to facility policy.
- Ensure that there is a nonskid surface or mat in the shower or tub.
- For patients who have impaired mobility or activity intolerance, use a shower chair in the shower or tub.
- Be sure that the shower or tub is safe. Most hospitals and long-term care facilities have grab bars and handrails in the bathrooms.
- To avoid burns, verify water temperature for clients with impaired cognition or decreased sensory perception. Water should be 110°F to 115°F (43°C to 46°C).
- Provide a call device for the patient to obtain help if needed; point out the emergency call device if there is one in the bathroom (usually it is a red button or cord on the wall).

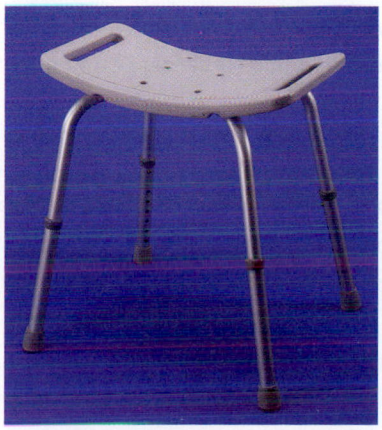

Shower chair

Home Care

- Encourage clients and families to install hand bars on the sides of the bathtub and on the wall next to the tub. Most hospitals and long-term care facilities have grab bars and handrails in the bathrooms, but these may need to be installed in the home.
- Advise parents never to leave a child alone in the tub or shower and to have a way to unlock the bathroom door from outside the room.
- Advise older adults or those who are ill not to lock the bathroom door while bathing so that help can be summoned if needed (e.g., if they become faint or fall).
- Help families to obtain benches for transferring into the bathtub, or use a plastic chair in the shower.
- Ensure that there is a nonskid surface or mat in the shower or tub.

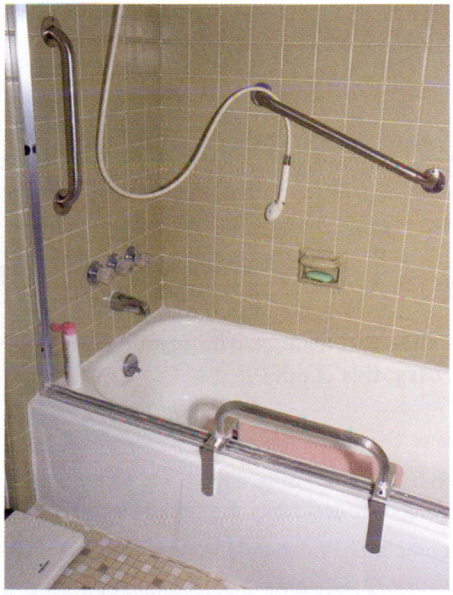

Bathtub with handrail and grab bars

Clinical Insight 25-2 ➤ Bathing a Patient With Dementia

- Focus on the patient, not the task; provide choices.
- Distract with food or by playing relaxing music.
- Use a gentler type of shower head for rinsing. *A strong spray may frighten the patient.*
- Avoid sensory overload: Turn down lights, warm the room, play soft music, speak calmly. *People with dementia have trouble processing information. Overloading the senses may trigger aggression.*
- Ensure continuity of care. *The patient can build a relationship with the caregiver and reduce fear.*
- Encourage the patient to wash her own face if able. *Makes her feel like an active participant; preserves some independence.*
- Bathe at a regular time—preferably the same time that the patient bathed at home.
- Explain the procedure simply, using short sentences.
- Provide privacy. *Patients with dementia do not necessarily lose their modesty and sense of privacy.*
- Let the patient know before you touch her or spray her with any fluids. *Sudden actions are often frightening to patients with dementia.*
- Do not rush. *The patient will feel the tension and may become agitated.*
- Be creative; try bathing one part of the body each day.
- Teach techniques to caregivers at home (e.g., being flexible with time, using a towel bath, etc.)
- Also refer to the What If . . . ? section of Procedure 25-1.

ASSESSMENT GUIDELINES AND TOOLS

Focused Assessment

Guidelines for Assessing Hygiene

Assessment of Functional Abilities

The Katz Index of Independence in Activities of Daily Living (ADL) is used extensively to assess functional abilities in activities of daily living (bathing/hygiene, dressing/grooming, feeding, toileting). To use the Katz ADL Index,

Go to Chapter 25, **Tables, Boxes, Figures: ESG Table 25-1,** on Davis *Plus* or **go directly to http://consultgerirn.org/uploads/File/trythis/try_this_2.pdf**

Observe Self-Care Abilities

When bathing, dressing, eating, and toileting, which of the following best describes the patient's ability?

- Is completely independent; requires no assistance.
- Requires a device or special equipment (e.g., a walker, a large-handle spoon).
- Requires help, supervision, or teaching from another person.
- Requires help, from another person, as well as a device or special equipment.
- Is totally dependent; does not participate in the activity (e.g., total bed bath).

The Environment

- Is the room temperature comfortable?
- Are the siderails up, when indicated? Is the bed in low position?
- Are bed wheels locked?
- Are bed linens clean and wrinkle free?
- Is the patient's call device within reach?
- Is the overbed table clean and uncluttered?
- Is the walking space uncluttered?
- Are there unpleasant odors?

Skin

Subjective Data

Patients may be sensitive about skin problems or poor hygiene practices, so direct your questions to the patient in a nonjudgmental, respectful manner. General questions to ask include the following:

- How often do you prefer to bathe?
- How do you usually care for your skin?
- What soaps, lotions, or other skin care products do you use?
- Do you have difficulty controlling body odor?
- Have you ever had an allergic skin reaction to food, medications, plants, skin care products, or other materials?
- What problems have you had with your skin in the past?
- What problems are you having with your skin now?
- For each problem identified, ask:

  What symptoms are you having (e.g., any rash or itching)?

  Where is the problem located?
- How long have you had this problem?
- What have you done to provide relief from the symptoms?
- Do you use any prescription, over-the-counter (OTC), or herbal remedies to treat this problem?
- Have you seen a healthcare provider about this problem?
- Was a diagnosis made? If so, what was it?
- How has this problem affected your life?

Focused Assessment

Guidelines for Assessing Hygiene—cont'd

- How can I best help you with your skin care?
- Also ask about the presence of diseases or other factors that are known to cause skin problems; for example, decreased mobility, decreased circulation, incontinence, inadequate nutrition, or deficient knowledge.

Objective Data

- Note the skin's overall cleanliness, condition, color, texture, turgor, hydration, and temperature.
- Observe for rashes, lumps, lesions, and cracking.
- Look for drainage from wounds or around tubes.
- Observe for four significant color changes: pallor, erythema, jaundice, and cyanosis.

Feet

Subjective Data

Ask the patient the following questions or obtain the data from his records:

- What is your normal foot care routine?
- What type of footwear do you usually wear? Observe what the patient is wearing.
- Have you had any foot problems; what treatments have you had for them?
- Do you examine your feet on a regular basis?
- Do you have diabetes mellitus or peripheral vascular disease?

Objective Data

Compare findings for both feet:

- Observe for cleanliness and skin integrity. Note open areas, drainage, or redness.
- Inspect for swelling, inflammation, or infection.
- Palpate for edema.
- Check the skin between the toes for cracks or signs of a fungal infection.
- Notice the color and temperature of the feet; are they the same bilaterally? The color and temperature provide data about circulation and oxygenation. For example, cold, dusky feet may indicate impaired circulation or tissue perfusion secondary to a peripheral vascular disease.
- Check capillary refill. How many seconds does it take for the color to return after you apply pressure?
- Note the presence of foot odors, if any.

Nails

Subjective Data

Ask about the patient's usual nail care practices, history of nail problems, and their treatments.

Objective Data

Inspect the nails for the following:

- Shape, contour, and cleanliness
- Presence of broken nails, hangnails, or cracked cuticles
- Hands: Do the fingernails appear neatly manicured, or does the patient bite the nails?
- Feet: Are the toenails trimmed appropriately, straight across?
- Presence of redness or swelling at the nail base or sides

Oral Cavity

Subjective Data

- Usual hygiene practices
- History of periodontal disease or other oral problems
- Financial or insurance problems that limit access to dental care
- Nutritional status and dietary habits (e.g., intake of refined sugars)
- Medications, such as anticonvulsants or diuretics
- Medical treatments, such as radiation therapy, oxygen therapy, and nasogastric tubes
- Other factors known to cause oral problems (smoking, alcohol use, NPO status, dehydration, mouth breathing)
- Self-care deficits (e.g., cognitive impairment, activity intolerance, impaired mobility, depression, lack of knowledge, lack of motivation)

Objective Data

- Observe the lips, which should be pink and moist without lesions.
- Inspect the oral mucosa and gums, which should also be pink, moist, smooth, and free of lesions.
- Healthy gums should have a well-defined margin at each tooth. There should be no visible bleeding.
- Instruct the patient to stick out his tongue and to move it around. It should move freely. The tongue should be symmetrical and pink, with a slightly rough surface.
- Assess the teeth for the presence of any loose, missing, or decaying teeth.
- Examine the hard and soft palates for color, lesions, patches, or petechiae.
- Note any unusual mouth odors or halitosis.

Hair

Subjective Data

- Use of special products or medicated shampoos
- History of hair problems or current conditions needing treatment (e.g., pediculosis)
- History or presence of disease or therapy that affects the hair (e.g., chemotherapy)
- Factors influencing the patient's ability to manage hair and scalp care (e.g., Impaired Mobility)
- Personal or cultural preferences for styling of the hair

Continued

Focused Assessment

Guidelines for Assessing Hygiene—cont'd

Objective Data

- Note the condition, cleanliness, texture, and oiliness of the hair.
- Inspect the scalp for dandruff, pediculosis (head lice), alopecia (hair loss), secretions, or lesions.

Eyes

Subjective Data

- If the patient wears glasses, ask when he uses them (e.g., for reading, for driving) and ask how well he sees without them.
- If the patient wears contact lenses, determine:
- The type of lens (hard, soft, long-wearing, disposable).
- How often he wears them (daily, occasionally) and for how long at a time. Are they worn during sleep?
- History of, or present, problems with lens usage (e.g., cleaning, removal).
- Usual practices for cleaning and storage.
- History of, or current, problems with the eyes (e.g., redness, tearing, irritation, dryness or "scratchy feeling").

Objective Data

- Inspect the eyes for redness, lesions, swelling, crusting, excessive tearing, or discharge.
- Check the color of the conjunctivae.

CLINICALREASONING

Applying the Full-Spectrum Nursing Model

PATIENT SITUATION

Alice Baker is a frail elderly woman, 93 years old, who lives in a nursing home. She has almost total Self-Care Deficit related to her weakness, painful joints, and dementia. Her mental and physical conditions are not likely to improve. Imagine that your charge nurse has instructed you to provide a complete bed bath and other hygiene care for Ms. Baker. When you enter her room with bath supplies and say, "Good morning, Ms. Baker; it's time for your bath," she screams, "Go away from me. I just had a bath. I don't want a bath." You discuss this with the charge nurse, who says, "She has not had a bath, and she needs one today. You will need to do it whether she likes it or not." You tend to agree that Ms. Baker needs a bath because her clothing and linens have food stains, and she smells of urine and perspiration.

THINKING

1. *Theoretical Knowledge:*
   a. What benefits does a bath have for Ms. Baker?
   b. What are the disadvantages of bathing a patient with dementia who is resisting the bath?
2. *Critical Thinking (Considering Alternatives, Deciding What to Do):*
   a. What do you think Ms. Baker is feeling and experiencing, and how does that help you know what to do?
   b. What are some alternatives to a complete bed bath that would achieve the same purposes?

DOING

3. *Practical Knowledge:* Imagine that you have, indeed, decided that Ms. Baker needs a bath. Which type bath you will give her? What supplies will you need, and where will you find them in the clinical agency you have attended most recently?

CARING

4. *Self-Knowledge:* What is your greatest concern about bathing Ms. Baker; what is the cause of your concern?

Critical Thinking and Clinical Reasoning

1. You are caring for Mrs. Little, a 57-year-old woman who has been experiencing severe arthritic pain for the past 2 years. She rates her pain at an 8 or 9 on a 10-point pain-rating scale. During your assessment, you notice that Mrs. Little has a moderate body odor, long and untrimmed fingernails and toenails, oily hair, and unshaven legs and axillae. Mrs. Little readily admits that she has neglected her hygiene practices.
   a. What is the first hygiene-related nursing diagnosis (problem and etiology) that comes to your mind for Mrs. Little?

b. What data do you have to support a diagnosis of Bathing Self-Care Deficit? What data do you have to support an etiology of "immobility secondary to pain"?
c. With the information in the scenario, how would you rate her Self-Care Deficit: mild, moderate, severe, or total?
d. Anything you could do to help relieve Mrs. Little's pain would facilitate her self-care abilities. However, to plan interventions in which you will assist with her hygiene care, what further patient data do you need?
e. Suppose you assess Mrs. Little further and determine that she has arthritis in multiple joints, including her hands, shoulders, back, knees, and feet. You also determine that she will need a complete bath, either tub or shower, but that she can brush her own teeth if someone provides the necessary supplies. Could you delegate her A.M. hygiene care to an experienced nursing assistive personnel (NAP)? If so, what instructions would you give the NAP?

2. Mr. Thomson is an 87-year-old African American man admitted 2 days ago after being found unconscious in his small apartment. Although Mr. Thomson denies being diabetic, his admission blood sugar was 653 mg/dL. His lower legs are swollen, red, and weeping a clear fluid. His toenails are long, thick, and yellow, and there is a small open sore on the great toe of his left foot. Mr. Thomson's skin is dry and scaly, his hair matted, and he has a strong odor of perspiration and urine. He is uncircumcised. He refuses help with hygiene, saying, "I've taken care of myself for 87 years, and I'll keep doing it. I take my bath once a week on Saturday evening. Now go away!"
   a. What theoretical knowledge will you need in order to know what to assess and how to provide his hygiene care?
   b. Self-knowledge is important in this case as well. What things in this situation would make caring for Mr. Thomson especially difficult for you? What biases, values, or attitudes might interfere with your ability to give your best care?
3. Recall the Meet Your Patients scenario in your textbook. The remaining critical-thinking questions refer to that scenario:

   Your instructor has assigned you to assist the following patients with their hygiene. You must assess the needs of each person, gather information on their bathing habits and preferences, plan nursing measures necessary to meet individual needs, and together with a NAP, provide care.

   The first person on your assignment is Mrs. Williams, a 76-year-old Indian American woman who was admitted yesterday after suffering a stroke that paralyzed her right side. Since the stroke, she has been unable to speak clearly and becomes frustrated as she attempts to communicate her needs. Her daughter says Mrs. Williams is a proud, independent, and tidy woman who has been living alone since her husband's death last year. She has been driving her car, cleaning the house, doing her grocery shopping, and maintaining the yard and garden. She wears eyeglasses for reading and driving and has a hearing aid, although she rarely uses it.

   The second person on your assignment is Mr. Gold, a 68-year-old man of Orthodox Jewish religion, admitted last week after he experienced a massive heart attack. Although his eyes are open, he is unresponsive to external stimuli. Because of Impaired Swallowing, Mr. Gold is unable to take food or fluid orally; his family has chosen to have a feeding tube placed to ensure adequate nutrition and hydration. His oral mucous membranes and lips are dry and crusty. He is incontinent of urine and stool. Mr. Gold's son, Ira, tells you that throughout his life Mr. Gold adhered to Orthodox Jewish law. The son requests that, in honor of his father, certain aspects of these laws be included in the care plan.

   The following questions are about Mrs. Williams:
   a. To assess Mrs. Williams' self-care abilities, what important patient data do you still need?
   b. What problem has resulted from her stroke that will make it difficult for you to find out about Mrs. Williams' hygiene preferences and practices?
   c. From what you know of the patient situation, why do you think Mrs. Williams is becoming frustrated?
   d. How do you think you would react if this were to happen to you?
   e. How could you provide opportunities for Mrs. Williams to maintain her independence?
4. The following questions are about Mr. Gold:
   a. What additional theoretical knowledge do you need to meet Mr. Gold's religious and cultural needs when providing hygiene care?
   b. Where could you obtain such information?
   c. If you decide to delegate Mr. Gold's bed bath to a NAP, how could you incorporate his religious and cultural needs into your delegation decisions?

5. For each of the following concepts, use critical thinking to describe how or why it is important to nursing, patient care, or facilitating hygiene. Note that these are *not* to be merely definitions.
Personal hygiene

Delegation of tasks
Cultural differences
Skin integrity
Life span variables
Self-Care Deficits
The nursing process
Patient teaching
Bathing
Oral care
Environment and comfort
Hair care
Nail care

What Are the Main Points in This Chapter?

- Current guidelines are changing the way nurses provide hygiene. The long-held tradition of using a basin, soap, and water to bathe hospitalized patients is no longer the recommended standard of practice.
- Recent recommendations include (1) the use of disposable, single-patient-use basins to reduce risk of bacterial contamination and (2) avoiding the use of unfiltered tap water in hospitals, unless the water lines are known to not contain biofilm. Alternatives include prepackaged bathing products and the use of sterile or distilled water or filtered water from faucets.
- Personal hygiene contributes to physical and psychological well-being by promoting comfort, improving self-image, and decreasing infection and disease.
- Although a patient may need assistance with hygiene measures, the goal is to encourage as much independence with these tasks as possible.
- Numerous factors influence individual hygiene practices, including personal preferences, cultural/religious/spiritual values and beliefs, economic status, living environment, developmental or knowledge level, and physical and emotional health.
- Maintain a respectful, nonjudgmental attitude about cultural and spiritual differences. Avoid the temptation to impose personal values about hygiene practices onto patients.
- Consider patients' personal hygiene preferences, and incorporate them into the care plan whenever possible. This reflects caring and promotes maximum participation and independence with ADLs.
- Although many hygiene measures can be delegated to the NAP, the nurse retains full responsibility for each patient and must instruct the NAP about the patient's limitations and restrictions, amount of assistance necessary, use of any assistive devices, any specific safety precautions to be undertaken, and any other factors influencing the patient's hygiene practices.
- The nurse should assess a patient's functional status regularly.
- Teaching patients about hygiene is a primary function of the professional nurse.
- Intact skin is the body's first line of defense to keep pathogenic microorganisms from entering the body and causing infection.
- Bathing removes perspiration and bacteria from the skin surface. It promotes relaxation and comfort, improves circulation, reduces odor, and enhances well-being by increasing self-image. However, it can be stressful for some patients.
- You should choose the type of bath to meet the patient's needs (e.g., assist bath, total bed bath, bag bath, and so on).
- Bathing is stressful to some patients (e.g., the frail elderly, people with dementia, the morbidly obese). You should focus on the patient's needs for warmth, safety, and comfort, and adapt the bathing procedure to help reduce stress.
- Despite common myths, it does not take a lot of water to get a person clean, and not all patients need a complete bath every day.
- A complete bath includes perineal care.
- Careful assessment of the feet allows for early detection of common foot problems, such as calluses, corns, tinea pedis, ingrown toenail, or foot odor.
- Because dirt and debris can collect under the nails and serve as a source of infection, nail care is an important part of hygiene, especially in patients with diabetes mellitus or peripheral neuropathy.
- To maintain healthy mucous membranes, teeth, and gums, and to prevent tooth loss and gum disease, regular dental checkups and daily mouth care,

including brushing and flossing the teeth, are necessary.

- For critically ill and frail elderly patients, as well as those using ventilators, special attention to oral hygiene helps to reduce the risk for pneumonia.
- Oral hygiene is challenging for patients with dementia, but it must not be neglected.
- The condition of the hair is a measure of an individual's overall health. Shampooing and daily brushing of the hair massages the scalp, stimulates the circulation, and distributes the natural oils.
- The eyes normally require very little care; however, when necessary, they may be gently cleansed from the inner to the outer canthus.
- Unconscious or critically ill patients who no longer have a blink reflex may need eye care at least every 2 to 4 hours. Keeping the eyes lubricated protects them from corneal abrasions and drying.
- Some contact lenses can be worn for only about 12 hours at a time; others may be worn for up to 30 days. Some are disposable; some are not. All types must be cleaned carefully and regularly.
- Hearing aids are expensive and should be properly handled and stored. They should not be immersed in water.
- When reinserting an artificial (prosthetic) eye, first be certain that it is wet.
- Usually no special care is required for the nose. Excess secretions can be removed by gentle blowing with both nostrils open.
- Clean, wrinkle-free bed linens help to promote comfort and a sense of well-being.
- Room temperature, adequate ventilation, low noise level, and neat and clean surroundings all contribute to a comfortable patient environment.

Knowledge Map

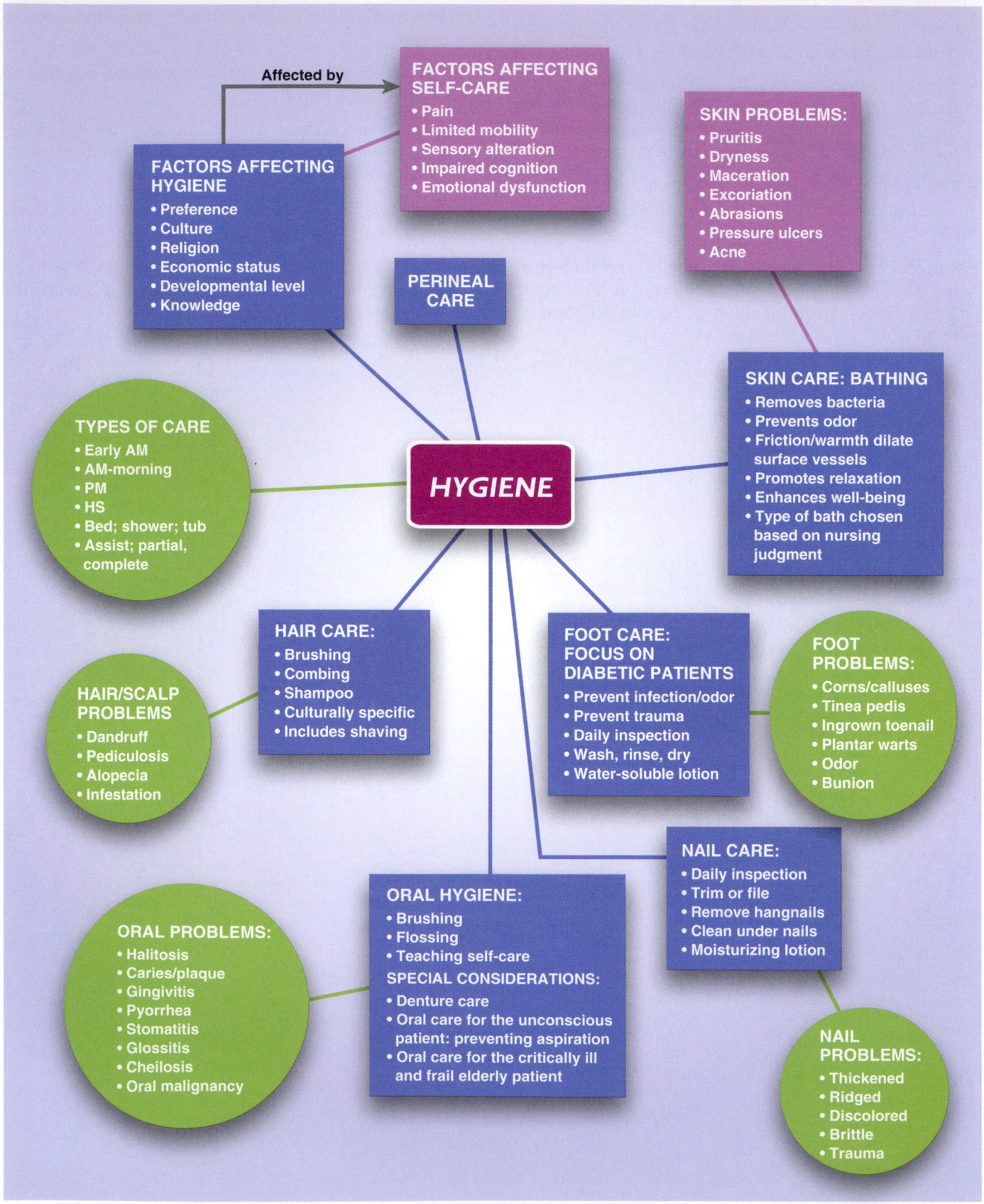

CHAPTER 26

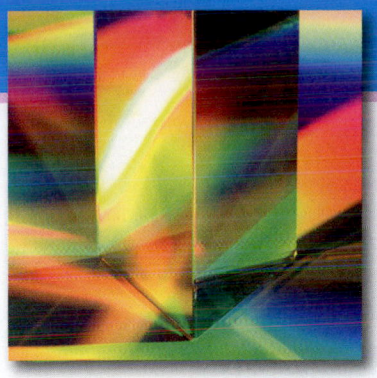

Administering Medications

STUDENT RESOURCES

*The questions and exercises in Volume 2 allow you to practice the kind of thinking you will use as a full-spectrum nurse. Critical-thinking questions usually have more than one correct answer, so we do not provide "answers" for these features. It is more important to develop your nursing judgment than to just cover content. You will learn by discussing the questions with your peers. If you are still unsure, consult your instructor. You will find Response Sheets (for writing your response to the questions) on Davis*Plus.

To explore learning resources for this chapter,

Go to Davis*Plus* at DavisPl.us/Wilkinson3.

Chapter Resources for Chapter 26:

- **Response sheets for all learning activities**
- **Resources for Caregivers and Health Professionals**
- **Reading More About Administering Medications (suggested readings)**
- **Concept Map of chapter content**

Interactive Case Studies

NCLEX-Style and Chapter Review Questions

CHAPTER OVERVIEW

For a podcast of an overview of this chapter,

Go to Student Resources, Chapter 26, **Podcast—Chapter Overview,** on Davis*Plus*.

Caring for the Nguyens

Kim Phan, the 3-year old grandson of Nam and Yen Nguyen, has been tired and observed to be sitting down a great deal at preschool. Last week, he developed coughing, wheezing, shortness of breath, nasal congestion, and extreme fatigue. The pediatrician at the Family Medicine Center diagnosed asthma. He prescribed a 5-day tapering course of prednisone, a leukotriene inhibitor (Singulair) 4 mg orally daily at bedtime, and periodic treatments with albuterol through a home nebulizer system.

Nam's mother, Mai Nguyen, became very upset when she saw the bottle of prednisone elixir. She was even more upset when she learned that Kim received an injection of the medicine in the office. She advised Yen not to give Kim the medicine because she said it causes weak bones and stunts growth. Yen has called the clinic asking for advice on how to handle this problem.

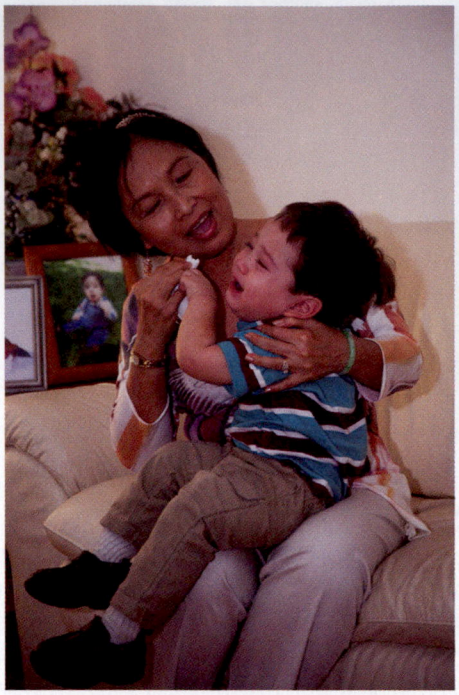

A. What theoretical knowledge do you need to answer these concerns?

B. What are some reliable sources where you might find this information?

C. What rationale could you offer to Yen to explain the safety of the prednisone prescription? You will need to use a variety of references to answer this question.

D. Yen asks you to explain why Kim received both a shot and pills. How would you respond?

E. Why is Kim receiving a leukotriene inhibitor (Singulair) orally and albuterol by nebulizer? Look up the medications, and use your knowledge of different routes of administration.

Practical Knowledge knowing how

The practical knowledge you will need to administer medications safely and effectively includes procedures and guidelines for calculating and measuring dosages and administering medications by a variety of routes.

PROCEDURES

Procedures in this section will assist you to prepare, measure, and administer various types of medications, to locate injection sites, and to handle needles safely. Use the following Medication Guidelines for all types and routes.

Medication Guidelines: ■ Steps to Follow for All Medications (Regardless of Type or Route)

➤ For steps to follow in *all* procedures, refer to the Universal Steps for All Procedures found on the inside back cover.

➤ **Key Point:** ***Regardless of the type or route of the medication you are giving, you should always follow the steps below.***

Equipment

- Medication administration record (MAR)
- Medication drawer or portable cart with, as needed, keys to the medication drawer
- Gloves for the procedure, as needed
- Other supplies and equipment needed for the specific procedure (e.g., water, antiseptic wipes)

Delegation

As a registered nurse (RN), you can usually delegate administration of medications (except for intravenous [IV] medications) to a licensed practical nurse/licensed vocational nurse (LPN/LVN). You cannot delegate this task to nursing assistive personnel (NAP). You can instruct a NAP in the therapeutic effects and side effects of medications and to report any effects observed.

Nurse practice acts governing medication administration vary from state to state, and policies vary among healthcare agencies. In some states, with additional education and training, LPN/LVNs can administer IV medications and NAPs can administer some medications. You must know the scope of practice described in your state's nurse practice act. The RN is always responsible for evaluating client responses, which include both therapeutic effects and side effects.

Pre-Procedure Assessments

- Assess your knowledge of the medication (e.g., drug action, purpose, recommended dosage, time of onset and peak action, common side effects, contraindications, drug interactions, and nursing implications).
- Determine whether the prescribed dosage is appropriate for the patient's age and weight.
  Dosages are generally decreased for children because of both age and weight. Usually dosing for elderly patients is not based on weight but on renal function. Both groups have less efficient liver and renal function, increasing the length of time a drug stays in the body before being excreted.
- Check for any history of allergies to medications or food.
  Some medications (e.g., penicillin and cephalosporin) have cross-sensitivity; that is, a patient with a penicillin allergy is at high risk for also being allergic to cephalosporin. Medications can also have cross-sensitivity with certain foods. For more information about how drugs interact with other drugs or with food,

Go to Chapter 26, **Tables, Boxes, Figures: ESG Table 26-5, Drug-Drug and Food-Drug Interactions,** on Davis*Plus*.

- At least the first time you administer medications to a patient, assess his knowledge of the medications being given.
  The patient will be more likely to take the medication correctly if she understands why she is taking the medication.
- Assess for factors that could interfere with drug absorption (e.g., diarrhea, inadequate circulation, foods, impaired liver function, edema, inflammation, age-related changes, and other medication).
- Assess vital signs and check lab studies specific to the medication to determine whether the medication can be safely administered.
  Medications are metabolized more slowly in a person with decreased liver function.
- Assess for situations in which it would not be reasonable to administer the medication (e.g., oral medications prescribed for a patient who is NPO, vomiting, swallowing difficulties, sedated).
  If the medication does not seem reasonable, question the prescriber.

➤ When performing the procedure, always identify your patient according to agency policy, using two identifiers, and be attentive to standard precautions, hand hygiene, patient safety and privacy, body mechanics, and documentation.

Procedure Steps

1. **Check the MAR** for the patient's name and identification number, medication, dose, route, time, and drug allergies. The rights of medication administration are: the right patient, right drug, right dose, right route, right time, and right documentation. At the beginning of your shift, check the MAR to determine when medications are due **(1st check)**.
   Medication prescriptions may change even during your shift; checking the MAR helps ensure that you do not miss medication changes.
2. **Verify the prescription.** It should include the patient's name, patient identifier, medication name, dose, route, time, and patient allergies.
   You must note whether it has changed (e.g., since the last time you gave the drug). Clarify any discrepancies before giving the medication.
3. **Follow agency policies** for medication administration, including the time frame. Most agencies allow medications to be given 30 minutes before or 30 minutes after the time indicated on the MAR. Do not prepour medications.
   The time of administration is important for some medications. For example, if an anti-infective agent is given early or late, a therapeutic blood level may not be maintained.
4. **Perform hand hygiene.**
   Hand hygiene minimizes transmission of microorganisms.
5. **Access the patient's medication** drawer, unlock the medication cart, or log onto the medication dispensing computer.
6. **Obtain the narcotic cabinet key** (or code), when administering a narcotic or barbiturate, and sign out the medication, including the patient's name, drug, dose, and other pertinent information per agency policy. Note the drug count when removing a narcotic.
   Federal law governs administration of controlled substances. All narcotics and barbiturates are counted and signed by an outgoing and oncoming nurse every shift.
7. **Select the prescribed medication.** Read the label and compare medication with the MAR for the first five rights (patient, drug, dose, route, time); check for drug allergies:
   - An inpatient should be wearing an identification band with the drug allergies identified.
   - Allergies should be clearly marked in the chart and on the MAR or in the electronic health record (EHR).
   - Ask the patient about allergies the first time you administer a medication and before giving a newly prescribed medication.

(continued on next page)

Medication Guidelines: ■ Steps to Follow for All Medications (Regardless of Type or Route) (continued)

These actions ensure that the correct drug is being given to the correct patient at the correct time in the correct dose by the correct route.

Key Point: ***Correct drug includes the correct form of the drug (e.g., oral, IV).***

8. **Calculate the medication dosage.** Double-check it. If you are unable to measure the dose exactly, contact the pharmacist.

9. **Check the expiration date** (on the label or on the box) of all medications.
   A medication that has expired is no longer guaranteed to be effective.

10. **Do a second check** after preparing the medications, to verify the correct patient medication, dose, route, and time **(2nd check)**.
    Verifies the first five rights of medication administration.

11. **Lock the medication cart.** Never leave an unlocked medication cart unattended.
    This guards against pilferage and protects children, older adults with dementia, or anyone wanting to open the cart.

12. **Administer the medications.**
    a. Take the medication and MAR or a hand-held portable device with the EHR into the patient's room.
    You must be able to do the final check in the patient's room and verify that you are administering the correct medication to the correct patient.
    b. Identify the patient using two forms of identification, according to agency policy: Check the identification bracelet, have the patient state her name, compare the patient to a posted picture of her, and check the patient's date of birth against the MAR.
    Agencies have different means of identifying patients. The Joint Commission requires two forms of identification.

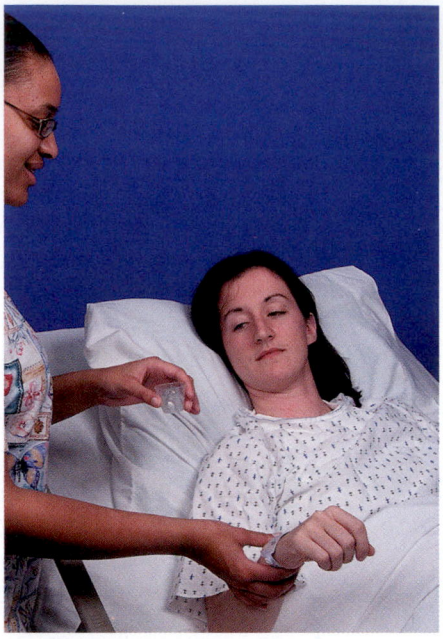

    c. Do a check of the rights of medication: right patient, right medication, right dose, right route, and right time **(3rd check)**.
    Checks for the rights of medication are always required to prevent medication errors. Although it is not actually an "error" until the patient has taken a medication, you may be required to file a report for a "near miss" that was detected during the pre-administration checking process.
    d. Perform any necessary assessments, such as checking the pulse or blood pressure.
    Some medications can be given only if physical findings or vital signs are within certain parameters. For example, antihypertensive medications may need to be held if the blood pressure is lower than the patient's normal baseline.
    e. Explain to the patient that you are there to administer the medication; teach her about the medication.
    Patient teaching increases the patient's understanding of and compliance with treatment. Also, the patient may identify potential errors in medication administration.

    ✚ If the patient questions a medication, double-check the medication to be sure you are giving the correct drug and dosage.

    f. Administer the medication using appropriate technique (see the procedures for administering medications by the specified route).
    g. Remain with the patient until you are sure that she has taken the medication.
    If you leave a medication at the bedside, someone else (e.g., another patient or a child) might take it, or the patient might discard it.
    h. Document the medication given in the patient's medication record (date, dose, route, and your name).
    Your initials on the MAR means that you administered the medication to the patient. If the documentation is not in the patient's record, there is a risk that another nurse will assume the medication was not given and administer it again.

? What if . . .

■ **The patient tells you the tablet you are ready to give him is a different color from what he normally takes of a certain prescribed medication?**

Determine why the tablet is different from what the patient is used to taking to be sure you are giving the correct drug and dose. Always verify the identity of the drug, especially when it is called into question by the patient who is familiar with the medication he normally takes.

Double-checking whenever you are uncertain about a medication you are about to administer helps prevent medication errors—it is possible you have the wrong drug or dosage.

- **The label on the medication shows an expiration date that has passed?**

  Do not give the medication. Send it back to the pharmacy for replacement.
  Expired medication can lose its potency.

- **The patient refuses to take the prescribed medication?**

  Discuss with the patient his concerns about the medication. Hold the dose and notify the prescriber of the patient's refusal and explain the patient's concerns.
  The patient has a right to refuse medication.

- **You cannot decipher the prescriber's handwritten medication order?**

  Hold the dose and contact the prescriber for clarification. Never administer medication if you are unable to read the entire order.
  Handwriting that is hard to read is a common cause of preventable error. Electronic prescribing can help to avoid this.

- **Your patient's medication is not available from the pharmacy at the time the dose is due?**

  Do not borrow the medication from another patient's supply. Administer only medication prescribed for that particular patient. Notify the pharmacy of the need to immediately dispense the medication.
  Using another patient's medication increases the risk for error because drug dilution or dosage might vary among patients; or the drug names might sound similar, but might be different medications. Also the safety system for charges and refills is bypassed when doses are borrowed from other patients, resulting in missing doses or erroneous charges.

Evaluation

- Evaluate the therapeutic effects of the medication (e.g., check blood pressure after administering an antihypertensive medication, or check pain level after an analgesic).
- Be alert for any adverse reactions, side effects, or allergic reactions. If present, notify the appropriate care provider.

Patient Teaching

- Describe how the drug is prescribed and when the patient should take the medication.
- Discuss the importance of taking the medication as prescribed.
- Explain the need for any laboratory tests for monitoring the medication, such as tests to measure drug level in the blood, if appropriate.
- Explain the purpose, common side effects, and drug interactions of the medications the patient is taking.
- Teach the patient to observe for side effects that signal the need to contact the prescriber.
- Discuss ways to minimize the side effects of a medication, such as avoiding the sun when taking a medication that causes photosensitivity or rising slowly when taking a medication that causes orthostatic hypotension.
- Discuss potential cultural issues related to taking the medication (e.g., In some Hispanic/Latino cultures, a patient may refuse a medication that is considered "hot" if he believes a "cold" treatment is needed).
- Teach the patient to self-administer medications (e.g., ear drops), as appropriate.

Home Care

- Assess the client's ability to safely self-administer medications.
- Determine the client's financial ability to obtain medications.
- Instruct the client about safe storage of medications.
- Provide instructions for use of each medication.
- Determine whether the client or caregiver has had past problems or present concerns about taking the medications as prescribed.
- If problems have occurred in the past or there are present concerns, discuss possible remedies. For example, you might teach the client or caregiver to use a medication storage container with compartments for the times and days of the week.

Documentation

- Chart the medication, time, dose, and route given, preadministration assessments, and your signature.
- Do not document before giving the drug; do not document for anyone else; do not ask another nurse to document a drug you have given. Document only *after* administering the medication.
- Chart all therapeutic and adverse effects of the medication. Chart your nursing interventions and teaching of potential adverse effects.
- Record the scheduled medications on the MAR. Record prn medications in the nursing notes and on the MAR, including the reason the medication was given and the patient's response to the medication.
- If the patient is unable or refuses to take the medication, document on the MAR that the medication was not administered and the reason, and inform the physician.
- For parenteral medications, chart the site of injection.

(continued on next page)

Medication Guidelines: ■ Steps to Follow for All Medications (Regardless of Type or Route) (continued)

Sample EHR documentation

t, I Room: Code Status: Alerts:
Sex:F Age:47 Y Diet:ADA Diet High Fiber, Lo...
Drug Allergies: Codeine
Food Allergies: Shellfish
Primary Physician:
Env Allergies: Iodine
Isolation: HELP ?

Pt Sel | Logged In: Hiam, Judith | Documenting In Current Date/Time | Log Off

Patient Charting | Vital Signs | Order Entry | Order Review | Patient Teaching | Patient CARD | Patient Data | M.A.R. | Care Plans | Reports

Select a View...
Show All | Scheduled | Show PRNs | Show Infusions

Scheduled Medications... (Click on Appropriate time to Chart Medication Action...)

Betamethasone Otic Drops AD 0.1% 1-2gtts BID Routine	08:00 Given @ 16:08	16:00 Given @ 16:07
Insulin, Humulin R SubQ Per SS Units Q4H PER SS Routine	07:00 Given BG: 162 @ 20:41	11:00
	16:00	21:00

PRN Medications... (Click on Medication Name to Chart Medication Action...)

Tylenol Suppository SUPP 650 MG Routine	Given @ 20:07	Given @ 20:08

Infusions... (Click on Medication Name to Chart Medication Action...)

Dextrose 5% in Water (D5W) 100 mL/hr Routine

Practice Resources

Institute for Safe Medication Practices (n.d.); The Joint Commission (n.d.); U.S. Food and Drug Administration (2012, updated 2013).

Thinking About the Procedure

To practice applying clinical reasoning to this procedure,

Go to *Davis's Nursing Skills Videos*, **Medication Guidelines.**

For suggested questions and responses,

Go to Chapter 26, **Thinking About the Procedure Questions and Suggested Responses,** on Davis*Plus*.

Procedure 26-1 ■ Administering Oral Medication

➤ For steps to follow in *all* procedures, refer to the Universal Steps for All Procedures found on the inside back cover. Also refer to Medication Guidelines: Steps to Follow for All Medications (Regardless of Type or Route).

Equipment

- Desired liquid for swallowing medications
- Disposable medication cup
- Drinking straw, if needed
- Procedure gloves, if you will need to place a tablet in the patient's mouth
- For enteral medications:
  –Water (for diluting and flushing the feeding tube)
  –60-mL catheter-tip syringe
  –Clean gloves
- Stethoscope *(e.g., to check the apical pulse before administering some cardiac medications)*

Delegation

- As a rule, you can delegate this skill to an LPN/LVN, depending on the medication, but not to a NAP, except under special policies and situations.

Pre-Procedure Assessments

- Assess the patient's condition to determine whether there are contraindications to oral medications or to the specific medication; for example, the ability to swallow.
  Impaired swallowing increases the risk for aspiration.

- Check fluid needs and restrictions. If the patient is NPO (nothing by mouth), check with the prescriber to determine whether the medication should be given by another route or can be given with small sips of water.
  A prescriber may decide it is medically necessary to administer oral medication to a patient who is NPO. If there is a fluid restriction, you need to consider how much fluid you can give with medication. Give additional fluid to a patient with dehydration; offer only sips for the patient with a fluid restriction.
- For enteral medications, check that the NG tube is in the stomach and is patent.

➤ When performing the procedure, always identify your patient according to agency policy, using two identifiers, and be attentive to standard precautions, hand hygiene, patient safety and privacy, body mechanics, and documentation.

Procedure Steps

1. Prepare the medication for administration.

For Tablet or Capsule

a. If you are pouring from a multidose container, do not touch the medication. Pour the tablet into the cap of the container, then into the medication cup.

b. If the medication is unit-dose, do not open the package. Place the entire unit-dose package into the cup.

c. Many institutions allow combining all tablets or oral caplets scheduled for the same time for the same patient into the same cup. However, even if the agency protocol permits dispensing from a single container, you will need separate cups for medications that require pre-administration assessment (e.g., checking the apical pulse rate prior to administering digoxin).
If a medication is held because of a pre-administration assessment finding, you can identify it more readily when it has been poured into a separate cup.

d. You may break scored tablets with a knife or a tablet cutter if necessary.
Only scored tablets may be broken. Breaking an unscored tablet would deliver an imprecise dose.

e. If a patient has difficulty swallowing, check to see whether the medication can be crushed. If so, use a mortar and pestle to grind it. If the medication is in a unit-dose package, grind it while it is still inside the package. Mix the ground medication with a small amount of soft food, such as applesauce or pudding.
Crushing some medications (e.g., capsules, enteric-coated tablets, and sustained-release formulas) may alter their effectiveness or result in an overdose due to rapid absorption.

For Liquid Medications

f. Check to see whether you must shake the liquid before opening the container.
Some liquids, such as suspensions, will precipitate and need to be shaken to mix the active ingredient with the suspension liquid.

g. Remove the bottle cap, and place it flat side down on the cart or counter.

h. Hold the bottle with the label in the palm of your hand.
Keeping the label on the upward side of the bottle prevents the liquid from dripping down onto the label and obscuring it. ▼

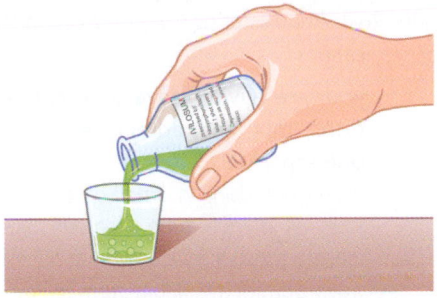

i. Hold or place the plastic medication cup at eye level, and pour the desired amount of medication. Read the dosage where the lowest part of the concave surface (meniscus) of the fluid is on the line. You can, instead, place the cup on a level surface, pour the medication, then hold the cup at eye level to read the amount.
Measuring liquids above or below eye level will cause you to read the dose incorrectly and pour too much or too little medication.

j. As you finish pouring medication, slightly twist the bottle to prevent the medication from dripping down the lip of the bottle. If medication does drip down over the lip, wipe the outside of the lip with a tissue or paper towel.
Wiping the outside of the bottle helps prevent contamination, particularly for thicker solutions, such as elixirs or syrups containing sugar.

2. Administer the medication.

a. Assist the patient to a high-Fowler's position, if possible.
An upright position facilitates swallowing and prevents choking.

b. ***Powder:*** Mix with liquid at the bedside, and give the mixture to the patient to drink.
Some powders thicken very quickly and must be mixed immediately before administration.

c. ***Lozenge:*** Instruct the patient not to chew or swallow it whole.
Medication is absorbed through the oral mucosa and is generally inactivated by the acidity in the stomach.

d. ***Tablet or capsule:***

1) If the patient is able to hold the medication in her hand, place the tablet or medication cup in her hand.
Promotes independence and is easier for the patient.

2) Give the patient water or other liquid.
Giving the medication with liquid moistens the mouth and helps the patient swallow the tablet or capsule.

3) If the patient is unable to hold the tablet, don procedure gloves and place the medication cup up to her lips, and tip

(continued on next page)

Procedure 26-1 ■ Administering Oral Medication (continued)

the tablet or capsule into her mouth.
Encourage the patient to do as much as possible. Getting the tablet or capsule to the back of the mouth will assist in swallowing.

e. ***Sublingual medications:*** Have the patient place the tablet under the tongue and hold it there until it is completely dissolved.
Sublingual medications are made to be rapidly absorbed through the oral mucosa. The area under the tongue is very vascular, so sublingual medications act very rapidly. Sublingual medications are inactivated by gastric acid if swallowed. ➤

f. ***Buccal medications:*** Have the patient place the tablet between the cheek and gums.
Buccal medications act by being absorbed through the oral mucosa or by being dissolved and swallowed in the saliva. ➤

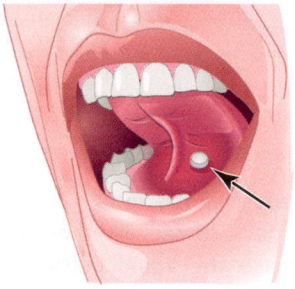

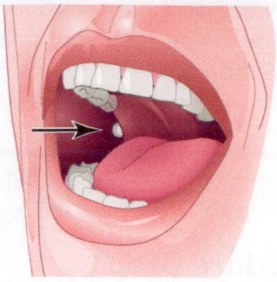

3. **Stay with the patient until** all medications have been swallowed or dissolved.
Some patients will "chipmunk" the medication in the side of the mouth without swallowing it, or spit it out. Staying at the bedside until the patient swallows oral medication ensures that the patient receives the dose.

Procedure 26-1A ■ Administering Medication Through an Enteral Tube

➤ For steps to follow in *all* procedures, refer to the Universal Steps for All Procedures found on the inside back cover. Also refer to Medication Guidelines: Steps to Follow for All Medications (Regardless of Type or Route).

- **If the patient is receiving a continuous tube feeding,** disconnect it before giving the medications. Leave the tube clamped for a few minutes after administering, according to agency protocol.
- **If the enteral tube is connected to suction,** you will usually discontinue the suction for 20 to 30 minutes after administration, and keep the tube clamped, to allow time for the drug to be absorbed.

➤ When performing the procedure, always identify your patient according to agency policy, using two identifiers, and be attentive to standard precautions, hand hygiene, patient safety and privacy, body mechanics, and documentation.

➤ *Note:* Follow Steps 1a through 1j of Procedure 26-1: Administering Oral Medication, then follow Steps 1 through 10, following. Also, follow precautions for administering enteral medications.

1. **Prepare the medication.**
   a. Give the liquid form of medication, if possible. If the solution is hypertonic, dilute with 10 to 30 mL of sterile water before instilling through a feeding tube.
   Hyperosmolar substances administered too rapidly into the gut can cause bloating, nausea, and osmotic diarrhea.
   b. If tablets or capsules must be given, verify that the medication can be crushed and given through an enteral tube.
   Some tablets (e.g., sustained-release or enteric-coated tablets) should not be crushed or capsules opened because doing so changes their action.
   c. Crush the tablet and mix it with approximately 20 mL of water or obtain a liquid medication. If you are giving several medications, mix and administer each one separately.
   If you are using a small-bore tube, such as a PEG tube, Keofeed NG feeding tube, or jejunostomy tube, always obtain the liquid form of the medication, because small-bore tubes clog easily. Ensure that the medication is diluted enough to pass easily through the tube. Instilling drugs one at a time allows you to identify each medication.
2. **Don nonsterile procedure gloves.**
Gloving maintains standard precautions.
3. **Place patient in a sitting (high-Fowler's) position,** if possible.
An upright position reduces the risk for aspiration and choking.
4. **For NG tubes, check tube** placement (see Chapter 27, Clinical Insight 27-7) by aspirating stomach contents or measuring the pH of the aspirate, if possible. Other, less accurate methods, are injecting air into the feeding tube and auscultating, or asking the patient to speak.

   Never rely on only one bedside method for checking tube placement; use a combination of methods.

   NG tubes can become displaced or positioned in the lungs. If medications are given through a misplaced NG tube, the patient may develop aspiration pneumonia.
5. **Check for residual volume** (see Chapter 27, Procedure 27-3).

6. **Flush the tube.** Based on the type of tube, use a piston tip or luer-lock syringe (usually a 30- to 60-mL syringe). Remove the bulb or plunger; attach the barrel to the tube; and pour in 20 to 30 mL of water.
Flushing ensures patency of the tube and also clears the tube of feeding solution that could clump with medication.

7. **Instill the medication** by using the barrel of the syringe as a funnel and allowing it to flow based on gravity. ▼

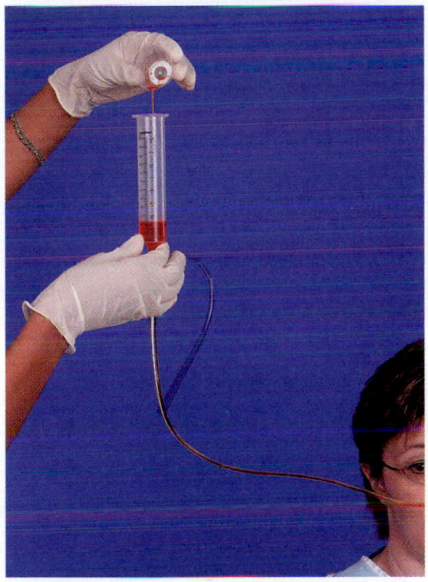

For Viscous Medication
Instill the medication by depressing the syringe plunger.

8. **Flush the medication through** the tube by instilling an additional 20 to 30 mL of water.
Flushing ensures that all the medication has been administered and prevents the tube from clogging.

9. **If there is more than one** medication, give each separately, flushing after each.
Some medications are less effective when given in combination, or there may be an additive effect if they have similar actions.

10. **Have the patient maintain a** sitting position for at least 30 minutes after you administer the medication.
An upright position minimizes the risk of aspiration. It takes at least 20 minutes for liquids to pass through the stomach.

? What if . . .

- **My patient is an older adult who is to receive medication through an enteral tube?**

Check level of consciousness, mentation, or alertness. Check for potential aspiration risk by checking the patient's swallow and gag reflexes.

- **My patient is a child who is to receive medication through an enteral tube?**

Use only medications that are prepared in liquid form.

Prevents occlusion of the tube.

Position an infant in a prone, side-lying, sitting, or reverse Trendelenburg position for 30 minutes to 1 hour following medication administration.
This position facilitates peristalsis and transport of medication through the intestine.

- **The prescribed medication should be given on an empty stomach?**

If the medication should be taken on an empty stomach, stop the feeding 30 minutes before giving the drug. Resume 30 minutes later.
These times allow for medication absorption to occur before the feedings resume.

Evaluation

For medications administered orally:

- Note whether the patient has difficulty swallowing, gags, or coughs while swallowing oral medication.
- Evaluate for gastric discomfort, nausea, vomiting, or diarrhea.
- Assess for signs of drug allergy or intolerance to the medication.

For medications administered through a feeding tube:

- In addition to the preceding assessments, assess that the NG tube is correctly placed and patent before and after administering the medication.

Patient Teaching

- Refer to Medication Guidelines: Steps to Follow for All Medication (Regardless of Type or Route).
- Discuss drug safety measures with the patient, including use of child-safety caps (or using an easy-open cap for an elderly population or with those likely to have difficulty opening containers of this type); keeping the medication in its original container; discarding expired medications; avoiding transferring medication to another container; and carefully reading the label and directions for each medication.
- Discuss the relationship between food and the medication, if needed. For example, is the medication to be taken with food or not? Does taking medication on an empty stomach contribute to nausea or gastric irritation? Does the medication interact with any foods? For more information about how drugs interact with food,

Go to Chapter 26, **Tables, Boxes, Figures: ESG Table 26-5, Drug-Drug and Food-Drug Interactions,** on Davis*Plus*.

For Enteral Medications

Cover the preceding topics for patient teaching about oral medications, plus the following:

- Discuss the importance of upright positioning for 20 to 30 minutes after taking medication through an enteral tube.
- Instruct the patient to immediately notify his healthcare provider if he chokes or has difficulty breathing during or shortly after medication is given by enteral tube. He should stop the medication immediately, and emergency care might be necessary.

(continued on next page)

Procedure 26-1 ■ Administering Oral Medication (continued)

Home Care

Advise clients who are receiving enteral medication at home to do the following:

- Notify the healthcare provider: (1) if any of the following lasts for more than a day: diarrhea, constipation, nausea, dark urine, bad-smelling urine, or dry mouth; (2) if the tube becomes clogged or seems to be moving farther out or in; or (3) if the feeding tube falls out or you cannot confirm that the end of the tube is in the stomach.
- To prevent a clogged feeding tube, flush the tube with water each time after giving a medication or a feeding.
- Brush your teeth at least twice daily, if an NG tube remains in place continuously.
- Clean daily the area where the NG tube goes into the nostrils. Use a cotton-tip applicator moistened with warm water. If your nose is sore, you might apply water-soluble lubricant.
- Change the nasal tape every other day or when it is loose or soiled.

Documentation

- Scheduled medications are often recorded only on the MAR.
- Document the drug, dosage, time, route, and your name as the healthcare provider administering the medication.
- Document any suspected drug reaction, intolerance, or patient response to the medication.
- For patients whose intake and output are being measured, document the amount of liquid medication and the water used for swallowing medication. Some patients may be on fluid restrictions, so record *all* intake. Follow your clinical facility protocol.

For Enteral Medications

Document the following:

- Patency, residual volume, and verification of placement.
- Any difficulty with administering the medications through the feeding tube.
- On the intake and output record, record the amount of liquid medication and the water used for flushing. Some providers order a specific amount of water to flush with each medication administration or feeding. Some healthcare facilities use a protocol amount of water to flush gastrostomy tubes. Follow the protocol in your clinical facility.

Sample documentation for a PRN oral medication:

mm/dd/yyyy 1800 *Placed client in Fowler's position. Administered Lasix 20 mg. PO tablet with 30 mL water. Patient tolerated medication with no swallowing difficulties.*
S. Smith, RN

Sample documentation for an enteral medication:

mm/dd/yyyy 1400 *Placed client in Fowler's position. GT placement confirmed with pH of 4.5 using gastric aspirate. Administered 10 mL of liquid medication and flushed with 20 mL of water. Tolerated medication with no complaints.*
S. Smith, RN

? What if . . .

- **My patient vomits shortly after taking oral medication?**
  Notify the prescriber for instructions about whether or not to repeat the dose.
- **My patient is unable to sit upright to take oral medication?**
  Assist the patient into a side-lying position and offer a straw to take water with capsules or tablets.
- **My patient has difficulty drinking from a cup?**
  Use a syringe without a needle to place the medication in his mouth. Place the patient in a side-lying or upright position. Place the syringe between the gum and cheek in the back corner of the mouth, and slowly push the plunger to administer the liquid.
- **My patient is NPO (nothing by mouth)?**
  Check with the prescriber to determine whether the medication should be given by another route or can be given with small sips of water.
- **My patient is on fluid restriction?**
  Use the smallest amount of water needed to swallow or dissolve tablets and to flush enteral tubes.
- **My patient is cognitively impaired?**
  Request the patient to open his mouth to see whether he has swallowed the medication; look under the tongue or side pocket near the inside of the cheek.

Thinking About the Procedure

To practice applying clinical reasoning to this procedure,

Go to the following *Davis's Nursing Skills Videos:*

Administering Oral Medications: Tablet or Capsule
Administering Oral Medications: Sublingual
Administering Oral Medications: Buccal
Administering Oral Medications: Liquid Medications

For questions and suggested responses,

Go to Chapter 26, **Thinking About the Procedure Questions and Suggested Responses,** on Davis*Plus*.

Practice Resources

Kelly, J., Eggleton, A., & Wright, D. (2011); Morris, H. (2012); Phillips, N., & Nay, R. (2008).

Procedure 26-2 ■ Administering Ophthalmic Medication

➤ For steps to follow in *all* procedures, refer to the Universal Steps for All Procedures found on the inside back cover. Also refer to the Medication Guidelines: Steps to Follow for All Medications (Regardless of Type or Route).

Equipment

- Eye drops or ointment
- Tissue

For irrigation, add:

- Prescribed eye irrigation solution (e.g., 500 to 1,000 mL of normal saline or lactated Ringer's solution are commonly used)
- IV tubing or eye irrigation insert, such as the Morgan lens (Follow manufacturer's directions for this specialized equipment.)
- Ocular anesthetic, according to protocol or provider's orders
- pH paper
- Basin and towel

Delegation

An RN can usually delegate eye instillations to an LPN/LVN. You usually cannot delegate this task to a NAP, unless the NAP has special training for a specific, defined situation (e.g., "medication aides" in some long-term-care settings). See Delegation, in Medication Guidelines: Steps to Follow for All Medication (Regardless of Type or Route).

Pre-Procedure Assessments

- Assess the patient's eyes for redness, discharge, or other signs of irritation.
- Determine whether the eyes need to be cleansed before administration of the medication.
  Excess tearing, debris, or excess mucus in the eye could interfere with the absorption, and thus effectiveness, of the medication.

Check the prescription for where to instill medication (*Note:* We do not advise using these abbreviations—they have been disallowed by The Joint Commission—but you may still see them written in prescriptions).

OD = right eye OS = left eye OU = both eyes

For irrigations also assess the following:

- Determine the cause of the eye problem—acid, alkaline, or other chemical burn or body fluid splash; or non-embedded foreign body.
  Irrigations are generally used to remove chemical or physical irritants, but they may be done following surgery or to treat a severe infection. Normal saline (NS) or lactated Ringer's is the solution generally recommended for high-volume eye irrigations because the pH of 6 to 7.5 is closest to the normal tear pH of 7.1. Volumes of 500 to 1,000 mL are generally used.
- Assess the patient's eyes for swelling, redness, drainage, or complaints of pain.
  A baseline assessment is useful for determining the need for and effectiveness of irrigation. Sclera should be smooth, white, and glistening.
- Determine the patient's level of discomfort and ability to cooperate with the procedure.
  Combative or otherwise uncooperative patients refusing instillation of medication can interfere with the efficiency of the procedure. If the patient cannot hold still for the procedure, he may need to be sedated.
- Assess the pain level.
  Debris, chemicals, and some liquids in the eye can be extremely painful. The eye may need to be anesthetized before irrigation or a general systemic pain medication given.

➤ When performing the procedure, always identify your patient according to agency policy, using two identifiers, and be attentive to standard precautions, hand hygiene, patient safety and privacy, body mechanics, and documentation.

(continued on next page)

Procedure 26-2 ■ Administering Ophthalmic Medication (continued)

Procedure Steps

1. **Assist the patient to a** high-Fowler's position with head slightly tilted back, if possible.

Do not tilt the head back if the patient has a neck injury or other contraindication. The medication can be given with the patient supine.

An upright position keeps eye drops in the eye and helps prevent eye drops from draining into lacrimal duct.

2. **Don procedure gloves.**
Gloving complies with standard precautions.

3. **Cleanse the edges of the eyelid** from the inner to outer canthus, if needed.
By following the principle of "clean to dirty," you avoid transferring debris into the nasolacrimal duct.

Procedure Variation: Instilling Eye Drops

(Follow Steps 1–3. Note, however, that some sources recommend that the patient lie supine for eye drops.)

4. **Gently rest your dominant** hand (the one with the eyedropper) on the patient's forehead.
Stabilizes the hand in the event the patient moves—prevents accidental injury to the eye.

5. **With your nondominant hand,** pull the lower lid down to expose the conjunctival sac.
Allows visualization of the area where you will administer the medication.

6. **Position the eyedropper** about 1.5 to 2.0 cm (½ to ¾ in.) above the patient's eye. Ask the patient to look up, and drop the prescribed number of drops into the conjunctival sac. Do not let the dropper touch the eye.
Keeping the dropper away from the globe of the eye reduces the risk of accidental injury to the eye and avoids contamination of the dropper. Having the patient look up helps to decrease the blink reflex.

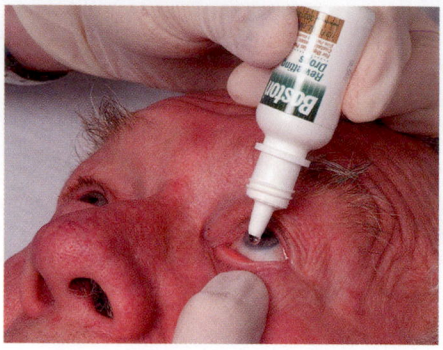

7. **Ask the patient to gently close** his eyes.
Closing the eyes helps to distribute the medication.

8. **If the medication has systemic** effects, press gently against the same side of the nose for 1 to 2 minutes to close the lacrimal ducts.
Reduces systemic absorption through the lacrimal duct.

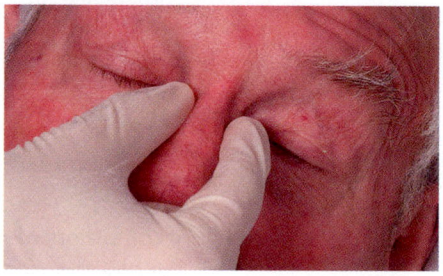

Procedure Variation: Administering Eye Ointment

(Follow Steps 1–3, then move to Step 9.)

9. **Gently rest your dominant** hand, the one with the eye ointment, on the patient's forehead.
Stabilizing your hand helps to prevent accidental injury to the eye.

10. **With your nondominant hand,** pull the lower lid down to expose the conjunctival sac.
Allows visualization of area where you will administer the medication.

11. **Ask the patient to look up** as you apply a thin strip of ointment—usually about 2 to 2.5 cm (1 in.)—in the conjunctival sac; twist your wrist to break off the strip of ointment. Do not let the tube touch the eye.
If the medication ribbon is not broken off, lifting the tube will pull the medication out of the conjunctival sac.

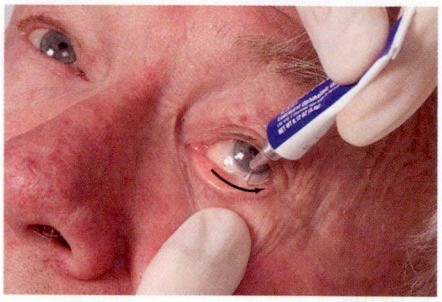

a. Ask the patient to gently close his eyes for 2 to 3 minutes. Alternatively, release the eyelids and have the client blink several times.
Helps to distribute the medication.

b. Explain to the patient that his vision will be blurred for a short amount of time after administration of the ointment.
The viscosity of the ointment can cause blurring.

What if . . .

- **My patient is a child who won't open his eye for the application?**

  Try distracting the child by turning on the television or offering an age-appropriate toy in view.
  Distraction and bribery are effective techniques for coaxing a child when cooperation is essential.

  Ask a family member to help you gain cooperation of the child.
  It might be fear or mistrust that is causing him to be unwilling to open his eyes.

- **My patient wears soft contact lenses?**

  Have the patient remove contact lenses before administering the medication and wait at least 15 minutes after instilling eye drops before reinserting the lenses.

Procedure 26-2A ■ Irrigating the Eyes

➤ When performing the procedure, always identify your patient according to agency policy, using two identifiers, and be attentive to standard precautions, hand hygiene, patient safety and privacy, body mechanics, and documentation.

Procedure Steps

1. **Assist the patient to a low-Fowler's position, with the head tilted toward the affected eye, if possible.**
   This position helps to drain the irrigating solution from the eye and prevents contamination of the unaffected eye.

2. **Place the towel and basin** under the patient's cheek to absorb the drainage.
   The patient will be more comfortable when he is clean and dry.

3. **Check the pH** by gently touching the pH paper to secretions in the conjunctival sac.
   A litmus test determines the correct irrigating solution and whether the irritant is alkaline or acidic. The normal pH of tears is approximately 7.1.

4. **Follow the agency protocol** or prescriber's order regarding use of ocular anesthetic drops.
   The ocular anesthetic will be washed out by the irrigation fluid, so it needs to be reinstilled every 2 to 3 minutes, or it can be added to the irrigation solution.

5. **Connect the solution and** tubing, and prime the tubing.
   Priming the tubing prevents blowing air across the cornea, which would be uncomfortable.

6. **Irrigate the eye.**
   a. Hold the tubing about 2.5 cm (1 in.) from eye.
   A safe distance helps prevent accidental trauma to the eye.
   b. Separate the eyelids with your thumb and index finger.
   It is easier to irrigate the cornea when the eyelids are separated.
   c. Direct the flow of solution over the eye from the inner canthus to the outer canthus.
   The inner canthus is considered clean, primarily because of the open duct in this area. Flowing irrigation solution in this manner follows the principle of "clean to dirty." ▼

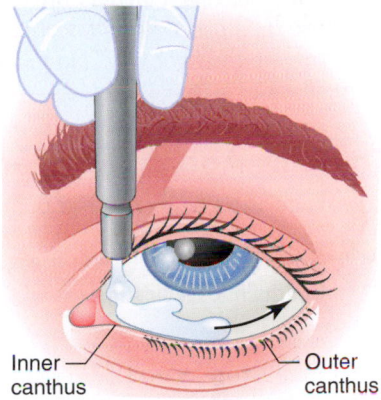

7. **Recheck pH, and continue** to irrigate the eye as needed.
   With alkaline or acidic chemical injuries, the pH of the eye needs to be returned to normal as soon as possible to prevent further eye injury.

Evaluation

- Examine the eyes for redness or drainage.
- Observe the patient's ability to follow instructions during the procedure.
- Observe the pain level during the procedure.
- After an irrigation, check for decrease in eye pain.

Patient Teaching

- Discuss how to prevent contaminating eye drops or ointment.
- Teach the best technique for instilling eye drops or ointment.
- Discuss the use of an eye drop guide, if the patient needs assistance with instilling drops.
- Discuss the signs and symptoms to report to the provider, including eye pain and increased redness or drainage.

For irrigations:

- Discuss the cause and prevention of eye injuries, including use of protective goggles.
- Discuss the need for follow-up treatment. If the patient will be instilling eye medications or applying eye patches, ensure that he demonstrates the correct technique.

Home Care

If a splash occurs to the eyes in the home, teach the client to immediately flood his eyes with cool water (as follows):

- Hold your eyelids open and put your head under a faucet or pour water from a clean container.
- Roll your eyes as much as possible while running water across your eyes.
- Flood your eyes for at least 20 minutes.
- Get medical help immediately after rinsing your eyes.

Documentation

- *For instillations:* Chart assessment data before, during, and after instillation. Record on the MAR, as for all medications.
- *For irrigations:* Chart the condition of the patient's eyes before the irrigation, including complaints of pain or burning. Document the eye pH, instillation of anesthetic drops, the type and amount of irrigation fluid used, the eye pH following irrigation, and the patient's response. Also record other treatment (e.g., instillation of lubricating and/or antibiotic ointment; application of eye patches).

(continued on next page)

Procedure 26-2 ■ Administering Ophthalmic Medication (continued)

Sample documentation

08/22/2016 1200. In preparation for discharge and after teaching, patient correctly self-administered Garamycin eye drops 1 gtt in right eye as prescribed. Patient closed her eyes and gently pressed against the right side of the nose for 1 minute after instillation. Stated, "I will not have a problem doing this at home. Thank you for teaching me the right way." No redness, discharge, or complaints of pain. ——— *S. Smith, RN*

For questions and suggested responses,

Go to Chapter 26, **Thinking About the Procedure Questions and Suggested Responses,** on Davis*Plus*.

Practice Resources

Centers for Disease Control and Prevention (CDC) (2010b); Glaucoma Research Foundation (2012); Heller, J. L. (2011, updated); Mason, I., & Stevens, S. (2010); Terrie, Y. (2012).

Thinking About the Procedure

To practice applying clinical reasoning to this procedure,

Go to *Davis's Nursing Skills Videos*, **Administering Ophthalmic Medication.**

Procedure 26-3 ■ Administering Otic Medication

➤ For steps to follow in *all* procedures, refer to the Universal Steps for All Procedures found on the inside back cover. Also refer to the Medication Guidelines: Steps to Follow for All Medications (Regardless of Type or Route).

Equipment

- Ear drops
- Dropper with flexible rubber tip
- Cotton-tipped applicators
- Cotton ball

Delegation

The RN can usually delegate administration of otic medications to an LPN/LVN. You usually cannot delegate this task to a NAP, unless allowed by the state's nurse practice act.

Pre-Procedure Assessments

- Assess the external ear and canal for erythema, drainage, and cerumen.
  You may need to clean the external ear to remove obstructions so that the medication can be distributed throughout the ear canal. Use the otoscope to evaluate the tympanic membrane if the drainage is bloody or the patient complains of pain or decreased hearing acuity. Use sterile technique if the tympanic membrane is ruptured.
- Assess for any ear pain or hearing impairment.
  Establishes a baseline that can be used to evaluate the effects of treatment.

➤ When performing the procedure, always identify your patient according to agency policy, using two identifiers, and be attentive to standard precautions, hand hygiene, patient safety and privacy, body mechanics, and documentation.

Procedure Steps

1. **Hold the ear drop bottle** in your hand to warm it, or place it in warm water (not hot). Gently shake the bottle before using the drops.
   Warm solution is more comfortable than cool. Also, placing cool solutions in the ear can cause dizziness. Gently shaking the bottle disperses the medication throughout the solution.
2. **Assist patient to a side-lying** position (or turn her head to the side), with the appropriate ear facing up.
   Facilitates administering the drops and prevents drops escaping from the ear.
3. **Clean the external ear** with a cotton-tipped applicator, if necessary.
   Cleaning the ear allows ear drops to reach all areas of the ear canal without trauma. Be careful not to push cerumen further into the ear canal.
4. **Fill the dropper** with the correct amount of medication.
5. **For infants and young children,** ask a parent or another caregiver to immobilize the child while you administer the medication.
   Mobilization and restraint reduce the risk for injury for the child who struggles during the procedure.
6. **Straighten the ear canal.**
   a. For a child younger than 3 years old, pull the pinna down and back. ▼

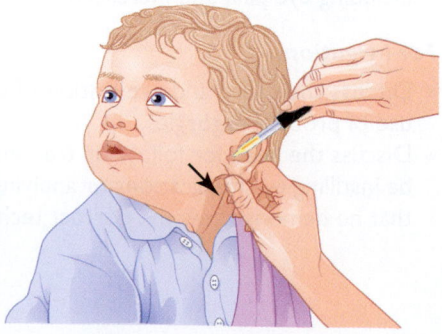

b. For children 3 years and older and adults, pull the pinna up and back.

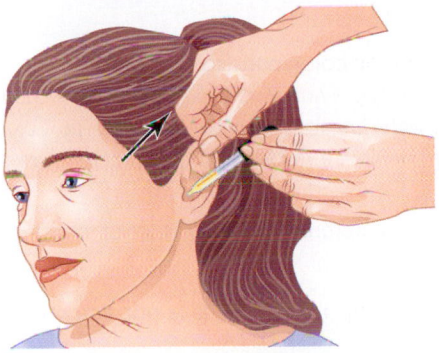

These positions straighten the ear canal for proper channeling of the medication.

7. **Instill the ordered number** of drops along the side of the ear canal, being careful not to touch the end of the dropper to any part of the ear.
   Avoiding contact between the dropper and the ear reduces the risk of contamination of the dropper.

8. **Gently tug on the external ear** after drops are instilled.
   Facilitates flow of medication into the auditory canal.

9. **Instruct the patient** to keep her head turned to the side for 5 to 10 minutes.
   Assists in distributing the medication and prevents drops from escaping the ear canal.

10. **Place a cotton ball**, or a piece of it, loosely at the opening of the auditory canal for 15 minutes.
    A cotton ball will absorb excess fluid and keep the medication from flowing out.

Keep in mind that cotton left near an infant can be a choking hazard and must be carefully supervised.

What if . . .

- **My patient is a child and rolls over so most of the otic medication flows back out of the ear?**

  Estimate the amount of the dosage that was lost. Replace it by repeating the procedure for instillation of the medication, except next time position the child securely until you are confident the medication has had time to penetrate the ear canal.

- **There is too much cerumen (ear wax) in the canal to instill otic drops?**

You can use special drops for softening the cerumen and allow for easier removal. Gentle irrigation with warm saline is effective, unless the patient has perforation of the tympanic membrane or myringotomy tubes.

You should not use a metal syringe (Pomeroy syringe) for the removal of cerumen because (1) this type of syringe is heavy and difficult to control and (2) may be associated with a higher risk of perforations of the tympanic membrane because of the pressure exerted.

Oral jet irrigators have been associated with some trauma, including tympanic membrane perforation.

You should not attempt to remove impaction by "ear candling," which is the application of hot candle wax.

Evaluation

- Assess for discomfort or pain during the procedure and for relief afterward.
- Evaluate for wax buildup, redness, swelling, or drainage.

Documentation

- Assess the amount, color, character, and odor of drainage, if present.
- Note any swelling or redness in the ear canal.
- Document pain or discomfort and hearing loss.

Thinking About the Procedure

To practice applying clinical reasoning to this procedure,

Go to *Davis's Nursing Skills Videos*, **Administering Otic Medication.**

For suggested questions and responses,

Go to Chapter 26, **Thinking About the Procedure Questions and Suggested Responses,** on Davis*Plus*.

Procedure 26-4 ■ Administering Nasal Medication

➤ For steps to follow in *all* procedures, refer to the Universal Steps for All Procedures found on the inside back cover. Also refer to the Medication Guidelines: Steps to Follow for All Medications (Regardless of Type or Route).

Equipment

- Medication drops, spray, or aerosol
- Tissues

Delegation

As an RN, you can usually delegate administration of nasal instillations to an LPN/LVN. You usually cannot delegate this task to a NAP.

Pre-Procedure Assessments

- Check for nasal obstruction and congestion.
  Nasal obstruction or congestion can prevent the medication from reaching the nasal mucosa.
- Assess nasal discharge for color, consistency, and odor.
  The appearance of drainage is not always diagnostic of infection, especially for people with chronic sinus problems or polyps. Color can be indicative of the body's response to viral, bacterial, and allergic sources.
- *Assess nasal mucous membranes for redness, color, moisture, excoriation, or trauma.*
- Check the dropper tip to be sure it is not cracked or chipped.
  A cracked or chipped tip might interfere with drawing up the medication and scratch the nasal mucosa.

➤ When performing the procedure, always identify your patient according to agency policy, using two identifiers, and be attentive to standard precautions, hand hygiene, patient safety and privacy, body mechanics, and documentation.

Procedure Steps

1. **Explain to the patient** that the medication may cause some burning, tingling, or unusual taste.
   The taste of nasal medications can cause patients to become nauseated or vomit. The medication is more likely to cause burning or tingling if the nasal mucosa is inflamed.
2. **Ask the patient to gently blow** his nose and wash his hands afterward.
   Removing nasal discharge allows the medication to come into contact with the mucous membranes without traumatizing already inflamed mucosa.
3. **Don procedure gloves.**
   Prevents transmission of microorganisms.
4. **Position the patient.**

When Medicating the Frontal Sinuses With Spray

"Head down and forward." Remember: "To spray your nose, look at your toes!" If the patient can comfortably assume this position, ask him to lean forward or kneel on the bed with his head down. Administer the medication, and then ask the patient to tilt his head back to medicate the nasal passages.

Radionuclide studies have demonstrated that using nasal drops or sprays with the patient sitting and leaning the head back causes poor distribution of the medications into the nasal complex and sinuses. ▼

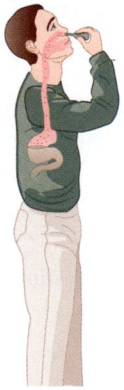

Wrong position

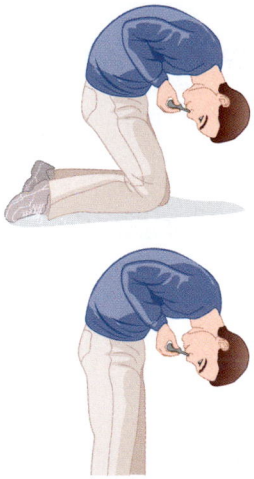

Correct positions

When Medicating the Ethmoid and Sphenoid Sinuses

Assist the patient into a supine position, tilt head back with his head over the edge of the bed. Support the patient's head. Alternatively, place a towel roll behind the patient's shoulders, and allow the head to drop back.

These positions help to prevent straining of the neck muscles and facilitate distribution of the medication to the ethmoid and sphenoid sinuses. ▼

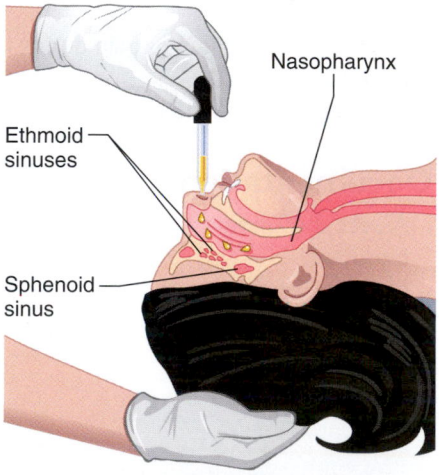

When Medicating the Frontal and Maxillary Sinuses With Drops

With patient supine, tilt the head back over the edge of the bed or place a pillow under the head and turn toward the affected side.

Titling the head promotes gravity to distribute the medication to the frontal sinuses.

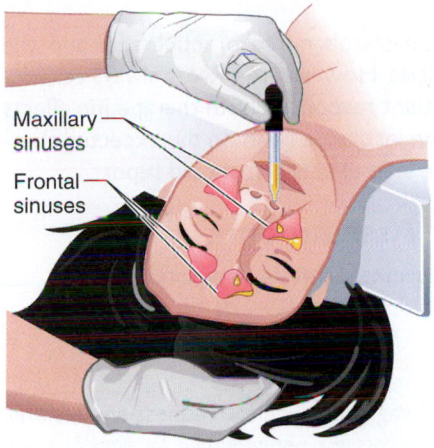

5. **Ask the patient to exhale** and then close one nostril.
   Blocking one nostril provides for deeper inhalation.

6. **Then ask the patient to breathe in** deeply through the nose and while he is breathing in, press down firmly and quickly once on the applicator. Ask patient to breathe out through the mouth. After spray, lean head backward for a few seconds. If a dropper is used, do not touch the sides of the nostril.
   Inhaling through the mouth prevents aspiration of the drops into the trachea and bronchi. Touching the dropper to the nostril will contaminate the dropper.

7. **Repeat for the other nostril.**

8. **If nose drops are used,** ask the patient to stay in the same position for 1 to 5 minutes (depending on the manufacturer's guidelines).
   Maintaining this position promotes better absorption by using gravity to disperse the medication throughout the nasal passages and sinuses instead of draining out the nose.

9. **Instruct the patient not to blow** his nose for several minutes.
   To prevent expelling the medication.

? What if . . .

- **My patient cannot assume the "head down and forward" position?**
  Help him to hold his head upright to administer the drops or spray.
- **My patient can taste the medicine after it is administered?**
  That means his head was not down enough or he did not inhale long enough. Instruct him to put his head back down and sniff again without the medicine.
- **My patient has an excoriated area on the inside septum?**
  Assess further, examining other areas of the nasal mucosa. Determine if the patient has a history of substance abuse or frequent nasal inhalations. Report the findings to the prescriber before administering nasal medication.
- **My patient begins to have nosebleeds after using nasal medication?**
  First, control the nosebleed. Then hold the medication and notify the prescriber. Assess for other signs of bleeding, bruising, or other petechiae.

Evaluation

Assess for a reduction of symptoms 15 to 20 minutes after administration.

Patient Teaching

- Teach the procedure for administering nasal drops or sprays, including proper positioning.
- Discuss the correct use of the medication and the adverse effects of overusing nasal decongestants.
- Explain the implications of the color of nasal secretions.

Documentation

Chart according to Medication Guidelines: Steps to Follow for All Medication (Regardless of Type or Route). For example, record the administration of the medication on the MAR.

For nasal instillation, document:

- Pre-medication assessment
- Type and amount of solution administered
- Discomfort the patient experienced during the procedure
- Patient's report of response to nasal administrations, such as nasal discharge, obstruction of nasal passage, bleeding, or other complication following the procedure

Sample documentation

mm/dd/yyyy 1340 *Client complained of nasal stuffiness. Administered mometasone (Nasonex) 2 sprays per nostril as ordered. Client noted nasal tingling following administration of this medication. Client left resting in recliner chair.* — H. Peralta, RN

Thinking About the Procedure

To practice applying clinical reasoning to this procedure,

Go to *Davis's Nursing Skills Videos*, **Administering Nasal Medication.**

For questions and suggested responses,

Go to Chapter 26, **Thinking About the Procedure Questions and Suggested Responses,** on Davis*Plus*.

Practice Resources

American Academy of Family Physicians (2004, updated 2011); CDC (2011a).

Procedure 26-5 ■ Administering Vaginal Medication

➤ For steps to follow in *all* procedures, refer to the Universal Steps for All Procedures found on the inside back cover. Also refer to the Medication Guidelines: Steps to Follow for All Medications (Regardless of Type or Route).

Equipment

- Medication: foam, jelly, cream, suppository, douche, or irrigating solution
- Applicator (if indicated)
- Perineal wash solution or wipes for perineal care as needed
- Water-soluble lubricant
- Toilet tissue
- Perineal pad
- Bath blanket
- **For irrigation:** you will also need a waterproof pad, bedpan, vaginal irrigation set (consists of a solution container, nozzle, tubing, and clamp; may be disposable) and IV pole.

Delegation

An RN can usually delegate the administration of vaginal medications to an LPN/LVN. Delegation of this task to a NAP will vary depending on the state's nurse practice acts and the healthcare facility policies. However, the RN is always responsible for evaluating patient responses, both therapeutic effects and side effects. You can instruct a NAP on the expected therapeutic effects and the side effects she should report.

Pre-Procedure Assessments

- Assess for vaginal burning, pruritus, and pain.
  A baseline assessment helps to determine the patient's level of comfort and later the effectiveness of treatment. Infections can cause vaginal burning, itching, and pain.
- Inspect the labia and vaginal orifice for redness and lesions.
  This is a good time to assess the perineal area for signs of sexually transmitted infection or other findings requiring healthcare.
- Check for vaginal discharge, including color, amount, consistency, and odor

➤ When performing the procedure, always identify your patient according to agency policy, using two identifiers, and be attentive to standard precautions, hand hygiene, patient safety and privacy, body mechanics, and documentation.

Procedure Steps

1. **Ask the patient to void** before you insert the vaginal medication.
   The increased pressure associated with a full bladder could cause discomfort during the instillation of vaginal medications.

2. **Position the patient** in a dorsal recumbent or Sims' position; drape the patient with a bath blanket so that only the perineum is exposed.
   a. **Dorsal recumbent position**—supine with knees flexed and legs rotated outward.
   b. **Sims' position**—semiprone on the left side with the right hip and knee flexed.
   These two positions allow for visualization during administration and promote retention of the medication following administration. Draping respects the patient's modesty.

3. **Prepare the medication.** Remove the wrapper from the suppository and place the suppository on the wrapper or in a medication cup; or fill the applicator according to the manufacturer's instructions. For irrigation, use a warm solution of approximately 105°F (40.5°C).
   Some suppositories come with applicators. Using a warm irrigation solution promotes patient comfort and prevents injury to the vaginal tissue. ▼

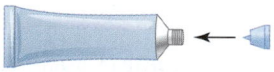

Invert cap and pierce end of medication tube

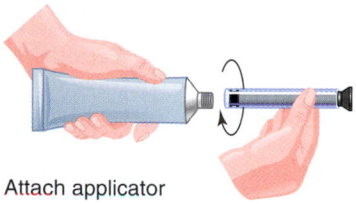

Attach applicator

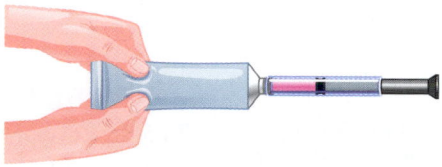

Squeeze medication into applicator

4. **Don procedure gloves.**
   Prevents contaminating your hands and spreading microorganisms.

5. **Inspect and clean around vaginal orifice.**
   Prevents the introduction of microorganisms into the vagina during medication administration.

6. **Administer the medication.**

   For a Suppository
   a. Apply water-soluble lubricant to the rounded end of the suppository and to your gloved index finger on your dominant hand.
   Eases insertion and prevents injury to the vaginal tissue.
   b. Separate the labia with your nondominant hand.
   Allows visualization of the vaginal orifice.
   c. Insert the suppository as far as possible along the posterior vaginal wall (about 8 cm, or 3 in.) or as far as it will go. If the suppository comes with an applicator, place the suppository in the end of the applicator, insert the applicator into the vagina, and press the plunger.
   The posterior vaginal wall is about 2.5 cm (1 in.) longer than the anterior wall. ▼

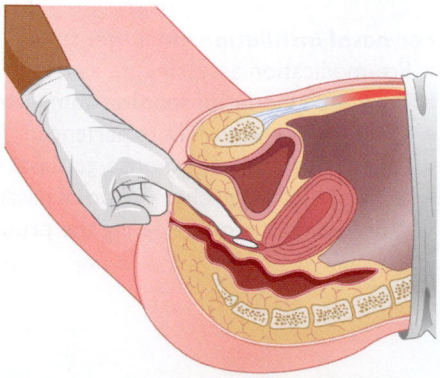

d. Ask the patient to remain in a supine position for 5 to 15 minutes. You may wish to elevate her hips on a pillow.
Lifting the hips promotes retention and absorption of the medication.

For Applicator Insertion of Cream, Foam, or Jelly

e. Separate the labia with your nondominant hand.
f. Insert the applicator approximately 8 cm (3 in.) into the vagina along the posterior vaginal wall.
g. Depress the plunger on the applicator, inserting the medication into the vagina.
h. Dispose of the applicator, or place it on a paper towel if the applicator is reusable. You will later wash it in the appropriate solution.
i. Instruct the patient to remain in a supine position for 5 to 15 minutes.
A flat position promotes retention and absorption of the medication.

For Irrigations

j. Hang the irrigation solution approximately 30 to 60 cm (1 to 2 ft) above the level of the patient's vagina.
Uses gravity to create enough pressure for continuous irrigation without increasing the pressure so much that it causes the patient discomfort and possibly damages the vaginal tissue.

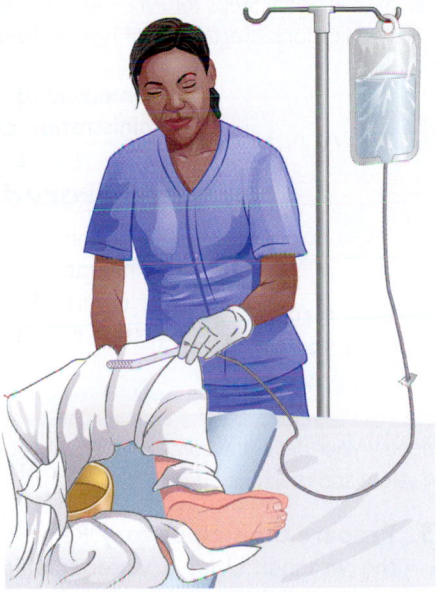

k. Assist the patient into a dorsal recumbent position, and position a waterproof pad and bedpan under the patient.
Positioning the patient on the bedpan and using a waterproof pad protects the bedding.
l. If using a vaginal irrigation set with tubing, open the clamp to allow the solution to completely fill the tubing.
Flushing the tubing prevents introducing air into the vagina, which can cause discomfort.
m. Lubricate the end of the irrigation nozzle.
Lubrication reduces discomfort and irritation to the vaginal mucosa.
n. Insert the nozzle approximately 8 cm (3 in.) into the vagina, directing it toward the sacrum.
o. Start the flow of the irrigation solution, and rotate the nozzle intermittently as solution flows.
The rotation ensures even distribution of the solution throughout the vagina.
p. After all irrigating solution has been used, remove the nozzle.
q. Assist the patient to a sitting position on the bedpan.
Promotes removal of all the irrigating solution by gravity.

7. **Remove the bedpan and clean** the perineum with perineal wash solution and a washcloth or wipes. Dry the perineum.
Drainage could cause skin irritation.

8. **Apply a perineal pad** if necessary for excessive drainage.

? What if . . .

- **The labia are reddened?**
Pour warm water (bottled or specially filtered tap water) over the labia with an irrigation bottle to soothe irritation and cleanse the area.

Evaluation

- Assess for complaints of vaginal burning, pruritis, or pain.
- Assess for purulent vaginal discharge.

Patient Teaching

- Discuss with the patient personal hygiene and pericare.
- Teach women that douching is not necessary for ordinary female hygiene and that it may even be harmful because it disturbs the normal pH and healthy balance of microorganisms in the vagina.

Documentation

- **For vaginal medications**, chart according to Medication Guidelines: Steps to Follow for All Medication (Regardless of Type or Route).
- **For vaginal irrigations**, chart assessment; the type and amount of solution administered; discomfort the patient experienced during the procedure; and the patient's report of decreased vaginal pain, itching, and/or burning following the procedure.

Sample documentation

mm/dd/yyyy 1500 Explained medication and procedure. Client placed in dorsal recumbent position with knees flexed at 90° angle. Vaginal suppository lubricated with water-soluble lubricant and inserted using two fingers. Instructed client to retain suppository as long as possible. Tolerated procedure well with no voiced complaints of pain or discomfort.
S. Snider, RN

Procedure 26-6 ■ Inserting a Rectal Suppository

➤ For steps to follow in *all* procedures, refer to the Universal Steps for All Procedures found on the inside back cover. Also refer to the Medication Guidelines: Steps to Follow for All Medications (Regardless of Type or Route).

Equipment

- Suppository
- Water-soluble lubricant
- Toilet tissue

Delegation

An RN can usually delegate administration of rectal medications to an LPN/LVN. Although in some institutions, you can delegate the administration of a glycerine suppository (nonmedicated) to a NAP, you generally cannot delegate administration of rectal medications to a NAP.

Pre-Procedure Assessments

- Determine the presence of contraindications for rectal administration, such as recent rectal surgery, rectal bleeding, or cardiac disease.
- Assess the rectal area for hemorrhoids or irritation.

➤ When performing the procedure, always identify your patient according to agency policy, using two identifiers, and be attentive to standard precautions, hand hygiene, patient safety and privacy, body mechanics, and documentation.

Procedure Steps

1. **Ask whether the patient needs** to defecate before the suppository insertion.
   Stool in the rectum interferes with insertion of medication against the rectal wall and therefore with retention of the medication.

2. **Assist patient to Sims' position**—lying on the left side with the right hip and knee flexed. Drape the patient, keeping her covered as much as possible.
   Sims' position allows visualization of the anus and promotes retention of the medication because the descending colon is on the left side. It also helps relax the external anal sphincter. Keeping the patient covered prevents chilling and maintains privacy.

3. **Don procedure gloves.**
   Gloving prevents exposure to feces and spread of microorganisms; maintains standard precautions.

4. **For an uncooperative patient,** such as a confused patient or a young child, ask someone to help immobilize the patient while you insert the suppository.
   Help holding the patient allows proper instillation of medication and prevents injury to the rectal mucosa.

5. **Prepare the suppository**: Remove the wrapper. Using a water-soluble lubricant, lubricate the smooth end of the suppository and the tip of glove on the index finger. If no lubricant is available, apply cool tap water to the rectal opening.
   Lubrication eases insertion and prevents friction damage to the rectal mucosa during insertion.

6. **Explain that there will be a cool** feeling from the lubricant and a feeling of pressure during insertion.
   The patient should not experience severe pain with the insertion of a suppository, but will feel the coolness of the lubricant and pressure as the suppository is inserted past the rectal sphincter.

7. **Using your nondominant hand,** separate the buttocks.
   Separation of the buttocks allows you to visualize the anus.

8. **Ask the adult patient to take deep** breaths in and out through the mouth.
   Deep breathing helps relax the rectal sphincter. Pushing a suppository through a constricted sphincter produces discomfort.

9. **Insert the suppository**:
   a. Using the index finger of your dominant hand, gently insert the lubricated smooth end first, or follow the manufacturer's instructions.
   Lubrication eases insertion. ▼

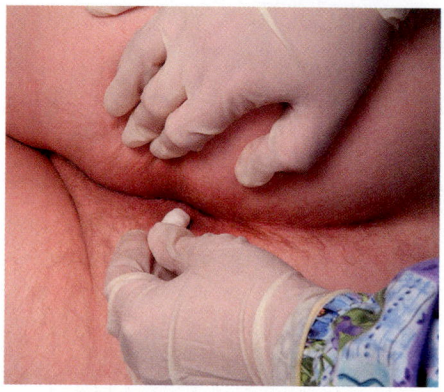

   b. ✚ Never force the suppository during insertion.
   Forcing the insertion of the suppository into a fecal mass would affect absorption. Forcing anything into the rectum may cause rectal irritation.

   c. Push the suppository past the internal sphincter and along the rectal wall (½ to 1 in. in infants and 1 to 3 in. in adults).
   The suppository must be in contact with the rectal wall for the medication to be absorbed. Inserting the suppository past the internal sphincter promotes retention. For a child,

inserting the suppository too far could damage the rectal mucosa.

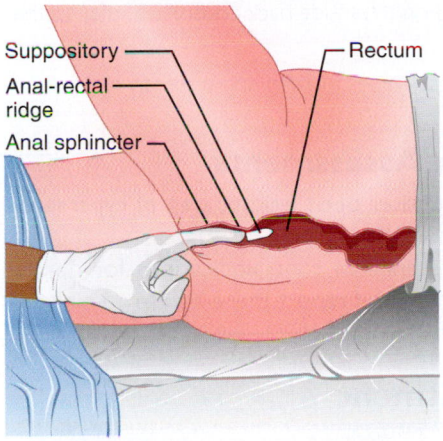

10. **Ask the patient to try to retain** the suppository if he is able. If he has difficulty retaining the suppository, hold his buttocks together for a short time.

11. **Wipe the patient's anus** with toilet tissue.
Wiping maintains hygiene and comfort.

12. **Explain to the patient need** to remain in the side-lying position for 5 to 10 minutes.
Sims' position promotes retention and absorption of the medication. Explanation promotes compliance.

13. **Discard used materials** into a biohazard receptacle and wash hands thoroughly.

14. **Leave the call device within** reach and bedpan handy, if the suppository was a laxative.
In case the patient has a sudden urge to defecate or cannot retain the suppository for the recommended time.

? What if . . .

- **The prescribed dose is only half of the suppository?**
  Cut the suppository lengthwise with a clean, single-edge razor blade.
- **My patient is a child. What is the best way to give a rectal suppository so the child doesn't expel it?**
  For pediatric patients, it may be necessary to gently hold the buttocks together for 5 to 10 minutes.
- **My patient is an older adult? Is there anything special I should know?**
  Older adults may have difficulty retaining a suppository because of poor sphincter control. You may need to put the bedpan under the patient while you are inserting the suppository.

Evaluation

- Assess for pain or burning during and after insertion of the medication.
- Determine that the patient retained the suppository for the desired length of time after insertion (reinsertion may be required).

Patient Teaching

Explain that suppositories may take up to 30 minutes to be absorbed, depending on the medication.

Documentation

- Refer to Medication Guidelines: Steps to Follow for All Medication (Regardless of Type or Route).
- Chart the condition of anal tissue if abnormalities are present, any complaints of discomfort that are outside of the expected feelings and experience, and the length of time that the suppository was retained.
- Chart responses to medication (e.g., symptom relief, side effects).

Sample documentation

06/01/16 2015 Patient temperature 103.2°F and complains of nausea. Tylenol grain X suppository given per rectum with patient in Sims' position. Instructed to remain in this position for 15 minutes. Voiced understanding. No rectal abnormalities observed. Tolerated procedure well with no complaints of pain or discomfort.——J. Kinsley, RN

Practice Resources

American Society of Health-System Pharmacists, Inc. (2001); Bradshaw, E., Collins, B., & Williams, J. (2009); Institute for Safe Medication Practice (n.d.).

Thinking About the Procedure

To practice applying clinical reasoning to this procedure,

Go to *Davis's Nursing Skills Videos*, **Inserting a Rectal Suppository.**

For questions and suggested responses,

Go to Chapter 26, **Thinking About the Procedure Questions and Suggested Responses** on Davis*Plus*.

Procedure 26-7 ■ Applying Medication to Skin

➤ For steps to follow in *all* procedures, refer to the Universal Steps for All Procedures found on the inside back cover. Also refer to the Medication Guidelines: Steps to Follow for All Medications (Regardless of Type or Route).

➤ **Note:** Follow agency policy or provider's prescription regarding whether to use prepackaged wipes or soap and water to cleanse the skin.

Delegation

An RN can usually delegate administration of most topical medications to an LPN/LVN. In some institutions you can delegate the administration of an over-the-counter medication to a NAP. Refer to agency policy regarding administration of topical medication.

Pre-Procedure Assessments

- Assess for skin irritation, open lesions, area of hypersensitivity, or other skin abnormality.
- Determine the presence of contraindications for dermal application. Document and report these before administering medication.

Procedure 26-7A ■ Applying Topical Lotion, Cream, and Ointment

➤ When performing the procedure, always identify your patient according to agency policy, using two identifiers, and be attentive to standard precautions, hand hygiene, patient safety and privacy, body mechanics, and documentation.

Procedure Steps

1. **Don clean procedure gloves.**
   Complies with universal precautions and protects your skin from the topical medication.
2. **Cleanse the skin** with cleansing wipes or soap and water (according to agency policy) and pat dry before applying
   Clean skin enhances absorption. Moisture on the skin can interfere with adherence of topical ointment, depending on the product used to suspend the medication.
3. **Warm the medication** in your gloved hands.
   This will be more comfortable for the patient and make the preparation easier to apply.
4. **Use gloved hands or an** applicator to apply and spread the medication evenly, following the direction of hair growth when coating the area.
   Excessive application may irritate the skin. Gloves will protect you so that you will not absorb the medication through your own skin. ▼

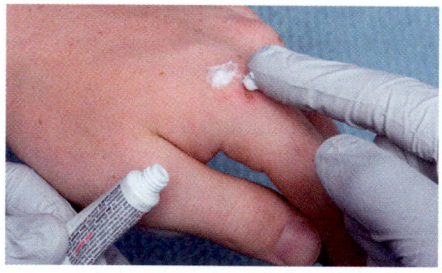

Procedure 26-7B ■ Applying Topical Aerosol Spray

➤ When performing the procedure, always identify your patient according to agency policy, using two identifiers, and be attentive to standard precautions, hand hygiene, patient safety and privacy, body mechanics, and documentation.

Procedure Steps

1. **Don clean procedure gloves.**
2. **Cleanse the skin** with cleansing wipe or soap and water (according to agency policy) and pat dry before applying to enhance absorption.
3. **Shake the container to mix** the contents.
   Active ingredients might not be evenly distributed throughout the aerosolized suspension and may settle at the bottom of the container.
4. **Hold the container at** the distance specified on the label (usually 6 to 12 in.), and spray over the prescribed area.
   This distance will prevent excess application to a local area.
5. **You will need to hold most** containers upright when spraying. If you are spraying near the patient's head, cover his face with a towel.
   This will prevent him from inhaling the spray.

Procedure 26-7C ■ Applying Prescribed Powder

➤ When performing the procedure, always identify your patient according to agency policy, using two identifiers, and be attentive to standard precautions, hand hygiene, patient safety and privacy, body mechanics, and documentation.

Procedure Steps

1. **Don clean procedure gloves.**
2. **Cleanse the skin** with a cleansing wipe or soap and water and pat dry before applying to enhance absorption.
   Powder applied to a moist surface creates a pasty solution, which may irritate the skin.
3. **Spread apart skinfolds**, and apply a very thin layer.
4. **Be careful that the patient does not inhale the powder.**
   Particulate matter, such as powder, can irritate lung tissue and lead to pneumonitis or other inflammatory processes.

Procedure 26-7D ■ Applying Transdermal Medication

➤ When performing the procedure, always identify your patient according to agency policy, using two identifiers, and be attentive to standard precautions, hand hygiene, patient safety and privacy, body mechanics, and documentation.

Procedure Steps

1. **Don clean procedure gloves.**
   Complies with universal precautions and protects your skin from the topical medication.

2. **Remove the previous patch,** folding the medicated side to the inside.
   This helps to prevent unintentional contact of the medication on a different area of the patient's skin.

3. **Dispose of the old patch** carefully in an appropriate receptacle, keeping it away from children and pets.
   Even a used patch has some active medication on it. Proper disposal is important to prevent medication exposure to others.

4. **Cleanse the skin of traces** of remaining medication. Allow the skin to dry.
   A clean, dry surface optimizes the effectiveness of adherence and absorption of the medication .

5. **Remove the new patch from** its protective covering, and then remove the clear, protective covering without touching the adhesive or the inside surface that contains the medication.▼

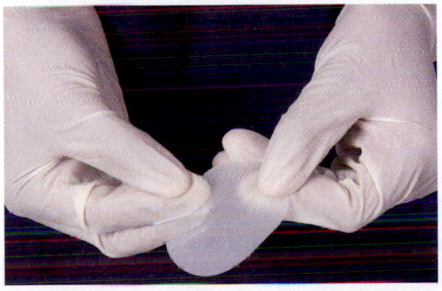

6. **Apply the patch to** a clean, dry, hairless (or little hair), intact skin area, pressing it down for about 10 seconds with your palm. Be sure the area is free of scars, lesions, and irritation.
   A smooth surface maximizes the contact between medication and the skin. Areas of the skin that are disrupted can become irritated by topical mediation. Other lesions involving thickened layers of skin should be avoided to avoid compromised absorption.

7. **Rotate application sites** with each new application. Common sites are the trunk, lower abdomen, lower back, and buttocks.
   Rotating sites prevents irritation to local areas of the skin

8. **Advise the patient *not*** to use a heating pad over the area.
   Heat can cause some ointments to irritate or even burn the skin.

9. **Write the date, the time,** and your initials on the new patch.
   Complete documentation of the dosage administered can reduce medication errors.

10. **Remove your gloves and** perform hand hygiene.

11. **Observe for local side effects,** such as skin irritation, itching, and allergic contact dermatitis.
    If an adverse response occurs at the local site, remove the patch, wipe the skin clean, and notify the prescriber.

? What if . . .

- **The medication is packaged as an ointment form with calibrated paper?**
  Wear gloves; apply the ointment in a continuous motion along those marks to measure the required dose. Fold the paper in half to distribute the ointment evenly on the patch.

- **My patient is a child who does not want the medication to be applied?**
  Hold the child securely while medication is applied. Then cover the site with a dressing to keep the child from disrupting the application of medication.

- **My patient is an older adult and has fragile skin?**
  Avoid areas where penetration of the cream or ointment is likely to be reduced or cause irritation. Be gentle with application of anything to the skin and diligent with your assessment of the skin response to medication. Avoid using tape; use tape alternatives.

Evaluation

- Assess for rash, excoriation, hives, redness, swelling, or signs of allergy or skin sensitivity to topical medication.
- Ask the patient if he feels burning, itching, pain, tenderness, or other sensation to skin where medication was applied.
- Assess for improvement in the patient's condition.

Patient Teaching

- Explain that topical medication may take up to 30 minutes to be absorbed, depending on the medication.
- Tell the patient to never ingest or inhale topical medication.
- Advise the patient to avoid touching his eyes after handling topical medication.
- Inform the patient not to use more medicine than prescribed or directed.

(continued on next page)

Procedure 26-7 ■ Applying Medication to Skin (continued)

Documentation

- Refer to Medication Guidelines: Steps to Follow for All Medication (Regardless of Type or Route).
- Record the skin condition if abnormalities are present and complaints of discomfort during or after administration.
- Document responses to medication (e.g., symptom relief, side effects).

Sample documentation

mm/dd/yyyy 0835 Transdermal nitroglycerine 74.6 mg patch applied to upper chest. Pt. instructed to leave patch intact for 12 hours. Patient reported mild, transient headache approximately 45 minutes after application of patch. No evidence of flushing, faintness, or dizziness. Patient denies chest pain. —— M. Finegold, RN

mm/dd/yyyy 0830 Fentanyl patch dated mm/dd/yyyy removed from upper left arm. Skin intact, no irritation noted. Fentanyl patch applied to the left anterior chest wall below the clavicle. Patient stated, "this patch really helps my back feel better." —— M. Finegold, RN

Thinking About the Procedure

To practice applying clinical reasoning to this procedure,

Go to *Davis's Nursing Skills Videos*, **Applying Transdermal Medication.**

For questions and suggested responses,

Go to Chapter 26, **Thinking About the Procedure Questions and Suggested Responses,** on Davis*Plus*.

Procedure 26-8 ■ Administering Metered-Dose Inhaler (MDI) Medication

➤ For steps to follow in *all* procedures, refer to the Universal Steps for All Procedures found on the inside back cover. Also refer to the Medication Guidelines: Steps to Follow for All Medications (Regardless of Type or Route).

Equipment

- Metered-dose inhaler
- Spacer
- Tissues

Pre-Procedure Assessments

Assess the respiratory status before administration of medication to establish a baseline for evaluating the effects of treatment.

Delegation

An RN can usually delegate administration of MDI medications to an LPN/LVN. You usually cannot delegate this task to a NAP, unless the NAP has special training for a specific defined situation (e.g., "medication aides" in some long-term care settings in some states). If the patient is having respiratory distress, you should not delegate this task. Refer to Medication Guidelines: Steps to Follow for All Medications (regardless of Type or Route).

➤ When performing the procedure, always identify your patient according to agency policy, using two identifiers, and be attentive to standard precautions, hand hygiene, patient safety and privacy, body mechanics, and documentation.

Procedure Steps

1. **Determine the number of** remaining inhalations of medication in the canister based on the start date and instructions for use. Do not use the old method of floating the canister in water, as it is not an accurate estimate. Replace the canister promptly when it is nearly empty.

Historically, patients have been instructed to float the canister in water to determine how much medication remains. However, propellants affect the weight of the canister and may lead to false reassurance that there is medication in an empty container.

Some MDI medications are used as rescue agents during asthma attacks or periods of dyspnea. It is important to always have medication available for use.

2. **Assist the patient to a seated** or high-Fowler's position if in bed.
   An upright position helps the patient take a deep inhalation when medication is administered.

3. **Ask the patient to rinse** out his mouth and spit the fluid out (not to swallow it).
   This helps to prevent transfer of bacteria from the mouth to the inhaler.

4. **Shake the inhaler.** Then remove the mouthpiece cap of the inhaler and insert the mouthpiece into the spacer while holding the canister upright.
   A spacer is the most efficient method to deliver inhaled medications. It should be used if the patient has difficulty coordinating the use of the inhaler, is using a corticosteroid, or if it is prescribed.

5. **Remove the cap from the spacer.**

6. **Ask the patient to breathe out** slowly and completely. If a patient is unable to use the MDI independently, time the use of the device with the patient's own respirations.
   Deep breathing helps the patient to time the dose with his natural breathing.

7. **Place the spacer mouthpiece** into the patient's mouth and have him seal his lips around the mouthpiece. Sharply press down on the inhaler canister to discharge one puff of medication into the spacer.

If No Spacer Is Used

If a spacer is not used, place the canister 1 to 2 inches (2.5 to 5.0 cm) from or directly into the mouth.

A good seal allows proper delivery of medication.

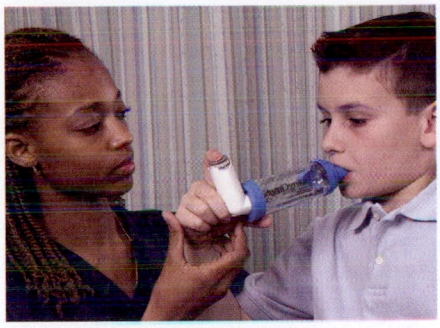

8. **Ask the patient to slowly inhale** and then hold his breath for as long as possible. Encourage the patient to hold his breath for 10 seconds if possible.
   When holding his breath the medication can be delivered deep into the lungs.

9. **If a second puff is needed,** wait at least 1 minute before repeating Steps 6 through 8.
   Pausing allows the medication to be absorbed and the canister to recharge.

10. **If a corticosteroid inhaler** was used, assist the patient to rinse out his mouth with water and spit out the rinse.
    Prolonged exposure of this medication to the oral mucosa is irritating and can lead to thrush in some patients.

11. **Wipe the mouthpiece** with a tissue or moist cloth and replace the cap. Periodically rinse the spacer, mouthpiece, and cap with water.
    Proper cleaning of the MDI keeps the dispenser from clogging.

The following illustrations summarize the steps for using an MDI.

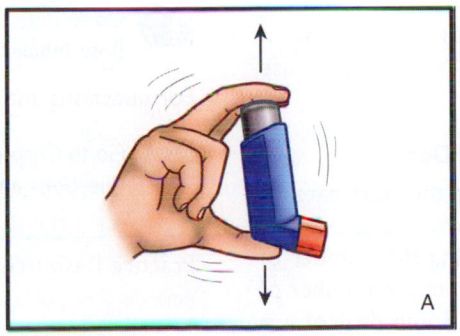

Shake canister.

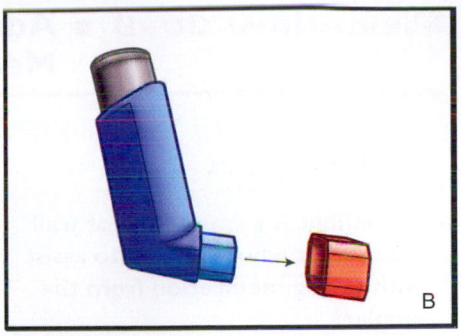

Remove cap. Discharge 2 puffs.

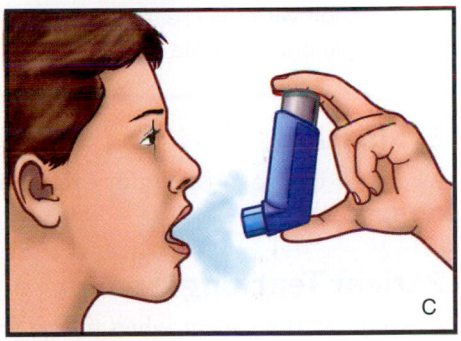

Deep breath out.

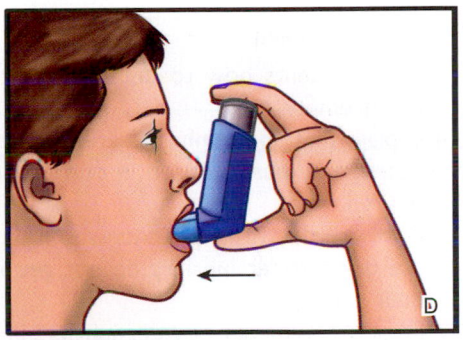

Press top. Inhale med slowly.

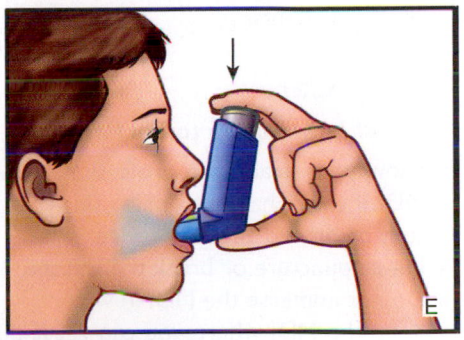

Hold breath. Exhale slowly.

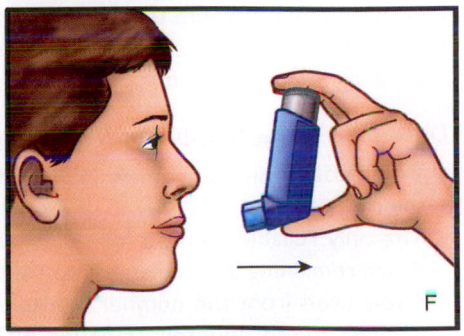

Remove inhaler from mouth.
Wait 1 minute before next puff.

(continued on next page)

Procedure 26-8 ■ Administering Metered-Dose Inhaler (MDI) Medication (continued)

? What if . . .

- **My patient is a small child or frail older adult who is unable to assist with taking medication from the inhaler?**

  You will need to time discharge of the medication with the client's inspiration if the patient is unable to administer the medication with his own deep breaths.

- **My patient uses an albuterol MDI with chlorofluorocarbon (CFC) as a propellant?**

  The FDA made a ruling, effective December 31, 2008, prohibiting use of CFCs in albuterol MDIs. If the patient has an inhaler containing this product, known to be detrimental to the ozone layer, the patient or caregiver can request an alternate prescription.

  Key Point: *In addition to the harmful effects of the propellant on the environment, the medication is also likely to be past its expiration date.*

Evaluation

Assess for change in respiratory status after medication administration.

Patient Teaching

- Explain to the patient when to use the inhaler and what side effects to anticipate.
- Teach and demonstrate to patients how to correctly use a spacer and MDI.
- Teach patients how to determine if the MDI canister is nearly empty.
- Explain that some inhalers are used in combination with others and must be used in correct order to receive the desired effect.
- Be aware that many patients who have not been taught to use dry powder inhalers do not get any medication into their lungs.
- Errors in using dry powder inhalers increase with age and illness severity. Carefully supervise older adults and seriously ill patients.

Home Care

General Information to Tell Patients

- Show your healthcare professional how you're using your MDI. If you're having trouble using your MDI, ask for tips or to recommend another device.
- Never puncture or break the canister.
- Do not immerse the MDI in water.
- Keep the MDI where you can get it quickly when needed, but out of children's reach.
- Store the MDI at room temperature. If it gets cold, warm it by rubbing the canister between your palms. Never use anything else to warm it.

Determining the Number of Remaining Doses

- When you begin using a new MDI, write the start date on the canister.
- The only reliable method for determining the number of doses remaining in a canister is to subtract the number of doses used from the number available. Some devices are equipped with counters. Floating MDIs in water is not accurate for assessing remaining doses and often will clog the valve.

Cleaning the MDI

- Clean your apparatus regularly to avoid drug buildup that might keep the medication from reaching the lungs. Specific maintenance procedures may vary with the manufacturer.
- Remove the metal canister that contains the medication by pulling it out.

Documentation

- Refer to Medication Guidelines: Steps to Follow for All Medications (regardless of Type or Route).
- Document the response to medications.

Sample documentation

mm/dd/yyyy 0800 Pt. c/o shortness of breath. RR 26 and labored. Combivent MDI 2 puffs administered with spacer. S. Smythe, RN

0815 RR 20 regular, even, comfortable. S. Smythe, RN

Thinking About the Procedure

To practice applying clinical reasoning to this procedure,

Go to *Davis's Nursing Skills Videos*, **Administering Metered-Dose Inhaler (MDI) Medication.**

For questions and suggested responses,

Go to Chapter 26, **Thinking About the Procedure Questions and Suggested Responses,** on Davis*Plus*.

Practice Resources

American Society of Health System Pharmacists, Inc. (n.d.); Gandhi, K., Dahiya, A., Taruna-Kalra, A., et al. (2012); Lareau, S., & Hodder, R. (2012); U.S. Food and Drug Administration (2013); Werner, R., & Morien, A. (2012).

Procedure 26-9 ■ Preparing, Drawing Up, and Mixing Medication

➤ For steps to follow in *all* procedures, refer to the Universal Steps for All Procedures found on the inside back cover. Also refer to the Medication Guidelines: Steps to Follow for All Medications (Regardless of Type or Route).

Equipment

- Medication vials, ampules, and/or prefilled syringe
- Alcohol prep pad (70% alcohol) or chlorhexidine gluconate (CHG)–alcohol product
- Syringe of the appropriate size for medication volume and viscosity
- Needle of the appropriate size for the site and viscosity to be aspirated through the vial access device (VAD)
- VAD, filter needle, or safety needle.
- Gauze pad or ampule snapper, if you are using ampules

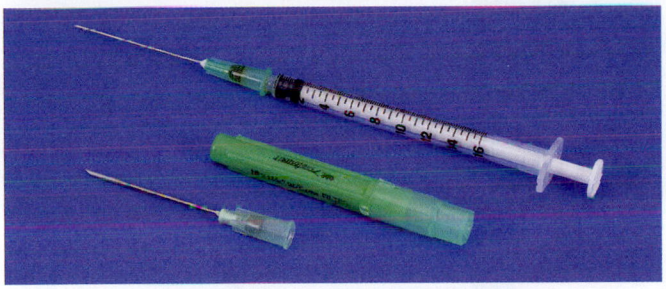

Top: Syringe with a regular needle. *Bottom:* Filter needle.

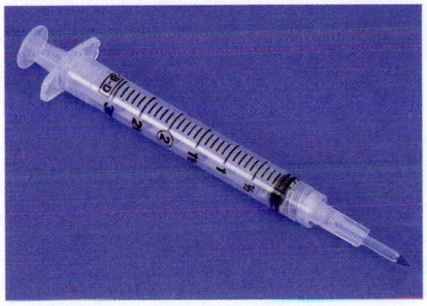

Vial access device.

Delegation

An RN can delegate administration of some parenteral medications to an LPN/LVN. You usually cannot delegate this task to a NAP. Nurse practice acts governing medication administration vary from state to state, and policies vary further among healthcare agencies. Nevertheless, the RN is always responsible for supervising and evaluating delegated care. You can instruct a NAP in the therapeutic effects expected from the medication.

Pre-Procedure Assessments

- Check the ampule or vial for intactness, cloudiness, particles, and color.
  A change in color, cloudiness, particles, or cracks indicate the medication is altered or contaminated and should not be used.
- Check the compatibility of the medications to be mixed.
  Some medications are either chemically or physically incompatible and cannot be mixed. Other medications may be compatible for only 20 to 30 minutes, so they must be given promptly after they are mixed. Although physically incompatible medications can frequently be identified by a change in appearance, such as precipitation, no such indication exists for chemically incompatible medications.
- Determine the total volume of medications and whether the total volume is appropriate for the administration site.
  Although the reason for mixing medications is to limit the number of injections a patient receives, the total volume of the injections must not be greater than what is appropriate for the site.

Procedure 26-9A ■ Drawing Up Medication From Ampules

➤ When performing the procedure, always identify your patient according to agency policy, using two identifiers, and be attentive to standard precautions, hand hygiene, patient safety and privacy, body mechanics, and documentation.

Procedure Steps

1. **Gently flick or tap the top** of the ampule with your index finger to remove medication trapped in the top of the ampule. Alternate method: Shake the ampule by quickly turning and snapping your wrist, like shaking down a mercury thermometer.
   Medication left in the top of the ampule may lead to administering an inadequate dose. All the medication must be in the bottom of the ampule before you open it.
2. **Wrap a 2 in. × 2 in. gauze pad** (or an unwrapped alcohol wipe) around the neck of the ampule, or use an ampule snapper. Snap the top off, breaking it away from you.
   Prevents you from accidentally cutting your fingers or spraying glass fragments toward you. Do not use an opened alcohol wipe

(continued on next page)

Procedure 26-9 ■ Preparing, Drawing Up, and Mixing Medication (continued)

to break the ampule, because it is not thick enough to prevent injury. ▼

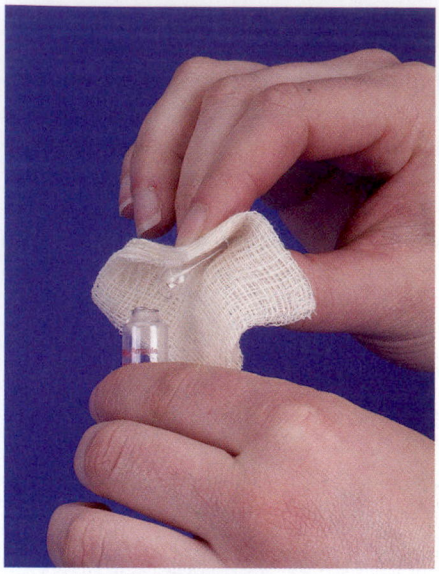

3. **Attach a filter needle** or filter straw to the syringe. If the syringe has a needle in place, remove both the needle and the cap, and place them on a sterile surface (e.g., a newly unwrapped alcohol pad still in the open wrapper), and attach the filter needle or straw.
   The American Society for Health System Pharmacists recommends filtering solutions drawn up from glass ampules to remove glass particles. Opening a glass ampule produces a spray of tiny fractured glass particles, which can enter the ampule and contaminate the contents.

4. **Withdraw the medication** from the ampule with a filter needle by using one of the following techniques. Be careful not to touch the neck of the ampule with the filter straw or needle while withdrawing medication.
   Touching the neck of the ampule with the needle or straw increases the risk of contamination.

   a. *Invert the ampule*, place the filter needle or straw tip in the liquid, and withdraw the prescribed amount of medication. Be careful not to insert needle through the medication into the air at the top of the inverted ampule.
   This method is particularly useful with small ampules. The medication's surface tension prevents the liquid from leaking from the inverted ampule. However, if you insert the needle too far (into the air pocket above the medication), the medication will run out. ▼

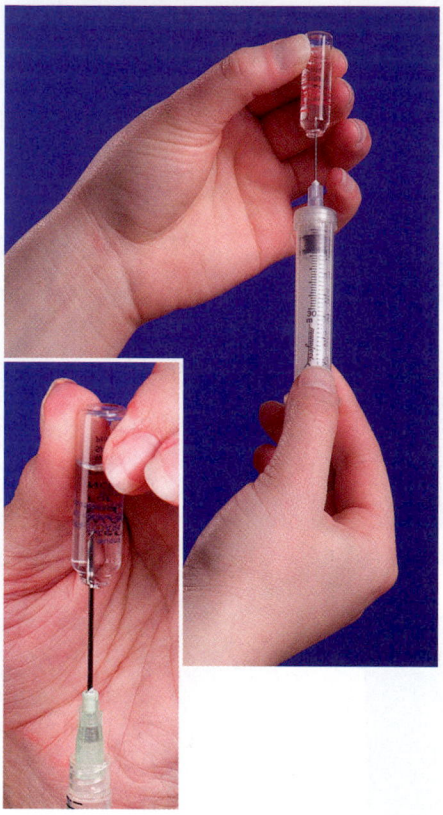

   b. *Alternatively, tip the ampule*, place a filter needle or straw in the liquid, and withdraw all medication. Reposition the ampule so that the needle or straw tip remains in the liquid.
   This method allows for easier stabilization of the ampule while you withdraw the medication, and may help keep you from contaminating the needle on the edge of the vial opening. ▼

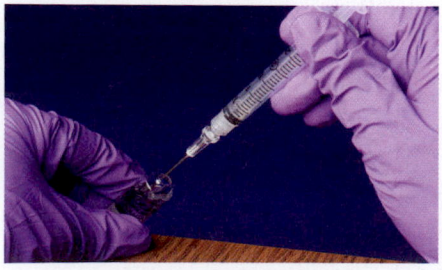

5. **Hold the syringe vertically**, and draw 0.2 mL of air into the syringe (see Clinical Insight 26-4). Draw up and measure the exact medication dose, plus 0.2 mL of air (the syringe plunger should be at 0.2 mL more than the prescribed dose).

6. **Remove the filter needle** or straw, and reattach the "saved" needle for administering the injection.

7. **Eject the 0.2 mL of air, and read** the dose. After all of the air is removed, if you need to eject some medication to make the dose correct, tip the syringe until it is horizontal to push out the medication.
   - *Pulling air into the syringe allows for an exact dose when the medication is injected; the air will clear the needle (after the medication) so that the patient receives all the medication that is in the syringe.*
   - *The syringe must be vertical to eject air. However, if you eject the medication while holding the syringe vertically, the drug will run down the needle and then track through the patient's tissue during the injection.*

For a filter needle

Use a filter needle only to withdraw, not to measure, medication. Do not eject medication from it.

Pushing the medication out through the filter needle could cause the filter to break and release the glass fragments.

Key Point: ***This is not the old "air lock" technique; you will eject the air before administering the medication to the patient.***

For medications that are irritating to tissues (e.g., parenteral iron)

You can leave the 0.2 mL of air in the syringe for injection. But be sure to account for the air when you read the dose markings on the syringe.

8. **Dispose of the top and bottom** of the ampule and the filter needle in a sharps container.
   Disposal into a puncture-proof container prevents accidental needlestick injury.

Procedure 26-9B ■ Drawing Up Medication From Vials

- When performing the procedure, always identify your patient according to agency policy, using two identifiers, and be attentive to standard precautions, hand hygiene, patient safety and privacy, body mechanics, and documentation.
- This procedure assumes you are using a vial access device (VAD), since that is preferred. Use a needle only when a filter needle is required.

Procedure Steps

1. **Mix the solution in the vial,** if necessary, by gently rolling the vial between your hands.
   Aqueous suspensions will settle to the bottom of the vial, so they need to be mixed. Rolling the vial between your hands will mix the medication without forming air bubbles. Shaking the vial traps air in the medication.

2. **Place the vial on a flat** work surface and thoroughly scrub the rubber top of the vial with an alcohol prep pad or CHG-alcohol product.
   The alcohol prep pad removes dust, grease, and microorganisms.

3. **If a needle is attached** to the syringe, remove it and place it on a sterile, opened alcohol pad. Then attach a VAD; do not touch the tip.
   VADs can be used only with single-use vials, unless the vial is designed for use with access pins, such as a Life-Shield vial.

4. **Remove and place the VAD cap** on a clean surface, or hold the cap open-side out between two fingers of your nondominant hand.
   This method prevents contamination of the cap and the needle during recapping.

5. **Draw air into the syringe** equal to the amount of medication to be withdrawn from the vial.
   Injection of air into the vial makes withdrawing the medication easier. For small unit-dose vials, you may not have to instill air prior to withdrawing the medication, but you will need to maintain backward pressure on the plunger until the needle is completely withdrawn. If you release the plunger, the negative pressure in the vial will pull the medication back into the vial.

6. **Insert the VAD** into the vial without coring and while maintaining sterile technique. Use a needle *only* if for some reason (e.g., the type of medication) requires a filter needle.
   a. Place the tip of the VAD or filter needle in the middle of the rubber top of the vial, with the bevel up at a 45° to 60° angle. ▼

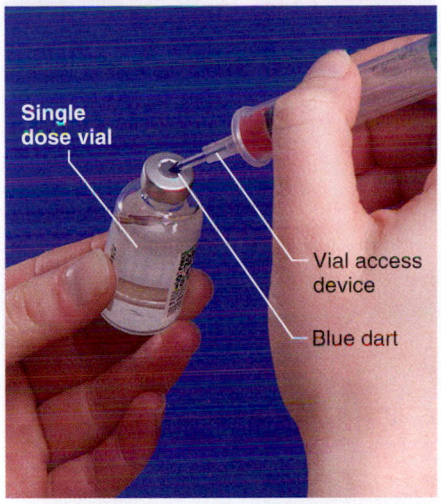

   b. While pushing the VAD into the rubber top, gradually bring the syringe (and VAD) upright to a 90° angle.
   This method helps prevent coring, which occurs when a small piece of the rubber top is trapped inside the VAD during insertion. Coring is more likely to occur with large-gauge needles and VADs. ▼

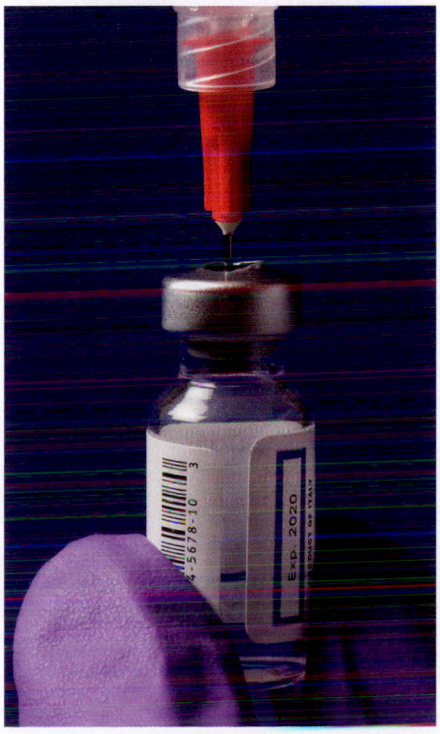

7. **With the tip of the VAD above** the fluid line, inject the air in the syringe into the air in the vial.
   Injecting air into the vial creates positive pressure, making the medication easier to withdraw. Injecting the air into the medication will create air bubbles, which interfere with dosage measurement. ▼

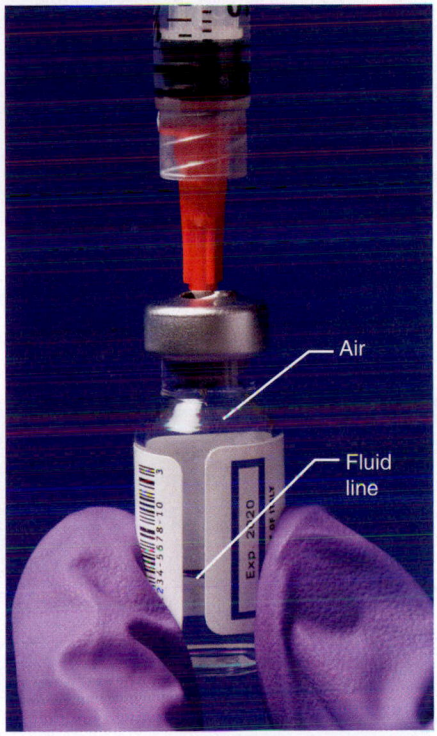

"Air to air."

8. **Invert the vial,** keep the VAD vertical in the medication, and slowly withdraw the medication.
   The vial needs to be inverted so that all the medication can be withdrawn. Keeping the VAD in the medication and slowly drawing the medication will help prevent you from drawing excess air into the syringe. ▼

(continued on next page)

Procedure 26-9 ■ Preparing, Drawing Up, and Mixing Medication (continued)

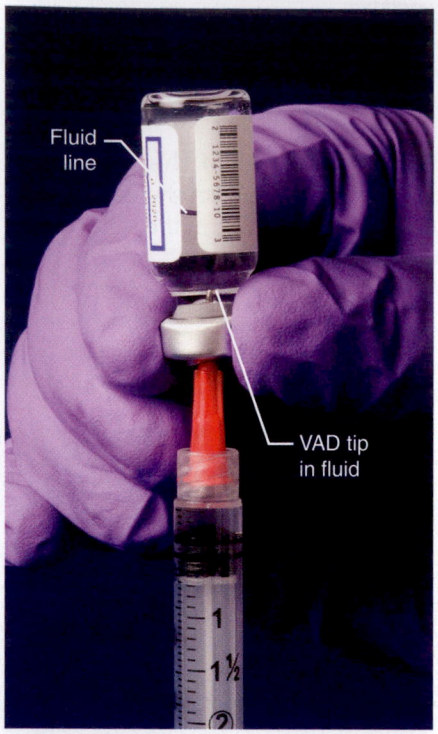

9. Keeping the VAD in the vial, remove any air from the syringe:▼

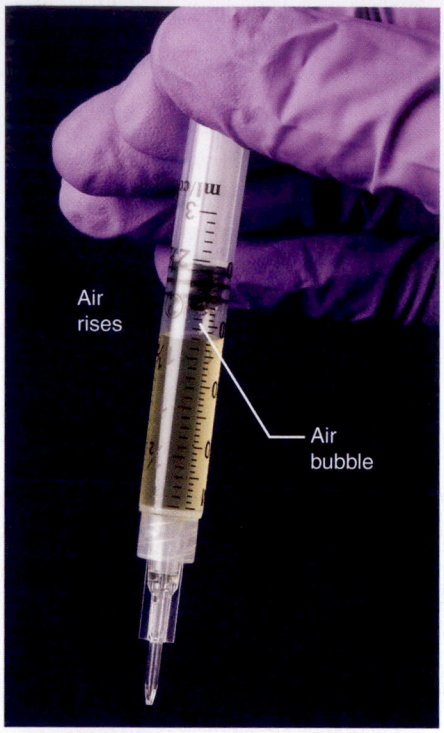

B, **Incorrect**—If tip is down, air is trapped at the plunger. ▲

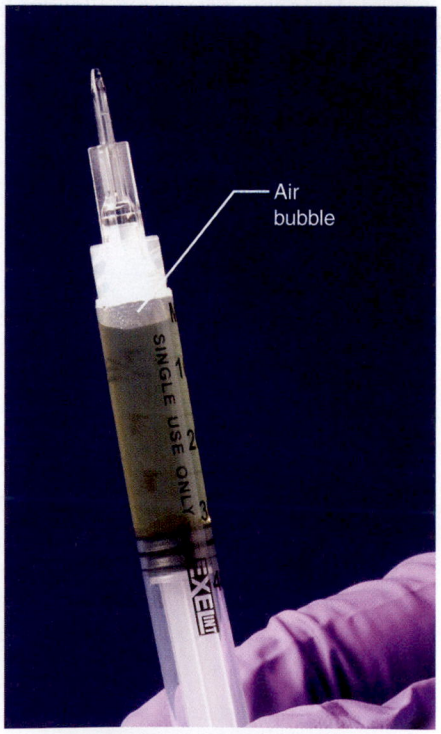

A, **Incorrect**—If syringe is not vertical, air is trapped near the hub.

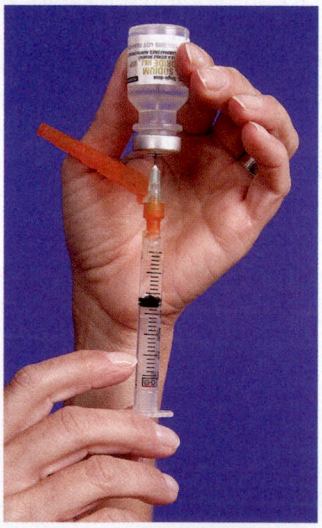

C, **Correct**—Syringe is vertical.

When the VAD is connecting the vial and syringe, a sterile unit is formed. The volume of air in the hub of the syringe and inside the needle/VAD, dead space, will be drawn back into the syringe. Air bubbles alter the dose of medication being administered, so they must be expelled. You can use a pen to tap the syringe if extra force is needed.

a. Carefully stabilize the vial and syringe, and firmly tap the syringe below the air bubbles. When air bubbles are at the hub of the syringe, make sure the syringe is vertical (straight up and down), and push the air back into the vial.

Remember that air rises, so if the syringe is tilted, air will be trapped in it.

b. If additional medication is necessary to obtain the correct dose, withdraw it before removing the VAD from the inverted vial.

When working with only one vial, you can withdraw and eject medication into the vial as many times as needed to expel bubbles from the syringe and obtain the correct dose.

10. When the dose is correct, withdraw the needle or VAD from the vial at a 90° angle.

A vertical angle prevents accidental contamination or bending of the needle.

11. Hold the syringe upright at eye level to recheck the medication dose.

Reading the syringe at an angle can result in inaccurate measurement.

12. Recap the VAD or vial access needle using a recapping device or the one-handed method. See Procedure 26-10.

Although recapping a sterile needle does not present a threat of bloodborne pathogen exposure, using a mechanical recapping device or the one-handed method helps develop safe habits.

13. Change the VAD or filter needle before you inject the medication:

a. Before changing the VAD or filter needle, draw back on the syringe plunger to remove all medication from dead space in the old needle (or VAD).

b. Remove the old needle (or VAD), and reattach a sterile needle for injection (see Clinical Insight 26-4).

You cannot eject medication through a filter needle; you cannot inject a patient with a VAD.

c. Hold the syringe vertically and expel the air. If it is necessary to expel some medication, hold the syringe horizontally to do so.

The difficulty with changing the needles is that you may slightly alter the dose. If you are planning to change the needles, draw slightly more than the ordered dose unless you are combining in one syringe. After changing the needle, re-measure the dose. Holding the syringe horizontally prevents medication from running down the needle and tracking into the patient's skin.

14. **Dispose of the vial, VAD,** or any recapped needles in a sharps container. *This prevents sharps injury to health-care workers or others in the vicinity. Proper disposal also reduces the risk of transmitting infectious organisms.*

Procedure 26-9C ■ Mixing Medication From Two Vials

➤ First review the Medication Guidelines: Steps to Follow for All Medications (Regardless of Type or Route); Procedure 26-9B (Drawing Up Medication From Vials); and Procedure 26-10A (Recapping Contaminated Needles).

Always use a VAD instead of a needle whenever possible. If you must use a needle, use a safety needle.

➤ When performing the procedure, always identify your patient according to agency policy, using two identifiers, and be attentive to standard precautions, hand hygiene, patient safety and privacy, body mechanics, and documentation.

Procedure Steps

1. **Scrub the tops of both vials** with an alcohol pad or CHG-alcohol product. *Note:* Some experts omit this step for single-dose vials.
   Not all pharmaceutical companies ensure the sterility of the rubber top on vials, even when they are first opened. However, be aware that once your fingers touch the alcohol pad, it is no longer sterile, either; therefore, you are not sterilizing, but rather are cleaning the vial top.

2. **Draw air into the syringe** in the same amount as the total medication doses for both vials (e.g., if the order is for 0.5 mL for vial A and 1 mL for vial B, then draw up 1.5 mL of air).

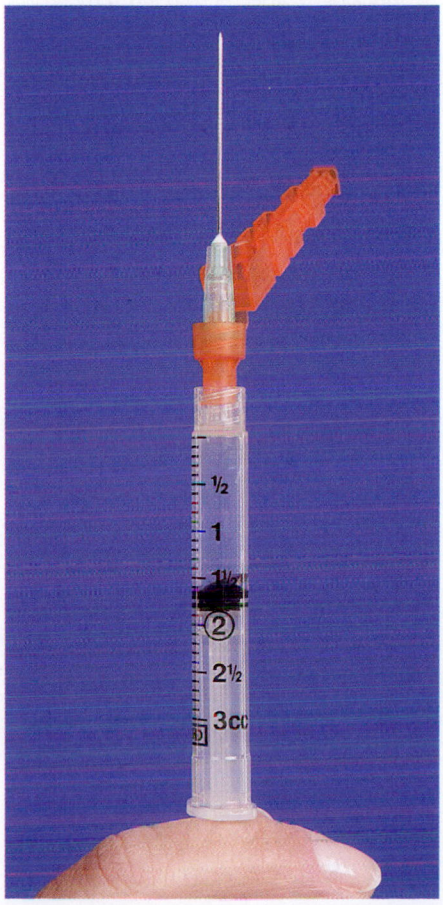

3. **Inject air into the vials.**
   a. Maintaining sterility, insert the vial access device [VAD] (or safety needle) into the vial in the middle of the rubber top of the vial with the bevel up at a 45° to 60° angle. While pushing the VAD (or needle) into the rubber top, gradually bring the needle upright to a 90° angle.

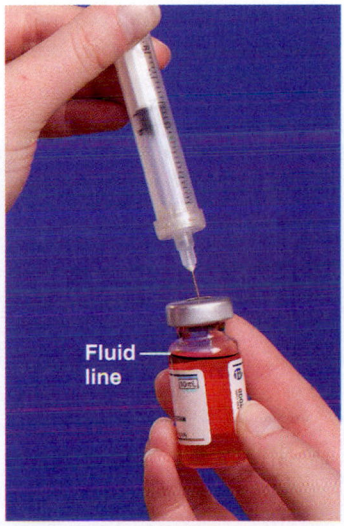

Vial A

This method helps prevent coring of the rubber top.

   b. Keeping the tip of the VAD (or safety needle) above the medication, inject an amount of air equal to the volume of drug to be withdrawn from the first vial (e.g., 0.5 mL for vial A in Step 2); then inject the rest of the air into the second vial (1.0 mL for vial B). Take care to prevent coring.
   Medication is easier to withdraw from a vial with positive pressure. For small unit-dose vials, it may be possible to withdraw the medication without instilling air, but you will need to maintain a slight backward pressure on the plunger until the needle is completely withdrawn. If you release the plunger, the negative pressure in the vial will pull the medication back in. Therefore, it is always safer to instill air.

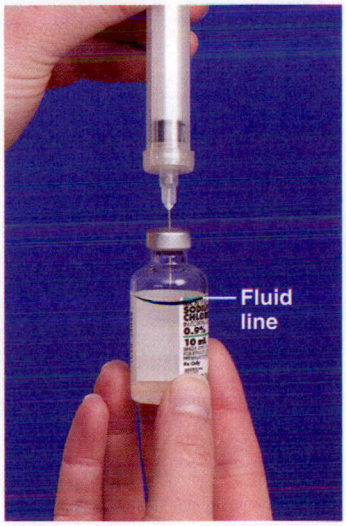

Vial B

Using One Multidose Vial and One Single-Dose Vial

You must withdraw medication from the multidose vial before withdrawing from the single-dose vial. However, the needle tip should stay above the medication at all times in Steps 3 and 4.
This is an extra precaution to prevent contamination of the multidose vial with medication from the single-dose vial.

When Mixing Two Types of Insulin

If you are mixing two types of insulin at Step 3, put air into the regular insulin last (see Clinical Insight 26-5 for mixing two types of insulin).

(continued on next page)

Procedure 26-9 ■ Preparing, Drawing Up, and Mixing Medication (continued)

4. **Without removing the VAD,** or needle, from the second vial (B), invert it and withdraw the ordered amount of medication. Expel any air bubbles, and measure the dose. Remove the VAD from the vial, then pull back on the plunger enough to pull all medication out of the VAD into the syringe (see Clinical Insight 26-4). Read the dose at eye level. Tip the syringe horizontally if you need to eject any medication.
   Allows you to withdraw all the medication. Keeping the needle in the medication and withdrawing the medication slowly helps prevent drawing excess air into the syringe and prevents bubbles. ▼

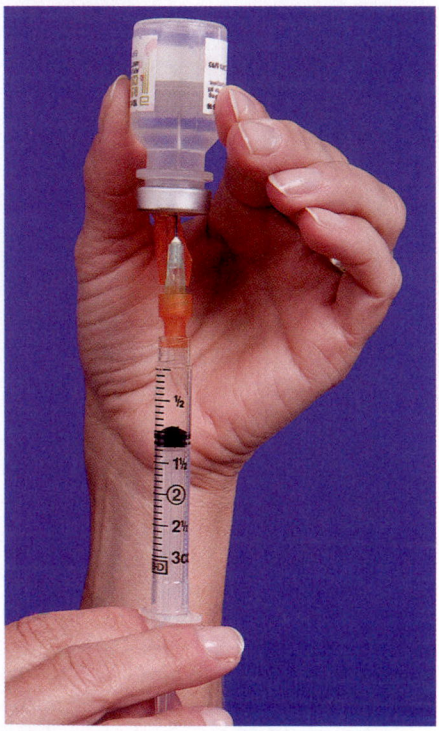

Vial B (Step 4)

5. **Insert the VAD or needle** into the first vial (A), invert, and withdraw the exact ordered amount of medication, holding the syringe vertical.
   - When finished, the plunger should be at the line for the total/combined dose for vials A and B. (Using the example in Step 2, you would have 1.5 mL of the mixed medications in the syringe.)
   - Be very careful not to withdraw excess medication; keep your index finger or thumb on the flange of the syringe to prevent medication being forced back by pressure. If this occurs, you must discard the medication in the syringe and start over.
   Because the medications are mixed, withdrawing extra from the second vial makes the entire mixture incorrect. If you eject excess medication from the syringe, you do not know how much of either medication you have ejected; so even if you have the correct amount of fluid (e.g., 1.5 mL in our example), you would not know how much of that is medication A and how much of it is medication B.

   You do not need to change the needle before Step 5 because even if one vial is a multidose vial, you would have withdrawn the medication from it first (in Step 4). It will not matter if you track medication into the single-dose vial. ▼

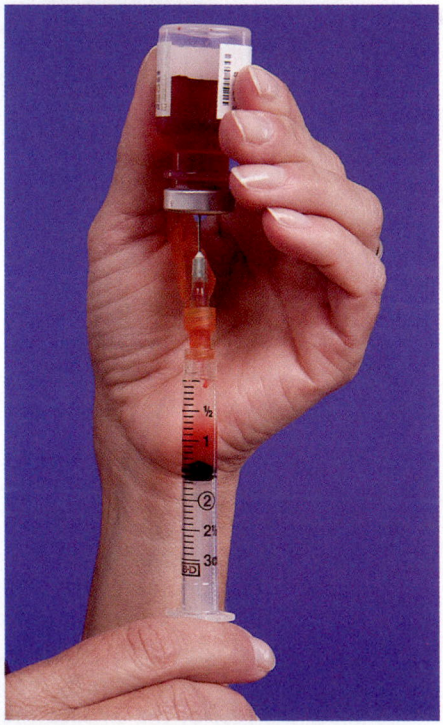

Vial A (Step 5)

6. **Recap the VAD** or access needle, using a needle capping device or the one-handed scoop method (see Procedure 26-10: Recapping Needles Using a One-Handed Technique).
   Although recapping a sterile needle does not present a threat of bloodborne pathogen exposure, using a mechanical recapping device or the one-handed method helps develop safe habits. As a rule, we do not recommend using the one-handed scoop for sterile needles; however, this needle will be discarded anyway, so if it is accidentally contaminated with a one-handed scoop, it will not be a major error.

7. **Remove the VAD** (or access needle), and attach a new sterile needle on the syringe for the injection.
   Obviously, you must replace a VAD with a needle for injection. In addition, if you used a needle instead of a VAD, by the time you are finished withdrawing both medications you will have put it through a rubber vial top at least three times. This dulls the needle. A sharp needle causes less trauma to the patient on injection. A new needle also prevents tracking of the medication through the skin and subcutaneous tissues.

8. **Hold the needle vertically** to expel all air and recheck the dosage (the total for both medications).
   Allows for more accurate accounting of the dose.

9. **If you have used a VAD or filter** needle, refer to Clinical Insight 26-4.

Procedure 26-9D ■ Mixing Medications From One Ampule and One Vial

- First review the Medication Guidelines: Steps to Follow for All Medications (Regardless of Type or Route); Procedure 26-9A (Drawing up Medications from Ampules); Procedure 26-9B (Drawing Up Medication From Vials); and Procedure 26-10A (Recapping Contaminated Needles).
- When performing the procedure, always identify your patient according to agency policy, using two identifiers, and be attentive to standard precautions, hand hygiene, patient safety and privacy, body mechanics, and documentation.

Procedure Steps

1. **Begin with the vial.** Scrub the stopper of the vial using an alcohol wipe or CHG-alcohol combination product.
   Protects against microbial contamination.

2. **Attach a VAD** and draw **the same volume of air** into the syringe as the dose prescribed for the medication in the vial.

3. **Keeping the tip of the VAD** or safety needle above the medication, inject the amount of air equal to the volume of drug to be withdrawn from the vial. The needle should be injecting air-to-air within the vial.
   Draw from the vial first because you do not need to add air to ampules before drawing up the medication. In addition, if it is a multidose vial, you would contaminate it with the medicine if you withdrew from the ampule first.

   Injecting air into the vial makes withdrawing the medication easier. For small unit-dose vials, it may be possible to withdraw the medication without instilling air, but you will need to maintain a slight backward pressure on the plunger until the needle is completely withdrawn. If you release the plunger, the negative pressure in the vial will pull the medication back into the vial. Therefore, it is safer always to instill air.

4. **Invert the vial.** Withdraw the prescribed volume (dosage) of medication, keeping the VAD tip in the fluid. See Procedure 26-9B.

5. **Expel any air bubbles** and measure the dose at eye level. Recheck the dosage, and withdraw more or eject the drug as needed.
   This prevents air from entering into the needle or VAD.

6. **After safely recapping** the VAD remove it from the syringe. You may place it on an opened, sterile alcohol pad if you need your hands to open the filter needle packaging.
   Keeps the needle sterile, if you are using one; you will reuse it. You would not reuse a VAD from this step on.

7. **Attach a filter needle** or filter straw to the syringe.
   The use of a 5-micrometer (μm) filter minimizes the possibility of withdrawing small glass fragments.

8. **Flick or tap the top** of the ampule (or snap your wrist) to remove medication from the neck of the ampule.
   Flicking the neck of the ampule will help the fluid to drain down into the main part of the ampule, thus reducing waste.

9. **Open the ampule** by wrapping the neck with a folded gauze pad or an unopened alcohol wipe or use an ampule snapper. Snap open away from you.
   Snapping outward prevents you from accidentally cutting your fingers or spraying glass fragments toward your face. Do not use an opened alcohol wipe to break the ampule, because it is not thick enough to prevent injury.

10. **Withdraw the exact prescribed** amount of medication from the ampule into the syringe (see Procedure 26-9A). Be very careful in drawing up the second medication; if the total amount of the two medications is incorrect, you must discard the syringe contents and start over.

11. **Draw 0.2 mL of air into the syringe.**
    The extra bit of air clears the filter needle (see Clinical Insight 26-4).

12. **Confirm the dose is correct** by holding the syringe vertically and checking the dose at eye level.
    Ensures the total volume in the syringe equals the ordered amount of both medications plus 0.2 mL of air from the needle.

13. **Recap the filter needle or straw,** using a needle capping device or the one-handed technique recommended in Procedure 26-10B.
    Although recapping a sterile needle does not present a threat of blood-borne pathogen exposure, using a mechanical recapping device or the one-handed method helps develop safe habits. Nevertheless, some scoop techniques pose a significant risk of contaminating the needle, so you must watch carefully that you maintain sterile technique.

14. **Remove the filter needle** or straw and discard it in a sharps container. Replace with a new sterile safety needle for administering the medication to the patient.
    This needle-recapping method prevents accidental needlestick injury. You cannot measure the dose accurately with a filter needle. You should not eject medication through the filter needle because of risk of breaking the filter. See Clinical Insight 26-4.

15. **After placing the administration** needle on the syringe, eject the 0.2 mL of air and check for the correct dose. If there is excess medication in the syringe, you must discard it and start over.

16. **Discard used needles** and ampules in a puncture-proof sharps container.

(continued on next page)

Procedure 26-9 ■ Preparing, Drawing Up, and Mixing Medication (continued)

Procedure 26-9E ■ Using a Prefilled Cartridge and Single-Dose Vial—For Intravenous Administration

- *Note:* It is best not to use this technique with multidose vials because there is a risk of contaminating the multidose vial with the cartridge medication.
- First review the Medication Guidelines: Steps to Follow for All Medications (Regardless of Type or Route). Review Procedures 26-9 and 26-10, as needed.
- When performing the procedure, always identify your patient according to agency policy, using two identifiers, and be attentive to standard precautions, hand hygiene, patient safety and privacy, body mechanics, and documentation.

Procedure Steps

1. **Scrub the rubber stopper** of the vial thoroughly with an alcohol prep pad or CHG-alcohol-based product.
2. **Assemble the prefilled cartridge** and holder (see Clinical Insight 26-2).
3. **Remove the needle cap** from the prefilled cartridge, expel the air, and measure the correct dose of medication.
   You must confirm that the dose of the first medication is correct before you mix it with the second medication.
4. **Holding the cartridge with** the needle up, draw in an amount of air equal to the volume of medication you need from the vial.
5. **While continuing to hold** the syringe with needle straight up (vertically), invert the vial and insert the needle into it until the tip of the needle shows in the air above the medication. Then inject the air into the vial. Maintain counter-pressure on the plunger so that air and/or medication do not flow back into the syringe.

Injecting air into the vial makes the medication easier to withdraw. ▼

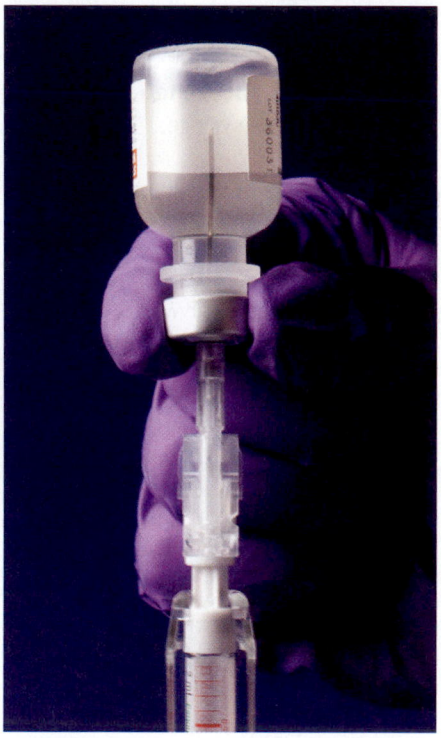

6. **While maintaining counter-pressure** on the plunger, pull the needle down into the fluid and allow the pressure in the vial to push the medication into the syringe. Withdraw the prescribed amount of vial medication, being careful not to withdraw any excess.
7. **The pressure will generally push** a little less than you need, so carefully withdraw the amount you need for a correct dose—again, do not withdraw any excess.
   Withdrawing excess medication will result in an altered mixed dose, so you would need to discard the syringe and start over.
8. **Recap the needle** (use a one-handed method) and if possible remove the needle from the prefilled syringe and replace it with a sterile injection cannula for IV administration. For an intramuscular (IM) injection, if the prefilled cartridge does not have a safety needle, you would need to transfer the medication to a new syringe with a sterile safety needle for injection.
   VADs and injection cannulas prevent needlestick injury. Unless there is a needle safety device for the prefilled syringe, it is not recommended for IM injections.

? What if . . .

- **I note particulate matter in the ampule or vial?**
  Discard the medication and order a new one.

Documentation

Document on the MAR.

Thinking About the Procedures

To practice applying clinical reasoning to this procedure,

Go to *Davis's Nursing Skills Videos,* **Drawing Up Medication From Ampules, Drawing Up Medication From Vials, Mixing Medication From Two Vials,** and **Mixing Medication From One Ampule and One Vial.**

For questions and suggested responses,

Go to Chapter 26, **Thinking About the Procedure Questions and Suggested Responses,** on Davis*Plus*.

Practice Resources

CDC (2010a, updated 2012); Denholm, B. (2013); Manchikanti, L., Falco, F., Benyamin, R., et al. (2012).

Procedure 26-10 ■ Recapping Needles Using a One-Handed Technique

➤ For steps to follow in *all* procedures, refer to the Universal Steps for All Procedures found on the inside back cover. Also refer to Medication Guidelines: Steps to Follow for All Medications (Regardless of Type or Route).

Equipment

- Mechanical recapping device, if available
- Needle cover
- Safety syringe, if available
- Other supplies depending on the method used. ▼

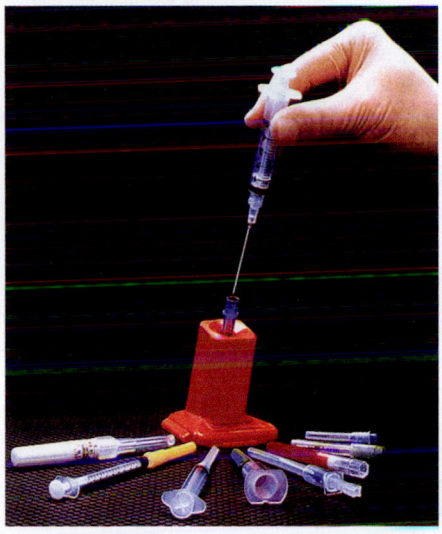

Needle recapping device.

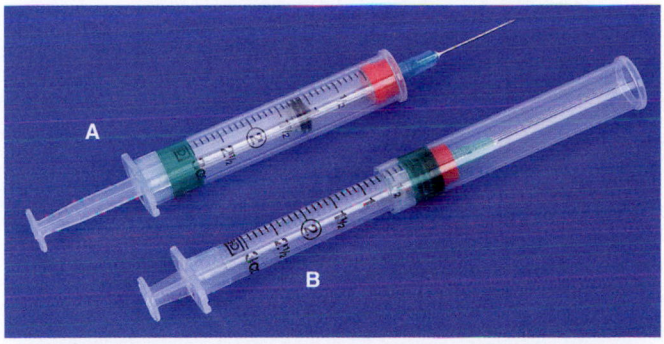

Safety syringe. *A*, Before injection. *B*, Cover slides up after injection.

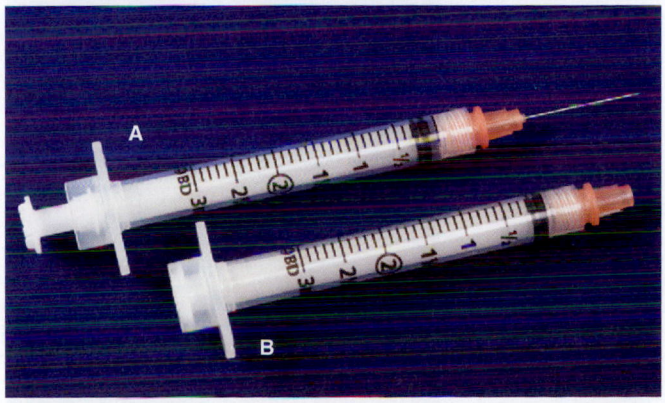

Safety syringe. *A*, Before injection. *B*, Needle retracted after injection.

Delegation

Delegation is not usually an issue because recapping needles is done in conjunction with administering parenteral medications, which you will usually not delegate. If you do delegate administration of parenteral medications to an LPN/LVN, you must supervise and evaluate recapping to ensure that the nurse uses proper technique.

Preparation

- **Assess the need to recap the needle.**
  Recap a contaminated needle only if doing so is absolutely unavoidable, according to Occupational Safety and Health Administration (OSHA) standards. As a rule, place a contaminated syringe and needle directly into a puncture-proof sharps container, without capping, bending, or breaking the needle.
- **Identify whether the needle is sterile or dirty.**
  Although a one-handed technique is used to recap both sterile and dirty needles, different considerations exist. When you use the one-handed method for recapping a sterile needle, it is easy to contaminate the needle without realizing it. You should modify the technique to help prevent that—the main consideration is to "protect" the needle. The danger in recapping a dirty needle is that you will stick yourself with it, exposing yourself to pathogens. The main consideration is to protect yourself.
- **Determine the availability of mechanical recapping device or safety syringe.**
  Always use a mechanical recapping device or safety syringe, if one is available. ◄

(continued on next page)

Procedure 26-10 ■ Recapping Needles Using a One-Handed Technique (continued)

Procedure 26-10A ■ Recapping Contaminated Needles

➤ When performing the procedure, always identify your patient according to agency policy, using two identifiers, and be attentive to standard precautions, hand hygiene, patient safety and privacy, body mechanics, and documentation.

Procedure Steps

1. **If you are using a safety needle,** engage the safety mechanism to cover the needle. (See Equipment.)
   OSHA regulations require the use of safety syringes to prevent needlestick injuries. You must engage the safety mechanism before placing the needle and syringe into the sharps container.
2. **Alternatively, place the needle** cap in mechanical recapping device, if one is available. (See Equipment.)
3. **If a mechanical recapping device** is not available, use the one-handed scoop method to recap the needle.
   a. Place the needle cover on a flat surface.
   Keeps the needle cover from rolling during the needle capping procedure. ▼

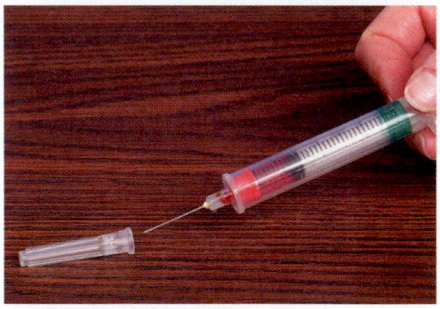

   b. Then, holding syringe in your dominant hand, scoop the needle cap onto the needle. Tip the syringe vertically to slip the cover over the needle. Do not hold onto the needle cap with your nondominant hand while scooping.
   A mechanical recapping device protects against accidental needlestick injury. If it is unavailable, the one-handed method of recapping will prevent accidental injuries when your own or the patient's safety is a concern. ▼

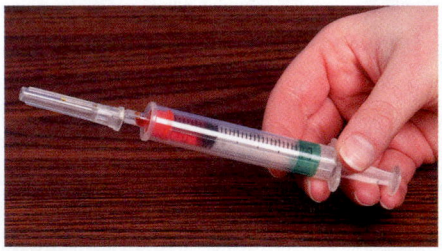

   c. Secure the needle cap by grasping it near the hub.
   Prevents an accidental stick if the needle goes through the needle cap. Needles are sharp enough to go through the needle cap if inserted at an angle. ▼

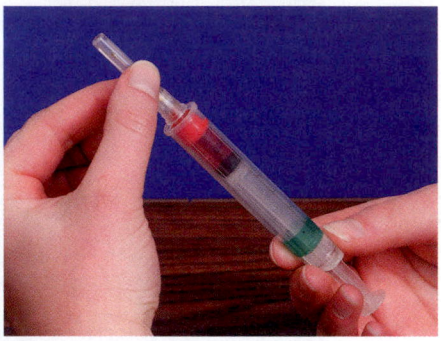

Procedure 26-10B ■ Recapping Sterile Needles

➤ When performing the procedure, always identify your patient according to agency policy, using two identifiers, and be attentive to standard precautions, hand hygiene, patient safety and privacy, body mechanics, and documentation.

➤ Use one of the following techniques to ensure that you do not contaminate a sterile needle. If you contaminate the needle, microorganisms will be introduced with the injection.

Procedure Steps

1. **Place the needle cap** in a mechanical recapping device, if one is available.
   The device is specially developed to provide safe recapping.
2. **Alternative method: Medication cup.** Place the cap into a small liquid medication cup with the open end facing up. You can then insert the sterile needle into the cap, keeping your free hand well away from the cup.
   This step performs the same function as a mechanical recapping device. The needle and cover need to be taller than the cup you are using, so that the open end of the cap protrudes above the cup. ➤

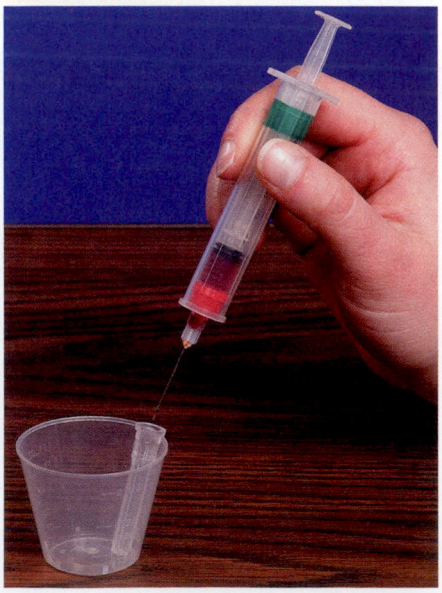

3. **Alternative method: Scoop technique.** Place the cap on a clean surface so that the end of the needle cap protrudes over the edge of the counter or shelf, and scoop with the needle; keep your free hand well away from the needle and cap as you are recapping.
This method prevents you from inadvertently hitting an unsterile surface with the needle.

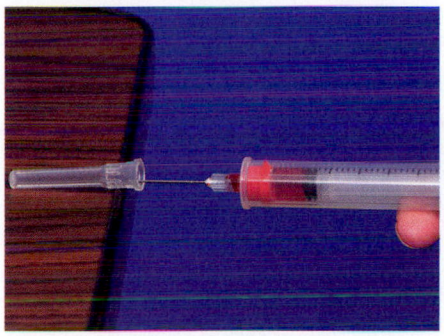

4. **Alternative method: Tubular container.** If the syringe is packaged in a hard plastic tubular container, stand the container on its large end; invert the needle cap; and place it in the top of the hard container. Insert the needle downward into the cap.

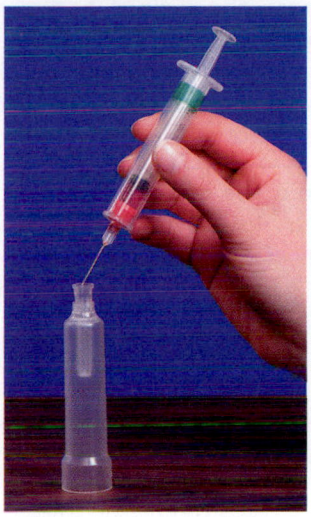

5. **Alternative method: Alcohol wipe.** Place the needle cap on a sterile surface, such as on an open alcohol prep pad, and use the one-handed scoop technique. Be very careful not to touch anything with the needle other than the inside of the needle cap.
The alcohol prep pad provides a sterile barrier. Because you must bring the needle parallel to the flat surface, and because the alcohol pad is so small, it is easy to contaminate the needle using this method.

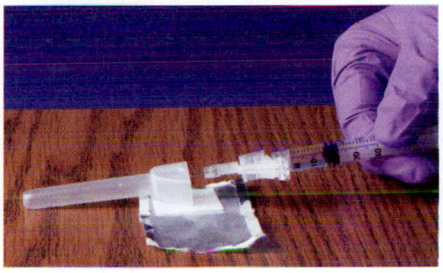

Documentation

No documentation needed for recapping needles.

Practice Resources

U.S. Department of Health and Human Services (USDHHS) (2012); Wagar, S., Siraj, M., Razzaq, Z., et al. (2011).

Procedure 26-11 ■ Administering Intradermal Medication

➤ For steps to follow in *all* procedures, refer to the Universal Steps for All Procedures found on the inside back cover. Also refer to Medication Guidelines: Steps to Follow for All Medications (Regardless of Type or Route).

Equipment

- Alcohol prep pad or CHG-alcohol product
- 2 in. × 2 in. gauze pad
- Pen (ink or felt)
- 1-mL syringe (tuberculin) with intradermal needle (25- to 28-gauge, ¼- to ⅝-inch with short bevel)

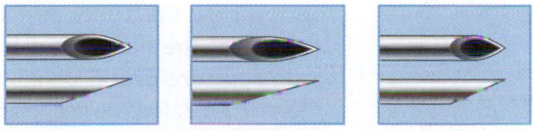

Regular bevel | Intermediate bevel | Short bevel

Delegation

As an RN, you can usually delegate administration of parenteral medications to an LPN/LVN. You usually cannot delegate this task to a NAP.

Pre-Procedure Assessments

- Assess for allergies, previous reaction to skin testing, and the skin for signs of irritation (e.g., bruising, swelling, tenderness).
Some skin tests, such as the tuberculin test, should not be repeated after positive test results.
Do not give intradermal skin tests if skin abnormalities are present. Also avoid giving them in areas where reading the results may be difficult, such as areas of heavy hair growth.

Preparation

- Have appropriate antidotes (usually epinephrine hydrochloride, a bronchodilator, and an antihistamine) readily available before the start of the procedure.
Because many intradermal injections are used for allergy testing, this is an important consideration.
- Know the location of resuscitation equipment (artificial airway, Ambu bag, and code cart)
Allergic reactions can be fatal.

➤ When performing the procedure, always identify your patient according to agency policy, using two identifiers, and be attentive to standard precautions, hand hygiene, patient safety and privacy, body mechanics, and documentation.

(continued on next page)

Procedure 26-11 ■ Administering Intradermal Medication (continued)

Procedure Steps

1. **Draw up the medication** from the vial (see Procedure 26-9B). The usual dose is 0.01 to 0.1 mL.
   Intradermal sites can only accommodate small volumes of medication.

2. **Select the site for injection.** Usual sites are the ventral surface of the forearm and upper back. The upper chest may also be used. If you need to review site locations,

   Go to Chapter 26, **Figure 26-23,** in Volume 1.

   Use areas where subcutaneous fat is less likely to interfere with administration and absorption. The forearm is the standard initial starting point because it has the least amount of subcutaneous tissue. The forearm and upper back usually have little hair, permitting easier visualization to interpret results accurately.

3. **Assist the patient to a** comfortable position. If you are using the forearm, instruct her to extend and supinate her arm on a flat surface. If you are using the upper back, ask the patient to lie prone or lean forward over a table or the back of a chair.
   This method stabilizes the injection site. The procedure will be more comfortable if the patient is able to relax his muscles. Tension, in general, increases pain perception.

4. **Don procedure gloves.**
   Procedure gloves are not required by OSHA for intradermal injections, but they are recommended by the CDC to prevent accidental exposure to bloodborne pathogens.

   Remember, gloves cannot prevent needlestick injuries.

5. **Scrub the injection site** with an alcohol prep pad or CHG-alcohol product pad. For an alcohol product, circle from the center of the site outward. For CHG products, use a back and forth motion. Allow the site to dry before administering the injection.
   Cleansing to remove microorganisms follows the principle of "clean to dirty." Alcohol can interfere with the test results if a small amount is introduced during the injection. Also, if the alcohol has not evaporated, it may cause the skin to sting during the injection.

6. **Grasp the syringe between** the thumb and index finger of your dominant hand, and uncap the needle.
   Enables you to administer the solution at the correct angle.

7. **Hold the client's skin taut** with your nondominant hand, by using one of the following methods:
   a. Place your hand under the client's arm and pull the skin tight with your thumb and fingers.
   b. Stretch the client's skin between your thumb and index finger.
   c. Pull the client's skin toward the wrist or down with one finger.
   A downward motion while stretching the skin eases needle insertion. Holding the skin tight can be difficult because of the low angle of administration.

8. **Continuing to hold the client's skin** taut with your nondominant hand, hold the syringe in your dominant hand with the needle bevel up and parallel to the client's skin at a 5° to 15° angle. Slowly insert the needle. There is some controversy about whether it is better to have the bevel down or up; however, the CDC recommends bevel up.
   The low angle of insertion is necessary to place the needle tip in the intradermal layer instead of the subcutaneous tissue. Having the bevel up likely decreases the chance of injecting the medication deeper into the subcutaneous tissue. Patients receiving intradermal injections report bevel up more comfortable. ▼

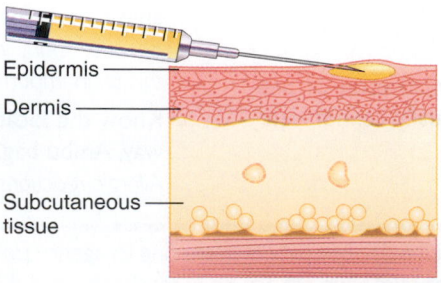

9. **Advance the needle** approximately 3 mm (⅛ in.) so that the entire bevel is covered. The bevel should be visible just under the skin.
   If the entire bevel is not inserted, the solution will leak out of the tissue. If you can see the bevel under the surface of the skin, you can be sure that the bevel is not in the subcutaneous tissue.

10. **Do not aspirate.** Hold the syringe stable with your nondominant hand.

11. **Release the taut skin and slowly inject the solution.** You should feel firm resistance. A pale wheal, about 6 to 10 mm (¼ in.) in diameter, will appear over the needle bevel.
    The dermis does not have room to absorb the solution, so a wheal forms, stretching the skin. Slow administration gives you time to terminate the injection should a systemic reaction occur. If a bleb (wheal) forms, you have administered the drug properly. The size of the bleb depends on the amount of medication you injected. ▼

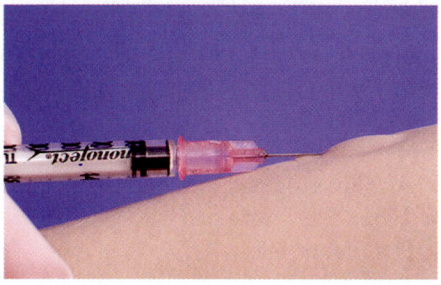

12. **Remove the needle** from the skin, engage the safety device, and dispose of the needle in a biohazard, puncture-proof container. If there is no safety device, place the uncapped syringe and needle directly in a biohazard, puncture-proof container.
    Prevents needlestick injuries.

13. **Gently blot any blood** with a dry gauze pad. Do not rub the skin or cover it with an adhesive bandage.
    Rubbing may cause the drug to leak out and alter absorption. An adhesive bandage can cause irritation and interfere with the skin test.

14. **With a pen, draw a 1-inch circle** around the bleb/wheal.
Marking the site helps you to identify any change in the size of the wheal at a later time.

? What if . . .

- **My patient has a history of a skin reaction to PPD testing?**
  Obtain details about the type and severity of the reaction. If the previous reaction involved ulceration at the site, further Mantoux testing is contraindicated. Report this to the prescriber.
- **My patient is pregnant, is receiving chemotherapy, or has severe eczema?**
  Defer tuberculosis skin testing and inform the prescriber.
- **My patient received a live vaccine at the time of tuberculosis skin testing?**
  Tuberculosis skin testing should be deferred for one month after live viral vaccines or other major viral infection.
- **My patient has topical anesthetic cream on the skin?**
  Use a site where the topical anesthetic cream was not applied or reschedule tuberculosis skin testing for another date.

Evaluation

- Reassess the client 5 and 15 minutes after administration for allergic reactions that may subsequently occur.
- Read the site within 48 to 72 hours of injection, depending on the test.
- Observe that a wheal (about 6 to 8 mm in diameter) forms at the site and that it gradually disappears.
- Observe for minimal bruising that may develop at the site of injection.

Patient Teaching

- Explain when the patient needs to have the intradermal injection read to determine whether the result is positive or negative.
- Explain that mild itching, swelling, or irritation may occur at the injection site and is normal.
  If the patient has antigens to the injected solution, a histamine response occurs, causing itching, swelling, or irritation. This response generally subsides within a week.
- Discuss the significance of a positive or negative skin test result. Explain that some signs of irritation may occur that do not mean a positive test result.
- Instruct the patient not to scratch, apply lotions or creams, cover the site with a bandage, or scrub the site.
  This might cause irritation and interfere with the test, which may produce false-positive results.

Documentation

- See the information in Medication Guidelines: Steps to Follow for All Medication (Regardless of Type or Route).
- Some medications require documentation of lot numbers (check agency policy).
- Chart when the test is to be read.

Sample documentation

mm/dd/yyyy 0800 *Explained purpose and procedure for Mantoux skin test. Client stated, "I need a PPD so that I can go to the long term care facility." 0.2 mL of tuberculin purified protein placed in left forearm per physician order. No reaction noted 5 minutes after procedure. Will read test at 0800 on mm/dd/yyyy.* M. Saleh, RN

Thinking About the Procedure

To practice applying clinical reasoning to this procedure,

Go to *Davis's Nursing Skills Videos*, **Administering Intradermal Medication.**

For questions and suggested responses,

Go to Chapter 26, **Thinking About the Procedure Questions and Suggested Responses,** on Davis*Plus*.

Practice Resources

National Center for HIV, STD, and TB Prevention, Division of Tuberculosis Elimination (2008, updated 2012); CDC (2011a).

Procedure 26-12 ■ Administering Subcutaneous Medication

➤ For steps to follow in *all* procedures, refer to the Universal Steps for All Procedures found on the inside back cover. Also refer to Medication Guidelines: Steps to Follow for All Medications (Regardless of Type or Route).

Equipment

- Syringe and needle appropriate for volume and site
- Alcohol prep pad or CHG-alcohol product
- Gauze pad (optional)

Delegation

As an RN, you can usually delegate administration of parenteral medications to an LPN/LVN. You usually cannot delegate this task to a NAP.

Pre-Procedure Assessments

- Check the selected site for inflammation, bruising, lumps, or other abnormalities that may contraindicate use of the site.
- Check the area for previous injection sites.
  Alternating among the arms, thighs, abdomen, and back changes the absorption rate of the medication. Absorption is fastest from the abdomen, then the arms, and lastly the thighs and back. Rotate sites within the same extremity or location, approximately 1 inch from the previous injection. Rotating the site helps prevent fat deposits and skin lumps.
- Do focused assessments for the specific medication being administered.

  Insulin—Check capillary blood sugar level, and determine when the patient will be having the next meal; check for signs of hypoglycemia or hyperglycemia.
  Insulin must be balanced with food intake to prevent the patient from developing hypoglycemia or hyperglycemia. Different insulins have specific rates of absorption, peak action, and duration. Some insulins, such as Humalog and regular insulin, are rapid acting. Before you administer rapid-acting insulin, the capillary blood sugar must be within the normal range or above, and the patient must be ready to eat. With Humalog, the patient's food tray should be in front of him before you administer the insulin.

  Heparin—Check activated partial thromboplastin time (aPTT) and for signs of overt bleeding (e.g., bleeding from gums, IV injection sites) and covert bleeding (e.g., blood in urine and stool)
  Heparin is an anticoagulant, so the major side effect is bleeding.

  Note: The aPTT will not be monitored as frequently with the low-molecular-weight heparins (LMWHs), because bleeding is less likely to occur.

➤ When performing the procedure, always identify your patient according to agency policy, using two identifiers, and be attentive to standard precautions, hand hygiene, patient safety and privacy, body mechanics, and documentation.

Procedure Steps

1. **Select an appropriate syringe** and needle.
   a. For insulin administration, you must use an insulin syringe—typically 0.3, 0.5, or 1.0 mL. Most insulin needles are 28- to 31-gauge. Needle length is often $^{3}/_{16}$- to 1-inch. For more information about giving insulin, see Clinical Insight 26-5.

   ✚ Although both insulin and tuberculin (TB) syringes come in a 1-mL size, they are not interchangeable. Insulin syringes are calibrated in units; they have a permanent (non-removable) needle and a very small amount of dead space.

   b. For other medications, for volumes less than 1 mL, use a tuberculin (TB) syringe with a 25- to 27-gauge, $^{3}/_{8}$- to $^{5}/_{8}$-inch needle.
   Because of the small increments on the TB syringe, small doses can be measured more accurately. ▼

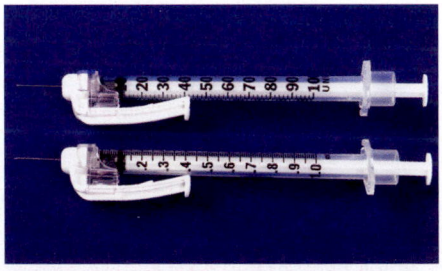

Top: Insulin syringe. *Bottom:* TB syringe.

   c. For administering a volume of 1 mL, you may use a 3-mL syringe with a 25- to 27-gauge, $^{3}/_{8}$- to $^{5}/_{8}$-inch needle.
   Although you can measure 1 mL with a TB syringe, it will be difficult to handle the syringe because the plunger will be pulled back as far as it can go. It is easy to pull it inadvertently out of the end of the syringe. Some medications are supplied in prefilled syringes. Examples are enoxaparin sodium (Lovenox) and the other LMWHs.

2. **Draw up the medication.** See Procedure 26-9.

3. **Select an injection site** with adequate subcutaneous tissue. If you need to review site locations,

   Go to Chapter 26, **Figure 26-25,** in Volume 1.

   Helps you avoid accidentally injecting into the muscle.
   a. The usual sites are the outer aspect of the upper arms, abdomen (at least 2 inches away from the umbilicus), anterior aspects of the thighs, and high on the buttocks near waist level.

These areas usually have good circulation and are easily accessible. The buttocks are more convenient when someone is giving the injection other than the patient.

b. The anterolateral and posterolateral abdomen ("love handles") sites are the only subcutaneous site used for administering heparin or LMWHs. For more information about giving heparin, see Clinical Insight 26-6.

The tissue 2 inches away from the umbilicus poses less risk of bleeding when an anticoagulant is administered.

4. **Position the patient** so that the injection site is accessible and the patient is able to relax the appropriate area. Check the site for inflammation, bruising, lumps, or other abnormalities.

Avoid areas with skin abnormalities, which may alter the absorption rates or increase patient discomfort during the injection.

5. **Don procedure gloves.**

To prevent exposure to bloodborne pathogens. You may prefer to don gloves before Step 4.

6. **Scrub the injection site** with an alcohol prep pad or CHG-alcohol product. Allow the site to dry before administering the injection. For alcohol, circle from the site outward; for CHG, use a back-and-forth motion. Do not go back over already scrubbed areas.

7. **Remove the needle cap.**

The needle cap is more difficult to remove when using a one-handed technique.

8. **With your nondominant hand,** pinch the tissue at the injection site, and determine the angle at which to inject the needle. Insert the needle using a 45° to 90° angle, depending on the amount of adipose tissue (the less adipose tissue, the lower the angle). If the adipose tissue pinches 2 inches or more (client is obese), use a longer needle and spread the skin taut instead of pinching.

Grasping and lifting the tissue prevents you from accidentally injecting into the muscle. Also, the subcutaneous injection must be given in the fatty tissue and not into intradermal layer. Traditionally, injections had been given using a 45° angle to ensure medication is deposited into the subcutaneous layer. ▼

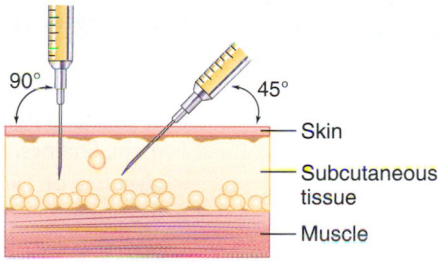

9. **Holding the syringe between** thumb and index finger of your dominant hand like a pencil or dart, insert the needle at the appropriate angle into the skinfold.

Quickly inserting the needle through the skin minimizes discomfort.

10. **Using the thumb or index finger** of your dominant hand, press the plunger slowly to inject the medication while stabilizing the syringe with your other hand. Alternatively, after inserting the needle, you can continue to hold the barrel with your dominant hand and use your nondominant hand to depress the plunger.

Slow administration allows the medication to disperse and decreases discomfort. Subcutaneous injections do not need to be aspirated beforehand, because accidental entry into a blood vessel is rare. Stabilize the syringe to avoid discomfort and tissue damage from the needle.

11. **Remove the needle** smoothly along the line of insertion.

Prevents pulling against the skin and tissue and thus minimizes discomfort.

12. **Gently blot the site with gauze** if needed. Do not massage the site unless directed to do so by prescription or policy.

Occasionally there will be blood at the site after the needle is removed. You might have nicked a surface blood vessel when you injected, and blood is following the needle track out to the surface. Massaging or rubbing the site will alter the rate of absorption of the medication.

13. **Engage the needle safety device,** and dispose of the needle in a biohazard container. If there is no safety device, place the uncapped syringe and needle directly into a biohazard, puncture-proof container.

A sharps container prevents needlestick injuries.

Evaluation

- Observe for minimal bruising that may develop at the site of injection.
- Reassess the patient for anticipated response and adverse reaction to medication.

  For insulin, observe for signs that patient's blood sugar level has returned to normal and for signs of hypoglycemia.

  For heparin, observe that patient has no signs of bleeding.

  For other medications, observe for side effects.

Patient Teaching

- Discuss possible lifestyle adaptations that the patient may need to undertake while receiving the medication (e.g., diet and exercise recommendations for managing diabetes mellitus).

Home Care

- Discuss with the client or caregiver the options for insulin administration to determine the most appropriate choice for the person administering the injections.

  Many options are available, including specially designed syringes that are easier to handle and read, pen injectors, and prefilled syringes.
- In the home environment, the client might not routinely use an alcohol wipe to cleanse the site. This is acceptable as long as the skin is clean.

  In the home environment there is less risk for superinfection with resistant strain organisms, and other hospital-acquired infections.

(continued on next page)

Procedure 26-12 ■ Administering Subcutaneous Medication (continued)

- Do not encourage reusing needles and syringes. However, if the client or caregiver believes they need to reuse syringes and needles in the home, teach them how to safely do so. Teach them the guidelines in Clinical Insight 26-1.

The very small insulin needles (30-gauge) bend very easily and are not recommended for reuse.

Determine whether reusing syringes is appropriate for the patient. Contraindications include inadequate hygiene, immunocompromised status, and difficulty handling equipment to prevent contamination of the needle.

Discuss safety concerns regarding subcutaneous medication administration in the home, such as how to dispose of biohazardous wastes correctly and where to obtain a puncture-proof biohazard container.

The patient or caregiver may use a large plastic bottle or a coffee can. Local regulations regarding disposal must be followed.

- Discuss with the patient the need to rotate sites and reasons for doing so. Recommend that he give injections at the same time of the day in the same body location about 1 inch from the previous injection site.
  Repeatedly giving the medication in the same site can cause abnormalities in the tissue and alter absorption rates.
- Remind the patient that when changing sites (thigh, arm, abdomen), the absorption rate may be altered.
- If the patient is receiving heparin or LMWHs, discuss the need to avoid nonsteroidal anti-inflammatory (NSAID) medications, such as acetylsalicylic acid (aspirin) and ibuprofen (Motrin, Advil).
  These drugs increase the risk of bleeding.
- For patients receiving heparin or LMWHs, discuss home safety and the need to avoid falls.
  The patient is at risk for bleeding and needs to follow safety guidelines to prevent injury.

Research shows that older females are more susceptible to hematomas after administration of LMWH (Nourbakhsh, Anvari, & Nugent, 2011). Nurses should carefully assess for abdominal bruising and complaints of abdominal pain.

Documentation

- Chart according to Medication Guidelines: Steps to Follow for All Medication (Regardless of Type or Route).
- Some agencies have a specific code for documenting subcutaneous injections, which allows exact site documentation on an outline of the body.
- In the nursing notes, document any related patient assessment findings, such as capillary blood sugar, signs of hypoglycemia or hyperglycemia, bruising, and so on.
- Document in the nursing notes as well as MAR any medication that was given PRN.

Sample EHR documentation

t, l Room: Code Status: Alerts:
Sex:F Age:47 Y Diet:ADA Diet High Fiber, Lo...
Drug Allergies: Codeine
Food Allergies: Shellfish
Primary Physician:
Env Allergies: Iodine
Isolation: HELP ?

Pt Sel | Logged In: Hiam, Judith | Documenting In Current Date/Time | Log Off

Patient Charting | Vital Signs | Order Entry | Order Review | Patient Teaching | Patient CARD | Patient Data | M.A.R. | Care Plans | Reports

Pharmacy | Laboratory | Radiology | PT/ST/OT | Nursing | Dietary

SubQ Per order Units

Insulin, Lente Human
Insulin, Lispro
Insulin, Lispro Protamine/Lispro
Insulin, Lispro Protamine/Lispro
Insulin, Novolin 70/30
Insulin, Novolin N
Insulin, Novolin R
Insulin, NovoLog
Insulin, NovoLog Mix 70/30
Insulin, NPH
Insulin, NPH/Regular 50/50
Insulin, NPH/Regular 70/30
Insulin, Regular
Insulin, Ultralente
Interferon Alfa 2b
Interferon Beta 1a
Interferon Beta 1b

Order Priority... Routine Now Stat!
Medication Route... SubQ
Medication Dose... Select...or Type Unit... Units
Medication Frequency As Needed (PRN)
Start Date/Time... Date: Today Time: 1000
Special Instructions... mm/dd/yyyy 1530 FSBS 162 Administered 2 units of Regular Insulin for blood sugar level of 162. Dose given in Left Upper Quadrant of abdomen. Will recheck blood sugar in one hour. Side rails up X2 and reminded client to call for assistance to get out of bed_____ B. Patel, RN

Add Order | Cancel

ORDER DESC					
Insulin, Regular SubQ	Per order	Units	One Time	Stat!	SS

Enter Orders... | Cancel Order...

Thinking About the Procedure

To practice applying clinical reasoning to this procedure,

Go to *Davis's Nursing Skills Videos*, **Administering Subcutaneous Medication.**

For questions and suggested responses,

Go to Chapter 26, **Thinking About the Procedure Questions and Suggested Responses,** on Davis*Plus*.

Practice Resources

Bartley, N. (2012); Nourbakhsh, E., Anvari, R, & Nugent, K. (2011); Pledger, J., Hicks, D., Kirkland, F., et al. (2012); Zaybak, A., & Khorshid, L. (2008).

Procedure 26-13 ■ Locating Intramuscular Injection Sites

➤ For steps to follow in *all* procedures, refer to the Universal Steps for All Procedures found on the inside back cover. Also refer to Medication Guidelines: Steps to Follow for All Medications (Regardless of Type or Route).

Delegation

As an RN, you can usually delegate administration of parenteral medications (including locating injection sites) to an LPN/LVN. You usually cannot delegate this task to a NAP. If you delegate the skill, you are responsible for evaluating the LPN/LVN's ability to locate injection sites correctly.

Pre-Procedure Assessment

Always palpate the landmarks and the muscle mass to ensure correct placement of the needle. Because patients' body shapes differ, the site locations will vary slightly.

Procedure 26-13A ■ Locating the Ventrogluteal Site

➤ When performing the procedure, always identify your patient according to agency policy, using two identifiers, and be attentive to standard precautions, hand hygiene, patient safety and privacy, body mechanics, and documentation.

Procedure Steps

1. **Ask the patient to assume a side-lying** position with the legs straight, if possible.
   This position makes the site easier to locate.

2. **Locate the greater trochanter,** anterior superior iliac spine, and the iliac crest. ➤

3. **Place the palm of your hand** on the greater trochanter, your index finger on the anterior superior iliac spine, and your middle finger pointing toward the iliac crest. (Use your right hand on the patient's left hip; use your left hand on the patient's right hip.) Note that if your hands are very large or very small, the location of the "triangle" will be higher or lower on the hip. Be sure you locate it well in the muscle mass.

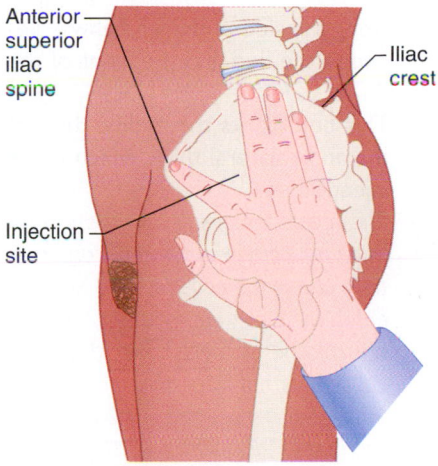

4. **The middle of the triangle** between your middle and index fingers is the injection site.
   This is a safe site for IM administration because it is not in close proximity to any major blood vessels or nerves. The landmarks are easy to find. This large muscle can take volumes up to 5 mL in the average adult. It is safe for patients of all ages and the preferred site for adults and children older than 7 to 12 months (there is some disagreement over the age; always palpate to assess adequacy of muscle mass, regardless of age). ▼

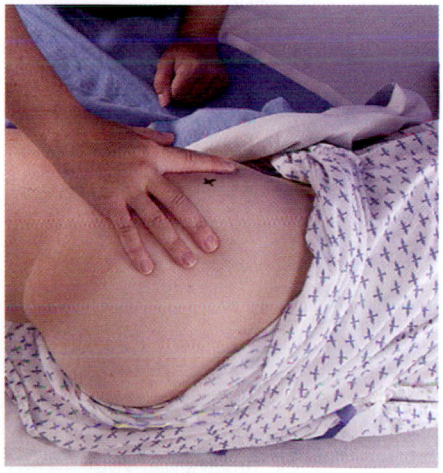

Procedure 26-13B ■ Locating the Deltoid Site

➤ When performing the procedure, always identify your patient according to agency policy, using two identifiers, and be attentive to standard precautions, hand hygiene, patient safety and privacy, body mechanics, and documentation.

Procedure Steps

1. **Completely expose the patient's** upper arm. Remove the garment; do not roll up the sleeve.
   Incomplete exposure of site and landmarks creates a risk of injecting into other than muscle tissue. This is a small site, and it is easy to make an error in location.

(continued on next page)

Procedure 26-13 ■ Locating Intramuscular Injection Sites (continued)

2. **Locate the lower edge** of the acromion process (knobby part of shoulder). This imaginary line forms the base of a triangle.▼

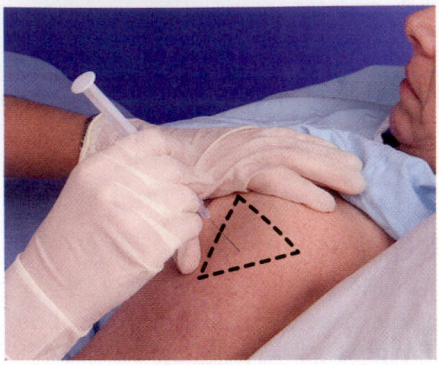

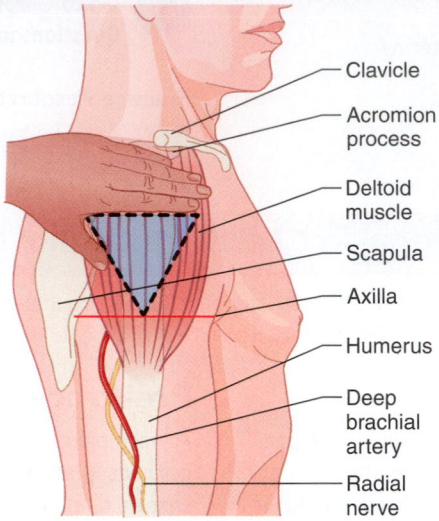

3. **Draw an imaginary line** from each end of the triangle base downward 1 to 2 in (3 to 5 cm) to the midpoint of the lateral arm.
4. **The deltoid site is in the center of the resulting** inverted triangle.
5. **An alternative approach** is to ◄ place four fingerbreadths across the deltoid muscle, with your top finger on the acromion process. The injection goes three fingerbreadths below the process in the midline of the upper arm.
   Locates the appropriate site while avoiding the radial nerve and deep brachial artery. Because it is a fairly small muscle, only 0.5 to 1 mL of medication can be administered.

Procedure 26-13C ■ Locating the Vastus Lateralis Site

➤ When performing the procedure, always identify your patient according to agency policy, using two identifiers, and be attentive to standard precautions, hand hygiene, patient safety and privacy, body mechanics, and documentation.

Procedure Steps

1. **Position the patient** lying supine or sitting.
   The patient may perceive the injection as less painful if supine because he cannot see the needle enter his leg. For some people this provokes anxiety and intensifies pain.
2. **Locate the greater trochanter** and the lateral femoral condyle.
3. **Place your hands on the thigh,** with one hand against the greater trochanter, and the other edge of hand against the lateral femoral condyle.
4. **Visualize a rectangle** between your hands across the anterolateral thigh.
   - The index fingers of your hands form the smaller ends of the rectangle.
   - The long sides of the rectangle are formed by (a) drawing an imaginary line down the center of the anterior thigh and (b) drawing another line along the side of the leg, halfway between the bed and the front of the thigh.
   - This box marks the middle third of the anterolateral thigh, which is the injection site.
     The rectus femoris lies on the top (or anterior) portion of the thigh and partially covers the edge of the vastus lateralis. Therefore, do not inject too near the midline of the anterior thigh. Because it is not near any major blood vessels or nerves, the vastus lateralis site is safe for patients of all ages and is the recommended site for children younger than 7 months.▼

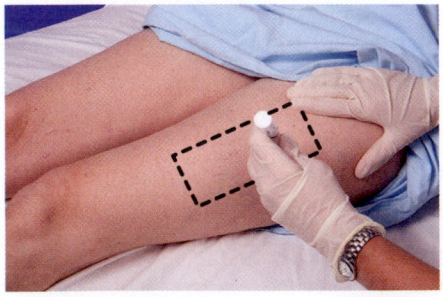

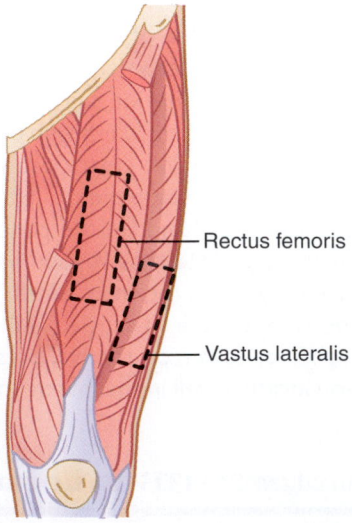

Procedure 26-13D ■ Locating the Rectus Femoris Site

➤ When performing the procedure, always identify your patient according to agency policy, using two identifiers, and be attentive to standard precautions, hand hygiene, patient safety and privacy, body mechanics, and documentation.

Procedure Steps

Use this site only if no other sites are accessible and no other medication routes are feasible.

1. **Position the patient** lying supine or sitting.
2. **Divide the top of the thigh** from the groin to the knee into thirds, and identify the middle third.
3. **Visualize a rectangle** in the middle of the anterior surface of the thigh. This is the location of the injection site. Also refer to the drawing of the adult thigh in Procedure 26-13C. ➤

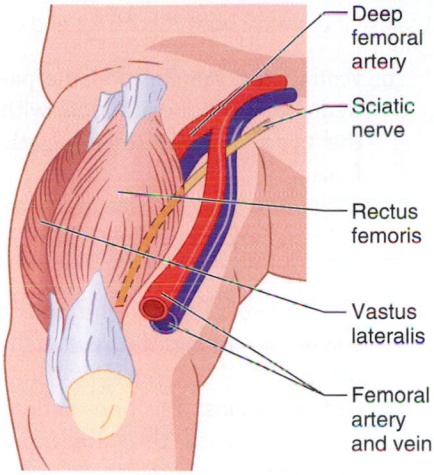

? What if . . .

- **My patient is a child. What is the best site to give an IM injection?**

  Because an infant's muscles are not fully developed, site selection is limited.

  For children who are walking, use the ventrogluteal site.

  For children who are not yet walking, use the vastus lateralis. Once the gluteal muscles are develop further, which occur with walking the ventrogluteal site can be used.

Thinking About the Procedure

To practice applying clinical reasoning to this procedure,

Go to *Davis's Nursing Skills Videos*, **Locating the Ventrogluteal Site; Locating the Deltoid Site; Locating the Vastus Lateralis Site;** and **Locating the Rectus Femoris Site.**

For questions and suggested responses,

Go to Chapter 26, **Thinking About the Procedure Questions and Suggested Responses,** on Davis*Plus*.

Procedure 26-14 ■ Administering an Intramuscular Injection

➤ For steps to follow in *all* procedures, refer to the Universal Steps for All Procedures found on the inside back cover. Also refer to Medication Guidelines: Steps to Follow for All Medications (Regardless of Type or Route).

➤ The z-track method is preferred for all IM injections, except in a rare instance in which it is contraindicated.

Equipment

- Syringe and needle appropriate for volume and site
- Alcohol prep pad or CHG-alcohol product
- Gauze pad or adhesive bandage
- Medication
- Procedure gloves
- Biohazard (sharps) container
- Small piece of gauze or cotton ball
- Small adhesive bandage

Delegation

As an RN, you can usually delegate administration of parenteral medications to an LPN/LVN. You cannot delegate this task to a NAP.

Pre-Procedure Assessments

- Identify the site of the previous injection.
- Assess the site for adequate muscle mass, bruises, edema, tenderness, redness, or other abnormalities.

  Muscle mass must be large enough to absorb the amount of medication prescribed. Abnormalities at the site increase patient discomfort and alter the absorption rate of the medication.
- Assess for factors that might affect absorption of the medication, such as decreased intramuscular blood flow, as found in shock or muscle atrophy.

  Decreased peripheral circulation or muscle atrophy decreases the absorption of the medication.

(continued on next page)

Procedure 26-14 ■ Administering an Intramuscular Injection (continued)

Procedure 26-14A ■ Intramuscular Injection: Traditional Method

➤ When performing the procedure, always identify your patient according to agency policy, using two identifiers, and be attentive to standard precautions, hand hygiene, patient safety and privacy, body mechanics, and documentation.

Procedure Steps

1. **Select the appropriate syringe** and needle.
   a. The usual syringe size is 1 to 3 mL, depending on volume of medication to be given. For doses less than 1 mL, you can use a tuberculin syringe with an intramuscular needle.
   b. The needle size is usually 21- to 25-gauge, 1½ inch in length for adults (or 1 in. for deltoid site), but a longer needle (3 in.) might be necessary to penetrate the muscle if the patient is obese.
   For IM administration, the needle gauge must be appropriate for the viscosity of the medication, and the needle must be long enough to deliver the medication into the muscle.
   c. Some medications are supplied in prefilled syringes, which are used for administration.

2. **Draw up the medication** (see Procedure 26-9A) or obtain prescribed unit dose and verify medication. If the volume for injection is more than 3 to 5 milliliters, divide the dose for separate injections.

3. **Don procedure gloves.**
   Procedure gloves are required by OSHA to prevent exposure to bloodborne pathogens. You may prefer to don gloves at Step 6, while waiting for the antiseptic to dry.

4. **Position the patient** so that the injection site is well exposed and the patient is able to relax the appropriate muscles. Be sure the lighting is adequate.
   When the patient's muscles are relaxed (and not tense), it is easier to perform the injection and it reduces patient discomfort during injection. You must be able to fully visualize and safely access the site.
   a. *Deltoid site:* Position the patient with the arm relaxed at the side or resting on a firm surface, and completely expose the upper arm.
   b. *Ventrogluteal site:* Position the patient on the opposite side, with the upper hip and knee slightly flexed.
   This position may cause the trochanter to become more prominent, making it easier to locate the site.
   c. *Vastus lateralis:* Position the patient supine or sitting, if the patient prefers.
   d. *Rectus femoris:* Position patient supine. Because this site often causes more discomfort than others, use it only if all other sites are inaccessible and no other route is feasible.
   e. ✚ *Dorsogluteal:* Do not use this site because of the muscle's proximity to the sciatic nerve and major blood vessels.

5. **Using appropriate landmarks,** identify the injection site (see Procedure 26-13). If the client is to receive more than one injection, rotate sites.
   Volumes of 1 to 5 mL may be given, depending on the muscle size (for adults, 0.5 to 1 mL in the deltoid; and typically 1 to 3 mL but up to 5 mL in the vastus lateralis site). If the volume for injection is more than 3 to 5 mL, then divide the dose for a separate injection. Rotating sites reduces discomfort and tissue trauma.

6. **Gently, but vigorously scrub the injection site.** Do not "go back over" already cleansed areas.
   a. If using an alcohol prep pad scrub by circling from the center of the site outward.
   b. If using a CHG-based antiseptic, use a back and forth motion.
   Cleanse to remove microorganisms; follow the principle of "clean to dirty."

7. **Place the wipe on the patient's** skin outside the injection site, with a corner pointing to the site. Allow the site to dry before administering the injection. Do not fan the site.
   Leaving the antiseptic prep pad on the skin with a corner pointing to the injection site helps identify the location for the injection. If the antiseptic has not evaporated, it may cause the skin to sting during injection.

8. **Remove the needle cap.**

9. **With your nondominant hand,** spread the skin taut between your thumb and index finger.
   It is quicker, easier, and less painful to insert a needle through the skin that is taut.

10. **Tell the patient what** you are going to do and that he will feel a prick as you insert the needle. Then hold the syringe between thumb and fingers of your dominant hand like a pencil or dart and insert the needle at a 90° angle to the skin surface. Insert fully.
    Quickly inserting the needle through the skin minimizes discomfort. A 90° angle is needed for the needle to penetrate through the subcutaneous and adipose tissue to the muscle.

11. **Stabilize the syringe** with your nondominant hand.
    This prevents the needle from moving around in the tissue, thereby causing discomfort and possible tissue trauma.

12. **Aspirate by pulling back** on the plunger and waiting for 5 to 10 seconds. If you obtain a blood return, remove the needle, discard the syringe, and prepare the medication again. If there is no blood return, continue with Step 13.
    Aspirating blood indicates that the needle is in a blood vessel. Injecting would result in administering the medication intravenously instead of intramuscularly. If the needle is in a small vessel, it may take a few seconds for the blood to appear in the syringe. **Key Point:** ***There are variations in practice regarding the requirement to aspirate for blood. Be sure to check with your instructor or the institution's protocol for the recommended method.***

13. **Using the thumb or index** finger of your dominant hand, press the plunger slowly to inject the medication (5 to 10 sec/mL).
Slow administration allows the medication to disperse and decreases discomfort.

14. **Remove the needle** smoothly along the line of insertion.
Removing the needle in this way prevents pulling against the skin and tissue and minimizes discomfort.

15. **Engage the safety needle** device, and dispose of the entire syringe in a biohazard container. If there is no safety device, place the uncapped syringe and needle directly into a biohazard puncture-proof container.
The biohazard sharps container prevents needlestick injuries.

16. **Gently blot the site** with a gauze pad, and apply an adhesive bandage as needed.
Apply pressure to stop the bleeding but do not massage or rub the site after IM injection. This can cause medication to disperse into the subcutaneous tissue where the needle was injected, which might be irritating to the tissue.

Procedure 26-14B ■ Intramuscular Injection: Z-Track Method

➤ When performing the procedure, always identify your patient according to agency policy, using two identifiers, and be attentive to standard precautions, hand hygiene, patient safety and privacy, body mechanics, and documentation.

Procedure Steps

1–8. Follow Procedure 26-14A, traditional method, preceding.

Step 5 Variation. For Z-Track Method, use the larger muscles:

a. *Ventrogluteal site:* Position patient on the side with upper hip and knee slightly flexed.
b. *Vastus lateralis:* Position patient supine or sitting.

9. **With the side of your** nondominant hand, displace the skin away from the injection site, about 2.5 to 3.5 cm (1 to 1.5 in.).
This displaces the skin and subcutaneous tissue over the muscle, so that when it is released after the injection, the medication is sealed in the muscle.

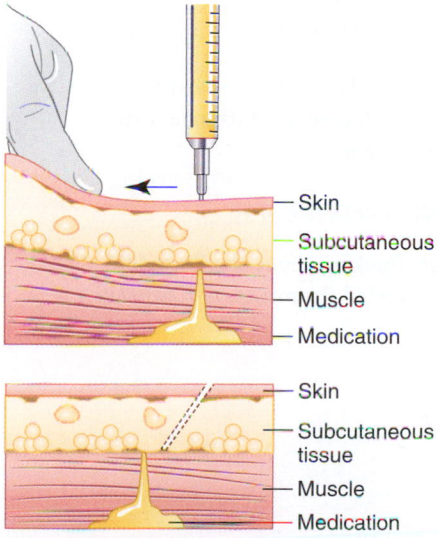

10. **Holding the syringe between** the thumb and fingers of your dominant hand like a pencil or dart, insert the needle at a 90° angle to the skin surface. Insert smoothly, quickly, and fully.
Quickly inserting the needle through the skin minimizes discomfort. A 90° angle is needed for the needle to penetrate through the subcutaneous and adipose tissue to the muscle.

11. **Stabilize the syringe** with the thumb and forefinger of your nondominant hand while continuing to displace the skin with your other three fingers. Do not release the skin to stabilize the syringe.
Stabilizing the needle reduces discomfort and possible tissue injury. You must keep the skin retracted to create a seal after the medication is injected and the skin released.

12. **Aspirate by pulling back slightly** on the plunger for 5 to 10 seconds. If you obtain a blood return, remove the needle, discard the syringe, and prepare the medication again.
Aspirating blood indicates that the needle has penetrated a vein. Continuing could result in administering the medication intravenously instead of intramuscularly. Practice varies on whether to aspirate, so follow institutional policy.

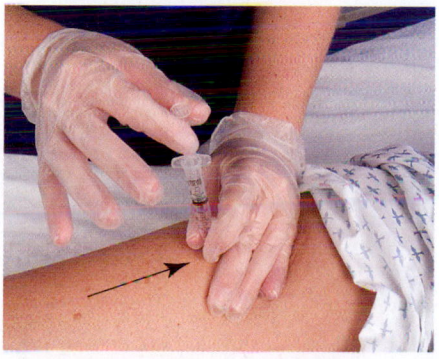

13. **Using the thumb or index** finger of your dominant hand, press the plunger slowly to inject the medication (5 to 10 sec/mL).
Slow administration allows the medication to disperse and decreases discomfort.

14. **Wait for 10 seconds**, then withdraw the needle smoothly along the line of insertion, then immediately release the skin.
Waiting before withdrawing the needle leaves a zigzag needle track that traps the medication in the muscle, preventing it from leaking up into the subcutaneous tissue.

15. **Engage the safety needle device**, and dispose of it in a biohazard container. If there is no safety device, place the uncapped syringe and needle directly in a biohazard puncture-proof container.

16. **Hold a cotton ball** or gauze pad with light pressure over the injection site. Do not massage the site. Apply an adhesive bandage if necessary.
Light pressure will stop superficial bleeding at the injection site. Massaging and rubbing can force medication into the subcutaneous tissues.

? What if . . .

- **My patient is unable to cooperate during the procedure?**
Ask another healthcare provider or family member to help keep the patient from moving during the injection or to help position the patient.

(continued on next page)

Procedure 26-14 ■ Administering an Intramuscular Injection (continued)

■ **My patient is a child; is there anything different about giving an IM injection?**

Adapt the procedure to decrease pain: Apply topical anesthetic cream (e.g., EMLA) or a topical cooling spray if time permits. If not, distract the child with conversation, or give him something to do, such as squeeze a hand. Or apply a cold compress over the site.

Adapt the way you spread the skin to inject: In infants and small children, grasp the muscle with your thumb and index finger; in obese children, spread the skin and then grasp the muscle.

Adapt the medication volume: Inject no more than 1 mL in a single injection, 0.5 mL in a small infant.

Be aware of the controversy about needle size: The CDC recommends 1- and 1¼-inch needles for children 1 year old or younger. Follow agency procedures.

■ **My patient is an older adult?**

Many older adults have decreased muscle mass, so use a shorter needle; spread the skin and grasp the muscle to localize and stabilize the site for injection.

Older adults tend to bleed from the site after injection because of reduced tissue elasticity. Apply a small pressure bandage if needed.

Evaluation

- Observe for minimal bruising or oozing that may occur at the site of injection.
- Observe for local reactions at site (e.g., pain, swelling, redness).

Home Care

- Discuss safety concerns with administering medication intramuscularly in the home, such as correct disposal of biohazardous wastes and where to obtain a puncture-proof biohazard container.
  The caregiver or patient can use a large plastic bottle. The local regulations must be followed for disposal.
- Discuss with the client the need to rotate sites.
  Repeatedly giving the medication in the same site can cause abnormalities in the tissue and alter absorption rates.

Documentation

- Refer to Medication Guidelines: Steps to Follow for All Medications (Regardless of Type or Route).
- Document related assessment findings, such as pain level or presence of nausea.
- Unless the medication is prn, you will typically document it only on the MAR.

Sample documentation for PRN medication:

mm/dd/yyyy 1600 Client reports of nausea after ambulating 150 feet with assistive device. Phenergan 25 mg administered IM in right ventrogluteal site. No complaints of pain or discomfort. See MAR
M. Santos, RN

mm/dd/yyyy 1700 Client reports "I don't feel like I'm going to vomit anymore."
M. Santos, RN

Practice Resources

Advisory Committee on Immunization Practices (ACIP) (n.d.); CDC (n.d.); Bartley, N. (2012); Walsh, L., & Brophy, K. (2011).

Thinking About the Procedure

To practice applying clinical reasoning to this procedure,

Go to *Davis's Nursing Skills Videos*, **Intramuscular Injection: Traditional Method** and **Intramuscular Injection: Z-Track Method.**

For questions and suggested responses,

Go to Chapter 26, **Thinking About the Procedure Questions and Suggested Responses,** on Davis*Plus*.

Procedure 26-15 ■ Adding Medications to Intravenous Fluids

➤ For steps to follow in *all* procedures, refer to the Universal Steps for All Procedures found on the inside back cover. Also refer to Medication Guidelines: Steps to Follow for All Medications (Regardless of Type or Route).

Equipment

- Prescribed IV solution
- Syringe for measuring medication
- Needleless access device or safety needle (if a VAD is not available)
- Antimicrobial swab
- Label with medication, dose, date, time, and your initials

Delegation

As an RN, you would not usually delegate adding medications to IV fluids to LPN/LVNs. Nurse Practice Acts governing IV medication administration vary from state to state, and policies can further vary among healthcare agencies regarding which additives may be added by LPN/LVNs. Even if you delegate the skill, you are always responsible for evaluating the patient's responses, both therapeutic effects and adverse effects.

Pre-Procedure Assessments

- Assess the patency of the IV site.
- Assess the appearance of the IV site.
- Check the medication insert or PDR for appropriate time or rate for infusion and for preparation.

Procedure 26-15A ■ Adding Medication to a New IV Bag or Bottle

➤ When performing the procedure, always identify your patient according to agency policy, using two identifiers, and be attentive to standard precautions, hand hygiene, patient safety and privacy, body mechanics, and documentation.

Procedure Steps

1. **Determine whether** the medication(s) are compatible with the IV solution and with each other.
   Not all medications or other additives can be mixed with the glucose or saline normally found in the primary IV bag. Multiple additives increase the possibility of incompatibility.
2. **Calculate or verify the amount** of medication to be instilled into the IV solution, and the rate of administration.
   Verifying the dose and the rate of infusion prevents medication errors.
3. **Remove any protective covers,** and inspect the bag or bottle for leaks, tears, or cracks. Inspect the fluid for clarity, color, and presence of any particulate matter. Check the expiration date.
   Double-checking the IV solution reduces the risk of infusing contaminated or expired solutions.
4. **Using the appropriate technique,** draw up the prescribed medication (see Procedures 26-9, as needed). Alternatively, insert a VAD transfer device into the medication vial.
   Medications can come in vials, ampules, or bags.
5. **Scrub all surfaces of the IV** additive port with an alcohol or CHG-alcohol combination product.
   Diligent scrubbing with antimicrobial products reduces the transmission of microorganisms and helps maintain the sterility of the solution.
6. **Remove the cap from** the syringe, insert the needle or the needleless access device into the injection port, and inject the medication into the bag, maintaining aseptic technique.▼

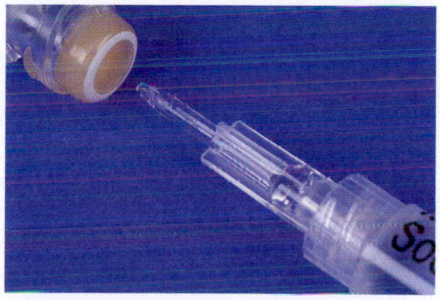

7. **Mix the IV solution and** medication by gently turning the bag from end to end.
   Ensures even distribution of the medication or additive into the solution.
8. **Place a label on the bag** so that it can be read when the bag is hung; include the medication name, dose, route, and your name. Be sure the label does not cover the solution label or volume marks.
   A label informs you and others of additives to IV solutions.▼

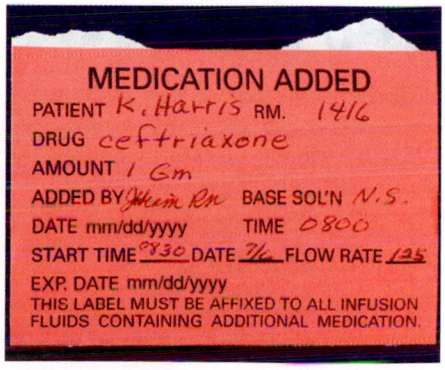
MEDICATION ADDED
PATIENT K. Harris RM. 1416
DRUG ceftriaxone
AMOUNT 1 Gm
ADDED BY [illegible] RN BASE SOL'N N.S.
DATE mm/dd/yyyy TIME 0800
START TIME 0930 DATE 7/6 FLOW RATE 125
EXP. DATE mm/dd/yyyy
THIS LABEL MUST BE AFFIXED TO ALL INFUSION FLUIDS CONTAINING ADDITIONAL MEDICATION.

9. **Dispose of used equipment,** syringe, or VAD appropriately.

(continued on next page)

Procedure 26-15 ■ Adding Medications to Intravenous Fluids (continued)

Procedure 26-15B ■ Adding Medication to an Infusing IV

➤ When performing the procedure, always identify your patient according to agency policy, using two identifiers, and be attentive to standard precautions, hand hygiene, patient safety and privacy, body mechanics, and documentation.

1. **Determine the compatibility** of the medication being added to the existing solution.
   Not all medications and solutions are compatible.

2. **Note the volume** in the existing IV bag and the amount needed for dilution of medication.
   Adequate solution is needed to dilute the medication.

3. **Clamp the running IV line.**
   Clamping prevents medication from directly infusing into the patient.

4. **Scrub all surfaces of the IV** additive port with the antimicrobial swab (alcohol or CHG-alcohol combination product).
   Vigorous scrubbing decreases the transmission of microorganisms and maintains the sterility of the solution.

5. **Remove the cap from** the syringe, insert the safety needle or the needleless VAD into the injection port, and inject the medication into the bag, maintaining aseptic technique. ➤

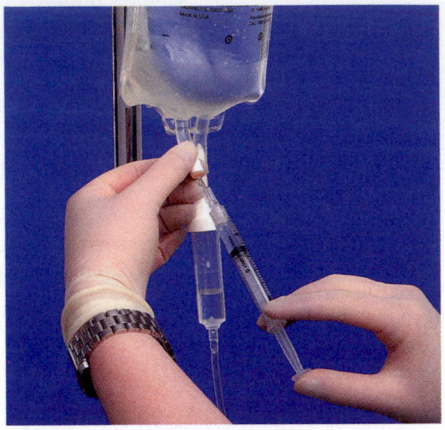

6. **Mix the IV solution and** medication by gently turning the bag from end to end. Keep the bag above the level of the patient's IV insertion site and do not invert the drip chamber.
   Turning the IV bag ensures even distribution of the medication or additive into the solution. Because of gravity, the height of the bag keeps blood from backing up in the IV tubing.

7. **Place the label on the bag** so that it can be read when the bag is hung. Be sure the label does not cover the solution label or volume marks.
   A label provides information regarding additives to IV solutions.

8. **Unclamp the IV line**, and run the IV at the prescribed rate.

9. **Dispose of used equipment**, syringe, needle, or VAD appropriately.

? What if . . .

- **The IV fluid infiltrates into a peripheral site.**

  Discontinue the infusion. Restart the peripheral IV, making sure you have good blood return and the line flushes easily. Some IVs are positional. This means the flow may be partially obstructed when the cannula in the vein lodges against the vein wall. In this case, the rate of the IV fluid to be delivered is likely to be compromised.

  If the tissue at the site of infiltration appears to be swollen and tender, you might apply a cool compress to the site. If the infusion contained irritating substances, such as calcium, dopamine, or various chemotherapy agents, you might need to contact the prescriber for an order to inject antidote medication into the intradermal layer.

Evaluation

- Check the IV line at least once every hour to ensure that the ordered or calculated rate is maintained.
- Assess the patient for complaints of pain at the infusion site.

Patient Teaching

- Discuss reasons the medication is being given intravenously.
- Let the patient know whether it is a continuous or intermittent infusion.
- Explain the need to report immediately any reactions to the medication, such as breathing problems, rashes, or pain at the IV insertion site.

Documentation

- Document information according to Medication Guidelines: Steps to Follow for All Procedures (Regardless of Type or Route).
- If you added medication to an existing IV setup, document related patient assessment findings, such as appearance of IV site and complaints of pain or discomfort during administration.
- Findings are usually documented on an IV flow record rather than in the nursing notes. Chart a nursing note only if there is something outside of the expected findings (e.g., if the IV has infiltrated).

Practice Resources

Infusion Nurses Society (INS) (2011a); Lavery, I. (2011).

Procedure 26-16 ■ Administering IV Push Medication

➤ For steps to follow in *all* procedures, refer to the Universal Steps for All Procedures found on the inside back cover. Also refer to Medication Guidelines: Steps to Follow for All Medications (Regardless of Type or Route).

Equipment

- Syringe appropriate for medication volume and the type of line (e.g., peripheral IV, PICC)
- If you are administering through an intermittent device:
  - Two 5- to 10-mL syringes, or one 10-mL syringe with 2 to 10 mL of normal saline or heparin for flushing the line. Heparin 100 units/mL rather than with saline solution is recommended (Bertolino, Pitassi, Tinelli, et al., 2012).
    Although either is acceptable, separate syringes pose less risk of contamination.
  - Depending on site and facility policy, one 5- to 10-mL syringe containing 2 to 5 mL of heparin flush (or saline) solution
    Evidence-based support and agency procedures differ: Some use saline to flush; others use heparin. New evidence recommends using heparin 100 units/mL (Bertolino, Pitassi, Tinelli, et al., 2012).
- Alcohol prep pad, or CHG-alcohol combination product and gauze pad
- Procedure gloves

Delegation

As an RN, you may, in some situations, be able to delegate administration of parenteral medications to an LPN/LVN. However, this is not a common practice.

Pre-Procedure Assessments

- Check the compatibility of the medication with the existing IV solution, if it is infusing.
  Medications can be physically or chemically incompatible with the IV solution. Physical incompatibility is often obvious because precipitation may occur. Chemical incompatibility is not obvious and may result in the medication's having a weaker or a stronger effect than anticipated.
- Assess the patency of the IV line.
  If the line is occluded, you will not be able to instill the medication.
- Check the site for redness, swelling, tenderness, and other signs of infiltration or phlebitis.
  Some medications are irritating and may be toxic to the tissue. If the IV line is infiltrated, the medication may leak into the tissue and cause injury. IV medications can also irritate the veins and cause phlebitis. Do not infuse a medication into a compromised site.

Procedure 26-16A ■ Administering IV Push Medications Through a Primary IV Line

➤ When performing the procedure, always identify your patient according to agency policy, using two identifiers, and be attentive to standard precautions, hand hygiene, patient safety and privacy, body mechanics, and documentation.

Procedure Steps

1. **Determine how fast the** medication may be administered and whether the medication needs to be diluted for administration. Also, check to be sure the medication is compatible with the solution infusing.
   IV push medications are frequently injected over 1 minute. Some must infuse over a longer time period, and some require diluting before administration. Giving an IV push medication too fast and/or undiluted can result in local or systemic adverse reactions.
2. **Prepare the medication** from a vial or ampule or obtain the prescribed unit dose and verify medication with the order (refer to Procedure 26-9). Dilute as needed. Temporarily pause the infusion pump to administer the medication. If the primary bag is infusing by gravity, simply clamp the tubing.
3. **Don procedure gloves** and thoroughly scrub all surfaces of the injection port closest to the patient with an alcohol prep pad or CHG-alcohol combination product.
   (1) Scrub time: Follow agency policy. Some facilities require nurses to cleanse the port for 1 minute when accessing venous access devices. (2) The port: Using the port closest to the patient minimizes the distance the medication must travel and gets it into the patient's circulation faster. You must use an injection port, which is self-sealing because if you puncture the plastic IV tubing, it will leak. (3) Scrub agent: Use povidone-iodine solution (Betadine) only if the patient is sensitive to alcohol or CHG-alcohol combination.
4. **Insert the medication syringe** into the injection port. If a needleless system is not available, use a syringe with a safety needle.
   Using a needleless system prevents needlestick injuries.
5. **Pinch or clamp the IV tubing** between the IV bag and the port.
   Occluding the tubing upline of the port prevents the medication from being injected back toward the IV bag. ▼

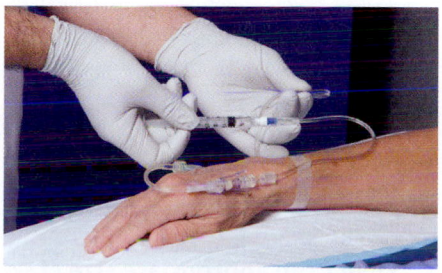

6. **Gently aspirate** by slowly pulling back on the plunger to check for a blood return. **NOTE:** Some newer connectors do not require or allow for aspiration. Follow institutional policy.
   (a) In tubing that allows for or requires aspiration, a blood return is one indication that the IV catheter is in the vein. An IV site may still be patent if no blood is returned, and an infiltrated IV line may have a blood return. Use the blood return as one indication of patency

(continued on next page)

Procedure 26-16 ■ Administering IV Push Medication (continued)

(Phillips, 2010). (b) Injecting an IV medication into an IV site that is not patent administers the medication into the local tissue at the IV site. Some medications will cause tissue irritation and even necrosis if infused into the subcutaneous tissue. In addition, the patient would not receive the immediate therapeutic benefit from the drug.

7. **If you have aspirated and obtained a blood return,** administer a small increment of the medication while observing for reactions to the medication.
Slow injection allows you to observe adverse reactions to the medication before all the medication has been injected. Administering IV push medications carries the highest potential risk to the patient because immediate, life-threatening reactions can occur.

8. **Administer another increment** of the medication (you may pinch the tubing while injecting medication and release it when not injecting; this is optional).

9. **Repeat Steps 7 and 8 until** the full dose of medication has been administered over the prescribed amount of time.
Medications require different administration times. Follow agency guidelines, physician orders, and pharmaceutical information regarding whether the medication needs to be diluted and the rate of administration.

10. **If you clamped the IV tubing** during the infusion, open it now and reset the pump at the correct infusion rate, if necessary.

11. **Dispose of used supplies safely** and according to agency procedures.

Procedure 26-16B ■ Administering IV Push Medications Through an Intermittent Device (IV Lock) When No Extension Tubing Is Attached to the Venous Access Device

➤ When performing the procedure, always identify your patient according to agency policy, using two identifiers, and be attentive to standard precautions, hand hygiene, patient safety and privacy, body mechanics, and documentation.

Procedure Steps

1. **Check the compatibility** of the medication with the intravenous solution, if one is infusing. Determine how fast the medication may be administered and whether the medication needs to be diluted for administration.
IV push medications are frequently injected over 1 minute. Some medications must be administered over a longer time period, and some medications must be diluted before administration. Giving an IV push medication too fast and/or undiluted can result in an adverse local or systemic reaction.

2. **Prepare the medication** from a vial or ampule. Dilute as needed. Refer to Procedure 26-9.

3. **Select the appropriate size** of syringe for flush solution.
Smaller syringes exert more pressure against the wall of the IV catheter than do larger syringes. Check with the IV catheter manufacturer for specific recommendations, and follow agency policy.

4. **Don procedure gloves.**

5. **Thoroughly scrub all surfaces** of the injection port closest to the patient with an alcohol prep pad or CHG-alcohol combination product. Use povidone-iodine solution (Betadine) only when the patient cannot tolerate an alcohol-based disinfectant.
Follow agency policy. Some facilities require nurses to scrub all surfaces of the port with an alcohol-based antimicrobial product for 1 minute when accessing venous access devices. Using the port closest to the patient minimizes the amount of medication in the IV line.

6. **Insert the flush syringe** into the injection port. Depending on the equipment, you may then need to aspirate for a blood return.
In tubing that allows for or requires aspiration, a blood return is an indication that the IV catheter is in the vein. An IV site may still be patent if no blood is returned; conversely, an infiltrated IV may have a blood return. Use the blood return as only one indication of patency.

7. **Administer a flush solution** (usually 1 to 3 mL) to clear the line if blood return is obtained. Use a forward pushing motion on the syringe, with a slow, steady injection technique. If blood is not returned, see the What If . . . ? section at the end of Procedure 26-16.
(a) Flush syringes may be prefilled; and in some cases, the amount to inject may be a part of agency policy. (b) Rapid flushing causes a jet effect that can cause the catheter tip to migrate to other venous locations; this should be avoided. (c) Injecting an IV medication into an IV site that is not patent administers the medication into the local tissue at the IV site. Some medications will cause tissue irritation and even necrosis if infused into the subcutaneous tissue.

8. **Continue to hold the injection** port; remove the flush syringe; and again scrub the port with the alcohol prep pad or CHG-alcohol combination product. Use povidone-iodine only when the patient is sensitive to alcohol-based disinfectants.
Cleansing the port reduces the risk of introducing microorganisms into the bloodstream.

9. **Attach the medication** syringe and inject the medication in small increments over the correct time interval. Use a slow, steady injection technique until the correct dose is instilled over the prescribed amount of time.

For example, if 1 mL of the medication is to be given over 1 minute, inject approximately 0.25 mL every 15 seconds.

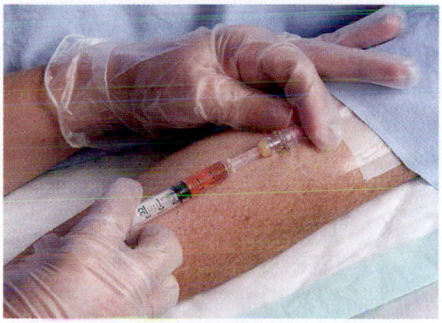

10. **Continuing to hold the injection port**, remove the medication syringe, and vigorously scrub all surfaces of the port with alcohol prep pad or CHG-alcohol–based product for at least 15 seconds. Attach the flush syringe.
Vigorous scrubbing reduces the chance of contamination of the port.

11. **Administer the flush solution** usually 1 to 3 mL, or according to prescription or agency policy.
Flushing ensures that all the medication has been administered and prevents occlusion of the IV catheter.

12. **Use a slow, steady injection** pressure technique when removing the syringe by placing your thumb or index finger to avoid movement of the plunger. (Follow equipment guidelines; you may not always need to do this.) Continue to administer the flush solution while withdrawing the syringe cannula from the injection port.
This positive-pressure technique prevents blood backflow into the IV catheter, which might cause an occlusion. Follow equipment guidelines because some injection ports maintain positive pressure by removing the syringe and then closing the clamp.

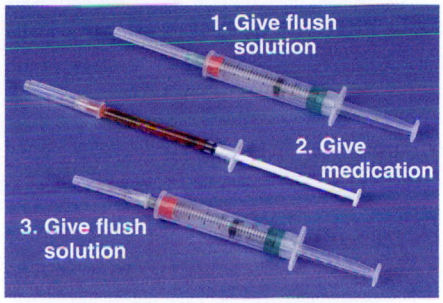

13. **Discard the flushing syringe** from the needleless connector into a safety disposal container.

Procedure 26-16C ■ Administering IV Push Medications Through an Intermittent Device With IV Extension Tubing

➤ When performing the procedure, always identify your patient according to agency policy, using two identifiers, and be attentive to standard precautions, hand hygiene, patient safety and privacy, body mechanics, and documentation.

Procedure Steps

1. **Check the compatibility** of the medication with the intravenous solution, if one is infusing. Determine how fast the medication may be administered and whether the medication needs to be diluted for administration.
IV push medications are frequently injected over 1 minute. Some must be administered over a longer time period, and some require diluting prior to administration. Giving an IV push medication too fast and/or undiluted can result in a local or systemic adverse reaction.

2. **Prepare the medication** from a vial or ampule. Dilute as needed. Refer to Procedure 26-9.

3. **Determine the volume** of any extension tubing attached to the access port.
The volume of extension sets can be greater than the IV push medication being given. If not accounted for, all the medication may be injected into the patient's bloodstream at once when the second flush solution is given.

4. **Don procedure gloves.**

5. **Scrub all surfaces of the injection port** with an antiseptic wipe.

6. **Insert the flush syringe** into the injection port. Depending on the equipment, you may then need to aspirate for a blood return as one sign of vein patency. Some equipment does not require or allow aspiration. If a needleless system is not available, use a syringe with a safety needle.
(a) In tubing that allows for or requires aspiration, a blood return is a sign that the IV catheter is in the vein. However an IV site may still be patent if no blood is returned. (b) Using a needleless system prevents needlestick injuries.

7. **Administer the flush** (commonly 1 to 3 mL) after establishing patency of the IV line. If blood appears in the tubing, administer the rest of the flush. If blood is not returned, assess patency by administering a small amount of the flush solution and monitoring for ease of administration, swelling at the IV site, or patient complaint of discomfort at the site.

8. **Again scrub the port.** Attach the medication syringe and inject a volume of medication equal to the volume of the extension set at the same rate as the flush solution.
   - When using a 5-mL syringe for peripheral lines and a 10-mL syringe for central lines, administer the flush solution briskly.
   - When you use a smaller syringe, use a slower rate to prevent excess pressure damaging the vein or shearing of the IV cannula.

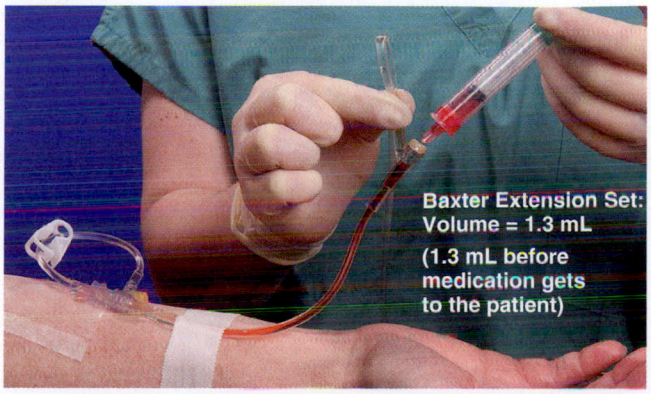

(continued on next page)

Procedure 26-16 ■ Administering IV Push Medication (continued)

The medication clears the line of saline solution and fills it with medication; it also flushes the IV catheter with saline as the medication pushes the saline through the catheter.

9. **Using a slow, steady injection** technique, administer the remainder of the medication over the prescribed time interval for the specific medication.
   Rapid flushing can create a jet effect that can cause the catheter tip to migrate to an unintended venous location.

10. **Continuing to hold the** injection port connector, remove the medication syringe, vigorously scrub all surfaces of the connector for at least 15 seconds, then attach the flush syringe. **Key Point:** ***The only time you should open the catheter hub is when the needleless connector or primary continuous IV set must be changed, usually at 96-hour intervals or as otherwise prescribed.***

11. **Administer the same amount** of flush solution at the same rate as the medication, using a slow, steady injection technique. For example, if the extension tubing has a volume of 1.3 mL, give the first 1.3 mL of the flush solution at the same rate as the medication. Then administer the remainder of the flush solution.
    (a) At this step, the extension tubing contains all the medication. Administering the flush solution all at once pushes the medication too fast (it will enter the vein all at once). (b) Once you have incrementally cleared the medication from the extension tubing and all the medication is already in the vein, then the rate no longer matters as far as the medication is concerned.

12. **Use a slow, steady injection** pressure technique when removing the syringe. Continue to administer the flush solution while withdrawing the syringe cannula from the injection port. Follow equipment instructions regarding the method and order of removing the syringe, closing the clamp, and maintaining positive pressure.

13. **Discard the flushing syringe** from the needleless connector into a safety disposal container.

? What if . . .

- **When using equipment requiring aspiration, no blood is returned?**

  Do not give IV push medication until you can verify the patency of the IV site. If the patency of the IV site is questionable, restart the IV at another site.

  Further assess the patency of the IV line by administering a small amount of the saline flush and monitoring for ease of administration, swelling at the IV site, or patient complaint of discomfort at the site.

  Another technique to determine patency is to lower the IV bag below the level of the IV site—a blood return should occur.

  If the IV catheter is a small gauge, a blood return may not always be aspirated.

- **There is resistance when flushing the line?**

  Never force the flush solution into the VAD; look for a closed clamp on the catheter or tubing. Or you may check to see if an inline filter is clogged. Do not proceed with the medication infusion until you are sure the catheter is still correctly positioned and that the fluid pathway is unobstructed.

- **The IV infusing a dextrose solution infiltrates into the surrounding tissue of a peripheral catheter?**

  Immediately stop the running fluid and remove the catheter. Initially apply a cool, moist compress to the site and later use heat to promote comfort.
  Infiltration can cause tissue injury, inflammation, and edema and may even lead to tissue necrosis and sloughing.

  Some medications, such as vasopressors (e.g., dopamine), might need intradermal injection of an antidote, such as phentolamine (Regitine), to reverse the effects of extravasation.
  If the IV fluid contains dextrose at greater than 10% concentration, calcium salts, potassium salts, sodium bicarbonate, blood, and parenteral nutrition, contact the primary care provider, who will likely prescribe injection of hyaluronidase (Amphadase) into the surrounding tissue.

Evaluation

- Assess the patient for complaints of pain or discomfort at the site.

Patient Teaching

- Discuss why the medication is being administered intravenously.
- Explain the need to report immediately any reaction to the medication.

Home Care

- Discuss with the client and/or caregiver how to care for the IV site, including flushing. Many IV push medications need to be administered by a nurse. However, cost-cutting efforts have led to short hospital stays, and some clients are now being taught to administer their own IV antibiotics at home.
- Explain how to identify problems with the IV site, such as infiltration and phlebitis.
- Determine whether the client has adequate facilities for storing the medication, such as refrigeration if needed.
- Discuss safety issues, such as keeping medications and needles and syringes secure and away from children and pets.

Documentation

Besides charting according to Medication Guidelines: Steps to Follow for All Medications (Regardless of Type or Route), document related patient assessment findings, such as the appearance of the IV site and patient complaints of pain or discomfort during IV administration. You will usually document on an IV flow record and/or MAR rather than in the nursing notes. Chart a nursing note only if there is a problem (e.g., if the patient experiences pain when you administer the medication).

Practice Resources

CDC (2011a); INS (2011a, 2011b); Phillips, D. (2010).

Thinking About the Procedure

To practice applying clinical reasoning to this procedure,

Go to *Davis's Nursing Skills Videos*, **Administering IV Push Medications Through a Primary IV Line, Administering IV Push Medications Through an Intermittent Device (IV Lock) When No Extension Tubing Is Attached to the Venous Access Device,** and **Administering IV Push Medications Through an Intermittent Device With IV Extension Tubing.**

For questions and suggested responses,

Go to Chapter 26, **Thinking About the Procedure Questions and Suggested Responses,** on Davis*Plus*.

Procedure 26-17 ■ Administering Medication by Intermittent Infusion

➤ For steps to follow in *all* procedures, refer to the Universal Steps for All Procedures found on the inside back cover. Also refer to Medication Guidelines: Steps to Follow for All Medications (Regardless of Type or Route). For step-by-step instructions in using volume-control devices (pumps), see Procedure 38-3.

Equipment

- Correct size syringe for measuring medication
- Needleless access cannula or safety needle
- Volume-control IV set (e.g., Buretrol, Volutrol, Soluset) or small bag of diluted medication with piggyback tubing
- Primary IV solution and tubing (unless one is already infusing)
- Antimicrobial swabs
- Labels for the IV tubing and medication administration system

Delegation

Nurse practice acts governing IV medication administration vary from state to state, and policies can further vary among healthcare agencies, regarding which medications or methods of administration the LPN/LVN may perform. You cannot delegate this procedure to a NAP.

Pre-Procedure Assessments

- Check the compatibility of the medication with the IV solution.
  Medications can be physically or chemically incompatible with the IV solution. Physical incompatibility will be obvious if precipitation occurs. Chemical incompatibility is not obvious and may result in the medication having a weaker or a stronger effect than anticipated.
- Assess the patency of the IV line.
  If the line is occluded or if the fluid has infiltrated the medication will not infuse.
- Check the site for redness, swelling, tenderness, and other signs of infiltration or phlebitis.
  Some medications are irritating to the tissue. If the IV fluid has infiltrated, medication would leak into the tissue and cause injury. IV medications can also irritate the veins and cause phlebitis. Do not infuse a medication into a compromised site.
- Determine the amount of IV solution needed to administer the specific medication.
  Most medications specify (on the order or on the label) specific dilution to prevent potential harm to the patient.
- Determine the time period over which the solution needs to be infused.
  Infusing a medication too slowly may result in an inadequate blood level to achieve therapeutic levels, and infusing a medication too rapidly can cause harm.
- Perform assessments that will provide a basis for evaluating the drug's effectiveness, such as checking blood pressure after administering an antihypertensive agent.

Procedure 26-17 ■ Administering Medication by Intermittent Infusion (continued)

Procedure 26-17A ■ Using a Volume-Control Administration Set

➤ For step-by-step instructions in using volume-control devices (pumps), see Procedure 38-3. If you have not already done so, affix a label to the secondary bag indicating the name and amount of medication, date and time given, and your name or initials.

➤ When performing the procedure, always identify your patient according to agency policy, using two identifiers, and be attentive to standard precautions, hand hygiene, patient safety and privacy, body mechanics, and documentation.

Procedure Steps

1. **Prepare the volume-control set.**
   a. Close both the upper and lower clamps on the tubing, if they are not already closed.
   Clamping prevents air bubbles from forming in the tubing.
   b. Open the clamp of the air vent on the volume-control chamber.
   Venting allows air to escape, which lets the IV solution enter the chamber.
   c. Maintaining sterile procedure, attach administration spike of the volume-control set to the primary IV bag.
   d. Fill the volume-control chamber with the desired amount of IV solution by opening the clamp between the bag and the volume-control chamber. When the correct amount of solution is in the chamber, close the clamp.
   The drip chamber provides solution for priming the tubing and diluting the IV medication.
   e. Prime the rest of the tubing by opening the clamp below the chamber and running the IV fluid until all the air has been expelled.
   Priming clears the IV tubing of air.
   f. Recheck the amount of fluid in the volume control chamber, and add more fluid to the desired amount, if needed.
   Priming the tubing alters the volume in the chamber. You must fill to the desired amount.
2. **With an alcohol or CHG**-alcohol swab, vigorously scrub all surfaces of the injection port closest to the patient.
   Vigorous cleansing is necessary to removes microorganisms and particles from the IV port, which could potentially enter the patient's bloodstream.
3. **Connect the end of the** volume-control IV line to the patient's IV site (e.g., directly to the IV catheter, to the extension tubing, or to the injection port closest to patient).
4. **Vigorously scrub the injection port** on the volume-control chamber, attach the medication syringe (preferably with a blunt, needleless device), and inject the medication into the solution in the chamber.
5. **Gently rotate the chamber** to mix the medication in the IV solution.
   Distributes the medication within the IV solution.
6. **Open the lower clamp**, and start the infusion at the correct flow rate.
   Unclamping allows the infusion of the medication. A correct flow rate infuses the medication over the correct amount of time and prevents a toxic reaction to it.
7. **Label the volume-control** chamber with the date, time, medication and doses added, and your initials, according to agency policy.
8. **When the medication has** finished infusing, add a small amount of the primary IV fluid to the chamber, and flush the tubing. For the flush volume, use twice the volume in the dead space of the tubing; check the tubing package for the amount.
   Flushing the line ensures all the medication is given to the patient and does not adhere to the tubing. ▼

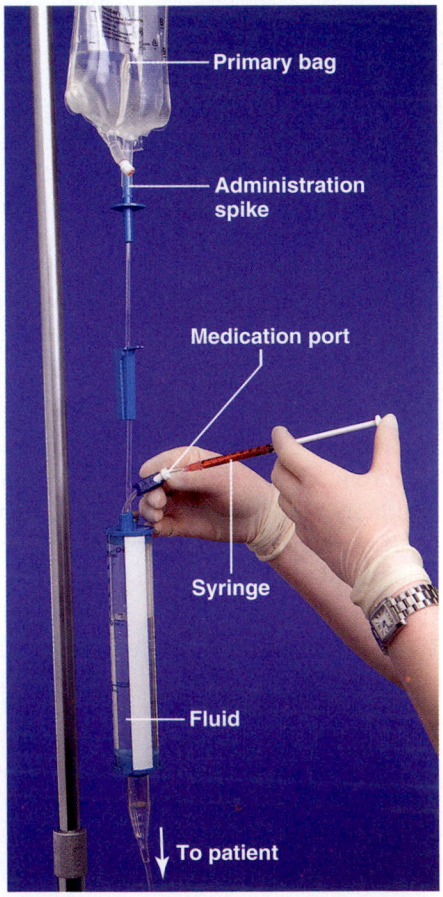

Thinking About the Procedure

To practice applying clinical reasoning to this procedure,

Go to *Davis's Nursing Skills Videos*, **Using a Volume-Control Administration Set.**

For questions and suggested responses,

Go to Chapter 26, **Thinking About the Procedure Questions and Suggested Responses,** on Davis*Plus*.

Procedure 26-17B ■ Using a Piggyback Administration Set With a Gravity Infusion

➤ When performing the procedure, always identify your patient according to agency policy, using two identifiers, and be attentive to standard precautions, hand hygiene, patient safety and privacy, body mechanics, and documentation.

Procedure Steps

1. **Obtain the medication.** IV medications usually are premixed and labeled in small bags by the pharmacy. Rarely, you may need to draw up the medication, and inject it into the piggyback solution (see Procedure 26-15). Date and initial the medication bag label. Verify that it has the patient's name, amount of medication, date, and time given.

2. **Obtain and attach** the piggyback tubing to the medication bag. Do not touch the spike.
   Tubing connects the piggyback to the primary line. Prevents contamination of tubing and solution. Piggyback tubing is short.

3. **Be sure the slide clamp is closed.** Squeeze the drip chamber, filling it one-third to one-half full.
   Clamping prevents excess air coming into the line when you are priming the tubing.

4. **Open the clamp and prime** the tubing, holding the end of the tubing lower than the bag of fluid. Do not let more than one drop of fluid escape from the end of the tubing. Close the clamp.

Alternative. "Backflushing" the Piggyback Line

a. Clamp the piggyback tubing.
b. Scrub all surfaces of the primary "Y" port, and attach the piggyback setup with the needleless connector.
c. Open the clamp on the piggyback tubing, and lower the bag below the primary bag to prime the piggyback line.
d. Once all the air is expelled from the piggyback tubing, clamp the tubing and finish the procedure.
   Priming removes air from the tubing and maintains sterility of the system. Medications are diluted in small amounts of fluid (usually 50 to 100 mL), so you cannot waste any medication. The backflush method ensures you will not do so.

5. **Label the piggyback tubing** with the time, the date, and your initials.
   Tubing used for intermittent infusions can be used for 48 to 72 hours, depending on facility policy; labeling allows the nurse to know when it must be changed.

6. **Hang the piggyback container** on the IV pole. Lower the primary IV container to hang below the level of the medication bag.
   Gravity causes the higher bag (the piggyback IV setup) to flow instead of the primary IV setup. When the piggyback IV solution has infused, the primary IV line will resume infusing.

7. **Open the clamp** of the piggyback line, and regulate the drip rate with the roller clamp on the primary line. Regulate to the prescribed infusion rate for the medication. ▼
   Because the piggyback is the only bag running, the primary roller clamp regulates the speed of the piggyback bag.

8. **When the medication is all infused**, clamp the piggyback tubing, and move the primary bag back to its original height. Use the roller clamp to reset the primary bag to its correct infusion rate.
   This ensures that the primary fluids infuse at their ordered rate rather than flowing at the rate the piggyback medication was flowing—which would probably be either faster or slower than the prescribed primary fluid rate.

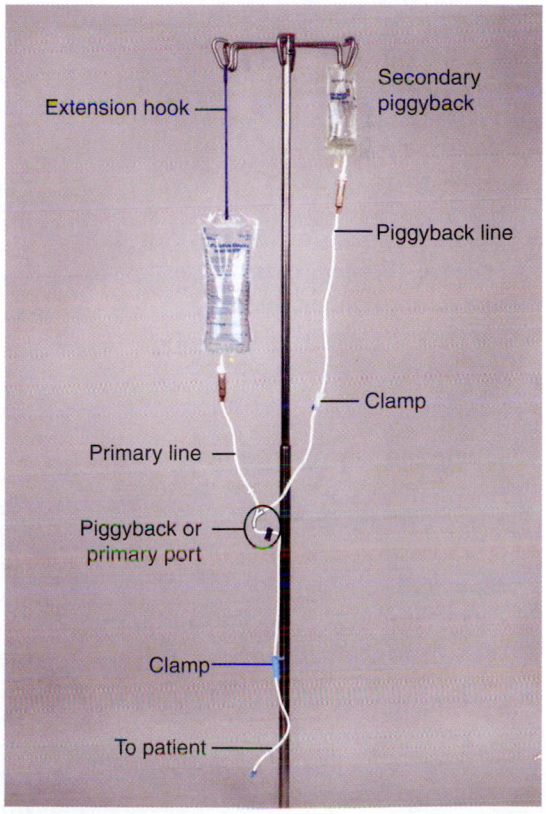

Thinking About the Procedure

To practice applying clinical reasoning to this procedure,

Go to *Davis's Nursing Skills Videos*, **Using a Piggyback Administration Set With a Gravity Infusion.**

For questions and suggested responses,

Go to Chapter 26, **Thinking About the Procedure Questions and Suggested Responses,** on Davis*Plus*.

(continued on next page)

Procedure 26-17 ■ Administering Medication by Intermittent Infusion (continued)

Procedure 26-17C ■ Using a Piggyback Administration Set with an Infusion Pump

- For step-by-step instructions in using intermittent infusion devices (pumps), also see Procedure 38-3.
- *Note:* This procedure describes the use of a one-piston infusion pump. The steps for using a two-piston pump vary slightly.
- When performing the procedure, always identify your patient according to agency policy, using two identifiers, and be attentive to standard precautions, hand hygiene, patient safety and privacy, body mechanics, and documentation.

Procedure Steps

1. **Obtain the medication.** IV medications usually are premixed in small bags and labeled by the pharmacy. If this is not the case, inject the medication into the prescribed piggyback solution (see Procedure 26-15). Date and initial the medication bag label. Verify that it has the patient's name, amount of medication, date, and time given.

2. **Be sure you have the correct secondary infusion tubing.** Hang the piggyback container on the IV pole. Attach the piggyback tubing to the medication bag. Do not touch the spike.
   Piggyback tubing is short; tandem tubing is much longer. Secondary tubing connects the piggyback to the primary line. Touching the spike would contaminate the tubing and solution.

3. **Be sure the slide clamp** is closed. Squeeze the drip chamber, filling it one-third to one-half full.
   Clamping prevents excess air coming into the line when you are priming the tubing.

4. **Open the clamp and prime** the tubing, holding the end of the tubing lower than the bag of fluid. Do not let more than one drop of fluid escape from the end of the tubing. Close the clamp.

Alternative. "Backflushing" the Piggyback Line

a. With the drip chamber one-third filled, air will be in the secondary tubing.
b. Pause the infusion pump.
c. Scrub all surfaces of the "Y" port on the primary line and attach the piggyback set-up with a needleless connector.
d. Open the clamp on the piggyback tubing, and lower the bag below the primary bag to prime the piggyback line. The fluid from the primary line will flow up through the secondary tubing until all air is removed from the tubing. Restart the pump.
e. Once the line is primed, clamp the tubing and finish the procedure.
   Priming removes air from the tubing and maintains sterility of the system. Medications are diluted in small amounts of fluid (usually 50 to 100 mL), so you cannot waste any medication. The backflush method ensures you will not do so.

5. **Label the piggyback tubing** with the time, the date, and your initials.
   Tubing used for intermittent infusions can be used for 48 to 72 hours, depending on facility policy; labeling allows the nurse to know when it must be changed.

6. **Lower the primary IV** container to hang below the level of the piggyback medication bag.
   The tubing system works such that the higher bag (the piggyback IV setup) flow instead of the primary IV setup.

7. **Program the pump** by selecting the secondary infusion button
   This converts the fluid infusing from the primary line to the secondary line.

8. **Program the rate and total volume** to be infused. (Some pumps allow you to select the medication and dose.)
   Ensures accurate infusion amount and restart of primary fluids.

9. **Scrub the port** of the primary line.
   Minimizes the introduction of microorganisms.

10. **Remove the cover from** the secondary tubing and connect it to the connection port of the primary line. (This was done at Step 4 if the blackflush priming method was used.)

11. **Open the clamp** on the secondary tubing.

12. **Press "start"** on infusion pump.

13. **Check drip chambers** to ensure that the secondary solution is infusing and the primary solution is not.
    This ensures that medication is infusing and patient does not receive an overload of fluids.

14. **Check the pump information** again to ensure the correct rate and volume.

15. **At the end of the infusion**, the primary IV line will resume infusing. Once the secondary infusion is complete, the pump programming will re-set to the previously programmed primary rate.
    This ensures that the primary fluids infuse at their ordered rate rather than flowing at the rate the piggyback medication was flowing—which would probably be either faster or slower than the prescribed primary fluid rate.

Thinking About the Procedure

To practice applying clinical reasoning to this procedure,

Go to *Davis's Nursing Skills Videos*, **Using a Piggyback Administration Set With an Infusion Pump.**

For questions and suggested responses,

Go to Chapter 26, **Thinking About the Procedure Questions and Suggested Responses,** on Davis*Plus*.

Evaluation

- Assess for pain or discomfort at the site.
- Intermittent infusions via a pump are generally infused over 30 to 60 minutes; therefore, you need to assess the patient as soon as the medication begins infusing and every 15 to 20 minutes until it is absorbed.

Patient Teaching

- Discuss why the medication is being administered intravenously.
- Explain the need to report immediately any reaction to the medication.
- Ask the patient to activate the call device if the infusion pump starts to alarm. Explain common reasons for the alarm to minimize anxiety.

Home Care

- Discuss with the client and/or caregiver how to care for the IV site. Only a nurse should add medications to the IV.
- Explain how to identify problems with the IV site, such as infiltration and phlebitis.
- Assess whether the client has adequate facilities for storing the medication, such as refrigeration if needed.
- Discuss safety issues, such as keeping medications, needles, and syringes secure and away from children and pets.

Documentation

- Chart information according to Medication Guidelines: Steps to Follow for All Medications (Regardless of Type or Route).
- Document related patient assessment findings, such as the appearance of the IV site and patient complaints of pain or discomfort during the administration.

Practice Resource

INS (2011a; 2011b); Wiegand, D. (2011).

Procedure 26-18 ■ Administering Medication Through a Central Venous Access Device (CVAD)

➤ For steps to follow in *all* procedures, refer to the Universal Steps for All Procedures found on the inside back cover. Also refer to Medication Guidelines: Steps to Follow for All Medications (Regardless of Type or Route).

Equipment

- Syringe appropriate for medication volume (10 mL or larger)

  ✚ Use of syringes smaller than 10 mL when flushing a CVAD can cause increase pressure and may rupture the CVAD.
- Needleless device or safety syringe with a filter needle for drawing up the medication (you would also need a sterile needle for injection)
- Two syringes for the flush solution
- Saline or heparin flush solution, as prescribed. New evidence supports flushing peripheral venous catheters with heparin 100 units/mL rather than with saline solution (Bertolino, Pitassi, Tinelli, et al., 2012).
- Prep pad: CHG-alcohol combination product or appropriate antiseptic solution and gauze pad
- One pair nonsterile procedure gloves

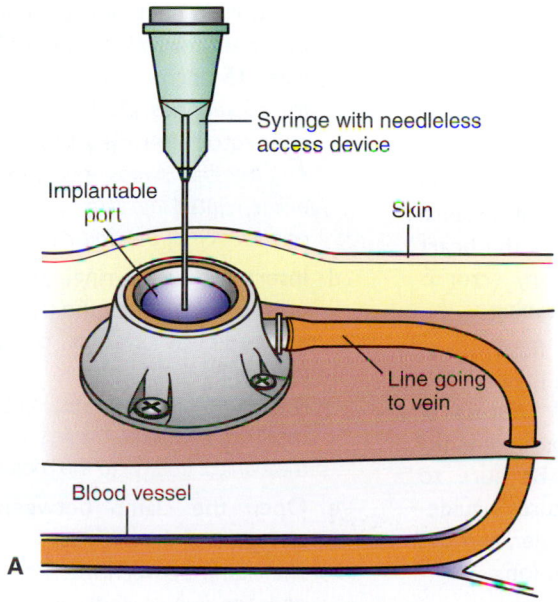

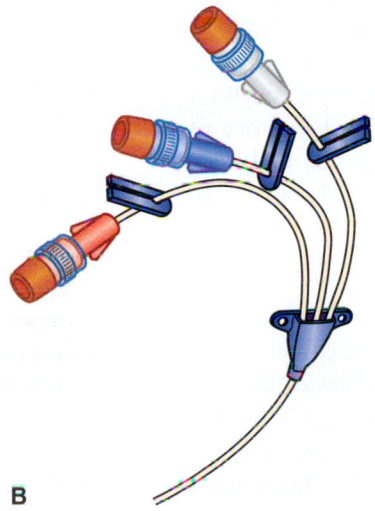

(continued on next page)

Procedure 26-18 ■ Administering Medication Through a Central Venous Access Device (CVAD) (continued)

Pre-Procedure Assessment

- Carefully palpate the area around the insertion site through the dressing. If the patient has tenderness, assess further for other signs of infection. Check the surrounding catheter insertion site for intact sutures, redness, swelling, warmth, or drainage.
  This can indicate catheter-related infection.
- Assess the patient's external chest wall for engorged veins at the surface of the skin. If the jugular's site is used, also assess for difficulty moving the neck or jaw, headache, or ear pain.
  This can indicate vein thrombosis.
- PICC line sites should be observed daily for swelling, tenderness, drainage, or streaking. Take site measurements at regular intervals during dressing changes and compare to pre-insertion arm circumference.
  May indicate problems with phlebitis and/or catheter sepsis.
- Conduct a comprehensive pain assessment, looking for unusual pain or discomfort.
  Pain can be associated with the catheter's position in the vein, especially if the line is not in an optimal position

➤ When performing the procedure, always identify your patient according to agency policy, using two identifiers, and be attentive to standard precautions, hand hygiene, patient safety and privacy, body mechanics, and documentation.

Procedure Steps

1. **Prepare the medication.**
   a. Check compatibility of the medication with the existing IV infusion.
   b. ✚ Verify the medication that can safely be administered through a central site. Double-check the infusion rate as well.
   Some medication might be incompatible with infusion solution or additives. Because dosage may be different for medications given centrally versus peripherally, and because the medication enters the heart almost instantly, any error is potentially life threatening.
   c. Draw up the medication using a needleless device or needle with a filter. Then change to a sterile safety needle or needleless device for administering the medication.
   Filter needles prevent small particles from entering into the line.
   d. Recap any needles throughout, using a needle-capping device or approved one-handed technique that has a low risk of contaminating the sterile needle (see Procedure 26-10B: Recapping Sterile Needles).
   Recapping prevents needlestick injury and, performed correctly, maintains the sterility of the needle.
   e. Dilute the medication, if needed. Fill the medication syringe to the exact volume to be infused; expel excess volume.
   f. Label the syringe with the contents, including medication name, dilution, time to be administered, route, and name of person constituting the medication.
   Excess volume of medication in the syringe is a risk for inadvertent overdosing.
2. **Flush the line.**
   a. Obtain heparinized or saline solution for flushing the CVAD, following the institution's protocol or the prescription.
   The usual concentration for heparin is 10 to 100 units/mL of solution for adults. The recommended volume of flush varies by institution. Most facilities recommend 3 to 5 mL of solution to flush the catheter, although some are flushed with 10 mL to flush the line. Some medication might be incompatible with infusion solution or additives.

   ✚ Dosage for centrally administered drugs is critical because the medication enters the heart almost instantly, so any error is potentially life threatening

   ✚ Using heparin flush in venous access devices is becoming more controversial because of the potential for heparin-induced thrombocytopenia. Be sure to follow the manufacturer's guidelines, prescriber's order, and the policy of your institution.

   b. Before flushing the CVAD, examine the syringe for bubbles. Remove them by flicking the syringe. Eject the air and bubbles, but be sure you have enough flush solution remaining in the syringe.
   Flicking causes the bubbles to rise to the top. Remove bubbles from the syringe before giving medication through the CVAD port to avoid injecting air into the patient's vein and causing an embolus.
   c. With clean procedure gloves, using pressure and friction, vigorously scrub all surfaces of the CVAD connectors as well as the luer-locking threads, and the luer-lock, including the extension "tail," with an alcohol wipe, CHG-alcohol combination product, or other antimicrobial product for at least 15 seconds. Then let it dry for 15 seconds. Do not touch this connector after cleansing.
   Antimicrobial swabs reduce the risk of line-related infection by decreasing colonization of the port and tubing.
   d. Insert the flush syringe at a vertical (90°) angle into the port using a needleless system or safety syringe.
   A 90° angle reduces stress on the access port, which may cause shearing or mechanical trauma to the material.
   e. Open the clamp between the syringe and the patient.
   The clamp between the access port and the tubing that goes to the

patient must be patent for medication to be injected through the CVAD.

f. Check for blood return, if necessary. Equipment differs regarding the need to aspirate, so follow agency protocols.
In some administration systems, aspiration is one indication that catheter placement is in the vein.

g. Inject saline or heparinized flush solution into the line, per agency protocol or provider's orders and type of catheter. Some catheter types (e.g., Groshong) do not require heparin in the flush solution. Close the clamp.
Saline or heparin flush is used, depending on the type of CVAD, institutional protocol, and manufacturer recommendations.
- *Saline is generally indicated when simple clearing of the line is needed.*
- *If blood is likely to backflow into the line, then heparin might be used in the flush solution in order to reduce the risk of clot formation.*
- *Most often heparin is used for implanted CVADs to reduce the risk of occlusion from a clot forming on the device.*
- *Different catheters require different volume of flush solutions. Some are more prone to clot formation, depending on whether they are open or closed system devices. The initial flush maintains patency of the line and removes any heparin that was left if the catheter was used previously.*

h. Never force the flush solution into the venous access device if you feel resistance. Look for a closed clamp on the catheter or tubing. Check to see if an inline filter is clogged.
Forcing fluid creates a risk of rupturing the catheter.

i. Disconnect the flush syringe.
CAUTION: Techniques of flushing and clamping may vary depending on the type of connector you are using. Consult agency protocols and manufacturer's instructions.

If using a needleless connector, in general, do the following:

If Using Negative Fluid Displacement Device

Use a positive-pressure technique:
- For a blunt cannula with split septum, or mechanical valve, withdraw the cannula before the syringe is completely empty, keeping your thumb on the syringe plunger.
- For a mechanical valve device with negative displacement, maintain pressure on the syringe plunger, close the clamp on the IV line between the needleless connector and the patient; and then disconnect the syringe.

If Using a Positive Fluid Displacement Device

Do not use a positive-pressure technique. Flush using a push-pause technique. Wait 10 seconds (or per manufacture guidelines) to allow fluid displacement to occur. Remove syringe, and only then may you clamp the catheter.
The positive-pressure technique would keep the internal mechanism from functioning properly.

For Neutral Fluid Displacement Devices

Any flushing technique can be used. The clamping and disconnecting sequence does not matter.
The clamping sequence is directly dependent upon the needleless connector being used and is critical for the final locking solution.

i. After removing the flush syringe from the port, discard it into a safety disposal container.

3. Administer medication through the CVAD.

a. Scrub all surfaces of the external ports, tubing, and connectors with a CHG-alcohol combination product for at least 15 seconds. Allow the port to dry for 15 more seconds or follow manufacturer's guidelines.
Antimicrobial swabs reduce the risk of line-related infection by decreasing colonization of the port and tubing.

b. Close the clamp to the infusion if a primary IV is running.
The medication could travel back up the line rather than infuse into the patient if the clamp is open.

c. Inject medication into the port, according to the medication order (infusion time).
Some medication is infused as a bolus; other medication is given over a period of time.

4. After scrubbing all surfaces of the port again with a CHG-alcohol product or other approved antiseptic, administer the second syringe of flush solution.
The flush prevents incompatible medication or fluid from mixing at later administrations and ensures that all of the medication clears the catheter and enters the bloodstream.

5. Clamp the tubing between the syringe and the CVAD port. If there is an infusing primary IV, make sure the tubing is open between the IV fluid and the patient.

? What if . . .

- **My patient is a child; how should I secure the line?**

  Dress infants and younger children in a one-piece undershirt that fastens between the legs and tape the line to the shirt, leaving a little bit of slack to allow for movement.

- **The line does not flush easily?**

  Make sure all clamps are unclamped. Check to see if the central line is kinked or twisted.

  After straightening lines, attempt to flush the central line again. If the flush solution cannot be injected easily from the syringe into the CVAD, do not force the flush.
  Too much flush pressure may dislodge a clot that has formed in the central line.

  Check to see if an inline filter is clogged.

  Assess the insertion site to see if the stabilization device or dressing may be causing the occlusion.

  Try to reposition the patient to lying down and turn to one side.

  You might also have the patient lift his arms above his head and then attempt to flush the central line.

  If it is still difficult to flush after repositioning, notify the provider.

- **The central line inadvertently comes out?**

  Hold firm, constant pressure on the site to control bleeding. Have a colleague notify the provider immediately.

(continued on next page)

Procedure 26-18 ■ Administering Medication Through a Central Venous Access Device (CVAD) (continued)

- **The central line is cracked or leaking?**
  Close the clamp between the break or leakage in the line and the patient's line insertion site. Wrap an alcohol wipe and gauze around the broken part of the line. Immediately change the tubing.
- **The clamp on the line is broken?**
  Change the tubing. Assure the clamp works properly on the new tubing. This essential for patient safety.
- **The central line gets caught on or pulled by the patient's clothing?**
  Loop the tubing over the dressing and secure with tape.
- **My patient is short of breath or complains of chest pain?**
  Notify the provider immediately.
  These symptoms could be a sign of fluid overload or other complications, such as a dislodged clot or embolism.
- **My patient feels pain in the neck or ear on the side where an implantable CVAD is located? Or the patient hears swishing noises or has palpitations?**
  Notify the provider immediately.
  In this case, the implanted device might be dislodged. Placement must be confirmed by x-ray.

Patient Evaluation

- Monitor for signs of catheter complications (e.g., shortness of breath, chest pain, and palpitations).
- Monitor for signs of catheter dislodgement (e.g., neck swelling or pain, bleeding at the site or within the line, palpitations, or gurgling noise).
- Assess for signs of catheter-related infection (e.g., fever, increased WBC count, redness, warmth at the site).
- Observe for leaking or blood backup at the injection ports, tubing connections, and the site.
- Observe for bleeding at the CVAD site.
- Assess for signs of allergic response or adverse effects to medication.

Patient Teaching

- Teach patients, families, and caregivers that the overall goal is to maintain a patent CVAD or PICC line that is free of infection, occlusion, or dislodgement.
- Avoid obtaining blood pressure readings in the arm where a PICC line is inserted.
- If a PICC line is in place, do not immerse the arm in water. The patient may shower if the site is covered by an occlusive dressing.
- Follow prescribed activity restrictions.
- Teach signs of catheter complications including line-related infection, thrombosis, and accidental dislodgement.
- Teach signs of catheter dislodgement to include pain or swelling in the neck or area near the ear of the affected side of the CVAD. Gurgling sounds might also indicate a problem with the placement of the CVAD.

Home Care

- The goals of home care for clients receiving medication through a CVAD or PICC line are medication safety and maintaining an infection-free line.
- Candidates for home IV therapy through a CVAD or PICC line are those who:
  - Have a family member or other caregiver who can competently provide or assist with care of the line.
  - Have telephone access—either via landline or cell phone.
  - Have access to reliable transportation in case of a line-related emergency.
  - Ideally, caregivers should be able to read instructions for home care.
- Procedures in the home environment are similar to the hospital setting, except clean technique is used instead of sterile.
- Home health supplies may be different than the ones used in the hospital.
- After discharge, follow-up care in the home environment is important to ensure safety.

Documentation

- Document any signs of allergic response to or adverse effects of medication.
- Note any signs of catheter complications or dislodgement
- Document signs of catheter-related infection.
- Record the date and time tubing and port cap are changed.
- Document all medications infused through the CVAD.

Sample Documenation

June 18, 2015 1200. PICC line insertion site clean and dry. No redness, swelling, or drainage. Arm circumference 16 inches; same as pre-insertion measurement. Pt reports no pain at site. Flushed with 10 mL of NS, no resistance noted. ——— Sue Creas, RN

Thinking About the Procedure

To practice applying clinical reasoning to this procedure,

Go to *Davis's Nursing Skills Videos*, **Administering Medication Through a Central Venous Access Device.**

For questions and suggested responses,

Go to Chapter 26, **Thinking About the Procedure Questions and Suggested Responses,** on Davis*Plus*.

Practice Resources

Bertolino, G., Pitassi, A., Tinelli, C., et al. (2012); CDC (2011b); INS (2011a, 2011b); Wiegand, D. (2011).

CLINICAL INSIGHTS

Clinical Insight 26-1 ➤ Reusing Needles and Syringes: Home Care

Assess for the Following:

- Is the patient capable of safely recapping a syringe: adequate vision, manual dexterity, and no obvious tremor?
- Are there contraindications to needle reuse (e.g., poor personal hygiene, an acute illness, open wounds on the hands, or decreased resistance to infection)?

Teach How to Use Needles Safely:

- Consult your healthcare provider before beginning this practice.
- Examine the needle carefully before reusing it. The new 30- and 31-gauge needles can easily be bent at the tip to form a hook, which can lacerate tissue or break off within the skin. Never reuse a needle that is deformed in any way.
- Recap the needle immediately after use if you plan to use it again.
- To recap a needle, hold the syringe in one hand, rest that arm or hand on a solid surface, and with the other, replace the cap with a straight motion of the thumb. Do *not* guide both the needle and cap to meet in midair, because this frequently results in needlestick injury.
- Do not mix insulin types if you reuse needles and syringes. Use one syringe for each insulin type. That means more injections, but certain insulins cannot be mixed without reducing their effectiveness.
- Dispose of needles safely. Do not bend or break a needle; doing so increases the chance of injury. Use a coffee can or other puncture-proof container with a lid to dispose of needles.

Teach Your Patient When to Discard A Needle:

- Discard needles when they become dull. Usually they cannot be used more than 10 times.
- When a needle hurts too much, it's time to discard it. Increased pain means that the silicone coating is wearing off.
- Do not reuse a needle if it has come in contact with anything other than the injection site.

Teach How to Clean and Store Needles:

- Do not use alcohol to cleanse the needle. Alcohol may remove the silicone coating that makes for less painful skin puncture. It is best not to clean the needle after use; just carefully recap it.
- You may store the syringe and needle at room temperature. The potential benefits or risks of refrigerating the syringe are unknown.

Teach How to Recognize and Avoid Infection:

- Be aware that reusing needles and syringes increases the risk of infection, although most insulin preparations have bacteriostatic additives that inhibit growth of bacteria commonly found on the skin.
- Inspect injection sites for redness or swelling. If these signs are present, do not reuse a needle; consult your healthcare provider.
- Never share syringes or needles with another person. This poses a risk of acquiring a bloodborne viral infection (e.g., hepatitis).

Clinical Insight 26-2 ➤ Using Prefilled Unit-Dose Systems

Prefilled systems are commonly used in a variety of health-care settings, and in self-administration. Depending on the system used, the need to remove the cartridge from the holder may create a needlestick risk for nurses.

Technique

1. Check each medication cartridge and dose carefully, because all of the cartridges look alike.
2. No medication preparation is necessary.
3. Insert the cartridge into the holder.
4. Swing or twist the plunger into place, depending on the type of syringe you use. Lock it securely at the needle end.
5. Attach the plunger, if necessary. (The system may come with plunger attached.)

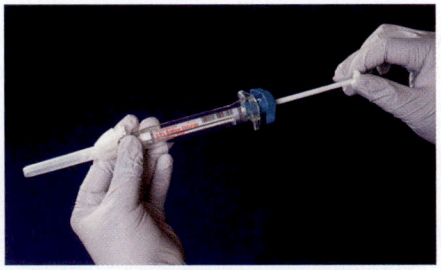

6. Expel air and excess medication.
7. Don gloves.
8. Administer the medication.
9. Dispose of the empty cartridge. Some types are available for reuse.

Technique Variations

The needle gauge or length is not correct for the patient. You can transfer the medication into a regular, disposable syringe, maintaining sterile technique. There are two ways you can do it.

Cartridge without removable needle:

1. Pull back on the plunger of the regular disposable syringe and keep a capped, sterile needle ready.
2. Insert the cartridge needle through the open tip of the disposable syringe.
3. Eject the medication into the regular syringe.
4. Replace the capped needle onto the regular syringe.
5. Eject the air and check for the correct dosage.

Cartridge with removable needle:
The capped needle can be removed from some prefilled cartridges, allowing the cartridge to be used as a vial. This allows you to safely draw the medications into a different (disposable) syringe, using a vial access device or safety needle. Do not inject air into a cartridge, because the excess pressure may eject the movable bottom.

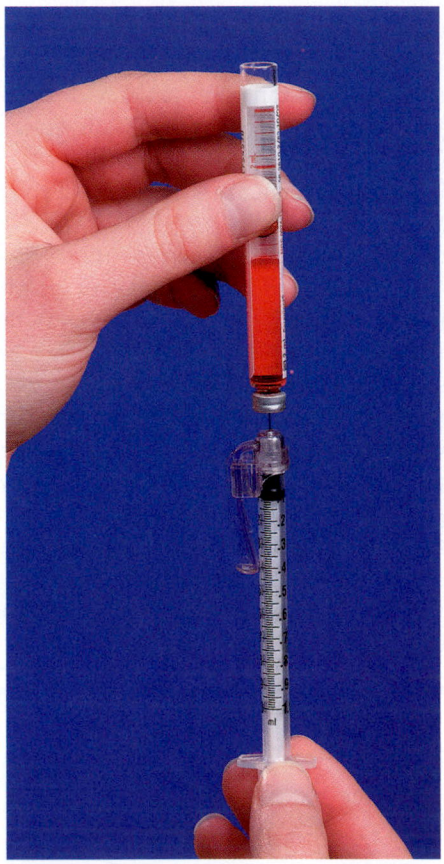

Clinical Insight 26-3 ➤ Reconstituting Medication

1. **Remove the caps of both the medication and diluent vials.**
2. **If a multidose vial is used, scrub the tops of both vials** with alcohol or other antiseptic wipe.

To clean the cap of dust and reduce the number of microorganisms.

3. **Use a VAD or, if agency policy allows, attach a filter needle to the syringe.**

To prevent withdrawing glass and rubber particles, which have been found in medications withdrawn from vials and ampules.

4. **Draw up the diluent into the syringe.**
   a. Draw air into the syringe in a volume equal to the amount of diluent you will be withdrawing.
   b. Insert the filter needle (or VAD) carefully through the center of the rubber cap and, keeping the bevel of the needle (or cannula) above the diluent, inject the air.

The air prevents negative pressure inside the vial when you withdraw the diluent, allowing you to withdraw the diluent easily. Keeping bevel above diluent helps prevent bubbles.

   c. Withdraw the diluent in the specified amount.

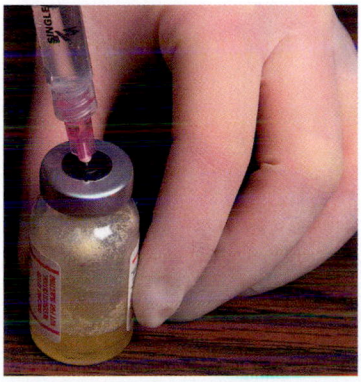

5. **Inject diluent into the medication vial** by inserting the VAD carefully through the center of the rubber cap and then injecting the diluent.
6. **Mix the medication, taking care not to create bubbles** (e.g., roll, do not shake, the vial). If medication does not mix easily, remove the needle or cannula from the vial, and place the syringe and needle on a sterile field (e.g., the wrapper the syringe came in) while you mix more. Alternatively, recap the sterile needle (see Procedure 26-10A).

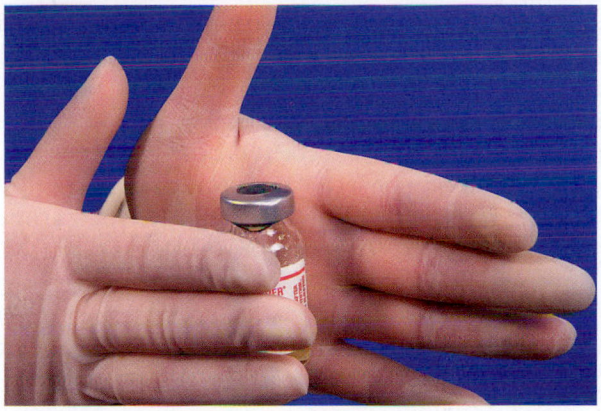

7. **Reinsert filter needle or VAD if it was removed** in Step 7, and withdraw the reconstituted medication into the syringe.
8. **Remove the filter needle or the cannula from the syringe**, and replace it with a sterile needle before measuring the medication.

This ensures that the dose is correct and minimizes discomfort. It also prevents tracking of medication through the tissues; filter needles are usually larger than you need for an injection. In addition, you should not eject fluid through a filter needle.

9. **Hold the syringe vertically, and carefully eject all air** from the syringe, but do not eject the medication. Read the dosage.
10. **If necessary, hold the syringe horizontally to eject unneeded medication** from the syringe to reach the prescribed dose.

Clinical Insight 26-4 ➤ Measuring Dosage When Changing Needles

Note: These are not the old "air lock" techniques.

Using a Nonfilter Needle

When drawing medication from a multidose vial, you may sometimes need to use two regular needles. Alternately, you may use a needleless reconstitution device that is designed with a dispensing spike instead of a needle on one end, and a luer-lock port on the other end that attaches to the syringe.

Equipment. One needle (or needless reconstitution device) for drawing up the medication; and one needle for injecting the medication into the patient.

1. **Using Needle #1, draw up the prescribed amount of medication.** When using a vial, inject air into the air pocket within the vial. Then withdraw the correct amount of medication from the vial. Be sure to keep the tip of the needle in the fluid in order to avoid aspirating air bubbles into the syringe.
2. **Remove bubbles; eject the air.** After drawing up the medication, tap on the barrel of the syringe to remove air bubbles, if necessary. Then eject the air from the syringe (keeping the syringe vertical) while retaining the correct amount of medication in the syringe. Check the volume closely at eye level.
3. **Remove the Needle #1 and discard it** into a needle-safe container. Put on a fresh needle (Needle #2) for injection.
4. **Using Needle #2**, pull back on the plunger, and draw an extra 0.2 mL of air to account for the air within the needle.
5. **Check the medication dosage.** Your plunger should be 0.2 mL more than the ordered dose.
6. **Still using Needle #2, when you inject the patient**, she will receive the correct dose. The air will drive the medication from the needle into the patient's tissues. This is important when giving irritating medications, such as iron. (This is called an air lock.)

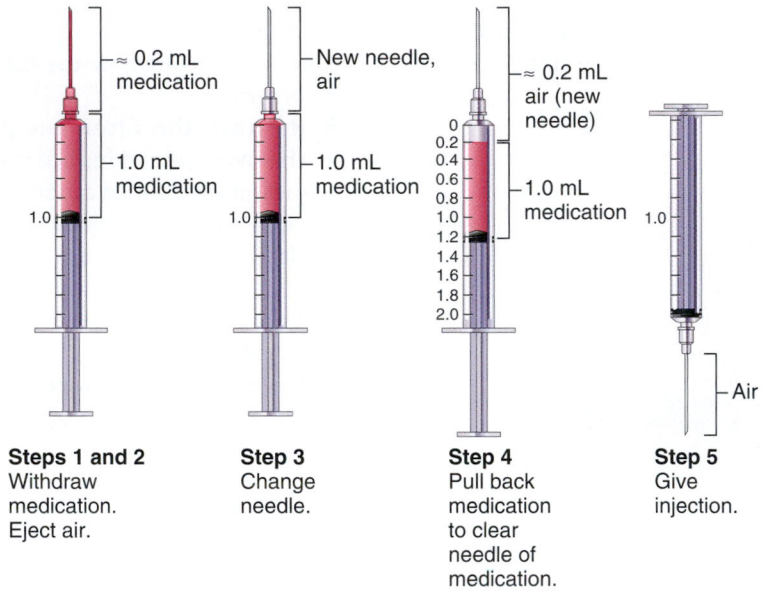

Nonfilter needles.

Using a Filter Needle

Always use a filter needle to withdraw medications, if one is available. You must change needles to give the injection, because:

- Filter needles are too large. To give the injection, you must use a needle of the correct gauge and length.
- You must eject air to measure the medication, but you should not push medication out of the syringe through the filter needle because it can break the filter and release glass (and other) fragments.

In the following method, pulling air into the syringe allows for exact dosage when the medication is injected. When ejected, the air will clear the needle so that the patient receives all the medication that is in the syringe.

Equipment. One filter needle (or filter cannula) and one regular needle.

1. **With the filter needle (or cannula)**, withdraw the exact amount of medication. Eject air bubbles (keeping the syringe vertical) as needed to obtain correct dose. Remember, you must not eject fluid through the filter needle.

Clinical Insight 26-4 ➤ Measuring Dosage When Changing Needles—cont'd

2. **Pull back on the plunger to withdraw all the medication from the filter needle (or filter cannula) into the syringe.** Depending on the size of the access cannula, this may be as much as 0.2 mL. It will now appear that you have more than the ordered dose in the syringe (but you do not; the air is taking up some of the space).
3. **Change to the needle you are going to use for injection.**
4. **Hold the syringe vertically, and eject air** until you see a drop of medication at the tip of the needle ("drop to the top").
5. **Measure the medication.** It should be at the correct syringe marking. If it is not, then tip the syringe horizontally, and eject the medication until the dose is correct.
6. **When you inject the patient, she will receive the correct dose** even though some medication will remain in the needle.
7. **If you are giving an irritating medication** (e.g., iron) draw 0.2 mL of air into the syringe before giving the injection. (This is called an air lock.)

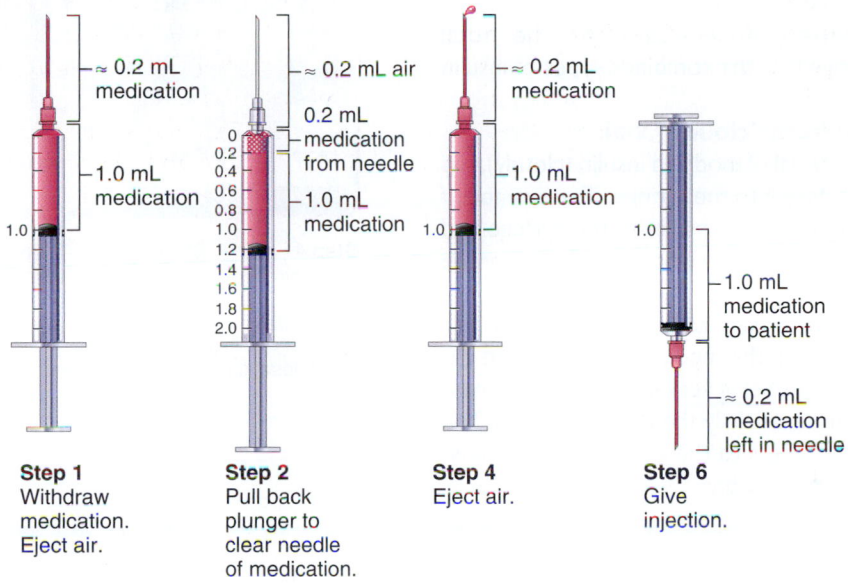

Filter needles.

Clinical Insight 26-5 ➤ Mixing Two Kinds of Insulin in One Syringe

What You Should Know

Various combinations of rapid-acting, intermediate-acting, and long-acting insulin may be prescribed. Some can be mixed; some cannot.

- Lente insulins (Lente and Lantus) can be mixed with each other, but not with neutral protamine Hagedorn (NPH).
- Even though they are compatible, do not mix Lente with regular insulin, except for patients who are already controlled on this mixture. Lente will bind with regular insulin, delaying the onset of action.
- A general rule is "clear before cloudy." Regular insulin is clear; all other types are cloudy. Therefore, you would draw up regular insulin into the syringe before Lente or NPH insulin, which are modified. If you draw up a modified type first, the needle may transfer it into the unmodified (regular) vial.

What You Should Do

Follow these steps when drawing up insulin from two vials into one syringe. The procedure assumes you are mixing regular (unmodified) insulin with a modified (e.g., NPH) insulin.

1. **Maintain sterile technique throughout.**
2. **Before preparing the insulin**—Rotate the vials between the palms of your hands for at least 1 minute, and invert them to ensure an adequate concentration. Do not shake the vials because this can create bubbles, which take up space and make it difficult to measure the dose precisely.
3. **Scrub vial stoppers** with alcohol or other antiseptic (they are usually multidose vials).
4. **Inject air into "cloudy" vial**—Using an insulin syringe and needle, inject an amount of air equal to the amount

(Continued)

Clinical Insight 26-5 ➤ Mixing Two Kinds of Insulin in One Syringe—cont'd

of insulin to be withdrawn from the vial of modified insulin (cloudy vial). Do not allow the needle tip to touch the insulin.

5. **Inject air into "clear" vial**—Using the same syringe, inject the appropriate amount of air into the vial of regular insulin (clear vial).
6. **Withdraw insulin from "clear" vial**—Do not withdraw the needle; withdraw the correct dose of regular insulin.
7. **Measure the dose of "clear"**—Remove the syringe from the regular insulin. Eject air, and remove all air bubbles to measure the correct dose.
8. **Calculate combined dose**—Calculate the total amount on the syringe that the combined types of insulin should measure.
9. **Withdraw insulin from "cloudy" vial.**
   a. Return to the (first) vial of modified insulin (cloudy), and draw the correct dose into the syringe. (For example, if you have 5 units of regular insulin in the syringe and you need 10 units of NPH, the plunger should be at the 15-unit mark when you have drawn up the NPH.)
   b. Recall that you have already added air to this vial in a previous step. Draw up the medication slowly and exactly to the total dose, being very careful not to create bubbles and to withdraw only the amount needed. You cannot return any excess to the vial because it is now a mixture of two medications.
10. **Administer the insulin mixture** within 5 minutes after preparation. Even NPH insulin will bind with regular insulin and delay the onset of its action.

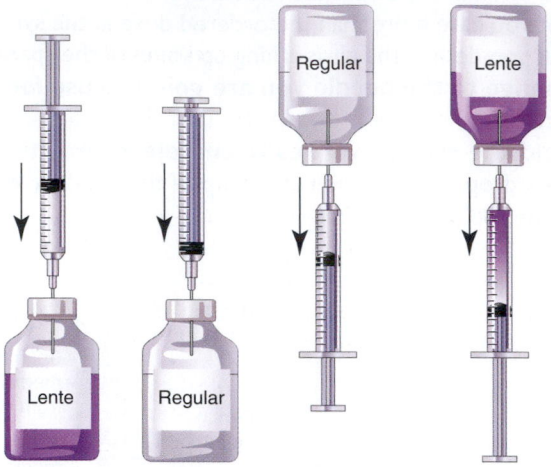

Step 4 Inject air (cloudy insulin vial). **Step 5** Inject air (clear insulin vial). **Step 6** Withdraw dose (clear vial). **Step 9** Withdraw dose (cloudy vial).

Total dose is mixture of clear and cloudy insulins.

Clinical Insight 26-6 ➤ Administering Anticoagulant Medication Subcutaneously

Because of the anticoagulant properties of heparin and enoxaparin (Lovenox), you will need to adapt your technique for subcutaneous injections in the following ways:

- Enoxaparin-prefilled syringes and graduated prefilled syringes are available with a system that shields the needle after injection.
- Use a ⅜-inch, 25- or 26-gauge needle.
- After drawing up the correct dose, add 0.2 mL of air to the syringe.
  To ensure that all of the medication is injected into the subcutaneous tissue and is not tracked into the superficial tissue.
- Do not expel the air bubble from the syringe before the injection.
  To avoid the loss of drug when using prefilled syringes.
- With your nondominant hand, pinch or spread the skin; insert the needle at a 90° angle, using your dominant hand.
  - If the patient has very little subcutaneous tissue, use a ⅝-inch needle and insert it at a 45° angle.
  - Introduce the whole length of the needle into a skinfold held between the thumb and forefinger; hold the skinfold throughout the injection.
- Alternate administration among sites on the abdomen. Give the injection subcutaneously deep on the abdomen, at least 2 inches away from the umbilicus.
- Do not aspirate before injecting.
  Doing so can traumatize tissue and cause bruising.
- Do not massage the site after injecting.
  Doing so can cause bleeding and bruising. It may also cause the heparin to be absorbed more rapidly than desired.
- Keep a record of the sites used. Most agencies have a chart of the body on which to record the sites injected.

Several mix-ups between heparin and insulin have been reported. To help avoid this, in addition to observing the "3 checks and 6 rights":

1. Do not store heparin and insulin vials beside each other.
2. Have another RN check your preparation before administering IV heparin or insulin.
3. Think critically (e.g., ask yourself if giving heparin—or insulin—makes sense given the patient's diagnosis) (Cohen, 2007; Mattox, 2012).

Clinical Insight 26-7 ➤ Taking Action After a Medication Error

First check the patient. Take his vital signs, and perform assessments related to the medication that was given.

- If you are unfamiliar with the side effects of the medication, consult a drug reference source.
- Verify that you have made a medication error, and identify the type of error.
- Notify the nurse in charge for guidance if this is your first error.
- Notify the prescriber and follow her orders for intervention.
- Document on the chart that the medication was given, but do not indicate that it was given in error. This alerts anyone reviewing the chart that an error was made.
- Complete an incident report according to the facility's policies. Ask for assistance if you are unfamiliar with the format or requirement of this form. It is important that the information you provide is factual and accurate.
- Do not document in the patient's chart that an incident report was filed. This alerts anyone reviewing the chart that an error was made and makes the incident report available for legal review in the event of a lawsuit.
- When you are calmer and can think clearly, critically review the error. Identify the influences that led to your making the error. Were you rushed? Did you check the prescription? Did you follow the rights of medication? Whatever the reason, use this situation as a learning experience to improve your practice.

TABLES: ABBREVIATIONS

Because abbreviations can be easily misread, it is better to write words in full, especially when you are working with medications. However, you might still see the following abbreviations, so you should be familiar with them. Be sure you are familiar with the list of abbreviations approved for use in your particular agency. Abbreviations should be used cautiously and avoided when possible.

Common Medication-Related Abbreviations

ABBREVIATION	EXPLANATION	ABBREVIATION	EXPLANATION
ac	before meals: Example: 0700, 1100, 1700 hours	mL	Milliliter
ad lib	as desired	OTC	over-the-counter
a.m.	Morning	oz	Ounce
bid	twice a day: 0900, 2100 hours	pc	after meals: Example: 0900, 1300, 1900 hours
c̄	With	p.m.	Evening
fl oz	fluid ounce	po or PO	by mouth
g, gm, or GM	Gram	prn	as needed
gtt	Drop	qh, qr (q1h, q1hr)	Every hour
h, hr	Hour	q2h, q2hr	every 2 hours: Example: 0800, 1000, 1200 hours, etc.
IM	Intramuscular	q3h, q3hr	every 3 hours: Example: 0900, 1200, 1500 hours, etc.
IV	Intravenous	q4h, q4hr	every 4 hours: Example: 0200, 0600, 1000, 1400, 1800, 2200 hours
IVPB	intravenous piggyback	q6h, q6hr	every 6 hours: Example 0600, 1200, 1800 hours, 2400.
Kg or kg	Kilogram	qid or QID	four times a day: Example 1000, 1400, 1800, 2200
KVO	keep vein open		
L or l	Liter		
mEq	Milliequivalent		

(Continued)

Common Medication-Related Abbreviations—cont'd

ABBREVIATION	EXPLANATION	ABBREVIATION	EXPLANATION
qs or QS	sufficient quantity	Tab or tab	Tablet
s̄	Without	T or Tbsp	Tablespoon
stat or STAT	at once	tid or TID	three times a day: 1000, 1400, 1800 hours
sup or supp	Suppository	t or tsp	Teaspoon
susp	Suspension		

Institute for Safe Medication Practices (ISMP) List of Error-Prone Abbreviations, Symbols, and Dose Designations

ABBREVIATIONS	INTENDED MEANING	MISINTERPRETATION	CORRECTION
µg	Microgram	Mistaken as "mg"	Use "mcg."
AD, AS, AU	Right ear, left ear, each ear	Mistaken as OD, OS, OU (right eye, left eye, each eye)	Use "right ear," "left ear," or "each ear."
OD, OS, OU	Right eye, left eye, each eye	Mistaken as AD, AS, AU (right ear, left ear, each ear)	Use "right eye," "left eye," or "each eye."
BT	Bedtime	Mistaken as "BID" (twice daily)	Use "bedtime."
cc	Cubic centimeters	Mistaken as "u" (units)	Use "mL."
D/C	Discharge or discontinue	Premature discontinuation of medications if D/C (intended to mean: "discharge") has been misinterpreted as "discontinued" when followed by a list of discharge medications	Use "discharge" and "discontinue."
ij	Injection	Mistaken as "IV" or "intrajugular"	Use "injection."
IN	Intranasal	Mistaken as "IM" or "IV"	Use "intranasal" or "NAS."
HS	Half-strength	Mistaken as bedtime	Use "half-strength."
hs	At bedtime, hours of sleep	Mistaken as half-strength	Use "bedtime."
*IU	International units	Mistaken as IV (intravenous) or 10 (ten)	Use "International units."
o.d. or OD	Once daily	Mistaken as "right eye" (OD-oculus dexter), leading to oral liquid medications administered in the eye	Use "daily."
OJ	Orange juice	Mistaken as OD or OS (right or left eye); drugs meant to be diluted in orange juice may be given in the eye	Use "orange juice."
per os	By mouth, orally	The "os" can be mistaken as "left eye" (OS-oculus sinister)	Use "PO," "by mouth," or "orally."
*q.d. or QD	Every day	Mistaken as q.i.d., especially if the period after the "q" or the tail of the "q" is misunderstood as an "i"	Use "daily."
qhs	Nightly at bedtime	Mistaken as "qhr" or every hour	Use "nightly."
qn	Nightly or at bedtime	Mistaken as "qh" (every hour)	Use "nightly" or "at bedtime."

Institute for Safe Medication Practices (ISMP) List of Error-Prone Abbreviations, Symbols, and Dose Designations—cont'd

ABBREVIATIONS	INTENDED MEANING	MISINTERPRETATION	CORRECTION
*q.o.d. or QOD	Every other day	Mistaken as "q.d." (daily) or "q.i.d." (four times daily) if the "o" is poorly written	Use "every other day."
qld	Daily	Mistaken as q.i.d. (four times daily)	Use "daily."
q6PM, etc.	Every evening at 6 PM	Mistaken as every 6 hours	Use "6 PM nightly" or "6 PM daily."
SC, SQ, subQ, or subq	Subcutaneous	SC mistaken as SL (sublingual); SQ mistaken as "5 every"; the "q" in "sub q" has been mistaken as "every (e.g., a heparin dose ordered sub q 2 hours before hours before surgery) surgery" misunderstood as every 2	Spell out "subcutaneous."
ss	Sliding scale (insulin)	Mistaken as "55"	Spell out "sliding scale"; use "one-half."
SSRI, SSI	Sliding scale regular insulin	Mistaken as selective-serotonin reuptake inhibitor; mistaken as Strong Solution of Iodine (Lugol's)	Spell out "sliding scale (insulin)."
i/d	One daily	Mistaken as "tid"	Use "1 daily."
TIW or tiw	3 times a week	Mistaken as "3 times a day" or "twice in a week"	Use "3 times weekly."
*U or u	Unit	Mistaken as the number 0 or 4, causing a 10-fold overdose or greater (e.g., 4U seen as "40" or 4u seen as "44"); mistaken as "cc" so dose given in volume instead of units (e.g., 4u seen as 4cc)	Use "unit."

DOSE DESIGNATIONS OR OTHER INFORMATION	INTENDED MEANING	MISINTERPRETATION	CORRECTION
*Trailing zero after decimal point (e.g., 1.0 mg)	1 mg	Mistaken as 10 mg if the decimal point is not seen expressed in whole numbers	Do not use trailing zeros for doses.
*No leading zero before a decimal dose (e.g., .5 mg)	0.5 mg	Mistaken as 5 mg if the decimal point is not seen	Use zero before a decimal point when the dose is less than a whole unit.
Drug name and drug dose run together (e.g., Inderal 40 mg)	Inderal 40 mg	Mistaken as Inderal 140 mg	Place adequate space between the drug name, dose, and unit of measurement.
Numeric dose and unit of measurement run together (e.g., 10 mg)	10 mg	The "m" can be mistaken for a zero, leading to a 10-fold dosing error	Place adequate space between the drug name, dose, and unit of measurement.
Abbreviations such as mg. or mL. with a period following the abbreviation	mg or mL	The period is unnecessary and could be mistaken as the number 1 if written poorly.	Use mg, mL, etc. without a period.
Large doses without properly placed commas (e.g., 100000 units or 1000000 units)	100,000 or 1,000,000 units	100000 has been mistaken for 10,000 or 1,000,000; 1,000,000 has been mistaken for 100,000.	Use commas for dosing units at or above 1,000 or use such words as 100 "thousand" or 1 "million" to improve readability.

(Continued)

Institute for Safe Medication Practices (ISMP) List of Error-Prone Abbreviations, Symbols, and Dose Designations—cont'd

DRUG NAME ABBREVIATIONS	INTENDED MEANING	MISINTERPRETATION	CORRECTION
NOTE: PHARMACIES DO NOT ACCEPT ORDERS FOR ABBREVIATED MEDICATIONS			
ARA A	vidarabine	Mistaken as cytarabine (ARA C)	Use the complete drug name.
AZR	zidovudine (Retrovir)	Mistaken as azathioprine or aztreonam	Use the complete drug name.
CPZ	prochlorperazine (Compazine)	Mistaken as chlorpromazine	Use complete drug name.
DPT	Demerol-Phenergan-Thorazine	Mistaken as diphtheria-pertussis-tetanus	Use complete drug name.
DTO	Diluted tincture of opium, or deodorized tincture of opium (Paregoric)	Mistaken as tincture of opium	Use complete drug name.
HCl	hydrochloric acid or hydrochloride	Mistaken as potassium chloride (The "H" is misinterpreted as "K.")	Use complete drug name unless expressed as a salt of a drug.
HCT	hydrocortisone	Mistaken as hydrochlorothiazide	Use complete drug name.
HCTZ	hydrochlorothiazide	Mistaken as hydrocortisone (seen as HCT 250 mg)	Use complete drug name.
*$MgSO_4$	magnesium sulfate	Mistaken as morphine sulfate	Use complete drug name.
*MS, MSO_4	morphine sulfate	Mistaken as magnesium sulfate	Use complete drug name.
MTX	methotrexate	Mistaken as mitoxantrone	Use complete drug name.
PCA	procainamide	Mistaken as patient-controlled analgesia	Use complete drug name.
PTU	propylthiouracil	Mistaken as mercaptopurine	Use complete drug name.
T3	Tylenol with codeine No. 3	Mistaken as liothyronine	Use complete drug name.
TAC	triamcinolone	Mistaken as tetracaine, adrenaline, cocaine	Use complete drug name.
TNK	TNKase	Mistaken as "TPA"	Use complete drug name.
$ZnSO_4$	zinc sulfate	Mistaken as morphine sulfate	Use complete drug name.
STEMMED DRUG NAMES	**INTENDED MEANING**	**MISINTERPRETATION**	**CORRECTION**
"nitro drip"	nitroglycerine infusion	Mistaken as sodium nitroprusside infusion	Use complete drug name.
"Norflox"	norfloxacin	Mistaken as Norflex	Use complete drug name.
"IV Vanc"	intravenous vancomycin	Mistaken as Invanz	Use complete drug name.

Institute for Safe Medication Practices (ISMP) List of Error-Prone Abbreviations, Symbols, and Dose Designations—cont'd

SYMBOLS	INTENDED MEANING	MISINTERPRETATION	CORRECTION
ʒ	dram	Symbol for dram mistaken as "3"	Use the metric system.
♏	Minim	Mistaken as "mL"	Use the metric system.
x3d	for 3 days	Mistaken as "3 doses"	Use "for 3 days."
< and >	greater than and less than	Mistaken as opposite of intended; mistakenly using incorrect symbols	Use "greater than" or "less than."
/ (slash mark)	separates two doses or indicates "per"	Mistaken as the number 1 (e.g., "25 units/10 units" misread as "25 units and 110" units)	Use "per" rather than a slash mark to separate doses.
@	at	Mistaken as "2"	Use "at."
&	and	Mistaken as "2"	Use "and."
+	plus or and	Mistaken as "4"	Use "and" or "plus."
°	hour	mistaken as zero (e.g., q2° seen as q 20)	Use "hr", "h", or "hour."

*Listed on The Joint Commission's "Do Not Use" List.
Source: Institute for Safe Medication Practices. (2004). *ISMP list of error-prone abbreviations, symbols, and dose designations.* Retrieved July 8, 2013, from, http://www.ismp.org/tools/errorproneabbreviations.pdf

MEASURING AND CALCULATING DOSAGE

Medications are not always available in the exact dosage the patient needs. Therefore, you must be proficient in calculating drug dosages to be sure your patients receive the correct amount of medication.

Drugs in solid form (e.g., tablets, powders) are measured by weight (e.g., milligrams, grains). Drugs used for irrigation, infusion, and injection are liquids (usually solutions), measured by volume, generally milliliters. A **solution** can be either a solid dissolved in a fluid, or a given volume of one liquid dissolved in a given volume of another liquid. Solution concentrations may be expressed as a proportion. A 1/100 solution is a solution of 1 gram of solid dissolved in 100 mL of fluid, or 1 mL of fluid mixed with 100 mL of another fluid.

When measuring and calculating, you can think of solutions as a quantity of "solid" drug dissolved in a quantity of "liquid" diluent. The diluent merely carries the medication. When you see a vial marked "50 mg/mL," for example, you will know this means that in each milliliter of diluent there are 50 mg (in weight) of the solid, active medication. Your task is to determine how many milliliters of liquid you need to give the patient the number of milligrams of active drug ordered.

Medication Measurement Systems

Medications are usually ordered and measured using the metric system; however, there are still a few medications that use the apothecary and household systems, so you need to learn how to work with all three systems.

Metric System

The metric system is the preferred system. The basic metric units of measurement are the **meter** (the unit for linear measurement), the **liter** (for capacity or volume), and the **gram** (for weight). A meter is a little longer than a yard, a liter a little larger than a quart, and a gram a little more than the weight of a steel paper clip. The metric system promotes accuracy by allowing for calculation of small drug dosages. A disadvantage of this system in the United States is its limited use among people outside of healthcare. The following are the metric units you will use in preparing medications.

Weights

1 mg (milligram) = 1000 mcg or (micrograms)
1 gm (gram) = 1000 mg (milligrams)
1 kg (kilogram) = 1000 g or gm (grams)

Volume

1000 mL (milliliters) = 1 L (Liter)
1000 (cubic centimeters) = 1 L (Liter)

The following are examples of medication orders using the metric system:

Milk of Magnesia 30 mL orally daily at bedtime
Ancef 1 gm IV q8hr

Apothecary System

The British apothecary system of measurement has been in use in the United States since colonial times. Only a few medications (e.g., aspirin) are measured using this system because it is less precise. Prescribers usually write apothecary measurements using Roman numerals, but you may also see them in Arabic numerals. The system uses fractions (e.g., gr ¼) instead of decimals (e.g., 0.25 gr). **Key Point:** ***Keep in mind the apothecary abbreviations are prone to misinterpretation and error because they are not often used.*** The following are the units used in preparing medications:

Volume

1 minim (m)	=	1 drop (gtt)
1 fluid dram (dr)	=	60 minims
1 fluid ounce (oz)	=	8 fluid drams

Weight

1 dram (dr)	=	27.34 grains (gr)
1 grain	=	60 milligrams (mg)

The following are Roman numerals you will use most often:

M	=	1000	X	=	10
D	=	500	V	=	5
C	=	100	II	=	1
L	=	50	II	=	2

The following are examples of medication orders using the apothecary system:

Aspirin grains V orally q4hr prn for fever greater than 101°F
Chloramphenicol otic 2 gtts in each ear tid daily

Many institutions are no longer using the apothecary system of measurement. If a prescription contains this unit of measurement, verify the intended dose with the prescriber and pharmacist.

Household Measurements

Because most people are familiar with the household system, it is easier to teach a patient about home medications using this system. However, nurses use it only occasionally because dosages measured in this system are usually only approximate. The following are household units of measurement with metric conversion:

Volume

1 tsp (t)	=	5 mL		
1 tablespoon (tbsp or T)	=	3 teaspoons (tsp)	=	15 mL
6 tsp or 2 T	=	1 ounce (oz)	=	30 mL
16 T or 8 oz	=	1 cup (c)	=	240 mL
16 T or 8 oz	=	1 glass	=	240 mL
2 C	=	1 pint (pt)	=	480 mL
2 pt	=	1 quart (qt)	=	946.4 mL
4 qt	=	1 gallon (gal)		

Weight

1 oz	=		=	28.35 gm
16 oz	=	1 pound (lb)	=	0.45 kg

Length

12 inches (in.)	=	1 foot (ft)	=	30.5 cm
3 feet (ft)	=	1 yard (yd)	=	91.4 cm

The following is an example of a medication order using the household system:

Amoxicillin 250 mg per 5 mL Give 1 tsp PO tid

Special Measurements: Units and mEq

Insulin, a drug used by diabetics to assist in the control of blood sugar, is measured in **units**, with 100 international units (U100) being the standard strength preparation. In this strength, 1 mL of the fluid medication contains 100 units of insulin. Heparin (an anticoagulant) and penicillin are also ordered in units.

Be aware that not all units are the same. You must always read the container label to know the number of units per milliliter.

The following are medication orders using units:

NPH insulin 14 units subcutaneous q morning
Heparin 4000 units subcutaneous bid (twice daily)

Milliequivalents (mEq) indicate the strength of the ion concentration in a drug. A milliequivalent is the number of grams of a solid contained in one milliliter of a solution. Electrolytes, such as potassium chloride (KCl), are measured in mEq. The following are medication orders using mEq:

KCl 20 mEq orally bid (twice daily)
D_5W 1000 mL with KCl 40 mEq q8hr

Note that units and mEq *cannot* be directly converted to the apothecary, metric, or household system.

Calculating Dosages

You should be able to calculate accurately using several different methods and formulas. Inaccurate calculations result in incorrect dosages and could harm the patient. One easy formula to remember is the following:

$$\frac{\text{Dose on hand}}{\text{Quantity (or volume) on hand}} = \frac{\text{Desired Dose}}{\text{Quantity (or volume) desired}} \quad \text{or} \quad \frac{DH}{QH} = \frac{DD}{X}$$

Or

$$\frac{DH}{QH} = \frac{DD}{X}$$

Remember: You must pay attention to *both* the milligrams (weight of the drug) marked on the medication container *and* the milliliters (amount of liquid in which the medication is dissolved). For example, suppose you have a prefilled syringe containing 50 mg of meperidine (Demerol) in 1 mL volume, but you wish to administer only 25 mg to the patient. How much of the liquid (how many mL) would you give?

$$\frac{DH}{QH} = \frac{DD}{X} \quad \text{or} \quad \frac{50\text{ mg}}{1\text{ mL}} = \frac{25\text{ mg}}{X}$$

Therefore (recalling your algebra),

50X = 25 mL,
so X = 25 divided by 50,
so X = 0.5 mL

Here is an alternative formula you can use for calculating dosages:

$$\frac{\text{Dose desired (DD)}}{\text{Dose on hand (DH)}} \times \text{quantity on hand (QH)} = \text{desired quantity}$$

ThinkLike a Nurse 26-1A

Mr. Pearson (Meet Your Patients, in Volume 1) has been ordered nifedipine (Procardia XL) 60 mg orally daily. You have available Procardia XL (extended-release nifedipine) 30-mg tablets. Calculate the number of tablets you will need for one dose. How many tablets per day?

Conversions Within One System

When a drug prescription is written in the same system as the preparation you have on hand, you can easily make conversions. For example, in the metric system, if you want to convert grams to milligrams, you simply multiply by 1000 (because 1 g = 1000 mg). So, if you have 2.5 grams,

2.5 gm × 1000 = 2500 mg

To change milligrams to grams, *divide* by 1000—move the decimal three places to the left. For example, if you wanted to know, in grams, the equivalent of 250 mg:

You know that 1000 mg = 1 g
By dividing: 250 mg ÷ 1000 mg = 0.25 g
Or by moving the decimal point three places to the left: 250.0 mg = 0.250 g

Use exactly the same procedures to convert liters (L) and milliliters (mL). For example, if you wanted to know how many milliliters are the equivalent of 0.25 L:

You know that 1 L = 1000 mL
By multiplying: 0.25 L × 1000 = 250 mL
By moving the decimal point three places to the right, 0.250 L = 250 mL (Notice that you must add a zero to *have* three places to the right.)

Within the apothecary system or the household system, use the equivalents and follow a similar process of multiplying and dividing (of course, you cannot just move the decimal in these systems). For example, suppose you have a dr ii (2 dram) tablet and you need to know how many grains you have (apothecary system). You know that 1 dram = 27.3 grains, so multiply:

2 drams (dr) × 27.3 grains (gr) = 54.6 gr,
rounded to 55 gr.

In the household system, suppose you have 4 tbsp of a liquid and you need to know what part of a cup that represents. You know that 1 cup = 16 tablespoons, so substitute the equivalent and divide:

16 tbsp = 1 cup

So,

4 tbsp = 16 ÷ 4 = 1/4 cup

KnowledgeCheck 26-1A

Lanoxin 0.25 mg orally daily is prescribed for a patient with congestive heart failure. The label on the package you have reads "Lanoxin 0.125 mg" How many tablets will you give? Use the "dose on hand (DOH)" formula.

Conversions Between Systems

You will sometimes need to make conversions from one measurement system to another. For example, you may need to convert pounds to kilograms because many medications are ordered as milligrams per kilograms (e.g., "Give 2 mg per kg of body weight"). The following are the basic methods for converting between systems. For an excellent summary of converting measurements within and between different systems,

Go to Chapter 26, the **Supplemental Materials, Measuring and Calculating Dosage,** on Davis*Plus*.

- **Metric and Apothecary—Weights**
  Grams and grains
  (Memorize: 1 g = 15 gr)
  To convert grams to grains—*multiply* the grams by 15
  To convert grains to grams—*divide* the grains by 15
  Grains and milligrams
  (Memorize: 1 gr = 60 mg)
  To convert grains to milligrams—*multiply* the grains by 60
  To convert milligrams to grains—*divide* the milligrams by 60
- **Metric and Apothecary and Household—Liquid Volume**
  Liters and ounces
  (Memorize: 1 L = 34.4 oz)
  To convert liters to ounces—*multiply* the liters by 33.4
  To convert ounces to liters—*divide* the ounces by 34.4
  Ounces and milliliters
  (Memorize: 1 oz = 30 mL)
  To convert ounces to milliliters—*multiply* the ounces by 30
  To convert milliliters to ounces—*divide* the milliliters by 30
  Milliliters and drops
  (Memorize: 1 mL = 15 drops or 15 minims)
  To convert milliliters to minims or drops—*multiply* milliliters by 15
  To convert minims and drops to milliliters—*divide* the minims or drops by 15

KnowledgeCheck 26-2A

Work the following conversions:

- How many drops in 4 mL?
- How many mL in 2 oz?
- Convert 16 oz to liters.
- You have 3 g. How many grains is this?
- You have 10 mg. How many grains is this?

How Should I Calculate Dosage for a Child?

You must be very careful when calculating medication dosages for children and infants. Most drug references list normal pediatric ranges, which can serve as additional verification.

You should rarely need to calculate a child's dosage on the basis of an adult dose, because medication prescriptions should specify the exact dosage for the individual child. However, when you must, you can use either the Body Surface Area Formula by using the nomogram for Children or Clark's Rule for Children to verify the safety of pediatric orders. To find a child's BSA using the nomogram, you must know the child's height and weight.

To use the nomogram, go to Chapter 26, **Tables, Boxes, Figures: ESG Figure 26-2: Nomogram,** on Davis*Plus*.

Orders for pediatric dosages are usually either calculated by the prescriber or stated in terms of "milligrams per kilogram of body weight." For example, you might have a prescription for "Erythromycin 30 mg/kg of body weight." You know that 1 kg equals 2.2 lb. If the child weighs 44 lb, then to convert to kilograms you divide 44 by 2.2; the child thus weighs 20 kg. So, 30 mg/kg would be 30 mg × 20, or 600 mg (the dosage for a 20-kg child).

For Clark's Rule, you would apply a formula using the child's weight in pounds. If you want to use Clark's Rule,

Go to Chapter 26, **Tables, Boxes, Figures: ESG Box 26-2,** on Davis*Plus*.

For a variety of Web-based dose calculators you can use,

Go to Manuel's Web site at http://www.manuelsweb.com/nrs_calculators.htm

Your electronic study guide (ESG) contains several practice problems for calculating adult and child dosages.

Go to Chapter 26, **Dosage Calculation Problems,** on Davis*Plus*.

If you cannot work the practice problems easily, you should obtain a dosage calculation book and practice the various formulas until you are proficient with conversion.

CLINICALREASONING
Applying the Full-Spectrum Nursing Model

PATIENT SITUATION

Leonard LeMonte is a 57-year-old African American man who has come to his primary care provider because of persistent headaches that increase in intensity over the course of a day. His overall health has been good, although he is approximately 50 to 60 pounds overweight. Past medical history is significant for borderline primary hypertension and non-insulin-dependent diabetes, type 2 (diet controlled). Mr. LeMonte tells you he works in a high-stress environment. He shares great concern with you that he fears losing his job and not being able to pay his bills and meet other financial commitments for his family. Mr. LeMonte tells you he has little time for hobbies or recreational outlets because he works so many hours.

THINKING

1. *Theoretical Knowledge (Facts and Principles):* You see in the chart that the provider prescribed repaglinide (Prandin), 2 mg tid (3 times/day), to treat Mr. LeMonte's diabetes. By what route is this medication given?
2. *Critical Thinking (Inquiry):* If you did not know the answer to the first question, specifically how did you get the information? State your source.

DOING

3. *Nursing Process (Assessment):* To evaluate Mr. LeMonte's responses to his diabetes medication, what questions do you need to ask him?
4. *Practical Knowledge (Skills):* Mr. LeMonte tells you that he forgot to take his Prandin this morning and also at lunchtime. What should you do?

CARING

5. *Self-Knowledge:* In what areas do you feel compassion for Mr. LeMonte, on which you might build a caring relationship?
6. *Self-Knowledge:* What do you identify as your strength in dealing with Mr. LeMonte's healthcare needs?
7. *Ethical Knowledge:* Mr. LeMonte tells you that he frequently skips doses of his Prandin because he can't afford the expense. He asks you not to tell his wife about this because he doesn't want her to worry. What will you do?

Critical Thinking and Clinical Reasoning

1. Your patient is prescribed Humulin R insulin 30 units subcutaneously. You have available in a multidose vial Humulin R insulin; the label reads "100 units per mL."
   a. What equipment and supplies do you need to administer this medication? Be specific.
   b. What practical knowledge (psychomotor skills) will you need?
   c. With regard to the psychomotor skills, what are the two aspects that require the most careful attention? Explain your thinking.
   d. What will you do to ensure that you have the correct dosage?
   e. What specific technique steps will you take to decrease the risk for infection?
   f. Suppose that after drawing the insulin into the syringe, you see that instead of the 30 units prescribed, you have only 20 units in the syringe. What will you do?
2. A physician orders heparin 4,000 units subcutaneous q12hr for Mr. Dale. You have on hand heparin 10,000 units/mL. How many milliliters should you draw up?

Patient Information for Exercises 3 Through 6 and 8

Recall the patients from Chapter 26, **Meet Your Patients,** in Volume 1. Exercises 3 through 6 and 8, following, refer to those patients. They are listed here for your convenience.

- Margaret Marks, an 82-year-old woman who has a fractured hip and experiences periods of confusion
- Cary Pearson, a 70-year-old man with feeding and swallowing difficulties who receives his medications through a gastrostomy tube
- Cyndi Early, a 32-year-old woman with diabetes who is scheduled for surgery at 1000 today
- James Bigler, a 44-year-old man who has had a repair of a compound fracture of the right arm and is receiving IV fluids and medications
- Rebecca Jones, an 84-year-old woman with compression fractures of two lumbar vertebrae resulting from a fall.

3. It is 0800, and you have begun organizing your medication pass for this shift by verifying the MAR entries against the provider's orders. You notice that Mr. Bigler has been prescribed Toradol 30 mg IM q6hr. His last dose was supposed to have been given at 0600, and there is no documentation that the medication was administered.
   a. What should you do?
   b. Should you assume the night shift nurse gave the medication but forgot to document that she had given it, and give the 0600 dose late? Why or why not?
   c. When should the next dose be given?
   d. If the night nurse did *not* give the medication as ordered, what type of medication error did she make? What factors that could have caused this error?
   e. Assuming that the nurse *did* give the medication as ordered at 0600, what error did the night nurse make? Which of the "rights of medication" was violated?
4. You receive the laboratory results for Cary Pearson's potassium level and find it to be 3.1 mEq/L. You notify the provider and receive a verbal order to add 20 milliequivalents of KCl to his IV of D_5 ½NS (5% dextrose in half-strength normal saline [0.45% saline]) to infuse at 125 mL/hr. The IV infusing is a new 1000-mL bag that is almost full.
   a. Write the prescription as you would write it on the order sheet.
   b. What information must you put on the additive label for this bag?
   c. Suppose the situation were slightly different. There is only 100 mL of IV fluid left in Mr. Pearson's IV bag when you call the provider, who prescribes, "Add 10 mEq to the IV, and infuse it at 125 mL/hr." Would you ask for clarification of this order? Why or why not?

d. Change the situation again. You have taken the order in this way: "Add 20 mEq of KCl to 1000 mL of D_5 ½NS and infuse at 125 mL/hr." You are preparing this medication and find that Mr. Pearson currently has 500 mL remaining in his IV. Should you add the KCl to this infusing IV or wait until you hang a new 1000-mL bag? If you do add it, how much KCl will you add? What is your rationale for your decision?

e. You begin preparing the infusion with the 20 mEq of KCl to be added and find you have available a vial containing KCl 40 mEq in a 10-mL vial. How many milliliters of KCl will you add to the bag of fluids?

5. Dr. Xi has ordered heparin 8000 units subcutaneous q12hr for Mrs. Marks.
   a. You have vials of heparin containing 10,000 units/mL. How many mL of heparin will you administer?
   b. To prevent tissue trauma and hematoma, and to help ensure adequate absorption, what precautions should you take while administering heparin?
   c. What syringe and needle will you select for administration, and why?
6. You are checking Mrs. Early's chart and find that the provider has prescribed a medication the patient lists as an allergy. What steps should you take?
7. A patient has been taking warfarin sodium (Coumadin) 3 mg daily for the past 3 years. She has tolerated the medication well, but recently she has noticed more bleeding tendencies, such as nosebleeds and hematuria (blood in the urine). You assess the patient and find that she has gross hematuria today and numerous bruises over her body. To answer the following questions, what theoretical knowledge do you need, and where can you find it? (*Note:* After you get the information you need, answer the following questions.)
   a. What could be causing these bleeding episodes?
   b. What laboratory test is indicated in this situation, and what do you expect the result to be?
   c. What actions should you take in this situation?
8. James Bigler has had a postoperative repair of a compound fracture of the right arm and is receiving IV fluids and medications, including opioid analgesics and antibiotics. He also has a herniated intervertebral disk and severe muscle spasms. He was given his first dose of an oral muscle relaxant, cyclobenzaprine (Flexeril) 10 mg, at midnight. At 0800 he received another dose. At 0900 he received an IV antibiotic, and, while awake, he has been self-administering his opioid analgesic using his patient-controlled analgesia (PCA) IV pump about every 4 hours in a low dose. Consider these facts:
   - The most common side effect of Flexeril is drowsiness. It has a half-life of 24 to 72 hours.
   - Common side effects of opioids are drowsiness, decreased respiratory rate and depth, decreased blood pressure, and constipation (if taken long term).
   - Aside from allergies, the most common adverse effect of Mr. Bigler's antibiotic is diarrhea.

   Mr. Bigler's muscle relaxant (Flexeril) is to be given every 8 hours. When you enter his room to give it again at 1600, you find that he is extremely sleepy. He will awaken when you shake him or speak to him, but he falls right back to sleep, and is slurring his words. These are new symptoms for him.
   a. Is there anything obvious about his medical diagnosis that might be producing these symptoms. If so, what?
   b. Which of his medications could cause these symptoms, and why?
   c. What would you do? Would you give the 1600 dose of cyclobenzaprine (Flexeril)?
9. Mrs. Thomas lives alone and until a few months ago was able to take care of herself. When her eyesight began to deteriorate, she experienced difficulty self-administering her medications.
   a. Discuss the assessment required to determine whether she is at risk for ineffective management of her medication regimen.
   b. Mrs. Thomas was prescribed lorazepam (Ativan) 1 mg orally. Is this prescription complete? If not, what is missing? What actions should you take?
   c. Mrs. Thomas has an order for digoxin (Lanoxin) 1.25 mg orally each a.m. You have available Lanoxin 0.25 mg, and you calculate that 5 tablets should be administered. You check a drug guide and find that the usual dose is 0.125 mg to 0.25 mg orally daily. What actions should you take?
10. Calculate dosages for the following medications that you will be administering during your medication pass today. Are there any orders you would question? If so, why?
    a. Cephalexin (Keflex) 500 mg IV q6hr. You have on hand Keflex 1 gram in 1 mL of solution.
    b. Furosemide (Lasix) 280 mg orally daily. You have 40-mg tablets of Lasix available.
    c. Meperidine (Demerol) 10 mg intramuscularly, to a child. You have Demerol 25 mg/mL available in a prefilled syringe. In addition to calculating the dosage, describe the equipment you would use to administer the Demerol to a child.

11. Describe the procedure for giving atropine sulfate 0.4 mg IM along with morphine 10 mg intramuscularly using the same syringe. The atropine is in a single-dose vial containing 0.4 mg of atropine in 0.5 mL of fluid. The morphine is in a prefilled 10 mg injectable cartridge containing 10 mg in 1 mL of fluid.
12. You have an order to give injectable phenytoin (Dilantin) and furosemide (Lasix). You would like to give them in the same syringe. What theoretical and practical knowledge do you need to decide whether you can do this?
13. For each of the following patient problems (1) state what you think might be the cause and (2) state one thing you might have done to prevent the problem.
    a. When you give Mrs. King an intramuscular injection in her ventrogluteal muscle, she complains of pain.
    b. Several weeks after receiving an intramuscular injection in the dorsogluteal site, Mr. Aguilar begins having pain in his left lower back and hip; the pain proceeds down his leg. He is beginning to limp when he walks.
    c. Several days after receiving a subcutaneous injection, Patti Deal's upper arm is red, hot, painful, and swollen. There is pus oozing from the injection site.
    d. Immediately after an intramuscular injection, a patient starts showing severe, unexpected symptoms.
14. For each of the following concepts, use critical thinking to describe how or why it is important to nursing, patient care, or administering medications. Note that these are *not* to be merely definitions.

Pharmacology
Drug classification systems (e.g., according to use or chemical traits)
The *United States Pharmacopoeia (USP)* and the *National Formulary* (U.S.)
Drug excretion
Therapeutic levels
Side effects and adverse reactions
The apothecary system
Household measurements
Units and milliequivalents
Standing orders
"Rights of medication" administration
Ventrogluteal site for intramuscular injection
Medication errors

What Are the Main Points in This Chapter?

- Drugs are classified according to their use, body systems, and chemical or pharmacological traits. Learning the classifications helps you to remember the characteristics of individual drugs.
- The form (preparation) of a drug affects its speed of onset, intensity of action, and route of administration.
- In the United States, the Food and Drug Administration (FDA) regulates the manufacturing, sale, and effectiveness of all medications. Various state and federal agencies and legislation also regulate the administration of medications.
- Controlled substances must be stored, handled, disposed of, and administered according to regulations established by the U.S. Drug Enforcement Agency (DEA).
- In general, IV medications are absorbed most rapidly, followed by intramuscular, subcutaneous, buccal, and oral medications.
- Metabolism is the chemical inactivation of a drug into a form that the body can excrete; drug metabolism takes place mainly in the liver.
- The primary route of drug excretion is from the kidneys; other routes are the liver, gastrointestinal tract, lungs, and exocrine glands.
- The therapeutic level of a drug is the concentration in the blood serum that produces the desired effect without toxicity.
- Medication effects can be primary (therapeutic and intended) or secondary (nontherapeutic and unintended). Secondary effects include side effects, adverse reactions, toxic reactions, allergic reactions, and idiosyncratic reactions.
- The metric system is preferred for medications; however, for a few medications, the apothecary and household systems are still used.
- You are legally responsible for the medications you administer. You must question orders you believe to be incorrect.
- To help prevent medication errors, observe the "three checks" (before and after pouring or drawing up a medication, and at the bedside) and "rights of medication" (right drug, right dose, right time, right route, and right patient, as well as right documentation immediately after giving the medication).
- If you make a medication error, it is absolutely necessary that you immediately assess the patient's vital signs and physical status; report findings to the primary care provider; and notify the nurse manager of your unit.
- The oral route is the one most commonly used; it is convenient and safe.
- Buccal and sublingual medications are held in the mouth so that they will be absorbed through the mucous membrane.

- For patients who cannot swallow or who have feeding tubes, you can give oral medications through enteric (e.g., NG and gastrostomy) tubes. The medications are given one at a time and the tube must be flushed before and after each medication.
- Topical medications may have local and systemic effects; transdermal patches are applied for their systemic effect.
- Nebulization is the production of a fine spray, fog, powder, or mist from a liquid drug.
- Parenteral medications require the use of sterile technique to prevent infection.
- Needle length and gauge are chosen based on the type of medication, the route of administration, and the amount of adipose and muscle tissue the patient has.
- Needleless systems and safety syringes reduce the likelihood of needlestick injury.
- Always dispose of needles in special "sharps" containers. If you must recap a needle, use a one-handed technique.
- The ventrogluteal site is the preferred intramuscular injection site for adults. Other sites are the vastus lateralis and the deltoid. Use the rectus femoris site only if no other sites are available, and never in infants and children. Do not use the dorsogluteal site.
- Experts agree the anterolateral thigh (vastus lateralis) is preferred for infants who are not walking and some recommend using it throughout childhood. Others recommend using the ventrogluteal site when the child starts walking and the gluteal muscle increase in mass. The deltoid can be used for older children if you are certain that the muscle mass is adequate.
- Medications may be given intravenously by adding the medication to a large-volume (primary infusion), by the IV push technique, or by intermittent (piggyback setup) infusion.
- You should report medication errors immediately after they occur; a risk management process for monitoring causative factors should be in place.
- The most common reasons for a patient to have a central venous access device (CVAD) are to:
  - Give long-term IV therapy
  - Provide total parenteral nutrition when the patient cannot eat normally
  - Have blood drawn without the trauma and complications of repeated venipuncture
  - Be used when peripheral IV placement is difficult

Knowledge Map

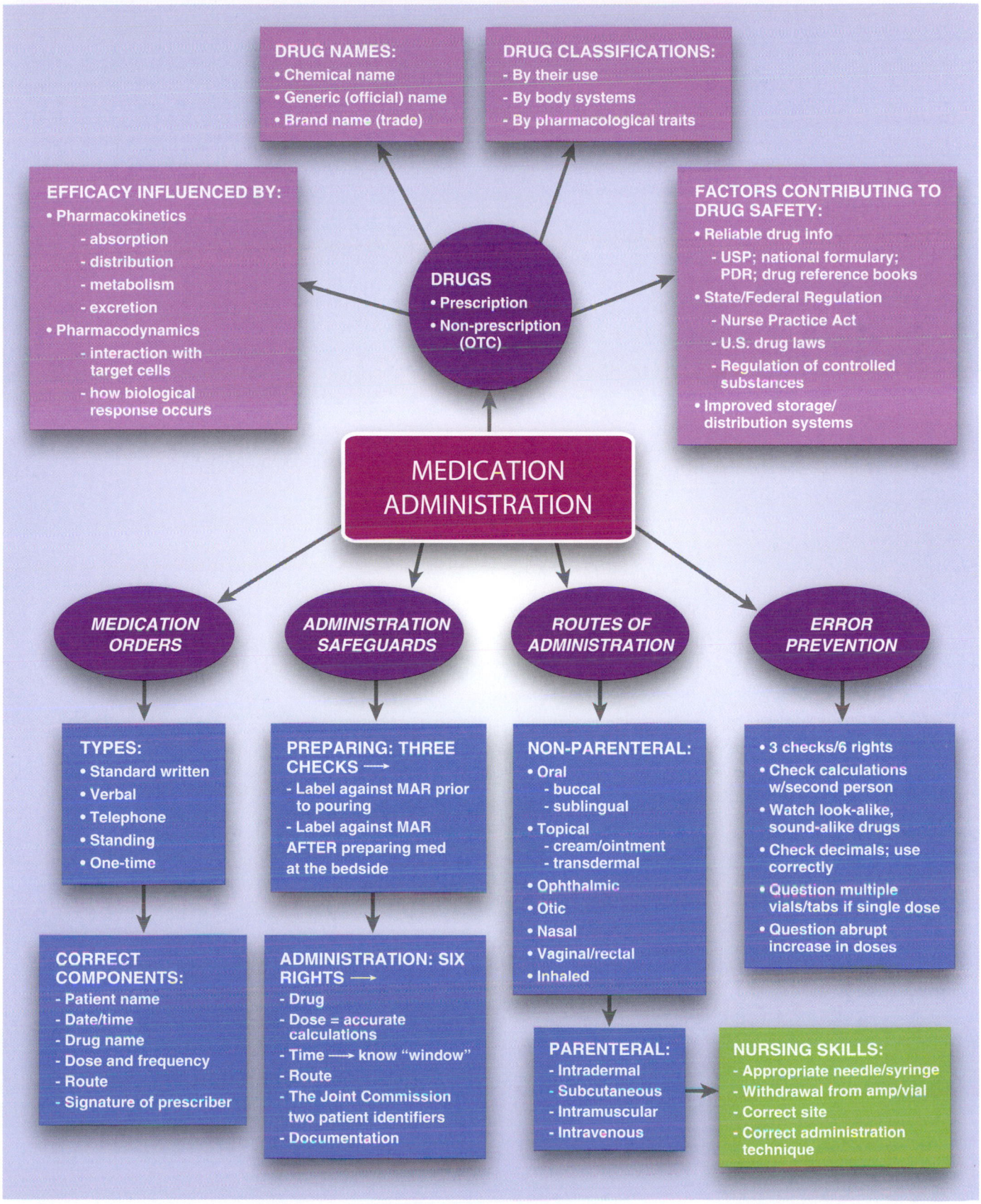

unit 4

Supporting Physiological Functioning

27 Nutrition

28 Urinary Elimination

29 Bowel Elimination

30 Sensation, Perception, & Cognition

31 Pain

32 Physical Activity & Mobility

33 Sexual Health

34 Sleep & Rest

35 Skin Integrity & Wound Healing

36 Oxygenation

37 Circulation

38 Fluids, Electrolytes, & Acid–Base Balance

CHAPTER 27

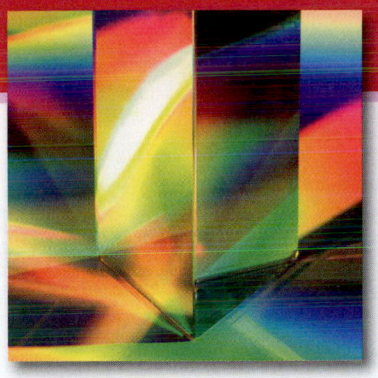

Nutrition

STUDENT RESOURCES

*The questions and exercises in Volume 2 allow you to practice the kind of thinking you will use as a full-spectrum nurse. Critical-thinking questions usually have more than one correct answer, so we do not provide "answers" for these features. It is more important to develop your nursing judgment than to just cover content. You will learn by discussing the questions with your peers. If you are still unsure, consult your instructor. You will find Response Sheets (for writing your responses to the questions) on Davis*Plus.

To explore learning resources for this chapter,

Go to Davis*Plus* at DavisPl.us/Wilkinson3.

Chapter Resources for Chapter 27:

- **Response sheets for all learning activities**
- **Resources for Caregivers and Health Professionals**
- **Reading More About Nutrition (suggested readings)**
- **Concept Map of chapter content**

Interactive Case Studies

NCLEX-Style and Chapter Review Questions

CHAPTER OVERVIEW

For a podcast of an overview of this chapter,

Go to Student Resources: Chapter 27, **Podcast—Chapter Overview,** on Davis*Plus*.

Caring for the Nguyens

Nam Nguyen has been diagnosed with hypertension, type 2 diabetes mellitus, obesity, osteoarthritis, and tobacco abuse. Zach Jackson has advised an 1,800-kcal diabetic diet with no added salt and a daily brisk 30-minute walk. Mr. Nguyen discusses these challenges with his daughter, Trinh.

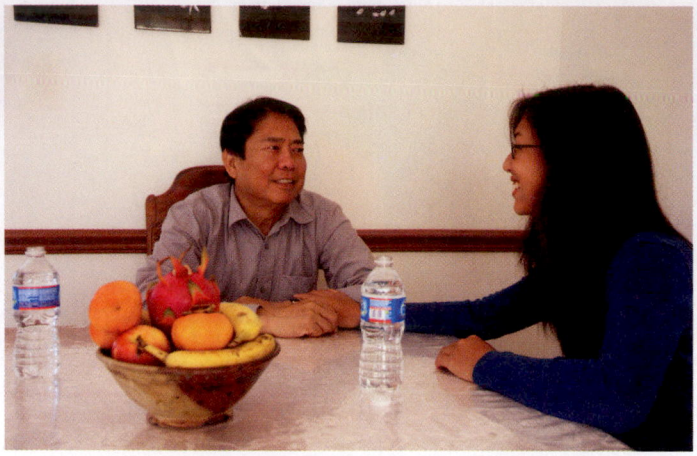

A. Why might Zach have selected this diet plan? Discuss the rationale for each component (i.e., 1,800 kcal, diabetic diet, no added salt).

B. Mr. Nguyen's diet is complex. He tells you he is overwhelmed by the many changes asked of him. How might Zach streamline his instructions about his diet?

C. Nam asks what is the best way for him to monitor his weight loss progress at home and how Zach Jackson will monitor his progress. How would you respond?

D. Identify teaching tools that might help Nam understand his diet.

Practical Knowledge knowing how

To apply concepts that support patient nutrition, you will need to master techniques for assessing nutritional status, feeding patients, administering supplemental feedings, and working with nasogastric (NG) and nasoenteric (NE) tubes.

PROCEDURES

Procedure 27-1 ■ Checking Fingerstick (Capillary) Blood Glucose Levels

➤ For steps to follow in *all* procedures, refer to the Universal Steps for All Procedures found on the inside back cover.

Equipment

- Blood glucose meter
- Test strip
- Sterile lancet (and injector, if available)
- Alcohol (or other antiseptic) pad, if required by policy
- 2 in. × 2 in. gauze pad or cotton ball
- Procedure gloves

Glucometers, fingerstick devices, and injectors should be assigned to individual patients. If this is not possible, you must clean and disinfect the devices between patients. If they are available, use single-use lancets that permanently retract upon puncture.

Store these supplies on a tray or cart outside patient's room. Do not carry supplies in your pocket. If there are unused supplies, leave them in the room; do not use them for another patient.

These measures help prevent needlestick injury and transmission of bloodborne pathogens (Centers for Disease Control and Prevention [CDC], 2005).

Delegation

Assess the patient first. If the patient's condition allows, you can delegate this procedure to a licensed practical nurse (LPN) or nursing assistive personnel (NAP) who has been adequately trained in performing the skill. Most patients perform this procedure independently at home.

Pre-Procedure Assessments

- Assess the patient's comprehension of the procedure.
  Allows you to tailor instructions to the individual patient.

- Assess potential puncture sites for bruising, inflammation, open lesions, poor circulation, or edema.
  Avoid such sites because of risk for infection and inaccurate results.
- Check for factors such as anticoagulant therapy, bleeding disorders, or low platelet count that place the patient at risk for bleeding after skin puncture.

➤ When performing the procedure, always identify your patient according to agency policy, using two identifiers, and be attentive to standard precautions, hand hygiene, patient safety and privacy, body mechanics, and documentation.

➤ *Note:* The steps of this procedure will vary, depending on the type of glucose meter used.

Procedure Steps

1. **Verify the medical prescription** for frequency and timing of testing.
   A prescription is necessary for testing. Timing and frequency of testing are crucial for accurate insulin dosing.

2. **Ask the patient to wash her hands** with soap and warm water, if able, and to dry completely using a clean towel.
   Reduces the risk for infection and dilates capillaries at the puncture site. Also ensures that the testing site is free of any sugar residue.

3. **Turn on the blood glucose meter.** Calibrate it according to the manufacturer's instructions.
   Calibration readies the meter for testing and checks it for accuracy of the machine.

4. **Check that the strip is the correct type** for the monitor. Check the expiration date on the container of reagent strips. If the strips are expired, replace them.
   Expired strips may alter test results. Different brands of monitors use different kinds of reagent strips.

5. **Don procedure gloves.**
   Gloving protects against exposure to blood.

6. **Remove the reagent strip** from the container and place it into the blood glucose meter. Then tightly seal the container.
   A tight seal protects reagent strips from exposure to air and light.

7. **Select and clean** a fingerstick site. If the patient is unable to do so, wash her hands with soap and water and dry them.
   Helps prevent infection by removing some surface microorganisms.

8. **Use a different site each time** you check the glucose.
   Adult and child: the lateral aspect of a finger (palmar surface, distal phalanx)
   Infant: heel or great toe
   The lateral aspect of the finger contains fewer nerve endings than the central fingertip, so it hurts less. Capillaries in infants are too small to obtain an adequate blood sample.

9. **Position the finger** (or heel or great toe for an infant) in a dependent position, and massage from the base toward the tip of the finger.
   A dependent position promotes blood flow to the site via gravity and pressure, ensuring an adequate specimen. The massaging action increases blood flow to the tip of the finger, which may prevent the need for repuncture.

10. **Prick the finger** (or other site) with the lancet:

Exposed-Blade Disposable Lancet

a. Remove the cover from the lancet, if there is a cover.
b. Place the back of the patient's hand on the table, or otherwise secure the finger (e.g., hold the finger and hand firmly).
c. Use a darting motion to puncture the site at a 90° angle to the skin.

Semi-Automatic Injector

d. Engage the sterile injector and remove the cover.
e. Place the disposable lancet firmly in the end of the injector.
f. Place the back of the patient's hand on the table, or otherwise secure the finger (e.g., hold the finger and hand firmly).
g. Position the end of the injector firmly against the skin, perpendicular (at a 90° angle) to the chosen puncture site.
h. Push the release switch, allowing the needle to pierce the skin.
   Proper positioning and stabilization of the site ensure that the lancet pierces to the correct depth. This prevents patient injury and allows for adequate blood sampling. Patients tend to pull away as you perform the puncture. ▼

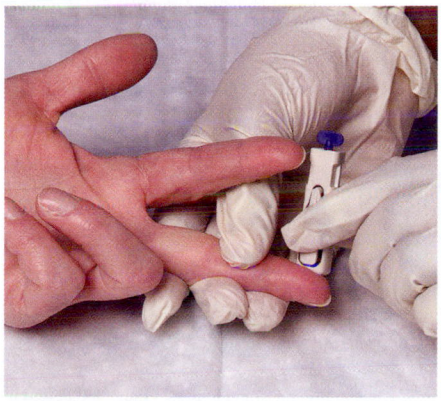

11. **Lightly squeeze the patient's** finger above the puncture site until a drop of blood has collected.
    Squeezing promotes a better blood sample for testing without causing injury to the puncture site.

12. **Place the reagent strip** test patch close to the drop of blood. Allow contact between the drop of blood and the test strip. Do not "smear" the blood over the reagent strip. ▼

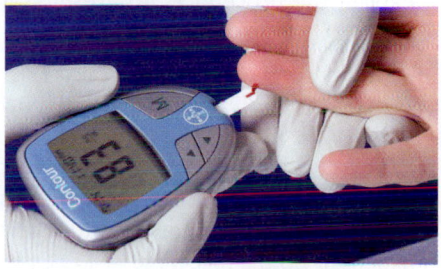

(continued on next page)

Procedure 27-1 ■ Checking Fingerstick (Capillary) Blood Glucose Levels (continued)

13. **Insert the strip into the meter**, if you have not already done so (follow the manufacturer's instructions); allow the blood sample to remain in contact with the test strip for the amount of time specified.
For some meters you insert the test strip before pricking the finger; with others you put the blood on the reagent strip and then insert the strip into the meter. The blood sample must be on the reagent strip for the specified amount of time to ensure accurate test results.

14. **Using a gauze pad, gently apply pressure** to the puncture site.
Pressure stops the bleeding by promoting coagulation.

15. **After the meter signals, read** the blood glucose level indicated on the digital display.▼

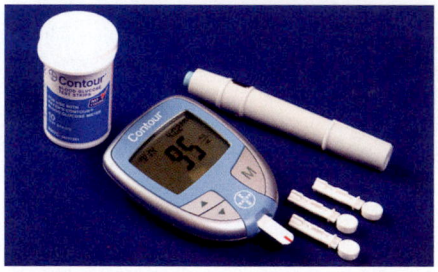

16. **Turn off the meter**. Dispose of the reagent strip, gauze pad, alcohol pad, and lancet in the proper containers (e.g., a sharps container for the lancet).
Proper disposal prevents sharps injury and the spread of infection via blood-borne pathogens.

17. **Remove your gloves**, and dispose of them in the covered trash receptacle or biohazards container. Perform hand hygiene.
Safe disposal reduces the transmission of pathogens.

? What if . . .

- **The patient has poor circulation or is a child or older adult?**
  Place a heel warmer or warm cloth on the site for about 10 minutes before obtaining the blood sample. Alternatively, position the patient's hand below the waist for 1 minute.
  Capillaries in infants are very small; older adults may have poor peripheral circulation. Warmth dilates the capillaries, and may help you obtain an adequate amount of blood; when dangling the extremities, gravity allows blood to pool in the extremity, making an ample specimen easier to obtain.
- **The patient is taking an anticoagulant such as warfarin sodium (Coumadin)?**
  After the procedure, hold pressure for 2 min and then apply a pressure bandage if needed. Recheck the site after 5 min to make sure bleeding has stopped.
- **The monitor shows an extremely unusual result or an error message?**
  Repeat the process using a different finger or site.
- **The patient uses a noninvasive method to measure blood glucose?**
  A new device called a continuous blood glucose monitor is available. It is worn like a wristwatch. Using an electrical current, it pulls fluid from the skin to give a blood glucose reading. It can take readings automatically every 20 min for up to 12 hr. Advise the patient to shave his arm if it is very hairy, or the reading may not be accurate. The patient should wear the device for a 3-hour warm-up before taking a reading, and should not bathe or swim during that time. The purpose of continuous monitoring is to track trends in blood glucose. It does not replace the patient's fingerstick method.

Evaluation

- Assess the puncture site for bleeding or bruising.
- Evaluate the patient's understanding of the procedure and the test results.
- Promptly notify the primary care provider of abnormal test results, or administer insulin based on test results, if prescribed.

Patient Teaching

- Explain the procedure, test results, and treatment to the patient.
  Information allows the patient to participate in his plan of care, and typically increases adherence to the therapeutic regimen.
- Discuss the importance of maintaining glycemic control.
- If the patient will be performing fingerstick blood glucose testing at home, teach the patient how to perform the procedure. Ask the patient to perform a return demonstration. Teach the patient to do the following:
  - Read the manufacturer's instructions carefully and call their toll-free number if he has any questions.
  - Always use the test strips that are recommended for the meter.
  - Take your meter to your health provider's office so she can make sure you are measuring your blood sugar correctly.
  - Perform quality control checks (read the instructions) to make sure the meter is measuring accurately.
  - Clean the meter according to the manufacturer's directions. Some meters will give you an electronic alert telling you when to clean them.

Home Care

- Assess the client's ability to perform fingerstick blood glucose monitoring independently.
  A change in the patient's condition may not allow the patient to perform testing. Certain conditions, such as arthritis and limited vision, may limit dexterity.
- Provide information about purchasing home glucose-monitoring equipment.
- Explain how to dispose of lancets in a labeled, puncture-proof container, such as an empty bleach container.

- Instruct caregivers to wear gloves when obtaining a blood sample for glucose monitoring.
- At home, patients should not cleanse their fingers with an alcohol wipe before puncturing it. However, they should wash their hands with soap and water and dry well.

Documentation

- Record the fingerstick blood glucose result in the progress notes or special flowsheet, including the date and time the test was performed.
- Note whether the physician was notified and record any treatment given.
- Document patient teaching.
- If the fingerstick is performed in response to patient symptoms, you may need to write a narrative note.

Sample documentation

8/12/16 1435 Patient reported feeling "cold and shaky." FBBS 62. Alert and able to swallow. Pt ate 5 saltine crackers with peanut butter and drank 3 ounces of orange juice. FSBS 92 at 1430. Will notify physician for further orders. ——— N. Jones, RN

Practice Resources

American Diabetes Association (n.d., 2011); CDC (2005); Glucose Monitoring (2008); Hortensius, J., Slingerland, C., Kleefstra, N., et al. (2011); U.S. Food and Drug Administration (2007b).

Thinking About the Procedure

To practice applying clinical reasoning to this procedure,

Go to *Davis's Nursing Skills Videos*, **Checking Fingerstick (Capillary) Blood Glucose Levels.**

For questions and suggested responses,

Go to Chapter 27, **Thinking About the Procedure Questions and Suggested Responses,** on Davis*Plus*.

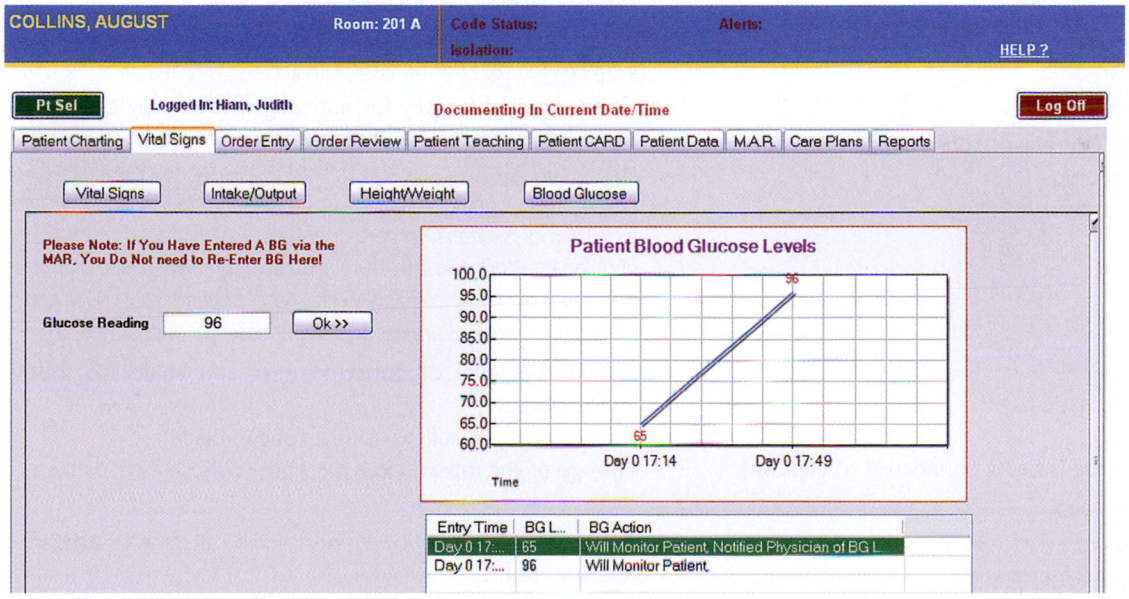

Procedure 27-2 ■ Inserting Nasogastric and Nasoenteric Tubes

➤ For steps to follow in *all* procedures, refer to the Universal Steps for All Procedures found on the inside back cover.

To watch an animated demonstration of inserting a nasogastric tube,

Go to **Animations: Inserting a Nasogastric Tube,** on DavisPlus.

Equipment

- Nasogastric tube (commonly 16 or 18 Fr for adults, but sometimes smaller) or nasoenteric (small bowel) tube (8 Fr, 10 Fr, or 12 Fr)
- Stylet or guidewire (for small-bore tubes), according to agency policy
- Procedure gloves
- Linen-saver pad or towel
- Water-soluble lubricant
- 50- to 60-mL catheter-tip syringe or bulb syringe for Salem sump tubes; 30-mL luer-lock syringe for small-bore feeding tubes
- Hypoallergenic tape (about 2.5 cm [1 in.] wide) or tube fixation device
- Indelible marker
- Skin adhesive
- Stethoscope
- Emesis basin
- Basin with warm water (for plastic tube) or ice (for rubber tube). Most tubes are plastic.
- Glass of water with a straw
- Penlight
- Tongue blade
- pH test strip
- Tissues
- Safety pin
- Gauze square or small plastic bag
- Rubber band
- Suction equipment (if tube is being connected to suction)

Delegation

This procedure should not be delegated because it requires knowledge of anatomy and physiology and the ability to adapt the procedure based on patient responses. You can, however, delegate associated oral hygiene needs.

Pre-Procedure Assessment

- Verify the medical prescription for type of tube to be placed and whether it is to be attached to suction or drainage.
- Confirm the patient's need for NG or NE intubation (e.g., surgery involving the gastrointestinal (GI) tract, impaired swallowing, or decreased level of consciousness).
  NG or NE intubation decreases the risk for aspiration in these patients. In many institutions, only specially trained nurses are allowed to place small-bowel feeding tubes.
- Assess each naris for patency, deviated septum, and skin breakdown. Ask the patient to close each nostril alternately and breathe. Select the nostril with the greatest air flow. Ask the patient to blow her nose, if not contraindicated.
  A septal defect or facial fracture may cause obstruction, placing the patient at risk for nasal membrane trauma if insertion is attempted through the affected naris.
- Check medical history for anticoagulant therapy, coagulopathy, nasal trauma, nasal surgery, epistaxis, or deviated septum.
  Patient history may place the patient at risk for injury during NG or NE insertion. Contraindications to NG insertion by a nurse include maxillofacial disorders, surgery, or trauma; esophageal tumors or surgery; laryngectomy; skull fracture; unstable high cervical spinal injuries; and esophageal varices (although these patients may have tubes placed by a medical professional via endoscope or fluoroscope).
- Assess the level of consciousness and ability to follow instructions.
- Assess for a gag reflex, using a tongue blade.
  Absence of gag reflex places the patient at risk for aspiration.

➤ When performing the procedure, always identify your patient according to agency policy, using two identifiers, and be attentive to standard precautions, hand hygiene, patient safety and privacy, body mechanics, and documentation.

Procedure Steps

1. Prepare the tube.

Plastic Tube

Wrap the tube around your index finger and then unwrap it and proceed or place in a basin of warm water for 10 minutes and proceed.

Rubber Tube

Place in a basin of ice for 10 minutes.

Small-Bore Tube

Insert a stylet or guidewire and secure into position, according to agency policy. (Small-bore tubes may come with the guidewire in them. If so, flush the tube with tap water to lubricate the wire for easy removal.) Leave the wire in place until the tube is positioned and its placement has been checked on x-ray film. Once the guidewire is removed, do not reinsert it. Agency policy determines which nurses are authorized to place small-bore tubes.

Warm water softens a plastic tube, and ice stiffens the rubber tube to make it easier to insert. (Most tubes are polyurethane or silicone-based.) Wrapping a plastic tube around your index finger helps the tube flex into a curve and aids in insertion. A guidewire facilitates passage of small-bore tube but can cause trauma if not secured in a proper position.

2. Assist the patient into a high-Fowler's position with pillow behind the head and shoulders. Raise the bed to a comfortable working level.
This position facilitates tube insertion and prevents aspiration should the patient vomit during tube insertion. Gravity

facilitates passage of the tube. Raising the bed reduces strain on the nurse's back.

3. **Measure the tube for placement.**

Nasogastric Tube

Measure the length of the tube to be inserted by measuring from the tip of the nose to the earlobe, and from the earlobe to the xiphoid process. Mark the length with tape or indelible ink.

This measurement indicates how far the tube must be inserted to reach the stomach.

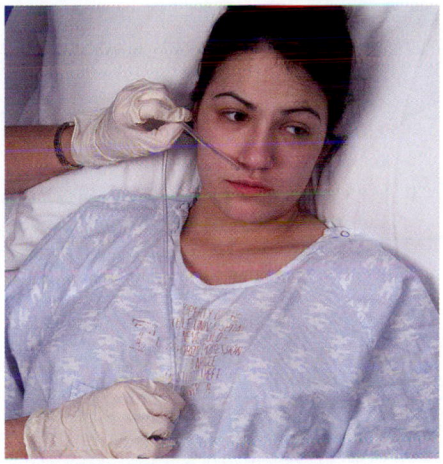

Nasoenteric Tube

Add 8 to 10 cm (3 to 4 in.) to the NG tube measurement, as directed, and mark the tube.

4. **If you are right-handed**, stand on the patient's right side; if you are left-handed, stand on the left side if. Drape a linen saver pad over the patient's chest, and hand her an emesis basin and facial tissues.

   Draping protects the patient's gown from becoming soiled during tube insertion.

5. **Prepare the fixation device.** Cut a 10-cm (4-in.) piece of hypoallergenic tape if securing tube with tape; split the bottom end lengthwise 2.5 cm (2 in.). If using a commercial feeding tube attachment device, have it ready at this time.

   To more readily secure the tube after insertion.

6. **Arrange a signal** by which the patient can communicate if she wants to stop (e.g., raising her hand).

   Relieves anxiety by giving the patient some control over the procedure.

7. **Don procedure gloves** if you have not already done so.

   Reduces the spread of pathogens.

8. **Wrap 10 to 15 cm (5 to 6 in.)** of the end of the tube tightly around your index finger, then release.

   Forms the tube into a curve that helps it conform more easily to the shape of the nasopharynx.

9. **Lubricate the distal 10 cm** (4 in.) of the tube with a water-soluble jelly.

   Lubrication eases the passage of the tube and prevents injury to the nasal mucosa. Water-soluble lubricant will dissolve if it is aspirated, whereas oil-based lubricants do not dissolve in the respiratory tract and cause inflammation and blockage of airways if they enter the lungs. Some nurses prefer water as a lubricant because aqueous jelly dries and can block and irritate nasal passages. Some tubes have a surface lubricant and require only that you dip them in room-temperature water.

10. **Hand the patient a glass** of water with a straw, if she is awake, alert, and able to swallow.

    Swallowing water during insertion eases passage.

11. **Instruct the patient** to hold her head straight up and extend her neck back against the pillow (slightly hyperextended). Begin inserting the tube.
    a. Grasp the end of the tube above the lubricant with the curved end pointing downward.
    b. Carefully insert the tube along the floor of the nasal passage, on the lateral side, aiming toward the ear.
    c. You will feel slight resistance when the tube reaches the nasopharynx; use gentle pressure, but do not force the tube to advance. The patient's eyes may tear; if so, provide tissues.
    d. Continue inserting the tube until just past the nasopharynx by gently rotating the tube toward the client's opposite naris.

    Hyperextending the neck straightens the curve where the nasal passage meets the pharynx (nasopharyngeal junction). Gentle insertion prevents trauma to the nasal mucosa. Tears are normal.

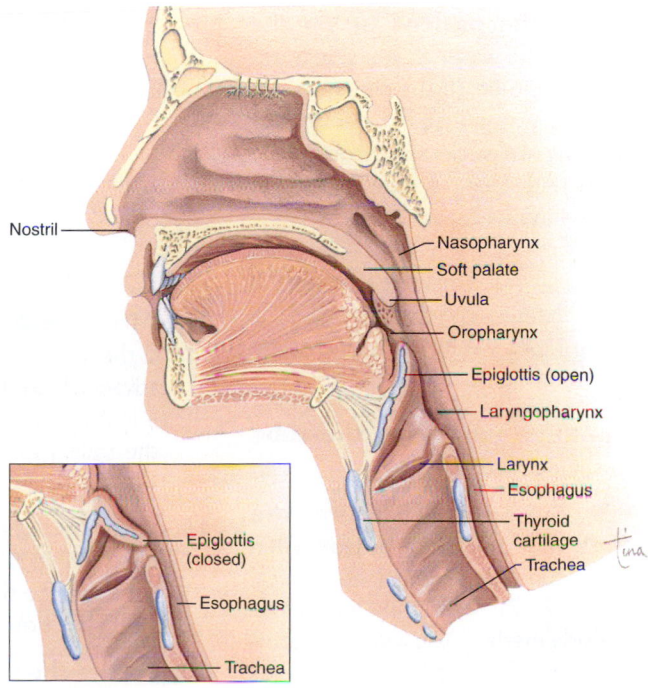

(continued on next page)

Procedure 27-2 ■ Inserting Nasogastric and Nasoenteric Tubes (continued)

12. **Pause for a moment** to allow the patient to relax, and perhaps use tissues. Explain that the next step requires her to swallow.
Stopping to relax can give the patient a feeling of control. Also, the rest can reduce gagging.

13. **Instruct the patient to flex** her head toward her chest, take a small sip of water, and swallow.
This maneuver closes the trachea and opens the esophagus.▼

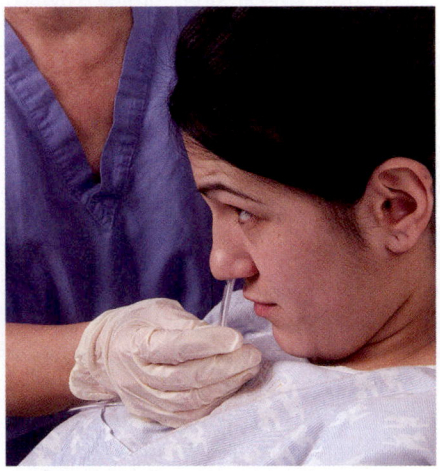

14. **Rotate the tube 180°.**
Rotation helps to redirect the tube so that it will not enter the patient's mouth.

15. **Direct the patient to sip** and swallow the water as you slowly advance the tube. (If the patient is not allowed water, instruct her to dry swallow or suck air through the straw.) Advance the tube 5 to 10 cm (2 to 4 in.) with each swallow.
Moving the tube with each swallow uses normal peristaltic movement to help advance the tube into the stomach. Swallowing closes the epiglottis so that the tube cannot advance into the trachea.

16. **Continue advancing the tube** to the desired distance.

17. **Temporarily secure the tube** with one piece of tape. Then verify tube placement (see Clinical Insight 27-7). Never rely on a single bedside method. You can use a combination of the following methods to verify placement at the bedside; however, radiographic verification is the only reliable method and should be done before medications or fluids are given through the tube for the first time (Joanna Briggs Institute, 2012).
If you do not secure the tube temporarily, it may move out of position—especially if you are waiting for placement to be confirmed by x-ray film.
    a. Inspect the posterior pharynx for presence of coiled tube.
    Visualization confirms that the tube has gone beyond the oropharynx.
    b. Aspirate gently to withdraw stomach contents; measure aspirate pH. The pH of stomach contents is normally 1 to 5.5.
    This may be difficult with small bore tubes. Refer to Clinical Insight 27-7, for rationale and further information about this method.
    c. Take note of the amount, color, and consistency of the aspirate. Gastric aspirates are cloudy tan, off-white, or greenish and may be curdled. Intestinal aspirates will be smaller in quantity, clear, and yellowish owing to the presence of bile, and not curdled.
    d. Inject air into the NG tube and listen with a stethoscope over the stomach. Use this only to confirm other methods because it is the least reliable method.
    If the tube is in the stomach, injecting 5 to 30 mL of air with the syringe should produce a gurgling sound.
    e. Ask the patient to speak.
    If she can do so, the tube is probably in the stomach. Use this only to confirm other methods; it is not reliable enough to use as the primary method of verification.

18. **After checking for placement,** if the tube is not in the stomach, advance it another 2.5 to 5 cm (2 to 4 inches) or as much as directed in the radiologic review. Repeat Steps 17a–e.

19. **After you confirm proper** placement, clamp the end of the tube or connect it to the drainage bag, feeding, or suction machine.

20. **Secure the tube using** one of the following methods.

Securing the Tube With 1-Inch (2.5 cm) Tape

a. Apply skin adhesive to the patient's nose, and allow it to dry.
A skin adhesive helps the tape to adhere and protects skin from breakdown.
b. Use the 5 cm (2 in.) piece of hypoallergenic tape, split lengthwise for 2.5 cm (1 in.) at one end.
A split tape can be wrapped around the tube in opposite directions to hold the tube in place more securely.
c. Apply the intact end of tape to the patient's nose.
d. Wrap the split strips around the tube where it exits the nose. Fold over the ends if adjustment is needed.

Securing the Tube With 1/2-Inch Tape

e. Use half-inch (1.3 cm) tape, 4 inches (10 cm) long. Apply one end of tape to the patient's nose and wrap the other end downward around the tube and then back up to secure on the opposite side of the nose (see photo).▼

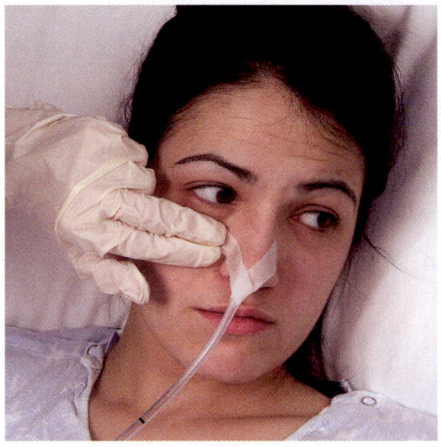

Securing the Tube With a Tube Fixation Device

f. Peel the backing off the pad and place the wide end of the pad over the bridge of the nose.
g. Position the connector around the NG or NE tube where it exits the nose.▼

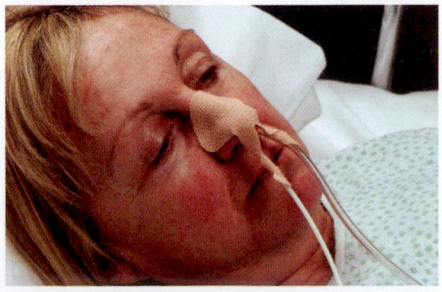

21. **Curve and tape the tube** to the patient's cheek (not necessary with some commercial tube fixation devices).
Securing the tube to the cheek reduces the tension on the naris.

22. **Fasten the tube to the patient's** gown: Tie a slipknot around the tube with a rubber band. Loop a rubber band in a slipknot near the connection. (Alternatively, wrap a short piece of tape around the tube to form a tab.) Then fasten the rubber band or the tab to the gown with a safety pin (or tape).
Reduces discomfort produced by the weight of the tube and prevents movement that may cause dislocation of the tube and irritation of the nose.

23. **Elevate the head of the bed** 30° unless contraindicated.

24. **Mark the tube with tape** where it enters the naris, or measure the length from the naris to the connector.
A marked tube allows you to easily notice whether tube placement has changed.

? What if . . .

- **The patient is confused, combative, or comatose?**
  - If the patient is comatose, place him into a semi-Fowler's position. Have a co-worker use a pillow to help position the patient's head forward for insertion.
  - If the patient is confused and combative, ask a coworker to assist you with insertion.
- **The patient gags, coughs, chokes, or vomits [at Steps 11 and 15]?**
  1. Stop advancing the tube. Ask the patient to take deep breaths and drink a few sips of water.
  Helps suppress the gag reflex.
  2. Instruct the patient to breathe easily and take some sips of water.
  3. If coughing continues, pull the tube back slightly.
  4. If gagging continues, use a tongue blade and penlight to check the tube position in the back of the throat.
  The tube may be coiled in the back of the throat.
  5. Continue to advance the tube to the desired distance.
- If the tube is coiled in the back of the throat, the patient coughs excessively during insertion, the tube does not advance with each swallow, or the patient develops respiratory distress (e.g., gasping, coughing, or cyanosis), withdraw the tube completely and allow the patient to rest before reinserting.
The tube may be in the patient's trachea.
- **You are unable to obtain an aspirate (at Step 17b) when confirming tube placement?**
  1. Use a 50-mL syringe and aspirate very slowly over at least 5 minutes.
  2. Flush the tube with air, then aspirate.
  3. Turn the patient to the left side, wait 20 minutes, then aspirate again.
  An aspirate might be difficult to obtain with small bore tubes.
- **The prescription states the tube needs to be in the jejunum?**
  1. To advance the tube into the jejunum after the tube has been placed in the stomach, position the patient on the right side.
  Positioning on the right side allows gravity to assist tube passage through the pyloric sphincter.
  2. Advance the tube 5 to 7.5 cm (2 to 3 in.) hourly, over several hours (up to 24 hours) until radiographic study confirms placement.
  Weighted tubes will advance by gravity and peristalsis if a loop of the designated length is made at the entrance to the naris. After reading the initial x-ray, the radiologist or primary physician can provide the measurement needed to advance the tube to the desired position. Note that specially trained nurses usually place these tubes at the bedside.
- **The procedure is anticipated to cause pain or discomfort?**
  Commercial hurricane spray or viscous lidocaine is sometimes used to aid in patient comfort. Some practitioners use them for all NG insertions.
  - You may insert 2% viscous lidocaine into the nasal passage using a syringe before tube placement, if prescribed by the primary provider.
  - Alternatively, you can apply an anesthetic spray to the nasal and oropharyngeal mucosa.
- **The patient is a child?**
  - Children usually require a smaller diameter tube.
  - Encourage parents to comfort infants and children and participate in their care.
  - You may need to apply restraints during insertion to prevent dislodging of the tube.
  - Monitor more frequently for complications.
  Small children are not able to communicate problems with the tube.

Evaluation

- Assess how well the patient tolerated the procedure (e.g., discomfort, gagging, coughing?)
- Note the color, consistency, and pH of NG or NE aspirate.
- Ask the patient whether she feels comfortable.
- Assess respiratory status.

Patient Teaching

- Explain that the sensation of the tube should decrease with time.
- Explain the importance of immediately reporting tension on the tube or displacement of the tape or fixation device.
- Discuss the need for frequent mouth care while the tube is in place.

Home Care

- Assess the client or caregiver's ability to maintain an PEG, or gastric button at home if long-term nutritional support is needed.

(continued on next page)

Procedure 27-2 ■ Inserting Nasogastric and Nasoenteric Tubes (continued)

- Assess the home environment to determine the client's risk for infection.
- Instruct the client or caregiver about aspirating stomach contents and measuring pH for NG tubes only.
- Teach the client or caregiver how to verify tube placement.
- Teach client or caregiver to assess the nare for skin breakdown.
- Reinforce the need for frequent mouth care.

Documentation

- Chart the date and time of insertion, size and type of the NG or NE tube and insertion site (which naris), length of tube from tip of the nose to the end of the tube, tolerance of the procedure, any abnormal findings, and methods for confirming NG or NE tube placement.
- Document description of gastric contents and respiratory status.
- NG or NE tube insertion is documented in the progress notes and flow sheets in most agencies.

Practice Resources

American Association of Critical-Care Nurses (AACCN) (2005a, revised 2009; 2005b, revised 2009); Rauen, C., Chulay, M., Bridges, E., et al. (2008); Shlamovitz, G. Z., & Shah, N. R. (2008); Wiegand, D. (2010); Wolfe, T., Fosnocht, D., & Linscott, M. (2000).

Thinking About the Procedure

To practice applying clinical reasoning to this procedure,

Go to *Davis's Nursing Skills Videos*, **Inserting Nasogastric and Nasoenteric Tubes.**

For questions and suggested responses,

Go to Chapter 27, **Thinking About the Procedure Questions and Suggested Responses,** on Davis*Plus*.

Procedure 27-3 ■ Administering Feedings Through Gastric and Enteric Tubes

➤ For steps to follow in *all* procedures, refer to the Universal Steps for All Procedures found on the inside back cover.

Equipment

- Prescribed feeding formula at room temperature
- Filtered water or prescribed diluent
- Tube feeding administration set with safety adapter that is not compatible with IV tubing, including bag for formula
- 60-mL luer-lock or catheter-tip syringe (two needed for syringe feeding)
- Connector to connect administration set to the feeding tube
- Stethoscope
- Enteral feeding infusion pump (if used). Recommended for all continuous feedings.
- IV pole
- Linen-saver pad
- Graduated container
- pH strip
- For gastrostomy and jejunostomy tubes: a small precut gauze dressing

Delegation

You can delegate the procedure to the NAP or LPN if the patient's condition is stable and the NAP's skills allow. You must verify peristalsis, tube placement, and feeding tube patency before the feeding is started. Remind the NAP to position the patient upright and to report patient discomfort and any difficulty with the infusion.

Pre-Procedure Assessment

- Check the length of the exposed tube: (1) Compare the length from the naris to the connector recorded after x-ray confirmation of placement; or (2) observe the mark that was made on it where it entered the nostril after insertion. Refer to Clinical Insight 27-7 for other bedside methods of verifying tube placement.
  These methods help confirm that the tube has not become displaced since radiography. If there is significant change in length, tube position must again be confirmed by radiography.
- Assess date and time of previous feeding bag set change. Bags should be changed every 24 hr or according to unit protocol.
- Assess for fluid volume excess or insufficiency by checking breath sounds, mucous membranes, skin turgor, edema, and intake and output.
- Obtain baseline weight and laboratory studies before starting the first feedings.
  Weight change is a sensitive measure reflecting fluid and nutritional status.
- Monitor vital signs before and after feedings.
  Vital signs may vary from baseline due to pain, impaction, or dehydration.
- Auscultate for bowel sounds before each feeding or every 4 to 8 hours for continuous feedings. Also check for distention, nausea, vomiting, and diarrhea.
  These symptoms may indicate intolerance of tube feedings. If GI motility is impaired, feedings accumulate in the stomach along with gastric secretions, predisposing the patient to reflux and aspiration. Some medications (e.g., opioids) also slow gastric emptying.
- Check patient history for food allergies.
  Helps prevent allergic reaction to ingredients in the feeding formula.
- For gastrostomy and jejunostomy tubes: Assess the exit site at every shift. Report redness or drainage to the primary care provider.
  Leaking of gastric or intestinal contents may cause skin breakdown.

➤ When performing the procedure, always identify your patient according to agency policy, using two identifiers, and be attentive to standard precautions, hand hygiene, patient safety and privacy, body mechanics, and documentation.

Procedure Steps

1. **Verify the feeding tube is in proper placement** prior to starting the procedure.
   Tube placement after insertion must be verified by radiography. For subsequent feedings, aspirate and measure gastric residual volume (GVR). For patients with a jejunostomy tube, do not measure the residual volume. See Clinical Insight 27-7 for methods for checking feeding tube placement.

2. **Elevate the head of the bed** (HOB) at least 30° to 45° unless contraindicated. If the patient cannot tolerate a backrest elevated position, use the reverse Trendelenburg position to elevate the HOB, unless contraindicated. And, place a linen saver pad under where the connection end of the feeding tube will be.
   A position in which the stomach is higher than the gut reduces the risk for aspiration of gastric contents, a serious risk factor for pneumonia or hypoxia. It also aids digestion.

3. **Check the prescription** for the type of feeding, rate of infusion, and frequency of feeding.
   A medical prescription is required for enteral feedings.

4. **Check the expiration date** of the tube feeding formula.
   Expired formula should be discarded.

5. **Prepare the formula.**
   a. Inspect the container of feeding solution. If the bag, bottle, or can has been opened or damaged in any way, don't use it.
   b. Shake the feeding formula thoroughly. Examine the solution. It should be uniform in color and consistency. Most often the formula is room temperature. Follow the manufacturer's instructions for safe storage.
   Because the formula goes directly into the stomach and is not warmed by the mouth and esophagus, cold formula may cause abdominal cramping and increase the risk for diarrhea.

6. **Prepare the equipment for** administration.
   a. Fill a disposable tube feeding container with a 4- to 6-hour supply of feeding formula. Or use a prefilled bottle with feeding formula. Follow similar procedure for flush bag if using a two-bag system.
   Limit hang-time to help prevent bacterial growth and prevent air from entering the GI tract.
   b. Label the container with the patient's name, room number, date, start time, formula type, feeding rate, and your initials. Write a warning using large, bold letters, for instance, "WARNING! For Enteral Use Only—NOT for IV Use."
   Labeling identifies the formula and prevents misconnection of the feeding tube into an IV line. Labeling also helps avoid administering formula past the expiration date.
   c. Be sure adapters and connectors used in the enteral system are incompatible with female luer-lock rigid connectors used for IV infusion.
   Prevents tube feeding misconnection with an IV line.
   d. Hang the tube-feeding container on an IV pole with the label facing forward. A prefilled container can safely hang for 24 to 36 hours (some agencies allow for 48 hours).
   Closed systems decrease the risk of contamination and prevent air from entering the GI tract.
   e. Open the administration set package. Make sure the tubing does not touch the floor.
   f. Close the clamp on the tubing before attaching the set to the container.
   g. Remove the cap from the end of safety connector. This adapter must not be fit with IV tubing. Do not touch the end of the connector or let it touch another surface.
   h. Insert the proximal end of the tubing (with the safety adaptor) into the cross-shaped opening of the port on the feeding tube bag. Twist the collar in a clockwise direction until it is securely fastened.▼

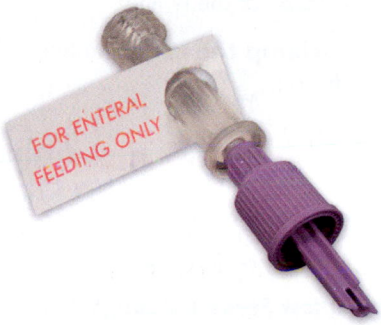

7. **Prime the tubing with the feeding solution.**

8. **Thread the administration set** tubing through the infusion pump according to the manufacturer's instructions. Be sure to close the roller clamp.
   Clamping the tube prevents air from entering the stomach or gastric contents from leaking out.▼

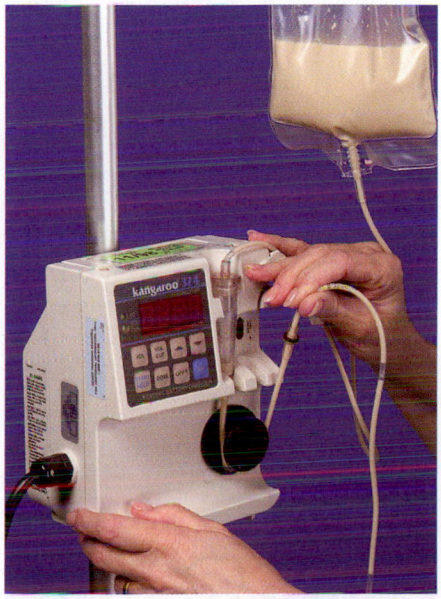

(continued on next page)

Procedure 27-3 ■ Administering Feedings Through Gastric and Enteric Tubes (continued)

9. **Connect the distal end of the tubing** primed with feeding solution to the connector or directly to the NG or NE tube.

10. **Turn on the infusion pump.** Set the correct infusion rate and volume to be infused. Follow the pump manufacturer's instructions.

    ✚ Trace the tubing from the bag back to the patient before starting the feeding to ensure that you have not inadvertently hooked the feeding bag or bottle to the IV line

11. **Unclamp the tube** and begin the infusion.

12. **When the feeding volume is complete**, stop the flow, flush the tube, and disconnect the feeding by turning off pump and closing the roller clamp.

13. **Disconnect the feeding tube** from the administration tubing.

14. **Flush feeding tube** with the prescribed amount of water—typically 50 to 100 mL.

15. **Cap the proximal end** of the feeding tube.
    Prevents spillage of gastric contents and stops air from entering the stomach.

16. **Keep the head of the bed elevated** at least 30° to 45° for 1 hour after administering the tube feeding.
    Elevation reduces the risk for aspiration of gastric contents.

17. **Provide or assist with regular oral hygiene** and encourage frequent gargling.
    Oral care reduces oropharyngeal discomfort from the tube.

18. **When you finish the procedure**, remember the Universal Steps that apply after all procedures. For example, leave the patient in a safe, comfortable position with the call device in easy reach.

Procedure 27-3A ■ Administering Feedings Through Gastric and Enteric Tubes Using an Open System: Syringe

Procedure Steps

First follow Steps 1 through 4, above. Then proceed as follows:

1. **Prepare the equipment** for administration.
   a. Don procedure gloves.
   b. Label the syringe with the patient's name, room number, date, time, formula type, feeding rate, start time, and your initials.

      ✚ Write a warning using large, bold letters, for instance, "WARNING! For Enteral Use Only—NOT for IV Use."

      Labeling identifies the formula and prevents misconnection of the feeding tube into an IV line. Labeling also helps avoid administering formula past the expiration date.
   c. Remove the plunger from the syringe.

2. **Clamp or pinch off** the end of the feeding tube to begin the feeding.
   Prevents air from entering the feeding tube.

3. **Attach the syringe to** the proximal end of the feeding tube.

4. **Fill the syringe** with the prescribed amount of formula.

5. **Unclamp the feeding tube**, and elevate the syringe. Do not elevate the syringe more than 18 inches (45 cm) above the insertion site. Allow the feeding to flow slowly.
   Gravity allows the formula to flow through the feeding tube. Rate of flow is determined by the height of the syringe. Feeding slowly prevents sudden stomach distention, which can lead to diarrhea, cramping, nausea, and vomiting. ▼

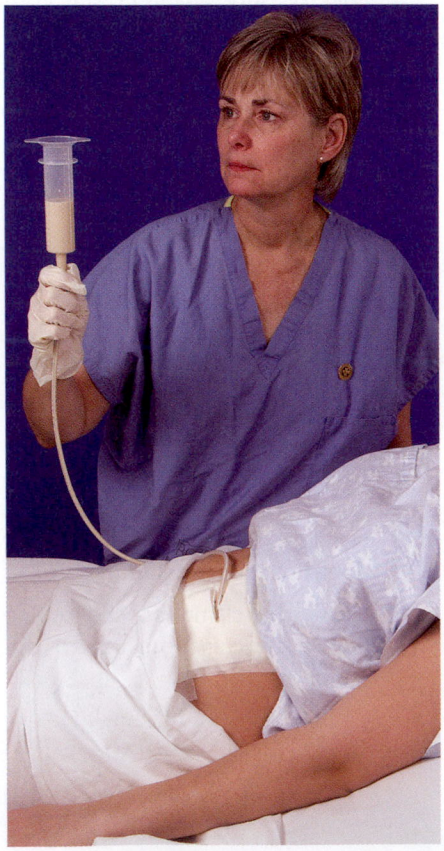

6. **When the syringe is nearly** empty, refill the syringe until the prescribed amount of feeding has been administered.
   If the tubing runs dry, air may enter the stomach and cause discomfort associated with gas.

7. **When the feeding volume** is infused, clamp or pinch the end of the feeding tube.

8. **Disconnect the syringe** from the feeding tube.

9. **Flush feeding tube** with the prescribed amount of water—typically 50 to 100 mL.

10. **Cap the proximal end** of the feeding tube.
    Prevents spillage of gastric contents and stops air from entering the stomach.

11. **Keep the head of the bed elevated** at least 30° to 45° for 1 hour after administering the tube feeding.
    Elevation reduces the risk for aspiration of gastric contents.

12. **Provide or assist with** regular oral hygiene and encourage frequent gargling.
    Oral care reduces oropharyngeal discomfort from the tube.

? What if . . .

- **When checking for residual, the volume is more than the formula flow rate for 1 hour or more than 150 mL?**

  Reinstill the gastric residual volume. Residual gastric contents should be reinfused in the absence of pain or abdominal distension.

  If the residual is >250 mL and if there is no abdominal pain or distension, continue the infusion. Recheck in 1 hour. If the residual is still >250 mL, stop the infusion for 4 hours and recheck. If still >250 mL, call healthcare provider (Bankhead, Boullata, Brantley, et al., 2009).

  If residual is <250 mL, restart the infusion at 50% original rate and monitor (Kenny & Goodman, 2010).

  If the gastric residual volume is ≥250 mL after a second gastric residual check, a promotility agent may be considered in adult clients (American Medical Directors Association (AMDA), 2010; American Society for Parenteral and Enteral Nutrition (A.S.P.E.N.), 2009a; Bankhead, Boullata, Brantley, et al., 2009).

  High residual volumes indicate delayed gastric emptying.

- **When checking for residual, none is obtained?**

  Use a large syringe (e.g., 60 mL) and inflate 20 mL of air into the tube, if agency policy permits; this may move the tube away from the gastric wall or clear the tube of any residual formula, medication, or water.

- **When irrigating the feeding tube, resistance is met? Or when instilling the feeding, the fluid does not flow?**

  Do not force the solution. Do not use any fluid other than water for flushing. Check for kinks in tubing and that the pump is working correctly. Turn the client onto his left side. Remove any enteral feeding solution remaining in the tube. Try instilling 5 mL of warm water into the tube and clamping the tube for 5 minutes. Then apply gentle negative pressure to the tube with a syringe. Try flushing with a smaller (e.g., 10 or 20 mL) syringe. If these measures fail, the tube may need to be removed and a new one inserted; contact the primary care provider.

  Note: *There are other methods, such as the alkalinized enzyme method; they require a medical prescription.*

  Forcing the solution may damage the tube. However, you can use a smaller syringe to exert slightly more pressure.

- **The patient has a cuffed tracheostomy tube?**

  Inflate the cuff before administering the feeding, and keep the cuff inflated for at least 15 minutes afterward, if the agency permits.

  Cuffing helps to prevent aspiration.

- **During the feeding, the patient vomits or complains of nausea or feeling too full?**

  Stop the feeding and assess the patient's condition. Flush the tube, wait an hour, then measure gastric contents and restart the feeding at a slower rate. You may need to obtain a medical order to decrease the volume of the feedings.

- **The patient has a jejunostomy tube?**

  Do not instill air into the tube or check for residual before feeding.

  The tube is in the jejunum rather than the stomach, and the jejunum isn't normally a reservoir; therefore, no residual volume is present in the jejunum. Gastrostomy and jejunostomy tubes are often placed through the upper abdominal wall; these tubes, of course, cannot inadvertently migrate into the airway. Injecting air into the tube is not necessary and introduces air into the GI tract, causing the patient discomfort from gas.

  Clean the insertion site daily with soap and water. You may apply a small, precut gauze dressing to the site.

  Helps prevent bacterial growth; prevents infection.

  Be aware that the delivery rate will likely be slower for jejunostomy tubes because of the loss of the stomach as a reservoir.

Evaluation

- Evaluate the patient's tolerance to the tube feeding; did the patient have any abdominal discomfort, nausea, vomiting, or diarrhea?
- Auscultate bowel sounds and vital signs every 4 hours.
- Check gastric residual volume every 4 hours.
- Monitor intake and output every 8 hours.
- Weigh patient at least 3 times per week.
- Assess the exit site for signs of skin breakdown.
- Assess characteristics and frequency of bowel movements.
- Check laboratory values to evaluate nutritional status.

Patient Teaching

- Demonstrate the procedure to the patient and caregiver if the patient will be continuing tube feedings at home.
- Explain the importance of flushing the feeding tube with tap water every 4 hours while the patient is awake to maintain tube patency and fluid and electrolyte balance.
- Discuss the importance of remaining upright for at least 1 hour after the feeding.

Home Care

- Provide written instructions.
- Be sure the client has a 7-day supply of enteral feedings.
- Identify with the client the person who will be responsible for care of the enteral tube and administration of feedings at home.
- Explain to the client and caregiver how to measure the prescribed amount of tube feeding formula and water for flushes by using household measuring equipment.
- Explain the importance of washing reusable equipment thoroughly with soap and water to prevent the spread of infection.
- Discuss how and where to purchase and store the formula.
- If home feedings are to be delivered by pump:
  - Facilitate a home care visit to provide training about the feeding pump.

(continued on next page)

Procedure 27-3 ■ Administering Feedings Through Gastric and Enteric Tubes (continued)

- Arrange for delivery of the feeding pump before discharge (or refer to the appropriate professional for this).
- Ensure that the client has a 7-day supply of disposable feeding sets and 50- or 60-mL syringes upon discharge.

Documentation

- Chart the type of tube feeding, rate and volume of infusion, amount of gastric residual volume (if any), and tolerance of procedure.
- Tube feeding intake is documented on the intake and output portion of the flowsheet in most agencies.
- Record all flushes as intake. Subtract any liquids that you aspirate and do not reinstill (e.g., when gastric residual is too high).

Practice Resources

AACCN (2005a, 2005b); American Medical Directors Association (2010); A.S.P.E.N. (2009a); Bankhead, Boullata, Brantley, et al. (2009); Griffiths, R., Thompson, D., Chau, J., et al. (2006); Rauen, C., Chulay, M., Bridges, E., et al. (2008); U.S. Preventative Services Task Force (USPSTF) (2009); Yantis, M. A., & Velander, R. (2011).

Thinking About the Procedure

To practice applying clinical reasoning to this procedure,

Go to *Davis's Nursing Skills*, **Administering Feedings Through Gastric and Enteric Tubes With Infusion Pump and Administering Feedings Through Gastric and Enteric Tubes Using an Open-System Syringe.**

For questions and suggested responses,

Go to Chapter 27, **Thinking About the Procedure Questions and Suggested Responses,** on Davis*Plus*.

Procedure 27-4 ■ Removing a Nasogastric or Nasoenteric Tube

➤ For steps to follow in *all* procedures, refer to the Universal Steps for All Procedures found on the inside back cover.

Equipment

- Linen-saver pad
- 60-mL luer-lock or catheter-tip syringe
- Nonsterile gloves
- Stethoscope
- Disposable plastic bag
- Emesis basin
- Gauze square

Delegation

This procedure should not be delegated to the LPN or NAP.

Pre-Procedure Assessments

- Auscultate the abdomen for the presence of bowel sounds.
  Bowel sounds and flatus confirm peristalsis, which indicates bowel function is present.
- Assess the patient's ability to consume an oral diet.
  Confirms readiness for discontinuing the NG or NE tube.
- Determine how long it has been since the patient's last enteral feeding.
  Wait at least 30 minutes after a feeding to remove the NG tube.

➤ When performing the procedure, always identify your patient according to agency policy, using two identifiers, and be attentive to standard precautions, hand hygiene, patient safety and privacy, body mechanics, and documentation.

Procedure Steps

1. **Check the patient's health** record to confirm removal of the tube. For feeding tubes, make sure tube feeding has been stopped at least 30 minutes before removal.
2. **Assist the patient to a sitting** or high-Fowler's position.
   Proper body alignment facilitates tube removal.
3. **Place the plastic bag and emesis** basin on the bed or within reach. Hand the patient facial tissue. Explain that the procedure may cause some gagging or nasal discomfort, but it will be brief.
   Patients often need to blow their nose after this procedure.
4. **Drape a linen-saver pad or towel** across the patient's chest, and don procedure gloves.
   Draping protects the gown and linens from soiling. Maintains universal precautions.
5. **Wash your hands and don nonsterile** gloves, if you have not already done so.
6. **If the NG tube is connected to** suction, turn off the suction and disconnect the tube.

7. **If you are right-handed**, stand on the patient's right side; and stand on the left side if left-handed.

8. **Attach the syringe** to the proximal end of the NG or NE tube and flush the tube with 10 mL of water, normal saline, or air.
Flushing clears the tube of feeding formula or gastric secretions that could cause irritation or be aspirated during tube removal.

9. **Unpin the tube** from the patient's gown, and then untape the tube from the patient's nose and cheek. Use an adhesive-remover pad to help loosen the tape as necessary.

10. **Clamp or pinch the end** of the tube in your hand. Hold gauze up to the patient's nose and be ready to grab the tube with the towel in the opposite hand upon removal.
This prevents gastric fluids from leaking out the end of the tube onto the nurse or patient.

11. **Ask the patient to take a deep** breath and hold it.
Breath holding closes the epiglottis to prevent aspiration.

12. **Withdraw the tube quickly**, steadily, and smoothly and place it in the plastic bag.
Rapid removal in one steady motion prevents tissue trauma. The plastic bag acts as a barrier to gastric fluids until the tube can be placed in the trash. Seeing and smelling the tube may cause the patient to become nauseated.

13. **Clean the patient's nares** and provide mouth care, if the patient cannot do so. Remove the tape residue from her nose with adhesive remover.
Promotes patient comfort and prevents infection.

14. **If the NG tube was connected** to suction, measure the drainage and note the character of the content. Dispose of the tube and drainage equipment in a biohazardous waste receptacle according to facility policy.
For patients receiving enteral feedings or gastric suction, record their intake and output. Proper equipment disposal prevents the spread of infection.

15. **Remove and dispose of gloves** in the nearest receptacle.

Evaluation

- Assess the nares for signs of skin breakdown or bleeding.
- Monitor the patient for signs of GI dysfunction, such as food intolerance, nausea, vomiting, and abdominal distention. Auscultate for bowel sounds.
GI dysfunction could necessitate reinsertion of the tube.
- Monitor intake and output every 8 hours.
- Weigh the patient regularly.
- Check laboratory values to evaluate nutritional status.

Patient Teaching

- Explain the importance of reporting nausea, vomiting, food intolerance, or abdominal distention to the physician.
- Explain the importance of and procedure for drinking fluids, if not contraindicated.

Home Care

- The procedure does not require special adaptation for home care, except that you might want to place the tube in a plastic zippered storage bag before discarding it in the trash receptacle.

Documentation

- Chart the date and time of removal as well as the patient's tolerance of the procedure.
- Document the amount of drainage if the tube was connected to suction.
- Note any complications following NG or NE tube removal, such as food intolerance, nausea, vomiting, and abdominal distention.

Sample documentation

4/13/16 1010 Explained to pt and wife NG tube was to be removed and procedure for removing NG tube. Pt stated, "I am ready to get this thing out." Untaped NG tube from gown and nose. Removed tube while asking pt to hold his breath. Pt tolerated procedure well without vomiting or bradycardia. Provided mouth care and facial cleansing. ——— A. Hiam, RN

4/13/16 1230 Taking clear liquids since NG tube was removed with no nausea, vomiting, or abdominal distention. Bowel sounds faint but audible in all 4 quadrants. ——— A. Hiam, RN

Practice Resources

National Institutes of Health (NIH) (n.d., last updated 2012)

Thinking About the Procedure

To practice applying clinical reasoning to this procedure,

Go to *Davis's Nursing Skills Videos*, **Removing a Nasogastric or Nasoenteric Tube.**

For questions and suggested responses,

Go to Chapter 27, **Thinking About the Procedure Questions and Suggested Responses,** on Davis*Plus*.

Procedure 27-5 ■ Administering Parenteral Nutrition

➤ For steps to follow in *all* procedures, refer to the Universal Steps for All Procedures found on the inside back cover.

Equipment

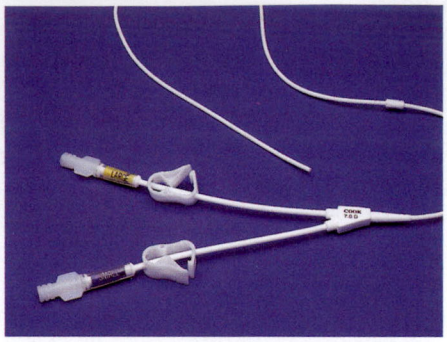

- Parenteral nutrition (PN) solution
  - Keep the PN refrigerated until 60 min before use; do not give cold. Do not hasten warming by placing in a microwave oven or hot water bath.
    Cold solution can cause pain, hypothermia, and venous spasm. Nutrients in PN solution are stable only for this short period of time. Nutrients could precipitate, causing catheter blockage or emboli.
  - Some pharmacies deliver the solution before infusion. Be sure the PN has not been mixed more than 24 hours beforehand. However, in home care you may find that solutions are mixed and delivered weekly.
- Procedure gloves
- Sterile gloves. (*Note*: If the central line has an injection cap and if IV tubing is connected onto the cap via luer-lock, some agencies do not require gloves.)
- Intravenous administration set, extension set if indicated (free of plasticizers, such as DEHP, when fat emulsion is to be infused)
- 0.22-micron filter (1.2-micron filter if solution contains albumin or lipids)
  A 0.22-micron filter will remove most particulates and microorganisms that might have been introduced during mixing, but it is too fine for larger-molecule lipids to infuse properly.
- Time tape
  Even though the PN is delivered by infusion pump, there have been numerous recalls of infusion pumps because of malfunction. This simple tape provides valuable information quickly and is an additional safety measure.
- 70% alcohol pads or chlorhexidine gluconate (CHG)-alcohol (e.g., 2% CHG in 70% isopropyl alcohol)
- Infusion pump
- 10-mL syringe and saline
- Blood glucose testing monitor
- Intake and output record
- Transparent dressing or sterile gauze and tape (if dressing is to be changed)
- Catheter stabilization device (e.g., StatLock)
  These are recommended for all catheters and must be changed with each dressing change.
- If the dressing is to be changed, you also need a transparent dressing or sterile gauze, tape, and a mask.

Delegation

Do not delegate this skill to the LPN or NAP because administration of parenteral nutrition requires advanced assessment and critical-thinking skills. The LPN or NAP can assist by monitoring vital signs, checking blood glucose, and verifying patient identity with you. Instruct them about complications associated with PN and ask them to inform you of any signs or symptoms or change in the patient's condition.

Pre-Procedure Assessments

- Assess nutrition status and nutritional needs (e.g., daily weights, intake and output [O], lab results). Patients requiring PN have complex nutritional needs, and actual nutritional status is assessed by a nurse or dietician specializing in nutritional support.
- Check the prescriber's orders for type and concentration of additives in each container and for rate of infusion. (Standardized order forms are recommended by the (A.S.P.E.N.).
- Check the patient's record to confirm that proper central venous catheter (CVC) tip placement has been established before the initial PN administration.
- Check agency policy.
  A few may require tubing and filter change with every bottle or bag. The CDC recommends changing the PN set every 72 hours and a fat emulsion set at least every 24 hours.
- Check the blood glucose level.
- Assess for apparent patency of the IV site.
  If PN is being administered continuously by pump and the infusion is running and there is no leakage from the insertion, you can begin the first few steps of the procedure. Actual patency is checked at Step 14.

➤ When performing the procedure, always identify your patient according to agency policy, using two identifiers, and be attentive to standard precautions, hand hygiene, patient safety and privacy, body mechanics, and documentation.

Procedure Steps

1. **Gather equipment** and place at the bedside.
   Promotes efficient use of time.

2. **Identify the patient**, using two identifiers, according to agency policy. Some institutions require, as an extra precaution, that two people identify the patient.

   Multiple patient identifiers help to avoid "wrong-patient" errors. PN solutions are mixed to meet individual needs.

3. **Explain to the patient** the procedure and the rationale for it.
Respects the patient's right to be informed.

4. **Perform hand hygiene.**
Reduces transmission of infectious microorganisms.

5. **Position the patient supine** in bed.

6. **Obtain and examine the PN** container. Check for leaks, cloudiness, or floating particles. Do not use if any of these are present. Some agencies require that two people examine the solution.

For Solutions Containing Lipids (3-in-1 Admixture)

Do not administer the admixture if it has a brown layer, oil droplets, or oil on the surface. This indicates that the emulsion has "broken," and the large lipid droplets can cause fat emboli if administered. Also note that this solution requires a 1.2-micron filter.
To reduce the risk of adverse events such as fat emboli.

7. **Compare the bag** to the patient's identification band; check for correct bag number, expiration date, and additives and their concentration. Compare with the original prescription. Have a coworker verify with you.
Ensures that the correct solution is administered. Check the expiration date to ensure that the solution will be discarded after that date and time. PN solutions are carefully calculated and prepared using the latest recommendations for sterile compounding of solutions. Therefore, you should not add any medications to the bag either before it is hung or while it is infusing.

8. **Connect the IV tubing to the PN** solution; prime the tubing. Note that priming may be done manually now or later (on the pump after the tubing is loaded into the pump), depending on the design of the pump.
Priming tubing removes air bubbles and prevents air from entering the patient's bloodstream, possibly causing air embolism. If there is PN already infusing, the old tubing must be removed from the pump and the rate regulated manually for the short period it takes to prime the new administration set.

When Using IV Tubing Without an Inline Filter

If the IV tubing does not have an inline filter, attach the filter and the extension tubing before priming. Attach the filter as close to the catheter site as possible.

9. Be sure to identify the correct port and IV line. Trace the PN tubing from the bag to the patient before starting the feeding.
Ensures that you have not inadvertently hooked the feeding bag or bottle to the IV line

10. **Place the IV tubing in** the infusion pump. (Prime the tubing if not done in Step 8.) Set the pump to the prescribed rate.

Administration via pump (preferably volumetric) helps prevent complications associated with too-rapid infusion. PN solutions must be administered by infusion pump with reliable, audible alarms. Catheter tip placement must be confirmed before initial PN administration.

11. **Identify the correct IV catheter** and lumen for the PN. This is usually a peripherally inserted central catheter (PICC) line or a centrally inserted venous line designated solely for PN. Never infuse PN into an IV line that is not central.
PN must be administered via a central venous catheter (e.g., subclavian catheter, internal jugular, or PICC) whose tip is positioned in the superior vena cava/right atrial juncture. Most guidelines state that a specific intravenous line be reserved for parenteral nutrition and not used for any other purpose. If a single-lumen catheter is used, it is used only for PN. If a multilumen catheter is used, one lumen will be dedicated for the PN, and blood and other fluids should not be given through that lumen.

12. **Clamp the catheter** and the old PN administration set, if still connected, before disconnecting the tubing.
   a. A clamp should be present on the central line catheters with valves built into the catheter itself.
   The central line for the PN should already be clamped if no PN is running. If a previous bag is running, always clamp the PN line near the patient before disconnecting. Clamping prevents air from entering the catheter when you open the connection.
   b. As an additional, optional safety measure, instruct the patient to perform the Valsalva maneuver just as you change the tubing.
   c. If Valsalva is contraindicated for a patient, instruct the patient to exhale at a specific time when the lumen is open.
   The Valsalva maneuver increases intrathoracic pressure and creates positive pressure in the central vessels, also helping prevent air embolism.

13. **Remove and discard gloves.** Perform hand hygiene.
In Steps 1 through 11, you were observing Universal Precautions. From this step forward, the emphasis is on preventing the introduction of microorganisms into the catheter lumen or the catheter insertion site.

14. **Don clean gloves (or sterile** gloves, if your agency policy requires them). Disconnect the old administration set. Using a chlorhexidine gluconate (CHG)–alcohol pad or a 70% alcohol pad, thoroughly cleanse all surfaces of the central line injection cap and extension leg (in a needleless system) or the luer-lock, including threads.
Because PN solutions are a good medium for growth of pathogens, and because the IV line enters the central circulation, the risk for sepsis is relatively high.

15. **Determine patency of the line.** Use a 10-mL syringe to aspirate for blood, looking for a brisk return with pulsating pressure; then flush with saline. If the PN is running continuously on a pump, there are no occlusion alarms, and the dressing is dry and intact, these are also signs—but not proof—of patency.

(continued on next page)

Procedure 27-5 ■ Administering Parenteral Nutrition (continued)

When PN is running continuously on a pump, the pump creates a constant fluid flow through the lumen to help keep it patent. There is some controversy about this step. Some experts prefer to aspirate for blood only for the first bag of a continuous infusion, and thereafter to flush without aspirating. As always, follow agency policy.

16. **Attach the infusion tubing** to the designated PN port and then turn the luer-lock to secure the connection. "Luer-slip" connections should not be used. Do not use tape. Trace the tubing from the patient back to the PN container to be certain you are using the correct lumen.
Securing the connection with a luer-lock connection prevents separation of the connection and decreases the risk for sepsis or embolism. Tape, even sterile tape, has been found to be a medium for bacterial colonization.

If the Previous Infusion Is Still Connected

Be sure the access line and the line to the "old" infusion bag are clamped (Step 11). Quickly disconnect from the central line, thoroughly cleanse the port, and connect the new infusion.

17. Trace the tubing from the bag back to the patient. Then start the infusion. Check again to make sure the catheter-tubing connection is secure. Infuse at the rate prescribed (depending on the patient's tolerance, PN is usually started at a rate of 40 to 50 mL/hr and then advanced 25 mL/hr every 6 hours).
PN solutions may contain as much as 70% dextrose. A gradual rate increase allows the patient's pancreatic beta cells time to increase their insulin output to handle the increased glucose load. For lower concentrations of dextrose, you can usually run the same rate for the complete 24-hour volume.

18. **Label the tubing** with the date and time of change (if it is new tubing or if you have changed the tubing).
Labeling allows other nurses to know when tubing is due to be changed and a new solution must be hung.

19. **Remove and discard gloves.** Perform hand hygiene.

? What if . . .

- **When you flush the catheter (at Step 15), you meet resistance?**
Examine the insertion site for leaking fluid or inflammation. Aspirate and try again to flush *gently*. Never forcibly flush against resistance. Remove syringe from luer-lock connection, then reconnect. Reposition the patient and ask him to cough. Roll the patient's shoulder or raise the arm on the same side the catheter is on. If these measures fail, notify the primary care provider.
Occlusion may be caused by a clot; drug precipitation; or catheter migration, kinking, or compression; or may be related to incomplete connection with the luer-lock. Forceful flushing may discharge a clot into circulation. Other measures to clear a catheter require a medical order.

- **The rate falls behind or the pump gives occlusion alarms?**
First check to be sure the pump is turned on, the bag is not empty, and all clamps are fully open. Change the filter if it is clogged. Perform the steps in the preceding item. If those measures do not work, change the pump and send it to biomedical engineering to be checked. Do not attempt to catch up by increasing the rate.
A slow rate may indicate a clogged filter or injection cap, a kinked catheter, or a malfunctioning pump. A clogged filter must be changed; you cannot run the PN without a filter.

- **The 24-hour total deviates from the prescribed infusion rate by 10% or more?**
Notify the primary provider or nutrition support team.

- **A PN solution must be discontinued abruptly for any reason?**
Notify the primary provider or nutrition support team. Another solution of 5% or 10% dextrose may be started.
The dextrose solution is started to prevent rebound hypoglycemia. Note that if it is a catheter complication that requires this discontinuation, 10% dextrose is the highest concentration that can be infused through a peripheral vein because infiltrated hyperosmolar fluid causes tissue injury.

- **The patient no longer needs parenteral nutrition?**
You may need to decrease the rate gradually, perhaps over 48 hours, before discontinuing the infusion completely. Be sure the patient either receives enteral nutrition or consumes food during the next few hours after stopping PN.
To prevent rebound hypoglycemia.

Evaluation

These are post-procedure evaluations. For ongoing monitoring, see Clinical Insight 27-8.

- Assess vital signs, I&O, and weight.
- Observe that the solution is infusing at the prescribed rate.
- Assess patient's tolerance to the infusion (e.g., observe for pulmonary edema; check lab results).
- Observe for skin rashes, flushing, color changes, or other signs of allergic reactions; notify the primary provider.

  Note: These are not common.
- Monitor blood glucose and do not increase the infusion rate until glycemic control is established.

Patient Teaching

- Inform the patient and family of the purpose and duration of the nutritional support.
- Teach them to recognize and report to the nurse symptoms of complications associated with PN.
- Teach the patient that the dressing must remain occlusive, and to notify nurse if it comes loose or gets wet.
- Teach the patient the importance of measures to prevent blood infections.

Home Care

- The home environment must provide dry storage space for supplies, a refrigerator for storing admixtures, a clean low-traffic area for procedure preparation, and electronic outlets for any electronic equipment.
- Teach safe disposal of supplies.
- Provide verbal and written instructions of the procedures; demonstrate and ask for a return demonstration. Role-play "what would you do if . . ." situations with the patient.
- Clients at home often administer their daily 24-hour total over 12 to 16 hours during the night. This allows them to disconnect from the infusion in the morning, flush the central line, and be free to pursue their usual activities during the day.
- Instruct about solution hang time and management of the access device.
  Depending on the anticipated length of therapy, patients may be sent home with a permanent venous access device.
- Provide 24-hour phone numbers for the primary care provider and home care agency.
- Home PN is less expensive than treatment in the hospital, and in many cases is associated with a lower risk of infection.
- Home nutritional support is usually under the direction of specialized nutrition support teams.

Documentation

- A special form may be used for documenting PN administration.
- Bag number, date and time hung, volume, type of fluid, rate of delivery, additives
- Date and time of dressing or tubing change (if performed)
- Patient's tolerance of procedure
- Pre- and post-administration assessment data, including complications and response to therapy
- Results of fingerstick blood glucose checks
- If insulin is required, type, amount, and route/site administered
- Weight
- I&O

Practice Resources

A.S.P.E.N. Board of Directors (2009a); A.S.P.E.N. Board of Directors & Task Force on Parenteral Nutrition Standardization (2007); A.S.P.E.N. Board of Directors & Task Force for the Revision of Safe Practices for Parenteral Nutrition (2004); Bankhead, R. Boullata, J., Brantley, S., et al. (2009); Infusion Nurses Society (INS) (2011); National Guideline Clearinghouse (NGC) (2006a, 2008b).

Procedure 27-6 ■ Administering Lipids

➤ For steps to follow in *all* procedures, refer to the Universal Steps for All Procedures found on the inside back cover.

➤ *Note:* If administering through a central line, refer to Procedure 27-5 for precautions associated with central lines.

➤ *Note:* This procedure is for administering fat emulsions. If you are administering an admixture with the parenteral nutrition solution, use Procedure 27-5.

Equipment

- Intravenous lipid solution (not refrigerated)
- Special tubing (infusion set) for lipids (must be without plasticizers [DEHP]). Set should be labeled to that effect)
- Needleless cannula (if using a split septum needleless connector that requires it)
- 70% isopropyl alcohol or chlorhexidine gluconate (CHG)-alcohol pads
- Procedure gloves
- Time tape
- Infusion pump
- I&O record
- If a filter is a used, it must be a 1.2-micron filter
  Lipid particles are large and will clog a smaller size.

Delegation

Do not delegate this skill to the LPN or NAP because administration of lipids requires advanced assessment and critical-thinking skills. The LPN or NAP can assist by monitoring vital signs and verifying patient identity with you. Instruct them about complications associated with lipids and ask them to inform you of any signs or symptoms or change in the patient's condition.

Pre-Procedure Assessments

- Assess for rash; eczema; dry, scaly skin; poor wound healing; and sparse hair.
  These are signs of essential fatty acid deficits.
- Check the history for anemia; coagulation disorders; and abnormal liver, pancreatic, or respiratory function.
  These factors predispose to fat emboli. Your role as a staff nurse is to be certain the PN prescriber is aware of these factors; they do not necessarily contraindicate giving the PN.
- Check peripheral IV site for erythema, infiltration, and patency. Check the central venous access site for erythema or other signs of infection.
- Take baseline vital signs just before infusing the lipids.
  An immediate reaction can occur upon starting the infusion. Note that not all guidelines require this action.

(continued on next page)

Procedure 27-6 ■ Administering Lipids (continued)

➤ When performing the procedure, always identify your patient according to agency policy, using two identifiers, and be attentive to standard precautions, hand hygiene, patient safety and privacy, body mechanics, and documentation.

Procedure Steps

1. **Review the prescriber's orders,** identify the patient, and explain the purpose of the procedure.
   Verifying helps to prevent dosage and wrong-patient errors. Explaining respects the patient's right to be informed and encourages cooperation.

2. **Gather equipment** and place at bedside. Adjust lighting as needed.
   Organization promotes efficient use of time.

3. **Perform hand hygiene** and don procedure gloves.
   Hand hygiene and gloving reduces transmission of infectious microorganisms.

4. **Position the patient supine** in bed.

5. **Be certain lipids are not cold.**
   Cold infusion can cause discomfort.

6. **Examine the container** for a layer of froth or for separation into fat globules or layers.
   Do not use the lipids if these occur.

7. **Label the container** with the patient's name, room number, date, time, rate, and start and stop times. Label the tubing with date and time. ***Note:*** *When lipids are infused with parenteral nutrition, the lipid infusion must be completed within 12 hours.*
   Labeling helps ensure that the patient receives the correct infusion.

8. **Compare the lipid container** to the patient's wrist band (bag number, expiration date); compare to the original prescription. Have a colleague verify.

9. **Determine patency of the IV** line.

10. **Cleanse the stopper** on the IV bottle with an antiseptic swab; allow to dry.

11. **Connect the special DEHP-free** lipids-infusion tubing to the container, twisting the spike as you insert it. **Key Point:** ***You must use new tubing for each bottle.***
    Twisting the spike helps ensure that particles from the stopper do not fall into the bottle. New tubing reduces the growth of microorganisms (the feeding provides a medium for fungal growth). DEHP is considered a toxin in the bloodstream.

12. **Place the primed tubing** in the pump and attach the tubing to the IV catheter lumen.

    ✚ Identify the correct IV line and port for the infusion. Trace the tubing from the bag back to the patient.
    Infusing enteral medication or feeding solution into an intravenous line could be life threatening.

    a. Thoroughly scrub the catheter injection port or hub and the luer-lock threads with an antiseptic wipe.
    b. If you are infusing lipids simultaneously with PN, attach the primed lipid tubing to the injection port/hub closest to the patient, below the tubing filter, or through a Y-connection at the catheter hub.
    c. Turn the luer-lock to secure the connection.
    d. ✚ *Note:* If a previous infusion has been running, clamp the catheter lumen and the old administration set tubing before disconnecting and changing the tubing.
    Prevents blood backup in the line.

13. **Begin the infusion.** Ideally, infuse slowly at first: 1.0 mL/min for adults and 0.1 mL/min for children (or as prescribed by the physician). Check again to be sure the catheter-tubing connection is secure.
    Slow infusion allows time to identify adverse reaction to the lipids and to stop the infusion before the patient has received a large volume. Nausea, vomiting, and elevated temperature have been reported when lipids are infused quickly.

14. **Take the vital signs** now, then every 10 minutes for 30 minutes. Observe for side effects (e.g., chills, fever, flushing, dyspnea, nausea, vomiting, headache, back pain).

15. **If no reactions occur,** adjust to the prescribed infusion rate and continue monitoring according to your agency's protocol.

16. **Remove gloves** and perform hand hygiene.

17. **When the infusion is finished,** discard the bottle and IV administration set.
    Formula contains sugars that are a medium for growth of pathogens.

? What if . . .

- **The entire bottle of lipids is not used?**
  Discard partially used bottles to prevent contamination.

Evaluation

- If ordered, monitor serum lipids 4 hours after discontinuing the infusion.
- Monitor the IV site for infection, inflammation, and infiltration.
- Monitor for symptoms of fat emboli.
- Monitor the IV line for patency.
- Monitor for allergic reactions (nausea, vomiting, headache, chest pain, back pain, fever).
- Monitor for lipid intolerance (triglyceride levels, liver function tests, hepatosplenomegaly, decreased coagulation, cyanosis, dyspnea).

Patient Teaching

- Inform the patient and family of the purpose and duration of the nutritional support.
- Teach the patient to recognize and report symptoms of complications associated with lipids infusion.

Home Care

- The home environment must provide dry storage space for supplies, a refrigerator for storing solutions, a clean low-traffic area for procedure preparation, and electronic outlets for any electronic equipment.
- Teach safe disposal of supplies.
- Provide verbal and written instructions for the procedures; demonstrate and ask for a return demonstration.
- Instruct about solution hang time and management of the access device.
- Provide 24-hour phone numbers for the primary care provider and home care agency.

Documentation

- A special form may be used for documenting lipids and PN administration.
- Lipid container number, date and time hung, volume, type of fluid, and rate of delivery
- Status of dressing, and date and time of dressing or tubing change (if performed)
- Patient's tolerance of the procedure and any problems encountered
- Pre- and post-administration assessment data and blood tests, if any
- Condition of the IV site
- Weight
- I&O

Practice Resources

A.S.P.E.N. Board of Directors (2009a); A.S.P.E.N. Board of Directors & Task Force on Parenteral Nutrition Standardization (2007); A.S.P.E.N. Board of Directors & Task Force for the Revision of Safe Practices for Parenteral Nutrition (2004); INS (2011); NGC (2006b, 2008b).

CLINICAL INSIGHTS

Clinical Insight 27-1 ➤ 10 Tips for Building Healthy Meals

	HEALTHY EATING TIP	HOW TO DO IT
1	Make half of your plate fruit and vegetables.	Choose vegetables rich in color; they are usually rich in nutrients. Good ones are sweet potatoes, beets, broccoli, spinach, and many others. Fresh fruits and vegetables are less expensive and more flavorful when bought in season.
2	Add lean protein to your meals.	High protein selections will help you to build muscle and reduce your carbohydrates. Be sure to eat lean beef, pork, or chicken; tofu; and beans. Seafood is a must at least twice a week.
3	Whole grains rule.	Like fiber, whole grains are more nutritious than refined or multigrain products. Try to cut out refined flour altogether. "If it's white, don't bite."
4	Dairy is a big deal.	To be sure you have essential nutrients, calcium, and vitamin D in your diet, plan your meal with fat-free or low-fat milk, soymilk, or low-fat yogurt.
5	Stay away from extra fat.	Stay clear of gravy, heavy sauces, salad dressings, and too much cheese on top of your food. It adds unneeded fat calories!
6	Take your time eating.	Eating slowly allows you to enjoy the taste and texture of your food. Savor your food by taking small bites and chewing thoroughly. Your body also has a chance to realize it is full before you eat too much.
7	Serve food on a smaller plate.	Serving food on a smaller plate is one good way to control portion size and keep from overeating.
8	Control your food. Don't let it control you.	Just say "no" to extra large portions. Choose healthier food options because you're worth it. Remember that nothing tastes as good as healthy feels!
9	Be open to trying new foods.	Eating a variety of foods is a good way to feed your body the essential vitamins and minerals it needs. Keep it interesting by trying different fresh foods without fillers, additives, or *trans*-fats.
10	Satisfying your sweet tooth doesn't have to be unhealthy.	Indulge in naturally sweet fruit. Serve it in an attractive way or use interesting spices to make it even more appealing.

Source: U.S. Department of Agriculture (USDA). (2011d, June). Build a healthy meal: Ten tips for healthy meals. 10 Tips Education Series, DG Tipsheet #7. Retrieved January 2013, from http://www.choosemyplate.gov/food-groups/downloads/TenTips/DGTipsheet7BuildAHealthyMeal.pdf

Clinical Insight 27-2 ➤ Skinfold Measurement

- Take measurements directly on the skin, not through clothing.
- Take each reading as soon as the jaws of the caliper come into contact with the skin and the reading has stabilized.
- In each site, take three readings in quick succession, and average the results to the nearest 0.1 mm. Note that the accuracy of this method varies with the technique.
- Add the averages of all skinfold sites to arrive at a total skinfold measurement.
- To determine the percentage body fat, compare the final calculated measurement with the values in the appropriate body fat and skinfolds table for the age and gender of the patient.

Measuring Triceps Skinfold

- Locate the midpoint on the posterior side of the dominant upper arm.
- With the client's arm hanging loosely at the side, palpate the measurement site at the midpoint to become familiar with distinguishing muscle from adipose soft tissue.
- From 1 cm above the midpoint, grasp a vertical pinch of skin and only the subcutaneous fat layer between the thumb and index finger. Gently pull the skinfold away from the underlying muscle.
- Place the skinfold caliper at the midpoint, and slowly release the jaw of the caliper while maintaining a grasp of the skinfold (see the figure).

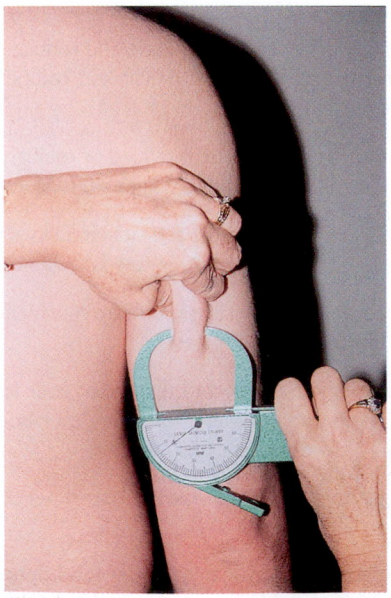

Triceps skinfold.

Measuring Subscapular Skinfold

- Follow the same procedure, except measure on the back, just under the shoulder blade. Grasp below the tip of the inferior angle of the scapula 45° to vertical.

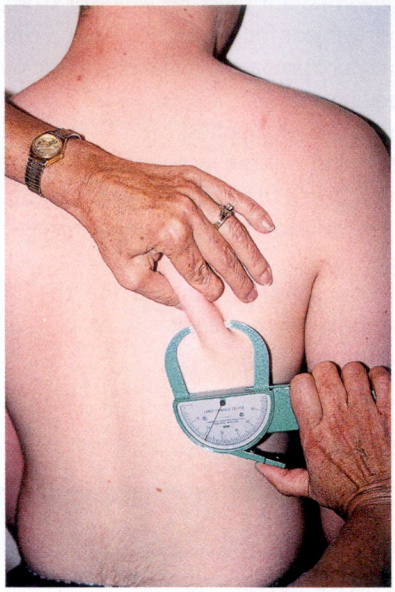

Subscapular skinfold.

Measuring Biceps Skinfold

- Follow the same procedure, except measure the muscle belly of the biceps. With the patient's arm hanging loosely at the side, grasp the skin and subcutaneous fat layer on the front of the upper arm, over the biceps, about level with the nipple.

Measuring Suprailiac Skinfold

- Follow the same procedure, except measure approximately 1 inch above the hipbone, above the iliac crest in the mid-axillary line.

Calculating Body Mass Index

Calculate the BMI using this formula:

$$\text{BMI} = \text{weight in kilograms} \div (\text{height in meters})^2$$

Clinical Insight 27-3 ➤ Measuring Circumferences to Evaluate Body Composition

Measuring Mid-Upper Arm Circumference

- Keeping the client's dominant arm parallel to the body, bend the elbow 90°.
- Using a tape measure, measure the distance between the **acromion** (the bony protrusion of the back of the upper shoulder) and the **olecranon process** (tip of the elbow).
- Mark the midpoint between these two landmarks.
- Ask the client to relax the arm, so that it hangs loose and parallel to the body.
- Position the tape around the upper arm at the marked midpoint. Make sure the tape is snug but not so tight as to indent or pinch the skin.
- Record the circumference to the nearest 0.1 cm.

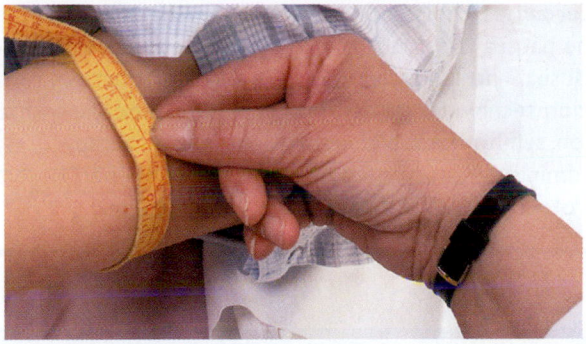

Calculating Waist-to-Hip Ratio (WHR)

WHR ratio greater than 1.0 in men and greater than 0.8 in women is considered obese.

- Use a tape measure to measure the circumference of the waist (at the umbilicus with stomach muscles relaxed).
- Use a tape measure to measure the circumference of the hips at their widest point.
- Calculate the waist-to-hip ratio using the following formula:

waist circumference (in.) ÷ hip circumference (in.)

Note: *Abdominal obesity is defined by World Health Organization (1999) as waist-to-hip ratio greater 0.85 in women, and greater than 0.9 in men.*

Example: Robert's waist measurement is 32 inches, and his hip measurement is 34 inches. His WHR is 32 ÷ 34 = 0.94.

Clinical Insight 27-4 ➤ Interventions for Patients With Impaired Swallowing

Provide Nutritional Support

Nutritional support includes the following activities from the NIC intervention Swallowing Therapy (Bulechek, Butcher, & Dochterman, 2012, pp. 707–708):

- Position the patient in a full upright, 90°, if possible.
- Provide/use assistive devices, as appropriate.
- Avoid use of drinking straws.
- Assist the patient to position head in forward flexion in preparation for swallowing (chin tuck).
- Assist patient to place food at the back of the mouth and on the unaffected side.
- Monitor the patient's tongue movements while she is eating. Frequently cue patient to chew and swallow. Patient may need to double swallow.
- Check mouth for pocketing of food after eating.
- Monitor body weight.
- Monitor body hydration (e.g., intake, output, skin turgor, mucous membranes).

Take Aspiration Precautions

(Bulechek, Butcher, & Dochterman, 2012, p. 145):

- Monitor level of consciousness, cough reflex, gag reflex, and swallowing ability.
- Position the patient upright 90° or as far as possible.
- Keep suction setup available.
- Feed in small amounts.
- Avoid liquids.
- Cut food into small pieces.
- Keep HOB elevated for 30 to 45 minutes after feeding [your text recommends 1 hour].

Clinical Insight 27-5 ➤ Interventions for Patients Who Have Nausea

- Identify the cause of the nausea (e.g., anxiety; pain; constipation; cough; dehydration; electrolyte disorders; treatments, such as surgery, radiotherapy, or chemotherapy; disease processes, such as peptic ulcer or pancreatitis).
- Keep tissues and water to rinse the mouth at the bedside.
- Maintain a calm environment.
- Provide cool, fresh air.
- Instruct the patient to wear loose clothing.
- Avoid wearing perfume. Discourage scented candles and other aromatic items while the patient is nauseated.
- Try serving cool or cold foods. Avoid greasy, warm, spicy, or aromatic foods. In some cases cold food is better tolerated. Allow the patient to eat what she finds appetizing and tolerates well. The sight and smell of hot food can induce nausea.
- Provide or assist with frequent oral hygiene.
- Ask the patient to sit in an upright position for 30 to 45 minutes after eating, unless contraindicated.
- Offer six small meals instead of three large ones.
- Instruct the patient to keep crackers by the side of the bed to eat before getting up if nausea occurs upon wakening. It can also help to eat lean meat or cheese before going to bed.
- Provide cool (not cold or iced) cola to drink. Drinks with sugar to calm the stomach.
- Have the patient suck on an ice cube, Popsicle, or sorbet, or even a piece of frozen fruit (pineapple, kiwi, or apple).
- Recommend a dietary consultation if nausea and vomiting persist.
- For malnourished patients, consult a dietitian. Consider dietary supplements; however, these are often poorly tolerated and may sometimes cause even more nausea.
- Assess for dehydration, if nausea and vomiting is severe or persistent; you may need to administer parenteral fluid and electrolytes.
- Certain psychological techniques may be effective when the nausea is related to anxiety, stress, or anticipation of nausea. The following may be helpful: distraction, relaxation techniques, guided imagery, systematic desensitization, self-hypnosis, biofeedback, and music therapy.
- Administer antiemetics as prescribed or per hospital protocol.

Clinical Insight 27-6 ➤ Assisting Patients With Meals

General Guidelines

- Recommend having one staff person for every two or three patients who need assistance, allowing about 20 to 30 minutes to feed a patient. Prolonged meal times do not promote appetite; nor does hurrying.
- Feeding assistants should be supervised by an RN or LPN.
- Do not interrupt meals with medications.
- Encourage family members to share mealtimes.
- If the patient's condition allows, encourage him to get out of bed for meals.
- Encourage residents in long-term care settings to eat meals in the dining room instead of in the bedroom (Leydon & Dahl, 2008).

Preparation

- Assess for rituals used before meals (blessings of food, and so on).
- Provide an opportunity for toileting, oral hygiene, and handwashing before meals.
- Assist the patient to eat and drink only as necessary; encourage independence.
- Provide privacy during meals if the patient is embarrassed; to further maintain dignity, use a napkin, not a bib, over the patient's clothes.
- Check for proper fit of dentures.
- Provide music during the meal if the patient wishes.
- Demonstrate the use of assistive devices and alternative methods for eating and drinking.

Assisting the Patient

- If the patient must eat in bed, place the head of the bed at the highest tolerable level, and adjust the overbed table to be in easy reach.
- If the patient can feed himself, prepare the food on the tray for him (e.g., open food containers, cut the meat, peel an orange, open the milk and butter containers, mash food if needed).
- If the client is visually impaired, identify the locations of the meal on the tray based on a clock face (e.g., "The coffee is at 1 o'clock above the plate on the right").

Feeding the Patient

- Feed the patient if she is unable to feed herself.
- Sit down while feeding the patient; do not rush.
- Position yourself so you can make eye contact.
- Be sure to provide adequate time for her to chew and swallow.
- If possible, ask her what food she would like next.
- Serve one food at a time; serve small amounts.
- Serve finger foods (e.g., fruit, bread) to promote independence.
- Cue older adults whenever possible with words or gestures.
- Have casual conversation with the patient while feeding her to make mealtime more pleasant and relaxed.

After the Meal

- Help the patient to wash hands or use the rest room.

Clinical Insight 27-6 ➤ Assisting Patients With Meals—cont'd

- Record the amount of food and fluid the patient consumed.
- Document feeding behaviors.
- Document changes in nutritional status.
- Document staffing and staff education, and availability of a supportive interdisciplinary team.

Assisting Older Adults With Dementia

As do all people, older adults with dementia differ in their abilities to eat and communicate. The following are general tips, but you should tailor interventions to each person's specific abilities to achieve the best results. In addition to many of the preceding interventions, try some of the following measures.

- Assess the patient's self-feeding abilities.
- Assess the patient's cognitive limitations and communication abilities.
- Assess for and treat pain.
- Minimize distractions: Turn off the TV; discourage people from entering the room.
- Help the patient to a comfortable chair if possible.
- Assist with oral hygiene and hand hygiene.
- Remove any unnecessary eating utensils; serve only one food at a time.
- Remove items that should not be eaten (e.g., packets of salt or pepper), and hot items that could be spilled.
- Cue the patient verbally to help with self-feeding (e.g., "take a bite," "chew," "swallow").
- Pantomime eating motions so the patient can imitate them.
- Place your hand over the patient's to begin and guide self-feeding (hand-over-hand).
- When assisting, sit at eye level and interact socially with the patient.
- Involve family members if they have assisted with feeding at home.
- Train and supervise NAPs in interacting with and feeding patients with dementia.
- Do not assist too soon—give the patient time to eat independently.
- Do not feed too fast. Feed at a rate that is safe and comfortable for the patient.

References

American Medical Directors Association (AMDA) (2010); Amella, E. (2008); Amella, E., & Lawrence, J. (2007); Bankhead, R., Boullata, J., Brantley, S., et al. (2009); Ebersole, P., Hess, P., Touhy, T., et al. (2009); NGC (2010).

Clinical Insight 27-7 ➤ Checking Feeding Tube Placement

Tube placement must be verified by x-ray before the initial feeding is given. Because none of the bedside methods is foolproof, always use pH measurement in combination with one of the other methods.

To Aspirate Stomach Contents:

- Don procedure gloves. This is a clean, not sterile, technique.
- Just before feeding, draw up 10 to 30 mL of air in a 30- to 60-mL syringe, insert the syringe in the distal end of the feeding tube, and inject air.
  To flush out formula, medications, and other substances. This also helps keep a small-bore tube from collapsing when you aspirate.
- With the same syringe, aspirate the air and 20 to 30 mL of stomach or intestinal contents. Use slow, gentle suction—over 3 to 5 minutes if necessary.
  It can take a long time to obtain enough fluid, especially from a small-bore tube.
- If you could not aspirate any fluid, inject another 20 mL of air and use a smaller syringe to aspirate again.
  Using a small (<10 mL) syringe for very small tubes creates less negative pressure and makes it less likely the tube will collapse.
- If you still do not aspirate fluid, repeat the procedure with this variation: Insert air with the large syringe; insert the small syringe into the end of the tubing, and leave it for 15 minutes to allow fluid to accumulate before aspirating.
- If you are still unsuccessful, reposition the patient and try again after 20 minutes.
  Repositioning may move the tube into a place where fluid has pooled.

Inspecting the Aspirate

- Aspirate stomach contents, as described above. Gastric contents are normally greenish brown and liquid. If the patient is receiving enteral feedings, gastric contents should be curdled and white or a greenish color; intestinal contents will be a more yellow (bile) color with no curdling.

Intestinal contents are usually yellow-green because of the influence of bile. The colors of gastric and pulmonary secretions are altered by a variety of conditions, so observation of the visual characteristics of feeding tube aspirates is of little value in differentiating between respiratory and GI placement (Joanna Briggs Institute, 2010a, 2010c).

(Continued)

Clinical Insight 27-7 ➤ Checking Feeding Tube Placement—cont'd

Measuring the Volume and pH of the Aspirate

- Aspirate stomach contents, as described above. Then measure the residual volume of the aspirate.
  Unexpected changes in volume of the aspirate can indicate poor GI motility. Gastric volumes will generally be larger than intestinal or esophageal volumes.
- Measure the pH of the aspirated fluid using nitrazine paper. See the accompanying figure.

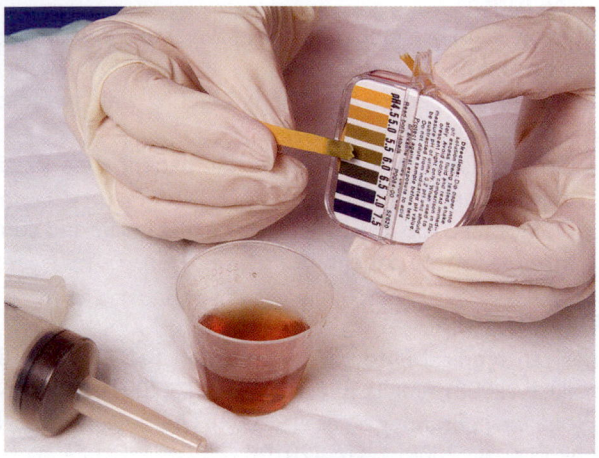

- The lower the pH, the more likely that the tube is in the stomach. The pH of gastric contents is typically 1 to 5.5. Measuring the pH is useful only if the fluid you aspirate is acidic, indicating gastric placement.
- Intestinal contents usually have a pH of 6 or greater.
- The pH of respiratory secretions is 7 or higher; however, respiratory secretions may occasionally have a pH as low as 6.
- Remember that many variables can make the gastric pH results unreliable (e.g., blood in the stomach, antacid medications).
- Measuring bilirubin, trypsin, and pepsin in the aspirate can also be used to diagnose placement of a feeding tube in the respiratory tract (Elpern, Killeen, Talla, et al., 2007; Peter & Gill, 2009).

Measuring and Observing the Length of the Tube that Extends From the Body

When the tube was inserted, it should have been marked with indelible marker where it exits the body (e.g., the naris), and the external length recorded. Compare the external length with previous measurements and with the mark made on the tube when it was inserted. If tube placement does not change, the external length should remain the same.

Injecting Air into the Feeding Tube

Although some professionals still inject air into the feeding tube, this method is the least accurate of the bedside methods.

- Draw 5 to 30 mL of air into a syringe; place the tip of the syringe in the end of the feeding tube.
- Place a stethoscope over the stomach.
- Listen with the stethoscope as you inject the air through the tube. If you hear a gurgling or whooshing sound in the left upper quadrant, the tube may be in the stomach. If the tube is in the lungs, you should hear no gurgling.

Ongoing Patient Assessments

The following require repeated assessments over time to be useful for confirming other methods of tube placement.

- ***Observe for respiratory distress.*** Note cyanosis or difficulty breathing, coughing, choking. These symptoms are a good indicator that the tube is in the respiratory tract; but keep in mind that the tube could instead be in the stomach and the symptoms caused by something else. Absence of symptoms does not necessarily indicate correct placement in the stomach. The tube might be in the airway and not be causing any respiratory symptoms.
- ***Assess whether the patient can speak.*** Keep in mind that some clients can speak even when the tube is in a lung.

Other Bedside Verification Methods

Capnometry and additional tests of gastric juices may also serve as measures to help verify that the tube is correctly placed. To find discussion of these methods,

Go to Chapter 27, **Checking Feeding Tube Placement,** in Volume 1.

Clinical Insight 27-8 ➤ Monitoring Patients Receiving Enteral Nutrition

Monitor the following:

- ***Position of the feeding tube.*** Periodically check the placement of the tube. As a rule, check on each shift or at each intermittent feeding. For double-lumen tubes, keep the air vent above the level of the patient's stomach so it will not act as a siphon and leak stomach contents.
- ***NG or NE tube insertion site.*** An NG or NE tube is secured by adhesive to the nose. Regularly check the skin, gently cleanse the area (with soap and water, as for normal washing; avoid harsh skin cleansers), and retape the tube as needed. Report tissue breakdown, epistaxis (nosebleed), or sinusitis, as they may signal a need for insertion of a percutaneous endoscopy gastrostomy (PEG) tube.
- ***Gastrostomy tube, PEG/PEJ insertion site.*** Inspect the insertion site for erythema or drainage, which are signs of infection. Clean it daily with soap and water.
- ***Fluid balance.*** Measure all intake and output.
- ***Weight.*** To assess the adequacy of the feeding, regularly weigh the patient. There is usually a medical prescription for frequency of weighing. Frequent weight checks allow adjustment of the feeding orders to achieve the desired goal.
- ***Tube feeding residual volume.*** To assess residual volume, aspirate the feeding tube to determine the amount of feeding remaining in the stomach. If the aspirate quantity is equal to or greater than the formula flow rate for 1 hour (or alternatively, a total of 150 mL), the patient may be receiving too much fluid or may have delayed gastric emptying. However, you should not automatically stop the feeding; if you obtain a single sample of an increased residual volume, recheck it in 1 hour. See Clinical Insight 28-7.
- ***Frequency of bowel movements.*** Bowel movements should occur regularly.
  - Constipation is usually due to inadequate water or fiber. Some commercial feedings contain fiber. You may add free water and perhaps fiber to other formulas.
  - Diarrhea may indicate intolerance of the formula, excessive feeding, or gastrointestinal disease.
- ***Bowel sounds.*** Check before each feeding, or every 4 to 8 hours for continuous feedings. Peristalsis must be present. Flatus is a better indication of complete bowel function than bowel sounds.
- ***Abdominal distention.*** Measure abdominal girth daily, at the umbilicus.
- ***Serum electrolyte levels.*** Monitor regularly (per protocol or prescription).
- ***Urine for sugar and acetone.*** This is sometimes done as a bedside screen for hyperglycemia. However, treatment is based on blood sugar levels.
- ***Skin turgor, hematocrit, and urine specific gravity.*** These are indicators of dehydration and overhydration, although skin turgor alone is not a reliable sign.
- ***Serum blood urea nitrogen (BUN) and sodium levels.*** This is especially important for high-protein formulas. Insufficient fluid intake combined with high protein intake may overload the kidneys so that nitrogenous wastes are not excreted adequately.

Clinical Insight 27-9 ➤ Preventing Infection in Patients Receiving Enteral Feedings

Contamination of the feeding can have serious consequences for a patient.

- Check dates on feeding solutions and supplies. Do not use any that are outdated.
- Use sterile equipment and supplies; once you have opened them, handle them as little as possible.
- Disposable feeding equipment is meant for one-time use. Do not wash and reuse.
- Use meticulous hand hygiene; wear nonsterile gloves.
- Replace feeding equipment after 24 hours.
- Store opened feeding solutions in the refrigerator in covered and labeled containers. Allow the solution to return to room temperature before giving it to the patient. Discard after 24 hours.
- Keep unopened solutions at room temperature.
- Follow agency policy regarding how long a solution may be left hanging. Usually:
  - Sterile feedings may be hung for up to 24 hours (or per unit policy).
  - Nonsterile feedings (i.e., reconstituted powder feedings) may hang for up to 4 hours (or per unit policy).
  - Label the feeding containers with the patient's name and the date and time hung; document the time in the patient record.
- Use sterile water for (1) patients who are immunocompromised, (2) patients receiving jejunal feeds, or (3) initially following a gastrostomy insertion.
- Never allow a feeding to hang below the height of the patient's stomach.
- Do not transfer sterile feedings into a second container.
- Replace the feeding tubes according to the manufacturer's recommendations (or agency policy if that is sooner).

References

Bankhead, R., Boullata, J., Brantley, S., et al. (2009).

Clinical Insight 27-10 ➤ Monitoring and Other Interventions for Patients Receiving Parenteral Nutrition

Monitoring

For patients receiving PN, you will need to monitor the following:

Catheter Insertion Site

- Assess catheter insertion site for swelling, redness, drainage, or tenderness (signs of infection (and/or phlebitis in PICC lines).
  The hypertonic PN creates a risk for phlebitis.
- Observe for swelling in the extremity on the same side of catheter insertion (sign of infiltration or phlebitis).
- Observe for catheter retraction from the vein; observe the length of the catheter from the insertion site to the hub at insertion and periodically.

Supplies and Equipment

- Monitor tubing connections to see that they are secure.
- Monitor to see that the dressing is secure and dry.
- Check the rate and amount infused at least hourly, to ensure the line is patent, the PN is flowing freely, and the pump is functioning properly.

Weight

- Regularly weigh the patient (according to medical order or agency policy, but commonly daily or 3 times per week).
  (1) Frequent weight checks allow for assessing the adequacy of the formula and making adjustments as needed to achieve the desired goal. (2) Because of the hypertonicity of the solutions, fluid overload can occur. Rapid weight increase is an indicator.

Glucose

Check blood glucose every 4 to 6 hours until stable, and then at least daily.

The high proportion of glucose in the formulas can cause hyperglycemia, the most common complication of PN. You may need to administer regular insulin according to a sliding scale (or the pharmacist may add it directly to the PN solution). The risk for hyperglycemia is less with 3:1 PN solutions.

Fluids

Monitor intake and output. Diuresis and dehydration can occur if hypertonic dextrose is infused too rapidly.

Lab Values

Patients receiving PN require regular lab studies (the following are examples and not a comprehensive list). The frequency of the studies depends on the patient's condition.

- Electrolytes, blood sugar, albumin, BUN, and creatinine (used for formula adjustment and to evaluate electrolyte balance and glucose metabolism).
- Albumin, transferrin, transthyretin (prealbumin), or retinol-binding protein (used to assess visceral protein status).
- 24-hour urine for urine urea nitrogen (weekly), to evaluate nitrogen balance.
- Complete blood count (CBC) and differential (to monitor changes in immune function).
- Liver function studies
- Serum zinc
- Plasma urea
- Plasma and urine osmolality
- Blood gases

Symptoms of Complications:

- *Electrolyte imbalances.* Symptoms depend on the electrolytes affected. Monitor lab values.
- *Sepsis.* Temperature greater than 100°F (37.8°C) orally, rapid pulse from baseline, chills, hypothermia, edema or erythema of skin, exudate from catheter insertion site, malaise, leukocytosis (increased white blood cell count), altered level of consciousness.
- *Air embolus.* Cyanosis, tachypnea, hypotension, heart murmur
- *Catheter dislodgement or thrombosis.* Swelling of arm or neck, pain, difficulty flushing catheter, difficulty infusing PN

Nutritional Status

- Calculate the daily calorie intake.
- Perform nutritional assessment at 2-week intervals.
- Possibly measure arm circumference and triceps skinfold thickness.
- Monitor serum albumin levels.
- Most agencies have specialized nutrition teams who will monitor these parameters.

Maintenance

- Change the dressing over the catheter every 24 hrs or according to agency policy; or when it becomes wet, soiled, or nonocclusive. Use sterile technique.
- Secure connections with luer-lock connectors; do not use tape.
- Change the filter every 24 hrs.
- Do not hang PN bottles for more than 12 hr (some guidelines and agency policies specify 24 hrs).
  Its high nutrient concentration makes PN solution ideal for bacterial growth.
- Use sterile aseptic technique when changing the dressing for a central line, as well as when changing the solution and tubing.
- Do not use the PN infusion line for administering any other medicines or solutions.
  To decrease the risk of contamination and infection.
- Infuse PN by pump with a reliable, audible alarm, to protect against "free flow."
- If an infusion falls behind schedule, do not increase the rate in an attempt to catch up. This can cause osmotic diuresis and dehydration.
- When PN is discontinued, it may be done gradually (perhaps over as many as 48 hours). To prevent a sudden drop in blood sugar.

SCREENING FOR NUTRITIONAL PROBLEMS

Clients who have risk factors for nutritional problems should be evaluated using one of the methods in this section: Subjective Global Assessment, Nutrition Screening Initiative (NSI), Nutrition Screening for Older Adults with Dementia, and Mini-Nutritional Assessment.

Focused Assessment

Subjective Global Assessment

Using the subjective global assessment (SGA) method, an experienced clinician examines the general medical history and physical examination to evaluate a client's nutritional status. There are six components pertinent to nutritional status:

1. *Weight history*—over previous 6 months
2. *Dietary history*—including a comparison of usual, recommended, and current intake, as well as changes in eating patterns over the past weeks or months
3. *Gastrointestinal symptoms history*—anorexia, nausea, vomiting, and diarrhea
4. *Energy level*—including activity level and functional abilities
5. *Existing disease*—evaluation of the metabolic demands of any disease states along with acute stressors that may alter those demands
6. *Physical examination data*—regarding loss of fat stores, muscle wasting, and the presence of edema and ascites

As a clinician, you would analyze these components to rate the client's nutritional status as normal, mild, moderate, or severe. The effectiveness of this method depends largely on the experience of the clinician (Bankhead, Boullata, Brantley, et al., 2009; Barone, Milosavljevic, & Gazibarich, 2003; Detsky, McLaughlin, Baker, et al., 1987). For a link to view this tool online and use with patients,

Go to Chapter 27, **Resources for Caregivers and Health Professionals, Subjective Global Assessment,** on Davis*Plus*.

Focused Assessment

Nutrition Screening Initiative (NSI), for Older Adults: Indications of Impaired Nutritional Status

Recognizing the importance of nutrition in our aging population, the American Academy of Family Physicians, the American Dietetic Association, and the National Council on Aging developed the Nutrition Screening Initiative (NSI) (1991). The NSI includes (1) a self-administered checklist to evaluate risk, (2) the Level I Screening Tool designed for health professionals, and (3) a Level II Screening Tool for use in healthcare facilities.

The NSI addresses nutritional concerns associated with chronic diseases that older adults frequently experience. The NSI requires collection and evaluation of data in four areas: clinical, dietary, body composition, and biochemical. In addition, it identifies indicators of impaired nutritional status (following).

MAJOR INDICATORS	MINOR INDICATORS	SYMPTOMS	PHYSICAL SIGNS	LAB VALUES
➤ Significant weight loss over time	➤ Concurrent syndromes	➤ Anorexia, nausea, or dysphagia	➤ Poor oral or dental status	➤ Reduced levels of serum albumin, transferrin, or prealbumin
➤ Significant high or low weight for height	➤ Alcoholism	➤ Early satiety	➤ Dehydration	➤ Folate deficiency
➤ Significant change in functional status	➤ Cognitive impairment	➤ Changed bowel habits	➤ Poorly healing wounds	➤ Iron deficiency
➤ Significant and inappropriate food intake	➤ Chronic renal insufficiency	➤ Fatigue or apathy	➤ Loss of subcutaneous fat or muscle mass	➤ Zinc deficiency
➤ Significant reduction in mid-arm circumference	➤ Multiple concurrent medications	➤ Memory loss	➤ Fluid retention	■ Reduced levels of ascorbic acid
➤ Significant decrease in skinfold	➤ Malabsorption syndromes			
➤ Osteoporosis or osteomalacia				
➤ Folate or vitamin B deficiency				

(Continued)

Focused Assessment

Nutrition Screening Initiative (NSI), for Older Adults: Indications of Impaired Nutritional Status—cont'd

To learn more about the NSI and for tools to use for nutritional screening of older adults,

Go to Chapter 27, **Tables, Boxes, Figures: ESG Figure 27-4, Nutrition Screening Initiative (for older adults): Determine Your Nutritional Health,** on Davis*Plus*.

Nutrition Screening for Older Adults with Dementia

For a tool to use in assessing nutritional status for patients with dementia,

Go to **Try This, Issue D11.1: Eating and Feeding Issues in Older Adults with Dementia: Part I: Assessment,** at http://www.hartfordign.org/Resources/Try_This_Series/

Focused Assessment

Mini Nutritional Assessment

The Mini Nutritional Assessment (MNA) is a quick and easy method of identifying individuals with nutritional risk or with malnutrition. (See the accompanying figure.) This tool was developed primarily for use with older clients. It consists of two parts. The first part screens for nutritional risk. The second part is completed only if the individual is identified to be at risk. The final score, which tallies the scores of both parts, is the Malnutrition Indicator Score. Indications of malnutrition require multidisciplinary follow-up.

References

Guigoz, Y. (2006); Rubenstein, L., Harker, J., Salva, A., et al. (2001); Vellas, B., Villars, H., Abellan, G., et al. (2006.)

To see and use the MNA,

Go to Chapter 27, **Tables, Boxes, Figures: ESG Figure 27-6, Mini Nutritional Assessment (MNA),** on Davis*Plus*.

Literature related to the MNA is regularly updated. For more information,

Go to the Nestlé Nutrition Institute Web site, which is regularly updated, at www.mna-elderly.com

FOCUSED NUTRITIONAL ASSESSMENT

If you identify nutritional problems or risks using the screening tools, you should perform a more in-depth nutritional assessment, such as the following.

Focused Assessment

Focused Nutritional Assessment

Nutritional History

Item	*Components*
Demographic data	Name, date, age, sex, date of birth, address, occupation, workplace
Chief complaint	Client's subjective statement of health problem, including onset and duration
Present illness and current health	Detailed data about chief complaint as it relates to nutrition status
	Recent diet changes and reasons
	Recent weight loss or gain and over what period of time
	Usual body weight: 20% above or below desirable weight?
	Change in appetite
	Unusual stress/trauma (surgery, job, family)
	Medications, prescriptions
	Alcohol, nicotine, caffeine consumption
Health history	Previous illnesses, trauma, major dental problems, or issues that could interfere with ability to shop, prepare food, chew, or swallow
	Allergies (i.e., environmental, foods, drugs)

Focused Assessment

Focused Nutritional Assessment—cont'd

	Eating disorders
	Chronic disease or surgery that affects gastrointestinal tract
	Substance abuse
	Nutritional programs
	Depression
Family health history	Genetic/familial disorders that could affect nutritional status: cardiovascular or gastrointestinal disorders, Crohn's disease, diabetes, cancer, sickle cell anemia, allergies, celiac disease, other food intolerances, obesity
Dietary history	Current food intake pattern using one of the following methods: 24-hour–7-day recall, as appropriate; food frequency questionnaire; food record; and comparison to dietary guidelines and Dietary Reference Intakes (DRIs)
	Special dietary considerations, restrictions
	Fad diets
	Vitamin and mineral supplements
	Commercial dietary supplements
	Nonconventional dietary supplements
	Food preferences, dislikes
	Dietary influences from ethnic, cultural, or religious practices
	Counseling needs (based on food knowledge)
Medication history	Recent use of steroids, immunosuppressants, chemotherapy, anticonvulsants, or oral contraceptives
Socioeconomic factors	Adequate food storage, refrigeration, food preparation, payments:
	Supplemental Security Income (SSI), food stamps, Women, Infants, and Children (WIC) program
	Who shops for, prepares, and cooks food?
	Location/availability of retail food/grocery store or availability of transportation
Personal factors	Stress/coping mechanisms, self-concept, social supports
	Daily activity level and exercise regimen

Nutrition-Focused Physical Examination

Correlate the following physical examination findings with the dietary history, screening methods, anthropometric measurements, and laboratory results.

I. The General Survey

Assess vital signs, height, weight, and overall impressions.

- ***Overall appearance.*** Does the client look ill? Does he appear adequately nourished? You will want to investigate any hunches as you move through the physical exam.
- ***Temperature.*** An increase in temperature raises the client's metabolic rate and need for fluid, is a sign of infection, and may decrease the client's appetite.
- ***Blood pressure (BP) and heart rate*** are affected by fluid status. An elevated BP may be related to fluid volume excess; a low BP may be a sign of dehydration. Heart rate usually increases when fluid volume is low.
- ***Height and weight.*** Calculate the body mass index (BMI) on the basis of these measures:

BMI = weight in kilograms ÷ (height in meters)^2

Classification of Body Mass Index Values

Classification	*BMI (kg/m^2)*	*Risk of Comorbidities*
Underweight*	<18.5	Low
Normal weight	18.5–24.9	Average
Pre-obese	25.0–29.9	Mildly increased
Class I obesity	30.0–34.9	Moderate
Class II obesity	35.0–39.9	Severe
Class III obesity	≥40.0	Very severe

**Note:* In adults in long-term care settings or with serious illness, nutritional support should be implemented for those with a BMI less than 21. In this population a BMI of less than 21 is associated with increased mortality (American Medical Directors Association, 2010).

(Continued)

Focused Assessment

Focused Nutritional Assessment—cont'd

II. Integumentary System

- ***Skin turgor*** is an indicator of fluid status. Poor skin turgor may result from dehydration. Swelling may result from overhydration.
- ***Skin integrity*** reflects overall nutritional status. Poor wound healing may suggest inadequate intake of protein, vitamin C, or zinc. Patients with uncontrolled diabetes or severely restricted diets often experience slow-healing wounds, especially in the feet and legs.
- ***Areas of warmth or erythema.*** These are signs of inflammation or infection.
- ***Other nutrition-related skin changes*** include red, swollen skin lesions (due to niacin deficiency); excessive bleeding seen as petechiae or ecchymosis (due to vitamin K or C deficiency); and xerosis (dry skin).
- ***Abnormal nail findings*** include spoon-shaped, brittle nails (due to iron deficiency); dull nails with transverse ridge (due to protein deficiency); pale, poor blanching, or mottled nails (due to vitamin A or C deficiency); bruising or bleeding beneath nails (due to protein or caloric deficiency); and splinter hemorrhages (due to vitamin C deficiency).
- ***Hair*** will grow slowly, thin, or break easily if protein is deficient.

III. The Head and Neck

The condition of the mouth, teeth, and gums has a major effect on a client's choice of food, ability to chew, and ability to swallow.

- ***Facial paralysis or drooping*** of one side of the face may be a result of stroke, injury, or nerve irritation, which also affects the ability to chew and swallow (dysphagia).
- ***Enlarged thyroid gland.*** Look for swelling of the thyroid, which may be related to hypothyroid or hyperthyroid states. Both disorders affect metabolic rate and energy requirements.
- ***Eyes.*** Nutritional deficits may cause the eyes to be red and dry and the conjunctiva pale.
- ***Lips and tongue.*** The lips may be chapped, red, or swollen. The tongue may be bright red, purple, or swollen or may have longitudinal furrows.
- ***Teeth and gums.*** Look for cavities, mottled or missing teeth, and spongy, bleeding, or receding gums.
- ***Lymph nodes.*** Palpate for enlarged or tender lymph nodes under the chin and along the neck. Nodes that are swollen can signal infection, such as a sore throat.

IV. Cardiovascular System

You will have gained initial information about the cardiovascular system by taking the vital signs. As you follow up and listen to the heart and check pulses, you should explore any abnormal vital signs.

- ***Bounding pulses*** are associated with fluid overload, fever, and hypertension.
- ***Weak, thready pulse*** may indicate dehydration, shock, or hypotension.
- ***Edema in the extremities*** may be a sign of fluid overload, inadequate protein stores, or electrolyte imbalance.

V. Abdominal Exam

- ***A scaphoid or concave abdomen*** indicates loss of subcutaneous fat, possibly caused by malnutrition.
- ***A round or protuberant abdomen*** points to obesity due to excess caloric and/or high fat intake.
- ***A generalized enlarged abdomen*** may signify **ascites** (fluid in the abdominal cavity) due to liver malfunction. Ascites results from three mechanisms: abnormal movement of protein and water into the abdomen; sodium and fluid retention; and decreased albumin production in the liver.
- ***Hyperactive bowel sounds*** are heard with gastrointestinal infection, laxative use, and malabsorption disorders.
- ***Hypoactive bowel sounds*** suggest sluggish motility in the GI tract.

VI. Musculoskeletal System

- ***Thin extremities with excess skinfolds*** may indicate muscle atrophy and fat loss related to malnutrition, especially protein and calories. This may also occur as a result of prolonged bed rest and inadequate food intake. Skinfold measurement is also useful in assessing muscle and fat stores.
- Look for any obvious ***swelling, deformities, or limitation in range of motion*** of the joints.
- ***Kyphosis*** of the spine may indicate osteoporosis and possible insufficient calcium intake.
- ***Joint pain*** on palpation or with movement is a sign of arthritis or gout. Arthritis may affect ability to shop for groceries, prepare food to eat, and use utensils for eating and drinking. Gout is often induced by diets high in **purines** (food substances that break down into uric acid), obesity, and excess alcohol intake.

Focused Assessment

Focused Nutritional Assessment—cont'd

VII. Neurological System

The neurological examination will give you insight into the client's ability to perform independent tasks.

- Look for ***altered level of consciousness or signs of behavioral disturbances and dementia*** through general conversation and appropriateness of answers to specific questions.
- Assess ***coordination and reflexes***.
- Assess for ***cognitive deficits or severe psychiatric disorders***. A client with cognitive deficits or severe psychiatric disorders may have difficulty preparing food or judging appropriate nutrient choices.
- Assess for ***motor or sensory deficits***. Clients with motor or sensory deficits may be unable to purchase, prepare, or eat a variety of foods.
- ***Confusion, weakness, diminished reflexes, paresthesia, and sensory loss*** may be cues to vitamin B deficiencies.
- ***Tetany or severe and generalized muscle spasm*** may indicate calcium or magnesium deficits.

VIII. What Are the Signs of Severe Malnutrition?

Malnutrition is a condition of impaired development or function caused by a long-term deficiency, excess, or imbalance in energy and/or nutrient intake.

- Symptoms of undernutrition due to insufficient food include reduced physical activity, weight loss, and reduced height.
- Children, older adults, and people with chronic illnesses such as cancer, HIV infection, and chronic obstructive pulmonary disease (COPD) are most likely to experience malnutrition. Malnutrition can occur with obesity.
- To assess for malnutrition in children, compare weight, height, and head circumference to the standards (norms) for the child's age.
- Other indicators in children include the presence of iron-deficiency anemia.
- In adolescents, look for a delay of stages of sexual maturation.

DIAGNOSTIC TESTING

Diagnostic Testing

Tests Reflecting Nutritional Status: Norms

Note: Norms are for adults (ages 19 to 65) unless otherwise noted.

Blood glucose	70 mg/dL to 100 mg/dL. Capillary blood sugar is frequently assessed at the bedside with a simple fingerstick. Serum blood glucose levels are assessed by drawing a venous blood sample. The level is measured in the laboratory.
	The American Diabetes Association (2011) recommends for diabetic patients a preprandial plasma glucose level of 70 to 130 mg/dL.
Serum albumin	3.4–4.8 g/dL
Prealbumin	12–42 mg/dL (age 6 years–adult)
Globulin	2.3–3.4 g/dL
Blood urea nitrogen (BUN)	5–18 mg/dL (children)
	8–21 mg/dL (age 14–adult); 10–31 mg/dL (adult older than 90)
Creatinine	0.5–1 mg/dL (female)
	0.6–1.2 mg/dL (male)
Hemoglobin	13.2–17.3 g/dL (male)
	11.7–15.5 g/dL (female)
	12.6–17.4 g/dL (male, older adult)
	11.7–16.1 g/dL (female, older adult)

CLINICALREASONING

Applying the Full-Spectrum Nursing Model

PATIENT SITUATION

Mrs. O is a 75-year-old retired schoolteacher who suffered a stroke 8 months ago. Since leaving the hospital, she has been living in a nursing home. Mrs. O has residual weakness on the right side—her dominant side—and has not mastered the use of tableware with her left hand. On admission to the nursing home 7 months ago, she weighed 150 pounds. Today she weighs only 125 pounds. Mrs. O refuses to go to the dining room for meals. The NAPs report that she eats a few bites of most foods, but never eats more than half of anything.

THINKING

1. *Theoretical Knowledge:*
   a. Based on Mrs. O's gender, age, and activity level, make a rough estimate of the number of kcal/day she needs.
   b. What are two other, more precise, ways you could determine Mrs. O's ideal body weight?
2. *Critical Thinking (Considering Alternatives):* What are some possible explanations for why Mrs. O is not eating all her food?

DOING

3. *Practical Knowledge:*
   a. Suppose you have decided to use the general ideal weight guide to determine Mrs. O's ideal weight. What, specifically, would you need to do? You do not need to actually calculate; just list the action steps.
   b. Suppose you have decided to determine Mrs. O's body mass index (BMI). What equipment would you need?
   c. What is the formula for calculating BMI from the height and weight?
4. *Nursing Process (Diagnosis):* Write a nursing diagnosis for Mrs. O. Use just the data provided in the situation. Assume her BMI is 20.

CARING

5. *Self-Knowledge:* What would you be feeling if you were in Mrs. O's situation?
6. *Ethical Knowledge:* What are one or two things you would do to help Mrs. O feel cared for and cared about?

Critical Thinking and Clinical Reasoning

1. Recall the employees (Isaac Schwartz and Sujing Lee) interviewed in the Meet Your Patient scenario in Volume 1. In addition, you now have two more patients, Wakenda Pierre and Luceno Jarin. Their information is provided below.
   - Isaac Schwartz, a 65-year-old accountant, works long hours. He describes a sedentary lifestyle, no tobacco use, infrequent alcohol use, no medical problems, and a nutritional history of skipping meals and daily consumption of restaurant food. You measure his height as 69 in. and weight as 245 lb.
   - Sujing Lee, a 29-year-old project manager, regularly works 65 hours per week. Sujing is 30 weeks pregnant. She does not smoke or drink and has never been hospitalized or had surgery. She has gained a total of 25 lb since becoming pregnant. Her diet consists mainly of traditional Chinese food. She eats three meals a day and always brings lunch from home. Lately she has felt "tired all the time." At the screening, she weighs 126 lb and measures 63 in. tall.
   - Wakenda Pierre is a 38-year-old administrative assistant. She exercises at the gym 4 to 5 days per week, smokes an occasional cigarette, has two to three drinks every night before dinner, struggles with keeping her blood pressure under control, and eats fast food for breakfast and lunch every day. She is 72 in. tall and weighs 165 lb.
   - Luceno Jarin is a 65-year-old business executive. He tells you he was diagnosed with type 2 diabetes mellitus 5 years ago. He is struggling to follow his prescribed diet. He drinks alcohol sporadically and walks briskly 30 minutes every day of the week. He is 67 in. tall and weighs 205 lb.

   a. Determine each client's BMI. Based on these results, what conclusions can you make about their weight status?

b. What are the likely causes of each person's weight status?
c. What additional work-up would be recommended for each individual?
d. What indications would lead you to believe that each client has adopted a healthier lifestyle?

2. The following are three clients admitted to the medical-surgical unit of your local hospital. On their admission, the primary nurse collected the following information.

	CLIENT 1	CLIENT 2	CLIENT 3
Weight	175 lb	100 lb	250 lb
Height	70 in.	59 in.	65 in.
Gender/Age	Male/40 years old	Female/18 years old	Male/65 years old
Usual Daily Caloric Intake	2,500 kcal	1,000 kcal	2,500 kcal
Usual Activity Level	Moderate	High	Light
Serum Albumin	Normal	Low	Normal
Serum Glucose	Normal	Low	High

a. Identify which client(s) is/are at risk for nutritional imbalance.
b. Which client is at risk for developing malnutrition?
c. What additional information would support this conclusion?
d. What nursing interventions would you initiate at this time?

3. After 3 days, you examine how well each of these clients is doing using the same parameters as admission day.

	CLIENT 1	CLIENT 2	CLIENT 3
Weight	170 lb	103 lb	250 lb
Current Daily Caloric Intake	2,500 kcal	1,500 kcal	1,500 kcal
Intake (mL)	2,000	2,000	1,000
Output (mL)	1,800	1,900	500
Current Activity Level	Up as tolerated	Up as tolerated	Bedrest
Serum Albumin	Normal	Low	Normal
Serum Glucose	Normal	Low	High

a. In comparison with the admission data, there are some changes. Which client's health status is a priority now, and why?
b. What is/are the most likely cause(s) of this concern?
c. Which nursing interventions should be initiated for this client while hospitalized? Focus on nutritional needs.
d. Identify appropriate education that should begin during hospitalization for this client.

4. For each of the following concepts, use critical thinking to describe how or why it is important to nursing, patient care, or nutrition. Note that these are *not* to be merely definitions.

Energy balance
Body mass index
Weight management
Body weight standards
Parenteral nutrition
Nutritional screening
Basal metabolic rate
Nutrients
Nutritional history
Enteral feedings
Special diets

What Are the Main Points in This Chapter?

- Reliable guidelines for designing a nutritious diet include the Dietary Reference Intakes (DRIs), the USDA Dietary Guidelines, and the nutrition facts panel found on packaged foods in the United States.
- ChooseMyPlate is a food guide that illustrates healthful dietary choices. It stresses six concepts for healthy eating: activity, moderation, personalization, proportionality, variety, and gradual improvement.
- Energy nutrients are carbohydrates, proteins, and fats (lipids). Other important nutrients are water and the micronutrients: fat-soluble vitamins, water-soluble vitamins, and minerals.
- Carbohydrates include simple sugars called monosaccharides and disaccharides and complex carbohydrates called polysaccharides.
- Glucose, a monosaccharide, is the primary source of energy for the brain, as well as for the body during moderate-to-intense physical activity.
- Proteins are made up of amino acids and are required for cell and tissue growth, maintenance, and repair. They also act as buffers in acid–base balance. Proteins are an energy source.
- Lipids, including fats and oils, are classified as glycerides, sterols, and phospholipids. They are essential components of cells, fuel the body at rest and during light activity, aid in absorption of fat-soluble vitamins, and promote a sense of satiety when eaten. Low-density lipoproteins (LDLs) are the "bad" cholesterol. High-density lipoproteins (HDLs) are the "good" cholesterol.
- Saturated fats and *trans*-fats are less healthful lipid choices than mono- and polyunsaturated fats. Saturated fats and *trans*-fats raise LDL cholesterol levels in the blood.
- The essential fatty acids omega-6 and omega-3 help protect against heart disease when they replace *trans*-fats in the diet. They are found mainly in vegetable oils, nuts, seeds, and fatty fish.
- Nutrients must be consumed at least at a minimal level in order to meet the body's physiological needs. This level is called Dietary Reference Intake (DRI).
- The fat-soluble vitamins are A, D, E, and K. Water-soluble vitamins are C and the B-complex vitamins.
- Minerals (e.g., calcium, iron, magnesium) are important for transmitting nerve impulses, regulating fluid balance, strengthening bones, and producing energy.
- The basal metabolic rate (BMR) is a measure of the energy required by resting tissue to maintain basic function.
- Factors influencing a client's nutritional status include developmental stage, pregnancy and lactation, education, lifestyle choices, vegetarianism, dieting for weight loss, culture, religion, disease processes, functional limitations, economic factors, and modified or special diets.
- Many people must follow a modified diet to assist in managing their illness. In addition, all inpatients must have a diet prescribed by their primary care provider.
- When examining an individual's nutritional balance, it is important to screen for nutritional problems. When risk factors are present, thoroughly assess nutritional history, physical findings, anthropometric measurements, imaging techniques, and biochemical values.
- A food record is the most accurate method of obtaining data about a client's actual food intake.
- The body mass index (BMI), skinfold measurements, and body part circumferences are estimates of body composition.
- Laboratory or biochemical indicators of nutritional status include blood glucose and serum protein levels or indices such as albumin, urea, and hemoglobin.
- Vitamin and mineral supplementation may be appropriate for some people, but they do not replace the need for a balanced diet.
- Government programs provide some assistance for clients who cannot afford to buy food.
- Nutritional requirements of older adults are similar to those for all adults, with a slight reduction in the need for calories, and the more likely need for nutrient supplementation. nutritional problems are also similar, but the incidence is higher among older adults.
- Nurses can help support nutrition for patients who have Self-Care Deficits or Impaired Swallowing by assisting patients with meals and providing swallowing therapy.
- Nutritional imbalance can range from either inadequate or excessive amounts of a single nutrient relative to overall caloric intake.
- Obesity is a major problem in the United States, both in children and adults.
- Interventions for underweight/undernutrition include measures to improve the patient's appetite, assisting with meals, and providing enteral and parenteral nutrition.
- Nasogastric tubes are inserted to lavage the stomach; collect a specimen of the stomach contents, or prevent nausea, vomiting, and gastric distention. They are also placed to facilitate enteral feeding.
- The most accurate way to check enteral tube placement is by radiographic (x-ray) verification. To check enteral tube placement at the bedside, you could also use a combination of techniques: aspirate stomach contents to observe color and measure the pH (normally 1 to 5.5 for stomach contents); the "whoosh test"; serial observations for respiratory distress, residual volume, length of tube extending outside the body; and capnometry. Do not rely on a single technique.
- Potential complications associated with enteral feedings include aspiration, infection, diarrhea, and electrolyte imbalance.
- Meticulous sterile technique when administering parenteral nutrition is critical because the solution is delivered into a large central vein; if infection occurs, sepsis is almost immediate.

Knowledge Map

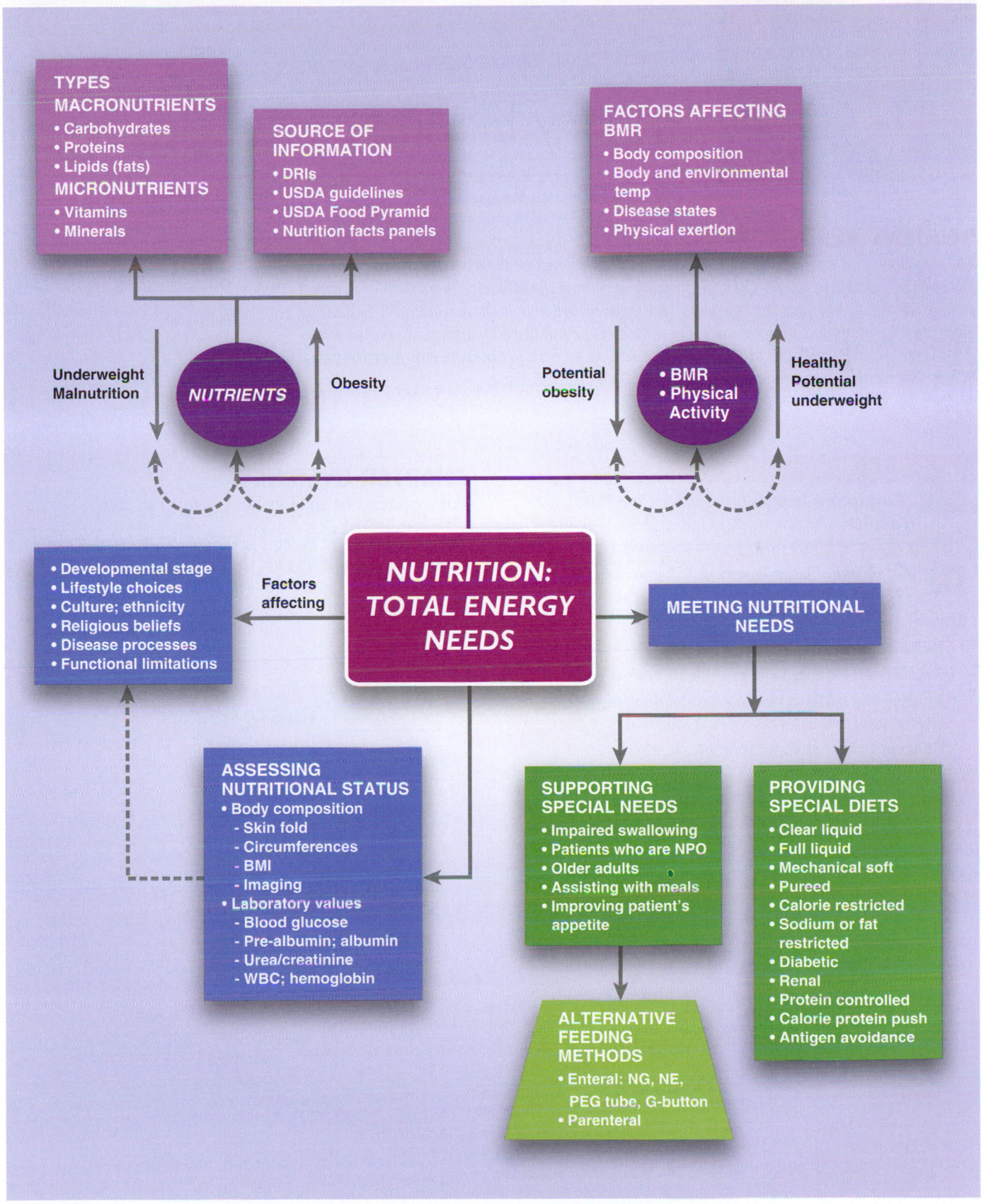

CHAPTER 28

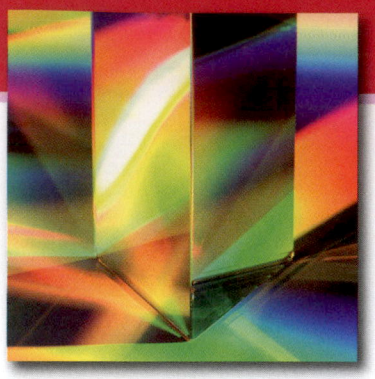

Urinary Elimination

STUDENT RESOURCES

*The questions and exercises in Volume 2 allow you to practice the kind of thinking you will use as a full-spectrum nurse. Critical-thinking questions usually have more than one correct answer, so we do not provide "answers" for these features. It is more important to develop your nursing judgment than to just cover content. You will learn by discussing the questions with your peers. If you are still unsure, consult your instructor. You will find Response Sheets (for writing your responses to the questions) on Davis*Plus.

To explore learning resources for this chapter,

Go to Davis*Plus* at DavisPl.us/Wilkinson3.

Chapter Resources for Chapter 28:

- **Response sheets for all learning activities**
- **Resources for Caregivers and Health Professionals**
- **Reading More About Urinary Elimination (suggested readings)**
- **Concept Map of chapter content**

Interactive Case Studies

NCLEX-Style and Chapter Review Questions

CHAPTER OVERVIEW

For a podcast of an overview of this chapter,

Go to Student Resources, Chapter 28, **Podcast—Chapter Overview**, on Davis*Plus*.

Caring for the Nguyens

At a recent visit to the Family Health Center, Nam and Yen Nguyen confide that Nam's mother, Mai Nguyen, has had several "accidents." She has denied the problem but Yen tells you that she helped her mother-in-law with laundry recently and many of the clothes smell of urine. They ask you how to approach Mai about this problem.

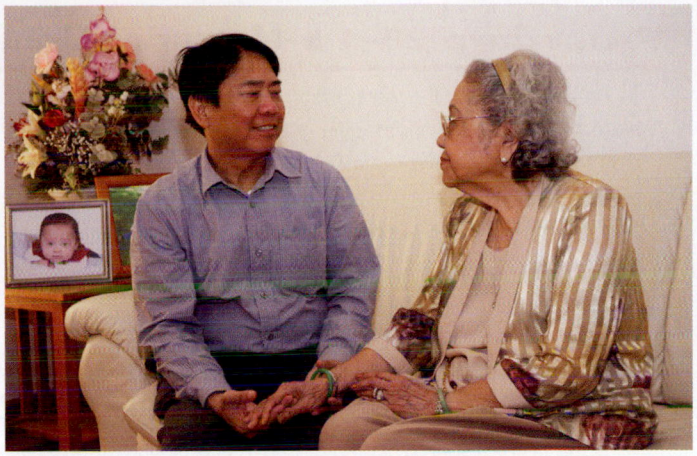

A. How would you respond?

B. What suggestions, if any, could you make to the Nguyens about treatment for Mai?

C. Yen says that she has been told that surgery is the best form of treatment. She asks you whether this is true. How would you answer her question?

Practical Knowledge knowing how

This section provides procedures and clinical insights you will need to support your patients' urinary function. You will also find assessment guidelines, information about diagnostic tests of urinary function, and standardized nursing language tables.

PROCEDURES

Procedure 28-1 ■ Measuring Urine

➤ For steps to follow in *all* procedures, refer to the Universal Steps for All Procedures found on the page facing the inside back cover. .

Equipment

- Bedpan or urinal
- Clean procedure gloves
- Graduated container
- Toilet paper, as indicated
- Washcloth or towel
- Hand sanitizer for patient's hands

Measuring Post-Void Residual Urine Volume With a Portable Bladder Scanner

- Portable bladder scanning device
- Ultrasound gel
- Clean gloves
- Tissues
- Antiseptic swabs or wipes

Delegation

Measuring urine, including post-void residual volume (PVR) using a portable bladder scanner, may be delegated to specially trained nursing assistive personnel (NAP) in some facilities. However, you must be sure that the NAP knows how to perform the procedure correctly, including proper cleansing of the bedpan/urinal and the graduated container according to the facility's policies. Also complete the following assessments and instruct the NAP when to stop the procedure and seek assistance from the nurse, and to report the results immediately. In some instances, you may choose to perform the bladder scan to ensure accuracy and expedite any necessary treatment.

Pre-Procedure Assessments

- Cognitive status

(continued on next page)

Procedure 28-1 ■ Measuring Urine (continued)

To determine whether the patient can be instructed to complete this procedure on her own and/or whether she can follow directions.

- Mobility status
  To determine whether the patient can be permitted to get out of the bed to use the toilet.
- Urinary status
  To determine the patient's ability to control bladder function.
- Post-void residual urine volume, ikkf needed.
  To determine the timing and amount of the last voiding.
  Note: A bladder scan should be done as soon as possible after voiding and within no more than 10 to 15 minutes.
- Palpate the bladder to assess for distention.

Procedure 28-1A ■ Measuring Urine Output From a Bedpan or Urinal

➤ When performing the procedure, always identify your patient according to agency policy, using two identifiers, and be attentive to standard precautions, hand hygiene, patient safety and privacy, body mechanics, and documentation.

Procedure Steps

1. **Perform hand hygiene** and don clean procedure gloves.
   Prevents transmission of bacteria.
2. **Place a bedpan or urinal** in the appropriate position.
   See Procedure 29-2 for placing a patient on the bedpan.
3. **Remove the bedpan or urinal**, being careful not to spill the urine. Reposition the patient and transport the urine to the bathroom.
4. **Pour the urine into a graduated** cylinder or calibrated measuring container while still wearing procedure gloves.
   a. Be sure that the measuring device is labeled with the correct patient information (in many institutions, labels are preprinted or barcoded).
   b. Do not use a measuring device for more than one patient.
5. **Place the measuring device** on a flat surface (e.g., shelf, table that is not used for food or personal care products), if available, and read the amount at eye level.
   When looking at fluid level from an angle, the meniscus may appear falsely low or high. Urine collection containers are considered "dirty" and should not be near to "clean" personal items.
6. **Observe the urine for color,** clarity, and odor.
7. **Discard the urine in the toilet.** If a specimen is required, transfer 30 to 60 mL of urine to the designated container.
8. **Clean the measuring container** and store in the patient's bathroom.
9. **Remove gloves.** Perform hand hygiene.
10. **Record the time and volume** on the intake and output (I&O) record.

Procedure 28-1B ■ Measuring Urine From an Indwelling Catheter

➤ When performing the procedure, always identify your patient according to agency policy, using two identifiers, and be attentive to standard precautions, hand hygiene, patient safety and privacy, body mechanics, and documentation.

Procedure Steps

1. **Wearing clean gloves**, place the drainage spout for the collection bag inside a calibrated measuring container. Avoid touching the spout to the inside of the container.
   Prevents transmission of bacteria.
2. **Unclamp the drainage spout**, and direct the flow of urine into the measuring device, still keeping the spout away from the sides of the container.
   Prevents contaminating the drainage spout. ➤

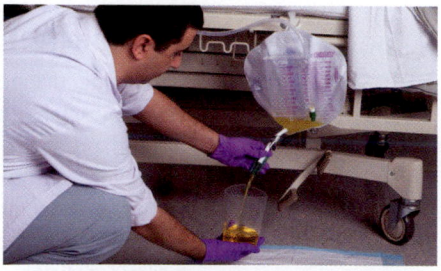

3. **Reclamp the spout** when the collection bag is empty.
4. **Wipe the drainage spout** with an alcohol pad or disinfecting wipe, and replace the spout into the slot on the collection bag.
   A clean spout reduces transmission of bacteria when the nurse touches it.
5. **Measure urine output** from the indwelling catheter at the end of each shift, or if the urine bag is getting full. ▼

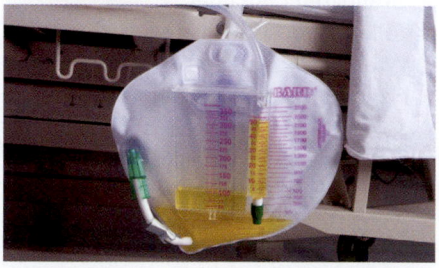

6. **Discard the urine in the toilet.**
7. **Remove gloves and wash your hands.**

Procedure 28-1C ■ Measuring Post-Void Residual Urine Volume With a Portable Bladder Scanner

➤ When performing the procedure, always identify your patient according to agency policy, using two identifiers, and be attentive to standard precautions, hand hygiene, patient safety and privacy, body mechanics, and documentation.

Procedure Steps

1. **Perform hand hygiene** and apply clean gloves.
   Prevents transmission of bacteria.

2. **Assist the patient to a supine** position. Uncover only the patient's lower abdomen and suprapubic area.

3. **Clean the scanner head** with antiseptic wipes.
   Prevents transmission of microorganisms between patients.

4. **Turn the device on.**

5. **Select the patient's gender.** If a woman has had a hysterectomy, follow manufacturer's directions for gender selection. In some cases, you will select the MALE icon for a woman who has undergone hysterectomy.
   The device is calibrated to adjust for uterus and bladder anatomy.

6. **Palpate the symphysis pubis** and then apply an ample quantity of warmed, ultrasound gel midline on the abdomen, approximately 2.5 to 4 cm (1 to 1.5 in.) above the symphysis pubis.
   The gel ensures proper transmission of the ultrasound. Warm gel is more comfortable for the patient.

7. **Position the scanner head** in the gel and aim it towards the bladder, pointing slightly downward toward the patient's coccyx.
   Proper placement allows for an accurate reading. ▼

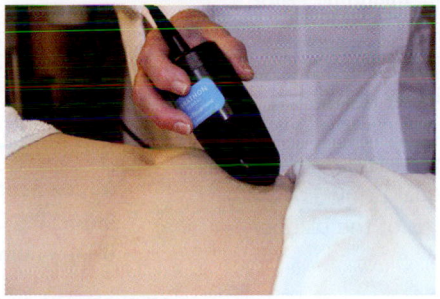

8. **Press and release the SCAN** button. Hold the scanner head steady until the scan is finished.
   An audible tone indicates the scan is complete.

9. **Read the bladder volume** measurement. Repeat the scan several times to ensure accuracy. *Note: Some scanners will also display an image of the bladder. The bladder image should be centered on the crossbars. If it is not, reposition the scanner head and repeat the scan.*
   Taking several readings ensures maximum accuracy. ▼

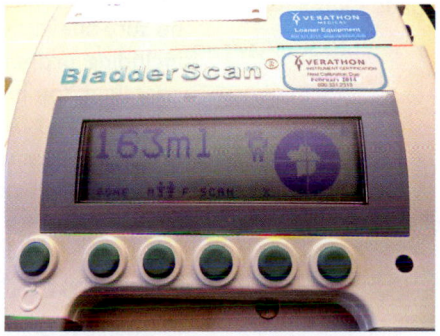

10. **Press DONE when finished.** Print the results by pressing PRINT.
    A printout provides for accurate documentation and may, in some facilities, be added to the patient record.

11. **Wipe the gel from** the patient's skin with tissue, cover the patient, and return the patient to a comfortable position.

12. **Clean the scanner head** with antiseptic. Remove gloves and perform hand hygiene.

? What if . . .

- **The provider orders hourly monitoring of the patient's urine output?**
  You will need to obtain a special collection bag with a small measuring chamber; document urine output on the I&O record every hour. Be sure that the cylinder does not overflow in the hour. Check the collection bag more frequently if the input is increased or if the patient has diuretic.

Evaluation

- Note any unusual characteristics of the urine (e.g., color, odor, presence of sediment or mucus).
- Note any difficulties with urination (e.g., pain, dribbling, difficulty beginning urination).
- Continue to assess that drainage from the indwelling catheter is not obstructed and that the drainage bag is below the level of the bladder.
- Assess for bladder distention.
  Bladder distention indicates poor bladder emptying. Utilize the bladder scanner to quantify the volume of urine in the bladder. A normal post-void residual volume is less than 50 to 100 mL.

Patient Teaching

Instruct the patient and/or primary caregiver to document fluid intake and urine output on the I&O record.

Home Care

Teach the client and/or the primary caregiver how to collect and measure urine, and how to document fluid intake and urine output on the I&O record.

(continued on next page)

Procedure 28-1 ■ Measuring Urine (continued)

Documentation

- Document urine volume and record the time and date the specimen was collected, per agency policy (e.g., in the nurse's notes or a patient graphic flow sheet, depending on the agency).
- Document the characteristics of the urine, including color, odor, particulate matter, blood, and clarity.
- Document any difficulty with voiding, including pain or burning with urination, frequency, or difficulty starting the urine flow.
- For PVR, document the time and amount of the last void prior to the scan and the amount of residual urine. Follow agency policy related to attaching a printout of the bladder scan to the patient record.

Sample documentation

12/15/16 1500 Voided 75 mL of clear, yellow urine with no odor, blood, or mucus. Pt states that he still feels full. Bladder palpated just above level of symphysis pubis. Bladder scan performed—350 mL of residual urine in bladder. Dr. Roy contacted and straight catheterization prescribed.
S. Tran, RN

Practice Resources

Rigby, D., & Housami, F. A. (2009); Siegel, J. D., Rhinehart, E., Jackson, M., et al. (2007).

Thinking About the Procedures

To practice applying clinical reasoning to these procedures,

Go to *Davis's Nursing Skills Videos*, **Measuring Urine Output from a Bedpan or Urinal, Measuring Urine from an Indwelling Catheter**, and **Measuring Post-Void Residual Urine Volume With a Portable Bladder Scanner.**

For questions and suggested responses,

Go to Chapter 28, Thinking About the Procedure Questions and Suggested Responses, on DavisPlus.

Procedure 28-2 ■ Obtaining a Urine Specimen for Testing

➤ For steps to follow in *all* procedures, refer to the Universal Steps for All Procedures found on the page facing the inside back cover.

Equipment

Collecting a Clean-Catch Urine Specimen

- Prepackaged collection kit
- If no kit is available:
  - Sterile specimen container
  - Antiseptic solution
  - Sterile cotton balls or 2 in. × 2 in. gauze pads
- Washcloth and towel, or perineal wipes
- Perineal wash solution
- Two pairs of clean procedure gloves
- Patient identification labels
- Bedpan or bedside commode for an immobile patient

Obtaining a Sterile Urine Specimen From a Catheter

- Clean gloves
- Antiseptic swab or wipe
- Sterile specimen container with a lid
- Patient identification label
- Sterile 5–10-mL syringe with a 21- to 25-gauge needleless access device

Collecting a 24-Hour Urine Specimen

Note: Some tests require using a double-storage container. Be sure to find out if you need a double-storage container and preservative, and if there are special instructions for collection of the sample.

- Basin and ice, possibly. Check with the laboratory to determine whether the specimen needs to be kept in a basin of ice during the 24-hour collection.
- Large collection container

Delegation

This procedure may be delegated to the NAP but you must be sure she knows how to perform the procedure correctly, including proper cleansing and maintaining sterility of the container. You must complete the following assessments and instruct the NAP to report any abnormalities seen in the urine (e.g., blood, foul odor, mucus) or any patient complaints of dysuria. Instruct the NAP to bring the specimen to you for inspection.

Pre-Procedure Assessment

- Cognitive status
  Knowing whether the patient can follow directions or not helps you to determine whether the patient learn to complete this procedure on her own.
- Mobility status
  Helps you to determine where the specimen will be collected (e.g., bed, commode, bedpan).
- Urinary status
  Patients with impaired ability to control urinary flow may not be able to collect a specimen in this manner.

Procedure 28-2A ■ Collecting a Clean-Catch Urine Specimen

➤ When performing the procedure, always identify your patient according to agency policy, using two identifiers, and be attentive to standard precautions, hand hygiene, patient safety and privacy, body mechanics, and documentation.

Procedure Steps

1. **Don procedure gloves.** Cleanse, or instruct the patient to cleanse, around the urinary meatus. Allow the area to dry.
   Cleansing prevents contamination of the specimen with surface bacteria.

2. **Remove soiled gloves**, perform hand hygiene, and don clean procedure gloves.

3. **Open the prepackaged kit** (if available), and remove the contents. Open the sterile specimen cup, being careful not to touch the inside of the lid or container and place within easy reach. Make sure to place the lid with the inside surface facing upward.

   Variation for Women

   a. Open the antiseptic towelette provided in the prepackaged kit. If there is no kit, pour the antiseptic solution over the cotton balls.
   b. To cleanse the perineum, spread the labia, wipe down one side of the meatus using one pad, and discard it. Then wipe the other side with a second pad. Wipe down the center over the urinary meatus with the third pad; then discard it. Use each towelette or cotton ball only once. Maintain separation of the labia until the specimen is obtained.
   Following the "clean to dirty" principle decreases the likelihood of contamination of the specimen and the urethra with feces. Antiseptic helps reduce the number of bacteria. ▼

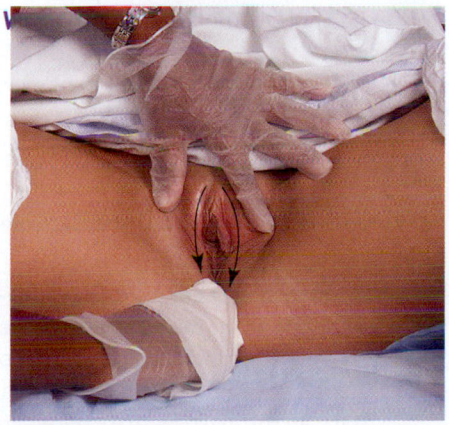

   Variation for Men

   c. If the penis is uncircumcised, retract the foreskin back from the end of the penis.
   Allows for better access when cleansing the area around the meatus.
   d. Use the towelette provided in the prepackaged kit or pour antiseptic solution over cotton balls. You might also use 2 in. × 2 in. gauze pad soaked with povidone-iodine to cleanse the periurethral area.

   ✚ Before using an iodine-based solution, be sure to check the patient's health history for allergy to iodine.

   e. With one hand, grasp the penis gently. With the other hand, cleanse the meatus in a circular motion from the meatus outward, and cleanse for a few inches down the shaft of the penis. Repeat this cleansing two more times, using each towelette or cotton ball only once.
   Cleansing the site helps in this manner prevent contaminating the specimen with bacteria.
   f. Keep one hand in place to retract the foreskin (if uncircumcised); or to hold the penis (for a patient who is unable to assist).

4. **Pick up the sterile specimen container** and hold it near the meatus. Instruct the patient to begin voiding.

5. **Allow a small stream of urine to pass**, and then without stopping the urine stream, place the specimen container into the stream, collecting approximately 30 to 60 mL. Check with the agency lab for specific advice as to how much urine to collect.
   Midstream urine collection prevents specimen contamination.

6. **Remove the container from the stream**, and allow the patient to finish emptying the bladder.
   Note: For men, if the penis is uncircumcised, replace the foreskin over the glans when the procedure is finished.

7. **Carefully replace the container lid**, touching only the outside of the cap and container. Avoid touching the rim of the cup to the genital area. Do not get toilet paper, feces, pubic hair, menstrual blood, or anything else in the urine sample.
   These measures maintain sterility of specimen and prevent cross-contamination.

8. **Label the container** with the correct patient information (in many institutions, labels are preprinted or barcoded). Place the container in a facility-specific carrier (usually a plastic bag) for transport to the lab.

9. **Remove your gloves and** perform hand hygiene.

10. **Assist the patient back to bed**, if applicable.

11. **Transport the specimen** to the lab in a timely manner.
    Delayed testing can cause inaccurate results (e.g., casts in the urine will break up if urine is allowed to sit for an extended period of time).

(continued on next page)

Procedure 28-2 ■ Obtaining a Urine Specimen for Testing (continued)

Procedure 28-2B ■ Obtaining a Sterile Urine Specimen From a Catheter

➤ When performing the procedure, always identify your patient according to agency policy, using two identifiers, and be attentive to standard precautions, hand hygiene, patient safety and privacy, body mechanics, and documentation.

Procedure Steps

1. **Don procedure gloves** and empty the drainage tube of urine into the collection bag.
2. **Clamp the drainage tube** below the level of the specimen port for 15 to 30 minutes to allow a fresh sample to collect. If the client's urine is flowing briskly, you may not need to clamp the catheter.
3. **Replace contaminated gloves** with a sterile pair, before scrubbing the specimen port with an antiseptic swab or wipe.
   Aseptic technique is used to obtain a catheter sample of urine (Loveday, Pratt, Wilson, et al., 2014)
4. **Insert the needleless access device** with a 10-mL syringe into the specimen port, and aspirate to withdraw the amount of urine you need. ➤

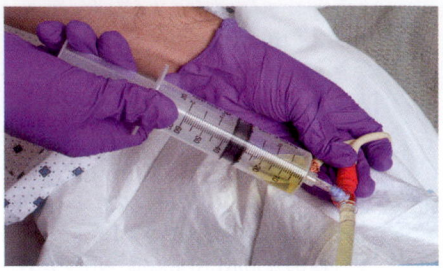

5. **Once you have the sample,** transfer the specimen into a sterile specimen container.
6. **Discard the needleless access device** and syringe in a safe container.
7. **Tightly cap** the specimen container.
8. **Remove the clamp** from the catheter. Remove gloves and disinfect the hands.

   ✚ Be sure to unclamp the tubing of the urinary collection bag after you obtain the sample.

   Urine backflow can cause bladder distention and lead to stasis-induced urinary tract infection.
9. **Label and package the specimen** with the correct patient identification according to agency policy.
   To avoid a wrong-patient error.
10. **Transport the specimen to the lab.** If immediate transport is not possible, refrigerate the sample per agency policy.

    ✚ Never disconnect the catheter from the drainage tube to obtain a sample. Interrupting the system creates a portal of entry for pathogens, thereby increasing the risk of contamination.

Procedure 28-2C ■ Collecting a 24-Hour Urine Specimen

➤ When performing the procedure, always identify your patient according to agency policy, using two identifiers, and be attentive to standard precautions, hand hygiene, patient safety and privacy, body mechanics, and documentation.

Procedure Steps

1. **Use a large collection container** (usually supplied by the lab), and collect all urine voided in the 24-hour period. If you need to use more than one container during the 24-hour period, use one container at a time. When it is full, collect the urine in the next container. Occasionally you will be asked to collect each voiding in a separate container.
2. **To begin collection,** have the patient void, and record the time. *Note: Discard this first voiding.*
   This marks the beginning of urine collection period.
3. **Collect all urine voided** during the next 24 hours. Just before the collection period ends, ask the patient to void again and add this last specimen to the collection container.
4. **Inform the patient and all staff** about the collection.
   Communication can help to prevent accidental discarding of urine.
5. **Post signs in prominent** locations, such as the patient's bathroom or entry door, to remind staff of the ongoing collection.
   Key Point: ***It is essential that none of the urine voided during the 24-hour period is accidentally discarded.***
6. **Apply a label on the specimen,** with the patient's name, date, and time the test ended on the storage container. Transport it to the lab in a timely lab, following agency protocol.

? What if . . .

- **A urine culture is ordered on the specimen?**

  Be sure to list current antibiotic therapy on the laboratory request form.
  This information is important to determine sensitivity of the microorganisms.
- **A clean-catch urine sample is needed for an immobile patient?**

  For the patient using a bedpan, raise the head of the bed to a semi-Fowler's position.
  Facilitates correct direction of urine flow down into the specimen container you are holding. In addition, this is the anatomical position for voiding.
- **You need to collect a urine sample from an infant?**
  1. Remove the paper covering adhesive patches on the back side of the specimen bag before applying it to the clean and dry perineal area. Start at the narrow area between the anus and vaginal or scrotal area. Press the adhesive sides firmly

against the skin while avoiding wrinkles in the skin against the patch.

2. It is easier to apply the lower portion of the bag first. The area must also be dry in order for the adhesive to stick to the skin. Since infants urinate frequently, it is best to work quickly to catch the specimen. Work upward to secure the bag around the entire genital area.
3. After the specimen bag is has been applied, put a diaper on the infant/child. Remember to check the collection bag every 15 to 30 minutes to see if there is a specimen. If the infant has not urinated in 2 to 3 hours, discard the bag, re-cleanse the area, and apply a new bag.

It is possible there was a leak in the seal between the skin and the adhesive sides of the specimen collection bag.

4. Once a specimen is obtained in the bag, remove it gently and pour the urine into a sterile specimen cup. Label it with the patient identifying information.▼

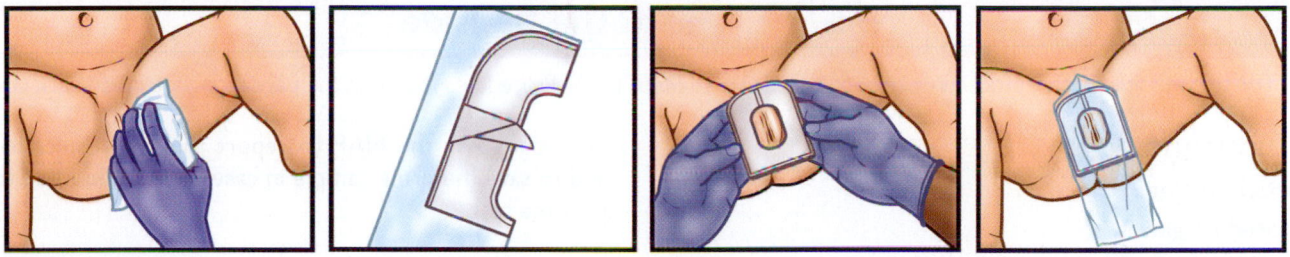

Evaluation

- Note any unusual characteristics of the urine (e.g., color, odor, clarity, crystals, blood, mucus).
- Note any difficulties with urination (e.g., pain, burning, dribbling, difficulty beginning).

Patient Teaching

- For clean-catch specimens, teach the patient the steps of the procedure, focusing on how to maintain sterility of the specimen. Explain that prepackaged antiseptic wipes cannot be flushed down the toilet.
- For the 24-hour urine specimen, explain the procedure to the patient, emphasizing the need to collect all urine during the 24-hour period. If the procedure is to be completed at home, tell the patient to refrigerate the urine specimen for up to 24 hours until it can be transported to the lab. Instruct the patient to place the specimen in a plastic bag, separate it from food items, and label it appropriately.
- For clean-catch and 24-hour urine specimens, instruct a menstruating woman that perineal cleansing is especially important. The woman may use a tampon to prevent leakage during specimen collection. Instruct her to notify the lab that she is menstruating.

Documentation

- Document urine volume in the patient record, per agency protocol, and the time and date that the specimen was collected.

  Some facilities use the Kardex to indicate the urine collection is either needed, in progress, or completed. Other facilities have nurses chart specimen collection in the nursing notes or electronic health records.
- Document the characteristics of the urine: color, odor, particulate matter, blood, clarity, or other qualities.
- Document any difficulty with voiding, including pain or burning with urination, frequency, or difficulty starting the urine flow.

Sample documentation ➤

mm/dd/yyyy 0800 *Order noted for clean-catch urine specimen. Explained to client the procedure for cleaning and obtaining urine specimen. Client stated "I must clean my bottom from front to back using the toilet in here. Then begin to void and stop voiding. Then void directly into this container." Assisted client to bedside commode. 100 mL of clear yellow urine without foul odor, blood, or particles collected. Pt. denies difficulty voiding, pain, and burning. Urine container labeled per protocol and sent to laboratory.*
L. Schaaf, RN

mm/dd/yyyy 1000 *Order noted for sterile urine specimen. Foley catheter clamped for 15 minutes. Port on Foley cleansed with antiseptic agent. 30 mL of pink tinged-urine without foul odor or sediment removed. Specimen labeled per protocol and sent to laboratory.*
L. Schaaf, RN

mm/dd/yyyy 1200 *Order noted for 24-hour urine collection. Explained procedure to client. Client stated, "I will call you when I void. This first void will be flushed and the test will begin. During the test, I will void in the white hat that is in the commode. Then every time that I void, I will call you to empty the urine into the big container. The big container for the urine must be kept cold with ice."*
L. Schaaf, RN

(continued on next page)

Procedure 28-2 ■ Obtaining a Urine Specimen for Testing (continued)

Practice Resources

Loveday, Pratt, Wilson, R.A., et al. (2014); St. Jude Children's Research Hospital (2004a, 2004b); Van Leeuwen, A. M., Poelhuis-Leth, D., & Bladh, M. L. (2011).

Go to *Davis's Nursing Skills Videos*, **Obtaining a Sterile Urine Specimen from a Catheter.**

Thinking About the Procedure

To practice applying clinical reasoning to Procedure 28-2B,

Go to Chapter 28, Thinking About the Procedure Questions and Suggested Responses, on Davis*Plus*.

For questions and suggested responses,

Procedure 28-3 ■ Testing Urine at the Bedside

➤ For steps to follow in *all* procedures, refer to the Universal Steps for All Procedures found on the page facing the inside back cover.

Equipment

Dipstick Testing

- Procedure gloves
- Dipstick testing kit

Refractometer Testing

- Refractometer
- Procedure gloves
- Distilled water
- Dropper
- Small urine sample

Delegation

You may delegate bedside urine testing to the NAP if you know that he has the knowledge and skill to perform the procedure. Ask the NAP to report the test results to you and to save the urine sample in case you should need to repeat the test.

Pre-Procedure Assessment

- Mobility status
  Knowing whether the patient can get out of bed or not helps you to determine where the specimen will be collected (e.g., toilet, bedside commode, bedpan).
- Urinary status
  Knowing whether the patient has an indwelling urinary catheter or not helps you to determine how the specimen will be collected.

Procedure 28-3A ■ Dipstick Testing of Urine

➤ When performing the procedure, always identify your patient according to agency policy, using two identifiers, and be attentive to standard precautions, hand hygiene, patient safety and privacy, body mechanics, and documentation.

Procedure Steps

1. **Read the instructions** and check the expiration date on the diagnostic kit.
2. **Wash your hands and** don procedure gloves.
   Hand hygiene and gloving prevents the transmission of bacteria.
3. **Have the patient void** into the collection container or obtain urine from the indwelling urinary catheter. See Procedures 28-1A and 28-1B for measuring urine.
4. **Obtain a test strip from the kit,** dip it into the urine, and begin timing. Follow the manufacturer's directions regarding the time needed for the reagent to develop.
5. **Compare the results to the color** chart at the specified time; record the findings. You will need good lighting to evaluate the results.

Procedure 28-3B ■ Measuring Specific Gravity of Urine

➤ When performing the procedure, always identify your patient according to agency policy, using two identifiers, and be attentive to standard precautions, hand hygiene, patient safety and privacy, body mechanics, and documentation.

Procedure Steps

1. **Clean the equipment lens** with distilled water and dry with a soft, nonabrasive cloth.
   To ensure accurate results.
2. **Calibrate the refractometer** before use, following the manufacturer's instructions. When calibrated, the refractometer should read 1.000.
3. **Perform hand hygiene** and don clean procedure gloves.
   Hand hygiene and gloving prevent the transmission of bacteria.
4. **Use fresh urine**; if you cannot perform the test within 1 hour, refrigerate the specimen.
5. **Wearing procedure gloves,** use the dropper to place one or two drops of urine on the prism surface (at the notched bottom of the cover).

6. **Hold the refractometer** horizontally, and turn toward the light. Rotate the eyepiece until the scale is in focus.
7. **Read the scale** at the point where the dividing line between bright and dark fields crosses the scale. The scale reads from 1.000 to 1.035 in increments of 0.001.
8. **Record the results.**
9. **When you are finished**, add a drop of distilled water to cleanse the prism. Dry the equipment with a soft, nonabrasive cloth.

? What If . . .

- **The diagnostic kit for dipstick testing is outdated?**

  Contact the pharmacy and/or work with the patient's caregiver to obtain a kit that is not expired.

Evaluation

- Characteristics of urine output (e.g., volume of output, color, clots, mucus).
- Abnormally concentrated or dilute urine

Patient Teaching

- Explain test procedures to the patient and the patient's caregiver and family members as indicated.

Home Care

- Teach the client or caregiver the steps of the procedure.
- Tell the client or caregiver that the urine must be tested within an hour or refrigerate the specimen to test later.
- Instruct the client or caregiver that the specimen should be tested as ordered by the healthcare provider.
- Teach the client or caregiver to record results on the flow sheet per agency protocol.

Documentation

- Document urine volume in the patient record, per agency protocol, and the time and date that the specimen was collected.

  Some agencies use the Kardex or a procedure checklist to indicate the urine collection is either needed, in progress, or completed. Other facilities have nurses chart specimen collection in the nursing notes.
- Document the urine specific gravity and pH and note the presence of hemoglobin, glucose, ketones, protein, white blood cells, bilirubin, casts, crystal, and nitrites.
- Chart other characteristics of the urine: color, odor, clarity, particulate matter, gross blood, mucus shreds, or other qualities.
- Record any difficulty with voiding, including pain or burning with urination, frequency, or difficulty starting the urine flow.

Sample documentation

3/4/16 1515 Pt voided in bedside commode. Urine is straw-colored with sediment. No unusual odor, blood, or mucus evident. No hemoglobin, glucose, ketones, protein, WBC, bilirubin, casts, or crystal nitrates noted on urine dipstick. Specific gravity 1.015, pH 6.6, and 3+ protein noted.
L. Schaaf, RN

Practice Resources

Chernecky, C. C., & Berger, B. J. (2013); Stuempfle, K. J., & Drury, D. G. (2003).

Procedure 28-4 ■ Inserting a Urinary Catheter

➤ For steps to follow in *all* procedures, refer to the Universal Steps for All Procedures found on the page facing the inside back cover.

Equipment

Intermittent Urinary Catheter (Straight Catheter)

- Washcloth and towel
- Periwash solution
- Procedure gloves, at least two pairs
- Catheter insertion kit containing:
  Sterile gloves
  Urinary catheter
  Antiseptic cleansing agent, forceps, and cotton balls or a packet of sterile antiseptic swabs or wipes
  Sterile waterproof drapes
  Sterile lubricant
  Urine receptacle
  Specimen container
- Extra pair of sterile gloves and extra sterile catheter
  Obtaining extra supplies prevents the need to leave the bedside to obtain additional supplies should the gloves or catheter become contaminated.
- Bath blanket
- Procedure lamp or flashlight
- Topical anesthetic gel [e.g., 2% lidocaine, (Xylocaine)] (according to agency policy and patient need) ▼

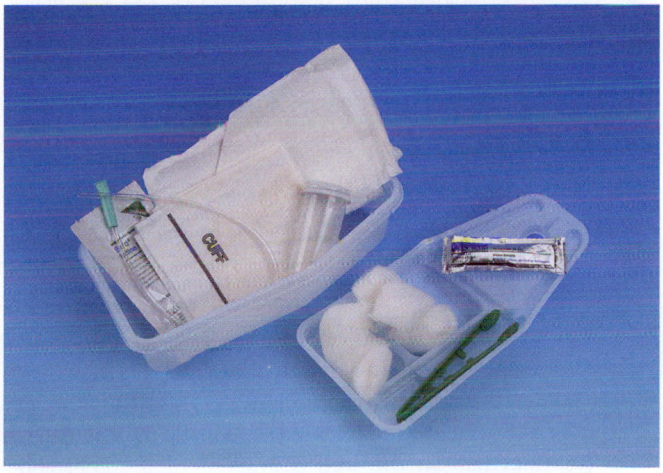

Straight catheter kit

(continued on next page)

Procedure 28-4 ■ Inserting a Urinary Catheter (continued)

Indwelling Urinary Catheter

An indwelling catheter is designed to remain in the urinary bladder. In addition to the supplies contained in a straight-catheter kit, an indwelling catheter kit will include the following:

- A double-lumen or triple-lumen catheter with a balloon tip for inflation instead of a single-lumen catheter
- A syringe prefilled with sterile water (to inflate the catheter balloon)
- Urine collection bag with drainage tubing attached; often the tubing is also attached to the catheter
- Commercial catheter securement device, such as a catheter tube holder or Velcro leg strap, if available. If not, hypoallergenic tape may be used.
- Safety pin and elastic band (if needed to secure the tubing to the bed; you can usually use the clamp on the drainage tubing) ▼

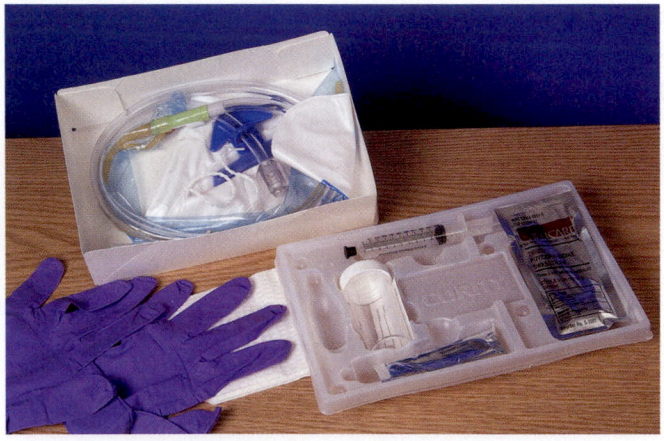

Indwelling catheter kit.

Delegation

In some institutions, NAPs receive special training to learn this skill. In such instances, you may delegate this task to the NAP. However, you must complete the following assessments and instruct the NAP when to stop the procedure and what abnormal findings to report. You must, from time to time, supervise to ensure that the procedure is being performed correctly.

Pre-Procedure Assessments

- Assess the patient's cognitive level.
  To determine whether the patient will be able to follow instructions.
- Assess for the presence of conditions that may impair the patient's ability to assume the necessary position.
  To determine whether you will need assistance to help the patient maintain the correct position.
- Assess the presence and degree of bladder distention.
  To establish a baseline against which to evaluate future data.
- Determine time of last voiding or last catheterization.
- Assess the general body size of the patient and size of the urinary meatus.
  To determine whether you need to choose a different size catheter.
- ✚ Determine whether the patient has an allergy to iodine (if that is the antiseptic solution in the kit). If so, use a different solution.
- Determine whether the patient is allergic to latex.
  Many catheters are made of latex.
- Note signs and symptoms of bladder infection (e.g., elevated temperature, urinary frequency, dysuria).
- Note conditions (e.g., enlarged prostate in men) that may make it difficult to pass the catheter.
- Assess the need for additional lighting.
  It is sometimes difficult to visualize a woman's urinary meatus. Supplemental, direct lighting helps.

Procedure 28-4A ■ Intermittent Urinary Catheterization

➤ When performing the procedure, always identify your patient according to agency policy, using two identifiers, and be attentive to standard precautions, hand hygiene, patient safety and privacy, body mechanics, and documentation.

➤ *Note:* The following steps are described for a *female* patient. If your patient is a male, refer to the procedure variation for Intermittent Urinary Catheterization (Straight Catheter) for a Male Patient, immediately following the Procedure Steps for females.

Procedure Steps

1. **If you are right-handed,** stand and work at the patient's right side; if you are left-handed, stand and work on the patient's left side.
2. **Place the patient supine** (dorsal recumbent), in a position to allow you to see the urinary meatus:
   a. Flex the patient's knees, and place her feet flat on the bed (dorsal recumbent position).
   b. Instruct the patient to relax her thighs and allow them to rotate externally. Obtain help if the patient is confused, unable to cooperate or follow directions, or unable to hold her legs in a correct position.
   The urinary meatus is sometimes difficult to visualize on women because it may resemble skinfolds or other anatomical landmarks in the area.
3. **Don clean procedure gloves.**
4. **Drape the patient.** Fold the blanket in a diamond shape, wrapping the corners around the patient's legs and folding the upper corner down over the perineum. (To review draping, see Procedure 25-4.) ▼

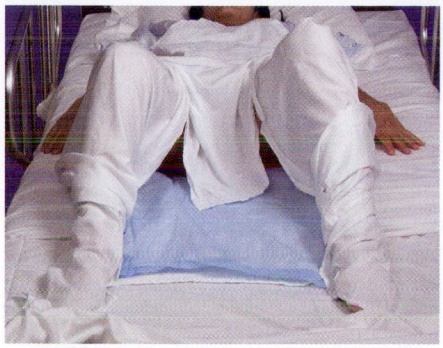

Providing privacy promotes comfort.

5. **Lift the corner of the privacy drape** to expose the perineum; position the procedure light to allow optimal visualization of the perineum, and then locate the urinary meatus.
   Locating the meatus during this step helps prevent delays at subsequent steps when it is important to maintain sterile technique.

6. **Cleanse the perineal area** with periwash solution; dry.
   Cleansing the perineum before inserting the catheter reduces the number of skin bacteria, thereby helping to prevent transmission of microorganisms into the bladder.

7. **Remove and discard gloves.** Perform hand hygiene.
   To prevent the transmission of microbes.

8. **Organize your work area.**
   a. Arrange the bedside table or overbed table within your reach.
   b. Open the sterile catheter kit according to manufacturer's instructions, and place it on the bedside or overbed table.
   c. Position a plastic bag or other trash receptacle so that you will not have to reach across the sterile field (between the patient's legs) to dispose of soiled cotton balls and so forth (e.g., a trashcan on the floor beside the bed; a trash bag on the bed near, but not between, the patient's feet; or the outer wrapping of the catheter kit).
   Carrying contaminated objects above a sterile field can contaminate the field.

9. **Place the sterile underpad and drape.** *Note: This step assumes the waterproof drape is packed as the top item in the kit. If your kit is different, see the What if... section.*
   These drapes provide sterile work surfaces and help prevent contaminating your gloves and sterile supplies.
   a. Place the sterile underpad: Remove the underpad from the kit carefully, allowing it to fall open as you remove it. Do not touch other kit items. Place it flat on the bed, shiny side down, and tuck the top edge under the buttocks, taking care to touch only the corners of the drape.
   b. Remove the sterile glove package, and don sterile gloves (see Procedure 23-7). *Note: Once you are wearing the sterile gloves, you may touch items inside the catheter kit, arranging the supplies as needed.*
   c. Place the fenestrated drape: This has a hole in the center. Pick up the drape, allowing it to unfold as you remove it, without touching any other objects from the kit. Place the drape over the perineum with the hole over the labia.▼

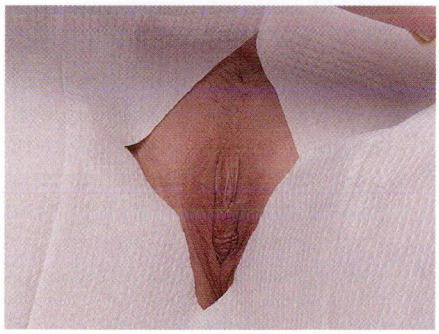

10. **Organize kit supplies on the sterile field,** and prepare the supplies in the kit.
    a. Open the antiseptic package and pour solution over the cotton balls.
    Note: Some kits contain a packet of sterile antiseptic swabs or wipes. Open the end of the packet where you feel the "sticks," leaving the swabs covered by the packet.
    b. Lay the forceps near the cotton balls.
    c. Open the specimen container if you need to collect a specimen.
    d. Remove any unneeded supplies, such as the urine specimen container, from the urine collection basin.
    e. Remove the plastic wrapper from the catheter, if it is covered.
    f. Open the packet or uncap the syringe filled with sterile lubricant.
    g. Squeeze sterile lubricant into the kit tray; roll the catheter slowly in the lubricant to generously lubricate the first 2.5 to 5 cm (1 to 2 in.). Leave the catheter tip in the lubricant or on the sterile field until ready to use.
    Lubrication allows for ease of insertion of the catheter. Prevents trauma to the mucosa.
    h. Touching only the box or sterile side of the wrapping, place the sterile catheter kit down onto the sterile field between the woman's legs.
    This approach allows you to reach supplies during catheter insertion. It also extends the sterile field created by the sterile underpad.

11. **Cleanse the urinary meatus.**
    a. Place your nondominant hand above the labia, and with your thumb and forefinger spread the patient's labia, pulling up (or anteriorly) at the same time, to expose the urinary meatus. Hold this position throughout the procedure—firm pressure is necessary. If the labia slip back over the urinary meatus, it is considered contaminated, and you will need to change gloves and repeat the cleansing procedure.
    When a woman is supine, gravity may cause tissues above the meatus to fall downward and obscure the meatus from sight. Once placed on the patient's perineal area, your hand is considered contaminated.
    b. With your dominant hand, pick up a moistened cotton ball with the forceps (or swab) and cleanse the perineal area, taking care not to contaminate your sterile glove.
    - Use one stroke and a new cotton ball or swab for each area.
    - Wipe from front to back (clitoris to anus).
    - *If there are five cotton balls or swabs:* Wipe in this order: far labium majora, near labium

(continued on next page)

Procedure 28-4 ■ Inserting a Urinary Catheter (continued)

majora, inside far labium, inside near labium, and directly down the center over the urinary meatus.

- *If there are only three cotton balls or swabs:* Cleanse only the inside far labium minora, inside near labium minora, and down the center of the urethral meatus.
- Discard the used cotton balls or swabs as you use them. Be careful not to move them across the open and sterile kit.
  Because the urethra is close to the anus in female patients, thorough cleansing of the perineum is very important to reduce contamination of the catheter and prevent bacteria from being introduced into the urethra. Following the "clean to dirty" principle prevents recontamination of the cleansed area.

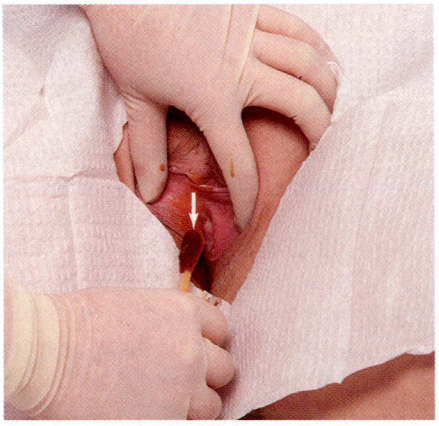

12. Prepare the urine receptacle. Place it 10 cm (4 in.) from the meatus (for women).
The end of the catheter will need to reach into the container to catch the draining urine.

13. Insert the catheter.

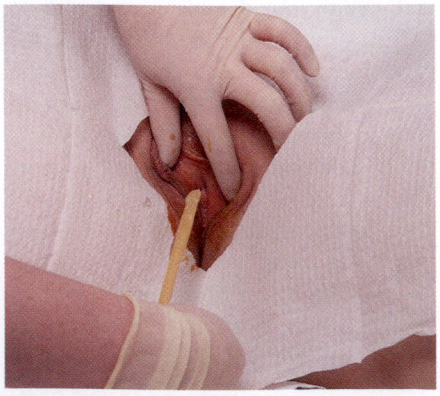

a. Grasp the catheter with your dominant hand, no more than 5 to 7.5 cm (2 to 3 in.) from the tip. Keep the rest of the catheter coiled in the palm of your hand. Slowly insert the end of the catheter into the meatus. Ask the patient to take slow, deep breaths until the initial discomfort has passed.
Bearing down helps relax the external sphincter and makes insertion easier and more comfortable. Holding the catheter close to the distal end will help to keep the tip stable and prevent it from being inserted into the vaginal opening. Deep breathing helps to relax the sphincters. Coiling the catheter in your hand keeps you from contaminating the catheter.

b. Ask the woman to bear down as though she is trying to void.

c. Continue inserting the catheter gently until urine flows, for a distance of 5 to 7.5 cm (2 to 3 in.). After you see urine, insert the catheter another 2.5 to 5 cm (1 to 2 in.).

> If you feel slight resistance as the catheter goes through the sphincters, twist the catheter slightly or apply gentle pressure, but do not force the catheter while inserting it. You might need to remove it and cautiously attempt the insertion action again using a new catheter.

Forcing may damage mucosa. Insert the catheter more deeply after urine flow to be sure the catheter is well into the bladder so that the bladder can empty completely. The catheter might not advance while inserted when it is misplaced in the vagina or if there is a stricture within the urethra or sphincter spasm.

d. If the catheter touches the labia or unsterile linens, or if you inadvertently place it in the vagina, it is contaminated and you must insert a new, sterile catheter. Leave the contaminated catheter in the vagina while you are inserting the new one into the meatus.
Leaving the catheter in the incorrect location serves as a visual landmark and helps you to avoid making the same mistake again.

14. Manage the catheter and/or urine collection device.

a. Continue to hold the catheter securely with your nondominant hand while the urine drains from the bladder.
Holding the catheter like this prevents the catheter from being expelled by bladder or urethral contractions.

b. If you are to collect a urine specimen, use your dominant hand to take the specimen container and put it into the flow of urine until you obtain the correct amount of urine. Cap the container, maintaining sterile technique. See Procedure 28-2B.

c. When the flow of urine has ceased and the bladder has been emptied, pinch the catheter and slowly withdraw it from the meatus. Discard the catheter in an appropriate receptacle.
Withdrawing slowly promotes adequate urinary drainage, preventing urinary stasis. Pinching prevents urine from dribbling out of the end of the catheter.

d. Remove the urine-filled receptacle, and set it aside outside the patient care area to be emptied when the procedure is finished.
Keeps the urine from spilling onto the bed.

15. Cleanse the patient's perineal area as needed; dry.
This removes residual antiseptic solution from the area, an especially important step if you used povidone-iodine (Betadine). Betadine left on intact healthy skin can cause irritation.

16. Remove and discard disposable supplies (e.g., drapes).

17. Remove your gloves and wash your hands.
Prevents transmission of bacteria.

18. Return the patient to a comfortable position.

Procedure Variation: Intermittent Urinary Catheterization (Straight Catheter) for a Male Patient

Procedure Steps	Nursing Action
1. Position the patient.	Position the patient supine, legs straight and slightly apart.
2. Drape the patient.	Cover the patient's upper body with a blanket; fold bed sheets down to expose the penis.
3. Don procedure gloves and cleanse the perineum.	After donning procedure gloves, wash the penis and perineal area with perineal wash solution; dry. If you are using a topical anesthetic gel (e.g., Xylocaine), use a syringe (no needle) to insert it into the urethra now. Remove and discard gloves.
4. Organize the work area.	Perform hand hygiene before starting. Open the sterile catheter kit and place on overhead table without contaminating the inside of the wrap. Position a trash receptacle nearby.
5. Place the sterile underpad and sterile drape.	Remove underpad from the kit before donning sterile gloves. Place the drape shiny side down between or across the patient's thighs.
6. Don sterile gloves.	Remove the sterile glove package, and don sterile gloves (see Procedure 23-7). *Note: Once you are wearing the sterile gloves, you may touch items inside the catheter kit, arranging the supplies as needed.*
7. Place the fenestrated drape.	Allow the fenestrated drape to fall open while removing it from the kit and without touching other kit items. Place the drape with the center hole over the penis.
8. Organize kit supplies on the sterile drape.	▪ Open the antiseptic package and pour over cotton balls or use antiseptic swabs or wipes. ▪ Open the sterile specimen container. ▪ Remove any unneeded supplies. ▪ Remove the wrapper from the catheter. ▪ Touching only the kit or inside of the wrapping, place the sterile catheter kit down onto the sterile field between the patient's legs.
9. Lubricate the catheter.	▪ Do not lubricate the catheter if you have already inserted a lubricant (lidocaine-based product) directly into the urethra. ▪ If the lubricant comes in a packet, squeeze it into the kit tray and roll the catheter slowly in it to generously lubricate 12.5 to 17.5 cm (5 to 7 in.) of the catheter. Leave the catheter tip in sterile lubricant or on the sterile field until ready to use. ▪ If your kit contains a prefilled syringe of lubricant, gently insert the tip of the syringe into the urethra and instill the lubricant.
10. Expose the urinary meatus.	▪ With your nondominant hand, grasp the penis, taking care not to contaminate the surrounding drape. This glove is no longer sterile. ▪ Hold the penis gently, but firmly, at a 90° angle to the body, exerting gentle traction. ▪ If the penis is uncircumcised, retract the foreskin to fully expose the meatus. If the foreskin accidentally falls over meatus and does not remain retracted or if you drop the penis during cleansing, you must change gloves and repeat the cleansing procedure.
11. Cleanse the urinary meatus.	▪ Continuing to hold the penis with your nondominant hand, hold the forceps in your dominant hand and pick up a cotton ball. Cleanse the glans in a series of circular motions, starting at the meatus and working partially down the shaft of the penis. ▪ Repeat with at least two more cotton balls or swabs. Discard the cotton balls or swabs as they are used. Do not move them across the open sterile kit and field.
12. Prepare the urine receptacle.	▪ Maintaining sterile technique, with your dominant hand place the plastic urine receptacle between the patient's thighs, close enough to the urinary meatus for the end of the catheter to rest inside the container as the urine drains. ▪ Hold the catheter 5 to 7.5 cm (2 to 3 in.) from the tip with remainder coiled in the palm of the hand and the distal end of the catheter is in the plastic container.
13. Insert the catheter into the urinary meatus.	▪ Ask the patient to bear down as though trying to void; slowly insert the end of the catheter into the meatus. Instruct the patient to take slow, deep breaths until the initial discomfort has passed. If you feel resistance, withdraw the catheter. Do not force against resistance. ▪ Continue inserting the catheter to about 17.5 to 22.5 cm (7 to 9 in.) or until urine flows. After you see urine, insert the catheter another 2.5 to 5 cm (1 to 2 in.).
14. Collect a specimen if needed.	If a urine specimen is to be collected, continue to grasp the penis, and use your dominant hand to place the specimen container into the flow of urine; cap container using sterile technique.
15. Manage the catheter.	When urine flow stops and the bladder has been emptied, pinch the catheter and slowly withdraw it from the meatus. Replace the foreskin. Discard the catheter in an appropriate receptacle.
16. Finish the procedure.	Remove gloves and perform hand hygiene. Return patient to a comfortable position.

(continued on next page)

Procedure 28-4 ■ Inserting a Urinary Catheter (continued)

Procedure 28-4B ■ Indwelling Urinary Catheterization

➤ When performing the procedure, always identify your patient according to agency policy, using two identifiers, and be attentive to standard precautions, hand hygiene, patient safety and privacy, body mechanics, and documentation.

➤ *Note:* The following steps are described for a ***male*** patient. If your patient is a female, refer to procedure variation for Indwelling Urinary Catheterization for a Female Patient, immediately following the Procedure Steps for males.

Procedure Steps

1. **Place the patient supine** with legs straight and slightly apart. If the patient is confused, unable to follow directions, or unable to hold his legs in correct position, obtain help with the procedure.

2. **If you are right-handed**, stand and work at the patient's right side; if you are left-handed, stand and work on the patient's left side.

3. **Drape the patient.** Cover the patient's upper body with a blanket; fold the bedsheets down to expose the penis.
   Covering the patient preserves modesty and enhances a feeling of security, while ensuring that you can visualize the urinary meatus.

4. **Don clean procedure gloves.** Cleanse the penis and perineal area with antiseptic solution; dry.
   Cleansing the area of skin bacteria reduces the risk of transmitting microbes into the bladder.

5. **If you are using topical anesthetic** gel, use a syringe (no needle) to insert it into the urethra.
   This is frequently used for men to provide local anesthesia. You insert it now because it takes 5 minutes for the gel to take effect at the time you are ready to insert the catheter.

6. **Remove and discard gloves.** Perform hand hygiene
   To prevent the transmission of microbes.

7. **Organize your work area:**
   a. Arrange the bedside table or overbed table within your reach.
   b. Open the sterile catheter kit according to the manufacturer's instructions, and place it on the bedside or overbed table.
   c. Position a plastic bag or other trash receptacle so that you will not have to reach across the sterile field to dispose of soiled cotton balls and so forth (e.g., a trash can on the floor beside the bed; a trash bag or the kit outer wrapper on the bed near, but not between, the patient's feet).
   Carrying contaminated objects above a sterile field can contaminate the field.

8. **Place the sterile underpad** and drape. *Note: This step assumes the waterproof drape is packed as the top item in the kit. If your kit is different, see the What If . . . section.*
   These drapes provide sterile work surfaces and help prevent contaminating your gloves and sterile supplies.
   a. Remove the underpad from the kit carefully. Drop the underpad shiny side down between or across the patient's thighs, touching only the corners.
   b. Remove the sterile glove package and don sterile gloves (see Procedure 23-7).
   Note: Once you are wearing the sterile gloves, you may touch any items inside the catheter kit, arranging the supplies as needed.
   c. Place the fenestrated drape: This has a hole in the center. Pick up the drape, allowing it to unfold as you remove it, without touching any other objects. Place it with the center hole over the penis.

9. **Organize the kit supplies** on the sterile field, and prepare the supplies in the kit.
   a. Pour antiseptic solution, such as Betadine, over the cotton balls. *Note:* Some kits contain a packet of sterile antiseptic swabs or wipes. Open the end of the packet where you can feel the "sticks," leaving the swabs covered by the remainder of the packet.
   b. Lay the forceps near the cotton balls.
   c. Open the specimen container, if you are to collect a specimen.
   d. Remove any unneeded supplies, such as the specimen container, from the kit.
   e. Remove the plastic wrapper from the catheter, if it is covered.
   f. Do not lubricate the catheter if you have already inserted a lubricant (xylocaine gel) directly into the urethra.

Variation: Lubricant in a Syringe

If the sterile lubricant in the kit is packaged in a syringe, you will insert the lubricant into the urethra at Step 11.

Variation: Lubricant in a Packet

If the lubricant comes in a packet, squeeze the lubricant into the kit tray and roll the catheter slowly in the lubricant. Generously lubricate 12.5 to 17.5 cm (5 to 7 in.) of the catheter. Leave the catheter tip in sterile lubricant or on the sterile field until ready to use.

   g. Attach the sterile water-filled syringe to the balloon port of the catheter.
   h. Touching only the box or sterile side of the wrapping, place the sterile catheter kit down onto the sterile field on top of the man's thighs. You may, as an alternative, set up the sterile field between his legs.
   Placement of supplies in this manner allows you to reach supplies during catheter insertion.
   i. If the bedside bag is preconnected to the catheter itself, leave the bag on or near the sterile field until after the catheter is inserted.

10. Cleanse the urinary meatus. ▼

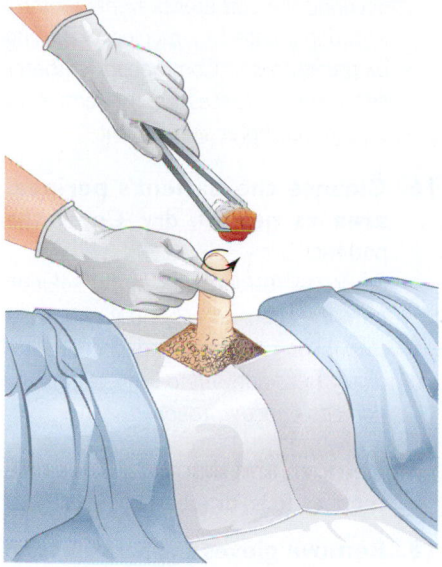

a. With your nondominant hand, reach through the opening in the fenestrated drape and grasp the penis, taking care not to contaminate the surrounding drape. This glove is no longer sterile. Hold the penis gently, but firmly, at a 90° angle to the body exerting gentle traction.
Supporting the shaft with the fingers straightens the urethra, easing insertion of the catheter.

b. If the penis is uncircumcised, retract the foreskin to fully expose the meatus. If the foreskin accidentally falls over the meatus or if you drop the penis during cleansing, you must change gloves and repeat the cleansing procedure.
Retracting the foreskin allows for full cleansing of the area.

c. Continuing to hold the penis with your nondominant hand, hold the forceps in your dominant hand and pick up a cotton ball. Cleanse the glans in a series of circular motions, starting at the meatus and working partially down the shaft of the penis.

d. Repeat with at least two more cotton balls or swabs. Discard the cotton balls or swabs as they are used. Do not move them across the open sterile kit and field.
Following the "clean to dirty" principle prevents recontamination of the cleansed area.

11. Lubricate the catheter if xylocaine gel was not instilled previously.

Lubricant Packaged in a Syringe

If the kit contains a prefilled syringe of lubricant, gently insert the tip of the syringe into the urethra and instill the lubricant.

Lubricant in a Packet

If the kit contains a single packet of lubricant, make sure you have already generously lubricated 12.5 to 17.5 cm (5 to 7 in.) of the catheter.

12. Insert the catheter. ▼

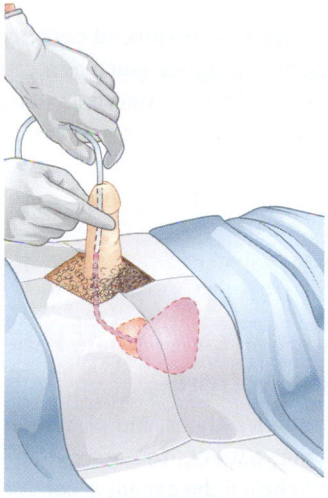

a. With your dominant hand, stabilize the catheter before inserting it by holding the catheter approximately 5 to 7.5 cm (2 to 3 in.) from the tip. Keep the rest of the catheter coiled in the palm of your hand if the catheter is not already preconnected.
Grasping the catheter close to the distal end aids in control and helps to avoid inadvertent contamination. Frequently the catheter and drainage bag are connected by the manufacturer.

b. With your nondominant hand, continue to hold the penis gently but firmly at a 90° angle to the body, exerting gentle traction.

c. Ask the patient to bear down as though trying to void; slowly insert the end of the catheter into the meatus. Ask the patient to take slow deep breaths until the initial discomfort has passed.
These strategies help the patient to relax the external sphincter and make insertion easier and more comfortable.

d. Continue inserting the catheter to about 17.5 to 22.5 cm (7 to 9 in.) or until urine flows. You will feel slight resistance at the level of the internal sphincter. Continue to advance almost to the bifurcation (Y connector).

You will commonly feel resistance at the prostatic sphincter. Hold the catheter firmly against the sphincter until the resistance eases. Then advance the catheter, but do not force it.

e. Lower the penis and replace the foreskin.
This prevents compromised circulation and painful swelling.

13. Manage the catheter.

a. Continue to hold the catheter securely with your nondominant hand to stabilize the catheter's position in the urethra. Use your other hand to pick up the water-filled syringe and inflate the catheter balloon.
Holding the catheter until the balloon is inflated decreases the chance that the catheter will be expelled by bladder or urethral contractions. The inflated balloon prevents the catheter from slipping out of the bladder. ▼

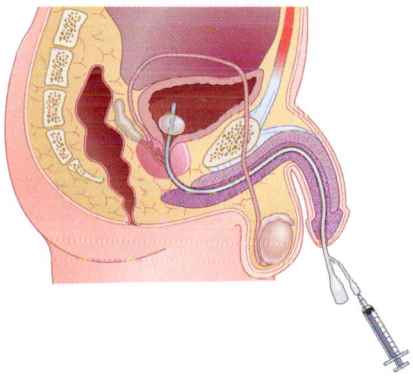

A Catheter placement, male.

(continued on next page)

Procedure 28-4 ■ Inserting a Urinary Catheter (continued)

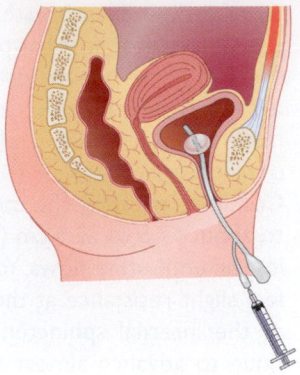

B Catheter placement, female.

b. If the patient complains of pain on inflation of the balloon, withdraw the water from the balloon, and reposition the catheter by advancing it 2.5 cm (1 in.).

Pain usually indicates that the balloon was in the urethra instead of in the bladder.

c. After the balloon is inflated, pull back gently on the catheter until you feel resistance. Lower the penis and replace the foreskin.

This indicates that the balloon is correctly positioned at the neck of the bladder.

14. **Connect the drainage bag** to the end of the catheter if it is not already preconnected. Hang the drainage bag on the side of the bed, below the level of the bladder.

Hanging the drainage bag below the bladder promotes adequate urinary drainage by gravity, preventing urinary stasis.

15. **Using a commercial catheter** securement device (such as a catheter tube holder or Velcro leg strap), if available, secure the catheter to the thigh or the abdomen. Otherwise, hypoallergenic tape may be used.

Securing the catheter prevents urethral irritation related to tugging or pulling of the catheter. Commercial catheter securement devices are preferable to tape for catheter securement.

16. **Cleanse the patient's perineal area** as needed; dry. Cover the patient.

Removes residual antiseptic solution from the area, an especially important step if you used povidone-iodine (Betadine). Betadine left on intact healthy skin can cause irritation.

17. **Remove and discard disposable** supplies (e.g., drapes).

18. **Remove gloves** and perform hand hygiene.

19. **Return the patient** to a comfortable position.

Procedure Variation: Indwelling Catheter Insertion for a Female Patient

Procedure Steps	Nursing Action
1. Position the patient.	Flex the patient's knees, and place her feet flat on the bed (dorsal recumbent position). Instruct the patient to relax her thighs and allow them to rotate externally. *Note:* Obtain help if the patient is confused, unable to follow directions, or unable to hold her legs in the correct position.
2. Drape the patient.	Fold the blanket in a diamond shape, wrapping the corners around the patient's legs and folding the upper corner down over the perineum (see Procedure 28-4A).
3. Cleanse the perineal area.	■ Don clean procedure gloves. ■ Lift the corner of the privacy drape to expose the perineum; ■ Position the procedure light to allow optimal visualization of the perineum and then locate the urinary meatus. ■ Cleanse the perineal area with antiseptic solution; dry. ■ Remove and discard gloves. Wash hands.
4. Organize the work area.	Arrange the bedside table or overbed table within your reach. Open the sterile catheter kit according to the directions, and place it on the table. Position a plastic bag or other trash receptacle so that you will not have to reach across the sterile field to dispose of soiled cotton balls and so forth.
5. Apply the sterile underpad and fenestrated drape.	■ Remove the sterile underpad from the kit before donning sterile gloves. Be sure not touch other kit items with bare hands. Touching only the corners, place the drape shiny side down under the patient's buttocks. ■ Carefully remove the sterile glove package from the kit and don sterile gloves. ■ Pick up the fenestrated drape; allow it to unfold without touching other objects; place over the perineum with the hole over the labia. ■ Remove the sterile glove package and don sterile gloves.
6. Organize the kit supplies on the sterile field.	■ Open the antiseptic packet and pour solution over the cotton balls, and position forceps nearby. Or if the kit comes with antiseptic swabs, open the packet so the sticks are convenient to grasp.

- Open the specimen container if a specimen is to be collected. Remove any unneeded supplies.
- Remove the plastic wrapper from the catheter, if it is covered. Squeeze the sterile lubricant into the kit tray. Roll the catheter slowly in the lubricant, being sure to generously lubricate the first 2.5 to 5 cm (1 to 2 in.) of the catheter. Leave the catheter tip in the sterile lubricant or on the sterile field until ready to use.
- Attach the sterile water-filled syringe to the balloon port of the catheter. Leave the syringe attached to the catheter.
- Touching only the box or sterile side of the wrapping, place the sterile catheter kit down onto the sterile field. You may, as an alternative, set up the sterile field between her legs.

7. Spread the labia and cleanse the urinary meatus.

- Place your nondominant hand above the labia, and, with thumb and forefinger, spread the patient's labia, pulling up at the same time to expose the urinary meatus. Use firm pressure to hold this position throughout the procedure. If the labia accidentally slip back over the meatus during cleansing, repeat the procedure.
- Wipe from the clitoris to the anus, wiping in the order of: far labium majora, near labium majora, inside far labium, inside near labium, and directly down the center over the urinary meatus.
- Discard cotton balls or swabs as they are used; do not move them across the open, sterile kit and field. Use only one stroke and a new cotton ball or swab for each area.

8. Insert the catheter.

Ask the woman to bear down as though she is trying to void. Grasp the catheter with your dominant hand, no more than 5 to 7.5 cm (2 to 3 in.) from the tip. Slowly insert the end of the catheter into the meatus. Ask the patient to take slow, deep breaths until the initial discomfort has passed.

9. Manage the catheter.

- Continue inserting the catheter gently until urine flows, for a distance of 5 to 7.5 cm (2 to 3 in.). After you see urine, insert the catheter another 2.5 to 5 cm (1 to 2 in.).
- If the catheter touches the labia or unsterile linens, or if you inadvertently place it in the vagina, it is contaminated and you must insert a new, sterile catheter. Leave the contaminated catheter in the vagina while you are inserting the new one into the meatus.
- After urine flows, stabilize the catheter in the urethra with your nondominant hand; use the dominant hand to pick up the sterile water-filled syringe and inflate the catheter balloon.

If the patient complains of pain when inflating the balloon, withdraw the water out of the balloon. Then reposition the catheter by advancing it 2.5 cm (1 in.).

10. Secure the catheter.

Using a commercial catheter securement device, if available, secure the catheter to the thigh.

11. Finish up.

Remove and discard disposable supplies. Remove and discard gloves. Return the patient to a comfortable position.

? What if . . .

- **The sterile gloves are packed as the top item in the catheter kit?**
  - Remove the sterile glove package and don sterile gloves (see Procedure 23-7). *Note:* Once you have donned the sterile gloves, you may touch any item inside the catheter kit, arranging the supplies as needed.
  - Place the sterile underpad: Grasp the edges of the sterile drape. Fold the entire edge down 5 to 7.5 cm (2 to 3 in.) and toward you, making a "cuff" to protect your gloves. Take care not to touch unsterile objects with your gloves or the drape.

For women: Carefully slide the drape under the patient's buttocks without contaminating your gloves. Ask the patient to raise her hips slightly if she can.

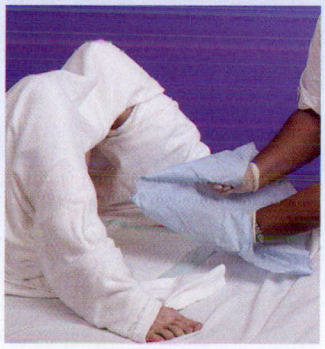

For men: Drop the sterile underpad across thighs.

  - Continue with the fenestrated drape as described in the standard procedures.
- **A woman is unable to maintain a dorsal recumbent position?**

  Use Sims' position (side-lying with the upper leg flexed at the hip). Cover the rectal area.

  Prevents contamination from the rectal area to the urethra.
- **A man has an erection during the procedure?**

  Treat the situation professionally. Take a break until the erection subsides. Never force the catheter.

  Forcing the catheter can cause urethral trauma.

(continued on next page)

Procedure 28-4 ■ Inserting a Urinary Catheter (continued)

Evaluation

- Note any difficulty with catheter insertion.
  This can indicate structural problems, especially in an older male patient with an enlarged prostate gland.
- Note the characteristics of the urine obtained (e.g., amount, color, odor, presence of sediment or mucus).
- Assess for absence of bladder distention.
  Palpating the bladder helps you to determine if it has been emptied. A portable bladder scanner may also be used to help you determine whether residual urine remains.
- For indwelling catheters, continue to monitor that drainage is not obstructed and that the drainage bag is below the level of the bladder.

Home Care

Indwelling Catheter

For inserting indwelling catheters in the home, teach clients:

- When to change the catheter
  Changing indwelling catheters at routine, fixed intervals is generally not recommended (Gould, Umscheid, Agarwal, et al., 2009). Clients should be taught to change catheters based on clinical indications, such as impaired urine drainage or encrustration.
- How to prevent catheter blockage (e.g., increase fluid intake)
  Fluids increase the urine volume, helping to reduce the deposit of sediment or other particles in the tubing.
- To empty the drainage bag frequently and to keep the bag below the level of the bladder
- How to prevent urinary tract infections (e.g., maintain a closed system, handwashing prior to handling catheter equipment, prevent blockage of urine outflow, adequate fluid intake, taking a shower rather than a bath.)
- How to prevent discomfort at the urethra
- Use of a leg bag
- To eat foods that help acidify the urine: meat, eggs, cheese, prunes, cranberries, and whole grains
- How to obtain additional supplies suitable for individual needs (Loveday, Pratt, Wilson, et al., 2014).

Documentation

- Document the time and date of the procedure.
- Document the size of catheter used.
- Record the amount of urine obtained on the I&O portion of the graphics sheet. Record the color of urine, odor, presence of mucus, blood, and so on, in the nursing notes.
- Record the patient's subjective statements.
- Document if you collected a specimen, and note the time it was sent to the lab.
- *For an indwelling catheter:* In addition, some facilities require that you record the amount of sterile water used to inflate the balloon.

Sample documentation

3/4/16 1010 Order noted for insertion of indwelling catheter. Explained the procedure to pt and reason for insertion. Pt verbalized understanding of the procedure and need for catheter. Placed pt in a dorsal recumbent position with blankets to keep pt warm and provide privacy. Perineal care completed. 14 Fr. Foley catheter inserted using sterile technique per protocol. Foley draining dark yellow urine with sediment and foul odor. No mucus or blood noted in urine. Bladder is not distended. Client returned to semi-Fowler's position. No needs noted at this time. Reminded pt to call nurse if there is any discomfort associated with urinary catheterization. Call light placed in pt's dominant hand.

C. Chin, RN

Practice Resources

Gould, Umscheid., Agarwal, et al., & Healthcare Infection Control Practices Advisory Committee (HICPAC) (2009); Herter, R., & Kazer, M. W. (2010); Loveday, Pratt, Wilson, R.A., et al. (2014); Pratt, R., & Pellowe, C. (2010); Smith, J. M. (2006); Wound, Ostomy, and Continence Nurses Society (WOCN) (2009).

Thinking About the Procedure

To practice applying clinical reasoning to these procedures,

Go to *Davis's Nursing Skills Videos*, **Intermittent Urinary Catheterization, and Indwelling Urinary Catheterization.**

For questions and suggested responses,

Go to Chapter 28, Thinking About the Procedure Questions and Suggested Responses, on Davis*Plus*.

Procedure 28-5 ■ Applying an External (Condom) Catheter

➤ For steps to follow in *all* procedures, refer to the Universal Steps for All Procedures found on the page facing the inside back cover.

Equipment

- Condom catheter
- Two pairs of clean procedure gloves
- Washcloth and towel
- Disposable basin of soap and purified water or antiseptic wash
- Bath blanket, if available
- Urine collection bag (e.g., bedside drainage bag or leg bag)
- Disposable tape measure
- Skin prep (per agency policy)
- Scissors
- Commercial leg strap

Delegation

You may delegate the application of a condom catheter to the NAP once you have assessed the NAP's skill level and completed the pre-procedure assessments. Instruct the NAP to report any alterations in the skin integrity along the shaft of the penis.

Pre-Procedure Assessments

- Assess the patient's cognitive status.
  Knowing whether the patient can follow directions helps you to determine how to approach the procedure and also to know if the patient may be prone to pulling on the catheter.
- Assess pattern of voiding (e.g., degree and time of incontinence).
  Knowing how often and how much the patient voids helps you to determine when the condom catheter should be applied.
- Assess the skin along the shaft of the penis, the glans, and the meatus (for swelling or excoriation).
  The condom catheter cannot be used on excoriated, irritated skin or over areas of impaired skin integrity.
- Note whether and how much the penis is retracted towards the body.
  There is an increased risk of nonadherence and leakage of urine in a patient with a retracted penis.
- Assess for the presence of neuropathy.
  Patients with neuropathies that affect sensation in the penis may not feel skin irritation from the condom catheter and will need to be assessed more frequently.

➤ When performing the procedure, always identify your patient according to agency policy, using two identifiers, and be attentive to standard precautions, hand hygiene, patient safety and privacy, body mechanics, and documentation.

Procedure Steps

1. **Determine appropriate size** of the external catheter by measuring the circumference of the penis using a disposable paper tape. Obtain a correctly sized catheter.
   A catheter that is too small impairs circulation. A catheter that is too large allows leakage of urine.
2. **Perform hand hygiene** and don clean procedure gloves.
   Hand hygiene and gloving prevent the transmission of bacteria.
3. **Organize supplies** and prepare the leg bag or bedside drainage bag for attachment to the condom catheter by removing it from the packaging and placing the end of the connecting tubing near the perineal area.
4. **Position the patient supine.** If the patient has difficulty breathing, raise the head of the bed to 30°.
5. **Fold down the bedcovers** to expose the penis, and drape the patient using the bath blanket.
   Covering the patient reduces patient embarrassment.
6. **Gently cleanse the penis** with soap and filtered water or antiseptic perineal wipes. Rinse and dry it thoroughly. If the patient is uncircumcised, retract the foreskin, cleanse the glans, and replace the foreskin. Excess hair along the shaft of the penis may be carefully clipped off with the scissors.
   Cleansing the penis not only helps to prevent infection but it also helps the condom catheter to adhere better to the shaft.
7. **Perform hand hygiene** and change procedure gloves.
8. **Apply skin prep** (if used by your agency), and allow it to dry. *Note: Some external condom catheters require the placement of the special adhesive strip onto the penis before the application of the condom. Follow the manufacturer's directions.*
9. **Hold the penis** in your nondominant hand. With your dominant hand, place the condom catheter at the end of the penis, and slowly unroll it along the shaft toward the patient's body. Leave 2.5 to 5 cm (1 to 2 in.) between the end of the penis and the drainage tube on the catheter.
   Careful unrolling in this manner helps to prevent irritation of the glans due to rubbing and allows for expansion of the penis if an erection were to occur.

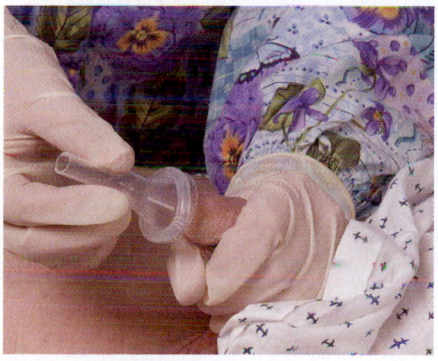

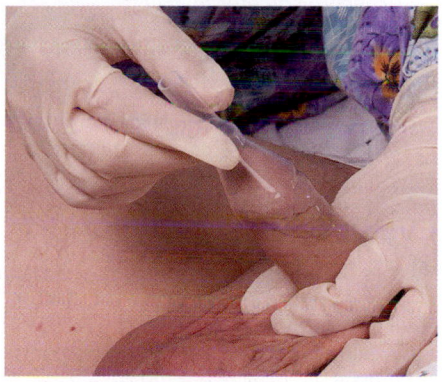

10. **Secure the condom catheter** in place on the penis.
    a. Ensure that the condom is not twisted.
       Twisting can obstruct urine flow.
    b. Do not use regular bandage or surgical dressing tape to hold an external condom catheter in place.
       Regular tape does not expand and could lead to decreased blood flow to the penis.

    Catheter With Internal Adhesive

    c. Gently grasp the penis and compress so that the entire shaft comes in contact with the condom.

    Catheter With External Adhesive Strip

    d. Wrap the strip around the outside of the condom in a spiral direction, taking care not to overlap the ends.
       Prevents constriction of blood flow to the penis.

(continued on next page)

Procedure 28-5 ■ Applying an External (Condom) Catheter (continued)

11. **Assess the proximal end** of the condom catheter. If a large portion of the condom is still rolled above the adhesive strip, you may need to clip the roll (Geng, Bonns, Eelen, et al., 2008; WOCN Continence Committee, 2008).
Clipping the roll prevents constriction of blood flow.

12. **Attach the tube end** of the condom catheter to a drainage system (e.g., a leg bag). Make sure there are no kinks in the tubing.
Kinks impede the flow of urine. Urine that does not drain away from the meatus can cause irritation and skin breakdown and possibly cause the condom catheter to fall off.

13. **Secure the catheter tubing** to the patient's thigh using a commercial leg strap. (Hypoallergenic tape may be used if a commercial leg strap is unavailable. Follow agency protocol.)
A leg strap controls movement of the tubing and accidental pulling on the condom catheter.

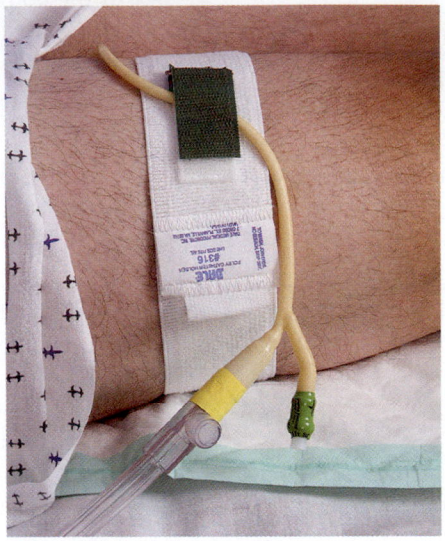

14. **Cover the patient** and return him to a comfortable position. Raise the siderails and lower the bed.

15. **Remove your gloves** and perform hand hygiene.

16. **Change the condom daily** or more often if needed.
This helps to prevent urinary tract infection and allows for inspection of the skin.

What if . . .

- **The urine flow becomes obstructed?**
Check the catheter and collecting tube for kinking; readjust if needed and make certain that the tubing is secured properly to the patient's thigh. Replace the catheter and tubing, if necessary.

Evaluation

Within 30 minutes of condom application, assess for:

- Urine flow (should not be obstructed)
- Swelling or discoloration of the penis
Swelling or discoloration might indicate that the condom is too tight.

Monitor:

- Penis for circulatory changes
- Position and patency of the drainage tubing
- Characteristics of the urine (e.g., amount, color, odor, bleeding)
- Patient comfort
- Leakage of urine

Home Care

- Clients and caregivers should wash their hands before and after any manipulation of the penis or apparatus.
- Daily bag decontamination with a diluted (1:10) bleach solution has been found effective in reducing bacteria.
- Teach the client and caregiver to recognize the signs and symptoms of skin irritation and excoriation, as well as the symptoms of urinary tract infection.
- Teach the client/caregiver to notify the care provider and discontinue use of the condom catheter if skin irritation or swelling occurs; if the urine becomes thick and cloudy, pink or red; if the urine has mucus in it; or if no urine has drained from the catheter in 6 to 8 hours.
- Change the external condom catheter every 24 hours.
- Keep the collecting bag below the level of the bladder.
- Regularly empty the collection bag before it becomes completely full.

Documentation

- Document the date and time of application of the external catheter in the nursing notes.
- Note any unusual findings related to the condition of the skin on the penis.
- Document characteristics of urine (e.g., color, odor, consistency, blood).

Practice Resources

Geng, V., Bonns, E., Eelen, P., et al. (2008); WOCN (2008).

Thinking About the Procedure

To practice applying clinical reasoning to this procedure,

Go to *Davis's Nursing Skills Videos*, **Applying an External Condom Catheter.**

For questions and suggested responses,

Go to Chapter 28, Thinking About the Procedure Questions and Suggested Responses, on Davis*Plus*.

Procedure 28-6 ■ Removing an Indwelling Catheter

➤ For steps to follow in *all* procedures, refer to the Universal Steps for All Procedures found on the page facing the inside back cover.

Equipment

- Syringe (5 to 30 mL, depending on balloon size)
- Clean procedure gloves
- Towel or drape
- Receptacle for the catheter, such as an emesis basin)
- Hygiene supplies (washcloth, warm filtered water or perineal wash solution, towel)

Delegation

In some institutions, unlicensed NAPs undergo special training to learn this skill. In such instances, you may delegate this task to the NAP. However, you must complete the following assessments and instruct the NAP about what abnormal findings to report.

Pre-Procedure Assessment

- Assess the patient's cognitive level.
  Knowing whether the patient can follow directions or not helps you to determine how to approach the procedure and also to know if the patient may be prone to pulling on the catheter or your hands when you are removing the catheter.
- Assess the condition of bladder (e.g., distention), perineum, and meatus (e.g., color, swelling, crusting, drainage, lesions).
  This information helps you to establish a baseline for later assessment.

➤ When performing the procedure, always identify your patient according to agency policy, using two identifiers, and be attentive to standard precautions, hand hygiene, patient safety and privacy, body mechanics, and documentation.

Procedure Steps

1. **Perform hand hygiene** before and after removing the catheter.
   For mechanical removal of microorganisms.
2. **Wear clean procedure gloves** during the removal.
   Gloving prevents transmission of bacteria.
3. **Explain** that this procedure is nearly always pain-free.
4. **Instruct** the patient to assume a supine position.
5. **Place the catheter receptacle** near the patient (e.g., on the bed).
6. **Place a waterproof drape** or towel.

Variation, Female

Place the drape between the patient's legs and up by the urethral meatus.

Variation, Male

Place the drape on his thighs.

These methods preserve modesty and a feeling of security, and prevent soiling of the bed.

7. **Obtain a sterile specimen** (see Procedure 28-2B), if needed. Some agencies require a culture and sensitivity test of the urine when an indwelling catheter is removed.
8. **Wash the perineum** with soapy water or periwash prior to removal of the catheter.
   The perineum and surface of the colonized with bacteria. Cleansing this area reduces the risk for urinary catheter-associated infection.
9. **Remove the device securing** the catheter to the patient
10. **Deflate the balloon completely** by inserting a syringe into the balloon valve and allowing the balloon to self-deflate. Allow at least 30 seconds for the balloon to deflate. *Note: Follow the manufacturer's directions for balloon deflation. If the direction is to attempt aspiration, it should be done slowly and gently.*
    Aspiration of the balloon may collapse the lumen and cause the formation of creases and ridges that may make removal of the catheter difficult (WOCN, 2009).
11. **Verify that the total fluid** volume has been removed by checking the balloon size written on the balloon port.
    If water remains in the balloon, removal of the catheter make cause urethral trauma.
12. **Ask the patient to relax** and take a few deep breaths as you slowly withdraw the catheter from the urethra. Pinch the catheter while removing it.
    Deep breathing helps the patient to relax the sphincters.
13. **Wrap the catheter in the towel** or drape or place in the catheter receptacle.
14. **Again cleanse the perineal area** with warm filtered water or perineal wash solution on gauze pads or perineal disposable wipes. A mild soap may also be used.
    Cleansing the perineum prevents transmission of bacteria.
15. **Measure the urine** and then empty it in the toilet; discard the catheter, drainage tube, and collection bag in the biohazard waste.
16. **Explain to the patient** the need to monitor the first few voidings after catheter removal. If the patient toilets independently, place a receptacle in the toilet or use a bedside commode. Ask the patient to notify the nurse when she voids and to save the urine.
17. **Remove and discard gloves**; perform hand hygiene.

(continued on next page)

Procedure 28-6 ■ Removing an Indwelling Catheter (continued)

18. **Record the date and time** of the procedure; the volume, color, and clarity of the urine; and your patient teaching.
19. **Return the patient to** a position of comfort.

? What if . . .

- **The balloon does not empty completely?**
  Do not pull on the catheter. Report to the charge nurse or the primary care provider before continuing the procedure.
  Pulling on the catheter could cause injury to the urethra.

Evaluation

- Observe for signs and symptoms of infection.
  Signs of a catheter-associated urinary tract infection include the presence of significant bacteriuria in a patient with signs or symptoms of a UTI such as fever, malaise, flank pain, dysuria, altered mental status, or hematuria.
- Observe the condition of the meatus.
- After removing the catheter, monitor the next few voidings. Place a collection container in the commode if the patient is ambulatory.
- Assess the characteristics of the urine at the time the catheter is removed. Then note the time of the first voiding and the amount voided, and observe the urine for color, amount, odor, and presence of blood.
- Compare voidings over the next 8 to 10 hours to the patient's intake.
- Monitor for bladder distention. A portable bladder-scanning device may be used to quantify any residual urine.

Patient Teaching

- Explain to the patient that you need to monitor the first few voidings after catheter removal to ensure that he does not have difficulty re-establishing bladder control.
- Teach the patient to notify you when he voids and to save the urine (if the patient toilets independently).

Home Care

For clients who will have catheters at home, teach the client and family the following:

- The steps for removing the catheter that you learned in this procedure
- To notify a healthcare provider if the client is unable to urinate within 8 hours after catheter removal, or if his abdomen becomes distended and painful
- The signs and symptoms of urinary tract infection
  Signs and symptoms of a urinary tract infection develop rapidly and can include a strong, persistent urge to urinate; a burning sensation when urinating; passing frequent, small amounts of urine; blood in the urine (hematuria); fever; flank pain; or an alteration in mental status.
- Increase fluid intake if not contraindicated by other health conditions.

The client should never remove a catheter unless trained by a healthcare provider. Remove the catheter only when prescribed by the provider.

Documentation

Document the following:

- Date and time the catheter was removed
- Amount of urine (on the I&O portion of the graphics sheet)
- Characteristics of urine (e.g., color, odor, cloudiness, turbidity, or blood)
- The time the specimen was sent to the lab
- The amount of fluid returned from balloon by self-deflation, amount of urine in drainage bag, and notification of first void
- Any unusual findings in your assessment of the perineum
- How the patient tolerated the procedure
- Patient teaching

Sample documentation

3/4/16 1010 Order noted for removal of indwelling catheter. Explained the procedure to patient. Pt stated, "I'm finally getting this thing out." Placed pt in a dorsal recumbent position with blanket to provide privacy. Perineal care completed. Allowed retention balloon to self-deflate, obtaining 10 mL of liquid. Removed catheter, using gentle pulling motion. Pt expressed no discomfort during removal. Perineal care again given. 250 mL of clear, yellow, strong-smelling urine noted in drainage bag. Instructed client to increase fluid intake, especially water, and to notify a nurse when she voids for the first time. ——— *C. Chin, RN*

Practice Resources

Geng, V., Cobussen-Boekhorst, H., Farrell, J., et al. (2012); Hooton, T. M., Bradley, S. F., Cardenas, D. D., et al. (2010); Parker, D., Callan., L., Harwood, J., et al. (2009a, b); Smith, J. M. (2006); WOCN (2009); Yates, A. (2008).

Thinking About the Procedure

To practice applying clinical reasoning to this procedure,

Go to *Davis's Nursing Skills Videos*, **Removing an Indwelling Urinary Catheter**

For questions and suggested responses,

Go to Chapter 28, Thinking About the Procedure Questions and Suggested Responses, on Davis*Plus*.

Procedure 28-7 ■ Irrigating the Bladder or Catheter

➤ For steps to follow in *all* procedures, refer to the Universal Steps for All Procedures found on the page facing the inside back cover.

Equipment

Intermittent Irrigation Through a Three-Way Catheter

- Bag of sterile irrigation solution
- Connecting tubing (to connect the bag to the irrigation port)
- IV pole
- Antiseptic swabs or wipes
- Bath blanket

Intermittent Irrigation via the Specimen Port Using a Syringe

- Sterile container
- Sterile 60-mL syringe with large-gauge needleless access device
- Sterile irrigation solution
- Two pairs of clean procedure gloves
- Antiseptic swabs or wipes

Continuous Bladder Irrigation

- Three-way (or triple-lumen) indwelling catheter in place
- Sterile irrigation solution at room temperature
- Connecting tubing
- Antiseptic swabs or wipes
- IV pole
- Bath blanket
- Measuring container
- Pair of clean procedure gloves

Delegation

Irrigation of an indwelling catheter requires nursing assessment and clinical decision-making. Because of the high potential for urinary tract infection, you should not delegate this procedure to the NAP. Bladder/catheter irrigation may be delegated with supervision to qualified LPNs who are trained in the procedure.

Pre-Procedure Assessment

- Note the characteristics of the urine (e.g., amount, color, odor, presence of clots or mucus).
- Assess for the presence and degree of bladder distension.
  This information helps you to establish a baseline for assessment.
- Note patient complaints of discomfort.
- Assess the patient's cognitive status.
  Helps you to determine whether the patient can follow directions and remain still during the procedure.
- Check the chart for the amount and type of sterile solution to use.
- Determine whether the irrigant is to remain in the bladder for any length of time.

Procedure 28-7A ■ Intermittent Bladder or Catheter Irrigation

➤ When performing the procedure, always identify your patient according to agency policy, using two identifiers, and be attentive to standard precautions, hand hygiene, patient safety and privacy, body mechanics, and documentation.

➤ *Note:* This is the procedure for the closed methods of irrigation. The "open" method is no longer recommended. Because of the risk for infection, you should never disconnect the drainage tubing from the catheter.

Procedure Steps

Procedure Variation Three-Way (Triple-Lumen) Indwelling Catheter

1. **Before starting irrigation**, prepare the connection tubing and irrigation solution warmed to room temperature.
   a. Close the clamp on the connection tubing.
   b. Spike the tubing into the appropriate portal on the irrigation solution bag, using aseptic technique.
   c. Invert the solution and hang it on an IV pole.
   d. Remove the protective cap from the distal end of the connection tubing. Hold the end of the tubing over the sink or trash receptacle. Open the roller clamp, and allow the solution to fill the tubing. Be sure to keep the end sterile.
   e. Reclamp the roller on the tubing to stop the flow of irrigation solution.
   f. Recap the tubing.
2. **Perform hand hygiene** and don procedure gloves.
   To reduce the transmission of microbes.
3. **Position the patient in the supine.**
4. **Drape the patient** so only the connection port on the indwelling catheter is visible.
   Protects patient privacy.
5. **Before beginning the flow** of irrigation solution, empty any urine that is in the drainage bag, and perform hand hygiene. Then document the volume on the I&O record.
   Starting the procedure with an empty drainage bag gives you a baseline for correct calculation of true urine output during irrigation.
6. **Scrub the catheter port** with antiseptic swabs or wipes.
7. **Connect the irrigation tubing** to the catheter port.
8. **Slowly open the roller clamp** on the irrigation tubing to the desired flow rate.
   Slow instillation prevents patient discomfort.
9. **Instill or irrigate** with the prescribed amount of irrigant. If the

(continued on next page)

Procedure 28-7 ■ Irrigating the Bladder or Catheter (continued)

irrigant is to remain in the bladder for a certain time period, clamp the drainage tubing for that time.

10. **When the correct amount** of irrigant has been used and/or the goals of the irrigation have been met, close the roller clamp on the irrigation tubing, leaving the tubing connected to the catheter for use during the next irrigation.
You can assess whether the goals of irrigation have been met by inspecting the color of the urine and assessing for presence of clots, mucus, or blood. Clamping the drainage tubing prevents immediate outflow.

11. **Remove gloves,** perform hand hygiene, and return the patient to a position of comfort.

Procedure Variation Two-Way Indwelling Catheter

12. **Don clean procedure gloves.** Empty any urine currently found in the bedside drainage bag.
Emptying the bag will ensure accurate output results.

13. **Perform hand hygiene** and then apply clean gloves.
Gloving prevents the transmission of microorganisms.

14. **Drape the patient** so that only the specimen removal port on the drainage tubing is exposed. Place a waterproof drape beneath the exposed port.
Draping ensures patient privacy and prevents soiling of the bed linens.

15. **Open the sterile irrigation** supplies. Pour approximately 100 mL of the irrigating solution, warmed to room temperature, into the sterile container, using aseptic technique.
Warm solution is more comfortable to the patient.

16. **Scrub all surfaces** of the specimen removal port with an antiseptic swab or wipe.
Cleaning the port reduces the risk of transmission of pathogens into the bladder.

17. **Draw up irrigation solution** into the syringe. Connect the syringe to the specimen port. For catheter irrigation, use a total of 15 to 20 mL; for bladder irrigation the amount is usually 30 to 60 mL, unless irrigation is prescribed postoperatively (in which case more irrigation might be needed).

18. **Clamp or pinch the drainage** tubing distal to the specimen port.
Clamping prevents irrigant from going down into the drainage bag instead of into the catheter and/or bladder.

19. **Inject the solution into the port.** Hold the specimen port slightly above the level of the bladder. If you meet resistance, have the patient turn slightly, and attempt a second time. If resistance continues, stop the procedure and notify the primary care provider.
Holding the port above the level of the bladder enhances gravitational flow of irrigant into the bladder. ➤

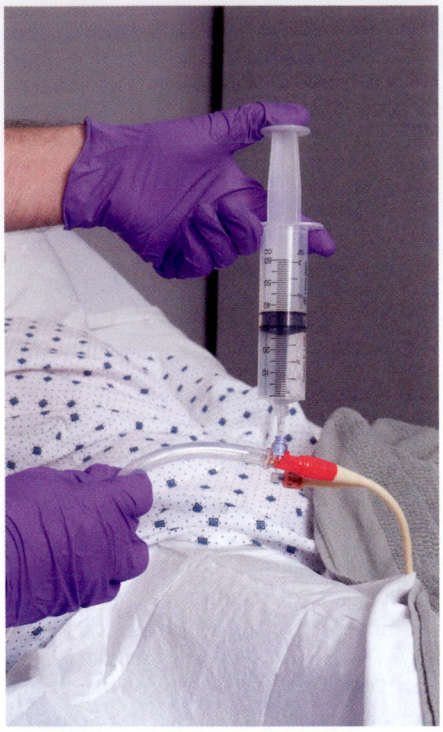

20. **When the irrigant has been** injected, remove the syringe. Refill the syringe if necessary.

21. **Unclamp or release** the drainage tubing, and allow the irrigant and urine to flow into the bedside drainage bag by gravity. (If the solution is to remain in the bladder for a prescribed time, leave the tubing clamped for that time period.)

22. **Repeat the procedure as necessary** until the prescribed amount has been instilled or until the goal of the irrigation is met (e.g., removal of clots and mucus, free flowing of urine).

23. **Remove gloves**, perform hand hygiene, and return the patient to a position of comfort.

Procedure 28-7B ■ Continuous Bladder Irrigation

➤ When performing the procedure, always identify your patient according to agency policy, using two identifiers, and be attentive to standard precautions, hand hygiene, patient safety and privacy, body mechanics, and documentation.

Procedure Steps

1. **If one is not already present,** insert a three-way (triple-lumen) indwelling catheter.
A triple-lumen catheter provides an access for the irrigation solution without disrupting the sterile drainage unit.

2. **Prepare the irrigation fluid** and tubing by warming it to room temperature:
   a. Close the clamp on the connecting tubing.
   b. Spike the tubing into the portal on the irrigation solution container, using aseptic technique.
   This prevents the introduction of microorganisms into the solution.
   c. Invert the container, and hang it on the IV pole.
   The elevated bag allows the solution to flow by gravity.
   d. Remove the protective cap from the distal end of the connecting tubing. Hold the end of the tubing over a sink or other receptacle. Open the roll clamp slowly, and allow the solution to fill the tubing

completely. Reclamp the tubing. Recap the tubing.
Priming the tubing flushes air from tubing, preventing bladder distension.

3. **Perform hand hygiene** and don clean procedure gloves.
These two actions prevent the spread of microorganisms.

4. **Place the patient supine** and drape him so that only the connection port on the indwelling catheter is visible.
Draping prevents exposure of the genital area and protects patient privacy.

5. **Place a waterproof barrier** drape under the irrigation port. Scrub the irrigation port with antiseptic swabs or wipes. Pinching the tubing and using aseptic technique, connect the end of the irrigation infusion tubing to the irrigation port of the catheter.

6. **Before beginning the flow** of irrigation solution, empty any urine that may be in the bedside drainage bag, and document the volume on the I&O record.
Starting the procedure with an empty bag gives you a baseline for correct calculation of true urine output during irrigation.

7. **Remove your gloves** and perform hand hygiene.
Gloving and hand hygiene prevent the transmission of microorganisms.

8. **Cover the patient**, and return him to a position of comfort.

9. **Open the roller clamp** on the tubing, and regulate the flow of the irrigation solution to meet the desired outcome for the irrigation.
The goal of continuous bladder irrigation for patients who have had a transurethral resection of the prostate is to keep the urine light pink to clear.

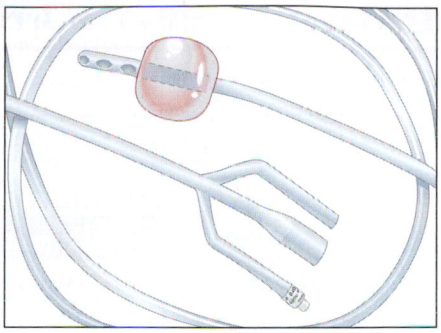

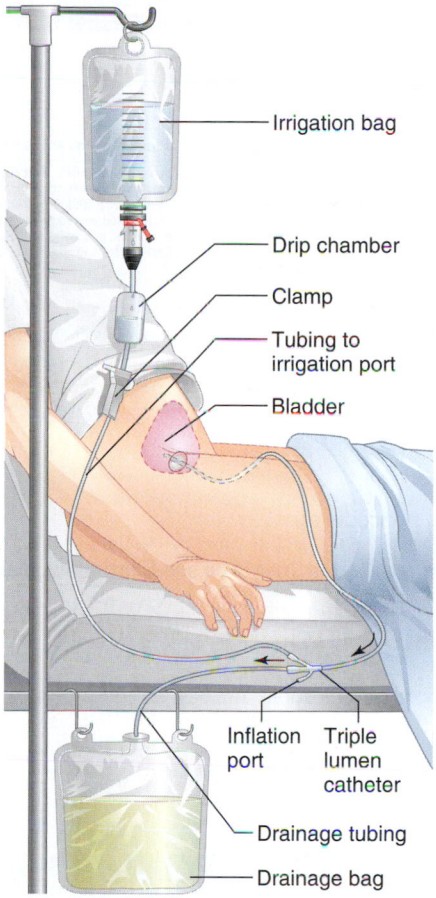

10. **Monitor the flow rate** for 1 to 2 minutes to ensure accuracy.
Monitoring the irrigation fluid for a minute or two prevents rapid introduction of solution into the bladder, which would cause patient discomfort.

? What if . . .

- **The draining irrigant solution and/or urine looks like it has red blood cells in it?**
  Stop the irrigation and report to the primary care provider.
  Increased red blood cells in the urine may indicate bladder irritation and possible trauma to the inner mucosal lining of the bladder.

- **You meet resistance when irrigating?**
  Ask the patient to turn slightly, and attempt a second time. If resistance continues, stop the procedure and notify the primary care provider.

Evaluation

- Note the flow rate of irrigant and/or inability to instill irrigant into the catheter.
- Note the characteristics of urine output (e.g., presence of output, color, amount, clots, mucus).
- Note patient report of discomfort (e.g., pain, spasms).
- Assess for development of bladder distention accompanied by lack of urine outflow. A portable bladder scanner may be used to quantify the amount of fluid retained in the bladder.

Home Care

For clients who will have continuous bladder irrigation at home, you will need to teach the family the necessary steps of the procedure. Also teach them to:

- Empty the urine collection device before beginning the procedure.
- Utilize strict aseptic technique when irrigating the bladder or catheter.
- Irrigate the catheter using the closed method, which carries the least risk for introducing bacteria into the bladder. The catheter and drainage tubing should never be disconnected.
- Identify signs and symptoms of urinary retention and urinary tract infection.
- Wash their hands before and after any manipulation of the catheter site or apparatus.
- Be certain to maintain unobstructed flow.
- For the syringe method, the client will need access to syringes and needleless access devices and a process to dispose of them properly.

Documentation

- Document the date and time of procedure, the type of irrigant, and the total volume infused.
- Document the characteristics of the urine (e.g., color, odor, clarity, sediment, presence of clots or mucus).
- Record evidence of catheter patency (e.g., flow of urine, absence of distention).

(continued on next page)

Procedure 28-7 ■ Irrigating the Bladder or Catheter (continued)

Sample documentation

Pt Sel | Logged In: Hiam, Judith | Documenting In Current Date/Time | Log Off

Patient Charting | Vital Signs | Order Entry | Order Review | Patient Teaching | Patient CARD | Patient Data | M.A.R. | Care Plans | Reports

Choose a Chart:
Admit/DC
Assessments
Treatments
Show All Charts

Admission Hx
Peds Admission Hx
Alcohol Screen
Adult DC Planner
Peds DC Planner
Adult DC Summary
Peds DC Summary
Drug Sceen
Smoking Cessation

Wounds/IVs/Ostomies/Drains/Tubes

Genito-Urinary Treatments

Urinary Treatments and Care

- [ ] Foley catheter maintained, patent and draining well
- [ ] Foley catheter inserted with sterile technique per protocol
- [ ] Foley catheter change per hospital protocol
- [ ] Foley catheter DC'd per order
- [ ] Condom catheter changed
- [ ] Leg bag changed
- [ ] Straight cath per orders for UA
- [ ] Straight cath by self
- [ ] Straight cath by nurse
- [x] Bladder irrigation per orders
- [ ] Bladder training in progress
- [ ] Foley clamped
- [ ] Foley unclamped, urine measured, reclamped
- [ ] Bladder scans for residuals
- [ ] Straight caths for residuals
- [ ] 24-hr Urine begun; (chart ending date/time)
- [ ] 24-hr Urine in progress; (chart ending date/time)
- [x] Teach rationale for nursing interventions

Patient Response

- [x] Tolerated procedure well
- [x] Compliant with Nsg regimen
- [x] Reports understanding of teaching

Urinary Treatments and Care Notes

mm/dd/yyyy 1415 Bladder irrigation per orders with 1 liter sterile saline solution. Urine with frank blood visible. Cleared to pale, straw-color at the completion of bladder irrigation. Mucous shreds and clots cleared. Pt. tolerated procedure without complaints of pain, discomfort, or burning. Catheter patency evidenced by free flow of urine and absence of distention.....M.M.Baker, RN

Practice Resources

Hagen, S., Sinclair, L., & Cross, S. (2010); Hooton, T. M., Bradley, S. F., Cardenas, D. D., et al. (2010); Loveday, Pratt, Wilson, R.A., et al. (2014); Lynn, P. B. (2011); WOCN (2009).

Thinking About the Procedure

To practice applying clinical reasoning to this procedure,

Go to *Davis's Nursing Skills Videos*, **Intermittent Bladder Irrigation** and **Continuous Bladder Irrigation.**

For questions and suggested responses,

Go to Chapter 28, Thinking About the Procedure Questions and Suggested Responses, on Davis*Plus*.

CLINICAL INSIGHTS

Clinical Insight 28-1 ➤ Caring for a Patient With an Indwelling Catheter

An indwelling catheter is connected to a drainage tube and collection bag, which constitute a closed system.

Goal 1: Prevent urinary tract infection.

- **Observe standard precautions** when providing catheter care.
- **Wear gloves when handling the catheter** or drainage system.
  Gloving prevents possible exposure to body fluids.
- **Clean around the meatus and perineum** before inserting or removing an indwelling urinary catheter; use aseptic technique and sterile equipment; perform strict and frequent catheter care (Gould, Umscheid, Agarwal, et al., 2009; Loveday, Pratt, Wilson, R.A., et al., 2014).
  Reduce the risk of urinary catheter-associated infection.
- **Maintain a closed system.** Do not disconnect the tubing or open the drainage system (e.g., to obtain specimens or measure the urine).
  A closed system minimizes the chance for pathogens to enter the system and infect the urinary tract.
- **Regularly check connections** between the catheter and drainage tubing and the drainage tube and collection bag.
  Loose connections cause leaks and serve as entry points for pathogens.
- **If the system becomes disconnected**, wipe the ends of both tubes with antiseptic (e.g., alcohol or chlorhexidine gluconate (CHG)–alcohol combination product) before reconnecting them.
- **If the catheter becomes soiled** from drainage or feces and after each bowel movement, cleanse it with mild soap and water by cleaning from the meatus outward. Rinse the catheter well, and pat it dry.
  This removes the medium for growth of microorganisms.
- **Empty the collection bag** at least every 8 hours and more frequently if urine output is high.
  This prevents stagnation of urine.

Clinical Insight 28-1 ➤ Caring for a Patient With an Indwelling Catheter—cont'd

- **Avoid touching the spout** to any surfaces when emptying the collection bag. If the spout is accidentally contaminated, cleanse it with an antiseptic (e.g., alcohol or CHG-alcohol combination product).
- **Keep collection bag below the level of the bladder**, but do not allow it to lie on the floor. Never place the bag on the bed.
  This prevents backflow of stagnant urine into the bladder. Assist the patient to take a shower regularly if his condition permits.
- **Teach the patient to report signs of UTI** (e.g., burning at the meatus); observe for cloudy, strong-smelling urine, chills, or fever.
- **Change the indwelling catheter** only when necessary (e.g., sediment collects in the tubing or catheter or when the urine does not drain well). Some agencies have a policy specifying that catheters be changed at specific intervals (e.g., monthly). However, this is not advisable because the more often a catheter is changed, the more likely an infection will develop

Goal 2: Maintain free flow of urine.

- **Keep the tubing and bag** below bladder level to prevent backflow.
  Urine drains by gravity in this system.
- **If the collecting bag must be higher** than the bladder at any time, you must clamp the catheter.
  Clamping prevents backflow of stagnant urine into the bladder.
- **Frequently inspect the tubing** to ensure that the urine flows freely.
  Kinks, coils, or compression of the catheter or tubing may impede flow and cause backup into the bladder.
- **If urine is not flowing**, check to be sure the patient is not lying on the tubing.

Goal 3: Prevent transmission of infection.

- Observe standard precautions when providing catheter care.
- **Wear gloves** when handling the catheter or drainage system.
  Gloving prevents possible exposure to body fluids.

Always perform hand hygiene before and after providing care to any patient, including one with an indwelling catheter.

Goal 4: Promote normal urine production.

Adequate urine production flushes pathogens out of the bladder, provides natural irrigation of the tubing, and prevents stasis of urine.

- **Encourage oral intake** of at least 8 to 10 glasses (approximately 2,000 to 2,500 mL) of fluid per day, unless contraindicated by other health problems (Turner & Dickens, 2011; WOCN, 2009). For patients who are unable to take oral liquid, provide an equivalent amount of parenteral or enteral fluids.
- **Monitor intake and** output at least every 8 hours. More frequent monitoring may be required if the patient is experiencing fluid and electrolyte problems.
- **For accurate determination of output**, empty the urine into a calibrated container.
  Although the urine collection bag has volume markings, they are only approximate.
- **Observe the urine output** for color and other characteristics. Report evidence of blood, sediment, or infection to the primary care provider.
- **Encourage the patient to be active** and out of bed as much as possible.

Goal 5: Maintain skin and mucosal integrity.

Perineal skin and mucosa can be irritated by feces and by movement or encrustation of the catheter.

- **Secure the tubing** by applying a commercial catheter securement device, such as a catheter tube holder or a Velcro strap, to the patient's thigh. Hypoallergenic tape may be used if a catheter securement device is unavailable. For men, if the catheter will remain in place for an extended period, secure the tubing to the abdomen to prevent damage to the penile–scrotal juncture.
  Failure to secure the tubing may cause significant injury to the bladder neck and urethra. Although the inflated balloon helps maintain the catheter in the bladder, you will need to secure the tubing to the leg to prevent traction on the bladder and urethral meatus.
- **Assist with routine hygiene care** as needed. Cleanse the area around the meatus with mild soap and filtered tap water or perineal wash solution daily, after each bowel movement, and more often if there is drainage or excessive sweating. Be sure to rinse well and pat dry.
  Routine hygiene care normally provides adequate cleanliness. Rinsing helps to avoid irritating the skin with soap residue.
- **Avoid using powders or lotions** in the perineal area.
  Topical products can be irritating to the skin.
- **Monitor the urethral meatus** and upper drainage tube.
  Encrustation, as evidenced by sandy particles at the meatus, is irritating to the mucosa and signals a need to change the catheter.

Clinical Insight 28-2 ➤ Caring for Patients With Urinary Incontinence

Most urinary incontinence (UI) is managed with skin care and behavioral interventions, but medications and other collaborative treatments are sometimes used.

Open Discussion about Incontinence

- Patients and families often do not raise the issue. Be direct and ask about continence using simple questions in a way that will not embarrass the patient, such as "Do you wear a pad to keep your clothes dry?" "Do you ever wet your clothing?"
- If you determine that the patient is incontinent, ask follow-up questions to identify the type of incontinence. For example: "Do you sometimes not make it to the toilet in time?" "Do you ever dribble urine when you sneeze or cough?"
- Encourage use of a bladder diary for at least 3 to 7 days, covering routine day-to-day activities as well as atypical situations.
- Advise patients to contact a healthcare provider if:
  - They have not been previously evaluated for this problem.
  - The urinary stream is weak.
  - There is burning, fever, chills, pain, or passing little urine for 1 to 2 days.
  - Urine is cloudy or unusually foul smelling.
  - Discharge occurs from the penis or vagina.
- Advise women who have a body mass index (BMI) >30 to lose weight (Rainsbury, Fabricius, & McLarty, 2011).
- Advise patients to take prescribed diuretics early in the morning. Diuretics taken at night can cause nocturia and lead to interrupted sleep.

Lifestyle Modification

Make the following recommendations to patients over for changes in lifestyle:

- **Increase daily oral fluids** to 8 to 10 glasses (or 2,000 to 2,500 mL), as tolerated. High fluid intake is good for flushing of the bladder. Limiting fluid intake has not been shown to be useful in preventing the development of incontinence (Townsend, Jura, Curhan, et al., 2011) and increases the risk for UTIs, constipation, and dehydration (Lucas, Bedretdinova, Bosch, et al., 2013).
- **Limit caffeine intake** to less than 100 mg. daily. This is about one cup of coffee or two 12-ounce cans of cola. Caffeine is a diuretic and a bladder stimulant.
- **Try limiting the intake** of alcohol, artificial sweeteners, spicy foods, and citrus fruits. These are thought to irritate the bladder.
- **Lose weight** (for persons with a BMI >30). Studies have shown this to be more effective for women than for men. Weight reduction by as little as 5% to 10% alleviates incontinence symptoms and improves the quality of life.
- **Stop smoking.** Smoking has been linked to stress UI and urge UI among women, and to urge UI in men.
- **Take prescribed diuretics early in the morning.** Diuretics taken at night can cause nocturia and lead to interrupted sleep.
- **Avoid constipation.** (See Chapter 29 for interventions to promote normal bowel elimination.) Fecal impaction and chronic constipation, especially in older adults, are associated with increased risk of UI.
- **Consider low-impact exercise.** High-impact exercise (e.g., running, jumping rope) is associated with increased stress UI.

Bladder Training

The goal of bladder training is to enable the patient to hold increasingly greater volumes of urine in the bladder and to increase the between voidings.

- Teach the mechanisms of urination.
- Teach distraction and relaxation strategies to help inhibit the urge to void. For example:
  - Instruct the patient to perform serial subtractions or become involved in an activity that requires concentration (e.g., a crossword puzzle) when she feels the urge to void.
  - Alternatively the patient might perform several rapid pelvic floor muscle contractions to quiet the sensations from the bladder.
  - Other techniques include deep breathing and guided imagery.
- **Scheduled voiding** is a form of bladder training involving timed voiding and habit retraining. The patient must be mentally and physically capable of self-toileting.
  - Assist the patient to the toilet, commode, or bedpan on a timed schedule. Initially this may be every 2 hours or even more often.
  - As a pattern develops and the person gains greater control, the length of time between voiding may be increased.
  - Scheduled voiding is usually combined with other techniques, including lifestyle adjustments and pelvic muscle exercises.
  - Ask the patient to keep a daily record of her adherence to the schedule and of the number of incontinence episodes.
  - When the patient can adhere to the schedule comfortably, the voiding interval can be increased by 15 to 30 minutes.

Pelvic Floor Muscle Exercises (PFMEs)

Teach patients the following routine to strengthen pelvic floor muscles:

- Imagine that you are urinating and wish to stop the flow; also tighten your rectum as though you are trying to keep from passing gas. The muscles you contract to interrupt flow are the pelvic floor muscles. *Note: Caution the patient against doing PFMEs while actually urinating because this may cause backflow of urine.*
- You should feel your rectum tighten. Women may also feel the vagina tighten. Your abdomen should not tighten—check by placing your hand lightly on your abdomen. Do not contract the thigh and gluteal muscles.
- Hold each contraction for 5 to 10 seconds and then rest for 5 to 10 seconds. Some people may be able to hold for only

Clinical Insight 28-2 ➤ Caring for Patients With Urinary Incontinence—cont'd

3 seconds at first. Count, "one-and-two-and-three. . . ." Keep contraction and relaxation times equal. That is, if you hold a contraction for 5 seconds, rest 5 seconds before the next contraction.

- A recommended daily exercise routine is to perform 10 to 15 PFMEs three times a day. Do not do all 30 to 45 exercises at one time; spread them out through the day.
- One way to remember to perform your exercises it to associate them with an activity. For example, do PFMEs at every stoplight or stop sign when you are in the car. Or, do some of these exercises every time you go to the bathroom—but not while you are urinating.

Supportive Interventions

Supportive interventions focus on helping the patient reach the toilet and perform toileting self-care.

- Ask where the toilet is and whether the patient can get there easily. If he cannot, it may be useful to place a commode near where the patient spends most of his time.
- Provide a bedside commode, raised toilet seat, bedpan, urinal, or other aids to make it easier to urinate independently. For some patients, a commode should be placed by the bedside on a large, absorbent, washable mat (to absorb any urine that leaks).
- Advise and assist the patient with gait and strength training to improve the person's ability to reach the toilet in time.
- When continence cannot be achieved, provide absorbent products with waterproof coverings. Meticulous skin care must be given when these are used. Under no circumstances should you refer to these as "diapers," as this is disrespectful of the patient's dignity.
- Men with urinary incontinence can use a drip collector, which is a small pocket of padding worn over the penis and held in place with underwear.

Practice Resources

Dowling-Castronovo, A., & Bradway, C. (2012); Goode, P. S., Burgio, K. L., Richter, H. E., et al. (2010); Lucas, M. G., Bedretdinova, D., Bosch, J., et al. (2013)

Clinical Insight 28-3 ➤ Caring for Patients With Urinary Diversions

The overall goals are for the patient to become comfortable with his changed body and to assume self-care.

- **Perform a thorough assessment.** A healthy stoma ranges in color from deep pink to brick red, regardless of skin color, and is shiny and moist at all times. A pale, dusky, or black stoma often indicates inadequate blood supply. Immediately document and report such findings to the surgeon.
- **Assess the skin surrounding the stoma for signs of irritation**, such as redness, tenderness, and skin breakdown.
  Key Point: *Skin care is critical. When the normally acid urine remains in contact with the skin, it becomes alkaline. Encrustations collect on the skin and the skin becomes macerated and excoriated. Skin breakdown may lead to infection, pain, and leakage.*
- **Be certain that the collection device fits** snugly against the skin. A moisture-proof skin barrier is usually placed around the stoma.
  Moisture on the skin can lead to irritation and maceration.
- **Barrier creams** may be prescribed for irritated skin; if fungal infection develops, nystatin may be prescribed.
- **Monitor the amount and type of drainage** from the stoma.
- **Empty the device frequently** during the day; connect it to a larger collection bag during the night when the patient is sleeping.
- **Be available to discuss the patient's reaction** to the stoma.
  Key Point: *Be careful your facial expressions do not convey disgust or disapproval when working with the patient and his stoma.*
- **Provide ample time** to explain stoma care and use of ostomy appliances.
  For most patients this is a life-long task; therefore, patient teaching is essential.

Patients with a continent urinary reservoir

These patients will also need instruction about catheterizing their reservoir to drain the urine. Once healed, the reservoir will need to be catheterized four or five times a day.

Patients with a neobladder

- These patients will not have a stoma, but will require bladder training once the postoperative retention catheter has been removed.
- The patient should be instructed to perform pelvic floor muscle exercises three times a day and empty the bladder on a schedule, as often as every two hours initially. Once bladder capacity builds, the interval between voidings may be increased.
- The patient will need to relax the pelvic muscles and bear down to release urine from the bladder. He may also need to use **Credé's maneuver**, applying manual pressure over the bladder to promote emptying.
- If the patient is unable to fully empty the bladder with these techniques, he may need to perform intermittent self-catheterization.

Clinical Insight 28-4 ➤ Teaching Clients About Clean, Intermittent Self-Catheterization

You will need to teach self-catheterization to clients who have compromised ability to spontaneously empty their bladders. In the home setting, this is a clean procedure rather than a sterile one. It is referred to as clean, intermittent self-catheterization (CISC).

Goals of intermittent self-catheterization

1. Completely empty the bladder.
2. Prevent urinary tract infections.

Teaching Considerations

- In teaching the steps of the procedure, consider the client's physical ability to manipulate the catheter equipment and reach the urethra (e.g., range of motion, fine motor skills, degree of sensation).
- Encourage the client to drink 8 to 10 eight-ounce glasses of fluid without caffeine each day to ensure a quantity of urine adequate to flush the bladder.
- Teach the client to report the signs and symptoms of urinary tract infection: burning, frequency, urgency, dull abdominal ache, fever, or malaise; or urine that contains sediment or becomes cloudy.

Older adults may experience confusion before the other signs and symptoms occur.

- Advise the client to contact a healthcare provider if there is bleeding, pain, or difficulty inserting the catheter.
- Some CISC catheters can be reused; some are disposable.
- Instruct the patient to wash her hands thoroughly before handling the equipment or performing the catheterization.
- Catheterize as often as needed. Most patients will need to catheterize 4 to 6 times daily.
- Discard a reusable catheter when it becomes difficult to clean or difficult to insert. A CISC catheter may be reused up to seven days (Newman & Willson, 2011).
- Recommendations for cleaning a reusable catheter include washing with soap and water, boiling or microwave sterilization, or soaking in an antiseptic solution. Running tap water forcefully through the catheter may remove encrustation or mucus deposits. Check for specific cleaning recommendations from the catheter manufacturer.

Procedure for Men

1. **Try to void before catheterization.** If you are unable to void or if the amount is less than 3 ounces (or the amount specified by your healthcare provider), then insert the catheter.
2. Assemble the catheter, lubricant, and drainage receptacle.
3. **Thoroughly wash** your hands with soap and water; cleanse the penis and the urethral opening.
4. **Lubricate** the catheter to 6 inches (15 cm).
5. **Stand over the toilet** or assume a comfortable position (e.g., sitting on the toilet).
6. **Hold the penis** perpendicular (at a right angle) to your body.
7. **Gently insert** and advance the catheter.
8. **When you meet resistance**, at the level of the prostate, take deep breaths to try to relax, and advance the catheter.
9. **When urine flow starts,** advance the catheter 1 inch (2.5 cm) more; return the penis to its natural position; hold the catheter in place until the urine flow stops and bladder is empty.
10. **Withdraw the catheter** slowly in small increments to be sure the entire bladder empties.
11. **Wash the catheter** with soap and water, if it is reusable (or follow the manufacturer's instructions for cleaning). Rinse and dry it well. If it is disposable, discard it immediately.
12. **Store catheters** in a clean, dry, secure place.
13. **Record the amount** of urine obtained.

Procedure for Women

1. **Try to void before catheterization.** If you are unable to void or if amount is less than 3 ounces (or the amount specified by your healthcare provider), then insert the catheter.
2. **Assemble the catheter,** lubricant, and drainage receptacle; a good light is important for women.
3. **Thoroughly wash hands** with soap and water.
4. **Cleanse your labia and urethra** with soap and water or with a moist towelette; rinse well. Cleanse and rinse from front to back.
5. **Lubricate the catheter** to about 1 inch (2.5 cm).
6. **Assume a comfortable position** for urinating. Some women perform CISC standing up with one foot on the toilet.
7. **Use a hand mirror** to locate the urethral opening, which is between the clitoris and the vagina.
8. **Spread your labia** with the second and fourth fingers; use the middle finger to feel for the urethral opening.
9. **Gently insert the catheter** into the opening, guiding it upward toward your umbilicus (belly button) until urine flows. This is usually 2 or 3 inches (5 to 8 cm) past the urethral opening.
10. **When urine flows,** advance the catheter another 1 inch (2.5 cm). Hold it in place until the urine stops and your bladder is empty.
11. **Withdraw the catheter slowly** in small increments, to be sure the entire bladder empties.
12. **If the catheter is reusable,** wash it with soap and water; rinse and dry it well (or follow the manufacturer's instructions for cleaning). If it is disposable, discard it immediately.
13. **Store catheters** in a clean, dry, secure place.
14. **Record the amount** of urine obtained.

Practice Resources

Joanna Briggs Institute (2011); Newman, D. K., & Willson, M. M. (2011).

ASSESSMENT GUIDELINES AND TOOLS

Focused Assessment

Urinary Elimination History Questions

Usual Urination Pattern

- How often do you urinate?
- Do you get up in the middle of the night to urinate?
- Do you have difficulty getting to the bathroom in time to urinate?
- Do you ever leak urine when you cough, laugh, or exercise?
- Do you ever leak urine on the way to the bathroom?
- Do you need to use pads or tissue in your underwear to catch urine?
- Do you have any difficulty starting to void?

Appearance of Urine

- How would you describe your urine?
- Have you noticed unusual odor with urination?

Changes in Urination Habits or Urine Appearance

- Have you experienced any changes in your voiding pattern recently?
- Have you experienced any changes in the appearance or odor of your urine?

History of Urination Problems

- Have you experienced any problems with urinary tract infections or kidney and bladder problems?
- Have you ever lost control of your urination?
- Have you ever had urinary tract surgery or diagnostic procedures?

Use of Urination Aids

- What aids, if any, do you use to help you urinate?
- What is your usual fluid intake over the course of a day?
- What medications are you taking? Have they had any effect on your urination pattern?

Lifestyle Questions

- Where is your bathroom located? Can you get to it easily?
- Can you manage your clothing when you go to the bathroom?
- How much fluid do you drink each day?
- How many caffeinated beverages do you drink?
- Do you smoke?
- Are you bothered with constipation?
- Do you do high-impact exercise (e.g., jogging)?

Presence of Urinary Diversions

- Have you ever had urinary tract surgery?
- If so, what and when?
- Gather data on the client's usual care of the stoma, use of appliances, and adjustment to the ostomy.

For Infants and Young Children

- Has the child been toilet-trained?
- What elimination routines have been established?

Focused Assessment

Guidelines for Physical Assessment for Urinary Elimination

Physical assessment for urinary elimination includes examination of the kidneys, bladder, urethra, and skin surrounding the genitals, as appropriate. For a complete discussion of physical examination of the genitourinary system, see Chapter 22, Procedures 22-17 and 22-18, in this volume.

The Kidneys

Technique	*Rationale*
The **costovertebral (CV) angle** is formed by the junction of the 12th rib and the spine on both sides of the back. Place one palm flat on the CV angle and lightly strike it with the closed fist of the other hand (see the accompanying figure).	You cannot usually palpate the kidneys. Instead, examine them by assessing for costovertebral angle tenderness (CVAT). If kidney inflammation is present, percussion of this angle produces pain.

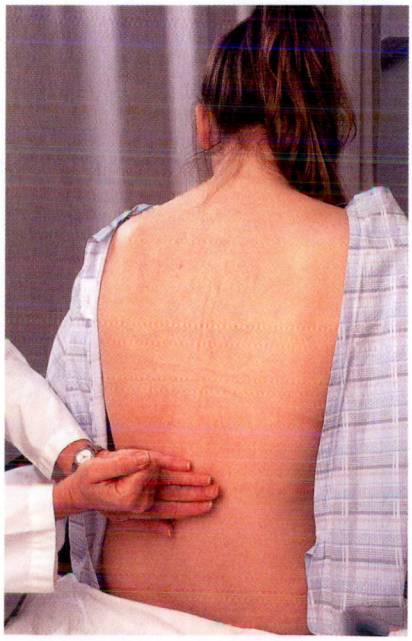

(Continued)

Focused Assessment

Guidelines for Physical Assessment for Urinary Elimination—cont'd

The Bladder

Inspect, palpate, and percuss the lower abdomen. Correlate your findings with data about the client's fluid intake and voiding.

➤ Inspect the lower abdomen.	An empty bladder, or one with limited urine, is small and sits below the symphysis pubis. In contrast, a distended bladder rises above the symphysis pubis. If it is very distended, you may be able to see a rounded swelling above the symphysis pubis.
➤ Lightly palpate the lower abdomen to define the bladder margin. Observe the patient's response to palpation, noting signs of tenderness or discomfort.	An empty bladder, or one with limited urine, will not be palpable.
➤ Percuss the area.	A distended bladder produces a dull sound as opposed to the normal tympanic sound of intestinal air.

The Urethra

➤ Inspect the urethral orifice. Look for erythema, discharge, swelling, or odor.	These are all signs of infection, trauma, or inflammation.

The Perineal Area

➤ Frequently inspect skin color, condition, texture, turgor, and presence of urine or stool.	Clients who have urine leakage or a urinary catheter are at risk for perineal skin problems. Ammonia in the urine may result in skin excoriation, skin breakdown, and subsequent infection. If both urine and stool are present on the skin, the likelihood of skin breakdown increases.

Diagnostic Testing

Urinalysis

Characteristic Findings	Expected	Variations
Color	A freshly voided sample is pale yellow to deep amber.	Urine becomes lighter in color and may even be clear if fluid intake is high or urine output is excessive. Urine becomes dark in color as it becomes more concentrated with decreased fluid intake or excessive fluid loss. Color is also affected by diet and medications.
pH	5.0–9.0	Indicates kidneys' ability to help maintain balanced hydrogen ion concentration in the blood. The pH increases (more alkaline) if the client eats dairy products or citrus fruits or has a vegetarian diet. The pH decreases (more acidic) if the client eats a high-protein diet or consumes cranberry juice.
Specific gravity	1.002–1.030	This is a reflection of the kidney's ability to concentrate urine. Specific gravity rises with limited fluid intake or dehydration. It may also rise with kidney disease. Specific gravity decreases as fluid intake increases.
Clarity	A freshly voided sample should be translucent. If the urine sits for a period of time, it will become cloudy.	Cloudiness in a freshly voided sample indicates the presence of other constituents in the urine. These may include bacteria, RBCs, WBCs, sperm, prostatic fluid, or vaginal discharge.
Odor	Fresh urine is mildly odorous.	Certain foods, such as garlic, onions, and asparagus, may give urine a distinctive odor. Bacteria will give urine an ammonia-like odor. A sweet syrup odor may indicate an inborn metabolic disorder (maple syrup urine disease).
Protein	<20 mg/dL	Proteinuria is the most common indicator of renal disease. Protein is increased in diabetic nephropathy, glomerulonephritis, nephrosis, and toxemia of pregnancy. May be increased in benign proteinuria secondary to stress or physical exercise.

Diagnostic Testing

Glucose	Negative	Glucose is found in the urine with elevated blood sugars and diabetes.
Ketones	Negative	Presence of ketones indicates impaired carbohydrate metabolism. Ketones may be detected with diabetes, fever, fasting, high-protein diets, starvation, vomiting, and during the postanesthesia period.
Hemoglobin	Negative on dipstick If RBCs are assessed via microscopic exam: <5 per high-power field	Hemoglobin may be detected with infection of the urinary tract, disease of the bladder, glomerulonephritis, pyelonephritis, trauma, nephrolithiasis, hemolytic reactions, or trauma. It also may be present in samples from women who are currently menstruating.
Bilirubin	Negative	Increased bilirubin occurs with liver disease.
Urobilinogen	Up to 1 mg/dL	Increase is found in cirrhosis, heart failure, liver disease, infectious mononucleosis, malaria, and pernicious anemia.
Nitrite	Negative	Nitrite is used to test for bacteriuria. Increased in the presence of nitrite-forming bacteria, such as *Escherichia coli*.
Leukocyte esterase	Negative If WBCs are assessed via microscopic exam: <5 per high-power field	Leukocytes are increased in bacterial infection, calculus formation, fungal or parasitic infection, glomerulonephritis, interstitial nephritis, or tumor.
Renal cells	None seen	Renal cells come from the lining of the collecting ducts. Their presence indicates damage to the tubular network.
Transitional cells	None seen	Transitional cells line the renal pelvis, ureter, bladder, and proximal urethra. Their presence is seen with infection, trauma, and malignancy.
Squamous cells	Rare	Typically insignificant: Squamous cells line the vagina and distal portion of the urethra.
Casts	Rare hyaline; otherwise negative	Large numbers of hyaline casts are seen in renal disease, hypertension, with diuretic use, and fever. Granular casts are seen in renal disease, viral infection, or lead intoxication.
Crystals	Absent in freshly voided sample	Crystals in the urine may indicate an old sample, stone formation in the urinary tract, gout, high dietary intake of oxalates, liver disease, or side effect of chemotherapy.
Bacteria, yeast, parasites	None seen	Microbes in the urine indicate an infection of the urinary tract.

Source: Adapted from Van Leeuwen, A. M., Poelhuis-Leth, D., & Bladh, M. L. (2011). *Davis's comprehensive handbook of laboratory & diagnostic tests—with nursing implications* (4th ed.). Philadelphia, PA: F.A. Davis.

Diagnostic Testing

Blood Studies: BUN and Creatinine

Normal Ranges

Blood urea nitrogen (BUN)	8–21 mg/dL
Creatinine	0.5–1.2 mg/dL

Levels may be increased in:

- Renal failure
- Impaired renal perfusion
- Kidney inflammation
- Kidney obstruction
- Dehydration
- Excessive protein intake
- Use of total parenteral nutrition (TPN)

Levels may be decreased in:

- Inadequate protein intake
- Malabsorption syndromes
- Liver disease

Source: Adapted from Van Leeuwen, A. M., Poelhuis-Leth, D., & Bladh, M. L. (2011). *Davis's comprehensive handbook of laboratory & diagnostic tests—with nursing implications* (4th ed.). Philadelphia, PA: F.A. Davis.

Diagnostic Testing

Studies of the Urinary System

Direct Visualization Studies

Cystoscopy

Direct visualization of the urethra, bladder, and ureteral orifices by insertion of a scope. May be used to obtain biopsies and treat pathology of visualized areas.

Preparation

- Instruct the patient that the procedure is performed under anesthesia. This anesthesia may be general, spinal, or local.
- Ensure that a signed consent form is on the chart.
- Restrict food and fluids for 8 hours if the patient is receiving general anesthesia. For local anesthesia, allow only clear liquids for 8 hours before the procedure.

Post-Procedure Care

- Monitor vital signs and intake and output (I&O).
- Observe the characteristics of urine after the procedure.
- Encourage increased fluid intake.
- Report suprapubic or flank pain, chills, or difficulty urinating.

Cystometry

This test is done to determine whether a muscle or nerve problem is causing problems with how well the bladder holds or releases urine. A catheter is inserted into the bladder and a pressure probe into the rectum. Warm fluid is injected and connected to cystometer, which measures how much the bladder can hold and the pressure in the bladder. Sometimes a gas or contrast material is used.

Preparation

- Ensure a signed consent form is on the chart.
- Explain that patient cooperation with positioning and activity is crucial during the test.
- There are no food or fluid restrictions before the test.

Post-Procedure Care

- Monitor vital signs and I&O.
- Encourage increased fluid intake.
- Report suprapubic or flank pain, chills, or difficulty urinating.

Indirect Visualization Studies

Intravenous Pyelogram (IVP) & Retrograde Pyelogram

An IVP uses intravenous radiopaque contrast medium to visualize the kidneys, ureters, bladder, and renal pelvis. It evaluates renal function by analyzing flow of contrast over time.

A retrograde pyelogram uses radiopaque contrast medium to visualize the renal collecting system. Contrast media is injected via a ureteral catheter inserted through a cystoscope.

Preparation

- Assess for history of allergies. Radiopaque dyes can be highly allergenic for some patient; therefore, this test is contraindicated for patients with allergies to shellfish or iodinated dye.
- Ensure baseline BUN and creatinine results are available. This test is contraindicated for patients who are in renal failure.
- Ensure that a signed consent form is on the chart.
- Restrict food and fluids for 8 hours prior to the procedure. Check agency protocols for specific guidelines, especially related to fluid intake.
- Some patients may require a laxative the evening before the surgery to clear the GI tract and improve visualization.
- Check to be sure diabetic patients who take insulin make an adjustment to the insulin dose when fasting for this examination.
- Determine the patient is not pregnant, breastfeeding, or with an intrauterine device (IUD) in place.
- Ask if the patient has had an X-ray test using barium contrast material (such as a barium enema) or have taken a medication containing bismuth (e. g., Pepto-Bismol) in the four days prior to the test. These can affect the test results.
- Check for a history of bleeding disorders or if the patient is taking any anticoagulant, aspirin, or other medications that affect blood clotting. It may be necessary to hold these medications prior to the procedure.

Post-Procedure Care

- Encourage increased fluid intake.
- Monitor vital signs and I&O.
- Observe for reactions to the contrast media: rash, nausea, hives.

Ultrasound

Using contrast media, computerized tomography (CT) scanning examines body sections from different angles using a narrow x-ray beam to produce a three-dimensional picture of the area of the body being scanned.

Preparation

- Ensure a signed consent form is on the chart.
- There are no food or fluid restrictions with renal ultrasound. A patient undergoing bladder ultrasound may be required to drink five to six glasses of fluid 90 minutes before the procedure to ensure a full bladder.

Post-Procedure Care

- No special care is required.

Computerized tomography

Using contrast media, a CT scan examines body sections from different angles using a narrow x-ray beam to produce a three-dimensional picture of the area of the body being scanned.

Diagnostic Testing

Preparation

- Obtain history of allergies. This test is contraindicated for patients with allergies to shellfish or iodinated dye.
- Ensure a signed consent form is on the chart.
- For a renal CT scan, food and fluids are usually restricted for 2 to 4 hours prior to the procedure.
- Remove all metal objects from the patient's body (e.g., eyeglasses, rings, safety pins).

Post-Procedure Care

- Monitor vital signs and I&O.
- Observe for reactions to the contrast media: rash, nausea, hives.

Renal biopsy

Removal of a piece of kidney tissue for microscopic evaluation, usually done with ultrasound guidance.

Preparation

- Ensure baseline coagulation studies and hemoglobin results are available.
- Ensure a signed consent form is on the chart.
- NPO 6 to 8 hours prior to an open biopsy procedure and at least 4 hours prior to a needle biopsy procedure. Protocols may vary among facilities.
- Instruct the patient that sedation and/or pain medication may be given.

Post-Procedure Care

- Monitor vital signs and I&O.
- The patient will be on bedrest for 6 to 24 hours as ordered.
- Monitor biopsy site for bleeding.
- Monitor urine for presence of blood.

Source: Adapted from Van Leeuwen, A. M., Poelhuis-Leth, D., & Bladh, M. L. (2011). *Davis's comprehensive handbook of laboratory & diagnostic tests—with nursing implications* (4th ed.). Philadelphia, PA: F.A. Davis.

CLINICALREASONING

Applying the Full-Spectrum Nursing Model

PATIENT SITUATION

You are providing care to an older-adult patient, Mrs. Patel, who has a number of health concerns, including diabetes and obesity. Mrs. Patel seeks healthcare because she is experiencing burning with urination, frequency, and urgency. You explain to her these are signs of a urinary tract infection. You discover while taking your nursing history that she also has difficulty with urinary continence. When asked about her toileting habits, she tells you she often doesn't "make it to the bathroom" even while at home. This has been going on for about 3 years. She has trouble getting up and walking upstairs to the bathroom because of a foot ulcer that doesn't seem to be healing well. Mrs. Patel's affect is flat with little expression. During your time with her, she seems to have little interest in talking about her health concerns. When you ask her about what she does to get out or socialize, she admits to being hesitant to go far because she is afraid of wetting without knowing it and carrying an odor that would be embarrassing to her.

THINKING

1. *Theoretical Knowledge (Recall of Facts and Principles):*
   a. What kind(s) of incontinence is this patient likely to have?
   b. What are this patient's risk factors for incontinence?
2. *Critical Thinking (Contextual Awareness):*
   a. What aspects of this situation have you experienced or observed before in your role as a caregiver?
   b. How might those past experiences affect your perception in this situation?

DOING

3. *Practical Knowledge (Patient Teaching):*
   a. How could you encourage this woman to seek healthcare for managing her urinary incontinence?
   b. What might you ask your patient to do in order to get a better idea of her bladder history and toileting habits?
   c. By looking at Mrs. Patel's bladder diary, you see a pattern suggestive of urinary incontinence. What other behavioral strategies might you suggest to improve her ability to have control of her bladder?

CARING

4. *Self-Knowledge:*
   a. Have you ever personally experienced urinary urgency when you had trouble getting to the bathroom in time? Reflect on this experience and examine how you might feel if you were incontinent much of the time.
   b. In what way(s) can you show compassion for the patient who has urinary incontinence?

Critical Thinking and Clinical Reasoning

1. You receive a report from the NAP that a patient with no history of urinary elimination problems has had 150 mL of oral liquids in 6 hours and has voided 100 mL of clear, dark amber urine. His vital signs at the start of the shift were as follows: blood pressure, 108/76 mm Hg; pulse, 72 beats/min; respirations, 18 breaths/min; temperature, 98.6°F (37.0°C). The most recent check revealed blood pressure, 112/80 mm Hg; pulse, 88 beats/min; respirations, 22 breaths/min; and temperature, 100.4°F (38.0°C).
   a. What conclusion might you draw about what has caused these symptoms?
   b. What actions should you take?
2. As you make patient rounds, you discover a collection bag for an indwelling catheter placed on the bed above the level of the patient's bladder.
   a. What should you do first? What assessments should you make?
   b. What teaching would be important in this situation?
3. Nursing assistive personnel (NAP) complain that Mr. Jones, a patient with dementia, keeps urinating in his trashcan and in the hallway.
   a. What special measures could be taken to assist Mr. Jones in finding the bathroom?
   b. What data could be helpful in developing a plan for Mr. Jones?
4. For each of the following concepts, use critical thinking to describe how or why it is important to nursing, patient care, or urinary elimination. Note that these are *not* to be merely definitions.

Blood pressure	Hydration
Kidney tubules	Specific gravity
Developmental stage	Urinary incontinence
Privacy	

What Are the Main Points in This Chapter?

- The urinary system consists of two kidneys, two ureters, the urinary bladder, and the urethra.
- The kidneys filter nitrogen and other metabolic wastes, toxins, excess ions, and water from the bloodstream and excrete them as urine.
- The bladder has a normal average storage capacity of 500 mL (1 pint), but it may distend, when needed, to a capacity twice that amount.
- Voiding occurs when contraction of the detrusor muscle pushes stored urine through the relaxed internal urethral sphincter into the urethra.
- The kidneys produce urine at a rate of approximately 60 mL per hour, or 1,500 mL per day. Most people urinate about five to six times per day.
- Voiding and control of urination require normal functioning of the bladder and the urethra, as well as an intact brain, spinal cord, and nerves supplying the bladder and urethra.
- As an adult ages, the number of functional nephrons gradually decreases, along with the ability to dilute and concentrate urine. The potential volume of the bladder also decreases as the bladder wall loses elasticity; thus, older adults need to urinate more frequently.
- Substances that contain caffeine act as diuretics and increase urine production.
- A diet high in salt causes water retention and decreases urine production.
- Medications with anticholinergic effects inhibit the free flow of urine and may contribute to urinary retention.
- An adequately hydrated adult produces clear yellow urine. Concentrated urine is darker in color, but dilute urine can appear colorless.

- A clean-catch urine specimen is preferred for many diagnostic tests. To collect this specimen, the client must cleanse the genitalia before voiding and collect the sample in midstream.
- Sterile urine specimens may be obtained by inserting a catheter into the bladder or withdrawing a sample from an indwelling catheter.
- Twenty-four-hour urine collection requires collection of all urine voided in the time period. The start time of the 24-hour collection begins when the first-voided urine is discarded.
- A routine urinalysis is one of the most commonly ordered laboratory tests. It is used as an overall screening test as well as an aid to diagnose renal, hepatic, and other diseases.
- Normal urine is free of bacteria, viruses, and fungi. Urinary tract infections are often caused by the introduction of *E. coli*, which normally live in the colon, into the urethra and bladder.
- Urinary retention is an inability to empty the bladder. It may occur because of obstruction, neurological problems, infection, surgery, medications, or anxiety.
- Urinary catheterization is the introduction of a pliable tube (catheter) into the bladder to allow drainage of urine.
- Urinary incontinence (UI) is a lack of voluntary control over urination. Nurses can independently perform the primary interventions to manage UI.
- A urinary diversion is required when the bladder must be removed or bypassed. There are three options: a conventional urostomy or ileal conduit, a continent urinary reservoir, or a neobladder.
- A patient with a urinary diversion requires physical and psychological care. The goal is to have the patient become comfortable with his changed body and assume self-care.

Knowledge Map

STRUCTURES:
Kidneys – filter; regulate
Nephrons – urine formation
Ureters – urine transport
Bladder – urine storage
Urethra – urine transport
Sphincters – flow control

FACTORS AFFECTING:
- Developmental stage: infants, elders
- Personal; sociocultural; environmental
  - time; privacy; loss of dignity
- Nutrition; hydration
- Activity
- Medications
- Surgery/anesthesia

PATHOLOGICAL CONDITIONS AFFECTING URINATION:
- UTI
- Calculi
- BPH
- Cardiovascular & metabolic diseases
- Neurogenic bladder
- Impairments: mobility, communication, cognition

URINATION

ASSESSING URINE:
- Intake and output
- Urine studies
  - analysis
  - specific gravity
  - dipstick
- Specimens from:
  - fresh-voided
  - clean-catch
  - sterile specimen
  - 24-hour collection

PROMOTING NORMAL URINATION:
- Provide privacy
- Position properly
- Establish toileting routines
- Provide adequate fluids/ nutrition
- Assist with voiding

COMMON URINARY PROBLEMS:
- Urinary tract infections
  - urethritis; cystitis; pyelonephritis
- Urinary retention
- Urinary incontinence:
  - urge
  - stress
  - overflow
  - functional
  - transient
  - reflex
  - enuresis
- Urinary diversions
  - cutaneous ureterostomy
  - ileal conduit
  - Kock pouch (continent urostomy)

URINARY CATHETERIZATION
- Straight catheter
- Indwelling catheter
- Suprapubic catheter

- Skin care
- Lifestyle changes
- Bladder training
- Scheduled voiding
- Kegels
- Biofeedback
- Anti-incontinent devices

CHAPTER 29

Bowel Elimination

STUDENT RESOURCES

*The questions and exercises in Volume 2 allow you to practice the kind of thinking you will use as a full-spectrum nurse. Critical-thinking questions usually have more than one correct answer, so we do not provide "answers" for these features. It is more important to develop your nursing judgment than to just cover content. You will learn by discussing the questions with your peers. If you are still unsure, consult your instructor. You will find Response Sheets (for writing your responses to the questions) on Davis*Plus.

To explore learning resources for this chapter,

Go to Davis*Plus* at DavisPl.us/Wilkinson3.

Chapter Resources for Chapter 29:

- **Response sheets for all learning activities**
- **Resources for Caregivers and Health Professionals**
- **Reading More About Bowel Elimination (suggested readings)**
- **Concept Map of chapter content**

Interactive Case Studies

NCLEX-Style and Chapter Review Questions

CHAPTER OVERVIEW

For a podcast of an overview of this chapter,

Go to Student Resources, Chapter 29, **Podcast—Chapter Overview,** on Davis*Plus*.

Caring for the Nguyens

Yen Nguyen arrives at the family health center for a scheduled appointment, accompanied by her grandson, Kim Phan. Recently, Yen has been constipated and has had several episodes of bleeding with bowel movements (BMs). She has read that a change in bowel habits is a sign of colon cancer and is worried about that. She brought her grandson along because he is also having bowel problems. Kim's bowel habits are erratic. At times he has a soft BM daily. However, he has also had bouts of constipation and diarrhea. Yen would like advice on her grandson's elimination status. As a critical thinker, you will begin by obtaining accurate, credible information.

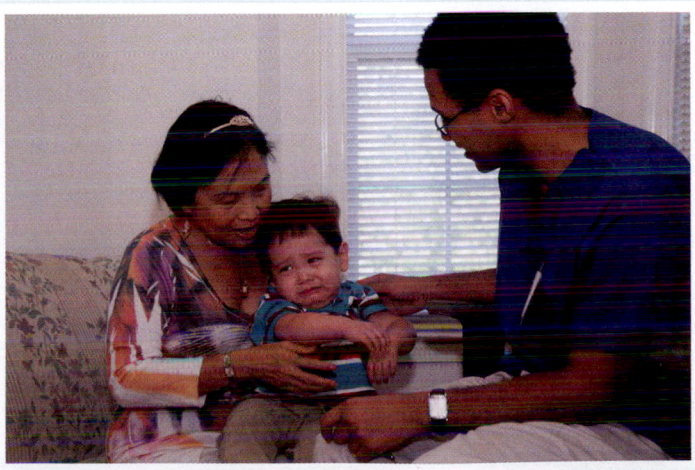

(Continued)

Caring for the Nguyens (continued)

A. What history questions would be appropriate to ask Yen regarding her bowel concerns? What data do you need? How can you get the data? Are the data accurate? What information is important; what is not? Write some specific questions, just as you would ask them in an interview.

B. What physical assessments would you conduct for Yen to add to, and possibly to validate, your subjective data?

C. Now you must consider the context. What factors must you consider when gathering a history on Kim?

D. The family nurse practitioner (FNP) examines Yen and determines that she has external hemorrhoids that have been bleeding because of recent straining at stool. The FNP prescribes rectal suppositories to decrease the swelling of the hemorrhoids and asks you to teach Yen about necessary lifestyle changes. What additional information will you need to gather to provide this teaching? Recall that you have already obtained a significant amount of information from the history questions. Again, think about context: Whatever the content of your teaching, Yen will be using that information to care for herself and her grandson in her home.

E. The FNP examines Kim and tells you that the examination is normal. Use your theoretical knowledge of bowel elimination and Kim's developmental stage to think of possible reasons for his erratic bowel pattern.

Practical Knowledge knowing how

To help you promote normal bowel elimination and support patients who have bowel elimination problems, this section applies concepts from Volume 1 to provide practical knowledge of procedures and clinical insights. You will also find assessment guidelines for assisting patients who are having diagnostic studies of the gastrointestinal system.

PROCEDURES

The procedures in this chapter will help you provide care to patients who have problems with bowel elimination.

Procedure 29-1 ■ Testing Stool for Occult Blood

➤ For steps to follow in *all* procedures, refer to the Universal Steps for All Procedures found on the inside back cover.

➤ *Note:* According to colorectal screening guidelines, all persons age 50 or older should be screened every 1 to 2 years for occult (hidden) blood in the stool. High-risk groups require initial screening at a younger age, and should perhaps undergo genetic testing. Some guidelines recommend that decisions should be made to screen those over age 75 only on an individual basis.

Equipment

- Clean gloves
- Tongue blade or other wooden applicator
- Clean, dry collection container to place in the commode, or a clean, dry bedpan
- Facility-specific fecal occult blood test (FOBT) slide or test paper
- Developing solution

Delegation

You can delegate the collection and testing of a stool sample for occult blood to the nursing assistive personnel (NAP) if the NAP has the necessary skills and the patient's condition is stable. Inform the NAP of any special considerations (e.g., the need to assist the patient with ambulation or the need for a bedpan). Instruct the NAP to inform you if there is visible blood in the stool and to show you the FOBT slide for evaluation of results when the test is complete.

Pre-Procedure Assessment

- Assess the patient's mobility status.
  Determines the patient's ability to participate in stool collection, the need for a bedpan or commode, and so forth.
- Assess the patient's dietary history for the past 24 to 48 hours.
  Some foods, such as red meat, chicken, fish, horseradish, turnips, or raw vegetables, may lead to a false-positive reading. Vitamin C in excess of 250 mg per day can produce a false-negative result (MEDLINE Plus, 2013).

- Assess medication history.
  If the patient is taking medications, such as salicylates, NSAIDs, iron, oxidizing drugs, reserpine, corticosteroids, anticoagulants, colchicines, and high doses of vitamin C, consult with a physician. These medications may cause a false-positive reading. If possible, they will be discontinued for 7 days before the test. If the patient must have them, then the results must be interpreted taking them into consideration.
- Assess for the presence of hemorrhoids.
  Any source of blood may cause a false-positive result for intestinal bleeding.
- If the patient is female, ask whether she is menstruating.
- Check the expiration date on the developing solution for the FOBT test slide.
- Assess the patient's or family's understanding of the need for the stool test.
  Provides a baseline for health teaching.

➤ When performing the procedure, always identify your patient according to agency policy, using two identifiers, and be attentive to standard precautions, hand hygiene, patient safety and privacy, body mechanics, and documentation.

Procedure Steps

1. **Determine whether the test** will be done by the nurse at the point of care (e.g., in the home or at the bedside) or by lab personnel.
   Because of the regulatory and billing practices in some settings, this test may be completed by lab personnel.
2. **Gather the necessary testing** supplies. Be sure you understand the directions for the testing kit you are using.
   This procedure gives instructions for using the FOBT slide method.
3. **Ask the patient to void** before collecting the stool specimen.
   Helps prevent contaminating the stool with urine.
4. **Perform hand hygiene and** don procedure gloves.
5. **Place a clean, dry container** for the stool specimen into the toilet or bedside commode in such a manner that any urine falls into the toilet and the fecal specimen falls into the container. Obtain a clean, dry bedpan for a patient who is immobile.
   Using a sample of stool that comes in contact with either urine or water may produce an inaccurate test result.
6. **Instruct the patient to defecate** into the container, or place the patient on the bedpan. Do not contaminate the specimen with toilet tissue.
7. **Once the specimen has been obtained** and the bedpan removed or the patient assisted to bed as necessary, perform hand hygiene, and don clean procedure gloves.
   Prevents the spread of intestinal bacteria.
8. **Explain the purpose of the test.** Explain to the patient that serial specimens may be needed.
   Testing serial specimens decreases the chances of a false-negative finding.
9. **Open the specimen side** of the FOBT slide. With a tongue depressor or other applicator, collect a small sample of stool and spread it thinly onto one "window" of the FOBT slide.
10. **With a different applicator** or the opposite end of the tongue blade, collect a second small sample of stool from a different location in the large sample. Spread the second sample thinly onto the second "window" of the slide.
    Reduces the possibility of a false-negative result.

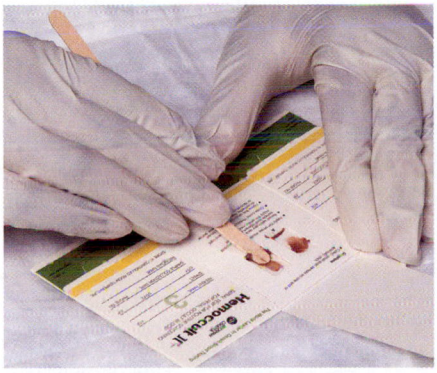

11. **Wrap the tongue depressor** in tissue and a paper towel; place it in a waste receptacle. Do not flush it.
    Prevents transfer of microorganisms. Flushing would likely clog the plumbing.
12. **Close the FOBT slide.**
    Prevents the transfer of microorganisms from the specimen smears on the slide.
13. **If the test is to be done by** laboratory personnel, transfer the specimen to a clean dry container, being careful not to contaminate the outside of the container with feces. Label the specimen in the presence of the patient according to agency policy, and place it into the proper receptacle for transportation to the lab.
14. **If you are to perform the test,** turn the slide over, and open the opposite side of the FOBT slide. Follow the directions on the package regarding the number of drops of the developing solution.
    Ensures an accurate reading.

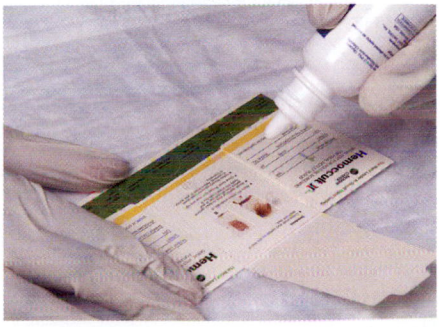

15. **Remove gloves and** perform hand hygiene.

(continued on next page)

Procedure 29-1 ■ Testing Stool for Occult Blood (continued)

Evaluation

- Observe the color of the paper inside the FOBT slide windows for 30 to 60 seconds.
- If the paper turns blue, consider the test for occult blood to be positive.

Patient Teaching

- Inform the patient of the reasons for performing the test.
- Explain the possible implications of a positive occult blood test, if one is obtained.

Home Care

- Determine the client's level of cognition and manual dexterity to assess his ability to follow instructions and physically perform the test.
- Explain necessary dietary and medication restrictions (see the Pre-Procedure Assessment section of this procedure).
- Instruct the client to collect the specimen in a clean, dry container. If an appropriate container is not available, the client may use the toilet.
- If defecating in the toilet, the client should flush it immediately prior to obtaining the sample. If commercial toilet bowl cleaners are in use, remove them from the tank, and flush twice. Then lay rice paper (from the kit) directly on the water; it is okay to get it wet. When using the probe to take the stool sample, take the sample from any area of stool that is above the water line.
- Protect the slide from heat, light, and household chemicals.
- Home collection slides come in a kit, connected together as a set of three. Instruct the client not to tear them apart.
- Emphasize to the client that each sample should be from separate bowel movements on separate days.
- After all three specimens have been collected over the course of at least 3 days, store the slide in a paper envelope to air-dry.
- The client must place the slides in the special mailing pouch that comes with the slides, if they are to be sent back to the lab. The slides should be returned to the care provider or lab no later than 14 days after the first sample was collected.

For additional instructions,

Go to the **Hemoccult** Web site at www.hemoccultfobt.com

Documentation

- Document the date and time of the specimen collection, both in the patient record and on the specimen container or FOBT kit.
- Note the appearance of the stool (e.g., color, odor) and the presence of blood, mucus, or other abnormal constituents.
- Note any rectal bleeding or discomfort during and after defecation.
- Document the test results on the appropriate agency form.
- Notify the appropriate care provider of the results.

Sample documentation

06/14/15 0915 Specimen taken from 2 separate sections of yellowish-brown soft stool containing mucus. No rectal bleeding or discomfort with defecation. Specimen sent to lab; test results pending. ——— S. Hoeszle, RN

Practice Resources

American Cancer Society (2013); Flitcroft, K. L., Irwig, L. M., Carter, S. M., et al. (2012); Gomella L., & Haist, S. (n.d.); Institute for Clinical Systems Improvement (ICSI) (2012); The Joint Commission Accreditation Program (2013); Siegel, J., Rhinehart, E., Jackson, M., et al. (2007).

Procedure 29-2 ■ Placing and Removing a Bedpan

➤ For steps to follow in *all* procedures, refer to the Universal Steps for All Procedures found on the inside back cover.

Equipment

- Bedpan
- Two pairs of clean gloves
- Toilet tissue
- Prepackaged disposable wipes
- Waterproof pad
- Bedpan cover

Delegation

You may delegate the placement and removal of a bedpan to the NAP after ensuring that the NAP has the necessary skills and that the patient's condition is stable. Complete the pre-procedure assessments, and inform the NAP of any special considerations (e.g., medical or surgical conditions that will necessitate the use of a fracture pan, extra care with turning or required positioning based on medical condition).

Pre-Procedure Assessments

- Assess the patient's level of consciousness, ability to follow directions, mobility status and physical status.
  Helps determine whether one or two persons are needed to complete the procedure
- Determine the patient's comfort level—note the presence of rectal or abdominal pain, hemorrhoids, or perianal irritation.
  Pain can cause difficulty with positioning and bearing down during defecation. Any unexplained pain should be evaluated by the primary care provider.
- Identify factors that will necessitate the use of a fracture pan. (Examples include a fractured pelvis; total hip replacement; lower back surgery; presence of casts, splints, or braces on lower limbs; or obesity.)

- Auscultate bowel sounds, and palpate for distention if indicated.
  The colon when full with fecal matter is a rounded, firm mass. A smooth, round mass above the symphysis pubis is a distended bladder.
- Review the patient's chart to determine the need to obtain a stool specimen.
  Promotes efficiency by allowing you to obtain a specimen container before placing the patient on the bedpan.

Procedure 29-2A ■ Placing a Bedpan

➤ When performing the procedure, always identify your patient according to agency policy, using two identifiers, and be attentive to standard precautions, hand hygiene, patient safety and privacy, body mechanics, and documentation.

Procedure Steps

1. **Obtain the necessary supplies,** and take them to the patient's room. Leave prepackaged disposable wipes at the bedside for use during bedpan removal.
   The patient will need to wash her hands after using the bedpan.

2. **If the bedpan is metal,** place it under warm, running water for a few seconds. Then dry it, making sure bedpan is not too hot.
   A warm bedpan allows the patient to be more comfortable and helps relax the anal sphincter. Most bedpans now are made of disposable plastic.

3. **Raise the siderail** on the opposite side from where you are working.
   Prevents patient from falling out of bed and gives the patient something to hold onto while moving around in bed.

4. **Raise the bed** to a comfortable working height.
   Allows you to use good body mechanics and prevents muscle strain.

5. **Prepare the patient** by folding down the covers to a point that will allow for placement of the bedpan, yet exposing only as much of her body as necessary.
   Privacy facilitates elimination by promoting relaxation.

6. **Perform hand hygiene** and don clean procedure gloves.
   Prevents the spread of microorganisms via contact with urine or feces.

7. **Observe for the presence of** dressings, drains, intravenous fluids, and traction; and be sure there is a linen saver pad in place.
   These appliances may hinder the patient from assisting with the procedure and may create the need for assistance from another caregiver.

Procedure Variation For the Patient Able to Move/Turn Independently in Bed

8. **Position the patient.**

Supine Position

a. Lower the head of the bed, placing the patient in a supine position.
b. Ask the patient to lift her hips. The patient may need to raise her knees to a flexed position, place her feet flat on the bed, and push up. You can also assist the patient to raise her hips by sliding a hand under the small of her back.

Semi-Fowler's Position

c. Place the bed in a semi-Fowler's position.
d. Ask the patient to raise her hips by pushing up on raised siderails or by using an overhead trapeze.

9. **Place the bedpan.**

Regular Bedpan

a. Place the bedpan under the patient's buttocks so that the wide, rounded end is toward the back.
   Sliding the pan against the patient's skin may cause damage to skin.

Fracture Pan

b. Place the wide, rounded end of the pan toward the front.

10. **Instruct or assist the patient** to lower her hips onto the bedpan. Move to Step 16.

Procedure Variation For the Patient Unable to Move/Turn Independently

11. **Ask for help** from another health-care worker if the patient's condition warrants.

12. **With the patient in the supine** position, lower the head of the bed.

13. **Assist the patient to** the side-lying position. Use a turn sheet, if necessary.

14. **Place the bedpan.**

Regular Bedpan

a. Place the bedpan under the patient's buttocks so that the wide, rounded end is toward the back. Do not push the pan under the patient's buttocks. ▼

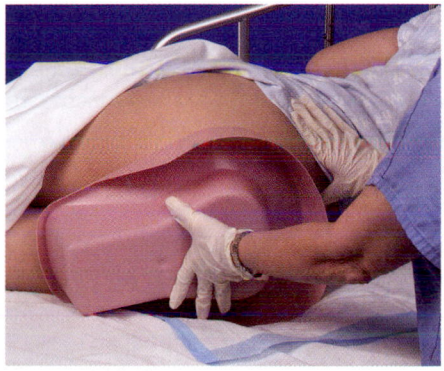

Fracture Pan

b. When using a fracture pan, place the wide, rounded end toward the front. ▼

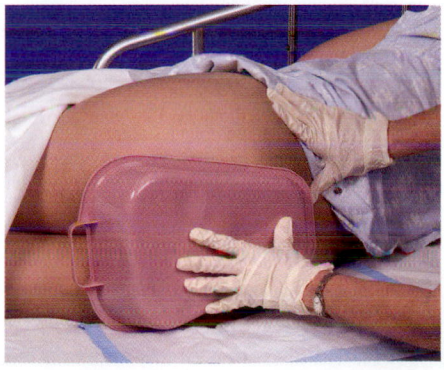

15. **Holding the bedpan in place,** slowly roll the patient back and onto the bedpan.

(continued on next page)

Procedure 29-2 ■ Placing and Removing a Bedpan (continued)

16. **Replace the covers**; raise the head of the bed to a position of comfort for the patient. Place a rolled towel, blanket, or small pillow under the sacrum (lumbar curve of the back).

17. **Place the call light** and toilet tissue within the patient's reach. Return the bed to its lowest position and raise the upper siderails.
Provides privacy, comfort, and safety.

18. **Remove your gloves** and perform hand hygiene.
Prevents the transmission of intestinal bacteria.

Procedure 29-2B ■ Removing a Bedpan

➤ When performing the procedure, always identify your patient according to agency policy, using two identifiers, and be attentive to standard precautions, hand hygiene, patient safety and privacy, body mechanics, and documentation.

Procedure Steps

1. **Don clean procedure gloves.** Open the prepackaged disposable wipes and place them near the work area.

2. **If the patient is immobile**, lower the head of the patient's bed. Pull down the covers only as far as needed to remove the bedpan.
Lowering the head of the bed is necessary only if the patient is immobile.

3. **Offer the patient toilet paper.** Assist patients who are unable to complete this task independently.

4. **Ask the mobile patient to raise her hips.** Stabilize and remove the bedpan. If the patient is unable to raise her hips, stabilize the bedpan and assist her to the side-lying position, and remove the bedpan.
Stabilizing the bedpan prevents spillage of contents.

5. **Cleanse the buttocks** with a warm, prepackaged disposable wipe. Allow to air dry.
Provides comfort and hygiene and decreases the risk of skin irritation and breakdown.

6. **Replace covers, and position** the patient for comfort. Offer the patient the second wipe to cleanse her hands.
Encourages independence with personal hygiene and decreases transmission of bacteria.

7. **Empty the bedpan** into the patient's toilet. Measure the output if that is part of the treatment plan. Clean the bedpan, following facility-specific guidelines.
If there is no toilet in the patient's room, cover the bedpan and carry it to the nearest toilet or soiled utility room for emptying.

8. **Remove the soiled gloves** and perform hand hygiene.
Prevents transmission of infectious microorganisms.

? What if . . .

Your patient is an older adult?

Offer a bedpan at set intervals, perhaps in conjunction with a turning schedule. For elderly clients with limited mobility you may wish to keep the bedpan readily available.
To minimize episodes of incontinence and/or falls. Trying to get out of bed to use the toilet is a common cause of falls

Evaluation

- Assess the amount and characteristics of any urine and/or stool.
- Observe the skin on the perineum and buttocks for redness and breakdown.

Home Care

Teach the patient's family the steps of this procedure.

Documentation

- Document the amount of urine voided if intake and output are being recorded.
- Note the presence of any unusual characteristics of either stool or urine, and include in the nursing notes. If there are no unusual characteristics, document the passage of stool or urine in the graphic records.

Practice Resources

Ayello, E., & Sibbald, R. (2008); Balas, M., Casey, C., & Happ, M. (2008); Gray-Micelli, D. (2008); Siegel, J., Rhinehart, E., Jackson, M., et al. (2007).

Thinking About the Procedure

To practice applying clinical reasoning to this procedure,

Go to *Davis's Nursing Skills Videos*, **Placing a Bedpan** and **Removing a Bedpan.**

For questions and suggested responses,

Go to Chapter 29, **Thinking About the Procedure Questions and Suggested Responses,** on Davis*Plus*.

Procedure 29-3 ■ Administering an Enema

➤ For steps to follow in *all* procedures, refer to the Universal Steps for All Procedures found on the inside back cover.

Equipment

- Enema administration container, correct enema solution, or prepackaged enema—depends on the type of enema ordered.
  - *Enema kit:* This may be a grouping of supplies that includes a small plastic bucket or a 1-liter plastic bag with attached tubing, disposable toweling, lubricant, and castile soap.
  - *Prepackaged enema solution:* If a prepackaged enema (e.g., Fleets) is ordered, you may need to obtain the preparation from the pharmacy or central supply department.
- Prepackaged disposable wipes and/or toilet tissue
- Bath blanket
- Waterproof pad
- Bedpan with cover or bedside commode, if needed
- Water-soluble lubricant
- Clean procedure gloves
- IV pole

Delegation

You may delegate this procedure to the NAP if the NAP is trained and the patient is stable. Complete the pre-procedure assessments, and instruct the NAP about conditions under which the procedure should be stopped (e.g., severe abdominal pain occurs, bleeding is seen, or the patient is unable to retain the solution). Instruct the NAP to report the results of the enema and show you any stool that appears to be abnormal (e.g., containing blood or pus).

Pre-Procedure Assessments

- Assess for history of bowel disorders (e.g., diverticulitis, ulcerative colitis, recent bowel surgery, abdominal pain, abdominal distention, hemorrhoids).
  Some disorders put the patient at risk for complications, such as mucosal irritation or perforation. Abdominal pain along with hypoactive bowel sounds and distention could indicate a bowel obstruction.
- Inspect the abdomen for the presence of distention.
  Establishes baseline for effectiveness of the enema.
- Review the patient's chart for the presence of increased intracranial pressure, glaucoma, or recent rectal or prostate surgery.
  These conditions contraindicate an enema.
- Review lab results, paying particular attention to blood urea nitrogen (BUN), creatinine, and electrolytes.
  Hypertonic and hypotonic enemas have been linked to fluid and electrolyte changes. Phosphate enemas (Fleets) have been associated with hyperphosphatemia and hypocalcemia.
- Note the date and time of the patient's last bowel movement, recent bowel movement pattern, and bowel sounds.
  Establishes baseline for evaluating bowel function.
- Assess the patient's cognitive level and mobility.
  Determines the patient's ability to follow instructions and the need for placing him on a bedpan for the enema.
- Assess the patient's rectal sphincter control.
  Determines whether you need to administer the enema with the patient on the bedpan. Also influences the amount of solution to instill.
- Assess for fecal impaction.
  May necessitate the need to obtain a prescription for a different type of enema.

Procedure 29-3A ■ Administering a Cleansing Enema

➤ When performing the procedure, always identify your patient according to agency policy, using two identifiers, and be attentive to standard precautions, hand hygiene, patient safety and privacy, body mechanics, and documentation.

Procedure Steps

1. **Place the bedpan nearby** or the commode near the bed.
   So you can reach the bedpan during the procedure; or so the patient can easily get to the commode.

2. **Open the enema supplies or kit.** Attach the tubing to the enema pail, if you are using a pail.
   The 1-liter enema bag comes with preconnected tubing.

3. **Close the clamp on the tubing,** and fill the container with 500 to 1,000 mL of warm solution. The water temperature should be lukewarm—105°F to 110°F (40°C to 43°C).

   ✚ Check the temperature with a bath thermometer. Never warm the enema solution in a microwave oven.

   a. For infants: Use 50 to 150 mL of solution.
   b. For toddlers: Use 250 to 350 mL of solution.
   c. For school-age children, use 300 to 500 mL of solution.
   Cold solution causes intestinal cramping. Very hot solution can damage the intestinal mucosa. Use the correct amount of solution to decrease the necessity of repeating the procedure.

4. **Add castile soap** (or the soap solution used by your facility) to the fluid at this time if a soapsuds enema has been prescribed.
   Soap causes mucosal irritation, which stimulates peristalsis and defecation.

(continued on next page)

Procedure 29-3 ■ Administering an Enema (continued)

5. **Hang the container** on the IV pole. Holding the end of the tubing over a sink or waste can, open the clamp and slowly allow the tubing to prime (fill) with solution. Reclamp the tubing when the tubing is filled.
Expresses air from the tubing. Air introduced into the bowel may cause intestinal distention and discomfort.

6. **Don clean procedure gloves.**
Prevents the transmission of intestinal bacteria.

7. **Position the patient:** Ask or assist the patient to turn, to a left side-lying position with the right knee flexed.
Allows the enema solution to fill the rectum and lower intestine following the natural flow of gravity.
   a. If the patient has shortness of breath associated with a respiratory condition, elevate the head of the bed very slightly. Avoid the semi-Fowler's position.
   The semi-Fowler's position increases the likelihood that gravity will cause the solution to leak out.
   b. Do not administer the enema with the patient on the toilet. The curved rectal tubing can scrape the rectal wall.
   c. If the patient has poor sphincter control, position him on the bedpan in a comfortable dorsal recumbent position.
   He will not be able to retain all of the enema solution.

8. **Place the waterproof pad** under the patient's buttocks or hips.
Prevents soiling of bed linens.

9. **Drape the patient** with the bath blanket, exposing only the buttocks and rectum. See Procedure 25-4 to review the procedure for draping.
Promotes patient privacy.

10. **Depending on the patient's** mobility status, place the bedpan flat on the bed, directly beneath the rectum, up against the patient's buttocks.

11. **Lubricate the tip of the enema** tubing generously.
Allows for ease of insertion, decreases patient discomfort, and helps prevent mucosal irritation.

12. **If necessary, lift the superior buttock** to expose the anus. Slowly and gently insert the tip of the tubing approximately 7 to 10 cm (3 to 4 in.) into the rectum. Have the patient take slow, deep breaths as you complete this step. If the tube does not pass with ease, do not force it. Allow a small amount of fluid to infuse and then try again, inserting the tube slowly.
Helps the patient to relax, provides additional lubrication, and decreases reflex tightening of the anal sphincter.

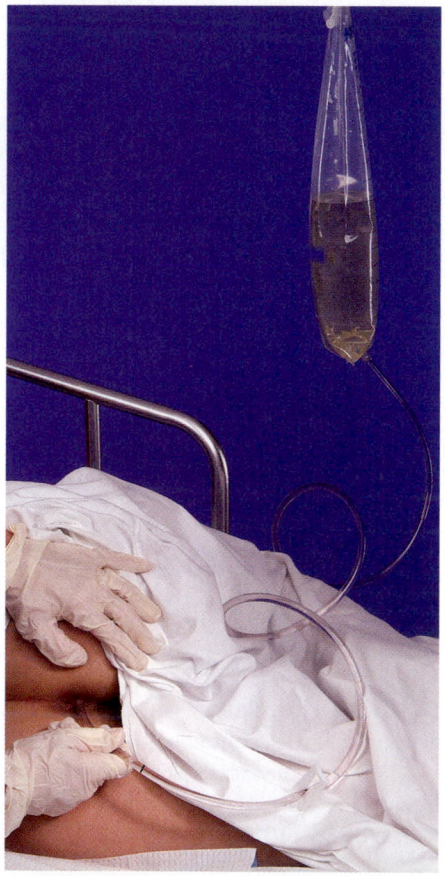

13. **Remove the container from the IV pole,** and hold it at the level of the patient's hips. Unclamp to begin instilling the solution.
Lowering the container slows the force of the instillation, decreasing pressure, cramping, discomfort, and reflex expulsion of the solution.

14. **Slowly raise the level** of the container, so that it is 30 to 45 cm (12 to 18 in.) above the level of the hips. Adjust the pole and re-hang the container. Continue a slow, steady instillation of the enema solution.
The height of the container determines the speed of the flow. A slow, steady rate of infusion decreases cramping and increases the patient's ability to retain the solution.

15. **Continuously monitor the patient** for pain or discomfort and ability to retain the solution. If the patient has difficulty with retaining the solution, lower the container, stop the flow for 15 to 30 seconds, and then resume the procedure.

If the patient feels pain or you meet with resistance at any time during the procedure, stop and consult with the primary care provider.

16. **When the correct amount** of solution has been instilled, clamp the tubing, and slowly remove it from the rectum. If there is stool on the tubing, wrap the end of the tubing in a disposable wipe or toilet tissue until it can be rinsed or disposed of. Remove the bedpan.
Prevents transmission of pathogens.

17. **Clean the rectal area,** cover the patient, and instruct him to hold the enema solution for approximately 5 to 15 minutes. Place the call light within reach.
Retention of the enema solution will distend the bowel and increase the stimulus to defecate. Leaving the solution in the bowel too long may result in fluid and electrolyte complications. Retaining hypertonic solutions may result in dehydration related to large amounts of fluids moving from the capillary bed into the bowel. Excessive retention of hypotonic solutions may cause fluid overload.

18. **Dispose of the enema supplies** or, if they are reusable, clean and store them in an appropriate location in the patient's room.
Maintains a pleasant environment and helps prevent transfer of pathogens.

19. **Remove your gloves and perform hand hygiene.**
Prevents transmission of intestinal pathogens.

20. **Depending on the patient's mobility**, assist him onto the bedpan, to the bedside commode, or to the toilet when he feels the need to defecate. Perform hand hygiene and use clean procedure gloves as necessary.

21. **After the patient has defecated**, remove the bedpan or assist the patient to bed; inspect the stool for color, consistency, and quantity.

Procedure 29-3B ■ Administering a Prepackaged Enema

➤ When performing the procedure, always identify your patient according to agency policy, using two identifiers, and be attentive to standard precautions, hand hygiene, patient safety and privacy, body mechanics, and documentation.

Procedure Steps

1. **Open the prepackaged enema.** Remove the plastic cap from the container. Clip the tip of the container if it does not have a hole in it. The tip of the enema container comes prelubricated. However, you may need to add extra lubricant.
Extra lubricant decreases discomfort and eases insertion of the tube into the rectum.

2. **Follow Steps 6 through 12 of Procedure 29-3A** (regarding gloving, positioning, draping, and inserting the enema tip).

3. **Tilt the container slightly** and slowly roll and squeeze the container until all of the solution is instilled.
Ensures that the container empties completely and that an adequate amount of solution is instilled.

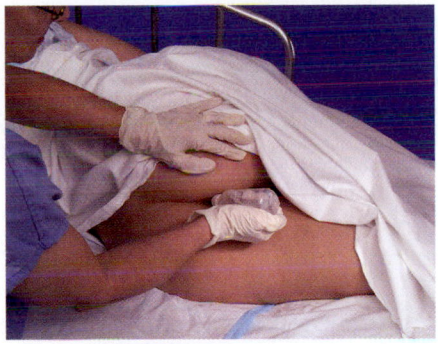

4. **Withdraw the container tip** from the rectum. Wipe the area with a disposable wipe or toilet tissue.
Prevents transmission of pathogens.

5. **Cover the patient, and instruct** him to hold the enema solution for approximately 5 to 10 minutes. Place the call light within reach.
Retention of the enema solution will distend the bowel and increase the stimulus to defecate. Retaining the solution for longer than the prescribed time has been associated with dehydration and electrolyte imbalances.

6. **Dispose of the empty container.**
Maintains a pleasant environment.

7. **Follow Steps 18 through 21 of Procedure 29-3A** (regarding equipment disposal, assisting the patient, and observations of stool).

Procedure 29-3C ■ Administering an Oil-Retention Enema

➤ When performing the procedure, always identify your patient according to agency policy, using two identifiers, and be attentive to standard precautions, hand hygiene, patient safety and privacy, body mechanics, and documentation.

➤ *Note:* An oil-retention enema may be administered to help a client pass hard stool; it also may be administered before digital removal of stool; or it may be given at least 1 hour before a cleansing enema. See Procedure 29-4 for digital removal of stool.

Procedure Steps

1. **Obtain a commercial** oil-retention enema kit; these kits include a small rectal tube. If a commercial kit is not available, use a small tube and about 90 to 120 mL of the prescribed solution.
A small tube allows for slower infusion, which minimizes cramping and thereby promotes retention.

2. **Warm the oil** to body temperature by running warm tap water over the container. Test a drop on your arm.
If the oil is too cold, it will cause cramping and expulsion of the oil. If it is too warm, it may injure the patient.

3. **Follow Steps 6 through 12 of Procedure 29-3A** (regarding gloving, positioning, draping, and inserting the enema tip).

4. **Instill the oil into the rectum.**
Softens stool and lubricates the rectum for easier passage of stool.

5. **Withdraw the container tip** from the rectum. Wipe the area with a disposable wipe or toilet tissue.

6. **Cover the patient and instruct** the patient to retain the oil for at least 30 minutes.

7. **Follow Steps 18 through 21 of Procedure 29-3A** (regarding equipment disposal, assisting the patient, and observations of stool).

(continued on next page)

Procedure 29-3 ■ Administering an Enema (continued)

Procedure 29-3D ■ Administering a Return-Flow Enema

➤ When performing the procedure, always identify your patient according to agency policy, using two identifiers, and be attentive to standard precautions, hand hygiene, patient safety and privacy, body mechanics, and documentation.

➤ *Note:* A return-flow enema (Harris flush) may be ordered to help a patient expel flatus and relieve abdominal distention.

Procedure Steps

1. **Obtain a rectal tube and solution** container (e.g., bag or pail).
2. **Prepare 100 to 200 mL** (for adults) of tap water or saline.
3. **Follow Steps 6 through 12 of Procedure 29-3A** (regarding gloving, positioning, draping, and inserting the enema tip).
4. **Instill all the solution** into the patient's rectum.
5. **Lower the tube and container** below the level of the rectum, and allow the solution to flow back into the container.
6. **Repeat this process several times**, or until the distention is relieved.
7. **Follow Steps 18 through 21 of Procedure 29-3A** (regarding equipment disposal, assisting the patient, and observations of stool).

? What if . . .

- **The solution for a return-flow enema becomes thick with fecal matter?**

  Discard it and begin again with new solution.

Evaluation

- Observe the amount, color, and consistency of the stool.
- Evaluate the patient's tolerance of the procedure (e.g., amount of cramping, discomfort).
- Determine whether the prescriber's orders require subsequent enema administration.
- Some bowel exams require repeated enemas or enemas administered until the returns are "clear." For the latter, you will need to examine the return and determine whether stool particles are still present. "Clear" does not mean absence of color, but rather absence of stool particles and transparency of the liquid.

Patient Teaching

- Teach the patient that dependence on enemas can disrupt the normal process that stimulates defecation.
- Teach dietary and lifestyle changes that promote regular elimination (e.g., increased fluid intake, diet high in fiber, increased exercise).

Home Care

- Show the patient the box for a prepackaged enema, and instruct him that he may purchase this type of enema at a local grocery or pharmacy.
- Assess the patient's ability to administer his own enema. If you determine that he will be unable to do so, encourage him to seek assistance and instruct the caregiver in the task.
- Teach the patient or caregiver proper handwashing. Encourage them to purchase nonsterile procedure gloves.

  Patients and caregivers may not be aware of the serious infections that can be caused by gram-negative intestinal bacteria.
- If the patient will be attempting to self-administer a cleansing enema, help him determine how and where to hang the container so that it is at the proper height.
- If a soapsuds enema is to be administered in the home setting, teach the patient which household soaps may be substituted for castile soap.

  Some soaps used in the home for cleaning purposes may be too harsh and irritating to the intestinal mucosa.

Documentation

- Document on the nursing notes type of enema given and, if applicable, the amount of the solution instilled; patient's tolerance of the procedure; characteristics and amount of stool.
- If the prescription is to administer enemas until the returns are clear, document the color of the return solution and the amount of stool seen.
- For prepackaged enemas, some facilities require documentation on the medication administration record (MAR) of the time given and the nurse's initials.

Sample documentation

06/04/2015 0825 Fleets enema administered (see MAR). Patient had no cramping; retained enema for 5 minutes. Passed moderate amount of solid, formed, brown stool with no mucus, but with streaks of bright red blood on the surface. _____ *R. Cline, RN*

Thinking About the Procedure

To practice applying clinical reasoning to this procedure,

Go to *Davis's Nursing Skills Videos*, **Administering a Cleansing Enema.**

For questions and suggested responses,

Go to Chapter 29, **Thinking About the Procedure Questions and Suggested Responses**, on Davis*Plus*.

Procedure 29-4 ■ Removing Stool Digitally

➤ For steps to follow in *all* procedures, refer to the Universal Steps for All Procedures found on the inside back cover.

Equipment

- Two pairs of clean procedure gloves
- Water-soluble lubricant (containing lidocaine, if agency policy permits)
- Bedpan and cover
- Prepackaged disposable wipes (or moistened towelettes)
- Bath blanket
- Waterproof pad

Delegation

This procedure should not be delegated to a NAP. Ongoing assessment of the patient by the professional nurse is required when stool is manually removed from the rectum. The nurse must monitor the patient for complications, such as bleeding and vagal nerve stimulation. Nursing judgment is necessary in determining the need to halt the procedure.

Pre-Procedure Assessments

- Assess the patient's baseline vital signs and history of heart disease. Be sure to monitor the patient's pulse before and during the procedure.
  Digital removal of stool can stimulate the vagus nerve, causing bradycardia. Patients who have a history of heart disease or dysrhythmia are at greater risk.
- Assess the patient's white blood cell (WBC) count.
  If the patient has a compromised immune status, evidenced by a low WBC count, you should discuss this procedure with the primary care provider to evaluate the risks and benefits of the procedure.
- Assess the patient's cognitive level and mobility.
  Determines the patient's ability to follow directions and turn in bed.
- Determine the time of the patient's last bowel movement.
  The longer stool remains in the lower bowel, the more water can be absorbed and the more likely it is that hard stool may form in the rectum.
- Assess the patient for history of fecal impaction.
  Can be a recurrent problem for immobile, disabled, or institutionalized patients.
- Assess stool consistency.
  Patients who are immobilized may become incontinent of watery stool. They may be able to pass small sections of hard stool or small quantities of watery stool. The latter, which may be intermittent or continuous, is a symptom of high colon impaction.
- Ask whether the patient has pain on defecation.
  Pain can cause the patient tends to suppress defecation, exacerbating the problem.
- Assess the patient's pattern of bowel movements, diet, exercise, mobility, and medications (e.g., iron supplements or opioid analgesics).
  Determine whether any of these factors contribute to the problem and add this information to the nursing care plan to help prevent recurrence.
- Assess bowel sounds and any abdominal distention.
  Peristalsis may be present without gastrointestinal patency. This creates abdominal distention, which can aggravate constipation.

Guidelines

- Prevention of fecal impaction is the best treatment, but if impaction has occurred, the stool must be removed. The procedure is both painful and embarrassing to your patient.
- Some practitioners may prescribe an oil-retention enema before the procedure to soften and moisten the stool, making removal easier.
- Many also advise that you follow digital removal of stool with either an oil-retention and/or tap water enema, to ensure evacuation of stool that may not have been reached by digital removal.
- Trim and file your fingernails if they extend past the end of your fingertips.

➤ When performing the procedure, always identify your patient according to agency policy, using two identifiers, and be attentive to standard precautions, hand hygiene, patient safety and privacy, body mechanics, and documentation.

Procedure Steps

1. **Determine whether lubricant** containing lidocaine is to be used, and obtain the correct lubricant.
   May decrease rectal discomfort for the patient.
2. **Drape the patient** with the bath blanket. Go to Procedure 24-4 to review the procedure for draping. Assist him to turn on his left side, with his right knee flexed toward his head. Place the waterproof pad halfway beneath his left hip.
   Provides privacy and exposes the anus for visualization. The pad protects the bed from being soiled.
3. **Don clean procedure gloves.** Some sources recommend double-gloving.
   Prevents the transmission of intestinal bacteria.
4. **Expose the buttocks.** Place a clean, dry bedpan on the waterproof pad next to the buttocks in line with the rectum.
5. **Open the packet of prepackaged disposable** wipes, or have toilet tissue ready to cleanse the rectal area when you complete the procedure.

(continued on next page)

Procedure 29-4 ■ Removing Stool Digitally (continued)

6. **Generously lubricate either** the gloved forefinger and/or middle finger on your dominant hand.
Helps prevent discomfort, pain, and mucosal injury.

7. **Slowly slide one lubricated** finger into the rectum. Observe for perianal irritation.
The patient may need skin care to reduce pain during additional bowel evacuation.

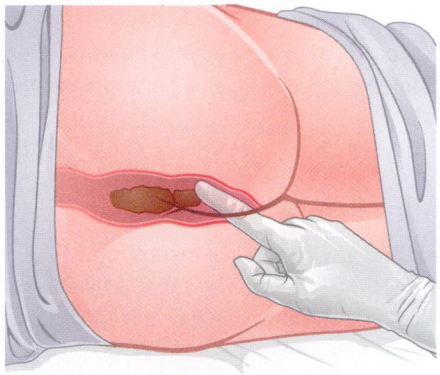

8. **Gently rotate your finger** around the mass and/or into the mass.
Assists in determining the amount and texture of the fecal bulk.

9. **Begin to break the stool** into smaller pieces. At this point, you may insert a second finger and gently "slice" apart the stool, using a scissoring motion. Remove pieces of stool via the rectum as they become separated, and place them in the bedpan.

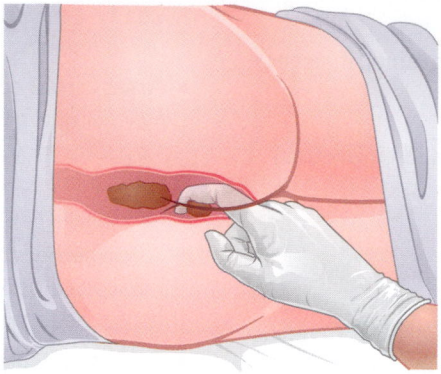

10. **As you proceed, instruct** the patient to take slow, deep breaths.
Helps the patient to relax his anal sphincter.

11. **Continue to manipulate** and remove pieces of stool, allowing the patient to rest at intervals. Reapply lubricant (containing lidocaine, if permitted) each time you reinsert your fingers.
Rest periods allow for assessment of and attention to the patient's comfort level and tolerance for the procedure.

12. **Assess the patient's heart rate** at regular intervals.
Bradycardia is a sign of vagal stimulation. Stop the procedure if the patient's heart rate falls or the rhythm changes from your initial assessment.

CAUTION: Some resources suggest that this procedure should be done in small steps (no more than four finger insertions in one session), giving a series of suppositories between stool removal episodes.

Prevents patient fatigue and pain. Reduces the risk of injury to the rectal tissue and vagal stimulation.

13. **When removal of stool** is complete, cover the bedpan and set it aside. Use a prepackaged disposable wipe and/or toilet tissue to cleanse the rectal area.
Provides personal hygiene and decreases transmission of pathogens.

14. **Assist the patient to return** to a position of comfort. Note the color, amount, and consistency of the stool, and dispose of it properly.

15. **Remove your gloves and** perform hand hygiene.
Prevents transmission of intestinal pathogens.

? What if . . .

- **The patient is an infant?**
When treating infants with fecal impactions, avoid enemas and mineral oils. Glycerin suppositories may be used to soften the stool before removal.

Evaluation

- Determine whether evacuation of the retained stool was complete. Perform a rectal exam to assess for presence of stool.
- Reassess vital signs, and compare the results to the initial assessment. Continue to monitor for 1 hour for bradycardia.
- Assess bowel sounds.
- Palpate the abdomen for tenderness and firmness.
- Ask the patient whether he feels relief from rectal pressure or abdominal discomfort.

Patient Teaching

Retained stool is most often the result of poor dietary habits, lack of fluid intake, lack of exercise, inattentiveness to the urge to defecate, and laxative abuse. Focus patient teaching on lifestyle changes that will facilitate a regular bowel elimination pattern.

Home Care

Home care should focus on preventing constipation that would require the digital removal of stool. Teach clients about high-fiber foods, adequate water intake, and the importance of exercise. Digital removal of stool may be necessary for some clients as part of a bowel program, for example patients who are paraplegic or tetraplegic (quadriplegic). You can teach this procedure to the caregiver in the home.

Documentation

- Document the bowel movement on the graphic record.
- Document the procedure and the patient's tolerance for the procedure in the nursing notes.
- Record the patient's pulse rate on the vital signs record.
- Document any unusual characteristics of the stool (e.g., black or green color, blood, or mucus).

Sample documentation

07/11/15 1815 Impacted stool removed digitally. No perianal irritation noted. Removed moderate amount (approximately 6 oz [170g]) dry, hard, gray-colored stool. Pulse 78 before removal; 84 after. Encouraged 8 oz of fluid every hour. —— C. Bryan, RNC

Practice Resources

National Guideline Clearinghouse (NGC) (1996, revised 2009, 2010); Obokhare, I. (2012); Siegel, J., Rhinehart, E., Jackson, M., et al. (2007).

Procedure 29-5 ■ Inserting a Rectal Tube

➤ For steps to follow in *all* procedures, refer to the Universal Steps for All Procedures found on the inside back cover.

Equipment

- 22- to 34-French rectal tube for adults. Choose the size according to the size of the client. For children or petite adults, a smaller size tube (12- to 18-Fr) may be required.
- Water-soluble lubricant
- Procedure gloves
- Toilet paper
- Skin care items (e.g., soap, skin cleanser, disposable wipes)
- Collecting device (waterproof pad, graduated cylinder partially filled with water, a urine collection bag nicked at the top to vent)
- Paper tape
- Stool specimen container if needed

Pre-Procedure Assessments

- Obtain baseline vital signs.
- Auscultate bowel sounds; percuss for tympany.
- Observe and palpate the degree of abdominal distention.
- Ask whether the patient is passing any flatus.
- Assess discomfort caused by flatulence.
- Assess the condition of perianal tissues.
- Assess the history of cardiac disease.
  Insertion of a rectal tube can stimulate the vagus nerve, causing bradycardia.

➤ When performing the procedure, always identify your patient according to agency policy, using two identifiers, and be attentive to standard precautions, hand hygiene, patient safety and privacy, body mechanics, and documentation.

Procedure Steps

1. **Wear procedure gloves.**
   Follows standard precautions.

2. **Ask the patient to lift his hips** or roll from side to side to place a waterproof pad.
   Protects against soiling of linens.

3. **Attach a collecting device** to the end of the rectal tube: Tape a plastic bag or urine collection bag around the distal end of the rectal tube and vent the upper side of the bag. Alternatively:

Use one of these alternatives:

- Insert the tube into the specimen container.
- Place the end of the tube in a graduated container partially filled with water.
  Collects small pieces of stool expelled with flatus. Venting the plastic bag prevents overinflation and bursting the bag. An advantage of using water in the container is that gas generates bubbles, and you will be able to assess the effectiveness of the rectal tube based on the amount of bubbling in the container.

4. **Place patient in left side-lying** position. Drape for privacy.
   Allows the tube to follow the normal curve of the rectum and sigmoid colon when inserted.

5. **Lubricate the tip** of the rectal tube.
   Prevents trauma to the rectal mucosa.

6. **Separate the buttocks** and ask the patient to take a deep breath. Gently insert the tube into the rectum.
   Adults: 10 to 12.5 cm (4 to 5 in.)
   Children: 5 to 10 cm (2 to 4 in.).
   Deep breaths relax the anal sphincter and ease tube insertion.

7. **For adults, tape the tube** in place; for children, hold it manually.

8. **Leave the rectal tube in** place for 15 to 20 minutes. If distention persists, you may reinsert the tube every 2 to 3 hours.
   Leaving the tube in place for more than 20 minutes may cause pressure necrosis of the mucosa; prolonged stimulation of the anal sphincter may result in loss of the neuromuscular response.

9. **Assist the patient to move** about in bed to promote gas expulsion. A knee–chest position is ideal.
   Because gas is lighter than fluid or solid, the position promotes passage of flatus. Unfortunately, many patients cannot tolerate this position.

10. **Remove the tube**, wipe the patient's buttocks with tissue, and assist to clean the rectal area as needed.
    Prevents transmission of microorganisms from feces; promotes patient comfort and skin integrity.

11. **Dispose of used equipment**; or clean it if it is to be reused. Follow agency procedures for cleaning.

(continued on next page)

Procedure 29-5 ■ Inserting a Rectal Tube (continued)

Evaluation

- Evaluate the patient's response to the procedure (e.g., vital signs, fatigue).
- Assess abdominal distention and abdominal comfort.

Patient Teaching

- Teach the patient that chewing gum, sucking on hard candy, using a straw, smoking, and drinking carbonated beverages increase air swallowing and abdominal distention.
- Teach factors that promote normal elimination (e.g., exercise, increased fluid intake, adequate dietary fiber).

Documentation

Record the following:

- Date and time tube was inserted
- Size of tube and characteristics of feces collected
- Abdominal distention before and after the procedure
- Pulse and respiratory rates before and after the procedure
- Tolerance of procedure and any complications
- Patient and family teaching

Procedure 29-6 ■ Changing an Ostomy Appliance

➤ For steps to follow in *all* procedures, refer to the Universal Steps for All Procedures found on the inside back cover.

➤ *Note:* Some pouches come with the wafer attached, some without. These instructions assume that the wafer is attached.

➤ *Note:* Also see Clinical Insight 29-2: Guidelines for Ostomy Care.

Also go to **Animations: Colostomy,** on Davis*Plus*.

Equipment

- Ostomy pouch
  - One-piece pouch with the wafer attached, or a two-piece system with a separate wafer and pouch
  - Clamp for pouches with an opening at the bottom (a new clamp is not used each time; usually one clamp is packaged with each box of pouches)
- Skin care items per agency protocol or recommended by the enterostomal therapist (e.g., pH balanced skin cleanser, skin prep, skin barrier wipe, adhesive remover, adhesive paste, and stoma paste if needed to fill and smooth skin surface)
- Stoma measuring guide (or precut template)
- Scissors
- Pen or pencil
- Two pairs of clean procedure gloves
- Prepackaged disposable wipes
- Toilet tissue
- 4 in. × 4 in. gauze pad
- Bedpan or container for **effluent** (fecal material)
- Plastic bag (for disposal of used pouch)
- Plastic bag for disposal of other contaminated articles
- Waterproof pad
- Ostomy deodorant
- Hypoallergenic paper tape (optional) or ostomy belt
- Bath blanket

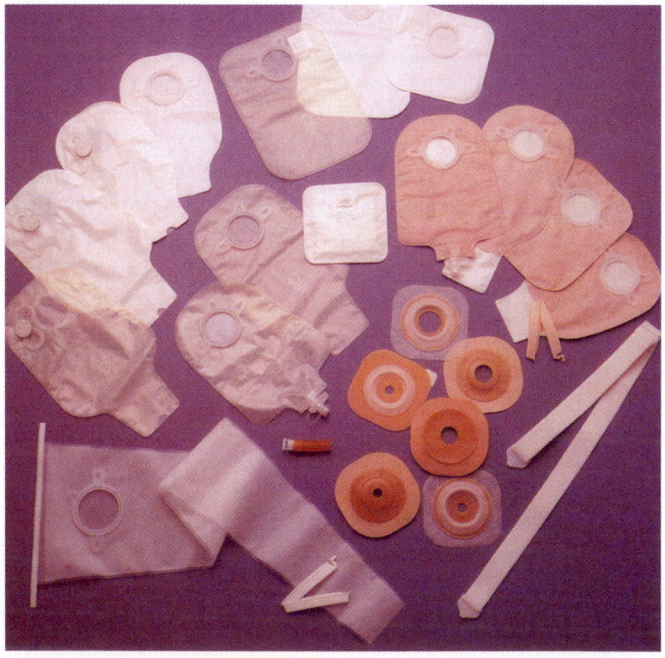

Delegation

During the immediate postoperative period, the professional nurse must assess the newly created stoma and peristomal skin area and use clinical judgment when changing a pouch. You may delegate to a NAP if it is a preexisting, stable stoma and if you are sure the NAP is qualified to perform the task. If you do delegate this task, instruct the NAP to report any changes or unusual findings (e.g., changes in stoma color, swelling, peristomal redness, excoriation, deviations from expected amount) and color and consistency of drainage from the stoma.

Pre-Procedure Assessments

- Assess the type of stoma (e.g., ileostomy, colostomy, urostomy), number of stomas, and location on the abdomen (e.g., is the stoma near structures that will impact care?). *Determines the type of pouch or system to use.*

- Assess stoma color, shape, size, and/or length of protrusion or retraction; stoma construction (end, loop, double barrel); direction of stoma lumen; and discharge. Does the stoma lie flat or does it protrude?
  The stoma should be moist and red or pink. Alterations in stoma color (purple, black, or blue) may indicate poor circulation and possible necrosis and should be reported to the primary provider. Protruding or retracted stomas will need special adjustments in wafer measurement and placement. It is normal for a new stoma to have yellow or blood-tinged mucus or dried blood on it.
- Assess peristomal skin for redness, rash, irritation, or excoriation. Observe the existing skin barrier and pouch for leakage and length of time in place. You may have to remove the pouch to observe the stoma fully, depending on the type of pouch (i.e., if the pouch is opaque). Notify the provider or an ostomy specialist immediately if you note peristomal skin abnormalities.
  Preserving peristomal skin is critical because skin excoriation may cause an ineffective seal between the wafer and the skin and leakage of effluent. This in turn causes more skin and tissue damage. Leakage may indicate the need for a different type of pouch system or sealant.
- Determine the changing schedule for the pouch.
  Pouches are usually changed every 3 to 5 days, preferably before leakage occurs. Frequency also depends on the type of stoma, the equipment used (e.g., one- or two-piece pouch), the effluent, the patient's preference, and the climate (i.e., pouches are changed more frequently during the summer). To decrease skin irritation, avoid changing the entire system. In a one-piece or two-piece pouching system, change the skin barrier only every 3 to 7 days, never daily.
- Observe abdominal shape and incision, if present.
  Abdominal shape determines the proper placement of the pouch. Because of stomal and abdominal characteristics, some patients may need convexity in their ostomy pouching system to avoid leakage.
- Assess the patient's willingness to look at the stoma, touch the appliance, and discuss or participate in the task.
  May indicate a readiness or desire to learn.
- Assess the patient's condition and self-care ability. Consider vision, dexterity or mobility, and cognitive ability.
  Helps determine best type of appliance to use.
- Auscultate for bowel sounds.
  Determines the presence of peristalsis.
- Observe for effluent from the stoma, and document your findings.
  Change the skin barrier pouch at times of lower effluent output. Avoid changing after meals, when the gastrocolic reflux increases chance of fecal effluent output. Mucous secretion is normal.
- Assess whether a new clamp will be needed or the one on the pouch can be used again.
- Consult a peristomal nurse or the primary care provider to determine whether an ostomy should be irrigated.
  Many patients with left-end colostomies may be safely irrigated as a method of continence management. An ileostomy, however, drains liquid containing high concentrations of sodium, chloride, potassium, magnesium, and bicarbonate.

Ileostomies should never be irrigated, except in cases of food blockage near the stomal outlet. Only a qualified person, such as an enterostomal therapy nurse, may perform a gentle lavage. For lavage procedure, see Procedure 29-7.

➤ When performing the procedure, always identify your patient according to agency policy, using two identifiers, and be attentive to standard precautions, hand hygiene, patient safety and privacy, body mechanics, and documentation.

Procedure Steps

1. **Perform hand hygiene** and don clean procedure gloves.
   Prevents transmission of pathogens.
2. **Fold down the bed covers** to expose the ostomy site. Place a clean towel across the patient's abdomen under the existing pouch.
   Helps prevent spilling effluent onto the patient.
3. **Position the patient** so that no skinfolds occur along the line of the stoma.
   Ensures an adequate seal between the wafer and the skin, preventing leakage.
4. **If the present ostomy pouch** is drainable, empty it into the bedpan.
   Pouches should be drained when they are one-third to one-half full because the weight of the contents may dislodge the skin seal; ostomy drainage is irritating to the skin. The pouch also collects flatus, which needs to be expelled because it can disrupt the skin seal.
   a. To calculate the amount of output in milliliters for an ostomy with a liquid effluent (e.g., ileostomy or urostomy), use a graduated measuring container.
   b. For pouches that you open by unrolling them at the bottom, you must remove a clamp to empty the pouch. Save this clamp for reuse.

   Note: Some pouches cannot be drained.
5. **Remove the appliance** by applying a silicone-based (hexamethyldisiloxane) adhesive remover, with one hand as you press the skin away from the wafer barrier with your other hand. Avoid pulling the appliance straight off. Begin at the top and work downward. ▼

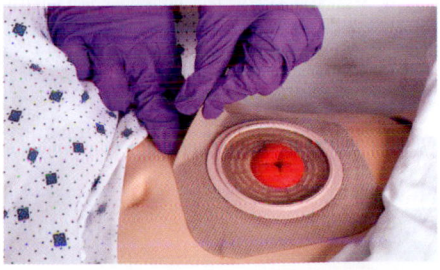

(continued on next page)

Procedure 29-6 ■ Changing an Ostomy Appliance (continued)

Silicone-based adhesive removers are preferred over alcohol- or oil-based products. Pulling the appliance from the skin tends to strip the loosely bound epidermal skin layers, making the skin more susceptible to moisture loss and irritation from effluent. Silicone-based products reduce the bind strength, whereas alcohol dissolves the adhesives; thus alcohol may cause dryness and irritation. It also causes pain if the skin is not intact. If you use an oil-based solvent, the new pouch will not adhere to the oily skin.

6. **Place the old pouch and wafer** in the plastic bag for disposal. If the pouch is not a drainable one, dispose of it according to agency protocol.
   Prevents transmission of infections caused by fecal bacteria.

7. **Inspect the stoma** and peristomal skin area for redness, rash, irritation, or excoriation (see Pre-Procedure Assessments).

8. **Cleanse the stoma** and surrounding skin using a skin cleansing agent with a pH of 5.5 that is designed to both cleanse and moisturize the skin.
   Removes old adhesive and any effluent that has leaked. Helps prevent skin irritation and/or breakdown and maintain skin moisture. Select cleansing agents that protect the stratum corneum lipids and proteins.

9. **Measure the size of the stoma.** You can accomplish this in several ways.
   a. Place a standard stoma measuring guide over the stoma.
   b. Reuse a previously cut template.
   c. Measure the stoma from side to side (approximating the circumference).
   The stoma may need to be remeasured frequently during the initial postoperative period because the size of the stoma may change as edema subsides. ➤

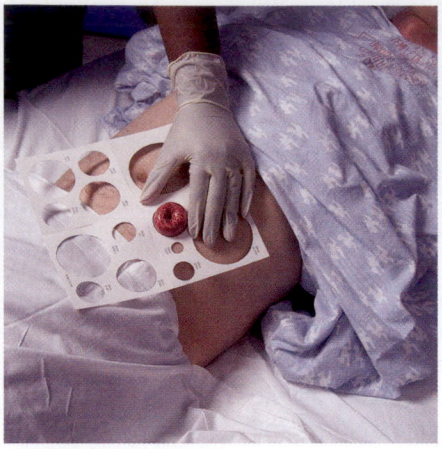

10. **Place a clean 4 in. × 4 in. gauze pad** over the stoma.
    Gauze will absorb any leaking effluent, keeping the skin clean and dry during application of the new pouch.

11. **Remove your gloves** and perform hand hygiene.
    Decreases the spread of intestinal bacteria.

12. **Trace the size of the opening** (obtained in Step 9) onto the paper on the back of the new wafer. Cut the opening. The opening in the wafer should be approximately 1/16 to 1/8 in. (1.5 to 3 mm) larger than the circumference of the stoma.
    Allows for skin movement with activity and prevents impaired circulation to the stoma.

13. **Peel the paper off the wafer.** Some resources suggest first holding the wafer between the palms of your hand to warm the adhesive ring.
    Enhances the integrity of the seal by making the ring more "sticky" so that it will bond better with the skin.

    Note: Some ostomy wafers come with an outer ring of tape attached. Do not remove the backing on this tape until the wafer is securely positioned.

14. **Don clean procedure gloves.**

15. **Apply ostomy skin care products** at this time using your clinical judgment, hospital protocol, or the recommendations of the enterostomal therapist (e.g., wipe around stoma with skin prep, apply skin barrier powder or paste, or apply extra adhesive paste).
    These products prevent or treat excoriated skin and/or ensure a tight seal between the wafer and the skin.

16. **Remove the gauze** from the stoma. Center the wafer opening around the stoma, and gently press it down. Make sure the bag is pointed toward the patient's feet. Press your hand firmly against the newly applied wafer and hold for 30 to 60 seconds.
    Heat from the hand activates the adhesive ring, making it adhere better thus promoting optimal wear time. Some sources also suggest taping down the edges of the wafer.

17. **Remove your gloves** and perform hand hygiene.

18. **Return the patient** to a comfortable position.

19. **Dispose of the used ostomy** pouch following your facility's policy for biohazardous waste.

? What if . . .

- **Your patient has a two-piece pouch?**
  After applying the wafer around the stoma with a good seal (Step 16), attach the bag following manufacturer's instructions.

- **Your patient's ostomy uses an open-ended pouch?**
  After applying the wafer securely around the stoma, fold the end of the pouch over the clamp, and close the clamp, listening for a "click" to ensure that it is secure.

- **When cleansing the stoma (Step 8), you notice that the stoma is bleeding?**
  Slight bleeding of the stoma is normal; report excessive bleeding to the primary care provider.

Evaluation

Make the following observations:

- Characteristics of stoma: color, size, presence of edema, and shape
- Presence of blisters, redness, or excoriation on peristomal skin
- Amount and characteristics of effluent: color, odor, consistency
- Whether the patient expressed a desire to participate in the task
- Whether the patient demonstrated nonverbal cues that she is ready to learn about the task (e.g., looking at the stoma)

Patient Teaching

Patient teaching is aimed at preparing the patient to complete this skill at home. She (or a caregiver) will need to be instructed in how to complete all the steps of the procedure.

Home Care

- Assess the patient's self-care ability and assist the client to establish a routine for changing the stoma wafer/pouch (see Clinical Insight 29-2).
- The client may need to stand in front of a mirror or sit to change her ostomy appliance if she is unable to view the stoma easily.
- Teach the client that slight bleeding is normal when the stoma is washed.
- The client should not use soaps and lotions containing oils. They decrease the adhesiveness of the wafer.
- The appliance and wafer cannot be flushed down the toilet.
- Teach the client to report changes in the color or size of the stoma and/or the presence of peristomal irritation or skin breakdown to the primary care provider.
- Provide information about ostomy supply vendors and community support groups, such as Ostomates.

Documentation

Document the following:

- Your assessment of the stoma and peristomal skin area
- Patient's tolerance of the procedure
- Type of appliance used, including the manufacturer and part number
- Use of any special ostomy skin care products
- Amount of liquid effluent (on the intake and output [I&O] portion of the graphics record)
- Patient teaching and the degree to which the patient participated in the procedure

Sample EHR documentation

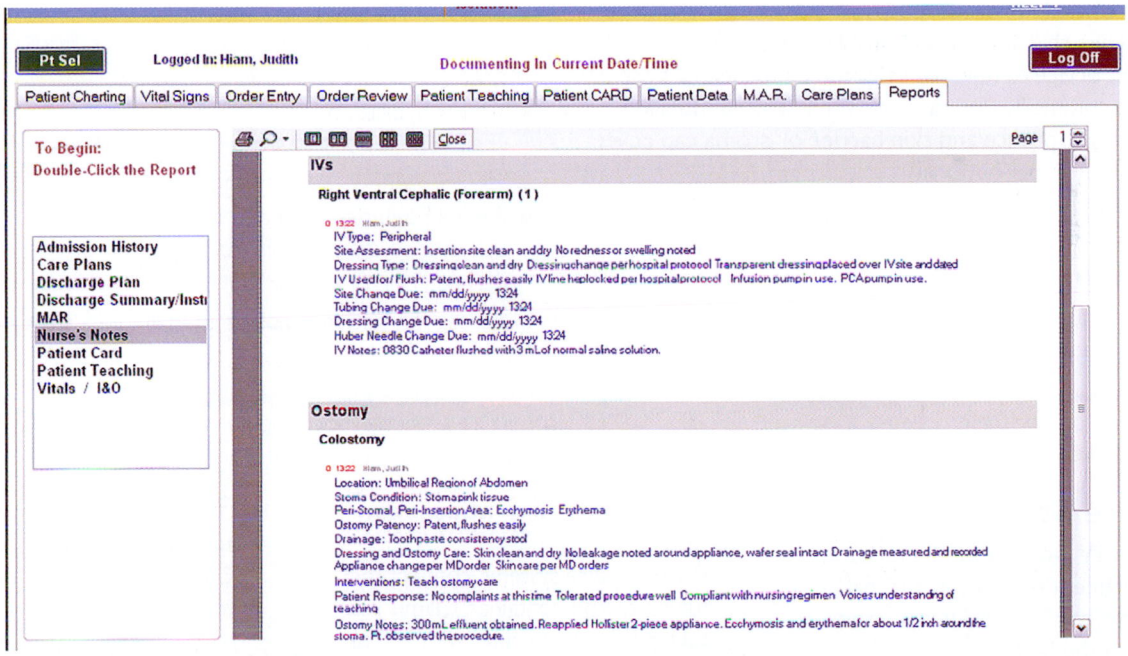

Practice Resources

Black, P. (2008); Burch, J., & Sica, J. (2008); Cronin, E. (2008); Goldberg, M., Aukett, L. K., Carmel, J., et al. (2010); Kent, M. (2008); Richbourg, L., Fellows, J., & Arroyave, W. (2008); Siegel, J., Rhinehart, E., Jackson, M., et al. (2007).

Thinking About the Procedure

To practice applying clinical reasoning to this procedure,

Go to *Davis's Nursing Skills Videos*, **Changing an Ostomy Appliance.**

For questions and suggested responses,

Go o to Chapter 29, **Thinking About the Procedure Questions and Suggested Responses,** on Davis*Plus*.

Procedure 29-7 ■ Irrigating a Colostomy

➤ For steps to follow in *all* procedures, refer to the Universal Steps for All Procedures found on the inside back cover.

➤ *Note:* Also see Clinical Insight 29-2: Guidelines for Ostomy Care.

Equipment

- Irrigation equipment
  - One-piece system with a fluid container connected to tubing with cone or two-piece system with a container separate from tubing with cone
  - Irrigation sleeve; a sleeve without adhesive backing requires a belt to hold it in place
  - Clamp for a sleeve with an opening at the top
  - Prescribed irrigating solution (usually 500 to 1,000 mL warm tap water, 100°F to 105°F (37.8°C to 40.6°C)
- IV pole or other equipment to hang the irrigation container
- Chair
- Water-soluble lubricant
- Silicone-based adhesive remover
- Skin cleansers and barriers as recommended by your agency
- Toilet tissue
- Prepackaged disposable wipes
- Waterproof pad
- Two pairs of clean procedure gloves
- Toilet facilities that include a flushable toilet and a hook or some other device to hold the irrigation container; or bedpan or bedside commode (for patients with impaired mobility)
- New ostomy appliance and skin barrier or stoma cap cover
- Ostomy deodorant (optional)
- Plastic bag for disposal of the used pouch

Delegation

The initial irrigation of a newly created colostomy requires nursing judgment and clinical decision making. Initially, this procedure should not be delegated to the NAP, although in some situations it may be delegated to an LPN, depending on agency policy.

Pre-Procedure Assessments

- Evaluate the defecation pattern (or absence) nature of stool, placement of stoma, abdominal distention, and nutritional pattern.
  Findings may indicate the need to irrigate to stimulate elimination function; consistency of stool varies along the length of the gastrointestinal (GI) tract.
- Assess the type of ostomy.
  Many patients with left-end colostomies may be safely irrigated as a method of continence management. However, do not irrigate an ileostomy.
- Assess the patient's usual bowel pattern.
  The purpose for irrigating a colostomy is to promote a regular pattern for bowel elimination.
- Assess for abdominal distention.
  Report distention to the primary care provider, as it may indicate excess gas or inflammation.
- Assess hydration.
  The colon may absorb some of the irrigation fluid if the patient is very dehydrated.
- Assess cognitive level and mobility.
  Determines the necessity for a bedpan or bedside commode. Also determines whether patient teaching will be effective.
- Assess the patient's ability to maintain a sitting position.

➤ When performing the procedure, always identify your patient according to agency policy, using two identifiers, and be attentive to standard precautions, hand hygiene, patient safety and privacy, body mechanics, and documentation.

Procedure Steps

1. **Place an IV pole near** the location of the procedure (e.g., in the bathroom, next to the bedside commode, or next to the bed).
   Allows you to work efficiently.

2. **Assist the patient to the bathroom** or commode, if possible. Ask the patient whether she prefers to sit directly on the toilet or on a chair in front of it. If the patient must remain in bed, elevate the head of the bed.
   Patients with impaired mobility can sit directly on or in front of the bedside commode, or they may remain in bed in the side-lying position.

3. **Prepare the irrigation container.**
   a. For two-piece systems, connect the tubing to the container. Clamp the tubing. Fill the container with 500 to 1,000 mL of warm tap water.

   ✚ Water that is too cold will cause cramping, nausea, and discomfort. Water that is too hot will damage the intestinal mucosa.

   Note: Some ostomy resources suggest that using 1,000 mL of water will promote a more effective irrigation of the entire colon and decrease the necessity to irrigate more than once a day.

   b. Unclamp the tubing to prime it and allow it to fill.
   Removes air from the tubing, preventing gas pains.

4. **Hang the solution container** on the IV pole. Adjust the pole so that it reaches the height of the patient's shoulder (approximately 45 cm [18 in.] above the stoma).
   The height of the container regulates the force of the flow.

5. **Perform hand hygiene** and don clean procedure gloves.
   Prevents the transmission of pathogens.

6. **Remove the existing colostomy** appliance (if the patient is wearing

one) following the steps in Procedure 29-6.
Use of ostomy skin care preparations may be needed when you replace the pouch.

7. **Dispose of the used colostomy** appliance properly. Empty the contents into the bedpan or toilet, and discard the pouch in a moisture-proof (e.g., plastic) bag.
Prevents transmission of intestinal bacteria.

8. **Assess the characteristics** of the stoma and the surrounding skin (see Clinical Insight 29-2).

9. **Apply the colostomy irrigation sleeve**, following the manufacturer's directions.
   - *If your patient is sitting on a toilet* or bedside commode, then the end of the sleeve should hang down past the patient's pubic area, but not down into the water. Place a waterproof pad under the sleeve over the patient's thighs.
   - *If your patient is in bed*, place the end of the sleeve into the bedpan.

   Prevents leakage and spilling of irrigation fluid and effluent.

10. **Generously lubricate the cone** at the end of the irrigation tubing with water-soluble lubricant.
Prevents irritation and damage to the stoma and intestinal lumen.

11. **Open the top of the irrigation** sleeve; insert the cone gently into the colostomy stoma, and hold it solidly in place.
Gentle insertion prevents damage to the mucosa.▼

12. **Open the clamp on the tubing**, and slowly begin the flow of water. The fluid should flow for about 10 to 15 minutes or as the patient can tolerate.
Proceeding slowly allows the patient to adjust to the distention of the bowel.

13. **If the patient complains** of discomfort, stop the flow for 15 to 30 seconds, and ask the patient take deep breaths.
Allows the patient to rest and adjust to the pressure of solution. Cramping may indicate that the bowel is ready to empty, the water is too cold, the flow is too fast, or the tube contains air.

14. **When the correct amount** of solution has instilled, clamp the tubing, and remove the cone from the stoma.

15. **Wrap the end of the cone** in tissue or paper towel until you can clean or dispose of it properly.
Prevents transmission of intestinal bacteria.

16. **Close the top of the irrigation** sleeve with a clamp.
Prevents spillage of irrigation fluid and feces.

17. **Wait for evacuation to occur:**
   - *If the patient is sitting*, ask her to remain sitting until most of the irrigation fluid and bowel contents have evacuated. Alternatively, you can clamp the end of the sleeve and ask the patient to ambulate to stimulate complete evacuation of stool.
   - *If the patient is in bed*, massaging the abdomen may also help stimulate return.

   This should take about 30 minutes on average. You might wait for about an hour to be certain all the fecal material has been returned.

18. **When evacuation is complete**, open the top clamp, and rinse and remove the irrigation sleeve. Set it aside.
The irrigation sleeve is reusable, but it should be rinsed promptly to make thorough cleansing easier in the following steps.

19. **Cleanse the stoma** and peristomal skin area with a warm prepackaged disposable wipe. Prep the skin and apply a new colostomy appliance, if the patient is wearing one, following the steps in Procedure 29-6. Otherwise, cover the stoma with a small gauze bandage.

20. **Clean the irrigation sleeve** with mild soap and water. Allow it to dry. Place the irrigation supplies in the proper place (e.g., in a plastic container or plastic bag).
The irrigation sleeve must be cleaned well to avoid odors and transmission of pathogens.

21. **Remove your gloves** and perform hand hygiene.
Prevents healthcare-associated infections.

22. **Assist the patient back to** a position of comfort.

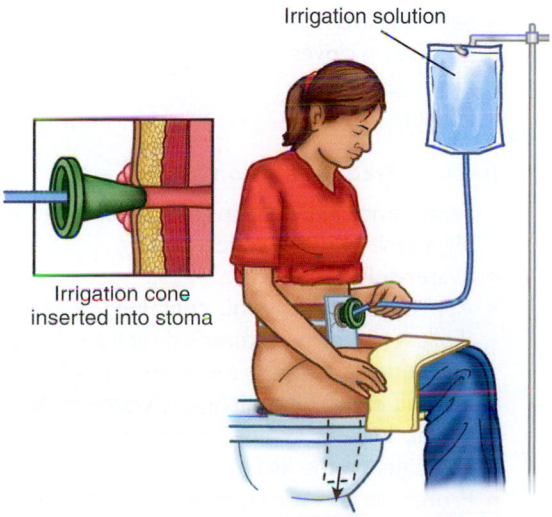

? What if . . .

- **Your patient has a colostomy sleeve without an adhesive backing?**

  Place the belt around the patient's waist, and attach the ends to the pouch flange on either side.

(continued on next page)

Procedure 29-7 ■ Irrigating a Colostomy (continued)

Evaluation

Observe the following:

- Characteristics of the stool: color, amount, consistency
- Signs of bleeding from stoma or bowel
- Presence or absence of abdominal distention
- Patient's tolerance of procedure (e.g., cramps, fatigue)
- Patient's ability to participate in the irrigation

Patient Teaching

- Teach the patient the purpose for the procedure.
- Explain that using sufficient fluid will decrease the need for multiple irrigations during the day.
- Teach the steps of the irrigation procedure to prepare the patient to complete the task at home.
- Explain that it takes approximately 6 to 8 weeks to achieve bowel regulation with irrigations.

Home Care

- Help the client determine where this procedure will be completed in the home setting.
- Make sure the client has resources for purchasing the supplies for the irrigation. Provide contact information.
- Help the client locate a place to hang the irrigation container. There may be a hook on the bathroom wall, for instance.
- If the irrigating solution does not flow well, the client should:
  Check the tubing for kinks.
  Change the position of the cone.
  Put the container at a slightly higher level.
- Explain and demonstrate how to care for the irrigation supplies (e.g., how to rinse and clean the sleeve and/or belt, if used).

Documentation

Document:

- Your assessment of the stoma and peristomal area
- The amount of irrigation solution used
- The date and time that you performed the irrigation
- Characteristics of the stool returned in the irrigation fluid
- Patient teaching

Sample documentation

06/14/15 0830 AM Ostomy irrigated with 750 ml warm tap water. Small amount of loose, formed, flakey stool returned in the fluid, with some undigested food apparent. No blood; very small amount of mucus. Stoma pink, peristomal area without redness. Explained procedure steps to patient as it was performed. Patient stated he will do some of the steps tomorrow. ——— C. Hiam, RNC

Practice Resources

Alverslid, I., Carlsson, E., Gylin, M., et al. (2012); Avent, Y. (2012); Black, P. (2008); Burch, J., & Sica, J. (2008); Cronin, E. (2008); Kent, D. (2008); Richbourg, L., Fellows, J., & Arroyave, W. (2007); Siegel, J., Rhinehart, E., Jackson, M., et al. (2007).

Thinking About the Procedure

To practice applying clinical reasoning to this procedure,

Go to *Davis's Nursing Skills Videos*, **Irrigating a Colostomy.**

For questions and suggested responses,

Go to Chapter 29, **Thinking About the Procedure Questions and Suggested Responses**, on Davis*Plus*.

Procedure 29-8 ■ Placing Fecal Drainage Devices

➤ For steps to follow in *all* procedures, refer to the Universal Steps for All Procedures found on the inside back cover.

Equipment

External Fecal Collection Device

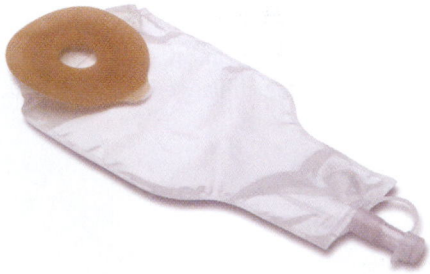

- pH-balanced soap and water or recommended skin cleanser
- Skin protection wipes (e.g., peristomal wipes to protect skin and improve adherence)
- Self-adhesive fecal containment device
- Procedure gloves
- Linen-saver pad
- Scissors

Internal Fecal Collection System

- Fecal device kit: Contains soft silicone catheter tube assembly, a syringe, and a collection bag.
- Water-soluble lubricant
- Approximately 100-mL container of tap water or saline. (Follow the manufacturer's directions for amount and type of solution.)
- 500 mL of lukewarm irrigant (water or saline)
- 60-mL luer-tip syringe and a catheter tip syringe (if not contained in the kit)
- Protective skin-care dressing (e.g., Stomahesive, DuoDerm)
- Tape

- Procedure gloves, mask, and goggles
- pH-balanced soap and water or recommended skin cleanser
- Scissors
- Linen-saver pad

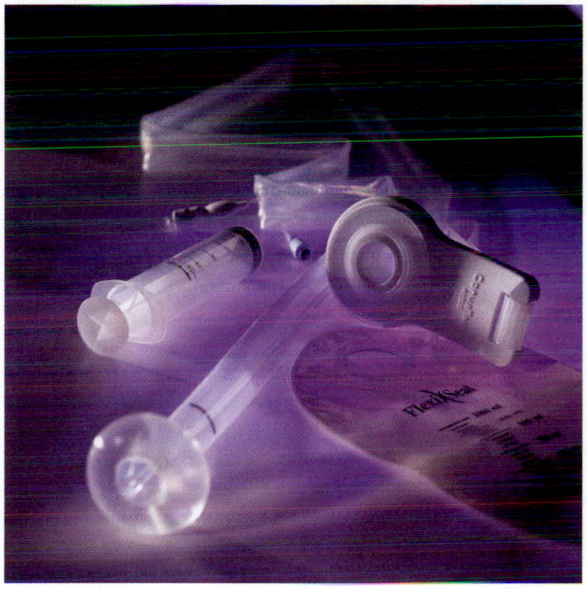

Delegation

Application of an external fecal collection system may be delegated to the NAP. Insertion of a internal fecal collection device is usually performed by a professional nurse, but may be delegated to an LPN depending on agency policy.

Pre-Procedure Assessments

- Assess the patient's bowel patterns.
  Fecal diversion is indicated when the patient is incontinent of liquid or semi-liquid stools (flowing).
- Assess for allergies to silicone. If the patient is sensitive or allergic to any of the materials in the device, it cannot be used.
- Inspect perirectal skin.
  External devices should not be used in patients with impaired skin integrity.

For Indwelling Devices, in Addition:

- Assess whether the patient has had a recent bowel movement.
  Patients who have not had a bowel movement for two or more days should be considered as having firm stool and will likely be given a bowel prep or enema before insertion of the indwelling device.
- Check for the presence of any indwelling anal or rectal device (e.g., thermometer for continuous temperature monitoring).
  The treatment plan may need to be changed. If suppositories or enemas are a part of the current treatment plan, collaborate with the prescriber, as these medication delivery mechanisms will need to be changed.

- Identify factors that increase your patient's risk for bleeding, including medications (anticoagulant and/or antiplatelet therapy) and lab results (PT, PTT, platelets).
  Patients with an increased risk of bleeding should be monitored carefully.
- Check the chart for contraindications to an indwelling fecal management system (e.g., proctitis, lacerations, rectal surgery in the past year, large or painful hemorrhoids).
  If your patient has a history of any of these problems, contact the primary care provider immediately. You may elect to use an external device, but an internal fecal catheter is contraindicated.
- Internal fecal catheters should not be used for children.

Procedure 29-8A ■ Applying an External Fecal Collection System

➤ When performing the procedure, always identify your patient according to agency policy, using two identifiers, and be attentive to standard precautions, hand hygiene, patient safety and privacy, body mechanics, and documentation.

Procedure Steps

1. **Recruit another nurse** or nursing assistant to help you. Assist the patient to a side-lying position and drape to expose the buttocks.
   For successful application (without leakage) it is best to have one caregiver position the patient and a second person apply the device.
2. **Don procedure gloves.**
   Observes standard precautions.
3. **Cleanse the perineal area** and dry well. If perianal hair is present, trim it away.
4. **Wipe the area with** skin protectant wipes
   To obtain a leak-proof seal, the device should be attached to clean, dry skin. The wipes protect the skin and improve adherence.
5. **Spread the buttocks apart** to expose the rectum.
6. **Remove the backing from the adhesive** on the fecal bag, then apply it, being careful to place the opening in the bag over the anus and to avoid gaps and creases.
   Careful application helps to obtain a leak-proof seal.
7. **Release the buttocks.** Connect the fecal incontinence pouch to a drainage bag.
8. **Hang drainage bag below the patient.**
   To collect and promote gravity drainage of fecal material.

(continued on next page)

Procedure 29-8 ■ Placing Fecal Drainage Devices (continued)

Procedure 29-8B ■ Inserting an Indwelling Fecal Drainage Device

➤ When performing the procedure, always identify your patient according to agency policy, using two identifiers, and be attentive to standard precautions, hand hygiene, patient safety and privacy, body mechanics, and documentation.

➤ *Note:* Because devices differ markedly, it is best to follow the manufacturer's instructions for placing the device. The following are generic instructions.

➤ *Note:* Also see Clinical Insight 29-1: Caring for a Patient With an Indwelling Fecal Drainage Device.

Procedure Steps

1. **Ensure that a primary care** provider has performed a digital rectal exam.
   To assess for contraindications and to check sphincter tone. When sphincter tone is compromised, the patient may not be able to retain the device.

2. **Don procedure gloves,** mask, and goggles.
   To protect from splatters when irrigating or disconnecting the device. Usually the devices are used for incontinence of loose, if not liquid, stool.

3. **Position the patient** in the left side-lying position.
   Allows access to the rectum.

4. **Remove any indwelling device.**
   The presence of a foreign body between the inflated balloon and rectum may damage rectal mucosa and a seal cannot be maintained.

5. **Depending on the type** of device, verify proper inflation and deflation of the intraluminal balloon. Attach the syringe, inflate with the recommended amount of air, deflate, and remove the syringe.

6. **Again depending on the device,** fill the retention cuff with 35 to 40 mL of water; disconnect syringe and check for leaks. After verifying function, slowly and completely aspirate all fluid from cuff and balloon and disconnect the syringe.

7. **Connect the indwelling tube** to the collection bag. Clamp and hang the bag lower than the level of the patient.

8. **Some systems have an** "introducer," which you must inflate with about 25 mL of air through a connector on the tube. Disconnect the syringe. ▼

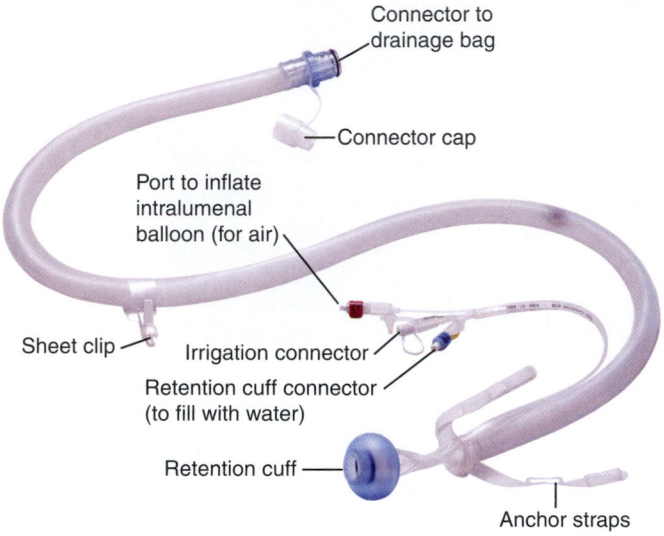

An indwelling fecal drainage device. (Courtesy of Hollister Incorporated, Libertyville, IL.)

9. **Insert your lubricated, gloved** index finger into the balloon cuff finger pocket (located above the position indicator line) and coat the balloon generously with lubricant.
   This allows for digital guidance during insertion.

10. **Gently insert the balloon end** of the catheter through the anal sphincter until the balloon is beyond the anus and well inside the rectal vault.
    This helps prevent accidental expulsion of the device.

11. **Inflate the retention cuff** with water or saline per the manufacturer's guidelines. Do not overfill. If the catheter will not accept the recommended amount of fluid, see the What If . . . ? section at the end of this procedure. ▼

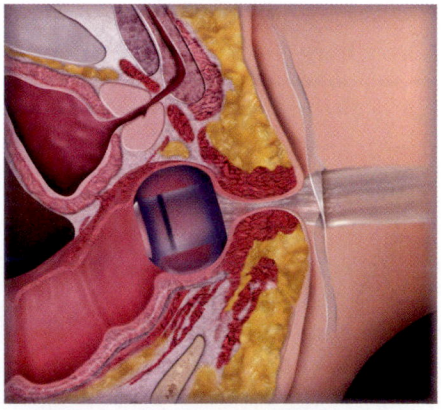

Indwelling fecal drainage device inserted in rectum, with retention cuff inflated. (Courtesy of Hollister Incorporated, Libertyville, IL.)

12. **Remove the syringe** from the inflation port and put gentle traction on the catheter.
To determine whether the balloon is securely in the rectum and appropriately positioned against the rectal floor.

13. **If you inflated an intraluminal** balloon or introducer in Step 8, you must now completely aspirate the air from it.

Do not leave an air-inflated intraluminal balloon inflated in an unattended patient.

An inflated balloon can cause tissue necrosis after a period of time.

14. **If the device has anchoring** straps, apply protective skin care dressing and tape one strap to each of the patient's buttocks.
Prevents internal migration of the tube and occlusion by twisting of the tube.

15. **Position the tubing along** the patient's leg, avoiding kinks and obstruction and position the collection bag lower than the patient.
Promotes flow of stool from the rectum to the collection bag.

16. **Dispose of used supplies** and perform hand hygiene.

? What if . . .

- **When irrigating, the catheter will not accept the recommended amount of fluid?**
  Deflate the balloon and reposition the catheter.
  The catheter is probably not positioned correctly. Do not use more than the recommended amount of fluid, as this would result in excessive pressure on the rectal vault and may cause mucosal or sphincter damage.

- **Rectal bleeding occurs with an internal fecal management device?**
  Discontinue the device and notify the physician.
  Bleeding may indicate pressure necrosis from the device.

Evaluation

- Confirm catheter/bowel lumen patency by irrigating the bowel according to manufacturer's instructions and physician order. Regular irrigation is required to facilitate evacuation through most devices.
  Stool needs to be of loose consistency to pass through the indwelling tube.
- Assess how well the patient tolerated the procedure.
- Note the color, consistency, and odor of stool.
- Monitor the amount of stool in the collection bag. When the collection bag is approximately two-thirds full, change it.
- Monitor for abdominal distention and pain.
- Regularly assess that connections are secure and that the device is not leaking.

  In addition, for indwelling devices monitor:
- Length of time the device is in place
  Not intended for use longer than 29 days.
- Rectal bleeding
  May indicate tissue necrosis, bowel perforation, or fistula formation; device must be removed.

Documentation

- Date, time, and type of collection device used
- Your assessment of the perineal skin
- Patient's tolerance of the procedure
- Characteristics and amount of stool in the collection bag (output)
- Patient/family teaching

Sample documentation

09/15/15 1435 After prepping skin, an external fecal collection device was applied. Patient tolerated procedure well. Rationale for device was explained. Pt and family verbalized they will report leaking, pain, or discomfort. Device is draining large amounts of brown liquid stool, with no visible mucus or blood.——— J. Smiley, RN

Practice Resources

Benoit R., & Watts, C. (2007); Keshava, A., Renwick, A., Stewart, P., et al. (2007); Pittman, J., Beeson, T., Terry, C., et al. (2012); Siegel, J., Rhinchart, E., Jackson, M., et al. (2007); Wishin, J., Gallagher, T., & McCann, E. (2008); Wound, Ostomy and Continence Nurses Society (2003, updated 2010).

Thinking About the Procedure

To practice applying clinical reasoning to this procedure,

Go to *Davis's Nursing Skills Videos*, **Applying an External Fecal Collection System.**

For questions and suggested responses,

Go to Chapter 29, **Thinking About the Procedure Questions and Suggested Responses,** on Davis*Plus*.

CLINICAL INSIGHTS

Clinical Insight 29-1 ➤ Caring for a Patient With an Indwelling Fecal Drainage Device

With an indwelling fecal drainage device, a catheter is present in the rectum and connected to a drainage tube and collection bag.

Nursing Goal 1: Prevent injury to rectal sphincter and/or rectal mucosa.

- Do not add air or fluid to the balloon port of the catheter.
- Check the catheter frequently for kinks or obstructions.
- Monitor for signs of complications and notify the health-care provider immediately if patient experiences rectal pain, rectal bleeding or abdominal distention and/or pain.
- Monitor stool for change in consistency (solid or soft-formed stool cannot pass through the catheter and will cause an obstruction).
- How to discontinue the catheter:
  1. Attach a 60-mL syringe to the balloon inflation port and deflate the retention balloon by pulling back on the plunger.
  2. Grasp the catheter as close to the patient as possible and slowly slide it out of the anus.
  3. Dispose of the device accordance to the agency policy for disposal of medical waste.

Nursing Goal 2: Maintain free flow of liquid stool.

- Monitor the patient for changes in stool consistency. If the stool is no longer liquid and flowing, the device must be discontinued.
- Make sure the tubing and bag remain below the level of the patient.
- Irrigate the tube as often as necessary to maintain patency:
  1. Fill a 60-mL syringe with room-temperature tap water.
  2. Attach it to the irrigation port of the catheter and flush by depressing the plunger.

Be sure you are using the irrigation port, NOT the balloon inflation port.

  3. Be sure to subtract the irrigation fluid from the stool volume to maintain an accurate record of I&O.
- Change the collection bag when it is three-fourths full.
  1. Remove the collection bag from the tubing. Snap the cap onto the used bag and dispose of according to agency policy for medical waste.
  2. Snap new collection bag securely onto the device.

Nursing Goal 3: Prevent transmission of pathogens to others.

- Follow the agency protocol for hand hygiene. Always wear clean procedure gloves when handling the fecal management device.
- Monitor stool cultures and implement isolation protocols as indicated. If a stool sample is ordered, you may obtain it from the collection bag:
  1. If the collection bag is more than 24 hours old, place a new collection bag before obtaining a sample.
  2. Cut the collection bag at the bottom and transfer stool to an appropriate container for transport to the lab.
  3. Apply a new collection bag to the connector at the end of the catheter.

Nursing Goal 4: Maintain perineal skin integrity or prevent wounds from being contaminated by stool.

- Monitor insertion site for leakage and signs of infection.
- If perineal wounds are present, keep clean and dry; notify the primary provider if signs of infection are present.
- Perform perineal care according to agency policy.

Clinical Insight 29-2 ➤ Guidelines for Ostomy Care

Assess stoma appearance.

- The stoma should be moist and red or pink. Immediately report to the surgeon a stoma that is pale, dusky, or black in color; dry; or with sloughing tissues.
  These are signs of inadequate blood supply to, and possible necrosis of, the portion of intestine that has been externalized.
- Protruding or retracted stomas will need special adjustments in wafer measurement and placement. It is normal for a new stoma to have yellow or blood-tinged mucus or dried blood on it.

Preserve peristomal skin.

- Preserving peristomal skin is critical because skin excoriation may cause an ineffective seal between the wafer and the skin. Leaking effluent will then cause skin and tissue damage. A different type of pouch system or sealant may be needed.
- Use recommended moisture-proof barrier creams and skin care products.

Plan for and change the pouch as scheduled.

- Change the skin barrier pouch at times of lower effluent.
- Avoid changing after meals, when the gastrocolic reflux increases chance of fecal effluent.
- Pouches are usually changed every 3 to 5 days, preferably before leakage occurs. Frequency also depends on the type of stoma, the type of equipment used, the effluent, the patient's preference, and the climate (e.g., pouches are changed more frequently during the summer).
- To decrease skin irritation, avoid changing the entire system. Try to change the skin barrier only every 3 to 7 days, never daily.

Assess the patient's self-care ability.

- Patients with poor vision may need to use magnification mirrors and yellow-tinted sunglasses to help reduce glare and improve contrast when they perform stoma care.
- Patients with immobility or spinal cord injury may need equipment that has a longer pouch that a seated patient can empty independently.
- Impaired dexterity or vision may warrant the use of a one-piece system or precut pouch and skin barrier. A two-piece system may be better for patients who need to keep the skin barrier in place for several days.
- Patients who are blind can be taught to change their own equipment.

Determine whether the ostomy should be irrigated.

- Consult a peristomal nurse or the primary care provider to determine whether an ostomy should be irrigated.
- Many patients with left-end colostomies may be safely irrigated as a method of continence management. An ileostomy, however, drains liquid containing high concentrations of sodium, chloride, potassium, magnesium, and bicarbonate.

Ileostomies should never be irrigated, except in cases of food blockage near the stomal outlet. Only a qualified person, such as an enterostomal therapy nurse, may perform a gentle lavage. For lavage, normal saline is preferred because excessive lavage could lead to a serious fluid and electrolyte imbalance.

Promote psychological adaptation.

- Be available to discuss the patient's reaction to the stoma. Your attitude and willingness to discuss the patient's body changes will help your patient begin adapting.
- Show acceptance when working with the patient and the stoma.
- Provide adequate ventilation and odor control when assessing the stoma or ostomy appliance.
- Provide ample time to explain stoma care and use of ostomy appliances. For most patients, this is a lifelong task.
- Teach the client about diet modifications.
- Encourage patients to return to their usual activities as much as possible.
- Encourage patients to discuss intimacy issues associated with the ostomy. Use the PLISSIT model (in Chapter 33) if necessary, and convey to them that sexual functioning is an appropriate topic to discuss. You may wish to use The United Ostomy Associations of America's *Intimacy After Ostomy Surgery Guide*, or give it to the patient (Turnbull, revised 2009).
- Refer the patient to the local ostomy association. Most of the counselors have ostomies and are able to share practical and personal information based on their own experience. To find the local chapter consult your phone book, or

Go to the **United Ostomy Associations of America** Web site at http://www.uoaa.org

ASSESSMENT GUIDELINES AND TOOLS

Focused Assessment

Bowel Elimination

Nursing History

Ask questions such as the following:

1. **Normal bowel pattern**
   - How often do you have a bowel movement (BM)?
   - What time of day do you usually have a BM?
   - Do you follow any routines to help you have a BM?
2. **Appearance of stool**
   - How would you describe your stool?
   - What color is your stool?
   - How would you describe the texture of your stool—hard, soft, or watery?
   - What shape is the stool?
   - Have you noticed unusual odor with your stool?
3. **Changes in bowel habits or stool appearance**
   - Have you had any changes in your bowel pattern recently?
   - Have you noticed any changes in the appearance, texture, or odor of your stool?
4. **For clients with a bowel diversion**, also gather data on the client's usual care of the stoma, use of appliances, and adjustment to the ostomy.
5. **History of elimination problems**
   - What has been your experience with bowel elimination problems?
   - Have you had any problems with constipation, diarrhea, or severe bloating or gas?
   - Have you ever lost control of your bowels?
   - Have you ever had bowel surgery or diagnostic procedures of the digestive tract?
6. **Use of bowel elimination aids**, including diet, exercise, medications, and remedies
   - What aids, if any, do you use to help you have a BM?
   - What foods help you maintain your bowel pattern?
   - What foods do you avoid? What effect do these foods have on you?
   - What is your usual fluid intake over the course of a day?
   - What is your usual exercise pattern?
   - What medications are you taking? Have they had any effect on your bowel elimination pattern?
   - What is your current stress level? What effect does stress have on your bowel elimination pattern?

Physical Assessment

Examine the abdomen, rectum, and anus.

- Recall that in abdominal assessment, the order of the exam is inspection, auscultation, percussion, and palpation.
- Observe the size, shape, and contour of the abdomen.
- Listen to bowel sounds. Describe them as follows:

  Normal—high-pitched, approximately 5 to 15 gurgles per minute.

  Hyperactive—very high-pitched, more frequent than normal.

  Hypoactive—low-pitched, infrequent, and quiet. Indicates decreased peristalsis.

  Absent—If after listening for 3 to 5 minutes, you hear no bowel sounds.
- When listening to bowel sounds, note the presence and timing of the sounds and the presence of any bruits.
- Percuss and palpate the abdomen for tenderness, presence of air or solid, and presence of masses.
- Inspect the anus for signs of hemorrhoids.
- Depending on the policies of your institution as well as your skill with assessment, you might also palpate the anus and rectum for the presence of stool or masses. For a complete discussion of physical examination of the abdomen, rectum, and anus, see Procedures 22-14 and 22-19.

DIAGNOSTIC TESTING

Diagnostic Testing

Direct Visualization Studies of the Gastrointestinal Tract

- Because all of the following studies are invasive procedures, you should ensure that the patient has signed an informed consent.
- All of the procedures require some degree of advance preparation, such as fasting. Check agency policy, because preparation may vary.
- Preparing the patient includes telling him what he will experience and feel during the procedure.
- When the patient is sedated (e.g., with midazolam or diazepam), an emergency medical cart ("crash cart") must be in the room during the procedure, and the patient monitored with pulse oximetry.
- All of the procedures require teaching for aftercare.
- For all tests, explain that rectal bleeding is normal for a few days if polyps were removed or a biopsy was taken.

Diagnostic Testing

Direct Visualization Studies of the Gastrointestinal Tract—cont'd

For more specific nursing responsibilities before, during, and after each test,

Go to Chapter 29, **Tables, Boxes, Figures: ESG Box 29-1, Direct Visualization Studies of the Gastrointestinal Tract: Nursing Care,** on Davis*Plus*.

Esophagogastroduodenoscopy (EGD)

Provides direct visualization of the upper GI system. A *fiberoptic endoscope*, a long, flexible tube with a light and lens, is introduced through the mouth and advanced for visualization of the esophagus, stomach, and duodenum. The physician may also perform tissue biopsies or coagulate bleeding sites through the endoscope.

Sigmoidoscopy

Allows visualization of the anal canal, rectum, and sigmoid colon. A rigid metal scope or a flexible fiberoptic scope may be used. The patient is usually not sedated. During the exam, the physician may perform a biopsy, remove polyps (small growths), or coagulate sources of bleeding in the area. A sigmoidoscopy is recommended as a screen for colon cancer for middle and older adults. Subsequent screening depends on the findings of the sigmoidoscopy as well as patient and family history; however, it is commonly done every 5 years.

Fiberoptic Colonoscopy

Provides direct visualization of the rectum, colon, entire large intestine, and distal small bowel. A flexible scope is inserted through the rectum and advanced to the cecum. Colonoscopy is useful in detecting lower GI disease. Many patients and healthcare providers choose a colonoscopy for cancer screening instead of a sigmoidoscopy, because colonoscopy provides greater visualization of the colon. This is the preferred test for clients with suspected problems above the level of the sigmoid colon. It may be done in a clinic or physician's office.

Source: American Cancer Society (2011). *Detailed guide: Colon and rectum cancer; Revised 06/25/13.* Retrieved from http://www.cancer.org/acs/groups/cid/documents/webcontent/003096-pdf.pdf; Van Leeuwen, A., Poelhuis-Leth, D., & Bladh, M. (2011). *Davis's comprehensive handbook of laboratory and diagnostic tests with nursing implications* (4th ed.). Philadelphia: F.A. Davis.

Diagnostic Testing

Indirect Visualization Studies of the Gastrointestinal Tract:

For nursing responsibilities before, during, and after each test,

Go to Chapter 29, **Tables, boxes, Figures: ESG Box 29-2, Indirect Visualization Studies of the Gastrointestinal Tract: Nursing Care,** on Davis*Plus*.

Abdominal Flat Plate

An anterior to posterior (AP) x-ray view of the abdomen is used to detect gallstones, fecal impaction, and distended bowel. This test requires no preparation and no special post-test care.

Barium Enema (BE)

A barium enema is a radiological examination of the rectum, colon, and distal small bowel. A rectal tube is inserted into the rectum or an existing ostomy. Barium (a contrast medium) is instilled. The patient must retain the barium through several position changes while air is instilled and radiographs are obtained. The test is especially useful for visualizing polyps, diverticula, and tumors. In addition, it may be used to reduce certain obstructions. As a rule, patients are not sedated. The test is invasive, so a signed informed consent is necessary.

Ultrasonography (Ultrasound)

Ultrasonography detects tissue abnormalities such as masses, cysts, edema, or stones. An ultrasound probe, called a transducer, is moved over the skin surface of the abdomen. The probe emits a sound wave that abdominal tissue and organs reflect back based on their density. The sound waves may be transformed into images visible on a computer screen.

Computed Tomography (CT) Scan

Computed tomography (CT) examines body sections from different angles using a narrow x-ray beam. It produces a three-dimensional picture of the area of the body being scanned. This test is useful in diagnosis of many abdominal disorders. A CT scan may be enhanced by injecting contrast dye that allows for improved visualization of circulatory function. The patient needs to lie very still during the procedure.

Magnetic Resonance Imaging (MRI)

Magnetic resonance imaging (MRI) produces cross-sectional images of the body. MRI utilizes a strong magnetic field and radio waves. This type of diagnostic test does not use ionizing radiation, so it is free of the hazards of x-rays. MRIs are very sensitive and may be used to detect edema, hemorrhage, blood flow, infarcts, tumors, and infections in organ structures. When used, the contrast medium is noniodinated, and it is administered intravenously to enhance contrast between normal and abnormal tissues. The patient must lie still in a narrow tube, sometimes for up to an hour.

Source: Van Leeuwen, A., Poelhuis-Leth, D., & Bladh, M. (2011). *Davis's comprehensive handbook of laboratory and diagnostic tests with nursing implications* (4th ed.). Philadelphia: F.A. Davis.

CLINICAL REASONING

Applying the Full-Spectrum Nursing Model

PATIENT SITUATION

Lucy Franklin is a frail, elderly woman, a long-time resident in a long-term care facility. She can no longer communicate and lies however the NAPs place her in bed, seldom moving. She is very thin, does not eat or drink, and is being fed entirely through a gastrostomy tube. She is incontinent of both stool and urine, and has recently started having copious diarrhea, probably from the tube feedings, but that has not been established definitely. The skin on Lucy's back, buttocks, and perineum is still intact, but it is quite red now. The healthcare team is considering various measures for controlling the diarrhea, but until that can be achieved, nurses want to protect her skin integrity.

THINKING

1. *Theoretical Knowledge:*
   a. Other than tube feedings, what else could be causing Lucy's diarrhea?
   b. In addition to Impaired Skin Integrity, what are some other risks associated with diarrhea?
   c. Why is fecal incontinence, especially with diarrhea, a risk factor for Impaired Skin Integrity?
2. *Critical Thinking:*
   a. *(Contextual Awareness):* What other factors in Lucy's situation do you think might make her even more vulnerable to Impaired Skin Integrity? If you do not yet have the theoretical knowledge you need, draw on your own experiences—and think carefully about everything you know about Lucy.
   b. *(Considering Alternatives):* A fecal incontinence pouch is being discussed as an intervention to preserve Lucy's skin integrity. Do you think it should be an external system or an internal system? Why?

DOING

3. *Practical Knowledge:*
   It has been decided that an external fecal collection system will be used. Describe the steps you will take to apply this system after you have made the necessary assessments.
4. *Nursing Process (Assessments):*
   What ongoing assessments will you need to make after the fecal collection system is applied?

CARING

5. *Self-Knowledge:*
   How comfortable would you be applying Lucy's fecal collection system? What aspects of the situation make you most uncomfortable?

Critical Thinking and Clinical Reasoning

1. Your neighbor is aware that you are a nursing student and calls you for advice. She has a 12-year-old daughter with diarrhea. "Everything runs through her," states the mother. There are also two other children in the house, ages 6 years and 18 months. Both have had watery stools this morning. Your neighbor explains that her husband has an ileostomy and has been hospitalized since yesterday. Your neighbor has no symptoms but is very worried. She asks, "Do we all need to go to the hospital?"
   a. Consider alternatives. What are the most likely explanations for the diarrhea?
   b. Based on your theoretical knowledge, how would you explain why her husband was hospitalized, while the rest of the family members, who have the same symptoms, remain at home?
   c. After reassuring her, what advice should you offer your neighbor about self-care for her and the children's elimination problem?
2. Consider the following patients:
   - A 54-year-old man diagnosed with colon cancer who now has a new sigmoid colostomy
   - A 21-year-old woman with Crohn's disease (an inflammatory bowel disorder) who has just had an ileostomy
   - A 36-year-old trauma victim who has a new double-barreled transverse colostomy

   a. How are these patients similar?
   b. In regard to their surgery, what nursing care priorities do these patients share?

c. How do the major concerns for these patients differ? (Consider the context. How are their surgical and self-care situations different?)

3. For each of the following concepts, use critical thinking to describe how or why it is important to nursing, patient care, or bowel elimination. Note that these are *not* to be merely definitions.
   Digestion (in the mouth, esophagus, stomach, and small intestine)
   Large intestine (colon)
   Rectum and anus
   Fluid intake
   Location of a bowel diversion
   Bowel sounds
   Providing privacy
   Diarrhea

What Are the Main Points in This Chapter?

- Bowel elimination is a normal process by which waste products are eliminated from the body.
- Feces are a mixture of insoluble fiber and other indigestible material, bacteria, and water.
- During defecation, the internal and external anal sphincters relax; the rectum contracts; and peristalsis increases in the sigmoid colon, propelling feces through the anus.
- The frequency of bowel movements (BMs) varies. As long as stools are passed without excessive urgency, with minimal effort and no straining, and without the use of laxatives, bowel function is regarded as normal.
- Adequate fiber, fluid, and exercise are required to maintain a person's normal bowel pattern.
- Factors affecting bowel function include developmental stage, personal and sociocultural factors, nutrition, hydration, activity level, stress, anesthesia, medications, pregnancy, surgery and other procedures, and pathological conditions.
- To promote regular defecation, provide privacy for the patient and allow time to use the toilet.
- Constipation is a decrease in frequency of BMs and the passage of dry, hard stool that requires more effort to pass.
- Bulking agents are the preferred medication for treating constipation.
- Habitual use of laxatives, with the exception of bulking agents, may cause reliance on medication for bowel elimination.
- Fecal impaction is detected by digital examination of the rectum. To treat a fecal impaction, enemas and/or digital removal of stool is required.
- An enema is the introduction of solution into the rectum to soften feces, distend the colon, and stimulate peristalsis and evacuation of feces.
- Monitor patients with diarrhea for intake and output, body weight, and vital signs to assess for fluid losses; provide hygiene measures to protect the skin.
- Bowel incontinence may be managed by providing assistance to the bathroom at regular intervals and at the times BMs are most likely to occur, and by beginning a bowel training program.
- External or internal fecal collection devices can be used to protect perianal skin or to collect large stool samples. They minimize odor, allow for accurate measurement of output, and improve patient comfort.
- A bowel diversion is a surgically created opening for elimination of digestive waste products.
- The **effluent** (fecal matter) of an ostomy ranges from liquid to solid, depending on the part of the bowel that is being diverted.
- A healthy stoma ranges in color from deep pink to brick red and is shiny and moist at all times.
- A client with a bowel diversion must adapt to the stoma for elimination and learn to care for the stoma.

Knowledge Map

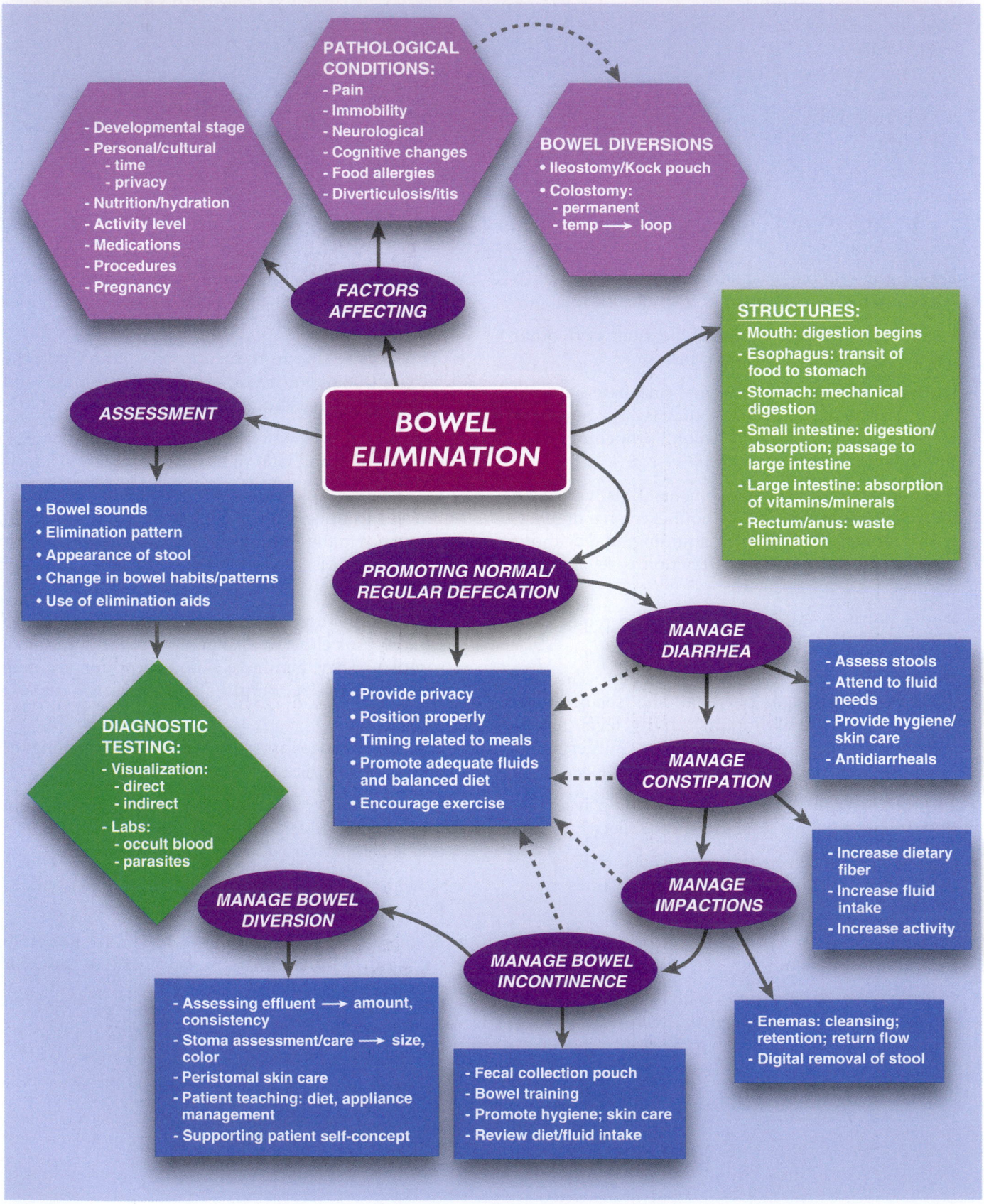

CHAPTER 30

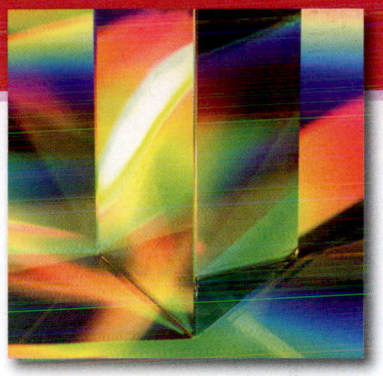

Sensation, Perception, & Cognition

STUDENT RESOURCES

*The questions and exercises in Volume 2 allow you to practice the kind of thinking you will use as a full-spectrum nurse. Critical-thinking questions usually have more than one correct answer, so we do not provide "answers" for these features. It is more important to develop your nursing judgment than to just cover content. You will learn by discussing the questions with your peers. If you are still unsure, consult your instructor. You will find Response Sheets (for writing your responses to the questions) on Davis*Plus.

To explore learning resources for this chapter,

Go to Davis*Plus* at DavisPl.us/Wilkinson3.

Chapter Resources for Chapter 30:

- **Response sheets for all learning activities**
- **Resources for Caregivers and Health Professionals**
- **Reading More About Sensation, Perception, & Cognition (suggested readings)**
- **Concept Map of chapter content**

Interactive Case Studies

NCLEX-Style and Chapter Review Questions

CHAPTER OVERVIEW

For a podcast of an overview of this chapter,

Go to Student Resources, Chapter 30, **Podcast—Chapter Overview,** on Davis*Plus*.

Caring for the Nguyens

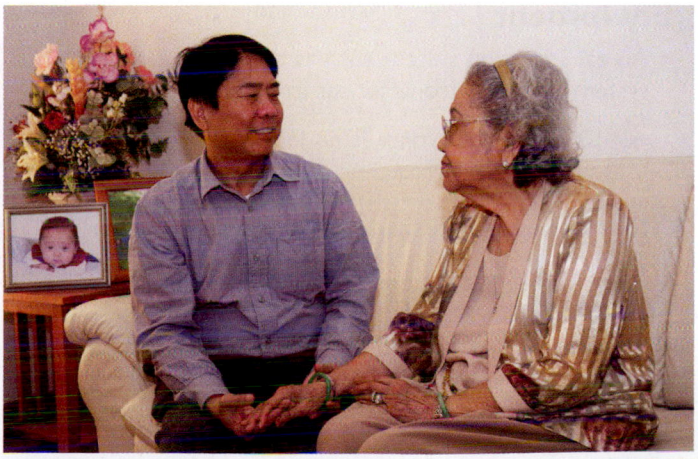

Mai Nguyen, Nam Nguyen's mother, has been experiencing blurred vision. At a recent ophthalmology appointment, she was told she has bilateral cataracts that will require surgical removal. She reports to the primary care clinic today, accompanied by Nam. Mai tells you, "I don't know what happened. I was pulling into a parking space at the grocery store, and the next thing you know, I hear this loud boom. I don't know how I did it, but I hit the car next to me. I just didn't see it."

Nam is very concerned and questions whether his mother should be allowed to drive. Mai is visibly upset. "I don't want to hurt anyone, but I don't want to lose all my freedom." Nam insisted on this appointment to discuss his concerns.

(Continued)

Caring for the Nguyens (continued)

A. What data will you need to gather from Mai and Nam?

B. What assessments will you need to perform?

C. How will cataract surgery most likely affect Mai? You will need to learn about the surgery and recovery to answer this question. Use a textbook, or, for a list of helpful Web sites you can access,

Go to Student Resources: Chapter 30, **Resources for Caregivers and Healthcare Professionals,** on Davis*Plus*.

D. What information would you offer to Mai and Nam?

Go to Student Resources: Chapter 30, **Caring for the Nguyens Response Sheet,** on Davis*Plus*.

Practical Knowledge knowing how

To provide support for patients with sensorineural alterations, you will need practical knowledge about assessing and diagnosing sensorineural functions. Nursing interventions involve caring for patients who have vision and hearing deficits. This section includes a procedure for otic irrigations, which may be used to correct hearing loss resulting from a cerumen-blocked ear canal. Some procedures to support sensory function, such as instilling medications and irrigating the eye, are presented in the procedures in Chapter 26 of this volume. For other interventions,

Go to **Chapter 26: Administering Medications,** and **Chapter 30: Sensation, Perception, & Cognition,** in Volume 1.

In this section you will also find techniques for communicating with patients who have visual or hearing deficits, as well as assessment guidelines.

PROCEDURES

Procedure 30-1 ■ Performing Otic Irrigation

➤ For steps to follow in *all* procedures, refer to the Universal Steps for All Procedures found on the inside back cover.

Equipment

- An ear irrigation system, such as the Welch Allyn ear wash system or an electronic jet ear irrigator

  Using a metal syringe is no longer recommended and is considered dangerous. *An ear irrigation system is also preferred over an Asepto or bulb syringe because of the better ability to control pressure and remove cerumen (Harkin, n.d.).*

- Asepto syringe, or rubber bulb syringe (if an ear irrigation system is not available)
- Irrigating solution (usually water, but may be an antiseptic solution), warmed to 98.6°F (37°C)
- Bath towel and moisture-resistant towel
- A headlight if one is available
- Emesis basin
- Otoscope
- Cotton balls
- Procedure gloves

Delegation

You must assess the client before performing this procedure and evaluate client responses during and after the procedure. The procedure requires knowledge of anatomy and physiology, use of an otoscope, and, sometimes, use of sterile technique. Therefore, you should not delegate otic irrigation to nursing assistive personnel (NAP).

Pre-Procedure Assessments

- Determine whether there are contraindications for ear irrigation.

  Contraindications include ruptured tympanic membrane, present or recent middle ear infection, prior surgery on the ear, cleft palate, or acute inflammation of the ear canal.

- **Assess the external ear for drainage.**

  Do not irrigate the ears if drainage is present. Drainage from the ear may be a sign of rupture of the tympanic membrane.

- Assess the external ear for cerumen.
  Impacted cerumen is the most common reason for performing an ear irrigation.
- Assess the external ear canal for redness, swelling, or foreign objects; visualize the tympanic membrane. If a foreign object is present, attempt to remove it before irrigation.
  Establishes the baseline. If you irrigate with a foreign object in the ear, it may cause the object to swell and become more difficult to remove. Also, if you cannot visualize the tympanic membrane, it may be perforated; if so, otic irrigation is contraindicated.
- Assess for pain or hearing loss.
  Establishes the baseline. Cerumen blockage in the ear canal may result in a conductive hearing loss.

➤ When performing the procedure, always identify your patient according to agency policy, using two identifiers, and be attentive to standard precautions, hand hygiene, patient safety and privacy, body mechanics, and documentation.

Procedure Steps

1. **Warm the irrigating solution** to body temperature (98.6°F [37°C]), and fill the reservoir of the irrigator.
   Placing cool solutions in the ear can cause dizziness.
2. **Assemble the irrigator** if necessary, and place a clean disposable tip on it.
3. **Assist the client into a** sitting or lying position, with the head tilted slightly toward the affected ear. Explain what you are going to do.
   Positioning facilitates administering the solution and allows fluid to run along the roof of the ear canal. Knowing what to expect may decrease patient anxiety and improve his ability to cooperate during the procedure.
4. **Don gloves;** put on the headlight.
   The gloves are needed because of the risk of exposure to body fluids. The headlight facilitates direct vision.
5. **Drape the client** with a plastic drape, and place a towel on the client's shoulder on the side being irrigated. Ask the client to hold an emesis basin under his ear to collect the irrigating fluid that drains out of the ear.
   Note: An emesis basin is not necessary if a comprehensive ear wash system is used.
   Drape and towel protect the client's clothing.
6. **Set the irrigator pressure** to the minimum level. Let it run for 20 to 30 seconds to prime the tubing or nozzle before irrigation. (If you must use an Asepto or rubber bulb syringe, fill the syringe with about 50 mL of the irrigating solution, and expel any remaining air.)
7. **Straighten the ear canal.**
   a. For a child younger than 3 years old, pull the pinna down and back.
   b. For older children and adults, pull the pinna upward and outward.
   Straightens the ear canal so that the solution can flow through the length of the canal.
8. **Instruct the client to notify** you if he experiences any pain or dizziness during the irrigation. Explain to the client that he may feel warmth, fullness, or pressure when the fluid reaches the tympanic membrane.
   Pain or dizziness may indicate a contraindication to the procedure.
9. **Place the tip of the nozzle** (or syringe) about 1 cm (½ in.) above the entrance of the ear canal, and direct the stream of irrigating solution gently along the top of the ear canal toward the back of the client's head.
   a. Do not occlude the ear canal with the nozzle.
   b. Instill the solution slowly.
   c. Allow the solution to flow out as it is instilled.
   d. Repeat these steps for 5 minutes or until you can see cerumen in the return solution.
   Directing the flow directly onto the tympanic membrane could injure the membrane. Strong pressure can cause discomfort and may even damage the tympanic membrane. ▼

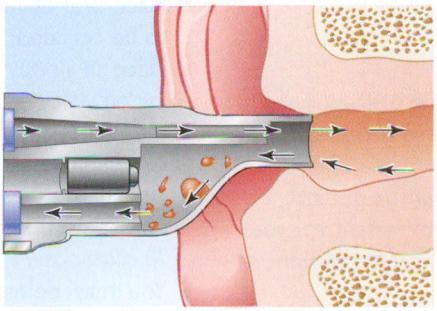

10. **Inspect the ear with** an otoscope to evaluate cerumen removal. See Procedure 19-7 if you need to review otoscopic examination.
    Allows visualization of the canal.
11. **Continue irrigating until** the examination indicates the canal is cleaned of cerumen and debris.
    The irrigating solution will soften the cerumen, easing removal. Blocking the canal prevents the outward flow of the solution.
12. **Place a cotton ball loosely** in the ear canal, and ask the client to lie on the side of the affected ear.
    The cotton ball will absorb excess fluid that drains by gravity.
13. **Clean and disinfect the irrigator,** according to the manufacturer's instructions or agency protocols. Dispose of the disposable tips.

? What if . . .

- **The cerumen is very hard or you have difficulty removing it?**
  The irrigating solution will help soften it, so you may attempt again after 15 minutes.
- **The patient is an infant or young child?**
  Ask another caregiver to immobilize the child during the irrigation.

(continued on next page)

Procedure 30-1 ■ Performing Otic Irrigation (continued)

Evaluation

- Observe the quantity and quality of ear cerumen you removed.
- Observe the appearance of the ear canal.
- Assess for complaints of pain or dizziness.
- Assess for improvement in hearing acuity.
- Reassess for drainage on the cotton ball.

Patient Teaching

- Avoid use of cotton-tipped swabs.
  They simply push cerumen deeper into the ear.
- Keep the ear dry for a few days. Use cotton balls coated with petroleum jelly when bathing.
  Exposure to a wet environment, such as a swimming pool, may increase the risk of bacterial or fungal infection. Petroleum jelly serves as a barrier to keep water from entering the ear.
- Clean ears daily with washcloth, soap, and water. If wax buildup is a problem, over-the-counter preparations (oils) can be used.
- Notify the primary care provider if you experience ear pain, vertigo, or "ringing in the ears."
  Ear irrigation is an invasive procedure and may result in otitis media, trauma to the external meatus, vertigo, tinnitus, and perforation of the tympanic membrane, although this is not common.

Home Care

- Provide the caregiver with instructions on ear care as stated above.
- Teach parents that it is best to avoid irrigation in young children unless absolutely necessary. Oil- or water-based ear drops may be used to treat a wax problem in a child, applying the oil when the child is asleep.

Documentation

- Document the ear solution used, the quantity, character, and odor of cerumen or drainage.
- Chart the condition of the ear canal and tympanic membrane after the irrigation.

Sample documentation

mm/dd/yyyy 1400 Pt c/o bilateral decreased hearing acuity. External ear canals occluded with dried cerumen. Irrigated with warm water using electronic jet ear irrigation system. Large amount of dry, brown cerumen removed with irrigation. External canals and tympanic membrane intact to otoscopic inspection after irrigation. —N. Ephrain, RN

Practice Resources

Burtin, M., & Doree, C. (2009); Chau, J., Lee, D., & Lo, S. (2012); Harkin, H. (n.d.); Roland, P. S., Smith, T. L, Schwartz, S. R., et al. (2008).

CLINICAL INSIGHTS

Clinical Insight 30-1 ➤ Seizure Precautions

Institute seizure precautions for patients with a new diagnosis of a seizure disorder or any seizure activity within the past 12 months; frequent seizure activity; history of head trauma (including surgery) within the past 3 years; withdrawal of anti-seizure medication or adjustment of the medication regimen.

The goal of seizure precautions is to protect the patient from injury and prevent serious complications.

Before a Seizure Event

- Explain to the patient the reasons for the precautions.
- If the patient has frequent or prolonged seizures, establish IV access.
  To provide a route to administer medications (e.g., diazepam [Valium]) in the event of a seizure. For intermittent episodes, you can use rectal diazepam (Diastat), lorazepam (Ativan), or midazolam (Versed).
- Obtain a bed with full-length siderails.
- Cover the headboard, footboard, and siderails with commercial pads or bath blankets. Tape the blankets in place.
  Padding protects the patient's limbs and head from injury if he has a seizure.
- Keep the rails raised and the bed in low position.
  To prevent falls and minimize injuries.
- Place oral or nasal suction equipment at the bedside. Test to be certain it is working.
- Place an airway at the bedside or tape to the wall, depending on your agency protocol.
- Make sure the family knows how to use a call bell.
  To summon help in the event of a seizure.
- Assign the patient to a room in close proximity to the nurses' station.
  To allow closer monitoring.
- You may delegate to the NAP the tasks of setting up seizure precautions.

Clinical Insight 30-1 ➤ Seizure Precautions—cont'd

When a Seizure Occurs

- If you are present when the patient reports having an aura, help him into bed, lower the head, and raise the siderails. If in another location, help him to the floor and put something soft under his head.
  To keep the head from being injured by hitting the floor, counter, or other hard object.
- Provide privacy.
- Stay with the patient.
- You may insert an oral airway.
  To keep the tongue from blocking the airway.
- Don't put anything into the patient's mouth and don't force the airway in place.
  This might break the teeth or cause other injury.
- Don't try to hold the jaw open or put your hands in the mouth.
  You may be bitten.
- Turn the patient on his side.
  This allows secretions to drain and the tongue to fall forward, keeping the airway patent.
- Loosen restrictive clothing.
- Move hard or sharp objects out of the way.
- Do not try to restrain the patient or control his movements.
  This might cause muscle and joint injury.
- If the seizure is prolonged or hypoxemia is present, administer oxygen as prescribed.
  To avoid hypoxia during the event.
- Usually little nursing action is required beyond preventing physical injury and maintaining a patent airway. The exception is with status epilepticus, in which the patient has repeated seizures without regaining consciousness. In that event, notify a physician immediately.
- Observe the characteristics of the seizure: how it started, location and duration of motor activity, type of movements (e.g., stiffening, jerking, twitching, loss of muscle tone), crying out, visual and auditory symptoms, tachycardia, pupil dilation, change in level of consciousness). Note the first symptom and how the seizure progressed.
  To help identify the area of the brain involved.
- You cannot delegate care of a patient who is having a seizure because nursing assessments and interventions are required. You can ask the NAP to obtain help.
- Administer prescribed antiseizure medication if the seizure is prolonged, typically >6 minutes.

After the Seizure

- Turn the patient on his side and apply suction, if needed.
  To allow secretions to drain and maintain a patent airway.
- Reorient and reassure the patient, and make him comfortable. If the patient was incontinent, change bedding and clothing.
- Examine for injuries.
- Keep the room quiet and the lighting dim.
- Stay with the patient, as he may be sleepy or confused.
- Do not give any food or drink until the patient is fully conscious and alert.
- Monitor vital signs and mental status every 15 to 30 minutes for 2 hours. You can delegate this activity to a NAP.
- Observe post-seizure behavior: Evaluate muscle strength, ability to speak, memory, and orientation.
- Pad the siderails, if not already done.
- Ask the patient whether he experienced an aura and what activities preceded the seizure.
  The type of aura helps locate the area in the brain where the seizure originated.
- Document what happened and your post-procedure assessment.

Lifestyle Management

Sleep deprivation lowers the threshold for seizure activity. The patient should have sufficient rest and a healthy diet. Advise the patient to visit his primary care provider regularly, take prescribed antiseizure medication on time, and avoid excess alcohol and any drugs that may interact with seizure medications.

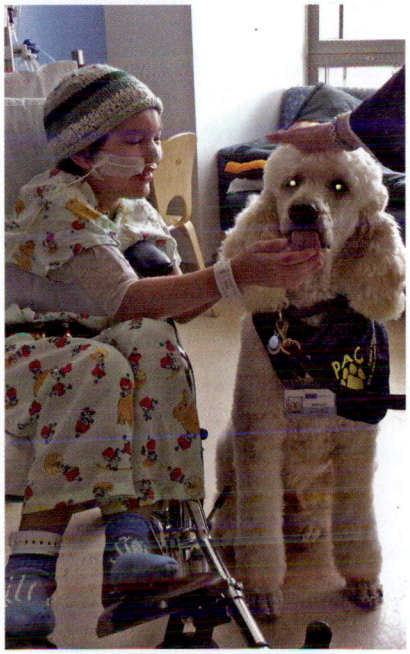

Living with epilepsy. Seizure dogs are trained to respond to seizures by alerting families for help and by lying next to the person to prevent injury.

References

American Association of Neuroscience Nurses (2007, revised 2009); Wiegand, L. (2011).

Clinical Insight 30-2 ➤ Communicating With Visually Impaired Clients

The Joint Commission (2010) requires that institutions address the communication needs of patients with impaired vision.

- Introduce yourself when you enter the room.
- Call the client by her name so that she can be certain you are addressing her.
- When you enter a room with a client who is visually impaired, describe the room, room layout, and activities that are occurring.
- Explain unfamiliar sounds, such as the paging system and monitor and pump alarms.
- If the client has limited vision, be sure to position yourself in the client's field of vision.
- Speak to the visually impaired person before you touch her so that she is prepared for your touch.
- Do not speak loudly unless the client has a hearing impairment.
- Let the client know when you are leaving the room.
- Use the words "see" and "look" as you would with a sighted person.
- Avoid expressions, such as "over there" or "right here." Guide the client to the location or place her hand on the object.

Clinical Insight 30-3 ➤ Communicating With Hearing-Impaired Clients

Healthcare agencies should address the communication needs of those with vision, speech, hearing, language, and cognitive impairments (The Joint Commission, 2010).

Assess the patient's method of receiving speech.

- If the patient wears a hearing aid, check to see that it is turned on.
- If not, does the patient read lips or use sign language? Remember that only about ⅓ of spoken words can be understood by speech reading.
- If possible, arrange a hearing evaluation for the client and construction of any required hearing aids.

Position yourself and minimize noise.

- Don't chew gum or eat while talking. Many clients use lip reading to help them interpret your speech.
- Make sure you are clearly visible to the client before you start speaking. Use touch to get the client's attention.
- Face the client directly; keep your hands away from your mouth.
- If the hearing deficit is predominantly in one ear, move closer to the less affected ear.
- Minimize environmental noise (e.g., turn off the TV).

Send the message.

- Speak slowly and articulate clearly, in a natural way. Don't shout. Shouting distorts your words.
- Don't drop your voice at the end of a sentence.
- Use simple, plain language, but longer phrases (e.g., "Would you like me to get you a drink of water?" instead of "Do you want a drink?")
- Use gestures to provide visual cues (e.g., act out what you want the patient to do).
- Use paper, pencil, or computer communication when necessary. Consider literacy skills.

Interpret the client's responses.

- Observe the client's verbal responses, facial expressions, and body language for clues to understanding. An inappropriate response indicates misunderstanding.
- Be aware the person may nod agreement or say "yes" even when she does not understand what is being said.
- Confirm that the client understood you by asking her to repeat what you said, especially if you are giving specific information, such as a time or place. Many numbers and words sound alike (e.g., "fifteen" and "fifty"; or "Prozac" and "Prograf").
- If the person does not understand what you've said, rephrase your statement. Don't repeat the same words.

For older adults: Use a low-pitched voice. The ability to hear high-pitched tones is lost first with aging.

ASSESSMENT GUIDELINES AND TOOLS

As a nurse, you should always consider your client's sensory–perceptual status. Sensory deficits and excess or inadequate stimulation have a significant influence on quality of life and may be especially troublesome for institutionalized clients.

Hearing Screening in Older Adults

To find a useful tool to screen hearing in older adults,

Go to the Hartford Institute for Geriatric Nursing, *Try this: Best practices in nursing care to older adults* at http://consultgerirn.org/uploads/File/trythis/try_this_12.pdf

Using this tool, a patient scores as follows. A total of 3 points indicates the need for further evaluation.

1 point for each of the following:

- Older than 70 years
- Male
- Did not attend 12th grade
- Cannot hear and understand (without seeing the face) what a person whispers from across the room.

2 points for each of the following:

- Has ever seen a doctor because of trouble hearing
- Unable to hear and understand (without seeing the face) a person talking in a normal voice from across the room.

Other Sensory Assessment Tools

Focused Assessment

Nursing History: Sensory Perceptual Status

Usual Sensory Function

Ask questions such as the following:

- How would you rate your vision?
- How would you evaluate your ability to see objects up close or at a distance?
- Do you have any difficulty hearing conversations or listening to the radio or television?
- Have you experienced any difficulty locating sounds?
- Do you experience ringing or buzzing in your ears?
- Do you enjoy the taste of food?
- Do you notice any difficulty with your ability to smell?
- Are you experiencing any pain or discomfort?
- Do you have any areas of numbness or tingling on your body?
- Do you have any difficulty with sensing hot or cold?
- Describe your level of coordination.
- What medications are you taking? Have they had any effect on your vision, hearing, sense of taste, smell, touch, or balance?
- What is your current stress level?
- What is your usual activity level?
- What is your preferred activity level?

Assess for Risk Factors for Impaired Sensory Function

- Developmental level (e.g., older adults)
- Health status (usual and current state of health, current health concerns (e.g., Ménière's disease), history of hospitalizations and surgeries)
- Medications (i.e., look up side effects to determine what, if any, effect the medications have on sensory function)
- Stress (current and usual stress level, major sources of stressors, usual coping mechanisms)
- Lifestyle (normal activity, noise, interaction levels, hobbies, and usual lifestyle)

History of Sensory Problems

Ask about the following:

- Have you experienced any problems with blurred vision, double vision, sensitivity to light, blind spots, objects moving in front of your eyes, or eye pain?
- Have you ever felt unable to follow a conversation because of difficulty hearing?
- Have you ever had problems with your ability to taste or smell?
- Have you ever had areas of numbness or tingling?
- Has anyone in your family ever been diagnosed with a stroke or circulation problem?
- Have you ever had episodes of confusion or disorientation?

Use of Sensory Aids, Including Diet, Exercise, Medications, and Remedies

- Does the client wear glasses or contact lenses at any time? If so, determine the following:

  When was the client's last eye exam?

  Are the glasses clean and in good repair? Are the glasses within easy reach?

  Are contact lenses in good condition? Is the client able to care for them?
- Does the client wear a hearing aid? If so, determine the following:

  Can the client hear adequately with the hearing aid in place?

  Are the batteries working?

  Is the hearing aid clean?

  How much help does the client need to place the aid in his ear?

(Continued)

Focused Assessment

- Does the client use a cane or walker? If so:
  - Has the cane or walker been properly fitted to the client?
  - How often does the client use the device when walking?
- What factors determine when the device will be used?

Assess Mental Status

- Assess behavior, appearance, response to stimuli, speech, memory, and judgment. If you need more specific instructions, see Procedure 21-16, Steps 1–10 and Questions for Evaluating Cognitive Status, at the end of the procedure.

- **For older adults**, a tool called the Mini-Cog is especially useful (Borson, Scanlan, Brush, et al., 2000). It consists of 3 memory questions and instructions to draw a clock face. To use this tool,

Go to http://consultgerirn.org/uploads/File/trythis/try_this_3.pdf

- Assess level of orientation: Have the client tell you his name, the date, and his current location. If he can answer these questions correctly, describe him as "awake, alert, and oriented to person, place, and time" (AA&O×3).
- Assess level of consciousness:

Alert	Is the patient awake and aware of the environment and himself, speaking clearly, making eye contact?
Confused	Are actions and speech inappropriate?
Lethargic	Is speech slow or sluggish? Are mental processes and movements sluggish?
Obtunded	This is a low level of awareness and response to environment. Document it if it occurs.
Stuporous	This occurs when the patient can be aroused by vigorous stimulation but seems confused during periods of arousal.
Comatose	In this state, there is no spontaneous movement, no verbalization, and only nonpurposeful movement with stimulation. (Huntley, 2008)

- Also see Chapter 22, Procedure 22-16, Assessing the Sensory-Neurological System, Glasgow Coma Scale, and Full Outline of UnResponsiveness Scale.

Assess Support Network for Clients With Sensory Deficit

- Are there support persons to help the client by assuming chores he can no longer perform?
- Are there people who provide comfort to ease the client's distress about sensory losses?
- Who can provide sensory stimulation?
- Who can help reorient and calm the client?
- Does the client need help with transportation in order to maintain social contact?

Focused Assessment

Bedside Assessment of Sensory Function

SENSE	ASSESSMENT PROCESS
Vision	Use the Snellen chart, or have the client read a newspaper.
	Observe for squinting.
Hearing	Perform the whisper test.
	Inspect the ear canals for hardened cerumen.
	Observe client conversations. Are there frequent requests for repeating information or misunderstandings?
	How loud is the client's radio or television?
	 *To screen hearing in older adults,* you will find a useful tool if you  Go to http://consultgerirn.org/uploads/File/trythis/try_this_12.pdf
Smell	Ask the client to close his eyes and identify common smells (e.g., coffee, vanilla, cloves, tobacco).
Taste	Ask the client to close his eyes and identify common tastes (e.g., salt, lemon, and sugar). Give water between tastes.
Tactile	With his eyes closed, touch the client with a wisp of cotton. Have him identify when you have touched him. Repeat this process with a sharp object, such as a needle.
	With his eyes closed, ask the client to identify where you are touching his body.
Kinesthesia	Have the client perform the Romberg test. See Procedure 22–7.
	Have the client perform alternating rapid motions, such as tapping heels or clapping.
	Observe the client's gait and movement.

CLINICAL REASONING

Applying the Full-Spectrum Nursing Model

PATIENT SITUATION

Clint Gossage is an 85-year-old man who lives at home alone. His wife moved to a nursing home a year ago. Although Mr. Gossage has many self-care deficits, he is still able to live at home, with regular visits from a home health nurse and community services to help with some meals and bathing. When you visit him, you notice that he shouts when talking to you, looks at you intently when you speak, and constantly asks you to repeat what you say. You examine his external ear canal and note that there is some hardened cerumen in the canal. He is not wearing a hearing aid. The patient record reveals tympanic membrane scarring and a diagnosis of conductive hearing loss.

THINKING

1. *Theoretical Knowledge:* Describe the pathophysiology of conductive hearing loss.
2. *Critical Thinking (Considering Alternatives):* Based on your knowledge of conductive hearing loss and your assessment of Mr. Gossage, what is the first follow-up question you would ask him about his hearing?

DOING

3. *Practical Knowledge:* At a subsequent visit, you discover that Mr. Gossage has impacted cerumen in his left ear. After obtaining a medical order, you prepare to perform an otic irrigation.
   a. To what temperature will you warm the solution?
   b. What position would you use for Mr. Gossage?
   c. Describe how you would place the tip of the syringe (or ear wash system) for irrigating.
   d. After the ear is cleared of cerumen and you have finished irrigating, what should you do next? And what position will you have Mr. Gossage assume when you do it?
4. *Nursing Process (Diagnosis):*
   a. Write a nursing diagnosis that focuses on Mr. Gossage's safety and that relates to hearing.
   b. Based on your nursing diagnosis, what safety measures would you recommend for Mr. Gossage's home? (Do not address the hearing aid issue here.)

CARING

5. *Ethical Knowledge:* Now think back to the first visit with Mr. Gossage. What are some reasons that he might not have been wearing a hearing aid? Consider physical changes associated with aging.

Critical Thinking and Clinical Reasoning

1. Review the following client scenarios.
   - **Margaret** is 84 years old. She is a retired schoolteacher who loves to read, work in her garden, and volunteer at the local children's hospital. She has developed macular degeneration and is progressively losing her sight.
   - **Rocky** is 55 years old. He is a former guitar player in a heavy-metal band. He now works in music production. He has significant hearing loss related to chronic exposure to loud music. Most recently he has developed tinnitus, which has exacerbated his hearing loss.
   - **Jesse** is 31 years old. He is a chef at a local four-star restaurant. He suffered a head injury in a motor vehicle accident and has lost his sense of smell.
   - **Natasha** is 26 years old. She is a licensed architect working for a firm in the downtown area. She has been taking birth control pills for 5 years. Recently she has been under a lot of stress. She began drinking lots of coffee, smoking cigarettes, and working long hours. She was admitted to the hospital with right-sided weakness and slurred speech. She is being evaluated for a cerebrovascular accident.
   - **Aahan** is 15 years old. He has cerebral palsy. As a result, he has a "scissor walk" and dysarthric speech. He has recently had a series of falls due to increasing problems with balance.

   a. For each client, write a nursing diagnosis to reflect his or her sensory perception problem. Write one other nursing diagnosis that might result from the sensory perception problem. Explain your thinking.
   b. Each of the clients is experiencing a sensory deficit. What interventions would be most appropriate to address each client's concerns?

c. Which client(s) is/are most likely to have difficulty adapting to the sensory deficit? How would you determine how each client is adapting?
d. Which client, if any, is most likely to be experiencing sensory overload?

2. Examine the clinical unit that you are visiting for your current clinical rotation. What unit factors contribute to the development of sensory overload?
3. What factors in the clinical unit contribute to the development of sensory deprivation?
4. For each of the following concepts, use critical thinking to describe how or why it is important to nursing, patient care, or sensory perception. Note that these are *not* to be merely definitions.

Sensory stimulation
Sensory overload
Sensory deprivation
Sensory deficits
Sensory aids

What Are the Main Points in This Chapter?

- The purpose of sensation is to allow the body to respond to changing situations and maintain homeostasis.
- A sensory experience involves four components: stimulus, reception, perception, and an arousal mechanism.
- Reception is the process of receiving stimuli from nerve endings in the skin and body.
- Perception is the ability to interpret the impulses transmitted from the receptors and give meaning to the stimuli.
- Humans respond to sensations when they are alert and receptive to stimulation. The response to a stimulus is based on intensity, contrast, adaptation, previous experience, illness, or injury.
- Sensory deprivation is caused by a deficiency of meaningful stimuli.
- Sensory deprivation can be due to environmental conditions or to interference with the reception or perception of stimuli.
- Sensory overload develops when either environmental or internal stimuli—or a combination of both—exceed a level that the client's sensory system can effectively process. It can also occur in clients with neurological or psychiatric disorders who are unable to adapt to continuing, nonmeaningful stimuli.
- Impaired vision and hearing are the sensory deficits most commonly encountered in nursing practice.
- The client with impaired vision, hearing, tactile sensation, olfactory sensation, or kinesthesia is at risk for injury.
- Visual and hearing changes may diminish the ability to communicate and may hamper social interaction.
- Developmental issues, culture, health status, medications, stress level, and individual preferences affect sensory perception.
- To assess sensory perceptual function, assess factors affecting sensory perception, mental status, recent changes in sensory stimulation, use of sensory aids, the client's environment, and the support network.
- Nursing strategies to address impaired sensory perception include activities to promote sensory function, prevent and treat sensory overload and deprivation, assist clients with sensory deficits, and communicate with clients with altered mental status.

Knowledge Map

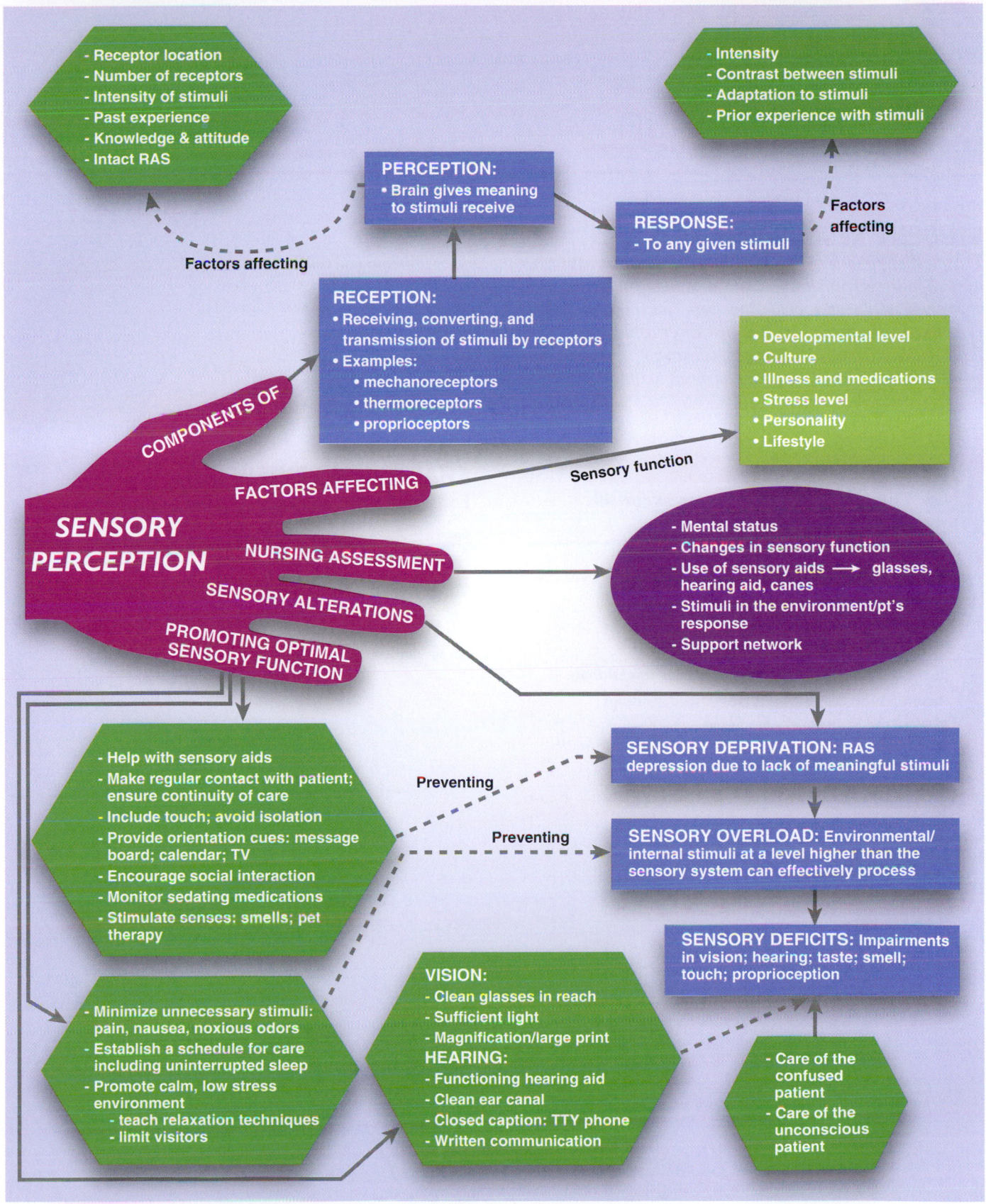

CHAPTER 31

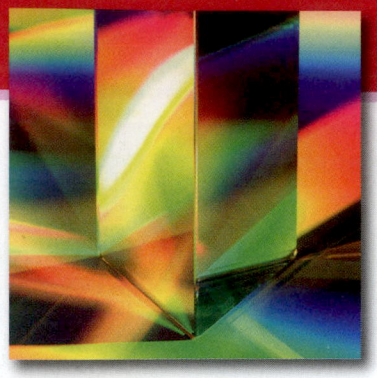

Pain

STUDENT RESOURCES

*The questions and exercises in Volume 2 allow you to practice the kind of thinking you will use as a full-spectrum nurse. Critical-thinking questions usually have more than one correct answer, so we do not provide "answers" for these features. It is more important to develop your nursing judgment than to just cover content. You will learn by discussing the questions with your peers. If you are still unsure, consult your instructor. You will find Response Sheets (for writing your responses to the questions) on Davis*Plus.

To explore learning resources for this chapter,

Go to Davis*Plus* at DavisPl.us/Wilkinson3.

Chapter Resources for Chapter 31:

- **Response Sheets for all learning activities**
- **Resources for Caregivers and Health Professionals**
- **Reading More About Pain (suggested readings)**
- **Concept Map of chapter content**

Interactive Case Studies

NCLEX-Style and Chapter Review Questions

CHAPTER OVERVIEW

For a podcast of an overview of this chapter,

Go to Student Resources, Chapter 31, **Podcast—Chapter Overview,** on Davis*Plus*.

Caring for the Nguyens

Review the introduction to the Nguyens at the front of this volume. Nam Nguyen has bilateral knee pain secondary to osteoarthritis. To develop a pain management plan, what patient data do you need to know?

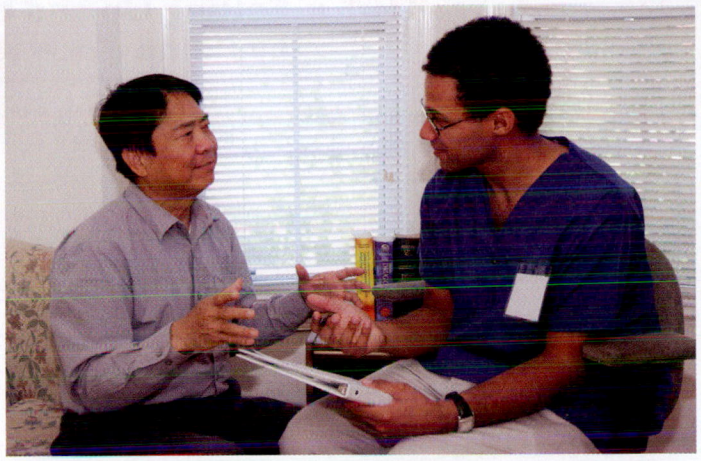

A. How will you get the data you need? What sources should you use?

B. What types of nursing knowledge (theoretical, practical, ethical, or self-knowledge) are needed to develop a pain management plan?

Practical Knowledge knowing how

When caring for patients with pain, you will need to be skilled in medication administration, including use of patient-controlled analgesia (PCA) pumps and caring for patients who have an epidural catheter.

PROCEDURES

Procedure 31-1 ■ Setting Up and Managing Patient-Controlled Analgesia by Pump

➤ For steps to follow in *all* procedures, refer to the Universal Steps for All Procedures found on the page facing the inside back cover.

Equipment

- PCA pump (infuser and central unit)
- Manufacturer's instructions for the pump
- Cartridge, syringe, or other type of sealed unit containing the medication
- Connecting tubing (to connect the PCA device to the patient's IV line)
- Maintenance IV supplies, as needed
- IV pole
- Antiseptic swab
- Flowsheet (electronic or paper)
- 1 pair of clean procedure gloves (if venipuncture is necessary)

Delegation

Because an opioid medication is delivered intravenously to the patient, this procedure is outside the scope of the practice of nursing assistive personnel (NAP) and should never be delegated. Furthermore, the NAP should not administer a dose for the patient, even if he asks her to do so. You can inform the NAP of expected side effects and ask her to report her observations to you.

Pre-Procedure Assessment

- Assess physical conditions that can affect respirations.
  Respiratory diseases (e.g., chronic obstructive pulmonary disease [COPD] and asthma) and conditions such as head injury and sleep apnea increase the risk for respiratory depression with opioid use.
- Assess level of consciousness and cognitive level.
  Determines whether the patient will be able to follow directions for self-dosing.
- Review lab values reflecting liver and kidney function, such as blood urea nitrogen (BUN), creatinine, and liver enzymes.
  Opioid analgesics are typically metabolized through the liver or kidneys.

(continued on next page)

Procedure 31-1 ■ Setting Up and Managing Patient-Controlled Analgesia by Pump (continued)

- **Assess the baseline respiratory rate, pulse, blood pressure, and oxygen saturation.**
  A change in vital signs (e.g., hypotension, respiratory rate below 8) may indicate adverse responses to opioid administration.
- **Be aware of the patient's age and weight.**
  Age is a factor when you are verifying the dose. Older patients and very young children are at increased risk for respiratory suppression, so may require lower doses.
- **Assess the patient's baseline pain level using a standardized pain assessment tool or numeric scale ranging from 0 to 10.**
  A quantified self-report is one of the most accurate measures of pain.
- **Assess the patient's manual dexterity.**
  Patients with impaired fine motor control or upper extremity injury may not be able to operate the self-dosing mechanism.
- **Review medications currently in use.**
  The risk of respiratory depression increases when a PCA pump is used in conjunction with other CNS depressants, such as diazepam (Valium).
- **Assess the extent of family involvement. Identify any family anxiety over the patient's pain. Reinforce that only the patient should use the PCA button.**
  Only the patient should administer the medication. "PCA by proxy" (someone other than the patient pushing the dosing button) is a major factor contributing to adverse patient outcomes (Wuhrman, Cooney, Dunwoody, et al., 2007).

➤ When performing the procedure, always identify your patient according to agency policy, using two identifiers, and be attentive to standard precautions, hand hygiene, patient safety and privacy, body mechanics, and documentation.

Procedure Steps

1. **Don clean procedure gloves,** and initiate IV therapy if the patient does not currently have an IV solution infusing. Refer to Procedure 38-1 as needed.
2. **Obtain the medication** and double-check it with the original prescription. You may need to remove air from the vial by pushing the injector into the vial. Connect the PCA tubing to the vial (or cartridge).
   Some vials may not be completely filled with medication. Ejecting the air makes it faster to prime the connecting tubing.
3. **Double-check your dose** calculation with another nurse before starting the infusion or wasting medication.
   To prevent medication errors in dosing.
   a. "On-demand" dose (the amount of drug to be delivered with each push of the button)
   b. The "lockout" interval (the number of minutes allowed between each administration of an on-demand dose [e.g., q10 min]). Even if the patient pushes the button more frequently, the PCA pump will not administer a dose until the preset time between doses has been met.
   c. Basal rate or continuous infusion (the amount of medication to be delivered automatically by the pump over 1 hour) should be used with caution. Giving the medication continuously without the patient having to push a button takes away some of the inherent safety of a PCA.
   d. One-time "bolus" (or *loading*) dose, which you administer after setting up the pump
   e. The 1-hour or 4-hour lockout interval (the maximum dose allowed in that time frame). For example, if the patient has a 4-mg on-demand dose with a 10-minute lockout interval, the patient can receive a maximum of six 4-mg doses per hour for a total of 24 mg/hr and a maximum dose of 96 mg in 4 hours.

   NOTE: PCA prescriptions are usually written in milligrams; however, pump settings may be in milliliters. In such cases, you must verify the concentration (milligrams per milliliter) to set the pump correctly.
4. **Prime the tubing; then clamp** the tubing above the connector.
   Priming prevents air from entering the pump and causing malfunction. Clamping prevents an accidental bolus of medication getting to the patient.
5. **Insert the cartridge or vial** into the pump, and lock the pump. Follow the manufacturer's instruction manual (e.g., some pumps can be set only if the door is closed and locked).
   Depending on the pump, it may be a syringe, a cartridge, or other sealed container that can be "locked" into the pump. Locking the pump prevents unauthorized access to the opioid and dosing features.
6. **Turn the pump on, and set** the parameters according to the prescriptions and your calculations. The settings may include:
   a. On demand
   b. Lockout interval
   c. Basal rate or continuous infusion —if applicable
   d. The 1-hour or 4-hour lockout dosage limit
   e. The one-time loading dose—if applicable
7. **Scrub the port on the IV** tubing closest to the patient, using alcohol or a chlorhexidine gluconate (CHG)–alcohol product; then connect the PCA pump tubing.
   Removes gross contamination and discourages growth of pathogens.
8. **Open the clamp and** administer the bolus (loading) dose if prescribed. Remain with the patient as the dose is delivered.
   A loading dose is usually larger than the basal and on-demand doses because

pain is likely to be more severe before the pump is initiated. Remaining with the patient allows you to observe for adverse effects.

9. **Close the pump door, and lock** the machine with the key.
10. **Check for flashing lights** or alarms that may indicate the need to correct settings.
11. **Be sure to release tubing clamps** if you previously clamped the tubing; press the start button to begin pump operation.
12. **Ensure that the battery life** is sufficient or, preferably, that the pump in plugged into an appropriate electrical outlet.
    To avoid battery failure.
13. **Place the control button** for on-demand doses within the patient's reach. Be sure the PCA cord is placed away from the call bell.
    To avoid error in self dosing with PCA. ➤

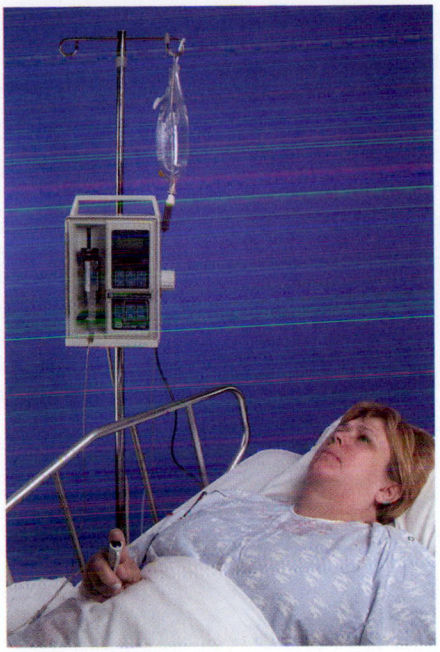

? What if . . .

- **The patient cannot verbally communicate pain status?**

  Use an alternate standardized pain tool, such as the FACES pain scale or a behavioral measure to determine pain level.

  Pain assessment in patients who are uncommunicative may include behavioral or physiological indicators to assess and monitor the effectiveness of pain medication.

- **The infusion infiltrates?**

  Discontinue the IV and establish another IV site. Follow facility policy for application of cold or warm compresses to the infiltrated area. Assess pain level. You may need to contact the prescriber for a bolus dose if the IV has been interrupted for an extended period or the patient has insufficient pain relief.

Evaluation

- Monitor the patient's pain level, sedation level, and respiratory rate at least every hour for the first 24 hours or according to facility policy after initiating PCA.
  Promotes the early detection of respiratory depression, oversedation, or inadequate pain control.
- Perform routine assessment of number and frequency of doses and pump settings per facility protocol.
- Check the IV site for redness, infiltration, or phlebitis.
- Check the IV tubing for patency (e.g., for kinks) to be sure the medication is infusing.

Patient Teaching

Patients who are candidates for use of PCA should be trained before surgery rather than in the immediate postoperative period, when the effects of anesthesia impair learning. Reinforce or teach the patient and family the following:

- Safe and correct use of the PCA pump
- The benefits of PCA for controlling pain
- The pump will deliver only the amount of medication prescribed. Pushing the button too many times will not result in overdosing.
- The patient cannot accidentally roll over on the button and unintentionally give additional medication.
- If pain is not being relieved, the patient should tell the nurse so adjustments can be made to the PCA.
- The pump will alarm when nearly empty, alerting nurses to change the syringe.
- The PCA button is to relieve pain—not to help the patient sleep.
- Signs and symptoms of allergic reaction and which ones to report
- How to rate pain using a standard pain scale
- The patient is the only one who may push the pain-dosing button. Explain why family members should not give "doses by proxy."

Documentation

You will usually document PCA initiation on a specialized checklist or flowsheet. Items charted include:

- Time the infusion was begun, including the drug, the patient demand dose, the loading dose, the basal dose if applicable, lockout interval, and hourly limit

(continued on next page)

Procedure 31-1 ■ Setting Up and Managing Patient-Controlled Analgesia by Pump (continued)

- Patient's baseline pain level and evaluation of subsequent pain level performed at intervals determined by facility policy
- Baseline respiratory rate, pulse, blood pressure, and oxygen saturation; routine evaluation of subsequent vital signs performed at intervals determined by facility policy
- Sedation level
- Continuous monitoring of vital signs, level of consciousness, and pain status, as well as the number and frequency of doses
- Unusual occurrences (e.g., oversedation, IV infiltration) in the nursing notes

Thinking About the Procedure

To practice applying clinical reasoning to this procedure,

Go to the *Nursing Fundamentals Videos*, **Setting up and Managing Patient-Controlled Analgesia by Pump**

For questions and suggested responses,

Go to Chapter 31, **Thinking About the Procedure Questions and Suggested Responses,** on Davis*Plus*.

Practice Resources

Best practices: Evidence-based nursing procedures (2008); Cohen, M. R., Weber, R. J., & Moss, J. (2006); d'Arcy, (2008a); Post-operative pain management. (2010).

CLINICAL INSIGHTS

Clinical Insight 31-1 ➤ Caring for the Patient With an Epidural Catheter

Nursing care of the patient with epidural analgesia focuses on safely administering analgesia, assessing pain while achieving maximum pain control, and preventing or identifying adverse reactions (Sawheney, 2012).

Epidural analgesia is contraindicated in patients who received anticoagulant therapy or other bleeding problems, infection at the insertion site or in the bloodstream, or increased intracranial pressure. Additionally, the patient with an allergy to local anesthetic or opioid must not receive this type of pain control. An epidural approach is typically not suited for those who have spinal defects, previous spinal surgery, or certain neurological conditions (e.g., multiple sclerosis) because any new or changed clinical symptoms may be difficult to distinguish.

Monitoring

- Closely monitor the patient's vital signs, especially for respiratory depression and hypotension (every hour for the first 24 hours, then every 4 hours if the patient is stable).

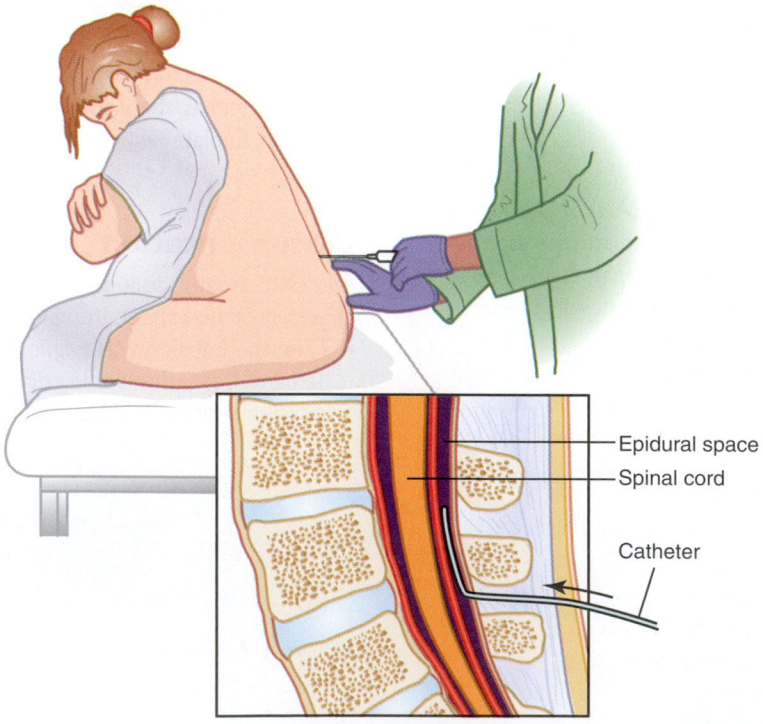

Clinical Insight 31-1 ➤ Caring for the Patient With an Epidural Catheter—cont'd

- Assess the degree of pain intensity using a pain rating scale (per institution's protocol) and degree of motor and sensory block.
- Monitor the site for leaking or drainage.
- Check connections for leaks. This can be fixed by carefully retightening connections. If the filter is cracked, replace with a new one using sterile technique.
- Assess for urine retention. Keep careful intake and output (I&O) records.
  Urinary retention is one side effect of epidural opioids.
- Observe for signs of headache in the patient as a result of dural puncture. Treatment consists of bedrest, analgesics, and liberal hydration. Caffeine is also helpful and may be administered IV. If unresolved after 72 hours, patient might receive an epidural blood patch.
- Observe for signs of catheter migration: nausea, a decrease in blood pressure, and a loss of motor function without a recognizable cause.
- Be alert to signs of local anesthesia toxicity occurring when anesthesia is injected directly into the bloodstream instead of the epidural space. The patient might report numbness or tingling around the mouth or ringing in the ears (tinnitus); or the nurse may assess irritability, tremors, seizures, or cardiac arrhythmias (Portenoy & McCaffery, 2011; Sawheney, 2012).

Prevention

- Clearly label solutions with "For epidural use only" using large font. Store IV and epidural medication in separate locations.
  Prevents errors in medication administration.
- Mark all lines *clearly*: Most epidural tubing is marked with a yellow stripe.
  Epidural lines must not be confused with IV solution for an arterial or venous catheter.
- Ensure the tape on the tubing connected to the patient is secure.
  To prevent catheter migration.
- Use strict aseptic technique when changing tubing, including mask and sterile gloves for access and maintenance procedures.

Discontinuing the Catheter

- If you are specially trained to remove an epidural catheter, first loosen the tape securing the catheter. While wearing clean gloves, apply slow, steady pressure to withdraw the catheter. Inspect the catheter on removal. You must be able to see the tip of the catheter. If not, a portion of the catheter may still be lodged in the patient's epidural space. Notify the anesthesia team immediately of this finding.
- If the catheter cannot be withdrawn with minimal force, try repositioning the patient to the same position for removal as the patient was in during insertion of the catheter.
- Cleanse the insertion site, and cover with a dry sterile dressing.

Clinical Insight 31-2 ➤ Guidelines for Assessing Pain

Assessing for Nonverbal Signs of Pain

When assessing for nonverbal signs of pain, keep the following guidelines in mind:

- **Facial expression, posture, and body position are reliable indicators of the intensity of pain.** Basic and common facial expressions that signal pain are lowering the brow, wincing, clenching jaws, and closing eyelids (Institute for Clinical Systems Improvement, 2005, updated 2011). Guarding a painful site or maintaining a tense position is also a sign of pain.
- **Changes in vital signs generally last only a short time.** The body seeks equilibrium; thus, after an hour or so, the vital signs typically return to baseline even though the patient may still be in pain. Continuous, severe pain may elevate the vital signs again from time to time, but they rarely remain elevated.
- **Key Point:** ***Normal vital signs do not mean that the patient is free of pain.***
- **Patients may be in pain even if they don't "act like" they are.** Unfortunately it has been well documented that healthcare professionals fail to assess pain and tend to underrate the pain the patient is experiencing (McCaffery & Pasero, 1999; McCaffery, Pasero, & Ferrell, 2007). They expect to see frowning, crying, or scowling. Patients who use laughter, distraction, or even sleep to cope with their pain are often undertreated.
  Key Point: ***To assess pain accurately, you must ask your patients and then believe them.***

Assessing Verbal Expressions of Pain

- **Assess for stoicism.** Some patients feel that they are being "bad" or "weak" if they express pain. Such patients

(Continued)

Clinical Insight 31-2 ➤ Guidelines for Assessing Pain—cont'd

may withdraw or become stoic. It is important that you establish a trusting relationship with them. Convey your concern, and acknowledge the person's pain. If the patient trusts you, she will feel free to verbalize thoughts and feelings.

- **Remember to assess for depression** (see Chapter 13 if you need to review). Approximately one-third to one-half of patients receiving treatment for pain also have depression (Hooten, Timming, Belgrade, et al., updated 2013). If depression is not treated aggressively, efforts to manage the pain may not be successful. Avoid the misconception, however, that pain is the cause of the depression and that controlling the pain will eliminate the depression. This is rarely the case.

Using Pain Scales

- **Use an interpreter if the patient speaks a different language.** Ask the interpreter to explain to the patient that it is important to manage pain and that you will be using a pain scale regularly to assess his pain. Have the interpreter translate and write out the explanation and directions for the pain scale so you can refer to these when you assess your patient. With written directions, patients can point to a face or numeric line to tell you about their pain when no one is present to translate.

ASSESSMENT GUIDELINES AND TOOLS

Focused Assessment

Pain Assessment

Taking a Pain History

Taking a pain history is the most effective way to perform an assessment. Each agency has a different assessment form for this history, but the questions typically will include the following:

Do you have pain now?

When did the pain begin?

Where is the pain located?

How do you rate your pain? (Use a pain scale.)

How would you describe your pain? Sharp? Dull? Achy? Burning?

How often do you have pain? Is it constant or intermittent?

Is there a rhythm or pattern to your pain? Is there anything you do that triggers the pain?

What makes the pain better? What makes it worse?

How many days this past week has pain interfered in your ability to do what you would like to do?

Does pain interfere with your ability to take care of yourself?

Does pain wake you up at night?

Does pain interrupt your concentration and reduce your ability to think clearly?

Does pain prevent you from participating in pleasurable activities, hobbies, and socializing with friends?

Have you experienced this type of pain in the past?

Do you have any other symptoms (such as nausea and vomiting) when you are experiencing pain?

Have you used any medications to treat the pain? If so, were they effective? How often do you need to take pain relievers?

What, if any, alternative treatments have you used for pain?

What past experiences or cultural factors, if any, influence the pain?

Observing for Nonverbal Indicators of Pain

Physiological (Involuntary) Responses

Sympathetic Responses (Acute Pain)

Increased systolic blood pressure

Increased heart rate and force of contraction

Increased respiratory rate

Increased alertness (resulting from dilated blood vessels to the brain)

Dilated pupils

Rapid speech

Parasympathetic Responses (Deep or Prolonged Pain)

Decreased systolic blood pressure, possible syncope

Decreased pulse rate

Changeable breathing patterns

Withdrawal

Constricted pupils

Slow, monotonous speech

Behavioral Responses (Voluntary)

Withdrawing from painful stimuli

Moaning

Facial grimacing

Crying

Agitation

Guarding the painful area

Focused Assessment

Psychological (Affective) Responses

- Anxiety
- Depression
- Anger
- Fear
- Exhaustion
- Hopelessness
- Irritability

Using Pain Scales

The most commonly used pain scales are the Visual Analog Scale (VAS), the Numerical Rating Scale (NRS), the Simple Descriptor Scale (SDS), and the Wong-Baker FACES rating scale.

The Visual Analog Scale

The Visual Analog Scale (VAS) is a 10-cm horizontal line in which "No pain" is written on the left side and "Worst pain imaginable" is written on the right. Patients point to a location on the line that reflects their current pain. Although this rating system is simple and quick, some patients have problems with the abstract nature of the scale.

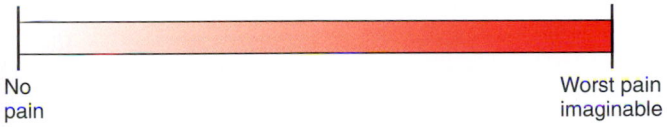

The Numerical Rating Scale

The Numerical Rating Scale (NRS) is a line numbered from 0 to 10. Zero indicates no pain at all, whereas a 10 indicates the worst possible pain. Patients choose a number from 0 to 10 to denote their level of pain. To use this scale, the patient must be able to count to 10. A scale of 0 to 5 may be more helpful for cognitively impaired patients.

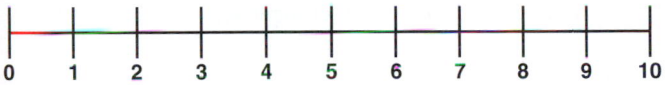

The Simple Descriptor Scale

The Simple Descriptor Scale (SDS) is a list of adjectives that describe different levels of pain intensity. The simplest version of this scale uses the words *mild, moderate,* and *severe*. An SDS with many words is not recommended; it is time consuming to describe and may not be understood by many patients.

The Wong-Baker FACES Pain Rating Scale

The FACES Scale uses simple illustrations of faces to depict various levels of pain. It requires no numerical or reading skill. Initially developed for use with children older than the age of 3, the scale has proved to be extremely useful for adults with communication and cognitive impairments as well.

Wong-Baker FACES Pain Rating Scale

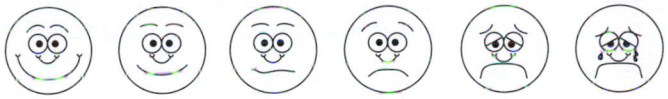

0	1	2	3	4	5
No hurt	Hurts little bit	Hurts little more	Hurts even more	Hurts whole lot	Hurts worst

Explain to the person that each face is for a person who feels happy because he has no pain (hurt) or sad because he has some or a lot of pain. Face 0 is very happy because he doesn't hurt at all. Face 2 hurts a little more. Face 3 hurts even more. Face 4 hurts a whole lot. Face 5 hurts as much as you can imagine, although you do not have to be crying to feel this bad. Ask the person to chose the face that best describes how he is feeling. Rating scale is recommended for persons age 3 and older.

From Hockenberry M. J., & Wilson D. (2009). *Wong's essentials of pediatric nursing* (8th ed.). St. Louis, MO: Mosby. Used with permission. Copyright Mosby.

Revised Faces Pain Scales

We commonly ask patients to rate their pain on a scale of 0 to 10. However, the Wong-Baker FACES Scale uses a 0 to 5 scale. To see a revised FACES scale adapted to a 10-point scoring system, see Spragud, L. J., Piira, T., & Baeyer, C. L. (2003). Children's self-report of pain intensity, *American Journal of Nursing, 103*(12), 62–64; or

Go to the **Pediatric Pain Sourcebook** on the International Association for the Study of Pain Web site at http://www.iasp-pain.org/Content/NavigationMenu/GeneralResourceLinks/FacesPainScaleRevised/default.htm

To see FACES scales using photos of children of various ethnicities,

Go to the **OUCHER! Web site** at www.oucher.org

Focused Assessment

Pain Relief Diary

Client Pain Relief Diary

For pain relief I am using:

Medications _____

Alternative therapy (relaxation, distraction, etc.) _____

I will call my physician if _____ (filled in by nurse before discharge)

My goals are a pain rating of _____

Date	Time	Number of pills	Pain scale 0 1 2 3 4 5 6 7 8 9 10	Goal met? Yes No	Activity

Focused Assessment

Richmond Agitation-Sedation Rating Scale

Sedation Rating Scale

Richmond agitation–sedation scale

Score	Term	Description
+4	Combative	Overtly combative or violent; immediate danger to staff
+3	Very agitated	Pulls on or removes tube(s) or catheter(s) or has aggressive behavior toward staff
+2	Agitated	Frequent nonpurposeful movement or patient–ventilator dyssynchrony
+1	Restless	Anxious or apprehensive but movements not aggressive or vigorous
0	Alert and calm	
-1	Drowsy	Not fully alert, but has sustained (more than 10 seconds) awakening, with eye contact, to voice
-2	Light sedation	Briefly (less than 10 seconds) awakens with eye contact to voice
-3	Moderate sedation	Any movement (but no eye contact) to voice
-4	Deep sedation	No response to voice, but any movement to physical stimulation
-5	Unarousable	No response to voice or physical stimulation

Sessler, C. N., Gosnell, M.S., Grap, M. J., et al. (2002). The Richmond Agitation–Sedation Scale: Validity and reliability in adult intensive care unit patients. *American Journal of Respiratory Critical Care Medicine, 166,* 1338–1344, Retrieved on March 24, 2012, from http://ajrccm.atsjournals.org/content/166/10/1338.full.pdf+html

CLINICAL REASONING

Applying the Full-Spectrum Nursing Model

PATIENT SITUATION

Dieter Schmidt is a 48-year-old with a 2-year history of cervical spine injury that began after a motor vehicle accident. Three years before the accident, Dieter fell through a roof to the cement basement when inspecting a building under construction. Presenting symptoms were neck pain when turning his head, biceps weakness, and pain down the arm with tingling into the fingertips. He is unable to sit for extended periods or walk distances. Initially he received treatment with medication, TENS to the site, physical therapy, and cervical fusion. Despite trying all treatments available to him, including surgery, Dieter continues to suffer chronic pain and fatigue. After prolonged suffering with no relief, Mr. Schmidt develops a cynical attitude toward healthcare. He begins missing more and more scheduled appointments for physical therapy. He describes stress he feels from the economic downturn impacting his land development business and fears bankruptcy. As a result, he has given up previous hobbies and most social activities. His relationships with his family and friends are increasingly strained as the pain persists over time.

THINKING

1. *Theoretical Knowledge:*
   What is the mechanism that explains how pain is transmitted in the spine?
2. *Critical Thinking (Considering Alternatives, Deciding What to Do):*
   a. When planning care for Dieter, what approach would you take in helping him to set goals for his rehabilitation?
   b. Why do you think Dieter displays a negative attitude and reduced compliance toward rehabilitative therapies?

DOING

3. *Practical Knowledge:*
   a. (*Nursing Process*: *Assessment*): What questions would you ask Dieter to assess the impact of pain on his daily living and quality of life?
   b. (*Nursing Process*: *Interventions*): In addition to drug therapy, what other measures might you teach your patient to do to control his pain and increase his comfort?

CARING

4. *Self-Knowledge:*
   Have you ever experienced chronic pain, such as back pain, fibromyalgia, arthritis, migraines, sports injuries, or other types? If so, how has it affected your daily life? Has your pain impacted your relationships? Has it interfered with your job or recreational activities? In what other ways would you say chronic pain has reduced the quality of your life?

Critical Thinking and Clinical Reasoning

1. Mrs. J is a 29-year-old woman with terminal metastatic breast cancer. She knows she is dying. She has a devoted husband and two children, ages 2 and 4. Her husband has been taking care of her at home, but she is currently hospitalized for intractable pain. She does not want to be heavily sedated because she wants to spend as much time with her family as she can. She has no pain management plan.
   a. What is it about the patient's situation that may intensify her pain?
   b. Would you suggest using alternative therapies? Why or why not?
2. Mr. L is a 39-year-old construction worker who fell from a roof at a construction site 8 months ago and is still having back pain from the accident. To manage pain, he is prescribed an oral opioid every 4 hours on a prn basis. He is still out of work and has great difficulty walking, so he spends most of the day in a recliner watching TV and drinking beer. Mr. L also sleeps most nights in the recliner. He states that the alcohol is the only thing that helps his pain. How would you alter his pain management plan to get better relief? What is your rationale for these changes?
3. How might you encourage a facility to enact a pain assessment strategy of pain as the fifth vital sign if this is not their current policy?

4. If you were delegating vital signs to nursing assistive personnel (NAP), what instructions would you give?
5. For each of the following concepts, use critical thinking to describe how or why it is important to nursing, patient care, or pain management. Note that these are *not* to be merely definitions.

Nociceptive pain	Opioid pain medications
Neuropathic pain	Adjuvant therapies
Unrelieved pain	Pain as the fifth vital sign
Fear of addiction	Pain scales
Nonpharmacological pain management	Pain flowsheets
Nonopioid pain medications	

What Are the Main Points in This Chapter?

- Pain is whatever the person says it is and exists whenever the person says it does.
- Pain has a protective function, warning us of potential or actual tissue damage and prompting us to take action.
- Pain can be classified by its origin, cause, duration, and quality.
- Pain begins when mechanical, thermal, or chemical stimuli activate nociceptors, which send pain impulses to the spinal cord.
- Fast pain impulses are carried on large-diameter A-delta fibers, whereas slow pain impulses are carried on thinner C fibers.
- Perception of pain occurs in the frontal cortex of the brain.
- Pain can be modulated by the endogenous analgesic system or by the gate control mechanism.
- Some of the factors that influence pain are emotional factors, life span variations, past pain experiences, sociocultural factors, inability to communicate, and cognitive impairment.
- Serious physiological as well as psychological problems can result from unrelieved pain.
- Nonpharmacological pain relief measures include cutaneous stimulation, immobilization, and cognitive–behavioral intervention.
- Pharmacological measures include nonopioid analgesics, opioid analgesics, and adjuvant analgesics.
- Local and regional anesthesia, nerve blocks, and ablation therapy can relieve short- and long-term pain.
- Surgical interruption of pain conduction pathways is an option for intractable pain. Options depend on the type and location of pain.
- Opioid addiction among individuals being treated for pain is rare.
- Pain should be considered the fifth vital sign and assessed when the patient is admitted to a healthcare facility, with each vital signs check, before and after an intervention, and when the patient reports pain.
- The patient's self-report is the most reliable indicator of pain, especially for those suffering chronic pain.
- Misconceptions about pain can interfere in pain management.
- Older adults are at risk for undertreatment of pain.
- Planning for the patient's pain management program includes discovering the patient's own goals, educating the patient and family, and developing a nursing plan of care.
- It is important to assess continually the effectiveness of pain management strategies.

Knowledge Map

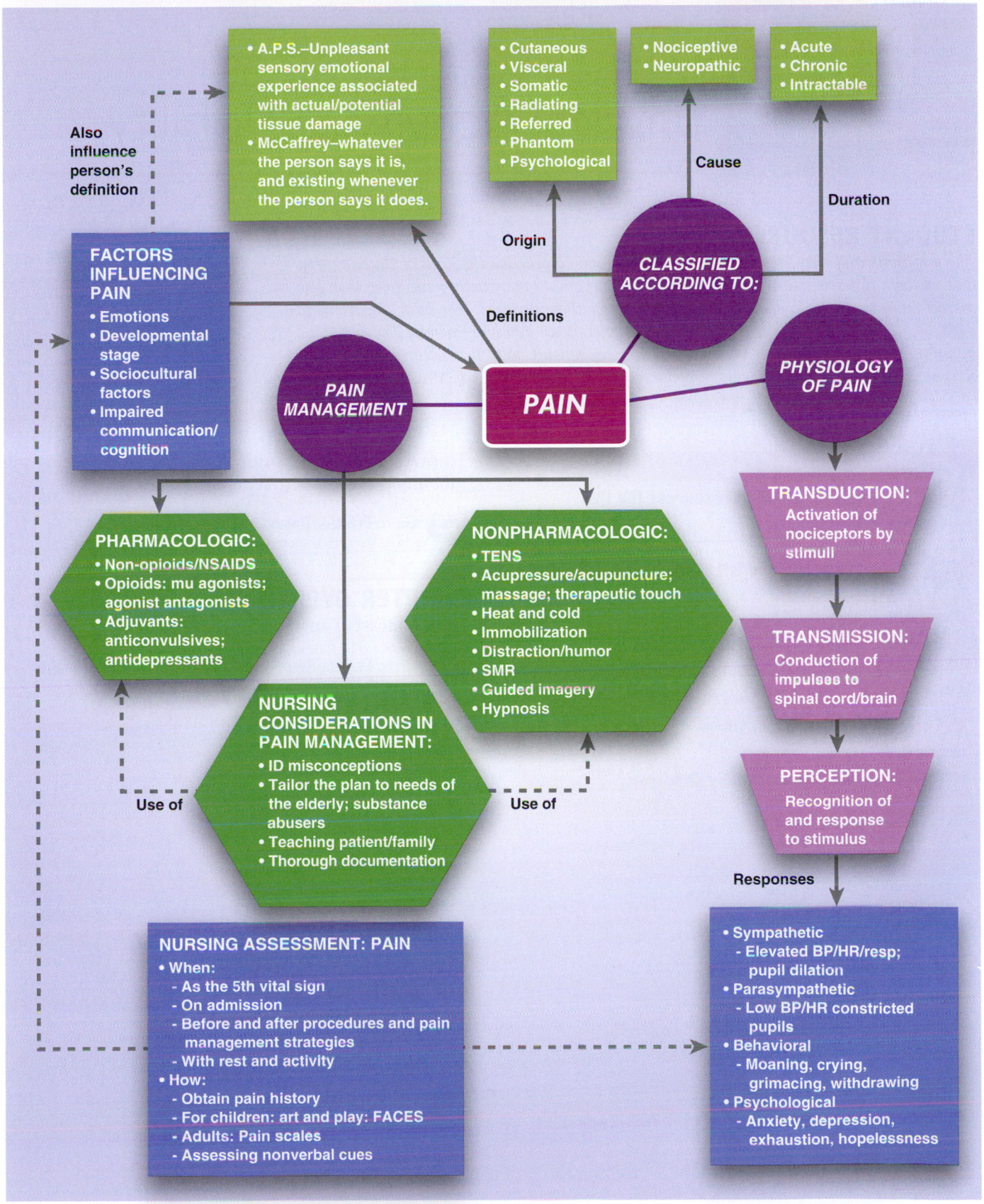

CHAPTER 32

Physical Activity & Mobility

STUDENT RESOURCES

*The questions and exercises in Volume 2 allow you to practice the kind of thinking you will use as a full-spectrum nurse. Critical-thinking questions usually have more than one correct answer, so we do not provide "answers" for these features. It is more important to develop your nursing judgment than to just cover content. You will learn by discussing the questions with your peers. If you are still unsure, consult your instructor. You will find Response Sheets (for writing your responses to the questions) on Davis*Plus.

To explore learning resources for this chapter,

Go to Davis*Plus* at DavisPl.us/Wilkinson3.

Chapter Resources for Chapter 32:
- **Response Sheets for all learning activities**
- **Resources for Caregivers and Health Professionals**
- **Reading More About Physical Activity & Mobility**
- **Concept Map of chapter content**

Interactive Case Studies

NCLEX-Style and Chapter Review Questions

To practice documentation for a patient experiencing mobility problems activity and exercise,

Go to **Practice Documentation,** on Davis*Plus*.

CHAPTER OVERVIEW

For a podcast of an overview of this chapter,

Go to Student Resources, Chapter 32, **Podcast—Chapter Overview,** on Davis*Plus*.

Caring for the Nguyens

As you may recall, Nam Nguyen has been advised to diet and exercise as part of the treatment plan for hypertension, type 2 diabetes mellitus, obesity, and osteoarthritis. Zach Jackson's exam has revealed no other cardiovascular problems.

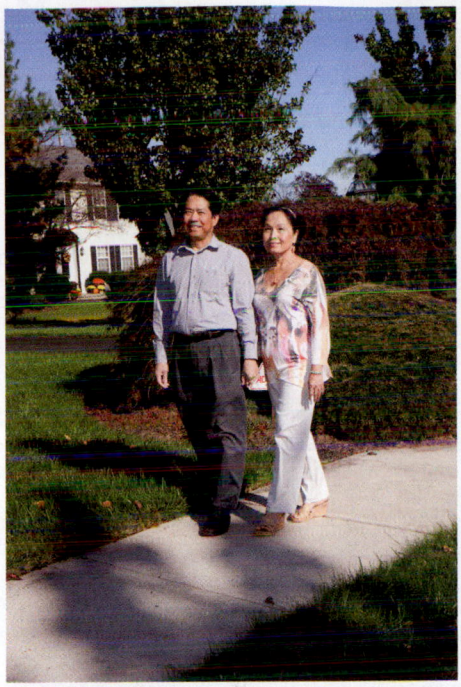

A. Design a fitness program for Nam. Describe the program in detail. Recall that Nam has been relatively sedentary.

B. Compare the type of program you would recommend for Nam with the type of program appropriate for his grandson, Kim.

C. What type of fitness program would be most appropriate for Mai Nguyen, Nam's mother? What additional information do you need to know to answer this question?

Practical Knowledge knowing how

In the next sections you will learn about procedures and techniques for positioning, moving, turning, transferring, and ambulating patients safely. Although the American Nurses Association (ANA, 2013) recommends that you use assistive equipment for all patient lifting and transferring, you may encounter situations in which equipment is not available or you do not have time to get it (e.g., in an emergency). In such situations, using good body mechanics may help you decrease the risk of injury to you and the patient.

PROCEDURES

Procedure 32-1 ■ Moving and Turning Patients in Bed

➤ For steps to follow in *all* procedures, refer to the Universal Steps for All Procedures found on the page facing the inside back cover.

Equipment

- Nonlatex gloves, if you may be exposed to body fluids
- Friction-reducing device, such as a transfer roller sheet or scoot sheet
- Pull or lift (draw) sheet
- Pillows, as needed

Delegation

You may ask nursing assistive personnel (NAP) to assist with moving a patient up in bed, turning a patient, or logrolling a patient after ensuring that the NAP has the necessary skills and that the patient's condition is stable. Complete the assessment, and inform the NAP of any special considerations when moving the patient.

(continued on next page)

Procedure 32-1 ■ Moving and Turning Patients in Bed (continued)

Pre-Procedure Assessment

Assess the following:

- Level of comfort
  If the patient is uncomfortable, you may need to administer an analgesic before moving.
- Level of consciousness, ability to follow directions, and ability to assist with the move
- Any restrictions in movement or position (ask the patient and check the provider's orders
- Physical size of the patient and the assistive devices available
- The patient's medical diagnoses. Identify problems that may affect positioning (e.g., respiratory or cardiac problems, pain).
- Presence of equipment such as IV setups, pumps, or casts and know what must be moved with the patient
  The preceding assessments all help determine how many assistants and equipment you need, the patient's ability to assist in the procedure, and how to proceed with the move safely.

Procedure 32-1A ■ Moving a Patient Up in Bed

➤ When performing the procedure, always identify your patient according to agency policy, using two identifiers, and be attentive to standard precautions, hand hygiene, patient safety and privacy, body mechanics, and documentation.

Procedure Steps

Key Point: ***Medicate the patient for pain, if needed, before moving the patient in bed.***

1. **Lock the bed wheels.** Lower the head of the bed, and place the patient in a supine position. Position one nurse on each side of the bed. Lower the siderails on the "working" side of the bed. Raise the height of the bed to waist level.
   Lowering the siderails and raising the bed allows you to move the patient while maintaining good body mechanics and working with gravity.

2. **Ensure that a friction-reducing** device, such as a transfer roller sheet, is in place under the drawsheet. If it is not in place, turn the patient from side to side to place the device under the drawsheet. You can improvise this device by placing a clean, unused plastic bag or plastic film under the drawsheet.
   A transfer roller sheet facilitates movement by reducing friction. This also helps to reduce back injury to the nurse.

   NOTE: This procedure uses a transfer roller sheet. This device is inexpensive and readily available. Scoot sheets further reduce the risk of back and musculoskeletal injury; however, their availability varies. Having a second person to help move a patient up in bed is the safest approach for staff and patients. Also follow the guidelines in Clinical Insight 32-1.

3. **Remove the pillow** from under the patient's head. Place it at the head of the bed.
   A pillow prevents patient from hitting his head on the head board.

4. **Instruct the patient to fold** his arms across his chest. If an overhead trapeze is in place, ask the patient to hold the trapeze with both hands if able. Have the patient bend his knees with feet flat on the bed.
   This position facilitates the patient's assistance with the move.

5. **Instruct the patient to flex** his neck.
   Protects the neck while moving.

6. **With a nurse positioned** on either side of the patient, grasp and roll the drawsheet close to the patient.

7. **Instruct the patient**, on the count of 3, to lift his trunk and push off with his heels toward the head of the bed.

8. **Position your feet with a wide** base of support. Point your feet toward the direction of the move. Flex your knees and hips.
   Allows you to maintain proper body mechanics and prevents injury while moving the patient. ➤

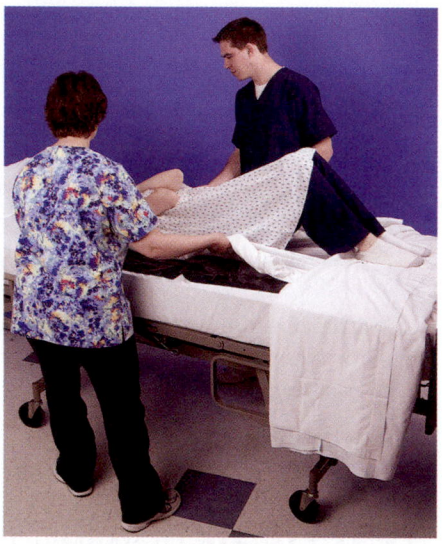

9. **Place your weight on your foot** nearest to the foot of the bed. Count to 3, and shift your weight forward toward the head of the bed.
   Shifting your weight allows you to use your momentum to move the patient, which helps protect your back from injury.

10. **Repeat until the patient** is positioned near the head of the bed. If you used a plastic bag or film to reduce friction, remove it now.
    Plastic is water impermeable, so it allows moisture to pool under the patient. This creates a risk for Impaired Skin Integrity.

11. **Straighten the drawsheet**, and tuck it in tightly at the sides of the bed.
A wrinkle-free sheet prevents uneven pressure, discomfort, and skin irritation.

12. **Place a pillow under** the patient's head, and assist him to a comfortable position.
Provides comfort and good body alignment.

13. **Place the bed in low position**, and raise the siderail.
Helps prevent falls.

14. **Place the call light** in a position where the patient can easily reach it.
Allows patient to call for help, if needed.

Procedure Variation for Use of an Approved Mechanical Lifting Device

15. **Lock the bed wheels.** Lower the head of the bed, and place the patient in a supine position. Position at least one nurse on each side of the bed. Lower the siderails. Raise the height of the bed.

16. **Using the drawsheet, turn** the patient to one side of the bed. Position the midline of the full body sling at the patient's back. Tightly roll the remaining half of the sling, and tuck the fabric under the drawsheet.

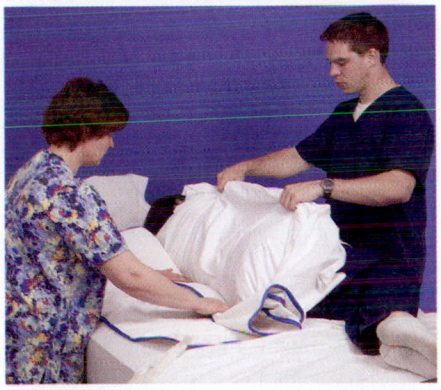

17. **With a second nurse positioned** on either side of the patient, use the drawsheet to turn the patient to the opposite side of the bed. Unroll the full body sling, and reposition the patient supine.

18. **Attach the sling** to the overbed lifting device or mechanical lift.

Be sure the fasteners are securely attached to the lifting device.

19. **Engage the lift** to raise the patient completely off the bed. Advance the lift toward the head of the bed until the patient is at the desired level.

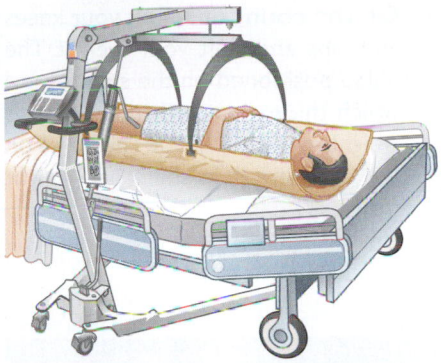

20. **Lower the lift**, and turn the patient to the desired position. You may leave the sling in place for future movement, or you may remove it by turning the patient from side to side.

NOTE: If a full body sling is not available, use a friction-reducing device, such as a transfer roller sheet, and at least three staff members.

Procedure 32-1B ■ Turning a Patient in Bed

➤ When performing the procedure, always identify your patient according to agency policy, using two identifiers, and be attentive to standard precautions, hand hygiene, patient safety and privacy, body mechanics, and documentation.

➤ *Note:* This procedure describes the use of a transfer roller sheet. This device is inexpensive and readily available.

Procedure Steps

1. **Lock the bed wheels.** Lower the head of the bed, and place the patient in a supine position. Position one nurse on each side of the bed. Lower the siderail on the side you are standing, but keep the opposite rail in the up position . Raise the height of the bed to waist level.
Lowering the siderails and raising the bed allow you to move the patient while maintaining good body mechanics and working with gravity to prevent injury.

2. **Position the patient for turning.**
   a. Remove the pillow from under the patient's head and place it at the head of the bed.
   b. Roll the patient side to side and place a friction-reducing device under the drawsheet. Smooth any wrinkles as needed. Tuck the friction-reducing device snuggly under the mattress. You can improvise this device by placing a large, clean plastic bag or plastic film under the drawsheet.
   c. Move the patient to the side of the bed you are turning him away from by rolling up the drawsheet close to the patient's body and pulling it.
   d. Align the patient's legs and head with the trunk.
This allows you to position the patient in the center of the bed after turning.

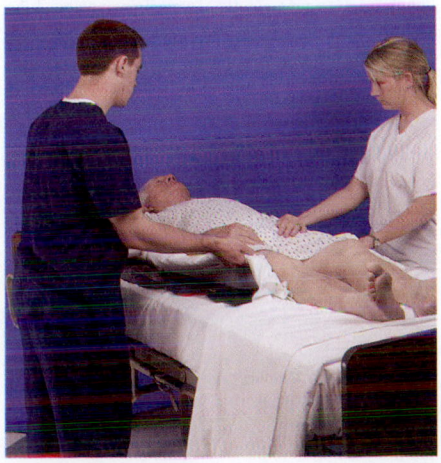

3. **Place the patient's near leg** and foot across the far leg (e.g., when turning the patient to his right, place his left leg over his right leg).

4. **Place the patient's near arm** (e.g., left when turning right) across his chest. And, position the patient's underneath arm up and away from his body.
Positioning the patient's legs and his near arm facilitates turning. Abducting and rotating the other arm prevents it from being caught under the patient during the turn.

5. **Each nurse positions her feet** with a wide base of support with one foot forward of the other. Bend from the hips, and grasp both ends of the drawsheet at the level of the patient's hip and the other at the level of the shoulder.
A wide base of support allows you to maintain good body mechanics while performing the move.

(continued on next page)

Procedure 32-1 ■ Moving and Turning Patients in Bed (continued)

6. **Instruct the patient** that the turn will occur on the count of 3.
Counting coordinates and facilitates patient cooperation with the move.

7. **On the count of 3, flex** your knees and hips and shift your weight. The nurse positioned on the side toward which the patient will turn shifts his weight to the back foot. The nurse on the opposite side shifts her weight forward.
Provides the best leverage to turn the patient.

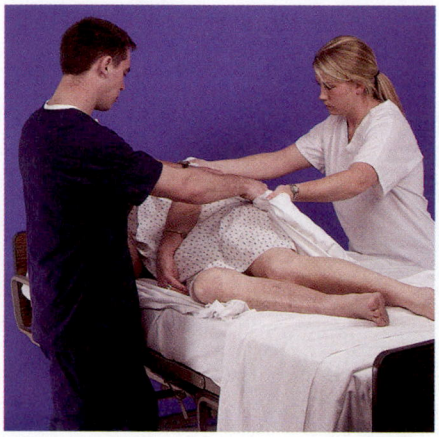

8. **If a plastic film is used**, remove it after you turn the patient.

9. **Position the dependent shoulder** forward. Place pillows behind the patient's back and between legs to maintain the patient in the lateral position. Replace the pillow under the patient's head.
Positioning ensures that patient is not putting excess pressure on the inferior shoulder. Pillows help maintain good body alignment.

Go to Chapter 32, **Table 32-2: Positioning a Bed-Bound Patient,** in Volume 1.

10. **Place the bed in low position,** and raise the siderail.
Helps ensure patient safety.

11. **Place the call light** in a position where the patient can easily reach it.
Allows patient to call for help, if needed.

Procedure 32-1C ■ Logrolling a Patient

➤ When performing the procedure, always identify your patient according to agency policy, using two identifiers, and be attentive to standard precautions, hand hygiene, patient safety and privacy, body mechanics, and documentation.

Procedure Steps

1. **Lock the bed wheels.** Lower the head of the bed with the patient supine. Lower the siderail on the side where you are standing, but keep the opposite rail in the up position. Raise the height of the bed to waist level.
Lowering the siderail and raising the bed allows you to move the patient while maintaining good body mechanics and working with gravity to prevent back injury.

2. **You should already have** a drawsheet with an underlying friction-reducing device, such as a transfer roller sheet, to move the patient to the side of the bed on which you are standing. (You can improvise this device by placing a clean, unused plastic bag or plastic film under the drawsheet.)

3. **Position one staff member** at the patient's head and shoulders; she is responsible for moving the head and neck as a unit. Position the other person at the patient's hips. If you need three staff members, position one at the shoulders, one at the waist, and the third at thigh level. One staff member must maintain the patient's head and neck in alignment. The other members assist with moving the rest of the body in alignment.

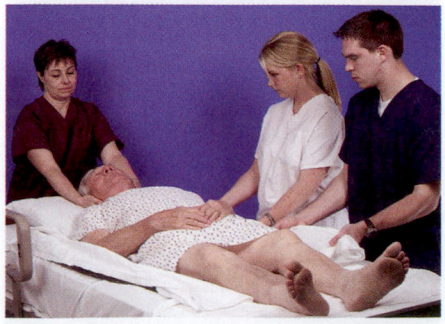

4. **Each nurse should position her** feet with a wide base of support with one foot slightly more forward than the other.
Facilitates proper body mechanics and minimizes risk of injury to staff members.

5. **Use the drawsheet** or transfer sheet to move the patient to the side of the bed on which the nurses are standing. The move must be smooth so that the patient's head and hips are kept in alignment. Position the patient's head with a pillow.
A transfer sheet maintains straight alignment of the spine.

6. **Instruct the patient to fold** his arms across his chest.

7. **Place a pillow** between the patient's knees.
A pillow prevents internal rotation of the hip and spine with movement. Maintains straight alignment of the spine.

8. **Raise the siderail,** and move to opposite side of the bed.
Siderails keep the patient from falling out of bed.

9. **Lower the siderail** on the "new" side of the bed, and face the patient. All nurses should position their feet with a wide base of support, with one foot forward of the other. Place your weight on the forward foot. Bend from the hips, and position your hands evenly along the length of the drawsheet.
Provides the best leverage to turn the patient while maintaining spine alignment.

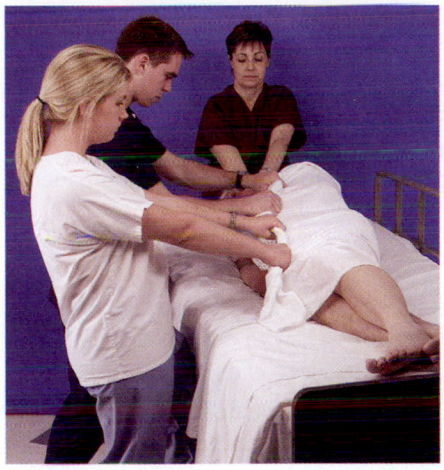

10. **All nurses flex their knees** and hips and shift their weight to the back foot on the count of 3. Be sure to support the head as the patient is rolled to his side.
Allows you to maintain straight alignment and body mechanics while performing the move.

11. **Place pillows to maintain** the patient in the lateral position.

Go to Chapter 32, **Table 32-2: Positioning a Bed-Bound Patient,** in Volume 1.

A pillow provides support and maintains proper alignment.

12. **Place the bed in low position,** and raise the siderail.

13. **Place the call light** in a position where the patient can easily reach it.
Allows patient to call for help, if needed.

What if . . .

- **Your facility has instituted a no-lift policy and you have to pull the patient up in bed?**
  Use assistive equipment, such as friction-reducing devices, mechanical lifts, air-powered mattresses, and/or lateral transfer devices to help prevent work-related injuries.
- **Your patient is obese or unable to assist (totally dependent) and you need to lift him?**
  Minimize manual lifting in all cases and eliminate it where feasible. Therefore, follow facility recommendations/protocols and use approved devices. You should be familiar with the lift devices in your facility.
- **The patient has had a total hip replacement and you have to turn or logroll your patient?**
  Maintain the affected leg in abduction, by using a pillow or abduction wedge between the legs.
  To ensure the hip will not become dislocated during turning.
- **The patient has a cast or is in traction and you have to turn or logroll your patient?**
  Designate a person to assist in the turning by guiding the affected extremity.
- **The patient has an external fixation device and you have to turn or logroll your patient?**
  Secure the device in place to keep it from moving when lifting or moving the limb as needed.
  By holding onto the device to secure it and keep it from moving, there is less movement of the healing bone, and therefore less trauma and pain.

Evaluation

- Assess the patient's comfort level after the position change.
- Assess body position and alignment after position change.
- Assess skin for pressure areas.

Patient Teaching

- Explain to the patient the importance of maintaining spine alignment.
- Explain to the patient the importance of frequent position changes.
- Instruct the patient to ask the nurse when she needs to be turned sooner than scheduled.
- Teach the patient how she can assist with moving and turning.

Home Care

- Instruct the family member or caregiver in the techniques for moving, turning, or logrolling the client.
- Discuss the shearing effects on the skin from sliding down in bed (see Chapter 35).
- Provide instruction on importance of changing position and maintaining proper body alignment.

Documentation

Repositioning and turning patients are considered routine aspects of care and are not usually charted every time they are done. However, document in the nursing notes any problems with positioning the patient or any areas of skin breakdown. You might also chart turning as an intervention when charting to a specific problem. For example, if the patient has Impaired Skin Integrity, you might describe the skin and chart, "Position changed hourly." Some facilities have flowsheets on which you indicate by a checkmark each time a patient is repositioned.

Practice Resources

Centers for Disease Control and Prevention (CDC) (n.d., updated 2012). Collins, J. W., Nelson, A., & Sublet, V. (2006); Nelson, A., & Baptiste, A. S. (2004); Waters, T. R., Nelson, A. N., Hughes, N., et al (2009).

(continued on next page)

Procedure 32-1 ■ Moving and Turning Patients in Bed (continued)

Thinking About the Procedure

To practice applying clinical reasoning to this procedure,

Go to *Davis's Nursing Skills Videos*, **Moving a Patient Up in Bed, Moving a Patient Up in Bed Using a Mechanical Lifting Device, Turning a Patient in Bed,** and **Logrolling a Patient.**

For questions and suggested responses,

Go to Chapter 32, **Thinking About the Procedure Questions and Suggested Responses,** on Davis*Plus*.

Procedure 32-2 ■ Transferring Patients

➤ For steps to follow in *all* procedures, refer to the Universal Steps for All Procedures found on the page facing the inside back cover.

Equipment

- Nonlatex gloves, if you may be exposed to body fluids
- Transfer board (for transferring from bed to stretcher, and sometimes bed to chair)
- Pull or lift (draw) sheet (for transfers)
- Gait transfer belt (for dangling and transferring from bed to chair)

Delegation

You may ask NAP to dangle, transfer a patient from bed to stretcher, or transfer a patient from bed to chair. Ensure that the NAP has the necessary skills and that the patient's condition is stable. Inform the NAP of any special considerations when dangling or transferring the patient and evaluate the patient after transfer.

Pre-Procedure Assessment

- Assess for any restrictions in movement or position by asking the patient and checking the physician's orders.
- Observe for the presence of equipment such as IV lines, drains, or catheters.
- Assess possible side effects of medications (e.g., dizziness and sedation). Assess the patient's level of consciousness, ability to follow directions, and ability to assist with the move.
- Assess the physical size of the patient and your own strength and ability to move the patient.
- Before transferring a patient to a chair, assess the patient's tolerance of dangling.
  The preceding assessments inform you about activity tolerance, readiness to get out of bed, and ability to participate in the transfer. They help you determine how many assistants you need, the appropriate transfer device, and how to proceed with the move while preventing injury and dislodging of equipment.
- Assess vital signs, and monitor for postural hypotension (light-headedness when sitting or standing up quickly from a recumbent position).
  If the patient is at risk for postural hypotension, you may need to allow additional time for the patient to change position.
- Assess the patient's level of comfort using a standardized pain scale.
  If the patient is experiencing pain, you may need to administer an analgesic before moving.

Procedure 32-2A ■ Transferring a Patient From Bed to Stretcher

➤ When performing the procedure, always identify your patient according to agency policy, using two identifiers, and be attentive to standard precautions, hand hygiene, patient safety and privacy, body mechanics, and documentation.

Procedure Steps

1. **Lock the wheels on the bed.** Position the bed so that it is flat (if the patient can tolerate being supine) and at the height of the stretcher.
   Locking the wheels ensures client safety during the transfer. Having the bed flat helps prevent injury to staff, because the patient is easier to move.
2. **Lower the siderails**, and position at least one nurse on each side of the bed. Move the patient to the side of the bed where the stretcher will be placed by rolling up the drawsheet close to the patient's body and pulling it toward the designated side. Align the patient's legs and head with her trunk.
   Positions patient to enable nurses to move her to the stretcher.
3. **Position the stretcher** next to the bed. Lock the stretcher wheels.
   Locking the wheels keeps the stretcher from moving during the transfer; prevents falls.
4. **Place the transfer board** against the patient's back.
   a. Place a friction-reducing device, such as a transfer roller sheet, over the transfer board. (You can improvise this device by placing a clean, unused plastic bag or plastic film under the drawsheet.)
   b. The nurse on the side opposite the stretcher uses the drawsheet to turn the patient away from the stretcher, while the other nurse places the transfer board against the patient's back halfway between bed and stretcher. Turn the

patient to her back and onto the transfer board.
Safely positions the transfer board under the patient, without friction.

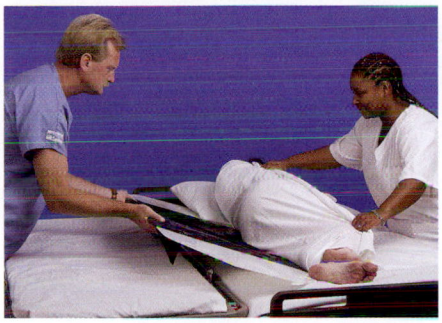

5. **Ensure the patient's feet** and shoulder are over the edge of the transfer board.
To prevent injury to the patient from the edge of the board.

6. **Ask the patient raise her head** if able. Use the drawsheet to slide her across the transfer board onto the stretcher.
Facilitates the move to the stretcher; prevents friction on patient's skin.

If Transferring a Patient From Bed to Stretcher With a Slipsheet

A slipsheet may be used instead of a transfer board. A slipsheet is a large, low-friction fabric that facilitates transfer.

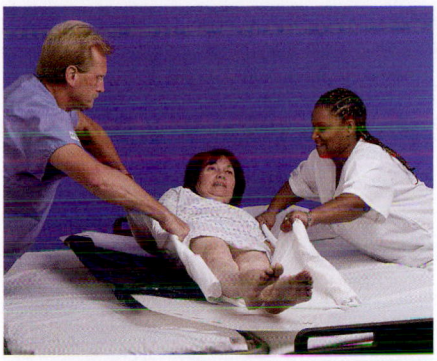

7. **Use the drawsheet to turn** the patient away from the bed; remove the board and roller sheet.

8. **Reposition the patient** on the stretcher for comfort and alignment.
Provides support and maintains proper alignment.

9. **Provide a blanket**, if needed for warmth or privacy.

10. **Fasten safety belts**, and raise the siderails on the stretcher.
Prevents falls.

11. **Lock the bed wheels. Position the bed** so that it is flat (if the patient can tolerate being supine) and at the height of the stretcher.
Ensures patient safety during the transfer. Helps prevent injury to staff because the patient is easier to move if the bed is flat.

12. **With the drawsheet, turn** the patient to the side opposite where the stretcher will be placed. Position the midline of the slipsheet under the patient. Roll the remaining half tightly, and tuck it under the patient.

13. **Turn the patient back over to the** side near to the stretcher; and pull the slipsheet through from under the patient.

14. **Place the patient supine**, and lower the siderail on the side where the stretcher will be placed.

15. **Move the stretcher** next to the bed and lock the wheels on the stretcher.

16. **Position at least two nurses** on the far side of the stretcher. Using the slipsheet, pull the patient onto the stretcher.

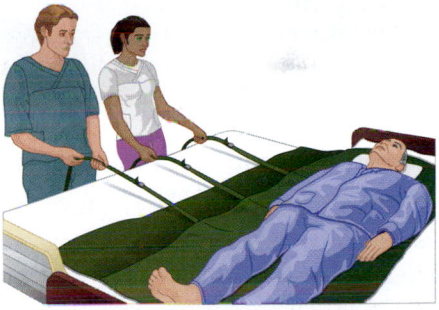

17. **Be sure to return the stretcher** to the locked position with the siderails raised for patient safety.

18. **Place the call light in reach** of the patient or position the patient where she can be seen by staff members at all times.

Procedure 32-2B ■ Dangling a Patient at the Side of the Bed

➤ When performing the procedure, always identify your patient according to agency policy, using two identifiers, and be attentive to standard precautions, hand hygiene, patient safety and privacy, body mechanics, and documentation.

Procedure Steps

1. **Lock the bed wheels.** Place the patient in a supine position, and raise the head of the bed to 90°. Keep the siderail elevated on the side opposite where you are standing.
Locking the wheels prevents the bed from moving as you move the patient. Raising the head of the bed prepares the patient to be dangled and requires less effort from you to help the patient sit erect.

2. **Apply a gait transfer belt** to the patient at waist level. Be sure the belt is snug but not uncomfortable. Place the bed in the low position.
Ensures patient safety and proper body mechanics.

3. **Instruct the patient to bend** his knees and turn the patient onto his side, if possible, keeping knees flexed.
Prepares the patient to be able to dangle his legs over side of bed.

4. **Stand at the side of the bed**, facing the patient and using a wide base of support. Place your foot closest to the head of the bed forward of the other foot. Lean forward, bending

(continued on next page)

Procedure 32-2 ■ Transferring Patients (continued)

at the hips, with your knees flexed. Instruct the patient to use his arm to push off the bed.
Allows you to maintain proper body mechanics and prevents injury.

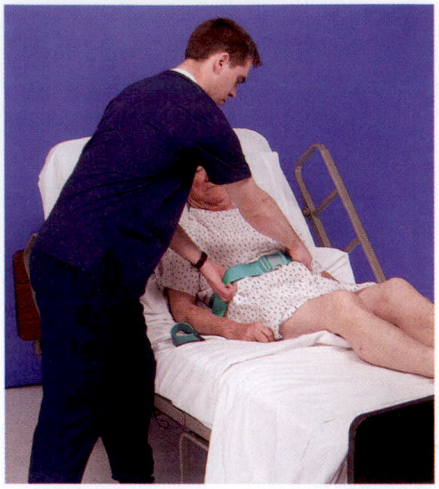

5. **Position your hands** on each side of the gait transfer belt.

6. **Rock onto your back foot** as you assist the patient toward you with the gait transfer belt, thereby moving the patient into a sitting position at the side of the bed.
Uses your body weight as leverage to reposition the patient, preventing injury to your back.

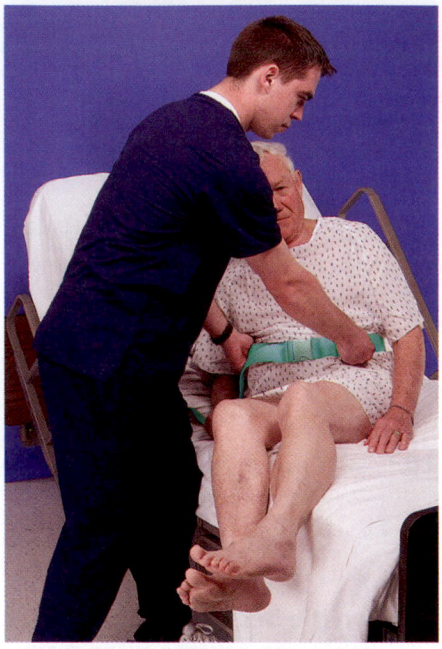

7. **Stay with the patient** as he dangles. Reassess comfort level and for dizziness.
Helps prevent falls.

Procedure 32-2C ■ Transferring a Patient From Bed to Chair

➤ When performing the procedure, always identify your patient according to agency policy, using two identifiers, and be attentive to standard precautions, hand hygiene, patient safety and privacy, body mechanics, and documentation.

Procedure Steps

1. **Position the chair** next to the bed. If possible, lock the chair.
Prevents the chair from moving during transfer. Ensures patient safety.

2. **Put nonskid footwear** on the patient.
Prevents the patient from slipping during transfer.

3. **Place the bed in a low position,** and lock the bed wheels.
Prevents the bed from moving during the transfer. Low position allows patient to place feet firmly on the floor.

4. **Apply a transfer belt.**
Facilitates transfer of the patient to the chair and helps prevent back injury to the nurse.

5. **Assist the patient to dangle** at the side of the bed (see Procedure 32-2B). Be sure the patient doesn't need support before releasing him.

6. **Stand toward the bed,** facing the patient. Brace your feet and knees against the patient's legs. Pay particular attention to any known weakness. Bend your hips and knees, and, keeping your back straight, hold onto the transfer belt on both sides. If two nurses are available to assist with the transfer, one nurse should be on each side of the patient.
Bracing provides stability. Bending the hips and knees allows you to use the major muscle groups and limit the risk of injury. Lifting the patient at waist level prevents injury to the arm or shoulder. ➤

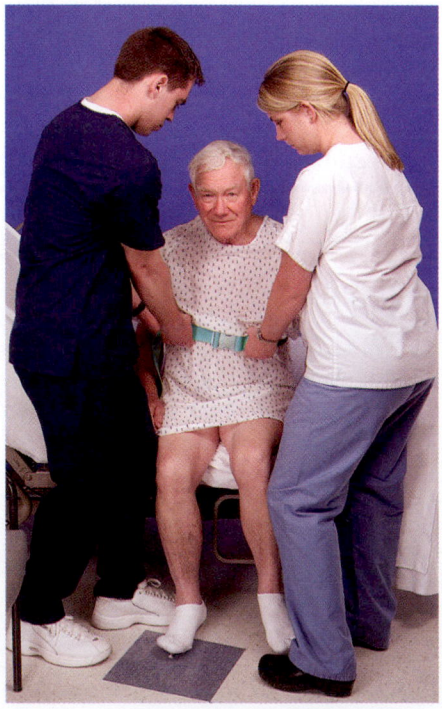

7. **Instruct the patient** to place his arms around you between the shoulders and waist (the location depends on your height and the height of the patient).
Having the patient hold you on your trunk prevents injury to your neck.

8. **Ask the patient to stand** as you move to an upright position by straightening your legs and hips.
Straightening your thighs and hips uses your large muscle groups and prevents injury to your back.

9. **Allow the patient to steady** himself for a moment. Ask whether he is feeling light-headed.
Provides the patient an opportunity to rest before further movement. Allows you to evaluate his tolerance to activity and ability to maintain an upright posture before continuing.

10. **Instruct the patient to pivot** and turn with you toward the chair.
Pivoting helps prevent twisting and straining the patient's back muscles.

11. **Assist the patient to position** himself in front of the chair. Have the patient flex his hips and knees, and as he lowers himself to the chair, reach for arms of the chair. Guide his motion while maintaining a firm hold on him and keeping your back straight.
Maintains good body mechanics and balance and ensures patient safety.

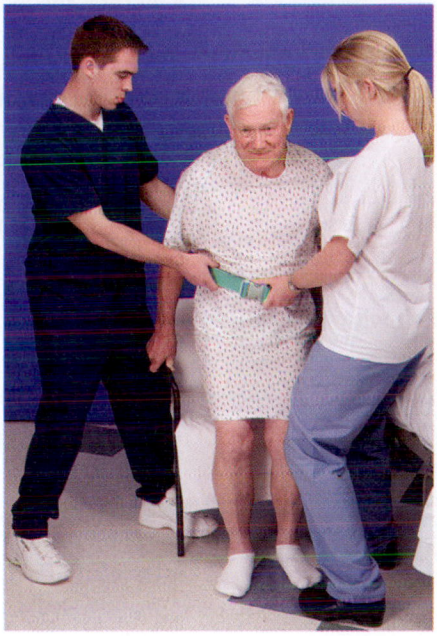

12. **Assist the patient** to a comfortable position in the chair.

13. **Provide a blanket** if needed for warmth or privacy.

14. **Place the call light in reach** of the patient or position the patient where he can be seen by staff members at all times.

? What if . . .

- **The patient is obese?**
  If the patient is obese or unable to assist, use a full body sling that allows the patient to assume a seated position. You may also use a powered standing assist lift, if one is available.
- **The patient has had hip surgery (replacement or fracture repair).**
  When assisting the patient out of bed, raise the bed to a higher position, allowing the patient to exit the bed without acute hip flexion.
  To avoid hip dislocation.
- **The patient becomes dizzy during the transfer?**
  Return the patient to sitting or recumbent position and assess his vital signs.
- **The patient has a weaker side, for example, from a cerebrovascular accident (CVA) or surgical procedure?**
  Instruct the patient to exit the bed from his unaffected side. Stand on the patient's weaker side.
  The stronger side should lead a transfer.

Evaluation

- Assess the level of patient participation in the transfer.
- Assess the patient's comfort level during the transfer and in the new position.
- Assess proper body position and alignment after his position change.
- Assess the patient's vital signs for postural hypotension after dangling or transferring to a chair.

Patient Teaching

- Explain the importance of frequent position changes and getting out of bed to avoid complications of immobility.

Home Care

- Instruct the family member or caregiver in the proper technique for assisting the client to dangle at the bedside or transfer to a chair.
- Provide instruction in the importance of changing position and maintaining proper body alignment.

Documentation

Patients are usually moved to a stretcher for transport to a test or procedure. The movement is a routine aspect of care and is not documented. When dangling or transferring a patient to a chair, document in the nursing notes how much assistance was required, the use of assistive devices, any problems with positioning the patient, how long the patient was out of bed, and how the patient tolerated the activity.

Practice Resources

Collins, J. W., Nelson, A., & Sublet, V. (2006); Occupational Safety and Health Administration, U.S. Department of Labor. (2009); Waters, T. R., Nelson, A. N., Hughes, N., et al. (2009).

Thinking About the Procedure

To practice applying clinical reasoning to this procedure,

Go to *Davis's Nursing Skills Videos*, **Transferring a Patient From Bed to Stretcher, Dangling a Patient at the Side of the Bed,** and **Transferring a Patient From Bed to Chair.**

For questions and suggested responses,

Go to Chapter 32, **Thinking About the Procedure Questions and Suggested Responses,** on Davis*Plus*.

Procedure 32-3 ■ Assisting With Ambulation

➤ For steps to follow in *all* procedures, refer to the Universal Steps for All Procedures found on the page facing the inside back cover.

Equipment

- Nonlatex gloves, if you may be exposed to body fluids
- Transfer belt
- Nonskid footwear

Delegation

You may ask nursing assistive personnel (NAP) to assist with ambulation. Ensure that the NAP has the necessary skills and that the patient's condition is stable. Inform the NAP of any special considerations when assisting a patient with ambulation and evaluate the patient after the activity.

Pre-Procedure Assessment

- Assess for any restrictions in movement or position by asking the patient and checking the physician's orders.
- Observe for the presence of equipment such as IV lines, drains, or catheters.
- Assess possible side effects of medications (e.g., dizziness and sedation).
- Assess the patient's level of consciousness, ability to follow directions, and ability to assist with the move.
- Assess the physical size of the patient and your own strength and ability to move the patient.
- Assess the patient's tolerance when dangling before beginning to ambulate.
  The preceding assessments inform you about activity tolerance, readiness to get out of bed, and ability to participate in the transfer. They help you determine how many assistants you need, the appropriate transfer device, and how to proceed with the move while preventing injury and dislodging of equipment.
- Assess vital signs, and monitor for postural hypotension.
  If the patient is at risk for postural hypotension, you may need to allow additional time for the patient to change position and plan for adequate help.
- Assess the patient's level of comfort using a standardized pain scale.
  If the patient is uncomfortable, you may need to administer an analgesic before moving.
- Assess for factors that may increase the risk of falls (elderly, muscle weakness, chronic disease, gait disturbance).
  Identifies patients at risk.

Procedure 32-3A ■ Assisting With Ambulation (One Nurse)

➤ When performing the procedure, always identify your patient according to agency policy, using two identifiers, and be attentive to standard precautions, hand hygiene, patient safety and privacy, body mechanics, and documentation.

Procedure Steps

1. **Put nonskid footwear** on the patient.
   Prevents the patient from slipping while transferring and ambulating.
2. **Apply the transfer belt.**
   Allows you to safely support the patient during the transfer and ambulation.
3. **Place the bed in a low position,** and lock the bed.
   Prevents the bed from moving during transfer. Makes it easier for the patient's feet to reach the floor.
4. **Assist the patient to dangle** at the side of the bed (see Procedure 32-2B, if you need to review).
5. **Face the patient.** Brace your feet and knees against the patient's feet and knees. Pay particular attention to any known weakness. Bend your hips and knees, and hold onto the transfer belt.
   Bracing provides stability of the patient's legs. Bending the hips and knees allows you to use the major muscle groups and limit injury. Lifting at the patient's waist level prevents injury to his arm or shoulder.
6. **Instruct the patient** to place his arms around you between the shoulders and waist (the location depends on your height and the height of the patient). Ask the patient to stand as you move to an upright position by straightening your legs and hips.
   Having the patient hold you on your trunk prevents injury to your neck. Straightening your thighs and hips uses your large muscle groups and promotes good body mechanics.
7. **Allow the patient to steady** himself for a moment.
   Allows the patient an opportunity to rest before further movement and to regain equilibrium before walking.
8. **Stand at the patient's side,** placing both hands on the transfer belt. If the patient is weak on one side, position yourself on the weaker side.
   By standing on the weaker side, the patient is freer to reach with the stronger arm and grip wall or bed rails with his strong-side hand, and use the stronger side for strength and balance. This position also keeps you clear of a cane or other assistive device, which would be used on the strong side, and allows you

to support the weaker side to prevent the patient from falling.

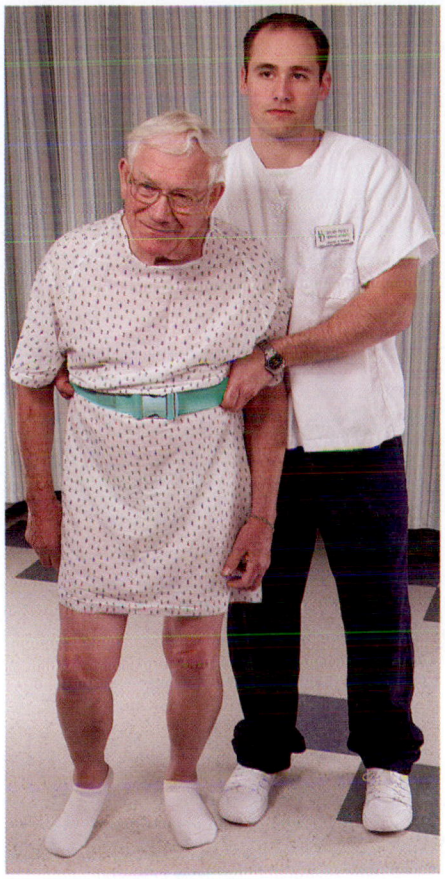

9. **Slowly guide the patient** forward. Observe for signs of fatigue or dizziness.
   Helps prevent falls.

10. **If the patient has an IV pole,** ask him to hold on to the pole on the side where you are standing. Assist the patient to advance the pole as you ambulate. Be sure the patient does not rely on the pole for support.
    Provides a grip for the patient and positions the IV pole near you so that you can assist the patient to move the pole.

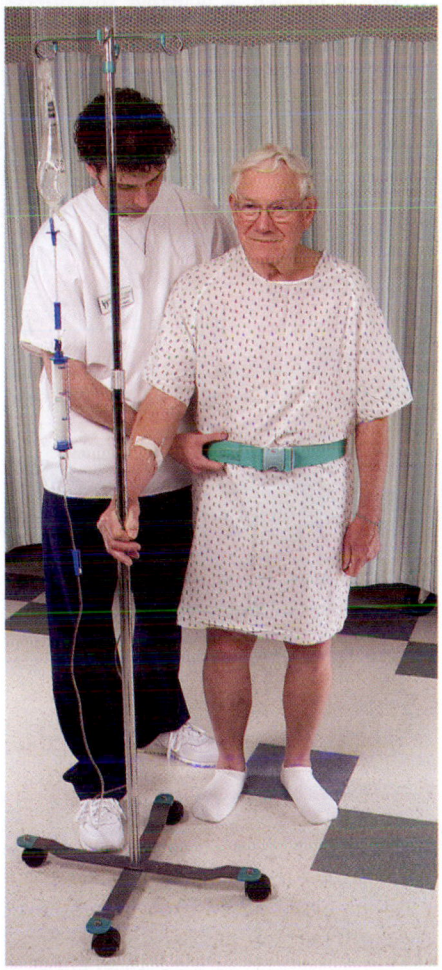

Procedure 32-3B ■ Assisting With Ambulation (Two Nurses)

➤ When performing the procedure, always identify your patient according to agency policy, using two identifiers, and be attentive to standard precautions, hand hygiene, patient safety and privacy, body mechanics, and documentation.

Procedure Steps

1. **Put nonskid footwear** on the patient.
   Prevents the patient from slipping during the transfer and ambulation.

2. **Apply the transfer belt.**
   Allows you to support client during transfer and ambulation.

3. **Place the bed in low position,** and lock the bed.
   Prevents the bed from moving during transfer and prevents the patient from falling.

4. **Assist the patient to dangle** at the side of the bed (see Procedure 32-2B, as needed).

5. **Each nurse should stand facing** the patient on opposite sides of the patient. Brace your feet and knees against the patient, paying particular attention to any known weakness. Bend from the hips and knees and hold onto the transfer belt.
   Bracing provides stability. Bending the hips and knees allows you to use the major muscle groups and limit injury. Lifting at the patient's waist level prevents injury to his arm or shoulder.

6. **Instruct the patient to place** his arms around each of you between the shoulders and waist (the location depends on your height and the height of the patient). Ask the patient to stand as each of you move to an upright position by straightening your legs and hips.

7. **Allow the patient to steady** himself for a moment.
   Allows the patient an opportunity to rest before further movement and to regain equilibrium. Allows you to evaluate the patient's tolerance to activity and ability to maintain an upright posture before ambulating.

8. **Each nurse stands at** the patient's sides, grasping hold of the transfer

(continued on next page)

Procedure 32-3 ■ Assisting With Ambulation (continued)

belt. If no belt is available, the nurses grasp each other's arms at the patient's waist.
Helps patient maintain an erect posture.▼

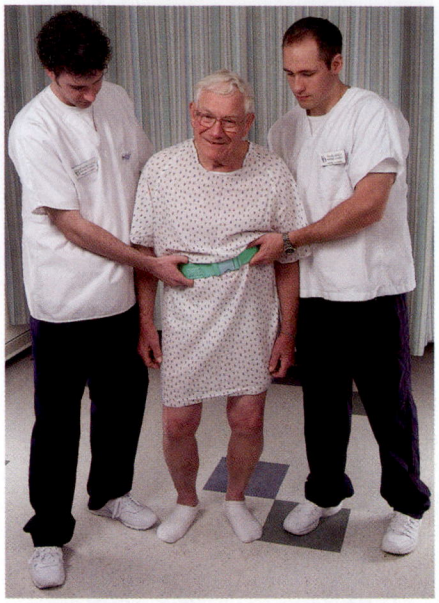

9. **Slowly guide the patient forward.** Observe for signs of fatigue or dizziness.
Ensures client safety.

10. **If the patient has an IV pole,** one nurse advances the IV pole along the side of the patient by holding the pole with the outside hand.

Remind the patient not to use the IV pole for support.
Positions the IV pole out of the path of the patient. Because the IV pole is on rollers, it will not support the patient if he starts to fall.

? What if . . .

- **The patient has a weaker side (e.g., from a stroke or musculoskeletal injury)?**

  If the patient has weakness on one side, provide additional support but allow him to use that side as he is able.
  This will force him to use his weaker side.

Evaluation

- Assess the level of patient participation in the transfer.
- Assess patient comfort with ambulation.
- Assess posture and base of support.
- Assess vital signs for postural hypotension.

Patient Teaching

- Instruct the patient to inform you if he feels dizzy or weak.
- Explain the importance of ambulation to prevent complications of immobility.

Home Care

- Teach family members or caregivers how to assist the client with ambulation.
- Provide instruction on importance of ambulation.

Documentation

Document in the nursing notes how much assistance was required, any problems with ambulation, and the distance walked.

Sample Documentation

11/11/15 0630 Pt assisted to ambulate to doorway in room. Required minimal assistance from one nurse. Placed in chair for 30 min and then assisted back to bed. Required maximum assist from two nurses to return to bed. ——— B. Bowen, RN

Practice Resources

Occupational Safety and Health Administration, U.S. Department of Labor (2009); Waters, T. R., Nelson, A. N., Hughes, N., et al. (2009).

Thinking About the Procedure

To practice applying clinical reasoning to this procedure,

Go to *Davis's Nursing Skills Videos*, **Assisting With Ambulation (One Nurse), and Assisting With Ambulation (Two Nurses).**

For questions and suggested responses,

Go to Chapter 32, **Thinking About the Procedure Questions and Suggested Responses,** on Davis*Plus*.

CLINICAL INSIGHTS

Clinical Insight 32-1 ➤ Applying Principles of Body Mechanics

Principles of body mechanics are the rules that enable you to move your body without causing injury. Use the following guidelines to decrease the risk of back and other injuries. Teach them to your patients as well.

The ANA states you should use mechanical equipment for lifting and transferring whenever possible and not rely on body mechanics alone to prevent injury.

Account for Patient Factors

- **Assess patient dependency levels** and select equipment after determining the patient's ability to assist in the transfer. You will also want to be aware of the patient's strength and ability to bear weight. Height and weight of the patient factor into how you transfer the patient safely.

Transferring Patients According to Dependency Level

PATIENT LEVEL OF DEPENDENCE	ASSISTIVE DEVICE
Complete dependence (immobile; no assistance)	Mechanical lift with full sling
Extensive dependence (holds on to device but with minimal strength)	Mechanical lift with full sling or stand/assist lift
Moderate dependence (no patient assist for lifting from floor)	Mechanical lift with full sling, or if transfer is manual, more than one helper might be needed
Patient assists with limited mobility	Transfer belt or gait belt
Limited dependence	Stand/assist lift or friction-reducing device

Source: Adapted from American Nurses Association (ANA). (2013). *Safe patient handling and mobility: Interprofessional national standards.* Silver Springs, MD: Author.

Make Use of Inanimate Objects and Get Help When Possible

- **Raise the height of the bed and over-the-bed table to waist level** when you are working with a patient.
- **Get help to move a heavy object** or patient. Assess the object or patient you are going to lift. If you have any doubt that you can do it by yourself, get help from a coworker.
- **Use assistive devices at all times** to limit the risk of back and musculoskeletal injury.
- **Maintain competency** in using all assistive and transfer devices.

Use Your Body Correctly

- **Use a wide base of support** (feet spread apart).
- **Minimize bending and twisting.** These movements increase the stress on the back. Instead, face the object or person, and bend at the hips or squat.
- **Squat to lift heavy objects** from the floor. (Squatting lowers your center of gravity.) Push against the strong hip and thigh muscles to raise yourself to a standing position. Avoid bending at the waist.
- **Use the muscles in your legs** as the power for lifting. Bend your knees, keep your back straight, and lift smoothly. Repeat the same movements for setting the object down.
- **Keep objects close to your body** when you lift, move, or carry them. The closer an object is to the center of gravity, the greater the stability and the less strain on the back.
- **Use both hands and arms** when you lift, move, or carry heavy objects.
- **Do not stand on tiptoes to reach** an object. If you must use a ladder or stepstool to reach for an object, make sure it is stable and adequate to position your body close to the object.
- **Push, slide, or pull heavy objects** whenever possible rather than lifting.
- **Maintain a good grip** on the patient or object you are moving before attempting to move it.
- **When possible, keep your elbows bent** when you carry an object.
- **Work with smooth and even movements.** Avoid sudden or jerky motions.

Clinical Insight 32-2 ➤ Using Common Positioning Devices

Applying a Trochanter Roll

Trochanter rolls prevent external hip rotation when the patient is in a supine position.

- Fold a towel or bath blanket lengthwise.
- Roll the towel or bath blanket tightly.
- Invert the roll. Turning the patient to one side, place the bath blanket or towel under the patient's hip and thigh. Repeat on the other side if needed.
- Roll the sheet or towel under until it is snug against the patient's hip and thigh.
  The patient's weight should keep the roll from moving and help to prevent external (outward) rotation of the hips.
- Make sure the roll does not extend as far as the knee.
  To avoid nerve compression and palsy that can lead to footdrop.

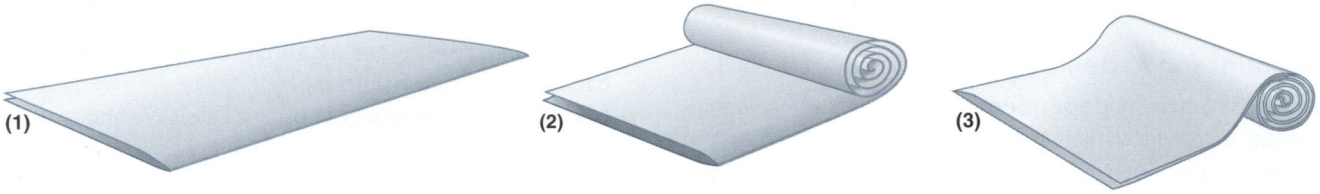

Alternate Method

- Alternately, you can place the patient on a sheet that has been folded so that the top edge is at the top of the hips, and the lower edge is about one-third the way down the thighs. Then place the rolled towels under the sheet and roll the sheet under tightly.

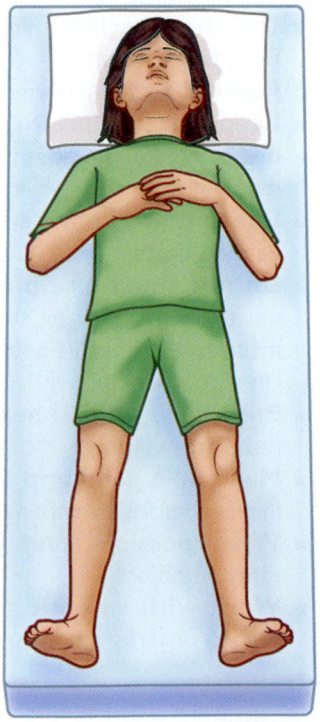

External rotation can occur without a trochanter roll.

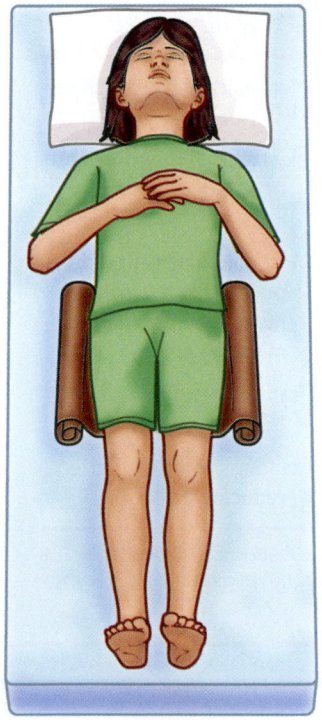

Proper alignment using a trochanter roll.

Clinical Insight 32-2 ➤ Using Common Positioning Devices—cont'd

Applying Hand Rolls

Hand rolls help prevent hand contractures.

- Place a rolled up washcloth or commercial hand roll in the patient's palm to maintain a neutral position.
- Secure the strap, if present.
- Roll soft gauze around the hand and secure with nonallergenic, adhesive tape to keep it from falling out of the patient's hand.
- Place another roll in the patient's other hand, if needed.

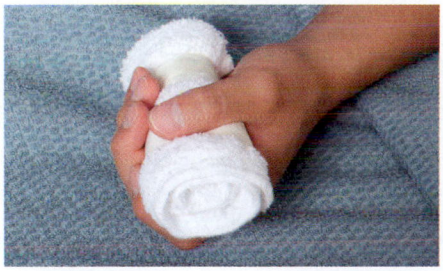

Applying Cradle Boots

Cradle boots prevent footdrop, hip rotation, and pressure on bony prominences, which lead to skin breakdown.

- Open the slit on the top surface of the boot.
- Place the patient's heel in the round cutout for the heel. If the patient is positioned on her side, you may put the boot on the bottom foot.
- Support the flexed top foot with a pillow.
- Apply the boot to the other foot, as needed.
- Position the patient's legs in neutral alignment with slight flexion.
  Neutral positioning prevents strain on hip ligaments.

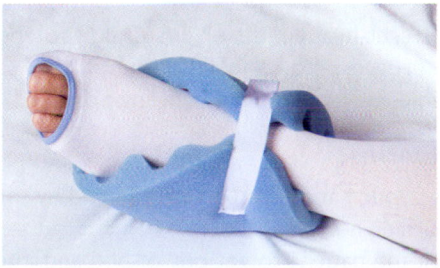

Applying Hip Abduction Pillow

Hip abduction pillows prevent internal hip rotation and hip adduction when the patient is in a supine position.

- Place the wedge-shaped, spongy pillow between the patient's legs when she is lying on her back.
- Slide it toward the groin so it touches the legs all along the inside of the thigh.
- Place both upper legs in the pillow's lateral indentations.
- Secure the straps to prevent the pillow from slipping down the mattress.

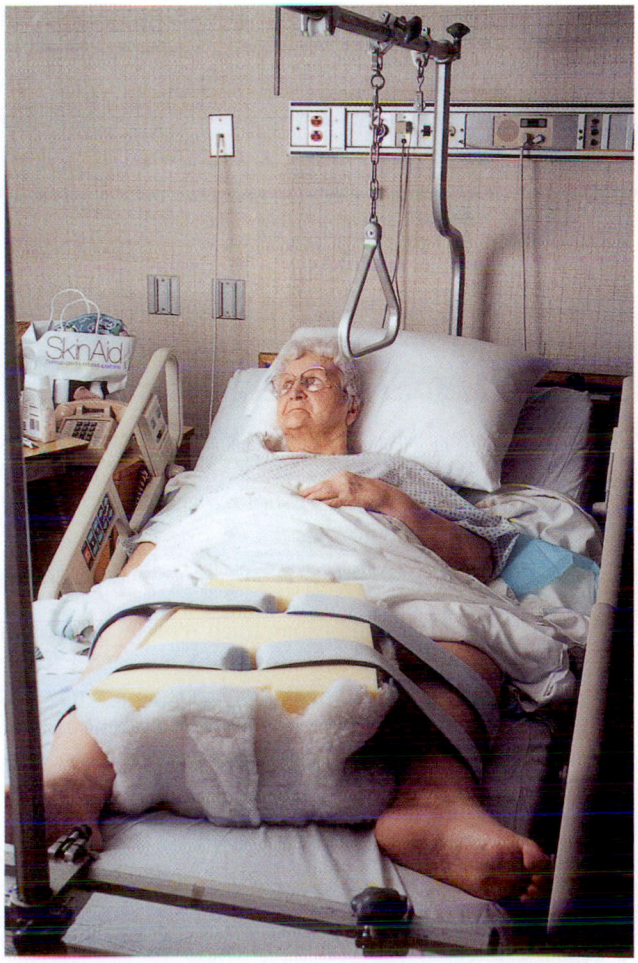

Clinical Insight 32-3 ➤ Tips for Performing Passive Range-of-Motion Exercises

Passive range of motion (PROM) is the movement of the joints through their full range of motion by another person. Nurses frequently perform PROM to maintain joint mobility.

- **Explain the purpose of PROM.** You may also wish to teach family members and caregivers about the importance of ROM exercises and enlist their help in exercising the patient when they visit.
- **Observe the patient as you perform PROM.** You may need to perform the exercises in several short segments if the patient tires easily or experiences discomfort.
- **Support the patient's limb** above and below the joint that is to be exercised.
- **Move the joint in a slow, smooth, rhythmic manner.** Avoid fast movements; they may cause muscle spasm.
- **Never force a joint.** Some patients may have limited ROM. Move each joint to the point of resistance. This should not be painful.
- **Perform PROM** at least twice daily. Move each joint through ROM three to five times with each session. Consider incorporating PROM into care activities, for example, while bathing or turning the patient.
- **Return the joint to a neutral position** when exercise is complete.
- **Encourage active exercise** whenever possible.

Thinking About the Procedure

To practice applying critical reasoning to this clinical insight,

Go to *Davis's Nursing Skills Videos*, **Performing Passive Range-of-Motion Exercises.**

For questions and suggested responses,

Go to Chapter 32, Thinking About the Procedure Questions and Suggested Responses, on Davis*Plus*.

Clinical Insight 32-4 ➤ Assisting With Physical Conditioning Exercises to Prepare for Ambulation

Patients who have been confined to bed for more than a week or who have sustained major injury require conditioning before they are able to resume walking. Conditioning exercises include the following.

Quadriceps and Gluteal Drills

- Ask the patient to tighten her thigh muscles by pushing downward with her knees and flexing her feet. Each leg may be done separately if moving both is contraindicated.
- Ask the patient to hold the position for a count of 5 and then relax.
- Repeat this process two to three times per hour during the waking hours.
- To exercise the gluteal muscles, ask the patient to pinch her buttocks together.
- Do this exercise when the patient exercises her quadriceps muscles.
- Instruct the patient not to hold her breath as she exercises.

Arm Exercises

- Install a trapeze bar on the patient's bed. Ask the patient to do pull-ups on the bar from a lying position. This exercises the biceps muscles.
- To exercise the triceps muscles, ask the patient to lift his upper body off the mattress by firmly pressing down with the palms.
- The patient can also do push-ups from a seated position at the side of the bed or from a stationary chair or wheelchair.

Dangling

- Dangling is a seated position at the side of the bed, feet resting on the floor.
- Provide a footstool if the patient's feet do not reach the floor.
- Assess for light-headedness or postural hypotension.
- Do not progress to ambulation until the patient is comfortable and stable in the dangling position.

Daily Activities

- Encourage your patient to be active in bed by repositioning and turning herself.
- Encourage the patient to get out of bed and into a chair before attempting to walk.
- Encourage the patient to perform as much of her activities of daily living (ADLs) as possible.
- ADLs exercise many of the muscle groups used in ambulation.

To see a nurse performing passive range-of-motion exercises,

Go to *Davis's Nursing Skills Videos*, **Physical Conditioning Exercises: Quadriceps, Gluteal, Arm, and Dangling.**

Clinical Insight 32-5 ➤ Sizing Walking Aids

Sizing Canes

- Ask the patient to stand erect, and place the cane tip 20 cm (4 in.) to the side of the foot.
- The top of the cane should reach the top of the hip joint so that the patient can hold the cane with her elbow flexed 30°.

Sizing Walkers

- Ask the patient to stand erect, holding onto the walker.
- The walker should extend from the floor to the hip joint so that the patient can comfortably hold the walker with 30° flexion of the elbow.

Sizing Crutches

To measure a patient for an axillary crutch, follow these guidelines:

- Ask the patient to lie down wearing the nonskid shoes that she will use when walking.
- Measure the distance between the heel and the anterior fold of the axilla, then add 2.5 cm (1 in.).
- Select a crutch that can be adjusted to this height.
- Have the patient stand, and position the crutch tip 10 to 15 cm (4 to 6 in.) to the side of the heel. Adjust the axillary crutch pad three fingerbreadths below the axilla.
- Adjust the handgrips so that the patient can comfortably grasp the bar while the elbow is slightly flexed. The patient's axilla should not rest on the crutchpad.

Clinical Insight 32-6 ➤ Teaching Patients to Use Canes, Walkers, and Crutches

Canes

After ensuring the cane is the proper size (refer to Clinical Insight 32-5), instruct the patient to do the following:

- Hold the cane on the stronger side.
- Distribute weight evenly between the feet and cane.
- Advance the cane and weaker leg simultaneously, then bring the stronger leg through.
- Avoid leaning over or on the cane.
- Maintain the integrity of the rubber tip for traction.

Walkers

After ensuring the walker is the proper size (refer to Clinical Insight 32-5), instruct the patient to:

- Stand between the back legs of the walker. Do not stand too far behind the walker.
- Pick up the walker, and advance it as you step ahead. Do not advance it so far as to lose balance.
- If one leg is weaker, move it forward as the walker moves forward.
- Pick up, rather than slide, the walker (unless it has wheels).

Crutches

After ensuring the crutches are the proper size (refer to Clinical Insight 32-5), do the following:

- When first teaching crutch walking, instruct the patient to stand near a wall with a chair behind him. Help the patient to stand and grip the crutches. Ask the patient to sway from side to side on the crutches to become accustomed to weight bearing by the arms.
- *Tripod position* is the basic crutch gait standing position. Place crutches 15 cm (6 in.) in front of the feet, with the crutch point 15 cm from the patient's center. In this position, a triangle is formed by the crutches and the body.
- Five crutch gaits exist (see accompanying chart): 2-point gait, 3-point gait, 4-point gait, swing-to gait, and swing-through gait.

To teach the patient how to go up and down stairs, instruct him to lead with the unaffected leg when going up the stairs and to lead with the affected leg coming down the stairs.

(Continued)

Clinical Insight 32-6 ➤ Teaching Patients to Use Canes, Walkers, and Crutches—cont'd

Navigating stairs with crutches can be dangerous. When possible, have the patient practice this technique before discharge. When having a patient practice, the nurse should always stand below the patient on the stairs to prevent falling.

NOTE: Read this table from bottom to top.

2-Point gait	3-Point gait	4-Point gait	Swing to	Swing through
• Partial weight bearing, both feet; faster, but less support than a 4-point gait	• Non-weight bearing; faster than a 4-point gait; can use with walker	• Partial weight bearing, both feet; patient must shift weight constantly	• Weight bearing, both feet; can use with walker	• Weight bearing; requires the most coordination and balance
4. Advance right foot and left crutch	**4.** Advance right foot	**4.** Advance right foot	**4.** Lift both feet; swing them forward, landing feet next to the crutches	**4.** Lift both feet; swing them forward, landing feet in front of the crutches
3. Advance left foot and right crutch	**3.** Advance left foot and both crutches	**3.** Advance left crutch	**3.** Advance both crutches	**3.** Advance both crutches
2. Advance right foot and left crutch	**2.** Advance right foot	**2.** Advance left foot	**2.** Lift both feet; swing them forward, landing feet next to the crutches	**2.** Lift both feet; swing them forward, landing feet in front of the crutches
1. Advance left foot and right crutch	**1.** Advance left foot and both crutches	**1.** Advance right crutch	**1.** Advance both crutches	**1.** Advance both crutches
Tripod position	Tripod position	Tripod position	Tripod position	Tripod position

Crutch gaits. The shaded area represents weight-bearing. The arrow shows movement.

ASSESSMENT GUIDELINES AND TOOLS

Focused Assessment

Assessing Activity and Exercise

Suggested History Questions

Usual Activity

Describe your typical daily activity level.

If the patient has very restricted activity, ask the following questions:

- Are you able to care for yourself in regard to hygiene, dressing, toileting, and getting out of bed?
- If the patient has ADL limitations: Who helps you with these daily activities?

If the patient does not indicate restricted activity, ask the following questions:

- What is your usual form of exercise?
- How often do you exercise?
- How long are your exercise sessions?
- How long have you been engaged in this type of activity?
- What types of exercise or sports have you participated in the past?
- Describe your activity level over the last 10 years.
- Are you exercising more or less than in the past?
- What factors have changed your activity level?

Fitness Goals

What aspects of exercise do you enjoy? What aspects of exercise do you dislike?

What do you think are the benefits of exercise?

How do you schedule your exercise?

What motivates you to exercise?

What are your current fitness goals?

Mobility Concerns

Do you have any pain or discomfort with activity?

Do you avoid any activities because of pain, discomfort, shortness of breath, or chest pain?

If the patient answered *yes* to either question, describe the following:

- Type of problem
- Onset of concern
- Frequency of problem
- Activities that trigger and relieve
- Severity and type of symptoms
- Effect of problem on day-to-day activities
- Treatments used to alleviate and how they worked

Underlying Health Concerns

Do you have any healthcare problem that affects your ability to engage in activity or exercise?

If so, describe the problem and the effect.

What medications do you take?

Have you ever been told you have a bone problem? If so, what was the nature of the problem?

Have you ever experienced a fracture, strain, or sprain? If so, where was the problem? When did it occur? How did it occur?

Have you ever had weakness of the muscles or problems coordinating movement?

Do you have any cardiac or respiratory problems that affect your ability to perform activities?

Have you ever experienced anxiety or depression that affected your ability to participate in activities?

Lifestyle

What kind of work do you do?

Describe your typical work activities.

How many hours per week do you work?

What other commitments do you have (school, family, other obligations)?

External Factors

Are there any restrictions in your home that limit your ability to be active?

Do you feel you need an assistive device?

Are you comfortable exercising outside your home or in your neighborhood?

Focused Physical Assessments for Activity and Body Alignment

With the patient standing, observe from the anterior, posterior, and lateral views. Check for the following:

Shoulders and hips are level.

Toes are pointed forward.

The spine is straight, with no abnormal curvatures noted.

The posture is not slumped.

Ask the patient to sit down; observe as he does so.

Does he have difficulty lowering his torso?

Can he control the movement?

Is he able to get into this position with ease?

When he sits, does he slump?

If the patient cannot stand or sit, assess his alignment in bed. Look for ability to move in bed, as well as the posture the patient maintains.

(Continued)

Focused Assessment

Assessing Activity and Exercise—cont'd

Joint Function

Assessing joint function includes inspection and palpation of the joints and assessment of range of motion.

Begin your assessment at the neck and systematically work your way through each of the joints.

At each joint observe for swelling, erythema, asymmetry, or obvious deformity.

Compare the size of the muscles above and below the joint and on each side of the body.

Palpate the joint for temperature and crepitus. Warmth over a joint indicates inflammation or infection. Be sure to compare body temperature over several joints and right to left. **Crepitus** is a grating sensation when the joint is moved. It can often be heard as well as felt. Crepitus is associated with degenerative joint disease or arthritic changes in the joint.

As you palpate the joint, move it through its range of motion.

Muscle Strength

Assess muscle strength by having the patient push and then pull against your hands.

Start at the neck, and test the strength of all major joints' range of motion.

To see a nurse using a performing passive range-of-motion exercises,

Go to *Davis's Nursing Skills Videos*, **Performing Passive Range-of-Motion Exercises.**

Gait

Gait is divided into two phases: stance and swing.

Stance-In the stance phase, the heel of one foot strikes the ground while the opposite foot pushes off and leaves the ground.

Swing—In the swing phase, the leg from behind moves in front of the body. When the right leg is in stance mode, the left leg is in swing mode.

You must observe the patient walking. Normal gait includes the following features:

- Head is erect, gaze forward.
- Heel strikes the ground before the toe.
- Opposite arm moves forward at the same time.
- Feet are dorsiflexed in the swing phase.
- Gait is coordinated and rhythmic.
- Weight is evenly distributed, with minimal swing from side to side.
- Movement starts and stops with ease.
- Movement is at a moderate pace.

If the patient uses an assistive device, such as a cane, crutch, or walker, pay attention to how he uses it. Ask the patient to ambulate a short distance with and without the device to determine if the device is actually providing stability.

Activity Tolerance

Assess and record vital signs before having the patient engage in 3 minutes of activity.

Select an activity appropriate for the patient. For example, if the patient uses a walker, ask the patient to walk down the hallway. For a patient without obvious health limitations, consider asking her to run in place for 3 minutes.

Observe the patient throughout the exercise. If she shows any signs of distress, stop the exercise, immediately take a set of vital signs, and repeat the vital signs every minute until they have returned to baseline.

If the patient can exercise continuously for 3 minutes, assess the patient at the end of the 3-minute period and at 1-minute intervals. Note the change in heart rate, blood pressure, and respiratory rate.

This type of approach is not appropriate for patients who easily become short of breath, develop chest pain, or are very unsteady on their feet. Instead, for example, limit your assessment to determining the amount of assistance the patient needs to turn in bed or get out of bed.

Muscle Mass and Strength

As you observe the patient, compare muscle mass on the right and left sides. If you notice an obvious discrepancy in size, measure the circumference of the limbs and compare.

To assess strength, ask the patient to push against your hand with the hands and feet. Once again, compare both sides.

For guidelines for assessing mobility in the home,

Go to Chapter 32, **Home Care: Home Assessment for a Patient With Mobility Concerns,** in Volume 1.

TABLES

Range of Motion at the Joints

JOINT	ILLUSTRATION
Neck (Pivot Joint) ***Flexion***—Move the head from upright midline position to the chin, resting the head on the chest. *Normal Range:* 45° from midline ***Extension***—Move the head from flexed to upright midline position. *Normal Range:* 45° from midline ***Hyperextension***—Move the head from upright midline position to as far back as possible. *Normal Range:* 10°	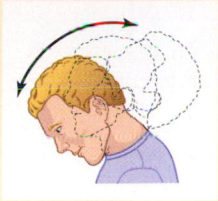
Lateral flexion—Tilt the head laterally from midline position toward the shoulder. *Normal Range:* 40° from midline	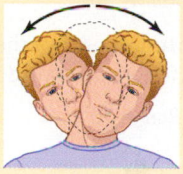
Rotation—Rotate the head in a circular motion from upright midline position to as far right or left as possible. *Normal Range:* 180°	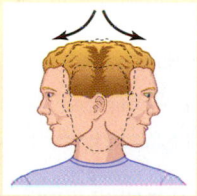
Shoulder (Ball-and-Socket Joint) ***Flexion***—Raise the arm from a neutral position at the side to alongside the head. *Normal Range:* 180° ***Extension***—Move the arm from flexed to a neutral position at the side of the body. *Normal Range:* 180° ***Hyperextension***—Move the arm, keeping the elbow straight, from a neutral position at the side of the bed to behind the body. *Normal Range:* 45°–60°	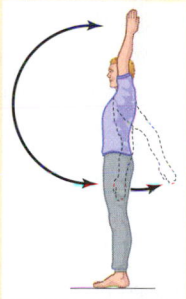
Abduction—Raise the arm laterally from a neutral position at the side of the body to a position at the side of the head, palm facing outward. *Normal Range:* 180° ***Adduction***—Move the arm downward from a position beside the head to across the front of the body as far as possible. *Normal Range:* 230°–320°	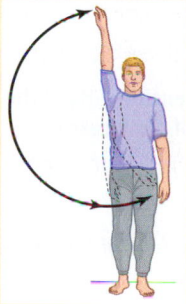

(Continued)

Range of Motion at the Joints—cont'd

JOINT	ILLUSTRATION
Circumduction—Circle the arm from the shoulder. *Normal Range:* 360°	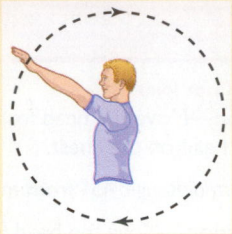
External rotation—Keeping arm held out to the side at shoulder level and bent to a right angle, fingers pointing down, move the arm upward so that the fingers point upward and are above the shoulder. *Normal Range:* 90° ***Internal rotation***—Move the arm forward and down to return to the starting position, fingers pointing down. *Normal Range:* 90°	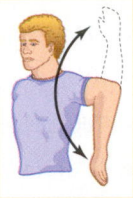
Elbow (Hinge Joint) ***Flexion***—Bend at the elbow to move the forearm from a straightened position up toward the shoulder. *Normal Range:* 150° ***Extension***—Straighten the arm by bringing the lower arm forward and down. *Normal Range:* 150°	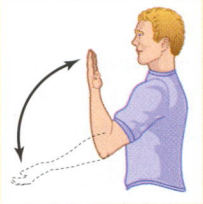
Rotation (for supination)—With the arm at the side, elbow bent, move the hand and forearm so that the palm is facing upward. *Normal Range:* 70°–90° ***Rotation (for pronation)***—With the arm at the side, elbow bent, move the hand and forearm so that the palm is facing downward. *Normal Range:* 70°–90°	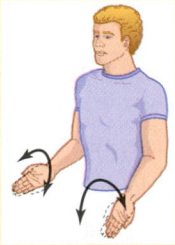
Wrist (Condyloid Joint) ***Flexion***—Bend the fingers of the hand toward the inner aspect of the forearm. *Normal Range:* 80°–90° ***Extension***—Straighten the wrist so that it is on the same plane as the forearm. *Normal Range:* 80°–90° ***Hyperextension***—Bend the wrist as far back as possible toward the outer aspect of the forearm. *Normal Range:* 70°–90°	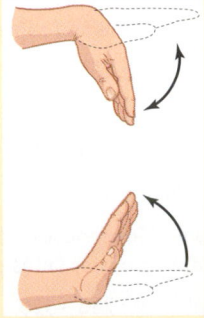
Abduction (radial flexion)—With the hand supinated, bend each wrist laterally toward the thumb side. *Normal Range:* 0–20° ***Adduction (ulnar flexion)***—With the hand supinated, bend each wrist laterally toward the fifth finger side. *Normal Range:* 30°–50°	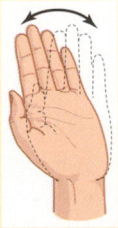

Range of Motion at the Joints—cont'd

JOINT	ILLUSTRATION
Hands and Fingers (Condyloid Joints: Interphalangeal Joints Are Hinges) ***Flexion***—Bend the fingers into a fist. *Normal Range:* 90° ***Extension***—Straighten the fingers. *Normal Range:* 90° ***Hyperextension***—Bend the fingers back. *Normal Range:* 30°	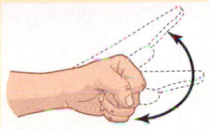
Abduction—Spread the fingers apart. *Normal Range:* 20° ***Adduction***—Bring the fingers together. *Normal Range:* 20°	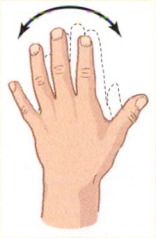
Thumb (Saddle Joint) ***Flexion***—Move the thumb across the palm of the hand toward the fifth finger. *Normal Range:* 90° ***Extension***—Move the thumb laterally away from the fingers. *Normal Range:* 90°	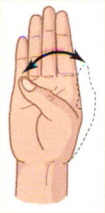
Opposition—Touch the thumb to the top of each finger of the same hand. *Normal Range:* NA	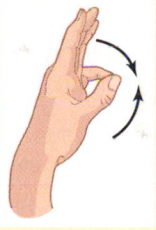
Hip (Ball-and-Socket Joint) ***Flexion***—Move the leg forward and up. *Normal Range:* Knee extended 90° ***Extension***—Move the leg back down beside the other. *Normal Range:* Knee flexed 120° ***Hyperextension***—Move the leg back behind the body. *Normal Range:* 30°–50°	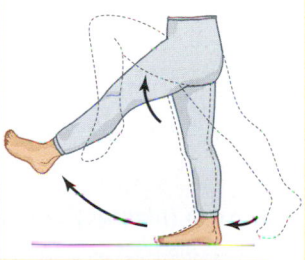 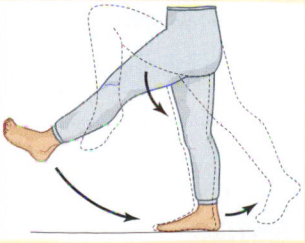

(Continued)

Range of Motion at the Joints—cont'd

JOINT	ILLUSTRATION
Abduction—Move the leg laterally. *Normal Range:* 45°–50° ***Adduction***—Sweep the leg inward across the midline. *Normal Range:* 20°–30° beyond the other leg	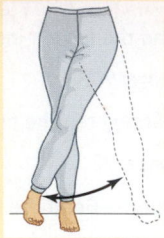
Circumduction—Circle the leg, keeping the knee straight. *Normal Range:* 360°	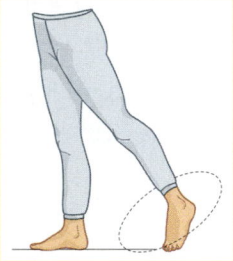
Internal rotation—Turn the foot and leg inward toward the other leg. *Normal Range:* 90° ***External rotation***—Turn the foot and leg outward, pointing the toes as far as possible away from the other leg. *Normal Range:* 90°	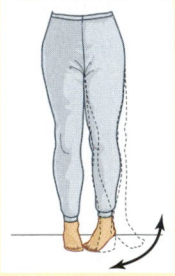
Knee (Hinge Joint) ***Flexion***—Bend at the knee, bringing the heel back toward the buttocks. *Normal Range:* 120°–130° ***Extension***—Straighten the knee, returning the leg to its original position. *Normal Range:* 120°–130°	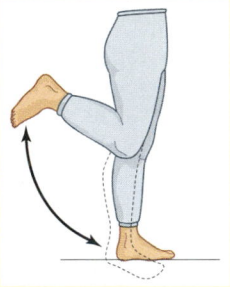
Ankle (Hinge Joint) ***Extension (plantar flexion)***—Point the toes and foot downward. *Normal Range:* 45°–50° ***Flexion (dorsiflexion)***—Pull the toes and foot upward. *Normal Range:* 20°	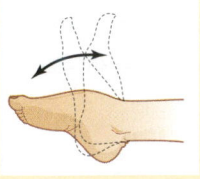
Foot (Gliding Joint) ***Eversion***—Turn the sole of the foot laterally. *Normal Range:* 5° ***Inversion***—Turn the sole of the foot medially. *Normal Range:* 5°	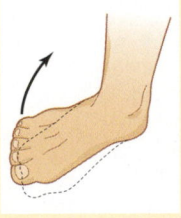

Range of Motion at the Joints—cont'd

JOINT	ILLUSTRATION
Toes (Hinge Joint except intertarsal joints, which are Gliding Joints) ***Flexion***—Curl the toes downward. *Normal Range:* 35°–60° ***Extension***—Straighten the toes. *Normal Range:* 35°–60°	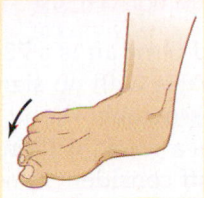
Abduction—Spread the toes apart. *Normal Range:* 0–15° ***Adduction***—Bring the toes together. *Normal Range:* 0–15°	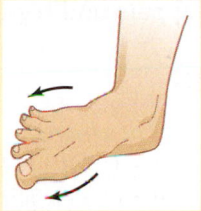
Trunk ***Flexion***—At the waist, bend forward toward the toes. *Normal Range:* 70°–90° ***Extension***—Straighten the trunk from the flexed position. *Normal Range:* 70°–90° ***Hyperextension***—Bend the trunk backward. *Normal Range:* 20°–30°	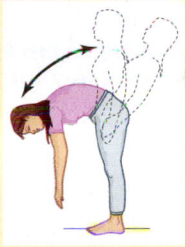
Lateral flexion—Bend the trunk to the side. *Normal Range:* 20°–40°	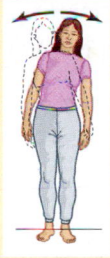
Rotation—Turn the upper body from side to side (twist at the waist). *Normal Range:* 30°–45°	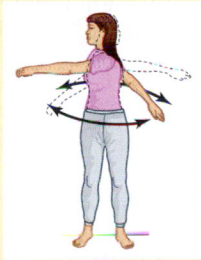

CLINICALREASONING

Applying the Full-Spectrum Nursing Model

PATIENT SITUATION

Mr. Ronald Ornduff is a 72-year-old retired man who lives with his wife in a one-story home. He has excellent general health with no significant health problems. Ronald typically walks with a moderate to fairly vigorous pace in his neighborhood or at the mall in the winter. He belongs to a health club and works out two or three times a week, walking on the treadmill, using the weight machines, or taking a basic conditioning class. Mr. Ornduff considers himself fit and of an acceptable weight for his age. When going outdoors to pick up the morning paper, he slipped on a patch of ice and fell. You are now caring for him 2 days after hip surgery. He is experiencing pain and seems fearful his injury could be the beginning of a decline in his health.

THINKING

1. *Theoretical Knowledge:*
   a. Based on Mr. Ornduff's age, physical condition, and activity level, make a rough estimate of the number of minutes/week of physical activity he should have after he recovers from surgery and resumes full mobility. What are the benefits of this physical activity?
   b. As a nurse planning the care for a patient after hip surgery, what complications of immobility should you assess for?
2. *Critical Thinking (Considering Alternatives):* What are some possible barriers for an older adult's participating in physical activity? What might you teach your patient to do to overcome those barriers?

DOING

3. *Practical Knowledge:*
   a. How might you position your patient after hip surgery?
   b. What equipment would you need to position your patient after surgery? Is there anything you can set up that will help your patient move around in bed when he can tolerate it?
   c. What type of physical activity would you recommend Mr. Ornduff incorporate into his exercise plan after he experiences full recovery from his surgery? What benefit will these exercises provide?
4. *Nursing Process (Diagnosis):* Write at least two nursing diagnoses for Mr. Ornduff. Use just the data provided in the situation. Assume he is 2 days post-op.

CARING

5. *Self-Knowledge:* What would you be feeling if you were in Mr. Ornduff's situation of being physically fit one day and suffering pain and immobility the next?
6. *Ethical Knowledge:* What are one or two things you would do to help Mr. Ornduff feel cared for and cared about?

Critical Thinking and Clinical Reasoning

1. In Volume 1, you were introduced (Meet Your Patient) to Helen Jillian, a 72-year-old woman with hypertension, high cholesterol levels, and chest pain. She is 61 inches tall and weighs 290 pounds. Ms. Jillian is admitted to the hospital for another episode of chest pain. You are assigned to care for her. Her physician has ordered her to be out of bed in the chair at least twice daily and to ambulate every day. How will you safely move this patient from bed to chair and assist her with ambulation? Work through that decision by answering the following questions.
   a. What aspects of this situation require the most careful attention (what are the risks; what could go wrong)?
   b. What steps can you take to prevent those difficulties?
2. Ms. Jillian is refusing to get out of bed. "I'm sick," she tells you. "If you make me get out of bed, I'll probably have chest pain." How would you respond to this statement?
3. Vince Fulk is an 85-year-old man who sustained a massive cerebrovascular accident (stroke). He is unresponsive and immobile. What activity or mobility interventions should you incorporate into his plan of care? What is your rationale for these interventions?

4. For each of the following concepts, use critical thinking to describe how or why it is important to nursing, patient care, or activity and exercise. Note that these are *not* to be merely definitions.

Body mechanics	Activity tolerance
Exercise	Assistive devices
Immobility	

What Are the Main Points in This Chapter?

- The skeletal system includes bones, cartilage, ligaments, and tendons. The skeleton forms the framework of the body and protects the internal organs.
- Movement depends on the interaction between the skeleton and the muscles. The ligaments, tendons, and cartilage serve as the interface between these two systems.
- Contraction of skeletal muscles causes the muscles to shorten, thus causing the bones to move at the joints.
- There are four natural curves to the spine. Proper posture maintains these natural curves in good alignment.
- In the human body, the center of gravity is below the umbilicus at the top of the pelvis. The feet provide the base of support.
- Range of motion (ROM) is the degree of maximum movement at a joint. Active range of motion (AROM) is when the patient independently moves his joints through flexion, extension, abduction, adduction, and circular rotation. Passive range of motion (PROM) is performed by another person when the patient is unable to do so for himself.
- Principles of body mechanics are the rules that allow you to move your body with proper alignment, strength, and balance without causing injury.
- The U.S. Department of Health and Human Services recommends a minimum of 150 minutes per week of moderate-intensity, or 75 minutes per week of vigorous-intensity aerobic physical activity, or an equivalent combination of moderate- and vigorous-intensity aerobic physical activity.
- A well-rounded exercise program focuses on flexibility and balance, resistance training, and aerobic conditioning.
- Regular physical activity each week, sustained for months and years, can produce long-term health benefits. Strong evidence links regular physical activity with a lower risk for early death, heart disease, stroke, type 2 diabetes, hypertension, colon and breast cancers, and depression.
- Together with a healthy diet, regular physical activity aids in weight management, better heart and lung function and muscular fitness, fall prevention, and improved memory and mental clarity in older adults.
- People who are physically active tend to feel better and have more energy. Sleep quality is improved. And, overall, for many people, physical activity promotes a sense of optimism and positive self-esteem.
- Factors that influence activity and exercise level include developmental stage, health concerns, nutrition, lifestyle, attitudes, and external factors.
- Severe illness associated with prolonged immobilization causes physiological changes in almost every body system.
- A nursing history focused on activity and exercise assesses usual activity, commitment to fitness goals, mobility concerns, underlying health concerns and injuries, lifestyle, attitude of hardiness and persistence, and external factors.
- Physical assessment that is focused on activity and exercise examines the musculoskeletal system and activity tolerance. Important data include vital signs, height, weight, body mass index, body alignment, joint function, gait, and activity tolerance.
- Patients require a change of position at least every 2 hours to prevent pressure injury, muscle discomfort, damage to superficial nerves and blood vessels, or contractures.
- Range-of-motion exercises maintain joint mobility and limit the complications of immobility.
- Patients who have been confined to bed for more than a week or who have sustained major injury require ROM and muscle strength conditioning before they are able to resume walking.
- Canes, braces, walkers, and crutches promote stability for patients to walk independently and more safely.

Knowledge Map

POSITIONING PATIENTS:
Why: prevents skin breakdown; contractions; discomfort
Ways to position:
- Fowler's
- Lateral
- Prone
- Sims
- Supine

Positioning devices:
- Adjustable beds; siderails
- Pillows
- Trapeze; footboard/foot cradle

MOVING PATIENTS:
In bed:
Moving up in bed; turning; logrolling for spinal surgery/injury
Transfer out of bed: to stretcher or wheelchair
Assistive devices:
- Transfer board
- Mechanical lift
- Transfer roller or belt

PROMOTING ACTIVITY:
Performing range of motion:
- Active
- Passive

Assisting with ambulation:
- Assess readiness; patient condition
- Obtain assistance/equipment
- Physical conditioning prior to

Ambulation aids:
- Cane
- Walker
- Braces
- Crutches

PRINCIPLES GUIDING CARE
- Use lifting devices
- Get adequate help
- Use good body mechanics
- Assess pt size/restrictions
- Control pt pain; explain activity interventions
- Avoid friction

ACTIVITY AND EXERCISE

Eliminating

HAZARDS OF IMMOBILITY:
- Muscle atrophy; stiff joints
- Decreased respiration depth; pooling secretions; pneumonia/atelectasis
- Venous pooling; clotting; orthostatic hypotension
- Glucose intolerance; reduced muscle mass; stress response
- Constipation; flatus; ileus
- Urinary stasis; calculi
- Depression; anxiety; sleep disturbances; apathy

Promoting

TYPES:
- Isometric
- Isokinetic
- Aerobic
- Anaerobic

PROGRAMS:
- Flexibility training
- Resistance training
- Aerobic conditioning

ACTIVITY EXERCISE

Bones, Muscles, & Neurological Control

Diseases Affecting

Factors Affecting

Body Mechanics

MOBILITY

SPECIFIC DISEASES:
- M/S: hip dysplasia, scoliosis
- Bone formation: OI
- Joint mobility: arthritis
- Bone integrity: osteoporosis/osteomyelitis
- Trauma
- Neuro: SCI, MS

- Developmental stage
- Nutritional status
- Lifestyle
- Stress
- Environmental/socioeconomic factors

COMPONENTS:
- Body alignment: posture; proper spinal curve position
- Balance: via alignment; line of gravity through center of gravity
- Coordination: neuromuscular pairing for smooth movement
- Joint mobility: ROM

CHAPTER 33

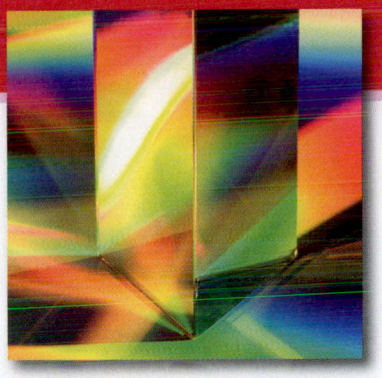

Sexual Health

STUDENT RESOURCES

*The questions and exercises in Volume 2 allow you to practice the kind of thinking you will use as a full-spectrum nurse. Critical-thinking questions usually have more than one correct answer, so we do not provide "answers" for these features. It is more important to develop your nursing judgment than to just cover content. You will learn by discussing the questions with your peers. If you are still unsure, consult your instructor. You will find Response Sheets (for writing your responses to the questions) on Davis*Plus.

To explore learning resources for this chapter,

Go to Davis*Plus* at DavisPl.us/Wilkinson3.

Chapter Resources for Chapter 33:

- **Response sheets for all learning activities**
- **Resources for Caregivers and Health Professionals**
- **Reading More About Sexual Health (suggested readings)**
- **Concept Map of chapter content**

Interactive Case Studies

NCLEX-Style and Chapter Questions

CHAPTER OVERVIEW

For a podcast of an overview of this chapter,

Go to Student Resources, Chapter 33, **Podcast—Chapter Overview,** on Davis*Plus*.

Caring for the Nguyens

As you may recall, Nam and Yen Nguyen are raising their 3-year-old grandson, Kim. Kim has made friends with Dinh, another little boy at preschool. Kim has asked whether they can play together. Yen works at the preschool and knows Dinh and his family. She is unsure whether she should allow her grandson to play with Dinh because she is uncomfortable with his family. Dinh was conceived via artificial insemination and is being raised by a lesbian couple. His parents are open about the relationship and voluntarily shared the conception information with Yen.

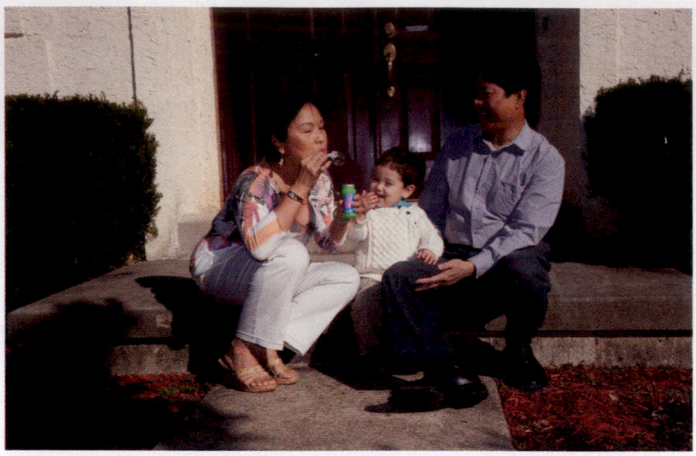

A. Yen calls the clinic to speak with you. She explains the situation and asks you whether you think it would be a problem to allow the boys to play together. She is concerned that being around this family may be a bad influence on Kim. How would you respond?

B. Yen remains concerned and presses you for more information. She is concerned that Kim's interest in Dinh may indicate that Kim has homosexual tendencies. How would you address her concerns?

C. Yen admits that Nam does not agree with her. "He told me that sexual orientation is genetic." How would you react to this statement?

Practical Knowledge knowing how

In this section you will find guidelines to assist you in assessing and planning care related to patients' sexual health.

CLINICAL INSIGHTS

Clinical Insight 33-1 ➤ Providing Care After Sexual Assault

- **Carefully collect information about the incident** and document findings in a fact-based manner, following your institution's protocol.
- **Be sensitive to the victim's fear, anxiety, and guilt** related to the event.
  Open discussion without communicating judgment or disapproval helps with fact finding for better care.
- **Assess the victim's emotional status,** including sexual identity, stress disorder, and risks for suicide and self-harm. Also discuss the potential for sexual and physical violence, including violence within relationships.
- **When collecting a nursing history for people with disabilities, be sure to screen for sexual violence.**
- **Administer prophylactic treatment** to patients who have been assaulted (vaginally, anally, or orally) to prevent sexually transmitted infections (STIs), such as chlamydia and gonorrhea. If there is a significant risk for HIV, prophylaxis may be prescribed within 72 hours of exposure.
- **Administer vaccines to prevent hepatitis B and human papillovirus (HPV),** as prescribed and according to your agency's policy.

Clinical Insight 33-1 ➤ Providing Care After Sexual Assault—cont'd

- **Administer emergency pregnancy prevention** (e.g., the "morning after" pill) to patients who have been vaginally assaulted even if penetration is uncertain, according to your agency's policy.
- **Document pregnancy status** with a urine or blood sample.
- **Teach follow-up care.** The victim should receive follow-up care within 1 week after the event to assess for healing of injuries and presence of STIs. Advise a female victim who has had vaginal penetration to obtain pregnancy testing again 2 weeks after the event.
- **Follow the current reporting requirements** for sexual assault in your state. Some states require reporting assault of children and adolescents, even if they do not consent to the reporting.
- **Know support services** available in your community for victims of abuse. Refer the victim to a sexual assault center for support, counseling, and additional information. Because of the long-term psychological and emotional consequences of sexual assault, most victims benefit from counseling.

Clinical Insight 33-2 ➤ Guidelines for Taking a Sexual History

1. **Provide privacy.**
   - Usually it is not enough merely to pull the curtains around the bed. Ask others who may be able to overhear private conversation behind the curtain to leave the room.
   - Talk to the client alone.
   - In some situations, it is also beneficial to talk to the partners as a unit, with the consent of both of course.
2. **Protect confidentiality.** Assure your client that information will not be shared with others, unless directly related to planning or delivering healthcare.
3. **Be relaxed in your approach**, and allow the client time to fully answer your questions. Your manner and attitude are critical in putting the client at ease.
4. **Make eye contact.** Do not act embarrassed or allow your body language to show your discomfort.
5. **Avoid communication stoppers**, such as:
   - "I'm only asking you these questions because I have to."
   - "I know that you probably won't want to tell me but . . ."
   - "You're not having any sexual problems, are you?"
6. **Consider a more inviting opening**, such as:
   - "Many people are embarrassed when asked questions about their sexuality, but whatever you tell me will remain confidential."
   - "Many people hesitate to talk about sexual problems. However, your sexual health is important to your overall health, and I would like to ask you a few questions about that."
7. **Be aware of verbal and nonverbal cues** that indicate concerns. Many people will cloak their concerns in comments such as, "I suppose that I won't need to worry about sexy lingerie any longer," or "Sex is for the young. I just have to accept that I'm sick and older now." Be careful that your response to such statements does not either negate or validate your patient's identity as a sexual being. Follow up with comments that encourage the client to provide more details (see Chapter 21 if you would like to review communication techniques).
8. **Realize the client may be embarrassed.** If the client is uncomfortable discussing topics about his own sexual health, reassure him by letting him know that some information, because of its private nature, may be difficult to discuss, but important.
9. **Encourage your client to use terminology that he is comfortable with.**
10. **Help the client feel comfortable.** Consider statements such as the following:
    - "Most people wonder how this surgery [or illness] may affect their sexual functioning."
    - "Whenever these medications are suggested, there are questions about sexual side effects."
    - "Have you thought about the kinds of adaptations you may have to make in your sex life after this surgery/treatment/illness?"
11. **Begin with a less sensitive topic** such as "When was your last menstrual period?" or "How is your relationship with your partner [spouse]?" Then you can move into more sensitive areas: "Many older women have some vaginal dryness that creates discomfort during intercourse. Do you have any concerns about this?"

Clinical Insight 33-3 ➤ Teaching Your Patient to Use a Condom

Using Male Condoms

The male condom is a sheath that covers the penis during sexual activity.

- Put the condom on before the penis touches the vagina, mouth, or anus.
- Inspect the package to ensure that the condom has not been damaged.
- Open the package without tearing the condom.
- Squeeze out the air at the tip of the condom, and unroll it over the erect penis, leaving some space at the tip to collect the ejaculate.
- After sex, to avoid breaking the condom, hold the condom at the rim as the penis is withdrawn. Discard the condom. Wash your hands.
- Use a new condom if you want to have sex again.

Using Female Condoms

The female condom is a plastic pouch that fits inside the vagina so that all vaginal tissue is protected from contact with the penis. The condom is inserted with the inner ring placed high in the vagina near the cervix and the outer ring on the labia.

- Insert the condom before the penis touches the vagina.
- Inspect the package to ensure that the condom has not been damaged.
- Open the package without tearing the condom.
- Put the inner ring and pouch inside the vagina.
- Push the inner ring as far into the vagina as it will go.
- Ensure that the outer ring stays outside the vagina.
- If needed, add lubricant to the inside of the condom.
- After sex, gently pull out the condom and discard.

Do

- Use latex condoms unless you or your partner are allergic to latex, or use polyurethane condoms.
- Treat condoms gently, and keep them out of the sun.
- Use only water-based lubricants to reduce friction and prevent tearing.
- Check the expiration date of the condom and packaging. Old condoms may be brittle and more likely to break.

Don't

- Don't store condoms in your wallet or other place where body heat can break down the latex.
- Don't use fingernails or teeth to open the condom wrapper; doing so can tear the condom.
- Don't reuse a condom.
- Don't use lotions or oils with condoms; these may cause breakage.

TABLES

Fertility Control Methods

FERTILITY CONTROL METHOD	ADVANTAGES	DISADVANTAGES
Abstinence—No sexual intercourse	100% effective Cost free	Lack of sexual expression May create stress in relationship.
Fertility awareness (natural family planning, rhythm method)—Intercourse only when a woman is thought to be in the infertile phase of her menstrual cycle	Cost free May be consistent with religious teachings No physical side effect	Requires cooperation of both partners. Menstrual cycle must be regular. Relatively high failure rate: Pregnancy may result. No protection against STIs
Withdrawal (coitus interruptus)—Removal of the penis from the vagina before ejaculation	Cost free	Requires discipline and mutual cooperation. Pre-ejaculatory fluid may contain sperm. Relatively high failure rate; pregnancy may result No protection against STIs

Fertility Control Methods—cont'd

FERTILITY CONTROL METHOD	ADVANTAGES	DISADVANTAGES
Male and female condoms	Obtained without a prescription Relatively inexpensive Protects against STIs	Must be put on before penetration; therefore, may diminish spontaneity of intercourse. May decrease sensation for both partners Cannot use certain types of condoms if either partner has latex allergy
Spermicides—Jelly, creams, or foams placed in the vagina	Obtained without a prescription More effective when used with a barrier (condom)	Significant pregnancy rate when used without a barrier (condom) No protection against STIs
Contraceptive sponge	May offer some protection against STIs Can be inserted into the vagina up to 24 hours before intercourse Inexpensive	Not fully effective against pregnancy
Vaginal ring	Highly effective in preventing pregnancy Does not have to be inserted before each act of intercourse—can be left in place for weeks to months, depending on the type	Requires a prescription because it is a hormonal method. Similar risks as birth control pills Costs similar to or greater than those of birth control pills Correct insertion is key factor in effectiveness of the method.
Oral contraceptives (birth control pills)	Very effective Do not interfere with intercourse Regulate menstrual flow Decrease menstrual cramps	Require a healthcare visit and prescription Significant cost Must be taken as prescribed to be effective Drug interactions No protection against STIs Carry some undesirable side effects Contraindicated for some women (e.g., those who smoke, who have significant varicose veins)
Depo-Provera injections	Last 3 months Highly effective Do not interfere with intercourse	Require a healthcare provider visit Amenorrhea (may be seen as an advantage) No protection against STIs
Intrauterine device (IUD)—A small piece of plastic that also may contain metal or a hormone: placed through the cervix into the uterus by a healthcare provider	Highly effective May remain in place for years Does not interfere with intercourse	Increased risk of pelvic inflammatory disease (PID) Must be inserted by a healthcare provider Increased menstrual flow and cramping No protection against STIs
Diaphragm—Latex dome-shaped cup with a flexible rim that is inserted in the vagina and fits over the cervix	Few side effects Quite effective if used properly with spermicide	Must be inserted prior to intercourse, thereby compromising spontaneity Must be removed about 6 hours after intercourse

(Continued)

Fertility Control Methods—cont'd

FERTILITY CONTROL METHOD	ADVANTAGES	DISADVANTAGES
		Must be used with a spermicide Increased risk of urinary tract infection (UTI) No protection against STIs
Hormonal implant—Small rod(s) containing hormones that are inserted under the skin, usually in the back of upper arm	One of the safest and most effective forms of birth control available (World Health Organization, 2006, updated 2010). Users do not have to think about their birth control every day or for every sexual intercourse. Menstrual periods are fewer and lighter for most women. Effective for 3 years Can be removed at any time Does not contain estrogen	No protection against STIs May be able to see the rod if the woman is very thin A small number of women have longer and heavier periods with breakthrough bleeding. May be limited availability More expensive than some other birth control methods Surgical procedure
Female sterilization (tubal ligation)	Effective Long-term cost-effectiveness May be reversible	May not be reversible No protection against STIs Usually not reversible
Male sterilization (vasectomy)	Effective Long-term cost-effectiveness Does not interfere with sexual performance May be reversible in some cases	Psychological effects No protection against STIs

ASSESSMENT GUIDELINES AND TOOLS

Focused Assessment

Guidelines and Questions for Taking a Sexual History

Topics to Include in a Sexual History

The topics to include in the sexual history depend on the nature of the patient's concern. The following topics are most commonly included:

- Reproductive history
- Sexual self-concept
- History of sexually transmitted infections
- History of sexual dysfunction
- Present sexual functioning
- Other factors that affect sexuality, such as medications and diseases
- Signs or symptoms of sexual abuse (see Procedure 9-1)
- Knowledge level about sex, reproduction, and contraception

Tailor your assessment to meet the client's needs. For example, Frank Thanee (Meet Your Patients, in Volume 1) is concerned about his family's reaction to his lifestyle and sexual orientation. In his situation, you would focus your assessment on his sexual self-concept, family relationships, present sexual functioning, and specific concerns about his heart and the impending family visit.

Questions to Ask Women

Menstrual Cycle

- How old were you when you started your menstrual periods?
- When was your last menstrual period?
- How often are your periods? How would you describe the flow? How long does your period last?
- Do you have any problems with your periods, such as cramping, breast pain, or heavy flow?

Focused Assessment

- Does your menstrual period ever prevent you from going to work or school or doing the activities you enjoy?
- What products do you use during your period, such as tampons and pads? Do you ever use douches, either during your period or at other times?

Cancer Screening

- When was your last Pap smear?
- Have you ever had an abnormal Pap smear? If so, how was it treated?
- Have you received a vaccine for HPV?
- Do you examine your breasts? If so, how often?
- Have you noticed asymmetry, lumps, or masses in your breasts? If so, describe them and show me where they are.
- When was your last mammogram? What were the results?
- Is there any history of breast cancer in your family?

Childbearing History

- How many living children do you have?
- How many times have you been pregnant?
- Have you ever had a miscarriage? An abortion?
- How many of your births were preterm (prior to 38 weeks)? Term?

Sexual Activity

- How often do you typically have sexual intercourse per month?
- Are you satisfied with the frequency or quality of sexual activity?
- Is there anything in your life that prevents you from sexual activity?
- Do you have any difficulty achieving orgasm?
- Is sexual intercourse ever painful for you?
- Are you sexually attracted to women? Have you had oral or genital sexual intercourse with women?

Questions to Ask Men

Sexual Activity

- How many times a month do you typically have sexual intercourse?
- Do you have any difficulty achieving or maintaining an erection or orgasm?
- Are you satisfied with the firmness of your erection?
- Do you experience either premature ejaculation or have difficulty achieving sexual orgasm?
- Are you sexually attracted to men? Have you had oral or anal intercourse with men?

Cancer Screening

- Have you been taught to examine your testicles? Do you practice testicular self-exam?
- Is there a history of testicular cancer in your family?

Questions to Ask Both Men and Women

Illnesses and Medications

- What types of illnesses have you been treated for in the past?
- Have you ever been hospitalized? Have you ever had surgery?
- What medications, herbal remedies, or over-the-counter medicines do you take?
- Has any medical treatment, surgery, or medication affected your sexual functioning?

Family Responsibilities

- Do you have children? If so, how many? How many are still at home? Dependent on you?
- Are you responsible for other children or adults? (This question may reveal whether the person continues to care for an adult, disabled child, or for grandchildren.)

Genitalia

- Have you noticed any redness, swelling, discharge, itching, or odor in your genital area?
- Have you noticed asymmetry, lumps, or masses in the genitals? If so, describe them and show me where they are.
- Have you ever been told you have a hernia?
- Have you ever had trauma to your genitals?
- Are you having any problems urinating?

Sexual Patterns

- Are you sexually active? If not, have you ever been?
- Do you have sex with men, women, or both?
- What types of sexual activity do you engage in? Oral, anal, or genital?
- How many partners do you currently have? How many partners have you had in the last 6 months?
- How would you describe your satisfaction with your current sexual relationship?
- What are your thoughts about how this procedure/illness may affect your sexual relationship?
- Have you experienced any recent changes in your sexual function—in your level of desire, your sexual activity, participation, or satisfaction?
- Do you have any concerns about your sexual function, including your level of desire, activity, participation, or satisfaction?

Contraception (as appropriate)

- Do you use birth control? If so, what type and how often?
- How satisfied are you with your method of contraception?

Sexually Transmitted Infections

- Have you ever been treated for an STI? If so, what type?
- Are you concerned about STIs or HIV?
- What precautions do you take to avoid STIs?

Abuse

- Have you ever been forced to have sex against your will?
- Have you ever been threatened or abused by a partner?
- Do you ever feel threatened by your partner?

For guidelines for your approach to taking a sexual history, see Clinical Insight 33-2.

CLINICALREASONING

Applying the Full-Spectrum Nursing Model

PATIENT SITUATION

Debra is perimenopausal at age 52, and her husband Roberto is 59. She has been feeling tired in the afternoon and moody at times. At her annual women's health visit, Debra tells you that she feels a lower level of sexual desire than she used to. Debra says, "I chalk it up to being very busy at work and yet still having so many demands on my time and energy with care of our three kids and housework." Debra is physically active, exercising four times a week, and is in good general health. She takes no medication and is within 15 pounds of her normal weight. Debra still has her period, but the flow is very heavy and cramping is more uncomfortable than it ever had been.

Recently, Debra has noticed that Roberto has been taking longer to achieve an erection, and his erection is not as firm as it used to be. He is in general good health except for high blood pressure and high blood cholesterol levels. He takes medication for both conditions.

THINKING

1. *Theoretical Knowledge (Factual Information):*
   a. What are the common physical and emotional manifestations occurring with perimenopause?
2. *Critical Thinking (Analyzing Alternatives, Deciding What to Do):*
   a. How would you respond to Debra when she asks for information and support regarding her husband's erectile dysfunction?
   b. Debra asks you whether her desire for sexual intimacy will continue to decline after she goes through "the change of life." Describe in detail what you would tell her.

DOING

3. *Practical Knowledge:*
   a. What general topics would you explore with Debra to assess her sexual history?
   b. What questions would you ask Roberto to assess his sexual history?

CARING

4. *Self-Knowledge:* What might you be feeling if you were in Debra's situation?
5. *Ethical Knowledge:* What are one or two things you would do to help Debra and Roberto feel cared for and cared about?

Critical Thinking and Clinical Reasoning

1. A 34-year-old married woman was hospitalized yesterday following an alleged rape. You are assigned to provide her nursing care. She will remain hospitalized for several days because of a head injury she suffered during the rape.
   a. How can you best approach this woman to establish a positive rapport?
   b. What fears is this patient likely to express?
   c. The patient's spouse is coming to visit. What concerns do you think that he may have?
   d. You begin to feel overwhelmed by this couple's emotions and questions. What can you do to help provide this couple with optimal care?
2. You are assigned a 26-year-old male patient who recently had a spinal cord injury. The doctors have talked to him about the possibility of regaining motor function and perhaps being able to walk again after intense therapy. What he now seems to be most concerned about is his relationship with his 25-year-old fiancée.
   a. What aspects of their relationship do you think he is concerned about?
   b. Do you have enough theoretical and patient information regarding his injury to answer all of his concerns?
   c. As you consider some of the changes in sexual functioning that may follow a spinal cord injury, what suggestions might you share with him?
   d. What clues would indicate that talking to the fiancée may be appropriate?

3. You are seeing Jessica, a 14-year-old girl, at the clinic. Her throat culture is positive for gonorrhea. The girl's mother has gone down to the coffee shop. The doctor has left a prescription for antibiotics. You are left to take care of the discharge from the clinic.
   a. How would you explain the culture results to Jessica?
   b. Jessica tells you that she cannot possibly have a sexually transmitted infection (STI) because she has not had sexual intercourse. How would you respond?
   c. Jessica tells you that she has had oral sex with her boyfriend, but no one else. What education regarding STIs and antibiotics would be appropriate?
   d. What information would you give the mother when she returns?
4. A 45-year-old married man with young children has just been informed that he is HIV positive. He is shocked by the news. He admits he had an extramarital relationship with a man 7 years ago.
   a. What concerns is he likely to have? As his nurse, what biases will you have to put aside to help him?
   b. What theoretical knowledge would you need at a later time to help him deal with questions about sexual activity?
   c. What patient information would you need to help him deal with questions about sexual activity?
5. Review the following scenarios from Meet Your Patients in Volume 1.
   - **Jocelyn Carter.** Two days after undergoing a fine-needle aspiration to evaluate a small breast mass, Jocelyn Carter's surgeon informed her that the mass was malignant. He recommended a mastectomy (removal of the breast). Today, she arrives alone at the surgery registration area at 0600. You ask how she is feeling, and she tells you that the past week has been a whirlwind of activity. "I had to arrange child care, cancel a business trip, and organize the house so that I could take a few days off to have the surgery. My husband is working overseas this fall, so he couldn't be here to help me. Honestly, I don't know how I'm feeling. I haven't had time to think about it." A few minutes later, as she waits in the surgery holding area, she begins to cry. You hold her hand and ask whether she would like to talk. She asks you, "Do you think my husband will still want me? I'm afraid he will be turned off when he looks at me now."
   - **Gabriel Thomas.** This patient comes to the outpatient clinic complaining of a throbbing headache for the past 3 days. He explains that he has tried several over-the-counter medicines and has had no relief. You check his blood pressure, and measure the reading at 240/130 mm Hg. When you ask whether he has ever been treated for high blood pressure, he replies, "Are you another one of these people trying to get me to take drugs that will ruin my sex life?"
   - **Frank Thanee.** Frank has heart disease, had a mitral valve replacement 3 days ago. He has been transferred to the cardiology floor for an additional day of hospitalization. His partner, Greg, has spent the last 3 days at the hospital and has just left to check on the apartment and feed their cat. Frank confides that he is worried about his parents' expected visit. "I've never been able to tell them about Greg. They wouldn't be able to understand it, never mind approve. I don't know how to handle this. What do you think I should do?"

   a. Write etiologies for each of the patients. The nursing diagnosis label is provided for you in each case.
      Jocelyn Carter—Ineffective Sexuality Patterns
      Gabriel Thomas—Ineffective Sexuality Patterns
      Frank Thanee—Sexual Dysfunction
   b. For each of the patients, instead of the sexuality diagnosis, identify another nursing diagnosis label that you should explore to see whether it fits the situation better. Consult a nursing diagnosis handbook, as needed.
      Jocelyn Carter:
      Gabriel Thomas:
      Frank Thanee:
6. For each of the following concepts, use critical thinking to describe how or why it is important to nursing, patient care, or sexual health. Note that these are *not* to be merely definitions.

Sexual health	Sexual expression
Gender	Sexually transmitted infections
Sexual orientation	Fertility control

7. An infant is born with ambiguous sex organs. The provider has informed the parents that they will need to make a decision regarding which gender they want to assign to the child. They also have the option of waiting and letting the child decide at a later date.
   a. What do you think the parents need to consider in making this decision?
   b. What emotional factors may be involved in this decision?

What Are the Main Points in This Chapter?

- Sexuality is a broad and complex aspect of the self, with physical, emotional, social, and spiritual dimensions.
- Sexuality involves how we feel about ourselves as individuals and how we interact with others and our environment.
- Gender, gender roles, gender identity, and sexual orientation contribute to expression of our sexuality throughout the life cycle.
- There are both typical and atypical forms of sexual expression.
- Culture, religion, lifestyle, sexual knowledge, and physical health all influence our attitudes toward sexuality, sexual behaviors, and intimate relationships.
- Sexual victimization is a societal and healthcare concern.
- Physical and psychological health status affects sexuality and sexual functioning.
- Sexual health is challenged by high-risk sexual behaviors, sexually transmitted infections (STI), negative interpersonal relationships, and sexual dysfunctions.
- Four phases of the sexual response cycle are excitement, plateau, orgasm, and resolution.
- A sexual history is a component of the nursing assessment.
- There are strategies you can use to help you gain comfort and competence in collecting sexual data.
- The PLISSIT model was developed as a guideline for counseling for sexual problems: Permission, Limited Information, Specific Suggestions, and Intensive Therapy.
- Sexual well-being may be enhanced through nursing interventions such as counseling for sexual problems; dealing with inappropriate sexual behavior; and teaching about body function and reproduction, self-care, contraception, and prevention of STIs.

Knowledge Map

Sexuality

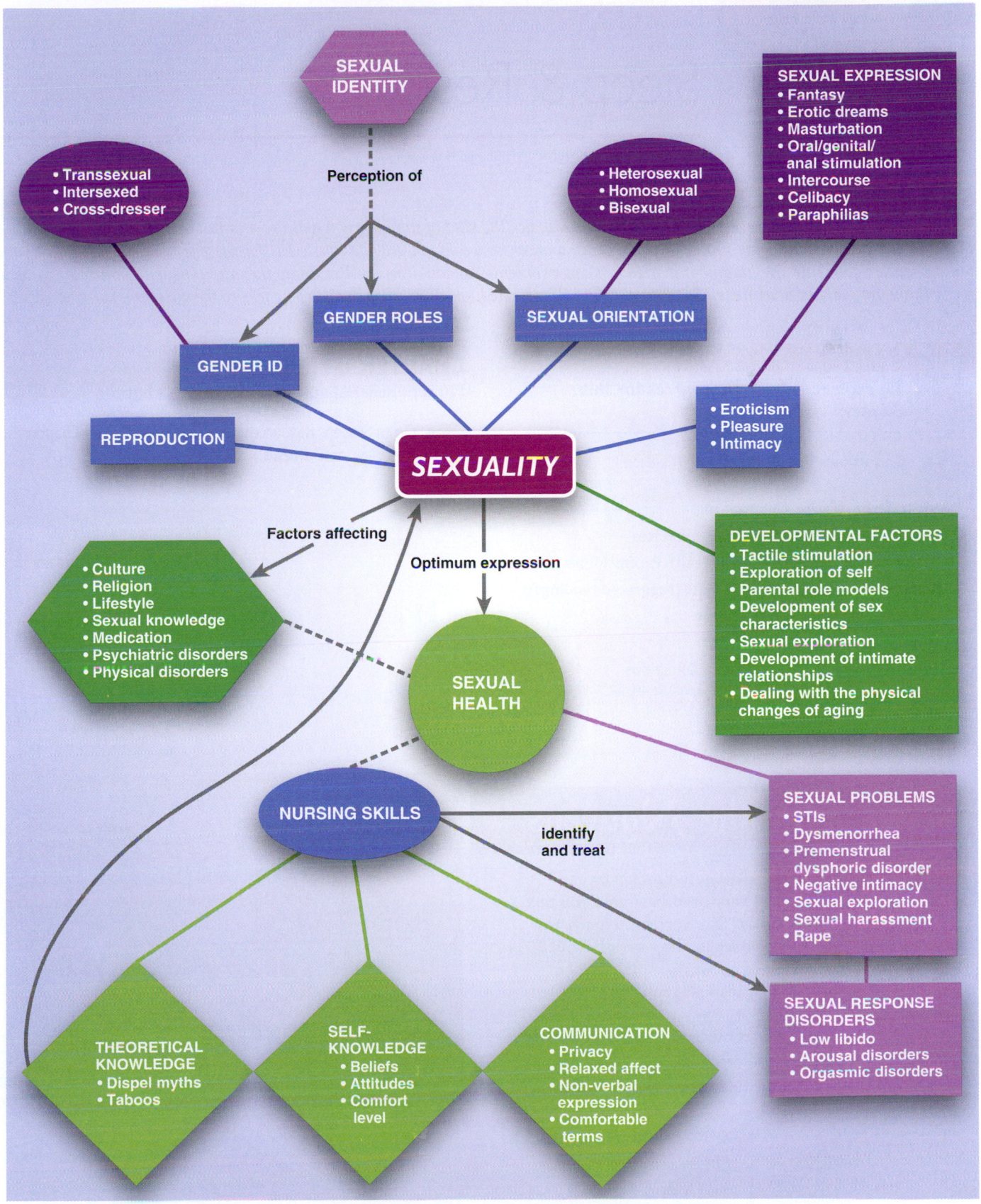

CHAPTER 34

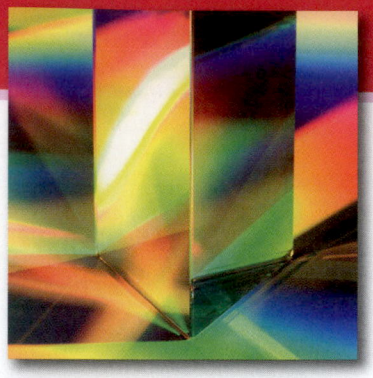

Sleep & Rest

STUDENT RESOURCES

*The questions and exercises in Volume 2 allow you to practice the kind of thinking you will use as a full-spectrum nurse. Critical-thinking questions usually have more than one correct answer, so we do not provide "answers" for these features. It is more important to develop your nursing judgment than to just cover content. You will learn by discussing the questions with your peers. If you are still unsure, consult your instructor. You will find Response Sheets (for writing your responses to the questions) on Davis*Plus.

To explore learning resources for this chapter,

Go to Davis*Plus* at DavisPl.us/Wilkinson3.

Chapter Resources for Chapter 34:
- **Response sheets for all learning exercises**
- **Resources for Caregivers and Health Professionals**
- **Reading More About Sleep & Rest (suggested readings)**
- **Concept Map of chapter content**

Interactive Case Studies

NCLEX-Style and Chapter Review Questions

CHAPTER OVERVIEW

For a podcast of an overview of this chapter,

Go to Student Resources, Chapter 34, **Podcast—Chapter Overview,** on Davis*Plus*.

Caring for the Nguyens

Yen Nguyen arrives at the clinic accompanied by her husband, Nam. She appears very tired. Nam tells you that she has been sleeping poorly. "She worries so much. She worries about Kim, our grandchild. She worries about our kids. Now she's worried about my mother. When we were going through that mammogram scare, she was even worse!"

Mrs. Nguyen shrugs her shoulders. "I can't help it. I'm like that. I've always been a worrier. But it's gotten worse lately. Now I worry and get so emotional. I lie in bed

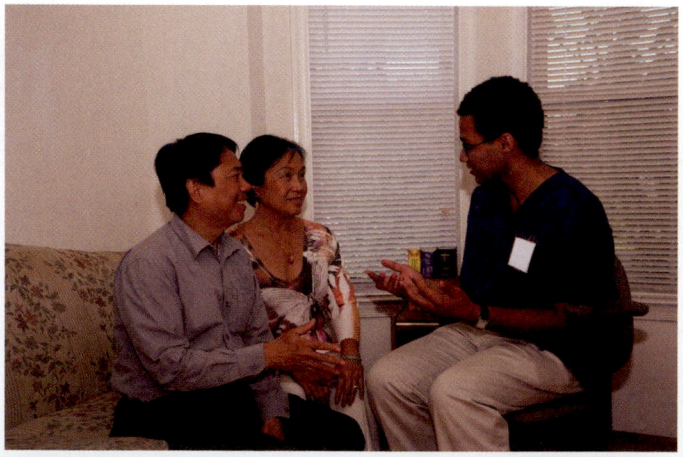

Caring for the Nguyens (continued)

thinking about all this stuff and end up in tears. Then, when I finally get to sleep, I wake up covered with sweat. I've tried extra soy for hot flashes, melatonin from the health food store, herbal tea, and even Benadryl—but nothing seems to work. I'm so tired. But when I get up, I have to deal with all these little kids at work. They're bouncing all over the place and noisy. I just get so short-tempered with them. That's not like me. I can't take this anymore."

A. *Patient data:* Clearly Mrs. Nguyen has a sleep problem. Underline the data that are defining characteristics (symptoms) of a sleep problem.

B. *Patient data:* Which data suggest ideas about the etiologies (causes) of Mrs. Nguyen's sleep problem?

C. *Nursing diagnosis:* Two NANDA-I sleep-related nursing diagnoses are Sleep Deprivation and Disturbed Sleep Pattern. You have already identified the patient's defining characteristics. Now, what *knowledge* do you need to decide which of these NANDA-I labels to use?

D. How could you obtain this knowledge?

E. Sleep Deprivation is defined as "prolonged periods of time without sleep" and Disturbed Sleep Pattern is defined as "time-limited disruption of sleep." Can you make the diagnoses on the basis of this knowledge? Why or why not?

F. Following are some of the defining characteristics for these two nursing diagnoses. Certainly there is some overlap between the two sets of symptoms. Nevertheless, which set seems to be a better fit for Mrs. Nguyen? Why?

Disturbed Sleep Pattern
- Verbal complaints of not feeling well rested
- Dissatisfaction with sleep
- Change in normal sleep pattern
- Decreased ability to function
- Reports being awakened
- Reports no difficulty falling asleep

Sleep Deprivation
- Daytime drowsiness
- Decreased ability to function
- Agitation
- Irritability
- Hallucinations
- Anxiety
- Inability to concentrate
- Apathy
- Slowed reactions
- Combativeness
- Fatigue
- Fleeting nystagmus
- Hand tremors
- Heightened sensitivity to pain
- Lethargy, listlessness, malaise
- Perceptual disorders (e.g., disturbed body sensation, delusions, feeling afloat)
- Restlessness
- Transient paranoia

G. Write a nursing diagnosis for Mrs. Nguyen.

Practical Knowledge knowing how

This section will help you learn to give a back massage, assist you in obtaining a sleep history, and provide standardized language to use in planning care for clients with sleep problems.

PROCEDURES

In the not-so-distant past, a relaxing back massage was a part of the evening care routine for every hospitalized patient. In this era of cost containment, this sleep enhancer has become a "nice but not essential" procedure in most agencies. Massage has therapeutic benefits, however. It promotes circulation, physical and emotional comfort, and sleep. Furthermore, it is an independent nursing activity for which you do not need a medical prescription (except in very rare circumstances). Try to offer a back rub whenever you can, and teach and encourage nursing assistive personnel (NAP) to do so as well. Refer to the following procedure.

Procedure 34-1 ■ Giving a Back Massage

➤ For steps to follow in *all* procedures, refer to the Universal Steps for All Procedures found on the page facing the inside back cover.

Equipment

Skin care lotion

Pre-Procedure Assessment

Check the skin for reddened areas or skin breakdown.

Delegation

You can delegate back massage to the NAP if the patient's condition and the NAP's skills allow. However, giving the back rub yourself provides an excellent opportunity to assess the patient, develop rapport, and provide emotional support.

➤ When performing the procedure, always identify your patient according to agency policy, using two identifiers, and be attentive to standard precautions, hand hygiene, patient safety and privacy, body mechanics, and documentation.

Procedure Steps

1. **Warm the lotion** by placing the bottle in warm water.
   Cold lotion can cause muscle contraction; warming the lotion helps relax the muscles.

2. **Raise the bed to working height.**
   Prevents back strain of the nurse.

3. **Position the patient comfortably** on her side or prone.
   a. Untie the patient's gown, and expose her back.
   b. Raise the siderail on the opposite side of the bed.
   c. Don procedure gloves.
   Siderails prevent the patient from falling off the bed when you turn her toward the side of the bed away from you.
   d. Wash the patient's back with warm water, if needed.
   Warm water will help relax the muscles while removing any sweat and soiling.

4. **Place lotion on your hands.**
   Placing the lotion directly on the back may cause the patient's muscles to tighten.

5. **Place your hands on either side** of the spine at the base of the neck. Using gentle, continuous pressure, rub down the length and then up the sides of the back.
   a. Repeat this motion several times.
   b. Never rub directly over the spine.
   The spine is a vulnerable area.▼

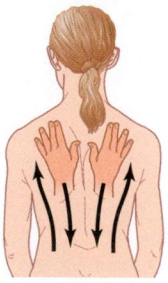

6. **Apply gentle thumb pressure** (using the fleshy part of your thumbs) on either side of the spine at the midback, pushing outward for about 2.5 cm (1 in.).
   a. Repeat from the midback to the base of the neck in a series of small, outward strokes.
   Strokes should be along the muscle length and not across the muscle to help stretch and relax it.
   b. Ask the patient whether the amount of pressure is comfortable. Be careful not to cause the patient discomfort, which might cause further muscle tightness.
   c. Always apply pressure away from the spine, not toward it.
   This gently stretches the muscles and helps prevent placing pressure on the spine.

d. If you are unable to massage both sides at the same time, work on one side and then the other.
Work as symmetrically as possible to increase muscle relaxation.▼

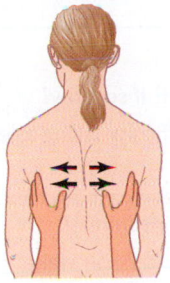

7. **Now go to the spots that felt** the tightest or that the patient states are tight. Work in small circles, using gentle thumb pressure.
Small circular movements can help release muscle "knots" and relax tightened muscles.▼

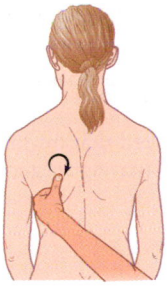

8. **Gently shake the scapulae.** Place your palm on one scapula, and gently shake it by quickly moving your palm back and forth. Repeat on the other side.
Movement of the scapula decreases when muscles tighten; gently vibrating the scapula helps loosen the muscles.▼

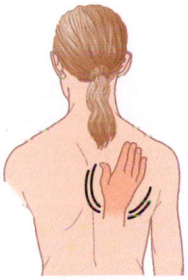

9. **Apply horizontal strokes** across the scapula, using your thumb. Using horizontal strokes from near the spine across the bottom of the scapula, push out all the way across the scapula from the spine. Move up and repeat until you have covered the entire scapula and top of the shoulder. Repeat on the other side.
This movement helps loosen the trapezius muscle.▼

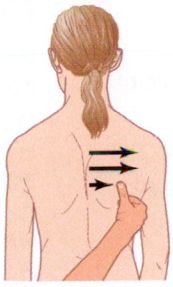

10. **If you find tender spots**, use the fleshy parts of your fingers in a small circular motion.

11. **Apply pressure in circles** using the heels of your hands down both sides of the spine. Beginning at the upper shoulder and working down to the lower back, apply pressure in medium-sized circles down the sides of the spine with the heels of your hands. Be cautious not to apply too much pressure. Assess patient for comfort.
The circular motion helps relax tightened areas in the paraspinal muscles.▼

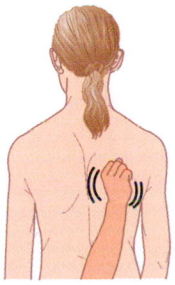

12. **Apply horizontal strokes** using the heels of your hands across the latissimus dorsi muscle. Using horizontal strokes from near the spine below the scapula, push out from the spine across to the ribs, and work down across the lower back with the heels of your hands.
This movement helps relax the latissimus dorsi muscle.

13. **Gently rub your hands up either side** of the spine from the base of the back to the base of the neck and then down the sides of the back. Repeat several times.
Long strokes help increase circulation and promote relaxation of the back muscles.

NOTE: If you are unable to do a complete back massage, ask the patient where she is most uncomfortable, and massage those areas. If the patient has general tightness, use the long strokes down each side of the spine and back up the sides.

Evaluation

Assess the patient's report of comfort, relaxation, and how soon she falls asleep.

Documentation

This is a routine aspect of care and is usually documented on a flowsheet.

Practice Resources

Dosey, B., & Keegan. L. (2009); Sports Injury Clinic (n.d.).

ASSESSMENT GUIDELINES AND TOOLS

This section will assist you in screening for sleep problems.

Questions for a Sleep History

A brief assessment for all patients should include questions about the following:

Usual Sleeping Pattern

- When do you go to sleep and wake up?
- How many hours do you sleep?
- Do you have a regular sleep schedule?
- How would you rate the quality of your sleep on a scale of 1 to 10, with 10 meaning "great"?
- Do you take a nap? If you do, for how long?
- How often do you waken during sleep, for example, to go to the bathroom?
- Do you feel adequately rested when you wake up?

Sleeping Environment

- Would you like a night-light?
- What room temperature do you prefer?
- What noise level do you prefer (for example, radio, television, absolute quiet)?

Bedtime Routines/Rituals

- What do you typically do in the hour before bedtime?
- What do you do to help you fall asleep?

Sleep Aids

- Do you need a special pillow or positioning aid?
- Do you take any sleep medications or other drugs, natural sleep aids, or homeopathic remedies that may affect sleep?

Sleep Changes or Problems

- Have your sleep patterns changed? If so, how?
- How often do you experience difficulty falling asleep? Staying asleep?
- Do you currently, or have you in the past, ever experienced a sleep disorder (e.g., narcolepsy, insomnia)?
- Do you remember your dreams after you wake? Do you ever have night terrors? Do you sleepwalk?
- Do you ever experience an unpleasant creeping feeling, crawling, or tingling, relieved only by moving the legs at night?
- Do you snore? Does your own snoring or grunting ever wake you or anyone in the room?
- Do you wear a cap at night? Do you require oxygen at night? Or any other medical aid or therapy while you sleep?
- Do you grind your teeth while you sleep? Do you wear a dental appliance to prevent grinding?
- Do you experience any kind of pain that makes it difficult for you to fall asleep or stay asleep?
- Is there anything that I have not asked that might help you sleep while you are in the hospital (having surgery, receiving home care)?

If the client reports experiencing satisfactory sleep, that is an adequate assessment, and you merely need to support her usual sleep patterns and rituals. When you suspect a sleep problem, you will perform a more in-depth assessment, such as a detailed sleep history or sleep diary.

Sleep Diary

A sleep diary provides specific information on the patient's sleep–wakefulness patterns over a long period. The diary is usually kept for 14 days and may include the following.

Note: If you work a night shift, adjust the time for sleep and waking in these questions accordingly.

Completed in the morning

1. Time you went to bed:_____
2. Approximate time you fell asleep:_____
3. Times you woke during the night:_____
4. Times you fell back to sleep:_____
5. Time you woke up in the morning:_____
6. Did you feel refreshed upon wakening?_____
7. What did you eat or drink just before bedtime? _____
8. What mental and physical activities did you engage in the 2 to 3 hours before bedtime?_____
9. Were you worried or anxious about anything when you went to bed?_____
10. Sleep medications you have taken:_____ Any repeated doses? _____ Times:_____

Completed in the evening

1. How sleepy did you feel during the day?
   ____ Sleepy; struggled to stay awake during the day
   ____ Somewhat tired
   ____ Fairly alert
   ____ Wide awake
2. Any naps during the day? _____ If so, for how long? _____
3. Frequency of pain medication taken and times _____
4. Exercise during the day? _____ If so, for how long? _____ What time of the day? _____
5. Number of alcoholic drinks _____ What time: _____
6. Number of caffeinated drinks _____ What time: _____
7. Number of tobacco products _____ What time: _____

CLINICAL REASONING

Applying the Full-Spectrum Nursing Model

PATIENT SITUATION

A 43-year-old healthy woman, Maria Lupe, is being seen for her annual women's health visit. She tells you she lies awake in bed for hours before falling asleep at night. Sometimes she falls asleep without problems but will wake up and then have trouble going back to sleep. After feeling as though she had been awake nearly all night, Maria wakes in the morning feeling exhausted. She tells you she feels tired all the time and can't seem to get things done during her time off because of her fatigue. Maria admits to feeling irritable with her coworkers and children. Because of her lack of rest, she doesn't have the desire to do things socially anymore.

THINKING

1. *Theoretical Knowledge:* The NANDA-I definition and defining characteristics of Insomnia differ slightly from the medical diagnosis of insomnia.
   a. What is insomnia, as defined medically (e.g., by the National Sleep Foundation)?
   b. What other health conditions might a medical diagnosis of insomnia be confused with?
   c. What factors either lead to or aggravate insomnia, as described medically?
2. *Critical Thinking (Contextual Awareness):*
   a. Obviously Maria has trouble sleeping. Based on the data you have, do you consider her difficulty sleeping significant enough to require consultation with her primary healthcare provider? Explain your thinking.

DOING

3. *Nursing Process (Assessments):*
   a. When conducting a sleep history for Maria, what questions would you ask her in order to (1) describe more fully her sleeping problem and (2) identify the cause of her sleeping problem?
   b. What would you suggest Maria do to help you gain more information about her sleeping problem?

4. *Nursing Process (Nursing Diagnosis):* Based on the data in the Patient Situation, would you use a nursing diagnosis of Sleep Deprivation or Insomnia for Maria? Explain your thinking. Use a nursing diagnosis handbook, as needed, to compare the defining characteristics of the two diagnoses.
5. *Nursing Process (Interventions):* How might you help your patient manage her Insomnia other than using prescription medication? What might you suggest?

CARING

6. *Self-Knowledge:*
   a. Have you ever had trouble falling or staying asleep? How did you feel at the time and in the morning? Describe your experience.
   b. How might you provide better emotional care and support to your patient after recalling your own episodes of sleeping difficulty?

Critical Thinking and Clinical Reasoning

1. You are a nurse working on a psychiatric unit. You are assigned to the care of Sheryl, a 23-year-old woman with the diagnosis of anorexia nervosa (a potentially life-threatening eating disorder characterized by an intense fear of weight gain and extremely restrictive food intake). Sheryl attends therapy each day, seems to be taking her medications, and is eating the required amount of food at each meal. But she continues to lose weight. The nurse working the night shift reports that Sheryl is unable to sleep at night; seems frightened, almost panicky; paces the hall; and cries. Sheryl is unwilling to talk about her inability to sleep, but you read in her chart that she was sexually abused during the night while she was in a foster home. As you are straightening up in her room, you find several of Sheryl's sleeping pills. Sheryl walks into the room and begs you to be her friend and not to tell anyone. She promises to take her pills that night.
   a. What do you think may be contributing to Sheryl's inability to sleep? Explain your reasoning.
   b. How do you *feel* about keeping Sheryl's secret? Why might you want to tell other caregivers about the sleeping pills? What reasons can you think of for *not* telling?
   c. For you to deal effectively with Sheryl's sleep problem, what theoretical knowledge would you need?
   d. Now assess your current theoretical knowledge. Do you need more knowledge about certain topics to help Sheryl? If so, where can you find out what you need to know?
2. Imagine that you are a registered nurse at a local nursing home. Gwen, a 74-year-old woman, has captured your heart. Gwen has severe rheumatoid arthritis with pain and joint deformities, so she cannot ambulate or perform activities of daily living independently. Gwen's family visits every weekend, and they always bring cookies or candy, usually chocolate. Gwen likes to eat these treats just before bedtime, right after her bedtime medications. She receives a stool softener, a sleeping pill, and a pain pill for her arthritis. Lately she has been awakening at least twice each night, seeming quite confused. She tells the day shift nurse that she needs another sleeping pill at bedtime because "I'm not sleeping as well as I used to, because I have to get up so many times to go to the bathroom." She also seems more sluggish than usual during the day. You will need to integrate all available information. Don't worry if you do not know much about arthritis or if there are other things you have not yet studied. Just try to reason out the questions based on the knowledge you *do* have.
   a. If you have not yet studied arthritis and urinary elimination, you may lack some theoretical knowledge you need to answer the following questions. What information do you need? Where would you go to get it?
   b. What are some reasons that Gwen might be awakening?
   c. What might be causing her confusion at night?
   d. Should you address the problem of having chocolate before bed? Why or why not?
   e. List as many different interventions as you can that you might use to address the problem of eating sweets before bed.
   f. Consider the consequences. How might her family react if you suggest that they bring something besides sweets?
   g. What teaching might you do with the family?
3. You are a home health nurse. One of your patients is a 55-year-old man named Grant. He is homebound because of complications of diabetes. He states that he sleeps during the day, taking several naps. His chief complaint today is a pain in his left foot. There are books about alternative medicine and bottles of vitamins

and minerals all over the house. He believes he can cure his diabetes with herbs. He refuses to take any medications that are prescribed for him by his physician.

a. Do you have enough information to conclude that Grant has a sleep problem? Explain your answer.
b. Examine the patient situation (context). What factors lead you to suspect that Grant may not be sleeping enough at night?
c. What would you do to find out whether Grant is getting enough sleep?
d. Imagine how you would feel about Grant's decision to forgo his medication and use herbal treatments.
e. What personal values and biases do you have that will affect the way you respond to Grant?

4. For each of the following concepts, use critical thinking to describe how or why it is important to nursing, patient care, or sleep and rest. Note that these are *not* to be merely definitions.

Sleep
Rest
Theoretical knowledge about the physiology of sleep
Circadian rhythm
Stages of sleep (e.g., REM sleep)
Sleep apnea
Sedatives
Sleep diary

What Are the Main Points in This Chapter?

- Sleep is a basic physiological need.
- Sleep and rest promote physical, mental, and spiritual well-being by restoring energy and reducing body demands while the body repairs itself.
- Illness can interfere with the ability to sleep and rest; conversely, people who suffer from sleep disorders have an increased susceptibility to illnesses.
- The hypothalamus and various neurotransmitters are involved in the physiology of sleep.
- Circadian rhythm is a biorhythm that is influenced by both internal and external stimuli, especially the light–dark patterns of day and night.
- The brain waves produced during REM sleep are similar to those of alert wakefulness. REM is characterized by rapid eye movements and dreaming.
- Duration of sleep varies according to age.
- Factors affecting sleep include developmental needs and stressors, work, exercise, foods, other lifestyle factors, use of medications, illness, pain, and the environment.
- Common sleep disorders include insomnia, sleep apnea, and narcolepsy.
- It is important to obtain information about the patient's usual sleep patterns and rituals; this may require use of a sleep diary.
- Nursing interventions to promote sleep include scheduling nursing care, creating a restful environment, promote comfort, and supporting bedtime rituals and routines.
- Pain is one of the main deterrents to sleep. Hormonal fluctuations and stress also contribute to sleep difficulties.
- Sleep medications, as a rule, should be used only as a temporary measure.
- Teaching patients and their families about the importance of rest and sleep is an important health promotion intervention.

Knowledge Map

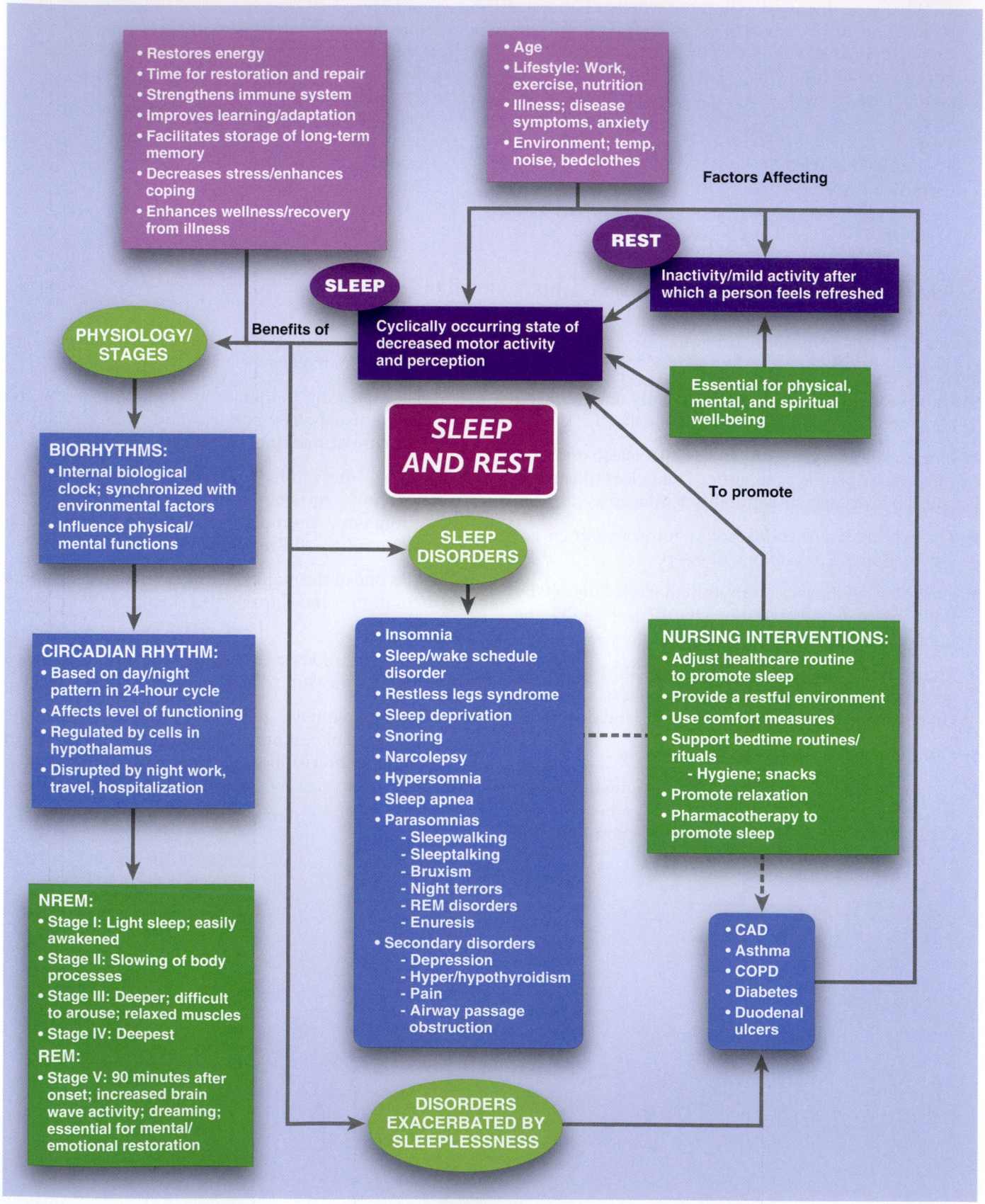

CHAPTER 35

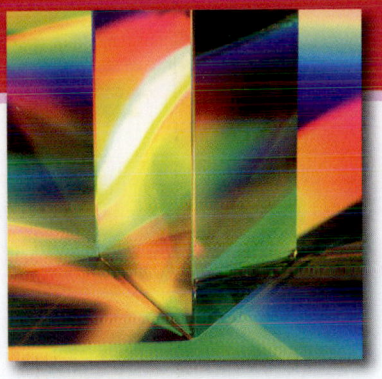

Skin Integrity & Wound Healing

STUDENT RESOURCES

*The questions and exercises in Volume 2 allow you to practice the kind of thinking you will use as a full-spectrum nurse. Critical-thinking questions usually have more than one correct answer, so we do not provide "answers" for these features. It is more important to develop your nursing judgment than to just cover content. You will learn by discussing the questions with your peers. If you are still unsure, consult your instructor. You will find Response Sheets (for writing your responses to the questions) on Davis*Plus.

To explore learning resources for this chapter,

Go to Davis*Plus* at DavisPl.us/Wilkinson3.

Chapter Resources for Chapter 35

- **Response sheets for all learning activities**
- **Resources for Caregivers and Health Professionals**
- **Reading More About Skin Integrity & Wound Healing (suggested readings)**
- **Concept Map of chapter content**

Interactive Case Studies

NCLEX-Style and Chapter Review Questions

CHAPTER OVERVIEW

For a podcast of an overview of this chapter,

Go to Student Resources, Chapter 35, **Podcast—Chapter Overview,** on Davis*Plus*.

Caring for the Nguyens

Kim Phan, Nam and Yen Nguyen's 3-year-old grandchild, fell at the neighborhood playground. He has abrasions on his knees, a deep puncture wound on his left hand, and a laceration on his scalp. Mr. and Mrs. Nguyen bring him to the clinic for assessment. He is crying loudly and moving all extremities. No treatment has been given.

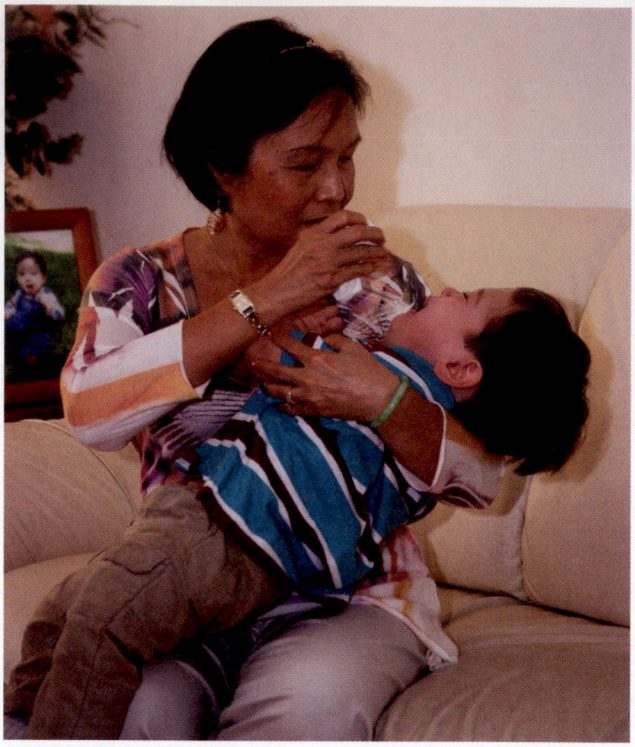

A. What should be your first course of action?

B. What kind of care will Kim need at the clinic?

C. You determine that the scalp laceration will need to be sutured. What actions should you take to prepare Kim for the suturing?

D. One week later Kim arrives at the clinic with his grandmother to have the sutures removed. The scalp laceration is dried and healed. When you inspect his other wounds, you notice that his left knee is erythematous, warm and painful to touch, and that there is a moderate amount of purulent drainage. What assessment questions should you ask?

E. Yen Nguyen tells you that Kim would not allow her to clean or dress the abraded knees. You cleanse the knee and remove several small pieces of gravel from the wound bed. The wound is yellow and malodorous. What kind of care will Yen need to provide to Kim to heal the left knee?

Practical Knowledge knowing how

As a nurse, you will care for many patients who have wounds or who are at risk for impaired skin integrity. You will need practical knowledge of wound assessment and wound care.

PROCEDURES

All wounds require a focused assessment. Assessment frequency depends on the condition of the wound, the work setting, the patient's overall condition and underlying disease process, the type of wound, and the type of treatment used for the wound. If you are providing wound care, you will assess the wound with every treatment.

Specific nursing interventions directed at maintaining skin integrity or healing wounds make use of procedures for obtaining wound cultures, cleansing wounds, and dressing wounds, for placing and removing wound closures, caring for wound drains, and applying binders and bandages, as well as Clinical Insights for applying local heat and cold therapy.

Procedure 35-1 ■ Obtaining a Wound Culture by Swab

➤ For steps to follow in *all* procedures, refer to the Universal Steps for All Procedures found on the page facing the inside back cover.

➤ *Note:* his procedure uses modified sterile technique because wound care is now usually performed using a clean approach rather than strict sterile technique.

Equipment

- Three pairs of clean nonsterile gloves
- Aerobic culturette tube with sterile calcium alginate or rayon swab
- Sterile 4 in. × 4 in. gauze in an impermeable tray or separate 4 × 4 packs and an impermeable barrier
- Sterile 0.9% (normal) saline solution for irrigation, warmed to body temperature when possible
  Cold solution lowers the temperature of the wound bed and slows the healing process.
- 20-mL syringe
- 19-gauge angiocatheter
- Gown and face shield
- Emesis basin
- Water-resistant disposable drapes

Delegation

This procedure requires knowledge of wound healing. It needs to be performed by a registered nurse. Do not delegate this skill to nursing assistive personnel (NAP).

Pre-Procedure Assessments

Note: If the wound is covered when you begin, you will make these assessments once you remove the soiled dressing *and* after cleansing the wound.

- Assess for pain.
  Wounds may be very painful, and wound irrigation may increase pain. Provide prescribed pain medication 30 minutes before performing the procedure, if indicated.
- Determine whether the wound requires sterile, modified sterile, or clean technique.
  Sterile technique is used for acute surgical wounds and for wounds that have undergone recent sharp debridement, or when the healthcare provider prescribes it. Chronic wounds are colonized with bacteria and may be cared for using clean technique, as in this procedure. To perform sterile wound irrigation, see Procedure 35-2.
- Assess the amount and type of tissue present in the wound bed.
  Granulating tissue is beefy red with a velvety appearance. It appears with the growth of new blood vessels and connective tissue. Pale pink tissue may indicate compromised blood supply to the wound bed. Necrotic tissue, which is black, brown, or yellow in appearance, is nonviable, and inhibits healing. Only red granulating tissue should be swabbed for a culture.
- Assess the type and amount of exudate.
  Exudate may be a sign of infection.
- Assess the wound for odor.
  A foul odor may indicate infection. Cleanse wounds before you assess for odor because some dressings interact with wound drainage to produce an odor.
- Assess the tissue surrounding the wound edge.
  Surrounding tissue that is red, warm, and/or edematous may indicate infection.

➤ When performing the procedure, always identify your patient according to agency policy, using two identifiers, and be attentive to standard precautions, hand hygiene, patient safety and privacy, body mechanics, and documentation.

Procedure Steps

➤ *Note:* Steps are for aerobic culture.

1. **Place the patient** in a comfortable position that provides easy access to the wound and will allow the irrigation solution to flow freely from the wound, with the assistance of gravity. Position a water-resistant disposable drape between the patient and the bed to protect the bedding from any possible runoff.
2. **After washing and drying hands,** don gown, face shield, and clean nonsterile gloves.
3. **Place an emesis basin** at the bottom of the wound to collect irrigation runoff. Avoid touching the wound with the basin.
   Prevents contamination of wound from the emesis basin; protects linens from runoff.
4. **Remove the soiled dressing.** Dispose of gloves and soiled dressing in a biohazard bag.
5. **Don clean gloves,** after performing hand hygiene.
6. **Using a 19-gauge angiocatheter,** remove the metal stylet needle and dispose into a sharps container. Attach the angiocatheter to a 35-mL syringe and fill with normal saline irrigation solution.
   Prevents contamination and needlestick injury. A 19-gauge angiocatheter with a 35-mL syringe provides 8 psi (pounds per square inch) of pressure and is effective for removing bacteria, necrotic tissue, exudate, and/or metabolic wastes.

   Note: This procedure follows guidelines established by the Agency for Healthcare Research Quality (AHRQ). Commercial irrigation kits containing a piston tip syringe may also be used. Their use is discussed in Procedure 35-2.

(continued on next page)

Procedure 35-1 ■ Obtaining a Wound Culture by Swab (continued)

7. **Holding the angiocatheter** tip 2 cm from the wound bed, gently irrigate the wound with a back-and-forth motion, moving from the superior aspect to the inferior aspect.
Irrigating from top to bottom prevents flow of contaminated solution over the cleansed area.

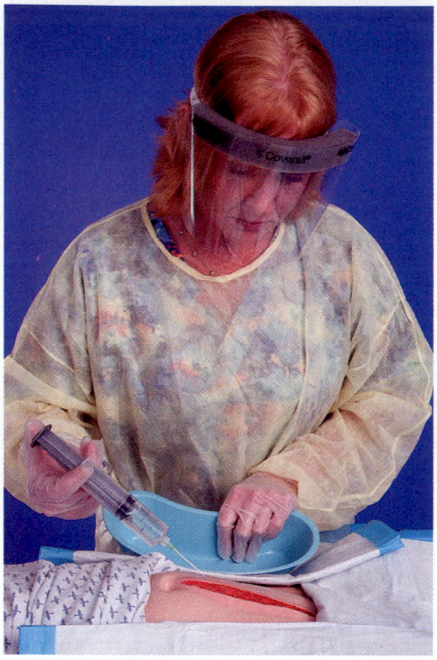

8. **Dispose of the syringe** and angiocatheter in the sharps container, and gloves in the biohazardous waste receptacle.
Prevents contamination and needlestick injury.

9. **Obtain an aerobic culturette tube** with calcium alginate or rayon swab (not cotton tip), and twist the top of the tube to loosen the swab.
Swab specimens are not suitable for anaerobic culture. Culture for anaerobic organisms may be obtained in tissue biopsy or needle aspiration specimens only.

10. **Don clean nonsterile gloves**, and locate an area of red, granulating tissue in the wound bed.

Using Levine Technique

a. Withdraw the swab from the culturette tube. Press the swab against the granulating area with sufficient pressure to express fluid from the wound tissue, and rotate the swab using a rolling motion.
Fluid from deeper within the wound bed is more indicative of the microbial colonization than culturing surface of a wound.

Using Z-Stroke Technique

b. Swab the wound from margin to margin in a 10-point, zigzag pattern, avoiding contact with the wound edge.
Provides a sampling in different areas of the wound bed.

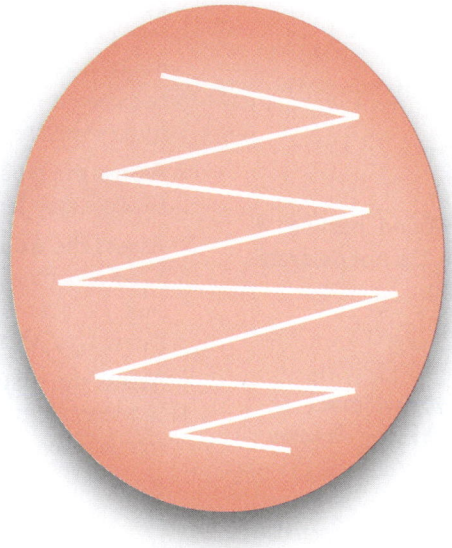

For Both Technique Variations

c. Do not allow the swab to touch anything other than the granulating area of the wound. Avoid wound edges.

d. Do not swab culture areas where slough or eschar is present.
These are areas of avascular or necrotic tissue and are contaminated with bacteria. Swab cultures detect only surface bacteria and are not a reliable means for diagnosing wound infection.

e. Do not roll the swab around in a pool of exudative material.
Pus is a collection of white blood cells that have already done their work, and includes the microorganisms that have already died. Obtaining a culture from this material would not produce reliable culture result. The culture specimen must be of "tissue" or "tissue fluid," not surface fluid or exudate.

f. Do not swab multiple sites with the same culturette. Use more than one culturette if several areas need to be cultured.

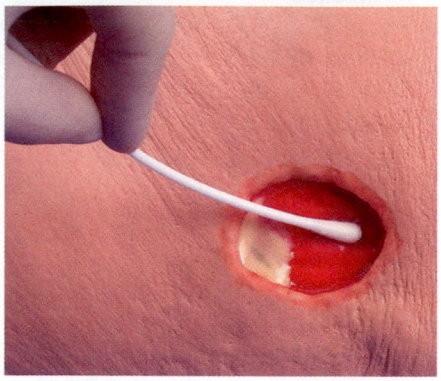

11. **Carefully insert the swab** back into the aerobic culturette tube, making sure it does not make contact with the opening of the tube upon reinsertion. Twist the cap to secure the tube.
Decreases risk of contamination; ensures that any microorganisms that grow in the culture are from the wound and were not introduced from the environment.

12. **Crush the ampule** of culture medium at the bottom of the tube. (*Note:* Inspect the culture tube to determine whether this step is required. In some systems it is not.)
The ampule contains medium for growth of microorganisms.

13. **Label the culturette tube** with the patient's name, patient identifier, birthdate, source of specimen, and date and time of collection.
Labeling ensures obtaining the results for the correct patient.

14. **Apply a clean dressing** to the wound, as needed.

15. **Arrange for transport** of the specimen for culture to the lab immediately. Do not refrigerate the specimen.

? What if . . .

- **You determined this wound requires sterile technique?**

  After removal of soiled dressing, apply sterile gloves for irrigating, obtaining culture, and applying new sterile dressing.

  Sterile technique is used for acute surgical wounds and for wounds that have undergone recent, sharp debridement, or when the healthcare provider prescribes it.

- **The culture tube is not sent to the lab within 72 hours?**

  If the culture swab is not sent to the lab within 48 to 72 hours, it must be discarded. Be sure to check the policy within your institution.

  The swab culture needs to be exposed to ideal laboratory conditions to allow microbial growth. If the culture sits on the unit too long, the culture medium might not produce reliable results. Most swab transport systems are validated for 48 to 72 hours after collection. However, if bacteria are suspected, the quicker the specimen is sent to the lab, the better.

- **The wound care and culture supplies are kept on a common treatment cart?**

  Common treatment carts should be left in the hall and not taken into individual rooms.

  When a mobile cart is rolled into a room, it is a source for possible cross-contamination.

Evaluation

- Assess the patient's pain level. Medicate according to prescriptions.
- Monitor lab reports for results of the swab culture.

Documentation

Document the following information (some agencies use a wound/skin flowsheet):

- Appearance and location of the wound and surrounding tissue. Note type, consistency and amount of exudate, and odor, if present, after irrigation.
- Patient's pain level before you obtained the culture.
- If the patient was medicated for pain, document the drug and dose used, time given, and patient response.
- Method by which the wound was cleansed before you obtained the swab culture
- Description of the area where the culture was obtained
- Dressing reapplied to wound, if applicable
- Education provided to the patient

Practice Resources

Association for the Advancement of Wound Care (AAWC) (2005, revised 2010); Baranoski, S., & Ayello, E. (2011); Benbow, M. (2010); Bonham, P.A. (2012); Cooper, R. (2010); Institute for Clinical Systems Improvement (ICSI) (2012); Levine, N. S., Lindberg, R. B., Mason, A. D., et al. (1976); McCulloch, J. M., & Kloth, L. C. (2010); National Guideline Clearinghouse (NGC) (2006, revised 2011); Non, L. R., (2012, updated); Rushing, J. (2007).

Thinking About the Procedure

To practice applying clinical reasoning to the procedure,

Go to *Davis's Nursing Skills Videos*, **Obtaining a Wound Culture by Swab.**

For questions and suggested responses,

Go to Chapter 35, **Thinking About the Procedure Questions and Suggested Responses,** on Davis*Plus*.

Procedure 35-2 ■ Performing a Sterile Wound Irrigation

➤ For steps to follow in *all* procedures, refer to the Universal Steps for All Procedures found on the page facing the inside back cover.

Equipment

- Nonsterile gloves
- Sterile gloves
- Gown and face shield
- Water-resistant, disposable drapes
- Tepid (body temperature) irrigation solution
- Cold solution lowers temperature of wound bed and slows the healing process.
- Sterile gauze
- Dressing supplies
- Biohazardous waste container
- Sterile impermeable barrier
- Sterile bowl

For Step 10A Variation:

- Sterile emesis basin
- 35-mL syringe
- 19-gauge angiocatheter (needle removed)

For Step 10B Variation:

- Sterile commercial irrigation kit containing a sterile basin and piston-tip syringe

Delegation

This is an invasive, sterile procedure that requires nursing assessment, judgment, evaluation, and teaching during the procedure. It requires knowledge of wound healing and should be

(continued on next page)

Procedure 35-2 ■ Performing a Sterile Wound Irrigation (continued)

performed by a registered nurse. Do not delegate this skill to nursing assistive personnel (NAP).

Pre-Procedure Assessments

Note: If the wound is covered when you begin, you will make these assessments when you remove the soiled dressing *and* after cleansing the wound.

- **Assess the amount and type of tissue present in the wound bed.**
  Granulating tissue is beefy red with a velvety appearance. It appears with the growth of new blood vessels and connective tissue. Pale pink tissue may indicate a delay in wound healing due to compromised blood supply to the wound bed or lack of proper nutrition. Necrotic tissue, which is black, brown, or yellow in appearance, is nonviable and inhibits healing and is a source of bacterial growth.
- **Determine whether the wound requires sterile, modified sterile, or clean technique for irrigation.**
  Irrigation helps wounds to heal because it removes bacteria, old drainage, and necrotic tissue from the wound bed. Sterile technique is used for acute surgical wounds, for wounds that have undergone recent sharp debridement, or when the health-care provider has ordered it. Chronic wounds are colonized with bacteria and may be irrigated with clean technique. Irrigation using clean technique is presented in Steps 1 through 8 of Procedure 35-1.
- **Assess the wound for signs of infection (erythema, induration, amount and type of drainage).**
  Exudate may be a sign of infection. Infected wounds require higher flow pressures for irrigation.
- **Assess the wound for odor.**
  A foul odor may indicate infection. Cleanse wounds before you assess for odor, because some dressings interact with wound drainage to produce an odor.
- **Assess the tissue surrounding the wound edge.**
  Surrounding tissue that is red, warm, and/or edematous may indicate infection. Tissue that is macerated (white and moist) indicates too much fluid is being held against the skin, usually from saturated dressings.
- **Assess for pain and the need to premedicate.**
  Wound irrigation may be very painful.

➤ When performing the procedure, always identify your patient according to agency policy, using two identifiers, and be attentive to standard precautions, hand hygiene, patient safety and privacy, body mechanics, and documentation.

Procedure Steps

1. **Administer pain medication** 30 minutes before the treatment, if necessary.
2. **Place the patient in a** comfortable position that provides easy access to the wound and will allow the irrigation solution to flow freely from the wound, with the assistance of gravity. Position a water-resistant disposable drape to protect the bedding from any possible runoff.
3. **After washing and drying** your hands, apply a gown, face shield, and clean nonsterile gloves.
   Personal protective equipment (PPE) provides a barrier against splattering that commonly occurs during wound irrigation.
4. **Remove the soiled dressing.** Dispose of gloves and soiled dressing in a biohazard bag.
   Soiled dressings contain body fluids and other contaminants and should be treated as biohazardous waste.
5. **Set up a sterile field** on a clean, dry surface. Add the following supplies to the field:
   Sterile gauze
   Sterile bowl
   Dressing supplies
   A sterile commercial irrigation kit, *or* a 19-gauge angiocatheter, 35-mL syringe, and sterile emesis basin.
   Setting up a sterile field at bedside provides easy access to equipment for irrigation and reduces the risk for contamination when retrieving supplies after getting started.▼

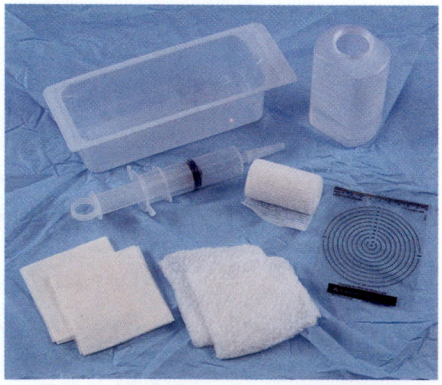

6. **Select irrigation solution** based on the wound assessment and goals of therapy. Sterile saline or sterile water is the solution of choice for irrigation, although commercial cleansers are increasingly used for irrigation for wounds with debris or in dirty, necrotic wounds.

   ✚ Do not use povidone-iodine (Betadine) if the patient has an iodine allergy.

   Cleansers contain surfactant (soap-like substance) that removes bacteria and cellular debris with less force and slow growth of bacteria, molds, and fungi. However, some antiseptic solutions can be harmful to healing tissues (e.g., hydrogen peroxide, acetic acid, povidone-iodine, bleach solutions, and sodium hypochlorite solutions [Dakin's solution]).
7. **Pour the tepid (room temperature)** irrigation solution into the sterile bowl.
   Local cooling of wound tissues impairs healing. This can occur if you irrigate with refrigerated solutions and change dressings frequently.

8. **Don sterile gloves.**
Gloving maintains sterile technique.

9. **Place the sterile basin** at the bottom of the wound to collect irrigation runoff.

10. **Fill the irrigation syringe.**

If Using an Angiocatheter

a. Attach the 19-gauge angiocatheter (with needle removed) to the 35-mL syringe, and fill with the irrigation solution.
A 19-gauge angiocatheter (with needle removed) and 35-mL syringe provides 8 psi of pressure and is effective for removing bacteria, necrotic tissue, exudate, and/or metabolic wastes.

If Using a Piston-Tip Syringe

b. Fill a piston-tip syringe with irrigation solution.

11. **Gently irrigate the wound.** Holding the angiocatheter tip or syringe tip 2 cm from the wound bed and use a back-and-forth motion, moving from the superior aspect to the inferior aspect.
Irrigating from top to bottom prevents flow of contaminated solution over cleansed area. Irrigating a clean, noninfected wound with gentle low-pressure (8 psi) reduces disruption of the healthy, healing tissue. Irrigating an infected wound with higher flow (but <15 psi) selectively debrides necrotic tissue while protecting healthy tissue.▼

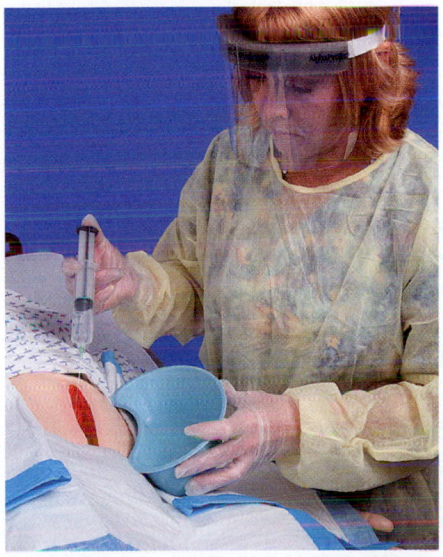

a. Ensure any undermining or tunneling is irrigated as well.
b. Repeat the irrigation until the solution returns clear.
Flushing removes exudate, debris, and some surface bacteria.

12. **Remove the basin** or sterile container from the base of the wound.

13. **Gently pat the skin surrounding** the wound dry with sterile gauze, beginning at the top of the wound and working downward.
Moisture on the surrounding tissue may lead to maceration and further breakdown of the wound margins.

14. **Dress the wound as prescribed.**

15. **Consider applying a** waterproof skin protectant around the wound if drainage is heavy.
Wound drainage contains irritating chemicals that can damage healthy tissues, especially at the wound edge and surrounding skin. Solutions used to keep the wound bed moist can also macerate or damage healthy skin if allowed to remain on intact skin.

16. **Dispose of the contaminated** irrigation fluid in a biohazardous receptacle.
Contaminated fluid should is biohazardous waste.

17. **Remove soiled drapes** from the patient area.

18. **Remove your gloves, face** shield, and gown. Dispose of these items appropriately.
Contaminants from the irrigation may be present on these items, and they should also be considered biohazardous.

19. **Reposition the patient** to a comfortable position. Change any linen that may have become wet during the procedure.

20. **Wash your hands.**
Hand hygiene prevents cross-contamination.

? What if . . .

- **The client has a wound covering a large area of the body?**
A general rule is that the larger the wound, the more solution needed to clean it.
The purpose of cleansing a wound is to remove bacteria and debris by flushing the wound.

- **Peroxide or another antiseptic solution is prescribed?**
First, identify the reason that the solution was ordered for the wound type. Then identify the length of time it is to be used. Weigh the benefit of using the solution with the potential risks to healing tissues. Finally, discuss any concerns with the healthcare provider.
Peroxide is indicated more for acute, traumatic wounds to remove dirt and other debris. Peroxide and other commercial antiseptics can damage fibroblasts and cause air embolism if used to forcefully irrigate or pack a tunneling wound. Fibroblasts produce collagen, the major structural protein of skin and healing tissues.

(continued on next page)

Procedure 35-2 ■ Performing a Sterile Wound Irrigation (continued)

Evaluation

- Determine whether the patient remains comfortable. If not, medicate according to prescriptions.
- Reassess the wound at regular intervals.

Patient Teaching

- Answer any questions the patient may have.
- Teach the patient about the expected healing process.
- Inform the patient and caregiver about signs and symptoms of infection and the need to report these findings.

Home Care

- Wound irrigation is commonly done in the home. In most cases, clean technique is used in the home setting.
- Irrigation solutions, such as saline, can be made and stored up to 7 days if refrigerated.
- Review with the family proper disposal of contaminated supplies.

Documentation

Document the following information (many agencies use a wound/skin flowsheet):

- Appearance and location of the wound, size, tissue in wound base, periwound tissue, type and amount of exudate, and odor, if present, after irrigation. A photograph is an accurate method for documenting the condition of a wound.
- The patient's pain level. If the patient was medicated for pain, document the drug and dose used, time given, and patient response.
- Method by which the wound was cleansed
- Dressing reapplied to the wound, if applicable
- Education provided to the patient

Sample documentation

mm/dd/yyyy 0800 Dressing change to sacral wound using modified sterile technique due to saturation of old dressing with serous drainage. Patient premedicated with Lortab 5 mg PO 30 minutes prior to dressing change. Wound irrigated with normal saline using 19-gauge needle-less angiocatheter and 35-cc syringe. Wound re-packed with saline-moistened fluffed gauze and ABD to cover. Healing Stage IV pressure ulcer with 100% granulation tissue to the wound bed; 4 X 3.5 cm, with 1 cm of undermining at 6:00; copious serous drainage though no odor was noted. Periwound is slightly macerated; therefore zinc- based barrier cream applied for protection. Patient reported no pain with procedure. Will continue to monitor and change dressing as needed.

L. Syzmanski, RN

Practice Resources

Fernandez, R., & Griffiths, R. (2012); ICSI (2012); Myers, B. A. (2011); Rolstad, B. S., & Ovington, L. G. (2011); Wilkins, R. G., & Unverdorben, M. (2013); Wound, Ostomy and Continence Nurses Society (WOCNS) (2010).

Procedure 35-3 ■ Taping a Dressing

➤ For steps to follow in *all* procedures, refer to the Universal Steps for All Procedures found on the page facing the inside back cover.

Equipment

- Nonsterile gloves
- Tape (cloth, plastic, foam, silk-like, etc.)

Delegation

As a nurse, you are responsible for assessing the wound and evaluating interventions. However, this procedure may be delegated to nursing assistive personnel (NAP).

Pre-Procedure Assessments

- Assess the degree of importance of the dressing.
  The more critical the dressing, the more adhesion required.
- Assess the characteristics of the dressing material, weight and conformability, and the device or tubing to be held.
  Heavier dressings require higher adhesion. Bulky dressings may need high conformability or greater adhesion.
- Assess the skin surface (i.e., dry, damp, diaphoretic, oily, hairy, edematous, fragile, or impaired skin integrity).
  Fragile skin may require less adhesion while damp or oily skin may require higher adhesion.
- Assess the anticipated wear time.
  Tape adhesion gets stronger over time. Breathable tapes can be used longer. Occlusive plastic tapes build up moisture and are used when adhesion is intended for a shorter period of time.

- Assess the patient's history and current medical conditions.
  Review allergies or sensitivities to tapes. Review medical conditions that may be affected by adhesives.
- Assess for activity level of the patient and the anticipated length of time the dressing will be needed.
  The more active the patient is, the more adhesion will be required.

➤ When performing the procedure, always identify your patient according to agency policy, using two identifiers, and be attentive to standard precautions, hand hygiene, patient safety and privacy, body mechanics, and documentation.

Procedure Steps

1. **Wash your hands. Don gloves.**
2. **Choose the type of tape** based on wound size, location, amount of drainage or edema, frequency of dressing changes, patient's activity level, and type of dressings used.
   Tapes come in many different adhesive types and backings. Select the tape based on individual characteristics.
   a. Choose tape of the width that is appropriate for the dressing. The larger the dressing, the wider the tape needed for securing.
   For example, a large abdominal dressing may require 3-inch tape, whereas a small incision on an extremity may need only ½-inch tape.
   b. Choose a tape that stretches if the area is at risk for distention, edema, hematoma formation, or movement.
   Skin distention under tape may cause blistering or skin tears.
3. **Tear strips that extend** 1 to 1½ inches beyond the dressing, depending on the size of the dressing.
   To anchor the dressing to the skin.
4. **Place the tape perpendicular** to the incision.
   Fewer skin tension injuries occur with perpendicular taping.
   a. When taping over joints, apply the tape at a right angle to the direction of joint movement, or at a right angle to a body crease. For example, tape a shoulder or knee horizontally, not lengthwise.
   b. Apply tape with an even amount tension on both sides, being careful not to pull at the edges.
   This reduces the risk of skin damage.
5. **Smooth tape in place** with your fingertips.
   To maximize the tape's adhesion to the skin surface.
6. **Replace tape if site becomes** edematous, or the skin is not intact. ▼

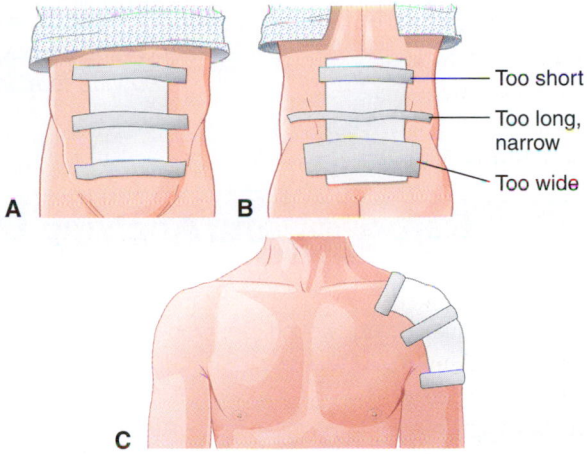

? What if . . .

- **The tape will not adhere to the patient's skin because of excess hair?**
  Remove the hair with clippers or scissors. Do not shave the site with a razor.
  Shaving can cause nicks or abrasions to the skin that could become a portal of entry for bacteria.
- **The patient's skin is diaphoretic or excessively oily?**
  Cleanse the skin with soap and water before the dressing change. Allow the skin to dry before applying the dressing and tape. You may also use polymer skin barriers to place a seal over the skin and allow the tape adhesive to adhere.

- **The patient has fragile skin (e.g., is an older adult)?**
  Use skin sealant preparations under adhesives. Use the least adhesive product possible.
  The junction between the epidermis and dermis on the older adult is not as strong as it is in a younger person.
- **The patient is allergic to tape adhesives?**
  Use hypoallergenic products.
  Circular wraps, ace bandages, or other such products may be used to secure dressings.

(continued on next page)

Procedure 35-3 ■ Taping a Dressing (continued)

Evaluation

- Verify type of tape that is appropriate for the patient and dressing.
- Note whether the tape adheres comfortably to the skin.
- Ensure that the patient verbalized understanding of the treatment.
- Inspect the dressing daily for intactness, edema, or hematoma.

Patient Teaching

- Teach the patient about the expected healing process.
- Educate the patient about the purpose of the procedure.
- Instruct the patient to keep the dressing dry.

Documentation

Document the following information (many agencies use a wound/skin flowsheet):

- Type of dressing and tape applied
- Location and characteristics of wound
- Education given to patient

Sample documentation

2/16/15 0800 Dressing applied to left hip incision using conformable cloth tape. Wound edges are well approximated with no drainage noted. Periwound skin is dry and intact without erythema, induration, or odor. Wound cleaned with normal saline using sterile technique. Educated patient about the purpose of the dressing and expected course for wound healing. Will continue to monitor ——— B. Hopkins, RN

Procedure 35-4 ■ Removing and Applying Dry Dressings

➤ For steps to follow in *all* procedures, refer to the Universal Steps for All Procedures found on the page facing the inside back cover.

➤ *Note:* This procedure uses clean technique because wound care is now usually performed using clean rather than sterile technique.

Equipment

- Three pairs of clean nonsterile gloves
- Normal saline solution for irrigation, warmed to body temperature when possible
  Cold solution lowers the temperature of wound bed and slows the healing process.
- Tray of sterile 4 in. × 4 in. gauze.
- Sterile gauze for dressings
- Tape
- Adhesive removal pads

Delegation

This procedure requires knowledge of wound healing. It should be performed by a registered nurse. Do not delegate this skill.

Pre-Procedure Assessments

Note: When you begin, the wound will likely be covered with a dressing. You will make these assessments when you remove the soiled dressing *and* after cleansing the wound.

- Assess for pain at least 30 minutes before performing the procedure.
  Wounds may be very painful. Provide pain medication 30 minutes before performing the procedure if needed, to allow the medication time to be distributed in target tissues. Changes in the quality or severity of pain are some symptoms linked with infection.
- Assess the type and amount of exudate.
  Exudate may be a sign of infection.
- Assess the wound for odor.
  A foul odor may indicate infection. Clean wounds before you assess for odor, because some dressings interact with wound drainage to produce an odor.
- Assess the tissue surrounding the wound edge.
  Surrounding tissue that is red, warm, and/or edematous may indicate infection.
- Determine the type of dressing needed.
  The type of dressing depends on the characteristics of the wound and the goal of treatment. Dry dressings are appropriate when there is no need to keep the wound bed moist, such as a wound healing by primary intention or a wound covered by eschar.

➤ When performing the procedure, always identify your patient according to agency policy, using two identifiers, and be attentive to standard precautions, hand hygiene, patient safety and privacy, body mechanics, and documentation.

Procedure Steps for Removing the Dressing

1. **Place the patient in a** comfortable position that provides easy access to the wound.
   Provides for patient comfort and proper nurse body mechanics during dressing change.

2. **Wash your hands**, and don clean nonsterile gloves.
   Handwashing is one of the most important measures for preventing infection transmission.

3. **Gently loosen the edges of the tape** of the old dressing at an angle parallel to the skin.
   a. Hold that edge with one hand and gently raise the edge until it is taut, but not pulling on the skin.
   b. Using your other hand, push down on the exposed skin at the point where the tape and skin meet. Push the skin off of the tape. Adhesive remover pads are advised to help prevent tearing of fragile skin
   The pull–push method will help prevent skin stripping from the adhesive and reduce discomfort and skin trauma as you remove the tape.

4. **Beginning at the edges** of the dressing, lift the dressing toward the center of the wound. If the dressing sticks, moisten it with normal saline before removing it completely.
   Moistening the dressing decreases the risk of bleeding and/or removal of granulating tissue.

5. **Assess the type and amount** of drainage on the soiled dressing.
   Allows for evaluation of wound healing. Purulent drainage is an indication of infection.

6. **Dispose of the soiled** dressing and gloves in a biohazard receptacle.
   Soiled dressings contain bodily fluids and other contaminants and should be disposed of as biohazardous waste.

7. **Remove the cover of a tray** of sterile 4 in. × 4 in. gauze. Moisten the gauze with sterile saline.
   The sterile container tray is impermeable and allows you to moisten the gauze while maintaining sterility. Gauze will not shed fibers into the wound (as do cotton balls). Fibers and any other foreign bodies in a wound promote inflammation and delay healing.

8. **Don clean nonsterile gloves.**

9. **Gather a gauze pad** by pulling the four corners up toward the middle. Use the center ball of the gauze to cleanse the wound.
   Forming a ball with the gauze pads prevents contamination of gloved hands during cleansing.

10. **Gently cleanse the wound** with the saline-moistened gauze by lightly wiping a section of the wound from the center toward the wound edge. Discard the gauze in a biohazard receptacle, and repeat in the next section using a new piece of gauze with each wiping pass.
    Removes surface bacteria and exudate.

11. **Discard the gloves** and soiled gauze into a biohazard bag.

12. **Reassess wound** for size, color of tissue present, amount and type of exudate, and odor.

Procedure Steps for Applying Dry Dressing

13. **Wash your hands**, or use an antiseptic hand rub at the bedside.

14. **Open sterile gauze packages** on a clean, dry surface.
    Maintains sterility of gauze.

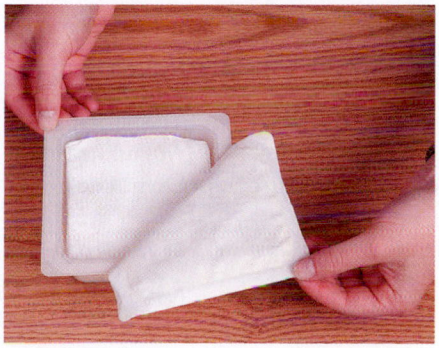

15. **Don clean nonsterile gloves.**

16. **Apply a layer of dry dressings** over the wound. If drainage is expected, use an additional layer of dressings.
    The first layer serves as a wick for drainage. A second layer is needed if increased absorption is required.

17. **Place strips of tape at the ends** of the dressing and evenly spaced over the remainder of the dressing. Use strips that are sufficiently long to secure the dressing in place. Tape the dressing around all edges, "window paning," if appropriate.
    Edges remain taped down and dressing stays intact.

18. **Remove gloves**, and discard them in a biohazard receptacle.

19. **Assist the patient** to a comfortable position.

? What if . . .

- **Signs of infection are noted with wound assessment?**
  Notify the healthcare provider. Cultures, wound care interventions, and potentially even antibiotics may be required.

- **The wound is not approximated?**
  Place the patient in a supine position, apply adhesive skin closures and cover with sterile saline dressings. Notify primary healthcare provider.
  This could indicate wound dehiscence.

- **The skin surrounding the incision is not intact?**
  Clean the area with sterile saline, dry thoroughly, and apply protective moisture barrier dressing. Consider using Montgomery straps.
  Montgomery straps are useful when dressings must be changed frequently because they do not cause trauma to the skin.

- **A drain or drainage tube is present?**
  Always clean the drain site after cleaning the primary incision site.
  Reduces the risk of cross-contamination.

(continued on next page)

Procedure 35-4 ■ Removing and Applying Dry Dressings (continued)

Evaluation

- Determine whether the dressing is clean, dry, and intact.
- Verify that the patient experienced minimal discomfort during the procedure.

Patient Teaching

- Teach the patient about the expected healing process.
- Inform the patient and caregiver about the signs and symptoms of infection and the need to report these findings.

Home Care

- Help the client to store dressings appropriately to keep them clean, for example, in a plastic container with a lid.
- Teach the client or caregivers to dispose of contaminated dressings and gloves by double-bagging them in moisture-proof bags (e.g., plastic grocery bags).
- Advise the client and family whether they can get the wound wet (e.g., during bathing). If it must be kept dry, demonstrate how to cover it with a waterproof barrier (e.g., a plastic bag).

Documentation

Document the following information (many agencies use a wound/skin flowsheet):

- Appearance and location of the wound, type and amount of exudate, and odor, if present, after cleansing
- The patient's pain level before the procedure. If the patient was medicated for pain, document the drug and dose used, time given, and patient response.
- Method of cleansing the wound
- Type of dressing applied to the wound
- Education provided to the patient

Sample documentation

10/22/15 1420 Pt with no report of pain. Gauze dressing removed from lateral aspect of right forearm without difficulty. No drainage noted on gauze. Surrounding skin intact. Abrasion on right, lateral forearm cleansed with normal saline. Sterile gauze dressing reapplied to wound and anchored with cloth tape. Pt instructed to report any change at wound site, such as bleeding, drainage, or increase in pain ——— D. Enferma, RN

Practice Resources

Armstrong, D. G., & Meyer, A. J. (updated 2014, January 28).

Thinking About the Procedure

To practice applying clinical reasoning to this procedure,

Go to *Davis's Nursing Skills Videos*, **Removing and Applying Dry Dressings.**

For questions and suggested responses,

Go to Chapter 35, **Thinking About the Procedure Questions and Suggested Responses,** on Davis*Plus*.

Procedure 35-5 ■ Removing and Applying Wet-to-Damp Dressings

➤ For steps to follow in *all* procedures, refer to the Universal Steps for All Procedures found on the page facing the inside back cover.

➤ *Note:* This procedure uses clean technique because wound care is now usually done using a clean or modified sterile approach rather than sterile technique. However, sterile technique is recommended for wounds that have recently had sharp debridement, have a drain, or are fresh surgical wounds. Sterile technique might also be used for patients with immunodeficiency.

Equipment

- Three pairs of clean nonsterile gloves
- Sterile or clean solution, typically saline or distilled water (in the hospital setting), warmed to body temperature when possible.
  Cold solution reduces the temperature of the wound bed and slows the healing process.
- Water-resistant disposable drapes
- Sterile fine-mesh gauze in a tray for dressing
- Surgipad
- Tape or Montgomery straps
- Adhesive removal pads

Delegation

This is an invasive procedure that requires knowledge of wound healing. It should be performed by a registered nurse. Do not delegate this skill to nursing assistive personnel (NAP).

Pre-Procedure Assessment

Note: When you begin, the wound will likely be covered with a dressing. You will make these assessments when you remove the soiled dressing *and* after cleansing the wound.

- Assess the amount and type of tissue present in the wound bed.

Granulating tissue is beefy red with a velvety appearance. It appears with the growth of new blood vessels and connective tissue. Pale pink tissue may indicate compromised blood supply to the wound bed. Necrotic tissue, which is black, brown, or yellow in appearance, is nonviable and inhibits healing.

- **Assess the type and amount of exudate.**
  Exudate may be a sign of infection.
- **Assess the wound for odor.**
  A foul odor may indicate infection. Clean wounds before you assess for odor, because some dressings interact with wound drainage to produce an odor.
- **Assess the tissue surrounding the wound edge.**
  Surrounding tissue that is red, warm, and/or edematous may indicate infection.
- **Assess for pain.**
  Wounds may be very painful. Assess for pain and provide prescribed pain medication 30 minutes before performing procedure, if needed. A change in the quality or intensity of pain may be a sign of infection.

➤ When performing the procedure, always identify your patient according to agency policy, using two identifiers, and be attentive to standard precautions, hand hygiene, patient safety and privacy, body mechanics, and documentation.

Procedure Steps for Removing the Wet-to-Damp Dressing

1. **Place the patient** in a comfortable position that provides easy access to the wound.
   Provides for patient comfort during dressing change.

2. **Wash your hands**, and don clean nonsterile gloves.
   Handwashing complies with standard precautions, helping to prevent transfer of pathogens.

3. **Gently loosen the edges** of the tape of the old dressing. Hold that edge with one hand and gently raise the edge until it is taut, but not pulling on the skin. Using your other hand, push down on the exposed skin at the point where the tape and skin meet. Push the skin off of the tape. Use adhesive remover pads to avoid tearing fragile skin.
   The pull–push method will help prevent skin stripping from the adhesive and reduce discomfort and skin trauma as you remove the tape.

4. **Beginning with the top layer,** lift the dressing from the corner toward the center of the wound. If the dressing sticks, moisten it with normal saline or bacteriostatic water before completely removing it. Remove first from one side of the wound, first toward the wound, and then from the other side. Continue to remove layers until you have removed the entire dressing.
   Moistening the dressing decreases the risk of bleeding and/or removal of granulating tissue.▼

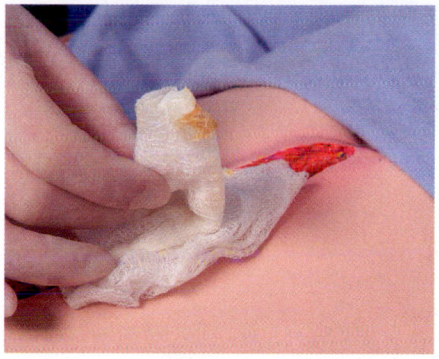

5. **Assess the type and amount** of drainage present on the soiled dressing.
   Type of drainage is an indication of the stage of healing. Purulent drainage is an indication of infection.

6. **Dispose of the soiled dressing** and gloves in a biohazard container. Wash your hands.
   Soiled dressings contain body fluid contaminants and should be disposed of as biohazardous waste.

7. **Remove the cover of a tray** of sterile 4 in. × 4 in. gauze. Moisten the gauze with sterile saline or water.
   The sterile container tray is impermeable and allows you to moisten the gauze while maintaining sterility. Gauze will not shed fibers into the wound (as do cotton balls). Fibers and any other foreign bodies in a wound promote inflammation and delay healing.

8. **Don clean procedure gloves.**
   Avoids introducing microorganisms into the wound.

9. **Gather a gauze pad** by pulling the four corners up toward the middle. Use the center of the gauze to cleanse the wound.
   Prevents contamination of your gloves during wound cleansing.

10. **Using gauze moistened** with saline or potable water gently wipe a section of the wound from the center toward the wound edge. Discard the gauze in a biohazard receptacle, and repeat in the next section using a new piece of gauze with each wiping pass.
    Removes surface bacteria and exudate. Prevents transfer of microorganisms from the skin to the wound.

11. **Reassess the wound** for location, amount of tissue present, exudate, and odor.
    Allows for determination of most effective treatment and type of dressing.

12. **Discard the gloves** and soiled gauze into a biohazard bag. Perform hand hygiene.
    Soiled gauze contains contaminants and should be disposed of as biohazardous waste.

Procedure Steps for Applying a Wet-to-Damp Dressing

13. **Open a sterile gauze pack tray** and a surgipad. The amount of gauze you use depends on the size of the wound.
    Maintains sterile field and supplies.

(continued on next page)

Procedure 35-5 ■ Removing and Applying Wet-to-Damp Dressings (continued)

14. **Moisten sterile gauze** with saline solution or potable water for irrigation.

15. **Don clean nonsterile** gloves.

16. **Squeeze out excess moisture** from the gauze. Apply a single layer of moist, fine-mesh gauze to the wound. Be sure to place gauze in all depressions or crevices of the wound. You may need to use forceps or a cotton applicator to ensure that you fill deep depressions or sinus tracts with gauze. "Fluff" the mesh gauze before placing in the wound so as it dries it acts as a wick for any drainage.
Maintains a moist environment for the wound bed.▼

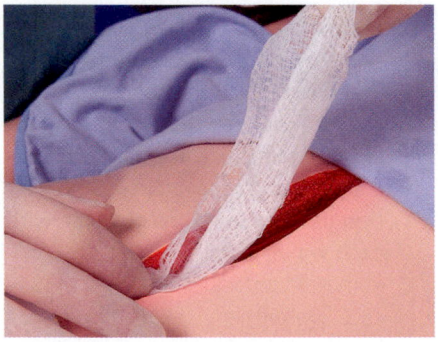

17. **Apply a secondary moist layer** over the first layer. Repeat this process until the wound is completely filled with moistened sterile gauze—but do not tightly *pack* the gauze into the wound. Do not extend the moist dressing onto the surrounding skin.
Packing the gauze tightly can restrict blood flow to the area. Moist dressings on the surrounding skin can cause maceration.

18. **Cover the moistened gauze** with a surgipad.
Protects the wound from external contaminants.▼

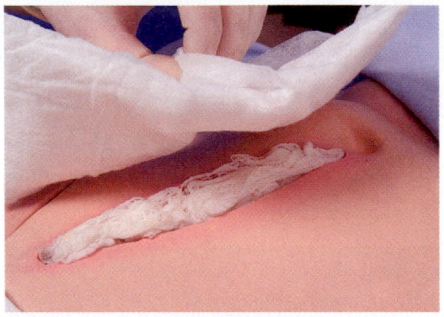

19. **Secure the dressing** with tape or Montgomery straps.
Montgomery straps are useful when dressings must be frequently changed because they do not cause trauma to the skin.▼

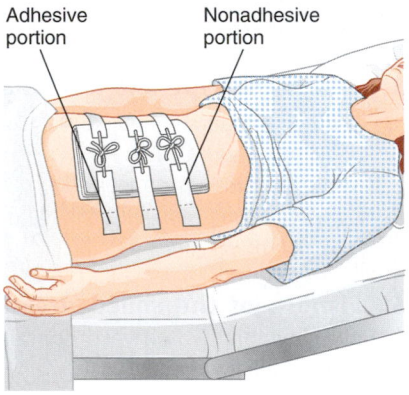

Montgomery straps

20. **Dispose of gloves** and materials in the biohazard waste receptacle. Perform hand hygiene and date and time the dressing.

21. **Assist the patient** to a comfortable position.

? What if . . .

- **Gauze becomes dry between dressing changes?**
  Moisten dressings with sterile saline before removing them; change dressing more frequently; consider using a semi-occlusive dressing.
  A moistened dressing prevents debridement of granulating tissue, maintains a moist environment, and prevents tissue injury. Dressings that become too dry will injure healthy tissue and impair healing.

- **The patient has multiple wounds?**
  The most infected wound should be treated last. Remember to always change your gloves in between wound dressing changes.
  The risk of cross-contamination is reduced when moving from clean to dirty and with fresh gloves.

Evaluation

- Evaluate whether the patient experiences pain with the procedure and afterward.
- Note whether the patient verbalizes understanding of the procedure.

Patient Teaching

- Teach the patient about the expected healing process.
- Inform the patient and caregiver about signs and symptoms of infection and the need to report these findings.

Home Care

- Help the client store dressings appropriately to keep them clean, for example, in a plastic container with a lid.
- Teach the client or caregivers to dispose of contaminated dressings and gloves by double-bagging them in moisture-proof bags (e.g., plastic grocery bags).
- Advise the client and family whether they can get the wound wet (e.g., during bathing). If it must be kept dry, demonstrate how to cover it with a waterproof barrier (e.g., a plastic bag).

Documentation

Document the following information (many agencies use a wound/skin flowsheet):

- Appearance and location of the wound, type and amount of exudate, and odor, if present, after cleansing
- The patient's pain level before and after the procedure
- Pain medication given including the dose, time, your name, and the patient's response.
- Method of cleansing the wound
- Type of dressing applied to the wound
- Education provided to the patient

Sample documentation

09/20/15 2120 Red granulating tissue noted throughout the wound bed of a stage IV pressure ulcer on sacrum. No tunneling or undermining observed. Minimal amount of serosanguineous drainage on old dressing. Wound cleansed with normal saline prior to application of new dressing. Wet-to-damp dressing applied. Pt tolerated procedure well with no verbalization of pain throughout procedure. Pt placed on 2-hr turn schedule and educated about pressure relief measures. Pt reports understanding.

W. Earl, RN

Practice Resources

Bhimji, S. (n.d., 2011, updated); WOCNS, (2010).

Thinking About the Procedure

To practice applying clinical reasoning to this procedure,

Go to *Davis's Nursing Skills Videos*, **Removing and Applying Wet-to-Damp Dressings.**

For questions and suggested responses,

Go to Chapter 35, **Thinking About the Procedure Questions and Suggested Responses,** on Davis*Plus*.

Procedure 35-6 ■ Applying a Negative Pressure Wound Therapy (NPWT) Device

➤ For steps to follow in *all* procedures, refer to the Universal Steps for All Procedures found on the page facing the inside back cover.

Equipment

- Suction unit (pump)
- Collection canister with connecting tubing
- Open-pore reticulated polyurethane foam dressing
- Semipermeable transparent adhesive dressing
- Skin preparation product or sealant (skin prep)
- Sterile 4 in. × 4 in. gauze
- Clean nonsterile gloves
- Two pairs of sterile gloves (if using sterile technique)
- Sterile scissors (if using sterile technique)
- Waterproof pad
- Bath blanket
- Goggles or safety glasses, mask, and protective gown
- 10- to 20-mL irrigation syringe
- Normal saline for irrigation
- Emesis basis
- Biohazard bag for contaminated materials

Procedure 35-6A Open-Pore Reticulated Polyurethane Form Therapy . . .

- GranuFoam (black), white or silver foam dressing
- Therapeutic regulated accurate care (TRAC) pad

Procedure 35-6B Gauze Dressing Application (i.e., Chariker–Jeter Dressing Method)

- Fenestrated drain
- Ostomy paste

Delegation

As a nurse, you are responsible for assessing the wound and evaluating interventions. You should not delegate application of a negative pressure wound therapy device to a NAP. However, you may ask the NAP to report to you any changes in the wound dressing, pressure in the unit, or alarms.

Pre-Procedure Assessments

- Assess the type of wound to be treated with negative pressure.

  Negative pressure wound therapy is used to promote wound healing by secondary or tertiary intention in acute, chronic, traumatic, and dehisced wounds; partial-thickness burns; or flaps and grafts. NPWT will prepare the wound bed for closure, reduce edema, promote granulation formation, and remove exudate and infective material.

- Determine if there is any contraindication to use of a NPWT: nonenteric or unexplored fistulas; necrotic tissue with eschar; untreated osteomyelitis; malignancy in the wound or in exposed blood vessels, anastomosis sites, organs, or nerves.
- Assess patients for active or prolonged bleeding; patients who are on anticoagulant therapy or platelet aggregation inhibitors; or patients with infected, damaged, irradiated, or sutured blood vessels.

  Patients who are at increased risk for bleeding should be closely monitored. These conditions could be fatal if negative pressure is

(continued on next page)

Procedure 35-6 ■ Applying a Negative Pressure Wound Therapy (NPWT) Device (continued)

applied and bleeding is uncontrolled (exsanguination could occur). Notify the healthcare provider of these conditions.

- **Assess the wound for bone fragments or sharp edges.**
  When NPWT is activated, mechanical stress is placed upon the wound. Sharp edges or bone may puncture protective barriers, vessels, or organs, causing injury, and bleeding, if uncontrolled, could be fatal.
- **Assess the wound for infection.**
  Monitor infected wounds closely, as they may require more frequent dressing changes than noninfected wounds.
- **Assess the wound for size (length, width, and depth in centimeters); location and depth of undermining or tunneling; amount, character, and odor of drainage; type and percentage of tissue present in wound bed (granulation, slough, fibrin, necrotic); and periwound condition (i.e., intact, denuded, erythema, induration, or maceration).**
  If no response or improvement in the wound condition occurs in 2 weeks, use of NPWT should be reevaluated.
- **Assess the patient's nutritional status.**
  Adequate protein stores are needed for wounds to heal. Evaluate the patient's albumin or prealbumin level before initiating therapy, as NPWT may deplete these levels and prevent healing.
- **Assess for pain.**
  Wound care is very painful. Poorly controlled wound pain can lead to wound bed hypoxia. This impairs wound healing and increases infection rates. Wound pain also negatively affects the patient's quality of life.

➤ When performing the procedure, always identify your patient according to agency policy, using two identifiers, and be attentive to standard precautions, hand hygiene, patient safety and privacy, body mechanics, and documentation.

➤ *Note:* The success of NPWT partially depends on the training and expertise of the clinician. Allow adequate time for this procedure. Experienced nurses need at least 15 to 30 minutes. You will need more time if problems arise, and even more if you are a novice.

➤ *Note:* This procedure assumes you are performing the initial application of V.A.C. therapy. If you are changing the dressing, first read the What If . . . section near the end of this procedure.

Procedure Steps

1. **Consider administering pain** medication before initiating negative pressure wound therapy.
   Allow sufficient time for the medication to take effect.

2. **Select the appropriate dressing** (per NPWT system used) to fill the entire wound cavity.
   Dressings should be placed directly against the wound surface to allow for equal suction/pressure throughout the wound bed.

3. **Obtain suction pump** unit as prescribed.
   Negative pressure wound therapy is provided by several different manufacturers. Use the unit and dressing method that is approved by your facility.
   a. Place the suction unit upright on a level surface.
   b. Remove the canister from the sterile package and insert it into the pump.
   c. Connect the tubing to the canister.
   d. Ensure the opposite end of the tubing remains clean before connecting with the tubing from the dressing.
   e. You may place the suction unit at the end of the bed or hang it on an IV pole.
   f. Do not place the unit on the floor. Ensure the unit is not knocked over, as drainage from the canister can back up and contaminate the pump's filter, blocking suction.

4. **Place the waterproof bag** or trash receptacle so you can reach it easily during the procedure.
   Convenient placement facilitates access to safe disposal of the dressing into a trash receptacle for biohazardous waste.

5. **Assist the patient** to a comfortable position that allows for easy access to the wound.
   Facilitates access to the wound site with less contamination and promotes good body mechanics for the nurse.

6. **Drape the patient** (use a bath blanket if needed) to expose only the wound area.
   Draping provides privacy and emotional comfort.

7. **Place a waterproof pad** as needed.
   An underpad protects the linens from moisture and drainage.

8. **Prepare a sterile or clean field,** and add all supplies: gloves, scissors, irrigation supplies, gauze pad, selected wound dressings, tubing, and/or connectors.

9. **Don sterile or clean procedure gloves.** Use a gown and protective eyewear.
   Using sterile/aseptic versus clean technique is based on the wound type, physician preference, or facility protocol. A safe rule to follow is to use sterile gloves for a fresh noninfected wound and clean gloves for other wounds.

10. **Irrigate the wound** with 10 to 30 mL of sterile saline or other prescribed solution before all dressing changes. Use a 35-mL syringe and a 19-gauge angiocatheter (needle removed) to direct the flow of the irrigation fluid from the clean end toward the dirty end of the wound.
    Irrigation facilitates loosening of adherent tissue and removes debris and exudate while adhering to infection control principles of clean-to-dirty.

11. **Remove the excess solution** from the wound. Clean and dry the periwound skin with sterile gauze

sponges, as needed. Consider a skin protectant around the wound edges.
Excess moisture predisposes skin to maceration and possible damage. Applying a skin protectant can assist the drape in sticking to the skin, and protecting the skin when the drape is removed (i.e., from stripping of skin by the adhesive).

12. **Remove soiled gloves** and don new sterile ones for the procedure.
Change gloves during patient care if the hands will move from a contaminated body site (e.g., perineal area or wound) to a clean body site.

13. **To apply appropriate dressing** per preferred negative pressure wound therapy unit, follow Procedure 35-6A or 35-6B.

Procedure 35-6A ■ Open-Pore Reticulated Polyurethane Foam Therapy (i.e., Vacuum-Assisted Closure [V.A.C.])

➤ When performing the procedure, always identify your patient according to agency policy, using two identifiers, and be attentive to standard precautions, hand hygiene, patient safety and privacy, body mechanics, and documentation.

Begin with Procedure Steps 1 through 13, at the beginning of Procedure 35-6. Then proceed as follows.

1. **Select the appropriate foam dressing**: black, white, or silver.
Black foam is sufficient for most wounds unless individual patient circumstances require white or silver. White foam is denser and will limit granulation formation. It may be used for painful or superficial wounds, tunneling/sinus tracts/undermining, or where granulation tissue growth needs to be limited. Silver dressings may act as a barrier to bacterial penetration in the wound bed. Silver may eradicate biofilms of colonized bacteria.

2. **Cut the foam dressing** to the appropriate size to fill the wound cavity. Do not cut the foam dressing over the wound. Rub the cut edges to remove any loose pieces.
If you cut the foam over the wound, particles may fall into the wound and create irritation.▼

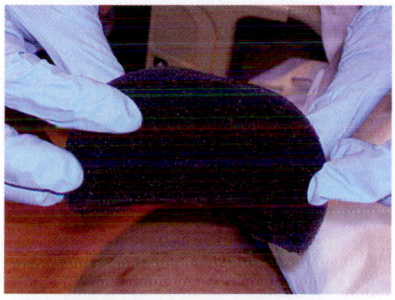

3. **Gently place the foam** dressing into the cavity without overlapping onto intact skin. Do not overfill the cavity or pack into deep crevices.
   a. Do not place foam into blind/unexplored tunnels.
   Forcing foam dressings into any area may damage tissue, alter the delivery of negative pressure, or hinder exudates or foam removal.
   b. ✚ Do not allow foam dressing to overlap onto healthy skin.
   Foam dressing becomes very wet during therapy and will macerate and damage intact skin.
   c. If you use more than one piece, note the total number of pieces that were placed into the wound so you can document them on the transparent dressing and in the patient record.
   An accurate record of the number of foam pieces is necessary to prevent retained material within the wound.

4. **Apply a liquid skin preparation** product to periwound, if needed.
Skin preps can protect the periwound skin from excess fluid, adhesive stripping, or other damage.

5. **Apply transparent film/drape** 3 to 5 cm (1 to 2 in.) from wound margins without pulling, stretching, or wrinkling the drape. Do not push down or compress foam while placing drape.
The occlusive dressing creates a seal to help create negative pressure within the wound. Tension from pulling, stretching, or wrinkling the dressing may lead to tissue injury. More pressure will be placed on the wound bed than necessary if you have flattened the foam before turning on the suction unit.

6. **Avoid placing dressings** that wrap all the way around an extremity. If necessary, place several smaller pieces of drape rather than one continuous piece.
When pressure is applied, a circumferential dressing may interfere with circulation, if wrapped too tightly.

7. **Identify a site over the dressing** for the suction track tubing apparatus.

8. **Pinch up a piece of drape** and cut at least a 2-cm round hole. Do not make a slit or X, as this may close off under pressure.▼

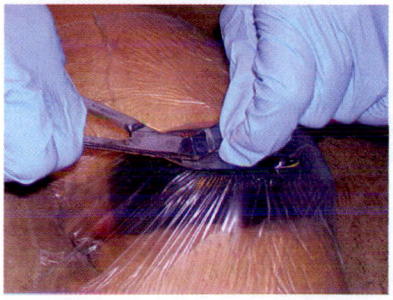

9. **Place the track adhesive** and suction device directly over the hole in the drape and apply gentle pressure to secure.
Negative pressure removes excess wound exudate from the wound bed.▼

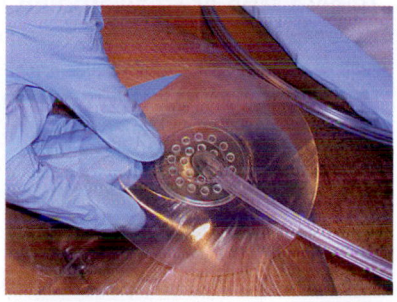

10. **Connect suction track tubing** to the canister tubing and open clamps. The canister is attached to a vacuum pump that provides either continuous or intermittent negative pressure, adjusted for the type of

(continued on next page)

Procedure 35-6 ■ Applying a Negative Pressure Wound Therapy (NPWT) Device (continued)

wound. Set suction to the prescribed pressure, which is typically in the range of –5 to –125 mm Hg (adjustable pressures, depending on the particular device used).
Suction draws excess exudate away from the wound and into an evacuation container.

11. **Connect tubing from the dressing** to the suction track tubing going to the collection canister.
Allows for collection and measurement of drainage.

12. **Position the tubing** and connector away from bony prominences and skin creases.
Prevents pressure injury to the skin.

13. **Ensure clamps are open** on all tubing.

14. **Turn on power to the pump** and set to the prescribed therapy settings to initiate therapy.
Therapy should be maintained for at least 22 out of 24 hours daily. Alternate wound care should be considered if the vacuum cannot be tolerated for this length of time.

15. **Listen for audible leaks** and observe dressing collapse or wrinkling as pressure is applied to the wound bed.
With an adequate seal, the dressing will collapse almost immediately. Any leak (i.e., between the dressing and drape, around tubing, at skin crevices, or at tubing connection sites) will prevent collapse.▼

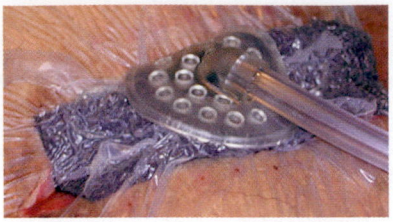

16. **Change the canister** at least once a week or when filled. Write the date on the canister.
This will help to know when it was changed last as well as how often it is being changed for fluid loss.

Procedure 35-6B ■ Gauze Dressing Application (i.e., Chariker–Jeter Method)

➤ When performing the procedure, always identify your patient according to agency policy, using two identifiers, and be attentive to standard precautions, hand hygiene, patient safety and privacy, body mechanics, and documentation.

Begin with Steps 1 through 13, at the beginning of Procedure 35-6. Then proceed as follows.

1. **Measure the length of drain** from wound margin, starting with the first hole perforation and pull back 1 cm.

2. **Moisten gauze** with normal saline.

3. **Wrap or "sandwich" the drain** in the moistened gauze and place in the wound base. Tuck gauze into any undermining areas to ensure contact with the wound bed.

4. **Apply a strip or small amount of ostomy paste** 1 cm from the wound edge and secure the drain as needed.
Paste is occlusive and will help maintain a seal between the drain and the transparent film dressing. Paste that is too close to the wound edge can get sucked into the drain, and occlude pressure.

5. **Apply liquid skin preparation** product to periwound, if needed. Extra drape, hydrocolloid, or transparent dressing may be used to protect fragile skin.
Skin preps can protect the periwound skin from excess fluid, adhesive stripping, or other damage.

6. **Apply transparent film** approximately 1.0 to 2.5 cm (½ to 1 in.) beyond the wound margin to intact skin. Pinch the film around the drain tubing to ensure a tight seal.

7. **Avoid wrapping dressings** around an extremity. If necessary, place several smaller pieces of drape rather than one continuous piece.
When pressure is applied, a circumferential dressing may interfere with circulation.

8. **Attach filter tubing** to the canister spout.

9. **Connect tubing** from the dressing to the evacuation tubing going to the collection canister.
Allows for collection and measurement of drainage.▼

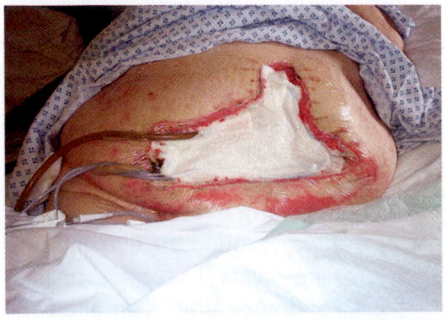

10. **Position the tubing** and connector away from bony prominences and skin creases.
Prevents pressure injury to the skin.

11. **Ensure clamps are open** on all tubing.

12. **Turn on power to pump** and set to the prescribed therapy settings to initiate therapy.
Therapy should be maintained for at least 22 out of 24 hours daily. Alternate wound care should be considered if suction cannot be tolerated for this length of time.

13. **Listen for audible leaks** and observe dressing collapse as pressure is applied to the wound bed.
With an adequate seal, the dressing will collapse almost immediately. Any leak (i.e., between the dressing and drape, around tubing, at skin crevices, or at tubing connection sites) will prevent collapse.

14. **Change the canister** at least once a week or when filled. Write the date on the canister.
This will help to know when it was changed last as well as how often it is being changed for fluid loss.

? What if . . .

- **You are changing the dressing instead of applying it for the first time.**

Follow the procedure steps below. *Note:* Dressings should be changed every 48 to 72 hours.
Dressings left in the wound longer than the recommended time frame can become difficult to remove if tissue grows into the foam, or can lead to infection or other adverse events.

a. Evaluate the need for analgesia.
b. Turn the suction pump unit off during the procedure.
c. Place a waterproof, biohazard pad under the body part requiring the dressing change.
d. Perform hand hygiene and don sterile or clean gloves as appropriate.
e. Remove the transparent dressing, using a push–pull method to gently pull up drape while pushing it slowly from the skin. Separating the drape from the skin in this manner will decrease the risk of tape stripping.
f. Gently remove gauze or foam dressing. If dressing is difficult to remove, instill normal saline onto the dressing for 15 to 30 minutes.
Dressing removal can damage new granulation tissue if tissue has grown into the dressing.
g. Count all pieces of gauze or foam dressing that were removed to ensure none remain in the wound bed. Ensure no dressing is left in tunneled or undermined areas.
Dressings are not bioabsorbable and can abscess if left in the wound.
h. Discard soiled dressings in a biohazardous waste receptacle.
i. Start at the beginning of Procedure 35-6 and perform Steps 1 through 13. Then, as instructed in Step 13, follow either Procedure 35-6A or 35-6B.

- **After 2 weeks, you see that the wound is not improving?**

Consult with the healthcare provider or a wound care specialist. Average length of therapy is usually 4 to 6 weeks. Therapy should be discontinued if the wound shows no improvement in 1 to 2 consecutive weeks, the patient is unwilling or unable to follow the medical plan, or the goal of therapy has been met.
The longer a wound is open, the longer it takes to heal, and places the patient at risk for complications. A steady decrease in wound size should be seen every week. If NPWT is not effective, alternate wound care should be evaluated.

- **You cannot find or remove a piece of foam?**

Notify the healthcare provider, as this may necessitate surgery.
The material could be retained in the patient and create an inflammatory response.

- **There is a foul odor when the dressing is removed?**

Clean the wound with normal saline to ensure odor is not emanating from the soiled dressing. If other signs of infection are present (i.e., fever, tenderness, redness, swelling, purulent drainage), notify the healthcare provider.

- **Suction cannot be maintained?**

Identify why the seal cannot be maintained. If the wound is very near the coccyx and gluteal fold, use a dollop of paste to help fill in the crack and maintain a seal. If the skin around the wound is moist, adhesive drape will not adhere to skin. Use a skin prep product or drape to protect the skin. If the tube is pulling away from the dressing or tension is being placed on the tube, anchor it with additional drape or tape several centimeters from the dressing or wound.

- **The canister is filling with blood?**

Immediately discontinue negative pressure therapy. The gauze or foam dressing will not stop the bleeding, so take measures to control bleeding (i.e., hold pressure on wound). Do not remove dressing until the treating healthcare provider is consulted.

- **Dressing does not collapse or the alarm sounds?**

a. Press firmly around the transparent dressing to seal.
b. Verify the machine is turned on, and all clamps are open and tubing is not kinked.
c. Check tubing and drape for leaks. Listen for leaks with a stethoscope or by moving your hand around the wound margins while applying slight pressure.
d. Additional small pieces of transparent dressing may be used to seal around hardware, skinfold, or creases.
e. Do not place multiple layers of drape or adhesive dressing.
Several layers may decrease the dressing's moisture vapor transmission rate, increasing the risk of maceration.
f. Never leave foam in place without an adequate seal for more than 2 hours. If an adequate seal cannot be achieved in that time, remove the foam and apply a saline moistened gauze dressing.

(continued on next page)

Procedure 35-6 ■ Applying a Negative Pressure Wound Therapy (NPWT) Device (continued)

Evaluation

- Note the patient's response to the procedure.
- Continue to monitor wound healing and changes in peri-wound tissues.
- Monitor dressing every 2 hours to ensure it is firm and collapsed in the wound bed while therapy is on.
- Monitor the seal of the dressing and pressure settings.
- Monitor for brisk or bright bleeding, evisceration or dehiscence, and symptoms of infection.
  These must be reported to the healthcare provider.

Home Care

- Refer the client to a home health agency for wound care.
- In limited circumstances, some patients or caregivers may be able to perform dressing changes. Determine their ability to perform dressing changes; teach and demonstrate as needed.
- Instruct the patient or family to visually check the dressing every 2 hours to ensure it is firm and collapsed in the wound bed.
- Review safety labeling, alarms, and pump instructions.
- Review conditions in which to seek medical care: bleeding, infection, unresolved alarms, or loss of suction.
- Review proper disposal of contaminated supplies.

Documentation

Document the following information:

- Date and time of dressing change
- Wound assessment: location of the wound, size (length, width, diameter), undermining or tunneling, amount and character of drainage, odor, wound bed including type and percentage of tissue seen, and periwound appearance
- Evaluation of therapy with evidence of healing
- Treatment selected: type of NPWT, type of gauze or foam, number of pieces placed in the wound
- Treatment settings: pressures, intermittent vs. continuous, or variable pressures
- Patient response to dressing change

Sample documentation for Procedure 35-6B: Chariker-Jeter Dressing Application

9/13/15. 1010 Patient reported pain rating 5 on a scale of 1 to 10. Administered hydrocodone 5.0 mg PO for pain at 0815 before initiation of negative wound pressure therapy. See MAR. Stage IV pressure ulcer to coccyx surgically debrided. Wound is 4 × 6 × 2 with no appreciable undermining. Wound bed is now clean of necrotic tissue with 100% pink tissue noted. Periwound has 2 cm of erythema to wound edges. Scant malodorous serosanguineous drainage. Using sterile technique, moistened saline gauze applied to wound bed with fenestrated drain. Ostomy paste applied at wound edge to assist in seal. Pump activated to 80 mm Hg continuous pressure. Patient rated pain in wound area as a 2 post-procedure. Plan: Begin dressing changes every 48 hours.
L. Opperta, RN

Practice Resources

Chariker, M. (2009); Gabriel, A., & Schraga, E. D. (2013, updated); McCulloch, J. M., & Kloth, L. C. (2010); Moore, C., & Young, J., 2011); NCG (2006, revised 2011); Sullivan, N., Snyder, D. L., Tipton, K., et al. (2009).

Thinking About the Procedure

To practice applying clinical reasoning to this procedure,

Go to *Davis's Nursing Skills Videos*, **Open-Pore Reticulated Polyurethane Foam Therapy (i.e., Vacuum-Assisted Closure [V.A.C.]).**

For questions and suggested responses,

Go to Chapter 35, **Thinking About the Procedure Questions and Suggested Responses,** on Davis*Plus*.

Procedure 35-7 ■ Applying and Removing a Transparent Film Dressing

➤ For steps to follow in *all* procedures, refer to the Universal Steps for All Procedures found on the page facing the inside back cover.

Equipment

- Clean nonsterile gloves
- Sterile gauze
- Normal saline solution or specified cleansing agent, warmed to body temperature when possible
  Cold solution lowers the temperature of the wound bed and slows the healing process.
- Scissors (if needed)
- Liquid skin preparation (if needed)
- Transparent film dressing

Delegation

Because assessment of the wound and knowledge of clean technique are important, you should not delegate this procedure to a NAP.

Pre-Procedure Assessment

- Assess the area to determine whether a transparent film dressing is appropriate.
  Transparent film dressings are indicated as primary dressings (dressings that touch the wound or area to be treated) to protect high-risk intact skin; for superficial or partial-thickness wounds that have little to no drainage (i.e., stage I or II pressure ulcers); and to assist in debriding eschar by autolysis. Films may be used as a secondary dressing to protect other types of dressings from bodily fluids (i.e., wounds near the perineum).
- Assess the wound to determine if use of a transparent film is contraindicated.
  Films are contraindicated in third-degree burns, arterial ulcers, and infected wounds. Films should not be used to fill dead space.
- Determine the size of the wound.
  Film dressings are available in many sizes. Select the appropriate size based on wound measurements, allowing for a 2.5 cm (1 in.) perimeter of intact skin around the wound for the adhesive to stick.
- Assess the periwound area.
  Film dressings should be attached to intact skin. The adhesive is not waterproof and will not adhere to wet or moist skin.

➤ When performing the procedure, always identify your patient according to agency policy, using two identifiers, and be attentive to standard precautions, hand hygiene, patient safety and privacy, body mechanics, and documentation.

Procedure Steps

1. **Place the patient in a** comfortable position that provides easy access to the wound.

Procedure Steps for Applying the Dressing

2. **If a dressing is present, wash your hands,** don clean nonsterile gloves, and remove the old dressing.
3. **Dispose of the soiled dressing** and gloves in the biohazard waste receptacle.
   Observe universal precautions, preventing transfer of pathogens.
4. **Don clean nonsterile gloves,** and cleanse the skin surrounding the wound with normal saline or a mild cleansing agent. Be sure to rinse the skin well if you use a cleanser. Allow the skin to dry.
   Cleansing prepares the skin for application of the dressing. Skin must be dry for the dressing to adhere.
5. **Cleanse the wound** as prescribed or according to agency procedure.
   Cleansing of wounds removes bacteria and necrotic debris from wound beds.
6. **Consider placing a skin barrier** around the wound before transparent film dressing application.
   Skin sealants may be applied to skin before tape to protect fragile skin from tears or epidermal stripping.
7. **Remove the center backing liner** from the transparent film dressing. ▼

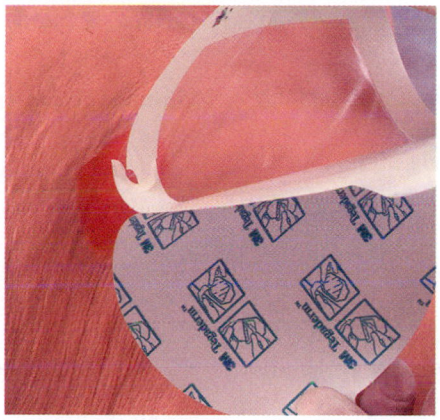

8. **Holding the dressing by the edges,** apply the transparent film to the wound without stretching or pulling the dressing or the skin.
   This reduces the risk of skin damage.
9. **Remove the edging liner** from the dressing.
10. **Gently smooth and secure** the dressing to skin.
    Allows the dressing to adhere fully to the patient's skin.
11. **Dispose of soiled equipment,** and remove your gloves.

Procedure Steps for Removing the Dressing

Transparent film dressings are typically changed every 3 days. Change dressing sooner if drainage extends beyond the edges of the wound onto periwound skin. To remove the dressing, do the following:

12. **Grasp one edge** of the film dressing.
13. **Gently lift the edge.**
14. **Stabilize the skin** underneath the elevated edge with your finger.
    Stabilizing the skin as the adhesive is taken off will prevent epidermal stripping.
15. **With the other hand,** slowly peel the dressing back over itself, "low and slow," in the direction of hair growth. Use of an adhesive removal pad is recommended especially for sensitive skin.
    Removing the dressing at an angle will increase the risk of pulling on the epidermis and causing mechanical trauma.
16. **As dressing is removed,** keep moving your finger as necessary to avoid newly exposed skin.

? What if . . .

- **The adhesive will not adhere to the patient's skin because of excess hair?**
  Hair may be removed with clippers/scissors. Do not shave the site with a razor.
  Shaving can cause nicks or abrasions to the skin that could become a portal of entry for bacteria.

(continued on next page)

Procedure 35-7 ■ Applying and Removing a Transparent Film Dressing (continued)

- **The patient's skin is diaphoretic or excessively oily?**

  Cleanse the skin with soap and water before the dressing change. Allow the skin to dry before continuing with the dressing. Also, polymer skin barriers may be used to place a seal over the skin and allow the tape adhesive to adhere.

- **The patient has fragile skin (e.g., an elderly patient)?**

  Skin sealant preparations may be used under adhesives.

  The junction between the epidermis and dermis on the older adult is not as strong as with a younger person. Less pressure or tension is needed to break those bonds and cause skin damage.

- **The dressing sticks to itself before it can be applied?**

  If a small portion of the dressing is stuck to itself, gently stretch or pull the edges in opposite directions. If a large portion is involved, throw the dressing away and start over.

  Transparent dressings can be difficult to apply because they are polyurethane sheets coated on one side with an acrylic, hypoallergenic adhesive and are flimsy in nature, making them clumsy to work with at times.

- **Purulent-appearing fluid has collected underneath the film dressing?**

  This does not necessarily mean the wound is infected. Remove the dressing and clean the wound per policy. Select an alternate dressing that will be more absorptive.

  Because films do not have absorptive capabilities, any drainage produced by the wound will pool underneath.

Evaluation

- Verify the transparent film dressing is appropriate for the wound.
- Determine whether the dressing adheres comfortably to skin.
- Ensure that patient verbalizes understanding of treatment.

Patient Teaching

- Teach the patient about the expected healing process.
- Teaching the patient about the use of transparent film dressings.
- Inform the patient and caregiver about signs and symptoms of infection and the need to report these findings.

Documentation

Document the following information (many agencies use a wound/skin flowsheet):

- Wound assessment: location of the wound, size (length × width × diameter) undermining or tunneling, amount and character of drainage, odor, wound bed including type and percentage of tissue seen, and periwound appearance
- Appearance and location of the wound, type and amount of exudate, and odor, if present, after cleansing
- The patient's pain level before the procedure. If the patient was medicated for pain, document the drug and dose used, time given, and the patient's response to analgesia.
- Method of cleansing the wound and surrounding skin
- Type of dressing applied to the wound
- Education provided to the patient

Sample documentation

2/22/15 2230 Transparent film dressing applied to stage I pressure ulcer on left lateral heel, 1 × 1 cm. Area is nonblanchable and painful to the touch. Cleaned with normal saline before dressing applied. Heel protectors placed bilaterally to keep heels suspended off the surface of the bed. Discussed pressure ulcer formation with patient, and the need to rotate positions and relieve heel pressure. Will continue to assist patient in turning every 2 hours.

M. K. Leonard, RN

Practice Resources

Association of periOperative Registered Nurses (AORN) (2013); Rolstad, B. S., & Ovington, L. G. (2011).

Procedure 35-8 ■ Applying a Hydrating Dressing (Hydrocolloid or Hydrogel)

➤ For steps to follow in *all* procedures, refer to the Universal Steps for All Procedures found on the page facing the inside back cover.

Equipment

- Clean nonsterile gloves
- Hydrating dressing 3 to 4 cm (1.5 in.) larger than the wound
- Moisture-proof bag

Obtain the following items, only if needed:

- Normal saline solution warmed to body temperature when possible
  Cold solution lowers the temperature of wound bed and slows the healing process.
- Emesis basin
- Sterile gauze for cleansing
- Disposable clippers or scissors (to trim hair or dressing)
- Skin prep
- Measuring device
- Tape

Delegation

This procedure requires knowledge of wound healing, dressings, and infection control and prevention. You should not delegate this procedure to a NAP.

Pre-Procedure Assessments

- Assess the area to determine whether a hydrating dressing is appropriate.
  Hydrating dressings are appropriate for wounds with minimal drainage. These dressings autolytically debride necrotic tissue from the wound bed. They may also be used to protect skin at risk for breakdown.
- Determine the size of the wound.
  Allows you to select a dressing of the appropriate size. Choosing a dressing size that extends beyond the ulcer ensures complete coverage.

➤ When performing the procedure, always identify your patient according to agency policy, using two identifiers, and be attentive to standard precautions, hand hygiene, patient safety and privacy, body mechanics, and documentation.

Procedure Steps

1. **Place the patient** in a comfortable position that provides easy access to the wound.
   Provides for patient comfort and proper nurse body mechanics during dressing change.

2. **If a dressing is present, wash your hands**, don clean nonsterile gloves, and remove the old dressing.
   Prevents transfer of pathogens.

3. **Dispose of the soiled dressing** and gloves in the biohazard waste receptacle.
   Dressings may contain body fluids and other contaminants, so they must be disposed of in moisture-proof containers.

4. **Wash your hands.** Don nonsterile gloves, and cleanse the skin surrounding the wound with normal saline or a mild cleansing agent. Be sure to rinse the skin well if you use a cleanser. Allow the skin to dry. Do not attempt to remove residue that is left on the skin from the old dressing.
   Cleansing and drying prepare the skin for application of the dressing. Removing residue irritates the surrounding skin.

5. **Apply skin prep** to the area covered by tape.
   Skin prep protects intact skin from breakdown from tape removal.

6. **Cleanse the wound as directed.** Wound cleansing may be performed with clean or sterile technique, depending on the type of wound.
   Cleansing the wound removes microbes and necrotic debris from wound bed. Studies show using either saline or tap water is similarly effective for cleansing.

7. **Remove soiled gloves**, and assess the condition of the wound. Note the size, location, type of tissue present, amount of exudate, and odor.
   Granulating tissue is beefy red with a velvety appearance. It appears with the growth of new blood vessels and connective tissue. Pale pink tissue may indicate compromised blood supply to the wound bed. Necrotic tissue, which is black, brown, or yellow in appearance, is nonviable and inhibits healing. A hydrocolloid dressing will interact with wound drainage to produce a thick, yellow gel that may have a foul odor. Clean the wound before assessing for exudate and odor.

8. **With the backing still intact,** cut the hydrating dressing, if necessary, to the desired shape and size. Size the hydrocolloid dressing so it will extend 3 to 4 cm (1.5 in.) beyond the wound margin on all sides and cover all areas of nonintact skin.
   Provides complete coverage of the wound.

9. **Don clean nonsterile gloves**, and remove the backing of the hydrocolloid dressing, starting at one edge. Place the exposed adhesive portion on the patient's skin. Position the dressing to cover the wound. ▼

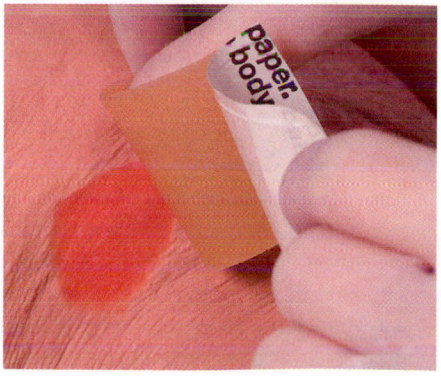

(continued on next page)

Procedure 35-8 ■ Applying a Hydrating Dressing (Hydrocolloid or Hydrogel) (continued)

10. **Gradually peel away** the remaining liner, and smooth the hydrocolloid dressing onto the skin by placing your hand on top of dressing and holding in place for 1 minute. *Warmth helps the dressing adhere to the skin.*▼

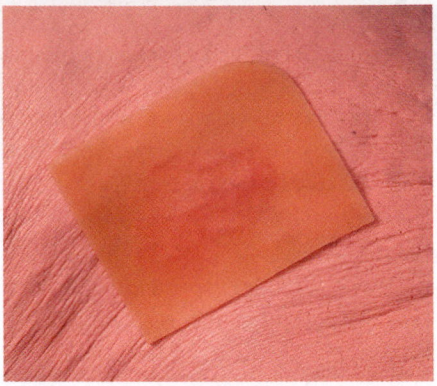

11. **Assist the patient to** a comfortable position, and remove your gloves. Wash your hands.

? What if . . .

- **Signs of infection are noted?**
  Notify healthcare provider. Cultures may be prescribed. A different type of dressing may be prescribed, as well.
- **The surrounding skin is not intact?**
  Choose a larger size hydrocolloid dressing to cover the nonintact area. Document your observations and report new findings to the healthcare provider.

Evaluation

- Verify that a hydrocolloid dressing is still appropriate for the wound.
- Note whether the dressing adheres comfortably to the skin.
- Ensure the patient verbalizes understanding of treatment.
- Inspect the dressing daily. Change it if it becomes dislodged, leaks, or wrinkles or if it develops an odor.

Patient Teaching

- Teach the patient about the expected healing process.
- Inform the patient and caregiver about signs and symptoms of infection and the need to report these findings.

Home Care

- Hydrating dressings may be required in the home setting. Teach caregivers to use the appropriate size and change the dressing if it begins to leak, develops an odor, or begins to separate from the skin.

Documentation

Document the following information (many agencies use wound care flowsheets):

- Appearance and location of the wound, type and amount of exudate, and odor, if present, after cleansing. Include wound measurements, if taken, and condition of surrounding skin.
- The patient's pain level before the procedure. If the patient was medicated for pain, document the drug and dose used, time given, and patient response.
- Method of cleansing the wound and surrounding skin
- Type of dressing applied to the wound
- Use of skin prep
- Education provided to the patient

Sample documentation

11/19/15 2230 Pt medicated with ibuprofen 600 mg by mouth for mild wound pain post-op. Pain rated as a 4 out of 10 prior to dressing change. Soiled hydrocolloid dressing removed from shear injury to left mid-scapular area. Wound cleansed with sterile saline and gauze. Shear is 3.5 X 4 cm and 100% covered with yellow slough. Moderate amount of nonodorous, serous drainage. Hydrocolloid reapplied as prescribed. Pain with no complaint of increase in pain. Educated pt. about autolytic action of hydrocolloid, plan of care, and expected outcomes for wound healing. ——— *S. Terril, RN*

Practice Resources

Dumville, J. C., O'Meara, S., Deshpande, S., et al. (2013); WOCNS (2010).

Thinking About the Procedure

To practice applying clinical reasoning to this procedure,

Go to *Davis's Nursing Skills Videos*, **Applying a Hydrating Dressing (Hydrocolloid or Hydrogel).**

For questions and suggested responses,

Go to Chapter 35, **Thinking About the Procedure Questions and Suggested Responses,** on Davis*Plus*.

Procedure 35-9 ■ Placing Skin Closures

➤ For steps to follow in *all* procedures, refer to the Universal Steps for All Procedures found on the page facing the inside back cover.

Equipment

- Adhesive skin closures
- Tincture of benzoin or skin protectant pads
- Forceps
- Normal saline
- Gauze
- Gloves (sterile if indicated)

Delegation

This procedure may be delegated to a NAP with the required training unless it is a new wound requiring sterile technique or has developed complications (e.g., dehiscence). Assessment of the incision line or wound is a licensed professional's responsibility and cannot be delegated.

Pre-Procedure Assessments

- Assess the type of wound to be closed.
  Adhesive closures are frequently used to keep surgical incisions well approximated. They may be used in conjunction with staples or sutures or following early staple/suture removal. Closures may be used to approximate the edges of lacerations or skin tears.
- Assess the wound for skin edge approximation.
  Wounds that are gaping or appear to have undermining should not be closed using adhesive closures.
- Assess the wound for drainage, amount, type, and odor.
  Wounds that are draining heavily might not be suitable for adhesive skin closures because the adhesive would not stick to the skin.
- Assess the periwound area or surrounding skin. Assessment should include skin color, texture, temperature, and integrity of the surrounding skin. Look for maceration (caused by heavy drainage), excoriation (from caustic effluent), stripping (from inappropriate adhesive removal), pustules, papules, or lesions.
  Adhesive closures should be placed only on intact skin.
- Assess the length of the wound, the location (over a joint), or if edema may occur, to determine the size of the skin closure used. Consider elastic skin closures if distention or movement is anticipated.
  Closures come in several different lengths, widths, and flexibility capabilities to meet elasticity and conformability needs.

➤ When performing the procedure, always identify your patient according to agency policy, using two identifiers, and be attentive to standard precautions, hand hygiene, patient safety and privacy, body mechanics, and documentation.

Procedure Steps

1. **Don clean nonsterile** gloves.
   Gloving prevents cross-contamination.
2. **Cleanse the skin** at least 5 cm (2 in.) around the wound with saline-moistened gauze. Pat the skin dry, allowing it to dry thoroughly.
   The skin surrounding the wound must be clean and dry in order for the strips to adhere.
3. **Apply a skin preparation product**, and allow it to dry (or follow agency procedures). Avoid benzoin on fragile skin.
   Because the strips are prone to peeling off with moisture, benzoin enhances adhesion of the strips.
4. **Do not allow skin preparation** product to come into contact with the wound.
   It may impair healing.
5. **Peel back package tabs** to access the adhesive closures.
6. **Remove the card** from the package using modified sterile technique as necessary.
   Careful technique should be followed when applying to a surgical wound to minimize contamination and promote healing.
7. **Grasp end of the skin closure** with forceps or gloved hand and peel strip from the card at a 90° angle.
   Closures lifted at a lesser angle or directly back on themselves may "curl," complicating handling.
8. **Starting at the middle** of the wound, apply strips perpendicular to the wound, drawing the wound edges together. Apply closures without tension; do not stretch or strap closures.
   a. Apply half of the closure to the wound margin and press firmly in place.
   b. Using fingers or forceps, ensure skin edges are approximated.
   c. Press free half firmly on the other side of the wound in a ladder fashion.
   d. Place the strips so that they extend at least 2 to 3 cm (¾ to 1 in.) on either side of the wound to ensure closure.
   e. Place the wound closure strips 3 mm (⅛ in.) apart along the wound. ▼

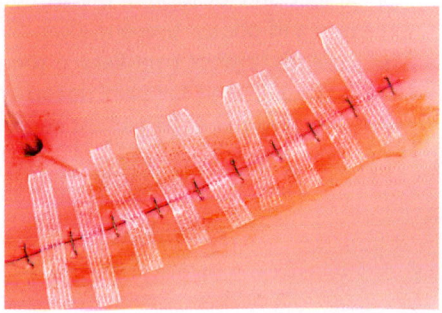

(continued on next page)

Procedure 35-9 ■ Placing Skin Closures (continued)

? What if . . .

- **A flap of skin rolls up on the edges?**

  Cleanse the wound with normal saline and reapproximate the edges of the skin flap with the intact epidermis. Apply skin closures across the flap.

- **The skin around the wound is swollen?**

  Apply skin closures without tension, and reapply as swelling increases.

  This prevents pulling on the skin that can delay healing or disrupt the approximated borders of the wound, which is more likely to lead to scarring.

- **Edges are not accurately approximated or tension has been placed on the skin?**

  Remove the closure over the affected area, peeling each side toward the wound, and reapply.

  Use of adhesive products can cause superficial skin damage if the skin is stretched during application or with edema formation. Tension blisters are the most common problem associated with taping.

Evaluation

- Verify that skin closures are appropriate for the wound.
- Note whether the closures adhere comfortably to the skin.
- Ensure the patient verbalized understanding of the treatment.
- Inspect the wound daily. Lifted closure edges may be trimmed or closures replaced if less than half of the strip remains.

Patient Teaching

- Teach the patient about the expected healing process.
- Inform the patient or caregiver about signs and symptoms of infection and the need to report these findings.
- Instruct patients not to pull or tug on the strips.
  Improper removal may damage the underlying skin or the wound itself.
- Instruct patients that they do not need to keep the strips dry. They can bathe and shower as directed by the health-care provider.
- Instruct the patient that adhesive strips are often kept in place until they begin to separate from the skin on their own.

Documentation

Document the following information (many agencies use specialized wound care flowsheets):

- Appearance and location of the wound, type and amount of exudates, and odor, if present, after cleansing
- The patient's level of pain before the procedure. If the patient was medicated for pain, document the drug and dose used, time given, and the patient response to analgesia.
- Method of cleansing the wound and surrounding skin
- Type of skin closures applied
- Education provided to the patient

Sample documentation

02/08/16 2040 Skin closures applied to surgical incision along right forearm. Wound edges are well approximated with slight erythema noted 4 mm from incisional site. Periwound skin is dry and intact with no drainage, induration, or odor noted. Wound cleansed with normal saline using sterile technique. Patient educated on the purpose of the closures and expected time and course of healing. Will continue to monitor. ———— S. Wong, RN

Practice Resources

Cole, E. (2007).

Thinking About the Procedure

To practice applying clinical reasoning to this procedure,

Go to *Davis's Nursing Skills Videos*, **Placing Skin Closures.**

For questions and suggested responses,

Go to Chapter 35, **Thinking About the Procedure Questions and Suggested Responses,** on Davis*Plus*.

Procedure 35-10 ■ Applying Binders

➤ For steps to follow in *all* procedures, refer to the Universal Steps for All Procedures found on the page facing the inside back cover.

Equipment

- Abdominal binder, triangular arm binder, or T-binder
- Clean nonsterile gloves
- Measuring tape

Delegation

This procedure may be delegated to a NAP. Assessment of the incision line or wound is a licensed professional's responsibility and cannot be delegated.

Pre-Procedure Assessments

- Assess the condition of the wound (if one is present). Note the amount and type of drainage. A wound must be dressed before it is bandaged; if there is a significant amount of exudate, you will need to apply a secondary dressing.
- Assess for pain, and check the circulation of the underlying body parts before and after applying the binder. Look for cool, pale, or cyanotic skin, tingling, and numbness.
- Determine whether the patient or family has the skills to reapply the binder when necessary.

➤ When performing the procedure, always identify your patient according to agency policy, using two identifiers, and be attentive to standard precautions, hand hygiene, patient safety and privacy, body mechanics, and documentation.

➤ Observe Steps 1 through 7, regardless of the type of binder you use:

Procedure Steps

1. **Choose a binder** of the proper size.
2. **Wash hands. Don nonsterile gloves.**
3. **Thoroughly clean and dry** the part to be covered.
   Moisture contributes to skin breakdown.
4. **Place the body part** in its natural comfortable position (e.g., with the joint slightly flexed) whenever possible.
   Prevents strain on ligaments and muscles.
5. **Pad between skin surfaces** (e.g., under the axilla) and over bony prominences.
   Prevents pressure and abrasion of the skin.
6. **Fasten from the bottom up**, especially for abdominal binders.

   ✚ Make sure the binder is secured with enough pressure to provide the needed support and control bleeding, but not so tightly as to compromise circulation or impair breathing.

   Fastening from the bottom up gives upward support
7. **Change binders** whenever they become soiled or wet.

Proceed to Step 8, 14, or 20, depending on the type of binder you are using.

Procedure Variation: Applying an Abdominal Binder

8. **Measure the patient** for the abdominal binder.
   a. Place the patient in supine position.
   b. With a measuring tape, encircle the abdomen at the level of the umbilicus. Note the measurement. This is the length of the binder. ▼

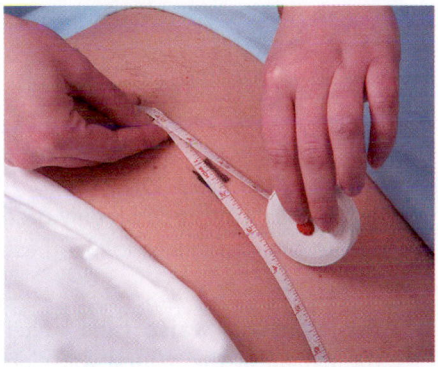

   c. Measure the distance from the costal margin to the top of the iliac crests. This is the width of the binder.
   d. Dispose of gloves and measuring tape, and wash your hands.
   e. Based on the measurements, obtain an abdominal binder.
9. **Assist the patient to roll** to one side. Roll one end of the binder to the center mark. Place the rolled section of the abdominal binder underneath the patient. Position the binder appropriately between the costal margin and iliac crest.
10. **Make sure the binder** does not slip upward or downward.
    If the binder is positioned too high, it could impair lung expansion and gas exchange. If it is positioned too low, the binder will not provide adequate support.
11. **Assist the patient to turn** to the other side as you unroll the binder from underneath him. ✚ Pad any pressure areas or skin abrasions to avoid pressure injury.
12. **With your dominant hand, grasp the end of the binder** on the side furthest from you, and steadily pull toward the center of the patient's abdomen. With your nondominant hand, grasp the end of binder closest to you, and pull toward the center. Overlap the ends of the binder so that the hook and loop fasteners (e.g., Velcro) meet. ▼

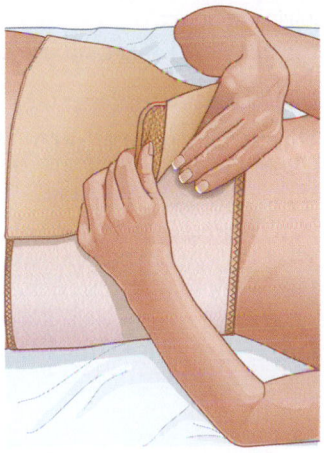

(continued on next page)

Procedure 35-10 ■ Applying Binders (continued)

13. **Assess the abdominal binder** every 2 to 3 hours. Observe that the binder has not shifted up or down or compromised the patient's breathing. Remove it to assess the underlying skin and dressings. Change wound dressings if they are soiled, or as prescribed.

Procedure Variation: Applying a Triangular Arm Binder

A triangular arm binder or sling is used to support the upper extremities. Obtain a commercial sling (consisting of a sleeve for the arm and a strap to go around the neck) or a triangular piece of fabric. To form a splint from a triangular cloth, follow these steps:

14. **Ask the patient to place** the affected arm in a natural position across the chest, elbow flexed slightly.
    Slight flexion prevents swelling of the hand and relieves pressure on the shoulder.

15. **Place one end of the triangle** over the shoulder of the uninjured arm, and allow the triangle to fall open so that the elbow of the injured arm is at the apex of the triangle.

16. **Move the sling** behind the injured arm.

17. **Pull up the lower corner** of the triangle over the injured arm to the shoulder of the injured arm.

18. **Tie the sling** with a square knot at the neck on the side of the arm requiring support.
    A square knot will not slip and is easy to untie.

19. **Adjust the injured arm** within the sling.
    To ensure patient comfort. ➤

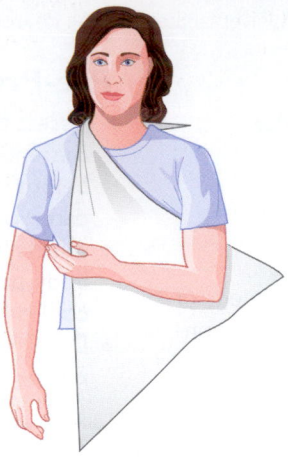

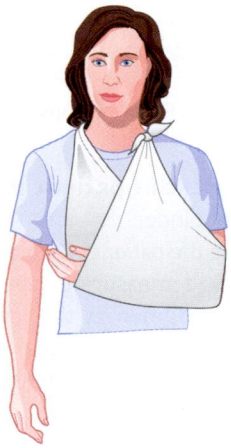

Procedure Variation: Applying a T-Binder

A T-binder is used to secure dressings or pads in the perineal area. A single T-binder is often used for women. A double T-binder is most commonly used for men. To apply a T-binder, follow these steps:

20. **Position the waist tails** under the patient at the natural waistline. Bring the right and left tails together, and secure them at the waist with pins or clips.

21. **For a single T-binder**, bring the center tail up between the legs of the patient. Secure the tail at the waist with pins or clips. ▼

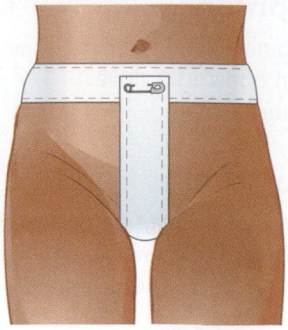

22. **For a double T-binder**, bring the tails up on either side of the penis. Secure the tail at the waist with pins or clips. ▼

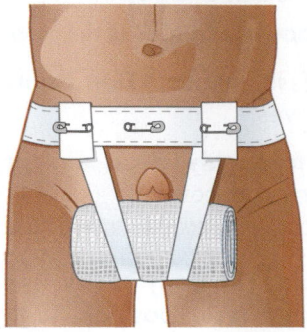

23. **Fasten the ties** at the waist using pins or clips.

? What if . . .

■ **The patient is obese?**

Obtain the appropriate size binder before applying. Do not try to position a binder that is too small for the patient. *A poorly fitting binder can constrict circulation, cause pressure points that can injure the skin, and can restrict movement of the chest for adequate breathing. A binder that is too tight is uncomfortable and it will not provide the proper support of an incision or wound needed for healing.*

Evaluation

- Evaluate whether the patient's physical condition has changed since using the binder.
- Assess circulation to be sure the binder is not secured too tightly. Check color, warmth, tingling, sensation, and capillary refill.
- Assess the depth of breathing to be sure the binder is not restricting ventilation.
- Check the skin under the binder to be sure there are no areas of irritation, pressure, or skin abrasion.
- Assess incisions or wounds under the binder to be sure they are not bleeding and are healing properly.
- Monitor comfort regularly.
- Assess the client's ability to perform ADLs while wearing the binder.

Home Care

- Teach the client and/or caregiver how to apply the binder in the proper position, snugly but not too tightly.
- Teach the family to inspect the site under the binder to be sure the skin is not pinched or with other points of pressure. This is especially crucial for older adults.
- Clean binders in warm, soapy water when soiled. Use a mesh laundry bag to keep the Velcro® straps from catching other clothing in the washer. Air dry thoroughly. Clients should have two binders at home—a clean one to wear while the other is laundered.
- Apply and remove binder to promote comfort and ensure good circulation. This also allows the patient and caregiver to inspect any incision or wound underneath.
- Binders for children at home could be decorated with permanent marking pens.
- Allow children to help with applying and removing the binder.

Documentation

Document the following information (many agencies use specialized wound care flowsheets):

- Appearance and location of the wound or incision under the binder, type and amount of exudates, and odor, if present, after cleansing
- Pain level before and after the procedure. If the patient was medicated for pain, document the drug and dose used, time given, and patient response.
- Type of binder applied
- Date and time the binder was applied and removed
- Any change in the appearance of the wound or skin in contact with the binder
- Education provided to the patient

Sample documentation

01/23/16 1230 Abdominal binder applied. Vertical abdominal incision with dressing dry and intact. No sign of active bleeding or wound drainage noted. Oral pain medication given approximately 30 minutes before applying binder (see MAR). Pt reported pain at level 3 on a scale of 1 to 10 while applying binder but improved to a 1 afterward. No report of pressure points. Pt instructed to call if the binder feels too tight or too loose. ——— C. Marano, RN

Procedure 35-11 ■ Applying Bandages

➤ For steps to follow in *all* procedures, refer to the Universal Steps for All Procedures found on the page facing the inside back cover.

Equipment

- Appropriate bandage dressing
- Clean nonsterile gloves (2 pairs)
- Gauze sponges
- Normal saline
- Primary dressing (as prescribed)
- Scissors
- Tape or metal closures

Delegation

This procedure may be delegated to a NAP who has the appropriate training. Assessment of the incision line or wound is a licensed professional's responsibility and cannot be delegated.

Pre-Procedure Assessment

- Determine the body part or area to be bandaged.
  This allows you to choose the correct width of gauze or elastic bandage to use.
- Assess the condition of the wound (if one is present). Assess size (length, width, and depth in centimeters); location and depth of undermining or tunneling; amount, character, and odor of drainage; type and percentage of tissue present in wound bed (granulation, slough, fibrin, necrotic); and periwound condition (intact, denuded, erythema, induration, or maceration)
  Wound dressings should be chosen based on the characteristics of the wound.
- Assess for pain, and check the circulation of the underlying body parts before and after applying the bandage. Look for cool, pale, or cyanotic skin, tingling, and numbness.
  Circulation to an extremity can be compromised if the bandage is too tight or the extremity swells after application.
- Determine whether the client or family has the skills to reapply the bandage when necessary.
  Teaching might be needed for home care.

(continued on next page)

Procedure 35-11 ■ Applying Bandages (continued)

➤ When performing the procedure, always identify your patient according to agency policy, using two identifiers, and be attentive to standard precautions, hand hygiene, patient safety and privacy, body mechanics, and documentation.

Procedure Steps

Observe the following steps, regardless of the type of bandage you use:

1. **Choose a bandage** of the proper width. For example, use a 2.5-cm (1-in.) wide bandage for a finger, a 5-cm (2-in.) wide bandage for an arm, and a wider bandage for a leg.
   Prevents pressure and abrasion of the skin.

2. **Thoroughly clean and dry** the part to be covered. Use a nontoxic cleansing solution, such as normal saline.
   Cleaning the wound removes debris, exudates, and bacteria. Drainage and moisture on the skin contribute to irritation.

3. **Remove excess moisture** by gently patting the wound and surrounding skin with gauze sponge.
   Drainage and moisture contribute to skin breakdown.

4. **Stand facing the patient.**
   In this position you can wrap the bandage evenly in the proper direction.

5. **Bandage the body part** in a comfortable position (e.g., with the joint slightly flexed), whenever possible.
   This prevents strain on ligaments and muscles. Movement of the extremity (extension) may cause skin damage if the bandage is too tight or the extremity is not properly positioned.

6. **Always work from distal** to proximal (or peripheral to central).
   This improves venous return and helps to prevent edema.

7. **If a wound is present,** apply a primary dressing, as prescribed, over the wound.
   A primary dressing is any dressing that is placed first in the wound bed. It provides exudates absorption, holds medications in place, provides antimicrobial coverage, or maintains a moist wound bed.

8. **Apply the bandage** with enough pressure to provide the needed support, but do not bandage too tightly. Make sure circulation to the area is not compromised.

9. **If possible, leave the fingers** (if you are bandaging an arm) or toes (if you are bandaging a leg or foot) exposed so that you can assess the circulation to the extremity. Begin the wrap along the pad of the foot or hand, just under the first bend of the toes or fingers (metatarsal or metacarpal joints).

10. **Begin the wrap** with the bandage against the skin. Unwind the bandage as if rolling it over the extremity.
    This helps to keep the bandage snug against the skin.

11. **Pad bony prominences** before bandaging if there are pressure concerns.

12. **Change bandages** whenever they become soiled or wet from external sources (stool, urine, etc.) and internal sources (drainage that has wicked on the outer surface of the bandage).
    Wound drainage contains chemicals, enzymes, and bacteria that can damage fragile healing tissues.

13. **After bandaging, assess** circulation and comfort regularly.

Proceed to Step 14, 16, 19, 25, or 28, depending on the type of bandaging you are using.

Procedure Variation Circular Turns

Use this technique to wrap a finger or toe, or as an anchor at the beginning and end of another wrapping technique.

14. **With one hand, hold one end** of the bandage in place. With the other hand, encircle the body part two times with the bandage—the second wrap should partially cover the first wrap. Continue to wrap the body part by overlapping two-thirds of the width of the bandage.

15. **Secure the bandage** with tape or metal clips when you are finished, if circular turns are not being combined with another technique. ▼

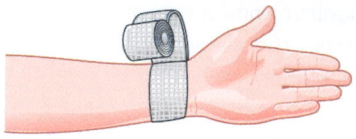

Procedure Variation Spiral Turns

Spiral turns are a variation of the circular turn technique. Spiral turns are most commonly used to wrap an extremity.

16. **Anchor the bandage** by making two circular turns—the second wrap completely covering the first one.

17. **Continue to wrap** the extremity by encircling the body part with each turn angled at approximately 30° so that you are overlapping the preceding wrap by two-thirds the width of the bandage.

18. **Complete the wrap** by making two circular turns and securing the bandage with tape or metal clips. ▼

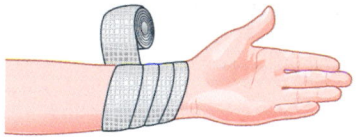

Procedure Variation Spiral Reverse Turns

Spiral reverse turns are used to bandage cylindrical body parts that are not uniform in size.

19. **Anchor the bandage** by making two circular turns.

20. **Bring the next wrap up** at a 30° angle.

21. **Place the thumb** of your nondominant hand on the wrap to hold the bandage. ➤

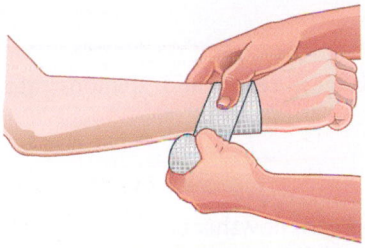

22. **Fold the bandage back on itself,** and continue to wrap at a 30° angle in the opposite direction.▼

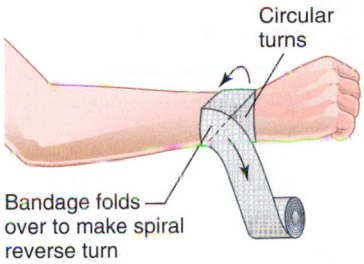

23. **Continue to wrap the bandage,** overlapping each turn by two-thirds. Align each bandage turn at the same position on the extremity.▼

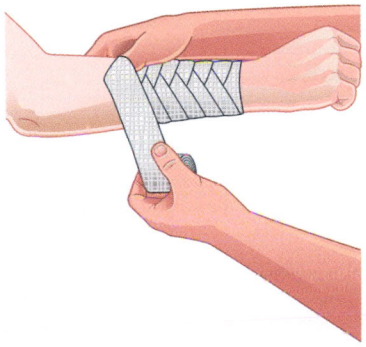

24. **Complete the wrap** by making two circular turns and securing the bandage with tape or metal clips.

Procedure Variation Figure-8 Turns

The figure-8 wrap is used on joints (e.g., ankle, elbow).

25. **Anchor the bandage** by making two circular turns.

26. **Wrap the bandage** by ascending above the joint and descending below the joint to form a figure 8. Continue to wrap the bandage, overlapping each turn by two-thirds. Align each bandage turn at the same position on the extremity.➤

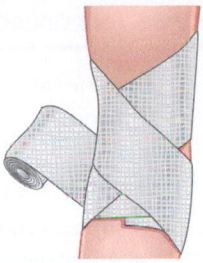

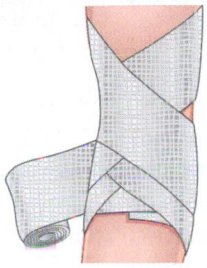

27. **Complete the wrap** by making two circular turns and securing the bandage with tape or metal clips.

Procedure Variation Recurrent Turns

28. **Anchor the bandage** by making two circular turns.

29. **Fold the bandage back on itself;** hold it against the body part with one hand. With the other hand, make a half turn perpendicular to the circle turns and central to the distal end being bandaged.▼

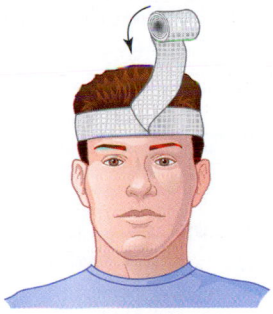

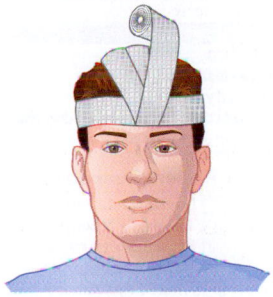

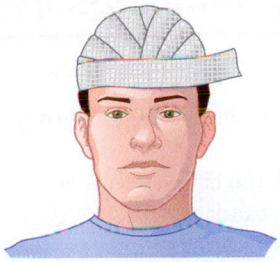

30. **Hold the central turn** with one hand, and fold the bandage back on itself; bring it over the distal end of the body part to the right of the center, overlapping the center turn by two-thirds the width of the bandage.

31. **Next, hold the bandage** at the center with one hand as you bring the bandage back over the end to the left of center. Continue holding and folding the bandage back on itself, alternating right and left until the body part is covered. Overlap by two-thirds the bandage width with each turn.

32. **Start and return each turn** to the midline or center of the body part, and angle it slightly more each time to continue covering the body part.

33. **Complete the bandage** by making two circular turns and securing the bandage with tape or metal clips.

? What if . . .

- **Drainage breaks through the outer bandage more frequently than expected?**

  Determine the cause of the drainage if possible (i.e., is it blood or serum?). Increased drainage may be a sign of infection and should be evaluated. You might need to change the dressing more often or an alternate, a more absorbent type of dressing may be needed.

  Wound exudates can harm healing tissues. Dressings that are saturated should be changed as soon as possible to prevent prolonged moisture exposure or maceration.

(continued on next page)

Procedure 35-11 ■ Applying Bandages (continued)

Evaluation

- Be sure the bandage is firmly wrapped without being too tight.
- Check the circulation is not compromised to the area distal of the bandage.
- Evaluate for numbness or pain around or distal to the bandaged area.

Patient Teaching

- Teach the patient about the expected healing process.
- Inform the patient and caregiver about signs and symptoms of infection and the need to report these findings.
- Instruct the patient and family about signs of circulation problems and how to remove the bandage if needed.

Home Care

- Refer the client to a home health agency for wound care.
- Some clients or caregivers may be able to perform dressing changes. Determine the client and/or caregiver's ability to perform dressing changes; teach and demonstrate as needed.

Documentation

Many agencies use wound care flowsheets.

- Appearance and location of the wound, type and amount of exudates, and odor, if present, after cleansing.
- Level of pain before the procedure. If the patient was medicated for pain, document the drug and dose used, time given, and patient response.
- Method of cleansing the wound and surrounding skin, if performed
- Application of primary and secondary dressings
- Education provided to the patient

Sample EHR documentation

6 Lateral Aspect, Left Posterior Forearm, proximal end — Cancel

☐ Wound Healed

Wound Category:
- ☐ Surgical
- ☐ Lesions
- ☐ Decubitus
- ☑ Burns
- ☐ Body Modifications

Wound Type:
- st Degree - (Superficial) Skin red in color; Area turns white when touched; No blisters; Painful.
- cond Degree - (Partial Thickness) Skin bright red in color; Area turns white when touched; Mottling;
- ird Degree - (Full Thickness): Skin bright red in color; Area may or may not turn white when touched
- urth Degree - (Full Thickness, Deep): Skin has charred patches; Charring may be black, brown or w

Length 4.8 cm
Width 2.4 cm
Depth cm

Wound Area:
- ☐ Skin is mottled (red/pink/white)
- ☐ Skin bright red in color
- ☐ Skin red in color
- ☑ Skin pink in color
- ☐ Fluid-filled blisters
- ☐ Wound edges are attached
- ☑ Undermining at wound edges

Wound Drainage/Exudate:
- ☐ Scant drainage/exudates
- ☐ Minimal drainage/exudates
- ☐ Draining serous fluid
- ☑ Draining serosanguinous fluid
- ☐ Draining blood-tinged fluid
- ☑ No odor
- ☐ Foul odor

Peri-Wound Area:

Dressing and Wound Care:
- ☐ No dressing, open to air
- ☑ Gauze dressing wraps
- ☐ Occlusive dressing
- ☐ Hydrocolloidal dressing
- ☐ Dressing clean, dry and intact
- ☐ Dressing reinforced, MD to perform 1st drsg change
- ☐ Wound cleansing & dressing change per MD orders

Solutions Used:
- ☐ None
- ☐ Neosporin
- ☐ Bacitracin
- ☑ Silvadene

Interventions:
- ☑ Increasing nutrition and hydration
- ☑ Burn recovery diet
- ☑ Keeping skin clean and dry
- ☐ Using paper tape
- ☐ Tape removal done slowly
- ☑ Pressure garments in use
- ☐ Face mask in use

Patient Response:
- ☐ No complaints at this time
- ☐ Tolerated procedure well
- ☑ Reports procedural pain
- ☐ Refused dressing change
- ☐ Refused Hydrotherapy
- ☑ Compliant with nursing regimen
- ☐ Non-compliant with nursing regimen

Notes:

mm/dd/yyyy 1200 Dressing change to left wrist burn site completed. Wound cleaned with normal saline. Wound bed with 50 % epithelial tissue and 50% fibrin. No signs of infection noted. Silvadene re-applied. Dry gauze dressing placed with gauze circular wrap bandage to cover. Patient reported no pain during procedure.

Practice Resources

Bergeron, J. D., Bizjak, G., Le Badour, G., et al. (2009); Rolstad, B. S., & Ovington, L. G. (2011).

Thinking About the Procedure

To practice applying clinical reasoning to this procedure,

Go to *Davis's Nursing Skills Videos*, **Applying Bandages.**

For questions and suggested responses,

Go to Chapter35, **Thinking About the Procedure Questions and Suggested Responses,** on Davis*Plus*.

Procedure 35-12 ■ Removing Sutures and Staples

➤ For steps to follow in *all* procedures, refer to the Universal Steps for All Procedures found on the page facing the inside back cover.

Equipment

- Nonsterile gloves
- Suture removal kit or sterile scissors and forceps (Procedure 35-12A)
- Staple remover (Procedure 35-12B)
- Gauze

Delegation

This procedure cannot be delegated to a NAP. Assessment of the incision line or wound is a registered nurse's responsibility and cannot be delegated. The procedure requires assessment and judgment during removal and may require stopping the procedure if complications occur.

Pre-Procedure Assessment

- Assess staples to ensure none have rotated or turned instead of lying flat along the incision.

Procedure 25-12A ■ Removing Sutures

➤ When performing the procedure, always identify your patient according to agency policy, using two identifiers, and be attentive to standard precautions, hand hygiene, patient safety and privacy, body mechanics, and documentation.

Procedure Steps

1. **Obtain a suture removal kit.**
2. **Wash hands.** Don nonsterile gloves
3. **Cleanse the wound** or suture line.
4. **Use the forceps** to pick up one end of the suture. ▼

Suture types

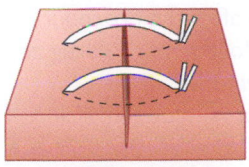

Plain interrupted

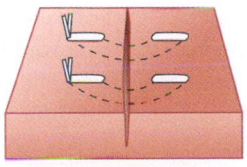

Mattress interrupted

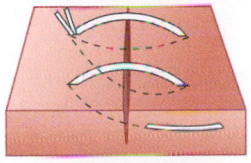

Plain continuous

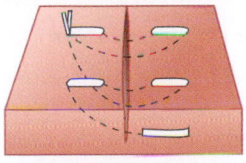

Mattress continuous

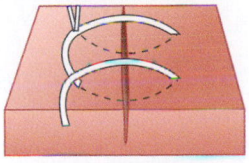

Blanket continuous

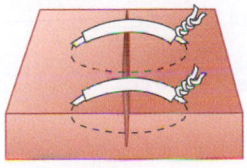

Retention

5. **Slide the small scissors** around the suture, and cut near the skin. *This helps you avoid pulling the exposed portion of the suture through the underlying tissue.*
6. **With the forceps, gently pull** the suture in the direction of the knotted side to remove it. ▼

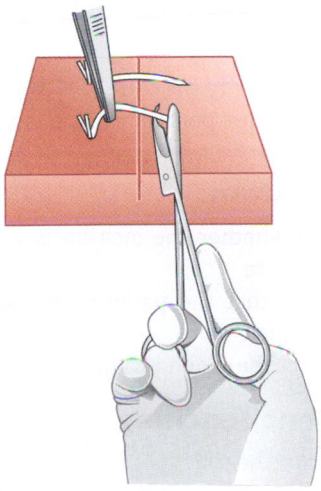

Removing interrupted sutures

7. **Apply a dressing** or adhesive skin closures if needed.
8. **Remove gloves** and perform hand hygiene.

(continued on next page)

Procedure 35-12 ■ Removing Sutures and Staples (continued)

Procedure 25-12B ■ Removing Staples

1. **Wash hands.** Don nonsterile gloves.
2. **After cleansing the wound** or incision, position the staple remover so that the lower jaw is on the bottom.
3. **Place both tips of the lower jaw** of the remover under the staple.

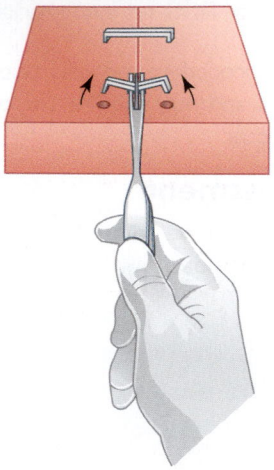

Removing staples

4. **Ensure the staple is** perpendicular to the plane of the skin. If not, reposition the staple with the tips of the lower jaw and apply gentle pressure, causing it to straighten the ends for easier removal.
5. **Lift slightly on the staple** ensuring that it stays perpendicular to the skin.
6. **Continue to lift slightly** as you gently squeeze the handles together to close.
   Spreads the ends of the staples apart, freeing them from the skin.
7. **Lift the reshaped staple** straight up from the skin.
8. **Remove every other staple**, and check the tension on the wound.
9. **If there is no significant pull** on the wound, remove the remaining staples.
   Where there are a large number of staples over an area of stress (abdomen, legs), the remaining staples are often removed a day or two later after assuring the incision remains intact.
10. **Place the removed staples** on a piece of gauze.
    Staples are small and can be easily lost. Keeping them in one place prevents this.
11. **Apply a dressing** or adhesive closures, if needed.
12. **Dispose of the removed staples** in the sharps container.
    Ends of the staples are sharp and should be handled with care.
13. **Remove gloves and wash hands.**

? What if . . .

- **A staple gets stuck?**
  Gently manipulate the staple with the remover until it is perpendicular to the skin.
  When the skin is stapled, the edges of the staple are crimped to hold the incision together. For the staple to be removed, those edges must be reshaped and straightened. If one edge of the staple is reshaped and the other is not, continuing to remove it can cause pain and tissue trauma.
- **The incision needs a dressing once the staples or sutures have been removed?**
  New surgical incisions should be covered with a sterile dressing the first 24 to 48 hours, but not necessarily after that time. Apply a dressing if you are concerned about soiling or per your institution's policy.
  In a healing incision, epithelial resurfacing is complete in 24 to 48 hours. Though only a few cells thick, this epithelium is enough to keep the wound closed and provide a bacterial barrier.

Evaluation

- Note whether the incision is well approximated after the procedure.
- Ensure that the patient verbalized understanding of the treatment.
- Inspect the wound daily.

Patient Teaching

- Instruct the patient of signs and symptoms of wound infections (i.e., redness, drainage) and the need to report these findings.
- Instruct the patient that he may be able to shower once sutures or staples are removed, if approved by the healthcare provider.

Documentation

Document the following information (many agencies use wound care flowsheets):

- Appearance and location of the wound, type and amount of exudates, and odor, if present, after cleansing
- The patient's level of pain before and after the procedure. If the patient was medicated for pain, document the drug and dose used, time given, and patient response.
- Method of cleansing the wound and surrounding skin, if performed
- Removal of staples or sutures
- Education provided to the patient

Sample documentation

02/23/16 1815 Staples removed from abdominal midline incision. Incision edges well approximated without erythema, drainage, or swelling. Dry dressing applied. Patient tolerated the procedure without discomfort. Discussed purpose of staple removal with patient. Will continue to monitor wound daily ——— *M. Dali, RN*

Practice Resources

Hin-Lun, L., & Hon-Ping, C. (2012).

Procedure 35-13 ■ Shortening a Wound Drain

➤ For steps to follow in *all* procedures, refer to the Universal Steps for All Procedures found on the page facing the inside back cover.

Equipment

- Nonsterile gloves
- Sterile gloves
- Sterile scissors
- Two safety pins or other clips (sterile)
- Sterile gauze

Delegation

Assessment of the incision line or wound and the drain is a registered nurse's responsibility and cannot be delegated. This procedure should not be delegated to a NAP. The risking for accidentally losing the drain into the body or pulling it out of the wound is too high.

Pre-Procedure Assessment

- Inspect the site around the drain, noting skin excoriation, tenderness, erythema, warmth to the touch, and drainage seeping from the wound.
  Could indicate a wound infection or irritation of the drain at the skin site. Excoriation can be the result of seeping drainage around the tube (e.g., if the tube diameter is not sufficient size to handle drainage output) or, more likely, an obstruction within the tubing.
- Assess the characteristics of the drainage, including color, volume of drainage, presence of blood, odor, pus, and any change in the type or amount of drainage through the tubing.
  A sudden decrease in drainage might indicate a blocked drain. Presence of fresh blood might be a sign of irritation within the wound. Pus and odor in the drainage could indicate wound infection.
- Check the suction apparatus to be sure it is functioning properly.
  A self-suction apparatus might need to be recompressed from time to time to maintain effective vacuum. Electric suction units can fail, delivering too much suction, which can lead to injury. Too little suction can contribute to insufficient drainage, which can lead to pressure on sutures if present, or cause the wound to become infected or heal more slowly.

➤ When performing the procedure, always identify your patient according to agency policy, using two identifiers, and be attentive to standard precautions, hand hygiene, patient safety and privacy, body mechanics, and documentation.

Procedure Steps

1. **After donning nonsterile gloves**, remove wound dressings.
2. **Remove soiled gloves** and discard in a moisture-proof biohazard collection container.
3. **Open sterile supplies** (scissors, etc.).
4. **Don sterile gloves**; use sterile scissors to cut halfway through a sterile gauze dressing (for later use) or use a sterile precut drain dressing.
5. **If the drain is sutured in place**, use sterile scissors to cut the suture.
6. **Firmly grasp the full width** of the drain at the level of the skin and pull it out by the prescribed amount (e.g., 5 cm [2 in.]).
7. **Insert a sterile safety pin** through the drain at the level of the skin. Hold the drain tightly between your fingers, and insert another pin above your fingers.
   The pin keeps the drain from disappearing into the wound. ➤

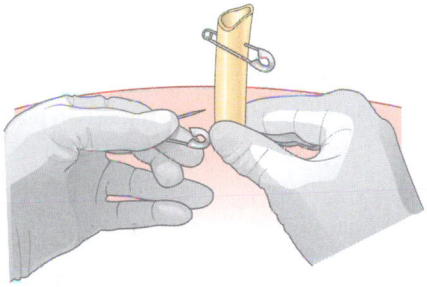

8. **Using sterile scissors, cut** the drain about 2.5 cm (1 in.) above the skin and pin. ▼

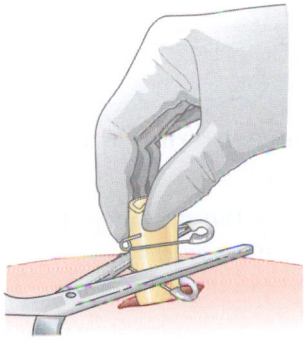

9. **Cleanse the wound**, using sterile gauze swabs and the prescribed cleaning solution. In some situations, you may use sterile forceps to manipulate the swabs.
10. **Apply precut sterile gauze** around the drain; then redress the wound. ▼

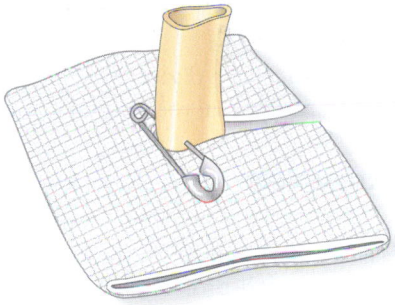

11. **Remove gloves** and discard in a biohazard container. Wash your hands.
12. **Leave the patient** in a safe and comfortable position.

? What if . . .

- **You shorten the drain too much?**
  Immediately notify the surgeon who placed the drain.
  The drain will need to be evaluated to be sure it remains intact, which it mostly likely will. Drainage tubing is secured under the skin surface and will probably not be dislodged with shortening.

(continued on next page)

Procedure 35-13 ■ Shortening a Wound Drain (continued)

Evaluation

- Assess the local area of skin around the drain after manipulating it.
- Note the patency of the drain after shortening it.
- Be sure the drain is secure after shortening.
- Evaluate for complications occurring related to shortening procedure.

Patient Teaching

- Patients should not shorten their own drains. Consult a healthcare provider if concerned about the length of tubing or drains.

Documentation

- Record the intervention.
- Note the amount and characteristics of the drainage.
- Document the appearance of the wound.
- Note any complications that occur with shortening a drain (e.g., manipulation of tubing causes bleeding or drainage at the site).

Sample documentation

10/11/15 0930 Penrose shortened by 2.5 cm per post-op orders. Drain intact and not draining. Skin surrounding Penrose slightly erythematous but not warm to touch. Pt. denies tenderness. Pt tolerated procedure without complication ——— M. Garcia, RN

Thinking About the Procedure

To practice applying clinical reasoning to this procedure

Go to *Davis's Nursing Skills Videos*, **Shortening a Wound Drain.**

For questions and suggested responses,

Go to Chapter 35, **Thinking About the Procedure Questions and Suggested Responses,** on Davis*Plus*.

Procedure 35-14 ■ Emptying a Closed-Wound Drainage System

➤ For steps to follow in *all* procedures, refer to the Universal Steps for All Procedures found on the page facing the inside back cover.

Equipment

- Drainage container with graduated markings
- Nonsterile gloves
- Biomedical waste disposal sink
- Biohazard disposal receptacle

Delegation

This procedure may be delegated to a NAP who is trained in the skill. Assessment of the wound and drainage characteristics is a licensed professional's responsibility and cannot be delegated.

Pre-Procedure Assessment

- Assess the appearance of the drainage tube site and sutures, if in place.
- Inspect for warmth, edema, redness, or pus where tubing penetrates the skin.
- Check to be sure the closed-wound drainage system is securely fastened at the connections and within the wound.
- Determine whether suction (electric, portable, or manual) is working properly.

➤ When performing the procedure, always identify your patient according to agency policy, using two identifiers, and be attentive to standard precautions, hand hygiene, patient safety and privacy, body mechanics, and documentation.

Procedure Steps

1. **Read the instructions** about the drainage device.
   Procedures vary among manufacturers and different systems.
2. **Don nonsterile gloves** and goggles or mask.
3. **Unpin the drainage device** from the patient's gown.
   The drainage device is often pinned to the patient's gown to prevent it from dislodging.

4. **Open the drainage port**, and empty the drainage into a small graduated container.

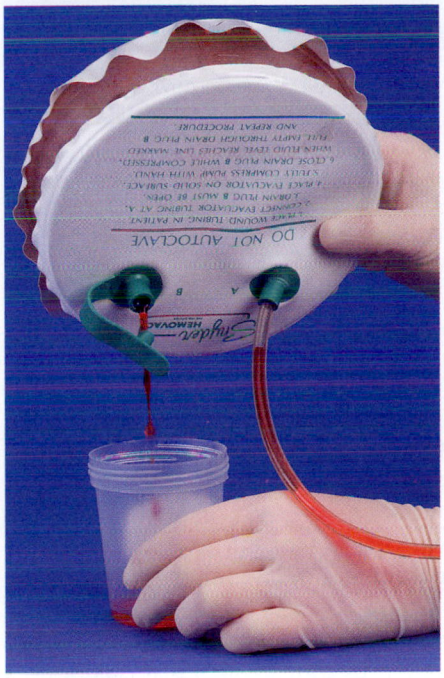

5. **With the port still open**, place the collection device on a firm, flat surface (e.g., the over bed table).
6. **Use the palm of one hand** to press down on the device and eject air from it. Do not stand directly over the air vent. Do not touch the drainage port.
   It can splash or bubble.
7. **Use your other hand to scrub** the port and plug with an alcohol-based antiseptic or povidone-iodine swab (Betadine), if the patient is not allergic to iodine.

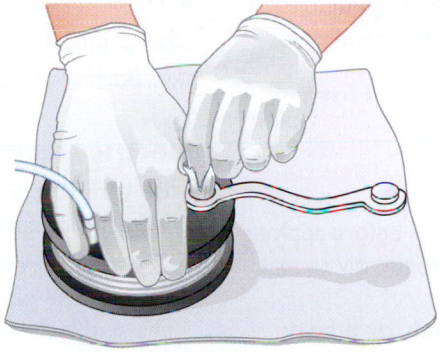

8. **Continuing to press down** on the device, replace the plug in the port. Do not touch the open port or the part of the plug that goes into the port.
   Creates a constant, negative pressure vacuum to facilitate suction.
9. **Re-pin the drainage device** to the patient's gown.
   Pinning keeps it secure and prevents it from accidentally dislodging.
10. **Measure the drainage** in the graduated container; discard drainage in the disposable container or sink for biohazardous material. Wash the graduated container. Do not stand in front of an air vent while doing so.
    Forced air in the room can cause the drainage to splash or bubble, introducing biohazardous material into the environmental air.
11. **Remove your gloves.** Perform hand hygiene.
12. **Document** in the patient's record.

? What if . . .

- **The wound drainage spills?**
  Don nonsterile gloves and protective clothing. Keep people away from the spill area. If sharps are present, remove with forceps. Contain the spill with absorbent pads and place all used materials in a red biohazard bag. Use an approved disinfectant. When finished place all materials including gloves and gowns in the bag and dispose of in the biohazard area.
  Proper handling of contaminated biomedical materials is important to prevent transmission of infectious organisms.

Home Care

- Teach family members who are emptying drainage systems at home to wear gloves and avoid touching the drainage port.

Documentation

- Note the date and time the drainage system is emptied.
- Record the volume lost. Report excess fluid loss to the healthcare provider.
- Describe the appearance of drainage, including presence of blood or purulent material.

Sample documentation

03/12/2016 0750 Hemovac drained 18 mL serosanguineous fluid over 12 hours. No odor or purulent material noted at drainage site. ——— R. Ferretti, RN

Practice Resources

Altman, G. B. (2012).

Thinking About the Procedure

To practice applying clinical reasoning to this procedure,

Go to *Davis's Nursing Skills Videos*, **Emptying a Closed-Wound Drainage System.**

For questions and suggested responses,

Go to Chapter 34, **Thinking About the Procedure Questions and Suggested Responses,** on *DavisPlus*.

CLINICAL INSIGHTS

Clinical Insight 35-1 ➤ Applying Local Heat Therapy

Preparation

- Determine whether there are any contraindications to the treatment, such as impaired circulation, bleeding, wound complications, or inability to tolerate the treatment.
- Explain the application and rationale to the patient.

Moist Heat (Irrigations, Compresses, Hot Soaks)

If skin is intact:

- Soak a washcloth or towel in warm water (105°F to 115°F [40°C to 46°C]), and wring out the excess before applying to the skin. Reapply and change water frequently to maintain a constant temperature.

For open areas, use a compress, a soak, or a bath:

- To make a compress, soak gauze in the heated solution (105°F to 115°F [40°C to 46°C]), and then apply it to the wound. Usually, you will use sterile gloves, gauze, and solution.
- Reapply compresses or towels, and change the water frequently to maintain a constant temperature.
  Heat disperses quickly.
- **For a soak** you will need to immerse the affected area. Sterilized tubs are often used for this procedure.
- **A sitz bath** soaks the patient's perineal area. A special tub or chair may be used. Because of infection control concerns, disposable sitz baths are preferred. Check that the water temperature is from 105°F to 110°F (40°C to 43°C). Instruct the patient to soak for 15 minutes.

Dry Heat (Electric Heating Pads, Disposable Hot Packs, Hot Water Bags)

Aquathermia pads (also called K-pads) are plastic or vinyl pads that circulate water in the interior.

- Connect the pad via tubing to the electric heating unit, which constantly exchanges water that has been heated to the specified temperature.
- Fill the reservoir about two-thirds full of distilled water.
- Set the temperature control to 98°F to 105°F (37°C to 40.5°C).
- Cover the pad with a towel, and apply it to the body part.
  To prevent tissue injury.

Disposable Hot Packs and Hot Water Bags or Bottles

- Use water that is 115°F to 125°F (46°C to 52°C).
- Fill the bag about two-thirds full of warm tap water, expel the air from the bag, and close the top.
- Tip the bag upside down to test for leaking.
- Wrap the bag in a towel, and place it on the patient.

- Never place a heat source directly on the patient's skin. Burns can occur.

Electric Heating Pads

- Be sure that the body part is dry or that the pad has a waterproof cover.

Safety Precautions for Electric Heating Pads

- Do not use pins (e.g., to hold a cover in place) or other sharp objects on the pad.
  The pin could go through a wire and cause an electric shock.
- Tell the patient to report any discomfort during the treatment
- For home use, warn the patient about the danger of burns from high settings. Use pads with a switch that cannot be turned up.
- Avoid direct contact with the heating device. Cover the heat source with a washcloth, towel, or fitted sleeve.
- Do not place the heating device (pad, bag) under the patient; place it over the body part.
  Helps prevent burns.
- Apply heat intermittently, leaving it on for no more than 15 minutes at a time in an area.
  This helps prevent tissue injury (e.g., burns, impaired circulation). It also makes the therapy more effective by preventing the rebound phenomenon: At the time the heat reaches maximum therapeutic effect, the opposite effect (vasoconstriction) begins.
- Check the skin frequently for extreme redness or blistering.
- Assess for hypotension and faintness. If they occur, discontinue the treatment. Have the patient lie down for several minutes, and check her BP. When the faint feeling passes, assist her to sit up slowly. Recheck the blood pressure (BP) in the sitting position. If the BP remains low, encourage her to remain seated. If the patient is ambulatory, have her dangle her feet for several minutes before getting up.

Clinical Insight 35-2 ➤ Applying Local Cold Therapy

Preparation

- Determine whether there are any contraindications to the treatment, such as impaired circulation, bleeding, wound complications, or inability to tolerate the treatment.
- Explain the application and rationale to the patient.
- Assess for indications for cold application (e.g., fever above 104°F [40°C]). Measure the patient's temperature.

Cooling Baths

A cooling bath is often used to treat a high fever (above 104°F [40°C]). It promotes heat loss through conduction and vaporization.

- Prepare a pan of water with a temperature from 65°F to 90°F (18°C to 32°C).
- You may add a fan to increase heat loss if the temperature is markedly elevated.
- Slowly sponge the face, arms, legs, back, and buttocks with the cool water. Do not dry the areas; cover with a damp towel.
- Take about 30 minutes to complete the bath.
  Cooling the body too rapidly will cause shivering, which will increase heat production.
- You may also place ice bags or cold packs on the forehead in the axillae and the groin.
- Assess the patient constantly during a cooling bath.
  If the patient begins to shiver, the temperature may actually begin to rise.

Cold Compresses

- Apply a cool, damp cloth or towel to the body part.
- Renew the compress or cloth frequently.
  The temperature of the compress or cloth will rapidly rise toward body temperature.

Ice Collars, Ice Bags, Commercially Prepared Cold Packs, Aquapads

- You can make an ice bag out of a nonsterile glove or small plastic bag by filling it with ice chips and tying a knot in the top.
- Fill the ice bag with ice chips or an alcohol-based solution.
- Cover ice bags or packs with a towel or soft cover.
- Apply to the skin for a maximum of 15 minutes, and then remove. You may reapply the cold pack in 1 hour.

Safety Precautions for Cooling Devices

- Measure water temperature with a bath thermometer.
- Tell the patient to report any discomfort during the treatment.
- Avoid direct contact with the cooling device. Cover the cold pack with a washcloth, towel, or fitted sleeve.
- Apply cold intermittently, leaving it on for no more than 15 minutes at a time in an area.
  Helps to prevent tissue injury (e.g., impaired circulation). It also makes the therapy more effective by preventing the rebound phenomenon: At the time the cold reaches maximum therapeutic effect, the opposite effect (vasodilation) begins.
- Observe for tissue damage: bluish purple mottled appearance of the skin, numbness, and sometimes blisters and pain.
- Monitor for elevated blood pressure.

ASSESSMENT GUIDELINES AND TOOLS

Focused Assessment

History Questions for Skin and Wound Assessment

- What is your typical activity level?
- Do you ever use a wheelchair or mobile device to get around? Do you require assistance to get out of bed or a chair?
- Tell me about your usual diet.
- How much liquid do you drink each day?
- Do you have any areas of numbness and tingling?
- Have you had any recent changes in your skin?
- Do you have any sores or open areas? If so, how long have you had the wound?
- Have you ever had difficulty with wound healing?
- What kinds of healthcare problems have you been experiencing?
- What medications—prescribed, herbal, or over the counter—are you taking?
- What is your typical hygiene routine?
- Do you ever lose control of your bladder or bowels?
- Do you smoke?
- How much time do you spend outdoors?
- Do you have diabetes? If so, how often do you check your feet? How often do you see a podiatrist? What is your average blood sugar?

Focused Assessment

Physical Examination: Wound Assessment

All Wounds

Assess all wounds for the following:

Location

Describe the location of the wound in anatomical terms. For example, you would describe an incision from cardiac surgery as a midsternal incision extending from the manubrium to the xiphoid process.

Size

- Measure the length and width of the wound in centimeters.
- To measure wound depth, gently insert a sterile cotton-tip applicator into the deepest part of the wound. Measure the applicator from the skin level to the tip.
- If possible, use photo documentation, indicating the dimensions on the photo. This is especially useful in the case of a wound with an irregular border.

Appearance

Your description of the appearance of the wound should be very detailed. You must describe:

- ***Type of wound*** *(open or closed)*
- ***If the wound is sutured***, examine the closure. Are the wound edges approximated? Is there tension on any aspect of the wound? Are the stitches intact?
- ***The color of the wound.*** Redness and inflammation for the first 2 to 3 days is normal, but erythema or swelling beyond that time may indicate infection.
- ***Condition of the wound bed (in an open wound).*** A beefy red, moist appearance is evidence of healing. A pale color or dry texture indicates a delay in healing.
- ***Examine for necrosis, slough, and eschar.*** Examine for a tunnel or sinus tract in the wound bed; if there is one, inspect and probe it for depth and characteristics.
- ***The skin surrounding the wound.*** Observe for skin discoloration, hematoma, or additional injury to the surrounding tissue. Observe for maceration, tunneling, crepitus, blistering, or erythema. Examine the edges of the wound for epithelial tissue and contraction. Look for undermining beneath the wound margins.

Drainage

- ***Presence of drainage or exudate.*** Describe the color, consistency, amount, and odor.
- ***Assess the quantity of wound drainage*** by weighing dressings before they are applied and again when they have been removed. The change in weight reflects the amount of drainage that they have absorbed.
- ***If a drain is present***, measure the amount of fluid in the collection container.
- ***Odor*** may indicate fistula formation or contamination with bacteria. If a new odor develops, assess carefully for presence of a fistula.

Patient Responses

Ask your patients about pain, discomfort, or itching related to the wound or wound care.

Assessing an Untreated Wound

Your assessment should determine what, if any, additional professional support is necessary. Assess the following same aspects as for treated wounds above: location, size, appearance, description of drainage, condition of wound margins, condition of surrounding skin, and effect of the wound on the patient. In addition, assess the following:

- ***Bleeding.*** If bleeding is profuse, apply direct pressure to the site. If bleeding continues after you apply pressure for 5 minutes or if blood is spurting from the wound, call the physician immediately.
- ***Severity of the wound.*** A gaping wound or a deep wound with fat, fascia, or muscle exposed will need additional care.
- ***Last tetanus immunization.*** Immunization should be given if (1) the last immunization was 10 years ago or longer, (2) the wound is contaminated with dirt or debris and the tetanus injection was given more than 5 years ago, or (3) it is uncertain when the patient last received an immunization.
- ***Whether the wound was caused by a bite.*** Determine whether the wound was caused by any type of bite, animal or human. A deep bite wound usually requires additional observation and/or antibiotics.
- ***Pain.*** Assess for pain. Any wound causing severe pain requires a comprehensive evaluation.
- ***Numbness or loss of movement.*** If any deficit is detected, the patient will need immediate evaluation.
- ***Presence of chronic medical conditions.*** Examples include diabetes, malnutrition, immunocompromise, a bleeding disorder. Patients with conditions that affect wound healing will need ongoing evaluation.

BRADEN SCALE FOR PREDICTING PRESSURE SORE RISK

Patient's Name _____ Evaluator's Name _____ Date of Assessment

SENSORY PERCEPTION ability to respond meaningfully to pressure-related discomfort	**1. Completely Limited** Unresponsive (does not moan, flinch, or grasp) to painful stimuli, due to diminished level of consciousness or sedation. OR limited ability to feel pain over most of body.	**2. Very Limited** Responds only to painful stimuli. Cannot communicate discomfort except by moaning or restlessness OR has a sensory impairment which limits the ability to feel pain or discomfort over 1/2 of body.	**3. Slightly Limited** Responds to verbal commands, but cannot always communicate discomfort or the need to be turned. OR has some sensory impairment which limits ability to feel pain or discomfort in 1 or 2 extremities.	**4. No Impairment** Responds to verbal commands. Has no sensory deficit which would limit ability to feel or voice pain or discomfort.				
MOISTURE degree to which skin is exposed to moisture	**1. Constantly Moist** Skin is kept moist almost constantly by perspiration, urine, etc. Dampness is detected every time patient is moved or turned.	**2. Very Moist** Skin is often, but not always moist. Linen must be changed at least once a shift.	**3. Occasionally Moist:** Skin is occasionally moist, requiring an extra linen change approximately once a day.	**4. Rarely Moist** Skin is usually dry, linen only requires changing at routine intervals.				
ACTIVITY degree of physical activity	**1. Bedfast** Confined to bed.	**2. Chairfast** Ability to walk severely limited or non-existent. Cannot bear own weight and/or must be assisted into chair or wheelchair.	**3. Walks Occasionally** Walks occasionally during day, but for very short distances, with or without assistance. Spends majority of each shift in bed or chair.	**4. Walks Frequently** Walks outside room at least twice a day and inside room at least once every two hours during waking hours.				
MOBILITY ability to change and control body position	**1. Completely Immobile** Does not make even slight changes in body or extremity position without assistance.	**2. Very Limited** Makes occasional slight changes in body or extremity position but unable to make frequent or significant changes independently.	**3. Slightly Limited** Makes frequent though slight changes in body or extremity position independently.	**4. No Limitation** Makes major and frequent changes in position without assistance.				
NUTRITION usual food intake pattern	**1. Very Poor** Never eats a complete meal. Rarely eats more than 1/2 of any food offered. Eats 2 servings or less of protein (meat or dairy products) per day. Takes fluids poorly. Does not take a liquid dietary supplement OR is NPO and/or maintained on clear liquids or IVs for more than 5 days.	**2. Probably Inadequate** Rarely eats a complete meal and generally eats only about 1/2 of any food offered. Protein intake includes only 3 servings of meat or dairy products per day. Occasionally will take a dietary supplement. OR receives less than optimum amount of liquid diet or tube feeding.	**3. Adequate** Eats over half of most meals. Eats a total of 4 servings of protein (meat, dairy products per day. Occasionally will refuse a meal, but will usually take a supplement when offered OR is on a tube feeding or TPN regimen which probably meets most of nutritional needs.	**4. Excellent** Eats most of every meal. Never refuses a meal. Usually eats a total of 4 or more servings of meat and dairy products. Occasionally eats between meals. Does not require supplementation.				
FRICTION & SHEAR	**1. Problem** Requires moderate to maximum assistance in moving. Complete lifting without sliding against sheets is impossible. Frequently slides down in bed or chair, requiring frequent repositioning with maximum assistance. Spasticity, contractures or agitation leads to almost constant friction.	**2. Potential Problem** Moves feebly or requires minimum assistance. During a move skin probably slides to some extent against sheets, chair, restraints or other devices. Maintains relatively good position in chair or bed most of the time but occasionally slides down.	**3. No Apparent Problem** Moves in bed and in chair independently and has sufficient muscle strength to lift up completely during move. Maintains good position in bed or chair.					
				Total Score				

© Copyright Barbara Braden and Nancy Bergstrom, 1988 All rights reserved

Source: U.S. Department of Health and Human Services. (1992). *Clinical practice guideline. Pressure ulcers in adults: Prediction and prevention* (pp. 16–17). PPPPUA Publication No. 92-0047. Rockville, MD: Public Health Service. Copyright © Barbara Braden and Nancy Bergstrom, 1988. Reprinted with permission.

The Norton Scale for Assessing Risk of Pressure Ulcers

Norton Scale for Assessing Risk of Pressure Ulcers

	Physical Condition	Mental Condition	Activity	Mobility	Incontinent	
	Good 4 Fair 3 Poor 2 Very bad 1	Alert 4 Apathetic 3 Confused 2 Stupor 1	Ambulant 4 Walk/help 3 Chair-bound 2 Bed 1	Full 4 Slightly limited 3 Very limited 2 Immobile 1	Not 4 Occasional 3 Usually/urine 2 Doubly 1	Total Score
Name/Date						

The Norton Scale uses five criteria to assess patients' risk for pressure ulcers. Scores of 14 or less indicate liability to ulcers; scores of <12 indicate very high risk.

Source: Norton, D., McLaren, R., & Exton-Smith, A. N. (1975). *An investigation of geriatric nursing problems in hospitals.* Edinburgh, Scotland: Churchill Livingstone. Used with permission.

The PUSH Tool for Evaluation of Pressure Ulcers

PUSH Tool - Version 3.0

Patient Name:_____ Patient ID#:_____

Ulcer Location: _____ Date:_____

DIRECTIONS:
Observe and measure the pressure ulcer. Categorize the ulcer with respect to surface area, exudate, and type of wound tissue. Record a sub-score for each of these ulcer characteristics. Add the sub-scores to obtain the total score. A comparison of total scores measured over time provides an indication of the improvement or deterioration in pressure ulcer healing.

Length x Width	**0** 0 cm^2	**1** <0.3 cm^2	**2** 0.3 - 0.6 cm^2	**3** 0.7 - 1.0 cm^2	**4** 1.1 - 2.0 cm^2	**5** 2.1 - 3.0 cm^2	**Subscore**
		6 3.1 - 4.0 cm^2	**7** 4.1 - 8.0 cm^2	**8** 8.1 - 12.0 cm^2	**9** 12.1 - 24.0 cm^2	**10** > 24 cm^2	
Exudate Amount	**0** None	**1** Light	**2** Moderate	**3** Heavy			**Subscore**
Tissue Type	**0** Closed	**1** Epithelial Tissue	**2** Granulation Tissue	**3** Slough	**4** Necrotic Tissue		**Subscore**
							Total Score

Length x Width: Measure the greatest length (head to toe) and the greatest width (side to side) using a centimeter ruler. Multiply these two measurements (length • width) to obtain an estimate of surface area in square centimeters (cm^2). **Caveat**: Do not guess! Always use a centimeter ruler and always use the same method each time the ulcer is measured.
Exudate Amount: Estimate the amount of exudate (drainage) present after removal of the dressing and before applying any topical agent to the ulcer. Estimate the exudate (drainage) as none, light, moderate, or heavy.
Tissue Type: This refers to the types of tissue that are present in the wound (ulcer) bed. Score as a "4" if there is any necrotic tissue present. Score as a "3" if there is any amount of slough present and necrotic tissue is absent. Score as a "2" if the wound is clean and contains granulation tissue. A superficial wound that is reepithelializing is scored as a "1". When the wound is closed, score as a "0".

4 - Necrotic Tissue (Eschar): black, brown, or tan tissue that adheres firmly to the wound bed or ulcer edges and may be either firmer or softer than surrounding skin.
3 - Slough: yellow or white tissue that adheres to the ulcer bed in strings or thick clumps, or is mucinous.
2 - Granulation Tissue: pink or beefy red tissue with a shiny, moist, granular appearance.
1 - Epithelial Tissue: for superficial ulcers, new pink or shiny tissue (skin) that grows in from the edges or as islands on the ulcer surface.
0 - Closed/Resurfaced: the wound is completely covered with epithelium (new skin).

Note: Refer to the NPUAP Website (www.npuap.org) for further information regarding development and use of the PUSH Tool.

Version 3.0: 9/15/98
© National Pressure Ulcer Advisory Panel

PRESSURE ULCER HEALING CHART

(use a separate page for each pressure ulcer)

Patient Name:_____ Patient ID#:_____

Ulcer Location: _____ Date:_____

Directions: Observe and measure pressure ulcers at regular intervals using the PUSH Tool. Date and record PUSH Sub-scale and Total Scores on the Pressure Ulcer Healing Record below.

	PRESSURE ULCER HEALING RECORD													
DATE														
Length × Width														
Exudate Amount														
Tissue Type														
Total Score														

Graph the PUSH Total Score on the Pressure Ulcer Healing Graph below.

PUSH Total Score	PRESSURE ULCER HEALING GRAPH													
17														
16														
15														
14														
13														
12														
11														
10														
9														
8														
7														
6														
5														
4														
3														
2														
1														
Healed 0														
DATE:														

Version 3.0: 9/15/98

© National Pressure Ulcer Advisory Panel

Source: National Pressure Ulcer Advisory Panel (NPUAP). (1998). Pressure ulcer scale for healing (PUSH) Tool, version 3.0. Retrieved from http://www.npuap.org/wp-content/uploads/2012/03/push3.pdf

DIAGNOSTIC TESTING

Diagnostic Testing

Tests for Assessing Wounds

Test	Normal Range	Comments
Leukocyte (WBC) count	4,500–11,000/mm^3	Usually done as a part of a complete blood count (CBC) but may be ordered as an independent test. White blood cells (WBCs) may increase when a wound develops; continued elevation may signal infection. A low WBC count may delay wound healing. Leukocytes are responsible for an inflammatory reaction at the wound site, phagocytosis of bacteria and cellular debris, and the creation of antibodies.
Serum protein *Serum albumin* *Serum prealbumin*	6.0–8.0 g/dL 3.4–4.8 g/dL 12–42 mg/dL	Low serum levels indicate limited nutritional stores that delay wound healing or place the patient at high risk for pressure ulcers. Serum protein may be monitored as an indicator of the ability to heal a wound or prevent a pressure ulcer. Serum protein and albumin levels are closely related. However, both fluctuate slowly. A more accurate measure of a patient's immediate protein stores is reflected in the prealbumin level.
Erythrocyte sedimentation rate (ESR)	<50 years old: 0–15 mm/hr; >50 years old: 0–20 mm/hr	In the presence of an inflammatory and necrotic process, blood proteins are altered. This test indicates whether the RBCs stick together, become heavier, and settle at the bottom of a lab tube when held vertically.
Coagulation studies: Partial thromboplastin time, activated (aPTT)	Varies with respect to equipment and reagents used. Critical values: >70 seconds or <53 seconds	Prolonged coagulation times may result in excessive blood loss or ongoing bleeding in the wound bed. Shortened coagulation times increase the risk for blood clot formation problems, such as deep vein thrombosis, pulmonary embolus, or stroke.
Prothrombin time (clotting time)	Critical values: >20 seconds (uncoagulated) or 3 times normal control (anticoagulated)	Altered coagulation may result from anticoagulant medications, a concurrent illness, trauma, or reaction to transfusions.
International normalized ratio (INR)	<2.0 for patients not receiving anticoagulation therapy; 2.0–3.0 for those receiving coagulation therapy	A standardized test to evaluate clotting times, considered the gold standard.
Wound cultures	Negative; no growth of pathogens	Wound cultures may be prescribed to determine the types of bacteria present in the wound. Cultures may be obtained by swab, aspiration, or tissue biopsy. A positive culture may not indicate an infection as chronic wounds are colonized with bacteria.
Tissue biopsy	Negative; no growth of pathogens	Wounds are not considered infected unless the bacteria count exceeds 100,000 organisms per gram of tissue. Exception: The presence of beta-hemolytic streptococci in any number indicates infection.

STANDARDIZED LANGUAGE

Standardized Language

Selected Standardized Outcomes and Interventions for Skin and Wound Diagnoses

Patient Situation (Data/Defining Characteristics)	NANDA-I Diagnosis	NOC Outcomes	Selected Indicators	Selected NIC Interventions and Specific Activities
Mrs. Whitefeather is 95 years old. She has cancer and has stopped eating and become very thin. Recently she has become too weak to move about in bed without help. However, her skin is intact with no redness, even over her bony prominences. She has a very low score on the Braden pressure ulcer assessment scale.	Risk for Impaired Skin Integrity	Tissue Integrity: Skin & Mucous Membranes *Other outcomes:* ➤ Immobility Consequences: Physiological ➤ Nutritional Status: Food & Fluid Intake ➤ Nutritional Status: Nutrient Intake	(5–Not compromised) Hydration Tissue perfusion Skin integrity (5–None) Erythema Blanching Skin lesions	*Bedrest Care* ➤ Keep bed linen clean, dry, and wrinkle free. ➤ Facilitate small shifts of body weight. *Pressure Ulcer Prevention* ➤ Monitor any reddened areas closely. ➤ Turn every 1–2 hours, as appropriate. ➤ Turn with care (e.g., avoid shearing) to prevent injury to fragile skin. ➤ Post a turning schedule at the bedside, as appropriate. ➤ Avoid massaging over bony prominences. ➤ Utilize specialty beds and mattresses, as appropriate. ➤ Avoid use of "donut" types of devices in the sacral area. ***Other Interventions*** ➤ Nutrition Management ➤ Positioning ➤ Pressure Management ➤ Skin Surveillance
Eddie Allen is 4 years old. He has a severe case of poison ivy, which has made blisters on his skin. He has been scratching and has bleeding, excoriated areas over his limbs, face, and trunk.	Impaired Skin Integrity	Tissue Integrity: Skin & Mucous Membranes *Other outcomes:* ➤ Infection ➤ Immune Hypersensitivity Response	(4–Mildly compromised) Skin integrity (4–Mild) Skin lesions Erythema (3–Moderate) Itching Localized inflammatory response	*Wound Care* ➤ Monitor characteristics of the wound, including drainage, color, size, and odor. ➤ Cleanse with normal saline or a nontoxic cleanser, as appropriate. ➤ Apply an appropriate ointment to the skin/lesion, as appropriate. ➤ Instruct the child and family member(s) about wound care procedures and signs of infection. ***Other Interventions*** ➤ Pruritus ➤ Management ➤ Skin Surveillance ➤ Wound Irrigation

Standardized Language

Selected Standardized Outcomes and Interventions for Skin and Wound Diagnoses—cont'd

Patient Situation (Data/Defining Characteristics)	NANDA-I Diagnosis	NOC Outcomes	Selected Indicators	Selected NIC Interventions and Specific Activities
Allie Newton has a stage II pressure ulcer on her left heel.	Impaired Tissue Integrity	Wound Healing: Secondary Intention *Other outcomes:* Tissue Integrity: Skin & Mucous Membranes	(4–Substantial) Granulation Decreased wound size (4–Limited) Purulent drainage Surrounding skin erythema Wound inflammation Foul wound odor	*Pressure Ulcer Care* ➤ Debride the ulcer, as needed. ➤ Cleanse the ulcer with the appropriate nontoxic solution, working in a circular motion from the center. ➤ Cleanse the skin around the ulcer with mild soap and water. ➤ Monitor for infection in the wound. ➤ Position every 1–2 hours to avoid prolonged pressure. ***Other Interventions*** ➤ Wound Care ➤ Pressure Management ➤ Infection Protection ➤ Medication ➤ Administration

Sources: Bulechek, G., Butcher, H., & Dochtermann, J. (Eds.). (2013). *Nursing interventions classification (NIC)* (6th ed.). St. Louis, MO: C.V. Mosby. Used with permission; Johnson, M., Moorhead, S., Bulechek, G., et al. (2012). *NOC, and NIC linkages to NANDA-I and clinical conditions.* (3rd ed.). St. Louis, MO: C.V. Mosby; Moorhead, S., Johnson, M., Maas, M., et al. (Eds.). (2013). *Nursing outcomes classification (NOC)* (5th ed.). St. Louis, MO: C.V. Mosby; and NANDA International. (2012). *Nursing diagnoses: Definitions and classification 2012–2014.* Philadelphia: Author.

CLINICALREASONING
Applying the Full-Spectrum Nursing Model

PATIENT SITUATION

Tio Santos is a 66-year-old obese man with diabetes and hypertension who is being seen for a wound on his right foot that doesn't seem to be healing. He injured his foot when repairing drywall at home. He is otherwise relatively sedentary at home. The wound is oozing, swollen, tender, and warm to the touch. Mr. Santos is now running a low-grade fever of 100.4°F at home. He tells you his foot is very painful, especially with any weight-bearing, and throbs when he is sitting or lying still. You measure the wound bed to be 6 cm × 4 cm and note purulent exudate at the distal edge. He is referred to an outpatient wound care center for treatment.

THINKING

1. *Theoretical Knowledge:*
   a. What is the Braden scale and why might it be used for Mr. Santos?
   b. What risk factors for delayed wound healing does Mr. Santos have?
2. *Critical Thinking (Considering Alternatives, Deciding What to Do):*
   a. To care for Mr. Santos's wound, should you use sterile gloves, clean nonsterile gloves, or no gloves? Explain your thinking.

DOING

3. *Practical Knowledge (Assessment):*
   a. What symptoms of infection does Mr. Santos have?
   b. To be certain the wound is infected what would you need to know or do?

CARING

4. *Self-Knowledge:* Imagine you have had a wound on your foot for 6 weeks. It has not healed and you have all Mr. Santos's symptoms and, in fact, are in his situation. What would be the most troublesome symptom in your daily life? What would worry you the most?

Critical Thinking and Clinical Reasoning

1. You are caring for a 22-year-old man who is paralyzed from the waist down secondary to an automobile accident. He has been admitted to the hospital with a urinary tract infection manifested by a fever of 102°F (39°C) and lethargy. His family reports he has been withdrawn and sits in his wheelchair watching TV all day long.
   a. What risk factors does this patient have for skin breakdown?
   b. What locations of his body should you be most concerned about in regard to pressure ulcer formation?
   c. What actions should you take to decrease the risk of pressure ulcers in this man? What further information do you need?
2. A 63-year-old man is admitted to your unit after an emergency appendectomy. His appendix was ruptured, and the surgeon has left the wound open to heal by secondary intention. A Jackson–Pratt drain is in place in the wound bed. A moderate amount of purosanguineous drainage is visible in the drain. The surgeon has ordered saline-moistened gauze packing every 4 hours.
   a. What actions should you take as you prepare to do the first dressing change?
   b. How will you secure the dressing?
3. For the following patients, write a NANDA-I diagnosis related to skin integrity. Include problem, etiology, and defining characteristics. If you do not have enough data for one of those components, state what additional data you need.
   a. Mrs. Whitefeather is 95 years old. She has cancer, and she has stopped eating and has become very thin. Recently she has become too weak to move about in bed without help. However, her skin is intact with no redness, even over her bony prominences. She has a very low score on the Braden pressure ulcer assessment scale.
   b. Eddie Allen is 4 years old. He has a severe case of poison ivy, and has blisters on his skin. He has been scratching and has bleeding, excoriated areas over his limbs, face, and trunk.
   c. Allie Newton has a stage II pressure ulcer on her left heel.
4. For each of the following concepts, use critical thinking to describe how or why it is important to nursing, patient care, or skin integrity and wound healing. Note that these are *not* to be merely definitions.

Shearing	Preventing pressure ulcers
Friction	Wound assessment
Pressure	Dressing changes
Wound healing process	

What Are the Main Points in This Chapter?

- The layers of the skin are the epidermis (outermost), the dermis, and the subcutaneous layer (innermost).
- The major functions of the skin are protection of the internal organs, unique identification of an individual, thermoregulation, metabolism of nutrients and metabolic waste products, and sensation.
- Age, mobility, nutrition, hydration, moisture underlying conditions, medications, contamination or infection, diminished sensation, cognitive impairment, hygiene, and lifestyle are factors that influence the ability to maintain intact skin and heal wounds.
- If there are no breaks in the skin, a wound is described as *closed*. A wound is considered *open* if there is a break in the skin or mucous membranes.
- Acute wounds may be intentional (e.g., surgical incisions) or unintentional (e.g., from trauma) and are expected to be of short duration.
- Wounds that exceed the anticipated length of recovery are classified as chronic wounds. Chronic wounds include pressure, arterial, venous, and diabetic ulcers. A chronic wound may linger for months or years.
- *Clean wounds* are uninfected wounds with minimal inflammation. *Clean-contaminated wounds* are surgical incisions that enter the gastrointestinal, respiratory, or genitourinary tracts. *Contaminated wounds* include open, traumatic wounds or surgical incisions in which a major break in asepsis occurred. *Infected wounds* are wounds with evidence of infection, such as presence of microorganisms.
- A wound that involves minimal or no tissue loss and has wound edges that are approximated are said to heal by primary intention.
- A wound that involves extensive tissue loss and has margins that cannot be approximated, or is infected, heals by secondary intention.
- Tertiary intention healing, or delayed primary closure, occurs when two surfaces of granulation tissue are brought together. Initially the wound is allowed to heal by secondary intention.
- Healing occurs in three stages. The *inflammatory phase* lasts from 1 to 5 days and consists of two major processes: hemostasis and inflammation. *The proliferative phase* occurs from days 5 to 21. It is characterized by cell development aimed at filling the wound defect and resurfacing the skin. The *maturation phase* begins in the second or third week and continues until the wound is completely healed.
- Wound closure methods include adhesive strips (Steri-Strips), absorbent sutures, surgical staples, and surgical glue.
- Drainage is the flow of fluids from a wound or cavity. It is often referred to as exudate (fluid that oozes as a result of inflammation).
- Complications of wound healing include hemorrhage, infection, dehiscence, evisceration, and fistula formation.
- Pressure ulcers are caused by unrelieved pressure over time that compromises blood flow to tissue, resulting in ischemia in the underlying tissue.
- A stage I pressure ulcer is an area of persistent redness and does not blanch.
- Stage II pressure ulcers involve partial-thickness skin loss of the epidermis, dermis, or both.
- A stage III pressure ulcer is characterized by full-thickness skin loss involving damage or necrosis of subcutaneous tissue, which may extend down to, but not through, the underlying fascia. The ulcer appears as a deep crater.
- Stage IV pressure ulcers involve full-thickness skin loss with extensive destruction; tissue necrosis; or damage to muscle, bone, or support structures. Undermining and sinus tracts (blind tracts underneath the epidermis) are common.
- Extrinsic factors leading to pressure ulcers are those that alter the skin and tissue integrity and blood supply (e.g., aging, low blood pressure, neurological injury, poor nutrition, edema, and fever).
- Extrinsic factors include friction and shearing, and exposure to moisture and pressure.
- Not all lower extremity ulcers are related to pressure. Some are caused by poor perfusion, such as venous stasis ulcers, diabetic foot ulcers, and arterial ulcers.
- An eschar is a black leathery covering of necrotic tissue. An ulcer covered by an eschar cannot be classified because it is impossible to determine the depth.
- The Braden, Norton, and PUSH scales evaluate risk for problems with skin integrity.
- When assessing a wound, note the following: the type of wound, the color of the wound and surrounding skin, the condition of the wound bed, drainage and odor, and the level of pain associated with the wound or wound care.

- Preventing pressure ulcers focuses on skin care, nutrition, turning and positioning, using therapeutic mattresses and cushions, and patient/family teaching.
- Five types of debridement are used: sharp, mechanical, enzymatic, autolytic, and biotherapy (maggot debridement).
- Wound care therapies to promote healing might include negative pressure wound therapy (NPWT), electrical stimulation, tissue growth factors, ultrasound, bioengineered skin substitutes, and surgical options.
- Primary dressings are ones that are placed in the wound bed and touch the wound. A secondary dressing covers or holds a primary dressing in place. Many dressings can act as both.
- Types of wound dressings are absorption, alginate, antimicrobial, collagen, gauze, foam dressings, hydrocolloid, hydrogel, skin sealants, and moisture barriers.
- Ideal wound irrigation pressures range from 4 pounds per square inch (psi) to 15 psi. Current recommendations are to use a 35-mL syringe attached to a 19-gauge angiocatheter. This will deliver the solution at approximately 8 psi.
- Heat application promotes vasodilatation, increases tissue metabolism, increases capillary permeability, reduces blood viscosity, and reduces muscle tension.
- The application of cold causes vasoconstriction, local anesthesia, reduced cell metabolism, increased blood viscosity, and decreased muscle tension.

Knowledge Map

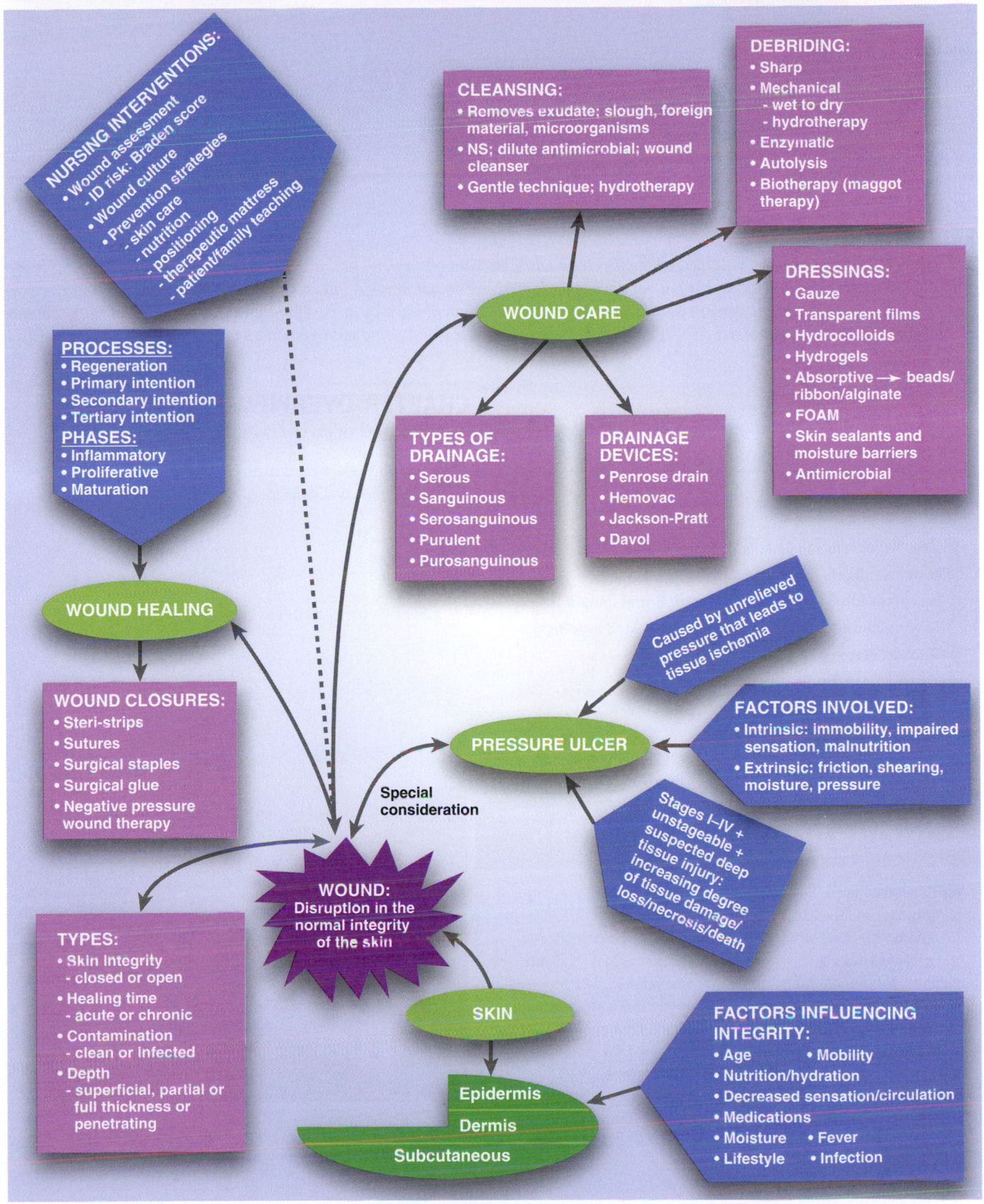

CHAPTER 36

Oxygenation

STUDENT RESOURCES

*The questions and exercises in Volume 2 allow you to practice the kind of thinking you will use as a full-spectrum nurse. Critical-thinking questions usually have more than one correct answer, so we do not provide "answers" for these features. It is more important to develop your nursing judgment than to just cover content. You will learn by discussing the questions with your peers. If you are still unsure, consult your instructor. You will find Response Sheets (for writing your responses to the questions) on Davis*Plus.

To explore learning resources for this chapter,

Go to Davis*Plus* at DavisPl.us/Wilkinson3.

Chapter Resources for Chapter 36:

- **Response sheets for all learning exercises**
- **Resources for Caregivers and Health Professionals**
- **Reading More About Oxygenation (suggested readings)**
- **Concept Map of chapter content**

Interactive Case Studies

NCLEX-Style and Chapter Review Questions

CHAPTER OVERVIEW

For a podcast of an overview of this chapter,

Go to Student Resources, Chapter 36, **Podcast—Chapter Overview,** on Davis*Plus*.

Caring for the Nguyens

Mai Nguyen, Nam's 76-year-old mother, has been complaining of fatigue and a persistent cough for approximately 2 weeks. Nam scheduled an appointment for her at the family clinic, where you are a nurse. Mrs. Nguyen appears disheveled. Her clothes are mismatched and rumpled, and her hair is tousled. Normally she is dressed neatly and wearing makeup. She has a hard time signing in at the desk and tells the receptionist she has a 1:00 p.m. appointment, but it is now 9:00 a.m. Mrs. Nguyen's vital signs are as follows: BP, 142/90 mm Hg; pulse, 94 beats/min and regular; respirations 24 breaths/min and labored; temperature, 99.6°F (37.5°C) oral.

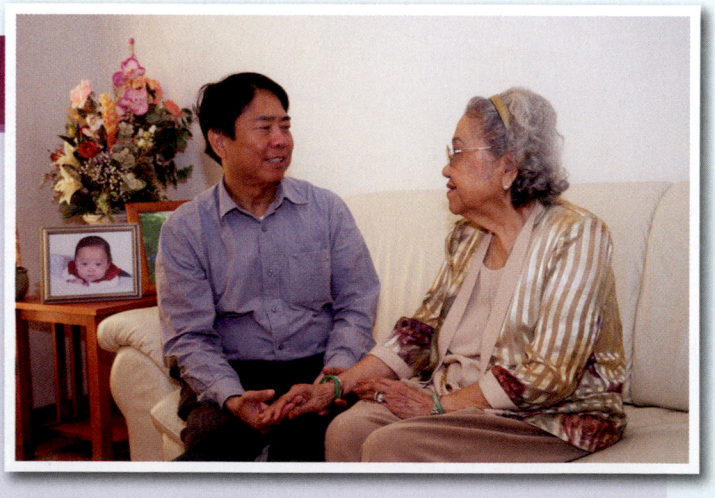

Caring for the Nguyens (continued)

A. What additional assessment data would be useful to gather at this time?

B. During her visit at the clinic, you notice that Mrs. Nguyen is very confused. Her weight has dropped 7 pounds since her visit last month, her mucous membranes are dry, and she is dyspneic with any activity. She is diagnosed with pneumonia. Because of her rapid decline, Mrs. Nguyen is admitted to the hospital to receive intravenous antibiotics. At the hospital, her initial pulse oximetry reading is 90%, and she is unable to cough up secretions. Write the most appropriate nursing diagnosis to focus interventions for Mrs. Nguyen.

C. What actions should you anticipate taking?

D. The hospitalist (hospital-based physician) writes prescriptions for IV fluids, antibiotics, suction prn, and continuous pulse oximetry. What additional prescriptions will you need to provide care for Mrs. Nguyen? What therapy would you suggest?

E. Mrs. Nguyen requires suctioning to help remove secretions. She has a weak cough and crackles and rhonchi throughout all lung fields. There are few secretions in her oropharynx, and she bites down on the catheter. What technique would you use to suction her? Explain your choice.

F. After 4 days in the hospital, Mrs. Nguyen is discharged to home. She asks the hospital nurse, "What can I do to make sure I never get that sick again?" How would you answer this question?

Practical Knowledge knowing how

As you perform the procedures, apply the concepts and other theoretical knowledge you learned in Volume 1. The registered nurse is responsible for assessing patients' oxygenation and their responses to procedures.

PROCEDURES

In this section you will find procedures necessary for supporting oxygenation. Some, but not all, of the procedures in this section can be delegated to qualified nursing assistive personnel (NAPs). Refer to the delegation notes in each procedure and to agency policies.

Procedure 36-1 ■ Collecting a Sputum Specimen

➤ For steps to follow in *all* procedures, refer to the Universal Steps for All Procedures found on the inside back cover.

Equipment

For all sputum specimens, you will need a patient identification label, a completed laboratory requisition form, and a small plastic bag with a biohazard label (or container designated by the agency) for delivering the specimen to the laboratory. Depending on how you obtain the specimen, you also need the following:

Procedure 36-1A: Collecting an Expectorated Sputum Specimen

- Sterile specimen container with lid
- Procedure gloves
- Glass of water
- Emesis basin
- Tissues
- Pillow (if abdominal or chest incision is present)

Procedure 36-1B: Collecting a Suctioned Sputum Specimen

- Sterile suction catheter or sterile suction kit
- Suction device (portable or wall)
- Sterile gloves
- Protective eyewear
- Inline sputum specimen container or trap
- Sterile saline solution
- Oxygen therapy equipment, if indicated
- Linen-saver pad or towel

Delegation

You can delegate collection of an expectorated sputum specimen to a NAP who has been adequately trained in performing the skill. Assess the patient's respiratory status

(continued on next page)

Procedure 36-1 ■ Collecting a Sputum Specimen (continued)

first; if the patient's condition is unstable, do not delegate the procedure. Do not delegate obtaining a specimen by tracheal suctioning.

Pre-Procedure Assessment

- **Assess the patient's comprehension of the procedure.**
  Understanding allays anxiety and promotes cooperation.
- **Assess breath sounds; respiratory rate, depth, and pattern; skin and nailbed color; and tissue perfusion.**
  You may need to delay sputum collection if the patient is in respiratory distress.
- **Assess ability to deep-breathe, cough, and expectorate.**
  If the patient is unable to deep-breathe, cough, and expectorate, suctioning may be necessary to obtain an adequate sputum specimen.
- **Determine when the patient last ate or had a tube feeding, especially for a specimen obtained by suction.**
  Specimen collection should be delayed for 1 to 2 hours after eating because the procedure may cause vomiting, which creates a risk for aspiration of stomach contents.
- **If suctioning is required to obtain the specimen, check for factors such as anticoagulant therapy, bleeding disorders, or low platelet count.**
  These factors place the patient at risk for bleeding when the suction catheter is introduced.

➤ When performing the procedure, always identify your patient according to agency policy, using two identifiers, and be attentive to standard precautions, hand hygiene, patient safety and privacy, body mechanics, and documentation.

Procedure Steps

1. **Verify the medical prescription** for type of sputum analysis.
   The type of sputum specimen determines the number of specimens required and the time of day the specimen should be collected. For example, specimens to confirm tuberculosis typically require three consecutive morning samples.
2. **Position the patient** according to the required specimen collection technique.
   a. For an *expectorated specimen*, assist the patient to high or semi-Fowler's position or to a sitting position at the edge of the bed.
   b. For a *suctioned specimen*, position the patient in high or semi-Fowler's position.
   These positions facilitate insertion of the suction catheter and the ability to cough. They also promote lung expansion, and prevent aspiration should the patient vomit during the procedure.
3. **Drape a towel or linen-saver pad** over the patient's chest. Ask the patient to rinse his mouth and gargle with water.
   A towel or pad protects the patient's gown from soiling during specimen collection. Rinsing the mouth removes flora that may contaminate the specimen; however, evidence is not conclusive on this point.
4. **If the patient has an abdominal** or chest incision, have the patient splint the incision with a pillow.
   Splinting the incision decreases discomfort when the patient coughs.

Procedure 36-1A ■ Collecting an Expectorated Sputum Specimen

Procedure Steps

Follow Steps 1 through 4, above.

5. **Provide the patient with** the specimen container. Advise the patient to avoid touching the inside of the container. If you must hold the container for her, first don procedure gloves.
   The inside of the container should remain sterile. Wear gloves because you may come in contact with secretions or airborne bacteria when the patient coughs and expectorates.▼

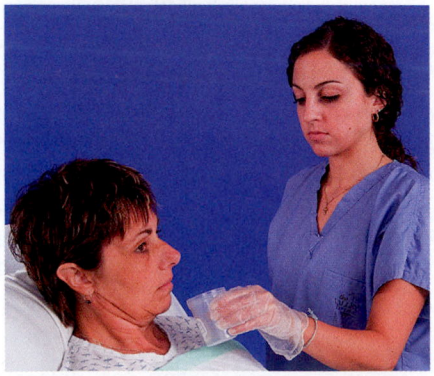

6. **Ask the patient to breathe** deeply for three or four breaths, and then ask him after a full inhalation to hold his breath and then cough.
   Deep breathing opens airways and stimulates the cough reflex. Coughing after a full inhalation creates enough force to mobilize secretions through the airways and into the pharynx.
7. **Instruct the patient to expectorate** the secretions directly into the specimen container.
   Prevents specimen contamination from outside organisms.

8. **Tell the patient to repeat deep breathing** and coughing until an adequate sample is obtained.
Typically 5 to 10 mL of sputum is required to ensure adequate sputum analysis.

9. **Don procedure gloves** if you are not already wearing them; cover the specimen container with the lid immediately after the specimen is collected.
Gloves protect you in the event the patient's coughing has contaminated the outside of the container. Covering the container immediately prevents spread of microorganisms.

10. **Label the specimen container** with patient identification, the name of the test, and collection date and time.
Correctly identifying the specimen ensures accurate diagnosis and treatment.

11. **Place the specimen in** a plastic bag with a biohazard label. Attach a completed laboratory requisition form.
The plastic bag protects healthcare workers from exposure to microorganisms. The laboratory requisition form ensures proper processing of the specimen.

12. **Send the specimen** to the laboratory immediately, or refrigerate it if transport might be delayed.
If bacterial cultures are delayed, contaminating organisms may grow, producing false culture results and possibly inappropriate treatment.

Procedure 36-1B ■ Collecting a Suctioned Sputum Specimen

Procedure Steps

Follow Steps 1 through 4, above

5. **Administer oxygen** to the patient, if indicated.
Suctioning may cause hypoxemia.

6. **Prepare the suction device**, and make sure it is functioning properly.

7. **Don protective eyewear.**
Protects your eyes from splattering of secretions during suctioning.

8. **Attach the suction tubing** to the male adapter of the inline sputum specimen container.

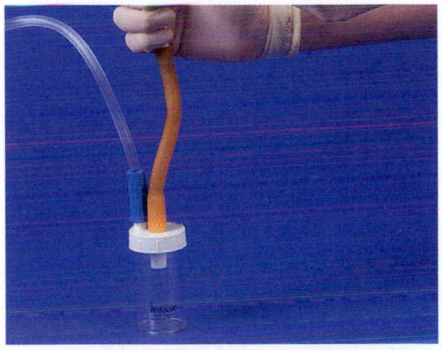

9. **Don sterile gloves.**
Protects the patient's sterile airways from contamination by outside organisms.

10. **Attach the sterile suction** to the flexible tubing on the sputum specimen container. The hand that touches the specimen container is no longer sterile.
Ensures that the sputum specimen goes directly into the specimen container instead of the suction tubing.

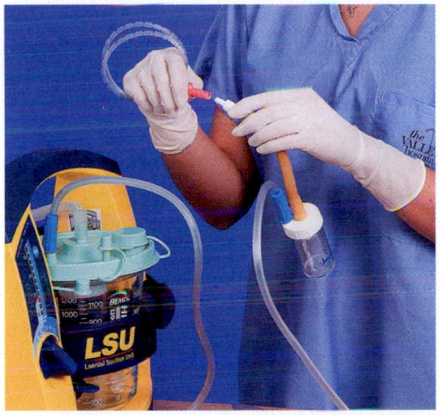

11. **Lubricate the suction catheter** with sterile saline solution.
Lubrication eases insertion and prevents trauma to mucosa.

12. **Insert the tip of the suction** catheter gently through the nasopharynx, endotracheal tube, or tracheostomy tube. Advance the tip into the trachea (see Procedure 36-6 or Procedure 36-8).
Gently insertion prevents airway trauma.

13. **When the patient begins** coughing, apply suction by placing your finger over the suction control port for 5 to 10 seconds to collect the specimen.
Applying suction for longer than 10 seconds can cause hypoxia.

14. **If an adequate specimen** (5 to 10 mL) is not obtained, allow the patient to rest for 1 or 2 minutes, and then repeat the procedure. Administer oxygen to the patient at this time, if indicated.
Allowing the patient to rest and administering oxygen prevent hypoxia. You must assess your patient continually during this procedure to ensure patient safety and respiratory status.

15. **When you have collected** an adequate specimen, discontinue suction, then gently remove the suction catheter.
Applying suction during catheter removal can damage the airway mucosa.

16. **Remove the suction catheter** from the specimen container, and dispose of the catheter in the appropriate container.
Disposal of contaminated supplies prevents the spread of infection.

17. **Remove the suction tubing** from the specimen container, and connect the rubber tubing on the specimen container to the plastic adapter.

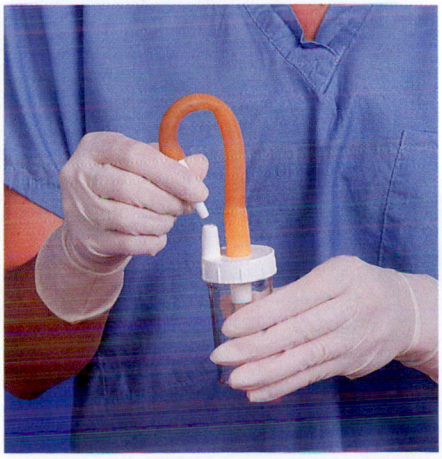

(continued on next page)

Procedure 36-1 ■ Collecting a Sputum Specimen (continued)

18. **If sputum comes in contact** with the outside of the specimen container, clean the outside with a disinfectant, according to agency policy.
Prevents spread of infection to staff members who must handle the specimen.

19. **After the patient expectorates,** offer tissues and provide mouth care.
Promotes patient comfort.

20. **Label the specimen container** with the patient's identification, the name of the test, and collection date and time.
Correctly identifying the specimen ensures accurate diagnosis and treatment.

21. **Place the specimen** in a plastic bag with a biohazard label. Attach a completed laboratory requisition form.
The biohazard bag protects healthcare workers from exposure to microorganisms. The laboratory requisition form ensures proper processing of the specimen.

22. **Send the specimen** to the laboratory immediately, or refrigerate it if transport might be delayed.
If bacterial cultures are delayed, contaminating organisms may grow, producing false culture results and possibly inappropriate treatment.

Evaluation

- Evaluate the patient's respiratory status during and after the procedure, especially if suctioning was necessary.
- Examine the color, consistency, and odor of the sputum specimen.
- Promptly report laboratory results to the primary care provider.
- Evaluate the patient's understanding of the procedure and test results.

Patient Teaching

- Explain proper collection techniques to avoid specimen contamination.
- Demonstrate proper coughing techniques to ensure an adequate specimen.
- Explain the importance of avoiding mouthwash before the procedure, as it may alter laboratory results.
- If the patient has an incision, show him how to splint his incision to avoid discomfort during coughing and expectoration.

Home Care

Explain how to collect an expectorated sputum specimen and the importance of sending the specimen to the laboratory immediately after collection.

Documentation

- Record the date and time the specimen was collected, the method of collection, and the type of specimen ordered.
- Note the amount, color, consistency, and odor of the specimen.
- Document the patient's tolerance of the procedure.

Sample documentation:

06/05/15 0700 Patient suctioned via tracheostomy. Sputum specimen obtained and sent for acid-fast bacillus (AFB) analysis. Specimen contained 15 mL of yellow, tenacious, odorless sputum. Patient became short of breath with suctioning. 100% O_2 administered via tracheostomy hood for 10 minutes after suctioning. Shortness of breath abated with treatment. O_2 returned to 40% ——— S. Ryan, RN

Practice Resources

Centers for Disease Control and Prevention (CDC) (2011); Texas Department of State Health Services, Laboratory Services Section Home (2009).

Procedure 36-2 ■ Monitoring Pulse Oximetry (Arterial Oxygen Saturation)

➤ For steps to follow in *all* procedures, refer to the Universal Steps for All Procedures found on the inside back cover.

Equipment

- Nail polish remover, if necessary
- Oximeter and probe sensor appropriate for patient age, size and weight, and for the desired location.
- Oximeter probe sensor appropriate for patient age, size, weight, and for the desired location

Delegation

Because it is noninvasive and simple to perform, the RN can delegate application of the pulse oximeter probe and measurement of arterial oxygen saturation (SaO_2) to a NAP or LPN who is adequately trained to perform the skill. Inform the NAP or LPN how often to take measurements, and instruct them to notify you immediately if Sa_{O_2} falls below 95%. Although this procedure can be delegated, it is the responsibility of the RN to interpret the results, assess the patient, and notify the primary care provider.

Pre-Procedure Assessment

- **Assess the need for Sa_{O_2} monitoring: low hemoglobin level; confusion, decreased level of consciousness, or respiratory distress; or risk factors, such as heart or pulmonary disease, recovering from anesthesia, or ventilator-dependent.**
  Sa_{O_2} monitoring helps detect oxygenation problems early. Monitoring is especially important in patients with risk factors. Patients with underlying pulmonary disease may have adapted to low oxygen saturation levels, so you may need to adjust the lower limit alarm and, if you have delegated the procedure, the level for notification for these patients.
- **Assess respiratory status, including breath sounds; respiratory rate, depth, and pattern; tissue perfusion; Sa_{O_2}; and skin and nailbed color.**
  Assessment findings may suggest a decrease in oxygen saturation and validate oximetry readings.
- **Determine the optimal location for the oximeter probe sensor, for example, the fingertip, earlobe, forehead, or bridge of the nose. Check the capillary refill and pulse at the pulse closest to the site.**
  To ensure accurate monitoring, choose a site that has adequate circulation, is free of artificial nails, and contains no moisture. Clinical Insight 36-1 offers suggestions on site placement based on patient factors.
- **Assess for factors that may interfere with pulse oximetry measurement, such as hypotension, hypothermia, and tremors.**
  The sensor requires adequate circulation to recognize hemoglobin molecules that absorb the emitted light. Tremors may produce artifact that may be misinterpreted by the oximeter, causing false readings.
- **Check patient history for allergy to adhesive.**
  An allergic reaction may occur if an adhesive-backed disposable probe sensor is used in a patient with a history of allergy to adhesives.

➤ When performing the procedure, always identify your patient according to agency policy, using two identifiers, and be attentive to standard precautions, hand hygiene, patient safety and privacy, body mechanics, and documentation.

➤ *Note:* This procedure explains how to apply a pulse oximeter. Refer to Clinical Insight 36-1 for tips for obtaining accurate pulse oximetry readings.

Procedure Steps

1. **Choose a sensor appropriate** for the patient's age, size, and weight and for the desired location.
   - If the patient is allergic to adhesive, use a clip-on probe sensor.
   - If the patient's peripheral circulation is compromised, use a nasal sensor.
     An appropriate type of sensor is more comfortable for the patient and ensures accurate readings.
2. **Prepare the site by cleansing** and drying it. If the finger is the site, remove nail polish or an acrylic nail, if present.
   Dirt and skin oils on the site can interfere with passage of light waves. Nail polish or acrylic nails may interfere with signal transmission, causing inaccurate Sa_{O_2} measurement. However, a recent study found that nail polish did not cause a clinically significant change in readings in healthy people (Chan, Chan, & Chan, 2013).
3. **Remove the protective backing** if you are using a disposable probe sensor that contains adhesive.
4. **Attach the probe sensor** to the chosen site. Make sure the photodetector and light-emitting diodes (LED) on the probe sensor face each other. Most probe sensors contain markings to facilitate correct placement.

When Using a Clip-on Probe Sensor

If you are using a clip-on probe sensor, warn the patient that he may feel a pinching sensation. Choose the site based on the status of circulation to the extremity and patient movement.
Inadequate circulation to the site and artifact caused by motion may alter Sa_{O_2} results. The photodetector diodes and LED must be properly placed to ensure accurate readings.

5. **Connect the sensor probe** to the oximeter and turn it on. Check the pulse rate displayed on the oximeter to see whether it correlates with the patient's radial pulse. (Be sure the pulse oximeter is plugged in to an electrical socket.)
   Correlation between the oximeter pulse display and the patient's radial pulse confirms accurate readings.
6. **Read the Sa_{O_2} measurement** on the digital display when it reaches a constant value, usually in 10 to 30 seconds, but may take up to 2 minutes.
   The oximeter requires time to detect the pulse, calculate oxygen saturation, and register an accurate reading.▼

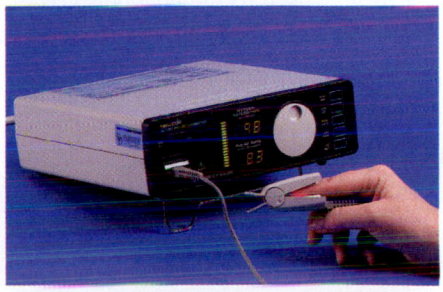

7. **Set and turn on the alarm** limits for Sa_{O_2} and pulse rate, according to the manufacturer's instructions, patient condition, and agency policy if continuous monitoring is necessary.
   Alarms must be set at appropriate levels to signify when Sa_{O_2} or pulse rate falls below predetermined levels. Alarms help ensure prompt recognition and treatment of hypoxia.

(continued on next page)

Procedure 36-2 ■ Monitoring Pulse Oximetry (Arterial Oxygen Saturation) (continued)

8. **Obtain readings as prescribed** or indicated by the patient's respiratory status.
   Some agencies require a prescription for pulse oximetry to ensure reimbursement.
9. **Rotate the site** if continuous monitoring is indicated.

   For an Adhesive Probe Sensor
   Rotate the site every 4 hours.

   For a Clip-on Probe Sensor
   Rotate the site every 2 hours.
   Probe sensors and prolonged pressure may irritate the skin; rotating the site prevents skin breakdown.
10. **Remove the probe sensor**, and turn off the oximeter when monitoring is no longer necessary.
    Some oximeters are battery powered; leaving them on after use depletes the battery.

Evaluation

- Evaluate the patient's understanding of the procedure and the obtained values.
- Compare pulse oximetry results with the patient's clinical presentation.
- Evaluate the effectiveness of therapy by comparing Sa_{O_2} results before, during, and after treatment.
- Assess the site every 4 hours if you are using an adhesive probe sensor or every 2 hours if you are using a clip-on probe sensor.

Patient Teaching

- Demonstrate the procedure to the patient and caregiver, especially if the patient will be continuing pulse oximetry at home.
- Explain to the patient and caregiver the significance of Sa_{O_2} results.
- Discuss the signs and symptoms of hypoxia (confusion, restlessness, shortness of breath, dyspnea, cyanosis, and somnolence) with the patient and caregiver.

Home Care

- Explain where to obtain a pulse oximeter.
- Tell the client and caregiver when to notify the primary provider of abnormal results or signs and symptoms of hypoxia.
- Help the client identify risk factors that decrease Sa_{O_2} levels.

Documentation

- Record the date and time of each pulse oximetry reading obtained. Most agencies use a flowsheet if frequent monitoring is necessary.
- Document whether readings are intermittent or continuous.
- If readings are continuous, record alarm parameters.
- Chart the patient's vital signs and Sa_{O_2} results, and indicate whether the patient is breathing room air or receiving oxygen therapy. For oxygen therapy, note the oxygen concentration and the mode of delivery.
- Document acute decreases in Sa_{O_2}, any precipitating factors, treatment interventions, and the patient's response.

Sample documentation

July 1, 2015 0300 Pt stated "short of breath." Crackles throughout lung fields. BP 140/92, apical pulse 110 beats/min, resp rate 32 breaths/min. Pulse oximetry applied to left index finger, and Sa_{O_2} 88% on room air. Places on O_2 at 4 L/min via nasal cannula. Dr. Jones notified. ——— Kate Jackson, RNC

Practice Resources

American Association of Critical-Care Nurses (AACN) (2010); Hill, E., & Stoneham, M. (2000); Rajkumar, A., Karmarkar, A., & Knott, J. (2006); Chan, E. D., Chan, M. M., & Chan , M. M. (2013).

Procedure 36-3 ■ Performing Percussion, Vibration, and Postural Drainage

➤ For steps to follow in *all* procedures, refer to the Universal Steps for All Procedures found on the inside back cover.

Equipment

- Bed capable of being placed in the Trendelenburg position
- Pillows
- Patient gown
- Facial tissues
- Emesis basin
- Sputum specimen container, if needed
- Suction equipment, if needed
- Stethoscope

Delegation

You should assess the patient to determine the need for the procedure and to evaluate whether the patient can tolerate the procedure. You should perform the initial procedure, but you can delegate subsequent treatments to a respiratory therapist or NAP who is adequately trained. Instruct the respiratory therapist or NAP to report any changes in the patient's condition immediately. The RN is responsible for ongoing assessment and monitoring of airway clearance and respiratory status.

Pre-Procedure Assessment

- Check the patient's chest x-ray results.
  Identifies which lung fields require treatment.
- Assess the patient's respiratory status, including respiratory rate, depth, and rhythm; breath sounds; color; and pulse oximetry results.
  Determines the need for and effectiveness of percussion, vibration, and postural drainage.
- Determine when the patient has last eaten.
  Postural drainage should not be performed for at least 2 hours after meals to prevent nausea, vomiting, and aspiration.
- Assess the patient for dysrhythmias, coagulopathy (a defect in blood clotting), hypertension, and pain or tenderness in the chest area being treated.
  If any of these are present, the procedure should be avoided because it might worsen these conditions.

➤ When performing the procedure, always identify your patient according to agency policy, using two identifiers, and be attentive to standard precautions, hand hygiene, patient safety and privacy, body mechanics, and documentation.

Procedure Steps

1. **Help the patient assume the appropriate** position, based on the lung field that requires drainage.
   Helps mobilize secretions in the affected lung field by gravity.
   a. ***Apical areas of the upper lobes.*** Ask the patient to sit at the edge of the bed, if possible. If needed, place a pillow at the base of the spine for support. If the patient is not able to sit at the edge of the bed, place him in high-Fowler's position. ▼

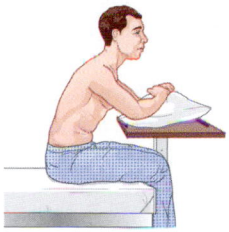

   b. ***Posterior section of the upper lobes.*** Position supine with a pillow under the hips and knees flexed. Have the patient rotate slightly away from the side that requires drainage. ▼

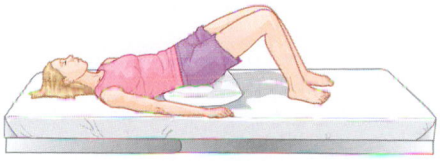

   c. ***Middle or lower lobes.*** Place the bed in the Trendelenburg position. Position the patient in Sims' position. To drain the left lung, position the patient on his right side. For the right lung, position the patient on his left side. ▼

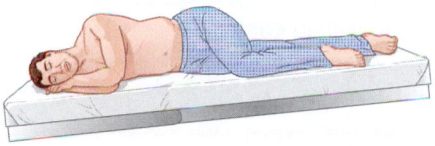

   d. ***Posterior lower lobes.*** Keeping the bed flat, position the patient prone with a pillow under her stomach. ▼

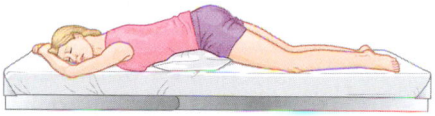

2. **Have the patient remain** in the desired position for 10 to 15 minutes, if tolerated.
   Allows adequate drainage of secretions by gravity from the desired lung field.
3. **Perform percussion** over the affected lung area while the patient is in the desired drainage position.
   Loosens and mobilizes secretions.
   a. Instruct the patient to breathe deeply and slowly.
   Relaxation helps the patient tolerate the procedure.
   b. Place a towel over the patient's skin or use the patient's gown to cover the area to be percussed.
   Protects the skin and promotes patient privacy and comfort.
   c. ✚ Avoid clapping over bony prominences, female breasts, or tender areas of the chest.
   Percussing over these areas may cause discomfort and compromise tissue integrity.
   d. Cup your hands, keeping your fingers flexed and your thumbs pressed against your index fingers.
   Cupping your hands promotes patient comfort during percussion.
   e. Place your cupped hands over the lung area that requires drainage.
   f. Percuss the lung area for 1 to 3 minutes by alternately striking your cupped hands rhythmically against the patient. ▼

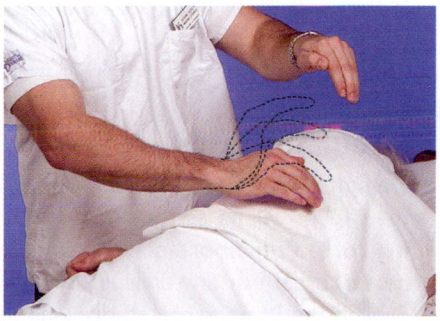

4. **Perform vibrations** while the patient remains in the desired drainage position. ▼

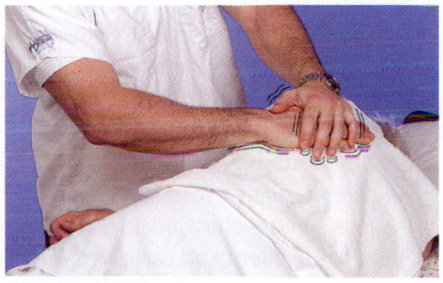

   a. Place the flat surface of one hand over the lung area that requires vibration. Place your other hand on top of that hand at a right angle.
   Using the flat surfaces of the hands provides a large surface area to

(continued on next page)

Procedure 36-3 ■ Performing Percussion, Vibration, and Postural Drainage (continued)

transmit vibrations through the chest. Placing one hand on top of the other provides better leverage for vibrating.

b. Instruct the patient to inhale slowly and deeply.
Promotes relaxation and lung expansion.

c. Instruct the patient to make a "fff" or "sss" sound as she exhales.

d. As the patient exhales, press your fingers and palms firmly against her chest wall.
Vibrating during exhalation enhances the downward movement of the rib cage that occurs during exhalation.

e. Push down, and gently vibrate with your hands over the lung area.
Vibration helps mobilize secretions.

f. Continue performing vibrations for three exhalations.

5. **After performing postural** drainage, percussion, and vibration, allow the patient to sit up. Ask her to cough at the end of a deep inspiration. Suction the patient if she is unable to expectorate secretions. If a sputum specimen is needed, collect it in a specimen container.
Coughing helps clear the airway of secretions.

6. **Repeat Steps 1 through 5** for each lung field that requires treatment. The entire treatment should not exceed 60 minutes.
Treating for longer than 60 minutes fatigues the patient.

7. **Provide mouth care.**
Cleanses the mouth of secretions and promotes patient comfort.

Evaluation

- Evaluate the effectiveness of percussion, vibration, and postural drainage.
- Auscultate breath sounds every 2 to 4 hours, as indicated.
- Monitor pulse oximetry and arterial blood gas (ABG) results.
- Evaluate the need for further treatment.

Patient Teaching

- Demonstrate percussion, vibration, and postural drainage if the patient will be continuing it at home.
- Reinforce the importance of immediately reporting shortness of breath or any difficulty breathing.
- Explain the importance of drinking fluids to help thin and mobilize secretions.
- Teach coughing and deep-breathing exercises.

Home Care

- Be sure the client/family/caregiver knows how often the procedure should be done. There should be a prescription from the primary care provider.
- Most clients will not have a bed that can be placed in the Trendelenburg position.
- Demonstrate how to position the client with hips elevated on pillows, higher than the chest, or, if the client is able, to assume a knee–chest position.
- Provide the client and caregiver with contact information of healthcare personnel who can be reached for advice or emergencies.

Documentation

- Document the date and time you performed percussion, vibration, and postural drainage.
- Note the positions used and the length of time the patient maintained each position.
- Note the anatomical locations in which you performed percussion and vibration.
- Document the patient's tolerance of the procedure, as well as any complications and the nursing interventions you used to treat the complication.
- Document the amount, color, odor, and consistency of sputum obtained during the procedure and whether you sent a sputum specimen to the lab.

Sample documentation

June 15, 2015 Percussion and vibration done over Right lower lobe. Expectorated 10 mL thick, yellow, odorless mucus. Specimen to lab. BP 142/78, HR 98 beats/min, respirations 24 breaths/min. Few crackles auscultated over Right lung base, Sao_2 98% on 2 L/min nasal cannula. —— Jeffrey Fine, RN

Practice Resources

Bilton, D. (2012); *Lippincott's Nursing Procedures* (2012).

Procedure 36-4 ■ Administering Oxygen

➤ For steps to follow in *all* procedures, refer to the Universal Steps for All Procedures found on the inside back cover.

Equipment

- Oxygen source
- Flow meter
- Oxygen tubing
- Nasal cannula, oxygen mask, or face tent
- Prefilled humidification device

Delegation

The RN is responsible for assessing respiratory function and initiating oxygen therapy. However, you may delegate reapplication and maintenance of oxygen therapy (e.g., adjusting the face mask) to appropriately trained assistive personnel when necessary.

Pre-Procedure Assessment

- Assess the patient's understanding of oxygen therapy.
- Assessment of the patient's respiratory status; includes respiratory rate, depth, and rhythm; breath sounds; color; capillary refill and pulse oximetry results.
  Determines the need for further treatment and effectiveness of oxygen therapy.
- Assess nares for patency (if a nasal cannula is being used) and behind the ears for signs of skin breakdown.

➤ When performing the procedure, always identify your patient according to agency policy, using two identifiers, and be attentive to standard precautions, hand hygiene, patient safety and privacy, body mechanics, and documentation.

➤ *Note:* Oxygen requires a medical prescription. In an emergency, administer oxygen to the patient to prevent respiratory distress, then notify the primary care provider for a prescription.

Procedure Steps

Also use Clinical Insight 36-3: Oxygen Therapy Safety Precautions.

1. **Attach the flow meter** to the wall oxygen source (the green meter on the wall).▼

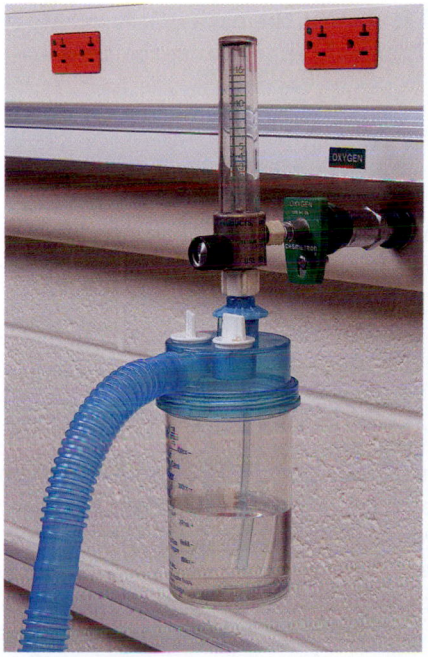

If Using a Portable Oxygen Tank

Attach the flow meter to the tank if it is not already connected. Once tubing is attached to the portable tank, check the amount of oxygen in the tank by looking at the meter.
The flow meter regulates the amount of oxygen delivered per minute.

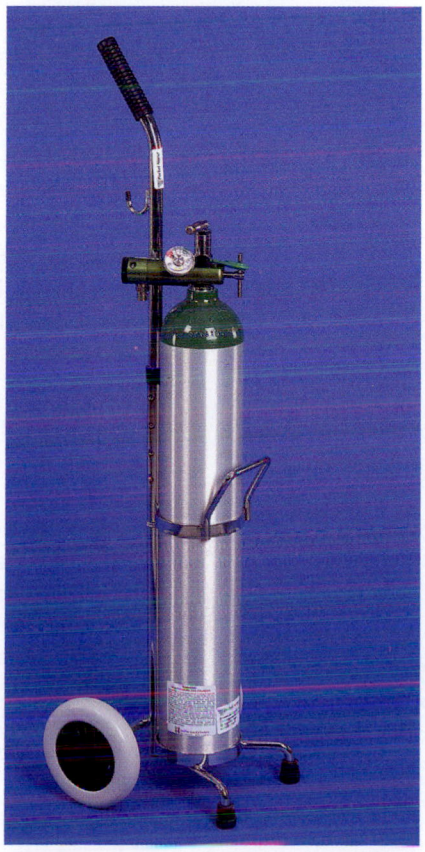

2. **Assemble the oxygen** equipment. (See the table at the end of this procedure for various oxygen delivery devices.)
3. **Attach the humidifier** to the flow meter. The humidifier is simply a small plastic container containing normal saline. If you are not using a humidifier, attach the adapter directly to the flow meter.
   The humidifier adds moisture in with the oxygen, which can dry the nasal or oral cavity.
4. **Turn on the oxygen** at the flow meter, and adjust the prescribed flow rate.

Procedure Variation for Nasal Cannula

Follow Steps 1 through 4.

5. **Attach the nasal cannula** tubing to the humidifier or the adapter.
6. **Place the nasal prongs** in the patient's nares—prongs curved downward—and then place the tubing around each ear.
   Properly positions the device for optimal oxygen delivery.

(continued on next page)

Procedure 36-4 ■ Administering Oxygen (continued)

7. **Use the slide adjustment device** to tighten the cannula in place under the patient's chin. It must fit securely, but not too tightly. Then proceed to Step 12.
The nasal cannula must fit securely to maximize the amount of oxygen inhaled by the patient. A good fit minimizes the amount of oxygen lost around the prongs.▼

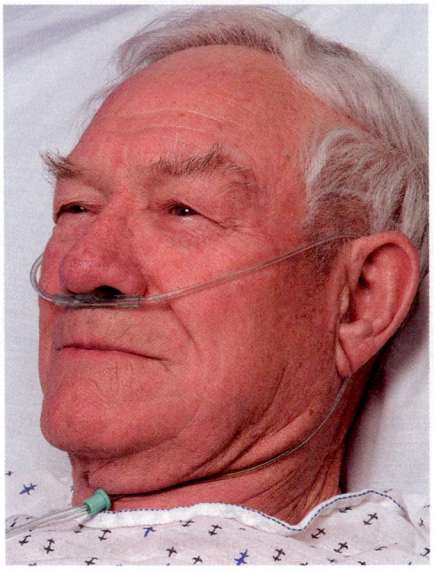

Procedure Variation for Face Mask
Follow Steps 1 through 4.

8. **Gently place the mask** on the patient's face, applying it from the bridge of the nose to under the chin.

9. **Secure the elastic band** around the back of the patient's head. Make sure the mask fits snugly but comfortably. Then proceed to Step 12.
The mask must fit snugly so that oxygen cannot escape around the edges of the mask. If the mask is too tight, it may cause skin breakdown.▼

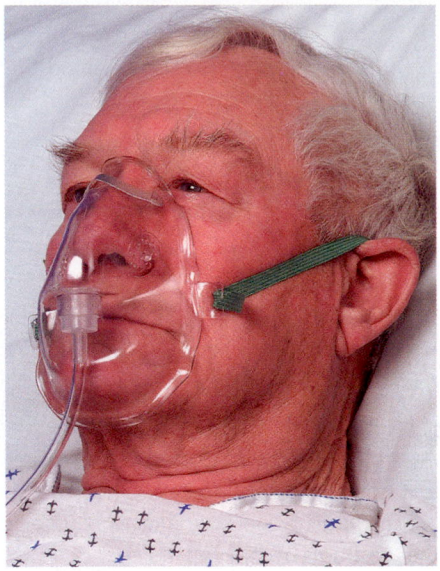

Procedure Variation for Face Tent
Follow Steps 1 through 4.

10. **Gently place the face tent** in front of the patient's face, making sure that it fits under the chin.

11. **Secure the elastic band** around the back of the patient's head.
To keep the face tent in place.▼

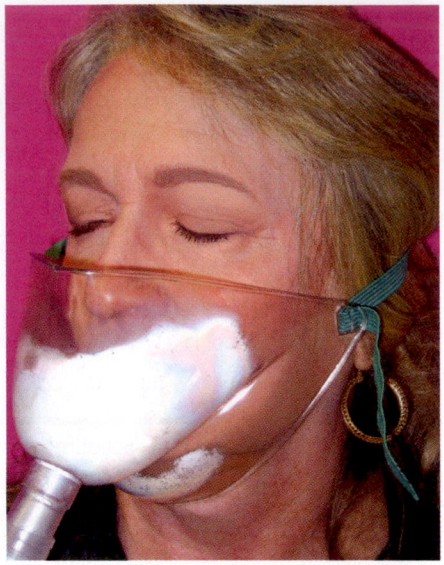

12. **Double-check that the oxygen** equipment is set up correctly and functioning properly.
Ensures that the oxygen is delivered at the prescribed rate. Oxygen delivered at an incorrect rate can cause patient injury.

13. **Assess the patient's respiratory** status before leaving the bedside.
To be certain it is safe to leave the patient.

Evaluation

- Assess respiratory rate, depth, and effort.
- Auscultate breath sounds before leaving the bedside, then monitor every 2 to 4 hours, and as indicated.
- Monitor pulse oximetry until respiratory status improves.
- Monitor ABG results if prescribed.
- Evaluate for skin breakdown, especially behind the ears, cheekbones, and under the chin—areas that are in contact with the oxygen delivery system.
- Notify the primary provider of respiratory status, oxygen, and response and any additional prescriptions needed.

Patient Teaching

- Demonstrate oxygen administration to the patient and caregiver if the patient will be continuing oxygen therapy at home. Allow for time to answer questions, and return demonstration of attaching and placing oxygen on.
- Explain the importance of immediately reporting shortness of breath or any difficulty breathing to the nursing staff before discharge. If the patient is at home, he will need to report the difficulty to the home health and/or primary care provider, and, if needed, to call 911.

Home Care

- Explain to the client and caregivers where to obtain oxygen equipment and what services are available. Make sure they choose a supplier who has 24-hour emergency services.
- Instruct the client and caregiver about oxygen therapy and its use as well as safety measures that they must institute. Safety measures include keeping oxygen away from items that may cause ignition such as lighters, cigarettes, fireplaces, heaters, etc.
- To demonstrate the oxygen is on, client can hold nasal prongs on the side of the cheek to feel air flow or over a glass of water to see air moving water.

- Teach the client and caregiver to clean the nasal cannula or face mask with soap and warm water when it becomes soiled, and allow the mask to air-dry.
- Provide contact information for healthcare personnel who can be reached for advice or emergencies.
- Explain the importance of immediately reporting shortness of breath or any difficulty breathing to the home health and/or primary care provider; and if needed, to call 911.
- In the home, liquid oxygen and oxygen concentrators are more commonly used than portable oxygen tanks. Liquid oxygen may be kept in small, portable containers; an oxygen concentrator removes nitrogen from room air and concentrates O_2. It requires a battery pack or electrical outlet for power. Oxygen concentrators can deliver a flow of 6 to 8 L/min.

Documentation

- Document the date, time, and reason oxygen therapy was initiated.
- Note the type of oxygen delivery system used, the amount of oxygen administered, and the patient's response to oxygen therapy.
- Document vital signs, pulse oximetry values, breath sounds, skin color, and respiratory effort.

Sample documentation

12/14/15 2015. Patient developed acute shortness of breath. RR 36/min & labored, P = 126 beats/min, and BP 212/110 mm Hg. Pulse ox 80% on room air. Crackles and expiratory wheezes auscultated throughout both lungs. Dr. Chow notified of patient's condition. Oxygen with partial rebreather mask @ 10 L/min and Lasix 40 mg IV prescribed and administered. Pulse ox using partial rebreather = 90%. S. Peters, RN

Practice Resources

Lippincott's Nursing Procedures (2012).

Oxygen Delivery Systems

DELIVERY METHOD	FIO_2	DISCUSSION	NURSING RESPONSIBILITIES
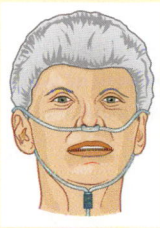 Nasal cannula	1 L/min = 24% 2 L/min = 28% 3 L/min = 32% 4 L/min = 36% 5 L/min = 40% 6 L/min = 44%	▪ Relatively comfortable. ▪ Patients can eat, talk, and cough with a nasal cannula in place. ▪ Works best if the patient breathes through his nose.	▪ Check frequently that the prongs are in the patient's nose. ▪ Assess for dryness of the nasal mucosa. ▪ Humidify flow at rates above 3 L/min (flow rates >3 L/min are drying). ▪ Encourage the patient to take slow, deep breaths so he will inhale more oxygen and less room air.
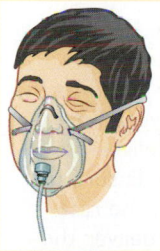 **Simple face mask:** A clear, flexible mask that covers the nose and mouth and delivers oxygen flow into the mask.	5–10 L/min = 40%–60% FIO_2	▪ Requires flow rates greater than 5 L/min to prevent accumulation and rebreathing of exhaled CO_2 from within the mask. ▪ Masks are not easily tolerated because they fit tightly and keep heat from radiating from the face, making patients feel hot. ▪ Talking is muffled by the mask, and it must be removed for the patient to eat or drink.	▪ Place face mask securely over the mouth and nose. ▪ Elastic straps fit around the head to hold the mask in place. Place the straps well above the ears to prevent skin irritation and breakdown. ▪ Place gauze or other soft material beneath the straps to prevent irritation. ▪ Check the skin around the mask frequently. ▪ Check the skin over the ears where the mask strap rubs. ▪ Encourage the patient to take slow, deep breaths, so he will inhale more oxygen and less room air.

(continued on next page)

Oxygen Delivery Systems—cont'd

DELIVERY METHOD	FIO_2	DISCUSSION	NURSING RESPONSIBILITIES
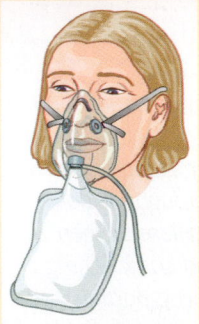 **Partial rebreather mask:** Uses the reservoir bag to capture some exhaled gas for rebreathing	6–15 L/min = 50%–90% FIO_2	▪ Allows higher FIO_2 levels to be delivered because O_2 is collected in the reservoir bag for inhalation. ▪ Exhalation ports allow most exhaled air to escape. ▪ Several types are available. ▪ Can deliver an FIO_2 above 50% at flow rates of 6–15 L/min. ▪ Patient rebreathes some exhaled air along with O_2.	▪ Maintain the flow at a high enough rate to prevent the reservoir bag from collapsing during inhalation. ▪ Encourage the patient to take slow, deep breaths, so he will inhale more oxygen and less room air.
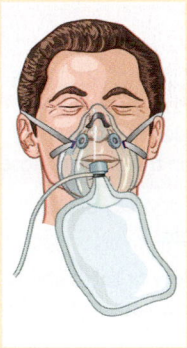 **Nonrebreather mask:** A type of reservoir bag mask; a valve keeps exhaled air from entering the reservoir bag.	6–15 L/min = 70%–100% FIO_2	▪ Contains only O_2, which allows higher FIO_2 delivery. An FIO_2 of 60%–100% can be delivered at flow rates of 6–15 L/min. ▪ This mask is the only external device capable of delivering an FIO_2 of 100% (in practice, it is rare to achieve a concentration above 75% because the mask does not seal perfectly with the face).	▪ Maintain the flow at a rate high enough to keep the reservoir at least one-third to one-half full during inhalation. ▪ Be sure the mask fits snugly so the patient will breathe in less room air.
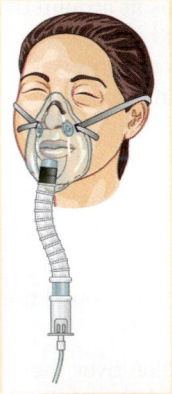 **Venturi mask:** A cone-shaped adapter that serves as a mixing valve to control the amount of O_2 and room air that flows through the mask.	24%–50% FIO_2	▪ The cone-shaped adapter at the base of the mask allows a precise FIO_2 to be delivered. This is very useful for patients with chronic lung disease. ▪ Exhalation ports keep CO_2 buildup to a minimum.	▪ The adapter indicates the required oxygen flow rate needed to deliver the desired FIO_2. Ensure that flow is set at the rate specified to deliver the FIO_2 desired.

Oxygen Delivery Systems—cont'd

DELIVERY METHOD	FIO_2	DISCUSSION	NURSING RESPONSIBILITIES
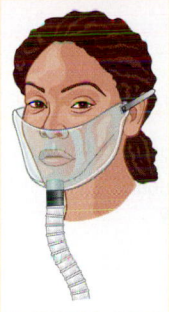 **Face tent:** A large, open plastic mask that fits under the chin. It is open at the top and is held in place with an elastic band around the head.	8–12 L/min = 30%–55% FIO_2	▪ Less reliable than a face mask for delivering precise FIO_2 levels. ▪ Allows moderate- to high-density aerosol delivery for humidification. ▪ Patients who feel claustrophobic in a face mask often tolerate a face tent.	▪ Check the skin over the ears where the mask strap rubs.
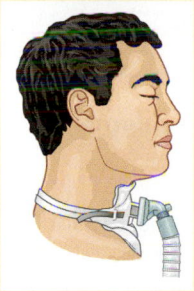 **Tracheostomy collar:** A small, cup-shaped device that fits over the tracheostomy opening and is held in place with elastic straps around the neck.	4–10 L/min = 24%–100% FIO_2	▪ It is possible to deliver both high FIO_2 and high humidity with a tracheostomy collar. ▪ Large-bore tubing is used to deliver humidification to the trachea; however, water frequently condenses inside the tubing and can be accidentally drained into the tracheostomy. Usually, a water trap of some sort is placed in the tubing to prevent this problem.	▪ Watch for water accumulation in the tubing.
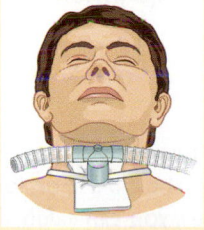 **T-piece:** A T-shaped plastic piece; the bottom of the T fits directly and tightly onto the tracheostomy tube.	4–10 L/min = 24%–100% FIO_2	▪ Oxygen and humidity are delivered into one side of the T and exhaled through the other side.	▪ Take care that the oxygen delivery tubing does not pull on the T-piece, which can dislodge the tracheostomy tube and create an airway emergency.

Thinking About the Procedure

To practice applying clinical reasoning to this procedure,

Go to *Davis's Nursing Skills Videos*, **Administering Oxygen.**

For questions and suggested responses,

Go to Chapter 36, **Thinking About the Procedure Questions and Suggested Responses,** on Davis*Plus*.

Procedure 36-5 ■ Performing Tracheostomy Care Using Sterile Technique

- For steps to follow in *all* procedures, refer to the Universal Steps for All Procedures found on the inside back cover.
- Also refer to Clinical Insight 36-4.
- Recall that the basic differences in sterile and modified sterile technique are that modified sterile technique uses a sterile catheter and supplies, but nonsterile procedure gloves.

Equipment

- Tracheostomy suction equipment (see Procedure 36-6)
- Tracheostomy care kit or the following sterile supplies: several cotton-tip applicators, two basins, a brush, sterile 4 in. × 4 in. gauze pads, sterile precut tracheostomy dressing
- Two pairs of sterile gloves (for modified sterile technique, use procedure gloves)
- Disposable inner cannula that is the same size as the tracheostomy, if available. Most tracheostomy tubes have disposable inner cannulas.
- Sterile normal saline solution (for modified sterile technique, you can use distilled or filtered water if agency policy allows)
- Hydrogen peroxide for cleaning of reusable inner cannula only
- Roll of twill tape or hook and loop fastener (Velcro) tracheostomy holder
- Bandage scissors
- Towel or linen-saver pad
- Overbed table
- Face shield and protective gown
- For modified sterile technique: disposable prepackaged wipes, or washcloth and distilled water and soap

Use only the sterile precut dressing, or open and refold a 4 in. × 4 in. gauze pad into a V-shape. Do not cut 4 in. × 4 in. gauze, and do not use cotton-filled gauze squares. The patient may aspirate the cotton or gauze fibers.

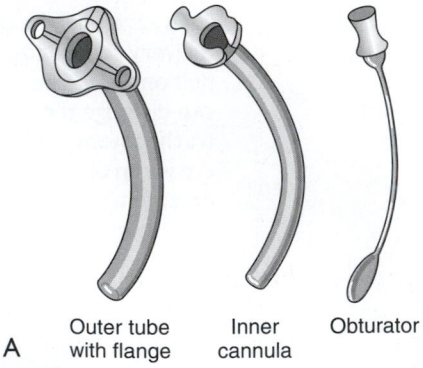

***A*, Nondisposable tracheostomy equipment**

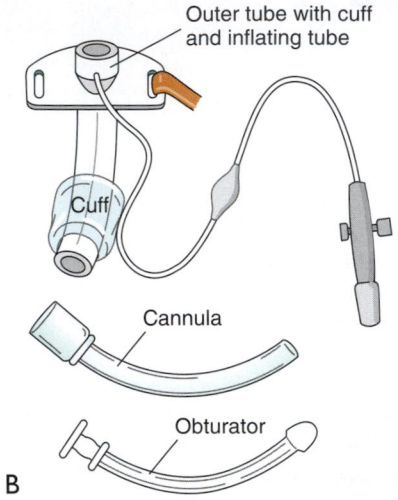

***B*, Disposable tracheostomy equipment**

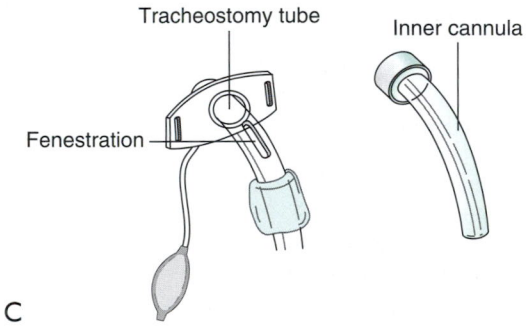

***C*, Fenestrated tracheostomy equipment**

Delegation

In acute care settings and with new tracheostomies, you should not delegate this procedure to the NAP. For long-standing and well-healed tracheostomies, you can safely delegate care to a NAP or LPN who is adequately trained to perform the skill. This varies by state. In some states only RNs can perform tracheostomy care. If you are not familiar with your state's nurse practice act, contact your state board of nursing.

Pre-Procedure Assessment

- Assess respiratory rate, depth, and rhythm; breath sounds; color; and pulse oximetry results.
  Helps determine whether the patient can tolerate tracheostomy care.
- Assess the tracheostomy site for drainage, redness, or swelling.
  Drainage, redness, or swelling may indicate infection.
- Determine when the patient last ate.
  It is best to schedule this procedure at least 3 hours after a meal to decrease the risk of the patient vomiting and aspirating stomach contents.

➤ When performing the procedure, always identify your patient according to agency policy, using two identifiers, and be attentive to standard precautions, hand hygiene, patient safety and privacy, body mechanics, and documentation.

➤ *Note:* Asterisks indicate steps that differ when using modified sterile technique.

Procedure Steps

1. **Position the patient** in semi-Fowler's position, and place a towel or linen-saver pad over the patient's chest.
   A semi-Fowler's position promotes lung expansion and prevents back strain for the nurse. A towel or linen-saver pad prevents soiling of the patient's gown.

*2. **Don sterile gloves, gown, and** face shield or mask.
   **(For modified sterile technique, don clean procedure gloves.)*

When Using One Sterile Glove

Put a sterile glove on your dominant hand and a clean glove on your other hand.

3. **Hyperoxygenate the patient as needed,** and suction the tracheostomy (see Procedure 36-6 or 36-7).
   Suctioning clears the tracheostomy of secretions that could occlude the outer cannula after the inner cannula is removed for care.

For a Passy–Muir Valve

Remove the Passy–Muir valve (PMV) before suctioning the patient to prepare for tracheostomy care. (A PMV is a device that is used to enable the patient with a tracheostomy to speak. It is attached to the end of the inner cannula at the tracheostomy site.)

4. **Remove and discard** the soiled tracheostomy dressing in the appropriate receptacle, and then remove and discard your gloves. Perform hand hygiene.

5. **Place the tracheostomy care** equipment on the overbed table, and prepare the equipment, using sterile technique.
   Ensures efficiency and helps maintain sterility during tracheostomy care.

*a. *Disposable inner cannula*—Pour sterile normal saline solution into the two sterile containers.
   **(For modified sterile technique, use filtered tap water or sterile normal saline, per agency policy).*

b. *Reusable inner cannula*—Pour hydrogen peroxide into one of the sterile solution containers, and pour normal saline solution into the other one. If the inner cannula is not disposable, use hydrogen peroxide to clean only the inner cannula. Use the sterile normal saline (or sterile water) to rinse the inner cannula and clean the faceplate and tracheostomy site.

*c. *Steps c through g apply to both types of cannula.* Open two 4 in. × 4 in. gauze packages. Wet the gauze in one package with sterile normal saline, and keep the second package dry. (For modified sterile technique, instead of sterile gauze you may use disposable prepackaged wipes).
   You will use the second package of gauze to dry the skin around the tracheostomy site after cleaning.

*d. Open one cotton-tip applicator package. Wet the applicators with normal saline solution. (For modified sterile technique, wet the applicators with filtered tap water or normal saline solution.)
   Prepares the applicators for cleaning the exposed surface of the outer cannula and the stoma site located under the faceplate of the tracheostomy tube, respectively.

e. Open the package containing a new disposable inner cannula.
   Allows for quick replacement of the inner cannula.

f. Open the package of Velcro tracheostomy ties, or cut a length of twill tape long enough to go around the patient's neck two times. Make sure to cut end of the tape on an angle.
   Allows for quick stabilization of the tracheostomy tube, preventing dislodgement. Cutting the twill tape on an angle allows for easy insertion through the faceplate eyelets.

g. Position a biohazard receptacle within reach.
   Allows you to dispose of contaminated supplies safely as you use them without leaving the patient or interrupting the procedure.

*6. **Don sterile gloves** (or a sterile glove on your dominant hand and a clean glove on your nondominant hand); keep the glove on your dominant hand sterile. Handle the sterile supplies with the dominant hand only.
   **(For modified sterile technique, don clean procedure gloves. Consider your dominant hand to be clean and handle supplies with that hand only.)*

7. **For patients receiving oxygen:** With your nondominant (nonsterile) hand, remove the oxygen or humidification source. Attach the oxygen source to the outer cannula, if possible. If not possible, have the respiratory therapist set up oxygen blow-by to use while you are cleaning the reusable inner cannula.
   Prevents oxygen desaturation in the patient during the procedure.

(continued on next page)

Procedure 36-5 ■ Performing Tracheostomy Care Using Sterile Technique (continued)

8. Unlock and remove the inner cannula with your nondominant hand, and care for it accordingly.

For a Disposable Inner Cannula

a. **Dispose of the inner cannula** in the biohazard receptacle according to agency policy. You should never clean and reuse a disposable inner cannula.
Prevents contamination by bacteria contained in the inner cannula.

*b. **With your dominant hand**, insert the new inner cannula into the patient's tracheostomy in the direction of the curvature. Following the manufacturer's instructions, lock the inner cannula in place securely to prevent it from dislodging. Remember to keep your dominant hand sterile.
**For modified sterile technique, keep dominant hand clean.*

For a Reusable Inner Cannula

c. If a reusable inner cannula was used, place the inner cannula into the basin filled with hydrogen peroxide.
Hydrogen peroxide helps loosen tenacious (sticky) secretions.

d. Pick up the reusable inner cannula from the container of hydrogen peroxide with your nonsterile hand, and scrub it with the sterile nylon brush, using your sterile dominant hand. ▼

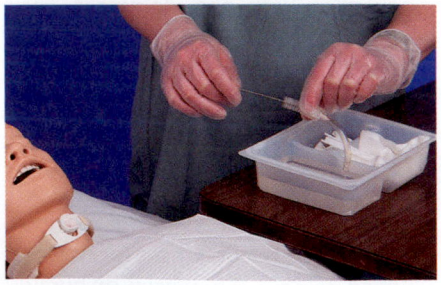

*e. Immerse the inner cannula in the container of sterile normal saline solution (for modified sterile procedure, tap water or normal saline), and agitate it until it is rinsed thoroughly.
Immersing the inner cannula in normal saline solution and agitating it removes the hydrogen peroxide (which can cause tissue irritation) and debris from the inner cannula.

*f. Tap the inner cannula against the side of the container. (For modified sterile technique, shake the cannula to remove water.)
Removes excess fluid so the patient does not aspirate it when you reinsert the cannula.

g. With your dominant hand, reinsert the inner cannula into the patient's tracheostomy in the direction of the curvature. Following the manufacturer's instructions, snap or lock the inner cannula in place securely to prevent it from dislodging. Remember to keep your dominant hand sterile.

For a Passy–Muir Valve

h. Swish the PMV in warm filtered tap water with mild soap.

i. Rinse the PMV thoroughly in warm filtered tap water.

j. DO NOT use hot water, peroxide, bleach, vinegar, alcohol, brushes, or cotton-tip applicators to clean PMV, as this could damage the valve.

k. Shake the PMV to remove excess fluid. If you are going to store the valve, be sure to air-dry the valve before placing it in a storage container.
Removes moisture, which can promote bacterial growth.

l. Set the PMV aside on clean surface to be replaced when the inner cannula is replaced.

For Patients Receiving Oxygen

m. Remove the humidification or oxygen source from the outer cannula, if indicated, using your nondominant hand.

n. Reinsert the inner cannula into the patient's tracheostomy in the direction of the curvature.

o. Following the manufacturer's instructions, lock the inner cannula in place securely. Remember to keep dominant hand sterile.
Lock the inner cannula in place securely to prevent it from dislodging.

p. Reattach the humidification or oxygen source, if indicated.
Provides the patient with needed humidity or oxygen and prevents oxygen desaturation.

***9. Clean the stoma** under the faceplate with cotton-tip applicators saturated with sterile normal saline solution, using a circular motion from the stoma site outward. Use each applicator only once, and then discard it.
*(If using modified sterile technique, applicators may be saturated with filtered tap water or you can use disposable prepackaged wipes.)
Prevents contamination of the cleaned area. ▼

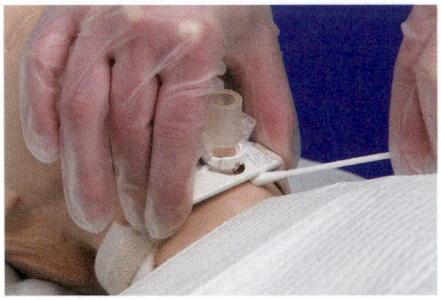

***10. Clean the top surface** of the faceplate and the skin around it with the gauze pads saturated with sterile normal saline solution. Use each gauze pad only once, and then discard it.
*(For modified sterile technique, use the gauze pads if they are contained in the tracheostomy kit, saturated with distilled or filtered tap water.)
Removes secretions that provide a prime medium for microbial growth; prevents contamination of cleaned areas.

11. Dry the skin and outer cannula surfaces by patting them lightly with the remaining dry gauze pad.
Clean, dry skin is needed to avoid skin breakdown and removes moisture, which can promote bacterial growth around the stoma site.

*12. **Seek assistance** from another staff member to help with changing the tracheostomy stabilizers.
Prevents accidental dislodging should the patient begin coughing during the procedure.

13. **Remove soiled tracheostomy stabilizers.**

Removing a Soiled Velcro Tracheostomy Holder

a. With an assistant stabilizing the tracheostomy tube, disengage the Velcro on both sides of the soiled holder, and remove it gently from the eyes of the faceplate. Discard the Velcro holder in the nearest biohazard receptacle.
Removing the soiled holder promotes hygiene and prevents the spread of infection.

Removing Soiled Twill Tape Tracheostomy Ties

b. With an assistant stabilizing the tracheostomy tube, cut the soiled tracheostomy ties using bandage scissors. *Do not* cut the tube of the tracheostomy balloon (if you do, the tracheostomy tube must be replaced). Remove the ties gently from the eyes of the faceplate, and discard them in the nearest biohazard receptacle.
The tracheostomy balloon helps stabilize the tracheostomy in the trachea and prevents an air leak. Cutting the tube to the balloon prevents the balloon from holding air. Removing the soiled holder promotes hygiene and prevents the spread of infection.

14. **Ask the patient to flex** his neck; if he is unable, ask the assistant to hold the patient's head forward, and apply new tracheostomy ties.
Flexing the neck provides the same neck circumference as when the patient coughs and thus ensures you do not place and secure the tracheostomy stabilizers too tightly.

For a Velcro Tracheostomy Holder

a. Thread one end of the Velcro through the eyelet of the faceplate, and fasten it.

b. Bring the holder around the back of the patient's neck.
The holder must be placed around the patient's neck to adequately secure the tracheostomy.

c. Thread the remaining end of the Velcro strap through the empty eyelet of the faceplate and fasten it, making sure that the holder fits securely.

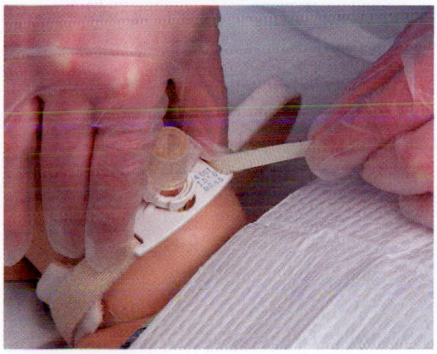

d. Place one finger under the stabilizer to make sure that it is securing the tracheostomy effectively but isn't too tight.
Securing the tracheostomy too tightly might place pressure on the jugular veins; interfere with coughing; or cause necrosis at the tracheostomy insertion site.

Using Twill Tape

e. Thread one end of the twill tape into one of the eyelets on the tracheostomy faceplate.

f. Continue to thread the twill tape through the eyelet, bringing both ends of the tape together.

g. Bring both ends of the twill tape around the back of the patient's neck.
To adequately secure the tracheostomy.

h. Thread the end of the twill tape that is closest to the patient's neck through the back of the eyelet on the faceplate.

i. Have your assistant place one finger under the twill tape while you tie the two ends together in a square knot.
Ensures you do not secure the tracheostomy too tightly.

j. Place one finger under the holder to make sure that the holder is securing the tracheostomy effectively but isn't too tight.
See Step 14d.

15. **Don a new pair of sterile gloves,** and insert a precut, sterile tracheostomy dressing under the faceplate and new tracheostomy stabilizers or fold a 4 in. × 4 in. gauze pad into a V shape (below).

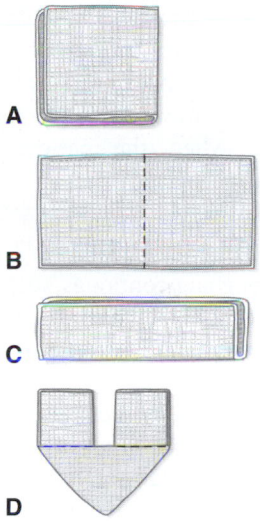

The new dressing absorbs secretions and prevents skin breakdown under the faceplate. Never cut the gauze to make a dressing because lint and fibers from the cut edge could enter the trachea and cause respiratory distress.

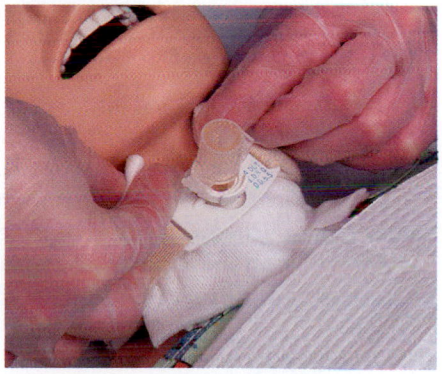

16. **Dispose of the used equipment** in the appropriate biohazard receptacle according to agency policy.
Helps prevent cross-contamination.

(continued on next page)

Procedure 36-5 ■ Performing Tracheostomy Care Using Sterile Technique (continued)

? What if . . .

- **Your patient begins coughing?**
  a. If the tracheostomy is still secured with ties or Velcro holder, wait to continue tracheostomy care until coughing has ended.
  b. If the tracheostomy is unsecured, stabilize the tube so that it does not become dislodged, being careful not to press too hard on the site. Continue with tracheostomy care when the patient finishes coughing.
  Pressing too hard at the tracheostomy site will stimulate the coughing reflex.
  c. If coughing continues, suspend tracheostomy care and suction the patient to remove any retained secretions.
  Retained secretions may cause increased airway irritation and coughing. Removing these secretions will reduce this irritation.

- **You do not have an assistant to hold the cannula in place while you replace the soiled tracheostomy ties?**

  Never cut the soiled tape before applying the clean tape. Always place the new tape/holders, be certain the tracheostomy is secured, and then cut off the soiled tape or holder.

- **The tracheostomy tube becomes dislodged?**
  a. To prevent this, plan ahead and always have another staff member with you to secure the tracheostomy tube while you change the tracheostomy ties or Velcro holder.
  b. If the tracheostomy tube slips out slightly but is still in the trachea site, gently push it back into the stoma and secure it.
  The pilot balloon will help to keep the tracheostomy tube from completely dislodging.
  c. If the tracheostomy tube becomes completely dislodged, stay with the patient and ask your assistant to call for the respiratory therapist or trained person in your facility to insert a new tracheostomy tube.

- **At Step 9, there are crusts around the stoma when you are cleaning the stoma?**

  Remove the crusts with a cotton-tip swab soaked in hydrogen peroxide; then rinse with a swab soaked in normal saline (or filtered tap water in modified sterile technique). Have the patient hold his breath while you remove crusts so he does not inhale them.

Evaluation

- Assess the area around the stoma site for signs of skin breakdown.
- Evaluate the patient's tolerance of the procedure. Note whether there were any signs of respiratory distress.

Patient Teaching

- Explain to the patient and his family that bloody secretions are normal for 2 to 3 days after tracheostomy tube insertion or for 24 hours after a tracheostomy tube change.
- Tell the patient and/or family to inform the nurse immediately if the tracheostomy tube becomes dislodged.
- Teach tracheostomy care to the patient and caregiver if the tracheostomy is expected to remain long term.

Home Care

- Clean technique can be used for tracheostomy care if the tracheostomy is more than 1 month old.
- Instruct the client and caregiver about home oxygen therapy and suctioning, if necessary.
- Demonstrate tracheostomy care to the caregiver, and ask for a return demonstration.
- Provide the client and caregiver with information about where to obtain tracheostomy care supplies.
- Supply the client and caregiver with contact information of healthcare personnel who can be reached for advice or emergencies.
- Recommend ways of adding moisture to the air, with a goal of maintaining a relative humidity of 50% (e.g., a large humidifier, house plants, wearing damp gauze over the stoma, closing the bathroom door and turning on the hot water to fill the room with steam).
- The stoma should be cleaned, using clean technique, at least twice daily (or more often, depending on the amount of secretions).
- Stress handwashing before and after doing any part of tracheostomy care.
- Remind client and caregiver not to use cotton or gauze.
  These can leave fibers that may get into the airway and increase the incidence of infection.

Documentation

- Document the date and time that you performed tracheostomy care.
- Note the color, amount, consistency, and odor of secretions.
- Note the condition of the stoma and skin around the stoma site, and the presence of drainage, redness, or swelling.
- Document respiratory rate, depth, and pattern; skin color; and breath sounds.

- Document the patient's tolerance of the procedure.
- If problems arose, document any interventions that were necessary.

Sample documentation

Note: Because this is only a partial computer screen, it may not show all the information you would need to record about the patient.

Thinking About the Procedure

To practice applying clinical reasoning to this procedure,

Go to *Davis's Nursing Skills Videos*, **Performing Tracheostomy Care Using Sterile Technique.**

For questions and suggested responses,

Go to Chapter 36, **Thinking About the Procedure Questions and Suggested Responses,** on Davis*Plus*

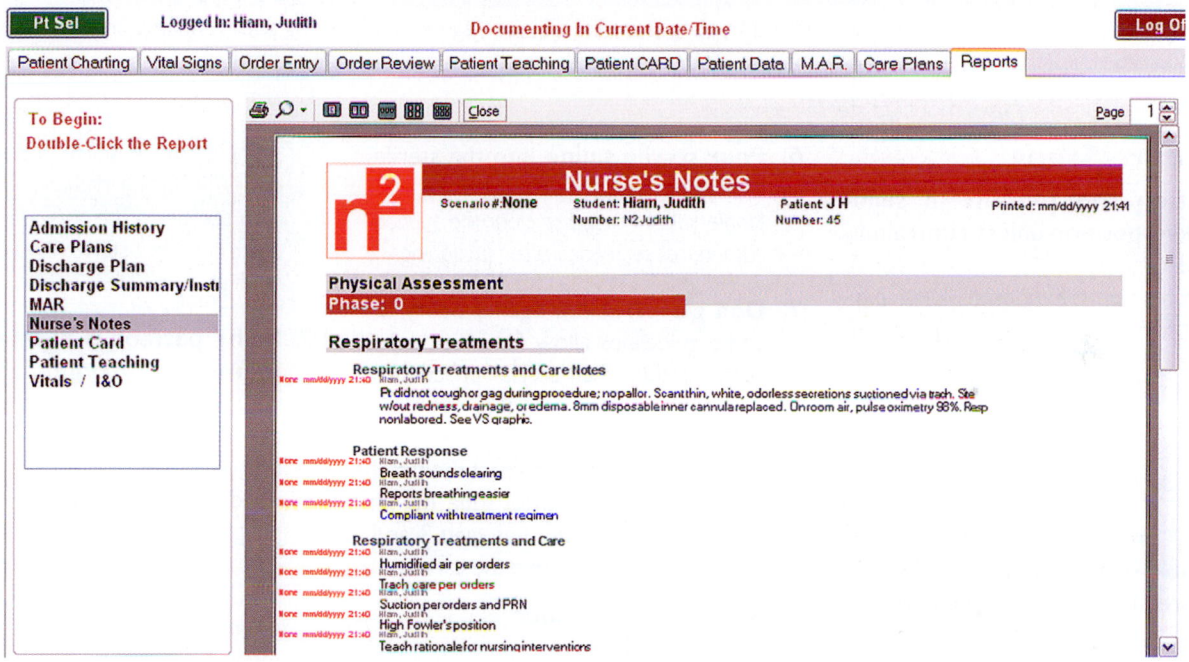

Practice Resources

Barnett, M. (2012); Johnston, J., Davis, S., & Sherman, J. (n.d.); Kozin, E., Straton, J., & Kapo, J. (2012); Mitchell, R. B., Hussey, H. M., Setzen, G., et al. (2013); National Guideline Clearinghouse (2011); Siddiqui, J., Sherren, P. B., & Birchall, M. A. (2013); Siegel, J., Rhinehart, E., Jackson, M., et al. (2007).

Procedure 36-6 ■ Performing Tracheostomy Suctioning (Open System)

➤ For steps to follow in *all* procedures, refer to the Universal Steps for All Procedures found on the inside back cover.

Equipment

- Portable or wall suction device with tubing and a collection canister
- Linen-saver pad or towel
- Resuscitation bag connected to oxygen source
- Sterile suction catheter kit: adults: 12 to 18 Fr; children: 8 to 10 Fr; infants: 5 to 8 Fr
- If a kit isn't available, collect the following: sterile gloves, sterile suction catheter of the appropriate size, and a sterile container.
- Pour-bottle of sterile, normal saline solution
- Sterile basin or container for fluids
- Prefilled 10-mL containers of normal saline solution
- Face shield or goggles
- Sterile gloves (or procedure gloves; follow agency policy)
- Protective gown

Delegation

As a rule you should not delegate tracheostomy suctioning to an LPN or NAP, because the procedure requires professional-level theoretical knowledge, assessment skills, and problem-solving ability. However, if the patient has a permanent tracheostomy tube in place and the patient will require long-term care, care can be delegated to trained personnel. Refer to individual state board of nursing for rules on delegating this procedure.

(continued on next page)

Procedure 36-6 ■ Performing Tracheostomy Suctioning (Open System) (continued)

Pre-Procedure Assessment

- Assess the respiratory rate, depth, and rhythm; breath sounds; color; and pulse oximetry results.
- Assess for signs that indicate the need for suctioning: restlessness, cyanosis, labored respirations, decreased oxygen saturation, increased heart and respiratory rates, visible secretions in the airway, increased peak airway pressures on the ventilator, decreasing SaO_2 or PaO_2, and adventitious breath sounds during auscultation.
  Suctioning should be performed only when necessary to prevent unnecessary oxygen desaturation and tissue trauma.

➤ When performing the procedure, always identify your patient according to agency policy, using two identifiers, and be attentive to standard precautions, hand hygiene, patient safety and privacy, body mechanics, and documentation.

➤ *Note:* This procedure uses modified sterile technique.

Procedure Steps

1. **Position the patient** in semi-Fowler's position unless contraindicated.
   Promotes lung expansion and oxygenation.

2. **Place the linen-saver pad** or towel on the patient's chest.
   Prevents soiling of the patient's gown during suctioning.

3. **Turn on the wall suction** or portable suction machine, and adjust the pressure regulator according to agency policy, using the lowest possible suction pressure. Typically, this is:
   Adults: 100 to 150 mm Hg
   Children: 100 to 120 mm Hg
   Infants: 50 to 95 mm Hg
   Using the appropriate pressure prevents tissue trauma and ensures successful suctioning. Higher pressures are associated with hypoxemia, tissue trauma, and atelectasis, yet do not improve removal of secretions.

4. **Don a nonsterile glove** and face shield or goggles. Test the suction equipment by occluding the connection tubing. Remove and discard the glove. Perform hand hygiene.
   Protective clothing protects you from contamination with secretions that may splash during suctioning. Testing the suction ensures proper functioning before you insert suction catheter.

5. **Open the suction catheter kit** or (if a kit isn't available) the gathered equipment. Maintain sterility of the inside of the suction kit or the gathered equipment.
   This prevents contaminating the airway when you introduce the suction catheter.

6. **Pour sterile saline** into the sterile container.
   Sterile saline is used to clear the suction catheter of secretions after suctioning.

7. **Don gloves.** Follow agency policy, as some guidelines allow for clean nonsterile rather than sterile procedure gloves; follow agency policy. Premeasure the catheter insertion distance for 0.5 to 1 cm (¼ to ½ in.) past the distal end of the endotracheal tube (ETT); the ETT normally sits between 3 and 7 cm (1 to 2¾ in.) above the carina.

   If Using Sterile Technique

   a. Don sterile gloves. Consider your dominant hand sterile and your nondominant hand unsterile.

   If Using Modified Sterile Technique

   b. Don clean nonsterile gloves. Consider your dominant hand clean and your nondominant hand contaminated.
   Keeping your dominant hand sterile (or clean, depending on the technique) prevents contamination of the suction catheter.

8. **Pick up the suction catheter** with your dominant hand, and attach it to the connection tubing. Do not touch the connection tubing with your sterile (or clean) glove.
   Prepares the suction catheter for use.

9. **Put the tip of the suction** catheter into the sterile container of normal saline solution, and suction a small amount through the suction catheter. Apply suction by placing a finger over the suction control port of the suction catheter.
   Lubricates the catheter and helps ensure that the suction equipment is functioning properly. Sterile saline is necessary to clear the suction catheter of secretions after suctioning. The outside of the saline container is not sterile; it would contaminate your dominant hand.

10. **If the patient is receiving supplemental oxygen**, hyperoxygenate the patient according to agency policy. If the patient does not require oxygen, you do not need to hyperoxygenate.
    Helps prevent hypoxia and related complications (cardiac arrhythmias, seizures, arrest) during suctioning. Suctioning clears secretions, but it also removes oxygen from airways.

    If the Patient Requires Mechanical Ventilation

    a. Press the 100% O_2 button on the ventilator. Some agencies require the nurse to manually hyperoxygenate the patient; follow agency policy.
    Ventilators typically have a button that allows you to hyperoxygenate the patient for a total of 2 minutes. Once this time period elapses, the ventilator automatically resumes its previous settings.

    If the Patient Does Not Require Mechanical Ventilation

    b. Obtain the assistance of a second provider.
    c. Have your partner attach the resuscitation bag to the tracheostomy tube, and hyperoxygenate the patient by compressing the resuscitation bag three to five times as the patient inhales. Remove the resuscitation bag, and place it next to the patient when finished.

You must perform hyperoxygenation manually if the patient does not require mechanical ventilation.▼

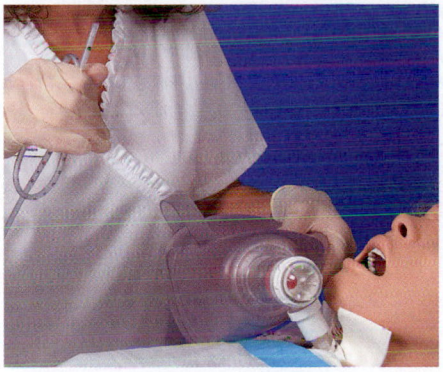

11. **Perform suctioning.**
    a. Lubricate the suction catheter tip with the normal saline solution.
    Lubrication eases passage of the suction catheter through the tracheostomy tube.
    b. Using your dominant hand, gently but quickly insert the suction catheter into the tracheostomy tube.▼

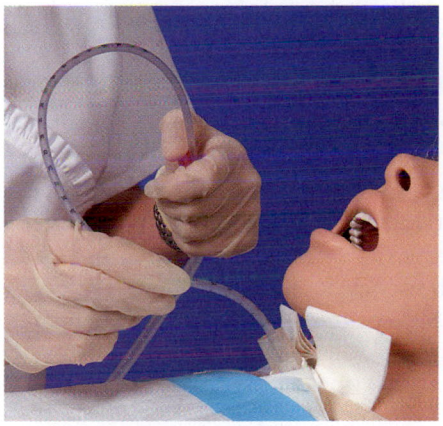

    c. ✚ Advance the suction catheter, with suction off, gently aiming downward, and being careful not to force the catheter. Insert to the premeasured length: no farther than the **carina tracheae** (the ridge at the lower end of the trachea that separates the openings of the two mainstem bronchi); do not insert more than 6 inches (15 cm), and do not force against any resistance.
    Forcing the catheter during insertion may cause tissue trauma.
    d. Apply suction while you withdraw the catheter; rotate the catheter (roll it between your thumb and forefinger) as you remove it. Make sure to apply suction for no longer than 15 seconds.
    Applying suction for longer than 15 seconds causes hypoxia and may cause tissue trauma.

12. **Repeat suctioning as needed.**
    Several passes with the suction catheter may be needed to clear the airway of secretions.
    a. Allow at least 30-second intervals between suctioning.
    b. Hyperoxygenate the patient between each pass.
    c. Limit total suctioning time to 5 minutes.

13. **Replace the oxygen source** if it was removed during suctioning.
    To prevent hypoxia.

14. **Coil the suction catheter** in your dominant hand (alternatively, wrap it around your dominant hand). Pull the sterile (or clean) glove off over the coiled catheter. Discard the glove containing the catheter in a fluid-resistant receptacle designated by your agency.
    Prevents contaminating the environment with secretions.

15. **Perform hand hygiene**, don clean procedure gloves.

16. **Using your nondominant hand**, clear the connecting tubing of secretions by placing the tip into the container of sterile saline.
    Prepares the tubing for later reuse.

17. **Turn off the** suction units (and the oxygen, if appropriate).

18. **Reposition the patient.**
    Promotes comfort and prevents skin breakdown.

? What if . . .

- **The patient has a cuffed tracheostomy tube?**
  Check to see that it is properly inflated before suctioning. Usually this is 20 to 25 mm Hg or less, but follow the manufacturer's instructions and use a cuff manometer. See Clinical Insight 36-4 to learn how to check cuff inflation.

Evaluation

- Assess the color, amount, and consistency of secretions.
- Evaluate the patient's tolerance of the procedure. (e.g., were there signs of respiratory distress during suctioning?)
- Evaluate the effectiveness of the procedure by comparing breath sounds, vital signs, and pulse oximetry before and after suctioning.

Patient Teaching

- Teach the patient and caregiver how to perform suctioning if the patient will be discharged with an artificial airway. Make sure they can successfully provide a return demonstration.
- Teach the caregiver strategies for managing the patient's airway at home.

Home Care

- Provide the family and caregiver information about where to obtain suction equipment, contact information for healthcare personnel who can be reached for advice or emergencies, and information about home oxygen therapy.
- Guidelines recommend clean technique for home care, and for repeated catheter use as long as the catheter is still clear.
- Teach the family and caregiver how to clean catheters for reuse (soak in hot, soapy water; rinse inside and out with clean water; air-dry; store in a dry container).

(continued on next page)

Procedure 36-6 ■ Performing Tracheostomy Suctioning (Open System) (continued)

Documentation

Document the following:

- Date, time, and reason you performed suctioning.
- The size of the suction catheter you used.
- Amount, color, consistency, and odor of secretions.
- Patient's respiratory status before and after the procedure.
- Patient's tolerance of the procedure.
- Any complications that occurred as a result of the procedure, and interventions you made in response.

Sample documentation

Sept. 18, 2015 0900 Pulse ox 93%, VS elevated, upper airway rhonchi auscultated. Hyperoxygenated with 100% O_2; suctioned moderate amount thick, yellow mucus with #12 Fr suction catheter. After procedure lungs clear, pulse ox 98%, VS WNL.——————Jackie Estes, RN

Practice Resources

Johnston, J., Davis, S., & Sherman, J. (n.d.); Kuriakose, A. (2008); Morrow, B., & Argent, A. (2008); NGC (2010); Rauen, C., Chulay, M., Bridges, E., et al. (2008).

Procedure 36-7 ■ Performing Tracheostomy or Endotracheal Suctioning (Inline Closed System)

➤ For steps to follow in *all* procedures, refer to the Universal Steps for All Procedures found on the inside back cover.

Equipment

For the once-a-day steps: Procedure gloves and inline suction catheter

When suctioning: Sterile normal saline

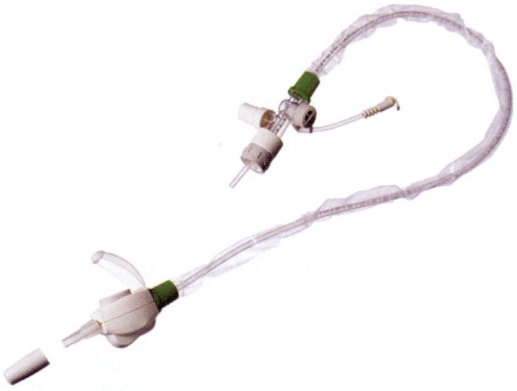

Inline suction catheter. (© Unomedical a/s, used with permission.)

Delegation

As a rule, you should not delegate tracheostomy or endotracheal suctioning to an LPN or NAP, because both procedures require professional-level theoretical knowledge, assessment skills, and problem-solving ability. Refer to the individual state board of nursing for rules on delegating this procedure.

Pre-Procedure Assessment

- Assess respiratory status, including respiratory rate, depth, and rhythm; breath sounds; color; and pulse oximetry results.
- Assess for restlessness, cyanosis, labored respirations, decreased oxygen saturation, increased heart and respiratory rates, visible secretions in the airway, and the presence of adventitious breath sounds during auscultation.

  These assessments help determine whether the patient requires suctioning. Suctioning should be performed only when necessary to prevent unnecessary oxygen desaturation and tissue trauma.

➤ When performing the procedure, always identify your patient according to agency policy, using two identifiers, and be attentive to standard precautions, hand hygiene, patient safety and privacy, body mechanics, and documentation.

➤ *Note:* This procedure uses modified sterile technique.

Daily Procedure Steps

An inline suction unit is available only for patients on a mechanical ventilator. Most agencies require the respiratory therapy department to set up the inline suction equipment. If this is not the agency's policy, you may need to perform these steps once per day:

1. **Open the inline suction** catheter package, using sterile technique.
2. **Remove the adapter** on the ventilator tubing.
3. **Attach the inline suction** catheter equipment to the ventilator tubing.
4. **Reconnect the adapter** on the ventilator tubing.
5. **Attach the other end** of the inline suction catheter to the connection tubing placed to suction.

Suctioning Procedure Steps

1. **Place the patient in semi-Fowler's** position, unless contraindicated.

   The suction catheter is contained within a sterile unit.
2. **Don clean procedure gloves.**

   You do not need to wear sterile gloves.

3. **Place a linen-saver pad** or towel on the patient's chest.

4. **If a lock is present** on the suction control port, unlock it.

5. **Turn on the wall suction** or portable suction machine, and adjust the pressure regulator according to agency policy or provider's prescription.
Using the appropriate pressure prevents tissue trauma and ensures successful suctioning.

6. **Pick up the catheter** with your dominant hand and use your nondominant hand for the suction port.
Using the dominant hand improves dexterity.

7. **Unlock the inline catheter** and gently insert the suction catheter into the airway by maneuvering the catheter within the sterile sleeve. ▼

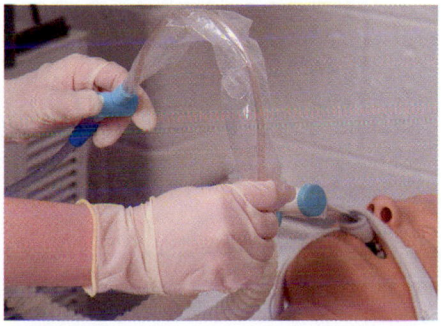

8. **Advance the suction catheter** into the airway, being careful not to force the catheter. Ask the patient to take slow, deep breaths if she can cooperate. Advance the catheter to the predetermined and premarked distance. Do not apply suction while advancing.
Forcing the catheter during insertion may cause airway trauma.

9. **Apply suction** by depressing the button over the suction control port as you withdraw the catheter. Make sure to apply suction for no longer than 15 seconds.
Applying suction for longer than 15 seconds causes hypoxia and may cause tissue trauma.

10. **Withdraw the inline suction** catheter completely into the sleeve. The indicator line on the catheter should appear through the sleeve.
The indicator line is a safety mechanism designed to make sure the suction catheter is withdrawn completely to prevent airway obstruction.

11. **Attach the prefilled 10-mL** container of normal saline solution to the saline port located on the inline equipment.
Provides a flush solution to clear the suction catheter of secretions.

12. **Squeeze the 10-mL container** while applying suction.
Clears the catheter of secretions, preparing the catheter for repeat use. If allowed to remain in the catheter or suction line, secretions may dry and harden, reducing line suction efficiency.

13. **Lock the suction regulator port.**
Prevents you from inadvertently applying suction.

? What if . . .

- **The patient experiences a dysrhythmia?**

  Stop suctioning and hyperoxygenate the patient. If a further attempt at suctioning promotes a dysrhythmia, notify the medical care provider.

For Evaluation, Patient Teaching, and Documentation, see Procedure 36-6. Typically, you would not be doing inline suctioning in the home.

Practice Resources

Cleveland Clinic (2009); Kuriakose, A. (2008); Morrow, B., & Argent, A. (2008); National Guideline Clearinghouse (2010); Restrepo, R. D., Brown, J. M., & Hughes, J. M. (2010).

Thinking About the Procedure

To practice applying clinical reasoning to this procedure,

Go to *Davis's Nursing Skills Videos*, **Performing Tracheostomy Suctioning (Inline Closed System).**

For questions and suggested responses,

Go to Chapter 36, **Thinking About the Procedure Questions and Suggested Responses,** on Davis*Plus*.

Procedure 36-8 ■ Performing Orotracheal and Nasotracheal Suctioning (Open System)

➤ For steps to follow in *all* procedures, refer to the Universal Steps for All Procedures found on the inside back cover.

Equipment

- Portable or wall suction device with connection tubing and a collection canister
- Linen-saver pad or towel
- Sterile, flexible, multiple-eyed suction catheter kit (12 to 18 Fr for adults, 8 to 10 Fr for children, and 5 to 8 Fr for infants). If a kit isn't available, collect the following: sterile gloves, sterile suction catheter of the appropriate size, and a sterile container for fluids
- Pour-bottle of sterile water or sterile normal saline solution
- Face shield or goggles and gown
- Water-soluble lubricant for NT suctioning
- Sputum trap, if a specimen is needed
- Nasopharyngeal airway when frequent NT suctioning is required
- Resuscitation bag with mask

Procedure 36-8 ■ Performing Orotracheal and Nasotracheal Suctioning (Open System) (continued)

Delegation

You should not delegate orotracheal and nasotracheal suctioning to an LPN or NAP, because these procedures require theoretical knowledge, assessment skills, and problem-solving ability.

Pre-Procedure Assessment

- Assess respiratory rate, depth, and rhythm; breath sounds; skin color; and pulse oximetry results.
- Assess for signs that indicate the need for suctioning: gurgling sounds during respiration, restlessness, labored respirations, decreased oxygen saturation, increased heart and respiratory rates, and the presence of adventitious breath sounds during auscultation.
  Suctioning removes oxygen from airways and can cause tissue trauma. It should be done only when essential (i.e., only when less invasive techniques have proved unsuccessful and when the secretions are causing physiological deterioration and/or distress).
- Assess the effectiveness of the cough.

➤ When performing the procedure, always identify your patient according to agency policy, using two identifiers, and be attentive to standard precautions, hand hygiene, patient safety and privacy, body mechanics, and documentation.

➤ *Note:* This procedure uses modified sterile technique. Although the oropharynx and nasopharynx are not sterile, you should keep the suction catheter free from other contaminants as much as possible. Some facilities do use sterile gloves for this procedure

Procedure Steps

1. **Position the patient.**

For Orotracheal Suctioning

a. Position the patient in semi-Fowler's position, with the head turned to face you.

For Nasotracheal Suctioning

b. Position the patient in semi-Fowler's position, with his neck hyperextended, unless contraindicated.
Hyperextending the neck makes it easier to insert the suction catheter. Upright position helps to prevent caregiver back strain.

2. **Place the linen-saver pad** or towel on the patient's chest.
Prevents soiling of the patient's gown during suctioning.

3. **Put on a face shield or goggles and gown.**
Protects you from contamination with secretions that may splash during suctioning.

4. **Turn on the wall suction** or portable suction machine, and adjust the pressure regulator according to agency policy. Guidelines from American Association for Respiratory Care (AARC) specify:
   Adults: 100 to 150 mm Hg
   Children: 100 to 120 mm Hg
   Infants: 80 to 100 mm Hg
   Neonates: 60 to 80 mm Hg
The suction regulator must be set appropriately to prevent tissue trauma and hypoxia and yet remove secretions effectively.

5. **Don a procedure glove** and test the suction equipment by occluding the connection tubing. Discard the glove and perform hand hygiene.
Testing the equipment ensures proper functioning before you insert the catheter in the patient's airway.

6. **Open the suction catheter kit** or, if a kit isn't available, the gathered equipment.

   Nasal approach: If you are using the nasal approach, open the water-soluble lubricant and a nasopharyngeal airway.

7. **Don gloves.** Follow agency policy, as some guidelines allow for clean nonsterile rather than sterile procedure gloves.

If Using Sterile Technique

a. Don sterile gloves. Consider your dominant hand sterile and your nondominant hand unsterile. Alternatively, put a sterile glove on your dominant hand and a clean procedure glove on your nondominant hand. Consider your dominant hand sterile and your nondominant hand nonsterile. (Note: if you consider both hands sterile, you must remove the cap from the sterile water before donning gloves.)

If Using Modified Sterile Technique

b. Don clean nonsterile gloves. Consider your dominant hand clean and your nondominant hand contaminated.
Keeping the dominant hand sterile prevents contaminating the upper airways with a nonsterile suction catheter. This is a modified sterile suction technique because the catheter enters the trachea via nose or the mouth—which are not sterile. However, take care to keep the catheter free from other contaminants.

8. **Pour sterile saline** into the sterile container, using your nondominant hand.
Sterile saline will be used to clear the suction catheter of secretions after suctioning.

9. **Pick up the suction catheter** with your dominant hand, and attach it to the connection tubing, maintaining sterility of your hand and the catheter.
Prepares the suction catheter for use.

10. **Put the tip of the suction** catheter into the sterile container of normal saline solution, and suction a small amount of normal saline solution through the suction catheter. Apply suction by placing a finger over the suction control port of the suction catheter.
Lubricates the catheter and helps ensure that the suction equipment is functioning properly.

11. **Ask the patient to take several slow, deep breaths.** If patient's oxygen saturation is <94%, or if he is

in any distress, you may need to give supplemental oxygen before, during, and after suctioning. See Procedure 36-4: Administering Oxygen.
Promotes relaxation and helps hyperoxygenate the patient before suctioning.

12. **Using your nondominant hand,** remove the oxygen delivery device, if present.

For Oral Approach, Patient Receiving Nasal Oxygen

a. If the patient is receiving nasal oxygen and you are doing orotracheal suctioning, you do not need to remove the oxygen source.

For Nasal Approach, Patient Receiving Nasal Oxygen

b. Remove the nasal oxygen and place the nasal cannula in the patient's mouth. See Procedure 36-4.
Placing the cannula in the patient's mouth makes it easier to access the nares for suctioning while still delivering oxygen to the patient (orally).

13. **Premeasure to approximate** the depth you should insert the suction catheter. For adults, insert the catheter about 15 cm (6 in.) for an oral approach, and 20 cm (8 in.) for a nasal approach. Be careful not to contaminate the catheter while you measure.
Prevents trauma at the carina and ensures suctioning of the full length of the trachea.

For Oral Approach

a. Measure the distance between the edge of the patient's mouth to the tip of the earlobe and down to the bottom of the neck. ▼

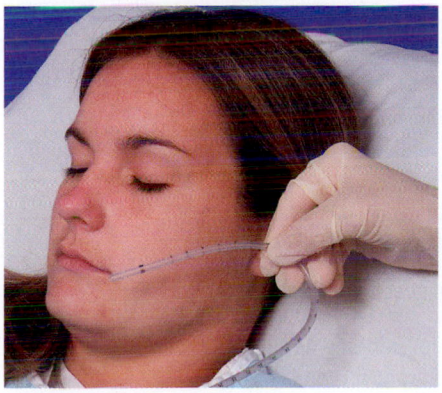

For Nasal Approach

b. Measure the distance from the tip of the nose to the tip of the earlobe and down to the bottom of the neck.

14. **If using nasal approach, insert nasopharyngeal** airway gently into the nostril, with the bevel toward the septum (center of the nose), advance the airway straight in, following the floor of the nose. See Procedure 36-13.
Do not force nasopharyngeal airway into the nostril as this may cause unnecessary edema and trauma.

15. **Lubricate and insert** the suction catheter.
Lubrication makes it easier to pass a suction catheter through the nares.

For Orotracheal Suctioning

a. Lubricate the suction catheter tip with normal saline solution.

b. Using your dominant hand, gently but quickly insert the suction catheter along the side of the patient's mouth or through the endotracheal tube into the oropharynx.
Quick insertion along the side of the mouth prevents gagging.

c. When the patient inhales, advance the suction catheter to the predetermined distance, being careful not to force the catheter.
Advancing the suction catheter during inhalation ensures that the catheter enters the trachea rather than the esophagus. Forcing the catheter during insertion may cause tissue trauma.

For Nasotracheal Suctioning

d. Lubricate the catheter tip with the water-soluble lubricant.
Water-soluble lubricant is preferred because it will dissolve if it accidentally enters the lungs, whereas an oil-based lubricant (e.g., petroleum jelly) won't dissolve in the respiratory tract and causes complications if it enters the lungs.

e. Using your dominant hand, gently but quickly insert the suction catheter into the nasotracheal tube and down to the pharynx. When the patient inhales, advance the suction catheter, gently aiming downward to the predetermined distance, being careful not to force the catheter.
Ensures that the catheter enters the trachea. Forcing the catheter during insertion may cause tissue trauma.

16. **Place a finger or thumb** over the suction control port of the catheter. Apply suction while you withdraw the catheter, using a continuous rotating motion. Apply suction for no longer than 15 seconds.
Using a continuous rotating motion and suctioning while withdrawing the catheter prevents trauma to any one area of the airway. Limiting suctioning to less than 15 seconds prevents hypoxia. ▼

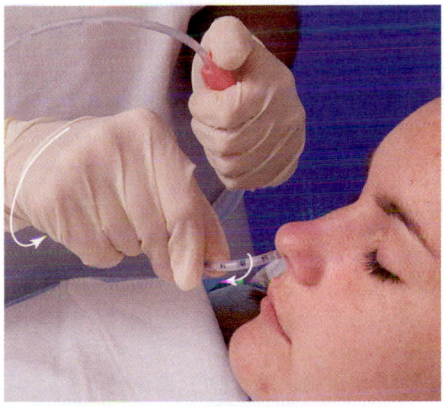

17. **After you withdraw** the catheter, clear it by placing the tip of the catheter into the container of sterile saline and applying suction. ▼

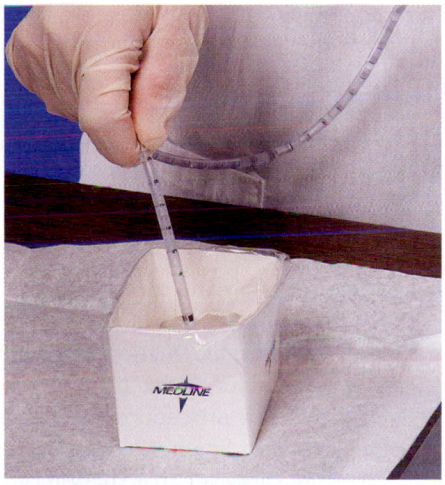

18. **Lubricate the catheter,** and repeat suctioning as needed, allowing intervals of at least 30 seconds between suctioning. Reapply oxygen between suctioning efforts, if required.
Several passes with the suction catheter may be needed to clear the airway of secretions. Total suctioning time should be limited to 5 minutes, however, to prevent trauma and hypoxia.

(continued on next page)

Procedure 36-8 ■ Performing Orotracheal and Nasotracheal Suctioning (Open System) (continued)

19. **Replace the oxygen source.**
Prevents hypoxia.

20. **Coil the suction catheter** in your dominant hand (alternatively, wrap it around your dominant hand). Hold the catheter while you pull the sterile glove off over it. Discard the glove containing the catheter in a biohazard receptacle (e.g., bag) designated by your agency.
These actions prevent contaminating the environment with secretions.

21. **Using your nondominant hand,** clear the connecting tubing of secretions by placing the tip into the container of sterile saline.

22. **Dispose of equipment,** and make sure new suction supplies are readily available for future suctioning.
The patient may require suctioning at any time, so equipment must be readily available.

23. **Provide mouth care.**
Promotes patient comfort and clears the mouth of any secretions the patient may have expectorated.

24. **Position the patient** in a comfortable position, and allow him to rest.
Comfort and rest help the patient recover from the stress of suctioning.

? What if . . .

- **The patient's oxygen saturation is less than 94%, or if he is in any distress?**

Administer supplemental oxygen before, during, and after suctioning. Notify the patient's primary provider if the patient does not respond to additional oxygen.

Evaluation

- Assess the color, consistency, and amount of secretions.
- Evaluate the patient's tolerance of the procedure. Note whether there were signs of respiratory distress during suctioning.
- Evaluate the effectiveness of the procedure by comparing breath sounds, vital signs, and pulse oximetry or blood gas data before and after the procedure.

Patient Teaching

- Explain the importance of administering supplemental oxygen or of taking several deep breaths before suctioning.
- Inform the patient that coughing typically increases with suctioning.
- Demonstrate orotracheal or nasotracheal suctioning to the caregiver, and ask for a return demonstration if suctioning will be required at home.

Home Care

- Instruct the family and caregiver about where to obtain suction equipment.
- Provide contact information of healthcare personnel who can be reached for advice or emergencies.
- Explain that the procedure can be performed using clean technique instead of sterile technique in the home.
- Instruct the caregiver that suction catheters can be cleaned for reuse by washing them with soapy water and then boiling them for 10 minutes. After they are cleaned, rinse the catheters with normal saline solution or tap water.
- Instruct to change the secretion collection container every 24 hours, or clean it according to home care agency guidelines every 24 hours.

Documentation

- Document the date, time, and reason you performed suctioning.
- Note the suction technique you used and the catheter size.
- Note the color, consistency, and odor of secretions.
- Document the patient's respiratory status before and after the procedure.
- Document the patient's tolerance of the procedure and any complications that occurred as a result of the procedure.
- Document any interventions you performed to address complications that occurred.

Sample documentation

July 31, 2015 0930 O_2 sat 89% on room air, bilateral rhonchi to bases auscultated, unproductive cough, heart rate 90, RR-18. Assistant nurse recruited for manual ventilation. Client placed in semi-Fowler's position, hyperventilated for 1 minute to 100% O_2 sat, oropharyngeal suctioning performed using sterile technique, resulting in moderate amounts of white, tenacious, yellow-tinged secretions. Improved breath sound with diminished rhonchi auscultated, O_2 sat at 97% on room air, heart rate 78, RR-14. Client smiles when asked how he feels. Bed in low position, call light and fluids in reach. ——— Kelton Jones, RN

Practice Resources

American Red Cross (n.d); Barnett, M. (2012); Restrepo, R. D., Brown, J. M., & Hughes, J. M. (2010).

Thinking About the Procedure

To practice applying clinical reasoning to this procedure,

Go to *Davis's Nursing Skills Videos*, **Performing Endotracheal Suctioning (Open System).**

For questions and suggested responses,

Go to Chapter 36, **Thinking About the Procedure Questions and Suggested Responses,** on Davis*Plus*

Procedure 36-9 ■ Performing Upper Airway Suctioning

➤ For steps to follow in *all* procedures, refer to the Universal Steps for All Procedures found on the inside back cover.

➤ *Note:* Upper airway suctioning may be done via the oropharyngeal or nasopharyngeal route. However, nasal suction is usually required only to improve oxygenation in infants because most adult airway obstruction occurs in the mouth and oropharynx.

Vigorous nasal suction can induce epistaxis (nosebleed) and further complicate an already difficult airway.

Equipment

- Portable or wall suction device with connection tubing and a collection canister
- Linen-saver pad or towel
- Sterile suction catheter kit (12 to 18 Fr for adults, 8 to 10 Fr for children, and 5 to 8 Fr for infants). If a kit isn't available, collect the following: sterile suction catheter of the appropriate size, and a sterile container. If you plan to suction both the oropharynx and the nasopharynx, you need a separate sterile catheter for each.
- Yankauer device can be used for oropharyngeal suction.
- Pour-bottle of sterile normal saline solution
- Sterile basin or other container for fluids
- Face shield or goggles and gown
- Procedure gloves
- Water-soluble lubricant for nasopharyngeal suctioning
- Sputum trap, if a specimen is needed
- Biohazard bag

Delegation

Do not delegate oropharyngeal and nasopharyngeal suctioning to an LPN or NAP, because these procedures require theoretical knowledge, assessment skills, and problem-solving ability. However, the NAP (and the client or family) can use a Yankauer tube to suction the oral cavity because there is less risk for trauma to mucosa than with oro- or nasopharyngeal suctioning.

Pre-Procedure Assessment

- Assess respiratory rate, depth, and rhythm; breath sounds; color; and pulse oximetry results. Note signs that indicate the need for suctioning: restlessness, cyanosis, labored respirations, decreased oxygen saturation, increased heart and respiratory rates, visible secretions in the airway, and the presence of adventitious breath sounds during auscultation. *You must be certain the patient requires suctioning. Suctioning should be performed only when necessary to prevent unnecessary oxygen desaturation and tissue trauma.*

➤ When performing the procedure, always identify your patient according to agency policy, using two identifiers, and be attentive to standard precautions, hand hygiene, patient safety and privacy, body mechanics, and documentation.

➤ *Note:* This procedure describes modified sterile technique: sterile supplies with clean procedure gloves. Although the oropharynx and nasopharynx are not sterile, you should keep the suction catheter free from other contaminants as much as possible. Some facilities do use sterile gloves for this procedure.

Procedure Steps

1. **Position the patient**. Explain that suctioning may stimulate coughing or gagging, but that coughing helps mobilize secretions.

Oropharyngeal Suctioning

Position the patient in a semi-Fowler's or high Fowler's position, with his head turned toward you.

Facilitates insertion of the suction catheter and prevents straining your back. It also promotes lung expansion and effective coughing.

For Nasopharyngeal Suctioning

Position the patient in semi-Fowler's or high Fowler's position with his neck hyperextended, unless contraindicated.

2. **Place the linen-saver pad** or towel on the patient's chest.
   Prevents soiling of the patient's gown during suctioning.

3. **Don a face shield or goggles and gown.**
   Protects you from contamination with secretions that may splash during suctioning. Not all guidelines specify wearing a gown for this procedure.

4. **Turn on the wall suction** or portable suction machine, and adjust the pressure regulator according to agency policy, typically:
   Adults: 100 to 150 mm Hg
   Children: 100 to 120 mm Hg
   Infants: 50 to 95 mm Hg
   The suction regulator must be set appropriately to prevent tissue trauma and hypoxia and to function effectively to remove secretions. Higher pressures are associated with hypoxemia, tissue trauma, and atelectasis, yet do not improve removal of secretions.

5. **Test the suction equipment** by occluding the connection tubing.
   Ensures proper functioning before use.

6. **Open the suction catheter kit** or the gathered equipment. If you are using the nasal approach, open the water-soluble lubricant.

7. **Don procedure gloves**; consider (and keep) your dominant hand clean; consider your nondominant hand to be contaminated.
   This is not a sterile suction procedure but care should be taken to keep the suction catheter free from other contaminants. Keeping the dominant hand clean prevents contaminating the upper airways with an unclean suction catheter.

8. **Pour sterile saline** into the sterile container, using your nondominant hand.
   Sterile saline is necessary to clear the suction catheter of secretions after suctioning. The outside of the saline container is not sterile; it would contaminate your dominant hand.

(continued on next page)

Procedure 36-9 ■ Performing Upper Airway Suctioning (continued)

9. **Pick up the suction catheter** with your dominant hand, and use your other hand to hold the connection tubing (to suction) while you attach it.

10. **Put the tip of the suction catheter** into the sterile container of normal saline solution, and suction a small amount of normal saline solution through the suction catheter. Apply suction by placing a finger over the suction control port. When using a Yankauer-type device, the suction is continuous and there is no port to occlude.
Ensures that the suction equipment is functioning properly. If you need to see a Yankauer device,

Go to **Figure 36-14,** in Volume 1.

11. **Approximate the depth** to which you will insert the suction catheter.

For Oropharyngeal Suctioning
Measure the distance between the edge of the patient's mouth and the tip of the patient's earlobe.
Determines the proper distance you should insert the suction catheter for oropharyngeal suctioning.

For Nasopharyngeal Suctioning
Measure the distance between the tip of the patient's nose and the tip of the patient's earlobe.
Helps determine the correct distance you should insert the suction catheter for nasopharyngeal suctioning.

12. ***For nasopharyngeal suctioning only:***
Using your nondominant hand, remove the oxygen delivery device, if present. Have the patient take several slow, deep breaths. If patient's oxygen saturation is <94%, or if he is in any distress, administers supplemental oxygen before, during, and after suctioning. See Procedure 36-4: Administering Oxygen.
Deep breathing helps to hyperoxygenate the patient and helps prevent hypoxia during suctioning.

13. **Lubricate and insert the suction catheter.**

For Oropharyngeal Suctioning
a. Lubricate the catheter tip with the normal saline solution.
b. Using your dominant hand, gently but quickly insert the suction catheter along the side of the patient's mouth into the oropharynx.
Inserting the suction catheter along the side of the mouth prevents gagging.

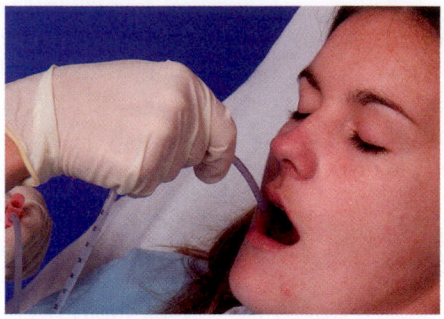

c. Advance the suction catheter quickly to the premeasured distance—usually 7.5 to 10 cm (3 to 4 in.) in the adult—being careful not to force the catheter.
Ensures that the suction catheter will reach the pharynx. Forcing the catheter during insertion may cause tissue trauma.

For Nasopharyngeal Suctioning
d. Lubricate the catheter tip with the water-soluble lubricant.
Eases passage of the suction catheter through the naris. Water-soluble lubricant is preferred because it will dissolve if it accidentally enters the lungs, whereas an oil-based lubricant (e.g., petroleum jelly or lotion) will not dissolve in the respiratory tract and causes complications if it enters the lungs.
e. Using your dominant hand, gently but quickly insert the suction catheter into the naris.
Prevents trauma to the naris.

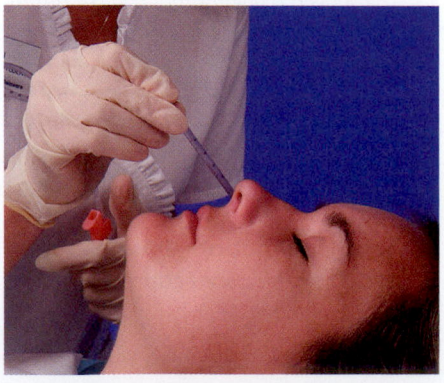

f. Advance the suction catheter, aiming downward to the premeasured distance—usually 13 to 15 cm (5 to 6 in.) in an adult—and being careful not to force the catheter. If you meet resistance, you may need to try the other naris.
Advancing the suction catheter the premeasured distance ensures that the suction catheter will reach the pharynx. Forcing the catheter during insertion may cause tissue trauma.

14. **Place a finger or thumb over** the suction control port of the suction catheter, and start suctioning the patient. Apply suction as you withdraw the catheter, using a continuous rotating motion.

Limit suctioning to 10 to 15 seconds.
Using a continuous rotating motion while withdrawing the catheter prevents trauma to any one area of the airway. Limiting suctioning to less than 10 to 15 seconds prevents hypoxia.

15. **After you withdraw** the catheter, clear it by placing the tip of the catheter into the container of sterile saline and applying suction.
Ensures patency of the catheter for repeat suctioning.

16. **Lubricate the catheter**, and repeat suctioning as needed, allowing at least 20-second intervals between suctioning.
Several passes with the suction catheter may be needed to clear the airway of secretions. The total suctioning time should be limited to 5 minutes, however, to prevent hypoxia and trauma to the mucosal membranes.

For Nasopharyngeal Suctioning
Each time you repeat suction, alternate nares.
Alternating nares prevents trauma that would occur if you used only one naris.

17. **Coil the suction catheter** in your dominant hand. Pull the sterile glove off over the coiled catheter. (Alternatively, wrap the catheter around your dominant, gloved hand, and hold the catheter as you re-

move the glove over it.) Discard the glove containing the catheter in a biohazard receptacle designated by your agency.
Coiling the catheter inside the glove prevents contamination with secretions.

18. **Using your nondominant hand,** clear the connecting tubing of secretions by placing the tip of the tube into the container of sterile saline.
Ensures patency and prepares the equipment for future use.

19. **Dispose of equipment** in biohazard waste container/bag, and make sure new suction supplies are readily available for future suctioning needs.
The patient may require suctioning at any time, so equipment must be readily available.

20. **Provide mouth care.**
Promotes patient comfort and clears the mouth of any secretions the patient may have expectorated.

21. **Discard your other glove** and remaining supplies.

22. **Position the patient** in a comfortable position, and allow him to rest.
Promoting comfort and allowing for a period of rest helps the patient recover from suctioning, which may be very tiring.

? What if . . .

- **The patient's oxygen saturation is less than 94%, or if he is in any distress?**

You may need to administer supplemental oxygen before, during, and after suctioning. See Procedure 36-4.

Evaluation

- Assess the color, consistency, and amount of secretions.
- Evaluate the patient's tolerance of the procedure. Note whether there were signs of respiratory distress during the procedure.
- Evaluate the effectiveness of the procedure by comparing breath sounds, vital signs, and pulse oximetry before and after the procedure.

Patient Teaching

- Explain the importance of administering supplemental oxygen to the patient before suctioning.
- Inform the patient that coughing typically increases with suctioning.
- Demonstrate oropharyngeal or nasopharyngeal suctioning to the caregiver, and ask for a return demonstration if suctioning will be required at home.

Home Care

- Instruct the family and caregiver where to obtain suction equipment.
- Provide contact information for healthcare personnel who can be reached for advice or emergencies.
- Explain that the procedure can be performed using clean technique instead of sterile technique in the home setting.
- Instruct the caregiver that suction catheters can be cleaned for reuse by washing them with soapy water and then boiling them for 10 minutes. After they are cleaned, rinse the catheters with normal saline solution or tap water.
- Teach to change the secretion collection container every 24 hours, or clean it according to home care agency guidelines every 24 hours.

Documentation

- Document the date, time, and reason you performed suctioning.
- Note the suction technique you used and the catheter size.
- Note color, consistency, and odor of secretions.
- Document the patient's respiratory status before and after the procedure.
- Document the patient's tolerance of the procedure and any complications that occurred as a result of the procedure, with resulting interventions.

Sample documentation

3/15/15 2200 Resp. labored, rate 28 breaths/min. Pulse oximetry on room air 92%. Breath sounds with rhonchi scattered throughout. Gurgling audible in upper airways. Patient unable to mobilize secretions with coughing. Suctioned by nasopharyngeal route using a 14-Fr. catheter. Approximately 30 mL thin, tan, odorless secretions obtained. After suctioning, resp. nonlabored, rate 20 breaths/min, and lungs clear on auscultation, with no gurgling audible. Pulse oximetry 96%. Patient tolerated procedure with no difficulty. ——— *C.F. Hiam, RN*

Practice Resources

McGrath, B. A., Bates, L., Atkinson, D., et al. (2012); Siegel, J., Rhinehart, E., Jackson, M., et al. (2007); Sole, M. L., Penoyer, D. A., Bennett, M. et al. (2011).

Thinking About the Procedure

To practice applying clinical reasoning to this procedure,

Go to *Davis's Nursing Skills Videos,* **Performing Upper Airway Suctioning: Oropharyngeal.**

For questions and suggested responses,

Go to Chapter 36, **Thinking About the Procedure Questions and Suggested Responses,** on Davis*Plus*.

Procedure 36-10 ■ Caring for Patients Requiring Mechanical Ventilation

➤ For steps to follow in *all* procedures, refer to the Universal Steps for All Procedures found on the inside back cover.

Ventilator Terminology

TERM	EXPLANATION
FIO_2	Fraction of inspired oxygen
Modes of ventilation	Describes the setting on the ventilator that assists the patient to breathe. Can be controlled (CMV), intermittent mandatory (IMV), or synchronized intermittent mandatory (SIMV).
Tidal volume	Amount of air delivered from the ventilator with each breath
Assist-control mode—also known as continuous mechanical ventilation (CMV)	The preset number of breaths per minute delivered by the machine. If the patient is able to initiate breaths, the machine will deliver a breath when the patient begins to inspire. If the patient is unable to breathe on his own, the machine will deliver the preset number of breaths in a rhythmic fashion.
Intermittent mandatory ventilation	A ventilator setting that delivers a minimum number of breaths per minute if the patient does not ventilate independently.
Synchronized intermittent mandatory ventilation (SIMV)	A ventilator setting that delivers a minimum number of ventilations per minute if the patient does not ventilate independently. The ventilator breaths are synchronized with the patient's breaths. This mode is used for weaning patients from the ventilator.
Pressure support	Provides positive pressure on inspiration to decrease the workload of breathing.
Continuous positive airway pressure (CPAP)	Provides positive pressure during inspiration and expiration to keep alveoli open in a spontaneously breathing patient.
Positive end expiratory pressure (PEEP)	Provides positive pressure on expiration to keep airways open for patients on CMV or SIMV mode ventilation.

Equipment

- Two oxygen sources
- Air source that provides 50 pounds per square inch (psi)
- Mechanical ventilator
- Humidification device
- Ventilator tubing, connectors, and adaptors
- Condensation collection device
- Inline thermometer
- Resuscitation bag with oxygen connection tubing
- Pulse oximetry device
- Procedure gloves, protective gown, and eye covering
- Sterile gloves, if you will perform suctioning
- Suction equipment (possibly)
- Sterile water for the humidifier. Some guidelines also recommend sterile water for rinsing the mouth.

Delegation

Care of a mechanically ventilated patient requires advanced knowledge of pulmonary anatomy and physiology and, therefore, should not be delegated to assistive personnel. In critical care settings, specially trained LPNs may provide care, but the RN is responsible for ensuring that procedures are implemented safely and effectively. RNs also provide ongoing assessment of the patient's ventilatory and oxygenation status. Patients requiring long-term ventilation are often cared for at home or in specialized long-term care units, where LPNs and family members may provide care.

Pre-Procedure Assessment

- Review the health record to make sure that mechanical ventilation is included in the options outlined in the patient's advance directive.
  The patient may not wish to pursue mechanical ventilation as a care option. If a patient who does not wish to be ventilated mechanically is currently on a ventilator, consult your hospital ethics committee.
- If the patient's condition allows, assess his understanding of mechanical ventilation therapy.
  Understanding helps allay anxiety and promotes cooperation.
- Assess respiratory rate, depth, and rhythm; breath sounds; color; and pulse oximetry results.
  Confirms the need for mechanical ventilation.
- Assess the oral cavity for bleeding, inflammation, odor, and presence of yeast or plaque.
  May indicate the need for more frequent oral care or for referral.
- Blood will probably be drawn for an ABG analysis
  To establish a baseline and, after that, to monitor response to therapy.

➤ When performing the procedure, always identify your patient according to agency policy, using two identifiers, and be attentive to standard precautions, hand hygiene, patient safety and privacy, body mechanics, and documentation.

Procedure Steps

Initial Ventilator Setup

1. **Prepare the resuscitation bag.**
   The resuscitation bag should be readily available to provide ventilation in the event of an emergency.▼

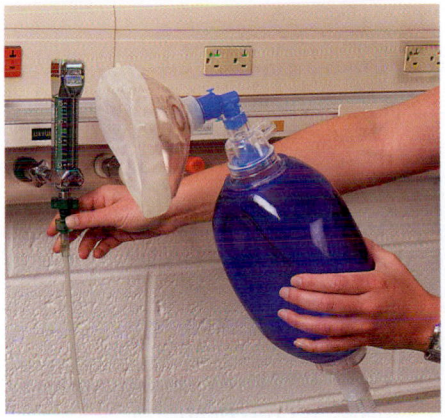

   a. Attach a flow meter to one of the oxygen sources.
      The flow meter helps regulate oxygen delivery.
   b. Attach an adapter to the flow meter, and connect the oxygen tubing to the adapter.
   c. Turn on the oxygen, and adjust the flow rate.

2. **Respiratory therapists** are responsible for setting up mechanical ventilation in most agencies. If you must assume the responsibility, refer to the manufacturer's instructions.

3. **Plug the ventilator into** a grounded electrical outlet and turn it on.

4. **Verify ventilator settings** and adjust as medically prescribed.
   Ventilator settings must be individualized according to the patient's need for respiratory support. Incorrect settings may cause harm (e.g., hypoxia or barotrauma) to the patient.▼

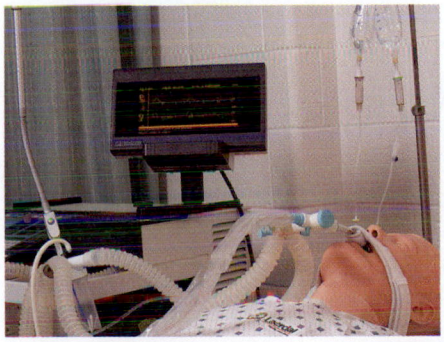

5. **Make sure that ventilator alarm** limits are set appropriately.
   Inappropriately set alarm limits can result in harm to the patient.

6. **Make sure the humidifier** is filled with sterile distilled water.

7. **Don gloves, gown, and eye protection** if you have not already done so.

8. **Attach the ventilator tubing** to the endotracheal tube or tracheostomy tube.

9. **Place the ventilator tubing** in the securing device.
   Prevents dislodging the endotracheal tube or tracheostomy when the patient moves.

10. **Attach a capnographic device,** if available.
    To measure levels of carbon dioxide. These data are used to confirm placement of the endotracheal tube and disconnection from or malfunction of the ventilator. Oxygen levels alone are not sufficient for the ventilated patient.

11. **Prepare the inline (closed)** suction equipment (see Procedure 36-7).

    Suctioning equipment should be readily available when the patient requires suctioning. Closed catheters are recommended to prevent ventilator-associated pneumonia.

After Initial Ventilator Setup

12. **Check respiratory status** and ABGs again about 30 minutes after setup. Also check whenever there are changes in the ventilator settings and as the patient's condition indicates.
    To be certain the patient is being adequately ventilated and not experiencing oxygen toxicity.

13. **Check the ventilator tubing** frequently for condensation. Drain the fluid into a collection device, or briefly disconnect the patient from the ventilator and empty the tubing into a waste receptacle, according to agency policy.

    ✚ Never drain the fluid into the humidifier.
    Condensation in the ventilator tubing can cause resistance to airflow. Moreover, the patient can aspirate it. The fluid should not be drained into the humidifier because the patient's secretions may have contaminated it.▼

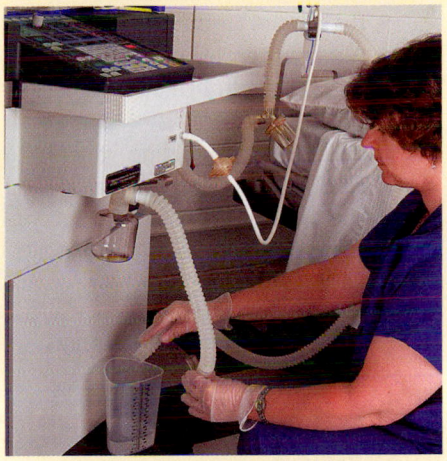

14. ✚ **Maintain the patient** in a semirecumbent position (head of bed elevated 30° to 45°). This is extremely important.
    To promote lung expansion, reduce gastric reflux, and prevent ventilator-associated pneumonia.

15. **Check ventilator** and humidifier settings regularly.

16. **Check the inline thermometer.**
    To ensure that the air being delivered to the patient is close to the body temperature to prevent scalding of the mucosal tissue or instead, cooling the patient (core temperature).

17. **Provide the patient with** an alternative form of communication, such as a letter board or white board.
    A patient being mechanically ventilated is unable to speak, which can produce extreme anxiety. The patient must have a way to express her needs and concerns.

18. **Reposition the patient** regularly (every 1 to 2 hours), being careful not to pull on the ventilator tubing.
    Repositioning protects skin integrity. However, pulling on the tubing creates pain. Patient comfort promotes relaxation, improving the effectiveness of the ventilator.

(continued on next page)

Procedure 36-10 ■ Caring for Patients Requiring Mechanical Ventilation (continued)

19. **Keep the patient's lips** moistened with a cool, damp cloth and water-based lubricant; and provide regular antiseptic oral care. A recommended regimen includes the following:
    - Brush the teeth twice a day for 3 or 4 minutes.
    - Use a soft toothbrush.
    - Rinse the mouth with sterile water, according to agency policy.
    - Moisturize oral mucosa and lips every 2 to 4 hours.
    - Use a chlorhexidine gluconate (0.12%) rinse twice a day during the perioperative period for patients who undergo cardiac surgery (adult patients).
    - Use mouthwash twice a day for adult patients. (AACN, 2008)

    Mouth care provides comfort and preserves integrity of the mucous membranes. Patients being mechanically ventilated, even for a short period, are at high risk for developing ventilator-associated pneumonia (VAP). VAP is not uncommon, and it is associated with high mortality rates. This regimen is thought to help prevent VAP.

20. **Make sure the call light** is always within reach, and answer call light and ventilator alarms promptly.
    Provides the patient with immediate access to help if a breathing problem occurs; reassures the patient and thus relieves anxiety.

21. **Monitor the tracheostomy** tube for proper cuff inflation (usually 20 to 25 mm Hg); see Clinical Insight 36-4.

22. **Check for gastric distention** and take measures to prevent aspiration.
    Aspiration creates high risk for pneumonia.

23. **Clean, disinfect, or change** ventilator tubing and equipment according to agency policy.
    There is no good evidence to indicate how often this should be done. Research so far indicates that tubing and equipment should not be routinely changed for infection control purposes (Han & Liu, 2010).

24. **Give sedatives or anti-anxiety** drugs as prescribed.

Evaluation

- After mechanical ventilation is instituted, assess for chest expansion and auscultate for bilateral breath sounds.
- Evaluate the patient's tolerance of mechanical ventilation. Verify that the patient is being adequately ventilated and that she is breathing in synchrony with the ventilator.
- Auscultate breath sounds every 2 to 4 hours, according to agency policy.
- When monitoring vital signs, count spontaneous breaths as well as those delivered by the ventilator.
- Monitor continuous pulse oximetry, capnography, and ABGs.

Patient Teaching

- Explain mechanical ventilation to the patient and family. Include information about the alarms they will hear.
- When appropriate, explain the weaning process to the patient and family.
- If the patient requires mechanical ventilation after discharge, make arrangements for a home ventilator, and teach the patient and caregiver how to use it.

Home Care

- Consult with your facility discharge planning program and/or case management for discharge plans.
- Explain to the family and caregiver where to obtain a home ventilator, resuscitation bag, and oxygen equipment and what services are available. Make sure they choose a supplier who has 24-hour emergency services available.
- Help the client and caregiver devise a backup plan for ventilating the client in the event of a power failure.
- Tell the caregiver to notify the utility company and area emergency personnel that the client is being maintained on a ventilator at home.
- Instruct the client and caregiver about oxygen therapy and its use as well as safety measures that they must institute.
- Teach the client and caregiver to clean the ventilator tubing with soap and warm water when it becomes soiled.
- Provide contact information of healthcare personnel who can be reached for advice or emergencies.

Documentation

- Document the date and time mechanical ventilation was initiated.
- Note the type of ventilator used and the prescribed settings used.
- Document the client's response to mechanical ventilation, including vital signs, breath sounds, ease of breathing, pulse oximetry, intake and output, skin color, and ABG and chest x-ray results.

Sample documentation

02/26/15 0800 Patient found difficult to arouse. Dr. Henry made aware. ABG obtained; results included: pH 7.28; PCO_2 78 mm Hg; PO_2 48 mm Hg. Dr. Henry in to evaluate patient. Anesthesia called to intubate patient. Medicated with Versed 5 mg IV and intubated orally with a 7.5-Fr. ET tube. Placed on mechanical ventilator: TV 700 mL; FIO_2 80%, respiratory rate 14 breaths/min. Portable chest x-ray confirms ideal placement of ET tube as well as white-out of both lung fields. ABGs to be obtained in 30 min. Pulse oximetry 90% since being placed on ventilator.

L. Houck, RN

Practice Resources

AACN (2008, 2010, 2008); Bozyk, P., & Hyzy, R. (2008); Coffin, W., Klompas, M., Classen, D., et al. (2008); Feider, L. L., Mitchell, P., & Bridges, E. (2010); Maselli, D., & Restrepo, M. (2011); Munro, C., Grap, M., Jones, D., et al. (2009).

Procedure 36-11 ■ Setting Up Disposable Chest Drainage Systems

➤ For steps to follow in *all* procedures, refer to the Universal Steps for All Procedures found on the inside back cover.

Equipment

- Two disposable closed drainage systems
- Chest tube insertion kit (common tube size for adults is 36 Fr). Should contain povidone-iodine, local anesthetic, syringe, needles, drapes, scalpel, suture, sterile drapes, chest tube, connecting tubing, and necessary instruments.
- 5-in-1 or Y-connector for two chest tubes, if not contained in insertion kit
- Sterile water (for water-seal system)
- Two rubber-tipped hemostats
- Sterile gloves, masks, and sterile gowns
- Dressings: sterile 4 in. × 4 in. gauze dressings, precut drain dressings, petroleum (or other recommended) gauze dressings, and large drainage dressings
- Tape: 2-in. silk tape, 1-in. silk tape (or nylon banding system)

For disposable dry-seal systems:

- 50-mL syringe and 45 mL of sterile water or saline. Some dry-seal CDUs include these.

Delegation

Some agencies permit only registered nurses in the critical care units to perform dressing changes. The physician must perform dressing changes on other units. You should not delegate this procedure, because it requires advanced knowledge of pulmonary anatomy and physiology. As needed, teach the LPN and NAP how to safely provide care for the patient with chest tubes. Instruct them to notify an RN immediately if the chest drainage system becomes disconnected, the chest tube becomes dislodged, sudden bleeding occurs, or the patient develops respiratory distress.

Pre-Procedure Assessment

- Ensure that the patient has venous access.
- Assess vital signs.
- Assess the level of consciousness, orientation, responsiveness, anxiety, and restlessness.
  These can indicate hypoxemia.
- Assess the patient's knowledge of chest tube therapy.
  Understanding helps allay fears and anxiety.
- Assess cardiac status; respiratory rate, depth, and rhythm; breath sounds; skin color; pulse oximetry; and ABG results.
  Provides a baseline for comparison after chest tube insertion. Evaluates chest tube functioning afterward.

➤ When performing the procedure, always identify your patient according to agency policy, using two identifiers, and be attentive to standard precautions, hand hygiene, patient safety and privacy, body mechanics, and documentation.

Procedure Steps

Steps for Preparing the CDU

1. **Obtain and prepare** the prescribed chest drainage unit (CDU).▼

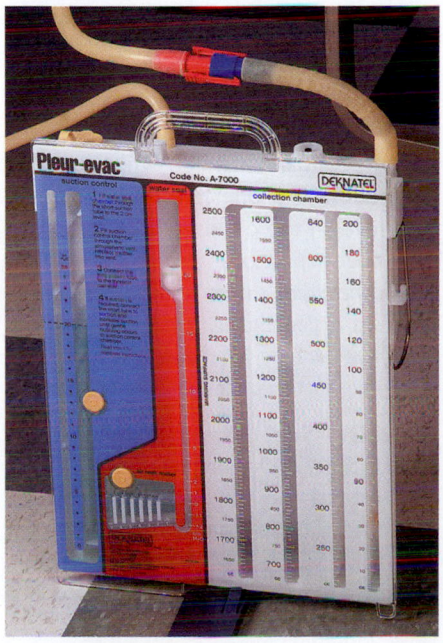

Disposable water-seal system.

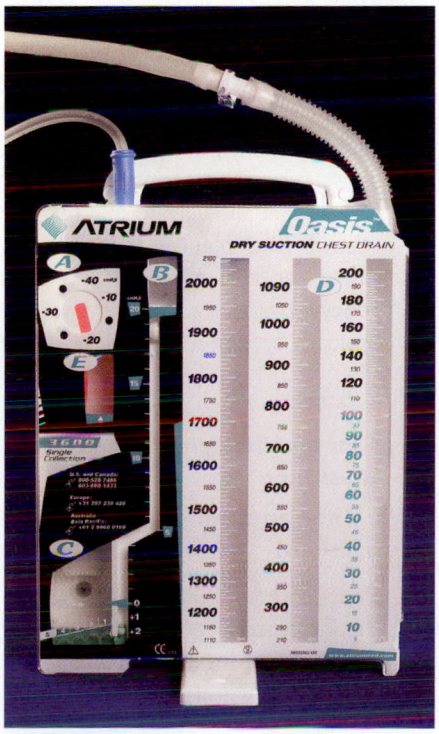

Disposable dry-seal system.

Procedure Variation for a Disposable Water-Seal CDU Without Suction

2. **Remove the cover** on the water-seal chamber, and, using the funnel provided, fill the second (water-seal) chamber with sterile water or normal saline. Fill the chamber to the 2-cm mark, or as indicated. (Note that some systems come prefilled.)
   The water-seal chamber allows air to exit from the pleural space during exhalation and prevents air from entering the pleural space during inspiration.
3. **Place the chest drainage unit** (CDU) upright, usually on the floor, and at least 30 cm (1 ft) below the patient's chest level.
4. **Replace the cover** on the water-seal chamber.
   Protects the chamber from contamination.

Go to Step 13.

(continued on next page)

Procedure 36-11 ■ Setting Up Disposable Chest Drainage Systems (continued)

Procedure Variation for a Disposable Water-Seal CDU With Suction

5. **Remove the cover** on the water-seal chamber. If it is not a prefilled system, use a syringe or the funnel provided to fill the water-seal chamber (second chamber) with sterile water or normal saline to the 2-cm mark.
   The water-seal chamber allows air to exit from the pleural space during exhalation and prevents air from entering the pleural space during inspiration.

6. **Add sterile water or normal** saline solution to the suction control chamber. Add the amount prescribed by the clinician, typically 20 cm (7 in.). Place the CDU upright, usually on the floor, and at least 30 cm (1 ft) below the patient's chest level.
   Suction is regulated by the height of fluid in the suction control chamber.

7. **Attach the tubing** from the suction control chamber to the suction source tubing. Turn on the wall (or other) suction source. A wall suction of –80 mm Hg is common.▼

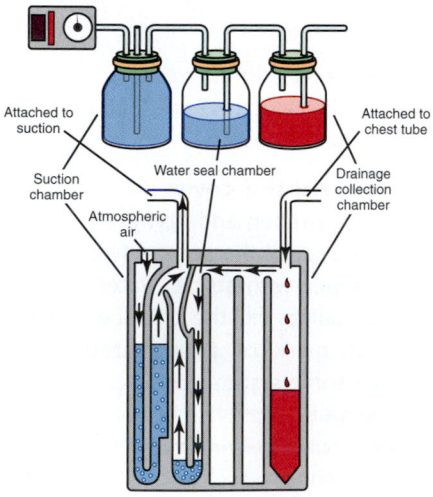

Comparison of glass bottles and disposable CDUs.

Go to Step 13.

Procedure Variation for a Disposable Dry-Seal CDU With Suction

8. **Remove the nonsterile** outer protective bag and the sterile inner wrapper following agency policy.

9. **Place the CDU upright**, usually on the floor, and at least 30 cm (1 ft) below the patient's chest level. Some CDUs have hangers for hanging at the bedside.

10. **If suction will be required**, attach the tubing from the suction control chamber to the connecting tubing attached to the suction source.

11. **Fill a syringe** with 45 mL of sterile water or saline (follow agency policy and the manufacturer's recommendation for type of fluid), or use the small bottle of sterile fluid in the CDU package. Fill the air leak monitor on the CDU by injecting the fluid via the needleless injection port on the back until it reaches the fill line.
    Once filled, the water may become colored for improved visibility of air leaks. Bubbles in this section of the CDU indicate an air leak.

Go to Step 13.

Procedure Variation for a Heimlich Valve

12. **When a patient has little or no** drainage and does not require suction, the chest tube may be connected to a Heimlich valve instead of a CDU. These valves are attached to the end of the chest tube and allow one-way flow of air out of the chest tube. They contain "flutter" leaflets that allow air to exit but not reenter the pleural space. These valves can also be used for emergency transport until a chest drainage system is available.

Go to Step 13.

Steps for Inserting and Connecting the Chest Tube

NOTE: **The remaining steps apply to all variations.**

13. **Position the patient** according to the indicated insertion site.
    - For removing air: second intercostal space at the midclavicular line
    - For fluid drainage: on the midaxillary line in the fifth or sixth intercostal space

14. **Open the chest tube insertion tray** and set up the sterile field. Using sterile technique, drop any necessary supplies on the field (e.g., 4 in. × 4 in. split gauze dressings, petroleum or other recommended gauze, syringes).

15. **Don a mask, gown, and sterile gloves** and organize the supplies you will need for dressing the chest tube insertion site.
    Protective clothing prevents contamination of the surgical site and protects you from splashing.

16. **Provide support to the patient** while the physician or nurse practitioner prepares the sterile field, anesthetizes the patient, and inserts and sutures the chest tube.

17. **As soon as the chest tube** is inserted, attach it to the CDU tubing, using a connector.
    Usually the nurse holds the nonsterile tubing that leads to the collection chamber and the physician attaches the sterile chest tube to it. Immediately attaching the chest tube to the drainage system prevents air from entering the pleural cavity.

18. **If suction is prescribed**, adjust the CDU suction to the level the clinician specifies, usually –20 cm H_2O. Also adjust the wall (or other) suction source, usually to –80 mm Hg.

For a Water-Seal Drainage Unit

Adjust the suction source (e.g., wall suction) until gentle bubbling occurs in the suction control chamber. When the tube is functioning properly, the height of the fluid level in the drainage tube fluctuates with the respiratory cycle.

NOTE: Increasing suction at the suction source increases airflow through the system and creates more bubbling, but it does not increase the amount of suction placed on the chest cavity.

For a Dry-Seal Drainage Unit

Adjust the CDU suction (e.g., to –20 cm H_2O) by turning the suction control dial on the CDU. Adjust the wall (or portable) suction pressure to –80 mm Hg or greater until the display on the suction-control chamber confirms adequate suction.

If Suction Is Not Prescribed

Leave the suction tubing on the drainage system open to maintain negative pressure. Follow the manufacturer's directions on the CDU, as models will differ.

Steps for Dressing the Chest Tube

19. **When the chest tube** is functioning properly, the physician or nurse practitioner will suture it in place. Then don a new pair of sterile gloves. Using sterile technique, wrap petroleum, saline-soaked, or other recommended gauze around the chest tube at the insertion site.
(Note: Sometimes the physician dresses the site.)
Theoretically, the moistened gauze creates a seal that prevents air from leaking around the site. However, continued use of petroleum gauze or ointments can macerate the skin, so use them with caution. Recent research suggests that saline-soaked, or even dry, gauze may be preferable to petroleum gauze; so follow your agency's policy.

20. **Place a precut, sterile split-drain** dressing over the gauze around the chest tube.
Absorbs drainage from the insertion site, thereby reducing skin irritation and possible breakdown. ▼

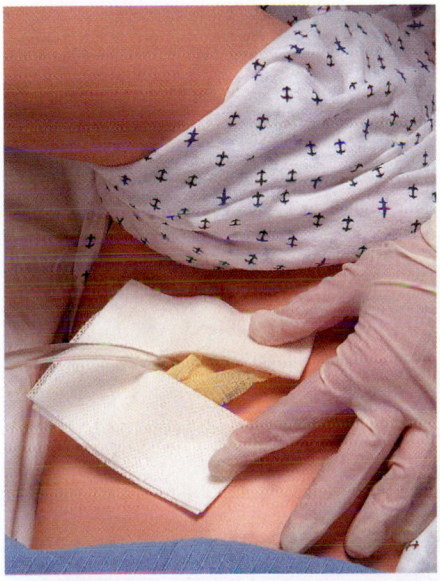

21. **Place a second sterile, precut** drain dressing over the first drain dressing with the opening facing in the opposite direction from the first.
The second drain dressing helps secure the first drain dressing and provides reinforcement against drainage.

22. **Place a large drainage dressing (e.g., ABD) over the two precut drain dressings.**
NOTE: Some guidelines recommend that instead of large amounts of tape and padding, a transparent dressing be used. This minimizes moisture collection around the site, allows nurses to inspect for leakage or infection, and does not restrict chest wall movement. Follow your agency's policy.
The large drainage dressing covers the insertion site, protecting it from outside sources of infection.

23. **Secure the dressing in place,** with wide tape, making sure to cover the dressing completely.
Creates an occlusive dressing that protects the chest tube from becoming dislodged and provides a seal over the insertion site, protecting it from outside sources of infection.

24. **Date, time, and initial the dressing.**
Informs other staff members when the dressing change was completed and by whom.

25. **Using the spiral taping** technique, wrap 1-in. cloth tape around the chest tube, starting above the connector and continuing below the connector. Reverse your wrapping by taping back up the tubing (using the spiral technique) until the wrapping is above the connector. The CDU may come with locking connections or bands; if so, use those.
Ensures a tight connection between the two tubings, thereby preventing an air leak at the connection site. ▼

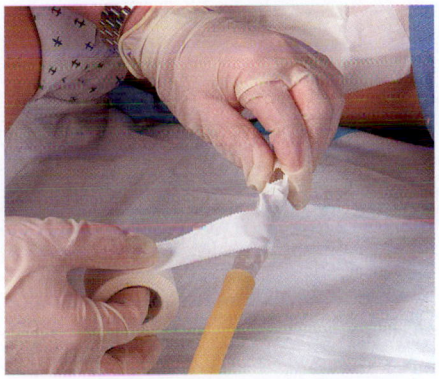

26. **Cut an 8-in.-long piece of 2-in. tape.** Loop one end around the top portion of the drainage tube, and secure the remaining end of the tape to the chest tube dressing.
Prevents pulling at the chest tube site when the patient moves.

27. **Make sure the drainage tubing** lies with no kinks from the chest tube to the drainage chamber.
Facilitates drainage and prevents fluid from accumulating in the pleural cavity. ▼

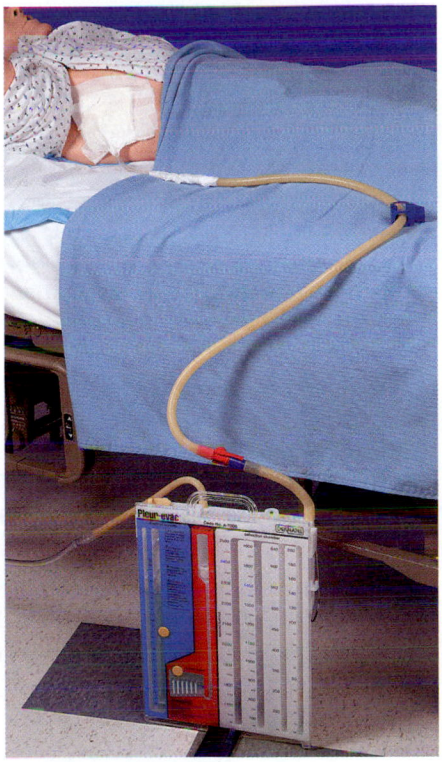

28. **Prepare the patient** for a portable chest x-ray exam.
A chest x-ray exam should be performed after the chest tube is inserted to ensure proper placement.

29. **Institute the following safety measures:**
   a. Place two rubber-tipped clamps at the patient's bedside for special situations.
   Rubber-tipped clamps are used to clamp the chest tube to check for an air leak, to change the drainage system, and to assess whether the chest tube can be safely removed.
   b. Place a petroleum gauze dressing at the bedside.
   In case the chest tube leaks or becomes dislodged, placing a petroleum gauze dressing over the insertion site

(continued on next page)

Procedure 36-11 ■ Setting Up Disposable Chest Drainage Systems (continued)

helps keep air from entering the pleural cavity

c. **Keep a spare disposable drainage system at the patient's bedside.** *To use in case the drainage system in use is accidentally upended or the drainage collection chamber becomes filled.* ➤

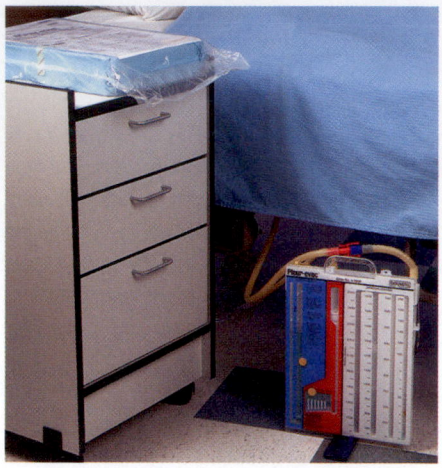

30. **Position the patient for comfort**, as indicated, but with the head of the bed elevated to at least 30°.
    - If the patient received a chest tube to relieve a pneumothorax, the preferred position is semi-Fowler's position.
    - If the chest tube was inserted to promote fluid drainage, high-Fowler's position is recommended.

Evaluation

- **Evaluate the patient's** tolerance to the chest tube insertion. Determine whether the patient's respiratory status has changed.
- Auscultate breath sounds every 2 hours.
- Check chest drainage every 15 minutes for the first 2 hours, and then check as prescribed. Observe type, color, and amount.
- Monitor the chest tube insertion site for drainage and subcutaneous emphysema at least every 4 hours.
  Crepitus is a sign that air is leaking into the subcutaneous tissues. Drainage is a sign that fluid is leaking around the insertion site. Both may indicate a compromise in tube patency.
- Confirm chest tube patency and determine whether bleeding is present.
- Monitor intake and output (I&O) every 8 hours.
- Check laboratory values to evaluate blood loss and oxygenation.
- Check the disposable chest drainage system for the presence of an air leak
  An air leak indicates that air is leaking from the chest and a tight seal has not yet formed over the site of injury.

Patient Teaching

- Teach the patient and family about chest tube insertion.
- Explain the importance of immediately reporting chest pain, shortness of breath, or tube dislodgement.

Home Care

- Explain to the client and caregiver how to care for the chest tube at home.
- Provide the client and caregiver with contact information should problems with the chest tube arise.

Documentation

- Assessment findings before, during, and after chest tube insertion (e.g., vital signs, breath sounds, cardiac status, pulse oximetry)
- Date and time of the chest tube insertion
- Name of the clinician who performed the procedure
- The location of the insertion site, the size of the chest tube, the type of drainage system, and the amount of suction applied, if any
- Any medications the patient received during the procedure
- Color and amount of drainage
- Chest tube output on the I&O portion of the flowsheet (in most agencies)
- Patient's tolerance to the procedure
- Presence of subcutaneous emphysema or air leak, if any
- Complications and any interventions preformed as a result of the complications
- Chest x-ray findings

Sample documentation

8/25/15 0230 Patient presented with acute shortness of breath, pulse ox 84%, respirations 40 breaths/min and shallow, heart rate 132 beats/min. BP 188/100 mm Hg. Breath sounds absent on right side. Patient received morphine sulfate 4 mg IVP. #36 Fr chest tube placed by Dr. Phan under sterile conditions in right anterior chest, midclavicular line, above the 2nd ICS. Chest tube attached to 20 cm of water pressure. Small air leak present, no crepitus. Portable chest x-ray obtained after procedure, revealed chest tube in good placement and right lung re-expanded. Vital signs post-insertion: pulse ox 94%; BP 153/90 mm Hg, heart rate 100 beats/min, and respiratory rate 24 breaths/min. Breath sounds audible bilaterally.——Pennie Bowen, RNC

Procedure 36-11 ■ Setting Up Disposable Chest Drainage Systems (continued)

Practice Resources

Carroll, P. (2012); Kane, C. J., York, N. L., & Minton, L. A. (2013); Maliakal, M. (2013); Siegel, J., Rhinehart, E., Jackson, M., et al. (2007).

Go to *Davis's Nursing Skills Videos*, **Setting Up Wet Seal Disposable Chest Drainage Systems** and **Setting Up Dry Seal Disposable Chest Drainage Systems.**

Thinking About the Procedure

To practice applying clinical reasoning to this procedure,

For questions and suggested responses,

Go to Chapter 36, **Thinking About the Procedure Questions and Suggested Responses,** on Davis*Plus*

Procedure 36-12 ■ Inserting an Oropharyngeal Airway

➤ For steps to follow in *all* procedures, refer to the Universal Steps for All Procedures found on the inside back cover.

The American Heart Association guidelines (2010) direct that you should insert an oropharyngeal airway only if you are trained in its use.

Equipment

- Oral airways in a variety of sizes
- Tongue blade
- Procedure gloves
- Suction equipment
- Resuscitation bag and oxygen source (depending on the patient's status)
- Padded tongue blade

Delegation

You should not delegate this procedure because it requires specialized knowledge, training, and assessment skills.

Pre-Procedure Assessments

- Determine the appropriate airway size by placing the airway on the outside of the patient's cheek. The length of the airway should extend from the front teeth to the end of the jawline.
- Assess breath sounds, respiratory rate and effort, skin color, and pulse oximetry findings.
  Findings confirm the need for the airway and provide a baseline for evaluating the effectiveness of the intervention.
- Assess for contraindications (e.g., patient is conscious or semiconscious; patient has loose teeth or recent oral surgery).
  An oropharyngeal airway may stimulate the gag reflex, causing vomiting or laryngospasm in a conscious patient.

➤ When performing the procedure, always identify your patient according to agency policy, using two identifiers, and be attentive to standard precautions, hand hygiene, patient safety and privacy, body mechanics, and documentation.

Procedure Steps

1. **Perform hand hygiene, and don** clean procedure gloves.
   Helps prevent transfer of microorganisms from the patient.
2. **Explain the procedure** to the patient, even if he appears to be unresponsive.
   Recall that hearing is the last sense lost, so the patient may be able to hear you. Information may help relieve the patient's anxiety, if present.
3. **Clear the mouth of any debris** or secretions. You may need to suction the mouth.
4. **Place the patient in supine** or semi-Fowler's position. Hyperextend the neck, unless contraindicated.
   Mild hyperextension allows the airway to slide naturally toward the pharynx.
5. **Gently open the mouth.** Remove dentures, if present.
   Dentures may cause further airway obstruction.

If Using Tongue Blade Technique

Open the patient's mouth and use the blade to depress the tongue.

If Using Crossed Fingers Technique

Place your thumb on the lower teeth. Cross your index finger over your thumb and place the finger on the upper teeth. Push the teeth apart.

6. **You may need to hold** the tongue down with a tongue blade as you insert the airway.
7. **Insert the airway** along the top of the tongue, in the upside-down position (the "C" faces upward toward the nose).
   Prevents pushing the tongue toward the pharynx.▼

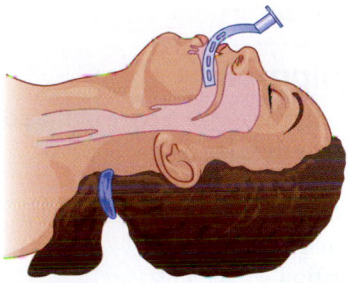

8. **As the airway approaches** the posterior wall of the pharynx, rotate the airway 180° so that the ends of the "C" turn downward over the back of the tongue. Continue to insert the

(continued on next page)

Procedure 36-12 ■ Inserting an Oropharyngeal Airway (continued)

airway until the front flange is flush with the lips. ▼

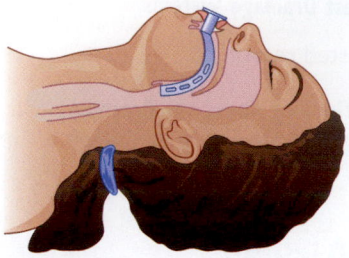

9. **Keep the patient's head tilted** slightly back and the chin elevated.
This position helps the oropharyngeal airway to function optimally.

10. **Do not tape the airway** in place.
You may need to remove the airway quickly for suctioning. Untaping would delay airway removal, increasing the risk of aspiration.

11. **Position the patient on her side.**
To minimize the risk of aspiration.

12. **Provide oral hygiene** at least every 2 to 4 hours. Remove and cleanse the airway at that time; use hydrogen peroxide and then rinse with water.

? What if . . . .

- **After inserting the airway, respirations are absent or inadequate?**
Use a mouth-to-mask technique, a handheld resuscitation bag, or an oxygen-powered breathing device to ventilate the patient. Have someone call for help.

Evaluation

- After inserting the airway, verify patency by auscultating for bilateral breath sounds.
- Check for bleeding or tooth damage in the mouth.
May be caused by airway insertion, especially if it must be done rapidly.
- Check to be certain the patient's lips and tongue are not caught between the teeth and the airway.
Prevents trauma to the soft tissues.
- Monitor the airway position frequently.
Ensures correct placement.
- Continually reassess the need for the airway. Remove it when the patient begins to cough or gag.
- Frequently assess oral mucous membranes when you remove the airway for care.
Prolonged airway use can cause tissue irritation or ulceration.
- Keep suction available at the bedside. Suction the oropharynx as needed by inserting the suction catheter alongside the airway.

Documentation

Document the following:

- Date and time of airway insertion
- Type and size of airway (oropharyngeal or nasopharyngeal)
- Assessments before and after the procedure, including breath sounds and focused respiratory assessment
- Any suctioning performed
- Patient's tolerance of the procedure
- Adverse reactions and interventions taken

Practice Resources

AACN (2010); American Heart Association (2010); Walls, R., & Murphy, M. (2012).

Procedure 36-13 ■ Inserting a Nasopharyngeal Airway

➤ For steps to follow in *all* procedures, refer to the Universal Steps for All Procedures found on the inside back cover.

The American Heart Association guidelines (2010) direct that you should insert a nasopharyngeal airway only if you are trained in its use.

Equipment

- Nasopharyngeal airway of the correct size
- Tongue blade
- Procedure gloves
- Water-soluble lubricant
- Penlight
- Suction equipment
- Resuscitation bag and oxygen source (depending on the patient's status)

Delegation

You should not delegate this procedure because it requires specialized knowledge, training, and assessment skills. Commonly, this procedure is performed by a respiratory therapist.

Pre-Procedure Assessments

- Determine the appropriate airway size: (1) Measure the diameter of the patient's nostril and use an airway that is slightly smaller than that; and (2) measure the distance from the tip of the patient's nose to the earlobe, and use an airway about 2.5 cm (1 in.) longer than that measurement. Airways are sized by their internal diameter. Generally, the larger the internal diameter, the longer the tube. Airways are available in a variety of pediatric and adult sizes.
  Small adult: 6 to 7 mm
  Medium adult: 7 to 8 mm
  Large adult: 8 to 9 mm

- Assess breath sounds, respiratory rate and effort, skin color, pulse oximetry findings.
  Findings confirm the need for the airway and provide a baseline for evaluating the effectiveness of the intervention.
- Assess for contraindications (e.g., anticoagulant therapy, hemorrhagic disorder, nasopharyngeal deformity, sepsis).
  Up to 30% of patients experience airway bleeding after insertion of a nasopharyngeal airway.

➤ When performing the procedure, always identify your patient according to agency policy, using two identifiers, and be attentive to standard precautions, hand hygiene, patient safety and privacy, body mechanics, and documentation.

Procedure Steps

1. **Perform hand hygiene** and don procedure gloves.
   Helps prevent transfer of microorganisms from the patient.
2. **Position the patient supine** or in semi-Fowler's position. Explain the procedure.
   A semi-Fowler's position facilitates airway insertions. Explaining may alleviate anxiety, enabling the patient to cooperate more with the procedure.
3. **Validate that the airway size** is correct. Hold the airway next to the patient's face. Measure airway from tip of nose to jawline below the ear, and use an airway about 2.5 cm (1 in.) longer than that. Airway should be slightly smaller than the nares.
4. **Lubricate the airway** with water-soluble lubricant.
   Prevents trauma to mucosa during insertion.
5. **Tilt the patient's head backward** to hyperextend the neck. Then push up the tip of the nose and gently insert the tip of the airway into the nose.
6. **Advance the airway** along the floor of the nostril into the posterior pharynx behind the tongue—until the outer flange rests on the nostril. If you meet resistance, rotate the tube slightly to enhance passage. Do not force against resistance.
   Forcing the tube can cause tissue trauma and airway kinking.
7. **Have the patient open her mouth.** Depress the tongue with a tongue blade and inspect the pharynx for proper placement of the tube tip. Use a penlight, if necessary, for better visualization.
   When the tube is fully inserted, the outer flange of the tube should rest on the nostril, and only the tip of the tube should be visible at the top of the posterior pharynx.▼

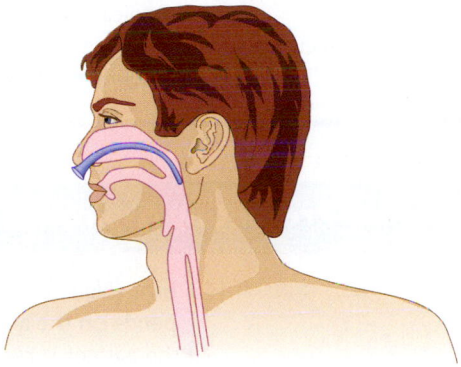

8. **Check for correct placement** and function: Close the patient's mouth, and place your finger close to the tube's opening to feel for air exchange.
9. **Auscultate the lungs** for the presence of bilateral breath sounds.
10. **Remove the airway** at least every 8 hours to check nasal mucous membranes for ulceration or irritation. Clean the airway at this time: Place in a basin, rinse with hydrogen peroxide, then rinse with water. Use a pipe cleaner to remove secretions, if necessary. Reinsert the airway in the other nostril.
    To avoid skin and mucous membrane irritation and breakdown and to prevent infection

? What if . . .

- **After you insert the airway, the patient coughs, gags, vomits, or has laryngospasm?**

  The tube may be too long. If the tip extends beyond the top of the posterior pharynx, remove it and insert a shorter one.

Evaluation

- Assess respiratory rate and effort.
- Assess breath sounds.
- Observe for bleeding of nasal mucosa; suction as necessary.
- If the patient is receiving artificial ventilation, monitor for gastric distention and hypoventilation.
- Provide frequent oral and nares care; assess the skin around the nostril.

Documentation

Document the following:

- Date and time of airway insertion
- Type and size of airway (nasopharyngeal)
- Assessments before and after the procedure, including breath sounds, focused respiratory assessment, and condition of the mucous membranes
- Suctioning, if performed
- Patient's tolerance of the procedure
- Adverse reactions and interventions taken
- Removal of the airway, cleaning, and replacement in the other nostril

Practice Resources

AACN (2010); American Heart Association (2010); American Red Cross (n.d.); Bullard, D., Brothers, K., Davis, C., et al. (2012); Walls, R., & Murphy, M. (2012).

CLINICAL INSIGHTS

Clinical Insight 36-1 ➤ Tips for Obtaining Accurate Pulse Oximetry Readings

Patient Movement. A nailbed is the most common site to place the probe. However, a tremor, twitch, shivering, or movement in bed can make pulse oximetry readings inaccurate. If the patient is unable to cooperate or control his movement, try using an ear probe or nasal sensor.

Acrylic Fingernails and Nail Polish. If the patient has acrylic nails, place the probe on a toe or earlobe. Many facilities stock individually packaged nail polish remover pads to remove nail polish before placing the probe.

Nail polish or acrylic nails may interfere with signal transmission, causing inaccurate Sa_{O_2} measurement. However, a recent study found that nail polish did not cause a clinically significant change in readings in healthy people (Chan, Chan, & Chan, 2013).

Dirt and Skin Oils. Dirt and oils on the site can interfere with passage of light waves.

Poor Perfusion. A low reading may result from poor perfusion of the area where the probe is placed.

- A bent elbow, for example, may cause a slight decrease in circulation to the nailbed. If Sa_{O_2} results are crucial to the patient's plan of care, use the earlobe to minimize the effect of movement on the reading.
- Keep the extremities warm to obtain a more accurate reading.

Vasoconstriction due to cool extremities may also limit circulation.

- If poor perfusion is related to a disease process, use the earlobe or nose as the monitoring site.

Lighting. Bright fluorescent lighting may influence the accuracy of the reading. Dim the lights or cover the probe with bed covers or a towel to reduce error.

Anemia, Carbon Monoxide, Intravascular Dyes, and Dark Skin Color. These must be considered when interpreting oximetry readings. Because these factors cannot be controlled, watch for trend changes in the readings.

Equipment Function. Look for a displayed waveform; a reading is meaningless without the waveform. If there is a weak signal or no signal, check the patient's vital signs. If vital signs are satisfactory, check the circulation to the site. If that is satisfactory, check equipment connections.

Accuracy of the Reading. If there is an instantaneous change in saturation (e.g., from 99% to 82%), suspect an error. This is not physiologically possible. For any suspected inaccuracy, check the reading using the equipment on a healthy person. If it seems accurate, check the patient's medications and history of circulatory disorders; also check items listed above. When in doubt, rely on your clinical judgment more than the reading from the machine.

Clinical Insight 36-2 ➤ Guidelines for Preventing Aspiration

To prevent aspiration, use the following guidelines.

For At-Risk Patients

Position the unconscious patient on his side to protect the airway.

Request medications in elixir or liquid form.

Break or crush pills, when appropriate.

Keep a suction setup available for routine and emergency use.

If the patient is intubated, keep the endotracheal or tracheostomy cuff inflated, and suction above the cuff before deflating the cuff.

Do not offer food or fluids if the patient is heavily sedated or in the initial recovery phase of anesthesia.

Enteral Feedings

Check the placement of the nasogastric tube before you administer enteral feedings.

Check gastric residual volume before administering the next enteral feeding. Hold the feeding if the residual volume is high. (*Note:* The amount of acceptable residual volume depends on the amount and frequency of feedings.)

If the patient is receiving continuous tube feedings, the head of the bed must remain elevated.

Also see Procedure 27-3 for step-by-step instructions for administering feedings through gastric and enteric tubes.

Oral Feedings

Position the patient upright or with the head of the bed elevated for feedings or meal.

Be sure the head of bed remains elevated for at least 30 minutes after each feeding or meal.

Offer small, frequent meals.

Avoid thin liquids, or use thickening agents.

Offer foods or liquids that can be formed into a bolus before they are swallowed.

Cut food into small pieces.

Clinical Insight 36-3 ➤ Oxygen Therapy Safety Precautions

- Post signs indicating that oxygen is in use.
- Do not permit smoking near oxygen delivery systems.
- Ensure that three-pronged plugs are used for electrical devices (to prevent sparks).
- Allow no open flames (e.g., candles) near oxygen.
- Do not use electrical equipment with frayed wires or loose connections.
- Do not use petroleum products, aerosol products, and products containing acetone where oxygen is in use. (These are flammable substances that are easily ignited.)
- Secure oxygen tanks to rigid stands.
- Secure portable oxygen cylinders in holders or carriers provided.

Clinical Insight 36-4 ➤ Caring for Patients With Endotracheal Airways

Assisting With Endotracheal Airway Insertion

- **Gather equipment.** You will need an oxygen source and a bag (e.g., Ambu or nonrebreather bag) to inflate the lungs, a laryngoscope, endotracheal tubes of various sizes, water-soluble lubricant, a syringe to inflate the cuff, and tape to secure the tube in place.
- **Keep suction at the bedside** to clear the mouth and airway if secretions are obstructing your view of the cords.
- **You will need a surgical tray** if a tracheostomy is performed to create the direct opening into the trachea.
- **Remain calm, and explain** to the patient that the airway will enable him to breathe effectively.
- **Once the airway is in place, listen to breath sounds** to establish that both lungs are ventilated.
- **Reassess breath sounds periodically.** After the airway is inserted, record the type and size, as well as the patient's response to the procedure.
- **Expect that a portable chest x-ray will be prescribed** to confirm correct placement.

Managing and Monitoring Endotracheal and Airways

The following are activities associated with the care of all types of endotracheal airways.

- **Have emergency equipment**, including a duplicate tracheostomy kit, extra cannula, and suction setup immediately available for reintubation if the tube should become dislodged.
- **Keep an extra cannula at the bedside**, as patients may accidentally decannulate.
- **Secure the endotracheal tube** with ties, Velcro tapes, or a commercial holder to prevent accidental displacement.
- **Provide tracheostomy care every 4 to 8 hours** (Mitchell, Hussey, Setzen, et al., 2013).
- **Change the endotracheal or tracheostomy ties every 24 hours.**
- **Secure the orotracheal tube** to the opposite side of the mouth with each change of tape or ties to prevent skin erosion and breakdown.
- **Inspect skin around the tube** or tracheal stoma for redness, swelling, drainage, or irritation at least every 8 hours.
- **Provide skin care** around the tube and tape or holder at least daily.
- **Perform regular oral care.**
- **Inflate the cuff of the tube with a minimal occlusive volume and monitor cuff pressures** to prevent pressure necrosis inside the trachea. (This is a joint responsibility with the respiratory therapist.) Maximum acceptable tube cuff pressure is 25 mm Hg. The following is a method for checking for minimal occluding volume:
  1. Place stethoscope on patient's neck over the carotid pulse.
  2. Attach a 10-mL syringe to the pilot balloon of the inflated cuff.
  3. Remove air from the cuff—(1 mL at a time) until you hear a slight leak at the peak of inspiration.
  4. When you hear the leak, inject 1 mL of air back into the cuff.
- **Monitor and document cuff pressure** once per shift and when the tube is changed or repositioned.
- **Note the centimeter reference marking** on the endotracheal tube to monitor for possible displacement.
- **Minimize pulling and traction** on the artificial airway by supporting all tubing connected to the airway and using flexible catheter mounts and swivels.
- If he is conscious, **remind the patient not to pull on the airway.**
- **Use a bite block** between the teeth to prevent the patient from occluding an orotracheal tube.
- **Provide 100% humidification** of inspired air. Check the oxygen setup regularly.
- **Routine saline instillation** to thin secretions is no longer recommended.
- **Ensure adequate hydration** with oral or IV fluids to keep the mucosa moist and thin secretions.
- **Suction the airway** when secretions collect. Remember, the patient probably can't cough effectively to clear secretions.

Clinical Insight 36-5 ➤ Managing Chest Tubes

Monitor Breathing, Gas Exchange, and Drainage

- Frequently assess breathing patterns, breathing effort, and breath sounds.
- Assess mental status, heart rate and rhythm, and pulse oximetry readings.
  These reflect adequacy of oxygenation.
- Monitor character, color, and amount of chest drainage. Immediately report sudden or large increases in drainage or new onset of bright red blood, along with an assessment of the patient's condition at that time.
  Drainage is usually greatest when the chest tube is initially inserted and decreases as the lung reexpands. You must replace the chest drainage unit (CDU) when the drainage compartment is almost full.

Prevent Complications or Intervene If They Occur

- Observe the dressing at least every 4 hours. Make sure that the dressing around the tube insertion site is occlusive (e.g., not wet or loose). Usually, petroleum gauze is wrapped around the insertion site to ensure occlusion.
- Inspect for excessive, abnormal, or foul-smelling drainage.
  This may indicate hemorrhage or infection.
- Palpate around the dressing for **subcutaneous emphysema** (air in the subcutaneous tissues).
  This may be caused by an incomplete seal at the chest tube insertion site.
- Assess for pain; medicate as needed.
- Reposition the patient every 2 hours and use pillows to keep the patient's weight off the chest tube.
  To prevent occlusion of the tube, promote drainage, and preserve skin integrity.
- Encourage the patient to use the arm on the affected side. Assist with range-of-motion exercises, if necessary.
  To maintain joint mobility.
- **Recollapse of the lung** can occur because of loss of negative pressure within the system. This is commonly caused by air leaks, disconnections, or breaks or cracks of the bottles or chambers. If any of these occur, immediately place the disconnected end nearest the patient into a bottle of sterile water or saline.
- Do not clamp the chest tube. Clamp chest tubes only for changing the drainage system. Limit the clamp time and monitor respiratory status constantly until the clamp is removed.
  Clamping can rapidly lead to a tension pneumothorax.
- If the tube is accidentally pulled out, immediately cover the wound with a dry, sterile dressing. Listen for air leaking out of the site. If you can hear air, tape the dressing loosely so that you do not occlude the site.
  If air cannot escape from the chest, a tension pneumothorax will occur, eventually compromising cardiovascular function.

Promote Lung Reexpansion

- Encourage the patient to be as active as his condition permits.
  Chest drainage systems are bulky, but with disposable systems, patients can still get out of bed and ambulate, but will need assistance to protect and monitor the system and the patient.
- Instruct the patient to perform deep breathing and coughing every 2 hours, unless contraindicated. Assist the patient to sit upright and splint the chest with a pillow or the hands, and provide analgesia as needed.
  These interventions help to minimize discomfort.

Key Points for Managing a One-Bottle System

- Keep the intake tube below the fluid level in the drainage bottle.
  To prevent drawing air into the pleural space with inhalation.
- Maintain the tubing about 2 cm below the water level. As tubing length below the water increases, more effort is required to exhale.
- Take precautions to see that the bottle is not accidentally tipped over, uncovering the long vent tube and allowing air to enter the pleural space.

Maintain the Drainage System

For All Types of CDUs:

- Make sure the drainage system is located below the insertion site.
  If the drainage system is higher than the insertion site, fluid may flow back into the pleural cavity, compromising the patient's respiratory status.
- Regularly inspect tubing to ensure that connections are airtight and tubing is not kinked or occluded.
  Kinks in the drainage tubing increase pressure in the pleural cavity and prevent fluid drainage.
- Monitor drainage.
  Blood or purulent matter can occlude the tubing.
- Inspect the air vent in the drainage system to make sure it is patent.
  If air builds up in the pleural cavity, pneumothorax may occur.
- Monitor to ensure the system is maintaining consistent negative pressure levels.
- Do not "milk" or strip the tubing.
  Doing so can create excess negative pressure and damage lung tissue
- Most systems will have some type of check system to ensure that the system is operating correctly. Always be sure to verify operation through the users' manual or with the product's vendor.
- To transport or ambulate a patient: (1) Keep the CDU upright below chest level; (2) disconnect the CDU from suction source and make sure the air vent is open.

Clinical Insight 36-5 ➤ Managing Chest Tubes—cont'd

Water-Seal Drainage Systems:

- Take precautions that the CDU is not tipped over (e.g., tape it to the floor).
- Observe for **tidaling** (fluctuations in the water-seal chamber's fluid level that correspond with respiration). The level will increase on inspiration and decrease on exhalation. This will be opposite for a patient on a mechanical ventilator.
- Bubbling in the bottom of the water-seal chamber indicates an air leak. When this occurs, check for poor tubing connections. A small amount of bubbling right after insertion or with exhalation or cough is normal.
- Check the water in the suction control chamber; replace as needed.
  The water can evaporate.
- ✚ If the chest tube disconnects from the drainage unit, establish a temporary water seal by immersing the open end of the chest tube in a bottle of sterile water to a depth of 2 cm until a new system can be connected. Cleanse the end of the patient connector on the drain system with alcohol and reconnect it if it has not been contaminated. If the patient connector on the drain system is contaminated, you must initiate a new CDU.

Dry-Seal Drainage Systems:

- Inspect the air vent in the drainage system to make sure it is patent.
  The air vent must remain patent to allow air to escape. If air builds up in the pleural cavity, pneumothorax may occur.
- Check the indicators on the CDU to be certain that suction is operating properly.
  A dry chest drainage system doesn't use water in the suction chamber. A valve inside the regulator continuously balances the forces of suction and the atmosphere. The valve automatically responds and adjusts to changes in patient air leaks and fluctuations in suction source vacuum to deliver accurate suction to the patient. Pressure can be set from –10 cm H_2O to –40 cm H_2O by adjusting the rotary dry suction dial.
- Observe for bubbling.
  If the water in a dry-seal CDU is bubbling, it means there is an air leak.

ASSESSMENT GUIDELINES AND TOOLS

Focused Assessment

Oxygenation

Part I. Questions to Assess Risk for Impaired Oxygenation

Demographic Data

- What is your age?
- Where do you live?
- What is your occupation?

Health History

- What healthcare problems are you currently being treated for?
- Have you ever been hospitalized or had surgery? If so, when and for what reason?
- Do you have a history of allergies or asthma?
- What medications do you currently take?
- What over-the-counter medications or alternative treatments do you use? What do you use them for?

Respiratory History

- Have you ever been diagnosed with a respiratory problem? If so, what was the diagnosis? When was the diagnosis made?
- Have you noticed any changes in your breathing?
- How often do you cough?
- When you do cough, is it productive?
- What do the secretions you cough up look like and smell like?
- How much sputum do you produce?
- How do you treat your cough? What effect did it have?
- Do you ever wheeze or feel short of breath?
- What causes you to wheeze or feel short of breath?
- Do body positions affect your breathing pattern?
- What position do you lie in when you sleep? Do you use more than one pillow?
- Do you ever wake up short of breath?

Environmental History

- Are there pets in the house?
- What response, if any, do you have to pets, dust, pollen, or plants?
- Are you exposed to smoke or fumes in the home and workplace?
- Are you exposed to respiratory irritants such as asbestos, chemicals, coal dust, fungus, molds, or soot in the home or workplace?
- What type of heating, air-conditioning, or air-filtering system do you have in the home or workplace?

(continued)

Focused Assessment

Lifestyle

- What is your current stress level? What are your major sources of stress?
- What is your usual diet? Is your current diet typical, or have you recently changed your eating habits?
- What is your usual activity level?
- What level of activity makes you feel short of breath?
- Do you smoke now, or have you ever smoked?
- If you smoke, how many packs per day and for how many years have you smoked?
- Do you smoke marijuana or use other substances?

Part II. Focused Physical Examination

Pulmonary System

- ***Inspect*** to observe respiratory patterns, signs of respiratory distress, chest structures and movement, skin and mucous membrane color, presence or absence of edema, sputum characteristics, and overall general appearance.
- ***Palpate*** skin temperature and areas of tenderness.
- ***Percuss*** over the lung fields (for consolidation or excess air pockets).
- ***Auscultate*** breath sounds and vascular sounds.
- ***Assess breathing patterns:*** eupnea, tachypnea, bradypnea, apnea, Kussmaul's breathing, Biot's breathing, and Cheyne-Stokes respirations.
- ***Assess cough and related symptoms:***

  Nasal congestion, sneezing, watery eyes, and nasal discharge suggest allergies.

  Fever, chest congention, noisy breath sounds, sputum production suggest a URI.

  Dyspnea, chest tightness, and wheezing suggest airway obstruction (e.g., asthma).
- ***Assess sputum:*** appearance, color, odor, amount, and timing.
- ***Obtain sputum samples*** as needed.
- ***Assess respiratory effort:*** Breathing should be effortless. Observe for shortness of breath, dyspnea, nasal flaring, head bobbing, retractions, use of accessory muscles during inspiration, grunting, needing to sit upright to breathe, paroxysmal nocturnal dyspnea, conversational dyspnea, stridor, and wheezing.

Key Point: *Ask every patient, not just those with oxygenation problems, whether they use tobacco and document their tobacco-use status regularly.*

DIAGNOSTIC TESTING

Diagnostic Testing

Lung Volumes and Capacities

The norms presented in this table are based on averages for a young adult man. The following are measured by spirometry.

Title	Definition	Significance
Tidal volume (V_T)	The amount of air moved into and out of the lungs with each normal breath. Normally around 500 mL.	In a healthy state, V_T increases when oxygen demand increases. Diseases that restrict lung inflation, create muscular weakness, or paralyze the diaphragm limit the ability of the body to increase tidal volume. When such disorders become severe, V_T will fall too low to support even resting oxygen demands.
Inspiratory reserve volume (IRV)	The maximum amount of air that can be inhaled above and beyond the normal tidal volume. Ranges from 2,000 to 3,000 mL.	IRV determines how much the tidal volume can increase when oxygen demands increase.
Expiratory reserve volume (ERV)	The maximum extra amount of air that can be forcefully exhaled after the end of a normal tidal expiration. Ranges from 1,000 to 1,500 mL.	Some diseases (e.g., emphysema) cause collapse of alveoli and airways, which traps extra air in the lungs. This "trapped" air cannot be exhaled and lowers ERV.
Residual volume (RV)	The amount of air remaining in the lungs after the most forceful exhalation. Ranges from 1,000 to 1,500 mL.	Diseases that reduce ERV lead to an increase in RV. As more air is trapped in the lungs and cannot be exhaled even with forceful attempts (ERV), it becomes part of the residual volume that is never completely exhaled.

Diagnostic Testing

Inspiratory capacity (IC)	The combination of the tidal volume and inspiratory reserve volume (V_T + IRV). Ranges from 2,500 to 3,500 mL.	This is the amount of air that can be inhaled with maximum effort. It reflects the capacity one has to inhale deeply.
Functional residual capacity (FRC)	The combination of expiratory reserve volume and residual volume (ERV + RV). Ranges from 2,000 to 3,000 mL. Exhalation of additional air requires effort to force more air out.	This is the amount of air that stays in the lungs at the end of a normal, passive quiet exhalation. Disorders that cause air trapping increase the FRC.
Vital capacity (VC)	The combination of inspiratory reserve volume and expiratory reserve volume (IRV + ERV). Ranges from 3,000 to 4,500 mL.	This is the maximum amount of air that can be forcefully exhaled after filling the lungs to their maximum level with the deepest possible inspiratory effort.

Diagnostic Testing

Tests Related to Oxygenation

Test	Purpose
Angiogram	A contrast dye is injected into a vein, and serial films are taken to assess patency of the vessels.
Arterial blood gases (ABG)	An analysis of arterial blood that evaluates the effectiveness of gas exchange
Bronchoscopy	Insertion of a flexible endoscope to examine the larynx, trachea, and bronchial tree
Cardiac catheterization	A catheter is passed into the heart to assess pressures, blood flow, and the size and patency of chambers.
Chest x-ray study (CXR)	Provides an anterior–posterior or lateral view of the heart and lungs, shows tissue density (e.g., to evaluate size, masses, fluid).
Creatine kinase-MB (CK-MB)	The MB isoenzyme is present only in the heart muscle. A serum measurement of the MB band is used to detect a myocardial infarction (MI). Levels rise with an acute MI.
Echocardiogram	An ultrasound evaluation of the heart that examines heart function and blood flow.
Electrocardiogram (ECG)	Electrodes placed on the extremities and chest wall conduct electrical activity from the heart. ECG illustrates heart rate, rhythm, and size and helps evaluate heart damage.
Hemoglobin (Hgb)	A serum measurement that affects the oxygen-carrying capacity of the blood. May be measured separately or as part of a complete blood count.
Holter monitor	A continuous ECG tracing used to correlate symptoms and cardiac activity. Typically the tracing lasts 48 hours to 7 days.
Pulmonary function studies	A series of tests to detect lung volume and capacity
Sputum culture	A microscopic evaluation of the sputum
Technetium scan	Technetium-99m sestamibi is injected intravenously. Approximately 90 to 120 minutes later, the heart is scanned. Areas of myocardial damage appear as "hot spots" on the scan.
Thoracentesis	Insertion of a large-bore needle through the chest wall into the pleural space to obtain fluid specimens, to instill medication, or to drain accumulations of fluid
Throat culture	A swab of the pharynx or tonsils is performed to assess pathogens present in the pharynx.
Treadmill test	Evaluates the effect of exercise on the heart and circulation via continuous ECG and vital sign monitoring during exercise.
Troponin	A serum evaluation of a complex of proteins is used to detect myocardial infarction (MI). Levels of these contractile proteins remain elevated for up to 7 days after MI.
Ventilation–perfusion scan	Used to assess for pulmonary embolus, this scan entails injection of a radioactive substance that allows blood flow to the lungs to be evaluated. A second substance is inhaled that maps out oxygen distribution in the lungs.
White blood cell (WBC) count	A serum measure to assess for the presence of infection

Diagnostic Testing

Reading a Tuberculin Skin Test Result

Size of Induration	Considered Positive For
>5 mm	People who have had recent close contact with someone with active TB
	People who have HIV or risk factors for HIV
	People with previous history of TB
>10 mm	IV drug users known to be HIV-negative
	People with medical conditions that increase the risk of progressing from latent TB to active TB (e.g., diabetes mellitus, use of steroids, chronic renal failure, some malignancies)
	Residents and employees of high-risk congregate settings: prisons, skilled nursing facilities (SNFs) and other long-term facilities, healthcare facilities, and homeless shelters
	Foreign-born persons recently arrived (i.e., within the past 5 yr) from countries having a high incidence of TB
	Low-income groups
	Children younger than 4 years of age or exposed to adults in high-risk categories
>15 mm	People who do not meet any of the above criteria

CLINICALREASONING

Applying the Full-Spectrum Nursing Model

PATIENT SITUATION

Haley, a 15-year-old female high school student, was admitted to the hospital with shortness of breath and right-sided chest pain when breathing. She states that she has had "the flu" for 3 days. She has a history of asthma since age 6, and smokes half a pack of cigarettes a day. Both her parents are heavy smokers as well. An IV was initiated, and she is receiving 800 mg of vancomycin (an antibiotic) intravenously every 12 hours. She is not on oxygen therapy, but receives 10 incentive spirometer treatments per hour while awake. Her heart rate is 80 beats/min, respiratory rate, 24 breaths/min, and blood pressure, 110/70 mm Hg. Her skin is pale but warm, and capillary refill time is 2 seconds. She has no clubbing of the fingers. She is urinating approximately 400 mL of clear yellow urine every 8 hours and maintaining a normal bowel elimination pattern. Laboratory results are:

Red blood cell count (RBCs): 3.56×10^6 (3.56 million/mm^3)
White blood cell count (WBCs): 11,800/mm^3
Hemoglobin: 11.2 g/dL
Hematocrit: 32.7%
Haley says, "I feel really tired, and too weak to even pick up a glass of water." Her cough produces white, thick sputum. Sputum culture on admission confirms a diagnosis of streptococcal pneumonia.

THINKING

1. *Theoretical Knowledge:*
   a. According to the CDC, should Haley have received a pneumonia immunization? Why or why not?
   b. What is clubbing of the fingers? You may wish to refer to Chapter 22 for review, or to a medical-surgical nursing text.
2. *Critical Thinking (Analyzing Assumptions):*
   Why is it a positive finding for Haley that she does not have clubbed fingers?

DOING

3. *Practical Knowledge:*
Twenty-four hours after the antibiotics were started, Haley's respiratory status becomes worse. She says, "It's so hard to breathe." It is decided to begin administering oxygen. Another sputum culture is prescribed. You are to collect a sputum specimen from the patient.
   a. What position should Haley assume for this procedure?
   b. What kind of protective clothing do you need for this procedure?
   c. You remove the lid from the specimen container. When you hand it to Haley, she touches the inside of the container with her fingers. What should you do?
   d. What would you tell Haley to do in order to expectorate the sputum specimen?
4. *Nursing Process (Assessment):*
In the admission data, what important information is missing with regard to her respiratory status?

CARING

5. *Self-Knowledge:*
Describe one or two patient care experiences you might draw upon to help you in caring for Haley. In what ways were those patients similar to Haley, and how might that help you?
6. *Ethical Knowledge:*
After you finish collecting the sputum specimen, what do you think Haley's biggest concern is right now?

Critical Thinking and Clinical Reasoning

1. Recall the three patients discussed in the Meet Your Patients scenario in your textbook in Volume 1:
   - Mary is a 4-year-old girl with a history of asthma. Her mother, Ms. Green, has brought her in for an asthma attack. Mary is sitting on her mother's lap and breathing rapidly through an open mouth. Her cough sounds congested and wheezy. The nurse practitioner has ordered a nebulized treatment containing albuterol (Proventil) and ipratropium bromide (Atrovent).
   - Mr. Chu is a 78-year-old man complaining of cough, sore throat, fatigue, and weakness. His temperature is 100.4°F (38°C), pulse is 90 beats/min, respirations are 26/min, and blood pressure (BP) is 166/82 mm Hg.
   - William is a 19-year-old male who has had a sudden onset of right-sided chest pain and shortness of breath. His chest x-ray revealed a right pneumothorax, and he is currently receiving 35% oxygen by face mask while waiting for an ambulance to transport him to the hospital for further evaluation.
   a. Which patients are experiencing problems with ventilation? Explain your answer.
   b. Which patient appears to be experiencing problems with hypoxia? Does the problem appear to be related to oxygenation or perfusion? Explain your answers.
   c. Mr. Chu has smoked two packs of cigarettes per day for 50 years. ABGs reveal a low P_{O_2} and a high P_{CO_2} consistent with chronic lung disease. He is diagnosed with an acute exacerbation of chronic bronchitis. He is placed on oral antibiotics and long-acting bronchodilators by metered-dose inhaler (MDI). What teaching could you offer to help Mr. Chu mobilize and expectorate secretions?
   d. Mary receives her nebulizer treatment and markedly improves. The physician has prescribed a variety of take-home medications that you must teach her mother about. The treatment plan includes a protocol based on peak expiratory flow monitoring. Discuss how you might involve Mary in her own care.
   e. William's chest x-ray film reveals a spontaneous pneumothorax. There is no apparent fluid in the pleural space. What chest tube systems can be used to treat his pneumothorax? Explain your thinking.
2. You are caring for a 68-year-old woman during the night shift. Earlier today she had an abdominal hysterectomy under general anesthesia. You note that her respiratory rate has steadily risen from 16 to 26 and that she has developed a mild, nonproductive cough. When you listen to her chest, you hear crackles throughout. She has a 40-pack-per-year cigarette smoking history. Identify an appropriate nursing diagnosis for this patient. Explain the reasons for your choice.
3. For each of the following concepts, use critical thinking to describe how or why it is important to nursing, patient care, or oxygenation. Note that these are not to be merely definitions.

Ventilation	Hypoventilation
Gas exchange	Hyperventilation
Artificial airways	Supplemental oxygen
Suctioning	Pulse oximetry
Negative pressure in the chest	

What Are the Main Points in This Chapter?

- The structures of the airways, lungs, chest cavity, heart, and blood vessels function together to supply oxygen to the tissues; thus, abnormalities in any of these structures can interfere with tissue oxygenation.
- Developmental stage, environment, lifestyle, smoking, medications, and pathological factors can interfere with ventilation, circulation, or gas exchange, leading to problems with tissue oxygenation.
- A health assessment related to oxygenation includes assessment of ventilation (breathing), circulation (blood flow), and gas exchange (exchange of oxygen and carbon dioxide). The length and focus of the assessment varies with the purpose and urgency of the clinical situation.
- A physical examination related to adequacy of oxygenation includes observations of adequacy of breathing, circulation, and gas exchange.
- Pulse oximetry and arterial blood gases are used to monitor oxygen saturation.
- Small changes in oxygen saturation are associated with large shifts in the amount of oxygen available to the tissues and organs.
- Interventions to promote optimal respiratory function include deep, regular breathing, supporting smoking cessation, flu and pneumonia immunizations for at-risk individuals, frequent position changes, incentive spirometry, and preventing aspiration.
- Deep breathing, coughing exercises, and hydration promote deep inhalation and forceful expulsion of secretions.
- Supplemental oxygen is used to prevent hypoxemia. It may be delivered by a variety of methods.
- Artificial airways provide an open airway for patients who cannot maintain their own airway. The most common artificial airways are oropharyngeal, nasopharyngeal, and endotracheal.
- Airways can be suctioned to remove secretions and maintain patency. Signs that indicate the need for suctioning include gurgling sounds during respiration, restlessness, labored respirations, decreased oxygen saturation, increased heart and respiratory rates, and adventitious breath sounds during auscultation.
- Mechanical ventilation with a positive pressure ventilator requires the patient to have an artificial airway.
- Chest tubes remove air or fluid from the pleural space so that the lungs can fully expand. Chest tubes should be clamped only for changing the drainage system; clamping can lead to tension pneumothorax.
- Respiratory medications promote ventilation and oxygenation by their effects on the respiratory system. The major types of respiratory medicines include bronchodilators, corticosteroids, cough preparations, decongestants, antihistamines, and mucolytics.

Knowledge Map

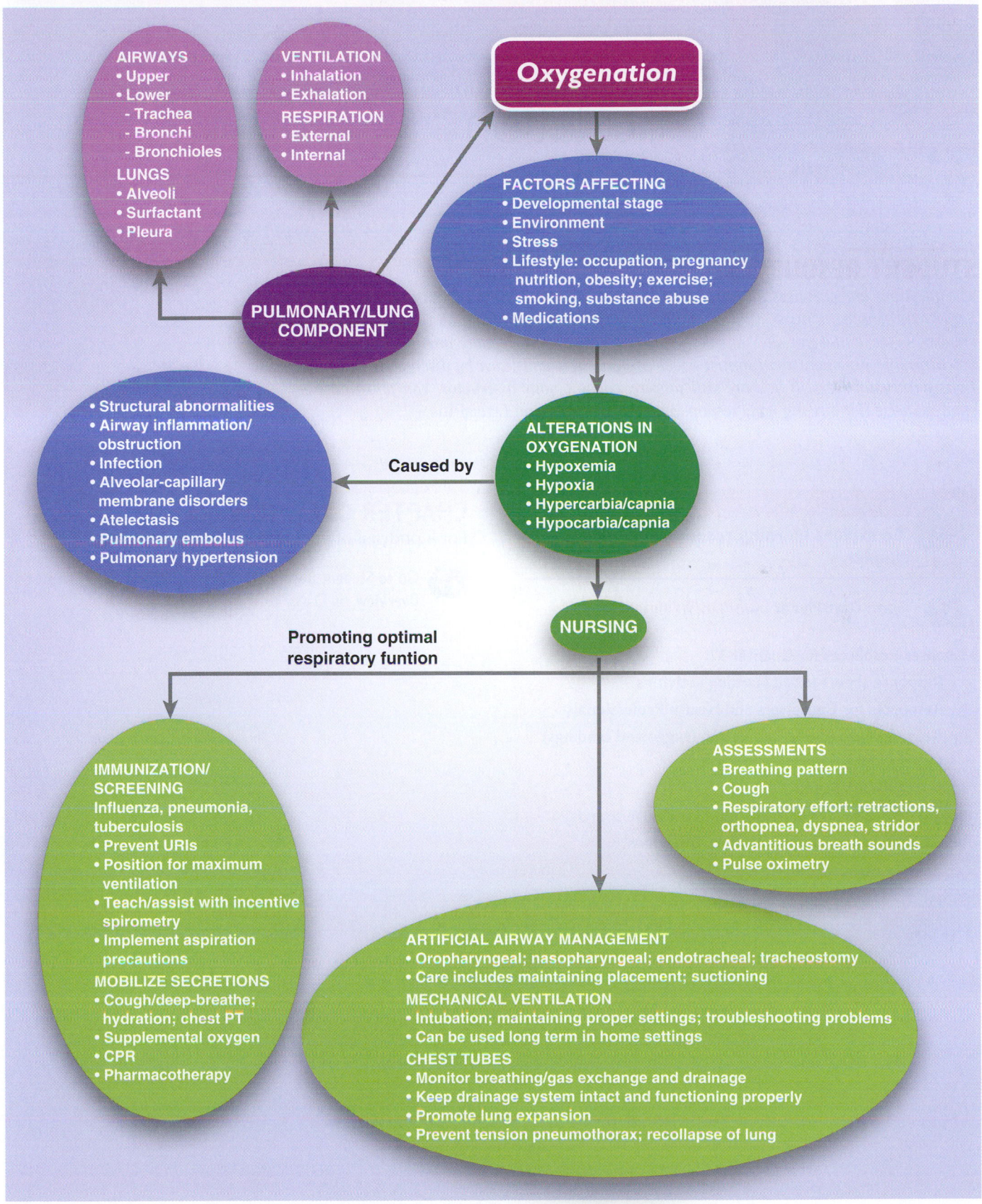

CHAPTER 37

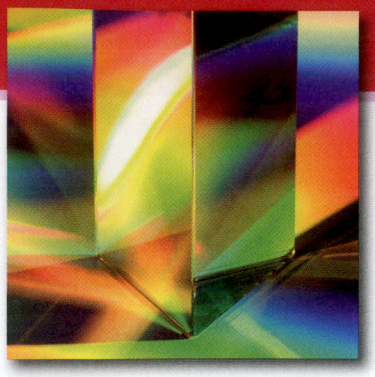

Circulation

STUDENT RESOURCES

*The questions and exercises in Volume 2 allow you to practice the kind of thinking you will use as a full-spectrum nurse. Critical-thinking questions usually have more than one correct answer, so we do not provide "answers" for these features. It is more important to develop your nursing judgment than to just cover content. You will learn by discussing the questions with your peers. If you are still unsure, consult your instructor. You will find Response Sheets (for writing your responses to the questions) on Davis*Plus.

To explore learning resources for this chapter,

Go to Davis*Plus* at DavisPl.us/Wilkinson3.

Chapter Resources for Chapter 37:

- **Response sheets for all learning activities**
- **Resources for Caregivers and Health Professionals**
- **Reading More About Circulation (suggested readings)**
- **Concept Map of chapter content**

Interactive Case Studies

Sound files (e.g., for heart and blood pressure sounds)

NCLEX-Style and Chapter Review Questions

CHAPTER OVERVIEW

For a podcast of an overview of this chapter,

Go to Student Resources, Chapter 37, **Podcast—Chapter Overview,** on Davis*Plus*.

Caring for the Nguyens

Mai Nguyen, Nam's 76-year-old mother, has been complaining she feels tired all the time; she just can't do what she normally does. She describes having a hard time catching her breath as she walks up stairs and goes about her day. Nam has noticed that his mother's ankles are more swollen than he has ever seen them. So he schedules an appointment for his mother at the family clinic where you are the nurse. Mrs. Nguyen appears pale and not her usual energetic self. Nam tells you that his mom is "not right" and seems to be confused about things at home, which is not like her. She has a history of chronic congestive heart failure.

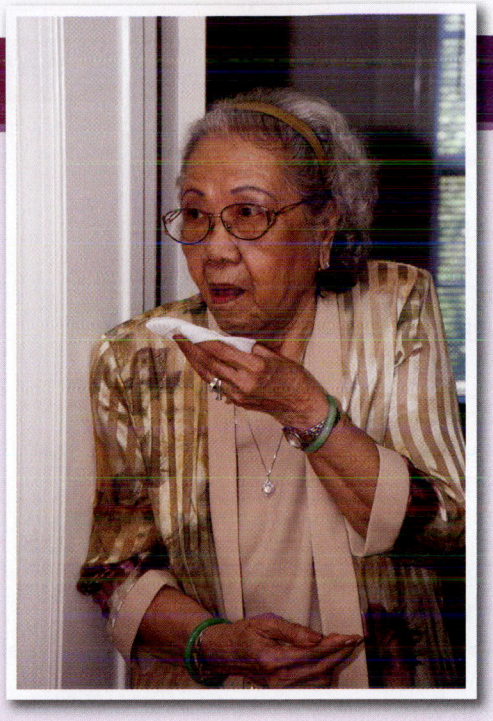

A. What additional health history data would be useful to gather at this time?

B. During her visit at the clinic, you observe that Mai has a cough. She spits a small amount of pink, frothy mucus into a tissue. Mrs. Nguyen's vital signs are as follows: BP, 142/90 mm Hg; pulse, 96 beats/min and with some irregular beats; respirations, 38 breaths/min and shallow; temperature, 97.8°F (36.5°C) oral.
- Which of these symptoms and vital signs is/are not within normal limits?
- For each abnormal finding, explain why you think it is occurring.

C. You decide to include a nursing diagnosis of Acute Confusion in Mrs. Nguyen's plan of care.
- What symptoms does she have that support this nursing diagnosis?
- What physiological changes are causing these symptoms?

D. In addition to angiotensin-converting enzyme (ACE) inhibitor, beta blocker, diuretic, and digoxin, what additional therapies do you anticipate the physician will prescribe?

E. Mrs. Nguyen asks you, "What can I do to make sure I never get this sick again?" How would you answer this question?

Practical Knowledge knowing how

PROCEDURES

In this section you will find the procedures necessary for supporting oxygenation. As you perform the procedures, apply the theoretical knowledge and concepts you obtained in Volume 1. The registered nurse is responsible for assessing patients' circulation and their responses to treatments and procedures.

Procedure 37-1 ■ Performing Cardiac Monitoring

➤ For steps to follow in *all* procedures, refer to the Universal Steps for All Procedures found on the inside back cover.

Equipment

- Alcohol pads
- Gauze dressing
- Washcloth
- Shaving supplies or scissors, if necessary
- Disposable electrodes

For hardwire monitoring, add:

- Cardiac monitor
- Cable with lead wires
- Safety pin
- 1-in. tape

For telemetry, add:

- Transmitter with lead wires (with a new battery inserted before each use)
- Pouch to carry transmitter

Delegation

You should not delegate this procedure to the LPN or NAP because it requires knowledge of anatomy, physiology, and advanced assessment techniques.

Pre-Procedure Assessment

- Assess cardiovascular status, including heart sounds, pulse rate, and blood pressure, and check for the presence of pain.
- Assess skin integrity of the chest before applying electrodes.
  Skin lesions contraindicate the application of leads to the affected area.
- Assess for history of dysrhythmias.
  Early recognition of dysrhythmias allows for prompt treatment, which improves patient outcomes.

➤ When performing the procedure, always identify your patient according to agency policy, using two identifiers, and be attentive to standard precautions, hand hygiene, patient safety and privacy, body mechanics, and documentation.

Procedure Steps

1. **Prepare the monitoring equipment.**

For Hardwire Monitoring

a. Plug the cardiac monitor into an electrical outlet, and turn it on.
Allows the monitor to warm up while you prepare the patient for monitoring.

b. Connect the cable with lead wires into the monitor.
The cable and lead wires must be properly connected to the monitor to obtain an accurate electrocardiogram (ECG) tracing. Most are color coded.

For Telemetry Monitoring

c. Insert a new battery into the transmitter.
A new battery should be inserted with each use to ensure transmitter function.

d. Turn on the transmitter.
Tests the unit to make sure that the battery is functional.

e. Connect the lead wires to the transmitter, if they are not permanently attached. Be sure to attach each one to its correct outlet.
The lead wires must be properly connected to the transmitter to obtain an accurate ECG tracing.

2. **Expose the patient's chest** and identify electrode sites based on the monitoring system being used and the patient's anatomy. Gently rub the placement sites with a washcloth or gauze pad until the skin reddens slightly.
The monitoring system will dictate lead placement. Sites over soft tissues or close to bone provide accurate waveforms; sites over bony prominences, thick muscles, and skinfolds can produce artifact.▼

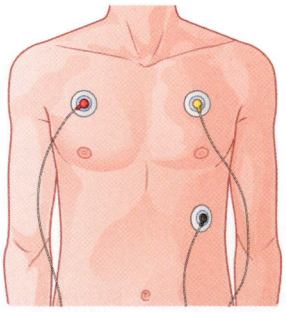

3. **If the patient's chest has dense** hair, shave or clip the hair with scissors at each electrode site.
Hair may interfere with electrical contact, preventing accurate ECG waveform transmission.

4. **With an alcohol pad** clean the areas chosen for electrode placement, and allow them to dry.
Alcohol removes oil on the skin that may prevent the electrodes from adhering.

5. **Remove the electrode backing** and make sure the gel is moist. Discard the electrode if the gel is dry. The number of electrodes needed will depend on the monitoring system being used. It will be three to five electrodes.
A dry electrode will not conduct electrical activity.

6. **Attach the lead wires** to the electrodes by snapping or clipping them in place.

7. **Apply the electrode** to the site by pressing it firmly. Repeat with the remaining electrodes.
Pressing the electrode firmly creates a tight seal, which ensures electrical contact.

8. **Secure the monitoring equipment.**

For Hardwire Monitoring

f. Wrap a piece of 1-in. tape around the cable, and secure it to the patient's gown with a safety pin.
Secures the cable so leads are not disconnected with patient movement.

For Telemetry Monitoring

g. Place the transmitter in the pouch, and tie it around the patient's neck. If there is no pouch, put the transmitter into a pocket on the robe or gown.
Allows the patient independence with ambulation.

9. **Check the patient's ECG** tracing on the monitor. If necessary, adjust the gain to increase the waveform size.
The ECG tracing should be large enough to accurately assess all of the waveform components.

For Telemetry Monitoring

You may need to call a monitoring room to verify ECG tracing and rhythm.

10. **Set the upper and lower** heart rate alarm limits according to agency policy or patient condition, and turn them on.

11. **Obtain a rhythm strip** by pressing the "record" button.
You must obtain a rhythm strip to document the patient's cardiac rhythm. ➤

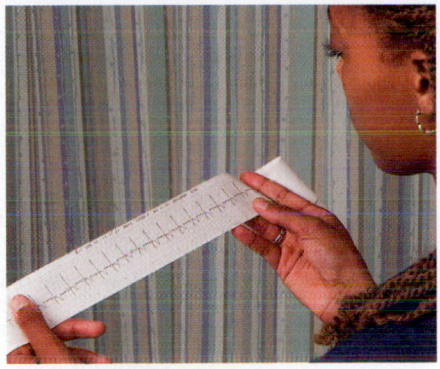

For Hardwire Monitoring

h. Press the "record" button on the bedside monitor.
The "record" button, located on the monitor at the bedside, allows you to print a rhythm strip immediately when cardiac symptoms occur.

For Telemetry Monitoring

i. Press the "record" button on the transmitter of the telemetry unit, or call the monitoring room to have the ECG trip printed.
The "record" button on the telemetry transmitter allows you or the patient to print a rhythm strip immediately when cardiac symptoms occur.

12. **Interpret the rhythm strip**, and then mount it (e.g., with transparent tape) in the patient's chart.
Provides a permanent record of heart activity; identifies rhythm abnormalities.

? What if . . .

- **The patient is diaphoretic?**
  Remove electrodes, clean the area with alcohol, allow the area to dry, and then reapply electrodes.
  To obtain an accurate ECG tracing.
- **The patient is receiving a cardiac medication?**
  Print a strip before and after giving medication. You may also need to call the telemetry station to have the ECG monitored.
  To assess and monitor effects of medication.
- **You are not getting a good reading on the monitor?**
  Recheck the leads; replace leads or move leads if necessary.

Evaluation

- Evaluate changes in the patient's cardiac rhythm.
- Check skin integrity, and replace the electrodes at least every 24 hours.
  Avoids skin irritation at the electrode sites. In addition, the gel begins to dry, so replacement ensures an adequate waveform.

Patient Teaching

- Explain the rationale for cardiac monitoring.
- Teach the patient that if he experiences symptoms (e.g., shortness of breath, chest pain, dizziness, palpitations) he should notify the nurse immediately so a rhythm strip can be recorded.
- Tell the patient being monitored by telemetry to remove the transmitter before showering. Ask the patient to inform you before removing it.
- Discuss home telemetry monitoring with the patient and caregiver if the patient requires telemetry monitoring after discharge.

Home Care

- Evaluate the client's and caregiver's ability to continue telemetry monitoring at home with help from an outside agency.
- Help the client and caregiver contact the monitoring agency and arrange for home telemetry monitoring.
- Explain to the caregiver and patient that the emergency medical service will be notified by the monitoring agency if a dysrhythmia develops.
- Instruct the caregiver and patient about proper lead placement and the need to rotate electrode sites to prevent skin breakdown.

Documentation

- Document the date and time that monitoring was instituted.
- Note the monitoring lead selected.
- Document a rhythm strip every 8 hours and with changes in the patient's condition according to agency policy. Label the rhythm strip (if the monitor does not label it for you) with the date, time, patient's name, and room number. Indicate on the strip when symptoms and treatment interventions occurred.
- Document the patient's response to treatment.

Practice Resources

Hancock, E. W., Deal, B. J., Mirvis, D. M., et al. (2009); Lieberman, K. (2008); Morrison, L. J., Neumar, R. W., Zimmerman, J. L., et al. (2013).

ASSESSMENT GUIDELINES & TOOLS

Focused Assessment

Assessing Circulation

Part I. Questions to Assess Risk for Impaired Circulation

Demographic Data

- What is your age?
- Where do you live?
- What is your occupation?

Health History

- Do you have current health problems? Describe.
- Do you have past health problems? Describe.
- Do you take medication for your heart, blood pressure, cholesterol, or erectile dysfunction, diabetes, breathing difficulty, or other conditions?
- Do you have chronic fatigue, heartburn, anxiety, swelling of the ankles, difficulty breathing, chest discomfort, palpitations, dizziness or fainting spells, dental problems, pain in the calf when walking that stops with rest, chronic cough or wheezing, shortness of breath, or unexplained weight loss?
- Do you take over-the-counter products, such as vitamins, supplements, or aspirin?
- Have you had surgery in the past?
- What else do you want to tell me about your physical or mental health history?

Family History

- Did your father or a brother develop coronary artery disease or have a heart attack before the age of 55?
- Did your mother or sister develop coronary artery disease or have a heart attack before the age of 65?

Cardiovascular History

- Have you ever had or been diagnosed with a heart attack, angina, coronary artery disease, peripheral artery disease, stroke, aortic aneurysm?
- Do you have high or low blood pressure? Do you feel dizzy if you stand up quickly?
- Do you have diabetes or prediabetes? Are you a normal weight?

Nutrition History

- In a typical day, how many servings of whole grains, fruits, vegetables, dairy products, eggs, nuts, and red meat or fish do you eat or drink per day?
- At how many meals per week do you east fast food or other high-fat food?
- How many sugar-sweetened soft drinks and sodas do you drink per day?
- How many meals per week do you eat out? Where?
- How many times per day do you add salt or eat salty foods?
- How many times per week do you skip a meal?

Lifestyle and Health Promotion Activities

- What is your current stress level? What are your major sources of stress? How do you relieve stress?
- What is you usual diet? Is your current diet typical, or have you recently changed your eating habits?
- What is your usual activity level? Do you exercise regularly? If so, how many minutes per week of moderate to vigorous physical activity do you get?
- Do you check your lipid profile (cholesterol and triglycerides) and blood sugar (fasting blood sugar and hemoglobin A_{1C}) on a regular basis?
- Do you smoke now, or have you ever smoked? If you smoke, how many packs per day and for how many years have you smoked?
- Do you use crack cocaine or other illicit substances?

Part II. Focused Physical Examination

Cardiovascular System

- Also review Procedure 22-13: Assessing the Heart and Vascular System.
- ***Inspect the neck*** for carotid and jugular pulsations. Palpate each carotid separately. Auscultate the carotid arteries and jugular veins for bruits and hums.
- ***Inspect the precordium*** for pulsations. Palpate for pulsations, lifts, heaves, and thrills.
- ***Auscultate for heart sounds.*** To hear examples of various heart sounds,

Go to Student Resources, **Sound Files,** on **Davis*Plus*.**

- ***Assess peripheral circulation:*** Palpate peripheral pulses, assess skin color and temperature, note hair distribution on extremities. Inspect for skin ulcers and edema of the feet and ankles.
- ***Inspect for venous valve competence.***
- ***Perform the capillary refill test*** anywhere you note signs of diminished blood flow.

DIAGNOSTIC TESTING

Diagnostic Testing

Tests Related to Circulation

Test	Purpose
Angiogram	A contrast dye is injected into a vein, and serial films are taken to assess patency of the vessels.
Arterial blood gases (ABG)	An analysis of arterial blood evaluates the effectiveness of gas exchange and perfusion.
Cardiac catheterization	A catheter is passed into the heart to assess pressures, blood flow, and the size and patency of chambers.
Chest x-ray study (CXR)	Provides an anterior–posterior or lateral view of the heart and lungs, shows tissue density (e.g., to evaluate size, masses, fluid).
Cholesterol, lipid profile	Indicates risk for cardiovascular disease long term.
Creatine kinase-MB (CK-MB)	The MB isoenzyme is present only in the heart muscle. A serum measurement of the MB band is used to detect a myocardial infarction (MI). Levels rise with an acute MI.
Echocardiogram	An ultrasound evaluation of the heart that examines heart function and blood flow
Electrocardiogram (ECG)	Electrodes placed on the extremities and chest wall conduct electrical activity from the heart. ECG illustrates heart rate, rhythm, and size and helps evaluate heart damage.
Hemoglobin (Hgb)	A serum measurement that affects the oxygen-carrying capacity of the blood. May be measured separately or as part of a complete blood count.
Holter monitor	A continuous ECG tracing used to correlate symptoms and cardiac activity. Typically the tracing lasts 48 hours to 7 days.
Technetium scan	Technetium-99m sestamibi is injected intravenously. Approximately 90 to 120 minutes later, the heart is scanned. Areas of myocardial damage appear as "hot spots" on the scan.
Treadmill test	Evaluates the effect of exercise on the heart and circulation via continuous ECG and vital sign monitoring during exercise.
Troponin	A serum evaluation of a complex of proteins is used to detect MI. Levels of these contractile proteins remain elevated for up to 7 days after MI.

CLINICALREASONING

Applying the Full-Spectrum Nursing Model

PATIENT SITUATION

Margarita, a 62-year-old director of management technology for a large company, was admitted to the hospital with shortness of breath, sudden and intense fatigue, and intense chest pressure that she describes as feeling like a steel band tightening around her rib cage. She reports the pain moved up to her jaw. The pain began suddenly but lasted approximately 5 to 7 minutes. During the episode, her husband tells you that Margarita acted as though she had a feeling of doom.

Margarita also has a history of sudden onset neck pain that seems to be triggered by heightened stress at work. Margarita is pale and clammy. She states she feels nauseated and has burning in her epigastric area. Her heart rate is 80 beats/minute, respiratory rate, 12 breaths/min, and blood pressure, 168/92 mm Hg. Skin is pale but warm, and capillary refill time is 4 seconds. Height is 5 ft 4 in. Weight is 156 lb. Body mass index (BMI) is 29.2. Waist circumference is 36 in.

The health history includes type 2 diabetes mellitus, high blood pressure, and tobacco use (half a pack of cigarettes a day). Margarita's mother had a heart attack in her 50s.

Lab work prior to admission:

Fasting lipids: total cholesterol, 288 mg/dL; LDL, 148 mg/dL; HDH, 44 mg/dL; triglycerides, 222 mg/dL
Serum glucose: 244 mg/dL
Hs-CRP: 3.1 mg/dL

THINKING

1 *Theoretical Knowledge:*
   a. What predisposing factors increase Margarita's risk for myocardial infarction?
   b. What does it mean to have infarcted myocardial tissue?
2 *Critical Thinking (Analyzing Assumptions):*
   Based on your knowledge of vascular causes of myocardial infarction, what are the most likely causes in this patient?

DOING

3. *Practical Knowledge:*
   After your patient's vital signs are stable and her pain is controlled, the emergency physician prescribes further diagnostic testing to determine the extent of damage to her heart.
   a. What tests would you expect your patient to have?
   b. You attempt to adhere electrodes for cardiac monitoring to Margarita's chest. The ECG tracing shows a great deal of artifact rather than a clear ECG tracing. What should you do to obtain an accurate tracing?
   c. You notice your patient is experience multiple "runs" of aberrant heartbeats. What should you do in response to the abnormal ECG tracing?
4. *Nursing Process (Assessment):*
   In the admission data, what important information is missing with regard to her cardiac status?

CARING

5. *Self-Knowledge:*
   Describe a personal experience involving someone in your own family or a friend who experienced a life-threatening event. How did you feel when your loved one was faced with a potentially life-altering heart condition? How might you draw upon this experience to help you in caring for Margarita?
6. *Ethical Knowledge:*
   a. After Margarita is finished with the last diagnostic test, what do you think her biggest concern is likely to be?
   b. Margarita tells you that she does not want anyone to know she has a heart problem. Yet her husband wants to tell other family members. How do you best respond to her concerns for privacy?

Critical Thinking and Clinical Reasoning

1. Recall the patient discussed in the Meet Your Patient scenario in Volume 1 of your textbook:
   Ms. Saunders is a 55-year-old accountant. She says she has been extremely tired, easily becomes short of breath, and is unable to complete her chores without frequent rest breaks. She is pale and seems tired. Her vital signs are as follows: temperature, 98.4°F (36.7°C); pulse, 86 beats/min; respirations, 24 breaths/min and unlabored; BP, 136/78 mm Hg; and pulse oximetry, 98% on room air. She is now waiting for her lab results, which include a complete blood count (CBC).

   Which of the following nursing diagnoses can you make, based on the patient data given here? Use a nursing diagnosis handbook and the standardized language table in this chapter of the ESG, as needed.

   Decreased Cardiac Output
   Risk for Decreased Cardiac Tissue Perfusion
   Ineffective Peripheral Tissue Perfusion
   Activity Intolerance
2. Ms. Saunders is diagnosed with severe anemia. She is hospitalized because her hemoglobin is 8.9 g/dL. How will this affect her oxygenation? What interventions would improve her fatigue?
3. For the following concept, use critical thinking to describe how or why it is important to nursing, patient care, or oxygenation. Note that this is *not* to be merely a definition.

   Perfusion

What Are the Main Points in This Chapter?

- The structures of the airways, lungs, chest cavity, heart, and blood vessels function together to supply oxygen to the tissues; thus, abnormalities in any of these structures can interfere with tissue oxygenation.
- Developmental stage, environment, individual characteristics, lifestyle, medications, and pathological factors can interfere with circulation and perfusion, leading to problems with tissue oxygenation.
- A health assessment related to circulation includes assessment of ventilation (breathing), circulation (blood flow), perfusion, and gas exchange (exchange of oxygen and carbon dioxide). The length and focus of the assessment varies with the purpose and urgency of the clinical situation.
- A physical examination related to adequacy of circulation includes observations of adequacy of circulation, and perfusion.
- Cardiovascular function is influenced by developmental stage, environment, lifestyle, substance abuse, medications, and pathophysiological conditions such as heart failure, coronary artery disease, and peripheral vascular disorders.
- The purposes of cardiac monitoring are to identify the patient's baseline rhythm and rate, recognize significant changes in the baseline rhythm and rate, and recognize life-threatening dysrhythmias that require immediate intervention.
- Promoting circulation ensures that oxygenated blood reaches tissues and organs and venous blood returns to the heart. Activities that promote venous return and peripheral arterial circulation and prevent clot formation assist with circulation.
- Cardiovascular drugs are used to enhance cardiac output, thus providing increased blood flow and oxygenation to organs and tissues. They include vasodilators, beta-adrenergic blocking agents, diuretics, and positive inotropes.

Knowledge Map

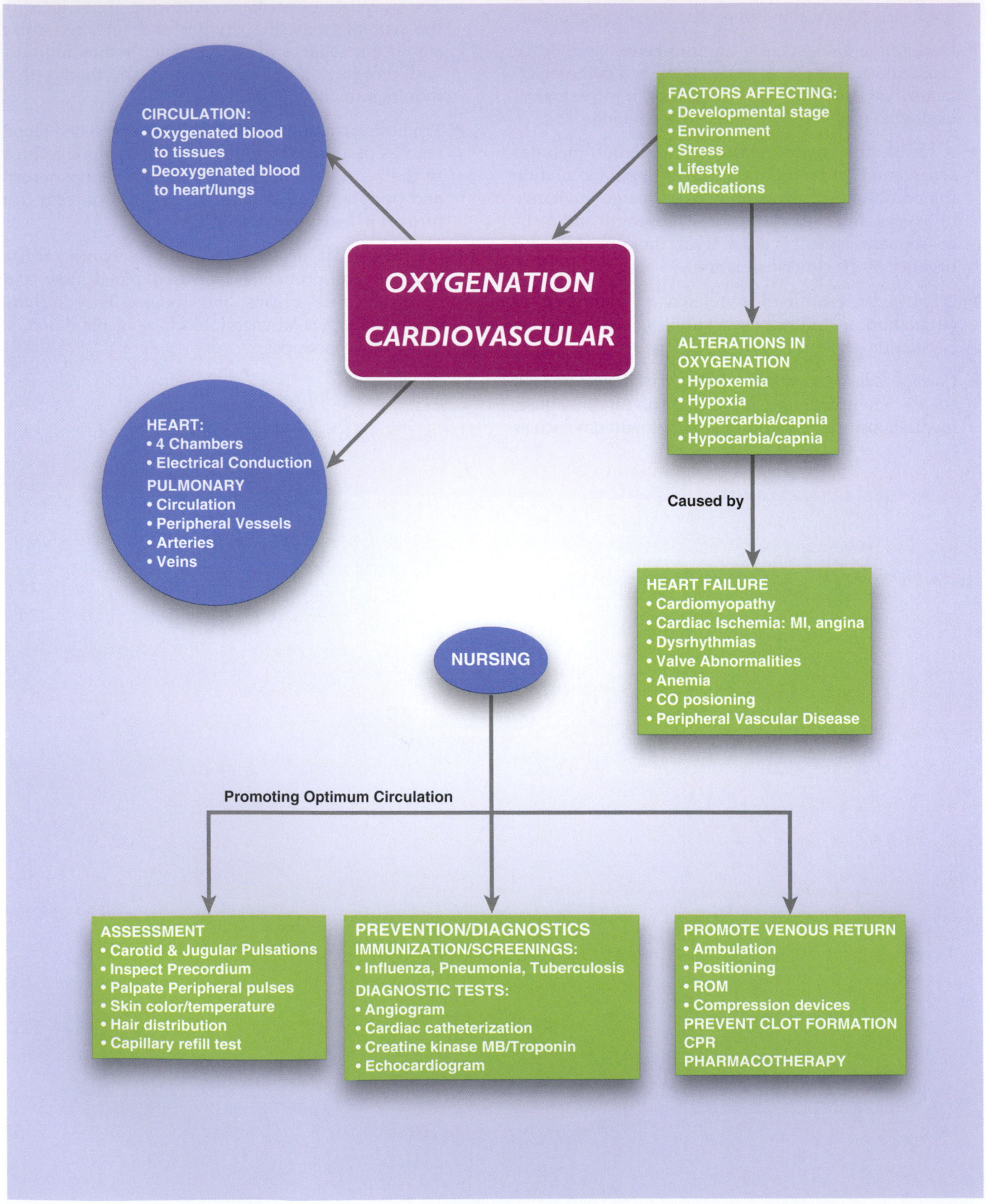

CHAPTER 38

Fluids, Electrolytes, & Acid–Base Balance

STUDENT RESOURCES

*The questions and exercises in Volume 2 allow you to practice the kind of thinking you will use as a full-spectrum nurse. Critical-thinking questions usually have more than one correct answer, so we do not provide "answers" for these features. It is more important to develop your nursing judgment than to just cover content. You will learn by discussing the questions with your peers. If you are still unsure, consult your instructor. You will find Response Sheets (for writing your responses to the questions) on Davis*Plus.

To explore learning resources for this chapter,

Go to Davis*Plus* at DavisPl.us/Wilkinson3.

Chapter Resources for Chapter 38:

- **Response sheets for all learning activities**
- **Resources for Caregivers and Health Professionals**
- **Reading More About Fluids, Electrolytes, & Acid–Base Balance (suggested readings)**
- **Concept Map of chapter content**

Interactive Case Studies

NCLEX-Style and Chapter Review Questions

CHAPTER OVERVIEW

For a podcast of an overview of this chapter,

Go to Student Resources, Chapter 38, **Podcast—Chapter Overview,** on Davis*Plus*.

Caring for the Nguyens

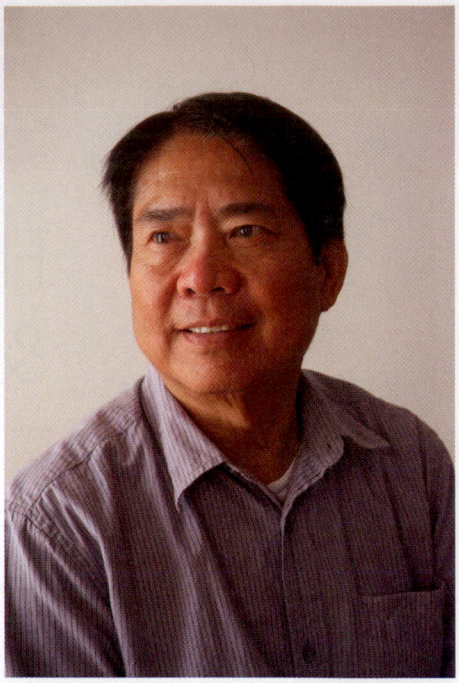

Nam Nguyen has been prescribed the following medicines:

lisinopril (Prinivil) 20 mg PO daily
hydrochlorothiazide (Diuril) 25 mg PO daily in the a.m.
metformin (Glucophage) 500 mg PO before breakfast and lunch

Today he had blood drawn for analysis. Following are the electrolyte panel results.

Sodium	136 mEq/L
Potassium	3.0 mEq/L
Chloride	96 mEq/L
Bicarbonate	24 mEq/L
BUN	18 mg/dL
Creatinine	0.8 mg/dL

A. Review the lab results. Compare Nam's lab work with the established norms for these values. Based on the lab results, what kind of assessment questions would be appropriate to ask Nam?

B. Use your pharmacology text to review Nam's medications. Which, if any, of these medicines might be contributing to Nam's lab results?

C. What teaching would be appropriate for Nam?

Practical Knowledge knowing how

To prevent, identify, and treat fluid, electrolyte, and acid–base problems, you will need to be skilled at initiating and managing intravenous infusions of fluids and blood, performing focused history and physical assessments, and interpreting arterial blood gas (ABG) values. When performing the procedures, apply the concepts and other theoretical knowledge you have learned.

PROCEDURES

Procedure 38-1 ■ Initiating a Peripheral Intravenous Infusion

➤ For steps to follow in *all* procedures, refer to the Universal Steps for All Procedures found on the inside back cover.

Equipment

- IV solution
- Administration set or IV lock and injection caps. (For a glass solution container, use vented tubing; for a plastic container you may use either vented or nonvented tubing.)
- Extension tubing with or without saline lock.
- Appropriately sized intravenous (IV) catheter
- Prefilled syringe to prime extension tubing.
- Clean, unsterile gloves
- Scissors
- Antiseptic swabs that contain solutions such as chlorhexidine (preferred by the Centers for Disease Control and Prevention [CDC], 2011) or 70% alcohol wipes.
- Tourniquet (non-latex, if available)
- Sterile manufactured catheter stabilization device or ½-in. tape.
- Transparent semipermeable occlusive dressing
- 1-in. nonallergenic tape, preferably clear
- Labels, time tape
- Linen-saver pad
- Arm board, if necessary

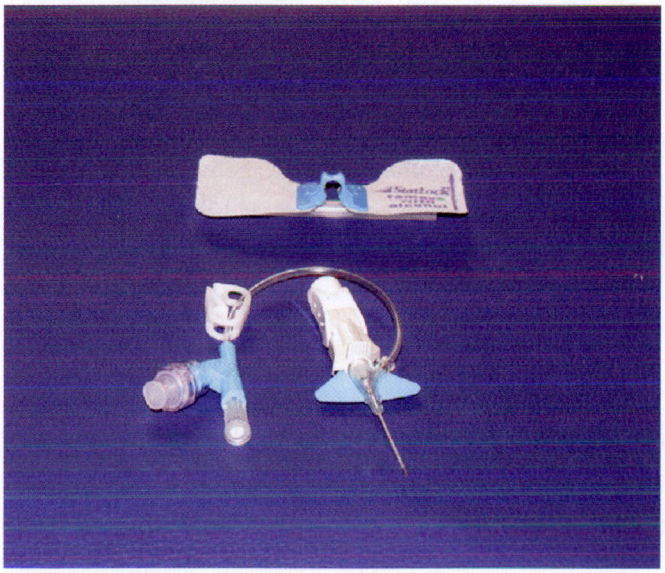

Delegation

In some states and agencies you can delegate peripheral IV catheter insertion to a licensed practical nurse (LPN) who is adequately trained in the skill.

Pre-Procedure Assessment

- Assess the patient's need for IV therapy by checking vital signs, laboratory values, urine output, skin turgor, breath sounds, and the condition of mucous membranes.
- Check for any situations that may contraindicate administering the prescribed fluids to the patient.
- Assess for allergy to tape.
- Assess the veins on the arms and hands for a potential insertion site.
  The upper extremities are preferred because of better blood flow, easier access, and less potential for complications than in other locations.
- Check the medical record for factors such as anticoagulant therapy, bleeding disorders, or low platelet count.
  These factors place the patient at risk of bleeding during IV catheter insertion.

➤ When performing the procedure, always identify your patient according to agency policy, using two identifiers, and be attentive to standard precautions, hand hygiene, patient safety and privacy, body mechanics, and documentation.

(continued on next page)

Procedure 38-1 ■ Initiating a Peripheral Intravenous Infusion (continued)

Procedure Steps

Note: Maintain scrupulous aseptic technique throughout this procedure.

Any microorganisms introduced can cause infection at the site, which could quickly migrate into the bloodstream and cause sepsis.

1. **Place the patient in** a comfortable position, the bed at a comfortable working height, and supplies within reach. Explain the procedure to the patient.
   Makes the procedure safer, easier, and decreases the risk for the nurse to develop back problems from improper body mechanics.

2. **Prepare the IV solution** and administration set or IV lock.
   a. Following the "rights" of medication administration, check the IV solution to make sure that you have the proper solution with the prescribed additives.
   IV solution is considered medication, and you should check it carefully to avoid administration and compatibility errors.
   b. Check the expiration date on the IV solution. Do not use IV solution after the expiration date.
   c. Check the IV solution for discoloration or particulate matter.
   Indicates contamination and should not be used.
   d. Label the IV solution container with the patient's name, date, and your initials. Place a time tape on the solution container with the prescribed infusion rate, time the infusion begins, and the time it is to be completed.
   Policies govern when solution containers, administration sets, dressings, and IV catheters need to be changed to avoid complications such as infection. Although not all agencies require a time tape, labeling infusion rates on the solution containers in this manner will alert others and makes it easy to see at a glance whether the solution is infusing on time.

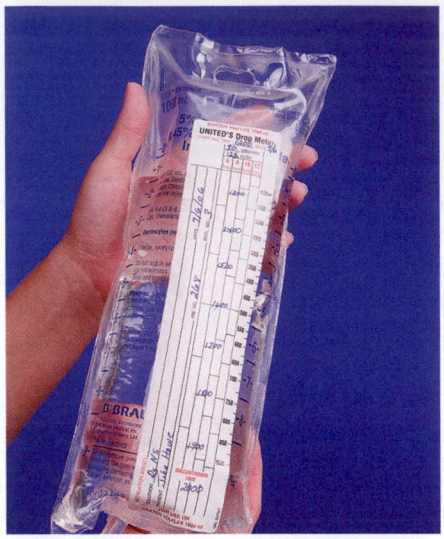

   e. Take the administration set from the package and close the roller clamp by rolling it downward. Label the tubing with the date and time.
   Ensures that fluid does not flow through inadvertently after the bag is spiked.
   f. Remove the protective cover from the solution container port.
   g. Remove the protective cover from the spike on the IV administration set, keeping the spike sterile. Insert the spike into the port of the solution container.

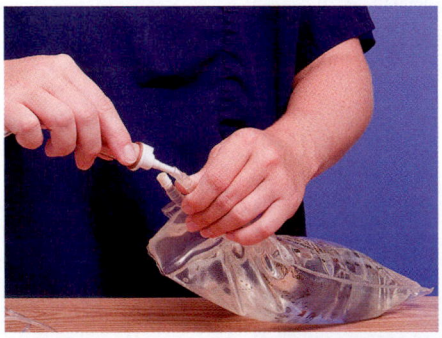

When Using a Glass Bottle

Clean the rubber stopper on the top of the bottle with an alcohol pad. Then insert the spike of the administration set through the stopper.

   h. Be certain the tubing is clamped. Hang the IV solution container on an IV pole.
   Clamping prevents leakage of fluid.
   i. Lightly compress the drip chamber, and allow it to fill up halfway.
   Overfilling the drip chamber will impair your ability to see the drips and adequately regulate the IV flow rate.

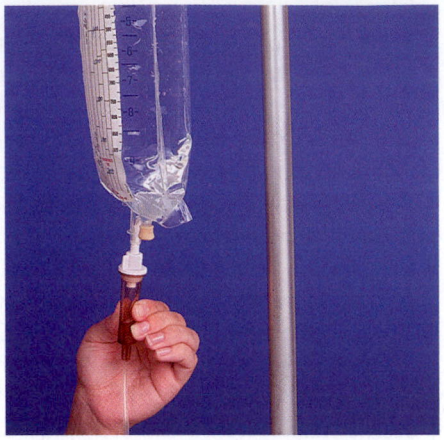

When Not Using Extension Tubing

Prime the tubing by opening the roller clamp and allowing the fluid to slowly fill the tubing. When tubing is filled, close the clamp.

When Using Extension Tubing

Either attach it to the end of the administration set now and prime it with the rest of the IV line, or prime it separately, as follows:

(1) Scrub the injection port of the extension tubing with an antiseptic pad and let it dry.
(2) Attach a flush syringe filled with normal saline to the injection port or to the non-luer-lock end and slowly push the fluid through the tubing until completely primed. (Consult packaging instructions for the amount of saline needed to flush the tubing.)
(3) Leave flush syringe attached to the extension tubing.
IV extension tubing makes it easier to convert an IV to a saline lock without disturbing the IV dressing and catheter. Manipulation of the IV catheter increases the risk of complications such as phlebitis, inflammation, infection, and infiltration.

j. Inspect the tubing for air. If air bubbles remain in the tubing, flick the tubing with a fingertip to mobilize them into the drip chamber. Recap the end of the tubing firmly.
Air in the tubing creates the potential for air embolism.

3. **Place a linen-saver pad** under the patient's arm.
Protects the bed from soiling during venipuncture.

4. **Place the patient's arm** in a dependent position.
Gravity helps fill and dilate the vein, making venipuncture easier.

5. **Apply a tourniquet** 10 to 20 cm (4 to 8 in.) above the selected site. Palpate the radial pulse. If no pulse is present, loosen the tourniquet, and reapply it with less tension.
Occluding the arterial flow diminishes venous filling, making venipuncture difficult.

6. **Locate a vein for inserting the IV** catheter. Select the best most distal vein on the hand or arm. Check with the medical provider before using an arm or hand that contains a dialysis graft or fistula, or the affected arm of a patient who has undergone a mastectomy. See Clinical Insight 38-3 for more guidelines.
Choose the most distal veins on the hand or arm so that you can perform subsequent venipunctures proximal to the previous site. This preserves veins for long-term therapy and prevents extravasation of fluid and medicines.

7. **Palpate the vein and press it** downward, making sure that it rebounds quickly. If the vein is not adequately dilated, ask the patient to open and close his fist; apply heat (e.g., a warm towel, a warming mitt); lightly tap the vein site; or stroke the extremity from distal to proximal, beginning below the selected venipuncture site. If available in your agency, use an infrared or other visualization device to assist in locating a vein.
These maneuvers bring blood to the local area to dilate the vein, making it easier to locate and making venipuncture easier.

8. **Loosen the tourniquet.** If excessive hair is present at the venipuncture site, clip it with a scissor.
Loosening the tourniquet restores blood flow and allows for patient comfort while preparing for venipuncture. Clipping the hair helps the dressings to adhere after catheter insertion. Shaving is not recommended because it may abrade the skin, providing a portal of entry for pathogens.

9. **Don clean nonsterile gloves.**
Provides protection from inadvertent exposure to blood. Note that some nurses don gloves routinely, even when preparing supplies and equipment. However, there is no risk for coming in contact with body fluids before this step, so strictly speaking, CDC standard precautions require gloves only from this step forward.

10. **Select an IV catheter** appropriate for the size of the vein, the solution to be infused, and the expected duration of therapy. Using aseptic technique, open the package touching only the outside of it.
Reduces the risk of extravasation and phlebitis. Always use the smallest diameter and shortest catheter that will deliver the desired solution flow. For most adults this will be a 20- to 24-gauge to minimize venous irritation and promote blood flow around the catheter. Aseptic handling reduces the risk of infection.

11. **Gently reapply the tourniquet** and scrub the site, using an antiseptic swab that contains chlorhexidine gluconate (preferred, CDC, 2011); if this is not available, use 70% alcohol wipes. Cleanse for 30 seconds, using friction.
Removes microorganisms from the skin so that they do not enter the venous system during venipuncture. Working "clean to dirty," or from the venipuncture site outward, avoids moving microorganisms toward the puncture site.

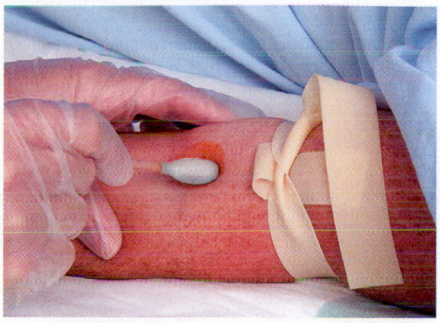

12. **Allow the antiseptic to air-dry.** Do not fan.
The antiseptic promotes adherence of the dressing. Fanning can cause contamination of the skin.

13. **Pick up the catheter and inspect the tip.**
There should be no burrs (rough spots, ridges) on the needle or peeling of the catheter material.

14. **Inform the patient** that you are about to insert the catheter and that it may be uncomfortable.
Keeping the patient informed promotes cooperation and lessens anxiety.

If Using a Wing-Tipped Catheter (Butterfly)

Grasp the catheter by the wings, using the thumb and forefinger of your dominant hand, making sure that the bevel is up. Remove the protective cap from the needle.
Stabilizes the catheter for insertion. Inserting the needle bevel up makes it less likely that you will pierce both vein walls (go "through" the vein) as well as making piercing the skin less painful for the patient.

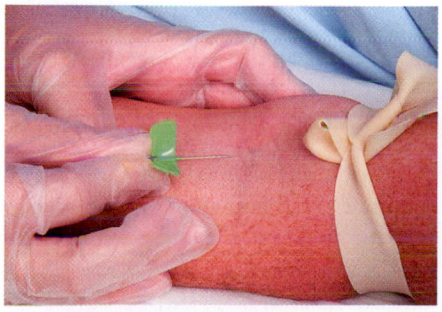

If Using an Over-the-Needle Catheter

Grasp the catheter by the hub, using the thumb and forefinger of your dominant hand, making sure that the bevel is up.

(continued on next page)

Procedure 38-1 ■ Initiating a Peripheral Intravenous Infusion (continued)

See Step 14 variation for an over-the-needle catheter, preceding.▼

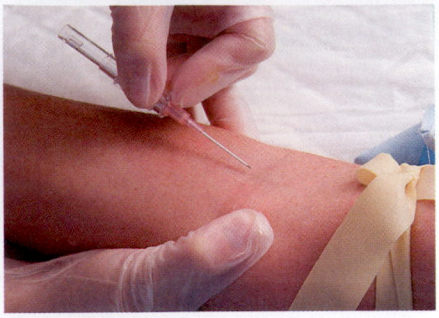

15. Using your nondominant hand, stabilize the vein by continuously pulling the skin taut below the puncture area (pull downward toward the hand or fingers). Do not press too hard, and make sure not to contaminate the insertion site.
Stabilizing the vein eases insertion and prevents damage to the underside of the vein as well as preventing the vein from rolling. Pressing too hard compresses blood flow in the vein and causes it to collapse.▼

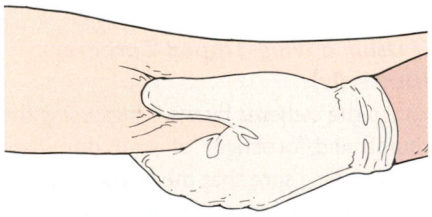

16. Holding the catheter at a 30° to 45° angle, pierce the skin directly over the vein. Penetrate all layers of the vein with one quick, smooth motion.
A 30° to 45° angle allows you to pierce the skin without inadvertently passing through the vein, and allows backflow of blood into the catheter.

17. Look for a flashback of blood into the chamber of the catheter or the tubing of the winged catheter.
The flashback of blood indicates that the vein has been entered, but only by the needle when using an over-the-needle catheter.

18. Lower the angle of the catheter and needle to skin level and advance them into the vein.

For a Wing-Tipped Catheter
Fully advance the catheter.

For an Over-the-Needle Catheter
Still maintaining traction on the skin with your nondominant hand, hold the catheter hub with your thumb and middle finger, and use your index finger to advance the catheter to at least half of its length before you begin withdrawing the needle. When a steady backflow of blood occurs, partially withdraw the needle while advancing the catheter fully into the vein. For an animated illustration of an over-the-needle IV catheter,

Go to **Animations: Insertion of an Over-the-Needle IV Catheter,** on DavisPlus.

Withdrawing the needle too early will result in the catheter not fully entering the vein, only the needle. There will be no bleeding from the catheter and infiltration will occur when starting the IV solution. The patient will also experience pain.▼

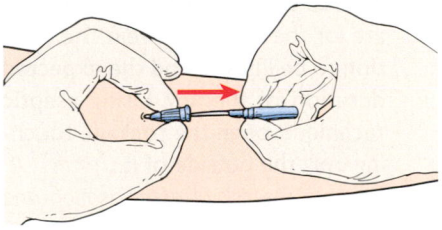

19. While holding the catheter in place with one hand, release the tourniquet and remove or retract the needle.

For an Over-the-Needle Catheter
Hold the catheter in place by placing light pressure on the catheter, away from the hub and venipuncture site.

Never attempt to reinsert the needle after it is withdrawn. This can damage the catheter and even cause bits of it to break off within the vein.

For a Winged Needle
Place a finger lightly on the same area plus a finger farther along the vein away from the needle so the needle does not go through the vein.
Releasing the tourniquet restores full circulation to the patient's extremity and prevents injury. Placing light pressure on the catheter or vein minimizes bleeding from the catheter or needle while you complete the procedure.

20. Quickly connect the administration set to the IV catheter, using aseptic technique.
To minimize bleeding and prevent infection.▼

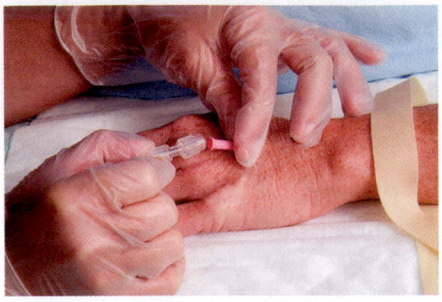

If Using a Peripheral IV Lock
Once the lock is connected, flush with normal saline and then disconnect the flush. A common amount is 1 to 2 mL, but tubing varies, so check package instructions for the exact amount needed.
Flushing the catheter both clears it and keeps it sterile.

21. While still holding the catheter in place, slowly open the roller clamp. Observe that flow is achieved. Adjust the drip to the prescribed flow rate.

22. Secure the connection between the tubing and the catheter. Many sets have luer-lock connections, so no further securing is needed. If not using luer-lock tubing, clasping devices and threaded devices can be used. Do not use tape.
Secure the connection to prevent separation of tubing from the hub.

Taping is not recommended because the junction is not visible under tape; therefore, the tubing could separate from the catheter without being discovered, possibly leading to air embolism, bleeding, or infection.

23. Stabilize the catheter. Use an agency-approved device. Catheter stabilization devices include manufactured devices (such as StatLok), or tape.

When Stabilizing With Tape
Place a narrow (¼-in.) strip of tape under the catheter hub and crisscross the ends over the hub to form a chevron. Apply tape only to the catheter hub, not to the catheter itself, and do not apply tape

directly to the site where the catheter enters the skin.
Luer-locks are designed to prevent accidental disengagement of tubing and catheter; they do not stabilize the catheter. Catheter stabilization is important to minimize catheter movement and help prevent complications such as phlebitis, inflammation, infiltration, and infection.

24. Dress the site, following agency policy. If needed, clean the site with an antiseptic swab and allow it to dry before applying the dressing.

If Using a Transparent Dressing (Preferred)

a. Open the package containing the dressing. Remove the protective backing from the dressing, making sure not to touch the sterile surface.
b. Cover the insertion site and the hub or winged portion of the catheter with the dressing. Do not cover the junction with the administration tubing.

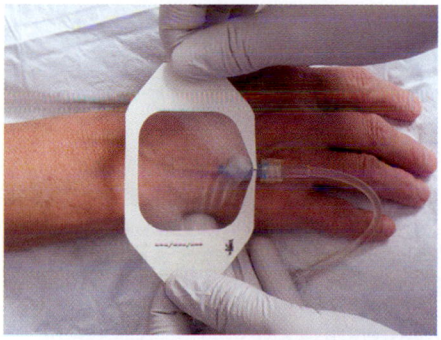

c. Gently pinch the transparent dressing around the catheter hub to secure the hub further. Smooth the remainder of the dressing so that it adheres to the skin.

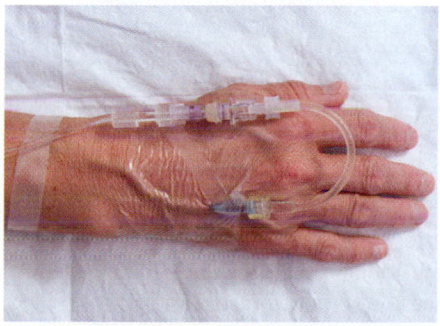

If You Must Use a Gauze Dressing

a. Fold a 2 in. × 2 in. sterile gauze dressing in half, cover it with 1-in. tape (about 3 in. long).
b. Place under the tubing/hub junction and press down on the tape.
Raises hub off the skin and prevents pressure on the skin.
c. Place a sterile gauze pad over the insertion site and catheter hub—but not over the catheter–hub junction.
d. Secure all edges with tape.

25. Label the dressing with the date and time of insertion, catheter size, and your initials.
A label lets nurses see at a glance how long the dressing has been in place.

26. Secure the IV administration tubing by looping and taping the tubing to the skin.
Helps prevent the IV catheter from becoming dislodged and decreases movement of the catheter, thereby decreasing the risk of phlebitis, inflammation and infiltration.

27. Place an arm board under the joint and secure it with tape, if the insertion site is located near a joint.
An arm board stabilizes the joint and helps prevent the catheter from becoming dislodged. However, avoid inserting an IV near a joint when possible, as there is increased potential for movement of the IV catheter, leading to an increased risk of complications. IVs placed in the antecubital fossa are difficult to assess for infiltration. Arm boards are not widely used because of the high acuity of inpatients, many of whom have central lines instead of peripheral IVs.

28. Dispose of all supplies, including sharps, into appropriate receptacles; raise the siderail; lower the bed; and be sure the patient call system is within reach. Wash your hands.
Prevents infection and ensure patient and staff safety.

? What if . . .

- **The patient is an older adult?**

Do not scrub skin too vigorously.
This can damage fragile surface tissue, creating a portal for pathogens.

Use a softer tourniquet and do not apply tightly; for well-dilated veins, do not use one at all.
This decreases the risk of rupture of fragile veins.

Use the smallest catheter possible to meet the infusion needs.
Insert the needle at an almost flat angle (10° to 20°).
In most older adults, veins are close to the skin surface.

Before penetrating the skin, apply traction to the vein below the insertion site.
For comfort and ease of insertion.

Insert the catheter on top of the vein; do not use the side access technique.
If bleeding occurs, hold gentle pressure longer than for younger patients.
A clot may take longer to form.

- **The patient is an infant younger than 2 months old?**

Allow the antiseptic to air-dry on the skin. Do not fan.
Increases the antiseptic's effectiveness; promotes patient comfort on puncture of the skin; promotes adherence of dressing. Fanning increases exposure to airborne microbes.

- **The patient is allergic to iodine or shellfish?**

Use 70% alcohol or chlorhexidine for 30 seconds to cleanse the site (not povidone-iodine or iodine).

- **You are not successful with the first venipuncture attempt?**

Use a new cannula and make a second attempt on the other arm; or if unsuccessful, higher up on the same arm. Do not make more than two attempts without seeking assistance.

- **When you insert the needle and catheter and connect the tubing, you see bright red blood quickly appear and start to advance up the tubing?**

You may have entered an artery. Remove the catheter and apply direct pressure for at least 5 minutes. Notify the primary care provider. Monitor the extremity distal to the insertion site for pulses, color, and temperature.

(continued on next page)

Procedure 38-1 ■ Initiating a Peripheral Intravenous Infusion (continued)

Evaluation

- Monitor the IV site and flow rate regularly (many agency standards require hourly) while IV fluid is infusing. Check for signs of infiltration, inflammation, and phlebitis.
- Monitor the patient's tolerance of IV therapy by auscultating breath sounds and monitoring vital signs, urine output, laboratory values, and neck vein distention. Report to the primary provider any signs of fluid overload, such as crackles, edema, shortness of breath, diminished urine output, increased blood pressure, increased heart rate with bounding pulse, and distended neck veins. Fluid overload can lead to pulmonary edema and heart failure.

Patient Teaching

- Instruct the patient about IV therapy.
- Teach the patient the importance of notifying staff immediately if the catheter or administration set becomes dislodged; the insertion site becomes tender, red, or swollen; or the patient notices moisture or fluid leakage.
- Explain the desired and adverse effects of IV therapy, and tell the patient to notify staff if he develops discomfort or breathing difficulty.
- Teach the patient measures to avoid dislodging the catheter.

Home Care

- Explain home IV therapy to the client and caregiver, and teach them how to identify complications.
- Provide the client with the name and phone numbers of people to contact in case problems arise with the catheter site or if there is a change in level of comfort.

Documentation

- Date and time of insertion, gauge and type of catheter, number of attempts, and location of the insertion site
- Tourniquet use (or nonuse)
- Blood return in catheter; whether the IV flushes, type and amount of flush solution used
- Dressing and tape type used
- Method of securing or stabilizing the IV line
- Type and rate of the IV fluid infusing
- Patient's tolerance of the procedure, any adverse reactions to the insertion or IV therapy, and the interventions required
- Patient teaching
- Often, IV care is documented on a flowsheet. Fluids infused are documented on the I&O record as well.

Sample documentation

06/07/16 0200. 20-gauge, winged catheter inserted in cephalic vein, with tourniquet, without difficulty on first attempt. Obtained blood return. Catheter flushed easily. Dressed site with a transparent, semipermeable dressing and clear tape. Catheter stabilized with fixation device. 1 L of D_5/NS hung at 125 mL/hr. Patient tolerated venipuncture with no difficulty. Instructed to notify nursing staff immediately if pain or swelling occurs at the site. Also instructed about precautions to take to avoid dislodging IV catheter and importance of notifying staff immediately should it become dislodged. ——S. Jiminez, RN

Practice Resources

Barclay, L., & Nghiem, H. (2011); Camp-Sorrel, D. (2010); CDC (2011a); Infusion Nurses Society (INS) (2011a); Masoorli, S. (2012); Moureau, N. (2008); Shlamovitz, G. (updated 2013a).

Thinking About the Procedure

To practice applying clinical reasoning to this procedure,

Go to *Davis's Nursing Skills Videos*, **Initiating a Peripheral Intravenous Infusion.**

For questions and suggested responses,

Go to Chapter 38, **Thinking About the Procedure Questions and Suggested Responses,** on Davis*Plus*.

Procedure 38-2 ■ Regulating the IV Flow Rate

➤ For steps to follow in *all* procedures, refer to the Universal Steps for All Procedures found on the inside back cover.

Equipment

- IV solution hanging on an IV pole and attached to an administration set
- Watch with a second hand or digital seconds
- Time tape

Delegation

Refer to your state nurse practice act and agency policy regarding delegation of this task to an LPN.

Pre-Procedure Assessment

- Assess the IV catheter for patency and date of insertion before starting the infusion and then regularly (many agencies specify hourly) while the IV fluid infuses.
  Decreases risk of complications related to incorrect infusion rate, expired infusion solution, tubing, or catheter dwell time.
- Assess the IV site for signs of phlebitis, infiltration, infection, or inflammation.
  You must change the IV catheter before regulating the flow rate if any of these complications occur.

- Confirm the patient's need for IV therapy by verifying the order and checking laboratory values, urine output, vital signs, and breath sounds.

Ensures that the patient still needs IV fluids and that the solution is correct. Laboratory values and assessment findings monitor the IV treatment plan. IV therapy creates a risk for fluid overload.

➤ When performing the procedure, always identify your patient according to agency policy, using two identifiers, and be attentive to standard precautions, hand hygiene, patient safety and privacy, body mechanics, and documentation.

Procedure Steps

1. **Follow all the "checks" and "rights"** of medication administration, including verifying the prescription. Check the solution to make sure that you have the proper IV fluid hanging with the prescribed additives, and that there is no discoloration of or particles or crystallization in the fluid. Also verify the infusion rate.
   IV solution is considered medication, and you should check it carefully to avoid administration and compatibility errors. Do not simply pull a bag of fluid from a shelf assuming that the shelf is labeled properly, as bags are often misplaced and this is a potential source of error.

2. **Calculate the hourly rate** if it is not specified in the order. Divide the volume to be infused by the number of hours it is to be infused. For example, if the physician prescribes 1,000 mL to run over the course of 4 hours, the infusion rate is 250 mL/hr.
   You must carefully calculate the infusion rate to ensure that the patient receives the correct volume of fluid.

   Note: If you are using a volume-control pump, you can omit Steps 3 and 4.

3. **Calculate the drip rate** by multiplying the number of milliliters to be infused in 60 minutes by the drop factor in drops [gtts]/per milliliter; then divide by 60 minutes:

$$\frac{\text{Hourly rate in mL} \times \text{(gtts/mL)}}{\text{60 minutes}} = \text{drip rate}$$

   For example, an hourly rate of 100 mL multiplied by 15 gtts/mL and divided by 60 minutes equals 25. Therefore, the drip rate equals 25 gtts/minute. Each administration set has a drip factor that is determined by the manufacturer. The ***drip factor*** *is the number of drops necessary to deliver 1 mL of solution. Microdrip tubing has a drip factor of 60 gtts/mL; blood administration tubing typically has a drip factor of 10 gtts/mL; macrodrip tubing has a drip factor of 15 gtts/mL.*

4. **Verify your calculations.**
   To prevent dosage errors, either have a second person verify your calculations or check them a second time yourself.

5. **Apply a time tape** when hanging a new bag to the IV solution container next to the volume markings. Mark the time tape with the time that the infusion was started. Continue to mark 1-hour intervals on the time tape until you reach the bottom of the container.
   The time tape allows all nurses to accurately monitor the rate of administration.

6. **Open the roller clamp** so that IV fluid begins to flow (when hanging a new bag).
   The roller clamp must be opened to allow the flow of fluid.

7. **Set the rate.**

   For Gravity Drip
   Using a watch placed next to the drip chamber, count the number of drops entering the drip chamber in 1 minute. Adjust the roller clamp by increasing or decreasing the flow until you achieve the prescribed drip rate.
   Timing the drip rate for 1 minute helps to accurately achieve the correct drip rate and having the watch next to what you are counting will ensure that you do not miss seeing any drops. ▼

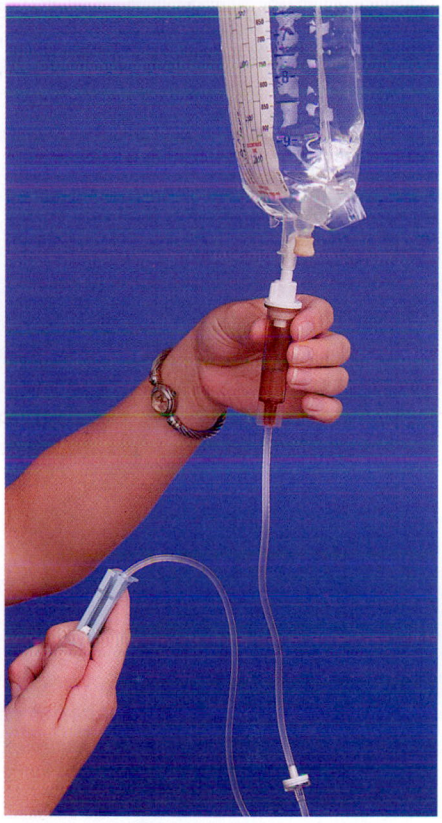

   For a Volume-Control Pump
   Program the ordered rate into the pump.
   IV solution is considered a medication and must infuse at the prescribed rate.

8. **Monitor manually regulated** infusion rates closely for the 15 minutes after you begin an infusion; then monitor at least hourly by counting drops per minute or reading the numbers on the pumps.
   Changes in the patient's position may speed up or slow down the infusion rate; frequent monitoring of the infusion rate ensures that the correct volume of fluid infuses over the correct length of time.

(continued on next page)

Procedure 38-2 ■ Regulating the IV Flow Rate (continued)

? What if . . .

- **The prescription for the IV flow rate changes?**
  Recalculate the new flow rate and adjust the drops/minute to obtain the desired new flow rate. Also, remove the old time tape and place a new time tape with the new rate of infusion.
- **When you check the rate, you discover that the IV has been running too slowly for the past hour?**
  Adjust to the correct rate, but do not attempt to catch up by adjusting the flow to a rate higher than prescribed. *Too rapid IV infusion can lead to fluid overload for patients with congestive heart failure or other cardiopulmonary problems.*
- **When you check the rate, you discover that the IV has been running too fast for the past hour?**
  Slow the rate and assess the patient for signs of fluid volume excess.

Evaluation

- Evaluate the patient's response to IV therapy by checking for signs of excessive or deficient fluid volume.
- Evaluate the IV site for signs of infiltration, inflammation, infection, and phlebitis.
- Check laboratory studies to help evaluate the effectiveness of IV therapy.
- Monitor for correct IV rate at least hourly.
- Evaluate the tubing for kinks, or patient lying on the tubing. *Kinked tubing will interfere with the flow rate.*

Patient Teaching

- Explain the desired and adverse effects of IV therapy.
- Discuss the importance of notifying staff immediately if the catheter or administration set becomes dislodged; if the insertion site becomes tender, red, or swollen; if the patient notices moisture or fluid leakage; or if he has difficulty breathing.
- Teach safety measures if the patient is permitted to ambulate while the IV is infusing.

Home Care

- Explain home IV therapy to the client and caregiver, and teach them how to identify complications.
- Provide the client and caregiver with the name and phone numbers of people to contact in case problems arise with the catheter, insertion site, or level of comfort.

Documentation

Often IV care is documented on a flowsheet, and includes the following.

- Date and time the infusion was started
- Type of IV fluid, rate of infusion, and IV catheter site
- Whether rate is manual or pump controlled
- Patient's tolerance of IV therapy, any complications, and the interventions taken
- Document the volume infused on the I&O record.

Practice Resources

INS (2011a); Phillips, L. (2010); Shlamovitz, G. (updated 2013a).

Procedure 38-3 ■ Setting Up and Using Volume-Control Pumps

➤ For steps to follow in *all* procedures, refer to the Universal Steps for All Procedures found on the inside back cover.

Equipment

- Nonsterile gloves
- Alcohol wipes or chlorhexidine/alcohol antiseptic product
- Volume-control pump and IV pole
- Administration set appropriate for the pump
- IV fluid or medicated solution
- Tape for IV fluid solution time tape

Delegation

You can delegate the task of setting up a volume-control pump to an LPN who is specially trained in IV therapy, if covered by the agency's policy. Do not delegate this task to nursing assistive personnel (NAP). Do, however, instruct the NAP to notify you of any pump alarms that sound.

Pre-Procedure Assessment

- Confirm the patient's need for IV therapy by checking vital signs, laboratory values, urine output, skin turgor, breath sounds, and the moisture of mucous membranes.
  IV therapy creates a risk for fluid overload and electrolyte imbalance, which may be revealed by assessment data.
- Assess the existing IV catheter for patency.
  Occlusion of the IV catheter prevents the infusion of IV fluid. If not patent, you will need to change the IV.
- Assess the IV site hourly for signs of phlebitis, infiltration, infection and inflammation.
  Complications of IV therapy retard the therapeutic benefit of the fluids, as well as increase medical concerns and treatment cost for the patient. You must change the IV catheter and site if any of these complications occur.

➤ When performing the procedure, always identify your patient according to agency policy, using two identifiers, and be attentive to standard precautions, hand hygiene, patient safety and privacy, body mechanics, and documentation.

Procedure Steps

1. **Calculate the infusion rate** by dividing the volume to be infused by the number of hours it is to be infused. For example, if the order states 1,000 mL to run over 8 hours, divide 1,000 mL by 8 hours to determine the infusion rate of 125 mL/hr.
This ensures that the patient receives the correct dose. Pumps are usually programmed in milliliters per hour instead of drops per minute.

2. **Verify your calculations.**
To prevent dosage errors, either ask a second person to verify your calculations or check them a second time yourself.

3. **Attach the pump to the IV pole,** and plug it into the nearest electrical outlet.

Check to be sure that the infusion pump has a safety sticker on it and that the cord and plug are intact.

Volume-control pumps need regular maintenance checks. Using an electrical outlet saves battery power if needed for transport or electrical outage. As with gravity flow, the IV solution container needs to remain above the pump to prevent occlusion and for proper drainage of the container.▼

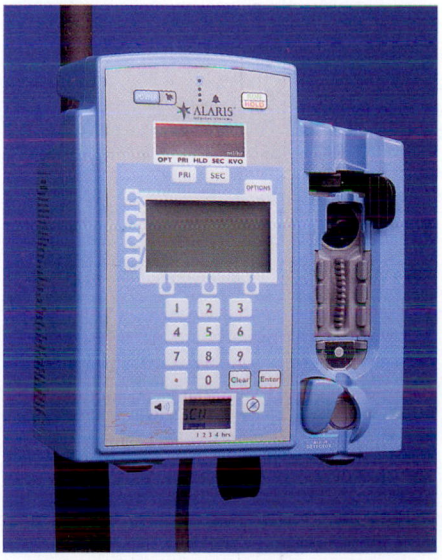

4. **Take the administration set** from the package, and close the clamp on it.
To prevent inadvertent loss of fluid.

5. **Attach a filter to the end** of the administration set, if required.
Filters are sometimes used to filter minute particles from the solution.

6. **Remove the protective covers,** and spike the port of the solution container with the administration set, maintaining sterility. Label the IV tubing and solution container with the date and time, and place a time tape on the solution container. Hang the container on the IV pole.
Labeling the administration set with the date and time informs the nursing staff when the administration set should be changed. The time tape allows you, and other nurses, to see at a glance whether the correct volume is infusing.

7. **Compress the drip chamber** of the administration set, and allow it to fill halfway. Consult the manufacturer's instructions for setup, as pumps differ. (On older gravity pumps, place the electronic eye on the drip chamber between the fluid level and the origin of the drop.)
Prepares the administration set for priming and prevents air from entering the tubing with the solution. Infusion pumps compress the tubing to move fluid; they measure the amount internally. On older gravity-type pumps, an electronic eye counts the number of drops to ensure the proper rate.

8. **Prime the administration set** with fluid by opening the roller clamp and allowing the fluid to flow slowly through the tubing. Recap the tubing and close the clamp.
Priming removes air from the tubing to prevent air embolus.

9. **Inspect the tubing** for air. If air bubbles remain in the tubing, flick the tubing with a fingertip to mobilize the bubbles into the drip chamber.
Air bubbles in the administration tubing interrupt flow and they can cause air emboli, which can be dangerous to the patient if they accumulate in the circulation.

10. **Turn on the pump, and load** the administration tubing into the pump according to the manufacturer's instructions.
Pumps differ. Consult the manufacturer's instructions.▼

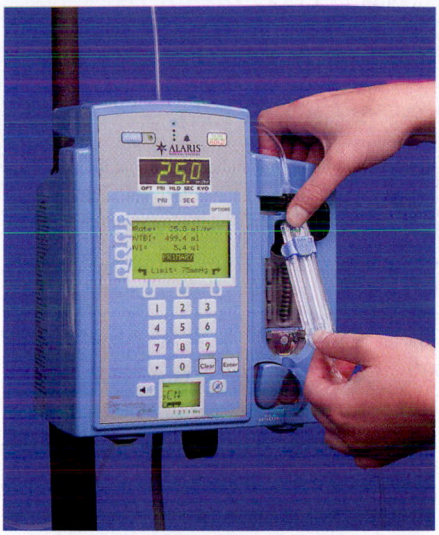

11. **Program the pump** with the prescribed information: total hours, infusion rate (hourly rate) and the volume to be infused (usually the total amount in the IV bag). *Note: Some pumps have only total hours and volume to infuse and do not have a feature that allows you to program in the infusion rate.*▼

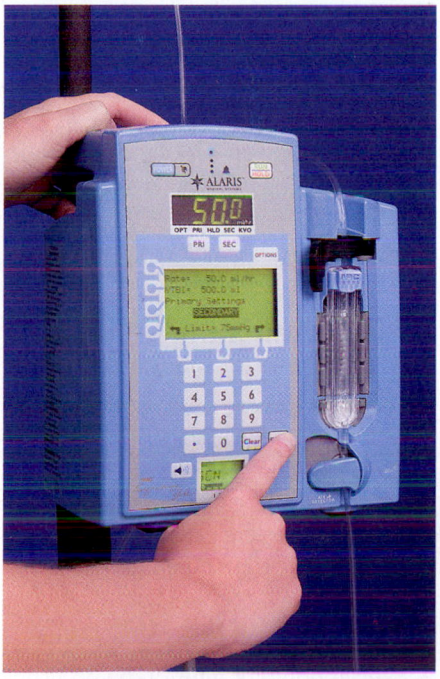

12. **Don clean nonsterile gloves,** check the IV site for patency, and scrub all surfaces of the primary line injection port or needleless connector, including the threads, with an antiseptic pad for at least 15 seconds. Allow it to dry.

(continued on next page)

Procedure 38-3 ■ Setting Up and Using Volume-Control Pumps (continued)

Clean nonsterile gloves protect from exposure to body fluids when you connect the tubing to the IV catheter or port. Scrubbing the port helps prevent infection.

13. **Connect the administration set** adapter to the injection port, keeping the connecting ends sterile.
Aseptic technique decreases the risk for contamination.

14. **Unclamp the administration set** tubing (open the roller clamp all the way), and press the start button on the pump.
Allows the IV fluid to flow through the administration set.

15. **Make sure the alarms** are turned on and audible.
The alarms must be functioning so that the pump can alert you of problems, such as kinks, air in the tubing, or catheter occlusion.

Key Point: ***Do not depend completely on the pump alarms to indicate IV patency. Pumps can infuse fluid, even if the line is clogged or infiltrated into the surrounding tissue.***

16. **Check the pump regularly** to make sure the correct volume is infusing. Checks are commonly done hourly.
Infusion pumps sometimes malfunction, so frequent monitoring is essential.

17. **At the end of your shift** (or at the time specified by your healthcare facility), clear the pump of the volume infused and record the volume on the patient's I&O form.
This helps the oncoming shift accurately monitor the fluid infused during their shift.

? What if . . .

- **In later evaluation you find the IV free flowing and not running via the pump setting?**

Immediately slow the IV fluid down. At the same time, begin assessing the patient: vital signs, mental awareness, lung sounds, pulse oximetry. Depending on the type of fluid running, you may need to make other assessments. Calculate the amount of IV fluid actually infused compared with the prescribed amount. Notify the provider and write out an occurrence report. If the pump is malfunctioning, set it aside, label it as "not working," and notify biomedical engineering so they can repair it.
Labeling the pump will prevent others from using it, until it can be repaired.

Evaluation

- Monitor the correct functioning of the pump regularly, perhaps hourly.
- Assess the IV site hourly for signs of phlebitis, infiltration, infection, and inflammation.
Complications of IV therapy interfere with the therapeutic benefit of the fluids and increase medical concerns, and treatment costs for the patient. You must change the IV catheter and document if any of these complications occur.

Patient Teaching

- Explain use of the IV infusion pump to the patient.
- Teach the patient the importance of notifying staff immediately if the infusion pump alarm sounds; the catheter or administration set becomes dislodged; the insertion site becomes tender, red, or swollen; or the dressing becomes wet.
- Teach the patient safety measures if he is able to ambulate while the infusion pump is in use.

Home Care

- Explain home IV infusion pump use to the client and caregiver, and teach them how to identify complications. Most home infusion pumps are smaller than institutional pumps.
- Provide the client with the name and phone numbers of people to contact in case problems arise with the catheter, insertion site, IV infusion pump, or other equipment.

Documentation

- Type and volume of IV fluid infusing, along with the infusion rate
- Use of the infusion pump, and patient's tolerance of IV therapy
- Any complications of IV therapy and the interventions taken
- Document volume infused on the patient's I&O record and/or an IV flowsheet.

Sample documentation

07/26/16 0600 Patient admitted from the ED with dehydration. NSS infusing at 250 mL/hr via infusion pump through an 18-gauge catheter. No signs of infiltration. No tenderness, redness, or swelling at the insertion site. Temp 102.6°F orally. HR 118 beats/min, RR 24 breaths/min, and BP 90/46 ——— R. Brill, RN

Practice Resources

Cummings, K., & McGowan, R. (2011); Phillips, L. (2010).

Thinking About the Procedure

To practice applying clinical reasoning to this procedure,

Go to *Davis's Nursing Skills Videos*, **Setting Up and Using Volume-Control Pumps.**

For questions and suggested responses,

Go to Chapter 38, **Thinking About the Procedure Questions and Suggested Responses,** on Davis*Plus*.

Procedure 38-4 ■ Changing IV Solutions and Tubing

➤ For steps to follow in *all* procedures, refer to the Universal Steps for All Procedures found on the inside back cover.

Equipment

- Nonsterile gloves
- Administration set
- IV solution
- IV pole
- Antiseptic swabs that contain solutions such as 70% alcohol or 2% chlorhexidine (chlorhexidine is not recommended in infants younger than age 2 months). You may use iodine-based products if alcohol or chlorhexidine are contraindicated and the patient is not allergic to iodine.
- 1-in. nonallergenic tape
- Time tape
- Watch with a second hand or digital seconds

Delegation

You can delegate the tasks of changing IV solutions and tubing to an LPN who is specially trained in IV therapy. The task should not be delegated to a NAP. However, do instruct the NAP to notify you of any problems that occur with IV therapy, such as the disconnecting of the administration set; catheter dislodging; or complaints of pain, swelling, or redness at the insertion site.

Pre-Procedure Assessments

- Assess the IV catheter for patency before changing the solution container or administration set.
- Assess the IV site for signs of phlebitis, infiltration, infection, or inflammation.
  If any of these complications occur, discontinue the IV and start a new IV at a different site.
- Check IV catheter insertion date.
  IV catheters are replaced per agency guidelines, which are based on the CDC recommendations of changing a peripheral IV site when clinically indicated (e.g., signs of phlebitis, infiltration, irritation).

Procedure 38-4A ■ Changing the IV Solution

➤ When performing the procedure, always identify your patient according to agency policy, using two identifiers, and be attentive to standard precautions, hand hygiene, patient safety and privacy, body mechanics, and documentation.

Procedure Steps

1. **Following the rights** of medication administration, prepare and label your next container of IV solution at least 1 hour before the present infusion is scheduled to finish.
   Preparing the next IV solution container reduces the risk of the present container running dry, thereby causing clots to form that would occlude the catheter.

2. **Close the roller clamp** on the infusing administration set.
   Prevents air from entering the tubing while changing the IV solution container.

3. **Wearing clean nonsterile gloves**, remove the old IV solution container from the IV pole. Remove the spike from the bag, keeping the spike sterile.
   The spike must remain sterile to prevent contamination of the new IV fluid. Clean nonsterile gloves protect you from exposure to body fluids.

4. **Remove the protective cover** from the new IV solution container port.

5. **Place the spike into the port** of the new solution container.

   For a Glass Bottle
   First scrub the rubber stopper on the top of the bottle with an antiseptic pad; then, insert the spike of the administration set through the rubber stopper.
   Cleansing the stopper removes particulate matter and microbes.

6. **Hang the IV solution** container on the IV pole.
   Allows the fluid to infuse by gravity.

7. **Inspect the tubing** to be sure that it is free of air bubbles and the drip chamber remains half-filled. Flick the tubing with a finger to mobilize the bubbles into the drip chamber.
   Prevents air from entering the system as the new solution is hung. If the drip chamber becomes too full, it will be difficult to impossible to count the drip rate properly and regulate the IV.

8. **Open the roller clamp** and adjust the drip rate, as prescribed.
   IV solution is considered a medication and must infuse at the prescribed rate for therapeutic effect and to prevent fluid overload.

9. **Affix the time tape** to the new IV solution container, if practiced within your agency. Mark the tape with the time the infusion was started, and mark 1-hour intervals on the tape until you reach the bottom of the container.
   The time tape allows you and other nurses to monitor the rate of administration easily.

10. **Dispose of used supplies** into appropriate receptacles, according to agency policy in line with CDC guidelines.

(continued on next page)

Procedure 38-4 ■ Changing IV Solutions and Tubing (continued)

Procedure 38-4B ■ Changing the IV Administration Tubing and Solution

➤ When performing the procedure, always identify your patient according to agency policy, using two identifiers, and be attentive to standard precautions, hand hygiene, patient safety and privacy, body mechanics, and documentation.

Procedure Steps

1. **Prepare the IV solution** and tubing as you would when initiating a new IV. (See Procedure 38-1, Step 2.)
2. **Hang the new administration** set on the IV pole.
3. **Close the roller clamp** on the old administration set.
   Stops the flow of fluid from the old container.
4. **Disconnect the old tubing**
   a. Wearing clean nonsterile gloves, place a sterile swab under the catheter hub.
   The swab absorbs any leakage from the catheter hub when you disconnect the tubing.
   b. Apply pressure to the vein about 3 inches above the insertion site, using the fourth or fifth finger of your nondominant hand. Hold the catheter hub firmly with the thumb and index finger of that hand, but do not apply downward pressure.
   Prevents blood from leaking out of the catheter during the tubing change. Holding the hub firmly keeps the catheter from moving about and traumatizing the vein.
   c. Then carefully remove the device securing the connection between the catheter and tubing. This may be as simple as unscrewing a luer-lock. The connection should not be covered by tape, but if it is, remove it so you can access the connection.
5. **Remove the protective cover** from the distal end of the new administration set.
   Cover keeps the distal end sterile until you are ready to connect it to the IV catheter.
6. **Continue to stabilize the IV** catheter with your nondominant hand while applying pressure over the vein. ▼

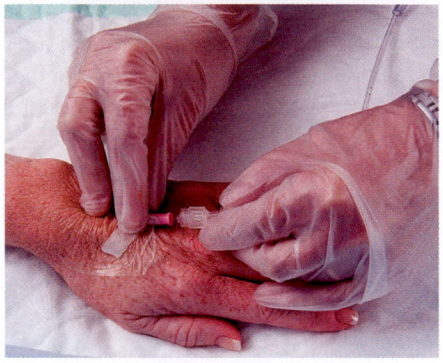

7. **Gently disengage the used** tubing from the IV catheter, and place it in a basin or other receptacle. Quickly insert the new tubing into the catheter hub.
   The CDC recommends IV tubing should be changed at 96-hours interval, but at least every 7 days, depending on agency policy and solution. Certain solutions (e.g., blood, blood products, fat emulsions) require more frequent tubing changes. Change it quickly to prevent microorganisms from entering the IV catheter.
8. **Open the roller clamp** on the new administration set, and allow the IV solution to infuse.
   This clears the IV catheter of blood, preventing catheter occlusion.
9. **Program and turn on** the volume-control pump. Or, for a gravity drip, use the roller clamp to adjust the flow to the prescribed rate.
   IV solution is considered a medication and must infuse at the prescribed rate.
10. **Cleanse the IV site** and secure the IV catheter and tubing connection.
    Removes microorganisms and media for growth; helps preserve the integrity of the intact line; and prevents air and microorganisms from entering the line.
11. **Loop and tape tubing** to patient's skin.
    Helps minimize catheter movement, which contributes to phlebitis.
12. **Label tubing and solution** with date, initials, rate, and time tape.
    Alerts staff to when tubing and solution was changed and to when they will need to be changed again to decrease the incidence of infection.
13. **Dispose of used supplies** into appropriate receptacles according to agency policy in line with CDC guidelines.

? What if . . .

- **The drip chamber becomes too full (over half) so that drops cannot be adequately counted?**
  Close the roller clamp, invert the bag or bottle, and squeeze the excess fluid back into the bag/bottle.
- **The tubing will not separate from the catheter connection when you attempt to disconnect it?**
  If the lock does not twist off, gently try using a hemostat ("mosquito" clamp) to twist the lock. Do not lock the hemostat; merely use it lightly as a grip. After the lock is off, if the tubing will not separate, use the hemostat to gently twist the tubing back and forth. If the catheter needs to be stabilized, wear a sterile glove or use a sterile hemostat.

Evaluation

- Assess the IV insertion site for signs of infiltration, inflammation, infection, and phlebitis.
- Evaluate the effectiveness of IV therapy by assessing the patient's hydration status or expected effect of the intravenous medication/solution.
- Monitor the IV rate regularly (usually hourly).

Patient Teaching

- Discuss the importance of notifying staff immediately if the catheter or administration set becomes dislodged; if the insertion site becomes tender, red, or swollen; or if the IV dressing becomes wet.

Home Care

- Explain home IV therapy to the client and caregiver; teach them how to identify complications.
- Obtain a return demonstration to ensure the caregiver is able to perform fluid and tubing changes, when necessary.

Documentation

- Fluid and tubing changes are usually documented on a flowsheet.
- Document the date and time the IV fluid and tubing were changed; type of IV fluid and rate of infusion; and the location and condition of the IV catheter insertion site.
- Any complications of IV therapy and the interventions taken.

Sample documentation

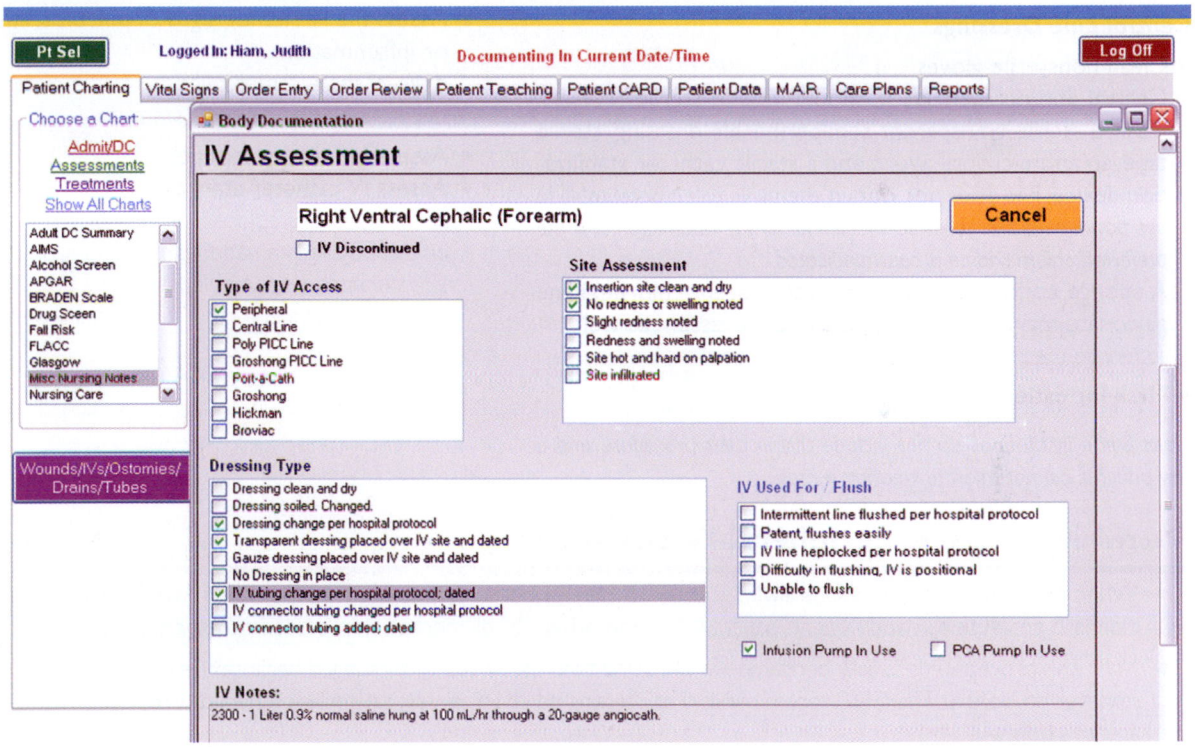

Practice Resources

CDC (2011b); INS (2011a).

Procedure 38-5 ■ Changing IV Dressings

➤ For steps to follow in *all* procedures, refer to the Universal Steps for All Procedures found on the inside back cover. For this procedure, also refer to Clinical Insights 23-1 through 23-6 if you need to review information about medical and surgical asepsis.

Equipment

Peripheral IV Dressings

- Clean nonsterile gloves
- Sterile transparent semipermeable dressing or dressing specified by institution
- Antiseptic swabs: alcohol or chlorhexidine (*Note: Use iodine-based products only if the preferred antiseptics cannot be used. Chlorhexidine is not recommended in infants younger than age 2 months.*)
- 1-inch nonallergenic tape or manufactured stabilization device

Central Line Dressings

- Clean nonsterile gloves
- Central line dressing kit. It should include sterile gloves, a mask, a sterile transparent semipermeable dressing, sterile tape, an antimicrobial agent, and a sterile catheter stabilization device. If it does not, obtain them. *Note: It is acceptable to use povidone-iodine followed by alcohol as the antimicrobial if the preferred chlorhexidine is contraindicated.*
- A sponge containing the antimicrobial agent chlorhexidine gluconate may be used as a part of the dressing, as well.
  To reduce the risk for catheter-related infection
- Mask for patient (possibly)

Note: Some institutions do not include this in their procedure and a few patients cannot tolerate wearing a mask.

Delegation

You can delegate the tasks of changing dressings to an LPN who is specially trained in IV therapy. The task should not be delegated to a NAP. Do, however, instruct the NAP to notify you of any problems that occur with dressing such as soiling, blood, leakage, or loosening.

Pre-Procedure Assessments

- Assess the IV catheter for patency before changing the dressing.
  Ensure that the IV is still working properly.
- Assess the IV site for signs of phlebitis, infiltration, infection, or inflammation.
  If any of these complications exist, the current IV will need to be discontinued and a new IV started.
- Assess for allergy to tape.
- Assess IV catheter start date.
  IV catheters are replaced per agency guidelines which are based on the CDC recommendations of changing a peripheral IV site at 96-hour intervals, but at least every 7 days. Changing more often than recommended actually increases the risk of infection.

Procedure 38-5A ■ Peripheral IV Dressings

➤ When performing the procedure, always identify your patient according to agency policy, using two identifiers, and be attentive to standard precautions, hand hygiene, patient safety and privacy, body mechanics, and documentation.

➤ *Note:* This procedure is usually performed at the same time the IV tubing is changed because the old dressing may need to be removed to do that. The CDC recommends that dressing be changed when damp, loosened, or visibly soiled. You should follow your agency's policy.

Procedure Steps

1. **Wearing clean nonsterile gloves,** stabilize the catheter with your nondominant hand, avoiding direct pressure on the catheter/hub junction, and carefully remove and discard the dressing and the catheter stabilization device.
   Remove the dressing gently to avoid dislodging the catheter.

2. **Inspect the insertion site.** Look for erythema and drainage, and note any tenderness. Remove procedure gloves and perform hand hygiene.
   If signs of infection, phlebitis, or infiltration are present, you must remove the IV catheter.

3. **Don a clean pair of nonsterile gloves.**

4. **Cleanse the insertion site,** and then allow the antiseptic to dry on the skin. Do not fan.

   If Using Chlorhexidine
   Apply using a back-and-forth motion and friction for at least 30 seconds. (Avoid using chlorhexidine in infants younger than age 2 months.)

   If Using Alcohol or 2% Tincture of Iodine
   Using a circular motion, start at the insertion site and work outward 2 to 3 inches. Do not go back over any cleansed area.
   Removes microorganisms from the skin to minimize the risk of their entering the venipuncture site. Allowing the antiseptic to dry increases its effectiveness.

5. **Perform hand hygiene** and change procedure gloves. Apply a new sterile catheter stabilization device and dressing. For illustrations, see Procedure 38-1.

If Using a Transparent Dressing

a. Open the package containing the sterile, semipermeable, transparent dressing. Remove the protective backing from the dressing, making sure not to touch the sterile surface.

b. Cover the insertion site and the hub or winged portion of the catheter with the dressing. Do not cover the junction with the tubing of the administration set.

c. Gently pinch the transparent dressing around the catheter hub to secure the hub. Smooth the remainder of the dressing so that it adheres to the skin.
Pinching the dressing around the hub prevents pressure of the hub on the underlying skin.

If You Must Use a Gauze Dressing

d. Fold a 2 in. × 2 in. sterile gauze dressing in half, cover it with 1-inch tape (about 3 inches long).

e. Place under the tubing/hub junction and press down on the tape.
Raises the hub to prevent pressure on the skin.

f. Place a sterile gauze pad over the insertion site and catheter hub—but not over the catheter/hub junction

g. Secure all edges with tape.

6. **Secure the connection between** the catheter and the tubing, but do not cover the catheter-tubing junction with tape.
Securing the connection helps maintain a closed system and prevents entry of microorganisms. You should not cover the junction with tape because removing the tape may interfere with your ability to disconnect the tubing from the hub quickly, should you need to do so. Removing tape requires much manipulation; the more the catheter is manipulated, the higher the risk for infection.

7. **Secure the IV administration** tubing by looping and taping the tubing to the skin.
Looping the tubing provides slack to prevent the IV catheter from becoming dislodged.

8. **Label the dressing with the date** and time of insertion, catheter size, and the date the dressing was changed and your initials.
Peripheral IV catheters should be replaced as clinically indicated (e.g., phlebitis, infiltration, irritation) to prevent complications. Labeling the dressing with the date and time of insertion helps communicate to other nurses the date of the IV insertion and dressing change.

9. **Discard all supplies** in the appropriate containers according to agency policy in line with CDC guidelines.

? What if . . .

- **The patient is immunocompromised? Or the peripheral midline catheter must be in the same site for an extended time?**

Use sterile gloves and a mask when changing the dressing and giving site care.

Thinking About the Procedure

To practice applying clinical reasoning to this procedure,

Go to *Davis's Nursing Skills Videos*, **Peripheral IV Dressings.**

For questions and suggested responses,

Go to Chapter 38, **Thinking About the Procedure Questions and Suggested Responses,** on Davis*Plus*.

Procedure 38-5B ■ Central Line Dressings

➤ When performing the procedure, always identify your patient according to agency policy, using two identifiers, and be attentive to standard precautions, hand hygiene, patient safety and privacy, body mechanics, and documentation.

➤ *Note:* This procedure focuses on dressing change. Refer to Clinical Insight 38-4 for assessments and maintenance of CVCs.

Procedure Steps

1. **Obtain a sterile central line** dressing kit (or equivalent supplies if there is no kit) and mask for the patient, if one is needed.
Because central lines have direct access to the central circulation, the risk of systemic infection is greater. Therefore, the procedure uses aseptic technique. All supplies must be sterile.

2. **Place the patient** in a semi-Fowler's position, if tolerated. Lower the siderail and adjust the bed to working height.
Semi-Fowler's position and bed adjustments facilitate site cleansing and dressing application and reduce strain on the nurse's back.

3. **Explain the procedure** and ask the patient to turn his head to the opposite side from the insertion site. If he cannot cooperate, place a mask on the patient.
Explanation may reduce anxiety and enhance cooperation; turning helps prevent contamination of the insertion site.

4. **Put on your mask** and clean nonsterile gloves. Carefully remove the old dressing and catheter stabilization device, if present.

5. **Inspect the site** for signs and symptoms of infection and other complications.
If a complication is suspected, notify the person who placed the central line.

(continued on next page)

Procedure 38-5 ■ Changing IV Dressings (continued)

6. **Remove and discard your gloves**, along with the soiled dressing. Wash your hands.

7. **Set up a sterile field** and open the dressing kit.
To prevent contamination of the insertion site and the sterile supplies.

8. **Don the sterile gloves** contained in the kit and arrange sterile supplies as needed.

9. **Scrub the insertion site** and surrounding skin with an antiseptic swab.

If Using Chlorhexidine
Use a back-and-forth motion with friction and scrub for at least 30 seconds.

If Using Povidone-Iodine and Alcohol
The kit should contain three swabs of each. Beginning with a povidone-iodine swab, start at the insertion site and work outward several inches ("dirty to clean"). Repeat with the other two povidone-iodine swabs. Then, using the same method, clean with the three alcohol swabs. With each swab, do not "go back over" an area you have just cleaned with that swab.
To rid the site of any potential infectious microorganisms, work "from clean to contaminated."

10. **Scrub the sutures (if any)**, and the catheter from insertion site to the hub or bifurcation, for at least 15 seconds with an alcohol swab or chlorhexidine/alcohol antiseptic product.

11. **Allow the site to dry**—do not fan.
Allows the antiseptic time to work completely and allows the dressing to stick properly. Povidone-iodine requires 1 minute to air-dry completely; chlorhexidine requires 30 seconds.

12. **Apply a new catheter** stabilization device, if one is used.

13. **Apply the transparent dressing** that comes in the kit.

If You Place Gauze Under the Catheter Hub
You may first place a small piece of folded sterile gauze under the catheter hub.
To reduce pressure on the skin under the hub.

If Chlorhexidine Gluconate Sponge Is Part of the Dressing
Apply the sponge directly over the catheter insertion site, ensuring that the sponge is in full contact with the skin. Then apply the transparent dressing over the sponge.
Reduces the risk for catheter-related infection, especially in units with high infection rates or in high-risk patients (CDC, 2011a; Timsit, Schwebel, Boudma, et al., 2009).

14. **Remove the drape**, if you used one.

15. **Loop the catheter gently** and secure it with tape to the skin. Avoid securing it to the dressing. Or, depending on type of CVC, place a piece of clear tape across the ends of the catheter lumens, near but not on the hubs.
Ensures that accidental tugging on the catheter does not dislodge the catheter. Do not cover the hubs, as you may need to access them.

16. **Label the dressing** with the date changed, time, and your initials.
Alerts staff to when the next dressing change will be due.

17. **Place the patient in** a comfortable position, raise the siderail, and be sure the call light is accessible.

18. **Remove your mask and gloves** and the patient's mask.

19. **Dispose of supplies** into the appropriate receptacles according to agency policy in line with CDC guidelines.

Thinking About the Procedure

To practice applying clinical reasoning to this procedure,

Go to *Davis's Nursing Skills Videos*, **Central Line Dressings.**

For questions and suggested responses,

Go to Chapter 38, **Thinking About the Procedure Questions and Suggested Responses,** on *DavisPlus*.

Procedure 38-5C ■ PICC Line Dressings

➤ When performing the procedure, always identify your patient according to agency policy, using two identifiers, and be attentive to standard precautions, hand hygiene, patient safety and privacy, body mechanics, and documentation.

Procedure Steps

1. **Obtain a sterile PICC** (central) line dressing kit (or equivalent supplies if there is no kit) and mask for the patient, if one is needed.
Because central lines have direct access to the central circulation, the risk of systemic infection is greater. Therefore, this procedure uses aseptic technique, even though the insertion site is peripheral. All supplies must be sterile.

2. **Place the patient in a** semi-Fowler's position, if tolerated. Lower the siderail and adjust the bed to working height.
Semi-Fowler's position and bed adjustments facilitate site cleansing and dressing application and reduce strain on the nurse's back.

3. **Explain the procedure** and ask the patient to turn his head to the opposite side from the insertion site. If the patient cannot cooperate, place a mask on him, if consistent with agency policy.
Explanation may reduce anxiety and enhance cooperation; turning helps prevent contamination of the insertion site from nasal and oral airborne secretions.

4. **Inspect the site** for signs and symptoms of infection and catheter migration.

5. **Put on your mask and** clean nonsterile gloves and carefully remove the old dressing by pulling towards the insertion site and catheter stabilization device, if present. Discard your gloves with the dressing.
The mask helps prevent contamination of the insertion site from the nurse's nasal and oral airborne secretions. Pulling toward the insertion site minimizes the possibility of dislodging the catheter.

6. **Perform hand hygiene**, open the kit, and remove and don the sterile gloves.

7. **If the kit contains a sterile drape,** unfold it and establish your sterile field. Transfer items from kit to your sterile field.
Ensures that strict sterile technique is maintained.

8. **Use a sterile tape measure** to compare the external length of the PICC with the baseline insertion length (if consistent with agency's policy).
Detects catheter migration, which may indicate that the PICC line is not in the correct location.

9. **Scrub the insertion site** and surrounding skin with an antiseptic solution. Ensure that blood or encrustations are removed from the site and catheter. (Refer to Procedure 38-5B: Central Line Dressings, Steps 9 and 10).
Minimizes the proliferation of microorganisms.

10. **Allow the site to air-dry.** If you are using a chlorhexadine gluconate sponge as part of the dressing, apply it directly over the catheter insertion site, ensuring that it is in direct contact with the skin.

11. **Apply a commercial stabilization** device, if applicable.

12. **Apply a transparent dressing** over catheter site. ▼

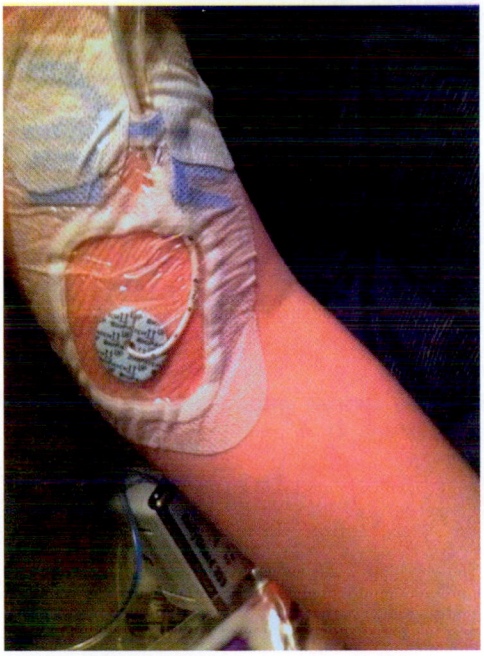

13. **Label the dressing** with the date, time, and your initials.
Used to identify the next scheduled dressing change.

14. **Loop and anchor the catheter, as needed;** secure it with tape.
Reduces the risk of accidental dislodgement.

15. **Place the patient** in a comfortable position, raise the siderails, and place the call light so it is accessible to patient.

16. **Dispose of used supplies** into the appropriate receptacles according to agency policy and consistent with CDC guidelines.

Evaluation

- Evaluate the IV insertion site and surrounding tissue for signs of infiltration, inflammation, infection, and phlebitis.
- Monitor the dressing for dampness, blood, soiling, or loosening.
If these occur, the dressing must be changed.

Patient Teaching

- Explain the importance of notifying staff if the IV dressing becomes soiled, dampened, or loosened.
- Remind the patient to notify staff immediately for bleeding, pain, or swelling around the catheter or dressing area or discomfort in the hand, arm, or shoulder on the same side as the catheter.

Home Care

- Explain home IV therapy to the client and caregiver; teach them how to identify complications.
- Obtain a return demonstration by the client or caregiver to ensure competent performance of fluid, tubing, and dressing changes when necessary.

(continued on next page)

Procedure 38-5 ■ Changing IV Dressings (continued)

Documentation

- Chart the date and time the dressing was changed. Document the location and condition of the IV catheter insertion site.
- Document any complications of IV therapy and the interventions taken.
- Document the dressing change on your IV record. Often, IV care is documented on a flowsheet.

Sample documentation

mm/dd/yyyy 2300 *New transparent semipermeable dressing applied over PICC insertion site in left forearm. No redness, tenderness, swelling, or exudates at the site.*
Mary Ramirez, RNC

Practice Resources

CDC (2011a); Hadaway, L. (2010); INS (2011a); Institute for Healthcare Improvement (IHI) (2012); The Joint Commission (2012); National Guideline Clearinghouse (NGC) (2011); Pronovost, P., Goeschel, A., Colantuoi, E., et al. (2010); Timsit, J-F., Schwebel, C., Boudma, L., et al. (2009).

Thinking About the Procedure

To practice applying clinical reasoning to this procedure,

Go to *Davis's Nursing Skills Videos*, **PICC Line Dressings.**

For questions and suggested responses,

Go to Chapter 38, **Thinking About the Procedure Questions and Suggested Responses** on Davis*Plus*.

Procedure 38-6 ■ Converting a Primary Line to a Peripheral IV Lock

➤ For steps to follow in *all* procedures, refer to the Universal Steps for All Procedures found on the inside back cover.

Equipment

- Clean nonsterile gloves
- Peripheral intermittent IV lock adapter
- Two syringes containing saline solution (one syringe with dilute heparin solution, if required by agency policy)
- Linen-saver pad
- Transparent semipermeable dressing
- Alcohol or chlorhexidine/alcohol or other antiseptic swab

Delegation

You can delegate the task of converting a primary IV line to an intermittent lock device to an LPN who is specially trained in IV therapy. The task should not be delegated to a NAP. However, you should instruct the NAP to notify you of any problems with the intermittent lock device, such as dislodging of the catheter or client complaints of pain, swelling, or redness at the insertion site.

Pre-Procedure Assessment

- Assess the patient's readiness to have the IV fluid discontinued (e.g., tolerating oral fluids, adequate urine output, and laboratory values within normal limits).
  If the patient's condition indicates that he still requires IV fluids, notify the primary care provider and do not discontinue the IV line.
- Assess for allergy to tape.
- Assess the IV site for signs of phlebitis, infiltration, extravasation, or infection.
  If complications are present or the IV has been in place longer than 96 hours or at least 7 days, remove the IV catheter instead of converting it to an intermittent lock.

➤ When performing the procedure, always identify your patient according to agency policy, using two identifiers, and be attentive to standard precautions, hand hygiene, patient safety and privacy, body mechanics, and documentation.

➤ Maintain sterility of supplies and equipment (e.g., do not touch catheter opening or ends of the IV lock; keep flush syringe connector sterile).

Procedure Steps

1. **Help the client assume** a comfortable position that provides access to the IV site.
   Promotes cooperation and facilitates your ability to perform the procedure.
2. **Lower siderails, raise the bed** to working height, and place linen-saver pad under extremity with the IV.
   Protects linens from blood and fluid that might leak from the vessel during catheter removal and ensures good body mechanics.
3. **Don clean nonsterile gloves.** Remove the IV lock from the package and flush the adapter with the first syringe of saline or dilute heparin, according to agency policy. Place the lock back loosely inside the sterile

package, keeping it sterile. **Continue with Step 5.**
Removes air from the lock.▼

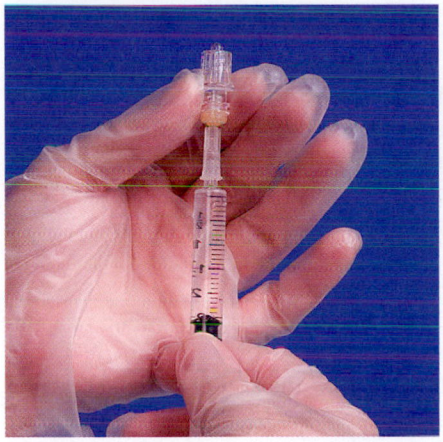

Procedure Variation for Primary Tubing Set-Up With Extension Tubing With a Lock

Merely discontinue the IV solution and disconnect the primary tubing from the extension tubing with lock. Then, flush extension tubing per agency policy and **skip to Step 13.**

4. **Carefully remove the IV dressing** and the tape that is securing the tubing.
   Provides access to the IV catheter.

5. **Close the roller clamp** on the administration set.
   Prevents loss of IV fluid during the procedure.

6. **With the side of your** nondominant hand, apply pressure over the vein just above the insertion site but not directly on the catheter–hub junction. At the same time, stabilize the catheter hub with your thumb and forefinger.
   Applying pressure over the vein stops blood from flowing from the catheter as you change the administration tubing.

7. **Gently disengage the used** tubing from the IV catheter. If the tubing does not separate from the catheter, see the What If . . . section at the end of Step 13.

8. **Quickly insert the lock adapter** into the IV catheter and turn it to lock it in place.
   Insert the adapter quickly to prevent bleeding from the IV catheter.▼

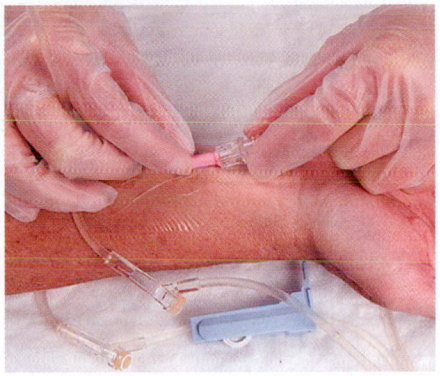

9. **Scrub the injection port** of the adapter with an antiseptic pad.
   Cleaning the port with antiseptic helps prevent contamination by microorganisms when the adapter is flushed.

10. **Insert the second syringe** containing saline or dilute heparin into the injection port of the adapter. Flush the catheter using the method recommended in your agency (e.g., push-stop-push or a slow, steady push).
    Some experts recommend a turbulence (push-stop-push method) on the theory that turbulence ensures patency of the IV catheter by clearing the catheter and helping prevent reflux of blood back into the catheter. Others believe this method has undesired effects and recommend, instead, a steady, slow push. There is no evidence to support the turbulence theory (INS, 2011a). In the meantime, follow agency policy regarding the flushing technique.▼

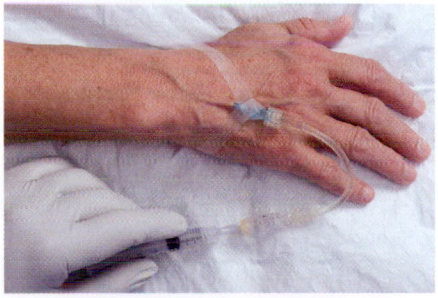

11. **Using aseptic technique**, cover the insertion site and catheter hub with a sterile transparent semipermeable dressing. Do not cover the junction of the catheter hub and the IV lock. See Procedure 38-5A for review of dressings.
    Secures the IV catheter and prevents contamination of the site.

12. **Label the dressing** with the date changed and your initials.

13. **Discard used supplies** into appropriate receptacles according to agency policy in line with CDC guidelines.
    Discarding used equipment properly keeps the healthcare environment safe.

? What if . . .

- **At Step 7, the tubing will not separate from the catheter?**

  First, if it is a luer-lock connection, be sure you have twisted the luer-lock "open." If so, place a hemostat ("mosquito" clamp) on the IV tubing and gently twist back and forth to loosen the connection. Then if the IV tubing still does not come loose, use the hemostat to gently twist the lock back and forth to loosen the connection. Do not lock the hemostat; merely use it lightly as a grip.
  Use of hemostat may help loosen tubing from the catheter, but placement is critical so that the IV catheter and connector are not damaged.

- **At Step 7, the IV catheter becomes dislodged while trying to disconnect the tubing?**

  If you can see as much as three-fourths of the catheter emerging from the site, you must remove it and start a new IV at a different site.
  Trying to re-advance the catheter might cause it to pierce through the vein as well as increase the risk of infection from reinserting a catheter that is no longer sterile. It also causes tissue trauma and increases the risk of phlebitis from catheter manipulation.

(continued on next page)

Procedure 38-6 ■ Converting a Primary Line to a Peripheral IV Lock (continued)

Evaluation

- Assess the patency of the catheter before each use according to institutional policy. Patency check and flushing are usually done every 8 to 24 hours.
- Evaluate the patient's tolerance to intermittent IV therapy.
- Inspect the insertion site for signs of complications.

Patient Teaching

Explain the importance of notifying staff if the IV site becomes red, painful, or swollen; or if the dressing becomes soiled, damp, or loosened (indicating that the catheter has become dislodged or the connection is loose). Include the family in the teaching, as the patient may not be able to assess his own IV therapy.

Home Care

- Explain home use of the intermittent lock to the patient and caregiver. Teach them how to flush the catheter before and after administering prescribed medications.
- Provide the patient and caregiver with the name and phone numbers of people to contact in case problems arise with the catheter or insertion site.

Documentation

- Chart the date and time the IV line was converted to an intermittent lock device.
- Note the size and location of the catheter, as well as the type and amount of flush solution used.
- Record on the I&O record the amount of IV fluid infused.
- Document the condition of the IV site and any complications noted.
- Often, IV care is documented on a flowsheet or the electronic patient record.

Sample documentation

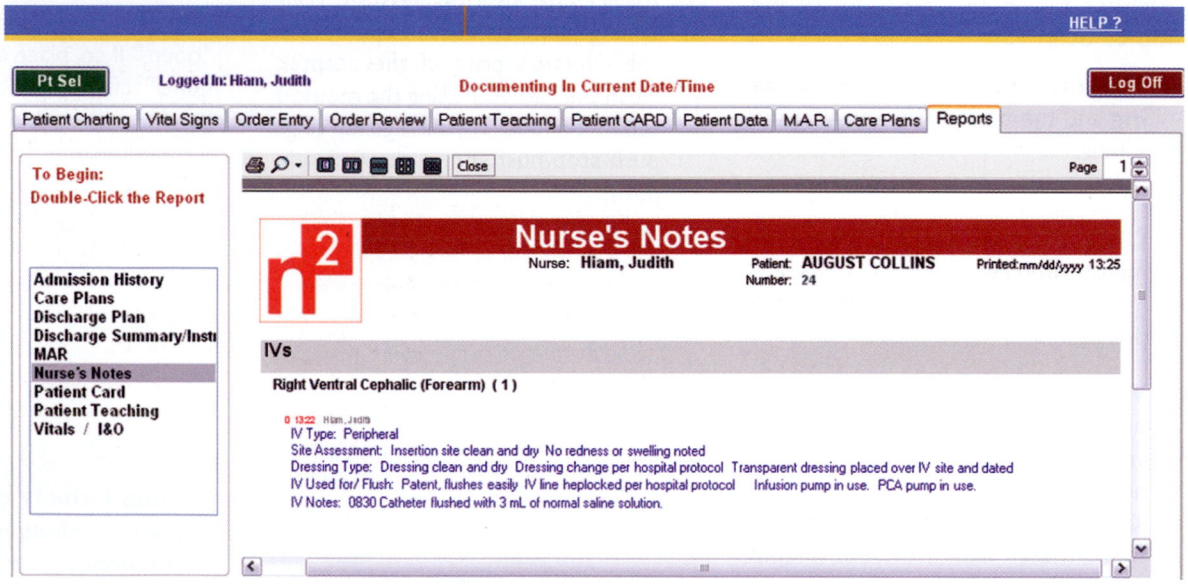

Practice Resources

CDC (2011); Hadaway, L. (2010); INS (2011a).

Procedure 38-7 ■ Discontinuing a Peripheral IV

➤ For steps to follow in *all* procedures, refer to the Universal Steps for All Procedures found on the inside back cover.

Equipment

- Clean nonsterile gloves
- Sterile 2 in. × 2 in. gauze dressings
- 1-in. tape or transparent semipermeable dressing
- Linen-saver pad

Delegation

You can delegate the task of discontinuing an IV to an LPN who is specially trained in IV therapy. The task should not be delegated to a NAP. However, you should instruct the NAP to notify you of any bleeding from the insertion site.

Pre-Procedure Assessment

- Assess the patient's readiness to have the IV fluid discontinued and verify the order. For example, determine whether he is tolerating oral fluids and has adequate urine output and whether laboratory values are within normal limits.
  If the patient's condition indicates that he still requires IV fluids, notify the physician and do not discontinue the IV line.

➤ When performing the procedure, always identify your patient according to agency policy, using two identifiers, and be attentive to standard precautions, hand hygiene, patient safety and privacy, body mechanics, and documentation.

Procedure Steps

1. **Assist the client to a** comfortable position and raise the bed to working height.
   Helps ensure patient cooperation with the procedure; supports good body mechanics for the nurse.

2. **Place a linen-saver pad** under the extremity with the IV.
   Protects linens from blood and fluid that might leak from the vein during catheter removal

3. **Don clean nonsterile gloves**, and close the roller clamp on the administration set.
   Closing the roller prevents IV fluid from spilling onto the bed or client during catheter removal. Procedure gloves protect you from body fluid exposure.

4. **Carefully remove the IV dressing**, catheter stabilization device, and the tape that is securing the tubing.
   Removing tape and dressings can be painful especially if over hair or sensitive or thin skin.

   If the IV Is Running Through an Extension Tubing or a Saline Lock
   Disconnect the administration set tubing and close the slide clamp on the extension tubing.

5. **Scrub the catheter–skin junction** with an alcohol prep pad or chlorhexidine/alcohol antiseptic product for at least 15 seconds.
   Removes microorganisms from the skin entry site.

6. **Apply a sterile 2 in. × 2 in. gauze** pad above the IV insertion site and gently remove the catheter, directing it straight along the vein. Do not press down on the gauze pad while removing the catheter.
   Directing the catheter along the vein prevents vein injury while you are removing the catheter.▼

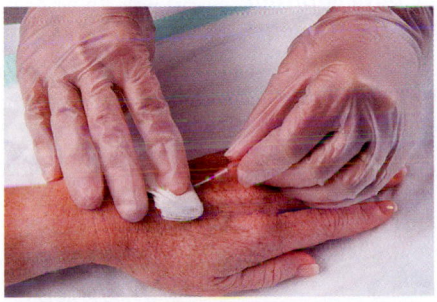

7. **Immediately apply firm pressure** with the gauze pad over the insertion site. Hold pressure for 1 to 3 minutes; hold longer if bleeding persists.
   This typically stops bleeding by hastening clot formation.

8. **Remove the soiled 2 in. × 2 in.** gauze pad, and replace it with a sterile 2 in. × 2 in. gauze pad folded over to form a pressure dressing. Secure it with 1-inch tape or a transparent semipermeable dressing.
   Protects the site from contamination.

9. **Return the bed to a low position.** Discard all supplies in the appropriate receptacles according to agency policy in line with CDC guidelines.

(continued on next page)

Procedure 38-7 ■ Discontinuing a Peripheral IV (continued)

Evaluation

- Assess the integrity of the removed catheter; compare the length with the original insertion length to ensure the entire catheter is removed. If a catheter defect is noted, report to the manufacturer and regulatory agencies and complete an incident report according to agency policy.
- Evaluate the patient's response to oral fluids after IV therapy is discontinued.
- Monitor for changes in the patient's condition to assess whether IV therapy should be re-established.

Patient Teaching

- Instruct the client and family to notify staff if bleeding or discomfort occurs at the insertion site.
- Teach the importance of drinking adequate amounts of fluid, within the prescribed treatment plan, to prevent dehydration. (Some patients have fluid restrictions.)

Documentation

- Chart the date and time that IV therapy was discontinued.
- Note the condition of the site, including the presence of any complications. If complications are present, document your interventions, including physician notification.
- Often you will record this procedure on a flow sheet or in the electronic patient record.

Sample documentation

mm/dd/yyyy 2100 RA#2, 22-gauge catheter discontinued. Site without redness, swelling, tenderness, or exudates. Pressure applied to site for 3 minutes. Bleeding stopped and sterile 2 × 2 gauze dressing applied. Informed patient to notify staff if bleeding or discomfort occurs.
S. Horowitz, RN

Practice Resources
CDC (2011); INS (2011a).

Thinking About the Procedure

To practice applying clinical reasoning to this procedure,

Go to *Davis's Nursing Skills Videos*, **Discontinuing a Peripheral IV.**

For questions and suggested responses,

Go to Chapter 38, **Thinking About the Procedure Questions and Suggested Responses,** on Davis*Plus*.

Procedure 38-8 ■ Administering a Blood Transfusion

➤ For steps to follow in *all* procedures, refer to the Universal Steps for All Procedures found on the inside back cover.

Equipment

- Clean nonsterile gloves
- Blood product
- Normal saline IV solution, 250 mL
  Key Point: ***Normal saline solution is the only solution that is compatible with blood products; other IV solutions cause hemolysis of blood cells.***
- Blood administration set (with a 200-micrometer filter and luer-lock connection). If there is no filter on the tubing, you must attach one.
- IV pole
- Watch with a second hand or digital seconds
- Thermometer
- Blood pressure cuff with sphygmomanometer
- Stethoscope

Delegation

Do not delegate this procedure to the LPN or NAP, because blood product administration requires advanced assessment and critical-thinking skills. The LPN and NAP can assist by monitoring vital signs. Instruct both about the complications associated with blood product administration, and instruct them to inform you if any occur.

Pre-Procedure Assessment

- Confirm the patient's need for blood products by assessing vital signs, urine output, and laboratory studies.
  Blood products may cause life-threatening complications; therefore, they should be administered only when needed.
- Check the patient's history for previous blood transfusions and reactions and verify her blood type.
  If the patient has a history of a blood transfusion reaction, precautions must be taken before she receives additional transfusions. For example, she may need premedication with acetaminophen, a corticosteroid, and diphenhydramine; specially treated blood products; and the use of a specialized administration set with greater filtering capabilities.
- Assess patency of the existing IV catheter, and make sure that it is the proper size for blood product administration.
  Nurses often use a 20-gauge catheter for blood administration. However, for routine transfusion, a 22-gauge or even a 24-gauge catheter can be used. You would need an 18- or 20-gauge catheter when large amounts of blood must be transfused rapidly. The primary consideration should be the size of the patient's veins and not an arbitrary catheter size.
- Assess for allergy to tape.

Procedure 38-8A ■ Administering Blood and Blood Products

➤ When performing the procedure, always identify your patient according to agency policy, using two identifiers, and be attentive to standard precautions, hand hygiene, patient safety and privacy, body mechanics, and documentation.

Procedure Steps

1. **Verify that informed consent** has been obtained.
   Informed consent is required for blood product administration, as for any invasive or risk-bearing procedure.

2. **Verify the medical prescription,** noting the indication, rate of infusion, and any medications. If there are any pretransfusion medications, administer them as prescribed.
   Helps prevent administration errors.

3. **Obtain a blood administration set** and 250 mL of IV normal saline solution.

4. **Obtain infusion pump,** if possible, and blood warmer, if necessary
   Having all supplies and equipment on hand minimizes delays in starting the transfusion.

5. **Obtain the blood product** from the blood bank, according to your institution's policy. Wear clean nonsterile gloves whenever handling blood products.
   Some blood banks require a pickup slip that verifies the presence of a functioning IV catheter, signed informed consent, and a prescription, because blood must be discarded after it has been out of refrigeration for 30 minutes.

6. **Verify that the blood product** matches the prescription. Inspect the blood. If you note any of the following abnormalities, return the blood to the blood bank and obtain a new bag:
   a. Pink plasma indicates hemolysis.
   b. The red cells should be red, not purple or black.
   c. There should be no large clots visible.
   d. There should be no leakage.

7. **Verify the patient and blood** product identification with another qualified staff member (as deemed by your institution).
   Only one of the staff members is required by The Joint Commission to be qualified to administer blood products; however, agency policies may specify those requirements.
   a. Use two patient coidentifiers (e.g., ask the patient to tell you her full name and date of birth) and compare it with the name and date of birth located on the blood bank form and patient ID band.
      Allowing the patient to confirm her identity and comparing the information against the blood bank form is a safety measure to ensure that the correct patient is receiving the correct blood product.
   b. Compare the patient name and hospital identification number on the patient's identification bracelet with the patient name and hospital identification number on the blood bank form attached to the blood product.
      Verifies that the correct patient is receiving the correct blood product.
   c. Compare the unit identification number located on the blood bank form with the identification number printed on the blood product container.
      Verifies that the blood bank has dispensed the correct blood product.▼

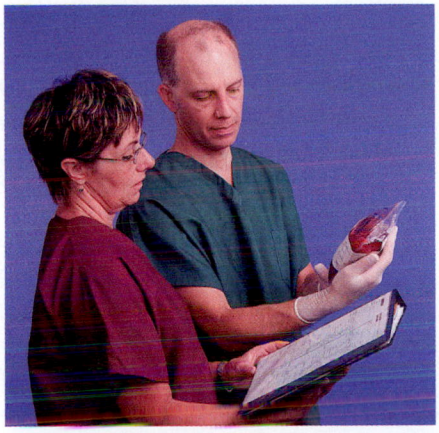

   d. Compare the patient's blood type listed on the blood bank form with the blood type listed on the blood product container.
      Verifies that the blood type of the product matches the patient's blood type.
   e. If all verifications are in agreement, both staff members should sign the blood bank form attached to the blood product container.

      ✚ Contact the blood bank immediately if any discrepancies occur during the identification process. If there are any discrepancies, do not administer the blood product.

      Signing the blood bank form confirms that the blood product was identified and verified by two qualified staff members.
   f. Document on the blood bank form the date and time that the transfusion was begun.
      Blood cannot be infused past the expiration time; documenting the start time alerts the nurse of the expiration time.
   g. Make sure that the blood bank form remains attached to the blood product container until administration is complete.
      Ensures product identity should a transfu sion reaction occur.

8. **Remove the blood** administration set from the package, and label the tubing with the date and time. Then, close all clamps on the administration set.
   Labeling the administration set with the date and time informs the nursing staff when the administration set should be changed.

9. **Remove the protective covers** from the normal saline solution container port and from one of the spikes located on the "Y" of the blood product administration set. Place the spike into the port of the solution container.

10. **Hang the normal saline solution** container on the IV pole.

11. **Compress the drip chamber** of the saline administration set, and allow it to fill halfway.
    Prevents air from entering the tubing with the solution.

12. **Open the roller clamp** and prime the administration set tubing with normal saline.
    Removes air from the tubing.

(continued on next page)

Procedure 38-8 ■ Administering a Blood Transfusion (continued)

13. **Close the roller clamp.** Inspect the tubing for air. If air bubbles are in the tubing, flick the tubing with a fingertip to mobilize the bubbles up into the drip chamber.
Air bubbles in the administration tubing can cause an air embolus.

14. **Gently invert the blood** product container several times, but do not shake the bag.
Mixes the blood product with the preservatives that are added to the container without causing trauma (lysis) to the cells.

15. **Remove the protective covers** from the blood spike on the blood tubing and the blood product port. Carefully spike the blood product container through the port.
Prevents inadvertent puncturing of the container.▼

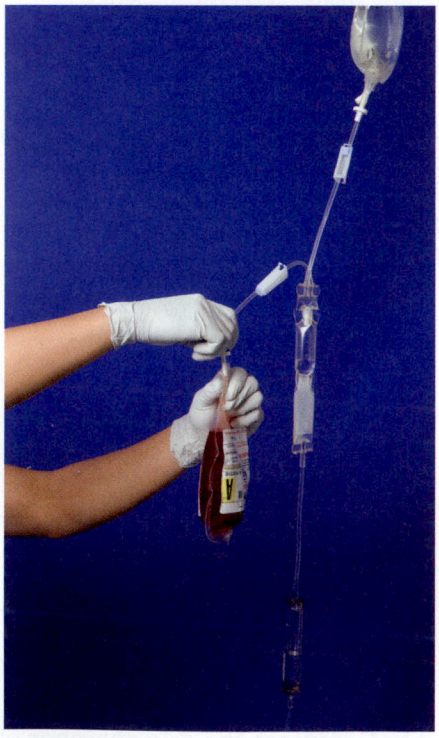

16. **Hang the blood product** bag on the IV pole, prime the short blood tubing by allowing the saline to backflow into the blood bag drip chamber. Then thread the line through the infusion pump.
Enables the blood to flow by gravity.

17. **Obtain and record** the patient's vital signs, including temperature, pulse, and blood pressure, before beginning the transfusion.
Establishes a baseline to help monitor for transfusion reactions.

18. **Using aseptic technique**, attach the distal end of the administration set to the IV catheter.
Prevents contamination of the IV catheter and administration set.

19. **Slowly open the roller clamp** closest to the blood product.
Allows the blood product to slowly fill that side of the "Y" of the administration set tubing.

20. **Set the infusion rate.** Start the rate slowly until 50 mL have infused; if there is no reaction, set it to prescribed rate.
A unit of blood cannot hang for more than 4 hours (some guidelines say 6 hours); otherwise, bacterial growth may occur.

For a Volume-Control Infusion Pump
Program the rate. Push "Start." Start the rate slowly until 50 mL have infused; if there is no reaction, set it to the prescribed rate.

For Gravity Flow
Using the roller clamp, adjust the drip rate. Keep in mind that blood administration sets have a drip factor of 10 gtts/mL.
Note: When using a 24-gauge needle, you will usually (but not always) use gravity infusion instead of a pump.
Forcing red blood cells through a smaller size catheter could result in some cell damage. Allowing the blood to flow by gravity allows time for the cells to change shape as they naturally do when flowing through small capillaries. However, only pumps that have been approved for blood transfusions should be used, because they prevent hemolysis (Galvey, Ibey, McConnell, et al., 2011).

21. **Remain with the patient** during the first 5 minutes, and then obtain vital signs.
Most severe blood transfusion reactions occur during the transfusion of the initial 50 mL of blood.

22. **Ensure that the patient's** call device is readily available, and have her alert you immediately of any signs or symptoms of a transfusion reaction, such as back pain, chills, itching, or shortness of breath.
If the patient alerts you immediately, you should be able to stop the transfusion in time to prevent serious complications.

23. **Obtain vital signs** again in 15 minutes (follow agency procedures), then again in 30 minutes, and then hourly while the transfusion infuses. Blood and blood product infusions must be completed within 4 to 6 hours.
Frequent monitoring alerts you to detect early signs of transfusion reaction or fluid overload.

24. **After the unit has infused,** close the roller clamp to the blood product container, and open the roller clamp to the normal saline solution to flush the administration set with normal saline solution.
Flushing the tubing with normal saline solution clears the tubing of any blood and avoids wasting any of the blood product.

25. **Close the roller clamp** to the normal saline, and then disconnect the blood administration set from the IV catheter, if an additional unit of blood has not been prescribed.

26. **If another unit of blood** is required, you may hang the second unit with the same administration set. However, administration sets and add-on filters need to be changed every 4 hours.
The same administration set can be used for two units of blood or per agency policy.

27. **Discard the empty blood** container and administration set in a biohazard receptacle, according to your institution's policy.
Promotes a safer healthcare environment.

? What if . . .

- **Two individuals are not available to verify that the blood and the patient are a match, and the blood must be hung now?**

In this instance, if it is available, an automated identification technology (e.g., bar coding) may be used.

Procedure 38-8B ■ Managing a Transfusion Reaction

➤ When performing the procedure, always identify your patient according to agency policy, using two identifiers, and be attentive to standard precautions, hand hygiene, patient safety and privacy, body mechanics, and documentation.

Procedure Steps

1. **If signs or symptoms of a transfusion reaction occur, stop the transfusion immediately. Do not flush the tubing.**
   Flushing the tubing causes the patient to receive the blood that remains in the tubing.

2. **Disconnect the administration set from the IV catheter. Call for help. Obtain vital signs, and auscultate heart and breath sounds.**
   Severe transfusion reactions may cause respiratory distress and shock; early recognition and treatment improve patient outcomes.

3. **Maintain patency of the IV catheter by hanging a new infusion of normal saline solution, using new tubing.**
   Maintaining a patent IV catheter with normal saline solution provides IV access in which emergency medication can be administered if necessary.

4. **Notify the primary provider as soon as you have stopped the blood, assessed the patient, and hung the new normal saline solution.**

5. **Place the administration set and blood product container, with the blood bank form attached, inside a biohazard bag. Send the bag to the blood bank immediately.**
   The remainder of the blood must be sent to the blood bank, where it can be analyzed to help determine the cause of the reaction.

6. **Obtain blood** (in the extremity opposite the transfusion site) and urine specimens according to your institution's policy.
   Blood banks typically require (1) a specimen for a type and crossmatch to compare with the pretransfusion type and crossmatch, (2) a specimen for free hemoglobin, and (3) a specimen for serum bilirubin level. A urine sample should also be sent to check for hemoglobinuria, a sign of acute hemolytic reactions.

7. **Continue to monitor vital signs frequently, at least every 15 minutes.**
   To quickly detect worsening of the patient's condition.

8. **Administer medications**, as prescribed.
   Medications will vary depending on the type of transfusion reaction.

? What if . . .

- **At Step 3, you do not have a new bag of normal saline to hang?**
  Clamp the normal saline line until you can obtain a new bag of normal saline, then disconnect the old normal saline. Do this as quickly as possible.
  Preserves the patency of the IV catheter.

Evaluation

- Evaluate the patient's response to the blood transfusion by checking for changes in blood pressure and oxygenation, improvement in color, or for signs of fluid overload.
- Monitor for signs and symptoms of transfusion reaction.
- Assess the IV insertion site for signs of infiltration, phlebitis, infection, or inflammation.
- Monitor laboratory studies, such as complete blood count, to help evaluate the effectiveness of therapy and/or transfusion reaction.

Patient Teaching

- Explain the signs and symptoms of transfusion reactions, and tell the client and family to notify staff immediately should they occur.
- Warn the client or family to notify staff immediately if tenderness, redness, or swelling occurs at the IV catheter insertion site.
- Explain the importance of notifying staff immediately if the administration set becomes disconnected from the IV catheter or the IV catheter becomes dislodged.

Documentation

- Chart the date, time, and reason the transfusion was started.
- Document transfusion vital signs according to institution policy (many institutions have a special form for transfusion vital signs).
- Record the amount of blood transfused on the I&O record.
- Chart any complications and the interventions taken.

Sample documentation

Mm/dd/yyyy 0600 1 unit (250 mL) PRBCs was hung at 0300 and infused through 20-gauge catheter in LA, for Hbg 8.3 mg/dL. Pretransfusion vital signs: T 98.9°F, BP 100/68 mm Hg, HR 114 beats/min, and RR, 22 breaths/min. See frequent vital sign sheet for other transfusion vital signs. Breath sounds remained clear throughout the transfusion. No evidence of reaction. Post-transfusion lab due at 1200. ——— L. Gilmore, RN

Practice Resources

American Association of Blood Banks (AABB) (n.d.); Agency for Healthcare Research and Quality (AHRQ)(2011); INS (2011a); The Joint Commission (2011); Kessler, C. (2013); Tolich, D., Blackmur, S., Stahorsky, K., et al. (2013).

(continued on next page)

Procedure 38-8 ■ Administering a Blood Transfusion (continued)

Thinking About the Procedure

To practice applying clinical reasoning to this procedure,

Go to *Davis's Nursing Skills Videos*, **Administering Blood and Blood Products.**

For questions and suggested responses,

Go to Chapter 38, **Thinking About the Procedure Questions** and **Suggested Responses** on Davis*Plus*.

Procedure 38-9 ■ Assisting With Percutaneous Central Venous Catheter Placement

➤ For steps to follow in *all* procedures, refer to the Universal Steps for All Procedures found on the inside back cover.

Equipment

- Sterile gloves (two or three pairs)
- Masks, hats, barrier gowns
- 10-mL vials of normal saline (three or four)
- Syringes with 1-in. needle (two or three)
- 25-gauge ⅝-in. and 18-gauge 1½-in. needles (two or three of each)
- Central venous catheter (CVC) kit containing: an introducer, antiseptic solution/swabs, sterile drapes, 10-mL syringe, 1% or 2% Xylocaine without epinephrine, suture, sterile scissors and needle holder, CVC kit (single- or multilumen)
- Injection caps
- Alcohol wipes

Delegation

Do not delegate this procedure because complex assessment and support skills are needed. The nurse must be alert to changes in the patient's condition and signs of developing complications. CVC placement at the bedside is associated with pneumothorax, hemothorax, cardiac tamponade, and air emboli.

Pre-Procedure Assessments

- Obtain baseline vital signs.
- Verify that informed consent has been given.
- Assess for allergy to tape.

➤ When performing the procedure, always identify your patient according to agency policy, using two identifiers, and be attentive to standard precautions, hand hygiene, patient safety and privacy, body mechanics, and documentation.

Procedure Steps

1. **Explain the procedure** to the patient.
   To relieve anxiety and increase the patient's ability to cooperate with the procedure.
2. **Verify informed consent** and obtain vital signs.
3. **Gather supplies and perform** meticulous hand hygiene.
   Promotes efficiency; removes contaminants to help prevent infection.
4. **Set up the sterile field** and add supplies. Position the table so it is easily accessible by the physician or advanced practice nurse (APN) during the procedure.
   Promotes efficiency and makes the procedure faster and therefore less burdensome for the patient.
5. **Position the patient** to facilitate the procedure, usually in the Trendelenburg position with a rolled towel between the shoulders.
   To prevent air embolism and dilate neck veins.
6. **Offer mask, gown, and sterile gloves** (and possibly hat, depending on agency policy) to the physician or APN after she performs hand hygiene.
   Maximum barrier precautions are required for central line placement.
7. **Don mask and then sterile gloves.**
   To prevent contamination of sterile areas and of the insertion site as you cleanse it. Don mask first to keep gloves sterile.
8. **Prep the marked site** with 2% chlorhexidine gluconate in 70% alcohol applicators, using a friction scrub.
   a. Use a back-and-forth motion to scrub an area at least 20 to 25 cm (8 to 10 in.) in diameter. Do not go back over an area with the same applicator.
   b. Repeat with three applicators. Total scrub should take at least 30 seconds (2 minutes for a moist site such as the femoral vein).
   c. Allow site to air-dry completely (about 2 minutes). Never wipe or blot dry.
   Insertion kits and agency policies may vary. Follow agency policy. If it does not conform to evidence-based guidelines, work for policy change.
9. **Drape the insertion site** with a large sterile drape, exposing only the prepared skin area. Use other large drapes to cover the patient from head to toe. If your agency does not have a policy that the patient wear a mask, have the patient turn his head in the opposite direction of insertion site.
   Creates a sterile field and decreases the chance of contamination by the patient's exhalations. Turning the head to the opposite side also helps to make it easier to advance the catheter when it passes through the subclavian site.

10. **Observe while the physician** or APN performs the following steps:
    a. Anesthetizes the area with lidocaine.
    b. Primes the central venous catheter with saline.
    c. Performs venipuncture with the insertion needle (in the internal jugular or subclavian site). The femoral site may be used in emergencies, but it is associated with a higher rate of complications than other sites.
    d. Attaches a syringe to the needle and aspirates for blood.
    To ensure the needle is in the vein.
    e. After obtaining blood return, removes syringe from the needle and inserts a guidewire through the needle.
    The guidewire guides the flexible catheter into the vein.
    f. Aspirates all air out of the catheter lumens and then flushes them with normal saline.
    To reduce the risk of air embolism.
    g. Places injection caps on each lumen.
    To prevent blood loss and maintain sterility of the lumens
    h. Sutures the catheter in place.
    To minimize movement and prevent catheter migration (in or out).

11. **Apply sterile transparent dressing** over the site after the physician or APN is finished.
    Minimizes contamination of the site. The most common route of infection is via migration of skin organisms at the insertion site into the cutaneous catheter tract with colonization of the catheter tip. Transparent dressing allows for observation of the site without removing the dressing and manipulating the catheter.

12. **If there are clamps** on the lumens, close them.

13. **Place tape over the lumens** near the ends, but not on the injection caps.
    To minimize movement of the catheter that increases the risk of dislodgement.

14. **Remove sterile drape** and assist the patient to a comfortable position.

15. **Dispose of used supplies** and equipment in the appropriate receptacles according to agency policy in line with CDC guidelines.

16. **Remove and dispose of mask** and gloves. Perform hand hygiene.
    Observes standard precaution guidelines.

Guidelines

- The patient and all staff in the room should wear a mask.
- A health professional who has received appropriate education (e.g., a nurse) should observe the CVC insertion to ensure that aseptic technique is maintained.
- This person should stop the procedure if aseptic technique errors are made.
- A central line checklist should be used during the procedure. You may be responsible for auditing the procedure and completing the checklist.

? What if . . .

- **In Step 9, a large sterile drape is not available?**

  Use two small drapes to cover the patient from head to toe.
  Evidence-based guidelines advise maximal barrier precautions for insertion of CVCs.

Evaluation

- Obtain vital signs.
- Auscultate the lungs and assess for respiratory distress, sharp chest pain, and coughing. Monitor for 24 hours for these signs.
  To detect pneumothorax or cardiac tamponade.
- Obtain a chest x-ray.
  To verify correct location of catheter tip in the distal third of the superior vena cava, as well as absence of thorax and cardiac puncture.
- Assess the patient daily to determine continuing need for the CVC.
  Risk of infection is closely related to the length of time the CVC is in place.
- For further evaluation and follow-up, refer to Clinical Insight 38-4: Caring for Patients With a Central Venous Access Device (CVAD): CVC and PICC, and Procedure 38-5B: Central Line Dressings.

Documentation

- Date and time of catheter insertion
- Catheter type and size
- Site location
- Assessments and interventions performed at insertion and immediately after
- Patient's tolerance of procedure (subjective and objective data)
- X-ray verification of catheter placement

Practice Resources

CDC (2011); Dumont, C., & Nesselrodt, D. (2012); INH (2011); Institute for Healthcare Improvement (IHI, 2012); Pronovost, P., Goeschel, C., Colantuoni, E., et al. (2010); Rhoads, J., & Meeker, B. (2008).

CLINICAL INSIGHTS

Clinical Insight 38-1 ➤ Assessing for Trousseau's and Chvostek's Signs

Positive Trousseau's and Chvostek's signs are signs of hypocalcemia. To check for these signs, follow these instructions.

Trousseau's Sign

Inflate a blood pressure cuff above systolic pressure. Flexion of the wrist and hand constitutes a positive sign.

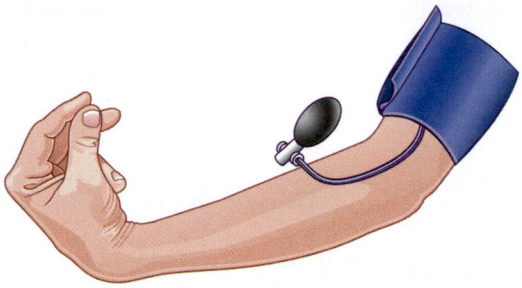

Chvostek's Sign

Tap the face in front of the ear and below the zygomatic bone (cheek bone). Facial twitching constitutes a positive sign.

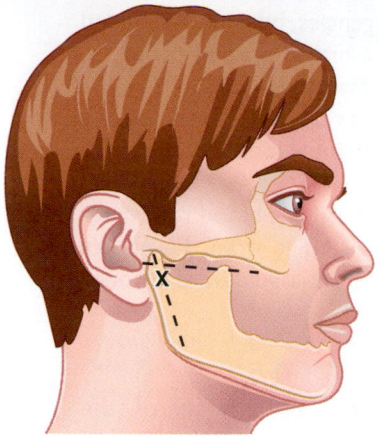

Clinical Insight 38-2 ➤ Guidelines for Measuring Intake and Output (I&O)

General Guidelines

Assessing

- Identify factors that can affect the patient's fluid intake or output (e.g., surgery, medical condition, or medications such as diuretics).
- Enlist the patient's help in keeping track of I&O if she is able.
- If you delegate the task of recording intake and output:
  - Be sure the assistive person understands its importance and knows how to perform the procedure correctly.
  - Be certain to evaluate the totals and the fluid sources. A patient or NAP can collect the data, but an RN must make the assessments.
- For accuracy, use a graduated container and hold it at eye level when measuring fluids.

Recording

- You will usually record measurements on a bedside I&O form and transfer the 8-hr total to a graphic sheet or the 24-hr I&O on the patient's record. You may sometimes need hourly measurements.
- Document your findings in milliliters (mL). Describe any fluid restrictions and the patient's compliance with them.

Measuring Intake

It is most accurate to premeasure fluids before they are consumed. However, if that is not possible, you can use the following estimates:

Equivalents

1 oz = 30 mL
1 teaspoon = 5 mL
1 tablespoon = 15 mL
1 home measuring cup of fluid = 8 oz (240 mL)
1 pint of fluid = 16 oz (480 mL)
1 quart of fluid = 32 oz (960 mL)

Various Containers

Record ice chips as fluid at half their volume (1 cup ice = ½ cup fluid)
Bowl (soup) = 180 mL
Creamer (small) = 30 mL
Custard cup = 100 mL
Drinking cup = 180 mL
Coffee mug = 240 mL
Gelatin cup = 100 mL
Ice cream serving = 120 mL
Juice glass = 120 mL
Paper cup, large = 200 mL

Clinical Insight 38-2 ➤ Guidelines for Measuring Intake and Output (I&O)—cont'd

Paper cup, small = 120 mL
Water glass = 200 mL
Water pitcher = 1,000 mL

Examples of fast-food drinks:
Child-size drink = 12 oz
Small drink = 16 oz
Medium drink = 21 oz
Large drink = 32 oz

Assessing

- Fluid intake includes the following:
  - Oral fluids, including the liquid in prepared foods
  - Soups
  - Everything that melts into liquid at room temperature (e.g., gelatin, custard, ice cream, and ice)
  - Liquid medications and fluids used to take tablets or capsules
  - IV fluids
  - Enteral or parenteral nutrition fluids
  - Instillations into the GI tract
  - Bladder irrigations
- Measure oral fluids according to agency policy.
- For increased accuracy, use a graduated cup to measure and record fluid amounts before the patient consumes them. Subtract from the total any fluid that the patient throws away or saves for future consumption.
- Wash the measuring cup after each use, except after measuring water.
- Measure and teach the patient to measure and record the amount of fluid he drinks with each meal, with medicine, and between meals.
- In the home, cups come in many different sizes, so do the following:
  - Use a measuring cup to measure how much the drinking cups and glasses hold.
  - Always use the same drinking cup or glass.
  - Explain that the labels on cans and bottles will help to determine precise fluid amounts.

Recording

- At least every 8 hours, record the type and amount of all fluids the patient has received and indicate the route (oral, parenteral, rectal, or enteric tube).
- Record all forms of intake except blood and blood products.

Measuring Output

Assessing

- Refer to Procedure 28-1 to review how to measure urine.

Fluid output includes everything that leaves the body in fluid form: urine, watery stool, vomitus, wound drainage, surgical drains, NG tubes, chest tubes, and any fluid aspirated from a body cavity.

- Use a calibrated container to measure fluids. Observe it at eye level and take the reading at the bottom of the fluid meniscus.
- Use a different graduated container for each patient; clean after use.
- Teach the patient to keep toilet paper out of the urine for accurate measurement.
- If irrigating an NG tube or the bladder, measure the amount instilled and subtract it from total output.
- You will need to empty wound drains or other devices to measure this volume.
- If a wound is draining, but the fluid is not collected in a drainage device, you may measure the amount of fluid lost by weighing dressings before and after they are applied. If measuring the exact volume is not crucial, you may evaluate the degree of saturation of the dressing.

Recording

- Record the type, route, and amount of all fluids the patient loses.
- Insensible fluid losses can't be easily quantified. However, unusual losses (e.g., saturated dressing, excessive perspiration, rapid breathing patterns, and large burn areas) should be objectively described in narrative charting.

Tips for Analyzing I&O

- Measure and record all intake and output.
- Determine if output is more or less than intake.
- Evaluate trends over for a period of 24 to 48 hours.
- To identify problems, when evaluating total urine output, ask how many times the patient voided. For example, was a total of 300 mL obtained from 2 voids, or from 10 voids of 30 mL each?
- Evaluate patterns and values outside the normal range (e.g., frequent voiding, infrequent voiding), keeping in mind the normal range for 24-hour intake and output.
- The amount of output is important, but consider color, color changes, and odor.
- Analyze intake and output holistically. Take into account the patient's usual pattern and amounts, age, medical problem, and type of surgical procedure.
- You must correlate I&O with daily weights to accurately determine overall fluid status (Collins & Claros, 2011; Crawford & Harris, 2012b).

Clinical Insight 38-3 ➤ Guidelines for Selecting a Peripheral Venipuncture Site

- As a general rule, select the most distal vein on an upper extremity.
- If available, use visualization technologies, such as portable ultrasound or imaging devices.
  This minimizes the number of needlesticks the patient must undergo.
- For adults, you will usually use veins in the hand or arm; for infants, veins in the scalp or dorsum of the foot can also be used.
- If possible, select a vein on the patient's nondominant hand or arm.
  Helps to preserve functional ability.
- Look for a vein that has a firm, round appearance with a relatively straight pathway. Do not use a red, hot, or hard vein.
- Avoid veins that are highly visible; they tend to roll.
- The cephalic vein of the arm is one of the best veins to use because it is relatively large, and the forearm provides a natural splint
- The dorsal veins of the hand are easy to access and are splinted by the metacarpals, but these veins are often quite small and fragile.

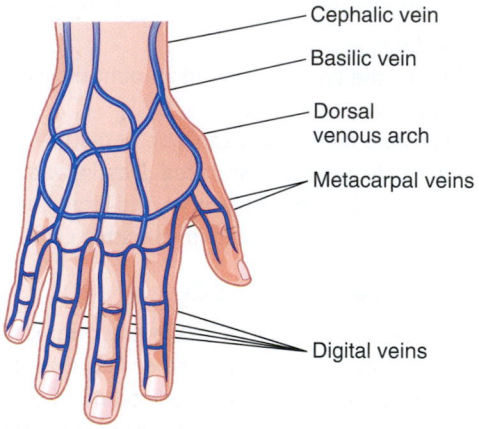

A Superficial veins of the hand

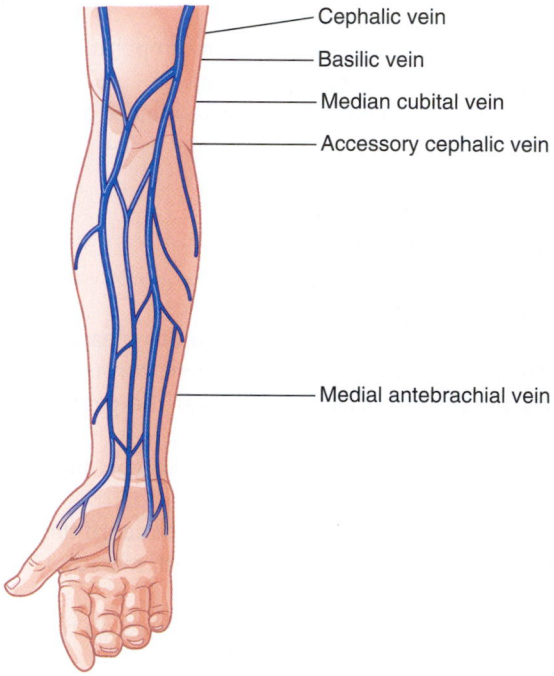

B Superficial veins of the forearm

- Avoid the antecubital veins if possible. If the patient flexes her arm, the IV catheter may become displaced, so you would probably need to splint her elbow to prevent that. Furthermore, if a PICC line is needed at a later time, you will still have the antecubital veins available for it.
- For these situations, you need to use the largest vein available, keeping other selection criteria in mind:
  - Hypertonic solutions, viscous solutions, or irritating medications
  - Rapid rates (also require a larger IV catheter)
- If the infusion is to be ongoing, begin the infusion with the best lowest vein and move proximal to the previous site (toward the heart) for subsequent insertions. Peripheral IV catheters are routinely changed at 96-hour intervals, but at least every 7 days. If you start the next IV below an already used site (i.e., to change the site or after a failed attempt at insertion), fluid may leak from the old site.
- Avoid areas at which the vein crosses over joints. If you must use such an area, splint the joint to limit movement.
  Splinting the joint helps preserve the vein for use, but it limits functional ability.
- Avoid areas with scarring, or with impaired circulation or neurological status (e.g., the affected arm following a mastectomy; an area with signs of infection, previous infiltration, or thrombosis; an arm with an arteriovenous fistula [shunt for dialysis]; or the affected side after cerebrovascular accident [stroke]). If you must use such an area, first obtain a medical prescription.
- Do not use veins in the legs and feet unless there is no other option.
  Peripheral circulation may not be adequate in the lower limbs, so there is increased danger of thrombus formation. In adults this location also interferes with mobility. Foot veins may be used for infants if the IV is taped securely.

Clinical Insight 38-4 ➤ Caring for Patients With a Central Venous Access Device (CVAD): CVC and PICC

Asepsis

- Use good hand hygiene and follow agency protocols for site care.
  To protect yourself and the patient.
- Use strict aseptic technique when manipulating injection ports, catheter hub and extension legs, needleless connectors, insertion site, and dressing. This includes sterile gloves and supplies, mask, and in some agencies a mask for the patient.
  To minimize line contamination and infection.
- Scrub injection ports, extension legs, and catheter hubs vigorously for at least 15 seconds, preferably with 70% alcohol or 2% chlorhexidine preparation, before accessing them.
- Appropriate antiseptics include alcohol and chlorhexidine gluconate (CHG). Do not use povidone-iodine and tincture of iodine to scrub ports unless there is some reason alcohol or CHG-alcohol combination products can't be used.
- Do not apply organic solvents, such as acetone or acetone-based products, to the skin before insertion of a catheter or during dressing changes.

Assessments

- Check the patient record for radiographic confirmation of correct tip location before beginning prescribed therapies.
- Inspect catheter–skin junction sites through the transparent dressing and palpate for tenderness daily. Do not remove transparent dressing except when dressing change is required. If site is dressed with gauze, you must remove it to inspect the site. Transparent dressings are preferred.
  A high-risk route of infection is via migration of skin organisms at the insertion site into the cutaneous catheter tract, with colonization of the catheter tip.
- Observe for excessive bleeding at the insertion site.
  You may need to obtain a prescription for a topical hemostatic agent and use with a pressure dressing.
- If symptoms of infection occur (e.g., fever without obvious cause; redness, edema, induration, exudates, or tenderness at the site), remove the dressing and inspect the site directly. Anticipate that blood cultures will be needed from both the peripheral site and the central catheter.
- Be aware that risk of infection is higher with femoral catheters and with multilumen catheters.
  Multilumen catheters require more manipulation, which encourages more colonization and bacterial growth within the catheter lumen.
- Assess for compromised catheter integrity (wet dressing; kinked, cracked, or leaking external catheter).
- Inspect catheter connections and pump function, including flow rate.
- Observe for symptoms of catheter migration to the right atrium or ventricle (i.e., mid- to lower sternal pain, dysrhythmias).
- If there are signs of complications, notify the medical provider.
- Assess the patient daily for indications that the CVC or PICC line is still needed.
  CVCs or PICC line should be removed as soon as possible because the infection rate is closely related to the length of time the catheter is in place.

Maintenance Interventions

- The site should be covered with a semipermeable transparent dressing, the catheter secured with a sterile commercially manufactured stabilizer (instead of tape), and the lumens anchored near the ports with clear tape.
- Keep dressings dry, intact, and air occlusive. Protocols generally require a dressing change every 5 to 7 days unless the integrity of the dressing is compromised (e.g., it is damp, loosened, or soiled) or if the site must be examined (e.g., because of pain or odor). A dressing change every 2 days is required if you must use gauze and tape dressings.
- Perform site care with each dressing change. Cleanse the catheter–skin junction with an appropriate antiseptic solution (e.g., 70% alcohol and CHG), apply a sterile stabilizer, and apply a new sterile dressing.
- Manipulate the catheter hub as little as possible.
  To minimize catheter movement, phlebitis, and contamination of the line. Less catheter manipulation is associated with fewer bloodstream infections.
- Flush catheters before and after any infusions or per agency protocol. This may be every 12 to 24 hours when not in use.
  - Flush volume should be twice the volume of the catheter and add-on devices (consult package label).
  - Use a syringe size recommended by the catheter manufacturer (10 mL is the smallest size recommended because of the pressure generated).
  - Type of flush solution depends on agency policy (saline versus heparin).
  - Use single-use, labeled syringes of flush solution to prevent cross-contamination.
  - If you have trouble flushing, the catheter may be kinked or malpositioned, the inline filter may be clogged, or a clamp may need to be released. You can correct these problems.
- Never flush against resistance.
  The catheter might be clogged and you would risk dislodging a small clot. This could also rupture the catheter.
- If the patient has a PICC line, take blood pressures on the alternate arm.
  Using the arm with the PICC can cause bleeding at the site, thrombus formation, retrograde blood flow, and increased risk of catheter occlusion.

Clinical Insight 38-4 ➤ Caring for Patients With a Central Venous Access Device (CVAD): CVC and PICC—cont'd

- If the patient is receiving parenteral nutrition, reserve and label one lumen just for that purpose.

Documentation

- Document routine assessments and the condition of the catheter–skin junction site. When site care is given, also document the patient's response and any actions taken to correct or prevent adverse reactions.

Related Information

For information about dressing changes, refer to Procedure 38-5B: Central Line Dressings. For information about administering medications through a CVAD, see Procedure 26-18: Administering Medication Through a Central Venous Access Device.

References

Infusion Nurses Society (INS). (2011a). Infusion nursing standards of practice. *Journal of Infusion Nursing, 34*(1S): S1–S84; Institute for Healthcare Improvement (IHI). (2012). How-to guide: Prevent central line-associated bloodstream infection. Retrieved from http://www.ihi.org/knowledge/Pages/Tools/HowtoGuidePreventCentralLineAssociatedBloodstreamInfection.aspx

Clinical Insight 38-5 ➤ Managing Infiltration and Extravasation

- At the first sign or symptom of infiltration or extravasation, stop the IV. Symptoms include slowed or stopped flow, swelling, tenderness, pallor, hardness, and coolness at the site.
- The patient may report a burning sensation in the area.

For a Central Venous Access Device: CVC OR PICC:

- Clamp and cap the catheter hub.
- Do not remove the catheter.
- Follow agency policy when you suspect infiltration or extravasation.
- If the patient has an implanted port, aspirate, remove the port access needle, and apply a dressing.
- Notify the provider who inserted the catheter, who may order an x-ray to help determine the cause of the problem.

For a Short Peripheral Catheter:

- Disconnect the tubing from the catheter hub; attach a 3- to 5-mL syringe and try to aspirate fluid from the catheter lumen. Use aseptic technique.
- Photograph the site to create a record of its condition, if agency policy allows.
- Wearing gloves, remove the catheter and hold a dry gauze pad over the site to stop the bleeding. Apply a dry dressing. Do not apply excessive pressure to the site.
- If you are to start a new IV, start it on the other arm, if possible. If it is not possible, start it in a more proximal location on the same arm.
- Measure the circumference of the arm and compare it with the opposite arm.
- Assess capillary refill, sensation, and motion distal to the infiltrated site.
- Apply cold or warm compresses depending on which fluid has escaped into the tissues.
  - For alkaloids (e.g., vincristine) and epipodophyllotoxins (e.g., etoposide), use heat.
  - For hypertonic fluids or medications, use cold.
  - For isotonic or hypotonic fluids or medications, choose either heat or cold, or alternate them, based on patient comfort.
- Apply compresses for 15 to 30 minutes every 4 to 6 hours; continue for 24 to 48 hours.
- Estimate the volume of fluid that escaped into the tissues; notify the prescriber.
- Some medications leaked into the surrounding tissue can cause damage and even necrosis. For instance, when dopamine extravasates, you might need to give a prescribed amount of antidote (e.g., regitine injected subcutaneously) as well as hydrocortisone and an anti-inflammatory to minimize tissue damage. Be sure to check the protocol at your facility.
- Elevate the extremity and advise the patient to rest.
- Document all fluids and medications involved, equipment being used (e.g., pump), size and type of the catheter, description of the site (including location, size, and color), methods used to assess the site before administering the fluids (e.g., aspiration), patient's signs and symptoms, interventions, notifications, and patient teaching.
- Complete an occurrence (or incident) report, as required by your facility.

References

Gahart, B. & Nazareno, A. (2013). *2013 Intravenous Medications, A Handbook for Nurses and Health Professionals* (29th ed). St. Louis: Elsevier-Mosby; Masoorli, S. (2012). Avoiding the pitfalls of IV therapy. Retrieved on September 11, 2013 from, http://ce.nurse.com/RetailCourseView.aspx?CourseNum=ce94-60&page=3&IsA=1.

ASSESSMENT GUIDELINES AND TOOLS

The following questions and guidelines will help you obtain subjective and objective data about patients' fluid, electrolyte, and acid–base balance.

Focused Assessment

Assessing Fluids, Electrolytes, and Acid–Base Balance

Nursing History

Demographic Data

Age, gender, height, weight, body mass index (BMI)

Past Medical History

- Have you ever been hospitalized or had surgery? If so, when and for what reason?
- What healthcare problems are you currently being treated for?
- Have you ever been diagnosed with kidney disease, high blood pressure, diabetes, or thyroid or parathyroid problems?

Current Health Concerns

- What symptoms are you currently experiencing?
- Have you recently experienced any of the following symptoms?

Excessive thirst	Difficulty breathing
Fever	Swelling of your hands, feet, or ankles
Excessive perspiration	Dizziness or feeling faint
Nausea, vomiting, or diarrhea	Muscle weakness
Dry skin or mucous membranes	Excessive fatigue
Dark, concentrated urine	Numbness, tingling, or cramping sensations
Limited amounts of urine	

- Is your weight stable? Have you had any recent changes in your weight?
- Do you believe you have any problems with fluid loss?

Food and Fluid Intake

- How much fluid do you usually drink in a 24-hour period?
- Do you believe you drink adequate amounts of fluid?
- Describe your usual diet.
- Have you recently changed your diet or fluid intake?
- Are you following a special diet?
- Have you ever been placed on a restricted diet?
- Have you experienced any recent changes in your appetite or thirst?
- Do you salt your food?
- Do you ever use salt substitute?

Fluid Elimination

- How often do you urinate in a 24-hour period? Has that changed recently?
- How often do you get up during the night to urinate?
- Have you noticed any recent changes in the amount or appearance of your urine?
- How often do you experience vomiting, diarrhea, or constipation? Describe your experience.
- Do you have any wounds? If so, where are they, and how did they happen? What is the color of drainage and how much drainage are you experiencing?
- Do you have any breaks in your skin? If so, describe the problem, and show me the area.

Medications

- What prescribed medications do you currently take?
- What over-the-counter medications or alternative treatments do you use? What do you use them for?
- How often do you take laxatives or antacids?
- What vitamins, herbals, or supplements do you take?

Lifestyle

- What is your usual activity level?
- What type of exercise do you engage in? How often?
- How much fluid do you consume before, during, and after exercise?
- Do you drink alcohol? If so, how much do you consume in a day, a week?
- Do you smoke? If so, how much? For how long?
- Do you use any illegal medications or drugs?

Physical Assessments

Skin

Assess the skin for the following:.

- ***Color and temperature*** may be cues to the presence of fever and circulation status.
- ***Moisture content*** offers some indication of fluid status. A diaphoretic client is losing fluid at a faster rate than a client with dry skin. Dry, scaling skin may indicate a fluid deficit. Any breaks in the skin are potential areas for fluid loss.
- ***Turgor*** varies with age, weight, and skin condition but does offer information on fluid status. Pinch the skin over the sternum. Normally skin immediately returns to its usual position. In fluid volume deficit or malnutrition the skin may remain "tented" for a period of time before returning to its original position. You must, however, correlate skin turgor with context and other clinical signs. For example, the skin loses elasticity with aging, so clients older than age 65 often have decreased turgor, which is normal for them.

Focused Assessment

Assessing Fluids, Electrolytes, and Acid–Base Balance—cont'd

- ***Edema*** in dependent areas is a cue for fluid volume excess. In an ambulatory client, assess the lower extremities and hands. In a bedridden client, edema will shift as the client is turned.
- ***To grade edema*** (on a scale +1 to +4, +1 represents minimal edema and +4 represents the most severe edema),

Go to Chapter 22, **Table 22-3: Assessing Edema,** in Volume 1.

Mucous Membranes

- Inspect the tongue and buccal mucosa. Mouth breathing alone usually does not change these areas.
- Dry, cracked, or dull mucous membranes are signs of fluid volume deficit.

Cardiovascular System

- ***Assess vital signs*** (see later section).
- If you suspect fluid volume deficit, ***assess for orthostatic hypotension:***
  - Assess blood pressure while client is lying or sitting.
  - Have the client rise to a seated or standing position, and reassess the blood pressure (BP).
  - A drop in systolic BP of >15 mm Hg is a sign of orthostatic hypotension.
- ***Check capillary refill.*** Delayed capillary refill is a sign of fluid volume deficit; rapid capillary refill indicates adequate circulation and volume. If capillary refill is delayed, evaluate feet and hands bilaterally. Delays in just one area indicate impaired circulation to the extremity rather than volume changes.
- ***Assess venous filling*** by observing the jugular and hand veins. Flat jugular or hand veins indicate low fluid volume. Distended vessels are a sign of overload.

Respiratory System

- ***Assess respiratory rate, depth, and pattern.*** The respiratory system rapidly responds to changes in pH. Similarly, alterations in gas exchange at the alveolar–capillary membrane may trigger pH changes.
- ***Assess breath sounds.*** Crackles or moist rales may indicate fluid overload. Areas of consolidation indicate impaired gas exchange.

Neurological System

- Assess level of consciousness and orientation.
- Assess neuromuscular irritability.
- Assess energy level and fatigue.
- Assess reflexes.

For specific neurological cues to alterations in fluid, electrolyte, or acid–base balance,

Go to Chapter 38, **Table 38-5: Electrolyte Imbalances,** and **Table 38-7: Acid–Base Imbalances,** in Volume 1.

Vital Signs

- ***Temperature.*** An elevated body temperature increases the loss of body fluids.
- In hypernatremia, body temperature elevates because less fluid is available for sweating.
- In uncomplicated fluid volume deficit, body temperature decreases.
- ***Pulse:***
  - Tachycardia is an early sign of fluid volume deficit.
  - Pulse rate is affected by fluid status and some electrolytes (primarily sodium, potassium, calcium, and magnesium).
  - Dysrhythmias are seen with potassium and magnesium imbalances.
- The pulse volume is directly affected by fluid status. As fluid volume increases, the pulse volume also increases. Similarly, a drop in fluid volume leads to a drop in pulse volume.
- ***Respiratory rate.*** Alterations in respiratory rate may cause acid–base imbalances or be associated with compensation for a metabolic disorder.
- ***Blood pressure:***
  - Blood pressure rises and falls with fluid volume.
  - Blood pressure is elevated by hypernatremia and fluid volume excess.
  - Respiratory acidosis causes increased heart rate, resulting in BP elevation.
  - High potassium intake may lower blood pressure.

Daily Weights

- Use the same balanced scale each day to monitor fluid status accurately.
- Weigh the client at the same time of day, making sure that the client is wearing the same amount of clothing.
- For clients undergoing hemodialysis (blood cleansing through an artificial kidney), weigh the client before and after dialysis treatments.
- You may institute weight monitoring as an independent nursing order.

Fluid Intake and Output

See Clinical Insight 38-2.

DIAGNOSTIC TESTING

Diagnostic Testing

Assessing Fluid, Electrolyte, and Acid–Base Balance

Venous Blood Sample	Normal Ranges
Sodium	135–145 mEq/L
Potassium	3.5–5.0 mEq/L
Chloride	97–107 mEq/L
Bicarbonate	22–26 mEq/L
BUN	10–31 mg/dL
Creatinine	0.5–1.2 mg/dL
Serum osmolality	275–295 mOsm/kg
Urine osmolality	250–900 mOsm/kg
Hematocrit	43%–49% in men
	38%–44% in menstruating women
Freshly Voided Urine Sample	
pH	5.0–9.0
Specific gravity	1.001–1.029
Arterial Blood Sample	
pH	7.35–7.45
P_{CO_2}	35–45 mm Hg
HCO_3^-	22–26 mEq/L

CLINICALREASONING

Applying the Full-Spectrum Nursing Model

PATIENT SITUATION

Darlene Malone, age 42, has been admitted to the emergency department with complaints of fatigue, extreme weakness, and heart palpitations. She says she has not seen a healthcare provider in nearly 10 years. Suddenly, she slumps and falls over. She is not breathing, has no pulse, and does not respond to verbal stimuli. She is resuscitated with CPR and IV epinephrine, and an endotracheal tube is placed. STAT lab results show a potassium level of 7.7 mEq/L, BUN of 102 mg/dL, and creatinine of 5 mg/dL. A physician diagnoses acute renal failure. Among other interventions, an IV is started to administer 10% calcium chloride solution, 1,000 mg, by slow IV push to counteract the toxic effects of hyperkalemia on the cell membranes. The nurse used a 20-gauge over-the-needle catheter in Ms. Malone's right cephalic vein, about 5 cm (2 in.) above her wrist.

THINKING

1. *Theoretical Knowledge:*
   a. Which lab results are abnormal? Are they high or low?
   b. Which lab results directly reflect her renal failure?
   c. What term correctly describes serum potassium of 7.7 mEq/L?
2. *Critical Thinking (Considering Alternatives):*
   a. What do you think is causing Ms. Malone to have hyperkalemia? You should be able to think this through and make a reasonable guess even if you have not studied pathophysiology.
   b. Ms. Malone is to be given 50 mEq of sodium bicarbonate by slow IV push for an acid–base imbalance that is often associated with hyperkalemia. Which imbalance do you think would be treated with sodium bicarbonate: metabolic acidosis or metabolic alkalosis?

DOING

3. *Practical Knowledge:*
   a. When you prepare to administer the sodium bicarbonate (in question 2b), you notice that the IV infusion is barely flowing and that the insertion site is swollen and pale. What is the first thing you should do?
   b. You aspirate the catheter and do not obtain a blood return. Ms. Malone absolutely must have this medication. Describe what you would do in the order you would do it.
4. *Nursing Process (Planning Goals):* The NOC outcome best suited to evaluating Ms. Malone's hyperkalemia is Electrolyte & Acid–Base Imbalance. Based on the function of this electrolyte, what is the primary indicator that you could use to evaluate her goal achievement for this problem?

CARING

5. *Self-Knowledge:* Ms. Malone will need dialysis to replace her inadequate renal function and control her serum potassium level. It is likely that her renal failure was brought on by years of illegal drug abuse. She has never held a full-time job and has not worked at all for the past 7 years. Her dialysis treatments will need to be paid for by Medicaid, which is funded by tax dollars. How do you feel about this—specifically, how do you feel about the issues of (a) a person's responsibility for her own health and (b) compassion for people who cannot afford to pay for healthcare? Focus on your own feelings, not on issues of what "should" be done.

Critical Thinking and Clinical Reasoning

1. Recall the Meet Your Patients scenario in Volume 1. When you review Jackson LaGuardia's chart to prepare for the clinical day, you find that he is in the emergency department (ED) with four other members of the LaGuardia family. All of them have come to the ED complaining of nausea, vomiting, and diarrhea related to severe gastroenteritis, a viral intestinal disorder. The family members include the following:
   8-month-old Jason, grandson of Jackson
   26-year-old Susanna, Jackson's daughter and Jason's mother
   60-year-old Jackson
   58-year-old Gemma, Jackson's wife
   82-year-old Martha, Jackson's mother
   Jason, Jackson, and Martha are being admitted to the hospital. However, Susanna and Gemma have been asked to follow up tomorrow in the urgent care clinic. The following questions pertain to this scenario.
   a. Martha LaGuardia's orders call for lactated Ringer's solution with 20 mEq KCl per liter to infuse at 150 mL/hr. After 4 hours of infusion, Martha begins to complain of shortness of breath and develops a cough. What do you suspect may be happening? What actions should you take?
   b. What theoretical knowledge will you use in caring for Ms. LaGuardia's immediate problem?
   c. Jason LaGuardia has been prescribed 250 mL of 0.9% saline solution over 8 hours. What type of equipment should you consider using?
   d. Calculate the drip rate for Jason's infusion if a gravity flow device is used. What further information do you need to perform this calculation?
   e. As you may recall, Jackson LaGuardia has end-stage renal disease. His lab work reveals a hemoglobin of 7.6 mg/dL and a hematocrit of 21%. He has been prescribed two units of packed red blood cells over 8 hours. Given his condition, for what fluid balance problem is he at risk? What additional parameters should you assess while he is receiving the transfusion?
2. You are asked to administer an antibiotic intravenously via piggyback. You are not familiar with the equipment that this facility uses. As a student, what approach should you take to solve this problem?
3. Identify techniques that you have observed that may contribute to contamination of an IV site.
4. Interpret the following ABG results. Explain your thinking.
   a. pH 7.47 P_{CO_2} 45 mm Hg HCO_3^- 32 mEq/L
   b. pH 7.32 P_{CO_2} 50 mm Hg HCO_3^- 25 mEq/L
   c. pH 7.30 P_{CO_2} 41 mm Hg HCO_3^- 18 mEq/L
   d. pH 7.45 P_{CO_2} 30 mm Hg HCO_3^- 22 mEq/L

5. For each of the following concepts, use critical thinking to describe how or why it is important to nursing; patient care; or fluids, electrolytes, and acid–base balance. Note that these are not to be merely definitions.
   Homeostasis
   Selectively permeable membranes
   Fluid imbalance
   Electrolyte imbalances
   Acid–base imbalances
   Parenteral fluid and electrolyte replacement

What Are the Main Points in This Chapter?

- Water is the largest single constituent of the body. Total body water content varies with age, gender, and the number of fat cells.
- Intracellular fluid (ICF) is contained within the cells. It is essential for cell function and metabolism and accounts for approximately 40% of body weight.
- Extracellular fluid (ECF) consists of three types of fluid: interstitial, intravascular, and transcellular fluid. ECF carries water, electrolytes, nutrients, and oxygen to the cells and removes the waste products of cell metabolism. ECF accounts for 20% of body weight.
- Electrolytes that carry a positive charge are called cations. These include sodium (Na^+), potassium (K^+), calcium (Ca^{2+}), and magnesium (Mg^{2+}). Electrolytes that carry a negative charge are called anions.
- Potassium and magnesium are the major cations in the ICF. Phosphate and sulfate are the major anions.
- The major electrolytes of ECF are sodium, chloride, and bicarbonate. Albumin is also present in the ECF.
- The functions of the major electrolytes include the following:
  - Sodium is essential to regulate fluid volume.
  - Chloride works with sodium to regulate osmotic pressure, and with the bicarbonate buffer system to regulate acid–base balance.
  - Potassium is essential for cellular metabolism.
  - Calcium is responsible for bone health and neuromuscular and cardiac function, and is an essential factor in blood clotting.
  - Magnesium is a mineral used in more than 300 biochemical reactions in the body.
  - Phosphorus is important in the formation of bones and teeth and has an inverse relationship with calcium.
- Osmosis, diffusion, filtration, and active transport are mechanisms used to maintain a balance between fluids and solutes in the body.
- General recommendations for total fluid intake are 2,700 mL per day for women and 3,700 mL per day for men.
- When the body is in a healthy state, fluid losses through urine, skin, insensible losses, and feces are equivalent to fluid intake.
- Fluid volume deficit occurs when there is a proportional loss of water and electrolytes from the ECF.
- Fluid volume excess involves excessive retention of sodium and water in the ECF.
- Bicarbonate is important in acid–base regulation and is regulated by the kidneys to maintain pH.
- The amount of acid or base present in a solution is measured as pH. The pH is reported on a scale of 1 to 14, with 1 to 6.9 being acidic, 7 neutral, and 7.1 to 14 basic, or alkaline. Normal blood pH is slightly alkalotic, between 7.35 and 7.45.
- A buffer system consists of a weak acid and a weak base. These molecules react with strong acids or bases to keep them from altering the pH by either absorbing free hydrogen ions or releasing free hydrogen ions. The principal buffer system in the ECF is the carbonic acid (H_2CO_3) and sodium bicarbonate ($NaHCO_3^-$) system.
- When the serum pH falls below 7.35, the patient is acidotic. When the serum pH increases above 7.45, the patient is alkalotic. Arterial blood gases (ABGs) are used to monitor acid–base balance.
- When the serum pH is too acidic (pH is low), the lungs remove carbon dioxide through rapid, deep breathing. If the serum pH is too alkaline (pH is high), the lungs try to conserve carbon dioxide through shallow respirations.
- The kidneys affect pH by regulating the amount of bicarbonate (base) that is kept in the body.

- Assessment of a client's fluid, electrolyte, and acid–base balance includes history; laboratory data; physical examination of the skin, mucous membranes, and neurological status; and assessment of cardiovascular and respiratory systems.
- Intake and output (I&O) are monitored to assess fluid status. To monitor, measure all fluids consumed and excreted in a 24-hour period.
- Tests used to monitor fluid, electrolyte, and acid–base balance include serum electrolytes and osmolality, complete blood count, urinalysis, and measurement of arterial blood gases.
- Nursing interventions for patients experiencing alterations in fluid, electrolyte, or acid–base balance include preventing imbalances modifying oral intake, providing parenteral replacement, and transfusing blood products.
- Intravenous fluids are classified as isotonic, hypotonic, and hypertonic solutions, based on their comparison to the osmolality of blood serum.
- Vascular access devices may provide access to peripheral or central veins.
- Intravenous equipment consists of the IV catheter, an administration set, extension tubing, and the IV solution.
- Nurses are responsible for using established formulas to calculate and maintain the correct rate of flow and for monitoring the client's response to the infusion.
- Assess for local IV site complications (e.g., infiltration, extravasation, infection, thrombus, and thrombophlebitis) and systemic complications (e.g. fluid volume excess, sepsis, and embolus).
- Meticulous aseptic technique is required for initiation and care of intravenous infusions, to prevent bloodstream infection.
- Blood products are infused when the client has experienced significant blood loss, diminished oxygen-carrying capacity, or a deficiency in one of the blood components.
- Nurses must administer the correct blood type to patients to prevent a hemolytic reaction.

Knowledge Map

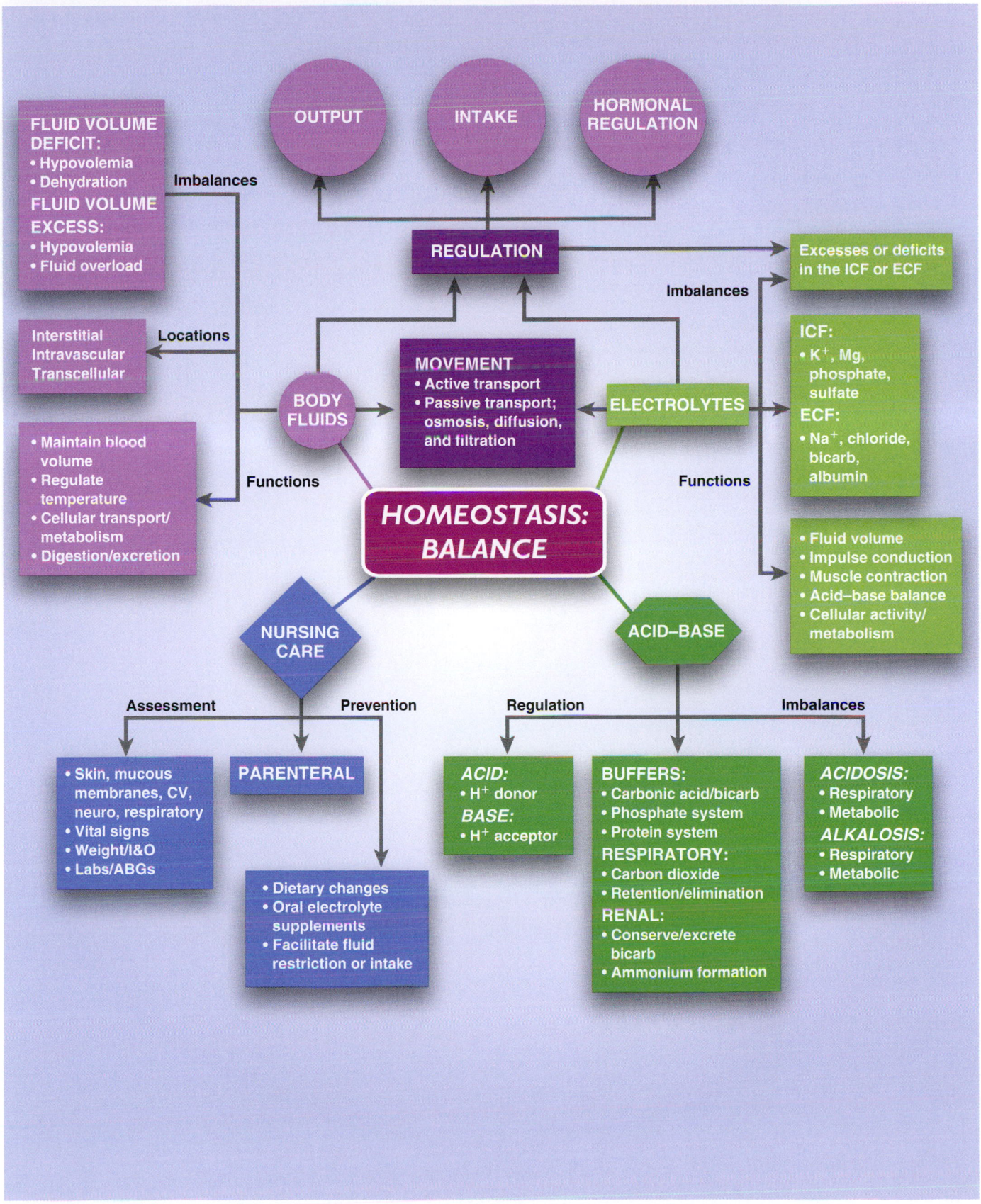

unit 5

Nursing Functions

39 Perioperative Care

40 Leading & Managing

41 Nursing Informatics

42 Promoting Health

CHAPTER 39

Perioperative Care

STUDENT RESOURCES

*The questions and exercises in Volume 2 allow you to practice the kind of thinking you will use as a full-spectrum nurse. Critical-thinking questions usually have more than one correct answer, so we do not provide "answers" for these features. It is more important to develop your nursing judgment than to just cover content. You will learn by discussing the questions with your peers. If you are still unsure, consult your instructor. You will find Response Sheets (for writing your responses to the questions) on Davis*Plus.

To explore learning resources for this chapter,

Go to Davis*Plus*, at DavisPl.us/Wilkinson3.

Chapter Resources for Chapter 39:
- **Response Sheets for all learning exercises**
- **Resources for Caregivers and Health Professionals**
- **Reading More About Perioperative Care**
- **Concept Map of chapter content**

Interactive Case Studies

NCLEX-Style and Chapter Review Questions

CHAPTER OVERVIEW

For a podcast of an overview of this chapter,

Go to Student Resources, Chapter 39, **Podcast—Chapter Overview,** on Davis*Plus*.

Caring for the Nguyens

Mai Nguyen, the 76-year-old mother of Nam Nguyen, has been experiencing blurred vision and decreased visual acuity. A local ophthalmologist diagnosed bilateral cataracts. The ophthalmologist has recommended cataract removal in the left eye, with insertion of an intraocular lens. He told Mrs. Nguyen to schedule the surgery "at your convenience" and explained that the surgery would be performed on an outpatient basis. The ophthalmologist gave Mrs. Nguyen a list of activities to prepare for the surgery, containing the following information:

- Schedule a date for your surgery. My receptionist will set up a time for your surgery. All surgeries are

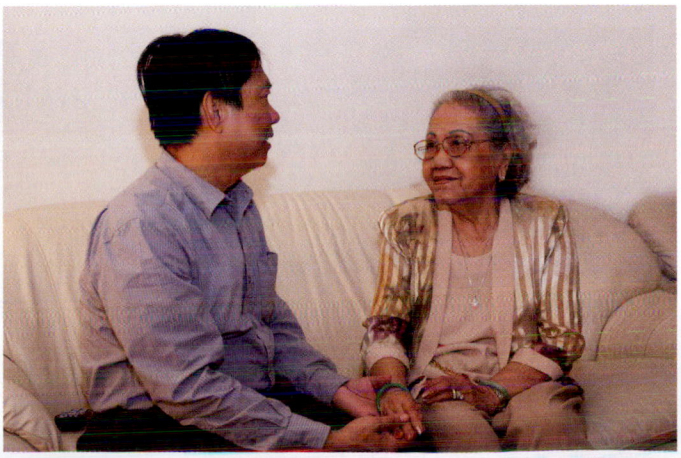

(Continued)

Caring for the Nguyens (continued)

performed at Western Medical Center Same-Day Surgery Department.
- Please arrange to be seen by your primary care provider 1 to 2 weeks prior to the surgery to receive clearance for surgery.
- Make an appointment with the Preoperative Center at Western Medical Center Same-Day Surgery Department 1 to 2 days before surgery.
- Arrange to have a ride to and from the surgery.

A. What preoperative testing is Mrs. Nguyen likely to undergo? Explain your rationale.

B. The preoperative list states that the client must be seen by the primary care provider to receive clearance for surgery. Why is this an essential part of the preoperative period?

C. What theoretical knowledge do you need to perform preoperative teaching for Mrs. Nguyen? How could you obtain that information? Be specific about your sources.

D. What content would you include in Mrs. Nguyen's preoperative teaching?

E. The ophthalmologist has planned anesthesia via conscious sedation. What factors, if any, might keep Mrs. Nguyen from receiving this form of anesthesia? What additional information do you need to answer this question?

Practical Knowledge knowing how

Perioperative care requires you to use the nursing process to ensure that the patient is in the best possible condition for surgery, is safe during surgery, and has the best possible outcomes postoperatively. Perioperative nursing care includes procedures and techniques designed for prevention and early detection of complications. Recall that full-spectrum nursing involves thinking, doing, and caring—all are equally important, in perioperative as well as other settings.

PROCEDURES

The procedures in this section will help you to prevent postoperative complications. Preoperative teaching of coughing, deep breathing, moving in bed, and leg exercises help to prevent thrombophlebitis, atelectasis, and pneumonia. Antiembolism stockings and sequential compression devices are designed to promote peripheral circulation and prevent thrombus formation. Gastrointestinal suction is used to relieve or prevent abdominal distention.

Procedure 39-1 ■ Teaching a Patient to Deep-Breathe, Cough, Move in Bed, and Perform Leg Exercises

➤ For steps to follow in *all* procedures, refer to the Universal Steps for All Procedures found on the inside back cover.

Equipment

For Teaching Deep Breathing and Coughing

- Folded blanket or a pillow (if teaching will include splinting of a surgical incision site)
- Tissues

For Moving in Bed

- Small pillow or folded blanket
- Pillows

Delegation

You or another RN should perform the initial teaching. You may delegate reinforcement of the teaching to a licensed vocational nurse (LVN), licensed practical nurse (LPN), or nursing assistive personnel (NAP).

Pre-Procedure Assessments

- Assess the patient's cognitive level and level of consciousness. *Helps assess the patient's ability to understand and follow directions and select the appropriate teaching method.*

- Assess the patient's pain level.
  Even preoperatively, pain must be well controlled to ensure full patient participation.
- Determine whether the surgical procedure and/or a physical disability will limit the patient's participation.
  For example, a fractured arm that has not yet been repaired will impair the patient's ability to hold a pillow for splinting.
- Determine whether the surgical procedure may entail special exercises or equipment. In addition, assess for any special equipment, such as braces, slings, or abductor wedges that may be needed when turning a patient in bed.

  Knee and hip surgeries often involve special exercises or equipment postoperatively. Consult the surgeon before teaching the patient any leg exercises. Spinal and neurological surgeries often limit movement in the postoperative period. For example, some spinal surgeries require the patient to logroll (move from head to toe as one unit). Some neurological procedures require limiting the amount of time the patient's head of bed is above 30°. Identify these restrictions preoperatively, and inform the patient and family about them during your teaching session.
- Assess the patient's belief about the ability of the surgical incision to remain intact.
  If the patient believes that the incision will not stay together if he coughs or moves, he is less likely to comply.

Procedure 39-1A ■ Teaching a Patient to Deep-Breathe and Cough

➤ When performing the procedure, always identify your patient according to agency policy, using two identifiers, and be attentive to standard precautions, hand hygiene, patient safety and privacy, body mechanics, and documentation.

Deep breathing and coughing expand the lungs, improve ventilation, promote gas exchange, and help prevent atelectasis and pneumonia. Coughing after deep breathing mobilizes secretions, which keeps airways and alveoli open and provides greater surface area for gas exchange.

Procedure Steps

1. **Assist the patient to a Fowler's** or semi-Fowler's position, with the shoulders relaxed.
   Allows for best chest and lung expansion.
2. **Assist the patient who will have** a chest or abdominal incision to practice splinting the site with a folded blanket or pillow (see the photo in column 2).
   Counterpressure supports the incision and decreases pain. ➤

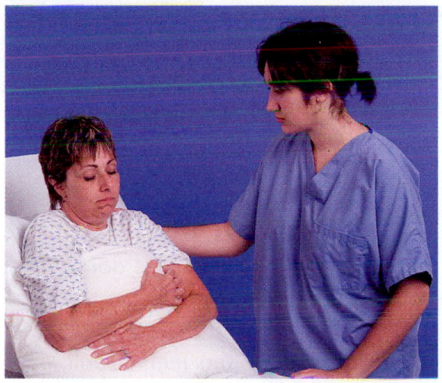

3. **Teach the patient diaphragmatic/** deep breathing. Tell the patient to:
   a. Place her hands anteriorly, along the lower end of the rib cage. The tips of the third fingers should touch at the midline.
   b. Slowly take a deep breath in through the nose. Tell the patient that she should feel her chest expanding as the diaphragm moves down.
   c. Hold her breath for 2 to 5 seconds.
   Stimulates surfactant production and helps prevent alveolar collapse.
   d. Slowly and completely exhale the breath through her mouth.
4. **Teach the patient to cough** in conjunction with diaphragmatic breathing. Instruct her to:
   a. Complete two or three cycles of diaphragmatic breathing.
   b. On the next breath in, have the patient lean forward and cough rapidly, through an open mouth, using the muscles of the abdomen, thighs, and buttocks. Cough several times on that breath.
   This information helps the patient to distinguish coughing from merely clearing her throat.

For a Patient Experiencing Weakness
If the patient is too weak to perform this maneuver, have the patient inhale deeply, bend forward slightly, and perform three or four "huffs" against an open glottis to move secretions forward.

Procedure 39-1B ■ Teaching a Patient to Move in Bed

➤ When performing the procedure, always identify your patient according to agency policy, using two identifiers, and be attentive to standard precautions, hand hygiene, patient safety and privacy, body mechanics, and documentation.

Moving in bed promotes blood circulation, stimulates respiratory function, and helps mobilize gas in the intestines.

Procedure Steps

1. **Start with the patient in** supine position, bedrails up. Then instruct the patient as follows.
2. **To turn to the left side:** Bend the right leg, sliding the foot flat along the bed and flexing the knee.
   Enables the patient to push herself over to the opposite side.

(continued on next page)

Procedure 39-1 ■ Teaching a Patient to Deep-Breathe, Cough, Move in Bed, and Perform Leg Exercises (continued)

3. **Reach the right arm across** the chest, and grasp the opposite bedrail.
   Helps the patient to turn, reduces the need to use the abdominal muscles for turning, and minimizes incision pain.

4. **Breathe deeply, and practice** splinting any potential abdominal or chest incisions. Provide as much assistance as the patient needs.
   Facilitates comfort during movement.

5. **Pull on the bedrail** while pushing off with the right foot.
   Assists patient to turn to the left.

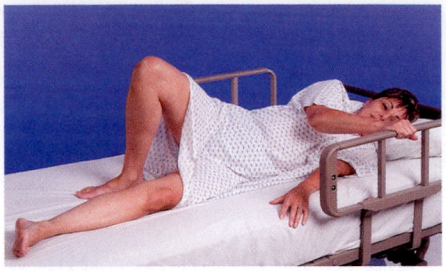

6. **If the patient cannot maintain** this position independently, place a folded pillow or blanket along her back for support.

7. **Teach the patient to change** positions every 2 hours, repeating the turning process with the opposite arm and leg. For patients who need pillows placed for support, you will need to assist with turning.

Procedure 39-1C ■ Teaching Leg Exercises

➤ When performing the procedure, always identify your patient according to agency policy, using two identifiers, and be attentive to standard precautions, hand hygiene, patient safety and privacy, body mechanics, and documentation.

Leg exercises flex and extend the leg muscles to increase peripheral circulation and help prevent thrombus formation. Thrombus formation is a common postoperative complication.

Procedure Steps

1. **Instruct the patient to lie supine** in the bed.
   Note: Although these exercises can be done when the patient is up in a chair, the effect will be diminished by the effects of gravity.

2. **Perform ankle circles.** Instruct the patient to:
   a. Start with one foot in the dorsiflexed position.
   b. Slowly rotate the ankle clockwise.
   c. After three rotations, repeat the procedure in a counterclockwise direction.
   d. Repeat this exercise at least three times in each direction, then switch and exercise the other ankle.

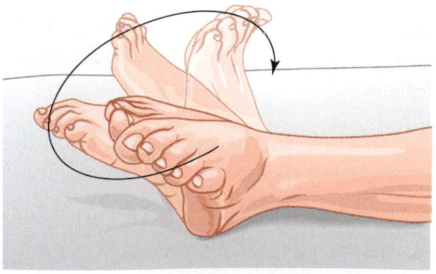

3. **Perform ankle pumps.** Instruct the patient to:
   a. Start with one foot, leg extended.
   b. Point the toe until her foot is plantar flexed.
   c. Pull the toes back toward her head until the foot is dorsiflexed; at the same time, press the back of the knee into the bed.
   d. Make sure she feels a pull, or a stretch, in the calf.
   e. Repeat the alternation between plantar and dorsiflexion several times.
   f. Repeat the cycle with the other foot.

4. **Perform leg exercises.** Instruct the patient to:
   a. Lie supine in the bed.
   b. Slowly begin bending one knee, sliding the sole of the foot along the bed until the knee is in a flexed position.

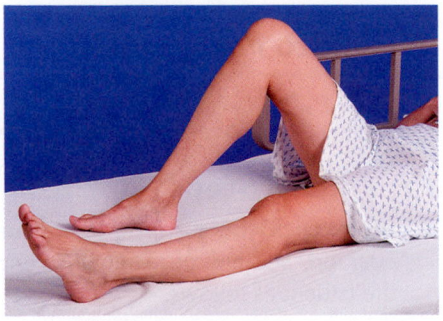

   c. Reverse the motion, extending the knee until the leg is once again flat on the bed.

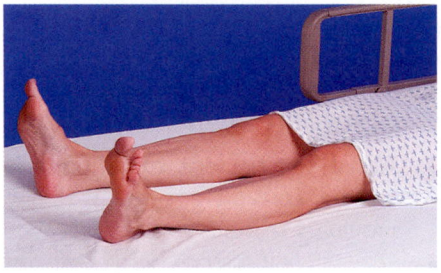

   d. Repeat several times.
   e. Repeat using the opposite leg.

? What if . . .

- **The patient has had knee, hip, or back surgery?**
  Leg exercises may be contraindicated in patients having knee, hip, or back surgery. Check the surgeon's prescriptions and/or collaborate with the physical therapist.

- **The patient has had nasal, ophthalmic, or neurological surgery?**
  Coughing and deep-breathing exercises are contraindicated.
  To avoid increasing intracranial pressure.

Evaluation

Make sure that the patient performs correctly a return demonstration of the procedures taught.

Documentation

In many healthcare facilities, checklists and charts have special areas in which to document patient teaching. Documentation should identify the person who completed the teaching, the person to whom the procedures were taught, what procedures were taught, and whether the patient understood the teaching. Also include the name and type of any printed materials given.

Sample electronic documentation

Note that because this is just one screen of a documentation system, not all of the information is visible. For example, you cannot see the date or the name of the nurse.

Practice Resources

Best Practices (2007).

Thinking About the Procedure

To practice applying clinical reasoning to this procedure,

Go to *Davis's Nursing Skills Videos*, **Teaching a Patient to Deep-Breathe and Cough, Teaching a Patient to Move in Bed,** and **Teaching Leg Exercises.**

For questions and suggested responses,

Go to Chapter 39, **Thinking About the Procedure Questions and Suggested Responses,** on Davis*Plus*.

Pt Sel | Logged In: Hiam, Judith | Documenting In Current Date/Time | Log Off

Patient Charting | Vital Signs | Order Entry | Order Review | Patient Teaching | Patient CARD | Patient Data | M.A.R. | Care Plans | Reports

Patient Teaching

Review Previous Teaching...

TEACHING TOPICS:
- Procedure
- Proper use of inhalers
- Respiratory
- Sexually Transmitted Disease
- Skin
- Smoking Cessation
- Street Drugs
- Surgery
- Vaccine
- Wound Care

TOPICS TAUGHT:
- [ ] Pre-Op Tests to expect
- [ ] Printed information given to patient
- [ ] Rationale for Incentive Spirometer use
- [ ] Rationale for SCD's
- [ ] Rationale for TED hose
- [ ] Reason for NPO status
- [x] Splinting incision for effective coughing
- [x] Turning, coughing, deep breathing
- [x] What to expect pre and post Op

PERSON(s) TAUGHT:
- [x] Patient
- [x] Spouse
- [ ] Parent
- [ ] Sibling
- [ ] Family Member
- [ ] Friend
- [ ] Significant Other

TEACHING METHOD(s):
- [x] Verbal Explanation and Discussion
- [ ] Printed Handout Given
- [ ] Video Shown
- [x] Demonstration
- [x] Return Demonstration Given

LEARNING BARRIERS:
- [x] No Barrier
- [ ] Patient in Pain
- [ ] Patient Fatigued
- [ ] Sensory Limits
- [ ] Cognitive Limits
- [ ] Needs Family Assistance
- [ ] Unable to Teach Patient

OUTCOME:
- [x] Verbalizes Understanding
- [ ] Verbalizes Need for further Teaching
- [x] Able to give return demonstration
- [ ] Unable to understand teaching
- [ ] Unable to give return demonstration
- [ ] Needs Practice to perfect demonstration

ADDITIONAL COMMENTS:

Add to BackPack... | Cancel Entry

Main Teaching Topic: | Topics Taught: | Person(s) Taught: | Method(s) U... | Learning Ba... | Outcome

Procedure 39-2 ■ Applying Antiembolism Stockings

➤ For steps to follow in *all* procedures, refer to the Universal Steps for All Procedures found on the inside back cover.

Equipment

- Measuring tape
- Antiembolism stockings
- Washcloth and towel (if needed to cleanse legs)
- Talcum powder (optional: check manufacturer's recommendations)

Delegation

You can delegate application of antiembolism stockings to nursing assistive personnel who have been trained in the task. Instruct the NAP as follows:

- Report the presence of any abnormalities on the lower extremities, such as lesions, sores, or redness, before applying the stockings.
- Instruct the patient to maintain a recumbent position for at least 15 minutes before applying the stockings.
- Do not massage the legs.
- Make sure there are no wrinkles in the stockings once they have been applied.

(continued on next page)

Procedure 39-2 ■ Applying Antiembolism Stockings (continued)

Pre-Procedure Assessment

- **Assess the level of consciousness and cognitive ability.**
  If the patient is unconscious or confused, you will need to call for assistance to hold and stabilize the lower extremities as you apply the stockings.
- **Assess for signs and symptoms of severe peripheral arterial disease, such as weak or absent pulses, discoloration or cyanosis, or gangrene.**
  Antiembolism stockings should not be used in patients with any of these findings because stockings compress the vessels and, therefore, further impede the already compromised arterial flow.
- **Assess skin condition. Note lesions, dermatitis, or major edema, as evidenced by shiny, taut skin.**
  If skin is overstretched by edema, antiembolism stockings may irritate or worsen skin conditions and cause skin breakdown.
- **Note the patient's position and length of time she has been in that position.**
  Place the patient supine for at least 15 minutes before stocking application. This prevents trapping of pooled venous blood.

➤ When performing the procedure, always identify your patient according to agency policy, using two identifiers, and be attentive to standard precautions, hand hygiene, patient safety and privacy, body mechanics, and documentation.

➤ If possible, apply stockings in the morning, before the patient gets out of bed.

Prevents venous distention and edema that occur when the patient is sitting or standing.

Procedure Steps

1. **Measure the patient's lower extremities** to obtain the correct size stockings. This is critical to their effectiveness.
   Stockings must be sized correctly in order to apply the correct amounts of pressure at the ankle, mid-calf, and upper thigh. If they are not tight enough, they will not improve venous return effectively. If they are too tight, they may compress the veins and impair circulation to the skin.

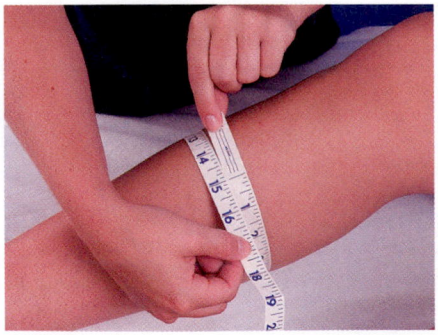

For Thigh-High Stockings

Note: Thigh-high elastic stockings have not been proved to be more effective in preventing thromboembolism than knee-high ones, and should probably be avoided because of the tendency to roll and have a tourniquet effect (Perry, Borchert, Burke, et al., 2012)

a. Measure the circumference of the upper thigh at the gluteal fold.
   The manufacturer of TED stockings recommends that thigh-high stockings not be applied if the thigh circumference exceeds 82 cm (32 in.). Use knee-high stockings instead.
b. Measure the calf circumference at the widest section.
c. Measure the distance from the gluteal fold to the base of the heel.

For Knee-High Stockings

a. Measure the circumference of the calf at the widest section.
b. Measure the distance from the base of the heel to the middle of the knee joint.
   Evidence is not conclusive, but increasingly supports the use of knee-high instead of thigh-high hose.

2. **Assist the patient to a supine** position, and instruct him to maintain that position for at least 15 minutes before you apply the stockings.
   Prevents trapping of pooled venous blood by the antiembolism stockings.
3. **Cleanse the patient's legs and** feet if necessary. Dry well.
   Removing surface dirt and bacteria will decrease the likelihood of infection and odor.
4. **Lightly dust the legs and feet** with talcum powder to ease the application of the stockings, if recommended by the manufacturer. **Key Point: *Do not use powder if the patient is or is likely to become diaphoretic. Powder eases the application of the stockings, but perspiration will cause the powder to clump.***
5. **Holding one stocking at the top** cuff in your dominant hand, slide your nondominant arm down and into the stocking until your hand reaches the heel of the stocking.
6. **Grasp the center of the heel** with your hand inside the stocking, and then slowly turn the stocking inside out to the level of the heel with your other hand.
   The elastic in the stockings is very strong; this method is the easiest way to fit it over the foot and calf.

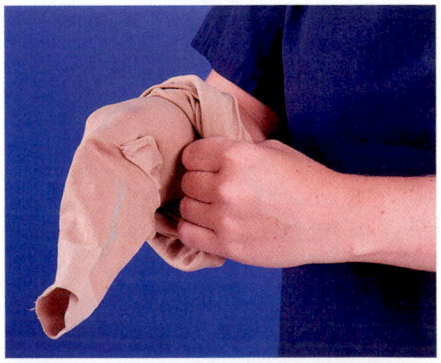

7. **Ask the patient to point his toes** as you grasp the turned foot of the stocking and ease it onto his foot and heel (like putting on a sock). Center the patient's heel in the heel of the stocking.
   Ensures that the pressure of the stocking is over the correct anatomical areas.
8. **Gradually pull the remainder** of the stocking up and over the leg,

turning it right side out as you proceed. Be certain the stocking is straight.

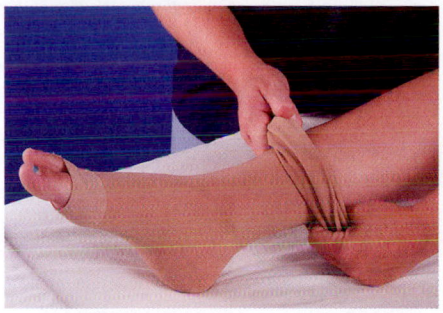

For Knee-High Stockings

a. Pull up to 2.5 to 5 cm (1 to 2 in.) below the knee

For Thigh-High Stockings

a. Pull up to the gluteal fold of the thigh, rotating inward so the gusset is centered over the femoral artery, slightly toward the inside of the leg.
Stockings apply varying amounts of compression between ankle, calf, and thigh areas. Keeping the stocking straight ensures that the pressure occurs over the correct areas.

9. **Smooth out any excess** material; keep stockings free of wrinkles and bunching.
Decreases the risk of skin breakdown and areas of inappropriate and potentially dangerous constriction.

10. **If the stockings have closed** toes, tug gently on the stocking toe to create a small space between the end of the toes and the stocking.
Prevents compression of small vessels in the toes, which may impede circulation.

11. **Repeat the procedure** on the other leg.

12. **Remove the stockings** and bathe and dry the legs daily.

13. **Launder the stockings** at least every 3 days; dry them on a flat surface.
Soiled stockings can irritate the skin; dry flat to prevent stretching.

? What if . . .

- **Both legs do not measure the same?**
  Order two different sizes of stockings and use one from each package to make two pairs.

Evaluation

- Evaluate patient comfort.
  Severe, continuous discomfort may indicate that the stockings are the wrong size.
- Check the stockings for wrinkles and/or rolling down at the top, especially when sitting.
  Wrinkles and rolling down can cause skin breakdown and areas of constriction.
- Evaluate and monitor skin condition.
  Elastic stockings should be removed for 20 to 30 minutes every 8 to 12 hours to allow you to inspect the patient's skin and evaluate the adequacy of his circulation.
- Evaluate the patient's ability to ambulate.
  It is important to reduce the time the patient is immobile due to pain, sedation, mechanical ventilation, and so on.
- Re-measure the legs regularly.
  To prevent complications related to swelling and weight gain.

Home Care

- Teach the client and/or caregiver to apply the stockings.
- Encourage the client to have two pairs of stockings on hand so that one pair can be used while the other is being laundered.
- Instruct the client to follow the manufacturer's directions for washing the stockings.
- Teach the client not to roll down the tops of the stockings.

Documentation

- Document leg measurements and size of the stockings used, to provide a baseline.
- Document the time and date applied.
- Note the condition of the skin, including any abnormalities.

Sample electronic documentation

Note that because this is just one screen of a documentation system, not all of the information is visible. For example, you cannot see the date or the name of the nurse.

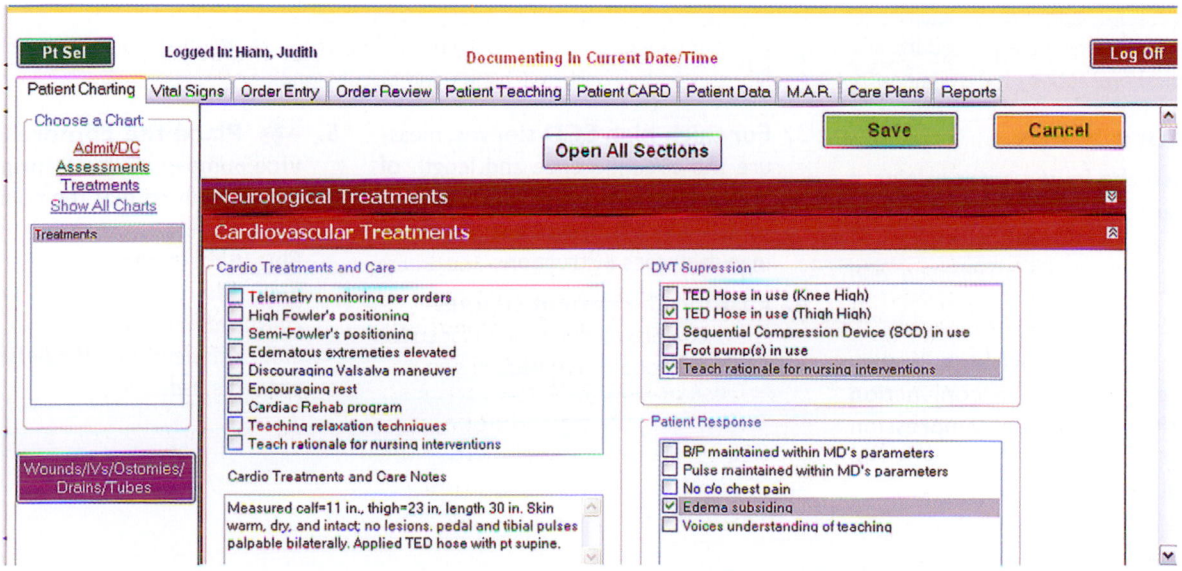

(continued on next page)

Procedure 39-2 ■ Applying Antiembolism Stockings (continued)

Practice Resources

American Association of Critical-Care Nurses (2010); Joanna Briggs Institute (2008a); Larry, C. (2003); National Guideline Clearinghouse (2008b); National Institute for Health and Clinical Excellence (NICE) (2007); Perry, D., Borchert, K., Burke, S., et al. (2012); Winslow, E., & Brosz, D. (2008).

Thinking About the Procedure

To practice applying clinical reasoning to this procedure,

Go to *Davis's Nursing Skills Videos*, **Applying Antiembolism Stockings**.

For questions and suggested responses,

Go to Chapter 39, **Thinking About the Procedure Questions and Suggested Responses,** on Davis*Plus*.

Procedure 39-3 ■ Applying Sequential Compression Devices

➤ For steps to follow in *all* procedures, refer to the Universal Steps for All Procedures found on the inside back cover.

Equipment

Note: Sequential compression devices may be referred to by several different brand names, including SCDS (sequential compression decompression stockings), Flowtrons, and PAS (pneumatic air stockings).

- Compression pump, motor, or machine
- Connecting tubing, if applicable (In some devices, the tubing is preconnected to the sleeves.)
- Compression sleeve (knee-high or thigh-high, depending on the order and the type of device)
- Elastic stockings (if also prescribed)
- Washcloth and towel as needed to cleanse the lower extremities
- Measuring tape

Delegation

You may delegate the application of the sequential compression device to a NAP who has had training in that task. Instruct the NAP to report any redness, irritation, or open areas on the lower extremities. Instruct the NAP to ensure that all cords and connecting tubing are in a place that will not create a fall risk for the patient or visitors. SCDs should not be removed for long periods of time because they are needed to support the patient's peripheral circulation.

Instruct the NAP to ensure that all cords and connecting tubing are in a place that will not create a fall risk for the patient or visitors.

Pre-Procedure Assessment

- Assess cognitive level and level of consciousness.
  Patients with altered cognition may be at higher risk for falls related to the presence of the connecting tubing and attachment to the compression pump. Patients who are unconscious will not be able to report a device that is creating too much pressure.
- Assess signs and symptoms of severe peripheral arterial disease, such as weak or absent pulses, discoloration or cyanosis, or gangrene.
  Increased compression of vessels by the sequential device may further impede arterial flow.
- Assess skin condition. Note lesions, dermatitis, or major edema, as evidenced by shiny, taut skin.
  If skin is overstretched by edema, the sequential compression sleeve may irritate or worsen skin conditions and cause skin breakdown.

➤ When performing the procedure, always identify your patient according to agency policy, using two identifiers, and be attentive to standard precautions, hand hygiene, patient safety and privacy, body mechanics, and documentation.

Procedure Steps

1. **Cleanse the lower extremities,** if necessary.
   Removes surface dirt and bacteria to decrease the likelihood of infection and odor.
2. **Apply elastic stockings** if they have been ordered in conjunction with the sequential compression device, following the steps in Procedure 39-2.
3. **For thigh-high SCD sleeves,** measure the circumference and length of both thighs to ensure that the sleeves are of the proper size. Follow the manufacturer's instructions.
4. **Position the patient supine.**
   Prevents venous pooling. Allows for easier application of the compression sleeve.
5. **Place the compression device** pump in a location near an electrical outlet so that the cord will not pose a fall risk.
   Plug in the pump.
   Note: Many compression pumps come equipped with hangers so you can hang the device at the bottom of the patient's bed.

6. Apply the compression sleeve.

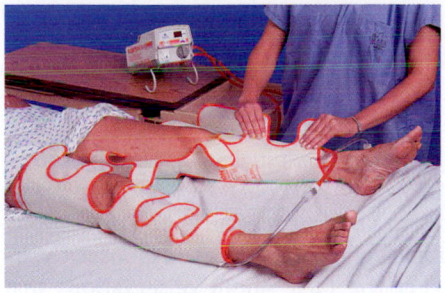

For Flowtron Brand (available in knee-length only)

a. Open the Velcro fasteners on the sleeve.

b. Place the sleeve under the lower leg below the knee, with the "air bladder" side down on the bed.

c. Bring the ends of the sleeve up, and wrap them around the lower leg, leaving one to two fingerbreadths of space between the leg and the sleeve.
Prevents excess pressure and overcompression.

For SCDS/PAS Brands

a. Open the Velcro fasteners on the sleeve.

b. For thigh-high sleeves, place the opened sleeve under the leg, ensuring that the knee opening is at the level of the knee joint and that the fastener will close on the anterior surface.
Ensures that compression occurs over the correct structures. Prevents restricted range of motion (ROM) of the knee joint.

c. Bring the ends of the sleeve up, and wrap them around the leg, leaving one to two fingerbreadths of space between the leg and the sleeve.
Prevents excess pressure and overcompression.

7. Connect the sleeve to the compression pump.

8. Turn the pump on and, if applicable, set the compression pressure on the pump device to the manufacturer's recommended setting. *Note: In some facilities, the compression pressure amount is preset and can be changed only by the central supply/equipment department.*

Evaluation

After applying the device, make the following ongoing assessments:

- Inflation and deflation of the sleeve
  Ensures that the device is actually working.
- Kinking or pinching of the connecting tubing
  Interferes with inflation of sleeves and may cause overheating or malfunction of the unit.
- Circulation, sensation, and motion of the foot, including skin color, pulses, temperature, capillary refill, motion, and sensation
- Patient comfort
  Increasing discomfort may indicate excess or incorrect pressure.
- Skin condition. Remove the compression sleeves at intervals so that you can inspect skin and evaluate the adequacy of circulation. *Note: If elastic stockings are being used in conjunction with the sequential compression device, follow the recommendations in Procedure 39-2.*
- Signs and symptoms of deep vein thrombosis
  Even with sequential compression device therapy, a patient can still develop thrombi.

Patient Teaching

Teach the patient to call for assistance when disconnecting the tubing from the compression pump to ambulate.
Prevents patient falls. The SCD tubing is a tripping hazard, and injuries from falls involving SCDs are likely to be more severe than injuries associated with general patient falls (Johnston & Davis, 2008).

Documentation

- Document the date and time you applied the device.
- Note the type and size (if applicable) of the compression sleeve used.
- Document the skin condition, including any abnormalities.

Sample documentation

11/11/16 1100. Knee-high SCD applied per order. Skin warm, dry, and intact at time of application. Peripheral pulses palpable. Pt's wife instructed on use of SCD. Pt unresponsive. No evidence of discomfort, no grimace or movement with application. ——— S. Bee, RN

Practice Resources

Johnston, J., & Davis, M. (2008); Markel, D., & Morris, G. (2002); Nelson, E. A., Mani, R., Thomas, K., et al. (2011).

Thinking About the Procedure

To practice applying clinical reasoning to this procedure,

Go to *Davis's Nursing Skills Videos*, **Applying Sequential Compression Devices**.

For questions and suggested responses,

Go to Chapter 39, **Thinking About the Procedure Questions and Suggested Responses,** on Davis*Plus*.

Procedure 39-4 ■ Managing Gastric Suction

➤ No Author. (2007). *Best practices: Evidence-based nursing procedures* (2nd ed). Philadelphia: Lippincott.

➤ For steps to follow in *all* procedures, refer to the Universal Steps for All Procedures found on the inside back cover.

Equipment

Procedure 39-4A Initial Equipment Setup

- Nonsterile procedure gloves
- Suction source (either a portable machine or piped-in wall source)
- Suction container and tubing
- Stopcock (to connect the NG tube to suction tubing)

Procedure 39-4B Emptying the Suction Container

- Clean nonsterile procedure gloves
- Graduated container
  To measure gastric output when emptying the suction container. Not needed if suction canister is marked for measuring.
- Alcohol wipes or chlorhexidine/alcohol antiseptic product

Procedure 39-4C Irrigating the Nasogastric Tubing

- Nonsterile procedure gloves
- Irrigating set (basin and bulb syringe or catheter-tipped syringe)
- Normal saline irrigant (unless another irrigant is prescribed)
- Linen-saver pads

Procedure 39-4D Providing Comfort Measures

- Nonsterile procedure gloves
- Emesis basin, cup, and water for mouth care
- Water-soluble lubricant
- Cotton-tip applicators
- Tissues or damp washcloth

Note: This procedure assumes an NG or other enteric tube is already in place and that its correct placement has already been verified. If you need to insert an NG tube or check placement, refer to Chapter 27. Tubes for gastric decompression are typically large-lumen tubes such as a Salem sump or Levin tube. See the table at the end of this procedure for more information about tubes.

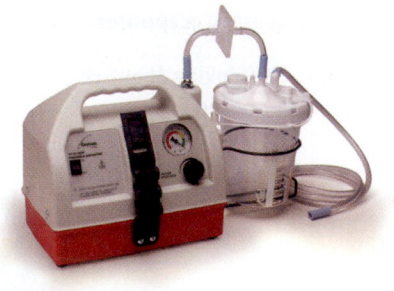

Portable suction source. (Courtesy of Allied Healthcare Products, St. Louis, MO.)

Delegation

A registered nurse should do the initial setup and any subsequent irrigation. You may delegate a NAP to empty and measure drainage and perform comfort measures. You must monitor equipment functioning and the patient's responses to the decompression. Instruct the NAP about observations that should be reported to you.

Pre-Procedure Assessments

- Determine that the NG tube has been inserted and placement has been verified.
- Verify the prescriber's order for type of tube and whether it is to be placed to suction or a drainage bag; also verify the type of suction to be used (low, high, continuous, intermittent).
- Auscultate for bowel sounds.
- Assess the patient's ability to cooperate with the procedure and understand explanations.
- Refer to the Evaluation section of this procedure. This procedure assumes an NG tube is already in place, so assessments are ongoing.

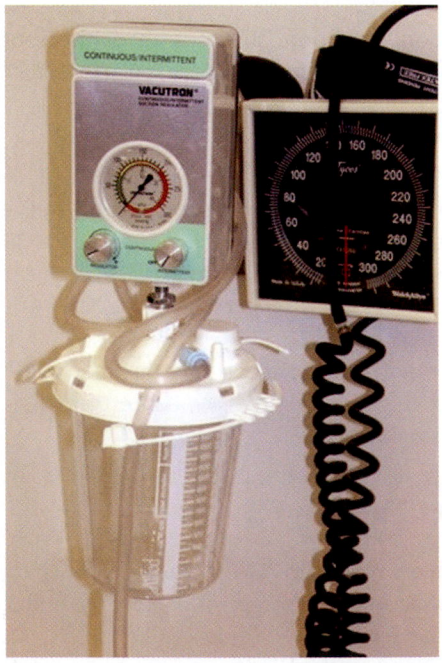

Wall suction unit.

Procedure 39-4A ■ Initial Equipment Setup

➤ When performing the procedure, always identify your patient according to agency policy, using two identifiers, and be attentive to standard precautions, hand hygiene, patient safety and privacy, body mechanics, and documentation.

Procedure Steps

1. **Place the collection container** in the holder (either on the portable suction machine or on the wall). Plug the power cord into a grounded outlet if using a portable suction machine.
2. **Connect the short tubing** between the container and the suction source. In some systems, the port will be marked "vacuum."
3. **Connect the long suction tubing** to the container (it may be marked "patient"); if one is available, connect a stopcock to the open end nearest the patient.
4. **Don nonsterile procedure gloves.**
   Helps prevent transfer of microorganisms.
5. **After the NG tube has been** inserted and placement verified, attach the end of the NG tube to the suction tubing.
   See Chapter 27 to review importance of tube placement. You must be certain the NG tube is in the stomach, not in the esophagus or airways.
6. **If the patient has a double-lumen** tube (e.g., Salem sump), instill 10 to 20 mL of air into the vent lumen to make sure it is patent. This should create a soft hissing sound.
7. **Check that the NG tube is secured** to the client's nose and gown (see Chapter 27 to review).
   Minimizes movement of the tube, helping to prevent irritation of the nares or other insertion site, as well as helping to keep the tube from migrating up out of the stomach.
8. **Turn on the suction source** to the prescribed amount. In an emergency when there is no order, always use low suction. Note the direction of the arrows and open the stopcock.
9. **Observe that drainage appears** in the collection container.
   It may take up to 5 minutes for air to be removed from the canister before the stomach contents will drain.▼

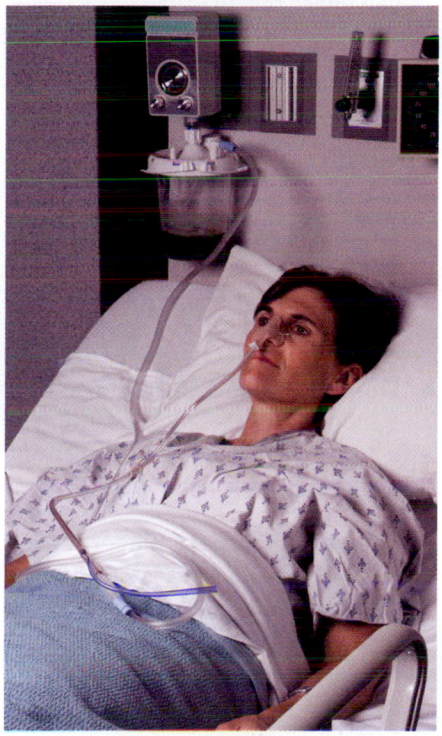

Procedure 39-4B ■ Emptying the Suction Container

➤ When performing the procedure, always identify your patient according to agency policy, using two identifiers, and be attentive to standard precautions, hand hygiene, patient safety and privacy, body mechanics, and documentation.

1. **Don clean nonsterile gloves.**
   Limits the transfer of microorganisms; protects your hands from contact with body secretions.
2. **Turn off the suction source** and close the stopcock on the tubing (or clamp the tubing, if there is no stopcock).
   Prevents suction flow during emptying of the container.
3. **Empty the suction canister.**

   For a suction container marked with measurements.
   Note the amount, color, and odor of the contents. Empty and rinse the container.

   For a suction container not marked incrementally.
   Remove the cap from the lid of the suction container and pour the drainage into a graduated measuring container. Note color, odor, and amount.
   A container with graduated markings enables you to monitor intake and output (I&O) accurately. Rinsing removes organic material that could be a reservoir for microorganisms.
4. **Wipe the port of the suction** container with an alcohol wipe. Place the suction container back in its holder and close the stopper on the lid.
5. **Turn on the suction source** to the prescribed amount. Note the direction of the arrows and turn the stopcock to the "On" position. If there is no stopcock, unclamp the tubing.
6. **Observe for proper functioning** of the suction and patency of the tubing.
   Prevents complications that would result from malfunction.
7. **Remove and discard your gloves.** Perform hand hygiene.

(continued on next page)

Procedure 39-4 ■ Managing Gastric Suction (continued)

Procedure 39-4C ■ Irrigating the Nasogastric Tubing

➤ When performing the procedure, always identify your patient according to agency policy, using two identifiers, and be attentive to standard precautions, hand hygiene, patient safety and privacy, body mechanics, and documentation.

1. **Place a linen-saver pad** on the bed under the NG tube.
2. **Open the irrigation set** and pour saline into the basin.
   Water is not used because it may cause electrolyte imbalances.
3. **Place patient at a 30° to 45°** elevation (unless contraindicated or not tolerated)
   This position helps avoid gastric reflux of irrigant.
4. **Don clean procedure gloves.**
   Limits the transfer of microorganisms; protects your hands from contact with body secretions.
5. **Check for correct placement** of the NG tube using at least two bedside methods (see Chapter 28 as needed).
   Prevents accidental instillation of irrigant into the airways.
6. **Fill the syringe with 10 to 30 mL** of saline and place it on the linen-saver pad.
7. **Clamp the NG tube** or turn off the stopcock connecting to the suction tubing. Then disconnect the NG tube from the suction tubing.
   Prevents backflow of drainage and soiling of linens and clothing.
8. **Hold the drainage tubing up** until suction clears it. Then place it on the linen-saver pad or hook it over the suction machine.
   Keeps secretions from soiling the bed linens or clothing.
9. **Turn off the suction machine.**
10. **Unclamp the NG tube** or turn on the stopcock.
11. **Unpin the NG tube** (or remove tape) from the patient's clothing.
12. **Attach the syringe and instill** the irrigant slowly into the NG tube. Do not force the solution. Be careful not to instill fluid into the air vent.
    Clears the NG tube of gastric contents to keep it patent and helps keep the tube from adhering to the gastric mucosa. Partially digested food, clotted blood, or tissue debris may clog the tube and prevent effective drainage.
13. **Lower the end of the NG tube** and then release the syringe bulb (or, depending on the type of syringe, pull back the plunger) to withdraw fluid. Instill and withdraw until fluid flows in and out freely.
    Uses the force of gravity with negative pressure to withdraw instilled fluid and gastric contents.

For a Double-Lumen NG Tube

Draw 30 mL of air into the syringe and inject it into the "pigtail" (the smaller-bore tube). Follow agency policy for this.
This clears the air-vent tube of any secretions. It must be patent in order to equalize pressure and prevent gastric tissue trauma at the drainage ports. The air also keeps the tube from draining fluid out of the stomach by capillary action.

14. **Reclamp the NG tube** or turn off the stopcock.
    Prevents backflow of drainage.
15. **Reconnect the NG tube** to the suction tube. Then release the clamp or turn on the stopcock.
16. **Reattach the NG tube** to the patient's clothing (with a pin or tape—see Chapter 27 as needed).
    Prevents pulling on and irritating the patient's nostril.
17. **Provide comfort measures** (e.g., mouth care).
18. **Remove and discard gloves.** Perform hand hygiene.

Procedure 39-4D ■ Providing Comfort Measures

➤ When performing the procedure, always identify your patient according to agency policy, using two identifiers, and be attentive to standard precautions, hand hygiene, patient safety and privacy, body mechanics, and documentation.

1. **Don clean nonsterile procedure gloves.**
2. **Provide mouth care** (see Procedures 25-6, 25-7, and 25-8 if you need to review). Use mouthwash as desired. Avoid using lemon-glycerine swabs. Apply water-soluble lubricant to the lips if they become dry and crusty.
   The patient most likely has a dry mouth from not receiving oral intake and from mouth breathing. Lemon-glycerine swabs cause even more drying of tissues.
3. **Remove nasal secretions** with a tissue or a damp washcloth. Moisten a cotton-tip applicator and wipe the inside of each nostril. If secretions are encrusted, moisten the applicator with hydrogen peroxide, then follow with an applicator moistened with water.
   To soften, dissolve, and remove secretions and prevent tissue irritation.
4. **Apply a small amount of** water-soluble lubricant to the inside of each nostril.
   Soothes and softens dried skin. Avoid petroleum-based lubricants, as complications may occur if they are inhaled.
5. **Check that the tape or tube** fixation device is secure. If it is not, replace it (see Procedure 27-2 as needed).
   Prevents irritation of the nasal skin and mucosa. Helps prevent migration of the NG tube from the stomach.

? What if . . .

- **Resistance is met when you irrigate the NG tube?**

  Check the tubing for kinks or evidence of obstruction. Have the patient turn to the left side.

  Turning to one side changes the position of the distal tip of the NG tube.

- **The patient complains that the NG tube is pulling against her nostril?**

  The tube may not be properly anchored to her clothing. Reattach the safety pin (or tape) closer to the nose so that there is more slack in the tube.

- **The NG tube causes excoriation of the nares?**

  Remove the tape or fixation device from the nose. Remove the residual adhesive from the skin. Apply skin sealant and anchor the tube so that the adhesive touches in a different place on the skin. Keep the excoriated areas clean and dry.

- **The NG tube does not drain?**

  Check tubing for kinks or blockage. Check the suction apparatus. If the collection container is higher than the patient's abdomen, lower it. If these aspects are working properly, irrigate the tube (see Procedure 39-4C, preceding). If the tube still is not draining and the patient is uncomfortable, document and notify the primary care provider. Encourage the patient to relax and breathe slowly through her nose. If the patient has abdominal distention, pain, or vomiting, notify the provider immediately.

If the container is too high, the negative pressure of low suction may not be enough to overcome the force of gravity. Abdominal distention, pain, or vomiting may mean the system is not working. Continued distention creates undue strain on the suture line. You should notify the care provider of these symptoms even when the mechanical aspects of the suction seem in working order.

Gastric Decompression Tubes

TYPE	LUMEN(S)	USE	MANAGEMENT	DISCUSSION
Levin	1, unvented	Decompression, feedings, or irrigation	Use low intermittent suction; may require irrigation.	If the tube opening(s) rest(s) against the gastric mucosa, the suction may irritate or injure the tissue.
Salem Sump	2	Decompression, suction, gastric lavage	Vented. May use high continuous suction.	The air vent helps keep the tube away from the gastric mucosa during suction.
Sengsten–Blakemore	3	Decompression; treatment of active bleeding from esophageal or gastric varices	Use low intermittent suction.	Gastric or esophageal balloons hold the tube in place.
Cantor	1, unvented	Decompression	Use intermittent suction.	Distal end is weighted with a balloon. Used in bowel obstruction. Rarely used because of the hazard posed by the mercury in the weighted balloon.
Miller–Abbott	2	Decompression	Use intermittent suction	Distal end weighted with a balloon. Used in bowel obstruction. Rarely used because it contains mercury in the weighted balloon.
Ewald or other very large-bore tube	May be passed orally for emergency evacuation of stomach contents to prevent absorption of ingested medications, poisons, or products. A piston tip syringe is placed on the end of the tube for manual suction. Typically the stomach is washed repeatedly with saline and all contents are withdrawn. Because of its large diameter, this type of tube is not tolerated by patients who are alert, and is not left in place after lavage is completed.			
Weighted Small-Bore Tubes (e.g., Keofeed)	For feedings only. Suction collapses the tube.			

(continued on next page)

Procedure 39-4 ■ Managing Gastric Suction (continued)

Evaluation and Maintenance

- Periodically assess placement of the tube by a combination of methods (i.e., checking pH of aspirate, by listening over the stomach with a stethoscope while injecting air into the tube, and by reviewing radiographic reports). See Chapter 26 for review, as needed.
- Monitor patency of the tube and the effectiveness of the suction. Check tube connections.
- Monitor patient comfort (e.g., sore throat).
  The continuing presence of a tube in the nose and throat is bothersome to patients. The major nuisance is the pressure of the tube against the internal mucous membranes, irritating the nostril, pharynx, and esophagus.
- Auscultate for bowel sounds; turn off suction while auscultating.
  Bowel sounds indicate the return of peristalsis and the success of gastric decompression. You may hear the sound of the suction apparatus and misinterpret it as bowel sounds.
- Monitor for gastric distention, vomiting, and abdominal pain.
  These symptoms probably indicate the suction is not working effectively. See the What If . . . section, preceding.
- Examine skin and mucous membranes around the insertion site (e.g., nares, abdomen).
- Follow agency policy or the primary care provider's prescription for irrigation of the gastric tube. It is common to irrigate with 10 to 30 mL of normal saline every 3 to 4 hours.
- Monitor the color of the drainage (should be green to gold). If there is blood in the drainage, notify the primary care provider.
- For clients undergoing prolonged GI suction, observe for signs and symptoms of hyponatremia and hypokalemia (i.e., fatigue, lethargy, confusion, seizures, muscle weakness, paresthesia, and cardiac dysrhythmias). Review lab results and report any symptoms to the primary care provider.
- Assess the patient's ability to move about in bed while attached to the suction source.

Patient Teaching

- Instruct the patient to notify you of any discomfort, and to not tug on or try to reposition the NG tube if it becomes uncomfortable.
- Instruct the patient to notify you if feeling nauseated.
  This could mean the tube is blocked and not draining effectively.

Home Care

Usually, gastric suction is performed in a hospital. If the client is to go home with gastric suction (e.g., a terminally ill person who has a bowel obstruction and wants to be in his or her own home), teach the family how to use the device before the person is discharged. Also arrange for home healthcare.

Documentation

- Record all drainage as output on the I&O record.
- Record the time, type, and volume of irrigations and the drainage returned.
- Be sure to include irrigation fluids as input on the I&O record.
- Note color, odor, and consistency of drainage.
- Document patient's emotional and physical responses to NG intubation.
- Document any evidence of tube or equipment malfunction.
- Document epigastric pain, discomfort, distention, or vomiting.

Sample electronic documentation

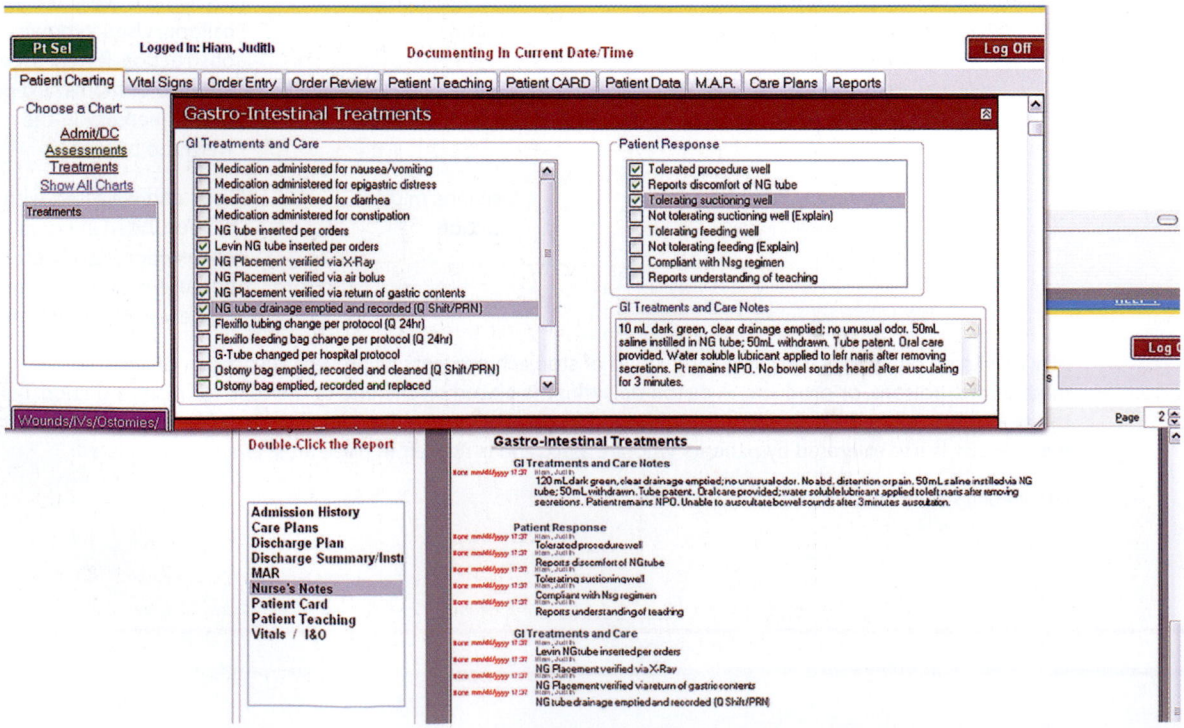

Practice Resources

Allied Healthcare Products, Inc. (n.d.); Bankhead, R., Boullata, J., Brantley, S., et al. (2009); *Best Practices* (2007); Green, S., Harris, C., & Singer, J. (2008); Sarasota Memorial Hospital (2008, reviewed 2011).

Thinking About the Procedure

To practice applying clinical reasoning to this procedure,

Go to *Davis's Nursing Skills Videos*, **Managing Gastric Suction: Initial Equipment Setup, Emptying the Suction Container, if Irrigating the Nasogastric Tubing.**

For questions and suggested responses,

Go to Chapter 39, **Thinking About the Procedure Questions and Suggested Responses,** on Davis*Plus*.

CLINICAL INSIGHTS

Clinical Insight 39-1 ➤ Preoperative Teaching

Explain What to Expect Before Surgery

- Explain the planned preoperative testing—lab tests, x-ray studies, ECG, and so on.
- Discuss skin preparation, including preoperative wash with an antibacterial product if this is included in the treatment plan.
- Discuss prescribed preoperative medications.
- Outline activities that will occur before surgery, such as insertion of an IV, placement of a urinary catheter, or cardiac monitoring.
- Review the preoperative restriction of fluid and food. Often the patient is to be NPO for at least 8 hours before the planned start of surgery. Some guidelines indicate that most children can drink clear liquids until 2 hours before surgery (Crenshaw, 2011, Joanna Briggs Institute, 2008a; "Practice Guidelines for Preoperative Fasting," 2011).
- If the patient is having surgery on the gastrointestinal (GI) tract, an additional bowel prep may be ordered (e.g., a low-residue diet beginning 1 week before surgery, and a liquid diet for the 48 hours preceding surgery). Patients having GI surgery also may have enemas before surgery. (If you need to review special diets, refer to Chapter 27.)
- Explain the need to remove jewelry, makeup, hearing aids, glasses, contact lenses, and any removable dental prostheses before being transported to the operating suite. It is best to have a family member take valuable belongings home for safekeeping.
- Tell the patient that a member of the anesthesia team will speak with him about the proposed anesthesia before surgery.
- Give the patient and family a tentative schedule for the operative day, including the time to arrive at the hospital or surgery center.

Explain What to Expect in the Operative Suite

- Inform the patient and family where they can go to wait during surgery.
- Discuss the preoperative holding area and activities that may occur there.
- Describe the operating room and the activities that the patient may anticipate before the surgery.
- Explain that the anesthesiologist or nurse anesthetist will monitor the patient and is responsible for keeping him comfortable with medications throughout the procedure.
- Describe the types of people who may be present in the operative suite. This is particularly important if the patient is not receiving a general anesthetic.

Explain What to Expect After Surgery

- Explain that the patient will initially be cared for in the postanesthesia care unit. After a period of observation, he will be transferred to the surgical unit. Note that some patients may be transferred directly to a critical care unit after surgery. If this is expected, tell the patient and family about this preoperatively.
- Family may visit after the patient has been admitted and assessed on the surgical unit.
- Tell the patient what to expect in terms of dressings, equipment, and monitoring devices.
- Describe the types of assessments that will be performed.
- Explain that pain medication will be given to keep the patient comfortable. If he experiences pain, he should tell the nursing staff.
- Discuss the usual progression of recovery, including activity level, deep breathing, coughing, leg exercises, and dietary intake.
- Discuss the anticipated length of stay.
- Teach the importance of deep breathing and coughing, especially after general anesthesia. Demonstrate how to splint the incision to facilitate deep breathing and coughing. Refer to Procedure 39-1A.
- Teach the patient how to move into and out of bed after surgery.
- Teach and emphasize the importance of leg exercises to minimize the risk of thrombus formation. Refer to Procedure 39-1C.
- If decreased activity or prolonged bedrest is anticipated, explain the use of antiembolism stockings or sequential compression devices.

Note: If the patient is to be discharged the day of surgery, inform him in advance about what to wear to the facility, and explain that he must arrange for a responsible adult to drive him home.

Clinical Insight 39-2 ➤ Preparing a Room for a Patient's Return From Surgery

In many institutions, the patient is transported to surgery using the bed that is in his hospital room, so these steps may vary.

- Put clean linens on the bed, including pads to protect the linen from drainage.
- Fold the linens back to the end of the bed.
- Raise the bed to stretcher height, and lock the wheels.
- Move furniture and equipment so that the stretcher can be placed directly against the bed.
- If needed, set up suction, oxygen, or other special equipment.
- Place the following equipment in the room:
  Stethoscope, manometer, thermometer (to measure vital signs)
  IV pole
  Emesis basin
  Tissues
  A clean gown, washcloth, and towel
  Extra pillows for positioning the patient

Clinical Insight 39-3 ➤ Creating an Operative Field

- A nonsterile team member (usually the circulating nurse) performs a surgical prep, using a scrub agent and "paint," to cleanse the operative site. Antiseptic agents must be approved by the U.S. Food and Drug Administration and by the agency's infection control professional. Chlorhexidine and povidone-iodine solutions are most commonly used.
- The area surrounding the operative site is then covered with sterile drapes so that only the operative area is exposed.

In the intraoperative period, sterile team members are the only persons allowed to enter the sterile field. The sterile field encompasses the patient and the area immediately surrounding the client. Creation of the sterile field proceeds as follows:

- Don head covering and shoe covers before entering the surgical suite.
- Perform a surgical scrub.
- Don sterile gown, gloves, and other surgical attire (e.g., mask).
- Cover the area surrounding the operative site with sterile drapes so that only the patient's operative area is exposed.
- Place sterile draping over the remainder of the patient's body.
- (In most cases) suspend a vertical drape at neck level so the client's head and airway are accessible to the anesthesiologist or nurse anesthetist (who is not sterile). For neurosurgery, even the head is draped, and the anesthesiologist or nurse anesthetist sits to the side of the head.

ASSESSMENT GUIDELINES AND TOOLS

Focused Assessment

Preoperative Assessment Topics

Include the following information in your preoperative assessment.

Health History—Discuss current and chronic health problems and prior hospitalizations or surgeries.

Physical Status—Identify any mobility concerns, and determine whether the client uses hearing aids, glasses, or contact lenses. Identify risk factors for venous thromboembolism (AORN, 2009, updated 2011):

- Venous stasis (such as occurs with bedrest, lengthy surgery, varicose veins, and heart failure)
- Vascular wall injury, which initiates clotting (e.g., surgery, IV catheter, irritating IV drugs, prior deep vein thrombus, smoking).
- Hypercoagulability (e.g., estrogen therapy, oral contraceptive use, cancer, dehydration, pregnancy)
- Older adults, especially those with other risk factors

Allergies—Check allergies to medications, food, tape, soaps, latex, or other substances.

Medications—Ask what prescribed medications and over-the-counter, herbal, or natural remedies the client takes (e.g., echinacea, ephedra, garlic, ginkgo biloba, ginseng, and St. John's wort). For more details about herbal products,

Go to Student Resources: Chapter 39, **Tables, Boxes, Figures: ESG Box 39-1, Examples of Risks Associated With Herbal Products,** on Davis*Plus*.

Mental Status—Note whether the client is able to respond to questions and offer a health history. Is he oriented? Does he appear anxious?

Knowledge—Understanding of the surgery and anesthesia. Ask the client to explain in his own words the planned surgery and postoperative course. Reinforce accurate statements, and correct any misconceptions.

Cultural and Spiritual Factors—Identify any cultural practices or spiritual beliefs that bring comfort to the client. Discuss how you can integrate these practices into the client's surgical experience.

Access to Social Resources—Identify the client's support network. Who is available to assist the client after surgery? Whom does the client rely on? Are those people aware of the client's upcoming surgery and condition?

Coping Strategies—Ask the client to identify the strategies he uses to cope with stress.

Use of Alcohol and Recreational Drugs—Inquire about the amount and frequency of alcohol use. Discuss the use of pain medications and recreational drugs. If the client uses these substances, identify the amount and frequency.

Focused Assessment

Example of a Preoperative Checklist

AORN *SAMPLE* Preoperative Assessment Form
(Facility Name and Address)

NOTE: *This record is a sample only. Clinical records should be customized to incorporate data fields that represent the setting, facility, procedure, and patient.* Reproductions and variations are encouraged, provided credit is given to AORN.

Addressograph

(Patient Information: name, age, gender, medical record number, date)

Date:_____

Structural Data:

Admitted via:
☐ Ambulatory ☐ Wheelchair ☐ Stretcher
☐ Other assistive devices:_____

Admitted from:
☐ Home ☐ Transferring hospital
☐ Acute rehab facility ☐ Extended/skilled care facility

Date of preoperative assessment:_____

Planned procedure:_____

Language(s) spoken: ☐ English ☐ Spanish ☐ Other:_____

☐ Patient's records, belongings, valuables secured (I115)
Belonging inventory: ☐ Watch ☐ Jewelry
☐ Contacts/glasses ☐ Dentures/partial(s) ☐ Hearing aid

Identity confirmed (I26): ☐ Yes ☐ No

Advance directive signed: ☐ Yes ☐ No
Location:_____

Operative procedure, surgical site, and laterality verified (I143): ☐ Yes ☐ No

Consent for planned procedures verified (I124): ☐ Yes ☐ No

NPO status verified (I138): ☐ Yes ☐ No
Since: (date/time)_____

Preadmission testing
☐ CBC_____ ☐ Urinalysis_____
☐ Potassium level_____ ☐ EKG_____
☐ CXR_____ ☐ Pregnancy test:_____
☐ Type and cross # of units:_____

Nursing Data Elements:

General health status: (check when present)
☐ Diabetes ☐ Cancer ☐ Obesity ☐ Pregnancy
☐ Hematologic disorders (anemia, sickle cell disease or conditions)

☐ Vital signs:
Temperature:_____ Pulse:_____ BP:_____
Respirations:_____ Height:_____ Weight:_____

☐ Allergies verified (note type of reaction) (I123)
Latex allergy: ☐ Yes ☐ No
Medications: ☐ Yes:_____ ☐ No
_____
_____
Food: ☐ Yes:_____ ☐ No
_____

☐ Daily medications (prescription, OTC, vitamins, alternative medication, herbal remedies, chemotherapy):
_____
_____
_____
Medications taken day of surgery:_____

☐ Alcohol/Drug social use:_____

☐ **Neurologic assessment:** ☐ Alert and oriented
☐ Speech intact ☐ Follows simple commands
☐ Risk of falls ☐ History of seizures
LOC: ☐ Alert/oriented ☐ Drowsy ☐ Sedated
☐ Asleep ☐ Unresponsive ☐ Disoriented
☐ Other:_____

☐ **Sensory assessment:**
☐ No limitations ☐ Hearing impairment ☐ Visual impairment

☐ **Cardiovascular assessment:**
☐ Pacemaker ☐ Implanted defibrillator
☐ Chest pain
☐ Peripheral edema: Location:_____
☐ DVT/PE risk:
☐ None ☐ Low ☐ Med ☐ High
_____
_____

☐ **Respiratory assessment:**
☐ Tracheotomy
☐ Intubated
☐ Chest tube
Respirations: ☐ Regular ☐ Labored
Smoking history ☐ Yes ☐ No
Packs/day:____ Years smoked:_____
Quit date:_____
☐ Cough ☐ Cold symptoms
☐ Current or recent respiratory infection
☐ Preexisting respiratory problems (specify):
_____
_____

☐ **Musculoskeletal assessment:**
☐ No limitations
☐ Paralysis
☐ Traction
☐ Limited ROM
☐ Amputation:_____
☐ Prosthesis:_____

Focused Assessment

Nursing Data Elements (continued):

☐ **Skin assessment:**
- ☐ Cool ☐ Warm ☐ Intact
- ☐ Dry ☐ Moist
- ☐ Body jewelry removed
- ☐ Makeup removed
- ☐ Tattoos: _____
- ☐ Rash: _____
- ☐ Bruises: _____
- ☐ Wounds: _____
- ☐ Ostomy: _____
- ☐ Catheter/Drain: _____
- ☐ Venous access device: _____

☐ **Gastrointestinal assessment:**

Last bowel movement (date/time): _____

Usual diet: _____

_____

Recent unexplained weight loss
- ☐ Yes: Amount: _____ Time frame: _____
- ☐ No

Problems chewing or swallowing
- ☐ Yes ☐ No

Special needs:
- ☐ Chewing ☐ Swallowing
- ☐ Appetite ☐ Diet preferences

☐ **Genitourinary/Gynecology assessment:**
- ☐ Voided on call to OR
  Time: _____ Amount: _____
- ☐ Urinary catheter: Amount in bag: _____
- ☐ Urinary incontinence

☐ **Psychosocial assessment:**
- ☐ Calm/relaxed ☐ Anxious ☐ Talkative
- ☐ Crying ☐ Restless ☐ Withdrawn
- ☐ Other: _____
- ☐ Concerns regarding surgery or hospitalization:
  _____
- ☐ Religious/cultural concerns/requests:
  _____
- ☐ Receives help from:
  - ☐ Children ☐ Support person
  - ☐ Other (specify):
  _____
- ☐ Patient cares for:
  - ☐ Children: Ages: _____
  - ☐ Self ☐ Spouse
  - ☐ Other (specify):
  _____

☐ Determine level of knowledge (I135):
- ☐ Barriers to learning: _____
- ☐ Motivation to learn
  - ☐ excellent ☐ average ☐ limited

☐ Abuse screening

Have you ever felt threatened verbally, emotionally, or physically in any of your relationships?
- ☐ Yes ☐ No

Have you been hit, slapped, kicked, or otherwise physically hurt by an intimate partner?
- ☐ Yes ☐ No

Are you afraid of your partner or anyone you live with?
- ☐ Yes ☐ No

If yes, describe and make appropriate referral

☐ **Pain assessment**
- ☐ Instructed on use of pain scale
- ☐ Pain assessment (0-10): _____
  Location: _____

☐ **Discharge planning**

Will require assistance after discharge
- ☐ Yes ☐ No

Discharge plan:
- ☐ Home
- ☐ Home nursing service
- ☐ Short-term care facility
- ☐ Extended care facility
- ☐ Other: _____

Individual who will escort patient home:

Name: _____

Phone number: _____

Relationship: _____

Comments:

_____

_____

_____

_____

_____

Preoperative nursing diagnoses
- ☐ Anxiety/fear (X4)
- ☐ Therapeutic regimen management ineffective (X33)
- ☐ Deficient knowledge (X30)
- ☐ Risk for injury (X29)
- ☐ Pain (X38)
- ☐ Other: _____

Comments:

RN Signature:
X

Source: Reprinted with permission from AORN Perioperative Patient-Focused Model. Copyright 2011 AORN, Inc, 2170 Paker Rd., Suite 300, Denver, CO 80231. All rights reserved.

Focused Assessment

Example of a Surgical Safety Checklist

World Health Organization

SURGICAL SAFETY CHECKLIST (FIRST EDITION)

Before induction of anaesthesia ▸▸▸▸▸▸▸▸▸ Before skin incision ▸▸▸▸▸▸▸▸▸▸▸▸▸▸ Before patient leaves operating room

SIGN IN

- ☐ **PATIENT HAS CONFIRMED**
  - IDENTITY
  - SITE
  - PROCEDURE
  - CONSENT
- ☐ **SITE MARKED/NOT APPLICABLE**
- ☐ **ANAESTHESIA SAFETY CHECK COMPLETED**
- ☐ **PULSE OXIMETER ON PATIENT AND FUNCTIONING**

DOES PATIENT HAVE A:

KNOWN ALLERGY?
- ☐ NO
- ☐ YES

DIFFICULT AIRWAY/ASPIRATION RISK?
- ☐ NO
- ☐ YES, AND EQUIPMENT/ASSISTANCE AVAILABLE

RISK OF >500ML BLOOD LOSS (7ML/KG IN CHILDREN)?
- ☐ NO
- ☐ YES, AND ADEQUATE INTRAVENOUS ACCESS AND FLUIDS PLANNED

TIME OUT

- ☐ **CONFIRM ALL TEAM MEMBERS HAVE INTRODUCED THEMSELVES BY NAME AND ROLE**
- ☐ **SURGEON, ANAESTHESIA PROFESSIONAL AND NURSE VERBALLY CONFIRM**
  - PATIENT
  - SITE
  - PROCEDURE

ANTICIPATED CRITICAL EVENTS

- ☐ **SURGEON REVIEWS:** WHAT ARE THE CRITICAL OR UNEXPECTED STEPS, OPERATIVE DURATION, ANTICIPATED BLOOD LOSS?
- ☐ **ANAESTHESIA TEAM REVIEWS:** ARE THERE ANY PATIENT-SPECIFIC CONCERNS?
- ☐ **NURSING TEAM REVIEWS:** HAS STERILITY (INCLUDING INDICATOR RESULTS) BEEN CONFIRMED? ARE THERE EQUIPMENT ISSUES OR ANY CONCERNS?

HAS ANTIBIOTIC PROPHYLAXIS BEEN GIVEN WITHIN THE LAST 60 MINUTES?
- ☐ YES
- ☐ NOT APPLICABLE

IS ESSENTIAL IMAGING DISPLAYED?
- ☐ YES
- ☐ NOT APPLICABLE

SIGN OUT

NURSE VERBALLY CONFIRMS WITH THE TEAM:

- ☐ **THE NAME OF THE PROCEDURE RECORDED**
- ☐ **THAT INSTRUMENT, SPONGE AND NEEDLE COUNTS ARE CORRECT** (OR NOT APPLICABLE)
- ☐ **HOW THE SPECIMEN IS LABELLED** (INCLUDING PATIENT NAME)
- ☐ **WHETHER THERE ARE ANY EQUIPMENT PROBLEMS TO BE ADDRESSED**
- ☐ **SURGEON, ANAESTHESIA PROFESSIONAL AND NURSE REVIEW THE KEY CONCERNS FOR RECOVERY AND MANAGEMENT OF THIS PATIENT**

THIS CHECKLIST IS NOT INTENDED TO BE COMPREHENSIVE. ADDITIONS AND MODIFICATIONS TO FIT LOCAL PRACTICE ARE ENCOURAGED.

Source: Reprinted with permission from the World Health Organization. Retrieved from http://www.who.int/patientsafety/safesurgery/tools_resources/SSSL_Checklist_finalJun08.pdf

Focused Assessment

Intraoperative Care Questionnaire

Common nursing interview questions include the following:

- What is your name?
- What type of surgery are you going to have today?
- Is someone here with you?
- Are you allergic to any medications, latex, or tape?
- When is the last time that you had anything to eat or drink?
- Do you have false teeth, contact lenses, or any other prostheses that need to be removed?
- Have you taken any medications today?
- Do you have any implants, such as metal plates or a pacemaker?
- Do you have any scratches, bruises, or other wounds on your body at this time?
- Are there any parts of your body that are painful, such as a stiff shoulder or leg?

Also see the WHO Surgical Safety Checklist, preceding.

Focused Assessment

Postanesthesia Assessment: Essential Elements

The postanesthesia care nurse performs a quick, focused initial assessment of the surgical patient in the presence of the anesthesia provider and circulating RN. After that, the nurse assesses the patient every 5 to 15 minutes. The AORN (2009, updated 2011) has identified the essential elements of assessment in the PACU.

- ***Vital signs***
  - Blood pressure, cuff or arterial
  - Respiratory rate, respiratory competence, and breath sounds
  - Respiratory adequacy, including skin color and condition
  - Temperature (record type of measurement used, for example, skin, tympanic, oral)
  - Pulse (apical and peripheral)
  - Oxygen saturation (e.g., pulse oximeter reading)
- ***Peripheral circulation*** (postoperative tissue perfusion), for example, peripheral pulses and sensation at extremities
- ***Neurological status***, including pupil response and intracranial pressure (if indicated)
- ***Mental status***, including level of consciousness, alertness, lucidity, orientation

Older adults make up nearly 40% of surgical patients, and dementia is among the most common surgical complications, including postoperative delirium.

- ***Intravenous therapy***, including patency, location of sites, rates of solution(s), and/or blood products infusing
- ***Allergies and sensitivities***
- ***Pain***
- ***Motor abilities***, including return of sensory and motor control in areas affected by local or regional anesthetics
- ***Skin integrity***
- ***Temperature regulation***
- ***Positioning***
- ***Surgical incision site***, including condition of suture line(s) if visible
- ***Nausea and vomiting***
- ***Fluid and electrolyte balance***
- ***Safety needs*** (e.g., siderails raised)
- ***Central venous pressure (CVP), pulmonary wedge pressure***
- ***Airway***: patency, presence of artificial airway, mechanical ventilator settings
- ***Condition of dressing(s)***
- ***Drainage***, including type; patency; and amount and type of drainage from dressings, tubes, and catheters

DIAGNOSTIC TESTING

Diagnostic Testing

Common Preoperative Screening Tests

Test	Uses
Urinalysis	To detect urinary tract infections (UTIs) and the presence of glucose or protein in the urine, which may indicate poorly controlled diabetes or renal disease
Complete blood	To detect irregularities in hemoglobin (Hgb) and count (CBC) hematocrit (Hct)
	A low Hgb level is an indication of anemia, which may place the client at risk if significant blood loss occurs
	Measures white blood cell (WBC) count as an indicator of immune function
	Measures platelet count, which affects clotting ability
ECG	To detect cardiac dysrhythmias (electrocardiogram) and other cardiac pathology
Chest x-ray	To detect for or evaluate underlying cardiopulmonary disease that examination may lead to postoperative complications
Blood type and crossmatch	To identify blood type in the event that blood transfusion is needed
Serum electrolytes	To detect sodium, potassium, chloride, magnesium, calcium, and pH imbalances, which affect cardiac and other organ function and fluid balance
Fasting blood sugar	To detect diabetes or poorly controlled diabetes
Comprehensive metabolic panel	Includes electrolytes, blood glucose, liver function tests (ALT, AST), serum albumin and protein, and renal function tests (BUN and creatinine); used to detect underlying health problems that may affect surgical risk or outcome

STANDARDIZED LANGUAGE

Standardized Language

Preoperative Patients: Selected Standardized Nursing Diagnoses, Outcomes, and Interventions

NURSING DIAGNOSES	SELECTED NOC OUTCOMES AND GOALS USING NOC INDICATORS	SELECTED NIC INTERVENTIONS AND NURSING ACTIVITIES (SHADED ACTIVITIES ARE ROUTINE NURSING MEASURES FOR ALL PREOPERATIVE PATIENTS)
Anxiety related to change in health status	***NOC outcomes:*** Anxiety Level Anxiety Self-Control ***NOC goals:*** Patient will exhibit: ➤ (5) No restlessness ➤ (4) Only mild muscle and facial tension ➤ (4) Only mild difficulty concentrating ➤ (5) No increased blood pressure, pulse rate, or respiratory rate ➤ (5) No physical signs of anxiety such as dilated pupils, sweating, and dizziness ➤ (3) Moderate verbalized anxiety ***Individualized goals:*** ➤ Identifies symptoms that are indicators of her anxiety. ➤ Communicates need for assistance.	*Anxiety Reduction* ➤ Use a calm, reassuring approach. ➤ Explain all procedures, including sensations likely to be experienced during the surgical procedure. ➤ Seek to understand the patient's perspective of the situation. ➤ Provide factual information [about the surgery]. ➤ Encourage verbalization of feelings perceptions, and fears [about surgery. This helps the patient feel supported and less anxious.] *Calming Technique* ➤ Maintain eye contact with patient. ➤ Maintain calm, deliberate manner. ➤ Identify significant others whose presence can assist patient. *Presence* ➤ Stay with the patient and provide assurance of safety and security during periods of anxiety. ➤ Listen to the patient's concerns. ➤ Touch patient to express concern, as appropriate. ➤ Be physically available as a helper.
Fear related to unknown outcome of surgery and fear of pain that may result	***NOC outcomes:*** Fear Level Fear Self-Control ***NOC goals:*** ➤ (5) Exhibits no restlessness or irritability. ➤ (5) Reports no difficulty concentrating. ➤ (5) No physical signs of fear: increased BP, radial pulse rate, respiratory rate, sweating, dilated pupils, pale skin ➤ (5) No verbalized fear ➤ (5) No crying ***Individualized goals:*** ➤ Does not exhibit physical signs of fear (e.g., pupil dilation; dry mouth; increased BP, pulse and respiratory rate). ➤ Reports understanding of pain control measures to be used during and after surgery.	*Anxiety Reduction* ➤ (See Anxiety diagnosis) *Coping Enhancement* ➤ Assist the patient in developing an objective appraisal of the event ➤ Evaluate the patient's decision-making ability. ➤ Encourage the use of spiritual resources, if desired. *Preparatory Sensory Information* ➤ Identify the typical sensations (what will be seen, felt, smelled, tasted, heard) the majority of patients describe as associated with each aspect of the procedure/treatment. ➤ Personalize the information by using personal pronouns. *Security Enhancement* ➤ Explain all tests and procedures to the patient/family. ➤ Assist the patient to use coping responses that have been successful in the past.

Standardized Language

Preoperative Patients: Selected Standardized Nursing Diagnoses, Outcomes, and Interventions—cont'd

NURSING DIAGNOSES	SELECTED NOC OUTCOMES AND GOALS USING NOC INDICATORS	SELECTED NIC INTERVENTIONS AND NURSING ACTIVITIES (SHADED ACTIVITIES ARE ROUTINE NURSING MEASURES FOR ALL PREOPERATIVE PATIENTS)
Deficient Knowledge of preoperative procedures and postoperative expectations **Knowledge-Related Diagnoses** (e.g., Ineffective Management of Therapeutic Regimen, or Risk for Infection)	***NOC outcomes:*** Knowledge: Disease Process Knowledge: Treatment Procedure(s) ***NOC goals:*** ➤ (3) Moderate knowledge of characteristics of specific disease ➤ (4) Substantial knowledge of strategies to minimize disease progression ➤ (4) Substantial knowledge of signs and symptoms of disease complications ***Individualized goals:*** ➤ Verbalizes rationale for pre- and postoperative interventions ➤ Describes or demonstrates postoperative expectations (i.e., deep breathing, turning/position changes)	*Teaching: Preoperative* ➤ Inform the patient/significant others how long surgery is expected to last. ➤ Determine the patient's previous surgical experiences and level of knowledge related to surgery. ➤ Provide time for the patient to ask questions and discuss concerns. ➤ Instruct the patient or caregiver [how to participate in the care (e.g., technique of splinting, coughing, and deep breathing)]. ➤ Describe preoperative routines (e.g., anesthesia, diet, bowel preparation, tests/labs, voiding, skin preparation, IV therapy, clothing, family waiting area, transportation to operating room). ➤ Describe any preoperative medications, the effects these will have on the patient, and the rationale for using them. ➤ Inform the patient and family of the scheduled date, time, and location of the surgery. ➤ Inform the patient and family how long the surgery is expected to last. ➤ Introduce the patient to the [perioperative] staff who will be involved in the . . . care, as appropriate. ➤ Discuss possible pain control measures. ➤ Describe postoperative routines and equipment (e.g., medications, respiratory treatments, tubes, machines, support hose, surgical dressings, ambulation, diet, family visitation) and explain their purpose. ➤ Instruct the patient in postoperative deep breathing exercises, splinting incision, coughing. ➤ Reinforce information provided by other healthcare team members, as appropriate. ➤ Instruct in a way that matches the patient's style of learning, including the use of holistic approaches and educational materials, as appropriate.
Disturbed Sleep Pattern related to anxiety about the upcoming surgery	***NOC outcome:*** Sleep ***NOC goals:*** ➤ (4) Mild interrupted sleep ➤ (5) Hours of sleep, not compromised ➤ (4) Sleeps through the night consistently, mildly compromised. ***Individualized goals:*** ➤ Reports minimal compromise in hours of sleep and sleep pattern. ➤ No difficulty falling and staying asleep reported or observed	*Sleep Enhancement* ➤ Determine the patient's sleep-activity pattern. ➤ Determine effects of patient's medications on sleep pattern. ➤ Adjust environment (light, noise, temperature, mattress, and bed) to promote sleep. ➤ Instruct the patient how to perform autogenic muscle relaxation or other nonpharmacological forms of sleep inducement. ➤ Initiate/implement comfort measures of massage, positioning, and affective touch.

Sources: Bulechek, G. M., Butcher, H. K., & Dochterman, J. M., et al. (Eds.) (2013). *Nursing interventions classification (NIC)* (6th ed.). St. Louis, MO: C.V. Mosby; Moorhead, S., Johnson, M., Maas, M., et al. (Eds.). (2013). *Nursing outcomes classification (NOC)* (5th ed.). St. Louis, MO: C.V. Mosby; NANDA International. (2012). *Nursing diagnoses: Definitions and classification 2012–2014*. Philadelphia: Author. Used with permission.

Standardized Language

Intraoperative Patients: Selected Standardized Nursing Diagnoses, Outcomes, and Interventions

NURSING DIAGNOSES (NANDA-I) AND COLLABORATIVE PROBLEMS	NOC OUTCOMES AND INDICATORS	NIC INTERVENTIONS AND ACTIVITIES (SHADED INTERVENTIONS ARE ROUTINELY PERFORMED FOR ALL SURGERY PATIENTS)
Nursing diagnosis: Risk for Aspiration related to depressed respirations and reflexes secondary to anesthesia ***Collaborative problem:*** Potential Complication of anesthesia: aspiration	***NOC outcome:*** Respiratory Status: Airway Patency ***NOC goal:*** (5) No choking or adventitious breath sounds	***Artificial Airway Management*** ➤ Institute endotracheal suctioning, as appropriate. ***Aspiration Precautions*** ➤ Monitor pulmonary status. ➤ Keep suction setup available. ➤ Maintain an airway. ***Sedation Management*** ➤ Ensure emergency resuscitation equipment is readily available, specifically a source to deliver 100% O_2, emergency medications, and a defibrillator. ➤ Initiate an IV line. ➤ Ensure availability of and administer antagonists as appropriate, per physician's order, or protocol ***Vomiting Management*** ➤ Position to prevent aspiration.
Nursing diagnosis: Risk for Imbalanced Body Temperature related to exposure in cool environment and administration of cool IV fluids	***NOC outcome:*** Thermoregulation ***NOC goals:*** ➤ (5) No hyperthermia ➤ (5) No hypothermia ➤ (4) Mild increased (or decreased) skin temperature	***Temperature Regulation: Perioperative*** ➤ Prewarm the patient with active warming device (e.g., forced air warming) for at least 15 minutes before start of anesthesia, as appropriate. ➤ Adjust ambient room temperature to minimize the risk of hypothermia (i.e., in addition to forced-air warming, when large surface areas are exposed, maintain room temperature at or above 73.4°F or 23°C). ➤ Minimize exposure of patient during surgical prepping and procedure, when possible. ➤ Warm or cool all irrigating, IV, and skin preparation solutions, as appropriate. ➤ Monitor for abnormal or unintentional increases or decreases in body temperature. ➤ Transport patient using warming device (e.g., heated [blanket or] isolette), as appropriate.
Collaborative problem: Potential Complication of surgery and anesthesia: hyperthermia		***Malignant Hyperthermia Precautions*** ➤ Maintain emergency equipment for malignant hyperthermia, per protocol. ➤ Notify surgical team of patient history or risk status. ➤ Place cooling water mattress under patient at risk for malignant hyperthermia at start of procedure. ***Vital Signs Monitoring*** ➤ Monitor blood pressure, pulse, temperature, and respiratory status, as appropriate. ➤ Monitor skin color, temperature, and moistness.

Standardized Language

Intraoperative Patients: Selected Standardized Nursing Diagnoses, Outcomes, and Interventions—cont'd

NURSING DIAGNOSES (NANDA-I) AND COLLABORATIVE PROBLEMS	NOC OUTCOMES AND INDICATORS	NIC INTERVENTIONS AND ACTIVITIES (SHADED INTERVENTIONS ARE ROUTINELY PERFORMED FOR ALL SURGERY PATIENTS)
Nursing diagnosis: Risk for Imbalanced Fluid Volume ***Collaborative problem:*** Potential complication of surgery: fluid and electrolyte imbalance	***NOC outcomes:*** Fluid Balance Urinary Elimination Vital Signs ***NOC goals:*** ➤ (4) Systolic and diastolic blood pressures, mild deviation from normal range ➤ (5) Mean arterial pressure not compromised ➤ (5) Central venous pressure not compromised ➤ (5) Pulmonary wedge pressure not compromised ➤ (4) Peripheral pulses mildly compromised ➤ (4) 24-hour intake and output balance mildly compromised ➤ (5) Adventitious breath sounds not present ➤ (5) Neck vein distension not present ➤ (5) Peripheral edema not present	***Fluid Management*** ➤ Maintain accurate intake and output record. ➤ Insert urinary catheter, if appropriate. ➤ Administer IV therapy, as prescribed. ➤ Monitor hemodynamic status, including CVP, MAP, PAP, and PCWP, if available. ➤ Arrange availability of blood products for transfusion, if necessary. ***Fluid Monitoring*** ➤ Determine possible risk factors for fluid imbalance (e.g., . . . renal pathologies, cardiac failure, liver dysfunction . . .). ➤ Monitor color, quantity, and specific gravity of urine. ➤ Monitor for distended neck veins, crackles in the lungs, peripheral edema, and weight gain. ➤ Monitor blood pressure, heart rate, and respiratory status. ➤ Monitor serum and urine electrolyte values. . . ***Intravenous (IV) Therapy*** ➤ Monitor IV flow rate and IV site during infusion. ➤ Monitor for IV patency before administration of IV medication.
Nursing diagnosis: Risk for Latex Allergy Response; or Latex Allergy Response related to multiple previous exposures to latex	***NOC outcomes:*** Immune Hypersensitivity Response Allergic Response: Localized ***NOC goals:*** (5) No localized inflammatory responses (5) Respiratory, cardiac, renal, and neurological functions not compromised (5) No localized rash, erythema, edema, or itching.	***Latex Precautions (Intraoperative)*** ➤ Place allergy band on patient [if not already done preoperatively]. ➤ Record allergy or risk in patient's medical record [or check to see that it was done]. ➤ Post sign indicating latex precautions. ➤ Survey environment and remove latex products. ➤ Monitor latex-free environment. ➤ Report information to physician, pharmacist, and other care providers, as indicated. ***Latex Precautions: (Preoperative)*** ➤ Question patient or appropriate other about history of neural tube defect (e.g., spina bifida) or congenital urological condition (e.g., exstrophy of the bladder). ➤ Question patient or appropriate other about history of systemic reactions to natural rubber latex (e.g., facial or scleral edema, tearing eyes, urticaria, rhinitis, and wheezing). ➤ Question patient or appropriate other about allergies to foods such as bananas, kiwi, avocado, mango, and chestnuts.

(continued)

Standardized Language

Intraoperative Patients: Selected Standardized Nursing Diagnoses, Outcomes, and Interventions—cont'd

NURSING DIAGNOSES (NANDA-I) AND COLLABORATIVE PROBLEMS	NOC OUTCOMES AND INDICATORS	NIC INTERVENTIONS AND ACTIVITIES (SHADED INTERVENTIONS ARE ROUTINELY PERFORMED FOR ALL SURGERY PATIENTS)
Nursing diagnosis: Risk for Perioperative Positioning Injury related to patient factors such as edema, emaciation, obesity, and sensory perceptual disturbances secondary to anesthesia ***Collaborative problem:*** Potential complication of surgery: neuromuscular, skeletal, or skin injury	***NOC outcomes:*** Circulation Status Mobility Neurological Status Physical Injury Severity Tissue Perfusion: Peripheral ***NOC goals:*** ➤ (4) PaO_2 mild deviation from normal range ➤ (4) $PaCO_2$ mild deviation from normal range ➤ (4) Pallor and dependent rubor mild ➤ (5) Joint movement not compromised ➤ (5) Spinal sensory/motor function not compromised ➤ (5) Central motor control not compromised ➤ (5) No burns, bruises, extremity or back sprains, impaired mobility ➤ (4) Capillary refill (fingers and toes) mild deviation from normal range ➤ (5) No numbness ➤ (5) All pulses no deviation from normal range ➤ (5) No skin breakdown	***Circulatory Precautions*** ➤ Perform a comprehensive appraisal of peripheral circulation (e.g., check peripheral pulses, edema, capillary refill, color, temperature of extremity, and ankle brachial index, if indicated). ***Positioning: Intraoperative*** ➤ Use assistive devices for immobilization. ➤ Lock wheels of stretcher and operating room bed. ➤ Use an adequate number of personnel to transfer patient. ➤ Support the head and neck during transfer. ➤ Immobilize or support any body part, as appropriate. ➤ Maintain patient's proper body alignment. ➤ Apply padding to bony prominences. ➤ Apply safety strap and arm restraint, as needed. ➤ Record position and devices used. ***Surgical Precautions*** ➤ Verify consent for surgery and other treatments, as appropriate. ➤ Verify with the patient or appropriate others the procedure and surgical site. ➤ Verify that patients identification band and blood band are correct. ➤ Verify the correct functioning of equipment. ➤ Monitor the accessories specific to the required surgical position e.g., supports, stirrups, fasteners). ➤ Assist in the transfer of the patient to the surgical table while monitoring devices. ➤ Count sponges, sharps, and instruments before, during, and after surgery, per agency policy; record results of counts. ➤ Provide an electrosurgical unit, grounding pad, and active electrode, as appropriate. ➤ Verify the integrity of electrical cords. ➤ Verify that the client is not in contact with metal. ➤ Verify absence of cardiac pacemaker, other electrical implant, or metal prostheses, contraindicating use of electrosurgical cautery. ➤ Inspect the patient's skin integrity at the site of [electrocautery] grounding pad. ➤ Verify that prep solutions are non-flammable or that flammable prep agents have evaporated prior to draping. ➤ Adjust coagulation and cutting currents, as instructed by physician or per agency policy. ➤ Inspect the patient's skin for injury [at conclusion of procedure]. ➤ (non-NIC) Monitor sterile technique throughout procedure.

Sources: Bulechek, G. M., Butcher, H. K., & Dochterman, J. M., et al. (Eds.) (2013). *Nursing interventions classification (NIC)* (6th ed.). St. Louis, MO: C.V. Mosby; Moorhead, S., Johnson, M., Maas, M., et al. (Eds.). (2013). *Nursing outcomes classification (NOC)* (5th ed.). St. Louis, MO: C.V. Mosby; NANDA International. (2012). *Nursing diagnoses: Definitions and classification 2012–2014*. Philadelphia: Author. Used with permission.

Standardized Language

Postoperative Patients: Selected Standardized Nursing Diagnoses, Outcomes, and Interventions

NURSING DIAGNOSES	OUTCOMES AND GOALS	NURSING INTERVENTIONS AND ACTIVITIES
These interventions are not routinely done for all patients. They are specific to patients who have the defining characteristics of each nursing diagnosis.		
Activity Intolerance r/t pain, the surgical procedure, and stressors of surgery	***NOC outcomes:*** Activity Tolerance Endurance Energy Conservation Psychomotor Energy ***NOC goals:*** ➤ O_2 saturation, heart rate, respiratory rate, systolic and diastolic blood pressure not compromised with activity ➤ Ease of breathing with activity not compromised ➤ Walking pace and distance not compromised ➤ Ease of performing activities of daily living (ADLs) not compromised ➤ Ability to speak with physical activity not compromised ➤ Energy restored after rest, not compromised ➤ Uses naps to restore energy, often demonstrated. ➤ Exhibits concentration, consistently demonstrated.	***NIC interventions:*** Activity Therapy Energy Management Exercise Promotion: Strength Training ***Nursing activities:*** ➤ Collaborate with [other disciplines] in planning and monitoring an activity program, as appropriate. ➤ Assist patient to choose activities . . . consistent with capabilities. ➤ Assist patient to focus on abilities rather than weaknesses. ➤ Encourage creative activities. . . . ➤ Instruct patient and family how to perform desired or prescribed activity. ➤ Refer to community centers, programs as appropriate. ➤ Arrange physical activities to reduce competition for oxygen supply to vital body functions (e.g., avoid activity immediately after meals). ➤ Avoid care activities during scheduled rest periods. ➤ Assist patient to sit on side of bed ("dangle"), if unable to transfer or walk. ➤ Monitor location and nature of pain during activity. ➤ Teach activity organization and time management techniques to prevent fatigue.
Acute Pain r/t (1) inflammation or injury in the surgical area, (2) abdominal distention secondary to decreased peristalsis, (3) muscle pain secondary to positioning and tension	***NOC outcomes:*** Pain Control Pain Level ***NOC goals:*** ➤ Consistently rates pain as controlled ➤ No moaning and crying ➤ No facial expressions of pain ➤ Describes causal factors, often demonstrated ➤ Uses preventive measures, consistently demonstrated. ➤ Uses nonanalgesic relief measures, often demonstrated. ➤ Uses analgesics as recommended, consistently demonstrated. ➤ Reports changes in pain symptoms to a health professional, consistently demonstrated. ***Other goals:*** No guarding of incision	***NIC interventions:*** Analgesic Administration Pain Management Patient-Controlled Analgesia Assistance ***Nursing activities:*** ➤ Perform a comprehensive assessment of pain to include location, characteristics, onset/duration, frequency, quality, intensity or severity of pain, and precipitating factors. ➤ Observe for nonverbal discomfort cues. ➤ Assure the patient attentive analgesic care. ➤ Consider cultural influences of responses to pain. ➤ Utilize developmentally appropriate assessment method. . . . ➤ Determine the needed frequency of making a pain assessment and implement monitoring plan. ➤ Provide information about the pain, such as causes, how long it will last, and anticipated discomforts from procedures. ➤ Control environmental factors that may influence the client's response to discomfort (e.g., room temperature . . . , noise). ➤ Provide the person optimal pain relief with prescribed analgesics.

(continued)

Standardized Language

Postoperative Patients: Selected Standardized Nursing Diagnoses, Outcomes, and Interventions—cont'd

NURSING DIAGNOSES	OUTCOMES AND GOALS	NURSING INTERVENTIONS AND ACTIVITIES
		➤ Implement patient-controlled analgesia as appropriate. ➤ Use pain control measures before pain becomes severe. ➤ Encourage patient to use adequate pain medication. ➤ Medicate before activity to increase participation, but evaluate the hazard of sedation. ➤ Teach nonpharmacological pain relief measures (e.g., guided imagery, progressive muscle relaxation). ➤ Utilize multidisciplinary approach to pain management.
Anxiety r/t change in health status, hospital environment	***NOC outcomes:*** Anxiety Level Anxiety Self-Control ***NOC goals:*** ➤ Consistently uses effective coping strategies. ➤ Often seeks information to reduce anxiety. ➤ Consistently uses relaxation techniques to reduce anxiety. ➤ Often maintains concentration. ➤ Verbalizes that anxiety is mild. ➤ Minimal restlessness, hand wringing, muscle tension, facial tension, difficulty concentrating. ➤ Mild changes in vital signs; no dilated pupils, sweating or dizziness ➤ Controls anxiety response consistently.	***NIC intervention:*** Anxiety Reduction ***Nursing activities:*** ➤ Use calm, reassuring approach. ➤ Assess for verbal and nonverbal signs of anxiety. ➤ Explain all procedures, including sensations likely to be experienced during the procedure. . . . ➤ Provide factual information concerning diagnosis, treatment, prognosis. ➤ Administer back rub or neck rub as appropriate. ➤ Listen attentively. ➤ Create trusting atmosphere. ➤ Help patient to identify situations that precipitate anxiety. ➤ [Assist the client to recognize that she is anxious]. ➤ Determine patient's decision-making ability. ➤ Encourage verbalization of feelings, perceptions, and fears [related to the surgical procedure]. ➤ Encourage family to stay with patient, as appropriate. ➤ Support use of appropriate defense mechanisms. ➤ Instruct the patient on the use of relaxation techniques.
Risk for Bleeding r/t side effects of surgery	***NOC outcomes:*** Blood Loss Severity Circulation Status ***NOC goals:*** ➤ (4) Systolic and diastolic blood pressure, mild deviation from normal. ➤ (5) Mean blood pressure not compromised. ➤ (5) Central venous pressure not compromised. ➤ (4)Urine output mildly compromised. ➤ (5) Hemoglobin and hematocrit are not compromised. ➤ (4) Mild Orthostatic hypotension present.	***NIC interventions:*** Bleeding Precautions Incision Site Care Surveillance ***Nursing activities:*** ➤ Monitor patient closely for hemorrhage. ➤ Note hemoglobin and hematocrit levels before and after blood loss as indicated. ➤ Monitor orthostatic vital signs, including blood pressure and pulse. ➤ Note characteristics of any drainage. ➤ Monitor the healing process at the incision site. ➤ Monitor for signs and symptoms of fluid and electrolyte imbalance. ➤ Monitor tissue perfusion, as appropriate. ➤ Activate rapid response team if indicated by patient bleeding or vital signs.

Standardized Language

Postoperative Patients: Selected Standardized Nursing Diagnoses, Outcomes, and Interventions—cont'd

NURSING DIAGNOSES	OUTCOMES AND GOALS	NURSING INTERVENTIONS AND ACTIVITIES
Nausea r/t manipulation of gastrointestinal tract, decreased peristalsis secondary to anesthesia	***NOC outcomes:*** Nausea & Vomiting Control Nausea & Vomiting: Disruptive Effects Nausea & Vomiting Severity Nutritional Status: Food & Fluid Intake ***NOC goals:*** ➤ (5) Reports nausea, retching, and vomiting controlled. ➤ (4) Mild or no intolerance of odors ➤ (4) Mild or no intolerance of movement ➤ (5) Recognizes onset of nausea. ➤ (5) Recognizes precipitating stimuli. ➤ (4) Frequency, intensity, and distress of nausea are mild. ➤ (5) Uses preventive measures often. ➤ (4) Only mild decrease in food and fluid intake ➤ (5) No weight loss ➤ (5) Reports bothersome side effects from antiemetics. ➤ (5) Reports failure of antiemetic treatment.	***NIC interventions:*** Nausea Management Medication Management ***Nursing activities:*** ➤ Provide information about the causes of nausea and how long it will last. ➤ Teach patient and/or family members the expected action and side effects of the [antiemetic] medication. ➤ Monitor recorded intake for nutritional content and calories. ➤ Encourage to monitor own nausea experience, including use of a symptom diary. ➤ Encourage patient to learn strategies for managing own nausea. ➤ Perform complete assessment of nausea, including frequency, duration, severity, and precipitating factors. . . . ➤ Observe for nonverbal cues of discomfort. . . . ➤ Evaluate past experiences with nausea (e.g., pregnancy and car sickness). ➤ Identify strategies that have been successful in relieving nausea. ➤ Teach the use of nonpharmacological techniques (e.g., guided imagery, self-hypnosis, relaxation, biofeedback, music therapy, distraction, acupressure) to manage nausea. ➤ Use frequent oral hygiene to promote comfort, unless it stimulates nausea. ➤ [Keep tissues and water to rinse the mouth nearby.] ➤ Give cold, clear liquid, odorless and colorless food, as appropriate. ➤ Instruct in high-carbohydrate and low-fat foods, as appropriate. ➤ Encourage eating small amounts of food that are appealing to the person. ➤ Encourage to drink cola, but not too cold; suck on an ice cube, sorbet, or a piece of frozen fruit. (non-NIC) ➤ Have the client sit in an upright position for 30 to 45 minutes after eating. (non-NIC) ➤ Control environmental factors that may evoke nausea (e.g., odors, sound, and unpleasant visual stimuli). ➤ Ensure that effective antiemetic drugs are given to prevent nausea when possible. . . .
Constipation r/t decreased activity, decreased food or fluid intake, decreased peristalsis secondary to anesthesia, pain medication	***NOC outcome:*** Bowel Elimination ***NOC goals:*** ➤ Elimination pattern not compromised ➤ Reports ease of stool passage not compromised.	***NIC interventions:*** Bowel Management Constipation/Impaction Management ***Nursing activities:*** ➤ Monitor for signs and symptoms of constipation. ➤ Note date of last bowel movement.

(continued)

Standardized Language

Postoperative Patients: Selected Standardized Nursing Diagnoses, Outcomes, and Interventions—cont'd

NURSING DIAGNOSES	OUTCOMES AND GOALS	NURSING INTERVENTIONS AND ACTIVITIES
	➤ Bowel sounds not compromised ➤ Muscle tone to evacuate stool not compromised ➤ Passes soft, formed stool in amount appropriate for diet. ➤ No pain with passage of stool ***Other:*** ➤ Bloating not present (non-NOC)	➤ Monitor bowel sounds. ➤ Monitor frequency, consistency, shape, volume, and color of bowel movements. ➤ Teach the patient about specific foods that assist in promoting bowel regularity. ➤ Insert a rectal suppository (or enema or irrigation), as appropriate. ➤ Evaluate medication profile for GI side effects (e.g., narcotic analgesics). ➤ Give warm liquids after meals, as appropriate. ➤ Encourage increased fluid intake, unless contraindicated. ➤ Instruct the client in foods high in fiber, as appropriate.
Urinary Retention r/t anesthesia, preoperative medications (anticholinergics), pain, fear, unfamiliar surroundings, client's position	***NOC outcome:*** Urinary Elimination ***NOC goals:*** ➤ Empties bladder completely, not compromised ➤ Fluid intake not compromised ➤ No hesitancy with urination ***Other:*** ➤ Bladder not palpable ➤ Reports subjective feeling of empty bladder. ➤ 24-hour intake and output balanced	***NIC interventions:*** Urinary Catheterization Urinary Retention Care ***Nursing activities:*** ➤ Perform comprehensive urinary assessment (e.g., urinary output, voiding pattern, cognitive function, preexisting urinary problems). ➤ Provide privacy for elimination. ➤ Use power of suggestion (run water, flush toilet). ➤ Provide enough time (10 minutes) for bladder emptying. ➤ Use spirits of wintergreen in bedpan or urinal. ➤ Insert urinary catheter as appropriate. ➤ Use percussion and palpation to estimate degree of bladder distention. (non-NIC) ➤ Catheterize for residual as appropriate.
Delayed Surgical Recovery (etiologies will vary with pathology) (*Note:* This diagnosis is broad and encompasses some of the other diagnoses. If the client has Delayed Surgical Recovery, you will not, for example, need a diagnosis of Nausea on the plan of care.)	***NOC outcomes:*** Ambulation Blood Loss Severity Endurance Hydration Infection Severity Nausea & Vomiting Severity Pain Level Post-Procedure Recovery Wound Healing: Primary Intention ***NOC goals:*** ➤ Decrease in systolic or diastolic blood pressure, mild. ➤ Energy restored after rest. ➤ Tissue perfusion not compromised. ➤ Ambulation tolerance in normal range ➤ No nausea, vomiting, shivering	***NIC interventions:*** Embolus Precautions Exercise Therapy: Ambulation Incision Site Care Nutrition Management Pain Management Self-Care Assistance ***Nursing activities:*** ➤ Inspect the incision site for redness, swelling, or signs of dehiscence. ➤ Monitor for postoperative complications. ➤ Monitor the healing process in the incision site. ➤ Provide incision care as needed. (non-NIC) ➤ Teach the client and family how to care for the incision, including signs and symptoms of infection. ➤ Facilitate early ambulation postoperatively.

Standardized Language

Postoperative Patients: Selected Standardized Nursing Diagnoses, Outcomes, and Interventions—cont'd

NURSING DIAGNOSES	OUTCOMES AND GOALS	NURSING INTERVENTIONS AND ACTIVITIES
	➤ No fever. ➤ Only mild pain ➤ No post-surgical bleeding ***Other:*** ➤ Ready for discharge within prescribed length of stay for surgery performed ➤ No postoperative complications (e.g., bleeding, infection, delayed wound healing, pneumonia)	➤ Instruct patient on diet requirements for disease state (e.g., for wound healing, encourage increased intake of protein, iron, and vitamin C, as appropriate). ➤ Determine number of calories and type of nutrients needed to meet nutrition requirements. ➤ Select and implement a variety of measures (e.g., pharmacological, nonpharmacological, interpersonal) to facilitate pain relief, as appropriate. ➤ Teach principles of pain management. ➤ Encourage independence, but intervene when the client is unable to perform.

Sources: Bulechek, G. M., Butcher, H. K., & Dochterman, J. M., et al. (Eds.) (2013). *Nursing interventions classification (NIC)* (6th ed.). St. Louis, MO: C.V. Mosby; Moorhead, S., Johnson, M., Maas, M., et al. (Eds.). (2013). *Nursing outcomes classification (NOC)* (5th ed.). St. Louis, MO: C.V. Mosby; NANDA International. (2012). *Nursing diagnoses: Definitions and classification 2012–2014*. Philadelphia: Author. Used with permission.

CLINICALREASONING

Applying the Full-Spectrum Nursing Model

PATIENT SITUATION

Recall Nishad Singh (Meet Your Patient, in Volume 1). He is a 68-year-old man who came to the emergency department (ED) with sudden onset of rectal bleeding. He had been "tired and dragging for several months." The ED nurse identified nursing diagnoses of Mild Anxiety, Pain, and Risk for Bleeding. Preoperatively, his vital signs were as follows:

BP: 138/88 mm Hg
Pulse: 104 beats/min and regular; 120 beats/min; 134 beats/min
Respiratory rate: 20 breaths/min
Temperature: 36.7°C (98.0°F)
Oxygen saturation: 98%

Mr. Singh was admitted to the hospital where he received an IV of 1,000 mL of lactated Ringer's solution and a unit of packed red blood cells. He was to undergo emergency colon resection surgery; however, a left hemicolectomy including the sigmoid colon and the anus was required. He spent 4 hours in the PACU, until his vital signs stabilized. Mr. Singh now has a colostomy high in his descending colon, with a stoma on his left abdomen slightly superior to the level of his umbilicus. He also has an abdominal incision that was made for exploration. On the next day after the surgery, the surgeon informed Mr. Singh that he has widespread adenocarcinoma (cancer) of the colon with metastasis to the liver. The nurse has identified these four nursing diagnoses (among others):

Deficient Knowledge (colostomy care) r/t lack of prior experience and no preparation prior to surgery
Fear r/t diagnosis of colon cancer, liver metastasis, and possible terminal illness
Pain secondary to surgical incision and manipulation of abdominal organs during the surgical procedure
Risk for Impaired Skin Integrity r/t irritation from fecal drainage and ostomy pouch

THINKING

1. *Theoretical Knowledge:*
   a. What is a left hemicolectomy? If you do not know the answer, consult an appropriate reference.
   b. What does "metastasis to the liver" mean? If you do not know the answer, consult an appropriate reference.
2. *Critical Thinking (Inquiry):*
   a. Why might Mr. Singh have needed a colostomy instead of having his transverse colon reconnected to the remaining lower colon or rectum? State the reference you used to answer this question.
   b. Why do you think Mr. Singh has a colostomy above the level of the umbilicus and not lower down in his abdomen? State the reference you used to answer this question.

DOING

3. *Practical Knowledge:* Mr. Singh returned from surgery with knee-high antiembolism stockings.
   a. You notice that the stockings have slid down and become wrinkled between his knees and ankles. After you straighten them and pull them up, the tops reach to about 7.6 cm (3 in.) below Mr. Singh's knees. What does this probably mean, and what should you do?
   b. Which of the following instructions should you give when delegating care of Mr. Singh's antiembolism stockings to the nursing assistant? (Mr. Singh's stockings have closed toes.)
      - Remove the stockings and bathe and dry the legs every 8 to 12 hours.
      - Massage the legs after removing Mr. Singh's stockings.
      - Before reapplying stockings, report the presence of any lesions, sores, or redness of the lower extremities.
      - Instruct the patient to remain supine for at least 15 minutes after removing the stockings.
      - Make sure there are no wrinkles in the stockings once they have been applied.
      - Tug gently on the end of the stocking to create a small space between the end of the toes and the stocking.
4. *Nursing Process (Nursing Diagnosis):* List Mr. Singh's four nursing diagnoses in order of priority. List the highest priority first. Explain how you decided the priorities.

CARING

5. *Self-Knowledge:*
   c. If you were assigned to care for Mr. Singh today, what aspect of care would you feel best prepared to give? Explain your thinking.
   d. What aspect of Mr. Singh's care would you be most uncomfortable providing? Explain your thinking.
6. *Ethical Knowledge:* You want to provide culturally competent care. What is the first thing you will need to do in order to address Mr. Singh's cultural needs? Review Chapter 15 if you need to.

Critical Thinking and Clinical Reasoning

1. You are speaking with several classmates about an upcoming surgical rotation. During the rotation, you will have a opportunity to work with a circulating nurse and a scrub nurse. One of your classmates says that she is very nervous. "I don't know whether I will be able to handle this rotation. I'm afraid I might not be able to watch the surgery. I've never really seen anything gross like that before." Another classmate confides that she is worried that she will contaminate everything and put the client at risk. What advice can you give them, and what actions can you take to prepare yourself for your experience in the OR?
2. You are working on a busy surgical unit on the evening shift. There is one NAP on the unit this evening. You are caring for the following clients:
   - Mr. Singh (Meet Your Patient, in Volume 1), who underwent a colon resection and colostomy for colon cancer. He is now in postoperative day 2 and is complaining of chest pain and shortness of breath.
   - Ms. Yasmin, a 52-year-old woman admitted to the unit from PACU 1 hour ago after total abdominal hysterectomy and bilateral salpingo-oophrectomy (TAH-BSO—removal of the uterus, ovaries, and fallopian tubes)
   - Steven Stellanski, a 16-year-old with trisomy 21 who underwent an emergency appendectomy early this morning.

   The PACU calls to inform you that they are ready to transport Mrs. Bauer back to the unit. She is an 87-year-old woman from the local skilled nursing facility who underwent an extensive debridement of a stage IV pressure ulcer on the coccyx. The PACU nurse tells you Mrs. Bauer is confused and agitated and will need close monitoring.
   a. What problem(s) does admission of this new patient present for you? To answer this question, identify the priority nursing activity for each of the three patients you already have, as well as for Mrs. Bauer.
   b. How will you handle this situation? Identify three options, and explain their advantages and disadvantages.
3. You will be caring for a 23-year-old client who underwent emergency surgery after an automobile accident. He has had no preoperative teaching. What concerns does this raise for you? How will you address these concerns?
4. For each of the following concepts, use critical thinking to describe how or why it is important to nursing, patient care, or perioperative nursing. Note that these are *not* to be merely definitions.

   Preoperative teaching
   Preoperative physical preparation
   Intraoperative safety measures
   Anesthesia
   Postoperative complications

What Are the Main Points in This Chapter?

- Perioperative nursing includes care of patients during the preoperative, intraoperative, and postoperative phases.
- Perioperative nursing requires the systematic integration and synthesis of the nursing process with established standards of practice.
- The Association of periOperative Registered Nurses (AORN) is the organization that developed the standards of care that inform perioperative nursing and the standardized language, the Perioperative Nursing Data Set (PNDS).
- "Never Events" are serious and costly errors resulting in severe consequences for the patient, and that are mostly preventable. Medicare will not reimburse institutions for care related to complications caused by never events.
- Surgical risk is associated with the type of surgery and the condition of the patient (e.g., age, general health, personal habits).
- During the preoperative period, it is essential to determine whether the client is physiologically, cognitively, and psychologically prepared for the intraoperative and postoperative phases of surgery.
- Preoperative care includes assessment, preoperative teaching, confirming that surgical consent has been obtained; preventing wrong patient, wrong site, wrong surgery; communicating with the surgical team; preparing the patient physically for surgery; transferring the patient to the operative suite; and preparing the postoperative room on the surgical unit.
- The surgical consent form is a witnessed legal document that ensures that the surgical patient has given informed consent for the surgical procedure. The physician is legally responsible for obtaining informed consent; however, the nurse sometimes obtains the patient's signature on the form after verifying that the patient has been informed.
- A great deal of perioperative nursing care is standardized, aimed at preventing potential complications, and applicable to all patients having surgery.
- General anesthesia produces rapid unconsciousness and loss of sensation. Regional anesthesia produces loss of pain sensation without loss of consciousness.
- Intraoperative care includes skin preparation, positioning the patient for surgery, and protective measures to ensure patient safety during surgery.
- The PACU RN integrates knowledge of common complications of surgery, well-established nursing diagnoses for the postoperative client, and data from an individualized comprehensive postoperative assessment to plan and implement appropriate outcomes and interventions for the client during the postoperative stage.
- Assessments during postoperative recovery are the same as those performed in the PACU, but they can be performed less frequently.
- Antiembolism stockings and sequential compression devices may be used to help prevent thrombophlebitis.
- Incentive spirometry may be used to help prevent atelectasis and pneumonia.
- Gastrointestinal suction may be used for gastric decompression after certain surgeries to prevent gastric distention, which can increase respiratory complications, place a strain on suture lines, and interfere with wound closure.

Knowledge Map

THE PERIOPERATIVE EXPERIENCE

PREOPERATIVE PHASE: Preparing the client for surgery

NURSING ASSESSMENTS:
- Health history: allergies, medications, alcohol/drug use
- Surgical risk factors
- Culture/spiritual factors
- Access to resources
- Coping strategies
- Understanding of surgery and anesthesia

PHYSICAL PREP:
- NPO
- Skin prep
- Bowel and bladder
- Pre-op medication
  - Routine meds
- Prosthesis management
- Antiembolism stockings

FACTORS AFFECTING SURGICAL RISK:
- Age
- Wounds present
- Preexisting conditions
- Mental status
- Medications: (e.g., anticoagulants; steroids)
- Personal/lifestyle habits
- Allergies

SURGERIES: CLASSIFIED BY:
- Body system involved
- Purpose (e.g., diagnostic, cosmetic)
- Urgency:
  - Emergency, urgent, elective
- Risk involved:
  - Major; minor

SAFETY: Signed/informed surgical consent

TEACHING:
- Based on the type of surgery
- Explanation of care pre, during and post surgery
- At patient's level; using appropriate language
- Written instructions; discussion

INTRAOPERATIVE PHASE

STERILE TEAM:
- Surgeon
- Surgical assistant
- Scrub person

CLEAN TEAM:
- Anesthesiologist
- Circulating nurse
- Technicians

ADMINISTRATION OF ANESTHESIA:
- General
- Conscious sedation
- Regional

SAFETY:
- Positioning
- Maintaining sterile fields
- Monitoring I&O
- Handling specimens
- Sponge/instrument count
- Documentation

POSTOPERATIVE PHASE

POST ANESTHESIA CARE UNIT: PACU
- Focused physical assessments
- Frequent monitoring:
  - Vital signs
  - Airway
  - LOC
  - Positioning
  - Wound/sutures
  - Dressings/drainage devices
  - IV therapy
  - Comfort

THE SURGICAL UNIT

- Continued frequent monitoring
- Patient/family teaching
  - Ambulation
  - Incentive spirometer
  - SCDs
  - Diet
  - Activity
  - Signs/symptoms to report
  - Follow-up appointment
- Prevention early detection of potential complications
  - Aspiration pneumonia/pneumonia
  - Atelectasis
  - DVT/PE
  - Hemorrhage
  - Hypovolemia
  - Nausea/vomiting; distention
  - Constipation/ileus
  - Urinary retention/infection
  - Renal failure
  - Dehydration
  - Evisceration
  - Infection

CHAPTER 40

Leading & Managing

STUDENT RESOURCES

The questions and exercises in Volume 2 allow you to practice the kind of thinking you will use as a full-spectrum nurse. Critical-thinking questions usually have more than one correct answer, so we do not provide "answers" for these features. It is more important to develop your nursing judgment than to just cover content. You will learn by discussing the questions with your peers. If you are still unsure, consult your instructor. You will find Response Sheets (for writing your response to the questions) on DavisPlus.

To explore learning resources for this chapter,

Go to Davis*Plus* at DavisPl.us/Wilkinson3.

Chapter Resources for Chapter 40:

- **Response sheets for all learning activities**
- **Resources for Caregivers and Health Professionals**
- **Reading More About Leading & Managing (suggested readings)**
- **Concept Map of chapter content**

Interactive Case Studies

NCLEX-Style and Chapter Review Questions

CHAPTER OVERVIEW

For a podcast of an overview of this chapter,

Go to Student Resources, Chapter 40, **Podcast—Chapter Overview,** on Davis*Plus*.

Caring for the Nguyens

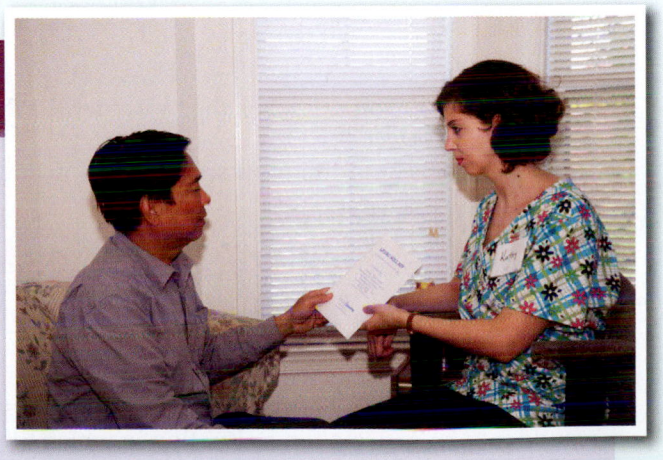

Anh Chu, Nam's aunt, is scheduled for outpatient cataract surgery later this week at the local hospital. Nam reports to the clinic wishing to discuss the plan for his aunt's surgery "with whoever is the boss." Nam is concerned that his aunt will not be staying at the hospital. "She's having surgery. I don't understand this! She's 78 years old. She's going to need help. This doesn't make sense. You have to change things. It won't be safe to do this as planned."

Nam tells you he has discussed his concerns with the ophthalmologist. He tells you that the ophthalmologist told him he was "overreacting. We always do it this way. You just don't understand." Nam is visibly upset. He

(Continued)

Caring for the Nguyens (continued)

believes that his aunt is receiving inadequate care. He appeals to you to help him take care of his aunt. "This is where Aunt Chu gets her care. You know her. You have to change this."

Anh Chu has been seen at the family clinic several times over the past few years. She takes a medication for osteoporosis and has been counseled about the need for exercise and weight loss. She has also begun to experience problems with "accidents," that is, urine leakage. She has never had surgery in the past, and her only hospitalizations have been for childbirth. Ms. Chu's husband recently passed away, and she has been living alone since then. Devise a plan to resolve this conflict with Nam.

CLINICALREASONING

Applying the Full-Spectrum Nursing Model

ORGANIZATIONAL SITUATION

A small, not-for-profit hospice center in a small community has received a generous memorial gift from the family of a client who recently died. The family asked only that the money be "put to the best possible use." Everyone in the facility has an opinion about the best use for the money.

The administrator wants to renovate their old, run-down headquarters. The financial officer wants to put the money in the bank "for a rainy day." The chaplain wants to add a small chapel to the building. The nurses want to create a food bank to help the poorest of their clients. The social workers want to buy a van to transport clients to healthcare providers. The staff has agreed that all the ideas have merit and all the needs are important. Unfortunately, there is enough money to meet only one of them.

The more the staff members discuss how to use this gift, the more insistent each group becomes about defending its own idea. At the last meeting it is clear that some are becoming angry and frustrated. A shouting match even occurs between the administrator and the financial officer.

THINKING

1. *Theoretical Knowledge:*
   Which is appropriate at this point, a problem-solving approach or informal negotiation? Explain your answer.

DOING

2. *Practical Knowledge:*
   If you were to conduct the informal negotiation, list the steps of the plan you would follow.

CARING

3. *Self-Knowledge:*
   Which idea do you think has the most merit? Why did you select the one you did?
4. *Ethical Knowledge:*
   Which groups or individuals seem to demonstrate the value of caring for clients? Explain your thinking.

Critical Thinking and Clinical Reasoning

1. Identify a personal or professional change that you would like to see take place, and outline the steps needed to implement the change.
2. Eleanor, an LPN returning to school to obtain her associate's degree in nursing, is faced with a multitude of responsibilities. A wife, a mother of two toddlers, and a full-time staff member at a local hospital, Eleanor suddenly finds herself in a situation in which there just are not enough hours in a day. She is convinced that becoming a registered nurse is an impossible goal. You are Eleanor's mentor. When you ask where she wants to be in 5 years, she answers, "At this moment, I think, on an island in Tahiti!"
   a. Help Eleanor develop a personal time inventory. To help her determine specifically what to include, make your own personal time inventory to share with her as an example.

b. Once Eleanor has finished her time plan, how would you advise her to use it to make better use of her time? Make specific suggestions.

3. What strategies could you use to better manage your time?
4. Why is it important to learn good time management habits while you are a student?
5. This is your first semester in the nursing program. Although you have attended college to complete the prerequisite courses, this seems to be so different. All of a sudden, you have to attend clinical rotations in addition to classes. And you have to prepare ahead of time for the clinical experience, often even going to the hospital the night before to obtain information related to your patients. You feel like you are drowning! What can you do?

Go to Chapter 40, **Table 40-4: Components of Time Management,** in Volume I.

Work through the table, asking yourself questions such as the following. Be very specific in your answers; give examples.

a. *Prioritizing:*
   - What tasks do you have to complete on a daily basis? Weekly? During the semester?
   - List the tasks in order of importance.
   - Which of the tasks do you have control over (e.g., scheduling a haircut or setting aside time to read the next assignment versus taking a test that is scheduled)?

b. *Assigning priorities:* Assign priorities to the tasks you have identified.

c. *Questioning effectiveness, efficiency:* Ask yourself, "How can I accomplish these tasks in the least amount of time but to the best of my ability?"

d. *Rechecking:* Review your plan. Mentally and physically recheck the plan. Revise the plan as needed.

e. *Self-reliance:* Carry out your plan. Use critical-thinking skills, and adapt the plan as needed so that you "go with the flow."

f. *Treating:* Be good to yourself, but commit yourself to time management and excellence. How can you do that? What treats will you give yourself?

6. For each of the following concepts, use critical thinking to describe how or why it is important to nursing, patient care, or managing or leading. Note that these are *not* to be merely definitions.

Leadership skills	Time management
Management skills	Resolving conflicts
Becoming a mentor	Delegating appropriately
Being a mentee	Understanding the change process

What Are the Main Points in This Chapter?

- Leadership is the ability to influence other people.
- Transformational leaders communicate their vision in a way that reduces negativity and inspires commitment in people.
- Three common behavioral leadership styles are authoritarian, democratic, and laissez-faire.
- A manager is an employee of an organization who has power, authority, and responsibility for planning and directing the work of others.
- Effective managers possess a combination of qualities: leadership skills, clinical expertise, and business sense.
- A manager's activities are generally organizational, interpersonal, and informational.
- Not all leaders should be managers, but all managers should be leaders.
- It is never too early in your career to develop a SWOT or SOAR analysis. Throughout your nursing program, revisit the analysis, and update it as you gain new knowledge and skills.
- A mentor is a role model who develops the novice nurse to be a professional by coaching, encouraging, supporting, and guiding him or her.
- Be mindful of nurses who demonstrate strong mentor qualities. Do not be afraid to ask for their support and guidance. Develop mentor qualities of your own, so you can also mentor a new student.
- At times throughout our nursing careers, we will all assume the role of follower.
- Followers need to be self-directing, actively participating experts who work on behalf of the organization.

- Sources of power include authority, reward, expertise, and coercion.
- Nurses have expertise, power, and authority over other healthcare workers. It is important that you understand your sources of power and use them wisely.
- Empowerment is the feeling of self-determination, competence, and recognition that your expertise and power within the healthcare system have meaning and positive impact.
- Evaluative feedback is a leadership responsibility that reinforces constructive and discourages undesirable behavior; provides recognition; and develops employee skills.
- Delegation of patient care tasks to other healthcare workers is one of the most important responsibilities of the registered nurse.
- Nurses must understand change and act as change agents within today's healthcare setting.
- Managing change involves recognizing and decreasing resistance.
- Conflict is inevitable, but it does not need to be destructive.
- One of a manager's responsibilities is to facilitate conflict resolution and, if necessary, function as an informal negotiator.
- Effective time management is essential to planning safe, effective patient care and demonstrating management skills.
- Time management includes goal setting and organizing and streamlining your work.
- Do not forget to get rest and "time off" when managing time.

Knowledge Map

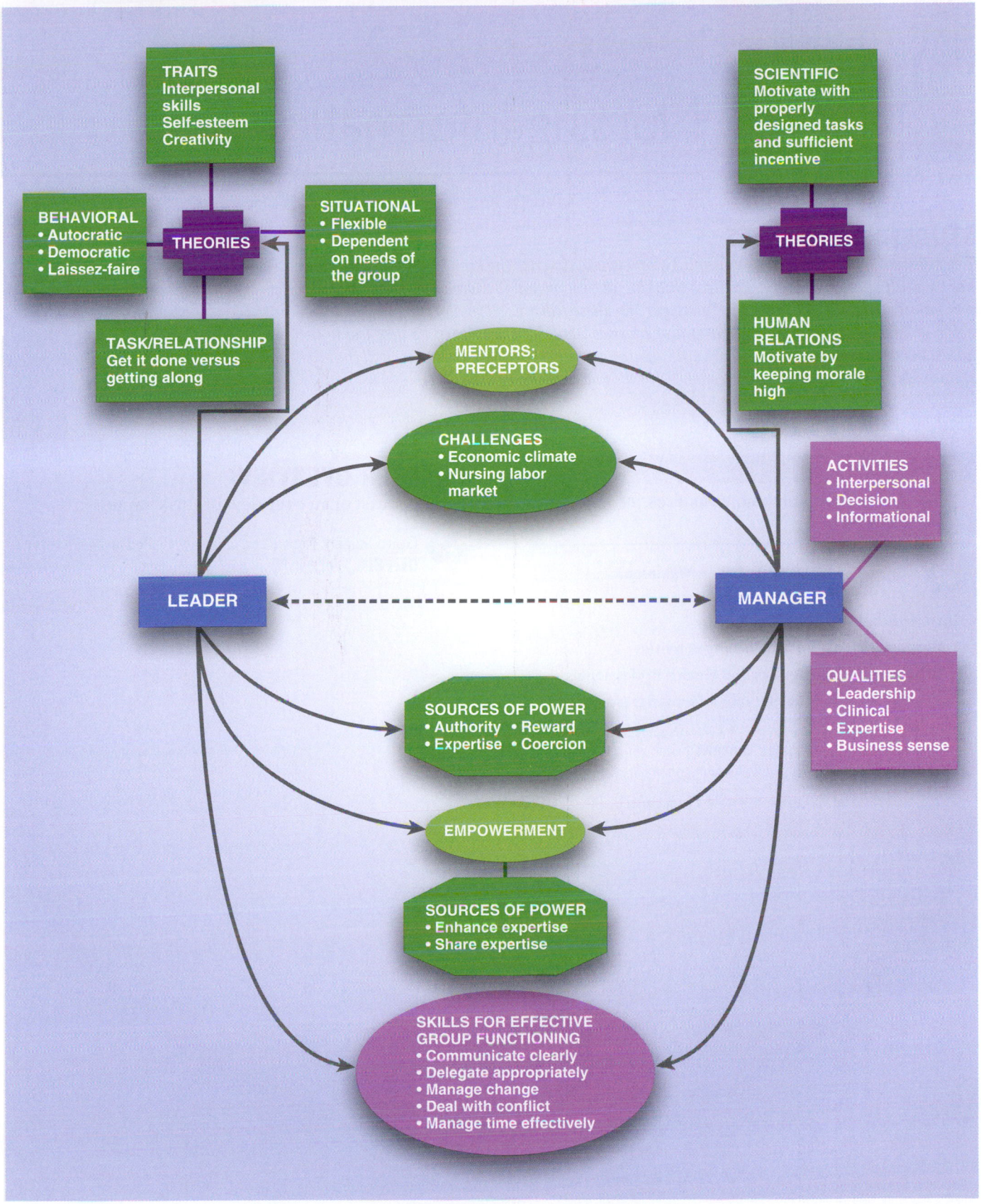

CHAPTER 41

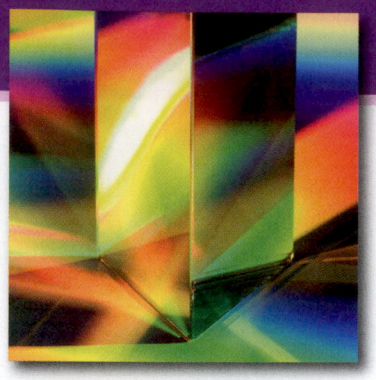

Nursing Informatics

STUDENT RESOURCES

*The questions and exercises in Volume 2 allow you to practice the kind of thinking you will use as a full-spectrum nurse. Critical-thinking questions usually have more than one correct answer, so we do not provide "answers" for these features. It is more important to develop your nursing judgment than to just cover content. You will learn by discussing the questions with your peers. If you are still unsure, consult your instructor. You will find Response Sheets (for writing your responses to the questions) on Davis*Plus.

To explore learning resources for this chapter,

Go to Davis*Plus* at DavisPl.us/Wilkinson3.

Chapter Resources for Chapter 41:

- **Response sheets for all learning activities**
- **Resources for Caregivers and Health Professionals**
- **Reading More About Nursing Informatics (suggested readings)**
- **Concept Map of chapter content**

Interactive Case Studies

NCLEX-Style and Chapter Review Questions

CHAPTER OVERVIEW

For a podcast of an overview of this chapter,

Go to Student Resources, Chapter 41, **Podcast—Chapter Overview,** on Davis*Plus*.

Caring for the Nguyens

Nam Nguyen, a patient you have been caring for at the Family Medicine Center, has been devastated by his recent diagnoses of type 2 diabetes mellitus and hypertension. "Oh my, this is bad. This stuff kills you. I don't understand what I did to cause this," he sighs. He is having difficulty following his medication regimen and says he doesn't understand what he is supposed to do. You have supplied him with information at each of his clinic visits as well as handouts, medication information, and a reminder sheet for his medicines. Nam asks you whether there is any information available on the Internet.

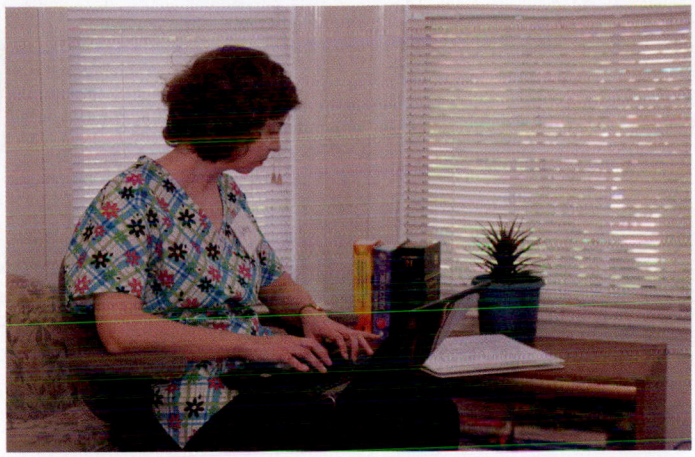

A. What advice would you give him about looking up medical information on the Internet?

B. What sources would you recommend to Nam?

Practical Knowledge knowing how

STANDARDIZED LANGUAGE

Standardized Language

American Nurses Association Recognized Languages for Nursing

Language	Description	Recognition Date
Diagnostic Related Group (DRG)	DRG is a classification system for most health conditions to establish a standardized reimbursement system for Medicare.	1983
NANDA International	2012–2014 Nursing Diagnoses Language includes 13 Domains with diagnostic labels with etiologies, risk factors, and defining characteristics.	1992
Nursing Interventions Classification (NIC)	The sixth edition contains 554 direct and indirect interventions assigned to one of seven domains and 30 classes. Each intervention includes a concept label, definition, and activities.	1992
Clinical Care Classification (CCC)	Developed by Virginia Saba, this language is used primarily by home health agencies and community settings. This language contains nursing diagnoses and interventions developed to code, index, classify, document, track, and analyze clinical care processes.	1992
Omaha System	This language also documents care in community and home care agencies. This system consists of four levels including 42 nursing diagnoses (patient assessment and problem classification), nursing interventions (delivery of care), and a problem-rating scale for outcomes.	1992
Nursing Outcomes Classification (NOC)	The fifth edition of NOC consists of 490 outcomes, including seven family-unit and six community-level outcomes. The NOC is a comprehensive standardized language designed to help clinicians evaluate the effectiveness of nursing interventions.	1997
Nursing Management Minimum Data Set (NMMDS)	This data set describes the healthcare and nursing environment associated with the diagnosis, intervention, and outcome segments from the administrative, management, and resource management perspectives. It is composed of 17 data elements in three categories: environment, nurse resources, and financial resources.	1998

(Continued)

Standardized Language

American Nurses Association Recognized Languages for Nursing—cont'd

Language	Description	Recognition Date
Perioperative Nursing Data Set (PNDS)	The PNDS language describes perioperative nursing practice and consists of 64 nursing diagnoses, 127 nursing interventions, and 29 patient outcomes. This was the first nursing language developed by a nursing specialty.	1999
Statistical Nomenclature of Medicine Clinical Terminology (SNOMED CT)	SNOMED CT is a reference terminology that includes clinical concepts used to describe assessment, diagnosis, intervention, and outcome. Although it includes nursing concepts, it is not developed specifically for nursing, but rather for a broad spectrum of healthcare domains.	2002
Nursing Minimum Data Sets (NMDS)	This data collection establishes comparability of nursing data across population settings, geographic areas, and times. It describes the nursing care of patients or clients and their families in a variety of settings, both institutional and noninstitutional.	1999
International Classification for Nursing Practice (ICNP)	ICNP describes nursing practice in various clinical settings worldwide using common language. It includes nursing phenomena or diagnoses, outcomes, and actions.	2000

CLINICALREASONING

Applying the Full-Spectrum Nursing Model

PATIENT SITUATION

Sarita, a nurse working in the surgical ICU, is ordering patient lab work and recording patient information in the electronic health record (EHR). While at the computer terminal, a physician walks over to her and requests an update on a postsurgery patient's condition. They go to the bedside to assess the patient's color and perfusion. Another nurse, Janelle, needs to order a STAT x-ray using the central computer in the unit. When Sarita goes back to the computer screen to order lab work and finish her documentation, Janelle has stepped in and is now accessing another patient's record.

THINKING

1. *Theoretical Knowledge:*
   a. Name five benefits of using an electronic health record for storing and retrieving patient data in a busy critical care unit.
   b. List five potential areas of difficulty in using this same electronic health record.
2. *Critical Thinking (Considering Alternatives):*
   a. Brainstorm about possible solutions for dealing with bottlenecks among staff using a centralized computer.

DOING

3. *Practical Knowledge:*
   a. Where would you look to find out who has accessed the patient record?

CARING

4. *Ethical Knowledge:*
   a. What violation has Sarita committed in this situation? What should she have done instead?
   b. What is the nurse's responsibility in protecting patient information in the electronic record? What kinds of things should the nurse do?

5. *Self-Knowledge:*
   a. Have you ever been so busy that you felt as though you just needed to take a "necessary" shortcut to save time? Describe your experience.

Go To Chapter 41, **Applying the Full-Spectrum Nursing Model Response Sheet,** on Davis*Plus*.

Critical Thinking and Clinical Reasoning

1. Refer to the following table. For each of the uses listed, what kind of information do you think the database should provide? That is, what kind of data would you need? For example, look at the first item under In Nursing Practice. For "Literature access and retrieval," you would use a database that contains information about journals, books, reports, and their content, perhaps CINAHL. For all of the following (Use in Nursing Practice), what kind of database would you use? What kind of information would you need? The first one is done for you.

   Work with your classmates. Share your knowledge and experience to answer these questions. Consult your instructor as needed.

USE	TYPE OF INFORMATION NEEDED
In Nursing Practice	
Literature access and retrieval (e.g., for evidence-based practice)	***Suggested response:*** CINAHL; information about books, journals, and their content; possibly the Internet
Care planning	***Clues:*** What information would you need for care planning? Where would you find it?
Client records (e.g., documenting, order entry, retrieving lab results)	
Telenursing (e.g., in home health)	
Case management	
In Nursing Education	
Literature access and retrieval	
Computer-assisted instruction (CAI) programs	
Classroom technology	
Distance learning	
Testing and grading	
Student records	
In Nursing Administration	
Quality assurance/improvement and utilization review	***Clues:*** What information would you need to evaluate the quality of care in your institution? Where would you find it?
Employee records (e.g., to track licenses, immunizations)	
Staffing patterns, hiring	
Buildings and facilities management	
Finance and budgets	
Accreditation reviews (e.g., monitoring quality control)	

(Continued)

USE	TYPE OF INFORMATION NEEDED
In Nursing Research	
Literature review	
Data collection	
Data analysis (both qualitative and quantitative)	
Research dissemination	
Applying for grants	

2. Search for "online nursing journals" on the Internet. Make a list of nursing journals that provide full-text articles that are available on the Internet, and at no charge. Hint:

Go to Chapter 41, **Resources for Caregivers and Health Professionals,** on Davis*Plus*.

3. For each of the following concepts, use critical thinking to describe how or why it is important to nursing, patients, or nursing informatics. Note that these are *not* to be merely definitions.

Nursing informatics	Connectivity
Data	Electronic mailing lists
Knowledge	Telehealth
Wisdom	Electronic health records
Evidence-based practice	Standardized nursing language
Computers	Literature databases
Hardware	World Wide Web
Storage media	Evaluating Web sites

What Are the Main Points in This Chapter?

- Whatever their roles—staff nurse, administrator, educator, researcher, primary care provider—nurses use data, information, and knowledge in their daily work.
- Informatics is the processing and management of data, information, and knowledge necessary for making practice decisions.
- The nursing informatics specialist uses nursing science, computer science, and information science to manage and communicate data, information, knowledge, and wisdom in nursing practice.
- A computer has four main functions: input, processing, output, and storage. Together they are known as information processing (or data processing).
- *Connectivity* is a term referring to the ways in which computers and other hardware communicate and share information.
- Some forms of electronic communication include electronic mail and text messaging, web conferencing and webinars, electronic distribution lists, social networking, interactive gaming and virtual learning, and telehealth applications.
- Electronic health records (EHRs) are a platform for communication among the interdisciplinary healthcare team regarding patient healthcare needs, patient data, plan for care.
- EHRs allow clinicians to create, store, edit, and retrieve patient charts via the Internet or local intranet software.
- An important benefit of EHRs is reduced errors resulting from illegible handwriting.
- EHRs equip providers with clinical support tools to conveniently access information to assist with clinical decision-making.

- Standardized languages within the EHR facilitate research to improve healthcare. They also aid in billing, recordkeeping, and scheduling follow-up care.
- It is important to use and protect passwords to guard the privacy of patient records.
- Computer illiteracy and discomfort with technology is a common reason for resisting use of an EHR. Many claim documentation in the system is time consuming, especially when less familiar with the system.
- Evidence-based practice requires the ability to organize and manage information to identify a clinical problem, search the literature, evaluate the evidence, and plan an intervention.
- An information literate person seeks authoritative, current, and reliable sources of information from trusted Internet sources.
- CINAHL and MEDLINE are two important databases to search for nursing literature.

Knowledge Map

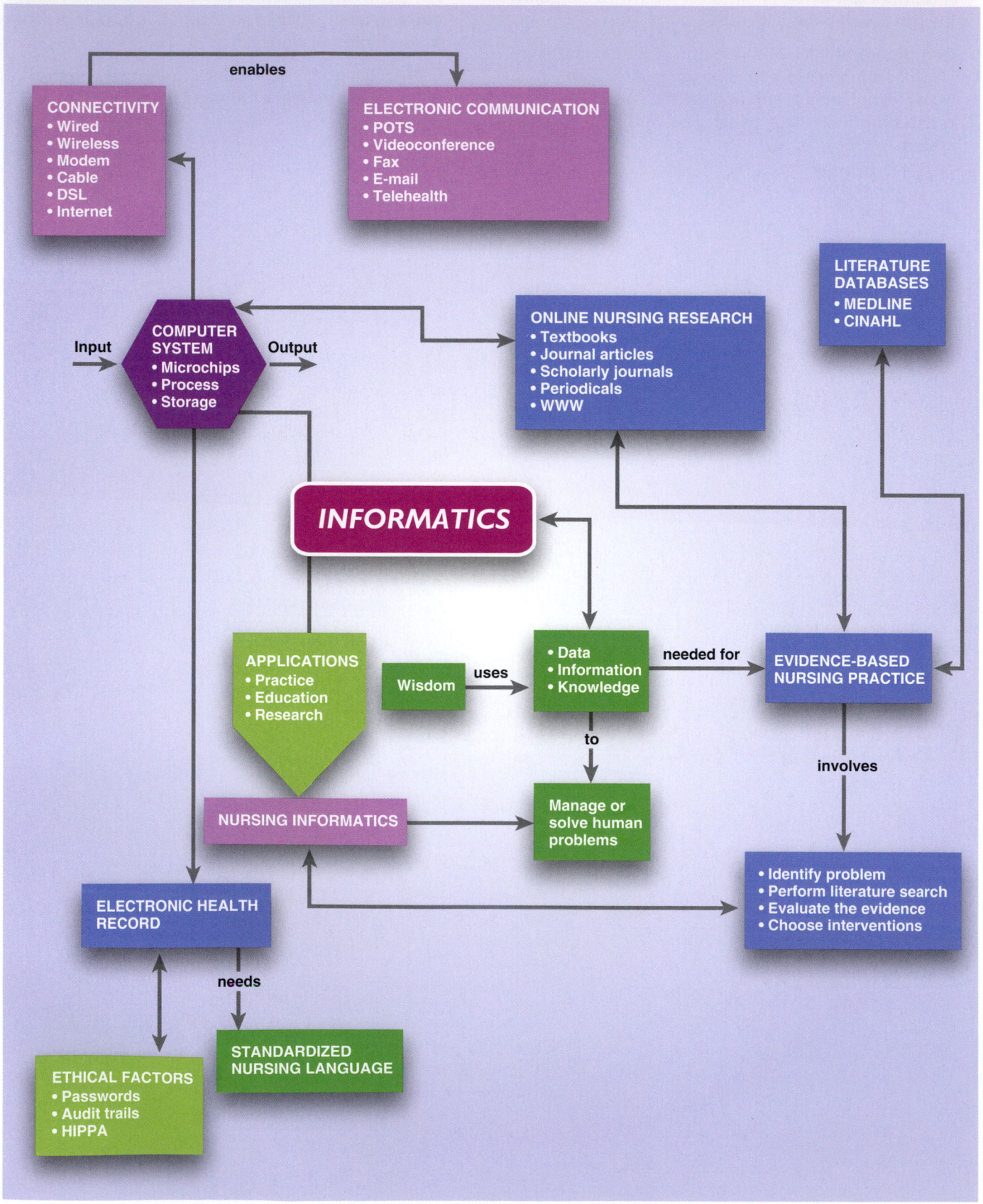

CHAPTER 42

Promoting Health

STUDENT RESOURCES

*The questions and exercises in Volume 2 allow you to practice the kind of thinking you will use as a full-spectrum nurse. Critical-thinking questions usually have more than one correct answer, so we do not provide "answers" for these features. It is more important to develop your nursing judgment than to just cover content. You will learn by discussing the questions with your peers. If you are still unsure, consult your instructor. You will find Response Sheets (for writing your responses to the questions) on Davis*Plus.

To explore learning resources for this chapter,

Go to Davis*Plus* at DavisPl.us/Wilkinson3.

Chapter Resources for Chapter 42:

- **Response sheets for all learning activities**
- **Resources for Caregivers and Health Professionals**
- **Reading More About Promoting Health (suggested readings)**
- **Concept Map of chapter content**

Interactive Case Studies

NCLE-Style and Chapter Review Questions

CHAPTER OVERVIEW

For a podcast of an overview of this chapter,

Go to Student Resources, Chapter 42, **Podcast—Chapter Overview,** on Davis*Plus*.

Caring for the Nguyens

Nam and Yen Nguyen; their 3-year-old grandson, Kim; and Mai, Nam's 76-year-old mother, are all patients at the Family Medicine Center. Zach Jackson, the family nurse practitioner at the center, asks you to devise a health promotion program for each member of the family.

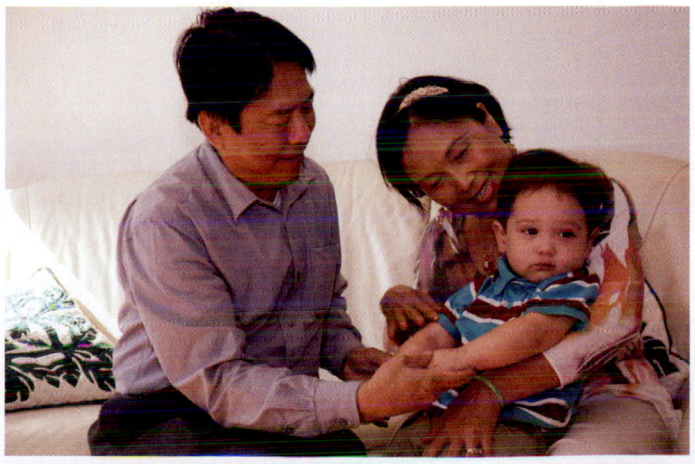

(Continued)

Caring for the Nguyens (continued)

A. What information should you gather before you begin?

B. How might you obtain this information?

C. How will the plans differ for each?

D. Review Meet the Nguyens in the front of this textbook; also review Nam's physical exam findings in Chapter 22. What health promotion strategies and health screenings should you recommend to Nam?

E. How would you begin to organize and prioritize a health promotion program for Nam?

F. Using therapeutic communication, give examples of appropriate questions to ask Nam about his health beliefs.

ASSESSMENT GUIDELINES AND TOOLS

Focused Assessment

Health Promotion: Physical Fitness Assessment

Cardiorespiratory Fitness

There are many different modes of testing, such as field tests (walking or running), motor-driven treadmills, stationary bicycles, and step testing.

- **Field tests** for running are good for children. A 9-year-old child should be able to complete a 1-mile run in approximately 10 minutes, and a 17-year-old boy should be able to complete a 1-mile run in approximately 7½ minutes (www.presidentschallenge.org).
- **The step test** is appropriate for most adults. Using a 12-inch bench, instruct the participant to step up and down at a rate of 24 steps per minute for 3 minutes. At the end of 3 minutes, he should check his heart rate. Stop testing immediately if the participant experiences any chest pain, shortness of breath, or light-headedness. Results depend on age and gender and are available below.

Step Test Evaluation Charts

3-Minute Step Heart Rate Test (Men)

Physical Condition	18–25 yr	26–35 yr	36–45 yr	46–55 yr	56–65 yr	65+ yrs
Excellent	<79	<81	<83	<87	<86	<88
Good	79–89	81–89	83–96	87–97	86–97	88–96
Above average	90–99	90–99	97–103	98–105	98–103	97–103
Average	100–105	100–107	104–112	106–116	104–112	104–113
Below average	106–116	108–117	113–119	117–122	113–120	114–120
Poor	117–128	118–128	120–130	123–132	121–129	121–130
Very poor	>128	>128	>130	>132	>129	>130

3-Minute Step Test (Women)

Physical Condition	18–25 yr	26–35 yr	36–45 yr	46–55 yr	56–65 yr	65+ yr
Excellent	<85	<88	<90	<94	<95	<90
Good	85–98	88–99	90–102	94–104	95–104	90–102
Above average	99–108	100–111	103–110	105–115	105–112	103–115
Average	109–117	112–119	111–118	116–120	113–118	116–122
Below average	118–126	120–126	119–128	121–129	119–128	123–128
Poor	127–140	127–138	129–140	130–135	129–139	129–134
Very poor	>140	>138	>140	>135	>139	>134

Muscular Fitness

- **Muscle strength** measures the amount of weight a muscle (or group of muscles) can move at one time. This is recorded as a ratio of weight pushed (or lifted) divided by body weight. For example, a woman weighing 150 pounds who is able to lift 86 pounds will have a ratio of 86 divided by 150, or 0.57.

Instruct the participant warm up and stretch before the test. Weight benches are ideal sites for testing upper body and leg strength.

Focused Assessment

Health Promotion: Physical Fitness Assessment—cont'd

Compare the ratio obtained with normative standards or with previous personal scores to evaluate improvement.

- **Muscle endurance** refers to the ability of a muscle to perform repeated movements. The push-up or curl-up (crunch) test may be performed to evaluate endurance. Ask the participant to perform as many push-ups or curl-ups as possible without pausing. The number of repetitions is the score. Once again, compare scores with norms or previous performance.

Flexibility

Flexibility is the ability to move a joint through its range of motion. **The sit-and-reach test** evaluates low back and hip [trunk] flexion.

- Ask the participant to sit on a floor mat with legs fully extended and feet flat against a box. Have her extend her arms and hands forward as far as possible and hold for a count of 3.
- Using a ruler, measure the distance in inches that the client can reach beyond the proximal edge of the box. If the client cannot reach the edge, measure the distance of the fingertips from the edge, and report it as a negative number.
- Norms for trunk flexion vary among men and women. The desired range for men is +1 to +5 inches, and for women it is +2 to +6 inches (Pender, Murdaugh, & Parsons, 2010).

Focused Assessment

Lifestyle and Risk Assessment

Lifestyle refers to the manner in which a person conducts his life. You can gather this information by interview or by using a variety of questionnaires. A health risk appraisal (HRA) is a questionnaire that evaluates risk for disease based on current demographic data, lifestyle, and health behaviors. The following is an example of an HRA.

Name _____ Age _____ Gender _____

Health View

In general, would you say your present health is?
- □ Excellent
- □ Very good
- □ Good
- □ Fair
- □ Poor

General Practices

1. **Physical activity.** How many days each week do you get at least 30 minutes of physical activity, such as brisk walking, cycling, active gardening, active dance, swimming, jogging, or active sports? _____
2. **Strength exercises.** How many days each week do you do strength-building exercises, such as weight lifting or isometric exercises? _____
3. **Smoking status.** Indicate your present smoking status.
   - □ Current smoker □ Ex-smoker
   - □ Nonsmoker, never smoked regularly.

   Environmental smoke. Do you live with or work with smokers and breathe secondhand smoke regularly?
   - □ Yes □ No
4. **Alcohol.** How many drinks do you typically have on a day you drink? *One drink is a bottle or can of beer (12 oz), a glass of wine or wine cooler (3.5 oz), or a shot glass of liquor (1.5 oz).*
   - □ Never drink.
   - □ Have no more than one drink in a day.
   - □ Have no more than two drinks in a day.
   - □ Sometimes have three or four drinks in a day.
   - □ Sometimes have five or more drinks in a day.
5. **Sleep.** How many hours of sleep do you usually get each night? _____

Eating Practices

6. **Breakfast.** How many days each week do you usually eat breakfast (more than just coffee and a roll)? _____
7. **Bread/grains.** How many servings of whole-grain breads and cereals do you eat daily? *One serving = 1 slice bread, ½ cup dry cereal, ½ cup cooked oatmeal or other whole-grain cereal or brown rice.* _____
8. **Fruits and vegetables.** How many servings of fruits and vegetables do you eat daily? *One serving = 1 medium fruit, 6 oz fruit or vegetable juice, 1 cup raw fruit or vegetables, ½ cup cooked fruit or vegetables.* _____
9. **Legumes.** How many times a week do you eat legumes (peas, beans, lentils, garbanzos)? *One serving = ½ cup cooked.* _____
10. **High-fat and high-cholesterol foods.** How often do you eat foods high in saturated fat and cholesterol (e.g., steak, hamburger, hot dog, sausage, bacon, cheese, fried chicken, French fries, ice cream, cheesecake, or other desserts)?
    - □ Daily
    - □ Eat these foods three or more times a week.
    - □ Seldom or never eat these foods.
11. **Nuts/seeds.** How many servings of nuts do you usually eat each week? *One serving = 1 oz or a small handful, or 2 tablespoons of natural nut butter.* _____
12. **Refined foods.** How often do you eat highly refined foods (soda pop, snack foods, chips, refined cereals, pastry, candy)?
    - □ Daily
    - □ Eat these foods three or more times a week.
    - □ Seldom or never eat refined foods.

(Continued)

Focused Assessment

Lifestyle and Risk Assessment—cont'd

13. **Water.** How many glasses (8 oz) of water do you typically drink each day? _____

14. **Weight.** How many pounds have you gained since you were 21 to 24 (enter 0 if you weigh the same, weigh less, or are younger than 21 years). _____

Mental/Social Health

15. **Happiness.** How happy have you been during the past month?
    - □ Very happy
    - □ Pretty happy
    - □ Not too happy
    - □ Very unhappy

16. **Mood/Feelings**
    - (a) During the past month, have you often been bothered by feeling down, depressed, or hopeless?
      □ Yes □ No
    - (b) During the past month, have you often been bothered by having little interest or pleasure in doing things?
      □ Yes □ No
    - (c) Have your feelings in the past month caused you significant distress or impaired your ability to function socially or at work (or school)?
      □ Yes □ No

17. **Stress and coping.** How much of the time do you feel stressed out and unable to cope with life?
    - □ Seldom or never
    - □ Occasionally
    - □ Much of the time
    - □ Most of the time

Social Support

18. **Support.** Do you have family or friends you can get help from if needed?
    □ Yes □ No

19. **Social Interaction.** Do you have frequent social contact with family or friends?
    □ Yes □ No

Community

20. **Community Support.** Do you meet regularly with a faith community or other group that gives you support, comfort, meaning, and direction in your life?
    □ Yes □ No

Safety

21. **Seat belts.** What percentage of the time do you wear seat belts when riding in a car? _____

22. **Smoke alarm.** Do you have a working smoke alarm on each floor of your home, including the area in which you sleep?
    □ Yes □ No □ Don't know for sure.

23. **Helmet.** When biking or rollerblading, do you always wear a helmet and protective gear?
    □ Yes □ No

24. **Substance use and driving.** Do you ever drive soon after drinking alcohol or taking drugs or ride with someone who has been using illicit substances, including alcohol?
    □ Yes □ No

Safer Sex

25. **Practice safer sex.**
    - (a) Are you in a monogamous relationship?
      □ Yes □ No
    - (b) Do you always use condoms, or abstain from sexual relations?
      □ Always □ Don't always practice safer sex

Preventive Exams

26. Do you keep current on recommended preventive exams (see list below) and immunizations?
    □ Yes □ No □ Don't know for sure.

Recommended Preventive Exams

- Periodic checkup, including blood pressure, height and weight, and cholesterol check as recommended by your doctor.
- Pap tests within last 1 to 3 years, for women 18 or older
- Mammogram within last 2 years, for women 40 or older
- Colorectal cancer screening for all persons 50 or older
- Prostate exam, for men 50 or older
- Flu and pneumonia immunizations, for everyone 65 or older

Height _____

Weight _____

Blood pressure _____

Blood cholesterol _____ (mg/dL)

Focused Assessment

Lifestyle and Risk Assessment—cont'd

Scoring

Your score is the number of good health indicators you meet out of the 17 possible listed (below) in this assessment. The higher your score, the healthier your lifestyle. The Average Health Style Score is 9.4

Health Indicator	Guidelines for Good Health
1. Physical activity	Get 30 or more minutes of physical activity most days of the week.
2. Strength training	Do strength-building exercises at least twice per week.
3. Not smoking	Avoid all tobacco use and frequent exposure to secondhand smoke.
4. Alcohol use	Alcohol is not recommended, but if you drink alcohol, limit to one to two drinks in a day.
5. Adequate rest	Get adequate rest, at least 7 to 8 hours of sleep daily for best health.
6. Breakfast daily	Eat a nutritious breakfast daily for optimal physical and mental performance.
7. Whole grains	Choose whole-grain breads and cereals, at least three or more servings/per day.
8. Fruits and vegetables	Eat at least five servings of fruits and vegetables daily.
9. Fats, cholesterol	Limit high-fat meats, whole milk, and butter. Vegetable oils are healthier than oils from animals.
10. Nuts	Nuts, such as almonds, contain healthy fats and protect against heart disease.
11. Healthy weight	Maintain a healthy weight by eating well and participating in regular, moderate-intensity physical activity.
12. Mental health	Develop effective coping skills, and maintain a happy, hopeful outlook.
13. Social support	Maintain good social support and frequent contact with family and friends.
14. Community	Participate regularly in a faith community or other group that provides meaning, direction, and support in your life.
15. Safety	Be safety conscious; wear safety belts in the car and helmets when biking.
16. Safer sex	Remain in a monogamous relationship, or always use condoms, or abstain.
17. Regular exams	Get regular exams, including age/gender recommended preventive exams.

Source: Adapted from Hall, C., & Rhodes, J. (2002, September). Employee wellness and beyond at Appleton Papers Inc. *Athletic Therapy Today*, 46–47.

Focused Assessment

Life Stress Review

Daily hassles, life events, and other stressors trigger physiological responses that may, over time, induce illness (Selye, 1976; Rahe, 1974). You will find one type of life change events assessment tool in Chapter 12, Assessment Guidelines and Tools, The Holmes-Rahe Social Readjustment Scale.

Alternatively, you might want to interview your patient to assess the following:

- His belief in his ability to control the experience (e.g., an impending decision, an illness)
- How deeply involved he feels in the activity that is producing stress (i.e., is it something he can change, or wants to change?)
- Whether he is able to view such a change as a challenge to grow

Focused Assessment

Selected Health Screening Activities

With regard to health screening guidelines, it is important to know:

1. Different agencies and groups generate different guidelines for type and frequency of screening. For example, the American Cancer Society has different Pap screening recommendations than does the U.S. Preventive Services Task Force; the American College of Obstetricians and Gynecologists may have yet another recommendation.
2. Most evidence-based guidelines make use of cost-benefit analysis to arrive at their recommendations.
3. Various third-party payors have different policies regarding the type and frequency of screening for which they will reimburse.
4. Guidelines and recommendations change often.

Clinicians must take all that into consideration when they decide which screening tests to offer to their patients.

Lipid screening. Adults age 20 years or older have a fasting lipid panel at least once every 5 years. If total cholesterol is 200 mg/dL or greater—or HDL is less than 40 mg/dL—frequent monitoring is required. Universal screening is recommended for children ages 9 to 11 years, regardless of risk factors for cardiovascular disease. (National Guideline Clearinghouse [NGC], 2011). For children age 2 to 8 years, screening is recommended if a parent, grandparent, aunt/uncle, or sibling has a history of myocardial infarction (MI), angina, stroke, coronary artery bypass graft (CABG)/stent/angioplasty, or a history of hyperlipidemia (NGC, 2011).

Dental health. Clients should have regular dental checkups to detect early signs of oral health problems such as tooth decay, gingivitis (gum disease), and oral cancers.

Colon cancer screening. Both men and women should have a fecal occult blood test every year beginning at age 50 and a screening colonoscopy based on risk factors. If there is a strong family history of colorectal cancer or polyps, screening should begin at an earlier age and be conducted more frequently (American Cancer Society, 2013).

Breast cancer screening. Breast self-examination (BSE) is an option for women 20 years and older. Women between the ages of 20 and 39 should have a clinical breast examination by a health professional every 3 years. Women who are age 40 and older should have a screening mammogram and a clinical breast examination by a healthcare professional every year. The clinical breast examination should be scheduled close to and preferably before the scheduled mammogram (American Cancer Society, 2012). Thermal mammography shows promise for breast cancer detection without using radiation.

Cervical cancer screening. A Papanicolaou (Pap) smear is used to detect cellular changes in the cervix. All women should begin cervical cancer screening at age 21. Women between the ages of 21 and 29 should have a Pap test every 3 years. They should not be tested for human papillomavirus (HPV) unless it is needed after an abnormal Pap test result. Women between the ages of 30 and 65 should have both a Pap test and an HPV test every 5 years. This is the preferred approach, but it is also okay to have a Pap test alone every 3 years. Women older than age 65 who have had regular screenings with normal results should not be screened for cervical cancer. Women who have been diagnosed with cervical pre-cancer should continue to be screened (American Cancer Society, 2013; NGC, 2013; Smith, Brooks, Cokkinides, et al. 2013).

Testicular cancer screening. Given the low prevalence of testicular cancer and the limited accuracy of self-examination, routine clinical examination is not advised in symptom-free males.

Prostate screening. Most agencies do not support routine testing for prostate cancer. However, healthcare professionals may consider offering the PSA and DRE yearly to men age 50 years and older at risk for prostate cancer and with at least a 10-year life expectancy—if there are risk factors, testing should begin at age 40 to 45 years (American Cancer Society, 2013).

Skin screening. During any health assessment or a specialized dermatological exam, a general survey of the skin using the ABCD criteria is a useful approach for assessing for skin malignancy: **A**symmetry, **B**order irregularity, **C**olor variability, **D**iameter greater than 6 mm. Rapidly changing lesions are also associated with an increased risk for cancer. Any suspicious lesions should be biopsied (U.S. Preventive Services Task Force [USPSTF], 2009).

STANDARDIZED LANGUAGE

Standardized Language

Examples of NANDA-I Health Promotion Diagnoses

- Readiness for Enhanced Breastfeeding
- Readiness for Enhanced Communication
- Readiness for Enhanced Community Coping
- Readiness for Enhanced Coping
- Readiness for Enhanced Family Coping
- Readiness for Enhanced Family Processes
- Readiness for Enhanced Fluid Balance
- Readiness for Enhanced Knowledge (specify)
- Readiness for Enhanced Nutrition
- Readiness for Enhanced Organized Infant Behavior
- Readiness for Enhanced Parenting
- Readiness for Enhanced Self-Concept
- Readiness for Enhanced Sleep
- Readiness for Enhanced Spiritual Well-Being
- Readiness for Enhanced Urinary Elimination

Source: NANDA International. (2012). *Nursing diagnosis: Definitions and classifications 2012–2014.* Philadelphia: Author. Used with permission.

Standardized Language

Selected NIC Health Promotion Interventions

NIC INTERVENTION	DEFINITION	EXAMPLES OF ACTIVITIES
Breast Examination	Performing activities to safeguard the health of the breasts and related areas	Advise regular mammograms as appropriate for age, condition, and risk.
Community Health Development	Assisting members of a community to identify a community's health concerns, mobilize resources, and implement solutions	Identify health concerns, strengths, and priorities with community partners.
Environmental Management: Worker Safety	Monitoring and manipulation of the worksite environment to promote safety and health of workers	Identify applicable OSHA standards and worksite compliance with standards.
Environmental Risk Protection	Preventing and detecting disease and injury in populations at risk from environmental hazards	Monitor incidents of illness and injury related to environmental hazards.
Exercise Promotion	Facilitation of regular physical activity to maintain or advance to a higher level of fitness and health	Appraise individual's health beliefs about physical exercise.
Family Planning: Contraception	Facilitation of pregnancy prevention by providing information about the physiology of reproduction and methods to control conception	Determine ability and motivation of patient and partner to correctly and regularly use contraception.
Health Education	Developing and providing instruction and learning experiences to facilitate voluntary adaptation of behavior conducive to health in individuals, families, groups, or communities	Target high-risk groups and age ranges that would benefit most from health education.
Health Policy Monitoring	Surveillance and influence of government and organization regulations, rules, and standards that affect nursing systems and practices to ensure quality care of patients	Compare requirements of policies and standards with current practices.
Health Screening	Detecting health risks or problems by means of history, examination, and other procedures	Complete appropriate Department of Health or other records for monitoring abnormal results, such as high blood pressure.
Health System Guidance	Facilitating a patient's location and use of appropriate health services	Inform the patient of accreditation and state health department requirements for judging the quality of a facility.
Immunization/Vaccination Management	Monitoring immunization status, facilitating access to immunizations, and providing immunizations to prevent communicable disease	Determine immunization status at every health care visit (including emergency department and hospital admission), and provide immunizations as needed.

(Continued)

Standardized Language

Selected NIC Health Promotion Interventions—cont'd

NIC INTERVENTION	DEFINITION	EXAMPLES OF ACTIVITIES
Oral Health Promotion	Promotion of oral hygiene and dental care for a patient with normal oral and dental health	Instruct and assist patient to perform oral hygiene after eating and as often as needed.
Parent Education: Childrearing Family	Assisting parents to understand and promote the physical, psychological, and social growth and development of their toddler, pre-school, or school-age child/children (also Parent Education: Adolescent and Parent Education: Infant)	Teach appropriate developmental tasks or goals for the child.
Patient Contracting	Negotiating and agreement with an individual that reinforces a specific behavior change	Encourage the individual to identify own goals, not those he/she believes the healthcare provider expects.
Program Development [Wellness]	Planning, implementing, and evaluating a coordinated set of activities designed to enhance wellness, or to prevent, reduce, or eliminate one or more health problems for a group or community	Assist the group or community in identifying significant health needs or problems.
Sleep Enhancement	Promoting restful sleep that meets body's needs for restoration	Determine patient's sleep/activity pattern.
Smoking Cessation Assistance	Helping another to stop smoking	Help patient identify reasons to quit and barriers to quitting.
Spiritual Growth Facilitation	Facilitation of growth in patient's capacity to identify, connect with, and call upon the source of meaning, purpose, comfort, strength, and hope in his/her life	Encourage conversation that assists the patient in sorting out spiritual concerns.
Sports-Injury Prevention: Youth	Reduce the risk of sports-related injury in young athletes	Monitor proper use and condition of safety equipment.
Substance Use Prevention	Prevention of an alcoholic or drug use lifestyle	Conduct programs in schools on the avoidance of drugs and alcohol as recreational activities.
Teaching: *Infant Nutrition* *Infant Safety* *Infant Stimulation* *Toddler Nutrition* *Toddler Safety* *Toilet Training*	Providing education to parent(s) concerning topics relevant to growth, development, and safety of infants and toddlers	*Note:* Teaching is integral to all health promotion/disease prevention activities, whether or not there is a special intervention label for the particular content.
Teaching: Safe Sex	Providing instructions concerning sexual protection during sexual activity	Create an accepting, nonjudgmental atmosphere.
Values Clarification	Assisting another to clarify her/his own values in order to facilitate effective decision making	Encourage consideration of values underlying choices and consequences of the choice.
Vehicle Safety Promotion	Assisting individuals, families, and communities to increase awareness of measures to reduce unintentional injuries in motorized and nonmotorized vehicles	Educate about the importance of proper and regular use of protective devices to decrease risk of injury (e.g., car seats, seat belts, helmets).

Sources: Bulechek, G. M., Butcher, H. K., & Dochterman, J. M. (Eds.). (2012). *Nursing interventions classification (NIC)* (6th ed.). St. Louis, MO: C.V. Mosby. Used with permission.

CLINICALREASONING

Applying the Full-Spectrum Nursing Model

PATIENT SITUATION

Shandra Shane is a single 37-year-old woman with three children, ages 12, 15, and 17. She is raising the children on her own, although her sister occasionally helps with transportation or advice about disciplining her teenage daughters. Ms. Shane is a night-shift worker at the hospital. Her typical schedule is 3 to 4 hours of sleep in the morning soon after she gets home and then a short nap in the early evening before going back to work. She smokes 1 to 1½ packs of cigarettes per day but tells you she has been trying to smoke less around her children. Her job stress is high, as the hospital is cutting back on the number of staff. Ms. Shane also takes care of her elderly mother, who has Alzheimer's and lives with her. Ms. Shane's outlet for stress is going out with friends and drinking beer on the weekend. She is seeking your professional guidance to lose some weight (about 60 pounds) and to feel more energetic.

THINKING

1. *Theoretical Knowledge:*
   List health behaviors that negatively influence health status.
2. *Critical Thinking (Contextual Awareness):*
   What factors in this situation would you consider threatening to Ms. Shane's health and could lead to disease later in life?

DOING

3. *Nursing Process (Planning/Intervention):*
   What suggestions might you make about Shandra's diet that could help her to lose weight? Why might these actions be effective for weight loss?
4. *Practical Knowledge:*
   What areas of her daily living other than her diet might you explore further and offer recommendations for improving to promote better health and prevent illness?

CARING

5. *Self-Knowledge:*
   Have you ever been in a situation in which you felt stressed, tired, and wanting gratification offered by food, nicotine, or alcohol? Describe your experience.
6. *Ethical Knowledge:*
   In what ways could you demonstrate genuine caring for Shandra?

Critical Thinking and Clinical Reasoning

1. While working in a physician's office, a 70-year-old woman is referred to you for counseling regarding health protection activities. She is hypertensive and obese.
   a. How does her age affect your assessments and communication?
   b. What type of learning aids might be needed?
   c. What health screenings are appropriate for this client?
2. Below is a group of clients who wish to enroll in a health promotion program.
   - Jennifer Kaska is 23 years old and was diagnosed with diabetes mellitus at the age of 12 years. She checks her blood sugar and administers insulin as needed. She runs 3 miles, 3 days per week.
   - Maurice Rosenthal is 47 years old with no known illness. He is 6 feet tall and weighs 240 pounds. His body mass index (BMI) is 33 kg/m^2, indicating obesity. He takes no routine medication, only acetaminophen for occasional headaches.
   - Clara Fenton is 83 years old and has been diagnosed with hypertension, emphysema, and osteoporosis. She takes 10 prescription medications daily in addition to a multivitamin and an occasional laxative.

   Discuss the pros and cons of providing a group program that includes all three of these clients.

3. L. F. is a 50-year-old man with heart disease. He had coronary artery bypass surgery 1 month ago. He has stopped going to his prescribed cardiac rehabilitation program because of the distance he must travel to the rehabilitation center. Discuss at least two approaches for working with this client.
4. Cecelia Kent is 32 years old. She takes no medications and has annual physical exams. She walks 4 to 5 miles, 5 days per week, and lifts light weights two to three times per week. She eats a low-fat, low-salt, low-sugar diet. She has never smoked, and drinks only limited alcohol.
   a. She asks you to recommend further health promotion activities. How would you respond?
   b. How could you incorporate Cecelia into a health promotion class that includes Jennifer Kaska, Maurice Rosenthal, and Clara Fenton (from question 2)?
5. For each of the following concepts, use critical thinking to describe how or why it is important to nursing, patient care, or health promotion. Note that these are *not* to be merely definitions.

Health promotion	Hardiness
Illness prevention	Health screenings
Lifestyle	Health education

What Are the Main Points in This Chapter?

- Health promotion refers to helping clients develop an optimal state of health.
- Intention is the difference between health promotion and health protection (illness prevention).
- There are three levels of activities for health protection: primary, secondary, and tertiary prevention. *Primary interventions* are designed to prevent or slow the onset of disease. *Secondary interventions* are designed to detect illnesses in early stages. *Tertiary interventions* focus on stopping the disease from progressing and on rehabilitation.
- The *Healthy People 2020* initiative is designed to achieve four overarching goals:
  - Attain high-quality, longer lives free of preventable disease, disability, injury, and premature death.
  - Achieve health equity, eliminate disparities, and improve the health of all groups.
  - Create social and physical environments that promote good health for all.
  - Promote quality of life, healthy development, and healthy behaviors all life stages.
- Pender's Health Promotion Model (HPM) identifies three groups of variables that affect health behavior: (1) individual characteristics and experiences; (2) behavior-specific cognitions and affect; and (3) behavioral outcome.
- A Wellness Wheel identifies six dimensions of health: emotional, intellectual, physical, spiritual, social/family, and occupational.
- The transtheoretical model of change identifies four stages of change: contemplation, determination, action, and maintenance.
- Health promotion activities for all age groups include nutrition, exercise, safety concerns, changing unhealthy lifestyles, immunizations, and screenings.
- Health promotion activities may be conducted in acute care facilities, the workplace, local communities, or schools.
- A health promotion assessment involves obtaining a health history, physical examination, fitness assessment, lifestyle and risk appraisal, life stress review, assessment of healthcare beliefs, nutritional assessment, and screening activities.
- Health screening activities are designed to detect disease at an early stage so that treatment can begin before there is an opportunity for disease to spread or reduce the quality of life.
- Health screening activities vary based on developmental stage and identified risk factors.
- Nurses promote health through role modeling, counseling, providing health education, and providing and facilitating support.

Knowledge Map

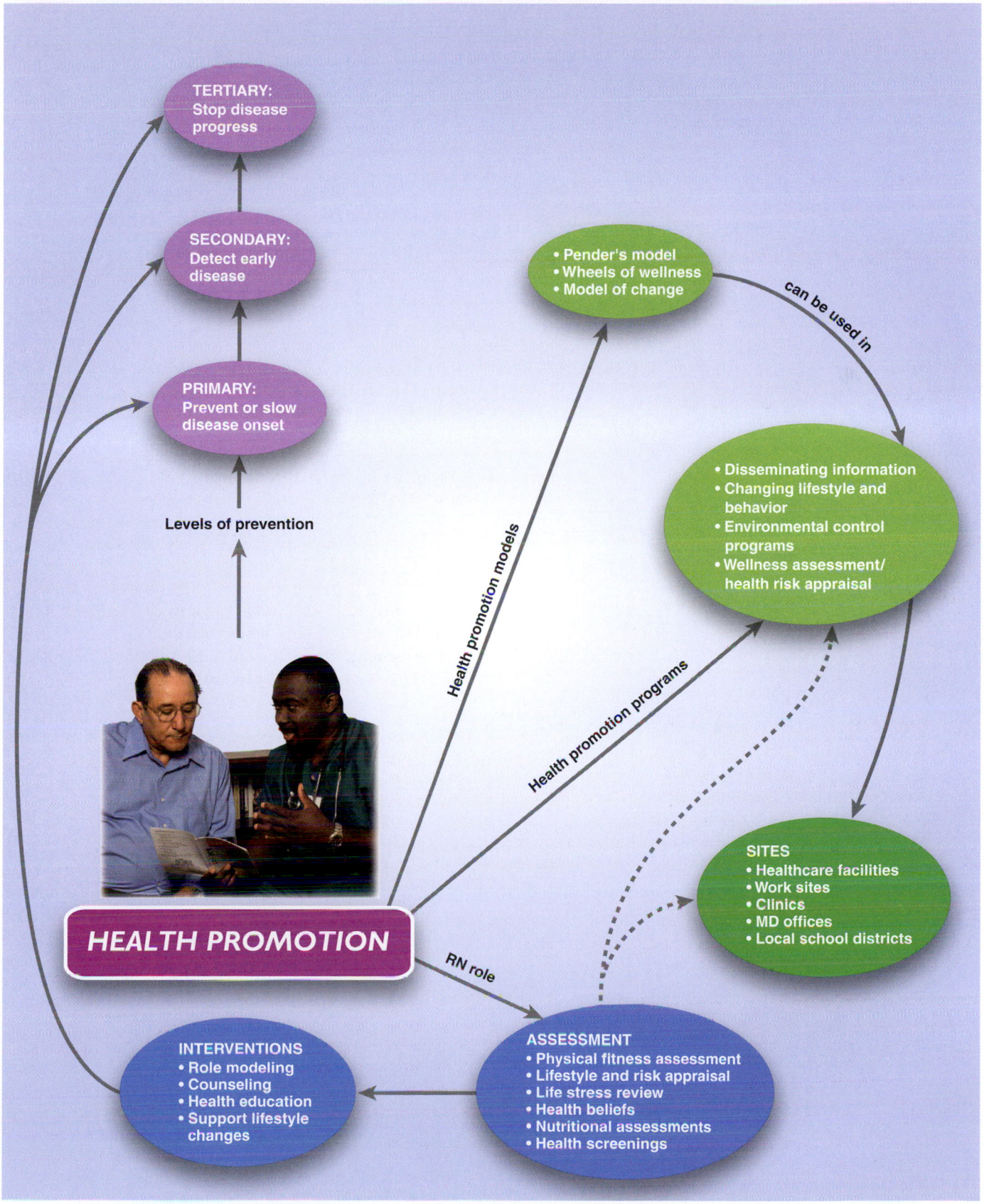

unit 6

The Context for Nurses' Work

43 Community & Home Health Nursing

44 Ethics & Values

45 Legal Accountability

46 Holistic Healing (on Davis*Plus*)

CHAPTER 43

Community & Home Health Nursing

STUDENT RESOURCES

*The questions and exercises in Volume 2 allow you to practice the kind of thinking you will use as a full-spectrum nurse. Critical-thinking questions usually have more than one correct answer, so we do not provide "answers" for these features. It is more important to develop your nursing judgment than to just cover content. You will learn by discussing the questions with your peers. If you are still unsure, consult your instructor. You will find Response Sheets (for writing your responses to the questions) on Davis*Plus.

To explore learning resources for this chapter,

Go to Davis*Plus* at DavisPl.us/Wilkinson3.

Chapter Resources for Community and Home Health Nursing

- **Response sheets for all learning exercises**
- **Resources for Caregivers and Health Professionals**
- **Reading More About Community & Home Health Nursing (suggested readings)**
- **Concept Map of chapter content**

Interactive Case Studies

NCLEX-Style and Chapter Review Questions

CHAPTER OVERVIEW

For a podcast of an overview of this chapter,

Go to Student Resources, Chapter 43, **Podcast—Chapter Overview,** on Davis*Plus*.

Caring for the Nguyens

Yen Nguyen works as preschool teacher in her community. Andre is a 4-year-old boy in her class. Over the past few months, she has noticed that Andre has many bruises in various stages of healing. He seems withdrawn and does not interact much with the other children. She is concerned that Andre might be a victim of child abuse, but she is reluctant to make that accusation, especially because her assistant doesn't seem to have noticed anything amiss.

Mrs. Nguyen talks to her husband, Nam, about her concerns: "I'm worried about a child at school, but I'm afraid to say anything. What if I'm wrong? I'd probably lose my job. But if I'm right and I don't say anything, I could still lose my job, and this boy could be hurt even worse." Nam suggests that she contact the clinic nurse at the Family Medicine Center for confidential advice on how to proceed.

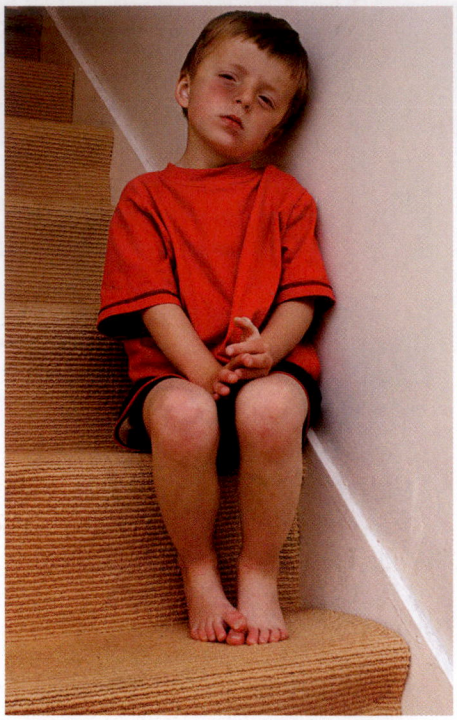

A. Imagine that you are the clinic nurse. Use the full-spectrum nursing model to identify at least 10 questions that you would need to answer to investigate Yen's concerns further.

B. *Self-knowledge:* What personal values do you have that would affect the manner in which you handle this situation? Explain.

C. *Ethical knowledge:* What is the most important ethical issue in this situation? That is, what is the most important goal? Note that there may be several moral and legal issues, but you are being asked to identify the *most* important one. Note also that we are not asking you what the nurse *can* do, but rather what the nurse ideally *should* do.

D. You share the questions you have with Yen. She believes that there is a real need to investigate child abuse. You advise her to call the local child protective services (CPS) agency. Based on your knowledge of community and public health nursing, what aspects of the community health role will the nurse from CPS use as she investigates this situation?

Practical Knowledge knowing how

Practical knowledge in community and home-care nursing requires you to apply the nursing process to both individuals and groups.

CLINICAL INSIGHTS

Clinical Insight 43-1 ➤ Safety Considerations in Home Care

Before the Visit

- **Plan ahead.** Know where you are headed. Use a map or global positioning system (GPS). Contact the client or family for directions if it is unclear where you are headed. File a visit plan with your office each day.
- **Dress in appropriate clothing** as dictated by your agency. Wear a nametag clearly identifying you and the agency. Wear shoes that will allow you to run if necessary.
- **Carry a cell phone.** Check to be sure it is charged. Program 911 into it in case of emergency.
- **Do not carry a purse**, multiple credit cards, or excess cash. Instead, use a waist or fanny pack and conceal it under clothing. Carry enough money for emergency transportation, telephone numbers for clients and home health agency, and emergency contact information.
- **Keep your car in good repair** and always have enough gasoline in the tank. Be prepared for inclement weather, and always carry an emergency car safety pack.
- **Do not get out of your car for any reason if driving in an area that might not be safe.** Carjacking involves minor car impact ("fender bender") as a strategy to get a person to exit the vehicle, leaving her vulnerable for attack, assault, or theft.
- **Observe your surroundings** as you drive to the visit. Notice the location of emergency services, local gas stations, and public places if help is required.
- **Carry mace or other items to aid in self-defense** in situations in which you feel threatened.
- **Park as close to your destination as possible.** If possible, park your car facing the direction you wish to go when you leave. Never enter dead-end streets or alleys.
- **Check your surroundings before you leave your car.** If you feel unsafe, leave the area immediately and call your office.
- **Lock the car. Leave no valuables in sight.**
- **Prepare your bag while you are still in the car.**
- **Carry your bag on one arm. In the opposite hand, carry your keys.** Always have them ready. You may need them if you decide to exit quickly. Also, you can use keys to defend yourself by placing the pointed ends of the keys between your fingers.
- **Walk directly to the client's house.** Walk in the middle of the sidewalk. Use common walkways. Avoid isolated and poorly lighted areas. Do not take shortcuts.
- **Knock or ring the doorbell before entering.** Never enter without being invited. If there is no answer at the door, call the patient using your cell phone, or return to a secure public pay phone and dial the client.
- **If for any reason you feel that the neighborhood is unsafe, do not get out of the car.** Instead, leave the neighborhood immediately and phone your agency.

At the Visit

- **Introduce yourself** and clearly identify your agency. Show your name badge.
- **Sit where you have access to an exit.** When you enter the home, observe all exits.
- **Notice who is present in the home. Request introductions.** This information is useful for planning care as well as for ensuring safety.
- **Leave immediately if you suspect substance use**, drug dealing, or drunken behavior.
- **Leave immediately if there is a violent domestic argument.** Do not attempt to intervene. When you return to your car, use your cell phone to dial 911, or drive to a phone booth in a safe location and place the call.
- **Request that animals be kept in another room** while you make your visit.
- **If weapons are visible, request that they be put away** immediately. Leave the home if this request is not met.
- **If household members interfere with the visit**, discuss the problem with the client. You may need to arrange a time to visit when they are not present.

After the Visit

- **Continue to observe the safety precautions** you used when getting to the visit. Do not let down your guard as you return to your car.
- **If you are in an unsafe neighborhood or poorly lighted area, leave immediately and do not consult the map** for directions to your next visit. Drive to a secure public location, and then consult the map.
- **Inform your agency** if you believe the home or neighborhood is potentially hazardous.
- **Request a security escort service** if future visits are required.
- **Document your assessments** and the care delivered.
- **Report abuse** if you suspect it in the home.

Other

You also need to protect yourself from infection and accidental injury, as you would in a hospital (see Clinical Insight 43-2).

- Use safe lifting techniques, especially because you might have to improvise more than in the hospital. There will probably be no one to assist with patient transfer, ambulation, or lifting. Mechanical lifts are likely not available.
- Do not dispose of loose sharps in household trash containers, toilets, or recycling bins. Place them immediately in a sharps disposal container. If a sharps container is not available, use a puncture- and leak-resistant plastic household container (e.g., a laundry detergent bottle or empty milk jug) (U.S. Food and Drug Administration, 2011).

Clinical Insight 43-2 ➤ Infection Control in the Home

The following suggestions can help you maintain infection control during a home visit.

Hand Hygiene

- Keep antibacterial cleanser and protective equipment approved by the Occupational Safety and Health Administration in your nursing bag.
- Perform hand hygiene using soap and warm water or an antibacterial handrub at the beginning and end of each visit and before and after any treatment.
- If the home conditions are very dirty or your hands become grossly soiled, wash your hands with soap and warm water as soon as possible after (if not during) the visit.

Supplies

- In homes that you know are not clean, limit the supplies you bring into the home. For example, leave your nursing bag in the car, and bring only the supplies you need for the visit.
- Some infection control experts believe the "bag technique" (i.e., placing a newspaper under the nursing bag before placing it on a surface) is not routinely needed, but should be used when home conditions warrant. If you use items from your nursing bag during the visit, always clean them with an approved antibacterial wipe before placing them back into your bag.
- If necessary, use a 1:10 dilution of chlorine bleach in water to disinfect surfaces or equipment in the home. Some equipment may need to be disinfected by boiling in a covered pan of water for 15 to 20 minutes. Do not boil plastic or rubber items.
- You can disinfect hard plastic items by wrapping them with a wet paper towel and placing them in a zippered plastic bag. Microwave the entire bag on high for 10 minutes.

Biohazard and Sharps Disposal

- Flush wound irrigation or potentially contaminated liquids down the toilet while wearing gloves and any other appropriate protective equipment.
- Double-bag dressings, equipment, or disposable supplies that have been contaminated with body secretions to prevent leakage. The bags should be labeled *Biohazard*.

Carry small biohazard sharps containers. Place syringes and sharps in the container without recapping. If clients or family must use syringes or sharps, you may wish to leave a sharps container in the home. An alternative solution is to have them use a metal coffee can with lid or a thick plastic milk jug with lid.

Client Teaching

- Provide instruction on home cleanliness, hygiene, handwashing, and food preparation, and instructions to avoid contact with persons who are ill, as needed.
- If the client is immunocompromised, teach the signs and symptoms of infection and the process for immediate notification of the primary care provider.

Special Situations

- If the patient has a multidrug-resistant infection or pulmonary tuberculosis, use appropriate barrier precautions. Leave reusable equipment (e.g., stethoscope, blood pressure cuff) in the home; and if possible, schedule these clients as the last appointment of the day.

STANDARDIZED LANGUAGE

This section provides guidelines for using NANDA-I, NOC, NIC, and the Omaha System to develop problem statements, goals, and nursing orders to use in planning care for aggregates and communities. If you need to review these three standardized languages,

Go to **Chapters 4, 5, and 6,** in Volume 1.

The Omaha System

The Omaha System is a problem-solving model for community health practice, education, and research. The taxonomy consists of *diagnostic labels* organized into four *domains* (categories), along with two sets of *modifiers*. Within those domains, the system classifies 42 client problems or areas of concern (see Omaha System: Domains and Examples of Problem Labels, following). As you can see, the problem labels in the environment domain are especially useful in community nursing. For the complete problem classification scheme,

Go to the **Omaha System Web site,** at http://www.omahasystem.org

Omaha Problem Classification Scheme

To create a diagnostic statement, choose an appropriate label, and add a modifier to it from each of the two sets in the accompanying box. For example, a group Environment diagnosis for workers in a meatpacking plant with lax safety standards might read *Deficit* in Group Workplace Safety. If only one worker were at risk (perhaps because of her inattention to safety rules), you could write *Potential Deficit in Individual* Workplace Safety.

Domain: Environment
Problems: Income, Sanitation, Residence, and Workplace Safety
Modifiers: (1) Health Promotion, Potential Deficit, or Deficit
(2) Family, Individual, or Group
Diagnostic Statements:
Deficit in Group Workplace Safety
Potential Deficit in Individual Workplace Safety

Omaha System: Domains and Examples of Problem Labels

Environmental Domain—The material resources, physical surroundings, and substances both internal and external to the client, home, neighborhood, and broader community

Problem (Diagnosis) Labels: Income, Sanitation, Residence, Neighborhood/Workplace Safety

Psychosocial Domain—Patterns of behavior, communication, relationships, and development.

Problem (Diagnosis) Labels: Social Contact, Role Change, Interpersonal Relationships, Spirituality, Grief, Mental Health, Sexuality, Caretaking/Parenting, Neglect, Abuse

Physiological Domain—Functional status of processes that maintain life.

Problem (Diagnosis) Labels: Hearing, Vision, Oral Health, Speech and Language, Pain, Respiration, Digestion-Hydration, Communicable/Infectious Condition

Health Related Behaviors Domain—Activities that maintain or promote wellness, promote recovery, or maximize rehabilitation potential.

Problem (Diagnosis) Labels: Nutrition, Personal Hygiene, Prescribed Medication Regimen, Sleep and Rest Patterns, Family Planning, Physical Activity

Problem Modifiers

Set 1—Health Promotion, Potential Deficit, Deficit

Set 2—Family, Individual, Group*

*Martin and Scheet (1992, p. 67) suggest that *Group* be added to these modifiers.

Source: Martin, K. S., & Scheet, N. J. (1992). *The Omaha System: Applications for community health nursing*. Philadelphia: W. B. Saunders, pp. 67–74. Used with permission.

Using the NOC and Omaha Systems to Write Aggregate Goals

NOC Outcomes

NOC standardized outcomes in the Community Health domain include the following (Moorhead, Johnson, Maas, et al., 2013):

- Community Competence
- Community Disaster Readiness
- Community Disaster Response
- Community Health Status
- Community Health Status: Immunity
- Community Risk Control: Chronic Disease
- Community Risk Control: Communicable Disease
- Community Risk Control: Lead Exposure
- Community Risk Control: Violence
- Community Violence Level

You can use these NOC labels to write goals by adding the appropriate NOC indicators and scales (see NOC Measurement Scales, in the Standardized Language section of Chapter 5, in this volume).

Omaha System Outcomes

Using the Omaha System, you will develop goals/outcomes from the words in the nursing diagnosis. Recall that all nursing diagnoses are identified as *individual, family,* or *group,* so a group nursing diagnosis will automatically indicate a group goal. For example, for the diagnosis Deficit in Group Workplace Safety, you would build the outcomes around the words "Group Workplace Safety." The Omaha system includes a five-point Problem Rating Scale for Outcomes (see the accompanying table) that describes what you expect to achieve in terms of the client's knowledge, behavior, and status.

Omaha Problem Rating Scale for Outcomes

CONCEPT	1	2	3	4	5
Knowledge					
The ability of the client to remember and interpret information	No knowledge	Minimal knowledge	Basic knowledge	Adequate knowledge	Superior knowledge
Behavior					
The client's observable responses, actions, or activities fitting the occasion or purpose	Never appropriate	Rarely appropriate	Inconsistently appropriate	Usually appropriate	Consistently appropriate
Status					
The condition of the client in relation to objective and subjective defining characteristics	Extreme signs/ symptoms	Severe signs/ symptoms	Moderate signs/ symptoms	Minimal signs/ symptoms	No signs/ symptoms

Source: The Omaha System. (2009, May 11, updated). *Solving clinical data-information: Problem rating scale for outcomes*. Retrieved from http://www.omahasystem.org/problemratingscaleforoutcomes.html

Using the above table, you would create expected outcomes by applying this scale to Group Workplace Safety, as follows.

Creating Outcomes for the Diagnosis Group Workplace Safety

Nursing Diagnosis: Deficit in Group Workplace Safety

RATING SCALE CONCEPT	PRESENT STATUS, BEFORE INTERVENTIONS	EXPECTED OUTCOME, AFTER INTERVENTIONS
Knowledge	(2) Minimal knowledge of workplace safety	(4) Adequate knowledge of workplace safety
Behavior	(2) Rarely appropriate safety behaviors	(4) Usually appropriate group safety behaviors
Status	(2) Severe signs/symptoms (e.g., frequent accidents or injuries)	(4) Minimal signs/symptoms (e.g., few accidents or injuries)

The outcomes in this table mean that after your interventions, you expect the group to have adequate knowledge of workplace safety, demonstrate usually appropriate behaviors (e.g., usually follow the safety rules), and demonstrate minimal accidents or injuries. To evaluate the client's progress, you would assign a scale number to the group's actual knowledge, behavior, and status *after interventions*.

Using the NIC and Omaha Interventions Labels for Community Health Care

The NIC Interventions Taxonomy

The NIC taxonomy includes 16 interventions specifically designed for community health (see the following box).

NIC Community Health Classes and Interventions

Class: Community Health Promotion—Interventions promote the health of the whole community

Interventions:

Case Management
Community Health Development
Fiscal Resource Management
Health Education
Health Policy Monitoring
Immunization/Vaccination Management
Program Development
Social Marketing

Class: Community Risk Management—Interventions that assist in detecting or preventing health risks to the whole community

Interventions:

Bioterrorism Preparedness
Community Disaster Preparedness
Communicable Disease Management
Environmental Management: Community
Environmental Management: Worker Safety
Environmental Risk Protection
Health Screening
Risk Identification
Surveillance: Community
Vehicle Safety Promotion

Source: Bulechek, G. M., Butcher, H. K., & Dochterman, J. M. (Eds.). (2013). *Nursing interventions classification (NIC)* (6th ed.). St. Louis, MO: C.V. Mosby. Used with permission from Elsevier Science.

The Omaha Interventions Taxonomy

The Omaha system taxonomy provides four "intervention categories" you can use in community-oriented nursing practice:

- **Health Teaching, Guidance, and Counseling.** These primary prevention activities include giving information; anticipating client problems; encouraging client action and responsibility for self-care; and assisting with coping, decision making, and problem-solving. As a community-oriented nurse, you should spend most of your time offering this level of intervention.
- **Treatments and Procedures.** These are secondary interventions directed toward preventing disease, identifying risk factors and early signs and symptoms, and decreasing or alleviating signs and symptoms.
- **Case Management.** Case management is a tertiary intervention that includes coordination, advocacy, and referral. These activities involve facilitating service delivery on behalf of the client, communicating with health and human service providers, promoting assertive client communication, and guiding the client toward appropriate community resources.

- **Surveillance.** These nursing activities include detection, measurement, critical analysis, and monitoring to indicate client status in relation to a given condition or phenomenon.

To write an intervention statement, you must combine one of those four "categories" of interventions with one of the 75 "targets" (objects of the nursing interventions), such as bowel care and nutrition. Then you must add patient-specific information to individualize the nursing order. See the accompanying box for intervention categories, examples of targets, and intervention statements (nursing orders). To see the entire set of intervention targets,

Go to the **Omaha System Web site,** at http://www.omahasystem.org/shminter.htm

You will notice that the targets can be used for individuals as well as groups. It is the designation of the nursing diagnosis as *individual, family,* or *group* that determines this.

Omaha Intervention Categories and Examples of Targets

Categories

I. Health Teaching, Guidance, and Counseling
II. Treatments and Procedures
III. Case Management
IV. Surveillance

Examples of Targets

Anatomy/physiology
Behavior modification
Communication
Discipline
Feeding procedures
Homemaking
Substance use
Wellness

Examples of Aggregate Targets

Caretaking/parenting skills
Day care/respite
Durable medical equipment
Education
Employment
Environment
Finances
Housing
Legal system
Transportation
Other community resource

Examples of Nursing Intervention Statements

Treatments and Procedures (II): Feeding procedures (Demonstrate to Mrs. Adams how to feed Mr. Adams at the next visit.)

Surveillance (IV): Feeding procedures (After teaching, observe a feeding. Monitor for choking.)

Source: The Omaha System. (2009, May 11, updated). Solving the clinical data-information scheme: Intervention scheme. Retrieved from http://www.omahasystem.org/interventionscheme.html

Clinical Care Classification System for Home Health Care

Clinical Care Classification: 21 Care Components (Version 2.5) Coded by Alphabetic Classes*

Code	Component	Code	Component
A	Activity	K	Physical Regulation
B	Bowel/Gastric	L	Respiratory
C	Cardiac	M	Role Relationship
D	Cognitive/NEURO	N	Safety
E	Coping	O	Self-Care
F	Fluid Volume	P	Self-Concept
G	Health Behavior	Q	Sensory
H	Medication	R	Skin Integrity
I	Metabolic	S	Tissue Perfusion
J	Nutritional	T	Urinary Elimination
		U	Life Cycle

*The Clinical Care Classification system is copyrighted, placed in public domain, and cannot be sold, but is available with written permission (Saba, V., 2012. *Clinical Care Classification (CCC) system manual.* New York: Springer, pp. 142–150).

An Example of CCC Nursing Diagnoses and Interventions

A—ACTIVITY COMPONENT *(1 of 21 Care Components)*—A cluster of elements that involve the use of energy in carrying out musculoskeletal and bodily actions.

01 Activity Alteration *(Major Nursing Diagnosis)*—Change in or modification of energy used by the body.

Subcategories that provide greater definition of the problem (of "01 Activity Alteration")

01.0 Activity Alteration
01.1 Activity Intolerance
01.2 Activity Intolerance Risk
01.3 Diversional Activity Deficit
01.4 Fatigue
01.5 Physical Mobility Impairment
01.6 Sleep Pattern Disturbance
01.7 Sleep Deprivation

Actions performed to carry out physiological or psychological daily activities:

Example: Teach Passive Range of Motion

Source: Saba, V. K. (2012.). About. Clinical Care Classification System. Version 2.5, (2nd ed.). New York: Springer. Retrieved September 13, 2013, from http://www.sabacare.com/Tables/Components.html

CLINICAL REASONING

Applying the Full-Spectrum Nursing Model

PATIENT SITUATION

Rachel, a freshman at State University, participated in a sorority rush activity during the second week of school. Nearly 150 other freshman girls attended the event to socialize in the Student Union. About 2 or 3 days later, Rachel learned six of the students at the party tested positive for the H1N1 virus and displayed signs of illness. Cite the resources you used to answer the following questions. Be sure they are of professional quality.

THINKING

1. *Theoretical Knowledge:*
   a. What is another name for the H1N1 virus?
   b. Name six common outward signs of an H1N1 infection that you might see in a college student.
2. *Critical Thinking (Contextual Awareness):*
   Why is it important to detect and treat H1N1 in a healthy population of young adults?

DOING

3. *Nursing Process (Assessment):*
   How might you assess the extent of the problem of H1N1 illness within the campus community?
4. *Practical Knowledge:*
   a. As the Community Health nurse, you design a *primary* intervention program to prevent an outbreak of H1N1 virus on campus. What might you do for this program?
   b. What interventions would you likely implement to deliver a *secondary* intervention program?
   c. Or a *tertiary* program?

CARING

5. *Self-Knowledge:*
   How would you feel if you were one of the first-detected cases or H1N1 illness spread across the college campus?

Critical Thinking and Clinical Reasoning

1. You are nearing completion of your fundamentals course. One night while you are preparing for your next clinical, the telephone rings. It is your neighbor, Tanya. Her 5-year-old daughter, Tiffany, attends kindergarten at the local public school. Tiffany came home with a letter from the school nurse stating that

another child in the class was ill with H1N1 and that all the students in the class had been exposed to this flu virus.

Tanya is concerned about the risks to Tiffany and the rest of the family. Tiffany was vaccinated against H1N1. Tanya is 8 months pregnant, and the family has no health insurance. She states that because you are a nursing student, she thought you might know what she should do or where she might go for assistance.

What are the key pieces of information (both theoretical knowledge and patient data) you need to solve your neighbor's situation?

2. You are a nurse in a public health clinic providing routine childhood immunizations. A 16-year-old mother comes into the clinic requesting "shots" for her newborn baby as well as a birth control "shot." She indicates that she has no money to pay for the shots because her 20-year-old boyfriend gave her only enough to get to the clinic. Which of the following is your nursing priority for this situation? What will you do next? Explain *how* you have chosen your priority diagnosis. On what did you base your choice?
   - Give the newborn the immunizations, and arrange for the client to meet with the social worker regarding securing healthcare coverage.
   - Educate the mother about birth control.
   - Take the client and child to a private room, and discuss the general health of the newborn and the plans for a healthcare provider to see the child. Also ask about the health needs of the mother.
   - Ask the mother whether she is being abused and report the incident if so.
3. Your assignment is to conduct a community assessment of your neighborhood. How will your membership in the community affect your assessment? What activities could you delete from the assessment?
4. You are driving home from nursing school clinical day and happen upon a car overturned along a deserted country road. You recall what you learned about the "Good Samaritan" laws. Under these circumstances, are you liable for the care you provide? What is your best course of intervention?
5. As a beginning home health nurse, you have been assigned to visit the following clients today:
   - Roland Escobar (Meet Your Patients, Volume 1), a 78-year-old man recovering from a cerebrovascular accident (stroke)
   - Sally Littlemoon, a 48-year-old woman with diabetes mellitus, blindness, and lower extremity cellulitis (a skin infection)
   - Beatrice Wayne, a 67-year-old woman who has undergone elective coronary artery bypass graft surgery (open-heart surgery)
   - Kent Churchill, an 80-year-old man with a recent hip fracture and surgical repair
   - Ms. Chana Padir, a 50-year-old woman with severe pain secondary to breast cancer with extensive metastases. She is receiving hospice care.

   a. Explore some alternatives for your schedule. How would you prepare to make these five visits in one day? How would you determine how to arrange your schedule?

   b. The report you receive from the home health supervisor includes the following information:
      - Ms. Littlemoon and Mr. Churchill require dressing changes.
      - Mr. Escobar and Ms. Wayne require teaching about their medications.
      - Mr. Escobar, Ms. Littlemoon, and Mr. Churchill require venipuncture for lab work.
      - Ms. Padir is having increasing pain.

      Based on this information, what else do you need to know and/or do before you begin your visits? What practical knowledge will you need to provide care for these clients?

   c. How might the care you deliver to Ms. Wayne differ from the care you give to Ms. Padir? To answer the question, consider the context for each woman. How are their situations different?

   d. When visiting Ms. Padir, you realize that her husband and children are very fearful of her impending death. They seem overwhelmed by the care she requires.

      What values and beliefs do you have about death and dying that might influence your care of the Padir family? (Review Chapters 15, 16, and 17 if necessary.)

      What must you consider to plan your interventions? How might you intervene?

   e. When you arrive at the home of Ms. Wayne, she is dressed and out of bed. She tells you she is able to get out of bed and ambulate about the house independently with very little pain. She can identify the medications she is receiving, their purpose, and their schedule for administration. Her chest wound is healing nicely, and her breath sounds are clear. She informs you that she is planning on going to her cabin in the mountains this upcoming weekend with her husband and children. What actions must you take with regard to continuing her home visits? Why?

      What rules/guidelines will influence your choice of action?

6. For each of the following concepts, use critical thinking and summarize how or why it is important to nursing, patient care, or community nursing. Note that these are *not* to be merely definitions.
   Community
   Aggregates
   Census tracts
   Vulnerable populations
   Healthy People 2020
   Windshield survey
   Primary intervention
   Secondary intervention
   Tertiary intervention
   Disaster preparedness
   Omaha system
7. For each of the following concepts, use critical thinking to describe how or why it is important to nurses, patient care, or nursing in the home. Note that these are *not* to be merely definitions.
   Delivering healthcare in the home setting
   Skilled services
   Caregiver role strain
   Preparing for the home visit
   Developing rapport at the home visit
   Assessment of the home environment
   Documentation of home healthcare services
   Clinical Care Classification System

What Are the Main Points in This Chapter?

- A community can be defined as a place with defined boundaries, a group of people with a common language, rituals, or customs.
- Each community determines the meaning of health and nursing activities to promote health.
- A vulnerable population is defined as an aggregate that is at increased risk of adverse health outcomes. Members of vulnerable groups have a higher probability of developing illness.
- The community nurse assesses three general dimensions of a community: structure, status, and process.
- Common practice areas for community-based nurses include schools, churches, prison systems, disaster relief services, occupational and public health clinics, and international relief organizations.
- Community health nursing focuses on the health of individuals, families, and groups and how their individual health affects the community as a whole.
- Public health nursing focuses on the community at large and the eventual effect of the community's health status on the health of individuals, families, and groups.
- Community-oriented nursing combines components of community and public health. Nurses practicing community-oriented nursing are fluid in their approach. Their focus is a comprehensive look at the individual, family, group, and community at large. Community-based nurses function as advocates, educators, collaborators, counselors, and effective communicators.
- Community-based nurses may provide care at three levels: primary (preventive), secondary (early detection and early treatment), and tertiary (halt disease progression). The focus is on primary prevention.
- The Omaha classification system is a commonly used documentation system for generating a care plan for a community or an individual within the community setting.
- A community health nurse might practice as a school nurse, public health nurse, parish or prison nurse, international health nurse, or disaster service.
- Home health care is delivered in the community setting.
- Home health nursing fosters client and family independence and promotes self-care.
- In the home setting, many factors, such as cleanliness and noise level, are not within the nurse's control. In addition, the home health nurse works without immediate on-site access to other healthcare professionals.
- Home health agencies may be public, voluntary, proprietary, or hospital-based agencies. They may

provide direct or indirect care and may specialize in certain types of clients.

- As a full-spectrum nurse working in home healthcare, you will function in the following roles: communicator, direct care provider, client/family educator, client advocate, and care coordinator (case manager).
- Hospice nurses work in hospitals, special hospice facilities, or the homes of patients who are dying. The goal of their care is to provide comfort and manage symptoms.
- Home healthcare is reimbursed by Medicare, by Medicaid, by private insurance, and through direct payment from the client. Medicare and Medicaid are the largest payors.
- To be eligible for continuing care under most government healthcare programs and private insurers, a client must be homebound and require skilled nursing care.
- Preparation for a home visit includes obtaining information from the referral, identifying the purpose of the visit, gathering required supplies, contacting the client to arrange the visit, and providing for your own safety.
- During a home visit, you will establish a rapport with the client and family, assess the needs of the client and caregivers, develop and discuss the plan of care and needed services with the client and caregivers, provide skilled care, and evaluate the need for continued services.
- Medicare requires specific client assessments using a form called the Outcome and Assessment Information Set (OASIS). It must be completed at the start of care, with each recertification (every 60 days), and at the termination of care.
- The Clinical Care Classification (CCC) system is a system of care and documentation used by most home-care agencies.
- Interventions to reduce Caregiver Role Strain include providing emotional support and arranging additional home and community services to support the client and caregiver.
- As a nurse delivering home care, you will need to follow standard precautions but recognize how infection control techniques may be modified to the home environment.
- In addition to infection control, nursing interventions usually include assisting with medication management, assessing and supporting home safety, and providing caregiver support.
- After a home visit you must document care, coordinate services for the client, and prepare for future visits.

Knowledge Map

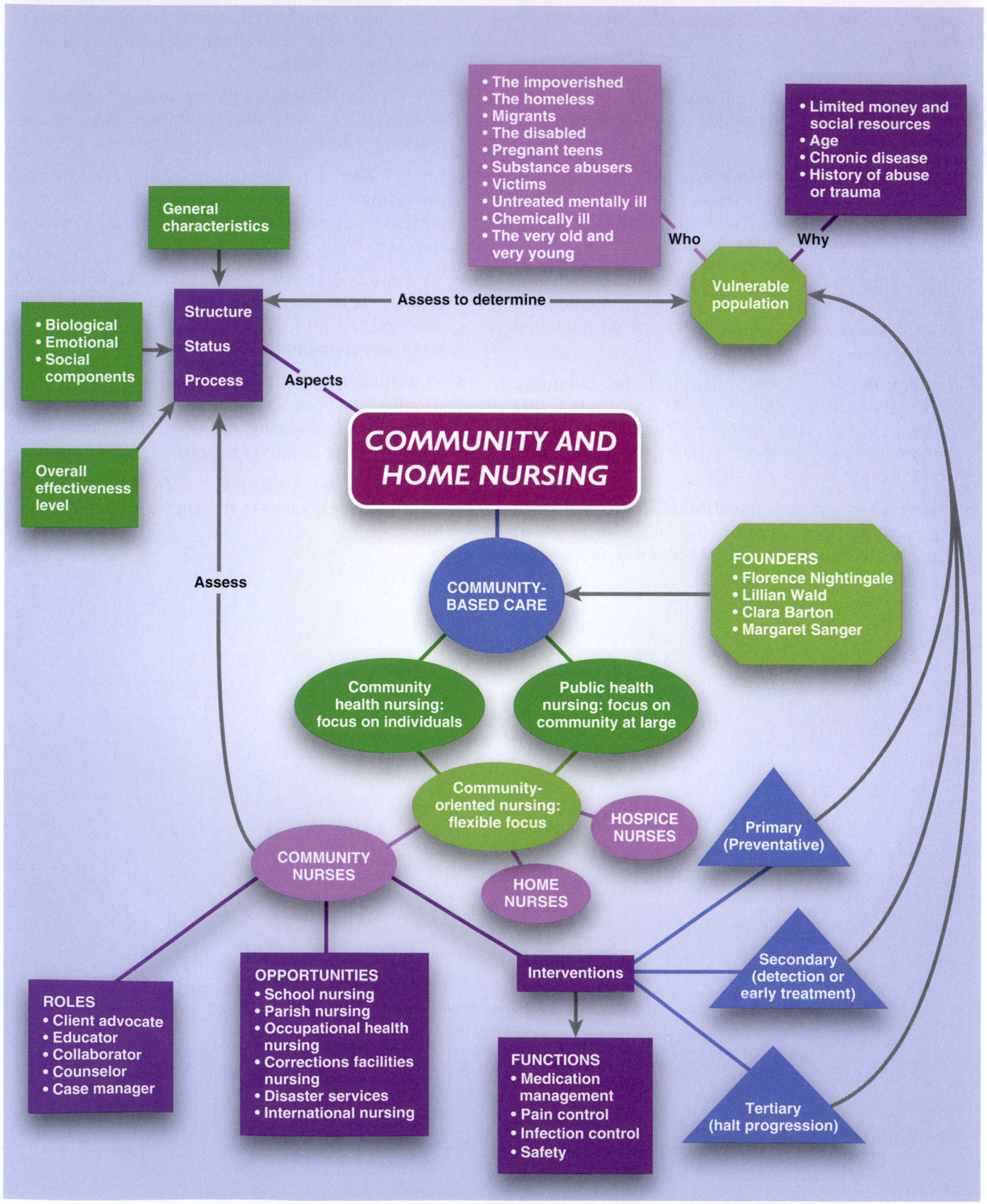

CHAPTER 44

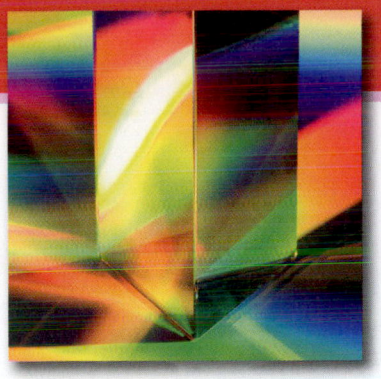

Ethics & Values

STUDENT RESOURCES

*The questions and exercises in Volume 2 allow you to practice the kind of thinking you will use as a full-spectrum nurse. Critical-thinking questions usually have more than one correct answer, so we do not provide "answers" for these features. It is more important to develop your nursing judgment than to just cover content. You will learn by discussing the questions with your peers. If you are still unsure, consult your instructor. You will find Response Sheets (for writing your responses to the questions) on Davis*Plus.

To explore learning resources for this chapter,

Go to Davis*Plus* at DavisPl.us/Wilkinson3.

Chapter Resources for Chapter 44:

- **Response sheets for all learning exercises**
- **Resources for Caregivers and Health Professionals**
- **Reading More About Ethics & Values (suggested readings)**
- **Concept Map of chapter content**

Interactive Case Studies

NCLEX-Style and Chapter Review Questions

CHAPTER OVERVIEW

For a podcast of an overview of this chapter,

Go to Student Resources, Chapter 44, **Podcast—Chapter Overview,** on Davis*Plus*.

Caring for the Nguyens

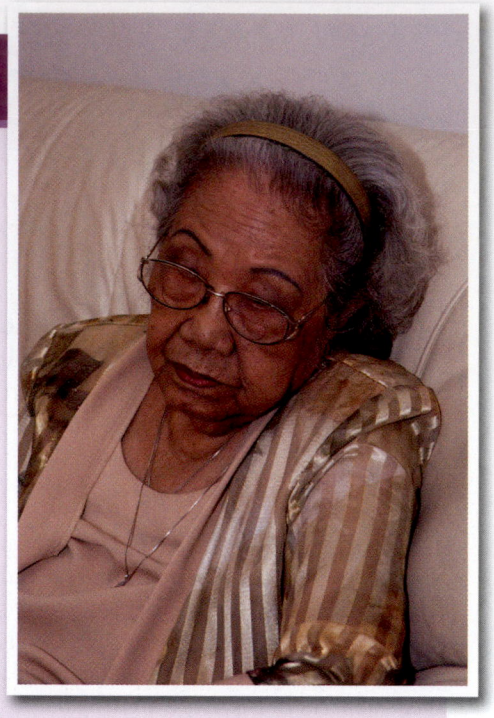

Mai Nguyen, Nam's mother, has hypertension. She is forgetful about taking her medicines. Since her husband died, she has experienced periods of depression. When asked about her medicines she often replies, "It doesn't really matter since my husband died. If I die, what difference will it make?"

Mai Nguyen was scheduled to have lunch with friends but did not arrive. When her friends called the house, they got no answer. At the end of lunch, one of Mai's friends decided to call Nam to inform him of her concerns about his mother. Nam found his mother unresponsive on the kitchen floor. He called 911, and she was brought to the hospital by ambulance. At the hospital, the emergency department (ED) doctor tells Nam that his mother has had a massive stroke (brain attack) brought on by uncontrolled hypertension. He asks Nam whether Mai has an advance directive or living will. Mai has neither. The physician asks Nam to consider what level of care to offer his mother. He tells Nam that comprehensive treatment would include intubation, mechanical ventilation, and tube feeding support. He feels it is unlikely that she will experience significant recovery from this stroke.

Nam tells you, "I want everything done for my mother. I lost my father this year, and I'm not going to lose her, too." Yen, Nam's wife, reminds you that Mai has been depressed since her husband died and has expressed a desire to die. Because Nam and Yen are not in agreement about the course of action, no decision is communicated. Mai's condition continues to deteriorate, and the ED physician feels he must intubate her, place her on a ventilator, and admit her to the ICU according to hospital protocol.

A. You are aware of Mai's statements and her poor compliance with treatment. What, if any, concerns do you have about this course of action?

B. Mai continues to decline. Nam is informed that the "only thing keeping his mother alive is the ventilator and IV medicines." Do you consider this heroic treatment?

C. How would you approach Mr. Nguyen to speak with him about how he is feeling?

D. Nam and Yen have asked to meet with the team providing care to Mai. They announce that they would like all the "heroic measures to end." They request that Mai be allowed to die. Could you participate in this care? What actions would you be comfortable with? What actions would you be uncomfortable with?

Practical Knowledge knowing how

Practical knowledge in nursing ethics primarily involves communication and problem-solving skills. We have included one model of ethical decision making as well as guidelines for patient advocacy for your quick reference in clinical situations.

CLINICAL INSIGHTS

Clinical Insight 44-1 ➤ Using the MORAL Model for Ethical Decision Making

- **M—Massage the dilemma.** Identify and define the issues in the dilemma. Consider the options of all the major players in the dilemma and their value systems. This includes patients, family members, nurses, physicians, religious representatives, and other interdisciplinary health-care members. Identify the information gaps.
- **O—Outline the options.** Examine all the options, including those that are less realistic and conflicting. This stage is designed only for considering options and not for making final decisions.
- **R—Resolve the dilemma.** Review issues and options, applying basic principles of ethics to each option. Decide the best option based on the views of all those concerned in the dilemma.
- **A—Act by applying the chosen option.** This step is usually the most difficult because it requires actual implementation, whereas the previous steps allow only for dialogue and discussion.
- **L—Look back and evaluate.** Reflect on the entire process and evaluate all steps, including the implementation. No process is complete without thorough evaluation. Ensure that those involved are able to follow through on the final option. If not, a second decision may be required and the process must begin again at the first step.

References

Tschundin, V. (2003). *Ethics in nursing: The caring relationship* (3rd ed.). Oxford, England: Butterworth & Heinemann.

Yoder-Wise, P. (2010). *Leading and managing in nursing* (5th ed.). St. Louis, MO: C. V. Mosby.

Clinical Insight 44-2 ➤ Guidelines for Advocacy

The following principles will help you to function effectively as an advocate.

- **Keep the ethical principle of patient autonomy always in mind.**
- **Know and document the facts** of the case.
- **Know the arguments** of those who oppose the patient. **Use role playing** to develop a strategy for responding to the arguments.
- **Have a sound base of support for your actions.** Be familiar with any policies or laws that apply.
- **Form a coalition of allies**, if you can. Get consultation. Communicate, inform, and clarify their collaborative roles.
- **Intervene high enough in the hierarchy** to get the job done. If the difficulty is with a physician or an organizational policy, merely going to the charge nurse will not be enough. You will need to communicate with nurse administrators or other agency administrators.
- **Demonstrate to the system** how it is defeating its own goals (e.g., for patient care).
- **Avoid getting into a power struggle** if possible (use the preceding steps first). If you must, decide how far you need to go and whether you are willing to go that far. You will need to enlist people with more power in the system than you have (e.g., family members, physicians, administrators).
- **Be aware of client vulnerability.** When possible, avoid confrontation. If there is risk for the client (as in a power contest), be sure the client is aware of his risks and possible gains; then let him choose how far to take the situation.
- **Have alternative actions.** Assess risks realistically. Weigh them against potential gains.

CLINICALREASONING

Applying the Full-Spectrum Nursing Model

PATIENT SITUATION

Read the following summary of the Kithari and Kirschner article:

Kothari, S., & Kirschner, K. (2006). Abandoning the Golden Rule: The problem with "putting ourselves in the patient's place." ***Topics in Stroke Rehabilitation, 13*****(4), 68–73.**

A large body of evidence documents the difficulties healthcare professionals have in predicting what their patient believes or wishes. These difficulties extend from the predictions of:

- Very specific patient wishes, such as for life-sustaining therapies
- More global assessments of patients' lives as a whole (for instance, their quality of life)

One explanation for this phenomenon is that healthcare professionals, either consciously or unconsciously, adopt "Golden Rule thinking." This refers to our attempts to understand another person's situation by imagining what we would believe or want under similar circumstances, in other words, "putting ourselves in the patient's place."

Although Golden Rule thinking would seem to be a promising strategy, studies show that it actually results in inaccurate presumptions of patients' wishes or beliefs. These presumptions, in turn, have significant clinical and ethical implications. That is, they cause healthcare professionals and families to make decisions for the patient that are, in reality, *not* what the patient would want. The thinking goes:

I should put myself in the patient's place.
If I were the patient, I would want X.
Therefore, the patient probably wants X.
Because the patient probably wants X, we will do X.

This thinking process can have different results: (1) The patient really does want X, so you have met his needs. (2) The patient really wanted Y, so you did not meet his needs.

THINKING

1. *Theoretical Knowledge:* What is the Golden Rule, or what does it say?
2. *Critical Thinking (Inquiry):* What is one thing that could be done ahead of time to prevent the need for Golden Rule thinking? Explain why that would work.

DOING

3. *Nursing Process (Assessment):* If you do not know what the patient would want, instead of thinking what *you* would want, how might you get an idea of what the patient might want?

CARING

4. *Self-Knowledge:* What is your earliest memory of being taught the Golden Rule?
5. *Ethical Knowledge:* Which ethical principle does the Golden Rule seem to try to follow: autonomy, nonmaleficence/beneficence, fidelity, veracity, or justice?

Critical Thinking and Clinical Reasoning

1. Some examples of ethical issues you may encounter are end-of-life issues, abortion or other reproductive issues, breaches of patient confidentiality, and incompetent or illegal practices of colleagues. Stop for a moment and think about a time when you have witnessed an ethical challenge in the clinical area.
   a. Describe the situation.
   b. How well equipped did you feel to handle the situation?
   c. What guided your thoughts and actions?
2. At the beginning of this chapter in Volume 1, Alan (Meet Your Patients), a teenager, had been injured in a soccer game. Without a blood transfusion, he may die, but because his family is of the Jehovah's Witnesses faith, Alan's parents have refused to sign permission for his transfusion. Taking each of the abilities required

for ethical agency, state whether or not you think these people have the abilities listed below: Alan, Alan's parents, the physician, the nurse. Explain your thinking. An ethical agent must be able to:

a. Perceive the difference between good and evil, right and wrong.
   Alan
   Parents
   Physician/surgeon
   Nurse
b. Understand abstract ethical principles.
   Alan
   Parents
   Physician/surgeon
   Nurse
c. Reason and apply ethical principles to make decisions, weigh alternatives, and plan ways to achieve goals.
   Alan
   Parents
   Physician/surgeon
   Nurse
d. Decide and choose freely.
   Alan
   Parents
   Physician/surgeon
   Nurse
e. Act according to his choice; this assumes both the power and the capability to act.
   Alan
   Parents
   Physician/surgeon
   Nurse

3. Consider Alan's situation again. Analyze the situation (a) using a deontological framework and ethical principles and then (b) using a utilitarian framework. Focus on this question: Is it ethical to try hard to influence the parents to consent to allow a blood transfusion?
   a. Deontology
   b. Utilitarianism
   c. Did you reach a different conclusion depending on the framework you selected?
4. You are a busy nurse caring for a caseload of eight patients. One patient is the mother of the hospital administrator. She had surgery 3 days ago and is progressing nicely, but she is very demanding and requires a great deal of assistance to be repositioned in bed and to move from bed to chair. She has frequent visitors, including children and young grandchildren. In the next room is a young Haitian woman whose bill is paid by Medicaid. She has a history of drug abuse and had surgery this morning. She speaks little English and seems very anxious. She is experiencing nausea and pain and needs a transfusion of a unit of packed red blood cells this evening. Her boyfriend is at the desk requesting to bring her 3-year-old daughter to the unit so that she may see her mother. The visiting policy says that children must be at least 12 years old to visit the unit. Consider what aspects of justice apply to this situation and how it might be most equitably handled. Focus on the principle of justice.
5. An example of the feminist ethical approach arises in deciding whether to allocate federal healthcare resources to younger people (e.g., education, day care, free immunizations) or to older adults (e.g., prescription drug insurance, long-term care). Feminist reasoning would be as follows:
   - In the United States, older women outnumber older men.
   - Older women tend to be poorer and are more likely to be alone than are men.
   - Therefore, if healthcare for older adults were to be rationed, it would negatively affect women more than it would men.
   - Thus, more healthcare resources should be allocated to older adults, especially women.

   a. Analyze this decision using a deontological framework. Explain your reasoning, as was done above.
   b. Analyze this decision using a consequentialist framework. Explain your reasoning.
6. Deception can take different forms, from intentional lying to nondisclosure of information or partial disclosure of information. Think about your duty to tell the truth. Is there ever a time when being completely honest is not the best nursing intervention? Do you consider withholding information the same as lying?

7. Review the following scenario. Examine your self-knowledge, and work through the steps of the values clarification process (choosing, prizing, and acting). A 40-year-old couple with no other children learn that their unborn child has Down syndrome. The couple needs to make a difficult decision because the mother is 18 weeks pregnant.
   a. How would you feel about this couple if they chose to have this child and insisted on doing everything possible to keep the baby alive even if it is born with severe handicaps?
   b. Do you think that your professional relationship with this couple would change if they chose to terminate the pregnancy?
   c. How can you help the couple clarify their values?
      (1) List alternatives.
      (2) Examine the possible consequences of the alternative choices.
      (3) Choose freely.
      (4) Feel good about the choice that has been made.
      (5) Affirm the choice to others.
      (6) Act on the choice.
      (7) Act with a consistent pattern.

What Are the Main Points in This Chapter?

- Ethics is a formal process for deciding right and wrong conduct in situations in which issues of values and morals arise.
- Nursing ethics refers to ethical questions that arise out of nursing practice.
- Morals are learned and internalized throughout the life span. Carol Gilligan proposed that moral development and reasoning are different between men and women.
- Ethical agency is the ability to make ethical choices and to be responsible for one's ethical actions. In practice, nurses sometimes make moral decisions that they are not able to carry out.
- Moral distress is the inability to carry out moral decisions.
- Whistleblowing occurs when a person identifies in the workplace an incompetent, unethical, or illegal situation or action of others, and then appeals to someone who may have the power to stop it.
- Nursing ethics problems arise from technological advances, the needs of a multicultural population, cost containment efforts in healthcare, the nature of nursing work, and the nature of the nursing profession.
- Nurses have complex obligations and multiple complex relationships within healthcare organizations (e.g., with employers, physicians, patients, families, and other nurses).
- Ethical decisions are affected by a person's developmental stage, values, ethical frameworks and principles, and professional guidelines.
- Attitudes are mental dispositions or feelings toward a person, object, or idea.
- A belief is something that one accepts as true.
- A value is a belief that you have about the worth of something; a value is highly prized and expressed through behaviors, feelings, and decisions.
- Values are transmitted through social interaction.
- Value neutrality means that we attempt to understand our own values regarding an issue and to know when to put them aside, if necessary, to become nonjudgmental.
- Six important ethical principles are autonomy, nonmaleficence, beneficence, fidelity, veracity, and justice.
- Consequentialist theories are ethical theories in which the rightness or wrongness of an action depends on the consequences of the act, rather than on the nature of the act itself.
- The principle of utility states that a "good" act is one that produces the greatest good for the greatest number of people.
- Deontological theories consider an action to be right or wrong independent of its consequences.
- Feminist ethics asserts that focusing on deontological principles distracts one from dealing with larger social issues and that objectivity is impossible.
- An ethics-of-care directs attention to a patient's specific situation viewed within the context of his or her life narrative. It emphasizes feelings, but not at the expense of some conventional ethical principles, such as autonomy, nonmaleficence, or beneficence.
- Nurses can obtain ethical guidance from professional codes of ethics, standards of practice, and the American Hospital Association's *Patient Care Partnership*.

- The principle of autonomy underlies informed consent—clients' right to decide for themselves whether or not they will agree to a proposed procedure or treatment.
- Specific ethical issues the nurse is likely to encounter may involve AIDS, abortion, allocation of resources, issues of confidentiality, end-of-life issues (e.g., advance directives, DNAR orders, life-sustaining treatments, informed consent, organ transplantation), and reproductive technologies.
- A **value** is a belief you have about the worth of something; it serves as a principle or a standard that influences your decision making.
- Values clarification is the process of becoming conscious of and naming one's values. Nurses can assist clients with values clarification.
- Not all moral problems are dilemmas. A dilemma is a particular kind of moral problem: It is a painful situation in which a choice must be made between two equally undesirable actions. There is no clearly right or wrong option.
- One method of working through an ethical problem is to perform assessment and diagnosis, as in the nursing process; then use the mnemonic MORAL: **M**assage the dilemma, **O**utline the options, **R**esolve the dilemma, **A**ct by applying the chosen option, and **L**ook back and evaluate.
- A good compromise preserves the integrity of all parties when there is disagreement among them in an ethical situation.
- Nurses should be patient advocates because (1) their professional role requires it, (2) they have special knowledge that the patient does not have, (3) they have a special relationship with patients, and (4) one aspect of the nursing role is to defend a patient's autonomous decisions.
- The nurse's role as an advocate is to inform, support, and communicate.

Knowledge Map

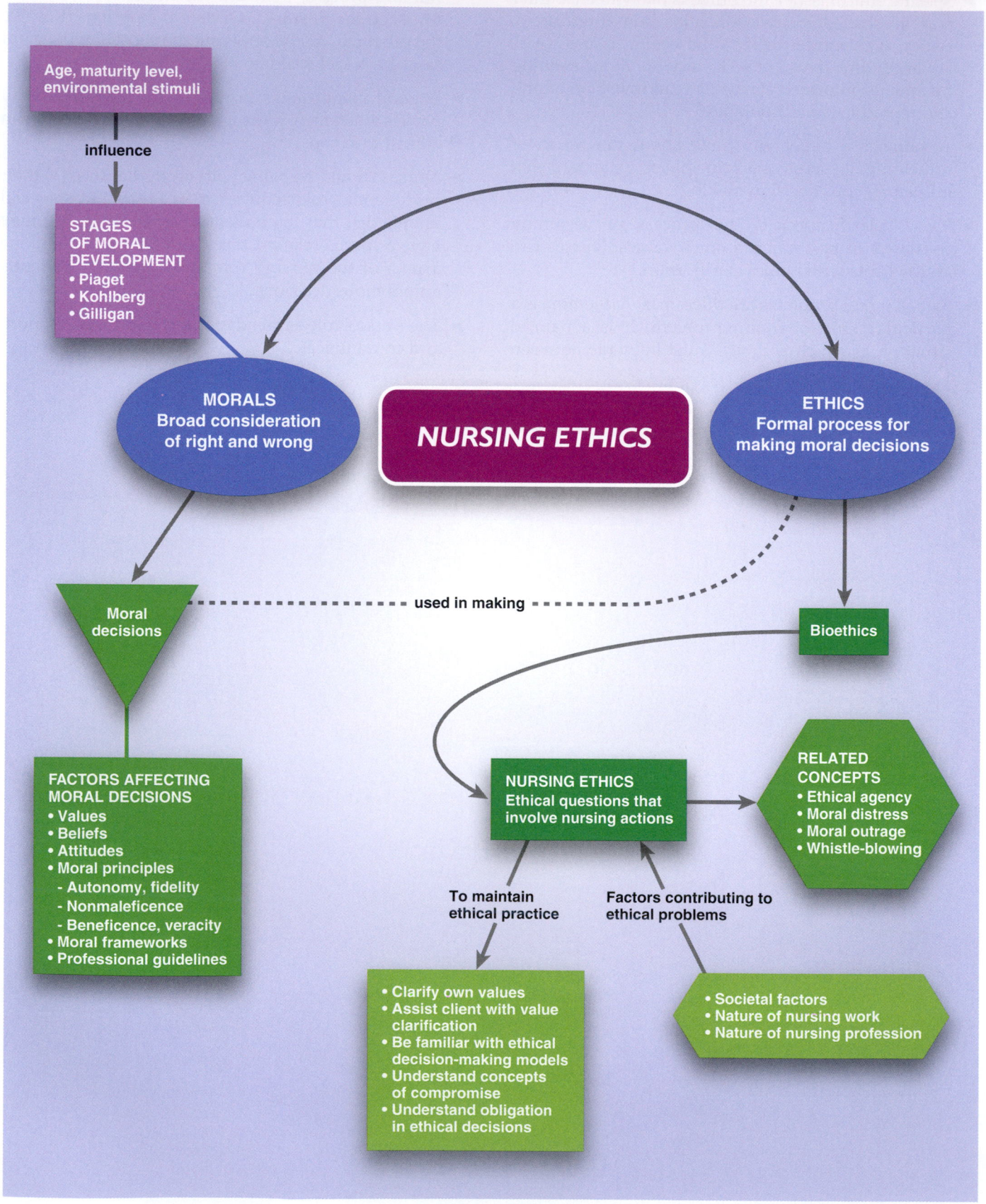

CHAPTER 45

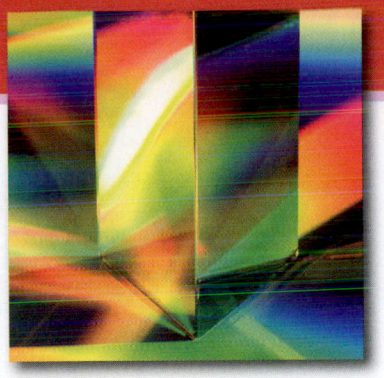

Legal Accountability

STUDENT RESOURCES

*The questions and exercises in Volume 2 allow you to practice the kind of thinking you will use as a full-spectrum nurse. Critical-thinking questions usually have more than one correct answer, so we do not provide "answers" for these features. It is more important to develop your nursing judgment than to just cover content. You will learn by discussing the questions with your peers. If you are still unsure, consult your instructor. You will find Response Sheets (for writing your responses to the questions) on Davis*Plus.

To explore learning resources for this chapter,

Go to Davis*Plus* at DavisPl.us/Wilkinson3.

Chapter Resources for Chapter 45:

- **Response sheets for all learning exercises**
- **Resources for Caregivers and Health Professionals**
- **Reading More About Legal Accountability (suggested readings)**
- **Concept Map of chapter content**

Interactive Case Studies

NCLEX-Style and Chapter Review Questions

CHAPTER OVERVIEW

For a podcast of an overview of this chapter,

Go to Student Resources, Chapter 45, **Podcast—Chapter Overview**, on Davis*Plus*.

Caring for the Nguyens

Nam and Yen Nguyen have requested an appointment with you, the nurse at the Family Medicine Clinic, to discuss advance directives. Their experience with Nam's mother, Mai, has created concerns about end-of-life care.

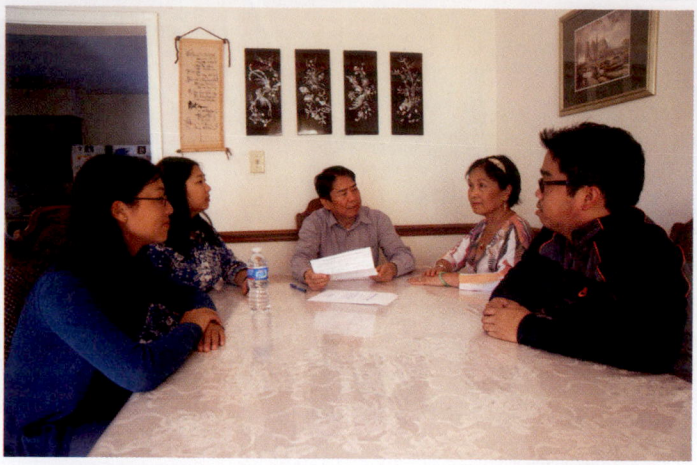

A. Nam asks you, "Do you think it's appropriate to create an advance directive at my age?" How would you respond?

B. Nam tells you that he believes in "natural death." He states, "I don't want extraordinary measures, and I never want to be resuscitated." Yen responds that she is extremely uncomfortable with blanket statements about treatment. "If he got hit by a car or had some accident, I would want you to do everything in your power to treat him. I couldn't carry out his wishes," she states. What actions should you take to help Nam and Yen resolve this discrepancy?

Practical Knowledge knowing how

CLINICAL INSIGHTS

Clinical Insight 45-1 ➤ Using Equipment Safely

The following will help you to ensure proper and safe use of equipment:

1. Obtain appropriate training on equipment use.
2. Follow the healthcare agency's protocols, policies, and procedures on the use of the equipment.
3. Follow the manufacturer's operating instructions.
4. Be sure medical equipment has been properly inspected.
5. Perform safety checks regularly and before each use.
6. Position and use equipment properly during treatment.
7. Know how the equipment functions; be alert to signs that it is not working properly.
8. Make sure rooms are not cluttered with equipment.
9. Follow agency policies regarding equipment brought from the patient's home (e.g., hair dryers, electric shavers, radios); usually these should be inspected for proper grounding and safe cords.
10. Remove and label equipment that is malfunctioning to prevent others from using it until it can be repaired or replaced.

Practice Resources

Mattox, E. (2012).

Clinical Insight 45-2 ➤ Tips for Avoiding Malpractice

- **Develop open, honest, respectful, caring relationships** with patients and families. Patients are more likely to sue if they are angry or feel that you were not caring and professional.
- **Careful, thorough documentation** is the best defense if a lawsuit does occur:
  - Use and document all steps of the nursing process.
  - Be especially thorough when documenting care for patients who will not comply with treatments or who complain a lot.
  - Courts assume that if care is not documented, it was not given.
- **Know and follow applicable laws:** (1) federal and state laws, (2) your state's nurse practice act (perform only the activities within your scope of practice and competence).
- **Know and follow agency policies and procedures.**
- **Know and follow standards of care** set forth in the state nurse practice act, by professional organizations, in professional literature, by agency policy, and so on.
- **Follow the "rights" of medication administration** (see Chapter 26).
- **Perform falls risk assessments**, document, and take measures to ensure patient safety.
- **Recognize "problem" patients.** Try to identify the basic problem or complaint and intervene to resolve it.
- **Follow medical orders**, but clarify them as needed. Do not implement a questionable order or one you do not understand.
- **Don't blame or criticize other healthcare providers** in the presence of patients (e.g., "Sorry the night shift didn't give you your pain medicine.")
- **Maintain patient privacy and confidentiality.**
- **Don't make statements that may appear to be an admission of guilt** (e.g., "Omigosh, I forgot to shut off that IV!"). Errors should not be included on the patient's health record, but instead in an incident report.
- **Stay competent in your area of practice**; for example, attend continuing education, webinars, and in-service programs to improve your knowledge and skills.
- **Don't accept a clinical assignment that you think you are not competent to perform.** Evaluate your assignment with your supervisor if there is a question.
- **Recognize significant assessment cues**, and notify primary care providers of changes in the patient's condition or patient complaints.
- **Document the time and content of telephone conversations with other healthcare providers.**
- **Send copies only**, never originals, of records and reports requested by other professionals.

Practice Resources

Austin, S. (2008); Banford, E. & Budake, A. (2012); Reising, D. (2012).

Clinical Insight 45-3 ➤ Guidelines for Documenting Care

Complete reporting and documentation must address the following:

1. Patient status (e.g., symptoms and responses to treatments)
2. The nursing care given
3. Physician and other provider prescriptions
4. Medications and treatments
5. Patient responses
6. Consultations with other members of the healthcare team regarding patient status

When documenting care, use the F-A-C-T mnemonic:

Factual
Accurate
Complete
Timely

Another way to remember how to document is to use the 5 Cs. Charting should be:

Complete
Clear
Correct
Comprehensive
Chronological

Practice Resources

Arnold, P. (2012); Austin, S. (2011); Helm, A. (2003, pp. 1-33).

CLINICALREASONING

Applying the Full-Spectrum Nursing Model

PATIENT SITUATION

A nurse employed by a temporary agency is assigned to a neurology unit for a 12-hour shift. On arrival, she discovers that the registered nurse (RN) assigned for the shift called in sick, leaving her with two nursing assistive personnel (NAPs) to provide patient care and administer medication, including controlled substances. The nursing supervisor informs her that she will be responsible for the unit with 22 patients, 12 of whom are acutely ill and require close observation and frequent care. The nursing supervisor is not available to work on the unit and has no additional RNs to provide patient care. The nurse decides not to accept the assignment, to report the decision and reasons to her agency supervisor, and to leave the neurology unit immediately before starting the shift.

THINKING

1. *Theoretical Knowledge:*
   a. In addition to protecting her nursing license, what other factors should the nurse have considered in deciding whether to stay or leave the unit?
   b. Because the nurse decided not to accept the assignment, would this have been considered abandonment?
   c. What standards, guidelines, and laws would apply to determine whether the nurse's behavior was in accordance with standards of practice?
2. *Critical Thinking (Contextual Awareness)*:
   a. Which statements in the ANA Nurses' Bill of Rights should the nurse have considered before deciding whether to accept the assignment?
   b. What factors in this situation could create legal problems for the nurse?

DOING

3. *Nursing Process (Planning/Intervention)*: The nurse's action (leaving the unit) might be viewed, under some laws in some situations, as abandonment of patients. What are some alternative actions the nurse might have taken to avoid that risk?

CARING

4. *Self-Knowledge:* Have you ever been in a situation in which you felt a moral obligation to help out but yet knew you would be in over your head? Describe your experience.
5. *Ethical Knowledge:* In your opinion, did the nurse do the right thing when she decided not to accept the assignment and to leave the nursing unit immediately? Explain your thinking.

Critical Thinking and Clinical Reasoning

1. Think about the Meet Your Nurse Role Model scenario you read at the beginning of the chapter in Volume 1. A nurse with 3 years of experience on a medical-surgical unit arrives to work and discovers that two of her colleagues called in sick, including the charge nurse. The nursing supervisor informs her that she will need to assume the charge nurse role, in addition to assuming care for three patients. Feeling frustrated, the nurse ponders whether she should just quit and find another job, but nevertheless accepts the assignment. Two hours into the shift, one of her patients begins to experience complications, requiring blood glucose checks every 2 hours and frequent monitoring. In addition, one of the nurses becomes ill and is replaced by a float nurse from the labor and delivery unit. The nurse contacts the nursing supervisor and requests additional assistance, but is told no other nurse is available and that the supervisor is involved with an emergency situation on another unit. The nurse begins to analyze this situation from a legal perspective to determine the best course of action.

   Use the critical-thinking model to identify questions to ask yourself in reflecting and deciding what to do.

Go to Chapter 2, **Table 2-1, Critical-Thinking Model,** in Volume 1.

   a. What questions do you need to ask about context?
   b. What knowledge do you need to make an informed and credible decision?
   c. What questions do you need to ask about considering alternatives?
   d. What questions do you need to ask about analyzing your assumptions?
   e. What questions do you need to ask about reflecting and deciding?

2. Analyze this passage:
Nursys is the national database for verification of nurse licensure, practice privileges, and disciplinary information for RNs and LVN/LPNs. The e-Notify feature of Nursys provides real-time information to employers about their nurse employees as the information is entered into Nursys (National Council of State Board of Nursing, 2012).
   - Do you think there is a need for Nursys?
   - What rights does it help protect?
3. Imagine that you are working in a large medical center in an area where there have been several robberies and assaults in the past 6 months, mostly late at night. Although the parking lot is nearly a block from the employees' exit and is not well lighted, there is only one security guard on duty outside the hospital after 2200. Despite repeated requests from employees all the way up the chain of command, no efforts are being made to improve lighting or to hire more security guards. What standards and laws might be helpful to the employees?
4. George Agnew, 75 years old, is admitted to the emergency department after being involved in a serious car accident. His wife is with him, and she is very upset—to the point of being hysterical. It is likely that Mr. Agnew will die, but physicians are considering whether he will need a ventilator in the next hour or so. You need to know Mr. Agnew's wishes on this issue, but he is not conscious. The charge nurse tells you not to ask Mrs. Agnew because it will just upset her more.
   a. What is happening in the situation that may influence the outcome?
   b. What factors may influence your behavior and others' behavior in this situation?
   c. What values or biases do you have that influence your behavior in this situation?
   d. Where might you get the information you need instead of asking Mrs. Agnew?
   e. What would you do? What legal support, if any, do you have?
5. Compare and contrast the following definitions of practical nursing and professional nursing taken from the Nurse Practice Act in Missouri and then discuss the differences in the scope of practice for the LPN/LVN and the RN. Identify two tasks/responsibilities that only the RN can perform.

   DEFINITION 1. Practical nursing is the performance for compensation of selected acts for the promotion of health and in the care of persons who are ill, injured, or experiencing alterations in normal health processes. Such performance requires substantial specialized skill, judgment, and knowledge. All such nursing care shall be given under the direction of a person licensed by a state regulatory board to prescribe medications and treatments or under the direction of a registered professional nurse. For the purposes of this chapter, the term "direction" shall mean guidance or supervision provided by a person licensed by a state regulatory board to prescribe medications and treatments or a registered professional nurse, including, but not limited to, oral, written, or otherwise communicated orders or directives for patient care. When practical nursing care is delivered pursuant to the direction of a person licensed by a state regulatory board to prescribe medications and treatments or under the direction of a registered professional nurse, such care may be delivered by a licensed practical nurse without direct physical oversight.

   DEFINITION 2. Professional nursing is the performance for compensation of any act which requires substantial specialized education, judgment, and skill based on knowledge and application of principles derived from the biological, physical, social. and nursing sciences, including, but not limited to:
   a. Responsibility for the teaching of health care and the prevention of illness to the patient and his or her family;
   b. Assessment, nursing diagnosis, nursing care, and counsel of persons who are ill, injured, or experiencing alterations in normal health processes;
   c. The administration of medications and treatments as prescribed by a person licensed by a state regulatory board to prescribe medications and treatments;
   d. The coordination and assistance in the delivery of a plan of health care with all members of a health team;
   e. The teaching and supervision of other persons in the performance of any of the foregoing. (Missouri Revised Statutes, 2013).
6. The patient was an older adult with various medical conditions and receiving multiple medications. The nurse determined the patient was a high fall risk, 8 on a scale of 0 to 10. The nurse decided to initiate the hospital's fall prevention plan, which meant raising the siderails and placing restraints on the patient without physician's orders. Hospital policy, however, did require a nurse who initiated restraints on a patient for fall prevention to notify a physician or physician's assistant within 1 hour after doing so.

   The next day another nurse, seeing that no orders for restraints had been received, removed the restraints. The patient was getting up out of bed on his own. His nursing neurological assessment showed signs of dementia and confusion. His oxygen saturation was low and his heartbeat was irregular. The physician was notified by phone but declined to order restraints. Later that evening the patient was found on the floor with a closed-head injury. He was transferred to a university hospital, where he died a few weeks later. The case was dismissed against the hospital (Sturgill v. Ashe Memorial Hosp., 2008).

a. In this case, the nurse was caring for a patient at high risk for fall but did not have a prescription to use restraints. Why do you think the court dismissed the case against the hospital?

b. What other action might the nurse have taken to prevent this patient's fall?

7. For each of the following concepts, use critical thinking to describe how or why it is important to nurses, patients, or legal issues. Note that these are *not* to be merely definitions.

Civil law
The U.S. Constitution Bill of Rights and the Patient Care Partnership
The ANA Code of Ethics; the ANA Standards of Practice; and the ANA Nurses' Bill of Rights
Patient advocacy
Battery
Vicarious liability

What Are the Main Points in This Chapter?

- The law is a binding practice, rule, or code of conduct that guides a community or society and is enforced by a controlling authority.
- Laws are primarily derived from four sources: (1) the Constitution, (2) statutes, (3) administrative bodies, and (4) the courts.
- The right of privacy comes from the Bill of Rights.
- A living will is prepared by an alert and oriented (competent) individual to give directions to others about the person's wishes regarding life-prolonging treatments if the person becomes unable to make those decisions.
- A durable power of attorney for healthcare identifies a person who will make healthcare decisions in the event the patient is unable to do so.
- State laws affecting nursing practice include mandatory reporting laws, Good Samaritan laws, safe harbor laws, and nurse practice acts.
- The ANA Code of Ethics describes the standards of professional responsibility for nurses and provides insight into ethical and acceptable behavior.
- The ANA Nurses' Bill of Rights identifies the rights nurses should expect from their workplace and work environment that are necessary for sound professional practice.
- A primary function of the medical malpractice system is to encourage healthcare providers to adhere to standards of practice and perform their responsibilities in a competent manner.
- Standards of practice look to what a reasonable and prudent nurse would do in the same or similar situation.
- Nurse practice acts are established by state boards of nursing to govern the practice of nursing.
- In most states, nurses are obligated legally to report suspected or actual patient abuse, impaired health professionals, and communicable diseases.
- State boards of nursing are empowered under the nurse practice act to approve prelicensure nursing education programs, determine the criteria for licensure, define the practice of nursing, and establish grounds for disciplinary actions against nurses.
- Criminal law deals with wrongs or offenses against society. Civil law deals with wrongs to individuals.
- Intentional torts include assault, battery, false imprisonment, fraud, and invasion of privacy.
- Quasi-intentional torts involve those actions that injure a person's reputation.
- Unintentional torts that involve healthcare professionals are negligence or malpractice.
- Negligence is a wrong committed against an individual by one who has failed to use ordinary care.
- Malpractice is negligence committed against an individual by a licensed professional involving a duty, breach of that duty, an injury, and damages.
- Litigation is the formal process where the legal issues, rights, and duties between the parties are heard and decided. The stages include (1) pleading and pretrial motions, (2) discovery, (3) alternative dispute resolution, (4) trial, and (5) appeal.
- Malpractice claims, in general, result from failure to maintain the standard of practice, including failure to assess, diagnose, plan, implement, and evaluate patient responses to care.
- Nurses can help reduce their legal risks by developing open, honest, respectful, caring relationships with patients and families; observing standards of care; and accurate documentation.
- You may witness a patient's signature on a consent form, but you are not legally responsible for explaining the treatments and options, nor for evaluating whether the provider has adequately explained them.

Knowledge Map

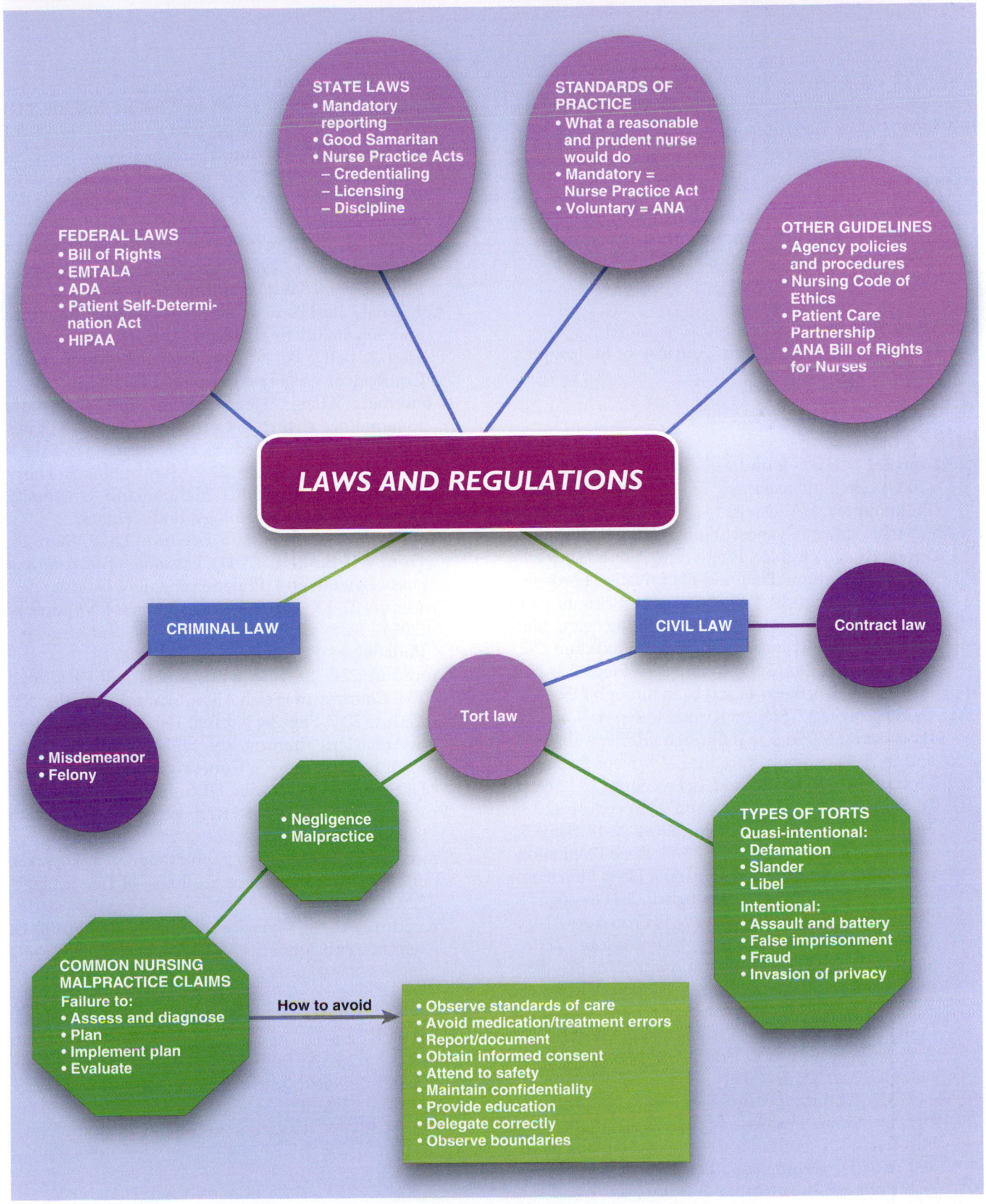

Credits

Note: Unless cited below, text credits appear within the text.

CHAPTER 11

Discharge Assessment/Instructions, Patient Education Form: Fisherman's Hospital, Marathon, FL. Used with permission.

CHAPTER 18

Do Not Resuscitate Orders: Courtesy of St. Joseph's Hospital Center.

CHAPTER 22

Abnormal Atlas: Jaundice: From L. Chapman. (2009).*Core components of maternal nursing*, Philadelphia: F.A. Davis.

Abnormal Atlas: Cyanosis,Vitiligo,Herpes Simplex, Venous Star, Petechiae, Ringworm, Alopecia Areata, Fungal Infection, Half-and-Half Nails, Lordosis, Scoliosis, Kyphosis, Propulsive gait, Scissors gait, Spastic gait, Steppage gait, Waddling gait, and Locations of direct and indirect hernias; Procedure 22-2, Step 1a and b, Step 7; Procedure 22-5, Steps 2 and 4; Procedure 22-6, Steps 4a and b, 5a through f, Step 6e (2), Step 6j, Step 7, Step 8d [1 and 2], Step 8e [1 and 2]; Procedure 22-7, Step 1a [i through iii], Steps 1b, 3e [1 and 2], 5, 6 [a and c]; Procedure 22-8, Steps 5a and b; Procedure 22-10, Steps 2 and 3a; Procedure 22-12, Step 5c, Steps 6 [a through c], 7b, and 9; Procedure 22-13, Steps 2, 1 [b and c], and8b; Procedure 22-14, Steps 5, 6, and 7 [c and d]; Procedure 22-14, Deep Palpitation (one-hand technique) and Bimanual Deep Palpation; Procedure 22-15, Steps 1 [c1 through d], 2b [1 through 7], 3 [a through b 2], 4a, 6c [1 and 2], 9; Procedure 22-15: Using a goniometer (image); Procedure 22-16, Steps 11c, 13a, 18a, 20, 21a through 22c, 22e, 23a through e, and 24; Procedure 22-17, Step 5 [a and c], 6, and 7 [1 and 2]; Procedure 22-18, Step 2 and 3 [b and c]: From P.M. Dillon. (2007). *Nursinghealth assessment: A critical thinking case studies approach* (2nd ed.). Philadelphia: F.A. Davis.

Abnormal Atlas: Port-Wine Stain, Capillary Hemangioma, Vesicles, Syphilitic Chancre, and Paronychia: From L. A. Goldsmith. (1997). *Adult and pediatric dermatology: A color guide to diagnosis and treatment*.Philadelphia: F. A. Davis.

Clinical Insight 22-1 a and b; Clinical Insight 22-3 a through e; Procedure 22-1, Various types of thermometers; Procedure 22-4, Step 1; Procedure 22-8, Step 4d; Procedure 22-2, Describing Skin Lesions; Procedure 22-9, Step 2b [1 and 2]; Procedure 22-11, Step 4a through c; Procedure 22-15, Step 8 [1 through 13]: From P. M. Dillon. (2003). *Nursinghealth assessment: A critical thinking case studies approach*. Philadelphia: F.A. Davis.

Abnormal Atlas: Pediculosis, Hordeolum, Pterygium, and Subconjunctival Hemorrhage; Procedure 22-5, Step 2, Bell's Palsy; Procedure 22-6, Step 8e(2): Courtesy of Wills Eye Hospital, Philadelphia.

Abnormal Atlas: Degenerative Joint Disease, Rheumatoid Arthritis, Genital Warts, and Herpes Vulvovaginitis; Procedure 22-5, Step 2, Cushing's Syndrome; Procedure 22-9, Step 4, Black Hairy Tongue: Courtesy MCP-Hahnemann University Department of Dermatology, Philadelphia.

Procedure 22-6, Step 3b, Procedure 22-12, Step 2b: From V. C. Scanlon. (2011). *Essentials of anatomy and physiology*(6th ed.). Philadelphia: F.A. Davis.

Procedure 22-13, Step 8: From L. Treas & J. Wilkinson. (2014). *Basic nursing: Concepts, skills and reasoning*. Philadelphia: F.A. Davis.

Procedure 22-7, Step 3e, Otitis Media and Perforated TM: Courtesy of Welch Allyn, Skaneateles Falls, NY.

Procedure 22-7, Step 3e, Normal TM, left ear: Courtesy of Ann Marie Ramsey, RN, MSN, CPNP.

Procedure 22-9, Step 3: Courtesy Robert A. Levine, DDS, and Sheryl Radin, DDS.

Procedure 22-9, Step 4, Red beefy tongue: From Custom Medical Stock Photo, Inc. Chicago, IL.

Procedure 22-9, Step 4, Geographic tongue, Leukoplakia, and Cancer of the tongue: Courtesy of Tina S. Liang, DMD.

Procedure 22-16, Glasgow Coma Scale: From G. Teasdale & B. Jennett. (1974). *Assessment of coma and impaired consciousness. Lancet*,81–84.

CHAPTER 23

Procedure 23-1A, Steps 3 and 5, Procedure 23-1B, Step 3: ©iStockphoto

Procedure 23-2, Step 1e: Courtesy of Moldex-Metric, Inc., Culver City, CA, www.moldex.com

CHAPTER 24

Procedure 24-1, Step 1: Infrared-Beam Detector, Cord-Activated Sensor: Courtesy of Smart Caregiver Corporation.

CHAPTER 25

Procedure 25-9, Step 10: Courtesy of EZ Access, Auburn, WA.

CHAPTER 26

Procedure 26-10, Equipment 1: Courtesy of Edward Lin, MD, Ingenious Technologies Corporation. Training video link: http://ingenious.com/NS/ns.htm

Procedure 26-17B, Step 7: Dr. Brian Oxhorn, Roseman University, Henderson, NV. Used with permission.

CHAPTER 27

Clinical Insight 27-1: United States Department of Agriculture (USDA). (2011, June).

Clinical Insight 27-2 a and b: From C. Lutz & K. Przytulski. (2006). *Nutrition and diet therapy* (4th ed.) Philadelphia: F.A. Davis.

Procedure 27-2, Step 11: V. C. Scanlon & T. Sanders. (2010). *Essentials of anatomy & physiology*(6thed.). Philadelphia: F.A. Davis

Procedure 27-2, Step 20g: Courtesy Dale Medical Products, Plainville, MA.

Procedure 27-3, Step 6i: Nestle Healthcare Nutrition Inc.

Procedure 27-5, Equipment: Permission for use granted by Cook Medical Incorporated, Bloomington, IN.

CHAPTER 28

Guidelines for Physical Assessment for Urinary Elimination: From P. Dillon. (2007). *Nursing health assessment*(2nded.). Philadelphia: F.A. Davis.

CHAPTER 29

Procedure 29-6, Equipment: From L. Williams & P. Hopper. (2003). *Understanding medical surgical nursing* (2nd ed.). Philadelphia: F.A. Davis.

Procedure 29-8, Equipment, and Procedure 29-8B, Step 8: Courtesy of Hollister Incorporated, Libertyville, IL.

CHAPTER 32

Clinical Insight 32-2, Applying Hip Abduction Pillow: From L. Williams & P. Hopper. (2003). *Understanding medical surgical nursing* (2nd ed.). Philadelphia: F.A. Davis.

CHAPTER 35

Procedure 35-6A, Steps 2, 8, 9, and 15: From J. Rhoads & B. J. Meeker. (2008). *Davis's guide to clinical nursing skills*. Philadelphia: F.A. Davis.

Procedure 35-6B, Step 10: Courtesy Talley Group Limited, Hampshire, England.

Braden Scale for Predicting Pressure Ulcer Score Risk: Copyright © Barbara Braden and Nancy Bergstrom, 1988. Reprinted with permission.

Norton Scalae for Assessing Risk of Pressure Ulcers: Copyright © D. Norton, R. McLaren, & A. N. Exton-Smith. 1975. Reprinted with permission.

The PUSH Tool for Evaluation of Pressure Ulcers: Copyright © D. National Pressure Ulcer Advisory Panel (NPUAP) 1998 Reprinted with permission.

CHAPTER 38

Procedure 38-1, Step 14 [1 and 2]: From J. Rhoads & B. J. Meeker. (2008). *Davis's guide to clinical nursing skills*. Philadelphia: F.A. Davis.

References Cited

CHAPTER 1

Aiken, L., Clarke, S., Sloane, D., et al. (2002). Hospital nurse staffing and patient mortality, nurse burnout, and job dissatisfaction. *JAMA, 288*, 1987–1993.

Aiken, L., Sloane, D., Cimiotti, J., et al. (2010). Implications of the California nurse staffing mandate for other states. *Health Service Research*. Retrieved October 18, 2012, from http://www.nursing.upenn.edu/chopr/Documents/Aiken.2010.CaliforniaStaffingRatios.pdf

American Association of Colleges of Nursing. (2011). *Nursing fact sheet*. Washington, DC: Author.

American Association of Colleges of Nursing. (2012). *Nursing fact sheet*. Washington, DC: Author.

American College of Nurse Practitioners (ACNP). (2012). *What is the difference between a skilled nursing facility and a nursing facility?* Retrieved October 8, 2012, from http://www.acnpweb.org/what-difference-between-skilled-nursing-facility-and-nursing-facility

American Health Care Association. (2012). *Trends in nursing facility characteristics*. Washington, DC: Author.

American Nurses Association (ANA). (2003). *Nursing's social policy statement*. Washington, DC: Author.

American Nurses Association (ANA). (2004). *Standards of clinical nursing practice* (3rd ed.). Washington, DC: American Nurses Publishing.

American Nurses Association (ANA). (2008). *ANA's health system reform agenda*. Silver Springs, MD: Author.

American Nurses Association (ANA). (2010). *Nursing: scope and standards of practice* (2nd ed.). Silver Springs, MD: Nursebook.org.

American Telehealth Association. (2011). *Telehealth nursing fact sheet*. Washington, DC: Author.

Anthony, M., Standing, T., & Hertz, J. (2001). Nurses' beliefs about their abilities to delegate within changing models of care. *Journal of Continuing Education in Nursing, 32*(5), 210–215.

Association of American Medical Colleges. (2011). *2011 State physician workforce data bank*. Retrieved November 21, 2012, from https://www.aamc.org/download/263512/data/statedata2011.pdf

Benner, P. (1984). *From novice to expert: Excellence and power in clinical nursing practice*. Menlo Park, CA: Addison-Wesley.

Benner, P., & Wrubel, J. (1989). *The primacy of caring*. Menlo Park, CA: Addison-Wesley.

Beverage, P. A. (2004). How LPNs can be part of the solution. *North Carolina Medical Journal, 65*(2), 96–97.

Blegen, M., Spetz, J., Vaughn, T., et al. (2011). Nurse staffing effects on patient outcomes: Safety-net and non-safety-net hospitals. *Med Care, 49*(4), 406–414.

Bodenheimer, T. S., & Grumbach, K. (2005). *Understanding health policy: A clinical approach* (4th ed.). Stamford, CT: Appleton & Lange.

Bright, M. A. (2002). *Holistic health and healing*. Philadelphia: F. A. Davis.

Brush, B. L., & Capezuti, E. (2001). Historical analysis of siderail use in American hospitals. *Journal of Nursing Scholarship, 33*(4), 381–385.

Brush, B., Lynaugh, G., Boschma, A., et al. (1999). *Nurses of all nations: A history of the International Council of Nurses, 1899–1999*. Hagerstown, MD: Lippincott Williams & Wilkins.

Bureau of Labor Statistics. (2012a). Licensed practical and licensed vocational nurses. *Occupational outlook handbook, 2012–2013 edition*, Retrieved October 1, 2012, from http://www.bls.gov/ooh/healthcare/licensed-practical-and-licensed-vocational-nurses.htm

Bureau of Labor Statistics. (2012b). Pharmacists. *Occupational outlook handbook, 2012–2013 edition*. Retrieved November 21, 2012, from http://www.bls.gov/ooh/healthcare/pharmacists.htm

Bureau of Labor Statistics. (2012c). Registered nurses. *Occupational outlook handbook, 2012–2013 edition*, Retrieved October 31, 2012, from http://www.bls.gov/ooh/healthcare/registered-nurses.htm

Capezuti, E. E., Wagner, L., Brush, B., et al. (2007). Consequences of an intervention to reduce restrictive side rail use in nursing homes. *Journal of the American Geriatrics Society, 55*(3), 334–341.

Carnegie, M. E. (1995). *The path we tread: Blacks in nursing 1854–1994* (3rd ed.). New York: National League for Nursing. Centers for Disease Control and Prevention (CDC), National.

Catalano, J. (2009). *Nursing now! Today's issues, tomorrow's trends* (5th ed.). Philadelphia: F. A. Davis.

Center for Health Statistics. (n.d., last updated 2012, May 16). *Nursing home care*. Retrieved October 1, 2012, from http://www.cdc.gov/nchs/fastats/nursingh.htm

Center for Medicare & Medicaid Services. (2010). *Nursing home data compendium*. Retrieved September 27, 2012, from www.cms.gov.

Chambers, P. (1958). *A doctor alone: A biography of Elizabeth Blackwell, the first woman doctor*. London: Abelard-Schuman.

Cohen, R., & Martinez, M. (2012). *Health insurance coverage: early release of estimates from the National Health Interview Survey, January–March, 2012*. National Center for Health Statistics. Retrieved September 19, 2012, from www.cdc.gov/nchs/data/nhis

Critical Care. (2007, July 21). Low hospital staff levels increase infection rates. Adapted by *Science Daily* from materials retrieved from *Critical Care*. Retrieved November 12, 2012, from http://www.sciencedaily.com/releases/2007/07/070719115825.htm

Cronenwett, L., Sherwood, G., Barnsteiner, J., et al. (2007). Quality and safety education for nurses. *Nursing Outlook, 55*(3), 122–131.

Darcé, K. (2007, November). Are retail clinics a healthy choice? Outlets opening in county could fill niche; physicians warn of drawbacks. *The San Diego Union-Tribune.* Retrieved November 3, 2012, from http://www.signonsandiego.com/news/business/20071107-9999-1n7clinics.html

Dey, J., Johnson, M., Pajerowski, W., et al. (2011). *Home health study report*. Retrieved September 15, 2012, from www.cms.gov

Dock, L. L., & Stewart, I. M. (1938). *A short history of nursing* (4th ed.). New York: Putnam.

Donahue, M. P. (1985). *Nursing: The finest art. An illustrated history*. St. Louis, MO: C. V. Mosby.

Dossey, B., Selanders, L., Beck, D., et al. (2005). *Florence Nightingale today: Healing, leadership, global action*. Washington, DC: Nursesbooks.org.

Enthoven, A. C. (2009). Integrated delivery system: the cure for fragmentation. *The American Journal of Managed Care, 15*, S284–S290.

Farlex. (2002). *The free dictionary*. Retrieved November 17, 2012, from http://medical-dictionary.thefreedictionary.com/health+care+rationing

Fuchs, V. R. (1998). *The future of health policy*. Cambridge, MA: Harvard University Press.

Fulcher, R., & Mullin, C. M. (2011, March). *A data-driven examination of the impact of associate and bachelor's degree programs on the nation's nursing workforce* (Policy Brief 2011-02PBL). Washington, DC: American Association of Community Colleges.

Gabr, H., & Mohamed, N. (2012). Job characteristics model to redesign nursing care delivery system in general surgical unit. *Academic Research International, 2*(1), 199–211.

Health Resources and Services Administration. (2004a). *Supply, demand, and use of licensed practical nurses*. Washington, DC: U.S. Department of Health and Human Services, Bureau of Health Professions. Retrieved November 3, 2012, from bhpr.hrsa.gov/healthworkforce/allreportsindex.html

Health Resources and Services Administration. (2004b). *The registered nurse population: Findings from the March 2004 national sample survey of registered nurses*. Washington, DC: U.S. Department of Health and Human Services, Bureau of Health Professions. Retrieved November 3, 2012, from http://bhpr.hrsa.gov/healthworkforce/rnsurveys/rnsurvey2004.pdf

Health Resources and Services Administration. (2010). *The registered nurse population: Findings from the March 2008 national sample survey of registered nurses*. Washington, DC: U.S. Department of Health and Human Services, Bureau of Health Professions. Retrieved September 28, 2012, from http://bhpr.hrsa.gov/healthworkforce/allreports.html

Henderson, V. (1966). *The nature of nursing*. New York: Macmillan.

History Channel. (2012). *Women in the Vietnam war*. Retrieved September 28, 2012, from http://www.history.com/topics/women-in-the-vietnam-war.

Hobbs, F. (2001). *The elderly population*. U.S. Census Bureau. Retrieved November 3, 2012, from http://www.census.gov/prod/1/pop/profile/95/24_ps.pdf

Holt, J. (2011). Hospital to ditch "team nursing." *Signalscv.com: The Santa Clara Valley Signal*. Retrieved November 12, 2012, from www.the-signal.com/archives/43785

Institute of Medicine. (2011). *The future of nursing: Leading change, advancing health*. Washington, DC: The National Academies Press.

International Council of Nurses. (n.d., last updated 2010, April 12). *ICN definition of nursing*. Retrieved September 15, 2012, from http://www.icn.ch/about-icn/icn-definition-of-nursing/

Jonas, S., & Kovner, A. R. (2008). *Health care delivery in the U.S.* (9th ed.). New York: Springer.

Kane, R., Shamliyan, T., Mueller, C., et al. (2007). The association of registered nurse staffing levels and patient outcomes: Systematic review and meta-analysis. *Medical Care, 45*(12), 1195–1204.

Kaufman, K. (2012). *Executive Summary: Findings from the Annual Survey of Schools of Nursing Academic Year 2010–2011*. Retrieved November 13, 2012, from http://www.nln.org/researchgrants/slides/exec_summary_1011.pdf

Kidder, M., & Cornelius, P. (2006). Licensure is not synonymous with professionalism. *Nurse Educator, 31*(10), 15–19.

Landon, B., Normand, S., Lessler, A., et al. (2006). Quality of care for the treatment of acute medical conditions in U.S. hospitals. *Archives of Internal Medicine, 166*, 2511–2517.

Laugesen, M., & Rice, T. (2003). Is the doctor in? The evolving role of organized medicine in health policy. *Journal of Health Politics, Policy and Law, 28*(2–3), 289–316.

MacWilliams, B., Schmidt, B., & Bleich, M. (2013). Men in nursing. *American Journal of Nursing, 113*(1), 38–44.

Mahaffey, E. H. (2002). The relevance of associate degree nursing education: Past, present, future. *Online Journal of Issues in Nursing, 7*(2), 3.

Master, K. (2009). *Role development in professional nursing* (2nd ed.). Sudbury, MA: Jones & Bartlett.

Meadus, R. J. (2000). Men in nursing: Barriers to recruitment. *Nursing Forum, 35*(3), 5.

Meleis, A. I. (1991). *Theoretical nursing: Development and progress*. Philadelphia: J. B. Lippincott.

Miller, B. K., Adams, D., & Beck, L. (1993). A behavioral inventory for professionalism in nursing. *Journal of Professional Nursing, 9*(5), 290–295.

National League for Nursing. (2010). *Nursing data review academic year 2007–2008*. New York: Author.

Natoli, C., Cheh, V., & Verghese, S. (2011). *Who will enroll in Medicaid in 2014? Lessons from Section 1115 Medicaid waivers*. Centers for Medicare & Medicaid Services. Retrieved November 17, 2012, from https://www.cms.gov/Research-Statistics-Data-and-Systems/Computer-Data-and-Systems/MedicaidDataSourcesGenInfo/Downloads/MAX_IB_1_080111.pdf

Nightingale, F. (1860). *Notes on nursing: What it is, and what it is not*. New York: D. Appleton and Company

Nightingale, F. (1876). *Notes on nursing for the labouring classes*. London: Harrison.

Penoyer, D. (2010). Nurse staffing and patient outcomes in critical care: A concise review. *Critical Care Medicine, 38*(7), 1521–1528.

Potera, C. (2007). In the news. Infections and deaths down, quality up. *American Journal of Nursing, 107*(4), 19.

Potetz, L., Cubanski, J., & Neuman, T. (2011). *Medicare spending and financing*. Menlo Park, CA: The Henry J. Kaiser Family Foundation.

Pullen, R. L., Jr. (2006). Why choose nursing education? *Men in Nursing, 1*(5), 36–39.

Quadagno, J. S. (2004). Physician sovereignty and the purchasers' revolt. *Journal of Health Politics, Policy and Law, 29*(4), 815–834.

Rockwell, L. H., Jr. (1994). The American Medical Association: A sordid history. *HealthE-Living News*. Retrieved September 15, 2012, from http://www.healthe-livingnews.com/articles/american_medical_association_sorbid_history.html

Safriet, B. J. (1994). Impediments to progress in healthcare work-force policy: License and practice laws. *Inquiry, 31*(3), 310–317.

Shapiro, S. E. (2002). Viewpoint: In favor of the bachelor's degree. *American Journal of Nursing, 102*(10), 11.

Spoelstra, S., Given, B., & Given, C. (2012). Fall prevention in hospitals: An integrative review. *Clinical Nursing Research, 21*(1), 92–112.

Starr, P. (1982). *The social transformation of American medicine.* New York: Basic Books.

Sterchi, L. S. (2007). Perceptions that affect physician-nurse collaboration in the perioperative setting. *AORN Journal, 86*(1), 45–57.

Stewart, I. M., & Austin, A. L. (1962). *A history of nursing* (5th ed.). New York: G. P. Putnam's Sons.

Stokowski, L.A. (2011). Overhauling nursing education. *Medscape.* Retrieved from http://www.medscape.com/viewarticle/736236

Sultz, H., & Young, K. (1997). *Health care USA: Understanding its organization and delivery.* Burlington, MA: Jones & Bartlett Learning.

Takase, M., Kershaw, E., & Burt, L. (2002). Does public image of nurses matter? *Journal of Professional Nursing, 18*(4), 196–205.

Tewes, R. (2009). Evolution of the health care system in the United States. *League of Women Voters.* Retrieved September 30, 2012, from http://www.lwvil.org/healthcare.asp

Tourangeau, A., Doran, D., Hall, L., et al. (2007). Impact of hospital nursing care on 30-day mortality for acute medical patients. *Journal of Advanced Nursing, 57*(1), 32–44.

Unruh, L., & Zhang, N. (2012). Nursing staffing and patient safety in hospitals: New variables and longitudinal approaches. *Nursing Research, 61*(1), 3–12.

U.S. Census Bureau. (2010). Age and sex composition: 2010. *2010 Census Briefs.* Retrieved September 19, 2012, from http://2010.census.gov/2010census/

U.S. Department of Health & Human Services. (2010). *Key features of the Affordable Care Act, by year.* Retrieved September 27, 2012, from http://www.healthcare.gov/law/timeline/full.html

Venes, D. (2013). *Taber's cyclopedic medical dictionary* (22nd ed.). Philadelphia: F. A. Davis.

Wawrzynski, M., & Davidhizar, R. (2006). The bachelor of science in nursing degree as entry level for practice: recapturing the vision in the United States. *Healthcare Manager, 25*(3), 263–266.

Wielawski, I. (2007). Fighting for more than member benefits. *American Journal of Nursing, 107*(6), 25–26.

Wilkinson, J. M. (1996). The C word: A curriculum for the future. *N&HC: Perspectives on Community, 17*(2), 72–77.

Wood, D. (2007). Major teaching hospital switches to team nursing. Retrieved November 12, 2012, from http://w3.rn.com/News/news_features_details.aspx?Id=9004

World Health Organization (WHO). (1984). *Health promotion: A discussion document on the concepts and principles.* Geneva, Switzerland: Author.

World Health Organization (WHO). (2007). Frequently asked questions. Preamble to the Constitution of the World Health Organization as adopted by the International Health Conference, New York, June 19–July 22, 1946; signed on July 22 by the representatives of 62 States (Official Records of the World Health Organization, no. 2, p. 100) and entered into force on April 7, 1948. Retrieved September 15, 2012, from http://www.who.int/suggestions/faq/en/

Yang, P-H, Hung, C-H, Chen, Y-M., et al. (2012). The impact of different nursing skill mix models on patient outcomes in a respiratory care center. *Worldviews on Evidence-Based Nursing, 9*(4), 227–233.

Yetter, D. (2010). Preserving a positive image of nursing in a complicated healthcare environment. *Nursing Made Incredibly Easy! 8*(2), 5–7.

CHAPTER 2

American Nurses Association (ANA). (2010). *Nursing: Scope and standards of practice* (2nd ed.). Silver Spring, MD: Nursebooks.org

American Philosophical Association. (1990). *Executive summary of: Critical thinking: A statement of expert consensus for purposes of educational assessment.* Millbrae, CA: The California Academic Press.

Assessment Technologies Institute. (2003). Critical thinking assessment developmental and statistical manual. Overland Park, KS: Assessment Technologies Institute.

Brookfield, S. D. (1991). *Developing critical thinkers.* San Francisco: Jossey-Bass.

Catlett, S., & Lovan, S. (2011). Being a good nurse and doing the right thing: A replication study. *Nursing Ethics, 18*(1), 54–63.

Davis, M. (2011). Concept mapping, mind mapping and argument mapping: What are the differences and do they matter? *Higher Education, 62*(3), 279–301.

Ennis, R. H. (2011). A Super-streamlined conception of critical thinking. Retrieved January 9, 2011, from http://www.criticalthinking.net/SSConcCTApr3.html

Heaslip, P. (1992). Creating the thinking practitioner: Critical thinking in clinical practice. [Unpublished manuscript]. (ERIC Document Reproduction Service No. ED 354 822).

McDonald, M. E. (2002). *Systematic assessment of learning outcomes: Developing multiple-choice exams.* Boston: Jones & Bartlett.

Moore, B. N., & Parker, R. (2009). *Critical thinking* (9th ed.). Columbus, OH: McGraw-Hill.

Paul, R. W. (1990). *Critical thinking.* Rohnert Park, CA: The Center for Critical Thinking and Moral Critique, Sonoma State University.

Paul, R. W. (1993). *Critical thinking: What every person needs to survive in a rapidly changing world* (3rd ed.). Santa Rosa, CA: Foundation for Critical Thinking.

Paul, R. W., Ennis, R. H., & Norris, S. (1996). In B. Fowler (Ed.), *Critical thinking definitions.* (Critical Thinking Across the Curriculum Project). Lee's Summit, MO: Longview Community College.

Raingruber, B., & Haffer, A. (2001). *Using your head to land on your feet.* Philadelphia: F. A. Davis.

Swanson, K. M. (1990). Providing care in the NICU: Sometimes an act of love. *Advances in Nursing, 13*, 60–73.

Wilkinson, J. M. (2011). *Nursing process & critical thinking* (5th ed.). Upper Saddle River, NJ: Prentice-Hall.

CHAPTER 3

American Nurses Association (ANA). (2001). *Code of ethics for nurses with interpretive statements.* Silver Spring, MD: Author. Retrieved June 29, 2012, from http://www.nursingworld.org/MainMenuCategories/EthicsStandards/CodeofEthicsforNurses/Code-of-Ethics.pdf

American Nurses Association (ANA). (2010). *Nursing: Scope and standards of practice* (2nd ed.). Silver Spring, MD: Nursebooks.org.

Cronenwett, L., Sherwood, G., Barnsteiner, J., et al. (2007). Quality and safety education for nurses. *Nursing Outlook, 55*(3), 122–131.

Dochterman, J. M., & Jones, D. A. (Eds.). (2003). *Unifying nursing languages: The harmonization of NANDA, NIC, and NOC.* Washington, DC: American Nurses Association, Nursesbooks.org

Gordon, M. (1994). *Analysis/nursing diagnosis: Process and application* (3rd ed., p. 70). St. Louis, MO: C. V. Mosby.

Gorman, L., & Sultan, D. (2008). *Psychosocial nursing for general patient care.* Philadelphia: F. A. Davis.

Graf, C. (2008). How to try this: The Lawton Instrumental Activities of Daily Living Scale. *American Journal of Nursing, 108*(4), 52–62.

The Joint Commission. (2012). *Hospital accreditation standards.* Oakbrook Terrace, IL: Author.

Karnofsky, D. A., & Burchenal, J. H. (1949). The clinical evaluation of chemotherapeutic agents in cancer. In C. M. MacLeod (Ed.), *Evaluation of chemotherapeutic agents.* New York: Columbia University Press. (Classic). Performance scale retrieved June 24, 2012, from http://www.acsu.buffalo.edu/~drstall/karnofsky.html. Posted September 30, 1997, by Robert S. Stall, MD.

Lawton, M. P., & Brody, E. M. (1969). Assessment of older people: Self-maintaining and instrumental activities of daily living. *The Gerontologist, 9*(3), 179–186.

Maslow, A. (1970). *Motivation and personality* (2nd ed.). New York: Harper & Row.

Maslow, A., & Lowery, R. (Eds.). (1998). *Toward a psychology of being* (3rd ed.). New York: Wiley & Sons.

NANDA International. (2012). *Nursing diagnoses definitions & classification 2012–2014.* Ames, IA: Wiley-Blackwell.

National Council of State Boards of Nursing (NCSBN). (2011). *Model nursing practice act and model nursing administrative rules.* Retrieved July 31, 2012, from https://www.ncsbn.org/Model_Nursing_Practice_Act_March2011.pdf

Orem, D. (1991). *Nursing: Concepts of practice* (4th ed., p. 126). St. Louis, MO: C. V. Mosby-Year Book.

Purnell, L. D., & Paulanka, B. J. (2008). *Transcultural health care: A culturally competent approach* (3rd ed.). Philadelphia: F. A. Davis.

Roy, C., & Andrews, H. (1991). *The Roy Adaptation Model: The definitive statement* (pp. 15–17). Norwalk, CT: Appleton & Lange.

Roy, C., & Andrews, A. (1999). *The Roy Adaptation Model* (2nd ed.). Norwalk, CT: Appleton and Lange.

Shelkey, M., & Wallace, M. (revised 2012). Katz index of independence in activities of daily living (ADL). *Try This: Best Practices in Nursing Care to Older Adults,* 2. Hartford Institute for Geriatric Nursing, New York University, College of Nursing. Retrieved June 29, 2012, from http://consultgerirn.org/uploads/File/trythis/try_this_2.pdf

Wilkinson, J. (2012). *Nursing process and critical thinking* (5th ed.). Upper Saddle River, NJ: Pearson Health Science.

CHAPTER 4

American Medical Association (AMA). (2010). *Current procedural terminology: CPT 2010. Professional edition.* Chicago: Author.

American Nurses Association (ANA). (1980). *ANA social policy statement.* Washington, DC: Author.

American Nurses Association (ANA). (2010). *Nursing: Scope and standards of practice* (2nd ed.). Silver Spring, MD: Nursebooks.org.

American Psychiatric Association (APA). (2000). *Diagnostic and statistical manual of mental disorders.* Arlington, VA: Author.

American Psychiatric Association (APA). (2013). *Diagnostic and statistical manual of mental disorders DSM-5.* Arlington, VA: American Psychiatric Association.

Bates, D. W., Ebell, M., Gotlieb, E., et al. (2003). A proposal for electronic medical records in U.S. primary care. *Journal of the American Medical Informatics Association, 10*(1), 1–10.

Beyea, S. (2000, May). Standardized nursing vocabularies and the perioperative nursing data set: Making clinical practice count. *CIN Plus, 3*(2), 1, 5, 6.

Carpenito, L. J. (2006). *Nursing diagnosis: Application to clinical practice* (11th ed.). Philadelphia: J. B. Lippincott.

Fry, V. (1953). The creative approach to nursing. *American Journal of Nursing, 98*(6), 44–47.

Gebbie, K. (1976). Development of a taxonomy of nursing diagnosis. In J. Walter, J. Walter, D. P. Pardee, & D. M. Molbo (Eds.), *Dynamics of problem-oriented approaches: Patient care and documentation.* Philadelphia: J. B. Lippincott.

Gordon, M. (1994). *Nursing diagnosis: Process and application* (3rd ed.). St. Louis, MO: C. V. Mosby.

Häyrinen, K., Lammintakanen, J., & Saranto, K. (2010). Evaluation of electronic nursing documentation—nursing process model and standardized terminologies as keys to visible and transparent nursing. *International Journal of Medical Informatics, 79*(8), 554–556.

International Council of Nurses. (2011). *International classification for nursing practice.* Geneva, Switzerland: Author. Retrieved July 2, 2010, from http://icnp.clinicaltemplates.org/icnp/download-langs/?product=PDF.

Lunney, M. (2008, January). Critical need to address accuracy of nurses' diagnoses. *Online Journal of Issues in Nursing, 13*(1).

Maslow, A. H. (1970). *Motivation and personality* (2nd ed.). New York: Harper & Row.

Maslow, A. (1971). *The farther reaches of human nature.* New York: The Viking Press.

Maslow, A., & Lowery, R. (Eds.). (1998). *Toward a psychology of being* (3rd ed.). New York: Wiley & Sons.

Müller-Stauber, M., Lavin, M. A., Needham, I., et al. (2006). Nursing diagnoses, interventions and outcomes—and impact on nursing practice: Systematic review. *Journal of Advanced Nursing, 56*(5j), 514–531.

NANDA International. (2012). *NANDA Nursing diagnoses: Definitions & classification 2012–2014.* Ames, IA: Wiley-Blackwell.

Shever, L. (2011). The impact of nursing surveillance on failure to rescue. *Research and Theory for Nursing Practice, 25*(2), 107–126.

Wilkinson, J. M. (2011). *Nursing process and critical thinking* (5th ed.). Upper Saddle River, NJ: Prentice-Hall.

World Health Organization (WHO). (1992). *Manual of the international classification of diseases and related health problems (ICD-10).* Geneva, Switzerland: Author.

CHAPTER 5

American Nurses Association (ANA). (2010). *Nursing: Scope and standards of practice* (2nd ed.). Silver Spring, MD: Author.

Camilleri, M. (2011). Opioid-induced constipation: Challenges and therapeutic opportunities. *The American Journal of Gastroenterology, 106*, 835–842.

Dahl, W. (2010). *Constipation myths* (Document FSH10-07). Gainesville: Department of Food Science and Human Nutrition, Florida Cooperative Extension Service, Institute of Food and Agricultural Sciences, University of Florida. Retrieved July 10, 2012, from http://edis.ifas.ufl.edu/pdffiles/fs/fs15500.pdf.

Fajardo, N., Cremonini, F., & Talley, N. (2006). Management of constipation in patients with cancer. *American Journal of Cancer, 5*(5), 319–330.

Gallagher, P., & O'Mahoney, D. (2009). Constipation in old age. *Best Practice & Research Clinical Gastroenterology, 23*(6), 875–887.

Green, C., & Wilkinson, J. (2004). *Maternal newborn nursing care plans*. St. Louis, MO: C. V. Mosby.

Harris, B. L. (1990). Becoming deprofessionalized: One aspect of the staff nurse's perspective on computer-mediated nursing care plans. *Advances in Nursing Science, 13*(2), 63–74.

Healthy People 2020. (2010). Washington, DC: U.S. Department of Health and Human Services. Retrieved July 8, 2012, from http://healthypeople.gov/2020/about/default.aspx

Johnson, M., Moorhead, S., Bulechek, G., et al. (2012). *NOC, and NIC linkages to NANDA-I and clinical conditions* (3rd ed., p. 196). St. Louis, MO: C. V. Mosby.

Jweinat, J. (2010). Hospital readmissions under the spotlight. *Journal of Healthcare Management, 55*(4). Retrieved July 7, 2012, from http://www.biomedsearch.com/article/Hospital-readmissions-under-spotlight/234418410.html.

Kossman, S., & Scheidenhelm, S. (2008). *CIN: Computers, Informatics, Nursing, 26*(2), 69–77.

Moorhead, S., Johnson, M., Maas, M., et al. (2012). *Nursing outcomes classification* (5th ed.). St. Louis, MO: C. V. Mosby/Elsevier.

Mueller, A., Johnston, M., Bligh, D., & Wilkinson, J. (2002). Viewpoint: Joining mind mapping and care planning to enhance student critical thinking and achieve holistic nursing care. *Nursing Diagnosis: The International Journal of Nursing Language and Classification, 13*(1), 24–27.

NANDA International. (2012). *Nursing diagnoses: Definitions & classification 2012–2014*. Ames, IA: Wiley-Blackwell.

NSW Department of Health. (2011). *Policy directive. Care coordination: Planning from admission to transfer of care in NSW public hospitals*. Sydney, Australia: Ministry of Health, NSW. Retrieved July 7, 2012, from http://www.health.nsw.gov.au/policies/pd/2011/pdf/PD2011_015.pdf

Rao, S., & Go, J. (2010). Update on the management of constipation in the elderly: New treatment options. *Clinical Interventions in Aging, 5*, 163–171.

Solomon, R., & Cherny, N. (2006). Constipation and diarrhea in patients with cancer. *The Cancer Journal, 12*(5), 355–364.

Tack, J., Müller-Lissner, S., Stanghellini, V., et al. (2011). Diagnosis and treatment of chronic constipation—a European perspective. *Neurogastroenterology & Motility, 23*(8), 697–710.

Walker, C., Hogstel, M., & Curry, L. (2007). Hospital discharge of older adults. *American Journal of Nursing, 107*(6), 60–71.

Wilkinson, J. M. (2011). *Nursing process & critical thinking* (5th ed.). Upper Saddle River, NJ: Prentice-Hall.

CHAPTER 6

Agency for Healthcare Research and Quality (AHRQ). (2003; updated 2008, June). Guideline summary. Preventing pressure ulcers and skin tears. In *Evidence-based geriatric nursing protocols for best practice*. Retrieved July 13, 2012, from http://www.guideline.gov/content.aspx?id=12262&search=pressure+ulcer#Section442

American Nurses Association (ANA). (2006). ANA recognized terminologies and data element sets. Retrieved July 10, 2012, from http://nursingworld.org/npii/terminologies.htm.

American Nurses Association (ANA). (2010). *Nursing: Scope and standards of practice* (2nd ed.). Silver Spring, MD: American Nurses Association.

Barton, M. B., Miller, T., Wolff, T., et al. (2007). How to read the new recommendation statement: Methods update from the U.S. Preventive Services Task Force. Originally published in *Annals of Internal Medicine, 147*, 123–127. Agency for Healthcare Research and Quality, Rockville, MD. Retrieved July 20, 2012, from http://www.uspreventiveservicestaskforce.org/uspstf07/methods/methupd.htm

Bulechek, G. M., Butcher, H. K., & Dochterman, J. C. (2012). *Nursing interventions classification (NIC)* (5th ed.). St. Louis, MO: C. V. Mosby.

Cronenwett, L. R. (2002). Research, practice and policy: Issues in evidence based care. *Online Journal of Issues in Nursing, 7*(2). Retrieved July 13, 2012, from www.nursingworld.org/MainMenuCategories/ANAMarketplace/ANAPeriodicals/OJIN/Columns/KeynotesofNote/EvidenceBasedCare.aspx

Cronenwett, L., Sherwood, G., Barnsteiner, J., et al. (2007). Quality and safety education for nurses. *Nursing Outlook, 55*(3), 122–131.

Fain, J. A. (2008). *Reading, understanding, and applying nursing research: A text and workbook* (3rd ed.). Philadelphia: F. A. Davis.

Field, M., & Lohr, K. (Eds.), & the Institute of Medicine. (1992). *Guidelines for clinical practice: From development to use*. Washington, DC: National Academies Press.

Frisch, N. C. (2001, May 31). Nursing as a context for alternative/complementary modalities. *Online Journal of Issues in Nursing, 6*(2), Manuscript 2, p. 2. Retrieved July 20, 2012, from http://www.nursingworld.org/MainMenuCategories/ANAMarketplace/ANAPeriodicals/OJIN/TableofContents/Volume62001/No2May01/AlternativeComplementaryModalities.aspx

Institute of Medicine. (2011, March). Clinical practice guidelines we can trust (Report Brief) Retrieved July 13, 2012, from http://www.iom.edu/~/media/Files/Report%20Files/2011/Clinical-Practice-Guidelines-We-Can-Trust/Clinical%20Practice%20Guidelines%202011%20Report%20Brief.pdf.

JBI. (2007). Topical skin care in aged care facilities. *Best Practice Information Sheet, 11*(3). The Joanna Briggs Institute. Retrieved July 10, 2011, from http://connect.jbiconnectplus.org/ViewSourceFile.aspx?0=4346

Johnson, M., Moorhead, S., Bulechek, G., et al. (2012). *NOC and NIC linkages to NANDA-I and clinical conditions* (3rd ed.). St. Louis, MO: C. V. Mosby.

Martin, K. (2005). *The Omaha System: A key to practice, documentation, and information management* (2nd ed.). Philadelphia: W. B. Saunders.

McCloskey, J. C., & Bulechek, G. M. (Eds.). (1992). *Nursing interventions classification (NIC)*. St. Louis, MO: C. V. Mosby.

Paradis, V., Cossette, S., Frasure-Smith, N., Heppell, S., & Guertin, M-C. (2010). The efficacy of a motivational nursing intervention based on the stges of change on self-care in heart failure patients. *Journal of Cardiovascular Nursing, 25*(2), 130–141.

Quality and Safety Education for Nurses. (2011). Quality and safety competencies. Retrieved April 9, 2011, from http://www.qsen.org/ksas_prelicensure.php.

Saba, V. K. (1995). Home Health Care Classifications (HHCCs): Nursing diagnoses and nursing interventions. In *An emerging framework: Data system advances for clinical nursing practice* (ANA Publication No. NP-94). Washington, DC: American Nurses Association (ANA). Also available at http://www.sabacare.com/

Saba, V. K. (2006). *Clinical care classification system manual: A guide to nursing documentation.* New York: Springer.

Titler, M. G., Mentes, J. C., Rakel, B. A., et al. (1999). From book to bedside: Putting evidence to use in the care of the elderly. *Joint Commission Journal of Quality Improvement, 25*, 545–556.

Wilkinson, J. M. (2011). *Nursing process & critical thinking* (5th ed.) Upper Saddle River, NJ: Prentice-Hall.

CHAPTER 7

American Nurses Association (ANA). (1996). *Registered professional nurses and unlicensed assistive personnel* (2nd ed.). Washington, DC: Author.

American Nurses Association (ANA). (2001). *Code of ethics for nurses with interpretive statements.* Washington, DC: Author.

American Nurses Association (ANA). (2007). Revised position statement: Registered nurses utilization of nursing assistive personnel in all settings. Retrieved July 22, 2012, from http://gm6.nursingworld.org/DocumentVault/Position-Statements/Unlicensed-Assistive-Personnel/Unlicensed AssistivePersonnel.txt

American Nurses Association (ANA). (2010). *Nursing: Scope and standards of practice* (2nd ed.). Silver Spring, MD: Author.

American Nurses Association (ANA) & the National Council of State Boards of Nursing (NCSBN). (2006). Joint statement on delegation. Retrieved July 22, 2012, from https://www.ncsbn.org/Delegation_joint_statement_NCSBN-ANA.pdf

Ayers, D. M. M., & Montgomery, M. (2008). Delegating the "right" way. *Nursing2008, 38*(4), 57–58.

Bulechek, G. M., Butcher, H. K., Dochterman, J. M., et al. (2012). *Nursing interventions classification (NIC)* (6th ed.). St. Louis, MO: Elsevier/Mosby.

Cronenwett, L., Sherwood, G., Barnsteiner, J., et al. (2007). Quality and safety education for nurses. *Nursing Outlook, 55*(3), 122–131.

Dickens, G., Stubbs, J., & Haw, C. (2008). Delegation of medication administration: An exploratory study. *Nursing Standard, 22*(22), 35–40.

Draper D., Felland, L., Liebhaber, A., & Melichar, L. (2008). *The role of nurses in hospital quality improvement* (HSC Research Brief No. 3). Retrieved July 23, 2012, from http://hschange.org/CONTENT/972/

Johnson, K., Hallsey, D., Meredith, R. L., et al. (2006). A nurse-driven system for improving patient quality outcomes. *Journal of Nursing Care Quality, 21*(2), 168–175.

National Council of State Boards of Nursing. (1995). *Delegation: Concepts and decision-making process* (National Council Position Paper). Chicago, IL: Author.

Potter, P., Deshields, T., & Kuhrik, M. (2010). Delegation practices between registered nurses and nursing assistive personnel. *Journal of Nursing Management, 18*(2), 157–165.

Schwiran, P., & Thede, L. (2011, February 15). Informatics: The standardized nursing terminologies: A national survey of nurses' experiences and attitudes—Survey I. *OJIN: The Online Journal of Issues in Nursing, 16*(2). doi:10.3912/OJIN.Vol16No02InfoCol01

Standing, T., & Anthony, M. K. (2008). Delegation: What it means to acute care nurses. *Applied Nursing Research, 21*(1), 8–14.

Thede, L., & Schwirian, P. (2013, March). Informatics: The standardized nursing terminologies: A national survey of nurses' experience and attitudes—SURVEY II: Participants' education for the use of standardized nursing terminology "labels." *OJIN: The Online Journal of Issues in Nursing, 18*(2). doi:10.3912/OJIN.Vol18No02InfoCol01.

U.S. Environmental Protection Agency (EPA). (2009). *Secondhand tobacco smoke and the health of your family.* Retrieved July 21, 2012, from http://www.epa.gov/smokefree/pdfs/trifold_brochure.pdf

Wilkinson, J. (2011). *Nursing process & critical thinking* (5th ed.). Upper Saddle River, NJ: Prentice-Hall.

CHAPTER 8

Alligood, M., & Marriner Tomey, A. (2009) *Nursing theorists and their work* (7th ed.). St. Louis, MO: C. V. Mosby.

American Nurses Association (ANA). (1981). *Guidelines for the investigative functions of nurses.* Washington, DC: Author.

American Nurses Association (ANA). (2010). *Nursing: Scope and standards of practice* (2nd ed.). Silver Spring, MD: Nursebooks.org

Benner, P. (1984). *From novice to expert. Excellence and power in clinical nursing practice.* Menlo Park, CA: Addison-Wesley.

Benner, P., & Wrubel, J. (1989). *The primacy of caring: Stress and coping in health and illness.* Menlo Park, CA: Addison-Wesley.

Brockopp, D. Y., & Hastongs-Tolsma, M. T. (2003). *Fundamentals of nursing research* (3rd ed.). Sudbury, MA: Jones & Bartlett.

Bulechek, G. M., Butcher, H. K., & Dochterman, J. M. (2008). *Nursing interventions classification (NIC)* (5th ed.). St. Louis, MO: C. V. Mosby.

Center for Evidence Based Medicine. (2009, April 7). Asking focused clinical questions. Retrieved August 3, 2012, from http://www.cebm.net/index.aspx?o=1036

Chinn, P., & Kramer, M. (1991). *Theory and nursing: A systematic approach.* St. Louis, MO: Mosby Year Book.

Chinn, P. L., & Kramer, M. K. (2007). *Theory and nursing: Integrated knowledge development* (7th ed.). St. Louis, MO: C. V. Mosby.

Code of Federal Regulations. (2009). *Title 45 Public Welfare, Part 46, Protection of Human Subjects.* Revised January 15, 2009. Retrieved August 3, 2012, from http://www.hhs.gov/ohrp/humansubjects/guidance/ohrpregulations.pdf

Cronenwett, L., Sherwood, G., Barnsteiner, J., et al. (2007). Quality and safety education for nurses. *Nursing Outlook, 55*(3), 122–131.

Dossey, B. M. (1999). *Florence Nightingale: Mystic, visionary, healer.* Springhouse, PA: Springhouse Corporation.

Educating nurses. (2012). Retrieved July 31, 2012, from http://www.educatingnurses.com

Fain, J. A. (2013). *Reading, understanding, and applying nursing research: A text and workbook* (4th ed.). Philadelphia: F. A. Davis.

Feil, N. (2003). *V/F validation* (Rev. ed.). Cincinnati, OH: Feil Productions. Also available from http://www.edwardfeilproductions.com/catalogue.html#books

Forchuk, C. (n.d.). University of Western Ontario Faculty of Nursing, Hildegard Peplau Nursing Theorist home page. Retrieved August 3, 2012, from http://publish.uwo.ca/~cforchuk/peplau/

Ghooi, R. (2011). The Nuremberg Code—a critique. *Perspectives in Clinical Research, 2*(2), 72–76.

Goode, C., Butcher, L., Cipperley, J., et al. (1996). *Research utilization: A study guide* (2nd ed.). Ida Grove, IA: Horn Video Productions.

Hall, L. E. (1966). Another view of nursing care and quality. In M. K. Straub (Ed.), *Continuity of patient care. The role of nursing*. Washington, DC: Catholic University of America Press.

Henderson, V. (1966). *The nature of nursing*. New York: Macmillan.

Horsley, J. A., Crane J., Crabtree, M. K., et al. (1983). *Using research to improve practice*. Orlando, FL: Grune & Stratton.

Imogene King—nursing theorist. (n.d.). *Nursing theory*. Retrieved July 31, 2012, from http://nursing-theory.org/nursing-theorists/Imogene-King.php

International Consortium of Parse Scholars. (n.d.). Retrieved August 3, 2012, from http://www.humanbecoming.org/

Johnson, D. E. (1968). Theory in nursing: Borrowed and unique. *Nursing Research, 11*, 206.

Johnson, D. E. (1980). The behavioral system for nursing. In J. P. Riehl & C. Roy (Eds.), *Conceptual models for nursing practice* (2nd ed., pp. 207–216). New York: Appleton-Century-Crofts.

King, I. M. (1971). *Toward a theory for nursing: General concepts of human behavior*. New York: John Wiley & Sons.

Kolcaba, K. Y. (1994). A theory of holistic comfort for nursing. *Journal of Advanced Nursing, 19*, 1178–1184.

Leininger, M. M. (1978). *Transcultural nursing: Concepts, theories and practices*. New York: John Wiley & Sons.

Leininger, M. M. (1981). The phenomenon of caring: Importance, research questions, and theoretical considerations. In *Caring: An essential* human *need* (Proceedings of the three National Caring Conferences, pp. 3–15). Thorofare, NJ: Charles B. Slack.

Levine, M. E. (1967). The four conservation principles of nursing. *Nursing Forum, 6*, 45–59.

Maslow, A. H. (1970). *Motivation and personality* (2nd ed.). New York: Harper & Row.

Maslow, A. (1971). *The farther reaches of human nature*. New York: The Viking Press.

Maslow, A., & Lowery, R. (Eds.). (1998). *Toward a psychology of being* (3rd ed.). New York: Wiley & Sons.

National Heart, Lung, and Blood Institute; National Institutes of Health. (2012). *Framingham Heart Study*. Retrieved August 3, 2012, from http://www.framinghamheartstudy.org/index.html.

National Institute of Nursing Research (NINR). (n.d.; page last updated 2012, May 4). Funding opportunities. Retrieved July 29, 2012, from http://www.ninr.nih.gov/ResearchAndFunding/DEA/OEP/FundingOpportunities/default.htm

National Institute of Nursing Research (NINR). (2006). *Areas of research emphasis, strategic plan* (pp. 16–23) (Publication No. 06-4832). Washington, DC: National Institutes of Health.

National Institute of Nursing Research (NINR). (2010). Weekly funding opportunities and notices, December 24, 2010, table of contents (TOC). Retrieved July 29, 2012, from http://grants1.nih.gov/grants/guide/WeeklyIndex.cfm/12-24-2010/

Neuman, B. M., & Young, R. J. (1972). A model for teaching total person approach to patient problems. *Nursing Research, 21*, 264–269.

Nieswiadomy, R. M. (2008). *Foundations of nursing research* (5th ed.). Upper Saddle River, NJ: Prentice-Hall.

Nightingale, F. (1859/1992). *Notes on nursing: What it is and what it is not*. Philadelphia: J. B. Lippincott.

The Nuremberg Code. (1949). *Trials of war criminals before the Nuremberg Military Tribunals Under Control Council Law, 10*(2), 181–182. Washington, DC: U.S. Government Printing Office. Retrieved July 30, 2012, from http://history.nih.gov/research/downloads/nuremberg.pdf.

Orlando, I. J. (1972). *The dynamic nurse-patient relationship: Function, process, and principles*. New York: G. P. Putnam's Sons.

Parse, R. R. (1981). *Man-living-health: A theory of nursing*. New York: John Wiley.

Pender, N. J., Murdaugh, C. L., & Parsons, M. A. (2011). *Health promotion in nursing practice* (6th ed.). Upper Saddle River, NJ: Prentice-Hall.

Peplau, H. E. (1952). *Interpersonal relations in nursing*. New York: G. P. Putnam's Sons.

Polit, D. F., & Beck, C. T. (2007). *Nursing research: Generating and assessing evidence* (8th ed.). Philadelphia: Lippincott Williams & Wilkins.

Rigdon, I. S., Clayton, B. D., & Dimond, M. (1987). Toward a theory of helpfulness for the elderly bereaved: An invitation to a new life. *Advances In Nursing Science, 9*(2), 32–43.

Rogers, M. (1970). *An introduction to the theoretical basis of nursing*. Philadelphia: F. A. Davis.

Roy, C. (n.d.; updated 2010, February 10). *The Roy Adaptation Model*. Chestnut Hill, MA: Boston College. Retrieved August 2, 2012, from http://www.bc.edu/schools/son/faculty/featured/theorist/Roy_Adaptation_Model.html

Sacket, D., Richardson, W., Rosenberg, W., et al. (1997). *Evidence-based medicine: How to practice and teach EBM*. New York: Churchill Livingstone.

Selye, H. (1993). *Neuroendocrinology and stress*. New York: New York Academy of Science.

Stilwell, S., Fineout-Overholt, E., Melnyk, G., et al. (2010). Evidence-based practice, step by step: Asking the clinical question: A key step in evidence-based practice. *American Journal of Nursing, 110*(3), 58–61.

University of Minnesota. (2004–2012). *The nun study*. Retrieved July 30, 2012, from https://www.healthstudies.umn.edu/nunstudy/faq.jsp

University of Southern California, Health Sciences, Los Angeles. (n.d.). Evidence based decision making, asking a good question (PICO). Retrieved August 3, 2012, from http://www.usc.edu/hsc/ebnet/ebframe/PICO.htm

Von Bertalanffy, L. (1976). *General system theory: Foundations, development and applications* (Rev. ed.). New York: George Braziller.

Walden University. (last updated October 31, 2011, October 31). Faye Glenn Abdellah's theory. Retrieved July 31, 2012, from http://currentnursing.com/nursing_theory/Abdellah.html

Watson, J. (1979). *Nursing: The philosophy and science of caring*. Boston: Little, Brown.

Watson, J. (1988). *Nursing: Human science and human care. A theory of nursing* (Publication No. 15–2236). New York: National League for Nursing Press.

Watson, J. (2012). Overview and evolution. In Theory of human caring [Web site]. Denver: University of Colorado Health Sciences Center School of Nursing. Retrieved July 29, 2012, from http://www.ucdenver.edu/academics/colleges/nursing/caring/humancaring/Pages/HumanCaring.aspx

Wiedenbach, E. (1964). *Clinical nursing: A helping art*. New York: Springer.

Wilson, H. S. (1993). *Introducing research in nursing* (2nd ed.). Redwood City, CA: Addison-Wesley Nursing.

Yura, H., & Torres, G. (1975). *Today's conceptual frameworks with the baccalaureate nursing programs* (NLN Publication No. 15-1558). New York: National League for Nursing.

CHAPTER 9

About teen depression [Fact sheet]. (n.d.). CRC Health Group. Retrieved August 30, 2012, from http://www.about-teen-depression.com/teen-depression.html

Adams S. M., Good M. W., & Defranco, G. M. (2009). Sudden infant death syndrome. *American Family Physician, 79*(10), 870–874.

Advisory Committee on Immunization Practices (ACIP). (2008). Prevention and control of influenza. Recommendations of the Advisory Committee on Immunization Practices (ACPI), 2007. *MMWR Recommendations and Reports, 57*(RR07), 1–60. Retrieved August 30, 2012, from http://www.cdc.gov/mmwr/preview/mmwrhtml/rr5707a1.htm

Agency for Healthcare Research and Quality (AHRQ). (2005, October; revised 2013, March). *Guideline synthesis: Screening for cervical cancer*. Rockville, MD: Agency for Healthcare Research and Quality. Retrieved March 23, 2013, from http://www.guideline.gov/syntheses/synthesis.aspx?id=43606&search=cervical+cancer

Agency for Healthcare Research and Quality (AHRQ). (2008). *National Healthcare Quality & Disparities Reports, 2008*. Retrieved September 9, 2012, from http://www.ahrq.gov/qual/qrdr08.htm

American Academy of Family Physicians (AAFP). (2006; updated 2010). *Toilet training your child*. Familydoctor.org. Retrieved August 30, 2012, from http://familydoctor.org/online/famdocen/home/children/parents/toilet/179.html

American Academy of Pediatrics (AAP). (2005). Policy statement: AAP Publications Reaffirmed, October 2004: Condom use by adolescents. *Pediatrics*, 2001; *107*, 1451–1455. Retrieved August 29, 2012, from http://pediatrics.aappublications.org/content/132/5/973.full.pdf

American Academy of Pediatrics (AAP). (2006). Policy statement. Active healthy living: Prevention of childhood obesity through increased physical activity. *Pediatrics, 117*(5), 1834–1842.

American Academy of Pediatrics (AAP). (2008). Preventive oral health intervention for pediatricians. *Pediatrics, 122*(6), 1387–1394.

American Academy of Pediatrics (AAP). (2011). Children's health topics. Car safety seats: A guide for families 2010. Retrieved August 30, 2012, from http://www.aap.org/en-us/about-the-aap/aap-press-room/Pages/AAP-Updates-Recommendation-on-Car-Seats.aspx

American Cancer Society. (n.d.; last revised 2012, June). American Cancer Society guidelines for the early detection of cancer. Retrieved August 31, 2012, from http://www.cancer.org/docroot/PED/content/PED_2_3X_ACS_Cancer_Detection_Guidelines_36.asp?sitearea+PED

American Cancer Society. (2013, December 31). How to perform a breast self-exam. Retrieved August 30, 2012, from http://www.cancer.org/docroot/CRI/content/CRI_2_6x_How_to_perform_a_breast_self_exam_5.asp

American College of Obstetricians and Gynecologists (ACOG). (2009). Interpreting the U.S. Preventive Services Task Force breast cancer screening recommendations for the general population. Retrieved August 31, 2012, from http://www.acog.org/About_ACOG/News_Room/News_Releases/2009/Interpreting_the_US_Preventive_Services_Task_Force

American Heart Association (AHA). (n.d; last updated 2012, June). Physical activity and children. Retrieved August 31, 2012, from http://www.heart.org/HEARTORG/GettingHealthy/PhysicalActivity/Physical-Activity-and-Children_UCM_304053_Article.jsp

American Heart Association (AHA). (2010). Understanding childhood obesity (statistical sourcebook). Retrieved September 6, 2012, from http://www.heart.org/idc/groups/heart-public/@wcm/@fc/documents/downloadable/ucm_304175.pdf

American Heart Association (AHA). (2011). Guideline for physical activity. Retrieved September 6, 2012, from http://www.heart.org/HEARTORG/GettingHealthy/PhysicalActivity/StartWalking/American-Heart-Association-Guidelines-for-Physical-Activity_UCM_307976_Article.jsp

American Heart Association (AHA). (2012). Overweight in children. Retrieved August 31, 2012, from http://www.heart.org/HEARTORG/GettingHealthy/WeightManagement/Obesity/Overweight-in-Children_UCM_304054_Article.jsp

American Lung Association (ALA). (2010; 2011, July). Trends in tobacco use. Retrieved August 31, 2012, from http://www.lungusa.org/finding-cures/our-research/trend-reports/Tobacco-Trend-Report.pdf

APGAR. (n.d.; last updated 2011, December 2). Medline Plus, U.S. National Library of Medicine, National Institutes of Health. Retrieved August 31, 2012, from http://www.nlm.nih.gov/medlineplus/ency/article/003402.htm

Balkaya, N., Memis, S., & Demirkiran, F. (2007). The effects of breast self-exam education on the performance of nursing and midwifery students: A 6-month follow-up study. *Journal of Cancer Education, 22*(2), 77–79.

Brodowski, M. L., Nolan, C. M., Gaudiosi, J. A., et al. (2008, April 4). Nonfatal maltreatment of infants-United States, October 2005–September 2006. *Morbidity and Mortality Weekly Report, 57*(13), 336–339. Retrieved August 31, 2012, from http://www.cdc.gov/mmwr/preview/mmwrhtml/mm5713a2.htm

Centers for Disease Control and Prevention (CDC). (n.d.a; last updated 2011, September 23). About BMI for children and teens. Retrieved August 31, 2012, from http://www.cdc.gov/healthyweight/assessing/bmi/childrens_bmi/about_childrens_bmi.html#My%20two%20children

Centers for Disease Control and Prevention (CDC). (n.d.a). Infant mortality statistics from the 2008 period linked birth/infant death data set. *National Vital Statistics Reports, 60*(5). Retrieved August 31, 2012, from http://www.cdc.gov/nchs/data/nvsr/nvsr60/nvsr60_05.pdf

Centers for Disease Control and Prevention (CDC). (2001; last reviewed 2012, January). Prevalence of obesity in the United States, 2009–2010. Retrieved August 31, 2012, from http://www.cdc.gov/obesity/data/adult.html

Centers for Disease Control and Prevention (CDC). (2006). The state of childhood asthma, United States, 1980–2005. *Advance Data from Vital and Health Statistics*, 381. Retrieved August 31, 2012, from http://www.cdc.gov/nchs/data/ad/ad381.pdf

Centers for Disease Control and Prevention (CDC). (2008). HIV/AIDS among persons aged 50 and older. Retrieved

August 31, 2012, from http://www.cdc.gov/hiv/topics/over50/resources/factsheets/pdf/over50.pdf

Centers for Disease Control and Prevention (CDC). (2010a). *State disparities in teenage birth rates in the United States* (NCHS Data Brief No. 46). Retrieved August 31, 2012, from http://www.cdc.gov/nchs/data/databriefs/db46.pdf

Centers for Disease Control and Prevention (CDC). (2010b). Summary health statistics for U.S. children: National health interview survey, 2010. *Vital and Health Statistics*, Series 10, No. 250. Retrieved August 31, 2012, from http://www.cdc.gov/nchs/data/series/sr_10/sr10_250.pdf

Centers for Disease Control and Prevention (CDC). (2011a; 2012, June 11). 2011 Child & adolescent immunization schedules. Department of Health and Human Services. Retrieved August 31, 2012, from http://www.cdc.gov/vaccines/schedules/hcp/child-adolescent.html

Centers for Disease Control and Prevention (CDC). (2011b). Sexual behavior, sexual attraction, and sexual identity in the United States: Data from the 2006–2008, National Survey of Family Growth. *Advance Data from Vital and Health Statistics, 36*. Retrieved August 31, 2012, from http://www.cdc.gov/nchs/products/ad.htm

Centers for Disease Control and Prevention (CDC). (2012a). Vital signs: Unintentional injury deaths among persons aged 0–19 Years—United States, 2000–2009. *Morbidity and Mortality Weekly Report, 61*(15), 270–276. Retrieved September 8, 2012, from http://www.cdc.gov/mmwr/preview/mmwrhtml/mm6115a5.htm?s_cid=mm6115a5_w

Centers for Disease Control and Prevention (CDC). (2012b). Youth risk behavior surveillance—United States 2011. *Morbidity and Mortality Weekly Report, 61*(4), 1–162.

Chandra, A., Mosher, W., & Copen, C. (2011). Sexual behavior, sexual attraction, and sexual identity in the United States: Data from the 2006–2008 national survey of family growth. Centers for Disease Control and Prevention (CDC). *Morbidity and Mortality Weekly Report, 64*(4), 1–162. Retrieved September 1, 2012, from http://www.cdc.gov/nchs/data/nhsr/nhsr036.pdf

Child Trends. (2012). Condom use. Retrieved September 6, 2012, from http://www.childtrendsdatabank.org/?q=node/264

Couser, N., Esmail, F., & Hutchinson, A. (2012). Vision screening in the pediatrician's office. *Open Journal of Ophthalmology, 2*, 9–13.

DeNoon, D. (2012). CDC: Little change in risky teen sex. Less racial disparity, little progress in safer teen sex. WebMd. Retrieved September 2, 2012, from http://teens.webmd.com/news/20120724/cdc-little-change-in-risky-teen-sex

Denver II. (1990). Available for purchase from Denver Developmental Materials, Inc., Denver, CO. Retrieved September 1, 2012, from http://www.denverii.com/home.html

Erikson, E. H. (1963). *Childhood and society* (2nd ed.). New York: W. W. Norton.

Fowler, J. W. (1981). *Stages of faith: The psychology of human development and the quest for meaning*. New York: Harper & Row.

Freud, A. (1966). *The ego and the mechanisms of defense*. New York: International Universities Press.

Garofalo, R., Herrick, A., Mustanski, B. S., et al. (2007). Tip of the iceberg: Young men who have sex with men, the Internet, and HIV risk. *American Journal of Public Health, 97*(6), 1113–1117.

Gavin, L., MacKay, A., Brown, K., et al. (2009). Sexual and reproductive health of persons aged 10–24 years—United States, 2002–2007. *MMWR Surveillance Summaries, 58*(SS06), 1–58.

Gemignani, M. (2011). Breast cancer screening: Why, when, and how many? *Clinical Obstetrics & Gynecology, 54*(1), 125–132.

General recommendations on immunization. Recommendations of the Advisory Committee on Immunization Practices (ACIP). (2011). *Morbidity and Mortality Weekly Report, 60*(RR02), 1–60. Retrieved September 1, 2012, from http://www.cdc.gov/mmwr/preview/mmwrhtml/rr6002a1.htm?s_cid=rr6002a1_e

Gilligan, C. (1993). *In a different voice: Psychological theory and women's development*. Cambridge, MA: Harvard University Press.

Goldschmidt, A. B., Stein, R. I., Saelens, B. E., & Theim, K. (2011). Practical approaches to the treatment of severe pediatric obesity. *Pediatric Clinics of North America, 58*(6), 1425–1438.

The guide to clinical preventive services 2010–2011 (AHRQ Publication No. 10-05145). (2010, August). Rockville, MD: Agency for Healthcare Research and Quality. Retrieved September 1, 2012, from http://www.ahrq.gov/clinic/pocketgd1011/pocketgd1011.pdf

Halpern-Felsher, B. (2008). Oral sexual behavior: Harm reduction or gateway behavior? *Journal of Adolescent Health, 43*(3), 207–208.

Havighurst, R. J. (1971). *Developmental tasks and education* (3rd ed.). New York: Longman.

Heron M., Hoyert D., Murphy S., Xu J., Kochanek K., & Tejada-Vera B. (2009). Deaths: Final data for 2006. *National Vital Statistics Report, 57*(14), 1–134.

Institute of Medicine, Food and Nutrition Board. (2010; updated 2012, June 13). *Dietary reference intakes for calcium and vitamin D*. Washington, DC: The National Academies of Sciences. Retrieved September 1, 2012 from, http://www.iom.edu/Reports/2010/Dietary-Reference-Intakes-for-Calcium-and-Vitamin-D.aspx

Kohlberg, L. (1968). Moral development. In D. Sills (Eds.), *International encyclopedia of social science*. New York: Macmillan.

Kohlberg, L. (1981). *Essays on moral development* (Vols. 1–3). San Francisco: Harper & Row.

Kösters, J. P., & Gøtzsche, P. C. (2004; updated 2009, October 8). Regular self-examination or clinical examination for early detection of breast cancer. *Cochrane Summaries*. Retrieved September 1, 2012, from http://summaries.cochrane.org/CD003373/regular-self-examination-or-clinical-examination-for-early-detection-of-breast-cancer

Leeb, R., Lewis, T., & Zolotor, A. (2011). A review of physical and mental health consequences of child abuse and neglect and implications for practice. *American Journal of Lifestyle Medicine, 5*(5), 454–468.

Lindberg, L., Jones, R., & Santelli, J. (2008). Noncoital sexual activities among adolescents. *Journal of Adolescent Health, 43*(3), 231–238.

Lippert, J., Shea, J., & Seagrave, M. (2008). Anorexia nervosa: Dying to be thin. *The Clinical Advisor, 11*(1), 67–70.

McFarlane, J. H., & Miller, A. (2005). Promoting community protection of adolescents. Juvenile Rights Project, Inc. Retrieved September 1, 2012, from http://www.jrplaw.org/Documents/CJA%20final%20part%201.pdf

Medline Plus, U.S. National Library of Medicine, National Institutes of Health. (Last updated 2012, August 27). APGAR. Retrieved August 30, 2012, from http://www.nlm.nih.gov/medlineplus/ency/article/003402.htm#top

Meissner, H., Klabunde, C., Han, P., Benard, V., & Breen, N. (2011). Breast cancer screening beliefs, recommendations and practices. *Cancer, 117*(14), 3101–3111.

Mersky, J., Topitzes, J., Reynolds, A. (2011). Unsafe at any age: Linking childhood and adolescent maltreatment to delinquency and crime. *Journal of Research in Crime and Delinquency, 49*(2), 295–318.

Moracco, K., Runyan, C., Bowling, J., et al. (2007). Women's experiences with violence: A national study. *Womens Health Issues, 17*(1), 3–12.

Murphy, S., Xu, J., and Kochanek, K. [U.S. Department of Health and Human Services, Centers for Disease Control and Prevention], (2012, January 11). Deaths: Preliminary data for 2010. *National Vital Statistics Report, 60*(4), 1–61. Retrieved September 1, 2012, from http://www.cdc.gov/nchs/data/nvsr/nvsr60/nvsr60_04.pdf

National Cancer Institute (NCI). (2008; last updated 2012, March). Breast cancer screening (PDQ). Retrieved September 1, 2012, from http://www.cancer.gov/cancertopics/pdq/screening/breast/HealthProfessional/page10

National Cancer Institute (NCI). (2009). What you need to know about breast cancer: Risk factors. Retrieved September 1, 2012, from http://www.cancer.gov/cancertopics/wyntk/breast/page4

National Center for Health Statistics (NCHS). (2011a). Adult obesity prevalence in Canada and the United States. Retrieved September 1, 2012, from http://www.cdc.gov/nchs/data/databriefs/db56.pdf

National Center for Health Statistics (NCHS). (2011b). Health, United States, 2011: With special feature on socioeconomic status and health. Retrieved September 1, 2012, from http://www.cdc.gov/nchs/data/hus/hus11.pdf

National Guideline Clearinghouse (NGC). (2007). *Guideline summary: Evaluation of suspected child physical abuse.* Rockville, MD: Agency for Healthcare Research and Quality. Retrieved September 1, 2012, from http://www.guideline.gov/content.aspx?id=11057

National Heart, Lung and Blood Institute. (2012). Integrated guidelines for cardiovascular health and risk reduction in children and adolescents. Retrieved September 3, 2012, from http://www.nhlbi.nih.gov/guidelines/cvd_ped/peds_guidelines_sum.pdf

National Institutes of Health (NIH). (2008). WHI follow up study confirms health risks of long-term combination hormone therapy outweigh benefits for postmenopausal women. *NIH News* Retrieved September 1, 2012, from http://www.nih.gov/news/health/mar2008/nhlbi-04.htm

Nelson, H., Bougatsos, C., & Blazina, I. (2012). *Screening women for intimate partner violence and elderly and vulnerable adults for abuse: Systematic review to update the 2004 U.S. Preventive Services Task Force Recommendation.* Rockville, MD: Agency for Healthcare Research and Quality. Retrieved September 1, 2012, from http://www.ncbi.nlm.nih.gov/pubmed/22675737

Office of Dietary Supplements, National Institutes of Health (2011). *Dietary supplement fact sheet: Vitamin D.* Retrieved September 1, 2012, from http://ods.od.nih.gov/factsheets/vitamind

Perry, R., Kayekjian, K., Braun, R., Cantu, M., Shoran, B., & Chung P. (2011). Adolescents' perspectives on the use of text messaging service for preventive sexual health promotion. *Journal of Adolescent Health, 51*(3), 220–225.

Piaget, J. (1952). *The origins of intelligence in children.* New York: International Universities Press.

Polan, E., & Taylor, D. (2010). *Journey across the life span: Human development and health promotion* (4th ed.). Philadelphia: F. A. Davis.

Reinberg, S. (2012, May 17). Drowning is leading cause of kids' accidental death: CDC. *HealthDay Reporter.*

Roberts, T., Auinger, P., & Ryan, S. (2004). Body piercing and high-risk behavior in adolescents. *Journal of Adolescent Health, 34*, 224–229.

Sadock, B., & Sadock, V. (2010). *Kaplan & Sadock's synopsis of psychiatry* (10th ed.). Philadelphia: Lippincott Williams & Wilkins.

Schnitzer, P. G., & Ewigman, B. G. (2008). Household composition and fatal unintentional injuries related to child maltreatment. *Journal of Nursing Scholarship, 40*(1), 91–97.

Scudder, L. (2007). Teens and body art—into the mainstream. *Medscape Education.* Retrieved September 6, 2012, from http://www.medscape.org/viewarticle/551430

Smith, R., Cokkinides, V., Brooks, D., Saslow, D., Shah M., & Brawley, O. (2011). Cancer screening in the United States, 2011: A review of current American Cancer Society guidelines and issues in cancer screening. *CA: A Cancer Journal for Clinicians, 61*(1), 8–30.

Smith, M., & Segal, J. (2012). Child abuse and neglect: Recognizing and preventing child abuse. *HealthGuide.org.* Retrieved September 9, 2012, from http://www.helpguide.org/mental/child_abuse_physical_emotional_sexual_neglect.htm

Substance Abuse and Mental Health Services Administration (SAMHSA), Office of Applied Studies, Department of Health and Human Services. (2010). *Results from the 2009 national survey on drug use and health: Volume 1: Summary of national findings.* Retrieved September 1, 2012, from http://www.oas.samhsa.gov/NSDUH/2k9NSDUH/2k9ResultsP.pdf

Tanner, J. (1962). *Growth at adolescence* (2nd ed.). Oxford: Blackwell.

Task force says men age 75 and older should not be screened for prostate cancer [Press release]. (2008, August 4). Rockville, MD: Agency for Healthcare Research and Quality. Retrieved September 1, 2012, from http://www.ahrq.gov/news/press/pr2008/tfproscanpr.htm

Townsend, M. (2011). *Psychiatric mental health nursing: Concepts of care* (7th ed.). Philadelphia: F. A. Davis.

U.S. Department of Health and Human Services (USDHHS). (2007–2008). Heads up: Concussion in youth sports [Centers for Disease Control and Prevention; National Center for Injury Prevention and Control]. Retrieved September 6, 2012, from http://www.cdc.gov/concussion/pdf/Heads_Up_Activity_Report_Final-a.pdf

U.S. Department of Health and Human Services (USDHHS). (2008). 2008 Physical activity guidelines for Americans. Retrieved September 2, 2012, from http://www.health.gov/paguidelines/pdf/paguide.pdf

U.S. Department of Health and Human Services (USDHHS). (2010a). Maternal, infant and child health. *Healthy People 2020.* Retrieved September 2, 2012, from http://www.healthypeople.gov/2020/topicsobjectives2020/default.aspx

U.S. Department of Health and Human Services (USDHHS). (2010b). Office of Disease Prevention and Health Promotion.

Healthy People 2020. Washington, DC. Retrieved September 9, 2012, from www.healthypeople.gov/

U.S. Department of Justice, Office of Justice Programs Bureau of Justice Statistics. (n.d., last reviewed 2012, August 23). Homicide trends in the U.S.: Intimate homicide. Retrieved August 31, 2012, from http://bjs.ojp.usdoj.gov/content/homicide/intimates.cfm

U.S. Environmental Protection Agency (EPA). (last updated 2010, October). Asthma. Indoor environmental asthma triggers. Retrieved September 2, 2012, from http://www.epa.gov/asthma/triggers.html

U.S. Preventive Services Task Force (USPSTF). (2004). Screening for family and intimate partner violence: Recommendation statement. *Annals of Internal Medicine, 140*(5), 382–386.

U.S. Preventive Services Task Force (USPSTF). (2009). *Screening for breast cancer: Clinical summary*. Rockville, MD: Agency for Healthcare Research and Quality. Retrieved September 1, 2012, from http://www.uspreventiveservicestaskforce.org/uspstf/uspsbrca.htm

U.S. Preventive Services Task Force (USPSTF). (2011a). Vision screening for children 1 to 5 years of age: U.S. Preventive Services Task Force recommendation statement. *Pediatrics, 127*(2), 340–346.

U.S. Preventive Services Task Force (USPSTF). (2011b). *Screening for testicular cancer: Recommendation statement*. Rockville, MD: Agency for Healthcare Research and Quality. Retrieved September 1, 2012, from http://www.uspreventiveservicestaskforce.org/uspstf/uspstest.htm

Waldrop, J. (2008). Stopping childhood obesity before it begins. *The Clinical Advisor, 11*(1), 35–36, 39–41.

Waugh, D. (1978). Moral development: Theory and process. In *Teaching and evaluating the affective domain in nursing programs* (pp. 17–30). Thorofare, NJ: Charles B. Slack.

Wilcox, W., & Dew, J. (2008, January). Protectors or perpetrators? Fathers, mothers, and child abuse and neglect. *Institute for American Values. Center for Marriage and Families* (Research Brief No. 7). Retrieved September 3, 2012, from http://www.americanvalues.org/pdfs/researchbrief7.pdf

Wilkinson, J. (2009). *Nursing diagnosis handbook* (9th ed.). Upper Saddle River, NJ: Prentice Hall.

Wood, J., Medina, S., Feudtner, C., et al. (2012). Local macroeconomic trends and hospital admissions for child abuse, 2000–2009. *Pediatrics, 2011*(3755).

CHAPTER 10

AARP Public Policy Institute. (2011). *Aging in place: A state survey of livability policies and practices*. Washington, DC: Author. Retrieved September 27, 2012, from http://assets.aarp.org/rgcenter/ppi/liv-com/aging-in-place-2011-full.pdf

Agency for Healthcare Research and Quality (AHRQ). (1996, November). *Clinical practice guidelines No. 19* (Publication No. 97-0702). Washington, DC: U.S. Department of Health and Human Services. Retrieved October 25, 2012, from http://www.ama-assn.org/resources/doc/public-health/aging_vs_dementia.pdf

Agency for Healthcare Research and Quality (AHRQ). (2005, October, revised 2013, March). *Guideline synthesis: Screening for cervical cancer*. Rockville, MD: Agency for Healthcare Research and Quality. Retrieved March 23, 2013, from http://www.guideline.gov/syntheses/synthesis.aspx?id=43606&search=cervical+cancer

Alley, D., Liebig, P., Pynoos, J., et al. (2007). Creating elder-friendly communities: Preparations for an aging society. *Journal of Gerontological Social Work, 49*(1/2), 1–18.

Al Omari, H., Kramer, K., Hronek, C., et al. (2005). The Wheat Valley assisted living culture: Rituals and rules. *Journal of Gerontological Nursing, 31*(1), 9–16.

Alzheimer's Association. (2008). Risk factors. Retrieved September 27, 2012, from http://www.alz.org/alzheimers_disease_causes_risk_factors.asp

American Cancer Society. (2013, last revised). American Cancer Society guidelines for the early detection of cancer. Retrieved February 20, 2013, from http://www.cancer.org/docroot/PED/content/PED_2_3X_ACS_Cancer_Detection_Guidelines_36.asp?sitearea+PED

American College of Obstetricians and Gynecologists (ACOG). (2009). Less frequent pap tests recommended [News release]. Retrieved October 25, 2012, from http://news.cancerconnect.com/acog-updates-cervical-cancer-screening-guidelines/

American College of Obstetricians and Gynecologists (ACOG). (2011). *Breast cancer screening* (ACOG Practice Bulletin No. 122). Washington, DC: Author. Retrieved September 27, 2012, from http://www.guideline.gov/content.aspx?id=34275

American College of Obstetricians and Gynecologists (ACOG). (2012). *Screening for cervical cancer* (ACOG Practice Bulletin No. 131, p. 17). Washington, DC: Author.

American Diabetes Association. (2011). *Diabetes statistics. Data from the 2011 national diabetes fact sheet*. Retrieved September 27, 2012, from http://www.diabetes.org/diabetes-basics/diabetes-statistics/

Badgwell, B., Giordano, S., Duan, Z., et al. (2008). Mammography before diagnosis among women age 80 years and older with breast cancer. *Journal of Clinical Oncology, 26*(15), 2482–2488.

Brodaty, H., Green, A., & Koschera, A. (2003). Meta-analysis of psychosocial interventions for caregivers of people with dementia. *Journal of the American Geriatrics Society, 51*, 657–664.

Centers for Disease Control and Prevention (CDC). (2011). How much physical activity do older adults need? Physical activity is essential to healthy aging. Retrieved December 6, 2012, from http://www.cdc.gov/physicalactivity/everyone/guidelines/olderadults.html

Centers for Disease Control and Prevention (CDC). (2012). Recommended adult immunization schedule, United States 2012. Department of Health and Human Services. Retrieved September 27, 2012, from http://www.cdc.gov/vaccines/schedules/downloads/adult/adult-schedule.pdf

Cherkas, L., Hunkin, J., Kato, B., et al. (2008). The association between physical activity in leisure time and leukocyte telomere length. *Archives of Internal Medicine, 168*(2), 154–158.

Chumbler, N. R., Mann, W. C., Wu, S., Schmid, A., & Kobb, R. (2004). The association of home-telehealth use and care coordination with improvement of functional and cognitive functioning in frail elderly men. *Telemedicine Journal & E-Health, 10*(2), 129–137.

Cumming, E., & Henry, W. (1961). Growing old, the process of disengagement. New York: Basic Books.

Erikson, E. H. (1963). *Childhood and society* (2nd ed.). New York: W. W. Norton.

Ertel, K., Glymour, M., & Berkman, L. F. (2008). Effects of social integration on preserving memory function in a nationally representative U.S. elderly population. *American Journal of Public Health, 98*(7), 1215–1220.

Federal Interagency Forum on Aging-Related Statistics. (2010). Older americans 2010: Key indicators of well-being. Retrieved September 27, 2012, from http://www.agingstats.gov/Main_Site/Data/Data_2010.aspx

Flaherty, J., Morley, J., Murphy, D., et al. (2002). The development of outpatient clinical glidepaths. *Journal of the American Geriatrics Society, 50,* 1886–1901.

Fletcher, K. (2012). Dementia: Nursing standard of practice protocol: Recognition and management of dementia. Hartford Institute for Geriatric Nursing. Retrieved October 4, 2012, from http://consultgerirn.org/topics/dementia/want_to_know_more

Folstein, M. F., Folstein, S., & McHugh P. R. (1975). Mini mental state: A practical method for grading the cognitive state of patients for the clinician. *Journal of Psychiatric Research, 12,* 189–198.

Fong, T., Jones, R., Rudolph, J., et al. (2010). Development and validation of a brief cognitive assessment tool. Archives of Internal Medicine. Frailty in older adults. (2006). *JAMA* patient page. *JAMA, 296*(18). Retrieved December 6, 2012, from http://archinte.jamanetwork.com/article.aspx?articleid=226801

Futterman, M. (2008). Over 80, it's anyone's race. *The Wall Street Journal,* pp. W1, W4.

Gellis, Z., Kenaley, B., McGinty, J., et al. (2012). Outcomes of a telehealth intervention for homebound older adults with heart or chronic respiratory failure: A randomized controlled trial. *The Gerontologist, 52*(4), 541–552.

Guide to clinical preventive services, 2010–2011 (AHRQ Publication No. 08–05122). (2010)., Rockville, MD: Agency for Healthcare Research and Quality. Retrieved September 27, 2012, from http://www.ahrq.gov/clinic/pocketgd1011/gcp10s2.htm

Harrell, R. (2011). *Housing for older adults: The impacts of the recession.* Washington, DC: AARP Public Policy Institute.

Havighurst, J. (1963). Successful aging. In R. H. Williams, C. Tibbitts, & W. Donahue (Eds.), *Processes of aging.* New York: Atherton Press.

Houser, A., Fox-Grage, W., & Gibson, M. J. (2012). *Across the states: Profiles of long term care and independent living* (9th ed.). Washington, DC: AARP Public Policy Institute.

Katz, S., Down, T., Cash, H., et al. (1970). Progress in the development of the index of ADL. *The Gerontologist, 10*(1), 20–30.

Katz index of independence in activities of daily living (ADL). (2007). Hartford Institute for Geriatric Nursing. New York University, College of Nursing. Retrieved September 27, 2012, from http://consultgerirn.org/uploads/File/trythis/try_this_2.pdf

Langlois, F., Vu, T., Chassé, K., et al. (2012). Benefits of physical exercise training on cognition and quality of life in frail older adults. *The Journals of Gerontology Series B: Psychological Sciences and Social Sciences.* doi:10.1093/geronb/gbs069

Laumann, E. O., Leitsch, S. A., & Waite, L. J. (2008). Elder mistreatment in the United States: Prevalence estimates from a nationally representative study. *Journal of Gerontology: Social Sciences, 63B*(4), S248–S254.

Liu, C. K., & Fielding, R. A. (2011). Exercise as an intervention for frailty. *Clinics in Geriatric Medicine, 27*(1), 101.

Lowry, F. (2012). *Unique injury pattern points to elder abuse.* Medscape Medical News from the Radiological Society of North America (RSNA) 98th Scientific Assembly and Annual Meeting. Retrieved December 6, 2012, from http://www.medscape.com/viewarticle/775363?src=mp

Macko, R., Benvenuti, F., Stanhope, S., et al. (2008). Adaptive physical activity improves mobility function and quality of life in chronic hemiparesis. *Journal of Rehabilitation Research and Development, 45*(2), 323–328.

Martin, F. C., & Brighton, P. (2008). Frailty: Different tools for different purposes? *Age and Ageing, 37,* 129–131.

Meijers, J., Halfens, R., Neyens, J., Luiking, Y., Verlaan, G., & Schols, J. (2012). Predicting falls in elderly receiving home care: The role of malnutrition and impaired mobility. *The Journal of Nutrition, Health & Aging,* 1–5.

Murphy, S., Xu, J., & Kochanek, K. (2012, January 11). [U.S. Department of Health and Human Services, Centers for Disease Control and Prevention] Deaths: Preliminary data for 2010. *National Vital Statistics Reports, 60*(4), 1–52. Retrieved October 22, 2012, from http://www.cdc.gov/nchs/data/nvsr/nvsr60/nvsr60_04.pdf

National Cancer Institute (NCI). (2008; last modified 2011, January). Breast cancer screening (PDQ®). Retrieved September 27, 2012, from http://www.cancer.gov/cancertopics/pdq/screening/breast/HealthProfessional/page10

National Center for Health Statistics. (2012). *Health, United States, 2011: With special feature on socioeconomic status and health.* Hyattsville, MD: Author.

National Guideline Clearinghouse (NGC). (2008, April; revised 2012, November). *Guideline synthesis: Screening and risk assessment for osteoporosis.* Rockville, MD: Agency for Healthcare Research and Quality. Retrieved December 6, 2012, from http://guideline.gov/syntheses/synthesis.aspx?f=rss&id=38658

National Guideline Clearinghouse (NGC). (2012, November). *Screening for cervical cancer.* Rockville, MD: Agency for Healthcare Research and Quality. Retrieved January 17, 2013, from http://guideline.gov/content.aspx?f=rss&id=38572&osrc=12#Section420

National Health Information Center. (2012). *Protect your health as you grow older.* Washington, DC. Retrieved December 6, 2012, from http://www.healthfinder.gov/prevention/PrintTopic.aspx?topicId=80

National Institute for Health and Clinical Excellence (NICE). (2006). *Supporting people with dementia and their careers in health and social care* (Clinical Guideline CG42). London: Author. Retrieved October 25, 2012, from http://www.nice.org.uk/guidance/cg42

Perls, T. (2006). The different paths to 100. *American Journal of Clinical Nutrition, 83*(Suppl.), 484S–487S.

Perls, T., Silver, M. H., & Lauerman, J. F. (1999). *Living to 100: Lessons in living to your maximum potential at any age.* New York: Basic Books.

Registered Nurses' Association of Ontario (RNAO). (2010). *Screening for delirium, dementia and depression in older adults, supplement.* Toronto, Ontario: Author.

Rockwood, K. (2005). What would make a definition of frailty successful? *Age and Ageing, 34,* 432–434.

Shephard, R. J. (2008, April). Maximal oxygen intake and independence in old age. *British Journal of Sports Medicine, 10.* Retrieved October 4, 2012, from http://bjsm.bmj.com/content/43/5/342.full?sid=5b6e0aa1-fef9-464b-bc32-7608b703d6ca

Smith, R., Cokkinides, V., & Eyre, H.; American Cancer Society. (2003). American Cancer Society guidelines for the early detection of cancer. *CA-Ca-A Cancer Journal for Clinicians, 53*, 27–43.

Smith, G. E., Lunde, A. M., Hathaway, J. C., & Vickers, K. S. (2007). Telehealth home monitoring of solitary persons with mild dementia. *American Journal of Alzheimer's Disease and Other Dementias, 22*(1), 20–26.

Snowdon, D. A. (2003). Healthy aging and dementia: Findings from the Nun Study. *Annals of Internal Medicine, 139*(5 Pt. 2), 450–454.

Stall, N., Nowaczynski, M., & Sinha, S. (2013). Back to the future: Home-based primary care for older homebound Canadians. Part 2: Where we are going. *Canadian Family Physician, 59*(3), 243–245.

Tahmaseb-McConatha, J., Volkwein-Caplan, K., & DiGregorio, N. (2011). Culture, aging and well-being: The importance of place and space. *International Journal Of Sport & Society, 2*(2), 41–48, *19*(2), 65–68.

Task force recommends against routine prostate cancer screening [Press release]. (2012, May 21). Rockville, MD: Agency for Healthcare Research and Quality. Retrieved October 25, 2012, from http://www.cancer.org/cancer/news/news/task-force-recommends-against-routine-prostate-cancer-screening

Tomita, M., Mann, W., Stanton, K., et al. (2007). Use of currently available smart home technology by frail elders. Process and outcomes. *Topics in Geriatric Rehabilitation, 23*(1), 24–34.

Total Living Choices. (2000–2012). Assisted living. Retrieved September 27, 2012, from http://www.tlchoices.com/default.asp

U.S. Census Bureau. (2007; revised 2012, September 19). Census Bureau releases new data on residents of adult correctional facilities, nursing homes, and other group quarters. Retrieved September 27, 2012, from http://www.census.gov/newsroom/releases/archives/american_community_survey_acs/cb07-cn11.html

U.S. Census Bureau. (2008). *2008 National population projections*. Washington, DC: Author. Retrieved September 27, 2012, from http://www.census.gov/population/www/projections/2008projections.html

U.S. Census 2010. (2011). *The older population: 2010*. Washington, DC: Author. Retrieved October 1, 2012, from http://www.census.gov/prod/cen2010/briefs/c2010br-09.pdf

U.S. Department of Health and Human Services (USDHHS). (2008). *Physical activity guidelines for Americans. At-a-glance: A fact sheet for professionals*. Retrieved September 27, 2012, from http://www.health.gov/paguidelines/factsheetprof.aspx

U.S. Department of Health and Human Services, Public Health Service, National Institutes of Health. (2003). *What's your aging IQ*. Retrieved September 27, 2012, from http://www.niapublications.org/tipsheets/pdf/Whats_Your_Aging_IQ.pdf

U.S. Preventive Services Task Force (USPSTF). (2002; updated 2009). *Screening for breast cancer: Systematic evidence review*. Rockville, MD: Agency for Healthcare Research and Quality. Retrieved September 27, 2012, from http://www.cdc.gov/cancer/breast/basic_info/screening.htm

U.S. Preventive Services Task Force (USPSTF). (2003a). Screening for dementia. Retrieved September 27, 2012, from http://www.uspreventiveservicestaskforce.org/uspstf/uspsdeme.htm

U.S. Preventive Services Task Force (USPSTF). (2003b). Screening for cervical cancer. What's new from the USPSTF. Retrieved March 12, 2011, from http://www.uspreventiveservicestaskforce.org/uspstf/uspscerv.htm

U.S. Preventive Services Task Force (USPSTF). (2009a, March). Screening for colorectal cancer. Topic Page. Retrieved September 27, 2012, from http://www.uspreventiveservicestaskforce.org/uspstf/uspscolo.htm

U.S. Preventive Services Task Force (USPSTF). (2009b). *Screening for breast cancer: Clinical summary*. Rockville, MD: Agency for Healthcare Research and Quality. Retrieved September 27, 2012, from http://www.ahrq.gov/clinic/uspstf09/breastcancer/brcansum.htm

U.S. Preventive Services Task Force (USPSTF). (2012a). *Screening for cervical cancer*. Rockville, MD: Agency for Healthcare Research and Quality. Retrieved February 20, 2013, from http://www.uspreventiveservicestaskforce.org/uspstf/uspscerv.htm

U.S. Preventive Services Task Force (USPSTF). (2012b). *Screening for prostate cancer: Recommendation statement*. Rockville, MD: Agency for Healthcare Research and Quality. Retrieved October 25, 2012, from http://www.uspreventiveservicestaskforce.org/prostatecancerscreening/prostatefinalrs.htm

U.S. Preventive Services Task Force (USPSTF). (2012c). *Screening for intimate partner violence and abuse of elderly and vulnerable adults: A U.S. Preventive Services Task Force recommendation statement*. Rockville, MD: Agency for Healthcare Research and Quality. Retrieved January 21, 2013, from http://www.uspreventiveservicestaskforce.org/uspstf12/ipvelder/ipvelderfinalrs.pdf

Villareal, D. T., Chode, S., Parimi, N., et al. (2011). Weight loss, exercise, or both and physical function in obese older adults. *New England Journal of Medicine, 364*(13), 1218–1229.

Vincent, G., & Victoria, A. (2010). *The next four decades: The older population in the United Stated: 2012 to 2050* (Current Population Reports P25-1138) Washington, DC: U.S. Census Bureau. Retrieved December 9, 2012, from http://www.census.gov/prod/2010pubs/p25-1138.pdf

Williams, K. N., Herman, R., Gajewski, B., et al. (2008). Elderspeak communication: Impact on dementia care. *American Journal of Alzheimer's Disease & Other Dementias*. doi:10.1177/1533317508318472

Wilson, D. M., & Palha, P. (2007). A systematic review of published research articles on health promotion at retirement. *Journal of Nursing Scholarship, Fourth Quarter*, 330–337.

Woodhouse, K. W., & O'Mahony, M. S. (1997). Frailty and ageing. *Age and Ageing, 26*, 245–246.

Young, L., Foster, L., Silander, A., et al. (2011). Home telehealth: Patient satisfaction, program functions, and challenges for the care coordinator. *Journal of Gerontological Nursing, 37*(11), 38–46.

Zimmerman, S., & Sloane, P. D. (2007). Improving practice through research in and about assisted living: Definition and classification of assisted living [Special issue]. *The Gerontologist, 47*(3), 33–39.

CHAPTER 11

Agency for Healthcare Research and Quality (AHRQ). (2009). Educating patients before they leave the hospital reduces readmissions, emergency department visits and saves money [Press release]. Retrieved November 24, 2012, from http://www.ahrq.gov/news/press/pr2009/redpr.htm

Albom, M. (1997). *Tuesdays with Morrie*. New York: Doubleday.

The American Geriatrics Society. (n.d.). *AGS/BGS clinical practice guideline: Prevention of falls in older persons*. American Geriatrics Society, British Geriatrics Society, and American Academy of Orthopaedic Surgeons Panel on Falls Prevention. Retrieved November 24, 2012, from http://www.americangeriatrics.org/health_care_professionals/clinical_practice/clinical_guidelines_recommendations/prevention_of_falls_summary_of_recommendations/

Benner, P., & Wrubel, J. (1989). *The primacy of caring*. Menlo Park, CA: Addison-Wesley.

Bettelheim, B. (1979). *Surviving and other essays*. New York: Alfred A. Knopf.

Centers for Disease Control and Prevention (CDC). (n.d.; last updated 2012, August 13). Chronic disease prevention and health promotion. Retrieved November 21, 2012, from http://www.cdc.gov/chronicdisease/overview/index.htm

Centers for Disease Control and Prevention (CDC). (2002). Prevalence of self-reported arthritis or chronic joint symptoms among adults—United States, 2001. *Morbidity and Mortality Weekly Report, 51*(42), 948. Retrieved November 24, 2012, from http://www.cdc.gov/mmwr/preview/mmwrhtml/mm5142a2.htm

Centers for Disease Control and Prevention (CDC). (2010; last updated 2012, November 15). Health effects of secondhand smoke. Retrieved November 24, 2012, from http://www.cdc.gov/tobacco/data_statistics/fact_sheets/secondhand_smoke/health_effects/index.htm

Centers for Medicare & Medicaid Services (CMS). (2011). *Chronic conditions among Medicare beneficiaries*. Baltimore: Chart Book.

Closson, B. L., Mattingly, L. J., Finne, K. M., & Larson, J. A. (2012). Telephone follow-up program evaluation: Application of Orem's self-care model. *Rehabilitation Nursing, 19*(5), 287–292.

Cockerham, W. (2011). *Medical sociology* (12th ed.). Upper Saddle River, NJ: Prentice Hall.

Dunn, H. L. (1959). High level wellness for man and society. *American Journal of Public Health, 49*(6), 786–788.

Frankl, V. (1959/1962/1984). *Man's search for meaning*. New York: Washington Square Press.

Frankl, V. (2004). *Man's search for meaning*. London: Rider.

Gemignani, M. L. (2011). Breast cancer screening: Why, when, and how many? *Clinical Obstetrics and Gynecology, 54*(1), 125–132.

Godress, J., Özgul, S., Owen, C., et al. (2005). Grief experiences of parents whose children suffer from mental illness. *Australian and New Zealand Journal of Psychiatry, 39*, 88–94.

Greenwald, J. L., Denham, C. R., & Jack, B. W. (2007). The hospital discharge: A review of a high risk care transition with highlights of a reengineered discharge process. *Journal of Patient Safety, 3*(2), 97–106.

Jaser, S. S., & White, L. E. (2011). Coping and resilience in adolescents with type 1 diabetes. *Child: Care, Health and Development, 37*(3), 335–342.

The Joint Commission (TJC). (2008). *2008 Hospital accreditation standards* (pp. 216–218, 366–367). Oakbrook Terrace, IL: Author.

The Joint Commission (TJC). (2012a). *2012 Hospital accreditation standards* (pp. 1–84). Oakbrook Terrace, IL: Author.

The Joint Commission (TJC). (2012b). 2012 National patient safety goals. Retrieved November 24, 2012, from http://www.jointcommission.org/standards_information/npsgs.aspx

Kim, J., Kim, S., Kim, H. C., et al. (2012). Effect of consumer-centered u-health service for the knowledge, skill, and attitude of the patients with chronic obstructive pulmonary disease. *Computers, Informatics, Nursing, 30*(12), 661–671.

Kokanovic, R., Petersen, A., & Klimidis, S. (2006). "Nobody can help me . . . I am living through it alone": Experiences of caring for people diagnosed with mental illness in ethno-cultural and linguistic minority communities. *Journal of Immigrant and Minority Health, 8*(2), 125–135.

Lewis, C. S. (1961). *A grief observed*. London: Faber and Faber.

Lifton, R., & Olson, E. (1974). *Living and dying*. New York: Praeger.

Lim, F., Foust, J., & VanCleave, J. (2011). Transitional care. In E. Capezuti, D. Zwicker, T. Fulmer, & M. Boltz (Eds.), *Evidence-based geriatric nursing protocols for best practice* (4th ed., pp. 682–702). New York: Springer.

McFetridge, B., Gillespie, M., Goode, D., & Melby, V. (2007). An exploration of the handover process of critically ill patients between nursing staff from the emergency department and the intensive care unit. *Nursing in Critical Care, 12*(6), 261–269.

Meissner, H. I., Klabunde, C. N., Han, P. K., et al. (2011). Breast cancer screening beliefs, recommendations and practices. *Cancer, 117*(14), 3101–3111.

Michael, Y., Lin, J., Whitlock, E., et al. (2010, December). *Interventions to prevent falls in older adults: An updated systematic review* (Evidence Synthesis No. 80; AHRQ Publication No. 11-05150-EF-1). Rockville, MD: Agency for Healthcare Research and Quality.

Moltmann, J. (1983). *The power of the powerless*. San Francisco: Harper & Row.

Myers, J., Sweeney, T., & Witmer, J. (2000). The wheel of wellness counseling for wellness: A holistic model for treatment planning. *Journal of Counseling & Development, 78*(3), 251–267.

Naylor, M., Brooten, D., Jones, R., et al. (1994). Comprehensive discharge planning for the hospitalized elderly. A randomized clinical trial. *Annals of Internal Medicine, 120*, 999–1006.

Neuman, B. (2002). The Neuman systems model. In B. Neuman, *The Neuman systems model* (4th ed.). Norwalk, CT: Appleton & Lange.

Nightingale, F. (1859/1992). *Notes on nursing: What it is, and what it is not*. Philadelphia: Lippincott.

The Ottawa Charter for Health Promotion. (1986). First International Conference on Health Promotion, Ottawa, 21 November 1986. World Health Organization (WHO). Retrieved November 24, 2012, from http://www.who.int/healthpromotion/conferences/previous/ottawa/en/

Parsons, T. (1975). The sick role and role of the physician reconsidered. *Milbank Memorial Fund Quarterly, 53*, 257–278.

Pearce, L. (2012). Power to the patients. *Nursing Standard, 26*(39), 23.

Peikes, D., Chen, A., Schore, J., & Brown, R. (2009). Effects of care coordination on hospitalization, quality of care, and health care expenditures among Medicare beneficiaries. *JAMA, 301*(6), 603–618.

Phillips, C. O., Wright, W. M., Kern, D. E., et al. (2004). Comprehensive discharge planning with postdischarge support for older patients with congestive heart failure—a meta-analysis. *JAMA, 291*, 1358–1367.

Reeve, C. (1998). *Still me*. New York: Random House.

Riesenberg, L. A., Leisch, J., & Cunningham, J. M. (2010). Nursing handoffs: A systematic review of the literature. *American Journal of Nursing, 110*(4), 24.

Rodin, D., & Stewart, D. E. (2012). Resilience in elderly survivors of child maltreatment. *SAGE Open, 2*(2), 1–9.

Seigel, B. (1986). *Love, medicine and miracles*. New York: Harper & Row.

Sheinfeld-Gorin, S., & Arnold, J. (2006). *Health promotion in practice*. San Francisco: Jossey-Bass.

Smith, P. (1992). *Living the disrupted life: A symphony of survival* (Unpublished doctoral dissertation). University of Kansas, Lawrence.

Stuck, A. E., Walthert, J. M., Nikolaus, T., et al. (1999). Risk factors for functional status decline in community living elderly people: A systematic literature review. *Social Science and Medicine, 48*(4), 445–469.

Suchman, E. A. (1972). Stages of illness and medical care. In E. G. Jaco (Ed.), *Patients, physicians, and illness* (2nd ed.). New York: Free Press.

Thompson, J., & Manore, M. (2012). *Nutrition: An applied approach* (3rd ed.). San Francisco: Benjamin/Cummings.

Townsend, M. (2012). *Psychiatric mental health nursing: Concepts of care in evidence-based practice* (7th ed.). Philadelphia: F. A. Davis.

U.S. Department of Health and Human Services (USDHHS). (2007). HHS initiative to assist hospitals in effective communication. *HHS Press Office*. Washington, DC.

U.S. Preventive Services Task Force (USPSTF). (2012). 2012 USPSTF recommendations on screening for cervical cancer. *PRACTICE, 61*(05), 278–282.

Valladares, A. (2001). *Against all hope: A memoir of life in Castro's gulag*. San Francisco: Encounter Books.

Vanauken, S. (1977). *A severe mercy*. New York: Bantam Books.

Watson, J. (1979). *Nursing: The philosophy and science of caring*. Boston: Little, Brown.

Wiktorsson, S., Runeson, B., Skoog, I., et al. (2010). Attempted suicide in the elderly: Characteristics of suicide attempters 70 years and older and a general population comparison group. *American Journal of Geriatric Psych, 18*(1), 57.

Wilber, T. (2000). *Grace and grit: Spirituality and healing in the life and death of Treya Killam Wilber* (Rev. ed.). Boston: Shambhala.

World Health Organization (WHO). (1948). Preamble to the constitution of the World Health Organization as adopted by the International Health Conference, New York, June 19–22, 1946 and entered into force on April 7, 1948.

CHAPTER 12

Alford, L. (2007). Findings of interest from immunology and psychoneuroimmunology. *Manual Therapy, 12*(2), 176–180. DOI: 10.1016/j.math.2006.06.007

Badger, J. (2008). Critical care nurse intern program: Addressing psychological reactions related to critical care nursing. *Critical Care Nursing Quarterly, 31*(2), 184–187. doi: 10.1097/01.CNQ.0000314479.87248.63

Barrett, B., Muller, H. M, Ward, A, et al. (2012). Meditation or exercise for preventing acute respiratory infection: A randomized controlled trial. *Annals of Family Medicine, 10*(4), 337–463. doi: 10.1370/afm.1376

Bennett, M., & Lengacher, C. (2007). Humor and laughter may influence health: IV. Humor and immune function. *Evidence-Based Complementary and Alternative Medicine, 6*(2), 159–164. http://dx.doi.org/10.1093/ecam/nem149

Bisson, J., Roberts, N. P., Andrew, M., et al. (2013, updated). Psychological treatment of post-traumatic stress disorder PTSD) in adults. *Cochrane Database of Systematic Reviews*, Issue 3. Art. No.: CD003388. doi: 10.1002/14651858.CD003388.pub4.

Blazer, D. G., Wu, L. T. (2011). The epidemiology of alcohol use disorders and subthreshold dependence in a middle-aged and elderly community sample. *American Journal of Geriatriatric Psychiatry, 19*, 685–694. doi: 10.1097/JGP.0b013e3182006a96

Bost, N., & Wallis, M. (2006). The effectiveness of a 15 minute weekly massage in reducing physical and psychological stress in nurses. *Australian Journal of Advanced Nursing, 23*(4), 28–33.

Brammer, L. M., & MacDonald, G. (2003). *The helping relationship: Process and skills* (8th ed.). Old Tappan, NJ: Pearson.

Bulechek, F., Butcher, H., & Dochterman, J. (2012). *Nursing interventions classification (NIC)*. (6th ed.). St. Louis, MO: C. V. Mosby.

Choi, H., & Riper, M. (2013). Siblings of children with Down syndrome: An integrative review. *MCN, The American Journal of Maternal/Child Nursing, 38*(2), 72–78. DOI: 10.1097/NMC.0b013e31826bad8e

Cousins, N. (1979). *Anatomy of an illness*. New York: Bantam Books.

Davidson, R., Kabat-Zinn, J., Schumacher, J., et al. (2003). Alterations in brain and immune function produced by mindfulness meditation. *Psychosomatic Medicine, 65*, 564–570.

du Pré, A. (1998). *Humor and the healing arts*. Mahwah, NJ: Lawrence Erlbaum.

Fagundes, C. P., Glaser, R., Johnson, S. L., et al. (2012, June). Basal cell carcinoma: Stressful life events and the tumor environment. *Archives of General Psychiatry, 69*(6), 618–626. doi:10.1001/archgenpsychiatry.2011.1535.

Gaylord, S. A., Paisson, O. S., Garland, El. L., et al. (2011). Mindfulness training reduces the severity of irritable bowel syndrome in women: Results of a randomized controlled trial. *The American Journal of Gastroenterology, 106*(9), 1678–88. doi: 10.1038/ajg.2011.184

Hall, L., Doran, D., & Pink, L. (2008). Outcomes of interventions to improve hospital nursing work environments. *The Journal of Nursing Administration, 38*(1), 40–46. doi: 10.1097/01.NNA.0000295631.72721.17

Hamer, M., Kivimaki, M., Stamatakis, G., et al. (2012, June 18). Psychological distress as a risk factor for death from cerebrovascular disease. *Canadian Medical Association Journal*. doi:10.1503/cmaj.111719.

Hegge, M., & Larson, V. (2008). Stressors and coping strategies of students in accelerated baccalaureate nursing programs. *Nurse Educator, 33*(1), 26–30. doi: 10.1097/01.NNE.0000299492.92624.95

Holmes, T., & Rahe, R. (1967). The social readjustment and rating scale. *Journal of Psychosomatic Research, 11*, 213–218.

Johnson, M., Moorhead, S., Bulechek, G., et al. (2012). *NOC, and NIC linkages to NANDA-I and clinical conditions* (3rd ed., p. 196). St. Louis, MO: C. V. Mosby.

Johnson, P. (2002). The use of humor and its influences on spirituality and coping in breast cancer survivors. *Oncology Nursing Forum, 29*(4), 691–695. DOI: 10.1200/JCO.2005.09.064

Kiecolt-Glaser, J. K., Christian, L., Preston, H., et al. (2010). Stress, inflammation, and yoga practice. *Psychosomatic Medicine, 72*(2), 113–121. doi: 10.1097/PSY.0b013e3181cb9377

Maddi, S. R., Koshaba, D. M., Fazel, M., et al. (2009, July 1). The personality construct of hardiness, IV. *Journal of Humanistic Psychology, 49*(3), 292–305. doi: 10.1177/0022167809331860

Maddi, S. (2002). The story of hardiness: Twenty years of theorizing, research and practice. *Consulting Psychology Journal, 54*, 173–185. http://dx.doi.org/10.1037/1061-4087.54.3.173

Maville, J., Bowen, J., & Genham, G. (2008). Effect of healing touch on stress perception and biological correlates. *Holistic Nursing Practice, 22*(2), 103–110. doi: 10.1097/01.HNP.0000312659.21513.f9

McCain, N. L., Gray, D. P., Elswick, R. K., Jr., et al. (2008). A randomized clinical trial of alternative stress management interventions in persons with HIV infection. *Journal of Consulting and Clinical Psychology, 76*(3), 431–441. doi: 10.1037/0022-006X.76.3.431

Moorhead, S., Johnson, M., & Maas, M., et al. (Eds.). (2012). *Nursing outcomes classification (NOC)* (5th ed.). St. Louis, MO: C. V. Mosby.

NANDA International. (2012). *Nursing diagnoses: Definitions & classification 2012–2014*. Ames, IA: Wiley-Blackwell.

Neeb, K. (2014). *Fundamentals of mental health nursing* (4th ed.). Philadelphia: F. A. Davis.

Ohio State University. (2013, August 22). The stress and cancer link: "Master-switch" stress gene enables cancer's spread. *ScienceDaily*. Retrieved October 26, 2014, from www.sciencedaily.com/releases/2013/08/130822194143.htm

Olson, R. (2003). Definitions of biofeedback. In M. S. Schwartz & F. Andrasik (Eds.), *Biofeedback: A practitioner's guide* (3rd ed.). New York: Guilford Press.

Pemberton, E., & Turpin, P. (2008). The effect of essential oils on work-related stress in intensive care unit nurses. *Holistic Nursing Practice, 22*(2), 97–102. doi: 10.1097/01.HNP.0000312658.13890.28

Quick, J., Saleh, K., Sime, W., et al. (2006). Symposium: Stress management skills for strong leadership: Is it worth dying for? *The Journal of Bone & Joint Surgery, 88–A*(1), 217–225. doi: 10.1007/s11999-008-0622-8

Richardson, S., Shaffer, J. A., Falzon, L., et al. (2012, September 12). Meta-analysis of perceived stress and its association with incident coronary heart disease. *American Journal of Cardiology*. doi: 10.1016/j.amjcard.2012.08.004

Riper, M. (2013). Siblings of children with Down syndrome: An integrative review. MCN, The *American Journal of Maternal/Child Nursing, 38*(2), 72–78. doi: 10.1097/NMC.0b013e31826bad8e

Scanlon, V., & Sanders, T. (2011). *Essentials of anatomy and physiology* (6th ed., pp. 239, 241). Philadelphia: F. A. Davis.

Selye, H. (1974). *Stress without distress*. Philadelphia: J. B. Lippincott.

Selye, H. (1976). *The stress of life* (Rev. ed.). New York: McGraw-Hill.

Slopen, N., Glynn, R. J., Lewis, T. T., et al. (2012, July 18). Job strain, job insecurity, and incident cardiovascular disease in the women's health study: Results from a 10-year prospective study. of America. *PLoS One, 7*(7), e40512. doi: 10.1371/journal.pone.0040512

So, P. S., Jiang, J. Y., & Qin, Y. (2008; online 2012, August 15). Touch therapies for pain relief in adults. *Cochrane Database of Systematic Reviews*, Issue 4. Art. No.: CD006535. doi:10.1002/14651858.CD006535.pub2.

Stuart, G.W. (2012). *Principles and practices of psychiatric nursing* (10th ed.). St. Louis, MO: Elsevier.

Sullivan, M., Hawes, K., Winchester, S., et al. (2008). Developmental origins theory from prematurity to adult disease. *JOGNN Journal of Obstetric, Gynecologic, & Neonatal Nursing, 37*(2), 158–164. DOI: JOGN216

Townsend, M. C. (2013). *Psychiatric mental health nursing* (8th ed.). Philadelphia: F. A. Davis.

U.S. Department of Health and Human Services (USDHHS). (2008). *2008 Physical activity guidelines for Americans*. Washington, DC: Author. Retrieved January 4, 2014, from http://www.health.gov/paguidelines/pdf/paguide.pdf

U.S. Department of Health and Human Services (USDHHS). (2010). Healthy People 2020 *framework: The vision, mission, and goals of* Healthy People 2020. Washington, DC: Author.

Wang, Y. P., & Andrade, L. H. (2013). Epidemiology of alcohol and drug use in the elderly. *Current Opinion in Psychiatry, 26*(4), 343–348.

CHAPTER 13

Agency for Healthcare Research and Quality. (2003, reaffirmed 2012, July). *Delirium: Proportion of patients meeting diagnostic criteria on the Confusion Assessment Method (CAM)*. Rockville, MD: Agency for Healthcare Research and Quality. Retrieved January 10, 2013, from http://www.qualitymeasures.ahrq.gov/content.aspx?id=27635

All about depression. (last updated 2010, June). Retrieved January 18, 2013, from http://www.allaboutdepression.com/gen_01.html#3

American Psychiatric Association (APA). (2013). *Diagnostic and statistical manual of mental disorders* (5th ed.). Arlington, VA: Author. Also available at http://psychiatryonline.org/

Arthurs, E., Steele, R. J., Hudson, M., et al. (2012). Are scores on English and French versions of the PHQ-9 comparable? An assessment of differential item functioning. *PloS one, 7*(12), e52028.

Baumann, L. C., & Dang, T. T. N. (2012). Helping patients with chronic conditions overcome barriers to self-care. *The Nurse Practitioner, 37*(3), 32.

Blanchflower, D. G., & Oswald, A. J. (2012). *Antidepressants and age in 27 European countries: Evidence of a U-shape in human well-being through life*. Unpublished manuscript, Dartmouth College, Hanover, NH.

Bourne, E. J. (2011). *The anxiety and phobia workbook* (5th ed.). Oakland, CA: New Harbinger.

Bracken, B. A. (Ed.). (1996). *Handbook of self-concept*. New York: John Wiley & Sons.

Bracken, B. A., & Panter, J. E. (2011). Using the Bracken Basic Concept Scale and Bracken Concept Development Program in the assessment and remediation of young children's concept development. *Psychology in the Schools, 48*(5), 464–475.

Breggin, P. (2009). *Medication madness: The role of psychiatric drugs in cases of violence, suicide, and crime*. New York: St. Martin's Press.

Brixval, C. S., Rayce, S. L., Rasmussen, M., Holstein, B. E., & Due, P. (2012). Overweight, body image and bullying—an epidemiological study of 11-to 15-years olds. *The European Journal of Public Health, 22*(1), 126–130.

Bulechek, G. M., Butcher, H. K., & Dochterman, J. M. (Eds.). (2012). *Nursing interventions classification (NIC)* (6th ed.). St. Louis, MO: C. V. Mosby.

Cargill, B. R., Clark, M. M., Pera, V., et al. (2012). Binge eating, body image, depression, and self-efficacy in an obese clinical population. *Obesity Research, 7*(4), 379–386.

Centers for Disease Control and Prevention (CDC). (2002). Hepatic toxicity possibly associated with kava-containing products—United States, Germany, and Switzerland, 1999–2002, *Morbidity and Mortality Weekly Report, 51*(47), 1065–1067. Retrieved January 18, 2013, from http://www.cdc.gov/mmwr/PDF/wk/mm5147.pdf

Centers for Disease Control and Prevention (CDC). (2012). Suicide. Facts at a glance. Retrieved January 10, 2013, from http://www.cdc.gov/violenceprevention/pdf/Suicide-DataSheet-a.pdf

Chen, T. M., Huang, F. Y., Chang, C., et al. (2006). Using the PHQ-9 for depression screening and treatment monitoring for Chinese Americans in primary care. *Psychiatric Services, 57*, 976–981.

Cheung, Y. B., Law, C. K., Chan, B., et al. (2006). Suicidal ideation and suicidal attempts in a population-based study of Chinese people: Risk attributable to hopelessness, depression, and social factors. *Journal of Affective Disorders, 90*(2–3), 193–199.

Compare, A., Germani, E., Proietti, R., & Janeway, D. (2011). Clinical psychology and cardiovascular disease: an up-to-date clinical practice review for assessment and treatment of anxiety and depression. *Clinical Practice and Epidemiology in Mental Health: CP & EMH, 7*, 148.

Crozier, F., & Hancock, L. E. (2012). Pediatric palliative care: Beyond the end of life. *Pediatric Nursing, 38*(4), 199.

Dickstein, E. (1977). Self and self-esteem: Theoretical foundations and their implications for research. *Human Development, 20*, 129–140.

Edwards, N. (2003). Differentiating the three D's: Delirium, dementia, and depression. *MEDSURG Nursing, 12*(6), 347.

Erikson, E. (1963). *Childhood and society* (2nd ed.). New York: W. W. Norton.

Fong, T. G., Tulebaev, S. R., & Inouye, S. K. (2009). Delirium in elderly adults: Diagnosis, prevention and treatment. *Nature Reviews Neurology, 5*(4), 210–220.

Goldston, D. B., Reboussin, B. A., & Daniel, S. S. (2006). Predictors of suicide attempts: State and trait components. *Journal of Abnormal Psychology, 115*(4), 842–849.

Gorman, L. M., & Sultan, D. E. (2008). *Psychosocial nursing for general patient care* (3rd ed.). Philadelphia: F. A. Davis.

Hamrin, V., Antenucci, M., & Magorno, M. (2012). Evaluation and management of pediatric and adolescent depression. *The Nurse Practitioner, 37*(3), 22.

Happ, M., Garrett, K., Thomas, D., et al. (2011). Nurse-patient communication interactions in the intensive care unit. *American Journal Of Critical Care, 20*(2), 28–40.

Hart, L. K., Freel, M. I., Haylock, P. J., et al. (2011). The Use of Healing Touch in Integrative Oncology. *Clinical Journal of Oncology Nursing, 15*(5), 519–525.

Hessel, J. A. (2009). Presence in nursing practice: A concept analysis. *Holistic Nursing Practice, 23*(5), 276.

Hulisz, D. T. (2008). Top herbal products: Efficacy and safety concerns. Retrieved January, 18, 2013, from http://www.medscape.org/viewprogram/8494

Jamison, K. R. (1997). *An unquiet mind: A memoir of moods and madness*. London: Picador.

Johnson, M., Bulechek, G., Dochterman, J., et al. (2012). *NOC, and NIC linkages to NANDA-I and clinical conditions: Supporting critical reasoning and quality care* (3rd ed.). St. Louis, MO: C. V. Mosby.

Judson, P., Dickson, E., Argenta, P., et al. (2011). A prospective, randomized trial of integrative medicine for women with ovarian cancer. *Gynecologic Oncology, 123*(2), 346–350.

Kozlowska, L., & Doboszynska, A. (2012). Nurses' nonverbal methods of communicating with patients in the terminal phase. *International Journal Of Palliative Nursing, 18*(1), 40–46.

Kroenke, K., Spitzer, R. L., & Williams, J. B. W. (2001). The PHQ-9. Validity of a brief depression severity measure. *Journal of General Internal Medicine, 16*(9), 606–613.

Kurlowicz, L. H. (2008). Depression. In E. Capezuti, D. Zwicker, M. Mezey, & T. Fulmer (Eds.), *Evidence-based geriatric nursing protocols for best practice* (3rd ed., pp. 57–82). New York: Springer.

Larson, B. K., Clark, T. C., Robinson, E. M., & Utter, J. (2012). Body satisfaction and sexual health behaviors among New Zealand secondary school students. *Sex Education, 12*(2), 187–198.

Leng, L. B. (2011). Overview of major depressive disorder. *The Singapore Family Physician, 37*(4), 18–21.

Lerner, N. B. (2012). The many faces of dementia. *Nursing Made Incredibly Easy, 10*(2), 26.

Lin, P. C., Lin, M. L., Huang, L. C., et al. (2011). Music therapy for patients receiving spine surgery. *Journal of Clinical Nursing, 20*(7–8), 960–968.

Maslow, A. (1968). *Toward a psychology of being* (2nd ed.). New York: Van Nostrand-Reinhold.

Maybury, B. C. (2008, March 10). Suicide prevention: Every nurse's responsibility. Retrieved January 18, 2013, from http://news.nurse.com/article/20080310/NY02/80305017

McCabe, M., & Ricciardelli, L. (2012). Parent, peer and media influences on body image and strategies to both increase and decrease body size among adolescent boys and girls. *Adolescence, 36*(142), 225–240.

Moorhead, S., Johnson, M., Maas, M. L., et al. (Eds.). (2013). *Nursing outcomes classification (NOC)* (5th ed.). St. Louis, MO: C. V. Mosby.

Morbidity and Mortality Weekly Report (MMWR). (2011). QuickStats: Age-adjusted death rates for the 10 leading causes of death—National Vital Statistics System, United States, 2008 and 2009. Atlanta, GA: Centers for Disease Control and Prevention. Retrieved January 18, 2012, from http://www.cdc.gov/mmwr/preview/mmwrhtml/mm6048a7.htm

Muehlenkamp, J. J., & Brausch, A. M. (2012). Body image as a mediator of non-suicidal self-injury in adolescents. *Journal of Adolescence, 35*(1), 1–9.

NANDA International. (2012). *Nursing diagnoses: Definitions and classification 2012–2014.* Philadelphia: Author.

National Guideline Clearinghouse (NGC). (2010; updated 2012, March). Major depression in adults in primary care. Retrieved January 18, 2013, from http://www.guideline.gov/content.aspx?id=37277

National Institute of Mental Health (NIMH). (n.d.; revised 2007, April). *Older adults: Depression and suicide fact sheet* (NIH Publication No. 4593). Retrieved January, 18, 2013, from http://www.nimh.nih.gov/health/publications/older-adults-depression-and-suicide-facts-fact-sheet/index.shtml

National Institute of Mental Health (NIMH). (n.d.). Suicide in the U.S.: Statistics and prevention [Page last reviewed September 27, 2010]. Retrieved January 10, 2013, from http://www.nimh.nih.gov/health/publications/suicide-in-the-us-statistics-and-prevention/index.shtml

Neeb, K. (2005). *Fundamentals of mental health nursing* (3rd ed., pp. 365–378). Philadelphia: F. A. Davis.

Nekanda_Trepka, C. J. S., Bishop, S., & Blackburn, I. M. (2011). Hopelessness and depression. *British Journal of Clinical Psychology, 22*(1), 49–60.

Peplau, H. (1963). A working definition of anxiety. In S. Burd & M. Marshall (Eds.), *Some clinical approaches to psychiatric nursing*. New York: Macmillan.

Piderman, K., Lapid, M., Stevens, S., et al. (2011). Spiritual well-being and spiritual practices in elderly depressed psychiatric inpatients. *The Journal of Pastoral Care & Counseling, JPCC, 65*(1–2), 3–31.

Plassman, B., Langa, K., Fisher, G., et al. (2007). Prevalence of dementia in the United States: The aging, demographics, and memory study. *Neuro-epidemiology, 29*, 125–132. Retrieved February 1, 2013, from http://content.karger.com/ProduktеDB/produkte.asp?doi=109998

Rund, D. A., & Hutzler, J. D. (1983). *Emergency psychiatry* (p. 144). St. Louis, MO: Mosby.

Schiller J. S., Lucas J. W., Ward B. W., et al. (2012, January). Summary health statistics for U.S. Adults: National health interview survey, 2010. *Vital and Health Statistics, Series 10*(252). Centers for Disease Control. Retrieved January 5, 2013, from http://www.cdc.gov/nchs/data/series/sr_10/sr10_252.pdf

Steptoe, A. (Ed.). (2007). *Depression and physical illness*. New York: Cambridge University Press.

Stuart, G. W. (2012). *Principles and practice of psychiatric nursing* (10th ed.). St. Louis, MO: C. V. Mosby.

Suls, J., & Howren, M. B. (2012). Understanding the physical-symptom experience: The distinctive contributions of anxiety and depression. *Current Directions in Psychological Science, 21*(2), 129–134.

Touhy, T., & Jett, K. (2009). *Ebersole and Hess' gerontological nursing & healthy aging* (3rd ed.). Philadelphia: F. A. Davis.

Townsend, M. C. (2010). *Essentials of psychiatric mental health nursing* (5th ed.). Philadelphia: F. A. Davis.

U.S. Preventive Services Task Force (USPSTF). (2009). Screening for depression in adults. Retrieved January 18, 2014, from http://www.uspreventiveservicestaskforce.org/uspstf/uspsaddepr.htm

Valente, S. (2010). Assessing patients for suicide risk. *Nursing2010, 40*(5), 36–40.

Walters-Brown, B., & Hall, J. M. (2012). Women's body image: Implications for mental health nursing interventions. *Issues in Mental Health Nursing, 33*(8), 553–559.

Wittstein, I. S. (2010). Depression, anxiety, and platelet reactivity in patients with coronary heart disease. *European Heart Journal, 31*(13), 1548–1550.

Woertman, L., & van den Brink, F. (2012). Body image and female sexual functioning and behavior: A review. *Journal of Sex Research, 49*(2–3), 184–211.

Yanez, B., Stanton, A. L., & Maly, R. C. (2012). Breast cancer treatment decision making among Latinas and non-Latina whites: A communication model predicting decisional outcomes and quality of life. *Health Psychology, 31*(5), 552–561.

CHAPTER 14

Backhouse, J., & Graham, A. (2012). Grandparents raising grandchildren: negogiating the complexities of role-identity conflict. *Child & Family Social Work, 17*(3), 306–315.

Bulechek, F., Butcher, H., & Dochterman, J. (2013). *Nursing interventions classification (NIC)*. (6th ed.). St. Louis, MO: C. V. Mosby.

Centers for Disease Control and Prevention (CDC). (2007, updated 2012, November 21).Vaccines & Immunizations. What would happen if we stopped vaccinations? Retrieved January 27, 2013, from http://www.cdc.gov/vaccines/vac-gen/whatifstop.htm

Centers for Disease Control and Prevention (CDC). (2010, updated 2012, November 21). Teen pregnancy prevention, 2010–2015. Retrieved January 26, 2013, from http://www.cdc.gov/teenpregnancy/PreventTeenPreg.htm

Centers for Disease Control and Prevention (CDC). (2012). Seasonal influenza (flu): 2012–2013 flu season. Retrieved January 25, 2013, from http://www.cdc.gov/flu/about/season/index.htm

Centers for Disease Control and Prevention (CDC). (2013). HIV among African Americans. Retrieved February 10, 2013, from http://www.cdc.gov/hiv/topics/aa/PDF/HIV_among_African_Americans_final.pdf

Children's Bureau. (2012). *Child maltreatment 2011*. Washington, DC: U.S. Department of Health & Human Services. Retrieved January 27, 2013, from http://www.acf.hhs.gov/programs/cb/research-data-technology/statistics-research/child-maltreatment

Conway, F. (2011). Emotional strain in caregiving among African American grandmothers raising their grandchildren. *Journal of Women & Aging, 23*(2), 113–128.

DeNavas-Wall, C., Proctor, B., & Smith, J. (2012). Income, poverty, and health insurance coverage in the United States: 2011. *U.S. Census Bureau, current population reports*. Washington, DC: U.S. Government Printing Office.

Dosser, I., & Kennedy, C. (2012). Family carers' experiences of support at the end of life: carers' and health professionals' views. *International Journal of Palliative Nursing, 18*(10), 491–497.

Friedman, M. M., Bowden, V. R., & Jones, E. G. (2003). *Family nursing: Research, theory, and practice* (5th ed.). Upper Saddle River, NJ: Prentice Hall.

Groh, D., Jason, L., Davis, M., et al. (2007). Friends, family, and alcohol abuse: An examination of general and alcohol-specific social support. *American Journal on Addictions, 16*(1), 49–55. doi:10.1080/10550490601080084

Hanson, S., Gedaly-Duff, V., & Kaakinen, J. R. (Eds.) (2005). *Family health care nursing: Theory, practice & research* (3rd ed.). Philadelphia: F. A. Davis.

Hill, R., & Hansen, D. (1960). The identification of conceptual frameworks utilized in family study. *Marriage and Family Living, 22*(4), 299–311.

Homer, S., Rew, L., & Brown, A. (2012). Risk-taking behaviors engaged in by early adolescents while on school property. *Issues in Comprehensive Pediatric Nursing, 35*(2), 90–110.

Huges, M. E., Waite, L. J., LaPierre, T. A., et al. (2007). All in the family: The impact of caring for grandchildren on grandparents' health. *The Journals of Gerontology Series B: Psychological Sciences and Social Sciences, 62*, S108–S119.

Johnson, M., Bulechek, G., Butcher, H., et al. (2012). *NANDA, NOC, and NIC linkages* (3rd ed.). St. Louis, MO: C. V. Mosby.

Kreider, R., & Ellis, R. (2011). *Living arrangements of children: 2009*. U.S. Census Bureau. Retrieved January 23, 2013 from http://www.census.gov/prod/2011pubs/p70-126.pdf

Land, H., & Guada, J. (2011). The Latina Caregiver Burden Scale: Assessing the factor structure for rapid clinical assessment. *Social Work Research, 35*(2), 95–106.

Leder, S., Grinstead, L. N., & Torres, E. (2007). Grandparents raising grandchildren: Stressors, social support, and health outcomes, *Journal of Family Nursing, 13*(3), 333–352.

Levine, C. (2011). The hospital nurse's assessment of family caregiver needs, Part 1. *American Journal of Nursing, 111*(10), 47–51.

Lofquist, D., Lugaila, T., O'Connell, M., et al. (2012). Households and families: 2010. *Census Briefs.* Retrieved January 23, 2013, from http://www.census.gov/prod/cen2010/briefs/c2010br-14.pdf

Luthy, K., Beckstrand, R., Callister, L., et al. (2012). Reasons parents exempt children from receiving immunizations. *Journal of School Nursing, 28*(2), 153–160.

McGoldrick, M., & Carter, E. (1985). The family life cycle: Its stages and dislocations. In J. Henslin (Ed.), *Marriage and family in a changing society* (4th ed., pp. 372–389). New York: Free Press.

Moorhead, S., Johnson, M., & Maas, M., et al. (Eds.). (2013). *Nursing outcomes classification (NOC)* (5th ed.). St. Louis, MO: C. V. Mosby.

Nguyen, M. (2009). Nurse's assessment of caregiver burden. *MEDSURG Nursing, 18*(3), 147–152.

Parker, K. (2012). The boomerang generation: feeling OK about living with mom and dad. *Pew Research Social & Demographic Trends*, Retrieved January 30, 2013, from http://www.pewsocialtrends.org/files/2012/03/PewSocialTrends-2012-BoomerangGeneration.pdf

Parker, K., & Patten, E. (2013). The sandwich generation: rising financial burdens for middle-aged americans. *Pew Research Social & Demographic Trends.* Retrieved January 31, 2013, from http://www.pewsocialtrends.org/2013/01/30/the-sandwich-generation/

Parsons, T., & Bales, R. F. (1955). *Family socialization and interaction process.* New York: Free Press.

Pazol, K., Warner, L., Gavin, L., et al. (2011). Vital signs: teen pregnancy—United States, 1991–2009. *Morbidity and Mortality Weekly Report, 60*(13), 414–420. Retrieved January 26, 2013, from http://www.cdc.gov/mmwr/preview/mmwrhtml/mm6013a5.htm?s_cid=mm6013a5_w

Petrovich, A. (2008). Lessons learned in the sandwich. *Journal of Women & Social Work, 23*(3), 223–230.

Pew Research Social & Demographic Trends. (2010). The return of the multi-generation family household. Retrieved January 30, 2013, from http://www.pewsocialtrends.org/files/2010/10/752-multi-generational-families.pdf

Pew Research Social & Demographic Trends. (2011). *A portrait of stepfamilies.* Washington, DC: Author. Retrieved January 31, 2013 from http://www.pewsocialtrends.org/2011/01/13/a-portrait-of-stepfamilies/

Pierce, C. (2012). Profiling the caregiver. *Gerontology Special Interest Section Quarterly, 35*(4), 1–4.

Prejean, J., Song, R., Hernandez, A., et al. (2011). Estimated HIV Incidence in the United States, 2006–2009. *PLoS ONE 6*(8), 1–13. Retrieved January 27, 2013, from http://www.plosone.org/article/info%3Adoi%2F10.1371%2Fjournal.pone.0017502

Rehabilitation Research and Training. (2012). *Annual Disability Statistical Compendium: 2012.* Retrieved January 25, 2013, from: http://www.researchondisability.org/docs/default-document-library/compendium_2012_rotatedpages.pdf?sfvrsn=4

Schumacher, L., MacNeil, R., Mobily, K., et al. (2012). The leisure journey for sandwich generation caretakers. *Therapeutic Recreational Journal, 46*(1), 42–59.

U.S. Census Bureau. (2012). Populations: Households, families, group quarters. *The 2012 Statistical Abstract.* Retrieved January 23, 2013, from http://www.census.gov/compendia/statab/cats/population/households_families_group_quarters.html

U.S. Equal Opportunity Commission. (2008). *ADA Amendments Act of 2008.* Retrieved January 25, 2013, from: http://www.eeoc.gov/laws/statutes/adaaa.cfm

van Eden-Moorefield, B., Palkey, K., Crosbe-Burnett, M., et al. (2012). Explaining couple cohesion in different types of gay families. *Journal of Family Issues, 33*(2), 182–201.

CHAPTER 15

Agency for Healthcare Research and Quality. (2012, March). *National healthcare disparities report I* (AHRQ Publication No. 12-0006) *2011.* Rockville, MD: U.S. Department of Health and Human Services, Agency for Healthcare Research and Quality. Retrieved February 23, 2013, from http://www.ahrq.gov/research/findings/nhqrdr/nhqrdr11/qrdr11.html

American Nurses Association (ANA). (1991). *Position statements: Cultural diversity in nursing practice.* Retrieved March 3, 2013, from http://www.nursingworld.org/MainMenuCategories/Policy-Advocacy/Positions-and-Resolutions/ANAPositionStatements/Position-Statements-Alphabetically/prtetcldv14444.html

American Nurses Association (ANA). (2010). *Nursing: Scope and standards of practice* (2nd ed.). Silver Spring, MD: Author.

Andrews, M. M., & Boyle, J. S. (2007). *Transcultural concepts in nursing care* (5th ed.). Philadelphia: Lippincott Williams & Wilkins

Andrews, M. M., & Boyle, J. S. (2011). *Transcultural concepts in nursing care* (6th ed.). Philadelphia: Lippincott Williams & Wilkins.

Baker, D. (2011). Conceptual parameters of acculturation within the Asian and Pacific Islander American populations: Applications for nursing practice and research. *Nursing Forum, 46*(2), 83–93.

Bates, M. S. (1996). *Biocultural dimensions of chronic pain.* Albany, NY: SUNY Press.

Buchan, S., Shakeel, M., Trinidade, A., et al. (2012). The use of complementary and alternative medicine by nurses. *British Journal of Nursing, 21*(11), 672–675.

Bulechek, G. M., Butcher, H. K., & Dochterman, J. M. (Eds.). (2013). *Nursing interventions classification (NIC)* (6th ed.). St. Louis, MO: C. V. Mosby.

Carballeira, N. (1997). The LIVE and LEARN model for cultural competent family services. *Continuum,* 7–12.

Carrion, I., Castañeda, H., Martinez-Tyson, D., et al. (2011). Barriers impeding access to primary oral health care among farmworker families in central Florida. *Social Work in Health Care, 50*(10), 828–844.

Centers for Disease Control and Prevention (CDC). (2011a; updated 2013). *Healthy People 2010* final review. Retrieved February 17, 2013, from http://www.cdc.gov/nchs/healthy_people/hp2010/hp2010_final_review.htm

Centers for Disease Control and Prevention (CDC). (2011b). *2011 national diabetes fact sheet.* Retrieved February 18, 2013, from http://www.cdc.gov/diabetes/pubs/estimates11.htm#6

Clingerman, E. (2011). Social justice: A framework for culturally competent care. *Journal of Transcultural Nursing, 22*(4), 334–341.

Davidhizar, R., & Giger, J. (1998). *Canadian transcultural nursing: Assessment and intervention.* St. Louis, MO: Mosby.

Deardorff, D. K. (2006). The identification and assessment of intercultural competence as a student outcome of internationalization at institutions of higher education in the United States. *Journal of Studies in International Education, 10* (3), 241–266.

Deardorff, D. K. (Ed). (2009). The SAGE handbook of intercultural competence. Thousand Oaks, CA: Sage - See more at: http://www.guninetwork.org/resources/he-articles/process-model-of-intercultural-competence#sthash.KiDy0yid.dpuf

Deliema, M., Gassoumis, Z., Homeier, D., et al. (2012). Determining prevalence and correlates of elder abuse using promotores: Low-income immigrant Latinos report high rates of abuse and neglect. *Journal of the American Geriatrics Society, 60*(7), 1333–1339.

Diamond, L., Wilson-Stronks, A., & Jacobs, E. (2010). Do hospitals measure up to the national culturally and linguistically appropriate services standards? *Medical Care, 48*(12), 1080–1087.

Galanti, G. (2008). *Caring for patients from different cultures* (4th ed.). Philadelphia: University of Pennsylvania Press.

Geissler, E. M. (1991). Transcultural nursing and nursing diagnosis. *Nursing and Health Care, 12*(4), 190–203.

Giger, J. (2012). *Transcultural nursing: Assessment and intervention* (6th ed.). St. Louis, MO: C. V. Mosby.

Giger, J. N., & Davidhizar, R. (2008). *Transcultural nursing: Assessment and intervention* (5th ed.). St. Louis, MO: C. V. Mosby.

Gupta, A. (2010). Racial differences in response to antihypertensive therapy: Does one size fits all? *International Journal of Preventive Medicine, 1*(4), 217–219.

Healthy People 2020. (n.d.a). Retrieved February 8, 2013, from http://www.healthypeople.gov/2020/TopicsObjectives2020/pdfs/HP2020_brochure_with_LHI_508.pdf

Healthy People 2020. (n.d.b). Disparities. Retrieved March 3, 2013, from http://healthypeople.gov/2020/about/DisparitiesAbout.aspx

Hicks, D. (2012). Cultural competence and the Hispanic population. *Medsurg Nursing, 2*(5), 314–315.

Hilmers, A., Hilmers, D., & Dave, J. (2012). Neighborhood disparities in access to healthy foods and their effects on environmental justice. *American Journal of Public Health, 102*(9), 1644–1654.

Jackson, A. K. (2007). Cultural competence in health visiting practice: A baseline survey. *Community Practitioner, 80*(2), 17–22.

Kersey-Matusiak, G. (2012). Culturally competent care: Are we there yet? *Nursing Management, 43*(4), 35–39.

Kroeber, A., & Kluckhohn, C. (1952). *Culture: A critical review of concepts and definitions*. New York: Random House.

Leininger, M. (1978). *Transcultural nursing: Concepts, theories, and practices*. New York: John Wiley & Sons.

Leininger, M. (Ed.). (1991). *Culture care diversity and universality: A theory of nursing*. New York: National League for Nursing Press.

Leininger, M. (1995). *Transcultural nursing: Concepts, theories, research and practice*. New York: McGraw-Hill.

Leininger, M. (2007). Theoretical questions and concerns: Response from the Theory of Culture Care Diversity and Universality perspective. *Nursing Science Quarterly, 20*(1), 9–13.

Leininger, M. M., & McFarland, M. R. (2002). *Transcultural nursing: Concepts, theories, research and practices* (3rd ed.). New York: McGraw-Hill.

Leininger, M. M., & McFarland, M. R. (2006). *Culture care diversity & universality: A worldwide nursing theory* (2nd ed.). Sudbury, MA: Jones & Bartlett.

Leppa, C. (2005). Transcultural communication within the health care subculture. In C. Munoz & J. Luckmann (Eds.), *Transcultural communication in health care* (2nd ed., pp. 93–105). Clifton Park, NY: Thomson Delmar Learning.

Lester, A., Henderson, G., & Taylor, J. (2012). Oral health disparities, barriers exist for America's elders. *Aging Today, 33*(3), 13–14.

Lipson, J., & Meleis, A. (1985). Culturally appropriate care: The case of immigrants. *Topics in Clinical Nursing, 7*(3), 48–56.

Long, J., Mareno, N., Shabo, R., et al. (2012). Overweight and obesity among White, Black, and Mexican American children: Implications for when to intervene. *Journal for Specialists in Pediatric Nursing, 17*(1), 41–50.

Mallidou, A., Cummings, G., Estabrooks, C., et al. (2011). Nurse specialty subcultures and patient outcomes in acute care hospitals: A multiple-group structural equation modeling. *International Journal of Nursing Studies, 48*(1), 81–93.

McMurry, T. (2011). The image of male nurses and nursing leadership mobility. *Nursing Forum, 46*(1), 22–28.

Minarik, P. A., Lipson, J. G., & Dibble, S. L. (Eds.). (1996). *Culture and nursing care: A pocket guide*. San Francisco: University of California San Francisco School of Nursing.

Munoz, C., & Luckmann, J. (2005). *Transcultural communication in health care* (2nd ed.). Clifton Park, NY: Thomson Delmar Learning.

Musolino, G., Burkhalter, S., Crookston, B., et al. (2010). Understanding and eliminating disparities in health care: Development and assessment of cultural competence for interdisciplinary health professionals at the University of Utah—a 3-year investigation. *Journal of Physical Therapy Education, 24*(1), 25–36.

Purnell, L. (2000). A description of the Purnell model for cultural competence. *Journal of Transcultural Nursing, 11*, 40–46.

Purnell, L. (2002). The Purnell model for cultural competence. *Journal of Transcultural Nursing, 13*(3), 193–196.

Purnell, L. D., & Paulanka, B. J. (2008). *Transcultural health care: A culturally competent approach* (3rd ed.). Philadelphia: F. A. Davis.

Reneau, M. (2013). Teaching nurses sight unseen: Comparing the cultural competency of online and on-campus BSN faculty. *Journal of Transcultural Nursing, 24*(1), 78–85.

Sequist, T., Fitzmaurice, G., Marshall R., et al. (2010). Cultural competency training and performance reports to improve diabetes care for black patients: A cluster randomized, controlled trial. *Annals of Internal Medicine, 152*(1), 40–46.

Serafica, R. (2011). Concept analysis of acculturation in Filipino immigrants within health context. *Nursing Forum, 46*(3), 128–136.

Shin, H., & Kominski, R. (2010). Language use in the United States: 2007. Retrieved February 23, 2013, from http://www.census.gov/hhes/socdemo/language/data/acs/ACS-12.pdf

Smith, L. (2013). Reaching for cultural competence. *Nursing 2013, 43*(6), 31–38.

Spector, R. E. (2004). *Cultural care guides to heritage assessment and health traditions* (3rd ed.). Upper Saddle River, NJ: Prentice Hall.

Spector, R. E. (2013). *Cultural diversity in health and illness* (8th ed.). Upper Saddle River, NJ: Pearson Education.

Starr, S., & Wallace, D. (2011). Client perceptions of cultural competence of community-based nurses. *Journal of Community Health Nursing, 28*(2), 57–69.

Suzuki, L. A., & Ponterotto, J. G. (2007). *Handbook of multicultural assessment: Clinical, psychological, and educational applications* (3rd ed.). San Francisco: Jossey-Bass.

Todd, K. (1996). Pain assessment and ethnicity. *Annals of Emergency Medicine, 27*(4), 421–423.

Transcultural Nursing Society. (2010). Standards of practice for culturally competent nursing care. Retrieved February 19, 2013, from http://www.tcns.org/files/Standards_of_Practice_for_Culturally_Compt_Nsg_Care-Revised.pdf

Urban Indian Health Commission. (2007). Invisible tribes: Urban Indian and their health in a changing world. Retrieved April 5, 2013, from http://www.uihi.org/wp-content/uploads/2009/09/UIHC_Report_FINAL.pdf

U.S. Census Bureau. (2010). 2010 Census questionnaire reference book. Retrieved February 9, 2013, from: http://www.census.gov/2010census/partners/pdf/langfiles/qrb_English.pdf

U.S. Census Bureau. (2012a). Hispanic origin. Retrieved February 8, 2013, from http://www.census.gov/population/hispanic/about/faq.html

U.S. Census Bureau. (2012b). U.S. Census Bureau projections show a slower growing, older, more diverse nation a half century from now. Retrieved February 8, 2013, from http://www.census.gov/newsroom/releases/archives/population/cb12-243.html

U.S. Department of Health and Human Services, Office of Minority Health. (2001). *National standards for culturally and linguistically appropriate services in health care: Final report.* Washington, DC: Author. Retrieved February 22, 2013, from http://minorityhealth.hhs.gov/assets/pdf/checked/finalreport.pdf

Vonarx, N. (2011). Haitian vodou as a health care system: Between magic, religion, and medicine. *Alternative Therapies, 17*(5), 44–51.

Weech-Maldonado, R., Elliott, M., Pradhan, R., et al. (2012). Moving towards culturally competent health systems: Organizational and market factors. *Social Science & Medicine, 75*(5), 815–822.

Wilkinson, J. M. (2011). *Nursing process & critical thinking* (5th ed.). Upper Saddle River, NJ: Pearson/Prentice-Hall.

Wilson-Stronks, A., Lee, K., Cordero, C., et al. (2008). *One size does not fit all: Meeting the health care needs of diverse populations.* Oakbrook Terrace, IL: The Joint Commission. Retrieved February 23, 2013, from http://www.jointcommission.org/assets/1/6/HLCOneSizeFinal.pdf

Zborowski, M. (1969). *People in pain.* San Francisco: Jossey-Bass.

CHAPTER 16

Abdel-Khalek, A. (2011). Islam and metal health: A few speculations. *Mental Health, Religion & Culture, 14*(2), 87–92.

American Nurses Association (ANA). (2010). *Code for nurses.* Washington, DC: American Nurses Publishing.

Aspen Reference Group. (2002). *Palliative care: Patient and family counseling manual* (2nd ed.). Clifton Park, NY: Thomson Delmar Learning.

Astrow, A., Wexler, A., Texeira, K., et al. (2007). Is failure to meet spiritual needs associated with cancer patients' perceptions of quality of care and their satisfaction with care? *Journal of Clinical Oncology, 25*(36), 5753–5737.

Balboni, M., Sullivan, A., Amobi, A., et al. (2013). Why is spiritual care infrequent at the end of life? Spiritual care perceptions among patients, nurses, and physicians and the role of training. *Journal of Clinical Oncology, 31*(4), 461–467.

Baldacchino, D. (2011). Teaching on spiritual care: the perceived impact on qualified nurses. *Nurse Education in Practice, 11*(1), 47–53.

BBC Religions. (2009). Rastafari at a glance. Retrieved March 21, 2013, from http://www.bbc.co.uk/religion/religions/rastafari/

Beckman, S., Boxley-Harges, S., Bruick-Sorge, C., et al. (2007). Five strategies that heighten nurses' awareness of spirituality to impact client care. *Holistic Nursing Practice, 21*(3), 135–139.

Bekelman, D., Rumsfeld, J., Havranek, E., et al. (2009). Symptom burden, depression, and spiritual well-being: A comparison of heart failure and advanced cancer patients. *Journal of General Internal Medicine, 24*(5), 592–598.

Bekke-Hansen, S., Pedersen, C., Thygesen, K., et al. (2012). Faith and use of complementary and alternative medicine among heart attack patients in a secular society. *Complementary Therapies in Medicine, 20*(5), 306–315.

Ben-Arye, E., Schiff, E., Vintal, H., et al. (2012). Integrating complementary medicine and supportive care: Patients' perspectives toward complementary medicine and spirituality. *Journal of Alternative & Complementary Medicine, 18*(9), 824–831.

Benson, H., Dusek, J. A., Sherwood, J. B., et al. (2006). Study of the therapeutic effects of intercessory prayer (STEP) in cardiac bypass patients: A multicenter randomized trial of uncertainty and certainty of receiving intercessory prayer. *American Heart Journal, 151*(4), 934–942.

Biro, A. (2012). Creating conditions for good nursing by attending to the spiritual. *Journal of Nursing Management,* 20(8), 1002–1011.

Blanchard, J., Dunlap, D., & Fitchett, G. (2012). Screening for spiritual distress in the oncology inpatient: a quality improvement pilot project between nurses and chaplains. *Journal of Nursing Management, 20*(8), 1076–1084.

Bodhi, B. (2007). The Buddhist way of life on the eightfold path. *Hindu Website.* Retrieved April 5, 2013, from http://www.hinduwebsite.com/buddhism/eightfoldpath.asp

Book of Common Prayer (1979). New York: Random House.

Boyd, D. (1974). *Rolling thunder.* New York: Random House.

Bronstein, L. (2012). What is reconstructionist Judaism? Retrieved March 26, 2013, from http://www.rrc.edu/resources/reconstructionist-resources/what-reconstructionist-judaism

Brussat, F., & Brussat, M. A. (1996). *Spiritual literacy: Reading the sacred in everyday life.* New York: Simon & Schuster.

Buck, H., Overcash, J., & McMillan, S. (2009). The geriatric cancer experience at the end of life: Testing an adapted model. *Oncology Nursing Forum, 36*(6), 664–673.

Bulechek, G. M., Butcher, H. K., Dochterman, J. M., et al. (Eds.). (2012). *Nursing interventions classification (NIC)* (6th ed.). St. Louis, MO: C. V. Mosby.

Byrne, M. (2007). Spirituality in palliative care: What language do we need? Learning from pastoral care. *International Journal of Palliative Nursing, 13*(3), 118–124.

Cavendish, R., Konecny, L., Mitzeliotis, C., et al. (2003). Spiritual care interventions of nurses using Nursing Interventions Classification (NIC) labels. *International Journal of Nursing Terminologies and Classifications, 14*(4), 113–124.

Cenkner, W. (1990). Hinduism. In J. A. Komonchak, M. Collins, & D. A. Lane (Eds.), *The new dictionary of theology* (pp. 466–469). Collegeville, MN: Liturgical Press.

Chan, M. (2010). Factors affecting nursing staff in practicing spiritual care. *Journal of Clinical Nursing, 19*(15–16), 2128–2136.

Cheatham, D. (2008). *Kinds of prayer—a brief review*. Retrieved March 18, 2013, from http://devotional.net.faithsite.com/uploads/147/95698.pdf

Christian Science. (2013). What is Christian Science? Retrieved March 15, 2013, from http://christianscience.com/what-is-christian-science

Cobb, M., Puchalski, C., & Rumbold, B. (2012). *Oxford textbook of spirituality in healthcare*. New York: Oxford University Press.

Cockell, N., & McSherry, W. (2012). Spiritual care in nursing: An overview of published international research. *Journal of Nursing Management, 20*(8), 958–969.

Collin, M. (2012). The search for a higher power among terminally ill people with no previous religion or belief. *International Journal of Palliative Nursing, 18*(8), 384–389.

Como, J. M. (2007). Spiritual practice: A literature review related to spiritual health and health outcomes. *Holistic Nursing Practice, 21*(5), 224–236.

Cotton, S., Zebracki, K., Rosenthal, S., et al. (2006). Religion/spirituality and adolescent health outcomes: A review. *Journal of Adolescent Health, 38*(4), 472–480.

Cronenwett, L., Sherwood, G., Barnsteiner, J., et al. (2007). Quality and safety education for nurses. *Nursing Outlook, 55*, 122–131. doi:10.1016/ joutlook.2007.02.006

Delgado, C. (2007). Meeting clients' spiritual needs. *Nursing Clinical of North America, 42*(2), 279–293.

Delisser, H. (2009). A practical approach to the family that expects a miracle. *Chest, 135*(6), 1643–1647. Retrieved March 25, 2013, from http://www.ncbi.nlm.nih.gov/pmc/articles/PMC2821292/

Doka, K. (2011). Religion and spirituality: Assessment and intervention. *Journal of Social Work in End-of-Life & Palliative Care, 7*(1), 99–109.

Dolarno, B. (2010). Spiritual nursing. *Nursing Update, 34*(4), 22–24.

Donahue, M. P. (1985). *Nursing: The finest art; An illustrated history*. St. Louis, MO: C. V. Mosby.

Draper, P. (2012). An integrative review of spiritual assessment: Implications for nursing management. *Journal of Nursing Management, 2*(8), 970–980.

Dunn, K., & Horgas, A. (2000). The prevalence of prayer as a spiritual self-care modality in elders. *Journal of Holistic Nursing, 18*(4), 337–351.

Dyer, C. (2012). Young Jehovah's Witness who refused a blood transfusion is allowed to die. *British Medical Journal, 344*(7861), 3.

Dyess, S. (2011). Faith: A concept analysis. *Journal of Advanced Nursing, 67*(12), 2723–2731.

Editors of Hinduism Today. (2007). *What is Hinduism: Modern adventures into a profound global faith*. Kapaa, HI: Himalayan Academy.

Ehman, J. (2011). Spiritual assessment and health care: A select bibliography of Medline-indexed articles published 2001–2011. Retrieved March 16, 2013, from http://www.uphs.upenn.edu/pastoral/cpe/Res_Bib_Spiritual_Asessment_MEDLINE.pdf

Elliott, B. A., Gessert, C. E., & Peden-McAlpine, C. (2007). Decision making by families of older adults with advanced cognitive impairment: Spirituality and meaning. *Journal of Gerontological Nursing, 33*(8), 49–55.

Ellison, C., Bradshaw, M., & Roberts, C. (2012). Spiritual and religious identities predict the use of complementary and alternative medicine among US adults. *Preventive Medicine, 54*(1), 9–12.

Esposito, J. L. (1990). Islam. In J. A. Komonchak, M. Collins, & D. A. Lane (Eds.), *The new dictionary of theology* (pp. 527–529). Collegeville, MN: Liturgical Press.

Esposito, J., Fasching, D., & Lewis, T. (2011). *World religions today* (4th ed.). New York: Oxford University Press.

Fowler, M. (2009). Religion, bioethics and nursing practice. *Nursing Ethnics, 16*(4), 393–405.

Gaskamp, C., Sutter, R., Meraviglia, M., et al. (2006). Evidence-based guideline: Promoting spirituality in the older adult. *Journal of Gerontological Nursing, 32*(11), 8–13.

Giske, T. (2012). How undergraduate nursing students learn to care for patients spiritually in clinical studies-a review of the literature. *Journal of Nursing Management, 20*(8), 1049–1057.

Gowri, A., & Hight, E. (2001). Spirituality and medical practice: Using the HOPE questions as a practical tool for spiritual assessment. *American Family Physician, 63*, 81–88.

Grudzen, C., Stone, S., Mohanty, S., et al. (2011). "I want to be taking my own last breath": Patients reflections on illness when presenting to the emergency department at the end of life. *Journal of Palliative Medicine, 14*(3), 293–296.

Hamptom, J. S., & Weinert, C. (2006). An exploration of spirituality in rural women with chronic illness. *Holistic Nursing Practice, 20I*(1), 27–33.

Hasan, U. (2012). Health, sickness, medicine, life and death in Muslim belief and practice. *European Journal of Palliative Care, 19*(5), 241–245.

Highfield, M. E. F. (1992). Spiritual healing of oncology patients: Nurse and patient perspectives. *Cancer Nursing, 15*(1), 1–8.

Highfield, M. E. F. (2000). Providing spiritual care to patients with cancer. *Clinical Journal of Oncology Nursing, 4*(3), 115–120.

Hodge, D., Horvath, V., Larkin, H., et al. (2012). Older adults' spiritual needs in health care settings: A qualitative meta-synthesis. *Research on Aging, 34*(2), 131–155.

Huang, C., Hsu, M., & Chen, T. (2012). An exploratory study of religious involvement as a moderator between anxiety, depressive symptoms and quality of life outcomes of older adults. *Journal of Clinical Nursing, 21*(5–6), 609–619.

Hubbartt, B., Corey, D., & Kautz, D. (2012). Prayer at the bedside. *International Journal for Human Caring, 16*(1), 42–47.

Huguelet, P., Mohr, S., Betrisey, C., et al. (2011). A randomized trial of spiritual assessment of outpatients with schizophrenia: Patients' and clinicans' experience. *Psychiatric Services, 62*(1), 79–86.

Hungelmann, J., Kenkel-Rossi, E., Klassen, L., et al. (1996). Focus on spiritual well-being: Harmonious interconnectedness of mind-body-spirit—use of the JAREL spiritual well-being scale. *Geriatric Nursing, 17*(6), 262.

Johannessen, B. (2011). Realization and development of self in CAM nurses and CAM treatment: A qualitative study. *International Journal for Human Caring, 15*(2), 14–20.

Jun, J., & Oh, K. (2013). Asian and Hispanic Americans cancer fatalism and colon cancer screening. *American Journal of Health Behaviors, 37*(20), 145–154.

Keddington, R. K. (2007). Caring for members of the church of Jesus Christ of Latter-Day Saints (Mormons) in the emergency department. *Journal of Emergency Nursing, 33*(3), 252–256.

Kirkwood, N. A. (2005). *A hospital handbook on multiculturalism* (Rev. ed.). Harrisburg, PA: Morehouse.

Kluckhohn, C., & Leighton, D. (1962). *The Navajo.* Garden City, NY: Doubleday.

Knierim, T. (n.d.). The noble eightfold path. Retrieved March 26, 2013, from http://www.thebigview.com/buddhism/eightfoldpath.html

Koenig, H., King, D., & Carson, V. (2012). *Handbook of religion and health* (2nd ed.). New York: Oxford University Press.

La Madrid, A. (2012). Waiting for a miracle. *Journal of Clinical Oncology, 30*(19), 2421–2422.

Lane, J. (1987). The care of the human spirit. *Journal of Professional Nursing, 3*(6), 332–337.

Last Chance Ministries. (2000; updated 2009, March 9). What is Rastafarianism? Retrieved March 21, 2013, from http://www.lastchanceministries.com/Rastafarianism.htm

Lazenby, J. (2010). On "spirituality," "religion," and "religions": A concept analysis. *Palliative & Supportive Care, 8*(4), 469–476.

Lee, D., & Higgens, P. A. (2010). Adjunctive therapies for the chronically critically ill. *AACN Advanced Critical Care, 21*(1), 92–106.

Levoy, G. (1997). *Callings: Finding and following an authentic life.* New York: Harmony Books.

Lewis, C. S. (1961). *A grief observed.* New York: Seabury Press.

Lindstrom, E., & Johnstone, R. (2010). Acute normovolemic hemodilution in a Jehovah's Witness patient: A case report. *AANA Journal, 78*(4), 326–330.

Mais, L. (2010). Perspectives on death and dying from an Atheist nurse. *Austin Atheist, 3*(1), 1–5.

McCaffrey, A. M., Eisenberg, D. M., Legedza, A. T. R., et al. (2004). Prayer for health concerns: Results of a national survey on prevalence and patterns of use. *Archives of Internal Medicine, 164*(8), 858–862.

McDonald, L. (Ed.). (2002). *The collected works of Florence Nightingale series.* Waterloo, Ontario: Wilfrid Laurier University Press.

McGrath, P. (2004). Reflections on serious illness as spiritual journey by survivors of haematological malignancies. *European Journal of Cancer Care, 13*, 227–237.

McGrew, T. (2013). Miracles. *The Stanford encyclopedia of philosophy.* Stanford, CA: Stanford University Press. Retrieved March 10, 2013, from http://plato.stanford.edu/entries/miracles/#ConDef

McSherry, W., & Jamieson, S. (2011). An online survey of nurses' perception of spirituality and spiritual care. *Journal of Clinical Nursing, 20*(11–12), 1757–1767.

Millspaugh, C. D. (2005). Assessment and response to spiritual pain: Part II. *Journal of Palliative Medicine, 8*(6), 1110–1117.

Moorhead, S., Johnson, M., Maas, M. L., et al. (Eds.). (2013). *Nursing outcomes classification (NOC)* (5th ed.). St. Louis, MO: C. V. Mosby.

NANDA International. (2012). *Nursing diagnoses: Definitions and classification 2012–2014.* Philadelphia: Wiley-Blackwell.

Nardi, D., & Rooda, L. (2011). Spirituality-based nursing practice by nursing students: An exploratory study. *Journal of Professional Nursing, 27*(4), 255–263.

Nath, J. (2010). "God is a vegetarian": The food, health and bio-spirituality of Hare Krishna, Buddist and Seventh-Day Adventist devotees. *Health Sociology Review, 19*(3), 356–368.

Nigosian, S. (2007). *World religions: A historical approach* (4th ed.). New York: Bedford/St. Martin's.

Noble, A., Rom, M., Newsome-Wicks, M., et al. (2009). Jewish laws, customs, and practice in labor, delivery, and postpartum care. *Journal of Transcultural Nursing, 20*(3), 323–333.

Olver, I., & Dutney, A. (2012). A randomized, blinded study of the impact of intercessory prayer on spiritual well-being in patients with cancer. *Alternative Therapies in Health & Medicine, 18*(5), 18–27.

Oxtoby, W. G., & Segal, A. G. (2007). *A concise introduction to world religions.* Cary, NC: Oxford University Press.

Palmer, R. F., Katerndahl, D., & Morgan-Kidd, J. (2004). A randomized trial of the effects of remote intercessory prayer: Interactions with personal beliefs on problem-specific outcomes and functional status. *The Journal of Alternative and Complementary Medicine, 10*(3), 438–448.

Pawlikowski, J. (1990). Judaism. In J. Komonchak, M. Collins, & D. A. Lane (Eds.), *The new dictionary of theology* (pp. 543–548). Collegeville, MN: Liturgical Press.

Posadzki, P. (2010). The transmission of affect: compassionate love in clinical and educational settings. *Integrative Medicine: A Clinician's Journal, 9*(5), 46–48.

Puchalski, C., & Ferrell, B. (2010). *Making health care whole: Integrating spirituality into patient care.* West Conshohocken, PA: Templeton Press.

Reeve, C. (1998). *Still me.* New York: Random House.

Reeve, C. (2002). *Nothing is impossible: Reflections on a new life.* New York: Random House.

Roberts, L., Ahmed, I., Hall, S., et al. (2011). Intercessory prayer for the alleviation of ill health (Review). *Cochrane Database of Systematic Reviews,* Issue 11. The Cochrane Collaborations: John Wiley & Sons, Ltd.

Ronaldson, S., Hayes, L., Aggar, C., et al. (2012). Spirituality and spiritual caring: nurses' perspectives and practice in palliative and acute care environments. *Journal of Clinical Nursing, 21*(15–16), 2126–2135.

Ross, R., Sawatphanait, W., & Tatirat, S. (2007). Finding peace (Kwam Sa-ngob Jai): A Buddhist way to live with HIV. *Journal of Holistic Nursing, 25*(4), 228–235.

Schaefer, J., Stonecipher, S., & Kane, I. (2012). Finding room for spirituality in healthcare. *Nursing2012, 42*(9), 14–16.

Schlitz, M., Hopf, H., Eskenazi, L., et al. (2012). Distant healing of surgical wounds: An exploratory study. *EXPLORE: The Journal of Science and Healing, 8*(4), 223–230.

Sessana, L., Finnell, D., & Jezewski, M. A. (2007). Spirituality in nursing and health-related literature: A concept analysis. *Journal of Holistic Nursing, 25*(4), 252–262.

Sessana, L., Finnell, D., Underhill, M., et al. (2011). Measures assessing spirituality as more than religiosity: A methodical review of nursing and health-related literature. *Journal of Advanced Nursing, 67*(8), 1677–1694.

Smyth, T., & Allen, S. (2011). Nurses' experience assessing the spirituality of terminally ill patients in acute clinical practice. *International Journal of Palliative Nursing, 17*(7), 337–343.

Spector, R. (2013). *Cultural diversity in health and illness* (8th ed.). Upper Saddle River, NJ: Pearson Education.

Stanley, C. (2011). *Handle with prayer: Unwrap the source of God's strength for living.* Colorado Springs, CO: David Cook.

Sternthal, M., Williams, D., Musick, M., et al. (2012). Religious practices, beliefs, and mental health: variations across ethnicity. *Ethnicity & Health, 17*(1–2), 171–185.

Swinton, J., Bain, V., Ingram, S., et al. (2011). Moving inwards, moving outwards, moving upwards: The role of spirituality during the early stages of breast cancer. *European Journal of Cancer Care, 20*(5), 640–652.

Swinton, J., & Pattison, S. (2010). Moving beyond clarity: Towards a thin, vague, and useful understanding of spirituality in nursing care. *Nursing Philosophy, 11*(4), 226–237.

Tait, E., Laditka, S., Laditka, J., et al. (2011). Praying for health by older adults in the United States: Differences by ethnicity, gender, and income. *Journal of Religion, Spirituality & Aging, 23*(10), 338–362.

Tate, J. (2011). The role of spirituality in the breast cancer experiences of African-American women. *Journal of Holistic Nursing, 29*(4), 249–255.

Taylor, E., & Carr, M. (2009). Nursing ethics in the Seventh-Day Adventist religion tradition. *Nursing Ethics, 16*(6), 707–718.

The Church of Jesus Christ of Latter-Day Saints. (2013). Mormonism 101: FAQ. Retreived March 15, 2013, from http://www.mormonnewsroom.org/article/mormonism-101#C15

The Joint Commission. (2010). *Advancing effective communication, cultural competence, and patient- and family-centered care: A roadmap for hospitals*. Oakbrook Terrace, IL: The Joint Commission. Retrieved March 9, 2013, from http://www.jointcommission.org/assets/1/6/aroadmapforhospitalsfinalversion727.pdf

Timmins, F., & McSherry, W. (2012). Spirituality: The Holy Grail of contemporary nursing practice. *Journal of Nursing Management, 20*(8), 951–957.

Trinkaus, M., Burman, D., Barmala, N., et al. (2011). Spirituality and use of complementary therapies for cure in advanced cancer. *Psycho-Oncology, 20*(7), 746–754.

Union for Reform Judaism. (2012). What is Reform Judaism? Retrieved March 26, 2013, from http://urj.org/about/reform/whatisreform/

Wachholtz, A., Pearce, M. J., & Koenig, H. (2007). Exploring the relationship between spirituality, coping, and pain. *Journal of Behavioral Medicine, 30*, 311–318.

Wachholtz, A., & Sambamoorthi, U. (2011). National trends in prayer use as a coping mechanism for health concerns: Changes from 2002 to 2007. *Psychology of Religion and Spirituality, 3*(2), 67–77.

Waldman, H., Perlman, S., & Chaudhry, R. (2010). Christian Science views on disability. *Exceptional Parent, 40*(8), 56–57.

Waldman, H., Perlman, S., & Chaudhry, R. (2012). Latter-Day Saints (Mormons): Their perceptions of individuals with disabilities. *Exceptional Parent, 42*(10), 20–21.

Warwick, A. (2012). Recovery following injury hinges upon expectation and hope. *Journal of Trauma Nursing, 19*(4), 251–254.

Weaver, H. (2012). Urban and indigenous: Challenges of being a Native American in the city. *Journal of Community Practice, 20*(4), 470–488.

Wilkins, A., & Mailoo, V. (2010). Care of the older person: A Hindu perspective. *Nursing & Residential Care, 12*(5), 249–251.

Williams-Orlando, C. (2012). Spirituality in integrative medicine. *Integrative Medicine: A Clinical's Journal, 11*(4), 34–40.

Wu, C., Weber, W., Kozak, L., et al. (2009). A survey of complementary and alternative (CAM) awareness among neurosurgeons in Washington State. *Journal of Alternative & Complementary Medicine, 15*(5), 551–555.

Yanez, B., Edmondson, D., Stanton, A., et al. (2009). Facets of spirituality as predictors of adjustments to cancer: Relative contributions of having faith and finding meaning. *Journal of Consulting and Clinical Psychology, 77*, 730–741.

Zumbro Valley Medical Society, Medicine and Religion Committee. (1978). *Religious aspects of medical care: A handbook of religious practices of all faiths* (2nd ed.). St. Louis, MO: The Catholic Hospital Association.

CHAPTER 17

Ahrens, T., Yancey, V., & Kollef, M. (2003). Improving family communications at the end of life: Implications for length of stay in the intensive care unit and resource use. *American Journal of Critical Care, 12*(4), 317–324.

American Association of Colleges of Nursing. (n.d.). *Peaceful death: Recommended competencies and curricular guidelines for end-of-life nursing care*. Washington, DC: Author. Retrieved May 4, 2013, from http://www.aacn.nche.edu/elnec/publications/peaceful-death

American Association of Colleges of Nursing. (2010; Updated 2013, April). *ELNEC fact sheet*. Retrieved April 17, 2013, from https://www.aacn.nche.edu/elnec/about/fact-sheet

American Nurses Association (ANA). (1994a). *Position statement: Active euthanasia*. Washington, DC: Author. Retrieved May 14, 2013, from http://www.nursingworld.org/MainMenuCategories/Policy-Advocacy/Positions-and-Resolutions/ANAPositionStatements/Archives/prteteuth14450.html

American Nurses Association (ANA). (1994b). *Position statement: Assisted suicide*. Washington, DC: Author. Retrieved May 14, 2013, from http://www.nursingworld.org/MainMenuCategories/Policy-Advocacy/Positions-and-Resolutions/ANAPositionStatements/Archives/prtetsuic14456.html

American Nurses Association (ANA). (2004). *Position statement: Nursing care and do-not-resuscitate decisions*. Washington, DC: Author. Retrieved May 14, 2013, from http://ana.nursingworld.org/MainMenuCategories/EthicsStandards/Ethics-Position-Statements/Copy%20of%20dnr0414405.aspx

American Nurses Association (ANA). (2010). *Revised position statement: Registered nurses' roles and responsibilities in providing expert care and counseling at the end of life*. Retrieved April 30, 2013, from http://www.nursingworld.org/MainMenuCategories/EthicsStandards/Ethics-Position-Statements/etpain14426.pdf

American Nurses Association (ANA). (2012). Revised position statement: Nursing care and do not resuscitate (DNR) and allow natural Death (AND) decisions. Retrieved April 19, 2013, from http://www.nursingworld.org/dnrposition

American Nurses Association (ANA). (2013). Euthanasia, assisted suicide, and aid in dying. Retrieved May 13, 2013, from, http://www.nursingworld.org/euthanasiaanddying

Balk, D. (2011). Adolescent development and bereavement: An introduction. *Prevention Researcher, 1*(3), 3–9.

Ball, C., Navsaria, P., Kirkpatrick, A., et al. (2010). The impact of country and culture on end-of-life care for injured patients: Results from an international survey. *Journal of Trauma, 69*(6), 1323–1334.

Beckstrand, R., Callister, L., Rawls, N., et al. (2011). Preventing suffering: Facilitating a peaceful death in children. *Communicating Nursing Research, 44*(2), 195.

Bednash, G., & Ferrell, B. (2000). *The end-of life nursing education consortium (2000). The ELNEC curriculum*. Washington, DC: American Association of Colleges of Nursing and City of Hope National Medical Center.

Boss, P., & Carnes, D. (2012). The myth of closure. *Family Process, 51*(4), 456–469.

Bowlby, J. (1982). *Attachment and loss* (Vols. 1–3). New York: Basic Books.

Boyle, D. K., Miller, P. A., & Forbes-Thompson, S. A. (2005). Communication and end-of-life care in the intensive care unit. Patient, family, and clinician outcomes. *Critical Care Nursing Quarterly, 28*(4), 302–316.

Boyle, J. S., Bunting, S. M., Hodnicki, D. R., et al. (2001). Critical thinking in African American mothers who care for adult children with HIV: A cultural analysis. *Journal of Transcultural Nursing, 12*(3), 193–202.

Breault, J. (2011). DNR, DNAR, or AND? Is language important? *The Oschner Journal, 11*(4), 302–306.

Brennan, C., Prince-Paul, M., & Wiencek, C. (2011). Providing a "good death" for oncology patients during the final hours of life in the intensive care unit. *AACN Advanced Critical Care, 22*(4), 379–396.

Briggs, D. A., & Pehrsson, D-E. (2008). Use of bibliotherapy in the treatment of grief and loss: A guide to current counseling practices. *Theory, Research & Practice, 71*, 32–42.

Brown, E. (2009). Helping bereaved children and young people. *British Journal of School Nursing, 4*(2), 68–73.

Bulechek, G., Butcher, H., & Dochterman, J. M. (2013). *Nursing interventions classification (NIC)* (6th ed.). St. Louis, MO: C. V. Mosby.

Burkle, C., Schipper, A., & Wijdicks, E. (2011). Brain death and the courts. *Neurology, 76*(9), 837–841.

Campbell, K. (2010). At the end of life dehydration is a comfort measure. Retrieved April 30, 2013, from http://www.hospiceotp.org/index.php?mact=News,cntnt01,print,0&cntnt01articleid=4&cntnt01showtemplate=false&cntnt01returnid=60

Clabots, S. (2012). Strategies to help initiate and maintain the end-of-life discussion with patients and family members. *Medsurg Nursing, 21*(4), 197–204.

Claxton, R., & Reynolds, C. (2012). Complicated Grief. *Journal of Palliative Medicine, 15*(7), 829–830.

College of American Pathologists. (last updated 2007). *Autopsy. Postmortem flow chart*. Northfield, IL: College of American Pathologists, Autopsy Committee. Retrieved May 12, 2013, from http://capstaging.cap.org/apps/docs/committees/autopsy/POSTMORTEM_FLOW_CHART.pdf

Corr, C., & Corr, D. (2013). *Death and dying, life and living* (7th ed.). Belmont, CA: Wadsworth, Cengage Learning

Covington, M. (2013). End-of-life care: implementing the Gold Standards Framework. *Nursing & Residential Care, 15*(3), 146–149.

DeSpelder, L., & Strickland, A. (1996). *The last dance*. Mountain View, CA: Mayfield.

Duffy, S., Jackson, F., Schim, S., et al. (2006). Cultural concepts at the end of life. *Nursing Older People, 18*(8), 10–14.

Duke, G., Yarbrough, S., & Pang, K. (2009). The Patient Self-Determination Act: 20 years revisited. *Journal of Nursing Law, 13*(4), 114–123.

Egan, K. A., & Arnold, R. L. (2003). Grief and bereavement care. *American Journal of Nursing, 103*(9), 42–52.

Eisenhandler, S. A. (2004). The arts of consolation: Commemoration and folkways of faith. *Generations, 28*(2), 37.

Emanuel, L., Ferris, F., von Gunten, C., et al. (2008). The last hours of living: Practical advice for clinicians CME/CE. From L. Emanuel, F. Ferris, C. von Gunten, et al. (2005), EPEC™-O: Education in Palliative and End-of-life Care for Oncology. (Module 6: Last Hours of Living © The EPEC Project™, Chicago, IL). Major funding provided by the National Cancer Institute; Supplemental funding provided by the Lance Armstrong Foundation. Retrieved April 16, 2013, from http://www.medscape.com/viewarticle/542262

End-of-Life Nursing Education Consortium (ELNEC). (2012). *History, statewide effort and recommendations for the future: Advancing palliative nursing care*. Long Beach, CA: Archstone Foundation.

Engel, G. L. (1961). Is grief a disease: A challenge for medical research. *Psychosomatic Medicine, 23*(1), 18–22.

Ferrell, B., & Coyle, N. (Eds.). (2010). *Textbook of palliative care nursing* (3rd ed.). Oxford: Oxford University Press.

Ferszt, G. G., & Leveillee, M. (2006). How do you distinguish between grief and depression? *Nursing2006, 36*(9), 60–61.

Fine, E., Reid, C., Shengelia, R., et al. (2010). Directly observed patient–physician discussions in palliative and end-of-life care: A systematic review of the literature. *Journal of Palliative Medicine, 13*(5), 595–603.

Florczak, K. L. (2008). The persistent yet ever changing nature of grieving a loss. *Nursing Science Quarterly, 21*(1), 7–11.

Friend, M. (2011). Physician-assisted suicide: Death with dignity? *Journal of Nursing Law, 14* (3–4), 110–116.

Galushko, M., Romotzky, V., & Voltz, R. (2012). Challenges in end-of-life communications. *Current Opinions in Supportive and Palliative Care, 6*(3), 355–364.

Ghesquiere, A., Shear, M., & Duan. (2013). Outcomes of bereavement care among widowed older adults with complicated grief and depression. *Journal of Primary Care & Community, 4*(2). doi:10.1177/2150131913481231

Germain, A., Shear, K., Walsh, C., et al. (2013). Dream content in complicated grief: A window into loss-related cognitive schema. *Death Studies, 37*(3), 269–284.

Goldring, E., & Leeuwenburgh, E. (2008). *Why did you die? Activities to help children cope with grief and loss*. Oakland, CA: Instant Help Books.

Gramling, R., Norton, S., Ladwig, S., et al. (2013). Direct observation of prognosis communication in palliative care: A descriptive study. *Journal of Pain & Symptom Management, 45*(2), 202–212.

Greenlee, S. (2013). *Grief entanglements: Understanding unresolved grief and what you can do about it*. Seattle, WA: CreateSpace Independent Publishing Platform.

Hamdan, S., Mazariegos, D., Melhem, N., et al. (2012). Effect of parental bereavement on health risk behaviors in youth. *JAMA Pediatrics, 166*(3), 216–223.

Hancock, K., Clayton, J., Parker, S., et al. (2007). Truth-telling in discussing prognosis in advanced life-limiting illnesses: A systematic review. *Palliative Medicine, 21*, 507–517.

Handbook of Non Drug Intervention Project Team, Handi. (2013). Bibliotherapy for depression. *Australian Family Physician, 42*(2), 199–200.

Harvey, J. (2001). Debunking myths about post-mortem care. *Nursing2001, 31*(7), 44–45.

Haylock, P. J. (2003). Nursing resources. TNEEL. A new approach to education in end-of-life care. *American Journal of Nursing, 103*(8), 99–100.

Health Care Chaplaincy. (updated 2013). *Handbook of patients' spiritual and cultural values for health care professionals*. Retrieved May 4, 2013, from http://www.healthcarechaplaincy.org/userimages/Cultural%20Sensitivity%20handbook%20from%20HealthCare%20Chaplaincy%20%20(3-12%202013).pdf

Heath, J., Oh, L., Clarke, N., et al. (2012). Complementary and alternative medicine use in children with cancer at the end of life. *Journal of Palliative Medicine, 15*(11), 1218–1221.

Hodgson, N. (2013). The palliative efficacy and mechanism of action of CAM modalities for advanced dementia care. *Journal of Pain and Symptom Management, 45*(2), 345.

Holtslander, L., & McMillan, S. (2011). Depressive symptoms, grief, and complicated grief among family caregivers of patients with advanced cancer three months into bereavement. *Oncology Nursing Forum, 38*(1), 60–65.

Hospice and Palliative Nurses Association. (2011). HPNA position statement, palliative sedation. Retrieved May 14, 2013, from http://www.hpna.org/DisplayPage.aspx?Title1=Position%20Statements

Hospice Foundation of America. (2005). *The dying process: A guide for caregivers.* Washington, DC: Author. Retrieved April 30, 2013, from http://www.optionsforeldercare.com/eldercarebooksandarticles/hospice_end_of_life_manual.pdf

Hudson, P. L. (2006). How well do family caregivers cope after caring for a relative with advanced disease and how can health professionals enhance their support? *Journal of Palliative Medicine, 9*(3), 694–703.

Institute of Medicine. (2013). Committee on transforming end-of-life care: First meeting. Retrieved April 17, 2013, from http://www.iom.edu/Activities/Aging/TransformingEndOfLife/2013-FEB-20.aspx

Johnson, M., Moorhead, S., Bulechek, G., et al. (2012). *NOC and NIC linkages to NANDA-I and clinical conditions* (3rd ed.). St. Louis, MO: C. V. Mosby.

Karnes, B. (1995). *Gone from my sight: The dying experience.* Stillwell, KS: Barbara Karnes Books.

Kelly, K., Malloy, P., Munevar, C., et al. (2010). Beyond bad news: Communication skills of nurses in palliative care. *Journal of Hospice and Palliative Nursing, 12*(3), 166–174.

Kraft, K. (2012). CAM for depression, anxiety, grief, and other symptoms in palliative care. *Progress in Palliative Care, 20*(5), 272–277.

Kruse, B. (2004). The meaning of letting go: The lived experience for caregivers of persons at the end of life. *Journal of Hospice and Palliative Nursing, 6*(4), 215–222.

Kübler-Ross, E. (1969). *On death and dying.* New York: HarperCollins.

Kübler-Ross, E. (1997). *On children and death.* New York: Touchstone Press.

Kurtz, S. F., Strong, C. W., & Gerasimow, D. (2007). The 2006 Revised Uniform Anatomical Gift Act—a law to save lives. *Health Law Analysis.* Retrieved May 3, 2013, from http://www.uniformlaws.org/Shared/Docs/UAGA/Kurtz%20Article%20February%202007.pdf

Lang, A., Fleiszer, A., Duhamel, F., et al. (2011). Perinatal loss and parental grief: The challenges of ambiguity and disenfranchised grief. *Omega: Journal of Death & Dying, 63*(2), 183–196.

Law, R. (2009). "Bridging worlds": Meeting the emotional needs of dying patients. *Journal of Advanced Nursing, 65*(12), 2630–2641.

Lobb, E., Kristjanson, L., Aoun, S., et al. (2010). Predictors of complicated grief: A systematic review of empirical studies. *Death Studies, 34*(8), 673–698.

Loike, J., Gillick, M., Mayer, S., et al. (2010). The critical role of religion: Caring for the dying patient from an Orthodox Jewish perspective. *Journal of Palliative Medicine, 13*(10), 1267–1271.

Lowey, S., Powers, B., & Sue, Y. (2013). Short of breath and dying: state of the science on opioid agents for the palliation of refractory dyspnea in older adults. *Journal of Gerontological Nursing, 39*(2), 43–52.

Lynn, J. (2000). *Promises to keep: Changing the way we provide end of life care.* Washington, DC: The National Coalition on Health Care, the Institute for Health Care Improvement.

MacKenzie, M. (2011). Preparatory grief in frail elderly adults. *Annals of Long Term Care, 19*(1), 22–26.

Mahon, M. (2010). (Ed.). Palliative care and end of life care. *Nursing Clinics of North America, 45*(3), 271–500.

Malloy, P., Virani, R., Kelly, K., et al. (2008). End-of-life care: Improving communication skills to enhance palliative care. *Medscape.* Retrieved April 27, 2013, from http://www.medscape.org/viewprogram/12632

Manzanec, P., & Tyler, M. K. (2003). Cultural considerations in end-of-life care. *American Journal of Nursing, 103*(3), 50–59.

Matzo, M., & Sherman, D. (2009). *Palliative care nursing: Quality care to the end of life* (3rd ed.). New York: Springer.

McGowan, C. (2011). Legal issues, legal aspects of end-of-life care. *Critical Care Nursing, 31*(5), 64–69.

Melvin, C. (2012). Professional compassion fatigue: What is the true cost of nurses caring for the dying? *International Journal of Palliative Nursing, 18*(12), 606–611.

Milberg, A., & Strang, P. (2011). Protection against perceptions of powerlessness and helplessness during palliative care: The family members' perspective. *Palliative & Supportive Care, 9*(3), 251–262.

Moorhead, S., Johnson, M., Maas, M., et al. (2013). *Nursing outcomes classification (NOC)* (5th ed.). St. Louis, MO: C. V. Mosby.

NANDA International. (2012). *NANDA nursing diagnoses: Definitions and classification 2012–2014.* Oxford: Wiley-Blackwell.

National Cancer Institute. (2011). Grief, bereavement, and coping with loss (PDQ®). Retrieved April 20, 2013, from http://www.cancer.gov/cancertopics/pdq/supportivecare/bereavement/Patient/page1/AllPages

National Caregiver Library. (n.d.). End of life issues. Retrieved May 13, 2013, from http://www.caregiverslibrary.org/caregivers-resources/grp-end-of-life-issues.aspx

National Conference of Commissioners on Uniform State Laws. (2009). Revised Uniform Anatomical Gift Act (2006) (amended in 2009). Retrieved April 19, 2013, from http://www.uniformlaws.org/shared/docs/anatomical_gift/uaga_final_aug09.pdf

National Hospice and Palliative Care Organization (NHPCO). (2011). Facts on hospice and palliative care. Graphs: Growth in patients and providers through 2011. Retrieved April 28, 2013, from http://www.nhpco.org/hospice-statistics-research-press-room/facts-hospice-and-palliative-care

National Office. (n.d.). Partnership for Caring. Download your state's advance directives. Retrieved May 12, 2013, from http://caringinfo.org/i4a/pages/index.cfm?pageid=3289

O'Connor, L., & Lunney, M. (1998). Care of the caregiver—Family member with a chronic illness. *Nursing Diagnosis, 9*(4), 152.

Ostler, T. (2010). Grief and coping in early childhood: The role of communication in the mourning process. *Zero to Three, 31*(1), 29–35.

Owens, D., Eby, K., Burson, S., et al. (2012). Primary palliative care clinic pilot project demonstrates benefits of a nurse practitioner-directed clinic providing primary and palliative care. *Journal of the American Academy of Nurse Practitioners, 24*(1), 52–58.

Pitorak, E. (2003). Care at the time of death. *American Journal of Nursing, 103*(7), 42–52.

President's Commission for the Study of Ethical Problems in Medicine and Biomedical and Behavioral Research. (1981). *Defining death: A report on the medical, legal, and ethical issues in the determination of death.* Washington, DC: U.S. Government Printing Office.

Prigerson, H., Frank, E., Kasl, S., et al. (1995). Complicated grief and bereavement-related depression as distinct disorders: Preliminary empirical validation in elderly bereaved spouses. *American Journal of Psychiatry, 152*(1), 22–30.

Prigerson, H., Horowitz, M., Jacobs, S., et al. (2009). Prolonged grief disorder: Psychometric validation of criteria proposed for DSM-V and ICD-11. Retrieved May 13, 2013, from http://www.plosmedicine.org/article/info%3Adoi%2F10.1371%2Fjournal.pmed.1000121

Prosser, R., Korman, D., & Feinstein, R. (2012). An orthodox perspective of the Jewish end-of-life experience. *Home Healthcare Nurse, 30*(10), 579–585.

Qaseem, A., Snow, V., Shekelle, P., et al. (2008). Evidence-based interventions to improve the palliative care of pain, dyspnea, and depression at the end of life: A clinical practice guideline from the American College of Physicians. *Annals of Internal Medicine, 148*(2), 141–146.

Rahim-Jamal, S., Sarte, A., Kozak, J., et al. (2011). Hospice residents' interest in complementary and alternative medicine (CAM) at end of life: A pilot study in hospice residences in British Columbia. *Journal of Palliative Care, 27*(2), 134–140.

Rando, T. (1984). *Grief, dying and death: Clinical interventions for caregivers.* Champaign, IL: Research Press.

Rando, T. (1986). *Loss and anticipatory grief.* Lexington, MA: Lexington Books.

Rando, T. (1993). *Treatment of complicated mourning.* Champaign, IL: Research Press.

Rando, T. (2000). *Clinical dimensions of anticipatory mourning: Theory and practice in working with the dying, their loved ones, and their caregivers.* Champaign, IL: Research Press.

Raus, K., Sterckx, S., & Mortier, F. (2011). Is continuous sedation at the end of life an ethically preferable alternative to physician assisted suicide? *American Journal of Bioethics, 11*(6), 32–40.

Reinhard, S., Given, B., Petlick, N., et al. (2008). Supporting family caregivers in providing support. In R. Hughes (Ed.), *Patient safety and quality: An evidence-based handbook for nurses* (Chapter 14). Rockville, MD: Agency for Healthcare Research and Quality. Retrieved April 25, 2013, from http://www.ncbi.nlm.nih.gov/books/NBK2665/

Riggs, D., & Willsmore, S. (2012). Experiences of disenfranchised grief from the unplanned termination of foster placement. *Adoption & Fostering, 36*(2), 57–66.

Robert Wood Johnson Foundation. (2012). Learning to learn. Retrieved April 17, 2013, from http://www.rwjf.org/en/about-rwjf/newsroom/newsroom-content/2012/05/learning-to-learn.html

Schwartz, J. (2003). Understanding and responding to patients' requests for assistance in dying. *Journal of Nursing Scholarship, 35*(4), 377–384.

Smith, M., Kerr, P., Galligan, H., et al. (2011). Elders' experiences of the death of an adult child. *Issues in Mental Health Nursing, 32*(9), 568–574.

Smith-Stoner, M., & Hand, M. (2012). Expanding the concept of patient care: Analysis of postmortem policies in California hospitals. *MedSurg Nursing, 21*(6), 360–366.

Songprakun, W., & McCann, T. (2012). Evaluation of a bibliotherapy manual for reducing psychological distress in people with depression: A randomized controlled trial. *Journal of Advanced Nursing, 68*(12), 2674–2684.

Stacy, K. (2012). Withdrawal of life-sustaining treatment: A case study. *Critical Care Nurse, 32*(3), 14–24.

Stroebe, M., Schut, H., & Van den Bout, J. (Eds.). (2013). *Complicated grief: Scientific foundations for health care professionals.* New York: Routledge.

Teno, J. M., Casey, V. A., Welch, L. C., et al. (2001). Patient-focused, family-centered end-of-life medical care: Views of the guidelines and bereaved family members. *Journal of Pain and Symptom Management, 22*, 738–751.

The Joint Commission (TJC). (2010). *Advancing effective communication, cultural competence, and patient-and family-centered care: A roadmap for hospitals.* Oakbrook Terrace, IL: Author.

The Joint Commission (TJC). (2013). *Hospital accreditation standards.* Oakbrook Terrace, IL: Author.

Theroux, P. (1997). *The book of eulogies: A collection of memorial tributes, poetry, essays, and letters of condolence.* New York: Scribner.

Traylor, E., Hayslip, B., Kaminski, P. L., et al. (2003). Relationships between grief and family system characteristics: A cross lagged longitudinal analysis. *Death Studies, 27*(7), 575–601.

U.S. Department of Health and Human Services. Dying, funerals & grief—by category. Retrieved May 30, 2013, from http://dying.about.com/od/livingafteradeath/ss/organdonate_3.htm

Valente, S. (2010). HIV, culture, and end-of-life issues. *JOCEPS: The Journal of Chi Eta Phi Sorority, 54*(1), 15–22.

Verheijde, J. L., Rady, M. Y., & McGregor, J. L. (2007). The United States Revised Uniform Anatomical Gift Act (2006), New challenges to balancing patient rights and physician responsibilities. *Philosophy, Ethics, and Humanities in Medicine.* Retrieved April 27, 2013, from http://www.ncbi.nlm.nih.gov/pmc/articles/PMC2001294/

Verheijde, J. L., Rady, M. Y., & McGregor, J. L. (2009). The Revised Uniform Anatomical Gift Act (2006) and constitutional civil rights in the United States. *Critical Care Medicine, 37*(5), 1830.

Von Gunten, C. F., Ferris, F. D., & Emanuel, L. L. (2000). Ensuring competency in end-of-life care: Communication and relational skills. *JAMA, 284*(23), 3051–3057.

Wakefield, J. (2012). Should prolonged grief be reclassified as a mental disorder in DSM-5? Reconsidering the empirical and conceptual arguments for complicated grief disorder. *Journal of Nervous & Mental Disease, 200*(6), 499–511.

Weissman, D., Quill, T., & Arnold, R. (2010). The family meeting: end of life goal setting and future planning. *Fast Facts and Concepts, No. 227.* Retrieved April 20, 2013, from http://www.eperc.mcw.edu/EPERC/FastFactsIndex/ff_227.htm

Wenzel, J., Shaha, M., & Klimmek, R. (2011). Working through grief and loss: Oncology nurses' perspectives on professional bereavement. *Oncology Nursing Forum, 38*(4), 272–282.

Widera, E., & Block, S. (2012). Managing grief and depression at the end of life. *American Family Physician, 86*(3), 259–264.

Wilson, F., Gott, M., & Ingleton, C. (2013). Perceived risks around choice and decision making at end-of-life: A literature review. *Palliative Medicine, 27*(1), 38–53.

Wittenberg-Lyles, E., Goldsmith, J., Oliver, D., et al. (2012). Targeting communication to decrease caregiver burden. *Seminars in Oncology Nursing, 28*(4), 262–270.

Worden, J. W. (2002). *Grief counseling and grief therapy: A handbook for the mental health practitioner* (3rd ed.). New York: Springer.

CHAPTER 18

American Nurses Association (ANA). (2010). *Nursing: Scope and standards of practice* (2nd ed.). Silver Spring, MD: Author.

AMNews. (2007, March 19). Hospital EMR not widespread yet. Retrieved June 1, 2013, from http://www.ama-assn.org/amednews/2007/03/19/bicb0319.htm

Barra, M., & Guttman, M. (2012). One less bell to answer: Improving clinical outcomes in an assisted living facility with bedside shift reports and hourly rounds. *UPNAAI Nursing Journal, 8*(1), 19–21, 23–26.

Blair, W., & Smith, B. (2012). Nursing documentation: frameworks and barriers. *Contemporary Nurse, 41*(2), 160–168.

Blank, L., Benyo, E., & Glover, J. (2012). Bridging the gap in transitional care: A closer look at medication reconciliation. *Geriatric Nursing, 33*(5), 401–409.

Blumenthal, D., & Tavenner, M. (2010). The "meaningful use" regulation for electronic health records. *The New England Journal of Medicine, 363*(6), 501–504.

Burke, W., & McLaughlin, D. (2013). Partnering for Change. *American Journal of Nursing, 113*(2), 47–51.

Cherry, B., Ford, E., & Peterson, L. (2011). Experiences with electronic health records: Early adopters in long-term care facilities. *Health Care Management Review, 36*(3), 265–274.

Children's Hospital of Wisconsin. (n.d.). SBARR basics. Retrieved June 4, 2013, from http://cupublic.chw.org/media/SBARR/sbarr_CHW_basics.htm

Currie, J. (2002). Improving the efficiency of patient handover. *Emergency Nurse, 10*(3), 24–28.

Collins, S., Stein, D., Vawdrey, D., et al. (2011) Content overlap in nurse and physician handoff artifacts and the potential role of electronic health records: A systematic review. *Journal of Biomedical Informatics, 44*(4), 704–712.

Dustin, C., Furukawa, M., & Hufstader, M. (2012). *Electronic health records systems and intent to attest to meaningful use among non-federal acute care hospitals in the United States: 2008–2011* (ONC Data Brief No. 1). Washington, DC: The Office of the National Coordinator for Health Information Technology, Retrievd June 3, 2013, from http://www.healthit.gov/media/pdf/ONC_Data_Brief_AHA_2011.pdf

Grbach, W., Vincent, L., & Struth, D. (2008). *Reformulating SBAR to "I-SBAR-R."* Washington, DC: QSEN Institute. Retrieved June 2, 2013, from http://qsen.org/reformulating-sbar-to-i-sbar-r/

Haig, K., Sutton, S., & Whittington, J. (2006). SBAR: A shared mental model for improving communication between clinicians. *Joint Commission Journal of Quality and Patient Safety, 32*(3), 167–175.

Hing, E., Burt, C., & Woodwell, D. (2006, October 26). *Electronic medical record use by office-based physicians and their practices: United States, 2006* (No. 393). Washington, DC: Centers for Disease Control Advance Data from Vital Health Statistics.

Hsiao, C., & Hing, E. (2012). *Use and characteristics of electronic health record systems among office-based physician practices: United States, 2001–2012* (NCHS Data Brief No. 111). Hyattsville, MD: National Center for Health Statistics. Retrieved June 3, 2013, from http://www.cdc.gov/nchs/data/databriefs/db111.htm

Huryk, L. (2010). Factors influencing nurses' attitudes toward healthcare information technology. *Journal of Nursing Management, 18*(5), 606–612.

The Joint Commission (TJC). (2008). *2008 hospital accreditation standards* (pp. 116–117). Oakbrook Terrace, IL: Author.

The Joint Commission (TJC). (2011). *2012 Comprehensive accreditation manual for hospitals: The official handbook.* Oak Brook, IL: The Joint Commission Resources.

The Joint Commission (TJC). (2012a). Facts about the official "Do Not Use" list of abbreviations. Retrieved June 7, 2013, from http://www.jointcommission.org/facts_about_the_official_/

The Joint Commission (TJC). (2012b). Joint Commission introduces new, customized tool to improve hand-off communications. *Joint Commission Online.* Retrieved June 1, 2013, from http://www.jointcommission.org/assets/1/23/jconline_June_27_12.pdf

The Joint Commission Center for Transforming Health Care. (2010; updated 2013, May). Improving transitions of care: hand-off communication. Retrieved June 3, 2013, from http://www.centerfortransforminghealthcare.org/assets/4/6/CTH_Hand-off_commun_set_final_2010.pdf

Kaiser Permanente of Colorado. (updated 2011, June 30). *SBAR technique for communication: A situational briefing model.* Cambridge, MA: Institute for Healthcare Improvement. Retrieved June 2, 2013, from http://www.ihi.org/IHI/Topics/PatientSafety/SafetyGeneral/Tools/SBARTechniquefor CommunicationASituationalBriefingModel.htm

Kerr, N. (2013). "Creating a protective picture": A grounded theory of RN decision making when using a charting-by-exception documentation system. *Medsurg Nursing, 22*(2), 110–118.

Kitch, B., Cooper, J., Zapol, W., et al. (2008). Handoffs causing patient harm: A survey of medical and surgical house staff. *The Joint Commission Journal on Quality and Patient Safety, 34*(10), 563–570.

Kohle-Ersher, A., Chatterjee, P., Osmanbeyoglu, H., et al. (2012). Evaluating the barriers to point-of-care documentation for nursing staff. *CIN: Computers, Informatics, Nursing, 30*(3), 126–133.

Kossman, S., & Scheidenhelm, S. (2008). Nurses' perceptions of the impact of electronic health records on work and patient outcomes. *CIN: Computers, Informatics, Nursing, 26*(2), 69–77.

Nelson, B., & Massey, R. (2010). Implementing an electronic change-of-shift report using transforming care at the bedside processes and methods. *Journal of Nursing Administration, 40*(4), 162–168.

Plemmons, S., Lipton, B. Fong, Y., et al. (2012). Measurable outcomes from standardized nursing documentation in an electronic health record. *ANIA-CARING Newsletter, 27*(2), 4–7.

Radtke, K. (2013). Improving patient satisfaction with nursing communication using bedside shift report. *Clinical Nurse Specialist: The Journal for Advanced Nursing Practice, 27*(1), 19–25.

Riesenberg, L., Leisch, J., & Cunningham, J. (2010). Nursing handoffs: A systematic review of the literature. *American Journal of Nursing, 110*(4), 24–34.

Schroeder, M. (2011). Looking to improve your bedside report? Try SBAR. *Nursing Made Incredibly Easy, 9*(5), 53–54.

Schroeder, S. (2006). Picking up the PACE: A new template for shift report. *Nursing2006, 36*(10), 22–23.

Spoerner, D. (2009). Check boxes are no substitute for narrative documentation. *American Journal of Critical Care, 18*(3), 192.

Triplett, P., & Schuveiller, C. (2011). Nurses' end-of-shift report process and implementation of a standardized report format tool and bedside handoff. *Critical Care Nurse, 31*(2), 43–44.

U.S. Department of Health and Human Services, Centers for Medicare & Medicaid Services. (updated 2012, February 27). Long term care minimum data sets (MDS). Retrieved June 7, 2013, from http://www.cms.gov/Research-Statistics-Data-and-Systems/Files-for-Order/IdentifiableDataFiles/LongTermCareMinimumDataSetMDS.html

U.S. Department of Health and Human Services, Centers for Medicare & Medicaid Services. (updated 2012, April 5). Outcome and Assessment Information Set (OASIS). Retrieved June 7, 2013, from http://www.cms.gov/Medicare/Quality-Initiatives-Patient-Assessment-Instruments/OASIS/index.html?redirect=/oasis/

Wakefield, D., Wakefield, B., Despins, L., et al. (2012). A review of verbal order policies in acute care hospitals. *The Joint Commission Journal on Quality & Patient Safety, 38*(1), 11–22.

Wang, N., Hailey, D., & Yu, P. (2011). Quality of nursing documentation and approaches to its evaluation: A mixed-method systematic review. *Journal of Advanced Nursing, 67*(9), 1858–1875.

Yee, T., Needleman, J., Pearson, M., et al. (2012). The influence of integrated electronic medical records and computerized nursing notes on nurses' time spent in documentation. *Computers, Informatics, Nursing, 30*(6), 287–292.

CHAPTER 19

Alsbaugh, L. (n.d.). A guide for nurses: Teaching healthcare effectively to patients. *Health Careers Journal.* Retrieved October 26, 2014, from http://www.healthcareersjournal.com/a-guide-for-nurses-teaching-healthcare-effectively-to-patients/

American Academy of Ambulatory Care Nursing. (n.d.). Guidelines for developing patient education materials. Retrieved October 26, 2014 from http://www.aaacn.org/guidelines-developing-patient-education-materials

American Hospital Association. (2003). *The patient care partnership.* Chicago, IL: Author. Retrieved October 26, 2014, from http://www.aha.org/aha/issues/Communicating-With-Patients/pt-care-partnership.html

American Nurses Association (ANA). (2001). *Code of ethics for nurses with interpretive statements.* Washington, DC: American Nurses Publishing. Retrieved August, 8, 2013, from http://www.nursingworld.org/MainMenuCategories/ThePracticeofProfessionalNursing/EthicsStandards/CodeofEthics.aspx

American Nurses Association (ANA). (2010). *Nursing: Scope and standards of practice* (2nd ed.) [Public comment draft, January 2010]. Silver Spring, MD: Nursebooks.org.

Badarudeen, S., & Sabharwal, S. (2010). Assessing readability of patient education materials: Current role in orthopaedics. *Clinical Orthopedic & Related Research, 468*(10), 2572–2580.

Bastable, S. B. (2014). *Nurse as educator: Principles of teaching and learning for nursing practice* (4th ed.). Boston: Jones & Bartlett.

Berkman, N. D., Sheridan, S. L., Donahue, K. E., et al. (2011). *Health literacy interventions and outcomes: An updated systematic review* (Evidence Report/Technology Assessment No. 199. [Prepared by RTI International—University of North Carolina Evidence-based Practice Center under Contract No. 290-2007-10056-I]; AHRQ Publication No. 11-E006). Rockville, MD: Agency for Healthcare Research and Quality. Retrieved August 10, 2013, from http://www.ahrq.gov/research/findings/evidence-based-reports/er199-abstract.htm

Bloom B. S., & Krathwohl, D. R. (1956). Taxonomy of educational objectives: The classification of educational goals. In *Handbook I: Cognitive domain.* New York: Longmans, Green.

Bloom, B. S., Mesia, B. B., & Krathwohl, D. R. (1964). Taxonomy of educational objectives (Vol. 1: *The Affective Domain* and Vol. 2: *The Cognitive Domain*). New York: David McKay.

Boston University School of Public Health. (last updated 2013, January). Health belief model. Retrieved August 12, 2013, from http://sph.bu.edu/otlt/MPH-Modules/SB/SB721-Models/SB721-Models2.html

Bridge, P. D., Jackson, M., & Robinson, L. (2009). The effectiveness of streaming video on medical student learning: A case study. *Medical Education Online, 14*, 11. doi: 10.3885/meo.2009.Res00311

Bulechek, G., Butcher, H., Dochterman, J. M., & Wagner, C. (2013). *Nursing intervention classification (NIC)* (6th ed.). St. Louis, MO: C. V. Mosby.

Deniard-Thompson, N. R., Steven, S. S., & Wofford, J. L. (2012). iPodTM technology for teaching patients about anticoagulation: A pilot study of mobile computer-assisted patient education. *Primary Health Care Research and Development, 13*(1), 42–47. doi:10.1017/S146342361100034X

Dickens, C., & Piano, M. R. (2013). Health literacy and nursing: An update. *American Journal of Nursing, 113*(6), 52–57. doi:10.1097/01.NAJ.0000431271.83277.2f

Edutopia. (2011, September). Twenty tips for creating a safe learning environment. Retrieved October 26, 2014, from http://www.edutopia.org/blog/20-tips-create-safe-learning-environment-rebecca-alber

Free, C., Phillips, G., Galli, L., et al. (2013). The effectiveness of mobile-health technology-based health behavior change or disease management interventions for health care consumers: A systematic review. *PLoS, 10*, e1001363. doi: 10.1371/journal.pmed.1001362

Hain, D., & Sandy, D. (2013). Partners in care: Patient empowerment through shared decision-making. *Nephrology Nursing Journal, 40*(2), 153–157.

Hoffman, J., Salzman, C., Garbaccio, C., et al. (2011). Use of on-demand video to provide patient education on spinal cord injury. *The Journal of Spinal Cord Medicine, 34*(4), 404–409. doi:10.1179/2045772311Y.0000000015

Jarrell, K., Alpers, R., & Wotring, R. (2011). Is knowledge deficit helpful or hindering nursing diagnosis? *Teaching and Learning in Nursing, 6*(2), 89–91. doi: http://dx.doi.org/10.1016/j.teln.2011.02.002

The Joint Commission. (2007). What did the doctor say? Improving health literacy to protect patient safety. Retrieved October 26, 2014, from http://www.jointcommission.org/What_Did_the_Doctor_Say/

The Joint Commission. (2010). *Advancing effective communication, cultural competence, and patient and family-centered care: A roadmap for hospitals.* Oak Brook, IL: Author. Retrieved October 26, 2014, from http://www.jointcommission.org/assets/1/6/ARoadmapforHospitalsfinalversion727.pdf

The Joint Commission. (2013). *Hospital accreditation standards, 2014.* Oak Brook, IL: Author.

Kessels, R. C. (2003). Patient's memory for medical information. *Journal of the Royal Society of Medicine, 96*(5), 219–222.

Krathwohl, D. R. (2002, Autumn). A revision of Bloom's taxonomy: An overview. *Theory Into Practice, 41*(4), 212–224. doi:10.1207/s15430421tip4104_2

London, F. (1999). *No time to teach*. Philadelphia: Lippincott.

Mitchell, S. E., Sadikova, E., Jack, B. W., et al. (2012). Health literacy and 30-day postdischarge hospital utilization. *Journal of Health Community, 17*(Suppl. 3), 325–338. doi: 10.1080/10810730.2012.715233

Moorhead, S., Johnson, M., Maas, M., & Swanson, E. (Eds.). (2013). *Nursing outcomes classification (NOC)* (5th ed.). St. Louis, MO: C. V. Mosby.

Muilenburg, L. Y., & Bergeb, Z. L. (2005). Student barriers to online learning: A factor analytic study. *Distance Education, 26*(1), 29–48. doi:10.1080/01587910500081269

Murray, M. D., Tu, W., Wu, J., et al. (2009). Factors associated with exacerbation of heart failure include treatment adherence and health literacy skills. *Clinical Pharmacologic Therapy, 85*(6), 651–658. doi: 10.1038/clpt.2009.7

NANDA International. (2012). *NANDA nursing diagnoses: Definitions and classification 2012–2014*. Philadelphia: Author.

National Network of Libraries of Medicine. (2008). Health literacy. Retrieved October 26, 2014 from http://nnlm.gov/outreach/consumer/hlthlit.html

Nielsen-Bohlman, L., Panzer, A. M., & Kindig, D. A.; Institute of Medicine of the National Academies (Eds.). (2004). *Health literacy: A prescription to end confusion*. Washington, DC: Institute of Medicine of the National Academies.

Nightingale, F. (1860/1992). *Notes on nursing: What it is and what it is not*. Philadelphia: Lippincott.

Osborn, C. Y., Paasche-Orlow, M. K., Bailey, S. C, et al. (2011). The mechanisms linking health literacy to behavior and health status. *American Journal of Health Behavior, 35*(1), 118–128.

Piaget, J. (1966). *Origins of intelligence in children*. New York: W. W. Norton.

Primeau, K., & Frith, K. (2013). Teaching patients with an intellectual disability. *Nursing2013, 43*(6), 68–69. doi: 10.1097/01.NURSE.0000429798.26483.2d

Ratzan, S. C., & Parker, R. M. (2000). Introduction. In C. R. Selden, M. Zorn, R. M. Ratzan, & S. C. Parker (Eds.), *National Library of Medicine current bibliographies in medicine: Health literacy* (Vol. NLM Publication No. CBM 2000-1). Bethesda, MD: National Institutes of Health, U.S. Department of Health and Human Services.

Sarkar, U., Karter, A., Liu, J., et al. (2010). The literacy divide: Health literacy and the use of an internet-based patient portal in an integrated health system—results from the Diabetes Study of Northern California (DISTANCE). *Journal of Health Communication: International, 15*(Suppl. 2), 183–196. doi: 10.1080/10810730.2010.499988

Tucker, J. M., Welk, G. J., & Beyler, N. K. (2011). Physical activity in U.S.: Adults' compliance with the Physical Activity Guidelines for Americans. *American Journal of Preventive Medicine, 40*(4), 454–461. doi:10.1016/j.amepre.2010.12.016.

U.S. Census Bureau. (2010). New census bureau report analyzes nation's linguistic diversity. *Newsroom*. Retrieved October 26, 2014, from http://www.census.gov/newsroom/releases/archives/american_community_survey_acs/cb10-cn58.html

U.S. Department of Health and Human Services, National Institutes of Health. (2013, February 13, updated). How to write easy-to-read health materials. *MedlinePlus*. Retrieved October 26, 2014, from http://www.nlm.nih.gov/medlineplus/etr.html

Wilson, E. A., Makoul, G., Bojarski, E. A., et al. (2012). A comparative analysis of print and multimedia health materials: A review of the literature. *Patient Education and Counseling, 89*, 7–14. http://dx.doi.org/10.1016/j.pec.2012.06.007

CHAPTER 20

Alexis, O. (2010). Providing best practice in manual pulse measurement. *British Journal of Nursing, 19*(4), 228–234.

American Association of Critical-Care Nurses (AACN). (2010). *AACN practice alert. Noninvasive blood pressure monitoring*. Retrieved October 26, 2014, from http://www.aacn.org/wd/practice/content/nibp-practice-alert.pcms?menu=practice

American Heart Association (AHA). (n.d.). High blood pressure. Retrieved October 26, 2014, from http://www.heart.org/HEARTORG/Conditions/HighBloodPressure/HighBloodPressureToolsResources/High-Blood-Pressure-Tools-Resources_UCM_002055_Article.jsp

American Heart Association (AHA). (2012). Home blood pressure monitoring. Retrieved October 26, 2014, from http://www.heart.org/HEARTORG/Conditions/HighBloodPressure/SymptomsDiagnosisMonitoringofHighBloodPressure/Home-Blood-PressureMonitoring_UCM_301874_Article.jsp

Amoore, D. (2010). Best practice in the measurement of body temperature. *Nursing Standard, 24*(42), 42–49. http://dx.doi.org/10.7748/ns2010.06.24.42.42.c7850

Aprahamian, N., Lee, L., Shannon, M., et al. (2009). Glass thermometer injuries: It is not just about the mercury. *Pediatric Emergency Care, 25*(10), 645–647. doi: 10.1097/PEC.0b013e3181b920cc

Barnason, S., Williams, J., Proehl, J., et al. (2012). Emergency nursing resource: Non-invasive temperature measurement in the emergency department. *Journal of Emergency Nursing, 38*(6), 523–530. doi: http://dx.doi.org/10.1016/j.jen.2012.05.012

Beard, R., & Day, M. W. (2008). Fever & hyperthermia. Learn to beat the heat. *Nursing2008, 38*(6), 28–31. doi: 10.1097/01.NURSE.0000320353.79079.a5

Bern, L., Brandt, M., & Mbelu, N. (2007). Differences in blood pressure values obtained with automated and manual methods in medical inpatients. *MedSurg Nursing, 16*(6), 356–361.

Best practices: Evidence-based nursing procedures (2nd ed., pp. 59–62). (2007). Philadelphia: Lippincott Williams & Wilkins.

British Hypertension Society, Hypertension Influence Team. (2006). *"Let's do it well" nurse learning pack*. Retrieved October 26, 2014, from http://www.bhsoc.org/pdfs/hit.pdf

Brook, R., Appel, L., Rubenfire, M., et al. (2013). AHA scientific statement. Beyond medications and diet: Alternative approaches to lowering blood pressure. *Hypertension, 61*(6), 1360–1383. doi: 10.1161/HYP.0b013e318293645f

Burke, L. (2010). Postoperative fever: A normal inflammatory response or cause for concern. *Journal of the Academy of Nurse Practitioners, 22*(4), 192–197. doi: 10.1111/j.1745-7599.2010.00492.x

Carlson, D., & White, T. (2012). Action STAT: Malignant hyperthermia. *Nursing2012, 42*(10), 72. doi: 10.1097/01.NURSE.0000419443.98792.4e

Centers for Disease Control and Prevention (CDC). (2006). Hypothermia-related deaths—United States, 1999–2002 and 2005. *Morbidity and Mortality Weekly Report, 55*(10), 282–284. Retrieved December 20, 2012, from http://www.cdc.gov/mmwr/preview/mmwrhtml/mm5510a5.htm

Centers for Disease Control and Prevention (CDC). (2008). Guideline for disinfection and sterilization in healthcare facilities, 2008. Retrieved November 28, 2012, from http://www.cdc.gov/hicpac/pdf/guidelines/Disinfection_Nov_2008.pdf

Centers for Disease Control and Prevention (CDC). (2010a). NIOSH fast facts: Protecting yourself from cold stress. Retrieved December 20, 2012, from http://www.cdc.gov/niosh/docs/2010-115/

Centers for Disease Control and Prevention (CDC). (2010b). NIOSH fast facts: Protecting yourself from heat stroke. Retrieved December 20, 2012, from http://www.cdc.gov/niosh/docs/2010-114/

Centers for Disease Control and Prevention (CDC). (2012). High blood pressure facts. Retrieved January 3, 2012, from http://www.cdc.gov/bloodpressure/facts.htm

Chester, J., & Rudolph, J. (2011). Vital signs in older patients: Age-related changes. *Journal of American Medical Directors Association, 12*(5), 337–343.

Cincinnati Children's Hospital Medical Center. (2011). *Best evidence statement (BESt). Axillary temperature taking tools: The evidence for change*. Cincinnati, OH: Author. Retrieved December 26, 2012, from http://guidelines.gov/content.aspx?id=33574

Davis, R. (2012). The big chill: Accidental hypothermia. *American Journal of Nursing, 112*(1), 38–39.

DeCurtis, M., Calzolari, F., Marciano, A., et al. (2008). Comparison between rectal and infrared skin temperature in the newborn. *Archives of Disease in Childhood—Fetal and Neonatal Edition, 93*, F55–F57.

Dourmap, C., Girerd, X., Marquand, A., et al. (2010). Systolic blood pressure is depending [*sic*] on the arm position when home blood pressure is measured with a wrist or an arm validated monitor. *Blood Pressure Monitoring, 15*(4), 181–183.

Dusek, J., Hibberd, P., Buczynski, B., et al. (2008). Stress management versus lifestyle modification on systolic hypertension and medication elimination: A randomized trial. *The Journal of Alternate and Complimentary Medicine, 14*(2), 129–138.

Elliott, M., & Coventry, A. (2012). Critical care: The eight vital signs of patient monitoring. *British Journal of Nursing, 21*(10), 621–625. Retrieved February 24, 2014, from http://publicationslist.org/data/m.elliott/ref-22/The%20eight%20vital%20signs%20of%20patient%20monitoring.pdf

Fadzil, F., Choon, D., & Arumugam, K. (2010). A comparative study on the accuracy of noninvasive thermometers. *Australian Family Physician, 39*(4), 237–239.

Farnell, S., Maxwell, L., Tan, S., et al. (2005). Temperature measurement: Comparison of non-invasive methods used in adult critical care. *Journal of Clinical Nursing, 14*(5), 632–639.

Frommelt, T., Ott, C., & Hays, V. (2008). Accuracy of different devices to measure temperature. *MedSurg Nursing, 17*(3), 171–182.

Garlsl, A. (2012). Unmonitored vital signs: disaster waiting to happen. *ED Legal Letter, 23*(6), 66–67.

Gomolin, I. H., Aung, M. M., Wolf-Klein, G., et al. (2005). Older is colder: Temperature range and variation in older people. *Journal of the American Geriatrics Society, 53*(12), 2170–2172.

Hebbar, K., Fortenberry, J., Rogers, K., et al. (2005). Comparison of temporal artery temperature measurements in pediatric intensive care unit patients. *Pediatric Critical Care Medicine, 6*(5), 557–561.

Helton, W., & Carter, J. (2011). The effect of investigator gender on lateral tympanic membrane temperature. *Laterality, 19*(2), 156–163.

Heusch, A. I., & McCarthy, P. W. (2005). The patient: A novel source of error in clinical temperature measurement using infrared aural thermometry. *Journal of Alternative & Complementary Medicine, 11*(3), 473–476.

Hwu, Y. J., Coates, V. E., & Lin, F. Y. (2000). A study of the effectiveness of different measuring times and counting methods of human radial pulse rates. *Journal of Clinical Nursing, 9*(1), 146–152.

Johnson, M., Bulechek, G., Butcher, H., et al. (2006). *Nursing diagnoses, outcomes, and interventions: NANDA, NIC, and NOC linkages* (2nd ed.). St. Louis, MO: C. V. Mosby.

Joint National Committee on Prevention, Detection, Evaluation, and Treatment of High Blood Pressure. (2004). *JNC 7 complete report. The seventh report of the Joint National Committee on Prevention, Detection, Evaluation, and Treatment of High Blood Pressure*. Bethesda, MD: National Institutes of Health. Retrieved December 20, 2012, from http://www.nhlbi.nih.gov/guidelines/hypertension/index.htm

Jordan, C., Yoder, B., Yuen, T., et al. (2013). A propective study of nighttime vital sign monitoring frequency and risk of clinical deterioration. *JAMA Internal Medicine*. doi:10.1001/jamainternmed.2013.7791. Retrieved July 30, 2013, from http://archinte.jamanetwork.com/article.aspx?articleid=1705722.

Keller, D. (2011). Antihypertensives at night cut cardiovascular risk best. *Medscape Medical News*. Retrieved January 11, 2013, from http://www.medscape.com/viewarticle/745516

Kennedy, S. (2007). Detecting changes in the respiratory status of ward patients. *Nursing Standard, 21*(49), 42–46.

Kennedy, K. J., Dreimanis, D. E., Beckingham, W. D., et al. (2003). Letters. *Staphylococcus aureus* and stethoscopes. *The Medical Journal of Australia, 178*(9), 468.

Kiekkas, P., Brokalaki, H., Theodorakopoulou, G., & Baltopoulos, G. I. (2008). Physical antipyresis in critically ill adults. *American Journal of Nursing, 108*(7), 40–50.

Lance, R., Link, M. E., Padua, M., et al. (2000). Comparison of different methods of obtaining orthostatic vital signs. *Clinical Nursing Research, 9*(4), 479–491.

Lange, J. (2012). *The nurse's role in promoting optimal health of older adults: Thriving in the wisdom years*. Philadelphia: F. A. Davis.

Lawson, L., Bridges, E. J., Ballou, I., et al. (2007). Accuracy and precision of noninvasive temperature measurement in adult intensive care patients. *American Journal of Critical Care, 16*(5), 485–496.

Lewis, A. M. (2007). Heatstroke in older adults. *American Journal of Nursing, 107*(6), 52–56.

Lockwood, C., Conroy-Hiller, T., & Page, T. (2004). Vital signs. *JBI Database of Systematic Reviews* (ID No. SR0115). Retrieved December 12, 2012, from http://onlinelibrary.wiley.com/doi/10.1111/j.1479-6988.2004.00012.x/abstract

Lowdermilk, D., Perry, S., Cashion, K., et al. (2012). *Maternity & women's health care* (10th ed.). St. Louis, MO: Elsevier.

Lu, S. H., & Dai, Y. T. (2009). Normal body temperature and the effects of age, sex, ambient temperature and body mass index on normal oral temperature: A prospective, comparative study. *International Journal of Nursing Studies, 46*, 661–668.

Ma, G., Sabin, N., & Dawes, M. A. (2008). A comparison of blood pressure measurement over a sleeved arm versus a bare arm. *Canadian Medical Association Journal, 178*(5), 585–589.

Mackowiak, P. A. (1998). Concepts of fever. *Archives of Internal Medicine, 158*(17), 1870–1881.

McCance, K. L., & Huether, S. E. (2010). *Pathophysiology: The biologic basis for disease in adults and children* (6th ed.). St. Louis, MO: C. V. Mosby.

McKay, D. W. (2008). Measuring blood pressure: A call to bare arms? *Canadian Medical Association Journal, 178*(5), 591–592.

Mercury-Free Health Care. (n.d.). Retrieved December 12, 2012, from http://www.mercuryfreehealthcare.org

Mininni, N., Mario, M., Kohler, W., et al. (2009). Pulse oximetry: An essential tool for the busy med-surg nurse; Faced with higher-acuity patients, med-surg nurses increasingly turn to pulse oximetry to detect deterioration early. *American Nurse Today, 4*(9), 31–33.

Mitchell, A., DeAlwis, N., Collins, J., et al. (2012). Stethoscope or 'Staphoscope'? *Journal of Hospital Infection, 76*(3), 278–279.

Mitchell-Brown, T. (2012). Malignant hyperthermia: Turn down the heat. *Nursing2012, 42*(5), 38–45.

Morton, P., & Rempher, K. (2009). Patient assessment: respiratory system. In P. Morton & D. Fontaine (Eds.), *Critical care nursing: A holistic approach*. Philadelphia: Lippincott.

Naccarato, M., Leviner, S., Proehl, J., et al. (2012). Emergency nursing resource: Orthostatic vital signs. *Journal of Emergency Room Nursing, 38*(5), 447–453.

NANDA International. (2009). *Nursing diagnoses: Definitions and classification 2009–2011*. Philadelphia: Author.

National Heart, Lung, and Blood Institute (NHLBI). (1996; revised 2005). *The fourth report on the diagnosis, evaluation, and treatment of high blood pressure in children and adolescents* (NIH Publication No. 05-5267). Washington, DC: U.S. Department of Health and Human Services. Retrieved December 20, 2012, from http://www.nhlbi.nih.gov/health/prof/heart/hbp/hbp_ped.pdf

National Heart, Lung, and Blood Institute (NHLBI). (2007). *A pocket guide to blood pressure measurement in children*. Washington, DC: National High Blood Pressure Education Program Working Group on High Blood Pressure in Children and Adolescents. National Institutes of Health. Retrieved December 20, 2012, from http://www.nhlbi.nih.gov/health/public/heart/hbp/bp_child_pocket/bp_child_pocket.pdf

National Institute of Health. (2011). *Genes that influence blood pressure*. Retrieved January 10, 2013, from http://www.nih.gov/researchmatters/september2011/09262011genes.htm

Nelson, D., Kennedy, B., Regnerus, C., et al. (2008). Accuracy of automated blood pressure monitors. *Journal of Dental Hygiene, 82*(4), 35.

Paes, B., Vermeulen, K., Brohet, R., et al. (2010). Accuracy of tympanic and infrared skin thermometers in children. *Archives of Disease in Childhood, 95*(12), 974–978.

Parkes, R. (2011). Rate of respiration: The forgotten vital sign. *Emergency Nurse, 19*(2), 12–18.

Perk, G., Stessman, J., Ginsberg, G., et al. (2003). Sex differences in the effect of heart rate on mortality in the elderly. *Journal of the American Geriatrics Society, 51*(9), 1260–1264.

Perloff, D., Grim, C., Flack, J., et al. (1993). *Human blood pressure determination by sphygmomanometry* (AHA Medical/Scientific Statement, Product Code: 88:2460–67). Dallas: American Heart Association.

Pickering, T., Hall, J., Appel, L., et al. (2005). Recommendations for blood pressure measurement in humans and experimental animals: Part 1: Blood pressure measurement in humans: A statement for professionals from the subcommittee of Professional and Public Education of the American Heart Association Council on High Blood Pressure Research. *Hypertension, 45*(1), 142–161.

Pinar, R., Ataalkin, S., & Watson, R. (1020). The effect of clothes on sphygmomanometric blood pressure measurement in hypertensive patients. *Journal of Clinical Nursing, 19*(13–14), 1861–1864. doi:10.1111/j.1365-2702.2010.03224.x

Polderman, K. (2009). Mechanisms of actions, physiological effects and complications of hypothermia. *Critical Care Medicine, 37*(Suppl. 7), S186–S202.

Pullen, R. (2010). Clinical queries. Using pulse oximetry accurately. *Nursing, 40*(4), 63.

Quatrara, B., Coffman, Z., Jenkins, T., et al. (2007). The effect of respiratory rate and ingestion of hot and cold beverages on the accuracy of oral temperatures measured by electronic thermometers. *MedSurg Nursing, 16*(2), 105–108.

Rabinowitz, R. P., Cookson, S. T., Wasserman, S. S., et al. (1996). Effects of anatomic site, oral stimulation, and body position on estimates of body temperature. *Archives of Internal Medicine, 156*(7), 777–780.

Ransome, S. (2005). Measuring BP at home. *British Journal of Primary Care Nursing, 2*(1), 48–49.

Rhinehart, E. (2001). Infection control in home care. *Emerging Infectious Diseases, 7*(2). Retrieved January 9, 2013, from http://www.cdc.gov/ncidod/eid/vol7no2/rhinehart.htm

Robinson, J. L., Jou, H., & Spady, D. W. (2005). Accuracy of parents in measuring body temperature with a tympanic thermometer. *Family Practice, 6*(1), 3.

Rothemich, S., Woolf, S., Johnson, R., et al. (2008). Effect on cessation counseling of documenting smoking status as a routine vital sign: An ACORN study. *Annals of Family Medicine, 6*(1), 60–68.

Ruppar, T., Dobbels, F., & Geest, S. (2012). Medication beliefs and antihypertensive adherence among older adults: A pilot study. *Geriatric Nursing, 33*(2), 89–95.

Russell, A., Secrest, J., & Schreeder, D. (2012). Stethoscopes as a source of hospital-acquired methicillin-resistant *Staphylococcus aureus*. *Journal of PeriAnesthesia Nursing, 27*(2), 82–87.

Rutala, W. A., & Weber, D. J. (2004). Disinfection and sterilization in health care facilities: What clinicians need to know. *Clinical Infectious Diseases, 39*, 702–709.

Schulman, C., & Staul, L. (2010). Standards for frequency of measurement and documentation of vital signs and physical assessments. *Critical Care Nurse, 30*(3), 74–76.

Siegel, J. D., Rhinehart, E., Jackson, M., et al. (2007). 2007 Guideline for isolation precautions: Preventing transmission of infectious agents in healthcare settings. Retrieved December 20, 2012, from http://www.cdc.gov/hicpac/pdf/isolation/isolation2007.pdf

Shindler, D. (2007). Practical cardiac auscultation. *Critical Care Quarterly, 30*(2), 166–180.

Smitherman, L., Janise, J., & Mathur, A. (2005). The use of folk remedies among children in an urban black community: Remedies for fever, colic, and teething. *Pediatrics, 115*(3), 297–304.

Sund-Levander, M., Forsberg, C., & Wahren, L. K. (2002). Normal oral, rectal, tympanic and axillary body temperature in adult men and women: A systematic literature review. *Scandinavian Journal of Caring Sciences, 16*(2), 122–128.

Sund-Levander, M., Grodzinsky, E., Loyd, D., et al. (2004). Errors in body temperature assessment related to individual variation, measuring technique and equipment. *International Journal of Nursing Practice, 10*(5), 216–223.

The Joint Commission. (2011). The fifth vital sign: Complying with pain management standard PC.01.02.07. *The Source, 9*(11), 1, 8–10.

Therapeutic Research Center. (2007). Thermometer comparison. *Healthcare Professional Information, 23*(231006). Stockton, CA: Author. Retrieved December 19, 2012, from http://pharmacistsletter.therapeuticresearch.com/pl/Browse.aspx?pt=6&fpt=31&dd=231006&pb=PL&cat=5719

Thompson, H., & Kagan, S. (2011). Clinical management of fever by nurses: Doing what works. *Journal of Advanced Nursing, 67*(2), 359–370.

Tomlinson, B. (2010). Accurately measuring blood pressure: Factors that contribute to false measurements. *Medsurg Nursing, 19*(2), 90–95.

Trim, J. (2005). Monitoring pulse. *Nursing Times, 101*(21), 30–31.

Turner, M., Burns, S. M., Chaney, C., et al. (2008). Measuring blood pressure accurately in an ambulatory cardiology clinic setting: Do patient position and timing really matter? *MedSurg Nursing, 17*(2), 93–98.

U.S. Department of Health and Human Services, Agency of Healthcare Research and Quality (AHRQ). (2008). *Patient safety and quality: An evidence-based handbook for nurses* (AHRQ Publication No. 08-0043). Retrieved January 3, 2013, from http://www.ahrq.gov/qual/nurseshdbk/

U.S. Environmental Protection Agency (EPA). (2001). Memorandum of understanding between the American Hospital Association & the U.S. Environmental Protection Agency. Retrieved January 10, 2013, from http://www.epa.gov/pbt/pubs/mou_news.pdf

U.S. Environmental Protection Agency (EPA). (2012). *Mercury recommended management and disposal options for mercury-containing products.* Retrieved November 12, 2012, from http://www.epa.gov/hg/mgmt_options.html#t2c11

Vital signs. (1999). *Best Practice, 3*(3), 1–6. Retrieved December 18, 2012, from http://connect.jbiconnectplus.org/ViewSourceFile.aspx?0=4309

Wall, R. (2009). Cleaning stethoscopes with ethanol-based cleaner vs isopropyl alcohol: Which is better? *Critical Care Alert, 17*(6), 42–43.

Washington, G. T., & Matney, J. L. (2008). Comparison of temperature measurement devices in post anesthesia patients. *Journal of PeriAnesthesia Nursing, 23*(1), 36–48.

Wood, M., Lund, R., & Stevenson, K. (2007). Bacterial contamination of stethoscopes with antimicrobial diaphragm covers. *American Journal of Infection Control, 35*(4), 263–266.

Worcester Polytechnic Institute (WPI). (2012). WPI awarded $1.9 million to develop sensors that can save wounded soldiers. Retrieved November 20, 2012, from http://www.wpi.edu/news/20123/armygrant.html

Wunderlich, C. A. (1871). *On the temperature in diseases* (2nd ed.). W. Bathurst Woodman (Trans.). London: The New Sydenham Society. Retrieved November 21, 2012, from http://books.google.com/books/about/On_the_Temperature_in_diseases.html?id=3-wHAAAAIAAJ

Zeng, W., Huang, F., Sheng, C., et al. (2012). Validation of the Kingyield BP210 wrist blood pressure monitor for home blood pressure monitoring according to the European Society of Hypertension-International Protocol. *Blood Pressure Monitoring, 17*(1), 42–44.

CHAPTER 21

Alpers, R. R., Jarrell, K., & Roxena, W. (2013). Is caring really teachable? *Teaching and Learning, 8*(2), 68–69. doi: http://dx.doi.org/10.1016/j.teln.2013.01.001

Alzheimer's Society. (2012, July). Communicating. Retrieved May 6, 2013, from http://www.alzheimers.org.uk/site/scripts/documents_info.php?documentID=130

Amer, K. (2013). *Quality and safety for transformational nursing. Core competencies.* Upper Saddle River, NJ: Pearson.

American Association of Critical-Care Nurses (AACN). (2005). *AACN standards for establishing and sustaining healthy work environment: A journey to excellence.* Aliso Viejo, CA: Author. Retrieved February 4, 2014, from http://www.aacn.org/WD/HWE/Docs/HWEStandards.pdf

American Heart Association. (2012). How should I communicate with heart and stroke patients? *Answers by Heart.* Retrieved October 26, 2014, from http://www.heart.org/idc/groups/heart-public/@wcm/@hcm/documents/downloadable/ucm_300665.pdf

American Nurses Association. (ANA). (2010). *Nursing: Scope and standards of practice* (2nd ed.). Silver Spring, MD: Nursebooks.org

American Speech-Language-Hearing Association. (n.d.). Information for AAC users. Retrieved October 26, 2014, from http://www.asha.org/public/speech/disorders/InfoAACUsers/

Benner, P. (1984). *From novice to expert. Excellence and power in clinical nursing practice.* Menlo Park, CA: Addison-Wesley.

Bulechek, G., Butcher, H., & Dochterman, J. (Eds.). (2012). *Nursing interventions classification (NIC)* (6th ed.). St. Louis, MO: C. V. Mosby.

Chapman, K. B. (2009). Improving communication among nurses, patients, and physicians. *American Journal of Nursing, 109*(11), 21–25. doi: 10.1097/01.NAJ.0000362013.53342.17

Cousin, G., Mast, M. S., Roter, D., et al. (2012). Concordance between physician communication style and patient attitudes predicts patient satisfaction. *Patient Education and Counseling, 87*(2), 193–197. doi: http://dx.doi.org/10.1016/j.pec.2011.08.004

Cronenwett, L., Sherwood, G., Barnsteiner, J., et al. (2007). Quality and safety education for nurses. *Nursing Outlook, 55*(3), 122–131. doi: http://dx.doi.org/10.1016/j.outlook.2007.02.006

De Meester, K., Verspuy, M., Monsiers, K. G., et al. (2013). SBAR improves nurse-physician communication and reduces unexpected death: A pre and post intervention study. *Resuscitation, 84*(9),1192–6. doi:10.1016/j.resuscitation.2013.03.016

Engel, M. (2006). *The other end of the stethoscope—33 insights for excellent patient care.* Orlando, FL: Ella Press.

Garon, M. (2012). Speaking up, being heard: Registered nurses' perception of workplace communication. *Journal of Nursing Management, 20*(3), 361–371. doi: 10.1111/j.1365-2834.2011.01296.x

Griffiths, J., Speed, S., & Keeley, P. (2012). A caring professional attitude: What service users and carers seek in graduate nurses and the challenge for educators. *Nurse Education Today, 32*(2), 121–127. doi: 10.1016/j.nedt.2011.06.005

Haig, K. M., Sutton, S., & Whittington, J. (2006). National Patient Safety Goals. SBAR: A shared mental model for improving communication between clinicians. *Joint Commission Journal on Quality and Patient Safety, 32*(3), 167–175.

Hall, E. T. (1992). *The hidden dimension*. Gloucester, MA: Peter Smith.

Hall, K. (2011). Professional boundaries: Building a trusting relationship with patients. *Home Healthcare Nurse, 29*(4), 210–217.

Hanna, A., & Suplee, P. (2012). Don't cross the line. Respecting professional boundaries. *Nursing2012, 42*(9), 40–48. doi: 10.1097/01.NURSE.0000419445.29116.e1

Holder, K., & Schenthal, S. (2007). Watch your step: Nursing and professional boundaries. *Nursing Management, 38*(2), 24–29.

The Joanna Briggs Institute. (2011). Effective communication between registered nurses and adult oncology patients in inpatient settings. *Best Practice, 15*(1), 1–4.

Johnson, M., Moorhead, S., Bulechek, G., et al. (2012). *Nursing diagnoses, outcomes, & interventions: NANDA, NOC, and NIC linkages* (3rd ed.). St. Louis, MO: Mosby.

The Joint Commission (TJC). (2010a). *Advancing effective communication, cultural competence, and family-centered care: A roadmap for hospitals*. Retrieved October 26, 2014, from http://www.jointcommission.org/assets/1/6/ARoadmapforHospitalsfinalversion727.pdf

The Joint Commission. (2010b). *Patient-centered communication standards for hospitals*. Oakbrook Terrace, IL: Author.

The Joint Commission (TJC). (2011, February 9). *R3: Requirement, rationale, reference, 1*. Retrieved October 14, 2014, from http://www.jointcommission.org/assets/1/18/r3%20report%20issue%201%2020111.pdf

The Joint Commission (TJC). (2013). *Critical access hospital: 2013 national patient safety goals*. Retrieved October 26, 2014, from http://www.jointcommission.org/cah_2013_npsg/

Institute for Healthcare Improvement. (2011; updated 2013). SBAR technique: A situational briefing model. Retrieved October 26, 2014, from http://www.ihi.org/knowledge/Pages/Tools/SBARTechniqueforCommunicationASituationalBriefingModel.aspx

Leebov, W. (2011, July 11). Nursing communication: How make sure patients feel our caring. Retrieved October 26, 2014, from http://allnurses.com/showthread.php?t=378288

Leonard, M., Graham, S., & Bonacum, D. (2004). The human factor: The critical importance of effective teamwork and communication in providing safe care. *Quality and Safety in Health Care, 13*(Suppl.), 85–90. doi: 10.1136/qshc.2004.010033

Military Health System, U.S. Department of Defense. (n.d.). Patient safety program: Situation, background, assessment, recommendation (SBAR) toolkit. Retrieved October 26, 2014, from http://www.health.mil/dodpatientsafety/ProductsandServices/Toolkits/SBAR.aspx

Miller, C. A. (2008). How to try this. Communication difficulties in hospitalized older adults with dementia. *American Journal of Nursing, 108*(3), 58–62.

Moorhead, S., Johnson, M., Maas, M., et al. (Eds.). (2012). *Nursing outcomes classification (NOC)* (5th ed.). St. Louis, MO: C. V. Mosby.

National Council of State Boards of Nursing. (2009). Professional oundaries—a nurse's guide to the importance of appropriate professional boundaries. Retrieved November 1, 2014 from https://www.ncsbn.org/ProfessionalBoundaries_Complete.pdf

Nurses Association of New Brunswick. (2011, February). Practice standard: The therapeutic nurse-client relationship. Retrieved October 26, 2014, from http://www.cno.org/learn-about-standards-guidelines/educational-tools/learning-modules/therapeutic-nurse-client-relationship/

Simoes, J., Jesus, L. M. T., & Voegeli, D. (2009, March). *Verbal communication with unconscious patients*. Paper presented at the Royal College of Nursing (RCN) International Nursing Research Conference, Cardiff, Wales.

Stein, L., Watts, D., & Howell, T. (1990). Sounding board: The doctor-nurse game revisited. *New England Journal of Medicine, 322*(8), 546–549.

Tannen, D. (2001). *You just don't understand: Women and men in conversation*. New York: HarperCollins.

Williams, K., Herman, R., Gajewski, B., et al. (2009). Elderspeak communication: Impact on dementia care. *American Journal of Alzheimer's Disease and Other Dementias, 24*(1), 11–20. doi: 10.1177/1533317508318472

Zembrzuski, C. (2013, revised). Communication difficulties: Assessment and interventions in hospitalized older adults with dementia. *Try This*, D7, 1–2. Hartford Institute for Geriatric Nursing, New York University College of Nursing, and the Alzheimer's Association. Retrieved October 26, 2014, from http://consultgerirn.org/uploads/File/trythis/try_this_d7.pdf

CHAPTER 22

Agency for Healthcare Research and Quality (AHRQ). (2005; revised 2013, March). *Guideline synthesis: Screening for cervical cancer*. Rockville, MD: Author. Retrieved March 25, 2013, from http://guideline.gov/syntheses/synthesis.aspx?id=43606.

American Cancer Society. (n.d.; last revised 2013a). American Cancer Society guidelines for the early detection of cancer. Retrieved February 20, 2013, from http://www.cancer.org/docroot/PED/content/PED_2_3X_ACS_Cancer_Detection_Guidelines_36.asp?sitearea+PED

American Cancer Society. (n.d.; last revised, 2013b). Detailed guide. Breast cancer: American Cancer Society recommendations for early breast cancer detection. Retrieved February 20, 2013, from http://www.cancer.org/docroot/CRI/content/CRI_2_4_3X_Can_breast_cancer_be_found_early_5.asp

American Congress of Obstetricians and Gynecologists (ACOG). (2009). Interpreting the U.S. Preventive Services Task Force breast cancer screening recommendations for the general population. Retrieved February 20, 2013, from http://www.acog.org/About%20ACOG/News%20Room/News%20Releases/2009/Interpreting%20the%20US%20Preventive%20Services%20Task%20Force.aspx

American Congress of Obstetricians and Gynecologists (ACOG). (2010a). Cervical cancer in adolescents: Screening, evaluation, and management. Retrieved February 20, 2013, from http://www.acog.org/Resources%20And%20Publications/Committee%20Opinions/Committee%20on%20Adolescent%20Health%20Care/Cervical%20Cancer%20in%20Adolescents%20-%20Screening%20Evaluation%20and%20Management.aspx

American Congress of Obstetricians and Gynecologists (ACOG). (2010b). *The initial reproductive health visit* (ACOG Practice Bulletin No. 140). Washington, DC: Author. Retrieved February 20, 2013, from http://www.acog.org/Resources%20And%20Publications/Committee%20Opinions/Committee%20on%20Adolescent%20Health%20Care/The%20Initial%20Reproductive%20Health%20Visit.aspx.

American Congress of Obstetricians and Gynecologists (ACOG). (2011). *Breast cancer screening* (ACOG Practice Bulletin No. 122). Washington, DC: Author.

Anderson, B., Kelly, A. M., Kerr, D., et al. (2008). Impact of patient and environmental factors on capillary refill time in adults. *American Journal of Emergency Medicine, 26*(1), 62–65.

Bates, C. K., Carroll, N., & Potter, J. (2011). The challenging pelvic examination. *Journal of General Internal Medicine, 26*(6), 651–657.

Centers for Disease Control and Prevention (CDC). (2009). Guideline for disinfection and sterilization in healthcare facilities, 2008. Retrieved February 20, 2013, from http://www.cdc.gov/hicpac/disinfection_sterilization/3_4surfacedisinfection.html

Centers for Disease Control and Prevention (CDC). (last updated 2012, April 27). *Defining overweight and obesity.* Atlanta, GA: Author. Retrieved January 30, 2013, from http://www.cdc.gov/obesity/adult/defining.html.

Centers for Disease Control and Prevention (CDC). (last updated September 13, 2011). *About BMI for children and teens.* Atlanta, GA: Author. Retrieved January 30, 2013, from http://www.cdc.gov/healthyweight/assessing/bmi/childrens_BMI/about_childrens_BMI.html

Chircop, A., Edgecombe, N., Hayward, K., Ducey-Gilbert, C., & Sheppard-LeMoine, D. (2013). Evaluating the integration of cultural competence skills into health and physical assessment tools: A survey of Canadian schools of nursing. *Journal of Transcultural Nursing, 24*(2), 195–203. doi:10.1177/1043659612472202

Fulmer, T. (1991). The geriatric nurse specialist role: A new model. *Nursing Management, 22*(3), 91–93.

Fulmer, T. (2007). How to try this. Fulmer SPICES. *American Journal of Nursing, 107*(10), 40–49.

Iyer, V. N., Mandrekar, J. N., Danielson, R. D., et al. (2009, August). Validity of the FOUR score coma scale in the medical intensive care unit. *Mayo Clinic Proceedings, 84*(8), 694–701. Retrieved March 30, 2013, from http://www.ncbi.nlm.nih.gov/pmc/articles/PMC2719522/

Linton, C. P. (2011). Describing the configuration of skin lesions. *Journal of the Dermatology Nurses' Association, 3*(6), 379.

Linton, C. P. (2012). Describing nail abnormalities. *Journal of the Dermatology Nurses' Association, 4*(2), 149.

Muniz, J., Sethi, R. K., Zaghi, J., Ziniel, S. I., & Sandora, T. J. (2012). Predictors of stethoscope disinfection among pediatric health care providers. *American Journal of Infection Control, 40*(10), 922–925.

National Guideline Clearinghouse (NGC). (2005; revised 2012). *Guideline synthesis: Screening for cervical cancer.* Rockville, MD: Agency for Healthcare Research and Quality. Retrieved February 21, 2013, from http://guideline.gov/content.aspx?id=38572&search=screening+for+cervical+cancer

National Guideline Clearinghouse (NGC). (2005; revised 2013, January). *Guideline synthesis: Management of overweight and obesity in children and adolescents.* Rockville, MD: Agency for Healthcare Research and Quality. Retrieved April 20, 2013, from http://guideline.gov/syntheses/synthesis.aspx?id=39378&search=overweight+and+obesity

National Heart, Lung, and Blood Institute (NHLBI), Obesity Education Initiative. (n.d.). Body mass index table. Retrieved February 21, 2013, from http://www.nhlbi.nih.gov/guidelines/obesity/bmi_tbl.htm

Rauen, C., Chulay, M., Bridges, E., et al. (2008). Seven evidence-based practice habits: Putting some sacred cows out to pasture. *Critical Care Nurse, 28*(2), 98–124.

Reddy, M. (2008). Skin and wound care: Important considerations in the older adult. *Advances in Skin & Wound Care, 21*(9), 424–436.

Rositch, A., Nowak, R., & Gravitt, P. (2014). Increased age and race-specific incidence of cervical cancer after correction for hysterectomy prevalence in the United States from 2000 to 2009. *Cancer, 120*(13), 2032–2038.

Russell, A., Secrest, J., & Schreeder, C. (2012). Stethoscopes as a source of hospital-acquired methicillin-resistant *Staphylococcus aureus. Journal of Peri-Anesthesia Nursing, 27*(2), 82–87.

Smith, R. A., Cokkinides, V., Brooks, D., et al. (2011). Cancer screening in the United States, 2011. *CA: A Cancer Journal for Clinicians, 61*(1), 8–30.

Smith, R. A., Duffy, S. W., & Tabár, L. (2012). Breast cancer screening: The evolving evidence. *Oncology, 26*(5), 471–475, 479–481, 485–486.

Tanner, J. (1962). *Growth at adolescence* (2nd ed.). Oxford: Blackwell Scientific.

U.S. Preventive Services Task Force (USPSTF). (2009). *Screening for breast cancer: Clinical summary.* Rockville, MD: Agency for Healthcare Research and Quality. Retrieved February 20, 2013, from http://www.ahrq.gov/clinic/uspstf09/breastcancer/brcansum.htm

CHAPTER 23

Agency for Healthcare Research and Quality. (2012a). *Prevention of healthcare-associated infections. closing the quality gap: Revisiting the state of the science* (Evidence Report Executive Summary No. 208; AHRQ Publication No. 12[13]-E012-1). Retrieved October 26, 2014, from http://www.effectivehealthcare.ahrq.gov/index.cfm/search-for-guides-reviews-and-reports/?pageaction=displayproduct&productid=1334

Agency for Healthcare Research and Quality. (2011). *Hospital-acquired infections dramatically increase trauma patients' risk of in-hospital death and hospital stay* (Research Activities, 372). Rockville, MD: Author. Retrieved October 26, 2014, from http://www.ahrq.gov/news/newsletters/research-activities/aug11/0811RA3.html

American Association of Critical-Care Nurses (AACN). (2013). American Association of Critical-Care Nurses practice alert: Bathing adult patients. Retrieved October 26, 2014, from http://www.aacn.org/wd/publishing/content/pressroom/pressreleases/2013/april-bathing-practice-alert-press-release.content?menu=AboutUscal-

American Nurses Association (ANA). (2010). *Nursing: Scope and standards of practice* (2nd ed.). Silver Spring, MD: Author.

American Society of Healthcare Engineering (ASHE). (n.d.). The environment of care and health care-associated infections: An engineering perspective. ASHE Monograph. Retrieved October 26, 2014, from http://www.fgiguidelines.org/pdfs/ASHE-FGI_Monograph-EOC_and_HAIs.pdf

American Society for Healthcare Engineering (ASHE) and the Association for Professionals in Infection Control & Epidemiology (APIC). (2011, April 7). Joint ASHE & APIC statement on recently presented research on electronic faucets. Retrieved October 26, 2014, from http://www.apic.org/Resource_/TinyMceFileManager/Practice_Guidance/APIC-ASHE-Statement-electronic-faucets.pdf

The Association of periOperative Registered Nurses (AORN). (2010a). In *Standards, recommended practices, and guidelines.* Denver, CO: Author.

The Association of periOperative Registered Nurses (AORN). (2010b). Recommended practices for surgical hand antisepsis/hand scrubs. In *Standards, recommended practices, and guidelines.* Denver, CO: Author.

The Association of periOperative Registered Nurses (AORN). (2012, June). Recommended practices for sterilization. In *Perioperative standards and recommended practices* (pp. 1–36). Denver, CO: Author.

The Association of periOperative Registered Nurses (AORN). (2013a). Recommended practices for prevention of transmissible infections in the perioperative practice setting. In *Perioperative standards and recommended practices* (pp. 331–364). Denver, CO: Author.

The Association of periOperative Registered Nurses (AORN). (2013b). Recommended practices for surgical hand antisepsis/hand scrubs. In *Perioperative standards and recommended practices.* Denver, CO: Author.

The Association of periOperative Registered Nurses (AORN). (2013c). Recommended practices for sterile technique. In *Perioperative standards and recommended practices* (pp. 91–120). Denver, CO: Author.

The Association of periOperative Registered Nurses (AORN). Recommended Practices Committee. (2004). Recommended practices for surgical hand: Antisepsis/hand scrubs. *AORN Journal, 79*(2), 416–431. doi: http://dx.doi.org/10.1016/S0001-2092(06)60619-4

Association for Practitioners in Infection Control and Epidemiology. (n.d.) Scientific guidelines. Retrieved October 26, 2014, from http://apic.org/Professional-Practice/Scientific-guidelines

Association for Professionals in Infection Control and Epidemiology (APIC). (2010). *Guide to the elimination of methicillin-resistant* Staphylococcus aureus *(MRSA) transmission in hospital settings* (2nd ed.). Washington, DC: Author. Retrieved June 10, 2013, from http://www.apic.org/Resource_/EliminationGuideForm/631fcd91-8773-4067-9f85-ab2a5b157eab/File/MRSA-elimination-guide-2010.pdf

Association for Surgical Technologists. (2008). AST recommended practices for creating the sterile field. Retrieved November 3, 2014, from http://www.ast.org/uploadedFiles/Main_Site/Content/About_Us/Standard_Creating_Sterile_Field.pdf

Association for Surgical Technologists. (2008). AST recommended practices for the surgical scrub. Retrieved November 2, 2014, from http://www.ast.org/uploadedFiles/Main_Site/Content/About_Us/Standard_Surgical_Attire_Surgical_Scrub.pdf

Bailey, R. R., Stuckey, D. R., Norman, B. A., et al. (2011). Economic value of dispensing home-based preoperative chlorhexidine bathing cloths to prevent surgical site infection. *Infection Control and Hospital Epidemiology, 32*(5), 465–471. doi: 10.1086/659763.

Bartley, J. M., Olmsted, R. M., & Haas, J. (2010). Current views of health care design. *Journal of Infection Control, 38,* S1–S12. doi: http://dx.doi.org/10.1016/j.ajic.2010.04.195

Bauman, R., Machunis-Masuoka, E., & Tizard, I. (2006). *Microbiology: Alternate edition with disease by body system* (3rd ed.). San Francisco: Benjamin Cummings.

Boyce, J. M., & Pittet, D. (2002, October 25). Guideline for hand hygiene in health-care settings. Recommendations of the Healthcare Infection Control Practices Advisory Committee, & the HICPAC/SHEA/APIC/IDSA Hand Hygiene Task Force. *Morbidity and Mortality Weekly Report, 51*(RR16), 1–44.

Broex, E. C. J., van Asselet, A. D. I., & Bruggeman, C. A. (2009). Surgical site infections: How high are the costs? *Journal of Hospital Infection, 72,* 193–201. doi: 10.1016/j.jhin.2009.03.020

Bulechek, G. M., Butcher, H. K., & Dochterman, J. M. (2013). *Nursing interventions classification (NIC)* (6th ed.). St. Louis, MO: C. V. Mosby.

Cardo, D., Dennehy, P. H., Halverson, P., et al. (2010). Moving toward elimination of healthcare-associated infection: A call to action. *Infection Control Hospital Epidemiology, 31*(11), 1101–5. doi:10.1086/656912

Centers for Disease Control and Prevention (CDC). (2013, April 19). Incidence and trends of infection with pathogens transmitted commonly through food—foodborne disease active surveillance network, 10 U.S. sites, 1996–2012. *Morbidity and Mortality Weekly Report, 62*(15), 283–287. Retrieved October 26, 2014, from http://www.cdc.gov/mmwr/preview/mmwrhtml/mm6215a2.htm?s_cid=mm6215a2_e

Centers for Disease Control and Prevention (CDC). (n.d.a; last updated 2013, February 5). Healthcare associated infections: The burden. Retrieved October 26, 2014, from www.cdc.gov/HAI/burden.html

Centers for Disease Control and Prevention (CDC). (n.d.b; last updated 2011, May 10). Vancomycin resistant enterococci (VRE) in healthcare settings. Retrieved October 26, 2014, http://www.cdc.gov/hai/organisms/vre/vre.html

Centers for Disease Control and Prevention (CDC). (n.d.c; updated 2012, March 6). *Clostridium difficile (C. diff)* in healthcare settings. Retrieved October 26, 2014, from http://www.cdc.gov/hai/organisms/cdiff/cdiff_infect.html

Centers for Disease Control and Prevention (CDC). (n.d.e; updated 2012, July 2). Antibiotic/antimicrobial resistance. Retrieved October 26, 2014, from http://www.cdc.gov/drugresistance/about.html

Centers for Disease Control and Prevention (CDC). (n.d.f; last modified 2014, May 24). Multidrug-resistant organisms in non-hospital healthcare settings. Retrieved October 26, 2014, from http://www.cdc.gov/ncidod/dhqp/ar_multidrugFAQ.html

Centers for Disease Control and Prevention (CDC). (2002). Guidelines for hand hygiene in health-care settings, Recommendations and reports, *Morbidity and Mortality Weekly Report, 51*(RR-16). Retrieved October 26, 2014, from http://www.cdc.gov/mmwr/preview/mmwrhtml/rr5116a1.htm

Centers for Disease Control and Prevention (CDC). (2008). Guideline for disinfection and sterilization in healthcare facilities, 2008. Infection Control Practices Advisory Committee (HICPAC). Retrieved February 10, 2014, from http://www.cdc.gov/hicpac/Disinfection_Sterilization/toc.html

Centers for Disease Control and Prevention (CDC). (2009). Guideline for prevention of catheter-associated urinary tract infections, 2009. Retrieved September 28, 2012, from http://www.cdc.gov/hicpac/cauti/001_cauti.html

Centers for Disease Control and Prevention (CDC). (2010). 2009 H1N1: Overview of a pandemic, impact of 2009 H1N1. Retrieved February 11, 2013, from http://www.cdc.gov/h1n1flu/yearinreview/yir5.htm

Cousins, N. (1979). *Anatomy of an illness.* New York: Bantam.

Davey, V. (2007). Disaster care. Questions and answers on pandemic influenza. *American Journal of Nursing, 107*(7), 50–57. doi: 10.1371/5028b6037259a

Dumont, C., & Nesselrodt, D. (2012). Preventing CLABSI. *Nursing2012, 42*(6), 41–47. doi: 10.1097/01.NURSE.0000414623.31647.f5.

Elixhauser, A., & Steiner, C. (2007). *Infections with methicillin-resistant* Staphylococcus aureus *(MRSA) in U.S. hospitals, 1993–2005* (HCUP Statistical Brief No. 35). Healthcare Cost and Utilization Project. Rockville, MD: Agency for Healthcare Research and Quality. Retrieved October 26, 2014, from http://www.hcup-us.ahrq.gov/reports/statbriefs/sb35.jsp

Flu.gov. (n.d.). Pandemic awareness. Retrieved October 26, 2014, from http://www.flu.gov/pandemic

Foxwell, A., Roberts, L., Lokuge, K., & Kelly, P. (2011). Transmission of influenza on international flights, May 2009. *Emerging Infectious Diseases, 17*(7). doi: 10.3201/eid1707.101135

Franco, G. P., de Barros, A. L., Nogueira-Martins, L. A., et al. (2003). Stress influence on genesis, onset and maintenance of cardiovascular diseases: Literature review. *Journal of Advanced Nursing, 43*(6), 548–554. doi: 10.1046/j.1365-2648.2003.02753.x

Garbutt, S. J. (2011). Hand hygiene in the OR: Using evidence-based practices. *OR Nurse 2011, 5*(2), 10–12. doi: 10.1097/01.ORN.0000394524.96696.d1

George, D. A., & Bhabra, M. (2010). A guide to scrubbing in: Student BMJ. *Medscape for Nurses.* Retrieved November 2, 2014, from http://www.medscape.com/viewarticle/725336_7

Halcomb, E. J., Griffiths, R., & Fernandez, R. (2008). Evidence synthesis. Role of MRSA reservoirs in the acute care setting. *International Journal of Evidence Based Healthcare, 6*(2), 50–62. doi: 10.1111/j.1744-1609.2007.00096.x.

Holcomb, S. S. (2008). MRSA infections. *Nursing2008, 38*(6), 33. doi: 10.1097/01.NURSE.0000320354.17197.1f.

Hutchins K., Karras, G., Erwin, J., et al. (2009). Ventilator-associated pneumonia and oral care: A successful quality improvement project. *American Journal of Infection Control, 7*, 590–597.

Jakobsson, J., Perlkvist, A., and Wann-Hansson, C. (2011). *Searching for evidence regarding using preoperative disinfection showers to prevent surgical site infections: A systematic review. Worldviews on Evidence-Based Nursing, 8*(3), 143–152.

Johns Hopkins Medicine. (2011, March 28). Latest hands-free electronic water faucets found to be hindrance, not help, in hospital infection control. Retrieved October 26, 2014, from http://www.newswise.com/articles/view/574922

Johnson, M., Bulechek, G. M., Dochterman, J. M., et al. (2012). *NANDA, NOC, and NIC linkages* (3rd ed.). St. Louis, MO: C. V. Mosby.

Johnson, D., Lineweaver, L., & Maze, L. M., (2009). Patients' bath basins as potential sources of infection: A multicenter sampling study. *American Journal of Critical Care, 18*(1), 31–38, 41. doi:10.4037/ajcc2009968

The Joint Commission. (2012, October). 2013, Hospital. National patient safety goals. Retrieved July 6, 2013, from http://www.jointcommission.org/assets/1/6/2013_HAP_NPSG_final_10-23.pdf

Kamel, C., McGahan, L., Polisena, J., et al. (2012). Preoperative skin antiseptic preparations surgical site infections: A systematic review. *Infection Control and Hospital Epidemiology, 33*(6), 608–617. doi: 10.1086/665723

Klevens, R. M., Morrison, M. A., Nadle, J., et al. (2007). Invasive methicillin-resistant *Staphylococcus aureus* infections in the United States. *JAMA, 298*(15), 1763–1771. doi:10.1001/jama.298.15.1763

Labeau, S. O., Witdouck, S. S., Vandijck, D. M., et al. (2010). Nurses' knowledge of evidence-based guidelines for the prevention of surgical site infection. *Worldviews on Evidence-Based Nursing,* 7(1), 16–24. doi: 10.1111/j.1741-6787.2009.00177.x

Lashley, F. (2006). Emerging infectious diseases at the beginning of the 21st century. *Online Journal of Issues in Nursing, 11*(1). doi: 10.3912/OJIN.Vol11No01Man01

Leung-Chen, P. (2008). Emerging infections. Everybody's crying MRSA. *American Journal of Nursing, 108*(8), 29–31.

Lo, E., Nicolle, L., Classen, D., et al. (2008). Strategies to prevent catheter-associated urinary tract infections in acute care hospitals, *Infection Control and Hospital Epidemiology, 29*(1), S41–S49. doi: 10.1086/675718

Maki, D. G. (2001). Engineering out the risk of infection with urinary catheters. *Emerging Infectious Diseases, 7*(2), 342–347.

McKibben, L., Horan, T., Tokars, M. D., et al.; the Healthcare Infection Control Practices Advisory Committee. (2005). Guidance on public reporting of healthcare-associated infections: Recommendations of the Healthcare Infection Control Practices Advisory Committee. *American Journal of Infection Control, 33*(4), 217–226. doi: http://dx.doi.org/10.1016/j.ajic.2005.04.001

Minnesota Department of Health. (n.d.). Components of personal protective equipment. Retrieved October 26, 2014, from http://www.health.state.mn.us/divs/idepc/dtopics/infectioncontrol/ppe/comp/index.html

Moorhead, S., Johnson, M., Maas, M. L., et al. (2013). *Nursing outcomes classification* (5th ed.). St. Louis, MO: C. V. Mosby.

NANDA International. (2012). *Nursing diagnoses: Definitions & classification 2012–2014.* Ames, IA: Wiley-Blackwell.

New York State Department of Health. (2011). Emergency preparedness Retrieved October 26, 2014, from http://www.health.state.ny.us/environmental/emergency/

New York State Department of Health Influenza Pandemic. (March 2011). Retrieved October 26, 2014, from http://www.health.ny.gov/diseases/communicable/influenza/pandemic/

Occupational Safety & Health Administration. U.S. Department of Labor. (n.d.; last reviewed 2009, January). Bloodborne pathogens and needlestick prevention. Post-exposure evaluation. Retrieved October 26, 2014, from https://www.osha.gov/SLTC/bloodbornepathogens/evaluation.html

Oman, K. S., Makic-Flynn, M. B., Fink, R., et al. (2012). Nurse-directed interventions to reduce catheter-associated urinary tract infections. *American Journal of Infection Control, 40*(6), 548–553. doi: 10.1016/j.ajic.2011.07.018

Ottum, A., Sethi, A. K., Jacobs, E. A., et al. (2012). Do patients feel comfortable asking healthcare workers to wash their hands? *Infection Control Hospital Epidemiology, 33*(12), 1282–1284. doi: 10.1086/668419

Peral, M. C., Huaman Martinez, M. A., & Valdez, J. C. (2009). Bacteriotherapy with lactobacillus plantarum in burns. *International Wound Journal, 6*(1), 73–81. doi: 10.1111/j.1742-481X.2008.00577.x

Pitout, J. D. D., & Laupland, K. B. (2008). Extended-spectrum B-lactamase-producing Enterobacteriaceae: An emerging public-health concern. *The Lancet Infectious Diseases, 8*(3), 159–166. doi:10.1016/S1473-3099(08)70041-0

Plan to protect you and your family. (2013, September 19, updated). Retrieved October 26, 2014, from http://www.ready.gov/emergency-planning-checklists

Pratt, R. J., Pellowe, C. M., Wilson, J. A., et al. (2007). Epic2: National evidence-based guidelines for preventing healthcare-associated infections in NHS hospitals in England. *Journal of Hospital Infection, 65*(Suppl. 1), S1–S64.

Rice, L. B. (2001). Emergence of vancomycin-resistant enterococci. *Emerging Infectious Diseases, 7*(2), 183–187.

Rupp, M. E., Fitzgerald, T., Puumala, S., et al. (2008). Prospective, controlled, cross-over trial of alcohol-based hand gel in critical care units. *Infection Control and Hospital Epidemiology, 29*(1), 8–15. doi: 10.1086/524333

Schneider, R., Alexander, C., Staggers, F., et al. (2005). Long-term effects of stress reduction on mortality in persons 55 years of age with systemic hypertension. *The American Journal of Cardiology, 95*(9), 1060–1064.

Siegel, J. D., Rhinehart, E., Jackson, M., et al. (2006). *Management of multidrug-resistant organisms in healthcare settings, 2006.* Retrieved October 26, 2014, from http://www.cdc.gov/hicpac/pdf/guidelines/MDROGuideline2006.pdf

Siegel, J. D., Rhinehart, E., Jackson, M., et al. (2007). *2007 guideline for isolation precautions: Preventing transmission of infectious agents in the healthcare setting.* Retrieved October 26, 2014, from http://www.cdc.gov/hicpac/pdf/isolation/Isolation2007.pdf

Simko, L. (2012). Breaking sterility: Dealing with procedural violations in healthcare. *Nursing2012, 42*(8), 22–26. doi: 10.1097/01.NURSE.0000415839.66736.4c

Smith, J. M. (2003). Indwelling catheter management: From habit-based to evidence-based practice. *Ostomy Wound Management, 49*(12), 34–45.

Smith, G., Vijaykrishna, D., Bahl, J., et al. (2009). Origins and evolutionary genomics of the 2009 swine-origin H1N1 influenza epidemic. *Nature, 459*, 1122–1125. doi:10.1038/nature08182

Sydnor, E. R., & Pert, T. M. (2011). Hospital epidemiology and infection control in acute care settings. *Clinical Microbiology Reviews, 24*(1), 141–173. doi:10.1128/CMR.00027-10

Tegethoff, M., Greene, N., Olsen, J., Schaffner, E., & Meinlschmidt, G. (2011). Stress during pregnancy and offspring pediatric disease: A national cohort study. *Environmental Health* Perspectives, *119*(11), 1647–1652. Retrieved from http://dx.doi.org/10.1289/ehp.1003253

Upshaw-Owens, M., & Bailey, C. A. (2012). Preventing hospital-associated infection: MRSA. *Medsurg Nursing, 21*(2), 77–81.

U.S. Department of Health & Human Services. (n.d.a). Pandemic flu planning checklists for individuals and families. Retrieved June 21, 2013, from http://www.gchd.us/Services/GeneralPrograms/EmergencyPreparedness/Pandemic%20Flu%20Checklist.pdf

U.S. Department of Health & Human Services. (n.d.b). Flu pandemics. Retrieved June 23, 2013, from http://www.flu.gov/individualfamily/about/pandemic/index.html

U.S. Department of Health & Human Services. (2011). National action plan to prevent hospital-associated infections: Road map to elimination. *Health.gov*. Retrieved February 8, 2014, from http://www.health.gov/hai/prevent_hai.asp#hai_measures

U.S. Department of Labor. (n.d.a). Occupational Safety and Health Standards: General description and discussion of the levels of protection and protective gear. 1910.120 App B. Retrieved September 23, 2012, from http://www.osha.gov/pls/oshaweb/owadisp.show_document?p_table=tablettp://www.os

U.S. Department of Labor. (n.d.b). (Lack of) personal protective equipment. Occupational Safety and Health Standards. 1910.1030(d)(3)(xii). Retrieved September 23, 2012, from http://www.osha.gov/SLTC/etools/hospital/hazards/ppe/ppe.html

Whyte, J. (2008). MRSA: Not a new crisis. *The Clinical Advisor, 11*(1), 100.

World Health Organization (WHO). (2011). Avian influenza in humans. Retrieved October 26, 2014, from http://www.who.int/influenza/human_animal_interface/avian_influenza/en/

World Health Organization (WHO). (2012, June 5). Save lives: Clean your hands. Retrieved October 26, 2014, from http://www.who.int/gpsc/5may/PSP_GPSC1_HH_5May2012/en/

CHAPTER 24

Ackley, B., & Ladwig, G. (2010). *Nursing diagnosis handbook* (9th ed.). St. Louis, MO: C. V. Mosby.

Adams P., Martinez M., Vickerie J., et al. (2011). Summary health statistics for the U.S. population: National Health Interview Survey, 2010. *Vital Health Statistics, 10*(251). Retrieved April 10, 2013, from http://www.cdc.gov/mmwr/preview/mmwrhtml/mm6104a8.htm

Adults. (n.d.). American Association of Poison Control Centers. Retrieved April 2, 2013, from http://www.aapcc.org/prevention/adults/

Aiken, L. H., Clarke, S. P., Sloane, D. M., et al. (2001). Nurses' reports on hospital care in five countries. *Health Affairs, 20*(3), 43–53.

Akyol, A. D. (2007). Falls in the elderly: What can be done? *International Nursing Review, 54*(2), 191–196.

American Academy of Neurology (AAN). (2008a, February). Get Up and Go Test. Retrieved April 1, 2013, from http://www.aan.com/practice/guideline/uploads/273.pdf

American Academy of Neurology (AAN). (2008b, February). Get Up and Go Test. Retrieved April 1, 2013, from http://www.aan.com/practice/guideline/uploads/274.pdf

American Academy of Pediatrics (AAP). (2011, updated 2013). Car seats: Information for families for 2013. Retrieved April 13, 2013, from http://www.healthychildren.org/English/safety-prevention/on-the-go/Pages/Car-Safety-Seats-Information-for-Families.aspx

American Nurses Association (ANA). (2001). Position statement: Reduction of patient restraint and seclusion in health care settings—10/17/01. Retrieved April 1, 2013, from http://www.nursingworld.org/restraintposition

American Nurses Association (ANA). (2002). Needlestick prevention guide. Retrieved April 1, 2013, from http://www.nursingworld.org/MainMenuCategories/WorkplaceSafety/Healthy-Work-Environment/SafeNeedles/NeedlestickPrevention.pdf

American Nurses Association (ANA). (2010). Health system reform: Nursing's goal of high quality, affordable care for all. Retrieved April 1, 2013, from http://www.nursingworld.org/MainMenuCategories/Policy-Advocacy/Positions-and-Resolutions/Issue-Briefs/Health-System-Reform.pdf

American Nurses Association (ANA). (2013). Safe patient handling and mobility. Retrieved April 1, 2013, from http://nursingworld.org/MainMenuCategories/WorkplaceSafety/Healthy-Work-Environment/SafePatient

American Red Cross. (2007). Be Red Cross ready. Conscious choking. Retrieved April 1, 2013, from http://www.redcross.org/flash/brr/English-html/conscious-choking.asp

American Red Cross. (2008). Re: Question re choking. Personal communication, August 26, 2008, from A. Adorante, Director of Preparedness, Health & Safety Services, American Red Cross, Kansas City, KS.

Akyol, A. D. (2007). Falls in the elderly: What can be done? *International Nursing Review, 54*(2), 191–196.

Berg, J., McConnell, R., Milam, J., et al. (2008). Rodent allergen in Los Angeles inner city homes of children with asthma. *Journal of Urban Health, 85*(1), 52–61.

Babysitters. (n.d.). American Association of Poison Control Centers. Retrieved April 2, 2013, from http://www.aapcc.org/prevention/babysitters/

Bronstein, A. (August 5, 2011). Carbon-monoxide-related deaths: United States, 2000–2009. *Morbidity and Mortality Weekly Report, 60*(30), 1014–1017. Retrieved April 1, 2013, from http://www.cdc.gov/mmwr/preview/mmwrhtml/mm6030a2.htm?s_cid=mm6030a2_e%0d%0a

Bulechek, G., Butcher, H., Dochterman, J., et al. (Eds.). (2012). *Nursing interventions classification (NIC)* (6th ed.). St. Louis, MO: C. V. Mosby.

Bureau of Labor Statistics. (2012). Economic news release. Nonfatal occupational injuries and illnesses requiring days away from work, 2011. Retrieved March 22, 2013, from http://www.bls.gov/news.release/osh2.nr0.htm

Capezuti, E., Wagner, L., Brush, B., et al. (2007). Consequences of an intervention to reduce restrictive side rail use in nursing homes. *Journal of the American Geriatrics Society, 55*(3), 334–342.

Centers for Disease Control and Prevention (CDC). (2005). Foodborne illness. Frequently asked questions. Retrieved April 2, 2013, from http://www.cdc.gov/ncidod/dbmd/diseaseinfo/files/foodborne_illness_FAQ.pdf

Centers for Disease Control and Prevention (CDC). (2011a, November). Prescription painkiller overdoses in the U.S. Retrieved April 1, 2013 from http://www.cdc.gov/vitalsigns/PainkillerOverdoses/index.html

Centers for disease Control and Prevention (CDC). (2011b, December). Bloodborne infectious diseases: HIV/AIDS, Hepatitis B, Hepatitis C. Preventing needlesticks and sharps injuries. National Institute for Occupational Safety and Health (NIOSH). Retrieved April 2, 2013, from http://www.cdc.gov/niosh/topics/bbp/sharps.html

Centers for Disease Control and Prevention (CDC). (2011c; last updated). Ticks. Retrieved May 12, 2011, from http://www.cdc.gov/ticks/index.html

Centers for Disease Control and Prevention, National Center for Injury Prevention and Control. (n.d.a; updated 2012, September). Web-based injury statistics query and reporting system (WISQARS). Retrieved April 1, 2013, from http://www.cdc.gov/HomeandRecreationalSafety/Falls/adultfalls.html

Centers for Disease Control and Prevention, National Center for Injury Prevention and Control. (n.d.b). Web-based injury statistics query and reporting system (WISQARS). 2007, United States: Unintentional injuries, all ages, all races, both sexes. Retrieved April 1, 2013, from http://www.cdc.gov/injury/wisqars/pdf/WISQARS-FactSheet20120425-a.pdf

Centers for Disease Control and Prevention, National Center for Injury Prevention and Control. (2006; updated 2013, March). *Child passenger safety: Fact sheet*. Retrieved April 2, 2013, from http://www.cdc.gov/MotorVehicleSafety/Child_Passenger_Safety/CPS-Factsheet.html

Centers for Disease Control and Prevention, National Center for Injury Prevention and Control. (2010a, updated July 2012). Injury prevention & control: Home and recreational safety: Unintentional poisoning. Web-based injury statistics query and reporting system (WISQARS). Retrieved April 1, 2013, from http://www.cdc.gov/HomeandRecreationalSafety/Poisoning/index.html

Centers for Disease Control and Prevention, National Center for Injury Prevention and Control (2010d; updated 2012, June 12). Child passenger safety. Retrieved April 1, 2013, from http://www.cdc.gov/features/passengersafety/

Centers for Disease Control and Prevention, National Center for Injury Prevention and Control. (2012). National action plan for child injury prevention. Atlanta. Retrieved April 2, 2013 from http://www.cdc.gov/safechild/pdf/National_Action_Plan_for_Child_Injury_Prevention.pdf

Centers for Disease Control and Prevention, National Center for Injury Prevention and Control. Web-based Injury Statistic Query and Reporting System (WISQARS) [online]. (2010b, updated June 29, 2012). *Poisoning in the United States: Fact sheet*. Retrieved April 1, 2013, from http://www.cdc.gov/HomeandRecreationalSafety/Poisoning/poisoning-factsheet.htm

Centers for Medicare & Medicaid Services. (2006a; modified 2011). Eliminating serious, preventable, and costly medical errors—never events [Press release]. Department of Health & Human Services. Retrieved April 2, 2013, from http://www.cms.hhs.gov/apps/media/press/release.asp?Counter=1863

Centers for Medicare & Medicaid Services. (2006b, December 8). Rules and regulations. Part IV. Department of Health and Human Services, CMMS, 42 CFR Part 482. Medicare and Medicaid programs; Hospital conditions of participation: Patients' rights; Final rule. *Federal Register, 71*(236), 71428.

Centers for Medicare & Medicaid Services. (2008, July 31). Medicare and Medicaid move aggressively to encourage greater patient safety in hospitals and reduce never events [Press release]. CMS Office of Public Affairs. Retrieved April 2, 2013, from http://www.cms.gov/About-CMS/Public-Affairs/MediaReleaseDatabase/Press-Releases/2008-Press-Releases-Items/2008-07-313.html

Centers for Medicare & Medicaid Services. (2011; modified 2013, January). HAC posting on Hospital Compare.

Retrieved April 2, 2013, from http://www.cms.gov/HospitalQualityInits/06_HACPost.asp

Chan, J., LeBel, J., & Webber, L. (2012). The dollars and sense of restraints and seclusion. *Journal of Law and Medicine, 20*(1), 73.

Choking—Infant under 1 year (n.d.a; updated March 2013, March). *MedlinePlus: Medical encyclopedia.* U.S. National Library of Medicine. Retrieved April 2, 2013, from http://www.nlm.nih.gov/MEDLINEPLUS/ency/article/000048.htm.

Choking—Adult or child over 1 year. (n.d.b; updated 2011, July). *MedlinePlus: Medical encyclopedia.* U.S. National Library of Medicine. Retrieved April 2, 2013, from http://www.nlm.nih.gov/MEDLINEPLUS/ency/article/000049.htm

Choking—Unconscious adult or child over 1 year. (n.d.c; updated 2011, July). *MedlinePlus: Medical encyclopedia.* U.S. National Library of Medicine. Retrieved April 2, 2013, from http://www.nlm.nih.gov/MEDLINEPLUS/ency/article/000051.htm

Compton, J., Copeland, K., Flanders, S., et al. (2012). Implementing SBAR across a large multi-hospital health system. *Joint Commission Journal on Quality and Patient Safety, 38*(6), 261–268.

Cooper, M., & Kulkarni, R. (2011, updated). Lightning injuries in emergency medicine. *Medscape reference.* Retrieved April 2, 2013, from http://emedicine.medscape.com/article/770642-overview

Cronenwett, L., Sherwood, G., Barnsteiner, J., et al. (2007). Quality and safety education for nurses. *Nursing Outlook, 55*(3), 122–131.

Cronenwett, L., Sherwood, G., & Gelmon, S. B. (2009). Improving quality and safety education: The QSEN Learning Collaborative. *Nursing Outlook, 57*(6), 304–312.

Degelau, J., Belz, M., Bungum, L., et al. (2012 April). *Prevention of falls (acute care). Health care protocol.* Bloomington, MN: Institute for Clinical Systems Improvement. Retrieved May 20, 2013, from http://guideline.gov/content.aspx?f=rss&id=36906

Deshpande, N., Metter, E., Bandinelli, S., et al. (2008a). Psychological, physical, and sensory correlates of fear of falling and consequent activity restriction in the elderly: The InCHIANTI study. *American Journal of Physical Medicine & Rehabilitation, 87*(5), 354–362.

Deshpande, N., Metter, E., Lauretani, F., et al. (2008b). Activity restriction induced by fear of falling and objective and subjective measures of physical function: A prospective cohort study. *Journal of the American Geriatrics Society, 56*(4), 615–620.

Doenges, M., Moorhouse, M., & Geissler-Murr, A. (2010). *Nursing diagnosis manual* (3rd ed.). Philadelphia: F. A. Davis.

Edelman, M., & Ficorelli, C. (2012). Patient safety. Keeping older adults safe at home. *Nursing2012, 42*(1), 65–66.

Evans, L., & Cotter, V. (2008). Avoiding restraints in patients with dementia. *American Journal of Nursing, 108*(3), 40–50.

Evergreen Industries & Obviously Enterprises. (2006). *The Internet consumer recycling guide. The world's shortest comprehensive recycling guide.* Retrieved April 2, 2013, from http://www.obviously.COM/recycle/guides/shortest.html

Field, J. M., Hazinski, M. F., Sayre, M. R., et al. (2010). Part 1: Executive Summary 2010 American Heart Association guidelines for cardiopulmonary resuscitation and emergency cardiovascular care. *Circulation, 122*(18, suppl. 3), S640–S656.

Flores, N. (2008). Dealing with an angry patient. *Nursing2008, 38*(5), 30–31.

FoodSafety.gov, U.S. Department of Health and Human Services. (n.d.). Keep food safe. Retrieved April 2, 2013, from http://www.foodsafety.gov/keep/index.html

Gates, S., Fisher, J., Cooke, M., et al. (2008). Multifactorial assessment and targeted intervention for preventing falls and injuries among older people in community and emergency care settings: Systematic review and meta-analysis. *BMJ, 336*, 130–133.

Gillespie, G. L., Gates, D. M., & Berry, P. (2013). Stressful incidents of physical violence against emergency nurses. *Online Journal of Issues in Nursing, 18*(1), 2.

Gomersall, J., Tufanaru, C., & White, S. (2012). The cost effectiveness of exercise for preventing falls in older people living in the community: A systematic review. *The Joanna Briggs International (JBI) Database of Systematic Reviews and Implementation Reports, 10*(57), 3949–3959.

Gray-Micelli, D., & Quigley, P. (2011). Preventing falls in acute care. In E. Capezuti, D. Zwicker, M. Mezey, et al. (Eds.), *Evidence-based geriatric nursing protocols for best practices* (4th ed., pp. 268–297). New York: Springer.

Grossman, V. (2003). Gang members in the ED. *American Journal of Nursing, 103*(2), 52–53.

Hendrich, A. (2007). How to try this. Predicting patient falls. *American Journal of Nursing, 107*(11), 50–59.

Hita-Contreras, F., Martínez-Amat, A., Lomas-Vega, R., et al. (2013). Predictive value of stabilometry and fear of falling on falls in postmenopausal women. *Climacteric, 16*(5), 584–589.

Hizel, S., Ozcebe, H., Sanli, C., et al. (2008). Children and firearms in Turkish homes. *Child: Care, Health & Development, 34*(1), 32–34.

Huang, A. R., Mallet, L., Rochefort, C. M., et al. (2012). Medication-related falls in the elderly: Causative factors and preventive strategies. *Drugs & Aging, 29*(5), 359–376.

Hughes, K., van Beurden, E., Eakin, E., et al. (2008). Older persons' perception of risk of falling: Implications for fall-prevention campaigns. *American Journal of Public Health, 98*(2), 351–357.

Holt, E., Theall, K., & Rabito, F. (2012). Individual, housing, and neighborhood correlates of asthma among young urban children. *Journal of Urban Health,* 90(1), 116–129.

Injury Center, Centers for Disease Control and Prevention (CDC). (n.d.; last updated 2013, March). Tips to prevent poisonings. Retrieved May 20, 2013, from http://www.cdc.gov/HomeandRecreationalSafety/Poisoning/preventiontips.htm

Institute for Clinical Systems Improvement (ICSI). (2008). Prevention of falls (acute care). Health care protocol. Bloomington, MN: Author. Retrieved April 2, 2013, from http://www.guideline.gov/content.aspx?id=36906

Institute for Healthcare Improvement. (n.d.). Overview of the 100,000 lives campaign. Retrieved April 2, 2013, from http://www.ihi.org/offerings/Initiatives/PastStrategicInitiatives/5MillionLivesCampaign/Pages/default.aspx

Institute of Medicine (IOM). (2001). *Crossing the quality chasm: A new health system for the 21st century.* Washington, DC: The National Academies Press. Retrieved April 2, 2013, from http://www.nap.edu/openbook.php?record_id=10027&page=R1

Institute of Medicine (IOM). (2011). *The future of nursing: Leading change, advancing health.* Washington, DC: The National

Academies Press. Retrieved April 2, 2013, from http://books.nap.edu/openbook.php?record_id=12956

Jellesmark, A., Herling, S. F., Egerod, I., et al. (2012). Fear of falling and changed functional ability following hip fracture among community-dwelling elderly people: An explanatory sequential mixed method study. *Disability and Rehabilitation, 34*(25), 2124–2131.

The Joanna Briggs Institute (2010). Interventions to reduce the incidence of falls in older adult patients in acute care hospitals. *Best Practice, 14*(1).

Johnson, M., Bulechek, G., Butcher, H., et al. (2012). *NANDA, NOC, and NIC linkages* (3rd ed.). St. Louis, MO: C. V. Mosby.

The Joint Commission. (2012). 2013 National Patient Safety Goals (NPSGs). Retrieved May 20, 2013, from http://www.jointcommission.org/assets/1/6/2013_HAP_NPSG_final_10-23.pdf

The Joint Commission. (2009). Restraint /Seclusion for hospitals that use The Joint Commission for deemed status purposes. Standards FAQ Details. Retrieved May 20, 2013, from http://www.jointcommission.org/standards_information/jcfaqdetails.aspx?StandardsFaqId=260&ProgramId=47

Kalisch, B. J., Tschannen, D., & Lee, K. H. (2012). Missed nursing care, staffing, and patient falls. *Journal of Nursing Care Quality, 27*(1), 6.

Kenny, R., Rubenstein, L., Tinetti, M., et al. (2011). Summary of the updated American geriatrics society/British geriatrics society clinical practice guideline for prevention of falls in older persons. *Journal of the American Geriatrics Society, 59*(1), 148–157.

Kit, B. K., Simon, A. E., Brody, D. J., et al. (2013). US prevalence and trends in tobacco smoke exposure among children and adolescents with asthma. *Pediatrics, 131*(3), 407–414.

Kochanek, K. D., Xu, J., Murphy, S. L., et al. (2012). Deaths: Final data for 2009. *National Vital Statistics Reports, 60*(3). Hyattsville, MD: National Center for Health Statistics. Retrieved May 20, 2013, from http://www.cdc.gov/nchs/data/nvsr/nvsr60/nvsr60_03.pdf

Lewiecki, E., & Miller, S. A. (2013). Suicide, guns, and public policy. *American Journal of Public Health, 103*(1), 27–31.

Malafarina, V., Úriz-Otano, F., Iniesta, R., et al. (2012). Risk factors for falls in elderly adults: Not only pharmacological effects. *Journal of the American Geriatric Society, 59*, 1883–1890.

Mobile device use while driving—United States and seven European countries, 2011. (2013). *Morbidity and Mortality Weekly Report, 62*(10), 177–182. Retrieved March 16, 2013, from http://www.cdc.gov/mmwr/pdf/wk/mm6210.pdf

Morbidity and Mortality Weekly Report. (2012, April 16). Vital signs: Unintentional injury deaths among persons aged 0–19 Years—United States, 2000–2009. *Centers for Disease Control and Prevention, 61*(15), 1–7. Retrieved April 2, 2013, from http://www.cdc.gov/mmwr/preview/mmwrhtml/mm61e0416a1.htm?s_cid=mm61e0416a1_w

Morbidity and Mortality Weekly Report Surveillance for Violent Deaths—National Violent Death Reporting System, 16 states, 2009: Surveillance summaries. (2012, September 14). *Centers for Disease Control and Prevention, 61*(ss06), 1–43. Retrieved May 20, 2013, from http://www.cdc.gov/mmwr/preview/mmwrhtml/ss6106a1.htm?s_cid=ss6106a1_w

Moorhead, S., Johnson, M., Maas, M., et al. (Eds.). (2012). *Nursing outcomes classification (NOC)* (5th ed.). St. Louis, MO: C. V. Mosby.

Morse, J. (2009). *Preventing patient falls: Establishing a fall intervention program* (2nd ed.). New York: Springer.

Morse, J. (2008). *Preventing patient falls* (2nd ed.). New York: Springer.

Morse, J. (2001, First Quarter). Preventing falls in the elderly. *Reflections on Nursing Leadership*, 26–27.

Myhre, M. C., Thoresen, S., Grøgaard, J. B., et al. (2012). Familial factors and child characteristics as predictors of injuries in toddlers: a prospective cohort study. *British Medical Journal, 2*(2).

NANDA International. (2012). *NANDA nursing diagnoses: Definitions and classification 2012–2014*. Ames, IA: Wiley-Blackwell.

National Ag Safety Database (NASD). (1998; reviewed 2002, April). How does safety rate on your farm or ranch? Check lists: Home safety 1, 2, and 3. Retrieved April 2, 2013, from http://nasdonline.org/document/1634/d001509/how-does-safety-rate-on-your-farm-or.html

National Cancer Institute. (n.d.). Secondhand smoke: Questions and answers [Factsheet]. Retrieved April 2, 2013, from http://www.cancer.gov/cancertopics/factsheet/Tobacco/ETS

National Capitol Poison Center. (n.d.). What is ipecac syrup? Retrieved April 1, 2013, from http://www.poison.org/prepared/ipecac.asp

National Center for Injury Prevention and Control (NCIPC). (2012). *Falls—Older adults*. Atlanta, GA:. Centers for Disease Control and Prevention. Retrieved March 28, 2013, from http://www.cdc.gov/HomeandRecreationalSafety/Falls/index.html

National Guideline Clearinghouse. (2003; updated 2008). *Preventing falls in acute care. In Evidence-based geriatric nursing protocols for best practice.* Rockville, MD: Agency for Healthcare Research and Quality (AHRQ). Retrieved March 25, 2013, from http://guideline.gov/content.aspx?id=12265&search=preventing+falls

National Guideline Clearinghouse. (2010). *Child passenger safety: An evidence-based review.* Rockville, MD: Agency for Healthcare Research and Quality (AHRQ). Retrieved May 26, 2013, from http://guideline.gov/content.aspx?f=rss&id=43768&osrc=12

National Institute for Occupational Safety and Health (NIOSH). (n.d.; updated 2010, December). *Safer medical device implementation in health care facilities*. Atlanta, GA: Centers for Disease Control and Prevention, Department of Health and Human Services. Retrieved April 2, 2013, from http://www.cdc.gov/niosh/topics/bbp/safer/

National Institute for Occupational Safety and Health (NIOSH). (2004). *Worker health chartbook 2004* (NIOSH Publication No. 2004–146). Atlanta, GA: Centers for Disease Control and Prevention, Department of Health and Human Services. Retrieved April 2, 2013, from http://www.cdc.gov/niosh/docs/2004-146/

National Institute for Occupational Safety and Health (NIOSH). (2003). *Protect your family: Reduce contamination at home* (DHHS [NIOSH] Publication No. 97-125). Atlanta, GA: Centers for Disease Control and Prevention, Department of Health and Human Services. Retrieved April 2, 2013, from http://www.cdc.gov/niosh/docs/97-125/

The National Rifle Association Headquarters. (n.d.). What is the Eddie Eagle GunSafe Program? Retrieved April 2, 2013, from http://eddieeagle.nra.org

The National Rifle Association Headquarters. (2011). Education & training programs. NRA gun safety rules. Retrieved April 2, 2013, from http://training.nra.org/nra-gun-safety-rules.aspx

National Safety Council. (2010). Summary from *Injury Facts*, 2020 edition. Retrieved April 2, 2013, from http://www.nsc.org/news_resources/injury_and_death_statistics/Documents/Summary_2010_Ed.pdf

National Safety Council. (2011). *NSC injury facts*. Itasca, IL: Author. Also available for purchase at http://www.nsc.org/news_resources/injury_and_death_statistics/Pages/InjuryDeathStatistics.aspx

O'Keefe, L. (2009). What to consider when positioning carseats for toddlers. *AAP News, 30*(4), 12. Retrieved April 2, 2013, from http://aapnews.aappublications.org/cgi/content/full/30/4/12-a

Page, K. (2012). Role of cockroach proteases in allergic disease. *Current Allergy and Asthma Reports, 12*(5), 448–455.

Papa, A., & Venella, J. (2013). Workplace violence in healthcare: strategies for advocacy. *Online Journal of Issues in Nursing, 18*(1), 5.

Park, M., & Tang, J. (2007). Changing the practice of physical restraint use in acute care. *Journal of Gerontological Nursing, 33*(2), 9–16.

Pham, J., Aswani, M. Rosen, M., et al. (2012). Reducing medical errors and adverse events. *Annual Review of Medicine, 63*, 447–463.

Plastic and Reconstructive Surgery. (2013, April 2). "Sharps" injuries pose serious hazard for surgeons, O.R. staff [News release]. Retrieved May 20, 2013, from http://www.philly.com/philly/health/topics/HealthDay675097_20130404__Sharps__Injuries_Pose_Serious_Hazard_for_Surgeons__O_R__Staff.html#SYsrdEua8sVMiIlI.99

Podsiadlo, D., & Richardson, S. (1991). The timed "Up and Go" Test: A test of basic functional mobility for frail elderly persons. *Journal of American Geriatric Society, 39*, 142–148.

Pope, C. A., Burnett, R., Turner, M., et al. (2012). S-097: Cardiovascular and lung cancer mortality associated with air pollution and cigarette smoke: Shape of the exposure-response relationship. *Epidemiology, 23*(Suppl. 5).

Sharkey, J. E., Van Leuven, K., & Radovich, P. (2012). Risks related to patient bed safety. *Journal of Nursing Care Quality, 27*(4), 346–351.

Shever, L., Titler, M., Kerr, P., et al. (2008). The effect of high nursing surveillance on hospital cost. *Journal of Nursing Scholarship, 40*(2), 161–169.

Stevens, J., & Sogolow, E. (2008, updated September 2012). *Preventing falls: What works*. Atlanta, GA: Centers for Disease Control and Prevention, National Center for Injury Prevention and Control. Retrieved April 2, 2013, from http://www.cdc.gov/ncipc/preventingfalls/CDCCompendium_030508.pdf

Stimpfel, A. W., & Aiken, L. H. (2013). Hospital staff nurses' shift length associated with safety and quality of care. *Journal of Nursing Care Quality, 28*(2), 122–129.

Talerico, K., & Capezuti, E. (2001). Myths and facts about side rails. *American Journal of Nursing, 101*(7), 43–48.

Taylor, J. L., & Rew, L. (2011). A systematic review of the literature: Workplace violence in the emergency department. *Journal of Clinical Nursing, 20*(7–8), 1072–1085.

Tilly, J., & Reed, P. (2008). Falls, wandering, and physical restraints: A review of interventions for individuals with dementia in assisted living and nursing homes. *Alzheimer's Care Today, 9*(1), 45–50.

U.S. Department of Health and Human Services (USDHHS). (2006). *The health consequences of involuntary exposure to tobacco smoke: A report of the Surgeon General*. Rockville, MD: Centers for Disease Control and Prevention (CDC), Coordinating Center for Health Promotion, National Center for Chronic Disease Prevention and Health Promotion, Office of Smoking and Health.

U.S. Department of Labor, Occupational Safety and Health Administration (OSHA). (n.d.). Bloodborne pathogens and needlestick prevention. Retrieved April 2, 2013, from http://www.osha.gov/SLTC/bloodbornepathogens/index.html

U.S. Department of Labor, Occupational Safety and Health Administration (OSHA). (2001). Enforcement procedures for the occupational exposure to bloodborne pathogens. CPL 02-02-069. Retrieved April 2, 2013, from http://www.osha.gov/pls/oshaweb/owadisp.show_document?p_table=directives&p_id=2570

U.S. Environmental Protection Agency (EPA). (2007). Methods of mosquito control. Retrieved April 2, 2013, from http://www.epa.gov/pesticides/health/mosquitoes/mosquito.htm

U.S. Environmental Protection Agency (EPA). (2008). Wastes. Retrieved May 12, 2011, from http://www.epa.gov/epawaste/

U.S. Food and Drug Administration (FDA). (n.d.). Food. Retrieved April 2, 2013, from http://www.fda.gov

Unruh, L. Y., & Zhang, N. J. (2012). Nurse staffing and patient safety in hospitals: New variable and longitudinal approaches. *Nursing Research, 61*(1), 3.

Vardaman, J., Cornell, P., Gondo, M., et al. (2012). Beyond communication: The role of standardized protocols in a changing health care environment. *Health Care Management Review, 37*(1), 88.

Viljanen, A., Kulmala, J., Rantakokko, M., et al. (2012). Fear of falling and coexisting sensory difficulties as predictors of mobility decline in older women. *The Journals of Gerontology Series A: Biological Sciences and Medical Sciences, 67*(11), 1230–1237.

Waljee, J., Sunitha, M., & Chung, K. (2013). Sharps injuries: The risks and relevance to plastic surgeons. *Plastic & Reconstructive Surgery, 131*(4), 784–791.

Watson, D. (2010). Never events in health care. *Association of Perioperative Registered Nurses (AORN), 91*(3), 378–382.

Weber, V., White, A., & McIlvried, R. (2008). An electronic medical record (EMR)-based intervention to reduce polypharmacy and falls in an ambulatory rural elderly population. *Journal of General Internal Medicine, 23*(4), 399–404.

Wijlhuizen, G., de Jong, R., & Hopman-Rock, M. (2007). Older persons afraid of falling reduce physical activity to prevent outdoor falls. *Preventive Medicine, 44*(3), 260–264.

Wilburn, S. (2004). Needlestick and sharps injury prevention. *Online Journal of Issues in Nursing, 9*(3), 104.

Wilkinson, J. (2013). *Prentice-Hall nursing diagnosis handbook* (10th ed.). Upper Saddle River, NJ: Prentice-Hall.

Woodrow, C., & Guest, D. E. (2012). Public violence, staff harassment and the wellbeing of nursing staff: an analysis of national survey data. *Health Services Management Research, 25*(1), 24–30.

CHAPTER 25

American Association of Critical-Care Nurses (AACN). (2007). AACN practice alert. Oral care in the critically ill. Retrieved April 20, 2013, from http://www.aacn.org/WD/Practice/Docs/PracticeAlerts/oral%20care%2004-2010%20final.pdf

American Dental Association (ADA). (n.d.). Cleaning your teeth and gums (oral hygiene). Retrieved April 22, 2013, from http://www.ada.org/2624.aspx

American Diabetes Association. (2013). Position statement. Standards of medical care in diabetes–2012. *Diabetes Care, 35*, S11–S63.

American Nurses Association (ANA). (2013). Safe patient handling and mobility. Retrieved April 1, 2013, from http://nursingworld.org/MainMenuCategories/WorkplaceSafety/Healthy-Work-Environment/SafePatient

Ames, N., Sulima, P., Yates, J., et al. (2011). Effects of systematic oral care in critically ill patients: A multicenter study. *American Journal of Critical Care, 20*(5), 103–114.

Bausch & Lomb. (2008). Official home page. Retrieved May 3, 2013, from http://www.bausch.com

Bausch & Lomb. (2009). Inserting and removing your GP contact lenses. Retrieved April 22, 2013, from http://www.bausch.com

Berry, A., Davidson, P., Nicholson, L., et al. (2012). Consensus based clinical guideline for oral hygiene in the critically ill. *Intensive and Critical Care Nursing, 27*, 180–185.

Bliss, D., Zehrer, C., Savik, K., et al. (2006). Incontinence-associated skin damage in nursing home residents: A secondary analysis of a prospective multicenter study. *Ostomy and Wound Management, 52*(12), 46–55.

Bloomfield, J., Pegram, A., & Jones, A. (2008). Recommended procedure for bedmaking in hospital. *Nursing Standard, 22*(23), 41–44.

Bulechek, G., Butcher, H., & Dochterman, J., et al., (2013). *Nursing interventions classification (NIC)* (6th ed.). St. Louis, MO: C. V. Mosby.

Cason, C., Tyner, T., Saunders, S., et al. (2007). Nurses' implementation of guidelines for ventilator-associated pneumonia from the Centers for Disease Control and Prevention (CDC). *American Journal of Critical Care, 16*(1), 28–38.

Clark, A., & John, L. (2006). Nosocomial infections and bath water: Any cause for concern? *Clinical Nurse Specialist, 20*, 119–123.

Collins, J., Nelson, A., & Sublet, V. (2006). *Safe lifting and movement of nursing home residents* (DHHS (NIOSH) Publication No. 2006-117). Altanta, GA: National Institute for Occupational Safety and Health. Retrieved June 15, 2011, from http://www.cdc.gov/niosh/docs/2006-117/pdfs/2006-117.pdf

Coughlan, M., & Healy, C. (2008). Nursing care, education and support for patients with neutropenia. *Nursing Standard, 22*(46), 35–41.

Courtney, M., Edwards, H., Chang, A., et al. (2012). Improved functional ability and independence in activities of daily living for older adults at high risk of hospital readmission: A randomized controlled trial. *Journal of Evaluation in Clinical Practice, 18*(1), 128–134.

Cuccio, L., Cerullo, E., Paradis, H., et al. (2012). An evidence-based oral care protocol to decrease ventilator-associated pneumonia. *Dimensions of Critical Care Nursing, 31*(5), 301–308.

Department of Veteran Affairs. (n.d.). Your VA hearing aid. Retrieved May 3, 2013, from http://www.ncrar.research.va.gov/ForVets/documents/HearingAidbook.pdf

D'Hondt, A., Kaasalainen, S., Prentice, D., et al. (2012). Bathing residents with dementia in long-term care: Critical incidents described by personal support workers. *International Journal of Older People Nursing, 7*(4), 253–263.

Doughty, D., Junkin, J., Kurz, P., et al. (2012). Incontinence-associated dermatitis: Consensus statements, evidence-based guidelines for prevention and treatment, and current challenges. *Journal of Wound Ostomy & Continence Nursing, 39*(3), 303.

Downey, L., & Lloyd, H. (2008). Bed bathing patients in hospital. *Nursing Standard, 22*(34), 35–40.

Erikson Labs Northwest. (n.d.). Handling your ocular prosthesis. Retrieved April 22, 2013, from http://www.ericksonlabs.com/v/Artificial_Eyes/care_handling.asp

EZ-Shampoo Instructions for use. (2005). EZ-Access, a division of Homecare Products, Inc., 1704 B Street N.W., Suite 110, Auburn, WA 98001–1650. Retrieved April 22, 2013, from http://mobilityexpress.com/images/products/Manual/EZ-SHAMPOO_Ins_c74f.pdf

Flori, L. (2007). Don't throw in the towel: Tips for bathing a patient who has dementia. *Nursing2007, 37*(7), 22–23.

Gray, M., Bliss, D., Doughty, D., et al. (2007). Incontinence-associated dermatitis: A consensus. *Journal of Wound, Ostomy and Continence Nursing, 34*(1), 45–54.

Haas, J., & Larson, E. (2008). Compliance with hand hygiene guidelines. *American Journal of Nursing, 108*(8), 40–44.

Harris D., Eilers J., Harriman, A., et al. (2008). Putting evidence into practice: Evidence-based interventions for the management of oral mucositis. *Clinical Journal of Oncology Nursing, 12*(1), 141–152.

Holman, C., Roberts, S., & Nicol, M. (2005). Promoting healthy sight and eye care. *Nursing Older People, 17*(1), 37–38.

Hospital Info. (2010). Artificial eye service (ocular prosthetics). Norfolk and Norwich University Hospitals, NHS Foundation Trust. Retrieved April 22, 2013, from http://www.nnuh.nhs.uk/Dept.asp?ID=517

Institute for Preventive Foot Health. (2012). *National foot health assessment 2012.* Retrieved June 6, 2012, from http://www.ipfh.org/images/research_materials/2012_National_Foot_Health_Assessment_June_2012.pdf

The Joanna Briggs Institute. (2004). Oral hygiene care for adults with dementia in residential aged care facilities. *Best Practice, 8*(4), 1–6. Retrieved May 3, 2013, from http://connect.jbiconnectplus.org

The Joanna Briggs Institute. (2007). Topical skin care in aged care facilities. *Best Practice, 11*(3), 1–3.

Johnson, D., Lineweaver, L., & Maze, L. (2009). Patients' bath basins as potential sources of infection: A multicenter sampling study. *American Journal of Critical Care, 18*, 31–40.

Johnson, M., Moorhead, S., Bulechek, G., et al. (2012). *NOC and NIC linkages to NANDA-I and clinical conditions* (3rd ed.). St. Louis, MO: C. V. Mosby.

Katz, S., Down, T., Cash, H., et al. (1970). Progress in the development of the Index of ADL. *The Gerontologist, 10*(1), 20–30. Copyright © The Gerontological Society of America. Retrieved May 3, 2013, from http://consultgerirn.org/uploads/File/trythis/try_this_2.pdf

Kayser-Jones, J., Bird, W., Paul, S., et al. (1995). An instrument to assess the oral health status of nursing home residents. Gerontologist, *35*(6), 814–824, 823. Copyright © The Gerontological Society of America. Reproduced by permission of the publisher. Retrieved December 21, 2008, April 30, 2013, from http://consultgerirn.org/uploads/File/trythis/try_this_18.pdf

Konno, R., Stern, C., & Gibb, H. (2013). The best evidence for assisted bathing of older people with dementia: a comprehensive systematic review. *The Joanna Briggs Institute (JBI) Database of Systematic Reviews and Implementation Reports, 11*(1), 123–212.

Landers, T., Abusalem, S., Coty, M. B., et al, (2012). Patient-centered hand hygiene: The next step in infection prevention. *American Journal of Infection Control, 40*(4, Suppl. 1), S11–S17.

Larkin, C. (2011). How to get an Alzheimer's patient to bathe. *Alzheimer's Reading Room*. Retrieved April 20, 2013, from http://www.alzheimersreadingroom.com/2011/04/how-to-get-alzheimers-patient-to-bathe.html

Larson, E., Ciliberti, T., Chantler, C., et al. (2004). Comparison of traditional and disposable bed baths in critically ill patients. *American Journal of Critical Care, 13*(3), 235–241.

Lorente, L., Lecuona, M., Jiménez, A., et al. (2012). Ventilator-associated pneumonia with or without toothbrushing: A randomized controlled trial. *European Journal of Clinical Microbiology & Infectious Diseases, 31*(10), 2621–2629.

Massachusetts Eye and Ear Infirmary. (n.d.; last updated 2009, January 5). Contact lens options. Retrieved May 3, 2013, from http://www.masseyeandear.org/specialties/ophthalmology/contact-lens/about/

Meade, C., Bursell, A., & Ketelsen, L. (2007). Effects of nursing rounds: On patients' call light use, satisfaction, and safety. *American Journal of Nursing, 107*(2), 58–70; quiz 70–71.

Mitchell, B., Wilson, F., McGregor, A., et al. (2012). *Evaluating environmental cleanliness in hospitals and other healthcare settings. What are the most effective and efficient methods to use?* Washington, DC: U.S. Department of Health and Human Services. Retrieved April 22, 2013, from http://www.dhhs.tas.gov.au/__data/assets/pdf_file/0007/126961/TIPCU_Environmental_Hygiene_Assessment_Report_2012.pdf

Moorhead, S., Johnson, M., Maas, M., et al. (Eds.). (2012). *Nursing outcomes classification (NOC)* (5th ed.). St. Louis, MO: C. V. Mosby.

NANDA International. (2012). *NAN DA nursing diagnoses: Definitions and classification, 2012–2014*. Oxford: Wiley-Blackwell.

National Guideline Clearinghouse (NGC). (2006; revised 2011). *Guideline synthesis: Prevention of pressure ulcers*. Rockville, MD: Agency for Healthcare Research and Quality. Retrieved April 20, 2013, from http://www.guideline.gov/syntheses/synthesis.aspx?id=25078&search=perineal+care.

National Guideline Clearinghouse (NGC). (2008a). *Clinical practice guideline for type 2 diabetes*. Rockville, MD: Agency for Healthcare Research and Quality. Retrieved June 19, 2013, from http://www.guideline.gov/content.aspx?id=36628&search=microvascular

National Guideline Clearinghouse (NGC). (2008b, December). *Guideline summary: Oral health: Nursing assessment and interventions*. Rockville, MD: Agency for Healthcare Research and Quality. Retrieved May 3, 2013, from http://www.guidelines.gov/content.aspx?id=15612&search=oral+health%3a+nursing+assessment+and+interventions.

National Institute on Deafness and Other Communication Disorders (NIDCD). (2007). *NIDCD fact sheet: Hearing aids*. Retrieved May 3, 2013, from http://www.nidcd.nih.gov/staticresources/health/hearing/HearingAids07.pdf

Neppelenbroek, K., Pavarina, A., Spolidorio, D., et al. (2008). Effectiveness of microwave disinfection of complete dentures on the treatment of *Candida*-related denture stomatitis. *Journal of Oral Rehabilitation, 35*(11), 836–846.

O'Flynn, J. (2007). Prospective sampling of patient bath basins in acute care setting: Qualitative evaluation of bacterial colonization. *American Journal of Infection Control 35*(5), E50–E51.

Pappas, P., Rex, J., Sobel, J., et al. (2009). Clinical practice guidelines for treatment of candidiasis: 2009 update by the Infectious Diseases Society of America. *Clinical Infectious Disease, 38*(2), 161–189. Retrieved May 3, 2013, http://www.guidelines.gov/content.aspx?id=14174&search=treatment+of+candidiasis

Peters, R. (2010). Artificial eyes of glass and plastic and suggestions regarding their care. *Center for Ocular Prosthetics*. Retrieved May 3, 2013, from http://www.fredharwin.com/ocular/index.php

Philip, P., Rogers, C., Kruger, E., et al. (2012). Oral hygiene care status of elderly with dementia and in residential aged care facilities. *Gerotontology, 29*(2), 306–311.

Plummer, E., & Albert, S. (2008). Diabetic foot care management in the elderly. *Clinics in Geriatric Medicine, 24*(3), 551–567, viii.

Powers, J., Peed, J., Burns, L., et al. (2012). Chlorhexidine bathing and microbial contamination in patients' bath basins. *American Journal of Critical Care, 21*(5), 338–342.

Procter & Gamble. (2008). How to shave. Trim and shape. Retrieved April 22, 2013, from http://www.gillette.com/en/us/mens-style/how-to-shave.aspx?utm_source=Bing&utm_medium=cpc&utm_term=for%2Bshaving%2B&utm_campaign=Gillette.BR_Search_Category%2BInterest_06.2010

Rasin, J., & Barrick, A. L. (2004). Bathing patients with dementia. *American Journal of Nursing, 104*(3), 30–33.

Ritz, J., Pashnik, B., Padula, C., et al. (2012). Effectiveness of 2 methods of chlorhexidine bathing. *Journal of Nursing Care Quality, 27*(2), 171–175.

Robles, R., Corcoles, G., Torres, L., et al. (2002). Frequency of the adverse events during [Spanish]. *Enfermia Intensive, 12*(2), 47–56.

Rönner, A. C., Berland, C. R., Runeman, B., et al. (2010). The hygienic effectiveness of 2 different skin cleansing procedures. *Journal of Wound Ostomy & Continence Nursing, 37*(3), 260.

Rose, M., & Drake, D. (2008). Best practices for skin care of the morbidly obese. *Bariatric Nursing and Surgical Patient Care, 3*(2), 129–134.

Rubin, C., Louthan, R. B., Wessels, E., et al. (2013). Chlorhexidine gluconate: To bathe or not to bathe? *Critical Care Nursing Quarterly, 36*(2), 233–236.

Rutala, W. A., & Weber, D. J.; HICPAC. (2008). *Guideline for disinfection and sterilization in healthcare facilities, 2008*. Atlanta, GA: Centers for Disease Control and Prevention. Retrieved July 17, 2014, from http://www.cdc.gov/hicpac/pdf/guidelines/Disinfection_Nov_2008.pdf

Salcido, R. (2012). Patient safety: It is in our hands. *Advances in Skin and Wound Care, 25*(8), 342.

Sergent, A. P., Slekovec, C., Pauchot, J., et al. (2012). Bacterial contamination of the hospital environment during wound dressing change. *Orthopaedics & Traumatology: Surgery & Research, 98*(4), 441–445.

7 Tips for the best shave ever. (updated 2011). *Men's Health*. Retrieved May 3, 2013, from http://www.mh.co.za/grooming/shave/7-tips-for-the-best-shave-ever.

Siegel, J., Rhinehart, E., Jackson, M., Chiarello, L.; the Healthcare Infection Control Practices Advisory Committee. (2007). *2007 Guideline for isolation precautions: Preventing transmission of infectious agents in the healthcare setting*. Retrieved May 3, 2013, from http://www.cdc.gov/hicpac/pdf/isolation/Isolation2007.pdf

Sievert, D., Armola, R., & Halm, M. (2011). Chlorhexidine gluconate bathing: Does it decrease hospital-acquired infections? *American Journal of Critical Care, 20*, 166–170.

Silva, M., Mima, E., Colombo, A., et al. (2012). Comparison of denture microwave disinfection and conventional antifungal therapy in the treatment of denture stomatitis: a randomized clinical study. *Oral Surgery, Oral Medicine, Oral Pathology and Oral Radiology, 114*(4), 469–479.

Slot, D., Dörfer, C., & Van der Weijden, G. (2008). The efficacy of interdental brushes on plaque and parameters of periodontal inflammation: A systematic review. *International Journal of Dental Hygiene, 26*(4), 253–264.

Thompson Healthcare, Inc. (2012). How to shampoo the hair of a person in bed. Retrieved April 22, 2013, from http://www.drugs.com/cg/how-to-shampoo-the-hair-of-a-person-in-bed.html

U.S. Food and Drug Administration. (2009, October). A new online guide to hearing aids. Retrieved May 3, 2013, from http://www.fda.gov/downloads/ForConsumers/ConsumerUpdates/UCM187245.pdf

U.S. Food and Drug Administration. (2013, April). FDA safety communication: Damaged or worn covers for medical bed mattresses pose risk of contamination and patient infection. Retrieved April 24, 2013, from http://www.fda.gov/MedicalDevices/Safety/AlertsandNotices/ucm348016.htm

Warchol, K. (2013). *Tips to reduce bathing and showering challenges—a therapist's role.* Milwaukee, WI: Crisis Prevention Institute (CPI). Retrieved April 20, 2013, from http://www.crisisprevention.com/Resources/Article-Library/Dementia-Care-Specialists-Articles/Behavior-Management/Tips-To-Reduce-Bathing-And-Showering-Challenges

Weening-Verbree, L., Huisman-de Waal, G., van Dusseldorp, L., et al. (2013). Oral health care in older people in long term care facilities: A systematic review of implementation strategies. *International Journal of Nursing Studies, 50*(4), 569–582.

White-Chu, E. F., & Reddy, M. (2011). Dry skin in the elderly: complexities of a common problem. *Clinics in Dermatology, 29*(1), 37–42.

Yao, L. Y., Chang, C. K., Maa, S. H., et al. (2011). Brushing teeth with purified water to reduce ventilator-associated pneumonia. *Journal of Nursing Research, 19*(4), 289–297.

CHAPTER 26

Advisory Committee on Immunization Practices (ACIP). (n.d.). Immunization schedules. Retrieved July 9, 2013, from http://www.cdc.gov/vaccines/schedules/hcp/index.html

Agac, E., & Gunes, U. (2011). Effect on pain of changing the needle prior to administering medicine intramuscularly: A randomized controlled trial. *Journal of Advanced Nursing, 67*(3), 563–568.

Amarasingham, R., Plantinga, L., Diener-West, M., et al. (2009). Clinical information technologies and inpatient outcomes: A multiple hospital study. *Archives of Internal Medicine, 169*, 108–114.

American Academy of Family Physicians (AAFP). (2004; updated 2011, February). Nasal sprays: How to use them correctly. *Family Doctor.* Retrieved July 9, 2012, from http://familydoctor.org/online/famdocen/home/common/allergies/treatment/104.html

American Society of Health-System Pharmacists, Inc. (n.d.). How to use rectal suppositories properly. Retrieved July 9, 2013, from http://www.safemedication.com/safemed/MedicationTipsTools/HowtoAdminister/HowtoUseRectalSuppositoriesProperly.aspx

Bartley, N. (2012). Administering intramuscular and subcutaneous injections in children. *World of Irish Nursing & Midwifery, 20*(8), 39–42.

Berryman, S., Jennings, J., Ragsdale, R., et al. (2012). Beers criteria for potentially inappropriate medication use in older adults. *MedSurg Nursing, 21*(3), 129–133.

Bertolino, G., Pitassi, A., Tinelli, C., et al. (2012). Intermittent flushing with heparin versus saline for maintenance of peripheral intravenous catheters in a medical department: A pragmatic cluster-randomized controlled study. *Worldviews on Evidence-Based Nursing, 9*(4), 221–226.

Bulechek, G., Butcher K., Dochterman, J., et al. (Eds.). (2013). *Nursing interventions classification (NIC)* (6th ed.). St. Louis, MO: Elsevier Mosby.

Castillo, S. L. M., & Werner-McCullough, M. (2012). *Student workbook to accompany calculating drug dosages* (3rd ed.). Philadelphia: F. A. Davis.

Centers for Disease Control and Prevention (CDC). (n.d.). Vaccine administration. Retrieved June 23, 2013, from http://www.cdc.gov/vaccines/pubs/pinkbook/downloads/appendices/d/vacc_admin.pdf

Centers for Disease Control and Prevention (CDC). (2010a, updated 2012). Administering vaccines: Dose, route, site, and needle size. Retrieved June 23, 2013, from http://www.immunize.org/catg.d/p3085.pdf

Centers for Disease Control and Prevention (CDC). (2010b). Eye safety. Retrieved July 9, 2013, from http://www.cdc.gov/niosh/topics/eye/

Centers for Disease Control and Prevention (CDC). (2011a). Medication administration questions. Retrieved July 9, 2013, from http://www.cdc.gov/injectionsafety/providers/provider_faqs_med-admin.html

Centers for Disease Control and Prevention (CDC). (2011b). Guidelines for the prevention of intravascular catheter related infections, 2011. Retrieved August 18, 2013, from http://www.cdc.gov/hicpac/pdf/guidelines/bsi-guidelines-2011.pdf

Centers for Disease Control and Prevention (CDC). (2012). Home healthcare workers: How to prevent needlestick and sharp injuries. Retrieved June 27, 2013, from http://www.cdc.gov/niosh/docs/2012-123/

Ching, J., Long, C., Williams, B., et al. (2013). Using lean to improve medication administration safety: In search of the "perfect dose." *Joint Commission Journal on Quality & Patient Safety, 39*(5), 194–204.

Cohen, M. (2007). *Preventing medication errors* (2nd ed.). Washington, DC: American Pharmacist Association.

Crawford, C., & Johnson, J. (2012). To aspirate or not: An integrated review of the evidence. *Nursing2012, 42*(3), 20–25.

Crawford, D. (2012). Maintaining good practice in the administration of medicines to children. *Nursing Children & Young People, 24*(4), 29–35.

Cummings, K., & McGowan, R. (2011). "Smart" infusion pumps are selectively intelligent. *Nursing2011, 41*(3), 58–59. Retrieved June 16, 2013, from http://www.fda.gov/MedicalDevices/Safety/AlertsandNotices/TipsandArticlesonDeviceSafety/ucm245160.htm

De Castillo, L., & Werner-McCullough, M. (2012). *Calculating drug dosages: An interactive approach to learning nursing math* (3rd ed.). Philadelphia: FA Davis.

Denholm, B. (2013). Repackaging medication from single-dose vials. *AORN Journal, 97*(3), 370–372.

DeYoung, J., Bauer, R., Brady, C., et al. (2011). Controlling blood glucose levels in hospital patients: Current recommendations. *American Nurse Today, 6*(5). Retrieved June 22, 2013, from http://www.americannursetoday.com/article.aspx?id=7802&fid=7770

Dougherty, L., Sque, M., & Crouch (2012). Decision-making processes used by nurses during intravenous drug preparation and administration. *Journal of Advanced Nursing, 68*(6), 1302–1311.

Dumont, C., & Nesselrodt, D. (2012). Preventing CLABSI. *Nursing2012, 42*(6), 41–47.

Elias, B., & Moss, J. (2011). Smart pump technology: What we have learned. *Computers in Informatics Nursing, 29*(3), 184–190.

Elliott, M., & Liu, Y. (2010). The nine rights of medication administration: An overview. *British Journal of Nursing, 19*(5), 300–305.

Fakih, M., Jones, K., Rey, J., et al. (2012). Peripheral venous catheter care in the emergency department: Education and feedback lead to marked improvements. *American Journal of Infection Control, 41*(6), 531–536.

Floyd, S., & Meyer, A. (2007). Intramuscular injections—what's best practice? *Nursing, 13*(6), 20–22.

Flynn, L., Liang, Y., Dickinson, G., et al. (2012). Nurses' practice environments, error interception practices, and inpatient medication errors. *Journal of Nursing Scholarship, 44*(2), 180–186.

Gandhi, K., Dahiya, A.,Taruna-Kalra, A., et al. (2012). Recent in transdermal drug delivery systems. *Journal of Pharmacy Research, 5*(8), 4329–4337.

Gangurde, M., Chordiya, M., Baste, N., Tamizharasi, S., & Upasani, C. (2012). Approaches and devices used in pulmonary drug deliver system: A review. *Asian Journal of Pharmaceutical Research & Health Care, 4*(1), 11–27.

Glaucoma Research Foundation. (2012). Eye drop tips. Retrieved July 9, 2013, from http://www.glaucoma.org/treatment/eyedrop-tips.php

Goedert, J. (2010, June 30). CPOE tester shows high error rates. *HDM Breaking News*.

Greenway, K. (2004). Using the ventral gluteal site for intramuscular injection. *Nursing Standard, 18*(29), 39–42.

Han, Y. Y., Carcillo, J. A., Venkataraman, S. T., et al. (2005). Unexpected increased mortality after implementation of a commercially sold computerized order entry system. *Pediatrics, 116*, 1506–1512.

Hayes, B., Klein-Schwartz, W., & Gonzales, L. (2009). Causes of therapeutic errors in older adults: Evaluation of national poison center data. *Journal of American Geriatrics Society, 57*(4), 653–658.

Heller, J. L. (2011, updated). Eye emergencies. *MedlinePlus*. Retrieved July 9, 2013, from http://www.nlm.nih.gov/medlineplus/ency/article/000054.htm

Infusion Nurses Society (INS). (2009). Infusion nursing standards of practice. *Journal of Infusion in Nursing, 29*(Suppl. 1), S1–S9.

Infusion Nurses Society (INS). (2011a). *Infusion nursing standards of practice*. Norwood, MA: Gardner Foundation.

Infusion Nurses Society (INS). (2011b). Infusion nursing standards of practice. *Journal of Infusion in Nursing, 34*(Suppl. 1), S1–S9, S41–S46.

Institute for Safe Medication Practices (ISMP). (n.d.). ISMP guidelines. Retrieved July 2, 2013, from https://www.ismp.org/default.asp

Institute for Safe Medication Practices (ISMP). (2004). IMSP list of error-prone abbreviations, symbols, and dose designations. Retrieved July 9, 2013, from http://www.ismp.org/tools/errorproneabbreviations.pdf

Institute for Safe Medication Practices (ISMP). (2013). ISMP medication safety alert! Retrieved August 27, 2013, from http://www.ismp.org/newsletters/acutecare/showarticle.asp?id=42

Ipp, M., Taddio, A., Sam, J., et al. (2007). Vaccine-related pain: Randomized controlled trial of two injection techniques. *Archives of Disease in Childhood, 92*(12), 1105–1108.

Jackson, L., Peterson, D., Nelson, J., et al. (2013). Vaccination site and risk of local reactions in children 1 through 6 years of age. *Pediatrics, 13*(2), 283–289.

The Joanna Briggs Institute. (2005). Strategies to reduce medication errors with reference to older adults. *Best Practice, 9*(4), 1–6.

Johnson, M., Bulchek, G., Moorhead, S., et al. (2012). *NOC and NIC Linkage to NANDA-I and Clinical Conditions* (3rd ed.). St. Louis, MO: Elsevier Mosby.

The Joint Commission (TJC). (n.d.). Sentinel event alert/topics library updates. Retrieved July 2, 2013, from http://www.jointcommission.org/daily_update/joint_commission_daily_update.aspx?k=721&b=&t=4&pg=1

The Joint Commission (TJC). (2008). Preventing pediatric medication errors. *Sentinel Event Alert*, 39. Retrieved August 6, 2013, from http://www.jointcommission.org/sentinel_event_alert_issue_39_preventing_pediatric_medication_errors/

The Joint Commission (TJC). (2010). *Summary data of sentinel events reviewed by The Joint Commission*. Oakbrook Terrace, IL: Author.

The Joint Commission (TJC). (2011). 2011–2012 National patient safety goals. Retrieved August 16, 2013, from http://www.jointcommission.org/assets/1/6/NPSG_EPs_Scoring_CAH_20110707.pdf

The Joint Commission (TJC). (2012). Hospital: 2013 national patient safety goals. Retrieved July 9, 2013, from http://www.jointcommission.org/standards_information/npsgs.aspx

Kelly, J., Eggleton, A., & Wright, D. (2011). An analysis of two incidents of medicine administration to a patient with dysphagia. *Journal of Clinical Nursing, 20*(1/2), 146–155.

Klejka, D. (2012). Shhh! Conducting a quiet zone pilot study for medication safety. *Nursing2012, 42*(9), 18–21.

Kliegman, R., Stanton, B., St. Geme, J., et al. (2011). *Nelson textbook of pediatrics* (19th ed.). St. Louis, MO: W. B. Saunders.

Lareau, S., & Hodder, R. (2012). Teaching inhaler use in chronic obstructive pulmonary disease patients. *Journal of the American Academy of Nurse Practitioner, 24*(2), 113–120.

Lavery, I. (2011). Intravenous therapy: Preparation and administration of IV medicines. *British Journal of Nursing, 2*(4), S28–S34.

Magaji, V., & Johnston, J. (2011). Inpatient management of hyperglycemia and diabetes. *Clinical Diabetes, 29*(1), 3–9.

Manchikanti, L, Falco, F., Beyamin, R., et al. (2012). Assessment of infection control practices for interventional techniques: A best evidence synthesis of safe injection practices and use of single-dose medication vials. *Pain Physician Journal, 15*, E573–E614.

Mandrack, M., Cohen, M., Featherling, J., et al. (2012). Nursing best practices using automated dispensing cabinets: Nurses' key role in improving medication safety. *MedSurg Nursing, 21*(3), 134–144.

Mason, I., & Stevens, S. (2010). Instilling eye drops and ointment in a baby or young child. *Community Eye Health Journal, 23*(72), 15.

Mattox, E. (2012). Strategies for improving patient safety: Linking task type to error type. *Critical Care Nurse, 32*(1), 52–78.

Mckay, M. (2012). Prevention of medical errors. *Advance for Nurses*. Retrieved June 15, 2013 from, http://nursing.advanceweb.com/Continuing-Education/CE-Articles/Prevention-of-Medical-Errors.aspx

Moorhead, S., Johnson, M., Maas, M., et al. (2013). *Nursing outcomes classification (NOC)* (5th ed.). St. Louis, Elsevier Mosby.

Morris, H. (2012). How to recognize dysphagia and provide support. *Nursing & Residential Care, 14*(10), 522–525.

NANDA International. (2012). *Nursing diagnoses: Definitions and classification 2012–2014*, Oxford: Wiley-Blackwell.

National Center for HIV, STD, and TB Prevention, Division of Tuberculosis Elimination. (2008; updated 2012, September 2). Mantoux tuberculosis skin test facilitator guide. Part one: Administering the Mantoux tuberculin skin test. Retrieved July 9, 2013, from http://www.cdc.gov/tb/education/Mantoux/part1.htm

National Coordinating Council for Medication Error Reporting and Prevention. (2012). Consumer information for safe medication use. Retrieved June 15, 2013, from http://www.nccmerp.org/consumerInfo.html

Needleless connectors for IV catheters. (2012). *American Journal of Nursing, 112*(11), 32–46.

Nourbakhsh, E., Anvari, R., & Nugent, K. (2011). Abdominal wall hematomas associated with low-molecular-weight heparins: An important complication in older adults. *Journal of the American Geriatrics Society, 59*(8), 1543–1545.

Occupational Safety and Health Administration (OSHA). (2011). *Protecting yourself when handling contaminated sharps* [Fact sheet]. Retrieved June 21, 2013, from http://www.osha.gov/OshDoc/data_BloodborneFacts/bbfact02.pdf

Olsen, D. (2012). Ethical issues: Putting the meds in the applesauce. *American Journal of Nursing, 112*(3), 67–69.

Perry, M. (2011). The problem of polypharmacy in the elderly. *Nurse Prescribing, 9*(7), 347–349.

Phillips, D. (2010). *Manual of IV therapeutics* (5th ed.). Philadelphia: F. A. Davis.

Phillips, N., & Nay, R. (2008). A systematic review of nursing administration of medication via enteral tubes in adults. *Journal of Clinical Nursing, 17*(17), 2257–2265.

Pledger, J., Hicks, D., Kirkland, F., et al. (2012). Importance of injection technique in diabetes. *Journal of Diabetes Nursing, 16*(4), 160–165.

Poon, E. G., Keohane, C. A., Yoon, C. S., et al. (2010, May 6). Effect of bar-code technology on the safety of medication administration. *New England Journal of Medicine, 362*(18), 1698–1707.

Pretorius, R., Gataric, G., Swedlund, S., et al. (2013). Reducing the risk of adverse events in older adults. *American Family Physician, 87*(5), 331–336.

Rosenthal, K. (2007). Avoiding common perils of drug administration. *Nursing, 37*(4), 20–21.

Roy, V., Gupta, P., & Srivastava, S. (2005). Medication errors: Causes & prevention. *Health Administrator, 19*(1), 60–64.

Rubin, J., Nash, P., & Safran, A. (2012, August). Medication error case settles for $8.25 million prior to trial. *Healthcare Risk Management*, 1–3.

Shanks, L. (2011). Medication Calculation Competency. *American Journal of Nursing, 111*(10), 67–69.

Sittig, D. F., & Singh, H. (2011). Defining health information technology–related errors: New developments since To Err Is Human. *Archives of Internal Medicine, 171*, 1281–1284.

State of Missouri Department of Health and Senior Service. (n.d.). Dispensing medications. Retrieved June 27, 2013, from http://health.mo.gov/living/lpha/phnursing/dispensingmeds.php

Terrie, Y. (2012). Relieving the discomfort of dry eye. *Pharmacy Times, 78*(4), 20, 22–23.

Trbovich, P. L., Pinkney, S., Cafazzo, J. A., et al. (2010, October 19). The impact of traditional and smart pump infusion technology on nurse medication administration performance in a simulated inpatient unit. *Quality and Safety in Health Care, 19*(5), 430–434.

Tzeng, H., Yin, C., & Schneider, T. (2013). Medication error-related issues in nursing practice. *MedSurg Nursing, 22*(1), 13–16, 50.

U.S. Department of Health and Human Services (USDHHS), National Institute for Occupational Safety and Health (NIOSH). (2011). *How to prevent needlestick and sharp injuries* (Publication No. 2012–123). Atlanta, GA: Centers for Disease Control and Prevention. Retrieved July 8, 2013, from http://www.cdc.gov/niosh/docs/2012-123/pdfs/2012-123.pdf

U.S. Department of Health and Human Services, National Diabetes Information Clearinghouse. (updated 2012, February 12). Types of insulin. Retrieved August 18, 2013, from http://diabetes.niddk.nih.gov/dm/pubs/medicines_ez/insert_C.aspx

U.S. Food and Drug Administration. (2012; updated 2013, February 5). Medication errors. Retrieved July 2, 2013 from http://www.fda.gov/drugs/drugsafety/medicationerrors/default.htm

U.S. Food and Drug Administration, Center of Evaluation and Research. (2013). Phase-out CFC metered-dose inhalers (MDI). Retrieved August 5, 2013, from http://www.fda.gov/Drugs/DrugSafety/InformationbyDrugClass/ucm063054.htm

Walden, A., & Vanglider, M. (2013). *To aspirate or not to aspirate? The latest evidence on intramuscular injection techniques*. Poster session presented at the 18th Annual Research Conference, University of North Georgia, Dahlonega. Retrieved June 23, 2013, from http://digitalcommons.northgeorgia.edu/ngresearchconf/2013/trialtrack/4/

Walsh, L., & Brophy, K. (2011). Staff nurses' sites of choice for administering intramuscular injections to adult patients in the acute care setting. *Journal of Advanced Nursing, 67*(5), 1034–1040.

Werner, R., & Morien, A. (2012). Topical medications: Another occupational hazard. *Massage & Bodywork, 27*(5), 48–51.

Zaybak, A., & Khorshid, L. (2008). Study on the effect of the duration of subcutaneous heparin injection on bruising and pain. *Journal of Clinical Nursing, 17*(3), 378–385.

Zwicker, D., & Fulmer, T. (2008). Reducing adverse drug events. In E. Capezuti, D. Zwicker, M. Mezey, & T. Fulmer (Eds.), *Evidence-based geriatric nursing protocols for best practice* (3rd ed.). New York: Springer.

Zwicker, M., & Fulmer, T. (updated 2012). MEDICATION—Nursing standard of practice protocol: Reducing adverse drug events. *Hartford Institute for Geriatric Nursing*. Retrieved June 19, 2013, from http://consultgerirn.org/topics/medication/want_to_know_more#item_5

CHAPTER 27

A Report of the Panel on Macronutrients, Subcommittees on Upper Reference Levels of Nutrients and Interpretation and Uses of Dietary Reference Intakes, and the Standing Committee on the Scientific Evaluation of Dietary Reference Intakes. (2005). Dietary Reference Intakes for energy, carbohydrate, fiber, fat, fatty acids, cholesterol, protein, and amino acids (macronutrients). National Academy of Science, Institute of Medicine, Retrieved July 1, 2013, from http://books.nap.edu/openbook.php?record_id=10490&page=R1

Academy of Nutrition and Dietetics. (2012). *Food and nutrition for older adults promoting health and wellness.* Chicago, IL: Author.

Agency for Healthcare Research and Quality (AHRQ). (2012, November). *Screening and diagnosing gestational diabetes mellitus.* Rockville, MD: Author. Retrieved June 27, 2013, from http://www.ahrq.gov/clinic/tp/gdmexuptp.htm

Agency for Healthcare Research and Quality (AHRQ). (2003, June). *Routine vitamin supplementation to prevent cancer and cardiovascular disease. What's new from the USPST.* (AHRQ Publication No. APPIP03–0012). Rockville, MD: Author. Retrieved July 3, 2013, from http://www.uspreventiveservicestaskforce.org/uspstf/uspsvita.htm

Alves, J., Gale, C., Mutrie, N., et al. (2009). A 6-month exercise intervention among inactive and overweight favela-residing women in Brazil: The Caranguejo exercise trial. *American Journal of Public Health, 99*(1), 76–80. doi: 10.2105/AJPH.2007.124495

Amella, E. J. (2008). Brief summary: Mealtime difficulties. In M. Mezey, I. Abraham, & D. A. Zwicker (Eds.), *Evidence-based geriatric nursing protocols for best practice* (2nd ed., pp. 337–351). New York: Springer. Retrieved July 3, 2013, from http://www.guideline.gov/content.aspx?id=12267

Amella, E., & Lawrence, J. F. (2007). Eating and feeding issues in older adults with dementia: Part II: Interventions. *Try This: Best Practices in Nursing Care for Hospitalized Older Adults With Dementia, D11.*2. The John A. Hartford Institute for Geriatric Nursing and the Alzheimer's Association. Retrieved October 26, 2014, from http://consultgerirn.org/uploads/File/trythis/try_this_d11_1.pdf

American Academy of Pediatrics (AAP). (2008). Breastfeeding, family physician supporting [Position paper]. Retrieved October 26, 2014, from http://www.aafp.org/online/en/home/policy/policies/b/breastfeedingpositionpaper.html

American Academy of Pediatrics (AAP). (2010). AAP publishes new recommendations for iron intake among infants, toddlers. Retrieved October 26, 2014, from http://www.aafp.org/news-now/clinical-care-research/20101020aapironrpt.html

American Association of Critical-Care Nurses (AACCN). (2005a; revised 2009, December). Practice alert. Verification of feeding tube placement. Retrieved October 26, 2014, from http://www.aacn.org/WD/Practice/Docs/PracticeAlerts/Verification_of_Feeding_Tube_Placement_05-2005.pdf

American Association of Critical-Care Nurses (AACCN). (2005b, revised 2009, December). Practice alert. Dye in enteral feeding. Retrieved October 26, 2014, from http://www.aacn.org/wd/practice/docs/practicealerts/dye_in_enteral_feeding_4-2005.pdf

American Association of Critical-Care Nurses (AACCN). (2010). *AACN procedure manual for critical care* (6th ed.). D. J. Wiegand (Ed.). St. Louis, MO: Elsevier Saunders.

American Diabetes Association. (2013, June 7, last reviewed Managing diabetes. Checking blood glucose. Retrieved July 3, 2013, from http://www.diabetes.org/living-with-diabetes/treatment-and-care/blood-glucose-control/checking-your-blood-glucose.html

American Diabetes Association. (2011). Summary of revisions to the 2011 clinical practice recommendations. *Diabetes Care, 34*(Suppl. 1), S3. doi:10.2337/dc11-S003

American Heart Association (AHA). (n.d.a; updated 2011, June 29). Fats and oils: AHA recommendation. Retrieved October 26, 2014, from http://www.heart.org/HEARTORG/GettingHealthy/FatsAndOils/Fats101/Fats-and-Oils-AHA-Recommendation_UCM_316375_Article.jsp

American Heart Association (AHA). (n.d.b). Fat substitutes. Retrieved October 26, 2014, from http://www.heart.org/HEARTORG/GettingHealthy/NutritionCenter/Fat-Substitutes_UCM_305978_Article.jsp

American Heart Association (AHA). (n.d.c, updated 2010, May 21). Consumer FAQ: "Better" fats (monounsaturated and polyunsaturated fats). Retrieved March 16, 2013, from http://www.heart.org/HEARTORG/GettingHealthy/NutritionCenter/Frequently-Asked-Questions-About-Better-Fats_UCM_305985_Article.jsp

American Medical Directors Association (AMDA). (2010). Altered nutritional status in the long-term care setting. Columbia, MD: Author. Retrieved March 14, 2013, from http://guideline.gov/content.aspx?id=32490&search=altered+nutritional+status

American Society for Parenteral and Enteral Nutrition (A.S.P.E.N.) Board of Directors. (2009a). Clinical guidelines for the use of parenteral and enteral nutrition in adult and pediatric patients, 2009. *Journal of Parenteral and Enteral Nutrition, 33*(3), 255–259. doi: 10.1177/0148607109333115

American Society for Parenteral and Enteral Nutrition (A.S.P.E.N.) Board of Directors. (2009b). Special report: Enteral nutrition practice recommendations. *Journal of Parenteral and Enteral Nutrition, 20*(10). doi:10.1177/0148607108330314

Annesi, J., & Whitaker, A. (2008). Relations of mood and exercise with weight loss in formerly sedentary obese women. *American Journal of Health Behavior,* 32(6), 676–683. doi: 10.5555/ajhb.2008.32.6.676

Annweiler, C., Rolland, Y., Schott, A. M., et al. (2012). Higher vitamin D dietary intake is associated with lower risk of Alzheimer's disease: A 7-year follow-up. *Journals of Gerontology: Series A, 67*(11), 1205–1211. doi: 10.1093/gerona/gls107

A.S.P.E.N. Board of Directors and Task Force on Parenteral Nutrition Standardization. (2007). A.S.P.E.N. statement on parenteral nutrition standardization. *Journal of Parenteral and Enteral Nutrition, 31*(5), 441–448. doi: 10.1177/0148607107031005441

A.S.P.E.N. Board of Directors and Task Force for the Revision of Safe Practices for Parenteral Nutrition. (2004). Safe practices for parenteral nutrition. *Journal of Parenteral and Enteral Nutrition, 28*(6), S39–S70. doi:10.1177/0148607104028006S39

Bankhead, R., Boullata, J., Brantley, S., et al. (2009). Monitoring enteral nutrition administration. In A.S.P.E.N. enteral nutrition practice recommendations. *JPEN: Journal of Parenteral and Enteral Nutrition, 33*(2),162–6.

Bankhead, R. Boullata, J., Brantley, S., et al.; American Society for Parenteral and Enteral Nutrition (A.S.P.E.N.), Board of Directors. (2009). Special report: Enteral nutrition practice recommendations. *Journal of Parenteral and Enteral Nutrition, 20*(10). doi:10.1177/0148607108330314

Barberger-Gateau, P., Raffaitin, C., Letenneur, L., et al. (2007). Dietary patterns and risk of dementia. The three-city cohort study. *Neurology, 69*, 1921–1930.

Barone, L., Milosavljevic, M., & Gazibarich, B. (2003). Assessing the older person: Is the MNA a more appropriate nutritional assessment tool than the SGA? *Journal of Nutritional Health Aging, 7*(1), 13–17.

Berkowitz, B., & Borchard, M. (2009). Advocating for the prevention of childhood obesity: A call to action for nursing. *Online Journal of Issues in Nursing, 14*(1), Manuscript 2. doi: 10.3912/OJIN.Vol14No1Man02

Boitano, M., Bojak, S., McCloskey, S., et al. (2010). Improving the safety and effectiveness of parenteral nutrition. *Nutrition in Clinical Practice, 25*(6), 663–671. doi: 10.1177/08845336 10385349

Buck, H. G., (2012). Real world symptom management: Nursing. *Nursing2012, 42*(3), 18–19. doi: 10.1097/01.NURSE. 0000411415.06409.c4

Bulechek, G., Butcher, H., & Dochterman, J. (2012). *Nursing interventions classification (NIC)* (6th ed.). St. Louis, MO: C. V. Mosby.

Centers for Disease Control and Prevention (CDC). (n.d.; updated 2011, August 17). *Health effects of overweight and obesity.* Atlanta, GA: U.S. Department of Health and Human Services, Centers for Disease Control and Prevention. Retrieved April 1, 2013, from http://www.cdc.gov/healthyweight/effects/index.html

Centers for Disease Control and Prevention (CDC). (n.d., updated 2011, September 13). *Body mass index.* Atlanta, GA: U.S. Department of Health and Human Services, Centers for Disease Control and Prevention. Retrieved April 1, 2013, from http://www.cdc.gov/healthyweight/assessing/bmi/index.html

Centers for Disease Control and Prevention (CDC). (2005). Recommended infection-control and safe injection practices to prevent patient-to-patient transmission of blood-borne pathogens. Diabetes care procedures & techniques. *Morbidity and Mortality Weekly Report, 54*(09), 220–223. Retrieved June 3, 2013, from http://www.cdc.gov/hepatitis/Populations/PDFs/diabetes_handout.pdf

Centers for Disease Control and Prevention (CDC). (2008; updated 2013, January). Overweight and obesity. Obesity prevalence. Retrieved July 3, 2013, from http://www.cdc.gov/nccdphp/dnpa/obesity/childhood/prevalence.htm

Centers for Disease Control and Prevention (CDC). (2009). Application of lower sodium intake recommendations to adults—United States, 1999–2006. *Morbidity and Mortality Weekly Report, 58*(11), 281–283. Retrieved January 3, 2013, from http://www.cdc.gov/mmwr/preview/mmwrhtml/mm5811a2.htm

Centers for Disease Control and Prevention. (2011). *National diabetes fact sheet: National estimates and general information on diabetes and prediabetes in the United States, 2011.* Atlanta, GA: U.S. Department of Health and Human Services, Centers for Disease Control and Prevention. Retrieved March 16, 2013, from http://www.cdc.gov/DIABETES//pubs/pdf/ndfs_2011.pdf

Cincinnati Children's Hospital Medical Center. (2011). *Best evidence statement (BESt). Confirmation of nasogastric/orogastric tube placement.* Cincinnati, OH: Author. Retrieved February 20, 2013, from http://www.guideline.gov/content.aspx?id=35117

Clark, R., Birks, J., Nexo, E., et al. (2007). Low vitamin B_{12} status and risk of cognitive decline in older adults. *American Journal of Clinical Nutrition, 86*(5), 1384–1391.

deRuyter, J. C., Olthof, M. R., Seidel, J. C., et al. (2012). A trial of sugar-free or sugar-sweetened beverages and body weight in children. *New England Journal of Medicine, 367*, 1397–1406. doi:10.1056/NEJMoa1203034.

Detsky, A., McLaughlin, J., Baker, J., et al. (1987). What is subjective global assessment? *Journal of Parenteral and Enteral Nutrition, 11*(1), 813–817.

DiMaria-Ghalili, R., & Guenter, P. (2008). The mini nutritional assessment. *American Journal of Nursing, 108*(2), 50–59; quiz 60. doi: 10.1097/01.NAJ.0000310340.60377.e8

Donnelly, J. E., Blair, S. N., Jakicic, J. M., et al. (2009, June). Appropriate physical activity intervention strategies for weight loss and prevention of weight regain for adults. American College of Sports Medicine Position Stand. *Medicine & Science in Sports & Exercise, 41*(2), 459–447. doi:10.1249/MSS.0b013e3181949333

Ebbeling, C. B., Feldman, H. A., Chomitz, V. R., et al. (2012, October 11). A randomized trial of sugar-sweetened beverages an adolescent body weight. *New England Journal of Medicine, 367*, 1407–1416. doi:10.1056/NEJMoa1203388

Ebersole, P., Hess, P., Touhy, T., et al. (2013). *Ebersole and Hess' gerontological nursing & healthy aging* (4th ed.). Philadelphia: Elsevier.

Editorial Board Palliative Care, Association of Comprehensive Cancer Centres (ACCC). (2006, January 12). *Practice guidelines: Nausea and vomiting*. Utrecht, the Netherlands: Author.

Elpern, E., Killeen, K., Talla, E., et al. (2007). Capnometry and air insufflations for assessing initial placement of gastric tubes. *American Journal of Critical Care, 16*(6), 544–550.

Estruch, R., Ros, E., Salas-Salvado, et al. (2013). Primary prevention of cardiovascular disease with a Mediterranean diet. *The New England Journal of Medicine.* doi:10.1056/NEJMoa1200303

Flicker, L. L., McCaul, K. A., Hankey, G. J., et al. (2010). Body mass index and survival in men and women aged 70 to 75. *Journal of the American Geriatrics Society, 58*(2), 234–241. DOI: 10.1111/j.1532-5415.2009.02677.x

Food and Nutrition Board, Institute of Medicine, National Academies. (1997–2011). Dietary Reference Intakes (DRIs): Recommended dietary allowances and adequate intakes, vitamins. Retrieved January 3, 2013, from http://www.iom.edu/Reports/2010/Dietary-Reference-Intakes-for-Calcium-and-Vitamin-D.aspx

Garibalia, S. E., & Forster, S. J. (2008). Dietary intake of older patients in hospital and at home: the validity of patient kept food diaries. *Journal of Nutrition, Health & Aging, 12*(2), 102–106. doi: 10.1007/BF02982561

Glucose monitoring. A guide to checking your blood sugar. (2008). *Advance for Nurse Practitioners, 16*(12), 28.

Griffiths, R., Thompson, D., Chau, J., et al. (2006). *Systematic reviews. Insertion and management of nasogastric tubes for adults.* The Joanna Briggs Institute. Retrieved April 3, 2013, from http://connect.jbiconnectplus.org/ViewSourceFile.aspx?0=5384

Guyton, A. C., & Hall, J. E. (2011). *Textbook of medical physiology* (12th ed.). Philadelphia: W. B. Saunders.

Hollis, J., Gullion, C., Stevens, V., et al.; Weight Loss Maintenance Trial Research Group. (2008). Weight loss during the intensive intervention phase of the weight-loss maintenance trial.

American Journal of Preventive Medicine, 35(2), 118–126. doi: 10.1016/j.amepre.2008.04.013

Honenyard, D. (2008). Dietary strategies for preventing cancer. *The Clinical Advisor, 11*(3), 23–25, 29–30.

Hortensius, J., Slingerland, R., Kleefstra, N. et al. (2011). Self-monitoring of blood glucose: The use of the first or the second drop of blood. *Diabetes Care, 34*(3), 556–560. doi: 10.2337/dc10-1694

Infusion Nurses Society (INS). (2011). Infusion nursing standards of practice. *Journal of Infusion Nursing, 34*(1S). Norwood, MA: Author.

Institute of Medicine. (2000). Dietary intakes of vitamin C, vitamin E, selenium, and carotenoids. *Pharmacist's Letter, 16*(5), 26–27. Washington, DC: The National Academies Press.

Institute for Safe Medication Practices (ISMP). (2010, July 15). Preventing catheter/tubing misconnections. *ISMP Medication Safety Alert*. Retrieved April 1, 2013, from http://www.ismp.org/newsletters/acutecare/articles/20100715.asp

Institute for Safe Medication Practices (ISMP). (2014, August 14). Urgent! Health systems need to plan now for upcoming changes in enteral feeding device connectors. *ISMP Medication Safety Alert!* Retrieved November 4, 2014, from Https://Www.Ismp.Org/Newsletters/Acutecare/Showarticle.Aspx?Id=86

Ip, S., Chung, M., Raman, G., et al. (2007). *Breastfeeding and maternal and infant health outcomes in developed countries* (Evidence Report/Technology Assessment No. 153; AHRQ Publication No. 07-E007). Rockville, MD: Agency for Healthcare Research and Quality.

The Joanna Briggs Institute. (2007). Effective dietary interventions for overweight and obese children. *Best Practice, 11*(1), 69–72.

The Joanna Briggs Institute. (2010). Methods for determining the correct nasogastric tube placement after insertion in adults. *Best Practice, 14*(1), 1–4. Retrieved March 3, 2013, from http://connect.jbiconnectplus.org/ViewSourceFile.aspx?0=5384

The Joanna Briggs Institute. (2012) Methods for determining the correct nasogastric tube placement after insertion in adults. *Best Practice, 14*(1), 2010.

Jockers, B. (2007). Vitamin D sufficiency: An approach to disease prevention. *The American Journal for Nurse Practitioners, 11*(10), 43–50.

Johnson, M., Bulechek, G., Dochterman, J. M., et al. (2012). *NOC and NIC linkages to NANDA-I and clinical conditions* (3rd ed.). St. Louis, MO: C. V. Mosby.

Kenny, D., Goodman, P. (2010). Care of the client with enteral tub feeding: An evidence based practice protocol. *Nursing Research, 59*(Suppl. 1), S22–S31. doi: 10.1097/NNR.0b013e3181c3bfe9

Lim, L. S., Hoeksema, L. J., Sherin, K.; the ACPM Prevention Practice Committee. (2009, April). Screening for osteoporosis in the adult U.S. population: ACPM position statement on preventive practice. *American Journal of Preventative Medicine, 36*(4), 366–375. doi:10.1016/j.amepre.2009.01.013

Lutz, C., & Przytulski, K. (2010). *Nutrition and diet therapy* (5th ed.). Philadelphia: F. A. Davis.

Marik, P. E., & Zaloga, G. P. (2004). Meta-analysis of parenteral versus enteral nutrition in patients with pancreatitis. *BMJ, 328*, 1407. doi.org/10.1136/bmj.38118.593900.55.

Marion County Children's Alliance. (2012, March 1). 5-2-1-0 brochure. Retrieved March 30, 2013, from http://www.mcchildrensalliance.org/5210/

Millin, C. J., & Brooks, M. (2012). Reduce—and report—enteral feeding tube misconnections. *Nursing2012, 40*(11), 59–60.

Mitrou, P., Kipnis, V., Thiébaut, A., et al. (2007). Mediterranean dietary pattern and prediction of all-cause mortality in a US population. *Archives of Internal Medicine, 167*(22), 2461–2468. doi:10.1001/archinte.167.22.2461

Moorhead, S., Johnson, M., Maas, M., et al. (2012). *Nursing outcomes classification (NOC)* (5th ed.). St. Louis, MO: C. V. Mosby.

NANDA International. (2012). *Nursing diagnoses: Definitions and classification 2012–2014*. Ames, IA: Wiley-Blackwell.

National Agricultural Library, U.S. Department of Agriculture. (n.d.). Dietary guidance, DRI tables. (1997–2011). Retrieved January 3, 2013 from http://iom.edu/Activities/Nutrition/SummaryDRIs/~/media/Files/Activity%20Files/Nutrition/DRIs/ULs%20for%20Vitamins%20and%20Elements.pdf

National Agricultural Library, U.S. Department of Agriculture. Dietary guidance, DRI tables. (2001). Retrieved January 3, 2013, from http://www.iom.edu/Global/News%20Announcements/~/media/48FAAA2FD9E74D95BBDA2236E7387B49.ashx

National Agricultural Library, U.S. Department of Agriculture. Dietary guidance, DRI tables. (last modified 2004, March 19). Retrieved January 7, 2013, from http://nutritionandaging.fiu.edu/DRI_and_DGs/DRI%20Table%203%20pages%209-13-2004.pdf

National Agricultural Library, U.S. Department of Agriculture. Dietary guidance, DRI tables. (2005). Retrieved January 3, 2013, from http://books.nap.edu/openbook.php?record_id=10490

National Association of Anorexia Nervosa and Associated Disorders. (n.d.). Eating disorders statistics. Retrieved January 3, 2013, from http://www.anad.org/get-information/about-eating-disorders/eating-disorders-statistics/

National Center for Health Statistics. (2012, October 10). Faststats. Overweight and obesity. In Centers for Disease Control and Prevention. Retrieved January 3, 2013, from http://www.cdc.gov/nchs/fastats/overwt.htm

National Digestive Diseases Information Clearinghouse (NDDIC). (2009, last updated 2012, April 23). Lactose intolerance. National Institute of Diabetes and Digestive and Kidney Diseases, National Institutes of Health. Retrieved January 3, 2013, from http://digestive.niddk.nih.gov/ddiseases/pubs/lactoseintolerance/#cause

National Guideline Clearinghouse (NGC). (2006). *Assessment and management of obesity and overweight in adults*. Rockville, MD: Agency for Healthcare Research and Quality. Retrieved January 3, 2013, from http://www.guideline.gov/syntheses/synthesis.aspx?id=25323

National Guideline Clearinghouse (NGC). (2008). Brief guideline summary: Prevention of bloodstream infections. In *Prevention and control of healthcare-associated infections in Massachusetts*. Rockville, MD: Agency for Healthcare Research and Quality. Retrieved January 3, 2013, from http://www.guideline.gov/content.aspx?id=12922

National Guideline Clearinghouse (NGC). (2009, April). *Guideline summary: Screening for osteoporosis in the adult U.S. population: ACPM position statement on preventive practice*. Rockville, MD: Agency for Healthcare Research and Quality. Retrieved January 3, 2013, from http://www.guideline.gov/summary/summary.aspx?view_id=1&doc_id=15270

National Guideline Clearinghouse (NGC). (2010). *Guideline summary: Altered nutritional status.* Rockville, MD: Agency for Healthcare Research and Quality. Retrieved December 20, 2012, from http://guideline.gov/content.aspx?id=32490&search=altered+nutritional+status

National Heart, Lung and Blood Institute (NHLBI). (n.d.). Classification of overweight and obesity by BMI, waist circumference, and associated risks. Retrieved January 3, 2013, from http://www.nhlbi.nih.gov/health/public/heart/obesity/lose_wt/bmi_dis.htm

National Heart, Lung and Blood Institute (NHLBI). (1998). Clinical guidelines on the identification, evaluation, and treatment of overweight and obesity in adults: The evidence report. Washington, DC: U.S. Department of Health & Human Services. Retrieved January 3, 2013, from http://www.nhlbi.nih.gov/guidelines/obesity/ob_gdlns.htm

National Institutes of Health (NIH). (n.d.a; last updated 2012, October 8). Nasogastric feeding tube. *MedlinePlus.* Retrieved December 25, 2012, from http://www.nlm.nih.gov/medlineplus/ency/patientinstructions/000182.htm

National Institutes of Health (NIH), Office of Dietary Supplements. (n.d.b). *Dietary supplement fact sheet: Zinc.* Retrieved December 14, 2012, from http://ods.od.nih.gov/factsheets/Zinc-HealthProfessional/

National Institutes of Health, Office of Dietary Supplements. (2010). Diet may protect against gene changes in smokers. *NIH News.* Retrieved March 16, 2013, from http://www.nih.gov/news/health/jan2010/nci-12.htm

National Institutes of Health, Office of Dietary Supplements. (2004). Dietary reference intakes for water and electrolytes; and Dietary reference intakes for trace elements. Retrieved January 7, 2013, from http://www.iom.edu/Global/News%20Announcements/~/media/442A08B899F44DF9AAD083D86164C75B.ashx

Naylor, P-J., & McKay, H. (2009). Prevention in the first place: Schools a setting for action on physical inactivity. *British Journal of Sports Medicine, 43,* 10–13.

Nestlé HealthCare Nutrition, Inc. The BE A. L. E. R. T.© poster is a joint effort of the American Society for Parenteral and Enteral Nutrition (A.S.P.E.N.) and Nestlé Health Care Nutrition, Inc. (2009). Be A. L. E. R. T.: Practice safe enteral feeding. Retrieved June 20, 2013, from http://www.nutritioncare.org/Professional_Resources/Patient_Safety/Patient_Safety

Newman, A. (2009, January 31). Obesity in older adults. *OJIN, 14*(1), Manuscript 3. Retrieved January 3, 2013, from http://www.nursingworld.org/MainMenuCategories/ANAMarketplace/ANAPeriodicals/OJIN/TableofContents/Vol142009/No1Jan09/Obesity-in-Older-Adults.aspx

Nutrition Screening Initiative (NSI). (1991). *Report of nutrition screening I: Toward a common view.* Washington, DC: Author.

Ogden, C. L., Carroll, M. D., Kit, B. K., et al. (2012, January). *Prevalence of obesity in the United States, 2009–2010* (NCHS Data Brief 82). Retrieved December 3, 2012, from http://www.cdc.gov/nchs/data/databriefs/db82.pdf

Orton, C. C. (2012). Vitamin B_{12} (cobalamin) deficiency in the older adult. *The Journal for Nurse Practitioners, 8*(7), 547–553. doi:10.1016/j.nurpra2011.10.009

Owen, C., Martin, R., Whincup, P., et al. (2007). Does breastfeeding influence risk of type 2 diabetes in later life? A quantitative analysis of published evidence. *American Journal of Clinical Nutrition, 84*(5), 1045–1054.

Peter, S., & Gill, F. (2009). Development of a clinical practice guideline for testing nasogastric tube placement. *Journal for Specialists in Pediatric Nursing, 14*(1), 3–11. doi: 10.1111/j.1744-6155.2008.00161.x

Rauen, C., Chulay, M., Bridges, E., et al. (2008). Seven evidence-based practice habits: Putting some sacred cows out to pasture. *Critical Care Nurse, 28*(3), 98–124.

Rosenbauer, J., Herzig, P., Kaiser, P., et al. (2007). Early nutrition and risk of type 1 diabetes mellitus—a nationwide case-control study in preschool children. *Experimental & Clinical Endocrinology & Diabetes, 115*(8), 502–508. doi: 10.1055/s-2007-973829

Ross, C. A., Taylor, C. L., Yaktine, A. L., et al. (Eds.). (2011). Committee to Review Dietary Reference Intakes for Vitamin D and Calcium. Institute of Medicine. Retrieved April 1, 2013, from http://www.nap.edu/openbook.php?record_id=13050

Scarmeas, N., Luchsinger, J., Mayeux, R., et al. (2007). Mediterranean diet and Alzheimer disease mortality. *Neurology, 69,* 1084–1093.

Schardt, D. (2008, March). Caffeine. The good, the bad, and the maybe. *Nutrition Action Health Letter.* Center for Science in the Public Interest. Retrieved January 3, 2013, from http://www.cspinet.org/nah/02_08/caffeine.pdf

Schlenker, E., & Roth, S. (2010). *Williams' essentials of nutrition & diet therapy* (10th ed.). St. Louis, MO: C. V. Mosby.

Shlamovitz, G. Z., & Shah, N. R. (2008). Nasogastric tube. *Emedicine.* Retrieved January 3, 2013, from http://emedicine.medscape.com/article/80925-overview

Simmons, S. (2013). Folic acid: Friend or foe? *Nursing2013, 43*(3), 55–60.

Simons, S. R., & Abdallah, L. M. (2012). Bedside assessment of enteral tube placement: Aligning practice with evidence. *American Journal of Nursing, 112*(2), 40–48.

Slinin, Y., Paudel, M., Taylor, B. C., et al. (2012). Association between serum 25(OH) vitamin D and the risk of cognitive decline in older women. *Journals of Gerontology, Series A, 67*(10), 1092–1098. doi: 10.1093/gerona/gls075

Smith-Spangler, C., Brandeau, M. L., Hunter, B. A., et al. (2012). Are organic foods safer or healthier than conventional alternatives? *Annals of Internal Medicine, 157*(5), 348–366. doi:10.7326/0003-4819-157-5-201209040-00007

Speroni, K., Earley, C., & Atherton, M. (2007). Evaluating the effectiveness of the Kids Living FitTM Program: A comparative study. *Journal of School Nursing, 23*(6), 329–336. doi: 10.1177/10594050702300605 01

Swinburn, B., Sacks, G., Lo, S., et al. (2009). Estimating the changes in energy flux that characterize the rise in obesity prevalence. *American Journal of Clinical Nutrition, 89*(6), 1723–1728. doi: 10.3945/ ajcn.2008.27061

Thompson, J., & Manore, M. (2012). *Nutrition: An applied approach* (3rd ed.). San Francisco: Benjamin Cummings.

Tufts University Nutrition. (2011, November). MyPlate for older adults. Retrieved December 23, 2012, from http://www.nutrition.tufts.edu/research/myplate-older-adults.

U.S. Department of Agriculture (USDA). (2011a, June). ChooseMyPlate.gov. Retrieved March 18, 2013, from http://www.choosemyplate.gov/

U.S. Department of Agriculture (USDA). (2011b, June). Healthy eating for vegetarians: Ten tips for vegetarians. *10 Tips Education Series, DG Tip sheet #8.* Retrieved April 3, 2013, from http://www.choosemyplate.gov/food-groups/downloads/TenTips/DGTipsheet8HealthyEatingForVegetarians.pdf

U.S. Department of Agriculture (USDA). (2011c, June). Be a healthy role model for children: Ten tips for setting good examples. *10 Tips Education Series, DG Tip sheet #12.* Retrieved January 3, 2013, from http://www.choosemyplate.gov/downloads/TenTips/DGTipsheet12BeAHealthyRoleModel.pdf

U.S. Department of Agriculture (USDA). (2011d, June). Build a healthy meal: Ten tips for healthy meals. *10 Tips Education Series, DG Tip sheet #7.* Retrieved April 3, 2013, from http://www.choosemyplate.gov/food-groups/downloads/TenTips/DGTipsheet7BuildAHealthyMeal.pdf

U.S. Department of Agriculture (USDA). (2011e, June). *ChooseMyPlate.gov: Weight management & calories.* Retrieved January 3, 2013, from http://www.choosemyplate.gov/STEPS/stepstoahealthierweight.html

U.S. Department of Agriculture. (2011f). Dietary Reference Intakes (DRIs): Tolerable upper intake levels, vitamins. Food and Nutrition Board, Institute of Medicine, National Academies. Retrieved January 3, 2013, from http://iom.edu/Activities/Nutrition/SummaryDRIs/~/media/Files/Activity%20Files/Nutrition/DRIs/ULs%20for%20Vitamins%20and%20Elements.pdf

U.S. Department of Agriculture. (2011g). Dietary Reference Intakes for calcium and vitamin D. Retrieved January 3, 2013, from http://fnic.nal.usda.gov/nal_display/index.php?info_center=4&tax_level=3&tax_subject=256&topic_id=1342&level3_id=5140

U.S. Department of Agriculture, Food and Nutrition Center. (2002–2005). Dietary guidance. DRI tables. Dietary reference intakes: Macronutrients. National Academy of Sciences. Institute of Medicine. Food and Nutrition Board. Retrieved from http://fnic.nal.usda.gov/dietary-guidance/dietary-reference-intakes/dri-tables

U.S. Department of Agriculture and U.S. Department of Health and Human Services. (2010). *Dietary guidelines for Americans, 2010* (7th ed.). Washington, DC: U.S. Government Printing Office.

U.S. Department of Health and Human Services (USDHHS). (2008). *2008 Physical activity guidelines for Americans.* ODPHP Publication No. U0036. In USDHHS, Office of Disease Prevention and Health Promotion. Retrieved January 3, 2013, from http://www.health.gov/paguidelines/guidelines/default.aspx

U.S. Department of Health and Human Services (USDHHS). (2010, last updated 2012, August 2). *Healthy People 2020, topics and objectives.* Nutrition and weight status. Retrieved January 3, 2013, from http://healthypeople.gov/2020/topicsobjectives2020/default.aspx

U.S. Department of Health and Human Services, Centers for Disease Control and Prevention, & National Center for Health Statistics. (2012). *Health, United States, 2011, with special feature on socioeconomic status and health. Publication* No. 2012-1232. Washington, DC: U.S. Government Printing Office. Retrieved January 3, 2013, from http://www.cdc.gov/nchs/data/hus/hus11.pdf#069

U.S. Food and Drug Administration (FDA). (2005). Luer lock misconnections can be deadly. Retrieved January 2, 2012, from http://www.premierinc.com/quality-safety/tools-services/safety/topics/tubing-misconnections/downloads/fda-luer-lock-misconnections.pdf

U.S. Food and Drug Administration (FDA). (2007a). A key to choosing healthful foods: Using the nutrition facts on the food label. Center for Food Safety and Applied Nutrition. Retrieved January 3, 2013, from http://www.fda.gov/downloads/Food/ResourcesForYou/Consumers/UCM079504.pdf

U.S. Food and Drug Administration (FDA). (2007b). Continuous 7-day glucose monitoring system. *Consumer update.* Retrieved January 3, 2013, from http://www.fda.gov/ForConsumers/ConsumerUpdates/ucm049062.htm

U.S. Preventive Services Task Force (USPSTF). (2009). Folic acid for the prevention of neural tube defects. *Clinical summary of U.S. Preventive Services Task Force recommendation. Agency for Healthcare Research and Quality.* Retrieved January 3, 2013, from http://www.ahrq.gov/clinic/uspstf09/folicacid/folicsum.htm

van Dam, R. M., Willett, W. C., Manson, J. E., et al. (2006). Coffee, caffeine, and risk of type 2 diabetes: A prospective cohort study in younger and middle-aged U.S. women. *Diabetes Care, 29*(2), 398–403. doi:10.2337/diacare.29.02.06.dc05-1512

Vegetarian Diet Information. (n.d.). U.S. Vegetarian dietary guideline. Retrieved April 3, 2013, from http://www.vegetarian-diet.info/vegetarian-dietary-guidelines.htm

Vogiatzoglou, A., Refsum, H., Johnston, C., et al. (2008). Vitamin B_{12} status and rate of brain volume loss in community-dwelling elderly. *Neurology, 71*(11), 826–832.

Wagner, C., & Greer, F.; the Section on Breastfeeding and Committee on Nutrition. (2008). Prevention of rickets and vitamin D deficiency in infants, children, and adolescents. *Pediatrics, 122*(5), 1142–1152. doi: 10.1542/peds.2008-1862.

Wamsteker, E. W., Geenen, R., Zelissen, P. M. J., et al. (2009). Unrealistic weight-loss goals among obese patients are associated with age and causal attributions. *Journal of the American Dietetic Association, 109*(11), 1903. doi:10.1016/j.jada.2009.08.012

Wolfe, T., Fosnocht, D., & Linscott, M. (2000). Atomized lidocaine as topical anesthesia for nasogastric tube placement: A randomized, double-blind, placebo-controlled trial. *Annals of Emergency Medicine, 35*(5), 421–425. DOI: http://dx.doi.org/10.1067/mem.2000.106988

World Health Organization (WHO). (n.d.). Global strategy on diet, physical activity, and health: Childhood overweight and obesity. Retrieved March 27, 2013, from http://www.who.int/dietphysicalactivity/childhood/en/

World Health Organization. (1999). *Definition, diagnosis, and classification of diabetes mellitus and its complications: Report of a WHO consultation. Part I: Diagnosis and classification of diabetes mellitus.* Geneva, Switzerland: Author.

World Health Organization (WHO). (2006a). BMI classification. Global database on body mass index. Retrieved January 3, 2013, from http://apps.who.int/bmi/index.jsp?introPage=intro_3.html

World Health Organization (WHO). (2006b). WHO child growth standards length/height-for-age, weight-for-age, weight-for-length, weight-for-height and body mass index-for-age. Retrieved January 3, 2013, from http://www.who.int/childgrowth/standards/Technical_report.pdf

Yackel, E. E. (2003). An activity calendar program for children who are overweight. *Pediatric Nursing, 29*(1), 17–22.

Yamakawa, M., Yorifuji, T., Inoue, S., et al. (2013, August 12). Breastfeeding and obesity among schoolchildren: A nationwide longitudinal survey in Japan. *JAMA Pediatrics.* doi: 10.1001/jamapediatrics.2013.2230

Yantis, M. A., & Velander, R. (2011). Untangling enteral nutrition guidelines. *Nursing2011, 41*(9), 33–39. doi: 10.1097/01.NURSE.0000405083.15784.83

CHAPTER 28

Beers, M. H., & Berkow, R. (Eds.). (2000). *The Merck manual of geriatrics* (3rd ed.). Whitehouse Station, NJ: Merck Research Laboratories.

Bernard, M. S., Hunter, K. F., & Moore, K. N. (2012). A review of strategies to decrease the duration of indwelling urethral catheters and potentially reduce the incidence of catheter-associated urinary tract infections. *Urologic Nursing, 32*(1), 29–37.

Brown, M. L., Pope, A. W., & Brown, E. J. (2011). Treatment of primary nocturnal enuresis in children: A review. *Child: Care, Health and Development, 37*(2), 153–160. doi: 10.1111/j.1365-2214.2010.01146.x

Buchko, B. L., & Robinson, L. E. (2012). An evidence-based approach to decrease early post-operative urinary retention following urogynecologic surgery. *Urologic Nursing, 32*(5), 260–264, 273.

Bulechek, G. M., Butcher, H. K., Dochterman, J. M., et al. (Eds.). (2013). *Nursing interventions classification (NIC)* (6th ed.). St. Louis, MO: Mosby.

Centers for Disease Control and Prevention (CDC). (2012). Catheter-associated urinary tract infection (CAUTI) event. Retrieved December 8, 2013, from http://www.cdc.gov/nhsn/pdfs/pscManual/7pscCAUTIcurrent.pdf

Chernecky, C. C., & Berger, B. J. (2013). *Laboratory tests and diagnostic procedures* (6th ed.). St. Louis, MO: Elsevier Saunders.

Dowling-Castronovo, A. (2013). Urinary incontinence assessment in older adults part 1–Transient urinary incontinence. *Try This: Best Practices in Nursing Care to Older Adults, 11.1*. Retrieved June 15, 2013, from http://consultgerirn.org/uploads/File/trythis/try_this_11_1.pdf

Dowling-Castronovo, A., & Bradway, C. (2012). Urinary incontinence. In M. Boltz, E. Capezuti, T. Fulmer, & D. Zwicker (Eds.), *Evidence-based geriatric nursing protocols for best practice* (4th ed., pp. 363–387). New York: Springer.

Engberg, S., Cohen, S., & Sereika, S. M. (2009). The efficacy of acupuncture in treating urge and mixed incontinence in women: A pilot study. *Journal of Wound, Ostomy, and Continence Nursing, 36*(6), 661–670. doi: 10.1097/WON.0b013e3181bd82dd

Gameiro, M. O., Moreira, E. H., Gameiro, F. O., et al. (2010). Vaginal weight cone versus assisted pelvic floor muscle training in the treatment of female urinary incontinence. A prospective, single-blind, randomized trial. *International Urogynecology Journal, 21*(4), 395–399. doi: 10.1007/s00192-009-1059-7

Geng, V., Bonns, E., Eelen, P., et al. (2008). *The male external catheter*. European Association of Urology Nurses. Retrieved June 15, 2013, from http://www.uroweb.org/fileadmin/EAUN/guidelines/EAUN_MEC_Guidelines_EN_2008_LR.pdf

Geng, V., Cobussen-Boekhorst, H., Farrell, J., et al. (2012, February). *Catheterisation: Indwelling catheters in adults*. European Association of Urology Nurses. Retrieved June 15, 2013, from http://www.uroweb.org/fileadmin/EAUN/guidelines/EAUN_Paris_Guideline_2012_LR_online_file.pdf

Glazener, C., Boachie, C., Buckley, B., et al. (2011). Urinary incontinence in men after formal one-to-one pelvic-floor muscle training following radical prostatectomy or transurethral resection of the prostate (MAPS): Two parallel randomised controlled trials. *Lancet, 378*(9788), 328–337. DOI: 10.3310/hta15240

Goode, P. S., Burgio, K. L., Richter, H. E., et al. (2010). Incontinence in older women. *JAMA, 303*(21), 2172–2181. Retrieved June 15, 2013, from http://dx.doi.org/10.1001/jama.2010.749

Gould, C. V., Umscheid, C. A., Agarwal, R. K., et al.; Healthcare Infection Control Practices Advisory Committee (HICPAC). (2009). *Guideline for prevention of catheter-associated urinary tract infections 2009*. Atlanta, GA: Centers for Disease Control and Prevention (CDC).

Grabe, M., Bjerklund-Johansen, T. E., Botto, H., et al. (2013, March). *Guidelines on urological infections*. European Association of Urology (EAU). Retrieved June 15, 2013, from http://www.uroweb.org/gls/pdf/18_Urological%20infections_LR.pdf

Griffiths, R., & Fernandez, R. (2009). Strategies for the removal of short-term indwelling urethral catheters in adults. *Cochrane Database of Systematic Reviews*, Issue 1. Art. No.: CD004011. doi: 10.1002/14651858.CD004011.pub3

Guay, D. R. (2009). Cranberry and urinary tract infections. *Drugs, 69*(7), 775–807. doi: 10.2165/00003495-200969070-00002

Hagen, S., Sinclair, L., & Cross, S. (2010). Washout policies in long-term indwelling urinary catheterisation in adults. *Cochrane Database of Systematic Reviews*, Issue 3. Art. No.: CD004012, doi: 10.1002/14651858.CD004012.pub4

Hayder, D., & Schnepp, W. (2010). Experiencing and managing urinary incontinence: A qualitative study. *Western Journal of Nursing Research, 32*(4), 480–496. doi: 10.1177/0193945909354903

Herbruck, L. F. (2008). Stress urinary incontinence: An overview of diagnosis and treatment options. *Urologic Nursing, 28*(3), 186–198.

Herter, R., & Kazer, M. W. (2010). Best practices in urinary catheter care. *Home Healthcare Nurse, 28*(6), 342–349. doi: 10.1097/NHH.0b013e3181df5d79

Hooton, T. M., Bradley, S. F., Cardenas, D. D., et al. (2010). Diagnosis, prevention, and treatment of catheter-associated urinary tract infection in adults: 2009 international clinical practice guidelines from the Infectious Diseases Society of America. *Clinical Infectious Diseases, 50*(5), 625–663. doi: 10.1086/650482

Institute for Healthcare Improvement. (2011). How-to guide: Prevent catheter-associated urinary tract infection. Retrieved December 9, 2013, from http://www.ihi.org/knowledge/Pages/Tools/HowtoGuidePreventCatheterAssociatedUrinaryTractInfection.aspx

The Joanna Briggs Institute. (2011, February). JBI Strategies to promote intermittent self-catheterization in adults with neurogenic bladders. *Best Practice, 1*(7), 1–4. Retrieved July 21, 2013, from http://connect.jbiconnectplus.org/ViewSourceFile.aspx?0=7118

Jepson, R. G., Williams, G., & Craig, J. C. (2012, October 17). Cranberries for preventing urinary tract infections (Review). *The Cochrane Library*. doi: 10.1002/14651858.CD001321.pub5

Joseph, A. C. (2006). Noninvasive therapies for treating post-prostatectomy urinary incontinence. *Urologic Nursing, 26*(4), 271–275, 269.

Lo, E., Nicolle, L., Classen, D., et al. (2008). Strategies to prevent catheter-associated urinary tract infections in acute care hospitals. *Infection Control and Hospital Epidemiology, 29*(Suppl. 1), S41–S50. doi: 10.1086/675718

Lucas, M. G., Bedretdinova, D., Bosch, J., et al. (2013, March). *Guidelines on urinary incontinence*. European Association of Urology. doi: 10.1016/j.eururo.2012.09.023

Lynn, P. B. (2011). *Taylor's clinical nursing skills: A nursing process approach* (3rd ed.). Philadelphia: Lippincott Williams & Wilkins.

Magers, T. L. (2013). Using evidence-based practice to reduce catheter-associated urinary tract infections. *American Journal of Nursing, 113*(6), 34–44. doi: 10.1097/01.NAJ.0000430923.07539.a7

Moola, S., & Konno, R. (2010). A systematic review of the management of short-term indwelling urethral catheters to prevent urinary tract infections. *JBI Library of Systematic Reviews, 8*(17), 695–729. Retrieved June 15, 2013, from http://connect.jbiconnectplus.org/ViewSourceFile.aspx?0=5381

Muzzi-Bjornson, L., & Macera, L. (2011). Preventing infection in elders with long-term indwelling urinary catheters. *Journal of the American Academy of Nurse Practitioners, 23*, 127–134. doi: 10.1111/j.1745-7599.2010.00588.x

NANDA International. (2012). *NANDA international nursing diagnoses: Definitions & classification, 2012–2014*. Oxford: Wiley-Blackwell.

National Institute for Health and Clinical Excellence. (2013, March corrected). *Urinary incontinence in women: The management of urinary incontinence in women* [Full guideline draft] (National Collaborating Centre for Women's and Children's Health, Author). Retrieved June 15, 2013, from http://www.nice.org.uk/nicemedia/live/13019/62658/62658.pdf

National Kidney and Urologic Diseases Information Clearinghouse. (2007; updated 2012, June 29). *Retention* (NIH Publication No. 08-6089). Retrieved December 10, 2013, from http://kidney.niddk.nih.gov/kudiseases/pubs/UrinaryRetention/

National Kidney and Urologic Diseases Information Clearinghouse. (2011, November). *Urinary tract infections in adults* (NIH Publication No. 12–2097). Retrieved June 15, 2013, from http://kidney.niddk.nih.gov/kudiseases/pubs/pdf/KU-03.pdf

Newman, D. K., & Willson, M. M. (2011). Review of intermittent catheterization and current best practices. *Urologic Nursing, 31*(1), 12–29,48.

O'Dell, K. K., & McGee, S. (2006). Acupuncture for urinary urgency in women over 50: What is the evidence? *Urologic Nursing, 26*(1), 23–29.

Parker, D., Callan, L., Harwood, J., et al. (2009a). Catheter-associated urinary tract infections: Fact sheet. *Journal of Wound, Ostomy, and Continence Nursing, 36*(2), 156–159.

Parker, D., Callan, L., Harwood, J., et al. (2009b). Nursing interventions to reduce the risk of catheter-associated urinary tract infection. Part 1: Catheter selection. *Journal of Wound, Ostomy, and Continence Nursing, 36*(1), 23–34. doi: 10.1097/01.WON.0000347656.94969.99

Pratt, R., & Pellowe, C. (2010). Good practice in management of patients with urethral catheters. *Nursing Older People, 22*(8), 25–29.

Price, N., Dawood, R., & Jackson, S. R. (2010). Pelvic floor exercise for urinary incontinence: A systematic literature review. *Maturitas, 67*(4), 309–315. doi: 10.1016/j.maturitas.2010.08.004

Rainsbury, P. G., Fabricius, M., & McLarty, E. (2011). Management of urinary incontinence in primary care. *InnovAiT, 4*(1), 23–30. doi: 10.1093/innovait/inq041

Rathnayake, T. (2011). *Urinary incontinence (post-prostatectomy): Management*. The Joanna Briggs Institute. Retrieved November 4, 2014, from http://connect.jbiconnectplus.org/ViewSourceFile.aspx?0=7115

Rigby, D., & Housami, F. A. (2009). Using bladder ultrasound to detect urinary retention in patients. *Nursing Times, 105*, 21. Retrieved July 21, 2013, from http://www.nursingtimes.net/nursing-practice/clinical-zones/continence/using-bladder-ultrasound-to-detect-urinary-retention-in-patients/5001853.article

Robinson, J. P. (2006). Pathology and management of postprostatectomy incontinence. In D. B. Doughty, *Urinary & fecal incontinence: Current management concepts* (3rd ed., pp. 255–265). St. Louis, MO: Mosby Elsevier.

Scanlon, V. C., & Sanders, T. (2011). *Essentials of anatomy and physiology* (6th ed.). Philadelphia: F. A. Davis.

Schröder, A., Abrams, P., Andersson K. E., et al. (2009, March). Incontinence in women. In *Guidelines on urinary incontinence* (pp. 28–43). Arnhem, the Netherlands: European Association of Urology.

Schumm, K., & Lam, T. B. (2010). Types of urethral catheters for management of short-term voiding problems in hospitalised adults. *Cochrane Database of Systematic Reviews*, Issue 11. Art. No.: CD004013. doi: 10.1002/14651858.CD004013.pub3

Seckel, M. A. (2013). Maintaining urinary catheters: What does the evidence say? *Nursing2013, 43*(2), 63–65. doi:10.1097/01.NURSE.0000425872.18314.db.

Shultz, J. M. (2012). Rethink urinary incontinence. *Nursing2012, 42*(11), 32–40.

Siegel, J. D., Rhinehart, E., Jackson, M., Chiarello, L.; Healthcare Infection Control Practices Advisory Committee. (2007). 2007 guideline for isolation precautions: Preventing transmission of infectious agents in healthcare settings. *American Journal of Infection Control, 35*(10, Suppl. 2), S65–S164. Retrieved July 22, 2013, from http://www.cdc.gov/hicpac/pdf/isolation/isolation2007.pdf

Sighinolfi, M. C., Rivalta, M., Mofferdin, A., et al. (2009). Potential effectiveness of pelvic floor rehabilitation treatment for postradical prostatectomy incontinence, climacturia, and erectile dysfunction: A case series. *Journal of Sexual Medicine, 6*(12), 3496–3499. doi: 10.1111/j.1743-6109.2009.01493.x

Smith, J. M. (2006). Current concepts in catheter management. In D. B. Doughty, *Urinary & fecal incontinence: Current management concepts* (3rd ed., pp. 269–307). St. Louis, MO: Mosby Elsevier.

St. Jude Children's Research Hospital. (2004a, June). *Collecting urine cultures from infant boys*. Retrieved June 15, 2013, from http://www.stjude.org/SJFile/sedation_collecting_urine_cultures_infant_boys.pdf

St. Jude Children's Research Hospital. (2004b, June). *Collecting urine cultures from infant girls*. Retrieved June 15, 2013, from https://www.stjude.org/SJFile/sedation_collecting_urine_cultures_infant_girls.pdf

Stuempfle, K. J., & Drury, D. G. (2003). Comparison of 3 methods to assess urine specific gravity in collegiate wrestlers. *Journal of Athletic Training, 38*(4), 315–319.

Thompson, J., & Manore, M. (2012). *Nutrition: An applied approach* (3rd ed.). San Francisco: Pearson Benjamin Cummings.

Townsend, M. K., Jura, Y. H., Curhan, G. C., et al. (2011). Fluid intake and risk of stress, urgency, and mixed urinary incontinence. *American Journal of Obstetrics & Gynecology, 205*(1), 73.e1–73.e6. doi: http://dx.doi.org/10.1016/j.ajog.2011.02.054

Turner, B., & Dickens, N. (2011). Long-term urethral catheterisation. *Nursing Standard, 25*(24), 49–56. doi: 10.7748/ns2011.02.25.24.49.c8344

Van Kampen, M., De Weerdt, W., Van Poppel, H., et al. (2000). Effect of pelvic-floor re-education on duration and degree of incontinence after radical prostatectomy: A randomised controlled trial. *Lancet, 355*(9198), 98–102.

Van Leeuwen, A. M., Poelhuis-Leth, D., & Bladh, M. L. (2011). *Davis's comprehensive handbook of laboratory & diagnostic tests—with nursing implications* (4th ed.). Philadelphia: F. A. Davis.

Vaughan, C. P., Goode, P. S., Burgio, K. L., et al. (2011). Urinary incontinence in older adults. *Mount Sinai Journal of Medicine, 78*(4), 558–570. doi: 10.1002/msj.20276

Wald, H. L., Fink, R. M., Makic, M. B., & Oman, K. S. (2012). Catheter-associated urinary tract infection prevention. In M. Boltz, E. Capezuti, T. Fulmer, & D. Zwicker (Eds.), *Evidence-based geriatric nursing protocols for best practice* (4th ed., pp. 388–408). New York: Springer.

Wilson, M. (2004). Urinary incontinence: A treatise on gender, sexuality, and culture. *Clinical Geriatric Medicine, 20*(3), 565–70.

Wound, Ostomy, and Continence Nurses Society (WOCN). (2003). Identifying and treating reversible causes of urinary incontinence. *Ostomy Wound Management, 49*(12), 28–33.

Wound, Ostomy, and Continence Nurses Society Continence Committee (WOCN). (2008, October). *External catheter fact sheet* [Fact sheet]. Retrieved June 15, 2013, from http://c.ymcdn.com/sites/www.wocn.org/resource/collection/6D79B935-1AA0-4791-886F-E361D29F152D/External_Catheter_-_FS_(2008).pdf

Wound, Ostomy, and Continence Nurses Society (WOCN). (2009). *Indwelling urinary catheters: Best practice for clinicians.* Mount Laurel, NJ: Author.

Yates, A. (2008). Urinary catheters part 4-removing an indwelling urinary catheter. *Nursing Times, 104*(42), 26–27.

Yu Ko, W. F., & Sawatzky, J. V. (2008). Understanding urinary incontinence after radical prostatectomy: A nursing framework. *Clinical Journal of Oncology Nursing, 12*(4), 647–654. doi: 10.1188/08.CJON.647-654

CHAPTER 29

Alverslid, I., Carlsson, E., Gylin, M., et al. (2012). Positive and negative aspects of colostomy irrigation: A patient and WOC nurse perspective. *Diabetes, 37*(5), 515–526.

American Cancer Society. (2011). Detailed guide: Colon and rectum cancer: Revised 03/2/2011. Retrieved June 25, 2013, from http://www.cancer.org/acs/groups/cid/documents/webcontent/003096-pdf.pdf

American Cancer Society. (2013). Cancer prevention & early detection facts & figures. Atlanta, GA: Author. Retrieved June 9, 2013, from http://www.cancer.org/acs/groups/content/@epidemiologysurveilance/documents/document/acspc-037535.pdf

Avent, Y. (2012). Understanding fecal diversions. *Nursing Made Incredibly Easy, 10*(5), 11–16.

Ayello, E., & Sibbald, R. (2008). Preventing pressure ulcers and skin tears. In E. Capezuti, D. Zwicker, M. Mezey, et al. (Eds.), *Evidence-based geriatric nursing protocols for best practice* (3rd ed., pp. 403–429). New York: Springer. Retrieved June 21, 2013, from http://www.guideline.gov/content.aspx?id=12262

Balas, M., Casey, C., & Happ, M. (2008). Comprehensive assessment and management of the critically ill. In E. Capezuti, D. Zwicker, M. Mezey, et al. (Eds.), *Evidence-based geriatric nursing protocols for best practice* (3rd ed., pp. 565–593). New York: Springer. Retrieved June 25, 2013, from http://www.guideline.gov/content.aspx?id=12253%20

Benoit R., & Watts, C. (2007). The effect of a pressure ulcer prevention program and the bowel management system in reducing pressure ulcer prevalence in an ICU setting. *Journal of Wound, Ostomy, & Continence Nursing, 34*(2), 163–175.

Black, P. (2008). Peristomal skin care: An overview of available products. *British Journal of Nursing, 16*, 1048–1056.

Bliss, D. Z., & Norton, C. (2010). Conservative management of fecal incontinence. *The American Journal of Nursing, 110*(9), 30–38.

Bliss, D. Z., Lewis, J., Hasselman, K., et al. (2011). Use and evaluation of disposable absorbent products for managing fecal incontinence by community-living people. *Journal of Wound, Ostomy, and Continence Nursing, 38*(3), 289.

Boyce, J. A., Assa'ad, A., Burks, A. W., et al. (2010). Guidelines for the diagnosis and management of food allergy in the United States: Report of the NIAID-sponsored expert panel. *The Journal of Allergy and Clinical Immunology, 126*(Supp. 6), S1.

Bulechek, F., Butcher, H., & Dochterman, J. (2012). *Nursing interventions classification (NIC)* (6th ed.). St. Louis, MO: C. V. Mosby.

Burch, J., & Sica, J. (2008). Common peristomal skin problems and potential treatment options. *British Journal of Nursing, 17*, S4–S11.

Claros, E., & Toner, F. (2012). Preventing, assessing, and managing constipation in older adults. *Nursing2013, 42*(12), 32–39.

Cronin, E. (2008). Colostomies and the use of colostomy appliances. *British Journal of Nursing, 17*, S12–S16.

Flitcroft, K. L., Irwig, L. M., Carter, S. M., et al. (2012). Colorectal cancer screening: Why immunochemical fecal occult blood tests may be the best option. *BMC Gastroenterology, 12*(1), 183.

Fritz, D., & Pitlick, M. (2012). Evidence about the prevention and management of constipation: Implications for comfort part 1. *Home Healthcare Nurse, 30*(9), 533–540.

Gallagher, P., O'Mahony, D., & Quigley, E. (2008). Management of chronic constipation in the elderly. *Drugs & Aging, 25*(10), 807–822.

Goldberg, M., Aukett, L. K., Carmel, J., et al. (2010). Management of the patient with a fecal ostomy: Best practice guideline for clinicians. *Journal of Wound Ostomy & Continence Nursing, 37*(6), 596–598.

Gomella, L., & Haist, S. (n.d.). Laboratory diagnosis: Chemistry, immunology, serology. *Clinician's pocket reference: The scut monkey* (11th ed., Chapter 4). New York: McGraw-Hill Professional.

Gray-Micelli, D. (2008). Preventing falls in acute care. In E. Capezuti, D. Zwicker, M. Mezey, et al. (Eds.), *Evidence-based geriatric nursing protocols for best practice* (3rd ed., pp. 161–198). New York: Springer. Retrieved June 25, 2013, from http://www.guideline.gov/content.aspx?id=12265&search=Accidental+fall+

Humes, D. J. (2012). Diagnosing and managing acute diverticulitis. *The Practitioner, 256*(1753), 21.

Institute for Clinical Systems Improvement (ICSI). (2012). *Colorectal cancer screening.* Bloomington, MN: Author. Retrieved June 23, 2013, from http://www.guideline.gov/content.aspx?id=37276

Jamshed, N., Lee, Z. E., & Olden, K. W. (2011). Diagnostic approach to chronic constipation in adults. *American Family Physician, 84*(3), 299.

The Joanna Briggs Institute. (2008). Management of constipation in older adults. *Best Practice, 12*(7), 33–36.

The Joint Commission Accreditation Program. (2013). Critical Access Hospital National Patient Safety Goals 2013. Retrieved June 25, 2013, from http://www.jointcommission.org/standards_information/npsgs.aspx

Kent, D. (2008). Changing an ostomy pouching system. *Nursing, 38*(12), 50–54.

Keshava, A., Renwick, A., Stewart, P., et al. (2007). A nonsurgical means of fecal diversion: The Zassi bowel management system. *Diseases of the Colon & Rectum, 50*, 1017–1022.

Leung, F. W., & Rao, S. S. (2011). Approach to fecal incontinence and constipation in older hospitalized patients. *Hospital Practice, 39*(1), 97–104.

Li, C. C., Rew, L., & Hwang, S. L. (2012). The relationship between spiritual wellbeing and psychosocial adjustment in Taiwanese patients with colorectal cancer and a colostomy. *Journal of Wound Ostomy & Continence Nursing, 39*(2), 161–169.

Linari, L. R., Schofield, L. C., & Horrom, K. A. (2011). Implementing a bowel program: Is a bowel program an effective way of preventing constipation and ileus following elective hip and knee arthroplasty surgery? *Orthopaedic Nursing, 30*(5), 317–321.

Lutz, C., & Przytulski, K. (2010). *Nutrition and diet therapy: Evidence-based applications* (5th ed.). Philadelphia: F. A. Davis.

Medline Plus. (2013). Stool guaiac test. U.S. National Library of Medicine, 8600 Rockville Pike, Bethesda, MD 20894. Retrieved July 10, 2013, from http://www.nlm.nih.gov/medlineplus/ency/article/003393.htm

Moorhead, S., Johnson, M., & Maas, M., et al. (Eds.). (2012). *Nursing outcomes classification (NOC)* (5th ed.). St. Louis, MO: C. V. Mosby.

NANDA International. (2012). *NANDA nursing diagnoses: Definitions and classification 2012–2014*. Ames, IA: Wiley-Blackwell.

National Guideline Clearinghouse (NGC). (1996; revised 2009). *Management of constipation*. Rockville, MD: Agency for Healthcare Research and Quality. Retrieved June 22, 2013, from http://www.guideline.gov/content.aspx?id=15434&search=digital+disimpaction

National Guideline Clearinghouse (NGC). (2010). Constipation in children and young people. Diagnosis and management of idiopathic childhood constipation in primary and secondary care. Rockville, MD: Agency for Healthcare Research and Quality. Retrieved June 25, 2013, from http://www.guideline.gov/content.aspx?id=23802

National Guideline Clearinghouse (NGC). (2012). Clinical Guidelines Committee of the American College of Physicians. *Screening for colorectal cancer: A guidance statement from the American College of Physicians*. Rockville, MD: Agency for Healthcare Research and Quality. Retrieved June 9, 2013, from http://www.guidelines.gov/content.aspx?id=38258

National Institute of Allergy and Infectious Diseases (NIAID). (2011; updated 2013, May). *Food allergy and intolerances: NIAID fact sheet: NIAID*. Retrieved June 9, 2013, from http://www.wrongdiagnosis.com/artic/food_allergy_and_intolerances_niaid_fact_sheet_niaid.htm

Obokhare, I. (2012). Fecal impaction: A cause for concern?. *Clinics in Colon and Rectal Surgery, 25*(1), 53–58.

Pitlick, M., & Fritz, D. (2013). Evidence about the pharmacological management of constipation, Part 2: Implications for palliative care. *Home Healthcare Nurse, 31*(4), 207–216.

Pittman, J., Beeson, T., Terry, C., et al. (2012). Methods of bowel management in critical care: A randomized controlled trial. *Journal of Wound Ostomy & Continence Nursing, 39*(6), 633–639.

Poletto, D., & Silva, D. M. G. V. D. (2013). Living with intestinal stoma: The construction of autonomy for care. *Revista Latino-Americana de Enfermagem, 21*(2), 531–538.

Rao, S. S., & Go, J. T. (2010). Update on the management of constipation in the elderly: New treatment options. *Clinical Interventions in Aging, 5*, 163.

Richbourg, L., Fellows, J., & Arroyave, W. (2008). Ostomy pouch wear time in the United States. *Journal of Wound Ostomy and Continence Nursing, 35*(5), 504–508.

Rohwer, K., Bliss, D. Z., & Savik, K. (2013). Incontinence-associated dermatitis in community-dwelling individuals with fecal incontinence. *Journal of Wound Ostomy & Continence Nursing, 40*(2), 181–184.

Salfi, S. F., & Holt, K. (2012). The role of probiotics in diarrheal management. *Holistic Nursing Practice, 26*(3), 142.

Scanlon, V., & Sanders, T. (2010). *Essentials of anatomy and physiology* (6th ed., p. 385). Philadelphia: F. A. Davis.

Shah, B. J., Chokhavatia, S., & Rose, S. (2012). Fecal Incontinence in the elderly: FAQ. *The American Journal of Gastroenterology, 107*, 1635–1646.

Shakil, A., Church, R., & Rao, S. (2008). Gastrointestinal complications of diabetes. *American Family Physician, 77*(12), 1697–1703.

Siegel, J., Rhinehart, E., Jackson, M., et al.; the Healthcare Infection Control Practices Advisory Committee. (2007). *Guideline for isolation precautions: Preventing transmission of infectious agents in healthcare settings, 2007*. Atlanta, GA: Centers for Disease Control and Prevention (CDC). Retrieved June 25, 2013, from http://www.cdc.gov/hicpac/pdf/isolation/Isolation2007.pdf

Song, H. J. (2012). Constipation in community-dwelling elders: Prevalence and associated factors. *Journal of Wound Ostomy & Continence Nursing, 39*(6), 640–645.

Trottier, M., Erebara, A., & Bozzo, P. (2012). Treating constipation during pregnancy. *Canadian Family Physician, 58*(8), 836–838.

Turnbull, G. (revised 2009). *Intimacy after ostomy surgery guide*. United Ostomy Associations of America, Inc. Retrieved October 5, 2013, from http://www.ostomy.org/ostomy_info/pubs/uoaa_sexuality_en.pdf

United Ostomy Associations of America. (2005; updated 2011). Ostomates food reference chart. In *Diet & nutrition guide*. Retrieved June 25, 2013, from http://www.uoaa.org/ostomy_info/pubs/uoa_diet_nutrition_en.pdf

Van Leeuwen, A., Poelhuis-Leth, D., & Bladh, M. (2011). *Davis's comprehensive handbook of laboratory and diagnostic tests with nursing implications* (4th ed.). Philadelphia: F. A. Davis.

Wishin, J., Gallagher, T., & McCann, E. (2008). Emerging options for the management of fecal incontinence in hospitalized patients. *Journal of Wound Ostomy & Continence Nursing, 35*(1), 104–110.

Wound, Ostomy and Continence Nurses Society. (2003; updated 2010). *Guideline for prevention and management of pressure ulcers*. Glenview, IL: Author.

CHAPTER 30

American Academy of Ophthalmology. (2009). Policy statement: Frequency of ocular examinations: November 2009. Retrieved March 13, 2014, from http://www.aao.org/about/policy/upload/Frequency-of-Ocular-Exams-2009.pdf

American Association of Neuroscience Nurses. (2007; revised 2009). *Care of the patient with seizures* (2nd ed.). Glenview, IL: Author. Retrieved March 13, 2014, from http://www.aann.org/pdf/cpg/aannseizures.pdf

Borson, S., Scanlan, J., Brush, M., et al. (2000). The Mini-Cog: A cognitive "vital signs" measure for dementia screening in multi-lingual elderly. *International Journal of Geriatric Psychiatry, 15*(11), 1021–1027. doi: 10.1002/1099-1166(200011)15:113.0.CO;2-6

Braun, C., Stangler, T., Narveson, J., et al. (2009). Animal-assisted therapy as a pain relief intervention for children. *Complementary Therapies in Clinical Practice, 15*(2), 105–109. doi: 10.1016/j.ctcp.2009.02.008

Bulechek, G., Butcher, H., & Dochterman, J. (2012). *Nursing interventions classification (NIC)* (6th ed.). St. Louis, MO: C. V. Mosby.

Burtin, M., & Doree, C. (2009). Ear drops for the removal of ear wax. *Cochrane Database of Systematic Reviews,* Issue 1. Art. No.: CD0043326. doi:10.1002/14651858.CD004326.pub2

Chau, J., Lee, D., & Lo, S. (2012). A systematic review of methods of eye irrigation for adults and children with ocular chemical burns. *Worldviews on Evidence-Based Nursing, 9*(3), 129–138. doi: 10.1111/j.1741-6787.2011.00220.x

Epilepsy Foundation of America. (n.d.). About epilepsy. Retrieved March 13, 2014, from http://www.epilepsyfoundation.org/about/

Flannery, R. B., Jr. (2005). Precipitants to psychiatric patient assaults on staff: Review of empirical findings, 1990–2003, and risk management implications. *Psychiatric Quarterly, 76*(4), 317–326. doi:10.1007/s11126-005-4965-y

Gleeson, M., & Higgins, A. (2009). Touch in mental health nursing: An exploratory study of nurses' views and perceptions. *Journal of Psychiatric & Mental Health Nursing, 16*(4), 382–389. doi: 10.1111/j.1365-2850.2009.01389.x

Gleeson, M., & Timmins, F. (2005). A review of the use and clinical effectiveness of touch as a nursing intervention. *Clinical Effectiveness in Nursing, 9*(1–2), 69–77. doi: 10.1016/j.cein.2004.12.002

Hardwick, M. E., Pulido, P. A., & Adelson, W. S. (2012). Nursing intervention using healing touch in bilateral total knee arthroplasty. *Orthopaedic Nursing, 31*(1), 5–11. doi:10.1097/NOR.0b013e31824195fb

Harkin, H. (n.d.). Ear care guidance from the NHS Modernisation Agency. Retrieved March 13, 2014, from http://www.wales.nhs.uk/sitesplus/documents/863/Package-for-GPs-no-PIL.PDF

Hooker, S. D., Freeman, L. H., & Stewart, P. (2002). Pet therapy research: A historical review. *Holistic Nursing Practice, 17*(1), 17–23.

Huntley, A. (2008). Documenting level of consciousness. *Nursing2008, 38*(8), 63–64. doi: 10.1097/01.NURSE.0000327505.69608.35.

Iwamoto, Y., & Hoshiyama, M. (2012, September). Time orientation during the day in the elderly with dementia. *Physical & Occupational Therapy in Geriatrics, 30*(3), 202–213. doi:10.3109/02703181.2012.713453

Johnson, M., Bulechek, G., Dochterman, J. M., et al. (2012). *NOC and NIC linkages to NANDA-I and clinical conditions* (3rd ed.). St. Louis, MO: C. V. Mosby.

The Joint Commission. (2010). *Advancing effective communication, cultural competence, and patient- and family-centered care: A roadmap for hospitals.* Oakbrook Terrace, IL: Author. Retrieved March 13, 2014, from http://www.jointcommission.org/assets/1/6/ARoadmapforHospitalsfinalversion727.pdf

Moorhead, S., Johnson, M., Maas, M., et al. (2012). *Nursing outcomes classification (NOC)* (5th ed.). St. Louis, MO: C. V. Mosby.

NANDA International. (2012). *Nursing diagnoses definitions & classification 2012–2014.* Ames, IA: Wiley-Blackwell.

O'Keeffe, E., Mukhtar, O., & O'Keeffe, S. (2010). Orientation to time as a guide to the presence and severity of cognitive impairment in older hospital patients. *Journal of Neurology and Neurosurgical Psychiatry, 82,* 500–504. doi:10.1136/jnnp.2010.214817

Polan, E., & Taylor, D. (2010). *Journey across the life span: Human development and health promotion* (4th ed.). Philadelphia: F. A. Davis.

Roland, P. S., Smith, T. L., Schwartz, S. R., et al. (2008). Clinical practice guideline: Cerumen impaction. *Otolaryngology—Head and Neck Surgery, 139,* S1–S21.

Scanlon, V., & Sanders, T. (2014). *Essentials of anatomy and physiology* (7th ed.). Philadelphia: F. A. Davis.

Wiegand, L. (2011). *AACN procedure manual for critical care* (6th ed.). Philadelphia: W. B. Saunders.

CHAPTER 31

Agency for Healthcare Policy and Research, Public Health Service (AHCPR), U.S. Department of Health and Human Services. (1994). *The clinical practice guideline for the management of cancer pain* (AHCPR Publication No. 94-0592). Rockville, MD: Author.

American Academy of Pediatrics (AAP), Committee on Psychological Aspects of Child and Family Health and American Task Force on Pain in Infants, Children, and Adolescents. (2001). The assessment and management of acute pain in infants, children and adolescents. *Pediatrics, 108*(3), 793–797.

American Geriatrics Society, Panel on Persistent Pain in Older Persons. (2009). Pharmacological management of persistent pain in older persons. *Journal of the American Geriatrics Society, 57*(8), 1331–1346. doi: 10.1111/j.1532-5415.2009.02376.x

American Medical Directors Association (AMDA). (2012). *Pain management in the long term care setting.* Columbia, MD: Author. Retrieved December 17, 2013, from http://www.guideline.gov/content.aspx?f=rss&id=45524&osrc=12

American Music Therapy Association. (n.d.). Music therapy and music-based interventions in the treatment and management of pain: Selected references and key findings. Retrieved January 13, 2013, from http://www.musictherapy.org/assets/1/7/MT_Pain_2010.pdf

American Pain Society. (1994). Part III: Pain terms, a current list with definitions and notes on usage. In H. Merskey, & N. Bogduk; IASP Task Force on Taxonomy (Eds.), *Classification of chronic pain* (2nd ed., p. 16). Seattle, WA: IASP Press.

American Pain Society. (2006). Pain: Current understanding of assessment, management, and treatments. Retrieved

October 16, 2012, from http://pain-topics.org/pdf/Pain_APS_2006.pdf

American Pain Society. (2009). *Principles of analgesic use in the treatment of acute pain and cancer pain* (6th ed.). Glenview, IL: APS Press.

American Society for Pain Management Nursing. (n.d.). Position papers. Retrieved January 16, 2013, from http://www.aspmn.org/Organization/position_papers.htm

Arnstein, P. (2010). *Clinical coach for effective pain management.* Philadelphia: F. A. Davis.

Baldridge, K., & Andrasik, F. (2010). Pain assessment in people with intellectual or developmental disabilities. *American Journal of Nursing, 110*(12), 28–37. doi: 10.1097/01.NAJ.0000391236.68263.90

Barnes, P. M., Bloom, B., & Nahin, R. L. (2008). *Complementary and alternative medicine use among adults and children: United States, 2007* (National Health Statistics Report, No. 12). Hyattsville, MD: National Center for Health Statistics.

Berdine, H. J. (2002). The fifth vital sign: Cornerstone of a new pain management strategy. *Disease and Management Outcomes, 10*(3), 155–156. doi: 10.2165/00115677-200210030-00003

Best practices: Evidence-based nursing procedures (pp. 117–124). (2008). Philadelphia: Lippincott Williams & Wilkins.

Bishop, F. L., Yardley. L., & Lewith, G. T. (2008). Treat or treatment: A qualitative study analyzing patients' use of complementary and alternative medicine. *American Journal of Public Health, 98*(9), 1700–1705. doi: 10.2105/AJPH.2007.110072

Bozimowski, G. (2012). Patient perceptions of pain management therapy: A comparison of real-time assessment of patient education and satisfaction and registered nurse perceptions. *Pain Management Nursing, 13*(4), 186–193. doi: 10.1016/j.pmn.2010.04.00

Bulechek, G., Butcher, G., & Dochterman, J. (Eds.). (2012). *Nursing interventions classification (NIC)* (6th ed.). St. Louis, MO: C. V. Mosby.

Cassileth, B., Trevisan, C., & Jyothirmai, G. (2007). Complementary therapies for cancer pain. *Current Pain & Headache Reports, 11*(4), 265–269.

Christo, P. J. (2009, January 30). *Clinical concepts in pain and aging*. Paper presented at the annual meeting of the American Academy of Pain Management (AAPM), Honolulu, HI.

Cohen, M. R., Weber, R. J., & Moss, J. (2006, April 1). Patient-controlled analgesia: Making it safer for patients. Institute for Safe Medicine Practice (ISMP). Retrieved March 14, 2013, from http://www.ismp.org/profdevelopment/PCAMonograph.pdf

Cole, L. C., & Lobiondo-Wood, G. (2012). Music as an adjuvant therapy in control of pain and symptoms in hospitalized adults: A systematic review. *Pain Management Nursing.* Advance online publication. pii: S1524-9042(12)00144-0. doi:10.1016/j.pmn.2012.08.010

D'Arcy, Y. (2008a, January). Keep your patient safe during PCA. *Nursing, 38*(1), 50–55.

D'Arcy, Y. (2008b, February). What you need to know about opioids. *Nursing, 38*(2), 26–28. doi: 10.1097/01.NURSE.0000309718.44432.42

Elkins, G., Johnson, A., & Fisher, W. (2012). Cognitive hypnotherapy for pain management. *American Journal of Clinical Hypnosis, 54*(4), 294–310. DOI: 10.1080/00029157.2011.654284

Ernst, E. (2008). *Complementary therapies for pain management: An evidence-based approach.* St. Louis, MO: Elsevier.

Evans, F. J. (1974). The placebo response in pain reduction. *Advances in Neurology, 4*, 289–296.

Flaherty, E. (2007; revised 2012). Pain assessment in older adults. *Try This: Best Practices in Nursing Care to Older Adults, 7*, 1–2 The Hartford Institute for Geriatric Nursing. The Hartford Institute for Geriatric Nursing, New York University College of Nursing. Retrieved May 7, 2013, from http://consultgerirn.org/uploads/File/trythis/try_this_2.pdf

Hart, J. (2008, April 1). Complementary therapies for chronic pain management. *Alternative and Complementary Therapies, 14*(2), 64–68. doi:10.1089/act.2010.16608

Herr, K., Bjoro, K., & Decker S. (2006). Tools for assessment of pain in nonverbal older adults with dementia: A state-of-the-science review. *Journal of Pain Symptom Management, 31*(2), 170–192. doi: http://dx.doi.org/10.1016/j.jpainsymman.2005.07.001

Herr, K., Coyne, P. J., Key, T., et al. (2006). Pain assessment in the nonverbal patient: Position statement with clinical practice recommendations. *Pain Management Nursing, 7*(2), 44–52. doi:10.1016/j.pmn.2006.02.003

Hockenberry, M. J., & Wilson, D. (2012). *Wong's essentials of pediatric nursing* (9th ed.). St. Louis, MO: C. V. Mosby.

Hooten, W. M, Timming, R., Belgrade, M., et. al.; Institute for Clinical Systems Improvement. (updated 2013, November). *Assessment and management of chronic pain* (6th ed.). Retrieved October 26, 2014, from https://www.icsi.org/_asset/bw798b/ChronicPain.pdf

Horgas, A. L. (2007). Assessing pain in older adults with dementia. *Try This: Best Practices for Nursing Care for Hospitalized Older Adults, D2*, 1–2. The Hartford Institute for Geriatric Nursing and the Alzheimer's Association. Retrieved October 26, 2014, from http://consultgerirn.org/uploads/File/trythis/try_this_d2.pdf

Horgas, A. L., Yoon, S. L., & Grall, M. (2012). Pain management. In M. Boltz, E. Capezuti, T. Fulmer, & D. Zwicker (Eds.), *Evidence-based geriatric nursing protocols for best practice.* (4th ed., pp. 246–267). New York: Springer.

International Association for the Study of Pain Subcommittee on Taxonomy; Merskey, H. (Eds.). (1986). Classification of chronic pain syndromes and definitions of pain terms. *Pain* (Suppl. 3), S1–S226.

Institute for Clinical Systems Improvement (ICSI). (2005, updated November, 2013, November). *Health care guideline: Assessment and management of chronic pain* (5th ed.). Bloomington, MN: Author. Retrieved October 26, 2014, from https://www.icsi.org/_asset/bw798b/ChronicPain-Interactive1111.pdf

Institute of Medicine. (2011, June). *Relieving pain in America a blueprint for transforming prevention, care, education, and research.* Retrieved October 26, 2014, from http://www.iom.edu/relievingpain

Jarzyna, D., Jungquist, C. R., Pasero, C., et al. (2011). American Society for Pain Management guidelines on monitoring for opioid-induced sedation and respiratory depression. *Pain Management Nursing, 12*(13), 118–145. doi: 10.1016/j.pmn.2011.06.008

Johnson, M., Moorhead, S., Bulechek, G., et al. (2012). *NOC and NIC linkages to NANDA-I and clinical conditions* (3rd ed.). St. Louis, MO: C. V. Mosby.

Lee, J. H., Choi, T. Y., Lee, M. S., et al. (2013). Acupuncture for acute low back pain: A systematic review. *Clinical Journal of Pain, 29*(2), 172–185. doi: 10.1097/AJP.0b013e31824909f9

Lewandowski, C. S., Good, M., & Draucker, C. B. (2005). Changes in the meaning of pain with the use of guided imagery. *Pain Management Nursing, 6*(2), 58–67. doi: http://dx.doi.org/10.1016/j.pmn.2005.01.002

Mailis-Gagnon, A. F., Sandoval, J. A., & Taylor, R. S. (2009, January 21). Spinal cord stimulation for chronic pain. *Cochrane Database of Systematic Reviews,* Issue 3. Art. No.: CD003783. doi:10.1002/14651858.CD003783.pub2.

McAuliffe, L., Brown, D., & Fetherstonhaugh, D. (2012). Pain and dementia: An overview of the literature. *International Journal of Older People Nursing, 7*(3), 219–226. doi: 10.1111/j.1748-3743.2012.00331.x

McCaffery, M. (1968). *Nursing practice theories related to cognition, bodily pain, and man-environment interactions.* Los Angeles: UCLA Students Store._

McCaffery, M., & Pasero, C. (1999). *Pain clinical manual* (2nd ed.). St. Louis, MO: C. V. Mosby.

McCaffery, M., Pasero, C., & Ferrell, B.R. (2007). Nurses' decisions about opioid dose. *The American Journal of Nursing, 107*(12), 35–39. doi: 10.1097/01.NAJ.0000301016.18877.19

McQuay, H. J., Derry, S., Eccleston, C., et al. (2012). Evidence for analgesic effect in acute pain—50 years on. *Pain, 153*(7),1364–1367 .doi: http://dx.doi.org.ezproxy.jccc.edu/10.1016/j.pain.2012.01.024

Merskey, H. (1979). Pain terms: A list with definitions and notes on usage recommended by the IASP Subcommittee on Taxonomy. *Pain, 6*(3), 249–252.

Merskey, H., & Bogduk, N. (Eds.). (1994). *Classification of chronic pain* (2nd ed., p. 971). Seattle, WA: International Association for the Study of Pain.

Molony, S. L., Kobayashi, M., Holleran, E. A., et al. (2005, March). Assessing pain as a fifth vital sign in long-term care facilities: Recommendations from the field. *Journal of Gerontological Nursing, 31*(3), 16–24.

Moorhead, S., Johnson, M., Maas, M., et al. (2012). *Nursing outcomes classification (NOC)* (5th ed.). St. Louis, MO: C. V. Mosby.

NANDA International. (2011). *Nursing diagnoses: Definitions and classification 2012–2014.* Oxford: Wiley-Blackwell.

National Guideline Clearinghouse (NGC). (2003; updated 2005, May 13). Assessment and management of pain. Rockville, MD: Agency for Healthcare Research and Quality. Retrieved March 11, 2013, from http://www.guideline.gov/summary/summary.aspx?doc_id=11507&nbr=005960&string

National Institutes of Health (NIH), National Institute on Drug Abuse. (2001; revised 2011, October). Research report series: Prescription drugs abuse and addiction. Retrieved March 13, 2013, from http://www.nida.nih.gov/ResearchReports/Prescription/prescription.html

O'Rourke, D. (2004). The measurement of pain in infants, children, and adolescents: From policy to practice. *Physical Therapy, 84*(6), 560–570.

Pasero, C. (1997). Pain ratings: The fifth vital sign. *American Journal of Nursing, 97*(2), 15–16.

Pasero, C., Manworren, R. C. B., & McCaffery, M. (2008). IV opioid range orders for acute pain management. *American Journal of Nursing, 107*(2), 52–60.

Pasero, C., & McCaffery, M. (2011). *Pain assessment and pharmacological management.* Philadelphia: Elsevier Mosby.

Patanwala, A. E., Edwards, C. J., Stolz, L., et al. (2012). Should morphine dosing be weight based for analgesia in the emergency department? *Journal of Opioid Management, 8*(1), 51–5. DOI: 10.5055/jom.2012.0096

Patterson, C. (2008). Six myths about opioid use. *Nursing2008, 38*(11), 60–61.

Portenoy, R. K., & McCafferty, M. (2011). Adjuvant analgesics. In *Pain assessment and pharmacological management.* Philadelphia: Elsevier Mosby.

Sawheney, M. (2012). Epidural analgesia: What nurses need to know. *Nursing2012, 42*(8), 36–42. doi: 10.1097/01.NURSE.0000418073.66125.98

Schneider, J. P. (2006–2007, Winter). Opioids, pain management, and addiction. *Pain Practitioner, 16*, 17–24.

Sessler, C. N., Gosnell, M. S., Carp, M. J., et al. (2002). The Richmond-Agitation Scale: Validity and reliability in adult intensive care unit patients. *American Journal of Respiratory Critical Care Medicine, 166*, 1338–1344. doi: 10.1164/rccm.2107138

Shin, S. Y., & Kolanowski. A. M. (2010). Best evidence of psychosocially focused nonpharmacologic therapies for symptom management in older adults with osteoarthritis. *Pain Management Nursing, 11*(4), 234–244. doi: 10.1016/j.pmn.2009.06.001

Slater, R., Cantarella, A., Fanck, L., et al. (2008, June 24). How well do clinical pain assessment tools reflect pain in infants? *PLoS Medicine, 5*(6), e129. Retrieved October 15, 2012, from http://www.asianhhm.com/Knowledge_bank/research_insights/clinical_pain_assessment_tools_reflect_pain.htm doi: 10.1371/journal.pmed.0050129

Spragud, L. J., Piira, T., & Baeyer, C. L. (2003). Children's self-report of pain intensity. *American Journal of Nursing, 103*(12), 62–64.

Takai, Y., Yamamoto-Mitani, N. Okamoto, Y., et al. (2010). Literature review of pain prevalence among older residents of nursing homes. *Pain Management Nursing, 11*(4), 209–223. doi: 10.1016/j.pmn.2010.08.006.

Topcu, S. Y., & Findik, U. Y. (2012). Effect of relaxation exercises on controlling postoperative pain. *Pain Management Nursing, 13*(1), 11–17. doi: 10.1016/j.pmn.2010.07.006

Warden, V., Hurley, A. C., & Volicer, L. (2003). Development and psychometric evaluation of the Pain Assessment in Advanced Dementia (PAINAD) scale. *Journal of the American Medical Directors Association, 4*(1), 9–15.

Webster, L. R., & Webster, R. M. (2005). Predicting aberrant behaviors in opioid-treated patients: Preliminary validation of the Opioid Risk Tool. *Pain Medicine, 6*(6), 432–442.

World Health Organization (WHO). (1990). *Cancer pain relief and palliative care: Report of a WHO expert committee* (WHO Technical Report series, No. 804, p. 34). Geneva, Switzerland: Author.

Wuhrman, E., Cooney, M. F., Dunwoody, C.J., et al. (2007). Authorized and unauthorized ("PCA by Proxy") dosing of analgesic infusion pumps: Position statement with clinical practice recommendations. *Pain Management Nursing, 8*(1), 4–11. doi: 10.1016/j.pmn.2007.01.002

CHAPTER 32

Ajnik, U., & Lorber, M. (2011). Influence of Parkinson's disease on quality of life of the patient. *Obzornik Zdravstvene Nege, 45*(3), 205–211.

American Nurses Association (ANA). (n.d.). *Handle with care fact sheet.* Retrieved November 1, from http://nursingworld.org/MainMenuCategories/WorkplaceSafety/Healthy-Work-Environment/SafePatient/Resources/FactSheet.html

American Nurses Association (ANA). (2013). *Safe patient handling and mobility interprofessional national standards.* Silver Springs, MD: Author.

Borg, G. (1998). *Borg's perceived exertion and pain scales*. Stockholm, Sweden: Human Kinetics;

Bucks, R. S., Cruise, K. E., Skinner, T. C., et al. (2011). Coping processes and health-related quality of life in Parkinson's disease. *International Journal of Geriatric Psychiatry, 26*(3), 247–255. doi:10.1002/gps.2520

Bulechek, G., Butcher, G., & Dochterman, J. (Eds.). (2012). *Nursing interventions classification (NIC)* (6th ed.). St. Louis, MO: C. V. Mosby.

Bunting-Perry, L. K. (2006, April). Palliative care in Parkinson's disease: Implications for neuroscience nursing. *Journal of Neuroscience Nursing, 38*(2), 106–113.

Caap-Ahlgren, M., Lannerheim, L., & Dehlin, O. (2002). Older Swedish women's experiences of living with symptoms related to Parkinson's disease. *Journal of Advanced Nursing, 39*(1), 87–95.

Caspersen, C. J., Powell, K. E., Christenson, G. M. (1985). Physical activity, exercise, and physical fitness: Definitions and distinctions for health-related research. *Public Health Report, 100*(2), 126–131.

Centers for Disease Control and Prevention. (CDC). (n.d.; updated 2014, February). Safe patient handling. *Workplace Safety and Health Topics*. Retrieved March 19, 2014, from http://www.cdc.gov/niosh/topics/safepatient/

Centers for Disease Control and Prevention (CDC). (2008; updated 2014). Physical activity for everyone. Retrieved March 23, 2014, from http://www.cdc.gov/physicalactivity/everyone/guidelines/olderadults.html

Collins, J. W., Nelson, A., & Sublet, V. (2006). *Safe lifting and movement of nursing home residents* (DHHS (NIOSH) Publication No. 2006-117). Washington, DC: Department of Health and Human Services.

Donnelly, J. E., Blair, S. N., Jakicic, J. M., et al. (2009, February). Appropriate physical activity intervention strategies for weight loss and prevention of weight regain for adults. Position Stand. American College of Sports Medicine (ACSM). *Medicine & Science in Sports & Exercise, 41*(2), 459–471. doi:10.1249/MSS.0b013e3181949333

Ehab, G., Barsnley, S., & Chellappa, R. (2012). Effect of physical exercise-movement strategies programme on mobility, falls, and quality of life in Parkinson's disease. *International Journal of Therapy & Rehabilitation, 19*(2), 88–96.

Foster, C. (2004). "Talk test" measures exercise intensity. *Medicine & Science in Sports & Exercise, 36*(9), 1632–1636.

Gray, B. B. (2012). Even women who exercise sit too much. *HealthDay News*. Retrieved March 23, 2014, from http://consumer.healthday.com/Article.asp?AID=670457

Gregory, P., Morgan, K., & Lynall, A. (2012). Improving sleep management in people with Parkinson's. *British Journal of Community Nursing, 17*(1), 14–20. doi: http://dx.doi.org/10.12968/bjcn.2012.17.1.14

Herlofson, K., & Larsen, J. P. (2003). The influence of fatigue on health-related quality of life in patients with Parkinson's disease. *Acta Neurologica Scandinavica, 107*, 1–6. doi: 10.1034/j.1600-0404.2003.02033.x

Howard, N. L. (2010). Patient handling: Fact vs. fiction. *American Nurse Today, 5*(7), 32–34.

Hsu, H., Chen, C., Huang, T., et al. (2009). Fatigue and related factors in patients with Parkinson's disease. *Journal of Nursing, 56*(5), 49–59.

Hsu, H., Huang, T., Weng, Y., et al. (2007). The inclination to depressive mood and related factors among patients with Parkinson's disease. *Journal of Evidence-Based Nursing, 3*(3), 195–204.

Jitramontree, N. (2010). Exercise promotion: Walking in elders. *Journal of Gerontological Nursing, 36*(11), 10–18. doi:10.3928/00989134-20101001-99

Koukouli, S., Vlachonikolis, I. G., & Philalithis, A. (2002). Sociodemographic factors and self-reported functional status: The significance of social support. *BMC Health Services Research, 2*, 20. Retrieved March 23, 2014, from http://www.biomedcentral.com/1472-6963/2/20

Moorhead, S., Johnson, M., Maas, M., et al. (2012). *Nursing outcomes classification (NOC)* (5th ed.). St. Louis, MO: C. V. Mosby.

The National Institutes of Health, National Institute on Aging. (2011; updated 2014, February 12). Exercise and physical activity: Your everyday guide from the National Institute on Aging. Retrieved March 23, 2014, from http://www.nia.nih.gov/HealthInformation/Publications/exercise.htm

The National Institutes of Health, National Institute on Aging. (2012, January). Exercise for your bone health. NIH Osteoporosis and Related Bone Diseases National Resource Center. Retrieved March 23, 2014, from http://www.niams.nih.gov/Health_Info/Bone/Bone_Health/Exercise/exercise_bone_health.pdf

National Osteoporosis Foundation. (n.d.a). Exercise for strong bones. Retrieved March 23, 2014, from http://www.nof.org/articles/238

National Osteoporosis Foundation. (n.d.b). Calcium and vitamin D: What you need to know.

Nelson, A., & Baptiste, A. (2004, September 30). Evidence-based practices for safe patient handling and movement. *Online Journal of Issues in Nursing, 9*(3). Retrieved March 23, 2014, from http://www.nursingworld.org/MainMenuCategories/ANAMarketplace/ANAPeriodicals/OJIN/TableofContents/Volume92004/No3Sept04/EvidenceBasedPractices.aspx

North American Menopause Society (NAMS). (2010, January). Management of osteoporosis in postmenopausal women: 2010 position statement of the North American Menopause Society. (2010). *Menopause, 17*(1), 25–54. doi:10.1097/gme.0b013e3181c617e6

Occupational Safety and Health Administration, U.S. Department of Labor. (2009). *Ergonomics for the prevention or musculoskeletal disorders: Guidelines for nursing homes* (OSHA 3182-2009). Retrieved March 23, 2014, from http://www.osha.gov/ergonomics/guidelines/nursinghome/final_nh_guidelines.pdf

Ogden, C. L., Carroll, M. D., Kit, B. K., et al. (2014). Prevalence of childhood and adult obesity in the United States, 2011–2012. *JAMA, 311*(8), 806–814. doi:10.1001/jama.2014.732

President's Council on Sports, Fitness, and Health. (2010, June). Exercise comes of age: Medicine for older adults. *Research Digest, 10*(3), 1–3. Retrieved April 16, 2013, from presidentschallenge.org/informed/digest/docs/june2010digest.pdf

Robinson, K., Dennison, A., Roalf, D., et al. (2005). Falling risk factors in Parkinson disease. *Neuro Rehabilitation, 20*(3), 169–182.

Swann, J. (2007). Rheumatoid arthritis: When the body rebels against itself. *Nursing & Residential Care, 9*(5), 222–224.

Sunvisson, H., & Ekman, S. (2001). Environmental influences on the experiences of people with Parkinson's disease. *Nursing Inquiry, 8*, 41–50.

Sunvisson, H., Ekman, S., Hagberg, H., & Lokk, J. (2001). An educational program for individuals with Parkinson's disease. *Scandinavian Journal of Caring Sciences, 15,* 311–317.

Taber's cyclopedic medical dictionary (22nd ed.). Philadelphia: F. A. Davis. Retrieved March 19, 2014, from http://www.tabers.com/tabersonline/view/Tabers-Dictionary/756143/0/mobility

U.S. Bureau of Labor Statistics, U.S. Department of Labor. (2013, November 26). Nonfatal occupational injuries and illnesses requiring days away from work, 2011. Retrieved March 19, 2014, from http://www.bls.gov/news.release/pdf/osh2.pdf

U.S. Department of Health and Human Services (USDHHS). (2008; updated 2011). 2008 physical activity guidelines for Americans. Retrieved March 23, 2014, from http://www.health.gov/paguidelines

U.S. Department of Health and Human Services (USDHHS). (2011). *Implementing Healthy People 2020.* Retrieved March 23, 2014, from http://www.healthypeople.gov/2020/implementing/default.aspx

U.S. Department of Health and Human Services (USDHHS). (2012). *National Center for Health Statistics. Health, United States, 2011: With special features on socioeconomic status and health.* Hyattsville, MD: Author.

Wade, D. T., Gage, H., Owen, C., Trend, P., Grossmith, C., & Kaye, J. (2003). Multidisciplinary rehabilitation for people with Parkinson's disease: A randomized controlled study. *Journal of Neurology Neurosurgery and Psychiatry, 74,* 158–162.

Waters, T. R., Nelson, A. N., Hughes, N., et al.; National Institute for Occupational Safety and Health (NIOSH), the Veterans Health Administration (VHA), the American Nurses Association (ANA). (2009, November). *Safe patient handling training for schools of nursing* (DHHS [NIOSH] Publication No. 2009-127). Retrieved March 23, 2014, from http://www.cdc.gov/niosh/docs/2009-127/pdfs/2009-127.pdf

CHAPTER 33

American Cancer Society. (2012a, revised 2013, November 5). Testicular self-exam. Retrieved November 1, 2014, from http://www.cancer.org/cancer/testicularcancer/moreinformation/doihavetesticularcancer/do-i-have-testicular-cancer-self-exam

American Cancer Society. (2012b; reviewed 2014, September 10). American Cancer Society recommendations for early breast cancer detection in women without breast symptoms. Retrieved November 1, 2014, from http://www.cancer.org/cancer/breastcancer/moreinformation/breastcancerearlydetection/breast-cancer-early-detection-acs-recs

American Geriatrics Society. (updated 2012c, May). Aging & health A to Z. Sexual problems. Retrieved November 1, 2014, from http://www.healthinaging.org/aging-and-health-a-to-z/topic:sexual-health/

American Psychiatric Association (APA). (2013a). *Diagnostic and statistical manual of mental disorders* (5th ed.). Washington, DC: Author.

American Psychiatric Association (APA). (2013b). *Gender dysphoria.* Retrieved July 23, 2013, from http://www.dsm5.org/Documents/Gender%20Dysphoria%20Fact%20Sheet.pdf

Annon, J. (1976). The PLISSIT model: A proposed conceptual scheme for the behavioural treatment of sexual problems. *Journal of Sex Education Therapy,* 2(1), 1–15.

Baird, D., & Eliasziw, M. (2011). Disparity in perceived illness intrusiveness and illness severity between cardiac patients and their spouses. *Journal of Cardiovascular Nursing, 26*(6), 481–486. doi: 10.1097/JCN.0b013e3182092c11

Bamford, S. (2012). Sexuality and intimacy in people with dementia. *Practice Nursing, 23*(9), 436–442.

Basson, R. (2001). Using a different model for female sexual response to address women's problematic low sexual desire. *Journal of Sex and Marital Therapy, 27,* 395–403.

Basson, R. (2008). Women's sexual function and dysfunction: Current uncertainties, future directions. *International Journal of Impotence Research, 20,* 466–478. doi:10.1038/ijir.2008.23

Bauer, M., McAuliffe, L., Nay, R., et al. (2013). Sexuality in older adults: Effect of an education intervention on attitudes and beliefs of residential aged care staff. *Educational Gerontology, 39*(2), 82–91. doi:10.1080/03601277.2012.682953

Bradford, B. R. (2012). Chemotherapy-induced infertility in patients with testicular cancer. *Oncology Nursing Forum, 39*(1), 27–30. doi: 10.1188/12.ONF.27-30

Bulechek, G., Butcher, H., & Dochterman, J. (2013). *Nursing interventions classification (NIC)* (6th ed.). St. Louis, MO: C. V. Mosby.

Centers for Disease Control and Prevention (CDC). (2012a). Risk youth behavior surveillance—U.S., 2011. *Morbidity and Mortality Weekly Report, 61*(4), 1–162. Retrieved July 24, 2013, from http://www.cdc.gov/mmwr/pdf/ss/ss6104.pdf

Centers for Disease Control and Prevention (CDC). (2012b; updated 2013, February 13). *Chlamydia—CDC fact sheet.* Retrieved July 28, 2013, from http://www.cdc.gov/std/Chlamydia/STDFact-Chlamydia.htm

Centers for Disease Control and Prevention (CDC). (2012c; updated 2013, February 11). *Gonorrhea—CDC fact sheet.* Retrieved July 28, 2013, from http://www.cdc.gov/std/Gonorrhea/STDFact-gonorrhea.htm

Centers for Disease Control and Prevention (CDC). (2012d; updated 2013, February 11). *Syphilis—CDC fact sheet.* Retrieved July 28, 2013, from http://www.cdc.gov/std/Syphilis/STDFact-Syphilis.htm

Centers for Disease Control and Prevention (CDC). (updated 2013a, June 6). Teen-age pregnancy. Retrieved July 24, 2013, from http://www.cdc.gov/teenpregnancy/

Centers for Disease Control and Prevention (CDC). (updated 2013b, July 25). *Genital HPV infection—fact sheet.* Retrieved July 28, 2013, from http://www.cdc.gov/std/HPV/STDFact-HPV.htm

Centers for Disease Control and Prevention. (2013c). CDC grand rounds: The growing threat of multidrug-resistant gonorrhea. *Morbidity and Mortality Weekly Report, 62*(6), 103–106.

Chinn, P. (2013). Lesbian, gay, bisexual, and transgender health: Disparities we can change. *Nurse Educator, 38*(3), 94–95.

Cooper, A., Skinner, J., Nherera, L., et al. (2007). *Clinical guidelines and evidence review for post myocardial infarction: Secondary prevention in primary care and secondary care for patients following a myocardial infarction (full NICE guideline).* National Collaborating Centre for Primary Care and Royal College of General Practitioners. Retrieved August 2, 2013, from http://www.nice.org.uk/cg48

Copen, C., Chandra, A., & Martinez, G. (2012). *Prevalence and timing of oral sex with opposite-sex partners among male and females, aged 15–24 years: United States, 2007–10* (National Health Statistics Report No. 56). Hyattsville, MD: National Center for Health Statistics.

Davies, H., Sridhar, S., Newkirk, L., et al., (2012). Gender differences in sexual behaviors of AD patients and their relationship to spousal caregiver well-being. *Aging & Mental Health, 16*(1), 89–101. doi: 10.1080/13607863.2011.609532

DeBusk, R., Drory, Y., Goldstein, I., et al. (2000). Management of sexual dysfunction in patients with cardiovascular disease: Recommendations of the Princeton consensus panel. *American Journal of Cardiology, 86*(2), 175–181.

Delamater, J. (2010). Sexual expression in later life: a review and synthesis. *Journal of Sex Research, 49*(2–3), 125–141. doi: 10.1080/00224499.2011.603168

Dickinson, T., Cook, M., Playle, J., et al. (2012). "Queer" treatments: Giving a voice to former patients who received treatments for their "sexual deviations." *Journal of Clinical Nursing, 21*(9/10), 1345–1354. doi: 10.1111/j.1365-2702.2011.03965.x

Doll, G. (2011). *Sexuality & Long-Term Care: Understanding and Supporting the Needs of Older Adults*. Baltimore: Health Professions Press.

Doll, G. (2013). Sexuality in nursing homes: Practice and policy. *Journal of Gerontological Nursing, 39*(7), 30–37. doi: 10.3928/00989134-20130418-01

Fulcher, M., & Coyle, E. (2011). Breadwinner and caregiver: A cross-sectional analysis of children's and emerging adults' visions of their future family roles. *British Journal of Developmental Psychology, 29*(2), 330–346. doi: 10.1111/j.2044-835X.2011.02026.x

Ginsberg, T. (2010). Male sexuality. *Clinics in Geriatric Medicine, 26*(2), 185–195.

Gollub, E., Cyrus-Cameron, E., Armstrong, K., et al. (2013). Basic body knowledge in street-recruited, active drug-using women enrolled in a "body empowerment" intervention trial. *AIDS Care, 25*(6), 732–737.

Hummer R., & Hamilton, E. (2010). Race and ethnicity in fragile families. *Future of Children, 20*(2), 113–131.

Hyde, J. S., & Delamater, J. D. (2010). *Understanding human sexuality* (11th ed.). Columbus OH: McGraw-Hill.

Jacobson, S. (2013). [Review of the book *Sexuality and long-term care: Understanding and supporting the needs of older adults* [by Gayle Appel Doll]. *Journal of Gerontological Social Work, 56*(4), 378–380.

Joller, P., Gupta, N., Seitz, D. P, et al. (2013, March). Approach to inappropriate sexual behaviour in people with dementia. *Canadian Family Physician, 59*(3), 255–260.

Katz, A. (2011). Sexually speaking. Breast cancer and women's sexuality: Acknowledging and discussing the consequences of treatment. *American Journal of Nursing, 111*(4), 63–66.

Kaufman, J.; American Academy of Pediatrics, Committee on Adolescence. (2008). Care of the adolescent sexual assault victim. *Pediatrics, 122*(2), 462–470. doi: 10.1542/peds.2008-1581

Kennedy-Malone, L., Fletcher, K., & Plank, L. (2004). *Management guidelines for nurse practitioners working with older adults*. Philadelphia: F. A. Davis.

Kennett, D., Humphreys, T., & Bramley, J. (2013). Sexual resourcefulness and gender roles as moderators of relationship satisfaction and consenting to unwanted sex in undergraduate women. *Canadian Journal of Human Sexuality, 22*(1), 51–61. doi: 10.3138/cjhs.933

Kinsey, A. (1998). *Sexual behavior in the human male*. Bloomington: Indiana University Press. (Original work published 1948)

Klein, F., Sepekoff, B., & Wolf, T. J. (1985, Spring). Sexual orientation: A multi-variable dynamic process. *Journal of Homosexuality, 11*(1–2), 35–49. doi: http://dx.doi.org/10.1300/J082v11n01_04

Laumann, E. O., Paik, A., Glasser, D. B., et al. (2006). A cross-national study of subjective sexual well-being among older women and men: Findings from the Global Study of Sexual Attitudes and Behaviors. *Archives of Sexual Behavior, 35*, 145–161. doi: 10.1007/s10508-005-9005-3

Levy, D., & Lo, J. (2013). Transgender, transsexual, and gender queer individuals with a Christian upbringing: The process of resolving conflict between gender identity and faith. *Journal of Religion & Spirituality in Social Work, 32*(1), 60–83. doi:10.1080/15426432.2013.749079

Lindau, S. T., Schumm, P., Laumann, E. O., et al. (2007). A study of sexuality and health among older adults in the United States. *New England Journal of Medicine, 357*(8), 762–774. doi: 10.1056/NEJMoa067423

Lim, F., Brown, D., Jr., & Jones, B. (2013). Lesbian, gay, bisexual, and transgender health: Fundamentals for nursing education. *Journal of Nursing Education, 52*(4), 198–203. doi: 10.3928/01484834-20130311-02

Mahieu, L., & Gastmans, C. (2012). Sexuality in institutionalized elderly persons: A systematic review of argument-based ethics literature. *International Psychogeriatrics, 24*(3), 346–357. doi: http://dx.doi.org/10.1017/S1041610211001542

Masters, W. H., & Johnson, V. E. (1966). *Human sexual response*. Philadelphia: Lippincott Williams & Wilkins.

Miner, M. M. (2006). Sexual activity after myocardial infarction: When to resume the use of erectogenic drugs. *Current Sexual Health Reports, 3*(1), 30–34. doi: 10.1007/s11930-006-0024-4

Moorhead, S., Johnson, M., Maas, M., et al. (Eds.). (2013). *Nursing outcomes classification (NOC)* (5th ed.). St. Louis, MO: C. V. Mosby.

Moser, D. K. (2007). The rust of life: Impact of anxiety on cardiac patients. *American Journal of Critical Care, 16*(4), 361–369.

Muller, J. E. (2000). Triggering of cardiac events by sexual activity: Findings from a case-crossover analysis. *American Journal of Cardiology, 86*(Suppl. 2A), 14F–18F.

Nagoshi, J., Brzuzy, S., & Terrell, H. (2012). Deconstructing the complex perceptions of gender roles, gender identity, and sexual orientation among transgender individuals. *Feminism & Psychology, 22*(4), 405–422. doi: 10.1177/0959353512461929

National Institute of Justice. (2010). Victims and perpetrators. Retrieved November 2, 2014, from http://www.nij.gov/nij/topics/crime/rape-sexual-violence/victims-perpetrators.htm

Parashar, S., Rumsfeld, J. S., Reid, K. J., et al. (2008). Impact of depression on sex differences in outcome after myocardial infarction. *Circulation: Cardiovascular Quality and Outcomes, 2*, 33–40.

Parker, M., & Yau, M. (2011). *Sexuality in women with spinal cord injury*. Occupational Therapy Australia, 24th National Conference and Exhibition, 29 June–1 July 2011 (#35501). *Australian Occupational Therapy Journal, 58*(Suppl. 127).

Paull, G., Arndt, P., Petkovski, D., et al. (2011). Sexuality and chronic cardiovascular disease—a neglected area of practice: The role of the occupational therapist in a cardiac rehabilitation setting. Occupational Therapy Australia, 24th National Conference and Exhibition, 29 June–1 July 2011 (#35503). *Australian Occupational Therapy Journal, 58*(Suppl. 127).

Penhollow, T. M., Young, M., & Denny, G. (2009, January/February). Predictors of quality of life, sexual intercourse, and sexual satisfaction in older adults. *American Journal of Health Education, 40*(1), 13–22. ERIC Number: EJ833251

Rennison, C. M., & Rand, M. R. (2008). *Crime victimization, 2007: Findings from the National Crime Victimization Survey.* Washington, DC: Bureau of Justice Statistics, U.S. Department of Justice. Retrieved November 2, 2014, from http://bjs.ojp.usdoj.gov/index.cfm?ty=dcdetail&iid=245

Rew, L. (2009). Vaginal douching increased the risk of sexually transmitted infections in high-risk adolescents. *Evidence Based Nursing, 12*(3), 88. doi:10.1136/ebn.12.3.88

Running, A., & Berndt, A. (2003). *Management guidelines for nurse practitioners working in family practice.* Philadelphia: F. A. Davis.

Schuler, M. (2013). "No one said this would be an issue . . ." Intimacy after ostomy surgery: Online exclusive. *Nursing2014, 43*(9), 1–4. doi: 10.1097/01.NURSE.0000432916.59376.1c

Sex after heart attack. (2013). *Harvard Health Letter, 37*(8), 5.

Sex after heart attack. (2013). *Mayo Health Clinic Letter, 31*(4), 7.

Stanley, M., Blaire, K. A., & Beare, P. G. (2005). *Gerontological nursing: Promoting successful aging with older adults* (3rd ed.). Philadelphia: F. A. Davis.

Steinke, E. E. (2002). A videotape intervention for sexual counseling after myocardial infarction. *Heart & Lung, 31*(5), 348–354.

Steinke, E. E. (2000). Sexual counseling after myocardial infarction. *American Journal of Nursing, 100*(12), 38–43.

Svedberg, P., Johansson, I., Persson, S., et al. (2012). Psychometric evaluation of the 25-item sex after MI knowledge test in a Swedish context. *Scandianavarian Journal of Caring Science, 26*(1), 203–208. doi: 10.1111/j.1471-6712.2011.00909.x

Syme, M., Klonoff, E., Macera, C., et al. (2013). Predicting sexual decline and dissatisfaction among older adults: The role of partnered and individual physical and mental health factors. *Journals of Gerontology Series B: Psychological Sciences and Social Sciences, 68*(3), 323–332. doi: 10.1093/geronb/gbs087

Taylor, A., & Gosney, M. (2011). Sexuality in older age: Essential considerations for healthcare professionals. *Age and Ageing, 40*(5), 538–543. doi: 10.1093/ageing/afr049

Tsitouras, P. (2011). Male menopause: Just the facts. *Clinical Geriatrics, 19*(8), 28–32.

University of California, Santa Barbara. (2012). Aging and the sexual response cycle. *SexInfoOnline.* Retrieved November 2, 2014, from http://www.soc.ucsb.edu/sexinfo/article/aging-and-sexual-response-cycle-0

Wallace, M. (updated 2012, July). Issues regarding sexuality, protocol: Sexuality in older adults. Hartford Institute for Geriatric Nursing. Retrieved November 2, 2014, from http://www.consultgerirn.org/topics/sexuality_issues_in_aging/want_to_know_more

Walsh B., Barnsteiner, J., De Leon Siantz, M., et al. (2012). Lesbian, gay, bisexual, transgendered, or intersexed content for nursing curricula. *Journal of Professional Nursing, 28*(2), 96–104. doi: http://dx.doi.org/10.1016/j.profnurs.2011.11.004

Wisnieski, D. (2013). Promoting healthy sexual behavior in adolescents. What the research says. *American Journal of Nursing, 113*(6), 67–70. doi: 10.1097/01.NAJ.0000431279.98524.f8

World Health Organization (WHO). (2006; updated 2010). Sexual and reproductive health. Defining sexual health. Retrieved November 2, 2014, from http://www.who.int/reproductivehealth/topics/sexual_health/sh_definitions/en/index.html#

World Health Organization (WHO). (2010; updated 2014, February). *Female genital mutilation* (WHO Fact Sheet No. 241). Retrieved November 2, 2014, from http://www.who.int/mediacentre/factsheets/fs241/en/

Yee, L. (2010). Aging and sexuality. *Australian Family Physician, 39*(10), 718–721.

CHAPTER 34

American Academy of Pediatrics Task Force on Sudden Infant Death Syndrome; Moon, R. Y. (2011). SIDS and other sleep-related infant deaths: Expansion of recommendations for a safe infant sleeping environment. *Pediatrics, 128,* 1030–1039. doi: 10.1542/peds.2011-2284

American Academy of Sleep Medicine. (2014, October 31). Insomnia increases risk of motor vehicle deaths, other fatal injuries. *ScienceDaily.* Retrieved November 17, 2014, from www.sciencedaily.com/releases/2014/10/141031121238.htm

American Psychiatric Association. (2013). *Diagnostic and statistical manual of mental disorders* (5th ed.). Washington, DC: Author.

Ball, E., & Caivano, C. K. (2008). Internal medicine: Guidance to the diagnosis and management of restless legs syndrome. *Southern Medical Journal, 101*(6), 631–634. doi: 10.1097/SMJ.0b013e3181705832

Birath, J. B., & Martin, J. L. (2007). Common sleep problems affecting older adults. *Annals of Long-Term Care, 12.* Retrieved November 3, 2014, from http://www.annalsoflongtermcare.com/article/8100

Broussard, J. L., Ehrmann, D. A., Van Cauter, E., et al. (2012). Impaired insulin signaling in human adipocytes after experimental sleep restriction: A randomized, crossover study. *Annals of Internal Medicine, 157*(8), 549–557. doi: 10.7326/0003-4819-157-8-201210160-0000

Budhiraja, R., Roth, T., Hudgel, D. W., et al. (2011). Prevalence and polysomnographic correlates of insomnia comorbid with medical disorders. *Sleep, 34*(7), 859–867. doi: http://dx.doi.org/10.5665/sleep.1114

Bulechek, G., Butcher, H., & Dochterman, J. (Eds.). (2012). *Nursing interventions classification (NIC)* (6th ed.). St. Louis, MO: C. V. Mosby.

Buxton, O. M., Ellenbogen, J. M., Wang, W., et al. (2012). Sleep disruption due to hospital noises: A prospective evaluation, *Annals of Internal Medicine, 157*(3), 170–179. doi:10.7326/0003-4819-157-3-201208070-00472

Centers for Disease Control and Prevention (CDC). (2010). Youth risk behavior surveillance—United States, 2009. *Morbidity and Mortality Weekly Report, 59*(46), SS-5.

Centers for Disease Control and Prevention (CDC). (2012). Suffocation deaths associated with use of infant sleep positioners—United States, 1997–2011. *Morbidity and Mortality Weekly Report, 61*(46), 933–937.

Centers for Disease Control and Prevention (CDC). (2013a, March 14). Sleep and sleep disorders. Retrieved March 27, 2014, from http://www.cdc.gov/features/sleep/

Centers for Disease Control and Prevention (CDC). (2013b, March 14). Insufficient sleep is a public health epidemic: Continued public health surveillance of sleep quality, duration, behaviors, and disorders is needed to monitor sleep difficulties and their health impact. Retrieved March 27, 2014, from http://www.cdc.gov/Features/dsSleep/

Centers for Disease Control and Prevention (CDC). (updated 2014, January 13). Insufficient sleep is a public health epidemic. Retrieved March 25, 2014, from http://www.cdc.gov/features/dssleep/index.html#References

Chee, M. W., & Chuah, L. Y. (2008). Functional neuroimaging insights into how sleep and sleep deprivation affect memory and cognition. *Current Opinion in Neurology, 21*(4), 417–423. doi: 10.1097/WCO.0b013e3283052cf7

Cohen, S., Doyle, W. J., Alper, C. M., et al. (2009). Sleep habits and susceptibility to the common cold. *Annals of Family Medicine, 169*(1), 62–67. doi: 10.1001/archinternmed.2008.505

Dosey, B., & Keegan, L. (2009). *Holistic nursing: A handbook for practice* (5th ed., pp. 361–364). Sudbury, MA: Jones & Bartlett Learning.

Epstein, L. J., Kristo, D., Strollo, P. J., Jr., et al. (2009). Clinical guideline for the evaluation, management and long-term care of obstructive sleep apnea in adults. *Journal of Clinical Sleep Medicine, 5*(3), 263–276.

Haesler, E. J. (2004). Effectiveness of strategies to manage sleep in residents of aged care facilities. *Joanna Briggs Institute Reports, 2*(4), 115–183. doi:10.1111/j.1479-6988.2004.00010.x

Hakin, F., Wang, Y., Zhang, S. X., et al. (2014). Fragmented sleep accelerates tumor growth and progression through recruitment of tumor-associated macrophages and TLR4 signaling. *Cancer Research, 74*(5), 1329–1337. doi:10.1158/0008-5472.CAN-13-3014

Hening, W. A. (2007). Current guidelines and standards of practice for restless legs syndrome. *American Journal of Medicine, 230*(Suppl. 1), S22–S27. doi: http://dx.doi.org/10.1016/j.amjmed.2006.11.004

Holcomb, S. S. (2006). Recommendations for assessing insomnia. *Nurse Practitioner, 31*(2), 55–60.

Holcomb, S. S. (2007). Putting insomnia to rest. *Nurse Practitioner, 32*(4), 28–34. doi: 10.1097/01.NPR.0000266511.55726.3b

Hui, L., Hua, F., Diandong, H., et al. (2007). Effects of sleep and sleep deprivation on immunoglobulins and complement in humans. *Brain, Behavior, & Immunity, 21*(3), 308–310. doi: 10.1016/j.bbi.2010.03.001

Institute of Medicine. (2006). *Sleep disorders and sleep deprivation: An unmet public health problem*. Washington, DC: The National Academies Press.

Johnson, M., Moorhead, S., Bulechek, G., et al. (2012). *Nursing diagnoses, outcomes, & interventions: NANDA, NOC, and NIC linkages* (3rd ed.) St. Louis, MO: Mosby.

The Joint Commission. (2011). Health care worker fatigue and patient safety. *The Joint Commission Sentinel Event Alert, 48*, 1–4. Retrieved March 27, 2014, from http://www.jointcommission.org/assets/1/18/sea_48.pdf

Laugsand, L. E., Strand, L. B., Vatten, L. J., et al. (2014). Insomnia symptoms and risk for unintentional fatal injuries—The HUNT Study. *SLEEP*. doi: 10.5665/sleep.4170

Mander, B. A., Tao, V., Lu, B., et al. (2013). Prefrontal atrophy, disrupted NREM slow waves and impaired hippocampal-dependent memory in aging. *National Neuroscience, 16*(3), 357–364. doi:10.1038/nn.3324

McBeth, J., Lacey, R. J., & Wilkie, R. (2014). Predictors of new-onset widespread pain in older adults: Results from a population-based prospective cohort study in the UK. *Arthritis & Rheumatology, 66*, 757–767. doi:10.1002/art.38284

McCance, K. L., & Huether, S. E. (2009). *Pathophysiology: The biologic basis for disease in adults and children* (6th ed.). St. Louis, MO: C. V. Mosby.

Meltzer, L. J., Davis, K. F., & Mindell, J. A. (2012). Patient and parent sleep in a children's hospital. *Pediatric Nursing, 38*(2), 64–71.

Moorhead, S., Johnson, M., & Maas, M., et al. (Eds.). (2012). *Nursing outcomes classification (NOC)* (5th ed.). St. Louis, MO: C. V. Mosby.

National Institutes of Health (NIH). (2010; reviewed 2012, December 3). Resting may boost memory. Retrieved April 7, 2013, from http://www.nih.gov/researchmatters/february2010/02082010rest.htm

National Institutes of Health (NIH). (2012a, Summer). Are you sleep deprived? Learn more about healthy sleep. *NIH Medline Plus, 7*(2), 16.

National Institutes of Health (NIH). (2012b, Summer). The importance of sleep. *NIH Medline Plus, 7*(2), 17.

National Institutes of Health (NIH). (2012c, Summer). Diagnosing sleep disorders. *NIH Medline Plus, 7*(2), 18.

National Institutes of Health (NIH). (2012d, Summer). Tips for getting a good night sleep. *NIH Medline Plus, 7*(2), 20.

National Institutes of Health (NIH). (2013, April). The benefits of slumber. *NIH News in Health*. Retrieved March 27, 2014, from http://newsinhealth.nih.gov/issue/Apr2013/Feature1

National Institute of Neurological Disorders and Stroke (NINDS). (2009; updated 2013, July 18). *Narcolepsy fact sheet*. National Institutes of Health. Retrieved March 27, 2014, from http://www.ninds.nih.gov/disorders/narcolepsy/detail_narcolepsy.htm

National Sleep Foundation. (n.d.). Restless leg syndrome (RLS) and sleep. Retrieved March 27, 2014, from http://www.sleepfoundation.org/article/sleep-related-problems/restless-legs-syndrome-rls-and-sleep

National Sleep Foundation. (2011). 2011 Sleep in America poll: Communications technology in the bedroom. Summary of findings. Retrieved November 2, 2014, from http://sleepfoundation.org/media-center/press-release/annual-sleep-america-poll-exploring-connections-communications-technology-use-

Ong, J. C., Stepanski, E. J., & Gramling, S. E. (2009, February 15). Pain coping strategies for tension-type headache: Possible implications for insomnia. *Journal of Clinical Sleep Medicine, 5*(1), 52–56.

Polan, E., & Taylor, D. (2010). *Journey across the life span* (4th ed.). Philadelphia: F. A. Davis.

Ranjbaran, Z., Keefer, L., Stepanski, E., et al. (2007). The relevance of sleep abnormalities to chronic inflammatory conditions. *Inflammatory Resource, 56*, 51–57.

Redeker, N. S., & McEnany, G. P. (2011). *Sleep disorders and sleep promotion in nursing practice*. New York: Springer.

Reeve, K., & Bales, B. (2010). Insomnia in adults: Etiology and management. *The Journal for Nurse Practitioners, 6*(1), 53–60. doi: http://dx.doi.org/10.1016/j.nurpra.2009.09.013

Roehrs, T. A., Harris, E., Randall, S., et al. (2012). Pain sensitivity and recovery from mild chronic sleep loss. *Sleep, 35*(12), 1667–1673. doi: http://dx.doi.org/10.5665/sleep.2240

Ruiter, M. (2012, June 11). *Top risk of stroke for normal-weight adults: Getting under 6 hours of sleep* [Abstract #0829]. Paper presented at Sleep 2012, the annual meeting of the Associated Professional Sleep Societies: Boston.

Roth, T., Roehrs, T., & Pies, R. (2007). Insomnia: Pathophysiology and implications for treatment. *Sleep Medicine Reviews, 11*(1), 71–79. doi: http://dx.doi.org/10.1016/j.smrv.2006.06.002

Schachter, S. C., Shafer, P. O., & Sirven, J. L. (2013). Sleep and epilepsy. Epilepsy Foundation. Retrieved March 27, 2014, from http://www.epilepsy.com/learn/triggers-seizures/lack-sleep-and-epilepsy

Smyth, C. A. (2008). Evaluating sleep quality in older adults. *American Journal of Nursing, 108*(5), 42–50.

Sports Injury Clinic. (n.d.) Sports massage for the lower back. Retrieved March 27, 2014, from http://www.sportsinjuryclinic.net/treatments-therapies/sports-massage/sports-massage-lower-back

U.S. Department of Health and Human Services, National Institutes of Health, and National Heart Lung and Blood Institute. (2005; revised 2011, August). Your guide to healthy sleep (NIH Publication No. 11–5271). Retrieved March 27, 2014, from http://www.nhlbi.nih.gov/health/public/sleep/healthy_sleep.pdf

U.S. Department of Health and Human Services, National Institutes of Health, and National Heart Lung and Blood Institute. (2010). What is restless legs syndrome? National Heart Lung and Blood Institute. Retrieved March 27, 2014, from http://www.nhlbi.nih.gov/health/health-topics/topics/rls/

Vinik, A. I., & Casellini, C. M. (2013). Guidelines in the management of diabetic nerve pain: Clinical utility of pregabalin. *Diabetes, Metabolic Syndrome, and Obesity, 6*, 57–78. doi:10.2147/DMSO.S24825.

Walker, M. P. (2009). The role of sleep in cognition and emotion. *Annals of the New York Academy of Science: The Year in Cognitive Neuroscience, 1156*, 168–197. doi:10.1111/j.1749-6632.2009.04416.x

Wilson, S. J., Nutt, D., J., Alford, C., et al. (2010, November). British Association for Psychopharmacology consensus statement on evidence-based treatment of insomnia, parasomnias and circadian rhythm disorders. *Journal of Psychopharmacology, 24*(11), 1577–1601. doi:10.1177/0269881110379307

CHAPTER 35

Aggarwal, V. K., Higuera, C., Deimemgian, G., et al. (2013). Swab cultures are not as effective as tissue cultures for the diagnosis of periprosthetic joint infection. *Clinical, Orthopaedic Related Research, 471*(10), 3196–3203. doi:10.1007/s11999-013-2974-y

Agency for Healthcare Research and Quality. (2009, July). *On-time pressure ulcer healing project*. Rockville, MD: Author. Retrieved November 2, 2014, from http://www.ahrq.gov/research/pressureulcerhealing/

Altman, G. B. (2012, June). Hemovac drain. *MedlinePlus*, U.S. National Library of Medicine, National Institutes of Health. Retrieved March 31, 2014, from http://www.nlm.nih.gov/medlineplus/ency/patientinstructions/000038.htm

Antokal, S., Brienza, D., Bryan, N., et al. (2012, November 20). Friction induced skin injuries: Are they pressure ulcers? *A National Pressure Ulcer Advisory Panel White Paper, 1*(1), 1–3. Retrieved March 31, 2014, from http://www.npuap.org/wp-content/uploads/2012/01/NPUAP-Friction-White-Paper.pdf

Armstrong, D. G., & Meyer, A. J. (2013; updated 2014, January 28). *Basic principles of wound management* (Topic 15912, v 5.0). Wolters Kluwer Health. Retrieved March 31, 2014, from http://www.uptodate.com/contents/basic-principles-of-wound-management

Armstrong, D. G., Ayello, E. A., Capitulo, K. L., et al. (2008). New opportunities to improve pressure ulcer prevention and treatment: Implications of the CMS inpatient hospital care present on admission indicators/hospital-acquired conditions policy—a consensus paper from the International Expert Wound Care Advisory Panel. *Advances in Skin Wound Care, 21*, 469–70, 472–478. doi:10.1097/01.WON.0000335960.68113.82

Association for the Advancement of Wound Care. (AAWC). (2005; revised 2010). *Association for the Advancement of Wound Care venous ulcer guideline* (p. 7). Malvern, PA: Author. Retrieved March 31, 2014, from https://www.guidelinecentral.com/guideline-library/summaries/association-advancement-wound-care

Association of periOperative Registered Nurses (AORN). (2013). *Perioperative standards and recommended practices*. Denver: AORN.

Ayello, E. A., & Sibbald, R. G. (2012, updated). *Nursing standard of practice protocol: Pressure ulcer prevention & skin tear prevention*. New York: Springer. Retrieved March 31, 2014, from http://consultgerirn.org/topics/pressure_ulcers_and_skin_tears/want_to_know_more

Baranoski, S., & Ayello, E. (2011). Wound culture and specimens. In S. Baranoski & E. Ayello, *Wound care essentials* (3rd ed., pp. 136–145). Philadelphia: Lippincott Williams & Wilkins.

Barker, A. L., Kamar, J., Tyndall, T. J., et al. (2013). Implementation of pressure ulcer prevention best practice recommendations in acute care: An observational study. *International Wound Journal, 10*, 313–320. doi:10.1111/j.1742-481X.2012.00979.x

Beeckman, D., Schoonhoven, L., Verhaeghe, S., et al. (2009). Prevention and treatment of incontinence-associated dermatitis: Literature review. *Journal of Advanced Nursing, 65*(6), 1141–1154. doi:10.1111/j.1365-2648.2009.04986.x

Benbow, M. (2010). Wound swabs and chronic wounds. *Practice Nurse, 39*(9), 27–30.

Bergeron, J. D., Bizjak, G., Le Badour, G., et al. (2009). *First responder* (8th ed.). Upper Saddle River, NJ: Prentice Hall.

Bhimji, S. (n.d.; 2013, updated). Wet to dry dressing changes. *Medline*. Retrieved March 31, 2014, from http://www.nlm.nih.gov/medlineplus/ency/patientinstructions/000315.htm

Bergstrom, N., Bennett, M. A., Carlson, C., et al. (1994). *Treatment of pressure ulcers* (Clinical Practice Guideline No 15; AHCPR Publication No. 95–0622). Rockville, MD: U.S. Department of Health and Human Services, Public Health Service, Agency for Health Care Policy and Research.

Black, J., Baharestani, M., Cuddigan, J., et al. (2007). National Pressure Ulcer Advisory Panel's updated pressure ulcer staging system. *Advances in Skin and Wound Care, 20*(5), 269–274.

Black, J. M., Cuddigan, J. E., Walko, M. A., et al. (2010, October). Medical device related pressure ulcers in hospitalized patients. *International Wound Journal, 7*(5), 358–365. doi:10.1111/j.1742-481X.2010.00699.x

Bonham, P. A. (2012). Swab cultures for diagnosing wound infections: A literature review and clinical guideline. *Journal of Wound Ostomy Continence Nursing, 36*(4), 389–395. doi:10.1097/WON.0b013e3181aaef7f

Brunner, M., Droegemueller, C., Rivers, S., et al. (2012). Prevention of incontinence-related skin breakdown for acute and critical care patients. *Urologic Nursing, 32*(4), 214–219.

Bulechek, F., Butcher, H., & Dochterman, J. (2013). *Nursing interventions classification (NIC)* (6th ed.). St. Louis, MO: C. V. Mosby.

Carney, A. Y. (2013). Hyperbaric oxygen therapy: An introduction. *Critical Care Nurse Quarterly, 36*(3), 274–279. doi:10.1097/CNQ.0b013e318294e936

Chariker, M. (2009). Moisture balance: Exploring options in negative pressure wound therapy. *Skin and Wound Care, 22*(Suppl. 1), 10–12. doi: 10.1097/01.ASW.0000323601.26712.78

Christina, M. L., Spagnolo, A. M., Casini, B., et al. (2014). The impact of aerators on water contamination by emerging gram-negative opportunists in at-risk hospital departments. *Infection Control and Hospital Epidemiology, 35*(2). doi:10.1086/674863

Cole, E. (2007). Wound closure using adhesive strips. *Nursing Standard, 22*(9), 48–49. doi: http://dx.doi.org/10.7748/ns2007.11.22.9.48.c6234

Collins, N., & Schnitzer, A. (2013). How dietary protein intake promotes wound healing. *Wound Care Advisor, 2*(6), 16–19. Retrieved November 2, 2014, from http://woundcareadvisor.com/wp-content/uploads/2013/11/Protein_N-D13.pdf

Convatec. (2012). Pressure ulcer management. Retrieved March 31, 2014, from http://www.convatec.com/wound-skin/wound-type/pressure-ulcers.aspx.

Cooper, R. (2010). Top tips for nurses taking a wound swab. *Wounds International,* 1(3). Retrieved March 31, 2014, from http://www.woundsinternational.com/practice-development/ten-top-tips-for-taking-a-wound-swab

DeGaspari, J. (2013). Not skin deep: Lower costs and better outcomes in wound care. *Healthcare Informatics.* Retrieved March 31, 2014, from http://www.healthcare-informatics.com/article/not-skin-deep-lower-costs-and-better-outcomes-wound-care

Dumville, J. C., O'Meara, S., Deshpande, S., et al. (2013). Alginate dressings for healing foot ulcers in people with diabetes mellitus. *Cochrane Database of Systematic Reviews,* Issue 6. Art. No.: CD009110. doi:10.1002/14651858.CD009110.pub3

Eskes, A., Ubbink, D. T., Lubbers, M., et al. (2011). Hyperbaric oxygen therapy for treating acute surgical and traumatic wounds: A review. *The Cochrane Library,* 2. doi:10.1002/14651858.CD008059.pub2

European Pressure Ulcer Advisory Panel and National Pressure Ulcer Advisory Panel. (2009). *Treatment of pressure ulcers: Quick reference guide.* Washington, DC: National Pressure Ulcer Advisory Panel. Retrieved March 31, 2014, from http://www.npuap.org/wp-content/uploads/2012/02/Final_Quick_Prevention_for_web_2010.pdf

Fernandez, R., & Griffiths, R. (2008). Water for wound cleansing. *Cochrane Database of Systematic Reviews,* Issue 2. Art. No.: CD003861. doi:10.1002/14651858.CD003861.pub2

Fernandez, R., & Griffiths, R. (2012). The effects of water compared with other solutions for wound cleansing. *Cochrane Database of Systematic Reviews,* Issue 2. Art. No.: CD003861. doi:10.1002/14651858.CD003861.pub3

Gabriel, A., & Schraga, E. D. (2013, updated). Wound irrigation. Retrieved March 31, 2014, from http://emedicine.medscape.com/article/1895071-overview

Hess, C. T. (2012b). Biofilm intervention pathway: An idealized algorithm. *Advances in Skin and Wound Care, 25*(10), 480. doi: 10.1097/01.ASW.0000421458.76031.bc

Hess, C. T. (2013a). Venous etiology clinical pathways integrated with evidence-based decisions: Part 1. *Advances in Skin & Wound Care, 26*(4), 192. doi: 10.1097/01.ASW.0000428866.80036.fd

Hess, C. T. (2013b). Venous etiology clinical pathways integrated with evidence-based decisions: Part 2. *Advances in Skin & Wound Care,* 26(5), 240. doi: 10.1097/01.ASW.0000427918.89626.97

Hin-Lun, L., & Hon-Ping, C. (2012). A simple technique for the retrieval of buried skin staples. *Burns, 38*(7), 1086–1088.

Immunization Action Coalition, U.S. Department of Health and Human Services, Centers for Disease Control and Prevention. (2012). Vaccine information statement: Td or Tdap vaccine, what you need to know. Retrieved January 11, 2014, from http://www.immunize.org/vis/td_tdap.pdf

Institute for Clinical Systems Improvement (ICSI). (2012). *Pressure ulcer prevention and treatment. Health care protocol.* Bloomington, MN: Author. Retrieved February 7, 2014, from https://www.icsi.org/_asset/6t7kxy/PressureUlcer.pdf

Institute for Healthcare Improvement. (2011). 5 Million Lives Campaign. How to guide: Prevent pressure ulcers. Retrieved April 2, 2014, from http://www.ihi.org/resources/Pages/Tools/HowtoGuidePreventPressureUlcers.aspx

The Joanna Briggs Institute. (2007). Topical skin care in aged care facilities. *Best Practice, 11*(3), 1–4.

The Joanna Briggs Institute. (2008a). Pressure ulcers: Management of pressure-related tissue damage. *Best Practice, 4*(3), 1–4. Retrieved November 2, from http://connect.jbiconnectplus.org/ViewSourceFile.aspx?0=431

The Joanna Briggs Institute. (2008b). Pressure ulcers: Prevention of pressure-related damage. *Best Practice, 4*(2), 1–4. Retrieved October 15, 2013, from http://connect.jbiconnectplus.org/ViewSourceFile.aspx?0=428

The Joanna Briggs Institute, Wound Healing and Management Group. (2012, November). Evidence summary: Wound infection: Biofilms and sharp debridement. *Wound Practice and Research, 20*(4), 209–211.

The Joanna Briggs Institute, Wound Healing and Management Node Group. (2013a). Evidence summary: Polyhexamethylene biguanide (PHMB) wound dressings. *Wound Practice Research, 21*(2), 83–85.

The Joanna Briggs Institute, Wound Healing and Management Group. (2013b). Evidence summary: Wound infection: Silver products and biofilms. *Wound Practice and Research, 21*(1), 48–49.

The Joanna Briggs Institute, Wound Healing and Management Node Group. (2013c). Evidence summary: Wound Infection: Iodophors and biofilms. *Wound Practice Research, 21*(2), 86–89.

The Joanna Briggs Institute, Wound Healing and Management Node Group. (2013d). Evidence summary: Wound Infection: Dressings—alginate. *Wound Practice Research, 21*(2), 90–92.

The Joanna Briggs Institute, Wound Healing and Management Node Group. (2013e). Evidence summary: Wound Infection: Debridement—autolytic. *Wound Practice Research, 21*(2), 94–95.

Johnson, M., Moorhead, S., Bulechek, G., et al. (2012). *NOC, and NIC linkages to NANDA-I and clinical conditions* (3rd ed.). St. Louis, MO: C. V. Mosby.

Kayser-Jones, J. S., Beard, R. L., & Sharpp, T. J. (2009). Dying with a stage IV pressure ulcer. *American Journal of Nursing, 109*(1), 40–49.

Lee, M. (2011, September). Application of negative pressure treatment to fistula wounds: A case study. *Wound Practice and Research, 19*(3), 114–117.

Levine, N. S., Lindberg, R. B., Mason, A. D., et al. (1976). The quantitative swab culture and smear: A quick, simple method for determining the number of viable aerobic bacteria on open wounds. *Journal of Trauma, 16*(2), 89–94.

Lyder, C. H., Wang, Y., Metersky, M., et al. (2012). Hospital-acquired pressure ulcers: Results from the national Medicare

Patient Safety Monitoring System study. *Journal of American Geriatrics Society, 60*(9), 1603–1608. doi:10.1111/j.1532-5415.2012.04106.x

Martindell, D. (2012). The safe use of negative-pressure wound therapy. *American Journal of Nursing, 112*(6), 59–63.

McCulloch, J. M., & Kloth, L. C. (2010). *Wound healing: Evidence-based management* (4th ed.). Philadelphia: F. A. Davis.

McInnes, E., Jammali-Blasi, A., Bell-Sye, S. E., et al. (2011). Support surfaces for pressure ulcer prevention. *Cochrane Database of Systematic Reviews,* Issue 4. Art. No.: CD001735. doi:10.1002/14651858.CD001735.pub4

Mills, E., Eyawo, O., Lockhart, I., et al. (2011). Smoking cessation reduces postoperative complications: Systemic review and meta-analysis. *The American Journal of Medicine, 124*(2), 144–154. doi: http://dx.doi.org/10.1016/j.amjmed.2010.09.013

Moore, Z. E., & Cowman, S. (2013). Wound cleansing for pressure ulcers. *Cochrane Database of Systematic Reviews,* Issue 3. Art. No.: CD004983.

Moore, C., & Young, J. (2011). Effectiveness of silver in wound care treatment. *Physical Therapy Reviews, 16*(3), 201–209.

Moorhead, S., Johnson, M., Maas, M., et al. (Eds.). (2013). *Nursing outcomes classification (NOC)* (5th ed.). St. Louis, MO: C. V. Mosby.

Mutluoglu, M., Uzun, G., Turhan, V., et al. (2012). How reliable are cultures of specimens from superficial swabs as compared with those of deep tissue in patients with diabetic foot ulcers? *Journal of Diabetes and Its Complications, 26*(3), 225–229. doi: 10.1016/j.jdiacomp.2012.03.015

Myers, B. A. (2011). *Wound management: Principles and practice* (3rd ed.). Upper Saddle River, NJ: Pearson Education.

NANDA International. (2012). *Nursing diagnoses: Definitions and classification 2012–2014.* Philadelphia: Author.

National Guideline Clearinghouse (NGC). (2006; revised 2014, February). *Guideline synthesis: Prevention of pressure ulcers.* Rockville, MD: Agency for Healthcare Research and Quality. Retrieved March 31, 2014, from http://www.guideline.gov/syntheses/synthesis.aspx?f=rss&id=47794

National Pressure Ulcer Advisory Panel (NPUAP). (n.d.). The facts about reverse staging in 2000, The NPUAP position statement. Retrieved April 1, 2014, from http://www.npuap.org/wp-content/uploads/2012/01/Reverse-Staging-Position-Statement%E2%80%A8.pdf

National Pressure Ulcer Advisory Panel (NPUAP). (1998). Pressure ulcer scale for healing (PUSH) tool (Version 3.0). Retrieved April 1, 2014, from http://www.npuap.org/wp-content/uploads/2012/03/push3.pdf

National Pressure Ulcer Advisory Panel (NPUAP). (2007). Pressure ulcer prevention points. Retrieved April 1, 2014, from http://www.npuap.org/wp-content/uploads/2012/03/PU_Prev_Points.pdf

National Pressure Ulcer Advisory Panel (NPUAC). (2010). Registered nurse competency-based curriculum: Pressure ulcer prevention. Revision of the 2001 Registered Nurse competency-based curriculum: Pressure ulcer prevention. Based on National Pressure Ulcer Advisory Panel and European Pressure Ulcer Advisory Panel. (2009) *Prevention and treatment of pressure ulcers: Clinical practice guideline.* Washington DC: Author. Retrieved March 31, 2014, from http://www.npuap.org/wp-content/uploads/2012/03/NPUAP-RN-Curr-landscape1.pdf

National Pressure Ulcer Advisory Panel, European Pressure Ulcer Advisory Panel. (2009). Pressure ulcer treatment recommendations. In *Prevention and treatment of pressure ulcers: Clinical practice guideline* (pp. 51–120). Washington, DC: Author. Retrieved October 15, 2013, from http://www.npuap.org/wp-content/uploads/2012/02/Final_Quick_Prevention_for_web_2010.pdf

Non, L. R. (2012, updated). Bacterial wound culture. Retrieved January 20, 2014, from http://emedicine.medscape.com/article/2103764-overview#aw2aab6b4

Norton, D., McLaren, R., & Exton-Smith, A. N. (1975). *An investigation of geriatric nursing problems in hospitals.* Edinburgh, England: Churchill Livingstone.

O'Meara, S., Cullum, N., Nelson, A, et al. (2012). Compression for venous leg ulcers. *Cochrane Database of Systematic Reviews,* Issue 11. Art. No.: CD000265. doi:10.1002/14651858.CD000265.pub3

Opletalova, K., Blaizot, X., Mourgeon, B., et al. (2012). Maggot therapy for wound debridement: A randomized multicenter trial. *Archives of Dermatology, 148*(4), 432–438. doi:10.1001/archdermatol.2011.1895

Panicker, V. N. (2009, November). A pilot study evaluating topical negative pressure using V1STA technology. *Wound Practice and Research, 17*(4), 194–200.

Perry, D., Borchert, K., Burke, S., et al. (2012). Pressure ulcer prevention and treatment protocol. Institute for Clinical Systems Improvement. Retrieved April 1, 2014, from https://www.icsi.org/_asset/6t7kxy/

Pieper, B., Langemo, D., & Cuddigan, J. (2009). Pressure ulcer pain: A systematic literature review and National Pressure Ulcer Advisory Panel white paper. *Ostomy Wound Management, 55*(2). Retrieved April 1, 2014, from http://www.npuap.org/wp-content/uploads/2012/01/Pieper_2009_Feb1.pdf

Posthauer, M. E. (2012, February). The role of nutrition in wound care. *Advances in Skin & Wound Care, 25*(2), 62–63. doi: 10.1097/01.ASW.0000411404.19016.ad

Robson, M. C., Cooper, D. M., Aslam, R., et al. (2006), Guidelines for the treatment of venous ulcers. *Wound Repair and Regeneration, 14,* 649–662. doi:10.1111/j.1524-475X.2006.00174

Rolstad, B. S., & Ovington, L. G. (2011). Principles of wound management. In R. A. Bryant & D. P. Nix (Eds.), *Acute and chronic wounds: Current management concepts* (4th ed.). St. Louis, MO: C. V. Mosby Elsevier.

Rushing, J. (2007). Clinical dos and don'ts: Obtaining a wound culture specimen. *Nursing2007, 37*(13), 18.

Russo, C. A., Steiner, C., & Spector, W. (2008). *Hospitalizations related to pressure ulcers among adults 18 and older, 2006* (HCUP Statistical Brief No. 64). Rockville, MD: Agency for Healthcare Research and Quality. Retrieved April 1, 2014, from http://www.hcup-us.ahrq.gov/reports/statbriefs/sb64.pdf

Salcido, R., & Popescu, A. (2012). Pressure ulcers and wound care. Retrieved April 1, 2014, from http://emedicine.medscape.com/article/319284-overview#aw2aab6b2

Schols, J. M., Heyman, H., & Meijer, E. W. (2009). Nutritional support in the treatment and prevention of pressure ulcers: An overview of studies with an arginine enriched oral nutritional supplement. *Journal of Tissue Viability, 18*(3), 72–79. doi: 10.1016/j.jtv.2009.03.002

Silverstein, P. (1992). Smoking and wound healing. *American Journal of Medicine, 93*(1A), 22S–24S.

Smith, M. E. B., Totten, A., Hickam, D. H., et al. (2013). Pressure ulcer treatment strategies: A systematic comparative effectiveness review. *Annals of Internal Medicine, 158*(1), 39–50. doi:10.7326/0003-4819-159-1-201307020-00007

Stechmiller, J. K., Cowan, L., Whitney, J. D., et al. (2008). Guidelines for the prevention of pressure ulcers. *Wound Repair and Regeneration, 16*, 151–168. doi:10.1111/j.1524-475X.2008.00356.x

Storm-Versioot, M., Vos, C., Ubbink, D., et al. (2010) Topical silver for preventing wound infection. *Cochrane Database Systematic Reviews*, Issue 3. Art. No.: CD006578. doi:10.1002/14651858.CD006578.pub2

Sullivan, N., Snyder, D. L., Tipton, K., et al. (2009, May 26). *Negative pressure wound therapy devices: Technology assessment report*. Rockville, MD: U.S. Department of Health and Human Services, Agency for Healthcare Research and Quality. Retrieved April 1, 2014, from http://www.ahrq.gov/research/findings/ta/negative-pressure-wound-therapy/negative-pressure-wound-therapy.pdf

U.S. Department of Health and Human Services. (2010; updated 2013). *Healthy People 2020* topics and objectives, older adults. Retrieved April 1, 2014, from http://www.healthypeople.gov/2020/topicsobjectives2020/objectiveslist.aspx?topicId=31

U.S. Department of Health and Human Services. (1992). *Clinical practice guideline. Pressure ulcers in adults: Prediction and prevention* (PPPPUA Publication No. 92-0047; pp. 16–17). Rockville, MD: Public Health Service.

Watret, L., & McClean, A. (2013). Cleansing diabetic foot wounds: Tap water or saline? *Wounds International, 4*(4), 1–4. Retrieved January 11, 2014, from http://www.woundsinternational.com/case-reports/cleansing-diabetic-foot-wounds-tap-water-or-saline/page-1

Wilkins, R. G., & Unverdorben, M. (2013). Wound cleaning and wound healing: A concise review. *Advances in Skin & Wound Care, 26*(4), 160–163. doi: 10.1097/01.ASW.0000428861.26671.41

Woo, K. Y. (2011). Exploring the effects of pain and stress on wound healing. *Advanced Skin Wound Care, 25*(1), 38–44. doi: 10.1097/01.ASW.0000410689.60105.7d

Woo, K. Y., Santos, V., & Gamba, M. (2013). *Understanding diabetic foot ulcers. Nursing2013, 43*(10), 36–41. doi: 10.1097/01.NURSE.0000434311.52768.1d

Wound, Ostomy and Continence Nurses Society (WOCN). (2010). *Guideline for prevention and management of pressure ulcers*. Mount Laurel, NJ: Author. Retrieved April 1, 2014, from http://www.guideline.gov/content.aspx?id=23868

Wound, Ostomy and Continence Nurses Society (WOCN). (2007; revised 2011). *Position statement: Pressure ulcer staging* (p. 52). Mount Laurel, NJ: Author. Retrieved January 11, 2013, from http://npuap.org/pr2.htm

Wound, Ostomy, and Continence Nurses Society. (n.d.). Wound, ostomy and continent nurses: A smart addition to the healthcare team. Retrieved January 17, 2014, from http://c.ymcdn.com/sites/www.wocn.org/resource/resmgr/smart_addition.pdf

Zulkowski, K. (2013). Skin bacteria: Implications for wound care. *Advances in Skin and Wound Care, 26*(5), 231–236. doi: 10.1097/01.ASW.0000429721.70911.7d

CHAPTER 36

Aehlert B. (2012). *ACLS quick review study guide* (4th ed.). St. Louis, MO: Mosby.

Allegranzi, B., & Pittet, D. (2009). Role of hand hygiene in healthcare-associated infection prevention. *Journal of Hospital Infection, 73*(4), 305–315.

American Academy of Pediatrics. (2011a). Committee on Infectious Diseases. Guideline summary. Recommendations for prevention and control of influenza in children, 2011–2012. *Pediatrics 2011, 128*(4), 813–825. Retrieved August 5, 2013, from http://www.guideline.gov/content.aspx?id=34977

American Academy of Pediatrics. (2011b). Pulse oximetery: A viable, readily available screening tool for infants with suspected critical congenital heart disease. *Healthy Children*. Retrieved July 16, 2013, from http://www.aap.org/en-us/about-the-aap/aap-press-room/Pages/Pulse-Oximetry-a-Viable,-Readily-Available-Screening-Tool-for-Infants-with-Suspected-Critical-Congenital-Heart-Disease.aspx

American Association of Critical-Care Nurses (AACN). (2010). *AACN procedure manual for critical care* (6th ed.). Philadelphia: W. B. Saunders.

American Association of Critical-Care Nurses (AACN). (2008). AACN practice alert. Ventilator associated pneumonia. Retrieved July 6, 2013, from http://www.aacn.org/WD/Practice/Docs/Ventilator_Associated_Pneumonia_1-2008.pdf

American Heart Association (AHA). (2010). Part 1: Executive summary 2010 American heart association guidelines for cardiopulmonary resuscitation and emergency cardiovascular care. *Circulation, 122*(18, Suppl. 3), S640–S656. Retrieved July 20, 2013, from http://circ.ahajournals.org/content/122/18_suppl_3/S640.full

American Lung Association (ALA). (2013). Six steps. Retrieved August 6, 2013, from http://www.lung.org/associations/states/hawaii/local-programs/asthma/six-steps/

American Lung Association (ALA). (n.d.). Secondhand smoke. Retrieved July 6, 2013, from http://www.lung.org/stop-smoking/about-smoking/health-effects/secondhand-smoke.html

American Lung Association (ALA). (2010). Trends in lung cancer morbidity and mortality. Retrieved July 6, 2013, from http://www.lungusa.org/finding-cures/our-research/trend-reports/lc-trend-report.pdf

American Lung Association (ALA). (2011). Trends in tobacco use. Research and Program Services Epidemiology and Statistics Unit. Retrieved July 2, 2013, from http://www.lung.org/finding-cures/our-research/trend-reports/Tobacco-Trend-Report.pdf

American Red Cross. (n.d.). Airway adjuncts. Retrieved August 5, 2013, from http://www.redcross.org/images/MEDIA_CustomProductCatalog/m4240191_AirwayAdjunctsFactandSkill.pdf

Barnett, M. (2012). Back to basics: Caring for people with a tracheostomy. *Nursing & Residential Care, 14*(8), 390–394.

Bilton, D. (2012). Chest physiotherapy techniques in bronchiectasis. *Clinics in Chest Medicine, 33*(2), 351–361.

Bozyk, P., & Hyzy, R. (2008). Modes of mechanical ventilation. *UpToDate for Patients*. Retrieved July 6, 2013, from http://www.uptodate.com/contents/modes-of-mechanical-ventilation

Bulechek, G., Butcher, H., & Dochterman, J. (2012). *Nursing interventions classification (NIC)* (6th ed.). St. Louis, MO: C. V. Mosby.

Bullard, D., Brothers, K., Davis, C., et al. (2012). Contraindications to nasopharyngeal airway insertion. *Nursing 2012, 42*(10), 66–67.

Bullen, C., Howe, C., Laugesen, M., et al. (2013). Electronic cigarettes for smoking cessation: A randomized controlled trial. *The Lancet*. Advance online publication. doi:10.1016/S0140-6736(13)61842-5

Carroll, P. (Ed.). (2012, Spring). Dressings for chest tubes. *Clinical Update.* Retrieved January 29, 2014, from http://www.atriummed.com/en/chest_drainage/clinical%20updates/clinicalupdatespring2012.pdf

Centers for Disease Control and Prevention (CDC). (2009). Cold and cough medicines: Information for parents. National Center for Preparedness, Detection, and Control of Infectious Diseases, Division of Healthcare Quality Promotion (DHQP). Retrieved July 15, 2013, from http://www.cdc.gov/features/pediatriccoldmeds/

Centers for Disease Control and Prevention (CDC). (2010). Respiratory syncytial virus infection (RSV): Infection and incidence. Retrieved July 21, 2013, from http://www.cdc.gov/rsv/about/infection.html

Centers for Disease Control and Prevention (CDC). (2011). Interim guidance on specimen collection, processing, and testing for patients with suspect influenza A (H3N2)v virus infection. Retrieved August 5, 2013, from http://www.cdc.gov/flu/swineflu/h3n2v-testing.htm

Centers for Disease Control and Prevention (CDC). (2012a). Work-related asthma—38 states and District of Columbia, 2006–2009. *Morbidity and Mortality Weekly Report, 61*(20), 375–378. Retrieved July 6, 2013, from http://www.cdc.gov/mmwr/preview/mmwrhtml/mm6120a4.htm

Centers for Disease Control and Prevention (CDC). (2012b). Vaccines and preventable diseases: PCV13 (pneumococcal conjugate) vaccine. Recommendations, scenarios and Q&As for health care professionals. Retrieved July 21, 2013, from http://www.cdc.gov/vaccines/vpd-vac/pneumo/vac-PCV13-adults.htm#recommendations

Centers for Disease Control and Prevention (CDC). (2013). Interim recommendations: Prevention and control of influenza with vaccines: Recommendations of the Advisory Committee on Immunization Practices (ACIP). Influenza prevention and control recommendations. Retrieved July 6, 2013, from http://www.cdc.gov/flu/professionals/acip/2013-interim-recommendations.htm

Chan, E. D., Chan, M. M., & Chan, M. M. (2013). Pulse oximetry: Understanding its basic principles facilitates appreciation of its limitations. *Respiratory Medicine, 107*(6), 789–799.

Chaney, S. E., & Sheriff, S. (2012). Evidence-based treatments for smoking cessation. *The Nurse Practitioner, 37*(4), 24–31.

Cleveland Clinic. (2009). Tracheal suction guidelines. Retrieved July 13, 2013, from http://my.clevelandclinic.org/services/tracheostomy/hic_tracheal_suction_guidelines.aspx

Coffin, W., Klompas, M., Classen, D., et al.; the Healthcare-Associated Infections Task Force. (2008). Guideline summary: Strategies to prevent ventilator-associated pneumonia in acute care hospitals. *Infection Control and Hospital Epidemiology, 29*(Suppl. 1), S31–S40. Retrieved July 2, 2013, from http://www.guideline.gov/content.aspx?id=13396

Cohen, H. A., Rozen, J., Kristal, H., et al. (2012). Effect of honey on nocturnal cough and sleep quality: A double-blind, randomized, placebo-controlled study. *Pediatrics, 130*(3), 465–471.

Dobbin, K., & Howard, V. (2011). Listen closely to detect healthcare-associated pneumonia. *Nursing2011, 41*(7), 59–62

Environmental Protection Agency (EPA). (2011). Health effects of exposure to secondhand smoke. Retrieved July 5, 2013, from http://www.epa.gov/smokefre/healtheffects.html

Feider, L. L., Mitchell, P., & Bridges, E. (2010). Oral care practices for orally intubated critically ill adults. *American Journal of Critical Care, 19*(2), 175–183.

Fiore, A. E., Uyeki, T. M., Broder, K., et al. (2010). Prevention and control of influenza with vaccines: Recommendations of the Advisory Committee on Immunization Practices (ACIP), 2010. *Morbidity and Mortality Weekly Report. Recommendations and Reports, 59*(RR-08), 1-62. Retrieved July 6, 2013, from http://www.cdc.gov/mmwr/preview/mmwrhtml/rr5908a1.htm

Fiore, M., Jaén, C., Baker, T., et al. (2008). *Treating tobacco use and dependence: 2008 update. Clinical practice guideline.* Rockville, MD: U.S. Department of Health and Human Services, Public Health Service. Retrieved July 21, 2013, from http://www.surgeongeneral.gov/tobacco/treating_tobacco_use08.pdf

Fuchs, P., Loeseken, C., Schubert, J. K., & Miekisch, W. (2010). Breath gas aldehydes as biomarkers of lung cancer. *International Journal of Cancer, 126*(11), 2663–2670.

Hall, J. E. (2011). *Guyton and Hall textbook of medical physiology* (12th ed.). New York: Saunders.

Han, J., & Liu, Y. (2010). Effect of ventilator circuit changes on ventilator-associated pneumonia: A systematic review and meta-analysis. *Respiratory Care, 55*(4), 467–474.

Hart, A., Patti, P., Noggie, B., et al. (2008). Acute respiratory infections and antimicrobial resistance. *American Journal of Nursing, 108*(6), 56–66.

HealthyPeople.gov. (2010). Tobacco use. Retrieved July 21, 2013, from http://healthypeople.gov/2020/topicsobjectives2020/overview.aspx?topicid=41

Hemilä, H., & Chalker, E. (2013). Vitamin C for preventing and treating the common cold. *Cochrane Database of Systematic Reviews,* Issue 5. Art. No.: CD000980. Retrieved July 15, 2013, from http://www.update-software.com/BCP/WileyPDF/EN/CD000980.pdf

Hill, E., & Stoneham, M. (2000). Practical applications of pulse oximetry. *Update in Anaesthesia, 11*(4). Retrieved July 17, 2013, from http://update.anaesthesiologists.org/wp-content/uploads/2008/12/Pulse-Oximetry-Practical-Applications.pdf

Johnson, M., Bulechek, G., Butcher, H., et al. (2012). *NANDA, NOC, and NIC linkages* (3rd ed.). St. Louis, MO: C. V. Mosby.

Johnston, J., Davis, S., & Sherman, J. (n.d.). Care of the child with a chronic tracheostomy. American Thoracic Society [Web site]. Retrieved July 21, 2013, from http://www.thoracic.org/education/care-of-the-child-with-chronic-tracheostomy/index.php

Jubran, A. (2009). Pulse oximetry. In G. Hedenstierna, J. Mancebo, L. Brochard, & M. R. Pinsky (Eds.), *Applied physiology in intensive care medicine* (2nd ed., pp. 45–48). New York: Springer.

Kane, C. J., York, N. L., & Minton, L. A. (2013). Chest tubes in the critically ill patient. *Dimensions of Critical Care Nursing, 32*(3), 111–117.

Kelly, D. M. (2012). *The organization of critical care nursing and outcomes of mechanically ventilated older adults* (Doctoral dissertation). Retrieved from http://repository.upenn.edu/dissertations/AAI3542907

Kinoshita, E., Hayashi, K., Katayama, H., et al. (2012). Anti-influenza virus effects of elderberry juice and its fractions. *Bioscience, Biotechnology, and Biochemistry, 76*(9), 1633–1638.

Kozin, E., Straton, J., & Kapo, J. (2012). Tracheostomy care. *Journal of Palliative Medicine, 15*(3), 359–360.

Kuriakose, A. (2008). Using the synergy model as best practice in endotracheal tube suctioning of critically ill patients. *Dimensions of Critical Care Nursing, 27*(1), 10–15.

Larsson, I., Sahlsten, M., Segesten, K., & Plos, K. (2011). Patients' perceptions of barriers for participation in nursing care. *Scandanavian Journal of Caring Sciences, 25*(3), 575–582.

Lipincott's nursing procedures (6th ed.). (2012). Philadelphia: Lippincott Williams & Wilkins.

Maddox, R., & Williams, C. K. (2012). Clinical experience with capnography monitoring for PCA patients. *Anesthesia Patient Safety Foundation Newsletter.*

Maliakal M. (2013). Patient education series: Chest tubes. *Nursing2013, 41*(7), 33–33.

Maselli, D., & Restrepo, M. (2011). Strategies in the prevention of ventilator-associated pneumonia. *Therapeutic Advances in Respiratory Disease, 5*(2), 131–141.

Mateoso, J., Gonzalez, N., Sadaba, M., et al. (2011). Nursing care in the prevention of ventilator-associated pneumonia. *Enferm intensive, 22*(1), 22–30.

MedlinePlus. (n.d.; last updated 10/9/2009). Chronic obstructive pulmonary disease. National Institutes of Health. Retrieved July 21, 2013, from http://www.nlm.nih.gov/medlineplus/ency/article/000091.htm

McGrath, B. A., Bates, L., Atkinson, D., et al. (2012). Multidisciplinary guidelines for the management of tracheostomy and laryngectomy airway emergencies. *Anaesthesia, 67*(9), 1025–1041.

Mitchell, R. B., Hussey, H. M., Setzen, G., et al. (2013). Clinical consensus statement tracheostomy care. *Otolaryngology—Head and Neck Surgery, 148*(1), 6–20.

Mogri, M., Desai, H., Webster, L., et al. (2009). Hypoxemia in patients on chronic opiate therapy with and without sleep apnea. *Sleep and Breathing, 13*(1), 49–57.

Monitoring your adult patient with bedside pulse oximetry. *Nursing2008, 38*(9), 42–44.

Moorhead, S., Johnson, M., Maas, M., et al. (2012). *Nursing outcomes classification (NOC)* (5th ed.). St. Louis, MO: C. V. Mosby.

Morrow, B., & Argent, A. (2008). A comprehensive review of pediatric endotracheal suctioning: Effects, indications, and clinical practice. *Pediatric Critical Care Medicine, 9*(5), 465–477.

Munro, C., Grap, M., Jones, D., et al. (2009). Chlorhexidine, toothbrushing, and preventing ventilator-associated pneumonia in critically ill adults. *American Journal of Critical Care, 18*, 425–437.

NANDA International. (2012). *NANDA nursing diagnoses: Definitions and classifications 2012–2014.* Ames, IA: Wiley-Blackwell.

National Guideline Clearinghouse (NGC). (2001; revised 2013, April). *Guideline synthesis: Treatment of tobacco dependence.* Rockville, MD: Agency for Healthcare Research and Quality. Retrieved July 6, 2013, from http://www.guideline.gov/syntheses/synthesis.aspx?id=43817&search=smoking+cessation

National Guideline Clearinghouse (NGC). (2011). Best evidence statement (BESt). Basic pediatric tracheostomy care. Rockville, MD: Agency for Healthcare Research and Quality. Retrieved July 17, 2013, from http://www.guideline.gov/content.aspx?id=34159&search=tracheostomy

National Guideline Clearinghouse (NGC). (2010). Endotracheal suctioning of mechanically ventilated patients with artificial airways. Rockville, MD: Agency for Healthcare Research and Quality. Retrieved July 17, 2013, from http://www.guideline.gov/content.aspx?id=23992&search=suctioning

Porth, C. M., & Matfin, G. (2010). *Pathophysiology: Concepts of altered states* (8th ed.). New York: Lippincott Williams & Wilkins.

Rajkumar, A., Karmarkar, A., & Knott, J. (2006). Pulse oximetry: An overview. *Journal of Perioperative Practice, 16*(10), 502–504.

Rauen, C., Chulay, M., Bridges, E., et al. (2008). Seven evidence-based practice habits: Putting some sacred cows out to pasture. *Critical Care Nurse, 28*(2), 98–124.

Rello, J., Afonso, E., Lisboa, T, et al. (2012). A care bundle approach for prevention of ventilator_associated pneumonia. *Clinical Microbiology and Infection, 19*(4), 363–369

Restrepo, R. D., Brown, J. M., & Hughes, J. M. (2010). AARC clinical practice guidelines. Endotracheal suctioning of mechanically ventilated patients with artificial airways. *Respiratory Care, 55*(6), 758–64.

Rice, V., & Stead, L. (2008). Nursing interventions for smoking cessation. *Cochrane Database of Systematic Reviews,* Issue 1. Art. No.: CD001188. doi:10.1002/14651858.CD001188.pub3. Retrieved July 13, 2013, from http://www.cochrane.org/reviews/en/ab001188.html

Rigotti, N. A., Clair, C., Munafò, M. R., et al. (2012). Interventions for smoking cessation in hospitalised patients. *Cochrane Database Systematic Reviews,* Issue 5. Art. No.: CD001837. doi:10.1002/14651858.CD001837.pub3. Retrieved July 6, 2013, from http://www.update-software.com/pdf/CD001837.pdf

Ross, S. M. (2012). African Geranium (EPs 7630), Part I: A proprietary root extract of *Pelargonium sidoides* (EPs 7630) is found to be effective in resolving symptoms associated with the common cold in adults. *Holistic Nursing Practice, 26*(2), 106–109.

Roy, A., Khanra, K., Mukherjee, A., et al. (2013). Asbestos: A potential food contaminant and associated safety risks to consumers. *Journal of Science, 3*(1), 241–243.

Schiller J., Lucas J., & Peregoy J. (2012). Summary health statistics for U.S. adults: National Health Interview Survey, 2011. National Center for Health Statistics. *Vital Health Statistics, 10*(256). Retrieved July 6, 201, from http://www.cdc.gov/nchs/data/series/sr_10/sr10_256.pdf

Siddiqui, J., Sherren, P. B., & Birchall, M. A. (2013). Evidence-based guidelines and protocols for the management of adult patients with a tracheostomy: A systematic review. *Critical Care, 17*(Suppl. 2), 166.

Siegel, J., Rhinehart, E., Jackson, M., et al.; the Healthcare Infection Control Practices Advisory Committee. (2007). 2007 guideline for isolation precautions: Preventing transmission of infectious agents in healthcare settings. Retrieved July 21, 2013, from http://www.cdc.gov/hicpac/pdf/isolation/Isolation2007.pdf

Sole, M. L., Penoyer, D. A., Bennett, M., et al. (2011). Oropharyngeal secretion volume in intubated patients: The importance of oral suctioning. *American Journal of Critical Care, 20*(6), e141–e145.

Stead, L. F., & Lancaster, T. (2012). Combined pharmacotherapy and behavioral interventions for smoking cessation. *Cochrane Database of Systematic Reviews,* Issue 10. Art. No.: CD008286. doi:10.1002/14651858.CD008286.pub2.

Stich, J., & Cassella, D. (2009). Getting inspired about oxygen delivery devices. *Nursing2009, 39*(9), 51–54.

Texas Department of State Health Services. Laboratory Services Section Home. (2009). Guidelines for specimen collection and submission: Mycobacteriology (AFB) collection, transport, and storage. Retrieved July 21, 2013, from http://www.dshs.state.tx.us/LAB/myco_guidelines.shtm

Thomas, J. (2012). Current drug information: Echinacea does not affect the course of the common cold. *AJP: The Australian Journal of Pharmacy, 93*(1102), 75.

U.S. Environmental Protection Agency. (2004). *Fact sheet: Revisions to the air quality index*. Retrieved July 4, 2013, from http://www.epa.gov/ttn/caaa/t1/fact_sheets/factsht.pdf

U.S. Food and Drug Administration/Consumer Health Information. (2013). Using over-the-counter cough and cold products in children. Retrieved July 15, 2013, from http://www.fda.gov/ForConsumers/ConsumerUpdates/ucm048515.htm#TipsforParentsandCaregivers

Valdez-Lowe, C., Ghareeb, S., & Artinian, N. (2009). Pulse oximetry in adults. *American Journal of Nursing, 109*(6), 52–58.

Vital Signs: Current cigarette smoking among adults aged ≥ 18 years—United States, 2005–2010. (2011). *Morbidity and Mortality Weekly Report, 60*. Advance online publication. Retrieved July 21, 2013, from http://www.cdc.gov/mmwr/preview/mmwrhtml/mm60e0906a1.htm?s_cid=mm60e0906a1_w

Walls, R., & Murphy, M. (2012). *Manual of emergency airway management* (4th ed.). Philadelphia: Lippincott Williams & Wilkins.

Williams, F., Blum, A., Forbes, B., et al. (2008). Adult smoking cessation strategies: A rural healthcare CE initiative. *American Journal for Nurse Practitioners, 12*(4), 44–52.

CHAPTER 37

Agency for Healthcare Research and Quality (AHRQ). (2009). U.S. Preventive Services Task Force. Aspirin for the prevention of cardiovascular disease. Retrieved July 31, 2013, from http://www.ahrq.gov/professionals/clinicians-providers/resources/aspprovider.html

American Heart Association (AHA). (2010). 2010 American Heart Association guidelines for cardiopulmonary resuscitation and emergency cardiovascular care science. *Circulation, 122*, S640–S656. Retrieved July 31, 2013, from http://circ.ahajournals.org/content/122/18_suppl_3/S640.full.pdf+html

American Heart Association (AHA). (2011a, November 14). Cigarette smoking and cardiovascular diseases. Retrieved July 31, 2013, from http://newsroom.heart.org/pr/aha/smoking-tip-sheet-nov-14-2011-217833.aspx

American Heart Association (AHA). (2011b, June 13). Heart failure medications. Retrieved July 31, 2013, from http://www.heart.org/HEARTORG/Conditions/HeartFailure/PreventionTreatmentofHeartFailure/Heart-Failure-Medications_UCM_306342_Article.jsp#.TsLKAmAqnL4

American Heart Association (AHA). (2011c, February 24). Hands Only CPR. Retrieved July 31, 2013, from http://www.heart.org/HEARTORG/CPRAndECC/HandsOnlyCPR/LearnMore/Learn-More_UCM_440810_FAQ.jsp

American Lung Association (ALA). (2011). Children and teens. Retrieved July 31, 2013, from http://www.lungusa.org/stop-smoking/about-smoking/facts-figures/children-teens-and-tobacco.html

Begum, M. N. (2013). To evaluate the effect of yoga on moderate degree hypertension and lipid profile. *National Journal of Integrated Research in Medicine, 4*(3), 109–114.

Bulechek, G., Butcher, H., & Dochterman, J. (2012). *Nursing interventions classification (NIC)* (6th ed.). St. Louis, MO: C. V. Mosby.

Centers for Disease Control (CDC). (2011). QuickStats: Age-adjusted death rates for the 10 leading causes of death—National Vital Statistics System, United States, 2008 and 2009. *Morbidity and Mortality Weekly Report, 60*(48), 1656–1656. Retrieved July 29, 2013, from http://www.cdc.gov/mmwr/preview/mmwrhtml/mm6048a7.htm

Centers for Disease Control and Prevention (CDC). (2012). Current cigarette smoking among adults—United States, 2011. *Morbidity and Mortality Weekly Report, 61*(44) 889–94. Retrieved July 29, 2013, from http://www.cdc.gov/mmwr/preview/mmwrhtml/mm6144a2.htm?s_cid=%20mm6144a2.htm_w

Deepa, T., Sethu, G., & Thirrunavukkarasu, N. (2012). Effect of yoga and meditation on mild to moderate essential hypertensives. *Journal of Clinical and Diagnostic Research, 6*(1), 21–26.

de Koning, L., Malik, V. S., Kellogg, M. D., et al. (2012). Sweetened beverage consumption, incident of coronary heart disease, and biomarkers of risk in men. Clinical perspective. *Circulation, 125*(14), 1735–1741.

Dumas, F., Rea, T. D., Fahrenbruch, C., et al. (2013). Chest compression alone cardiopulmonary resuscitation is associated with better long-term survival compared with standard cardiopulmonary resuscitation, clinical perspective. *Circulation, 127*(4), 435–441.

Hancock, E. W., Deal, B. J., Mirvis, D. M., et al. (2009). AHA/ACCF/HRS Recommendations for the standardization and interpretation of the electrocardiogram part V: Electrocardiogram changes associated with cardiac chamber hypertrophy. A scientific statement from the American Heart Association Electrocardiography and Arrhythmias Committee, Council on Clinical Cardiology; the American College of Cardiology Foundation; and the Heart Rhythm Society endorsed by the International Society for Computerized Electrocardiology. *Journal of the American College of Cardiology, 53*(11), 992–1002.

Healthy People 2020. (2010). Heart disease and stroke. Topics and objectives. Retrieved July 31, 2013, from http://www.healthypeople.gov/2020/topicsobjectives2020/overview.aspx?topicid=21

Johnson, M., Moorhead, S., Bulechek, G., et al. (2012). *NOC and NIC linkages to NANDA-I and clinical conditions*. St. Louis, MO: C. V. Mosby:

The Joint Commission (TJC). (2013). Specifications manual for national hospital inpatient quality measures, venous thromboembolism (VTE). Retrieved July 31, 2013, from http://www.jointcommission.org/specifications_manual_for_national_hospital_inpatient_quality_measures.aspx

Kokubo, Y., Iso, H., Saito, I., et al. (2013). The impact of green tea and coffee consumption on the reduced risk of stroke incidence in Japanese population: The Japan Public Health Center-Based Study Cohort. *Stroke, 44*(5), 1369–1374.

Kosova, E. C., Auinger, P., & Bremer, A. A. (2013). The relationships between sugar-sweetened beverage intake and cardiometabolic markers in young children. *Journal of the Academy of Nutrition and Dietetics, 113*(2), 219–227.

Lieberman, K. (2008). Interpreting 12-lead ECGs: A piece by piece analysis. *The Nurse Practitioner, 33*(10), 28–35.

Moorhead, S., Johnson, M., Maas, M., et al. (2012). *Nursing outcomes classification (NOC)* (5th ed.). St. Louis, MO: C. V. Mosby.

Morrison, L. J., Neumar, R. W., Zimmerman, J. L., et al. (2013). Strategies for improving survival after in-hospital cardiac arrest in the United States: 2013 Consensus recommendations: A consensus statement from the American Heart Association. *Circulation, 127*(14), 1538–1563.

Mizuno, J., & Monteiro, H. L. (2012). An assessment of a sequence of yoga exercises to patients with arterial hypertension. *Journal of Bodywork and Movement Therapies, 17*(1), 35–41.

Naib, B. A., & Salih, N. A. (2013). Accuracy of Color Duplex Imaging (CDI) in diagnosis deep vein thrombosis (DVT) versus Clinical Prediction Index. *International Journal of Science and Research (IJSR), 2*(6), 66–70.

NANDA International. (2012). *NANDA nursing diagnoses: Definitions and classifications 2012–2014.* Ames, IA: Wiley-Blackwell.

National Heart, Lung, and Blood Institute (NHLBI). (2011). Integrated guidelines for cardiovascular health and risk reduction in children and adolescents. Retrieved July 31, 2013, from http://www.nhlbi.nih.gov/guidelines/cvd_ped/

National Heart, Lung, and Blood Institute (NHLBI). (2002; updated 2012). Third report of the expert panel on detection, evaluation, and treatment of high blood cholesterol in adults (Adult Treatment Panel III). Retrieved July 31, 2013, from http://www.nhlbi.nih.gov/guidelines/cholesterol/

Overbaugh, K. (2009). Acute coronary syndrome. *American Journal of Nursing, 109*(5), 42–53.

Porth, C. M. (2010). *Pathophysiology: Concepts of altered states* (9th ed.). New York: Lippincott Williams & Wilkins.

Ray, K. K., Kastelein, J. J., Boekholdt, S. M., et al. (2014). The ACC/AHA 2013 guideline on the treatment of blood cholesterol to reduce atherosclerotic cardiovascular disease risk in adults: The good the bad and the uncertain: A comparison with ESC/EAS guidelines for the management of dyslipidaemias 2011. *European Heart Journal*, doi:10.1093/eurheartj/ehu107

Sayre, M., Berg, R., Cave, D., et al. (2008). Hands-only (compression-only) cardiopulmonary resuscitation: A call to action for bystander response to adults who experience out-of-hospital sudden cardiac arrest; A science advisory for the public from the American Heart Association Emergency Cardiovascular Care Committee. *Circulation, 117*, 2162–2167. Retrieved July 31, 2013, from http://circ.ahajournals.org/cgi/reprint/CIRCULATIONAHA.107.189380

Scanlon, V. C., & Sanders, T. (2011). *Essentials of anatomy and physiology* (6th ed.). Philadelphia: F. A. Davis.

Sinz, E., Navarro, K., & Soderberg, E. (2011). *Advanced cardiovascular life support: Provider manual.* Dallas: American Heart Association.

Stone, N., Robinson, J., Lichtenstein, A., et al. (2013). ACC/AHA Prevention Guideline: 2013 ACC/AHA Guideline on the Treatment of Blood Cholesterol to Reduce Atherosclerotic Cardiovascular Risk in Adults: A Report of the American College of Cardiology/American Heart Association Task Force on Practice Guidelines. *Circulation.* Advance online publication. Retrieved April 3, 2014, from http://circ.ahajournals.org/content/early/2013/11/11/01.cir.0000437738.63853.7a.citation

Sugiri, S. N., Hisatome, I., & Bahrudin, U. (2012). Carbohydrate diet links to higher risk of significant coronary artery disease in young Indonesian patients: Cardiometabolic Investigation study. *Biomedical Research, 23*(2), 159–165.

U.S. Preventive Services Task Force. (USPSTF). (2012). Screening for coronary heart disease with electrocardiography. *Medscape Education Clinical Briefs.* Retrieved July 31, 2013, from http://www.medscape.org/viewarticle/769006?src=cmemp

Van Beek, M. H., Mingels, M., Voshaar, R. C., et al. (2012). One-year follow up of cardiac anxiety after a myocardial infarction: A latent class analysis. *Journal of Psychosomatic Research, 73*(5), 362–368.

Woo, K., & Cowie, B. (2013). Understanding compression for venous leg ulcers. *Nursing2013, 43*(1), 66–68.

CHAPTER 38

American Association of Blood Banks (AABB). (n.d.). Blood FAQ. Retrieved September 12, 2013, from http://www.aabb.org/resources/bct/Pages/bloodfaq.aspx#a1

Agency for Healthcare Research (AHRQ). (2011). *Blood transfusion: Indications, administration and adverse reactions.* Rockville, MD: Author. Retrieved February 8, 2014, from http://www.guideline.gov/content.aspx?id=34955

American Medical Directors Association (AMDA). (2001; revised 2009). Guideline: Dehydration and fluid maintenance in the long-term care setting. Retrieved September 15, 2013, from http://www.guideline.gov/content.aspx?id=15590&search=dehydration+and+fluid+maintenance

Ayers P., & Warrington L. (2008). Diagnosis and treatment of simple acid–base disorders. *Nutrition in Clinical Practice, 23*(2), 122–127.

Barclay, L., & Nghiem, H. (2011). CDC updates IV catheter infection prevention guidelines. Medscape. Retrieved September 9, 2013, from, http://www.medscape.org/viewarticle/740412

Bulechek, G., Butcher, H., Dochterman, J., et al. (Eds.). (2013). *Nursing interventions classification (NIC)* (6th ed.). St. Louis, MO: C. V. Mosby.

Camp-Sorrell, D. (Ed.). (2010). *Access device guidelines: Recommendations for nursing practice and education* (3rd ed.). Pittsburgh, PA: Oncology Nursing Society.

Centers for Disease Control and Prevention (CDC). (2011a). 2011 guidelines for the prevention of intravascular catheter-related infections. Retrieved September 9, 2013, from, http://www.cdc.gov/hicpac/BSI/03-bsi-summary-of-recommendations-2011.html#rpmc

Centers for Disease Control and Prevention (CDC). (2011b). Replacement of administration sets. Retrieved September 9, 2013, from, http://www.cdc.gov/hicpac/bsi/07-bsi-background-info-2011.htmles-2011.html

Collins, M., & Claros, E. (2011). Recognizing the face of dehydration. *Nursing2011, 41*(8), 26–32.

Crawford, A., & Harris, H. (2011a). Balancing act: Hypomagnesemia & hypermagnesemia. *Nursing2011, 41*(10), 52–55.

Crawford, A., & Harris, H. (2011b). IV fluids. What nurses need to know. *Nursing2011, 41*(5), 30–39.

Crawford, A., & Harris, H. (2011c). Balancing act: Na+ Sodium K+ Potassium. *Nursing2011, 41*(7), 44–50.

Crawford, A., & Harris, H. (2012a). Balancing act: Calcium & phosphorus. *Nursing2012, 42*(1), 36–42

Crawford, A., & Harris, H. (2012b). SIADH: Fluid out of balance. *Nursing2012, 42*(9), 50–58.

Cummings, K., & McGowan, R. (2011). "Smart" pumps are selectively intelligent. *Nursing2011, 41*(3), 58–59.

David, K. (2007). IV fluids: do you know what's hanging and why? Retrieved September 19, 2013, from, http://www.modernmedicine.com/modern-medicine/news/iv-fluids-do-you-know-whats-hanging-and-why

Dumont, C., & Nesselrodt, D. (2012). Preventing CLABSI-central line-associated bloodstream infections. *Nursing2012, 42*(6), 41–46.

Fecher, I., & Knight, J. (2012). A framework for independent prescribing of intravenous fluids. *Emergency Nurse, 20*(7), 30–34.

Gahart, B., & Nazareno, A. (2013). *2013 intravenous medications: A handbook for nurses and health professionals* (29th ed.). St. Louis, MO: Elsevier-Mosby.

Galvey, J., Ibey, A., McConnell, G., et al. (2011). Infusion pumps for blood and blood products transfusions and administration. Retrieved September 14, 2013, from, http://resna.org/conference/proceedings/2011/CMBEC34/galvey-69501.pdf

Geiger, T., & Howard, S. (2007). Acetaminophen and diphenhydramine premedication for allergic and febrile nonhemolytic transfusion reactions: Good prophylaxis or bad practice? *Transfusion Medicine Review, 21*(1), 1–12. doi:10.1016/j.tmrv.2006.09.001. Retrieved February 11, 2014, from http://www.ncbi.nlm.nih.gov/pmc/articles/PMC1868404/

Hadaway, L. (2010). Don't disconnect IV administration sets [Weblog post]. *Lynn Hadaway Associates, Inc.* Retrieved October 10, 2013, from http://hadawayassociates.blogspot.com/2010/03/dont-disconnect-iv-administration-sets.html

Houck, D., & Whiteford, J. (2007). Transfusion with infusion pump for peripherally inserted central catheters and other vascular access devices. *Journal of Infusion, 30*(6), 341–344.

Infusion Nurses Society (INS). (2011a). Infusion nursing standards of practice. *Journal of Infusion Nursing, 34*(1), S57.

Institute for Healthcare Improvement (IHI). (2012). How-to guide: Prevent central line-associated bloodstream infection. Retrieved September 20, 2013, from http://www.ihi.org/knowledge/Pages/Tools/HowtoGuidePreventCentralLineAssociatedBloodstreamInfection.aspx

Institute of Medicine (IOM). (2004). *Dietary reference intakes for electrolytes and water.* Washington, DC: The National Academies Press.

Institute of Medicine of the National Academies. (2010; revised 2011). Dietary reference intakes for calcium and vitamin D. Retrieved February 4, 2014, from http://www.iom.edu/~/media/Files/Report%20Files/2010/Dietary-Reference-Intakes-for-Calcium-and-Vitamin-D/Vitamin%20D%20and%20Calcium%202010%20Report%20Brief.pdf

Jagger, J., Perry, J., Parker, G., et al. (2011). Blood exposure risk during peripheral I.V. catheter insertion and removal. *Nursing2011, 41*(12), 45–49.

The Joint Commission (TJC). (2011). Implementation guide for the patient blood management performance measures 2011. Retrieved September 20, 2013, from http://www.jointcommission.org/patient_blood_management_performance_measures_project/

The Joint Commission (TJC). (2012). Preventing central-line associated infection: A global challenge, a global perspective. Retrieved September 9, 2013, from http://www.jointcommission.org/assets/1/18/CLABSI_Monograph.pdf

The Joint Commission (TJC). (2013). 2013 Hospital national patient safety goals. Retrieved September 9, 2013, from http://www.jointcommission.org/assets/1/6/2013_HAP_NPSG_final_10-23.pdf

Kessler, C. (2013). Priming blood transfusion tubing: A critical review of the blood transfusion process. *Critical Care Nurse, 33*(3), 80–83.

Kraut, J., & Madias, N. (2011). Consequences and therapy of the metabolic acidosis of chronic kidney disease. *Pediatric Nephrology, 2*(1), 19–28.

Ladeserto, F., Chohan, H., Kasa, K., et al. (2009). Accuracy of daily weights and fluid balance in medical intensive care unit patients with the intervention of electronic medical records and electronic bedside weight measurements. *Chest Journal, 136*(4), 15S.

Lian, J (2013). Using ABG's to optimize Ventilation. *Nursing 2013, 43*(6), 46–53.

Masoorli, S. (2012). Avoiding the pitfalls of IV therapy. Retrieved September 11, 2013, from http://ce.nurse.com/RetailCourseView.aspx?CourseNum=ce94-60&page=3&IsA=1

Miller, C. (2012). *Nursing for wellness in older adults* (6th ed.). Philadelphia: Lippincott Williams & Wilkins.

Moorhead, S., Johnson, M., Maas, M., et al. (Eds.). (2013). *Nursing outcomes classification (NOC)* (5th ed.). St. Louis, MO: C. V. Mosby.

Moureau, N. (2008). Tips for inserting an I.V. device in an older adult. *Nursing2008, 38*(12), 12.

NANDA International. (2012). *Nursing diagnoses: Definitions and classifications 2012–2014.* Ames, IA: Wiley-Blackwell.

National Guideline Clearinghouse (NGC). (2010). Screening for osteoporosis in the adult U.S. population: ACPM position statement on preventive practice. Rockville, MD: Agency for Healthcare Research and Quality. Retrieved September 13, 2013, from http://www.guideline.gov/summary/summary.aspx?view_id=1&doc_id=15270

National Guideline Clearinghouse (NGC). (2011). Guidelines for the prevention of intravascular catheter-related infections, 2011. Retrieved September 20, 2013, from http://www.guideline.gov/content.aspx?id=34426

National Osteoporosis Foundation. (n.d.). Calcium and vitamin D: What you need to know. Retrieved September 13, 2013, from http://www.nof.org/articles/10

Niel-Neise, B., Stijnen, T., & van den Broek, P. (2010). Should in-line filters be used in peripheral intravenous catheters to prevent infusion-related phlebitis? A systematic review of randomized controlled trials. *Anesthesia & Analgesia, 110*(6), 1624–1629.

NIH MedlinePlus. (2011). New recommended daily amounts of calcium and vitamin D. Retrieved February 4, 2014, from http://www.nlm.nih.gov/medlineplus/magazine/issues/winter11/articles/winter11pg12.html

Nuttal, G., Abenstein, J., Stubbs, J., et al. (2013). Computerized bar code-based blood identification systems and near-miss transfusion episodes and transfusion errors. *Mayo Clinic Proceedings, 88*(4), 354–359.

Occupational Safety and Health Administration (OSHA). (2011). *Quick reference guide to the bloodborne pathogens standard.* Retrieved September 9, 2013, from https://www.osha.gov/SLTC/bloodbornepathogens/bloodborne_quickref.html

O'Grady, N., Alexander, M., Burns, L. et al. (2011). *Guidelines for the prevention of intravascular catheter-related infections, 2011.* Atlanta, GA: Centers for Disease Control and Prevention (CDC). Retrieved September 10, 2013, from http://www.cdc.gov/hicpac/pdf/guidelines/bsi-guidelines-2011.pdf

Phillips, L. (2010). *Manual of IV therapeutics* (5th ed.). Philadelphia: F. A. Davis.

Pronovost, P., Goeschel, C., Colantuoni, E., et al. (2010). Sustaining reductions in catheter related bloodstream infections in Michigan intensive care units: Observational study. *BMJ, 340*, c309. Retrieved September 20, 2013, from http://www.bmj.com/cgi/content/full/340/feb04_1/c309

Pruitt, B. (2010). Interpreting ABGs: An inside look at your patient's status. *Nursing2010, 40*(7), 31–36.

Rhoads, J., & Meeker, B. (2008). *Davis's guide to clinical nursing skills*. Philadelphia: F. A. Davis.

Scales, K., & Pilsworth, J. (2008). The importance of fluid balance in clinical practice. *Nursing Standard, 22*(47), 50–57.

Shepherd, A. (2011). Measuring and managing fluid balance. *NursingTimes.Net*. Retrieved September 8, 2013, from http://www.nursingtimes.net/nursing-practice/clinical-zones/nutrition/measuring-and-managing-fluid-balance/5032614.article

Shlamovitz, G. (updated 2013, May 22). Intravenous cannulation. *Medscape*. Retrieved September 14, 2013, from http://emedicine.medscape.com/article/1998177-overview

Timsit, J-F, Schwebel, C., Boudma, L., et al. (2009). Chlorhexidine-impregnated sponges and less frequent dressing changes for prevention of catheter-related infections in critically ill adults: A randomized controlled trial. *JAMA, 301*(12), 1231–1241, 1285–1287.

Tolich, D., Blackmur, S., Stahorsky, K., et al. (2013). Blood management: Best-practice transfusion strategies. *Nursing 2013, 43*(1), 40–48.

U.S. Department of Agriculture (USDA). (2011). Center for Nutrition Policy and Promotion. 2010 Dietary guidelines for Americans. Retrieved September 20, 2013, from http://www.cnpp.usda.gov/DGAs2010-PolicyDocument.htm

U.S. Department of Agriculture (USDA). (n.d.). Dietary Reference Intakes (DRIs): Recommended dietary allowances and adequate intake, elements. Retrieved September 13, 2013, from http://www.iom.edu/Activities/Nutrition/SummaryDRIs/~/media/Files/Activity%20Files/Nutrition/DRIs/5_Summary%20Table%20Tables%201-4.pdf

U.S. Department of Agriculture (USDA). (2011). Center for Nutrition Policy and Promotion. 2010 Dietary guidelines for Americans. Retrieved September 13, 2013, from http://www.cnpp.usda.gov/DGAs2010-PolicyDocument.htm

Van Leeuwen, A., Poelhuis-Leth, D., & Bladh, M. (2011). *Davis's comprehensive handbook of laboratory and diagnostic tests with nursing implications* (4th ed.). Philadelphia: F. A. Davis

Wilson, K. M. (2014). Choosing the right line for the right time. *Nursing2014, 43*(12), 66–68.

Wunderlich, R. (2013). Principles in the selection of intravenous solutions replacement: Sodium and water balance. *Journal of Infusion Nursing, 36*(2), 126–130.

CHAPTER 39

Agency for Healthcare Research and Quality (AHRQ). (2003, December). *AHRQ's patient safety initiative: Building foundations, reducing risk. Interim report to the Senate Committee on Appropriations* (AHRQ Publication No. 04-RG005). Rockville, MD: Author. Retrieved August 8, 2012, from http://www.ahrq.gov/qual/pscongrpt/

Agency for Healthcare Research and Quality (AHRQ). (2008). New AHRQ study finds surgical errors cost nearly $1.5 billion annually [Press release]. Retrieved August 8, 2012, from http://www.ahrq.gov/news/press/pr2008/surgerrpr.htm

Allied Healthcare Products, Inc. (n.d.). Product information and technical specification. Retrieved August 17, 2012, from http://www.alliedhpi.com/suction.htm

American Association of Critical-Care Nurses (AACN). (2010). AACN practice alert. Venous thrombosis prevention. Retrieved August 8, 2012, from http://www.aacn.org/WD/Practice/Docs/PracticeAlerts/VTE%20Prevention%2004-2010%20final.pdf

Association of periOperative Registered Nurses (AORN). (2009; updated 2011). *Perioperative standards and recommended practices*. Denver, CO: Author.

Bashaw, M., & Scott, D. (2012). Surgical risk factors in geriatric perioperative patients. *Association of periOperative Registered Nurses Journal, 96*(1), 59–71, doi:10.1016/j.aorn.2011.05.025.

Best practices: Evidence-based nursing procedures (2nd ed.). (2007). Philadelphia: Lippincott.

Boyce, J., & Pittet, D. (2002). Guideline for hand hygiene in health-care settings. Recommendations of the Healthcare Infection Control Practices Advisory Committee and the HICPAC/SHEA/APIC/IDSA Hand Hygiene Task Force. *Morbidity and Mortality Weekly Report, 51*(RR16), 1–44. Retrieved July 21, 2012, from http://www.cdc.gov/mmwr/preview/mmwrhtml/rr5116a1.htm

Brooks, P. (2012). Postoperative delirium in elderly patients. *American Journal of Nursing, 112*(9), 38–50.

Bulechek, G. M., Butcher, H. K., & Dochterman, J. M., et al. (Eds.). (2013). *Nursing interventions classification (NIC)* (6th ed.). St. Louis, MO: C. V. Mosby.

Buppert, C. (2012). How do I assess competence to give informed consent? *Medscape Nurses—Legal and Professional Issues for Nurses*. Retrieved August 18, 2012, from http://www.medscape.com/viewarticle/764904?src=rss

Centers for Disease Control and Prevention (CDC). (n.d.). (updated 2011). Having surgery? What you should know before you go. Retrieved July 11, 2012, from http://www.cdc.gov/features/SafeSurgery/

Centers for Diseases Control and Prevention (CDC). (2001). *Handwashing: Clean hands save lives*. Retrieved July 15, 2012, from http://www.cdc.gov/handwashing

Centers for Medicare & Medicaid Services. (2006, Updated 2011). Eliminating serious, preventable, and costly medical errors—never events [Press release]. Department of Health & Human Services. Retrieved August 7, 2012, from http://www.cms.gov/apps/media/press/release.asp?Counter=1863

Centers for Medicare & Medicaid Services. (2008, July 31). Medicare and Medicaid move aggressively to encourage greater patient safety in hospitals and reduce never events [Press release]. CMS Office of Public Affairs. Retrieved July 20, 2012, from http://www.cms.gov/apps/media/press/release.asp?Counter=3219&intNumPerPage=10&checkDate=&checkKey=2&srchType=2&numDays=0&srchOpt=0&srchData=never+events&keywordType=All&chkNewsType=1%2C+2%2C+3%2C+4%2C+5&intPage=&showAll=1&pYear=&year=0&desc=&cboOrder=date

Chow, W., Ko, C., Rosenthal, R., et al. (n.d.). ACS NSQIP®/AGS best practice guidelines: Optimal preoperative assessment of the geriatric surgical patient. Retrieved December 10, 2012, from http://site.acsnsqip.org/wp-content/uploads/2011/12/ACS-NSQIP-AGS-Geriatric-2012-Guidelines.pdf

Cohen, A., Tapson, V., Bergman, J-F., et al. (2008). Venous thromboembolism risk and prophylaxis in the acute hospital care setting (ENDORSE study): A multinational cross-sectional study. *The Lancet, 371*(9610), 387–394.

Crenshaw, J. T. (2011). Preoperative fasting: Will the evidence ever be put into practice? *American Journal of Nursing, 111*(10), 38–45.

Cronenwett, L., Sherwood, G., Pohl, J., et al. (2009). Quality and safety education for advanced nursing practice. *Nursing Outlook, 57*(6), 338–348.

Crowe, L., Chang, A., Fraser, J., et al. (2008). Systematic review of the effectiveness of nursing interventions in reducing or relieving post-operative pain. *International Journal of Evidence-Based Healthcare, 6*(4), 396–430.

Cullen, K., Hall, M., & Golosinskiy, A. (2009). *Ambulatory surgery in the United States, 2006* (National Health Statistics Report Number 11). Hyattsville, MD: National Center for Health Statistics. Retrieved July 20, 2012, from http://www.cdc.gov/nchs/data/nhsr/nhsr011.pdf

Cutshall, S.M., Wentworth, L., Engel, D., et al. (2010). Effect of massage therapy on pain, anxiety, and tension in cardiac surgical patients: A pilot study. *Complementary Therapies in Clinical Practice, 16*, 92–95.

Dale, A., Rothrock, J., & McEwen, D. (Eds.). (2011). *Alexander's care of the patient in surgery* (14th ed.). St. Louis, MO: C. V. Mosby.

Egol, K., & Strauss, E. (2009). Perioperative considerations in geriatric patients with hip fracture: What is the evidence? *Journal of Orthopedic Trauma, 23*, 386–394.

Green, S., Harris, C., & Singer, J. (2008). Gastrointestinal decontamination of the poisoned patient. *Pediatric Emergency Care, 24*, 176–178.

Haynes, A., Weiser, T., Berry, W., et al. (2009). A surgical safety checklist to reduce morbidity and mortality in a global population. *New England Journal of Medicine, 360*(5), 491–499.

Hendrickson, S., Wadhera, R., & ElBardissi, A. (2008). Development and pilot evaluation of a preoperative briefing protocol for cardiovascular surgery. *Journal of the American College of Surgeons, 208*(6), 1115–1123.

Hooper, V., Chard, R., Clifford, T., et al. (2010). ASPAN's evidence-based clinical practice guideline for the promotion of perioperative normothermia: Second edition. *Journal of PeriAnesthesia Nursing, 25*(6), 346–365. Retrieved July 11, 2012, from http://www.aspan.org/Portals/6/docs/ClinicalPractice/Guidelines/Normothermia_Guideline_12-10_JoPAN.pdf

Institute for Healthcare Improvement. (n.d.). Overview of the 100,000 Lives Campaign. Retrieved July 17, 2012, from http://www.ihi.org/offerings/Initiatives/PastStrategicInitiatives/5MillionLivesCampaign/Documents/Overview%20of%20the%20100K%20Campaign.pdf

Institute for Healthcare Improvement. (2011). Protecting 5 million lives. Retrieved August 17, 2012, from http://www.ihi.org/offerings/Initiatives/PastStrategicInitiatives/5MillionLivesCampaign/Pages/default.aspx

The Joanna Briggs Institute. (2007). Pre-operative hair removal to reduce surgical site infection. *Best Practice, 11*(4).

The Joanna Briggs Institute. (2008a). Preoperative fasting for preventing perioperative complications in children. *Best Practice, 12*(1), 29–32.

The Joanna Briggs Institute. (2008b). Graduated compression stockings for the prevention of post-operative venous thromboembolism. *Best Practice, 12*(4).

The Joanna Briggs Institute. (2010). Strategies for the management and prevention of hypothermia within the adult perioperative environment. *Best Practice, 14*(13).

Johnston, J., & Davis, M. (2008). When sequential-compression devices cause falls. *American Journal of Nursing, 108*(4), 37–38.

The Joint Commission (TJC). (2010). Advancing effective communication, cultural competence, and patient- and family-centered care. Retrieved August 17, 2012, from http://www.jointcommission.org/assets/1/6/ARoadmapforHospitalsfinalversion727.pdf

The Joint Commission (TJC). (2012). *National patient safety goals for 2012.* Retrieved August 17, 2012, from http://www.jointcommission.org/assets/1/6/NPSG_Chapter_Jan2012_HAP.pdf

Kaye, K., Sloane, R., Sexton, D., et al. (2006). Risk factors for surgical site infections in older people. *Journal of The American Geriatrics Society, 54*(3), 391–396. doi:http://dx.doi.org/10.1111

Larry, C. (Ed.). (2003). Applying anti-embolism stockings. Retrieved July 22, 2012, from http://www.newlook.com.sg/tutorial.asp

Makary, M., Mukherjee, A., Sexton, J., et al. (2007). Operating room briefings and wrong-site surgery. *Journal of the American College of Surgeons, 204*(2), 236–243.

Mangram, A., Horan, T., Pearson, M., et al. (1999). The Hospital Infection Control Practices Advisory Committee. Guideline for prevention of surgical site infection, 1999. *Infection Control and Hospital Epidemiology, 20*(4), 247–278. Retrieved August 17, 2012, from http://www.cdc.gov/hicpac/pdf/guidelines/SSI_1999.pdf

Markel, D., & Morris, G. (2002). Effect of external sequential compression devices on femoral venous blood flow. *Journal of the Southern Orthopaedic Association, 11*(1), 2–9.

Moorhead, S., Johnson, M., Maas, M., et al. (Eds.). (2013). *Nursing outcomes classification (NOC)* (5th ed.). St. Louis, MO: C. V. Mosby.

NANDA International. (2012). *Nursing diagnoses: Definitions and classification 2012–2014.* Philadelphia: Author.

National Guideline Clearinghouse (NGC). (2008a). *Guideline summary: Strategies to prevent surgical site infections in acute care hospitals.* Rockville, MD: Agency for Healthcare Research and Quality. Retrieved July 12, 2012, from http://www.guideline.gov/content.aspx?id=13399

National Guideline Clearinghouse (NCG). (2008b). *Nursing management for prevention of deep vein thrombosis (DVT)/venous thrombo-embolism (VTE) in hospitalized patients.* Rockville, MD: Agency for Healthcare Research and Quality Author. Retrieved July 25, 2012, from http://www.guideline.gov/content.aspx?id=15539&search=venous+thrombosis.

National Guideline Clearinghouse (NCG). (2011). *ACR Appropriateness Criteria routine admission and preoperative chest radiography.* Rockville, MD: Agency for Healthcare Research and Quality. Retrieved August 16, 2012, from http://www.guideline.gov/content.aspx?id=35150&search=chest+x+ray

National Institute for Health and Clinical Excellence (NICE). (2007). *Venous thrombolism. Reducing the risk in surgical inpatients. Methods, evidence & guidance.* London: National Collaborating Centre for Acute Care.

National Institute for Health and Clinical Excellence (NICE). (2008; updated 2011). *Surgical site infection: Prevention and treatment of surgical site infection* (NICE Clinical Guideline No. 74). Retrieved July 12, 2012, from http://www.nice.org.uk/CG74

National Priorities Partnership. (2011). Priorities for the national quality strategy. Washington, DC: National Quality Forum. Retrieved July 19, 2012, from http://www.qualityforum.org/Setting_Priorities/NPP/National_Priorities_Partnership.aspx

Nelson, E. A., Mani, R., Thomas, K., & Vowden, K. (2011). Intermittent pneumatic compression for treating venous leg ulcers. *Cochrane Database of Systematic Reviews*, Issue 2. Art.

No.: CD001899. Retrieved July 23, 2012, from http://www.ncbi.nlm.nih.gov/pubmed/21328252.

Peterson, C., & Kleiner, C. (2011). Evolution and revision of the perioperative nursing data set. *Journal of the Association of periOperative Registered Nurses*, 93(1), 127–132.

Practice guidelines for preoperative fasting and the use of pharmacologic agents to reduce the risk of pulmonary aspiration: Application to healthy patients undergoing elective procedures; An updated report by the American Society of Anesthesiologists Committee on Standards and Practice Parameters. (2011). *Anesthesiology, 114*(3), 495–511.

Quality and Safety Education for Nurses (QSEN). (2012). Quality and safety competencies. Retrieved August 3, 2012, from http://www.qsen.org/competencies.php.

Reid, J. H. (2011). Surgical never events should never happen. *Journal of Perioperative Practice, 21*(11), 373–378.

Sarasota Memorial Hospital. (Reviewed 2011). Nursing procedure: Gastric suction—GOMCO. *SMH Nursing Procedures*. Retrieved August 17, 2012, from http://home.smh.com/sections/services-procedures/medlib/nursing/NursPandP/suc04_gastric_042811.pdf

Siegel, J., Rhinehart, E., Jackson, M., et al.; the Healthcare Infection Control Practices Advisory Committee. (2007). *2007 Guideline for isolation precautions: Preventing transmission of infectious agents in healthcare settings*. Retrieved August 6, 2012, from http://www.cdc.gov/hicpac/pdf/isolation/Isolation2007.pdf

Venous thromboembolism in adult hospitalizations—United States, 2007–2009. (2012, June 8). *Mortality and Morbidity Weekly Report, 61*(22),401–404. Retrieved August 17, 2012, from http://www.cdc.gov/mmwr/preview/mmwrhtml/mm6122a1.htm?s_cid=mm6122a1_w

White, J., Khan, W., & Smitham, P. (2011). Perioperative implications of surgery in elderly patients with hip fractures: An evidence-based review. *Journal of Perioperative Practice, 21*(6), 192–197.

Winslow, E., & Brosz, D. (2008). Graduated compression stockings in hospitalized postoperative patients: Correctness of usage and size. *American Journal of Nursing, 108*(9), 40–51.

World Health Organization (WHO). (2009). Surgical safety checklist. Retrieved July 21, 2012, from http://whqlibdoc.who.int/publications/2009/9789241598590_eng_Checklist.pdf

CHAPTER 40

American Nurses Association (ANA). (2002). *Position statements: Registered nurse utilization of unlicensed assistive personnel*. Washington, DC: Author.

American Nurses Association (ANA). (2007). *Position statements: Registered nurses' utilization of nursing assistive personnel in all settings*. Washington, DC: Author.

American Nurses Association (ANA). (2010). *Nursing Professional Development: Scope and standards of practice*. Silver Spring, MD: Nursebooks.org

American Nurses Association (ANA). (2011). *Registered nurses in the U.S., nursing by the numbers*. Retrieved July 24, 2013, from http://www.nursingworld.org/NursingbytheNumbersFactSheet.aspx

American Nurses Association and National Council of State Boards of Nursing. (n.d.). *Joint statement on delegation*. Retrieved August 25, 2013, from https://www.ncsbn.org/Delegation_joint_statement_NCSBN-ANA.pdf

American Nurses Credentialing Center (ANCC). (2013). Program overview. Retrieved August 5, 2013, from http: www.nursecredentialing.org/Magnet/ProgramOverview.

Bacon, T. (2011). *The Elements of Power*. New York: AMACOM.

Barker, A. M. (1992). *Transformational nursing leadership: A vision for the future*. New York: National League for Nursing.

Bass, B. M., & Avolio, B. J. (1993). Transformational leadership: A response to critique. In M. M. Chemers & R. Ayman (Eds.), *Leadership theory and research: Perspectives and directions*. San Diego, CA: Academic Press.

Battilana, J., & Casciaro, T. (2013).The network secrets of great change agents. *Harvard Business Review, 19*(7), 62–68.

Birk, S. (2010). The 10 most common myths about leadership. *Healthcare Executive, 25*(6), 30–32, 34–36, 38.

Blake, R. R., Mouton, J. S., & Tapper, M. (1981). *Grid approaches for managerial leadership in nursing*. St. Louis, MO: C. V. Mosby.

Browne, M., & Kelley, S. (2010). *Asking the right questions: A guide to critical thinking* (9th ed.). Upper Saddle River, NJ: Prentice-Hall.

Cannon, S. (2013). Building on Maslow to meet director and staff needs. *Exchange, 211*, 8–11.

Carroll, L. (2010). *Alice in wonderland*. (Original work published 1865.) Retrieved from http://www.amazon.com/Alice-in-Wonderland ebook/dp/B003A83VUK/ref=sr_1_3?s=books&ie=UTF8&qid=1375985292&sr=1-3&keywords=alice+in+wonderland

The Center for Health Design. (2009). Pebble Project® Data Summary. Retrieved July 23, 2013, from http://www.healthdesign.org/pebble

Cipriano, P. (2010). Overview and summary: Delegation dilemmas; Standards and skills for practice. *Online Journal of Issues in Nursing, 15*, (2). Overview. Retrieved August 25, 2013, from http://www.nursingworld.org/MainMenuCategories/ANAMarketplace/ANAPeriodicals/OJIN/TableofContents/Vol152010/No2May2010/Overview-and-Summary-Delegation-.html

Dean, J. (2013). *Making habits, breaking habits*. Philadelphia: DeCapo Press.

Doody, O., & Doody, C. (2012). Transformational leadership in nursing practice. *British Journal of Nursing, 21*(20), 1212–1218.

Doolin, C., Quinn, L., Bryant, L., et al. (2011). Family presence during cardiopulmonary resuscitation using evidence-based knowledge to guide the advanced practice nurse in developing formal policy and practice guidelines. *Journal of the American Academy of Nurse Practitioners, 23*, 8–14.

Douglas, K. (2009). The naked truth: Staffing in health care needs an overhaul. *Nursing Economics, 27*(5), 332–334.

Duffield, C., Roche, M., Blay, N., et al. (2010). Nursing unit managers, staff retention and the work environment. *Journal of Clinical Nursing, 20*, 23–33.

Farrell, K., & Broude, C. (1987). *Winning the change game: How to implement information systems with fewer headaches and bigger paybacks*. Los Angeles: Breakthrough Enterprises.

Feather, R. (2009). Emotional intelligence in relation to nursing leadership: Does it matter? *Journal of Nursing Management, 17*, 376–382.

Fitton, R. A. (1997). *Leadership: Quotations from the world's greatest motivators*. Boulder, CO: Westview Press.

Flackman, B., Hansebo, G., & Kihlgren, A. (2009). Struggling to adapt: Caring for older persons while under the threat of organizational change and termination notice. *Nursing Inquiry, 16*(1), 82–91.

Fralic, M. F. (2000). What is leadership? *Journal of Nursing Administration, 30*(7/8), 340–341.

Furtado, L., Batista, C., & Silva, F. (2011). Leadership and job satisfaction among Azorean hospital nurses: an application of the situational leadership model. *Journal of Nursing Management, 19,* 1047–1057.

Gardiner. (2012). Lake Health TriPoint Medical Center teamwork and sustainable design helps define model of care and improve patient outcomes (2012). *Gardiner Solutions.* Retrieved August 6, 2013, from http://www.whgardiner.com/media/documents/website-tripoint-case-study.pdf

Ghannadian, F. (2013). What employers want, what we teach. *BizEd.* Retrieved September 4, 2013, from http://www.bizedmagazine.com/features/articles/what-employers-want-what-we-teach.asp

Gonzalez, M. (2012). *The mindful leadership: The 9 ways to self awareness.* Mississauga, Ontario: Jossey-Bass.

Graham, I. W. (2010). The search for the discipline of nursing. *Journal of Nursing Management, 18,* 355–362.

Grossman, S., & Valiga, T. (2012). *The new leadership challenge: Creating the future of nursing* (4th ed.). Philadelphia: F. A. Davis.

Hagemann, B., & Stroope, S. (2012). Conflict management lessons from the second grade. *Training & Development, 66*(7), 58–61.

Hamman, W., Beaudin-Seiler, B., & Beaubien, J. (2010). Understanding interdisciplinary health care teams: Using simulation design processes from the Air Carrier Advanced Qualification Program to identify and train critical teamwork skills. *Journal of Patient Safety, 6*(3), 137–146.

Haslam, S., Reicher, S., & Platow, M. (2011). *The new psychology of leadership: Identity, influence, & power.* New York: Psychology Press.

Havig, A., Skogstad, A., Kjekshus, L., et al. (2011). Leadership, staffing and quality of care in nursing homes. *BMC Health Services Research, 11,* 327. Retrieved August 6, 2013, from http://www.biomedcentral.com/1472-6963/11/327

Hendrich, A., Chow, M., Sklerczynski, B., et al. (2008). A 36–hospital time and motion study. How do medical-surgical nurses spend their time? *Permanence Journal, 12,* 25–34.

The Joint Commission. (2011). Sentinel event data—root causes by event type (2004–second quarter 2011). Retrieved July 23, 2013, from http://www.jointcommission.org/Sentinel_Event_Statistics/

Jones, R. D., & Rudd, R. D. (2007). Transactional, transformational, or laissez-faire: An assessment of college of agriculture academic program leaders (deans) leadership styles. *Proceedings of the 2007 AAAE Research Conference, 34,* 520–530.

Kean, S., Haycock-Stuart, E., Baggaley, S., et al. (2011). Followers and the co-construction of leadership. *Journal of Nursing Management, 19*(4), 507–516.

Kelly, P. (2012). *Nursing leadership and management* (3rd ed.). Clifton Park, NY: Delmar Cengage Learning.

Kotter, J. P. (1999). Leading change: The eight steps to transformation. In J. A. Conger, G. M. Spreitzer, & E. E. Lawler (Eds.), *The leader's change handbook.* San Francisco: Jossey-Bass.

Lansdale, B. M. (2002). *Cultivating inspired leaders: Making participatory management work.* West Hartford, CT: Kumarian Press.

Lapp, J. (2002, May). Thriving on change. *CARING Magazine,* 40–43.

Leach, L. S. (2005). Nurse executive transformational leadership and organizational commitment. *Journal of Nursing Administration, 35*(5), 228–237.

Lewin, K. (1951). *Field theory in social science: Selected theoretical papers.* New York: Harper & Row.

Lindy, C., & Schaefer, F. (2010). Negative workplace behaviours: An ethical dilemma for nurse managers. *Journal of Nursing Management, 18*(3), 285–292.

Lykins, L. (2011). Companies need emotionally intelligent leaders. *Journal of Corporate Recruiting Leader*ship, *6*(3), 6–8.

Magrane, D., Khan, O., Pigeon, Y., et al. (2010). Learning about teams by participating in teams. *Academic Medicine, 85*(8), 1303–1311.

Manser, T. (2009). Teamwork and patient safety in dynamic domains of healthcare: A review of the literature. *Acta Anaesthesiologica Scandinavia, 53*(2), 143–151.

Marquis, B., & Huston, C. (2012). *Leadership roles and management functions in nursing* (7th ed.). Philadelphia: Lippincott Williams & Wilkins.

Maslow, A. H. (1970). *Motivation and personality.* New York: Harper & Row.

McGregor, D. (1960). *The human side of enterprise.* New York: McGraw-Hill.

Mintzberg, H. (1989). *Mintzberg on management: Inside our strange world of organizations.* New York: Free Press.

Nash, J., & Taylor, E. (2011). Has it really been two years? A Pebble Project reflects on success. *Healthcare Design.* Retrieved August 6, 2013, from http://www.healthcaredesignmagazine.com/article/has-it-really-been-two-years-pebble-project-reflects-success

National Council of State Boards of Nursing (NCSBN). (2009). Joint statement on delegation. American Nurses Association and National Council State Boards of Nursing. Retrieved July 23, 2013, from https://www.ncsbn.org/1625.htm

Neumann, T. (2010). Delegation—better safe than sorry. *American Association of Occupational Health Nurses, 58*(8), 321–322.

Northouse, P. (2012). *Introduction to leadership: Concepts and practices.* Thousand Oaks, CA: Sage.

Northouse, P. (2013). *Leadership theory and practice.* Thousand Oaks, CA: Sage.

O'Brien, M. E. (2011). *Servant leadership in nursing.* Subdury, MA: Jones & Bartlett.

O'Leary, D. (2010). The impact of manager philosophy on knowledge management systems. *Intelligent Systems in Accounting, Finance and Management, 17*(2), 111–126.

Orr, B. (2013). Conducting a SWOT Analysis for program improvement. *US-China Education Review, 3*(6), 381–384.

Pavitt, C. (1999). Theorizing about the group communication-leadership relationship. In L. R. Frey (Ed.), *The handbook of group communication theory and research.* Thousand Oaks, CA: Sage.

Pethtel, O., & Chen, Y. (2013). Age differences in choice deferrals as functions of interattribute conflict and decision domain. *Educational Gerontology, 39*(10), 772–782.

Plawecki, L., & Amrheim, D. (2010). A question of delegation. *Journal of Gerontological Nursing, 36*(8), 18–21.

Poghosyan, L., Lucero, R., Rauch, L., et al. (2012). Nurse practitioner workforce: A substantial supply of primary care workers. *Nursing Economics, 30*(5), 268–274, 294.

Porter-O'Grady, T. (2011). *Quantum leadership information, advancing innovation, transforming healthcare.* Sudbury, MA: Jones & Bartlett.

Ricketts, K. G. (2010). Followership understanding the basics of teamwork. Retrieved July 23, 2013, from http://www2.ca.uky.edu/agc/pubs/cld1/cld15/cld15.PDF

Ripper, B. (2013, August 9). The big bad boss: Poor management costly. *The Business Times*. Retrieved August 11, 2013, from http://thebusinesstimes.com/the-big-bad-boss-poor-management-costly/

Robert Wood Johnson Foundation. (2009). Charting nursing's future archives. Part 1, Issue of charting nursing's future addresses the quality and safety gap. Case studies in transforming hospital nursing and building cultures of safety. Retrieved July 22, 2013, from http://www.rwjf.org/humancapital/product.jsp?id=45629

Robert Wood Johnson Foundation (2013). Progress on the nation's nursing workforce. Retrieved July 24, 2013, from http://www.rwjf.org/en/about-rwjf/newsroom/newsroom-content/2013/05/progress-on-the-nations-nursing-workforce.html

Ryder, J. (2013). Leadership begins at the end of your comfort zone. *Leadership, 42*(4), 20–38.

Sabir, M., Sohail, A., & Khan, A. (2011). Impact of leadership style on organization commitment: In a mediating role of employee values. *Journal of Economics and Behavioral Studies, 3*(2), 145–152.

Sadri, G. (2012). Emotional intelligence and leadership development. *Public Personnel Management, 41*(3), 535–548.

Salanova, M., Lorente, L, Chambel, M., et al. (2011). Linking transformational leadership to nurses' extra-role performance: The mediating role of self-efficacy and work engagement. *Journal of Advanced Nursing, 67*(10), 2256–2266.

Shingleton, J. (1994). The job market for '94 grads. In College Placement Council (Ed.), *Planning job choices* (pp. 19–26). Philadelphia: Author.

Sportsman, S., Wieck, L., Yoder-Wise, P., et al. (2010). Creating tomorrow's leaders today: The emerging nurse leaders program of the Texas Nurses Association. *The Journal of Continuing Education, 41*(6), 259–266.

Sprangel, J., Stravos, J., & Cole, M. (2011). Creating sustainable relationships using the strengths, opportunities, aspirations and results framework, trust, and environmentalism: A research-based case study. *International Journal of Training and Development, 15*(1), 39–57.

Stanley, D., & Sherratt, A. (2010). Lamp light on leadership: Clinical leadership and Florence Nightingale. *Journal of Nursing Management, 18*(2), 115–121.

Stavros, J., Cooperrider, D., & Kelley, L. (2007). SOAR: A new approach to strategic planning. *Fast Fundamentals*. The BK Whitepaper Series. Retrieved July 22, 2013, from http://www.scribd.com/doc/17330716/SOAR-A-New-Approach-to-Strategic-Planning-by-Jackie-Stavros-David-Cooperrider-and-D-Lynn-Kelley. Excerpted from *The change handbook* (2nd ed.). San Francisco: Berrett-Koehler.

Taylor, F. W. (2011). *The principles of scientific management*. Seattle, WA: Create Space Independent Publishing Platform. (Original work published 1911.)

U.S. Department of Health and Human Services (USDHHS), Health Resources and Service Administration, Bureau of Health Professions Division of Nursing. (2013). The U.S. nursing workforce: Trends in supply & education. Retrieved July 23, 2013, from http://bhpr.hrsa.gov/healthworkforce/reports/nursingworkforce/nursingworkforcefullreport.pdf

Villarreal, J. (2002). What employers want: The measure of importance of various skills for registered nurses (Paper No. 60). *Applied Research Projects*. Retrieved July 24, 2013, from https://digital.library.txstate.edu/handle/10877/3792

Watkins, N., Zook, J., Gray, W., et al. (2013). Accountable design for accountable care. Retrieved from http://mcgraw-hillresearchfoundation.org/2013/03/04/accountable-design-for-accountable-care-2/

Weydt, A. (2010). Developing delegation skills. *The Online Journal of Issues in Nursing, 15*(2), Manuscript 1. Retrieved August 25, 2013, from http://www.nursingworld.org/MainMenuCategories/ANAMarketplace/ANAPeriodicals/OJIN/TableofContents/Vol152010/No2May2010/Delegation-Skills.html

White, R., & Lippitt, R. (1960). *Autocracy and democracy: An experimental inquiry*. New York: Harper & Row.

Whitehead, D., Weiss, S., & Tappen, R. (2009). *Essentials of nursing leadership and management* (5th ed.). Philadelphia: F. A. Davis.

Zineldin, M., & Hytter, A. (2012). Leaders' negative emotions and leadership styles influencing subordinates' well-being. *The International Journal of Human Resource Management, 23*(4), 748–758. Retrieved August 6, 2013, from http://dx.doi.org/10.1080/09585192.2011.606114.

CHAPTER 41

Alliance for Nursing Informatics. (2009). The TIGER Initiative. Collaborating to integrate evidence and informatics in nursing practice and education: An executive summary. Retrieved June 22, 2013, from http://tigersummit.com/uploads/TIGER_Collaborative_Exec_Summary_040509.pdf

American Nurses Association (ANA). (2008). *Scope and standards of nursing informatics practice* (ANA Publication No. NIP21). Washington, DC: American Nurses Publishing/American Nurses Foundation.

American Nurses Association (ANA). (2010). *Nursing: Scope and standards of practice* (2nd ed.). Silver Spring, MD: Author. Retrieved March 30, 2013, from https://www.ania.org/

Association of College & Research Libraries. (n.d.). Information literacy competency standards for higher education. Retrieved July 1, 2013, from http://www.ala.org/acrl/standards/informationliteracycompetency

Bell, M. M. (2009, May). Bar code point of care systems: Benefits and pitfalls. *Pennsylvania Nurse*, 9–10.

Cannon-Diehl, M. R. (2009). Simulation in healthcare and nursing. *Critical Care Nursing Quarterly, 32*(2), 128–136. doi: 10.1097/CNQ.0b013e3181a27e0f

Duffy, M. (2012). Tablet technology for nurses. *American Journal of Nursing, 112*(9), 59–64.

DuLong, D. (2009). *The TIGER Initiative: Collaborating to integrate evidence and informatics into nursing practice and education: An executive summary* (pp. 1–30). Retrieved June 30, 2013, from http://www.tigersummit.com/uploads/TIGER_Collaborative_Exec_Summary_040509.pdf

Englebardt, S., & Nelson, R. (2002). Major theories supporting health care informatics. In S. Englebardt & R. Nelson, *Health care informatics: An interdisciplinary approach* (p. 13). St. Louis, MO: Elsevier.

Enrado, P. (2009, May 1). Tele-nurses help with 911 calls as cities cope with tight budgets. Retrieved November 2, 2014, from http://www.healthcareitnews.com/news/tele-nurses-help-911-calls-cities-cope-tight-budgets

Ford, E. W., Menachemi, N., Peterson, L. T., et al. (2009). Resistance is futile: But it is slowing the pace of EHR adoption nonetheless. *Journal of the American Medical Informatics Association, 16*(3), 274–281. doi:10.1197/jamia.M3042

Fowler, S. B., Sohler, P., & Zarillo, D. F. (2009). Bar-code technology for dedication administration: Medication errors and nurse satisfaction. *MedSurg Nursing, 18*(2), 103–109.

Gee, P. M., Greenwood, D. A., Kim, K. K., et al. (2012). Exploration of the e-patient phenomenon in nursing informatics. *Nursing Outlook, 60*(4), e9–e16. doi: 10.1016/j.outlook.2011.11.005

Graves, J., & Corcoran, S. (1989). The study of nursing informatics. *Image: The Journal of Nursing Scholarship, 21*(4), 227–230.

Hebert, C., Beaumont, J., Schwartz, G., et al. (2012, August 7). The influence of context on antimicrobial prescribing for febrile respiratory illness: A cohort study. *Annals of Internal Medicine, 157*(3), 160–169. doi:10.7326/0003-4819-157-3-201208070-00005

Huryk, L. (2012). Information systems and decision support systems. *American Journal of Nursing, 112*(1), 62–65. doi:10.1097/01.NAJ.0000410365.51061.81

Kossman, S. P., & Scheidenhelm, S. L. (2008). Nurses' perceptions of the impact of electronic health records on work and patient outcomes. *Computers, Informatics, Nursing, 26*(2), 69–77. doi: 10.1097/01.NCN.0000304775.40531.67

McBride, S., Delaney, J. M., & Tietze, M. (2012). Health information technology and nursing. *American Journal of Nursing, 112*(8), 36–44. doi: 10.1097/01.NAJ.0000418095.31317.1b

McShane, R. (2013). Should patients with dementia who wander be electronically tagged? Yes. *BMJ, 346*, f3603. doi:http://dx.doi.org/10.1136/bmj.f3603

Menachimi, N., and Collum, T. H. (2011). Benefits and drawbacks of electronic health record systems. *Risk Management and Healthcare Policy, 4*, 47–55. doi: 10.2147/RMHP.S12985

Mitchell, M. (2012). Nursing informatics. How mobile is your technology? *Nursing Management, 43*(9), 26–30. doi: 10.1097/01.NUMA.0000418776.69056.be

National Institutes of Health (NIH). (2013). The National Library of Medicine PubMed. Retrieved March 30, 2013, from http://www.ncbi.nlm.nih.gov/pubmed/

Nelson, R., & Joos, I. (1989, Fall). On language in nursing: From data to wisdom. *PLN Visions, 6*, 7.

Pew Research Center. (2013). Health online. Retrieved July 16, 2013, from http://pewinternet.org/~/media//Files/Reports/PIP_HealthOnline.pdf

Pipe, T. B., Cisar, N. S., Caruso, E., et al. (2008). Leadership strategies: Inspiring evidence-based practice at the individual, unit, and organizational levels. *Journal of Nursing Care Quality, 23*(5), 265–271. doi: 10.1097/01.NCQ.0000324592.76590.32

Prgomet, M., Georgiou, A., & Westbrook, J. I. (2009). The impact of mobile handheld technology on hospital physicians' work practices and patient care: A systematic review. *Journal of the American Medical Informatics Association, 18*(6), 792–801. doi: 10.1197/jamia.M3215

Quality and Safety Education for Nurses (QSEN). (n.d.). Informatics competencies. Retrieved November 2, 2104, from, http://qsen.org/competencies/pre-licensure-ksas/#informatics

Rippen, H., & Risk, A. (2000). e-Health code of ethics. *Journal of Medical Internet Research, 2*(1), e2. doi:10.2196/jmir.2.2.e9

Rogers, E. M. (2003). *Diffusion of innovations* (5th ed., pp. 282–285). New York: Free Press.

Schleyer, R. H., Burch, C. K., & Schoessler, M. T. (2011). Defining and integrating informatics competencies into a hospital nursing department. *CIN: Computers, Informatics, Nursing, 29*(3), 167–173. doi: 10.1097/NCN.0b013e3181f9db36

Taylor, H. (2008). Number of "cyberchondriacs" adults going online for health information has plateaued or declined. *Healthcare News, 8*(8), 1–6.

The TIGER Initiative (Technology Informatics Guiding Educational Reform). (n.d.). http://www.tigersummit.com/About_Us.html

Turisco, F., & Rhoads, J. (2008). Equipped for efficiency: Improving nursing care through technology. Retrieved November 2, 2014, from http://www.chcf.org/publications/2008/12/equipped-for-efficiency-improving-nursing-care-through-technology

U.S. Department of Health and Human Services (USDHHS). (n.d.). *Quick guide to health literacy*. Retrieved July 16, 2013, from http://www.health.gov/communication/literacy/quickguide/quickguide.pdf

U.S. Department of Health and Human Services (USDHHS). (2013, May 22). Doctors and hospitals' use of health IT more than doubles since 2012. Retrieved July 1, 2013, from http://www.hhs.gov/news/press/2013pres/05/20130522a.html

CHAPTER 42

Agency for Healthcare Research and Quality. (2010, September). *The guide to clinical preventive services 2010–2011: Recommendations of the U.S. Preventive Services Task Force* (AHRQ Publication No. 10-05145). Rockville, MD: Author.

American Academy of Family Physicians (AAFP). (2012, October). *Summary of recommendations for clinical preventive services*. Leawood, KS: Author. Retrieved November 2, 2014, from http://www.aafp.org/dam/AAFP/documents/patient_care/clinical_recommendations/October2012SCPS.pdf

American Cancer Society. (2012, updated 2014, September 10). Breast awareness and self-exam. Retrieved November, 2, 2014, from http://www.cancer.org/cancer/breastcancer/moreinformation/breastcancerearlydetection/breast-cancer-early-detection-acs-recs-bse

American Cancer Society. (2013, revised 2014, September 29). Guidelines for the early detection of cancer. Retrieved November 2, 2014, from http://www.cancer.org/healthy/findcancerearly/cancerscreeningguidelines/american-cancer-society-guidelines-for-the-early-detection-of-cancer

American College of Sports Medicine (ACSM). (2013). *ACSM'S guidelines for exercise testing and prescription* (9th ed.). New York: Lippincott Williams & Wilkins.

Ashwell, M., Gunn, P., & Gibson, S. (2012). Waist-o-height ratio is a better screening tool than waist circumference and BMI for adult cardiometabolic risk factors: Systematic review and meta_analysis. *Obesity Reviews, 13*(3), 275–286.

Berry, L. L., Mirabito, A. M., & Baun, W. B. (2010). What's the hard return on employee wellness programs. *Harvard Business Review, 88*(12), 104–112.

Bulechek, G., Butcher, H., & Dochterman, J. (2012). *Nursing interventions classification (NIC)* (6th ed.). St. Louis, MO: C. V. Mosby.

Centers for Disease Control and Prevention (CDC). (2010). Tobacco use—smoking and second hand smoke. *CDC Vital Signs*. Retrieved August 25, 2013, from http://www.cdc.gov/vitalsigns/TobaccoUse/Smoking/

Centers for Disease Control and Prevention (CDC). (2012a, August 10). Current tobacco use among middle and high school students—United States, 2011. *Morbidity and Mortality Weekly Report, 61*(31), 581–585. Retrieved August 14, 2013, from http://www.cdc.gov/mmwr/preview/mmwrhtml/mm6131a1.htm?s_cid=mm6131a1_e

Centers for Disease Control and Prevention (CDC). (2012b, September). Summary health statistics for U.S. adults: National Health Interview Survey, 2011. *Vital Health Statistics, 10*(256). Retrieved August 25, 2013, from http://www.cdc.gov/nchs/data/series/sr_10/sr10_256.pdf

Centers for Disease Control and Prevention (CDC). (2012c, January). Prevalence of obesity in the United States, 2009–2010. *National Center for Health Statistics, 82*. Retrieved August 25, 2013, from http://www.cdc.gov/nchs/data/databriefs/db82.pdf

Centers for Disease Control and Prevention (CDC). (2013). Deaths: Final data for 2011. *National Vital Statistics Report, 61*(4), 1–90. Retrieved August 8, 2013, from http://www.cdc.gov/nchs/data/nvsr/nvsr61/nvsr61_04.pdf

Cooley, M. E., Emmons, K. M., Haddad, R., et al. (2011). Patient_reported receipt of and interest in smoking_cessation interventions after a diagnosis of cancer. *Cancer, 117*(13), 2961–2969.

Cooley, M. E., Finn, K. T., Wang, Q., et al. (2013). Health behaviors, readiness to change, and interest in health promotion programs among smokers with lung cancer and their family members: A pilot study. *Cancer Nursing, 36*(2), 145–154.

Escolas, S. M., Pitts, B. L., Safer, M. A., et al. (2013). The protective value of hardiness on military posttraumatic stress symptoms. *Military Psychology, 25*(2), 116.

Ford, E. S., van Dam, R. M., & Fonarow, G. C. (2009). Trends in the prevalence of low risk factor burden for cardiovascular disease among United States adults. *Circulation*. Retrieved August 13, 2013, from http://circ.ahajournals.org/cgi/content/abstract/CIRCULATIONAHA.108.835728v1

Halls, C., & Rhodes, J. (2002, September). Employee wellness and beyond at Appleton Papers Inc. *Athletic Therapy Today*, 46–47.

Hettler, W. (1984). Wellness: Encouraging a lifetime pursuit of excellence. *Health Values: Achieving High Level Wellness, 8*, 13–17.

Hoffman, A. J., Brintnall, R. A., Brown, J. K., et al. (2013). Too sick not to exercise: Using a 6-week, home-based exercise intervention for cancer-related fatigue self-management for postsurgical non-small cell lung cancer patients. *Cancer Nursing, 36*(3), 175–188.

Jadelhack, R. (2012). Health promotion in nursing and cost-effectiveness, *Journal of Cultural Diversity, 19*(2), 65–68.

Kobasa, S. (1979). Stressful life events, personality, and health: An inquiry into hardiness. *Journal of Personality and Social Psychology, 37*(1), 1–11.

Leavell, H., & Clark, E. (1965). *Preventive medicine for doctors in the community*. New York: McGraw-Hill.

Lazarus, R. S. (1966). *Psychological stress and the coping process*. New York: McGraw-Hill.

Linn, H. H., Ezzati, M., Chang, H. Y., et al. (2009). Association between tobacco smoking and active tuberculosis in Taiwan: Prospective cohort study. *Journal of Respiratory Critical Care Medicine, 180*(5), 475–480.

Maddi, S. R., Koshaba, D. M., Fazel, M., et al. (2009, July 1). The personality construct of hardiness, IV. *Journal of Humanistic Psychology, 49*(3), 292–305.

Moorhead, S., Johnson, M., Maas, M., et al. (2012). *Nursing outcomes classification (NOC)* (5th ed.). St. Louis, MO: C. V. Mosby.

Morbidity & Mortality Weekly Report, 62(35), 729–730. Notes from the Field: Electronic Cigarette Use Among Middle and High School Students—United States, 2011–2012. Retrieved September 11, 2013, from http://www.cdc.gov/mmwr/preview/mmwrhtml/mm6235a6.htm?s_cid=mm6235a6_w

Myers, J., Sweeney, T., & Witmer, J. (2000). The wheel of wellness counseling for wellness: A holistic model for treatment planning. *Journal of Counseling & Development, 78*(3), 251–267.

NANDA International. (2012). *Nursing diagnosis: Definitions and classifications 2012–2014*. Philadelphia: Author.

National Cancer Institute. (2009, Reviewed 2012). Prostate-specific antigen (PSA) Test. Retrieved August 13, 2013, from http://www.cancer.gov/cancertopics/factsheet/detection/PSA

National Guideline Clearinghouse. (2011). Lipids and lipoproteins. In *Expert panel on integrated guidelines for cardiovascular health and risk reduction in children and adolescents* (pp. 184–281). Bethesda,MD: National Heart, Lung, and Blood Institute. Retrieved August 13, 2013, from http://www.guideline.gov/content.aspx?id=35583&search=cholesterol+and+lipid+children

Neuman, B. (1995). *The Neuman systems model* (3rd ed.). Stamford, CT: Appleton & Lange.

Pender, N. J., Murdaugh, C. L., & Parsons, M. A. (2010). *Health promotion in nursing practice* (6th ed.). Upper Saddle River, NJ: Prentice-Hall.

Pope, M. A., Burnett, R. T., Krewski, D., et al. (2009). Cardiovascular mortality and exposure to airborne fine particulate matter and cigarette smoke. Shape of the exposure-response relationship. *Circulation, 120*(6), 941–948. Retrieved August 13, 2013, from http://circ.ahajournals.org/cgi/content/abstract/120/11/941

Prochaska, J., & DiClemente, C. (1982). Transtheoretical therapy: Toward a more integrative model of change. *Psychotherapy: Theory, Research and Practice, 19*(3), 276–288.

Qureshi, N., Wilson, B., Santaguida, P., et al. (2009, August). *NIH State-of-the-Science Conference: Family history and improving health* (Evidence Report/Technology Assessment No. 186; prepared by the McMaster University Evidence-based Practice Center, under Contract No. 290-2007-10060-I; AHRQ Publication No. 09–E016). Rockville, MD: Agency for Healthcare Research and Quality. Retrieved August 13, 2013, from http://www.ahrq.gov/clinic/tp/famhimptp.htm

Rahe, R. (1974). Life change and subsequent illness reports. In E. K. Gunderson & R. H. Rahe (Eds.), *Life stress and illness*. Springfield, IL: Charles C Thomas.

Rositch, A., Nowak, R., & Gravitt, P. (2014). Increased age and race-specific incidence of cervical cancer after correction for hysterectomy prevalence in the United States from 2000 to 2009. *Cancer, 120*(13), 2032–2038.

Selye, H. (1976). *The stress of life*. New York: McGraw-Hill.

Smith, R. A., Brooks, D., Cokkinides, V., et al. (2013, March–April). Cancer screening in the United States, 2013. A review of current American Cancer Society guidelines, current issues in cancer screening, and new guidance on cervical cancer screening and lung cancer screening. *CA: Cancer Journal for Clinicians, 63*, 87–105.

Tria, T. M. (2013). Breast cancer screening update. *American Family Physician, 87*(4), 274–278.

U.S. Department of Health and Human Services (USDHHS). (2008). 2008 physical activity guidelines for Americans. Retrieved February 5, 2011, from http://www.health.gov/paguidelines/

U.S. Department of Health and Human Services (USDHHS), Office of Disease Prevention & Health Promotion and Human Services. (2009; last updated March 8). *Healthy People 2020* topics and objectives. Retrieved August 13, 2013, from http://www.healthypeople.gov/hp2020/Objectives/TopicAreas.aspx

U.S. Department of Health and Human Services (USDHHS), & U.S. Department of Agriculture. (2011). Dietary guidelines for Americans 2010. Retrieved August 13, 2013, from http://www.health.gov/dietaryguidelines/dga2010/DietaryGuidelines2010.pdf

U.S. Preventive Services Task Force. (USPSTF). (2009). Screening for skin cancer: U.S. Preventive Services Task Force recommendation statement. *Annals of Internal Medicine, 150*(3), 188–193. Retrieved August 13, 2013, from http://www.guideline.gov/content.aspx?id=13695

U.S. Preventive Services Task Force. (USPSTF). (2012). Screening for prostate cancer. U.S. Preventive Services Task Force recommendation statement. Retrieved August 25, 2013, from http://www.uspreventiveservicestaskforce.org/prostatecancerscreening/prostatefinalrs.htm#summary

U.S. Preventive Services Task Force. (USPSTF). (2013). *Screening and behavioral counseling interventions in primary care to reduce alcohol misuse: Recommendation statement* (AHRQ Publication No. 12-05171-EF-3). Retrieved August 25, 2013, from http://www.uspreventiveservicestaskforce.org/uspstf12/alcmisuse/alcmisusefinalrs.htm

Wallston, K. A., Wallston, B. S., & DeVellis, R. (1978; last modified 2007, June 15). Development of the multidimensional health locus of control (MHLC) scales. *Health Education Monographs, 6*, 160–170. (MHLC scales available at Vanderbilt University, Multidimensional health locus of control scales.) Retrieved August 13, 2013, from http://www.vanderbilt.edu/nursing/kwallston/mhlcscales.htm

Watson, J. (1979). *Nursing: The philosophy and science of caring.* Boston: Little, Brown.

Witmer, J., & Sweeney, T. (1992). A holistic model for wellness and prevention over the life span. *Journal of Counseling & Development, 71*, 140–148.

World Health Organization (WHO). (1948). Preamble to the Constitution of the World Health Organization as adopted by the International Health Conference, New York, June 19–22, 1946; signed on July 22, 1946 by the representatives of 61 states (Official Records of the World Health Organization, No. 2, p. 100) and entered into force on 7 April 1948.

World Health Organization (WHO). (1986). Ottawa charter for health promotion. First International Conference on Health Promotion, Ottawa, November 21, 1986. Retrieved August 25, 2013, from http://www.who.int/healthpromotion/conferences/previous/ottawa/en/

Youth risk behavior surveillance—United States, 2011. (2012). *MMWR Surveillance Surveys, 61*(4). Retrieved August 25, 2013 from http://www.cdc.gov/mmwr/pdf/ss/ss6104.pdf

CHAPTER 43

111th Congress, first session. (2010). H.R.3962, the Affordable Health Care for America Act. Retrieved September 3, 2013, from http://docs.house.gov/rules/health/111_ahcaa.pdf

Abbas, A. H. (2011, November 23). Children vaccination reminder via SMS alert. *International Conference on Research and Innovation in Information Systems*, 1–5. doi:10.1109/ICRIIS.2011.612575

Agency for Healthcare Research and Quality. (2011, December). *Human factors challenges in home health care: Research Activities, 376*. Rockville, MD: Author.

Allender, J. A., Rector, C., & Warner, K. (2010). *Community health nursing: Promoting and protecting the public's health* (7th ed.). New York: Wolters Kluwer Health, Lippincott Williams & Wilkins.

American Academy of Pediatrics (AAP). (2008). Role of the school nurse in providing school health services. *Pediatrics, 2*(5), 1052–2056. doi:10.1542/peds.2008-0382

American Nurses Association (ANA). (1986). *Standards of community health nursing practice.* Washington, DC: American Nurses Association Publishing.

American Nurses Association (ANA). (2008). *Home health nursing. Scope and standards of practice.* Silver Spring, MD: Author.

American Nurses Association (ANA). (2013a). *Correctional nursing: Scope and standards of practice* (2nd ed.). Silver Spring, MD: Author.

American Nurses Association (ANA). (2013b). *Public health nursing: Scope and standards of practice* (2nd ed.). Silver Spring, MD: Author.

American Nurses Association and the Health Ministries Association. (2012). *Faith community nursing: Scope and standards of practice* (2nd ed.). Silver Spring, MD: Author.

American Nurses Association (ANA) and the National Association of School Nurses (NASN). (2011). *School nursing: Scope and standards of practice* (2nd ed.). Silver Spring, MD: Author.

American Telemedicine Association. (2009). *ATA home telehealth toolkit*. Washington, DC: Author.

Barrett, B., Muller, H. M., Ward, A., et al. (2012). Meditation or exercise for preventing acute respiratory infection: A randomized controlled trial. *Annals of Family Medicine, 10*(4), 337–463. doi: 10.1370/afm.1376

Bercovitz, A., Sengupta, M., Jones, A., & Harris-Kojetin, L. D. (2010). *Complementary and alternative therapies in hospice: The National Home and Hospice Care Survey: United States, 2007* (National Health Statistics Report No. 33). Hyattsville, MD: National Center for Health Statistics.

Bradford, N., Armfield, N. R., Young, J., et al. (2013). The case for home based telehealth for pediatric palliative care: A systematic review. *BMC Palliative Care, 12*(4). doi:10.1186/1472-684X-12-4

Bulechek, G., Butcher, H., & Dochterman, J. (Eds). (2013). *Nursing interventions classification (NIC)* (6th ed.). St. Louis, MO: C. V. Mosby.

Caffrey, C., Sengupta, M., Moss, A., et al. (2011). *Home health care and discharged hospice care patients: United States, 2000 and 2007* (National Health Statistics Report No. 38). Hyattsville, MD: National Center for Health Statistics.

Centers for Disease Control and Prevention. (2010). *Community Health Assessment aNd Group Evaluation (CHANGE) Action Guide: Building a foundation of knowledge to prioritize community needs.* Atlanta, GA: U.S. Department of Health and Human Services. Retrieved November 2, 2014, from http://www.cdc.gov/healthycommunitiesprogram/tools/change.htm

Centers for Disease Control and Prevention (CDC). (modified 2011a). *Healthy homes.* Atlanta, GA: Author. Retrieved November 2, 2014, from http://www.cdc.gov/healthyhomes/

Centers for Disease Control and Prevention (CDC). (updated 2011b). *Reminder systems and strategies for increasing vaccination rates.* Atlanta, GA: Author. Retrieved November 2, 2014, from http://www.cdc.gov/vaccines/recs/reminder-sys.htm

Clemen-Stone, S., McGuire, S., & Eigsti, D. (2009). *Comprehensive community health nursing: Family, aggregate, and community* (6th ed.). New York: Elsevier.

Dawood, F. S., Jain, S., Finelli, L., et al. (2009). Emergence of a novel swine-origin influenza A (H1N1) virus in humans. *New England Journal of Medicine, 360,* 2605–2615. doi: 10.1056/NEJMoa0903810

Federal Emergency Management Agency (FEMA). (2004, August). *Are you ready? In depth guide to citizen preparedness. IS-22.* Jessup, MD: FEMA.

Gershon, R., Pogorzelska, M., Qureshi, K., et al. (2008). Home health care registered nurses and the risk of percutaneous injuries: A pilot study. *AJIC: American Journal of Infection Control, 36*(3), 165–172. doi: http://dx.doi.org/10.1016/j.ajic.2007.04.278

Huynh-Hohbaum, A-L., Villa, V., Aranda, M., et al. (2008). Evaluating a multicomponent caregiver intervention. *Home Health Care Services Quarterly, 27*(4), 299–325. doi:10.1080/01621420802589777

Jones, A. L., Harris-Kojetin, L., & Valverde, R. (2012). *Characteristics and use of home health care by men and women aged 65 and over* (National Health Statistics Report No. 52). Hyattsville, MD: National Center for Health Statistics. Retrieved November 2, 2014, from www.cdc.gov/nchs/data/nhsr/nhsr052.pdf

Jones-Cooper, S. N., & Walton-Moss, B. (2012). Using reminder/recall systems to improve influenza immunization rates in children with asthma. *Journal of Pediatric Health Care, 27*(5), 327–333. doi.org/10.1016/j.pedhc.2011.11.005

The Joint Commission (TJC). (2014). *2014 Home Care National Patient Safety Goals.* Retrieved November 4, 2013, from http://www.jointcommission.org/ome_2014_npsgs/

Kulbok, P. L., Thatcher, E., Park, E., et al. (2012, May). Evolving public health nursing roles: Focus on community participatory health promotion and prevention. *The Online Journal of Issues in Nursing, 17*(2). doi:10.3912/OJIN.Vol17No02Man01

Larsson, L. S., & Butterfield, P. (2002). Mapping the future of environmental health and nursing: Strategies for integrating national competencies into nursing practice. *Public Health Nursing, 19*(9), 301–308.

Lescure, F-X, Locher, G., Eveillard, M., et al. (2009). Community-acquired infection with healthcare-associated methicillin-resistant *Staphylococcus aureus*: The role of home nursing care. *Infection Control & Hospital Epidemiology, 27,* 1213–1218. doi: 10.1128/CMR.00081-09

Levine, C., Albert, S., Hokenstad, A., et al. (2006). "This case is closed": Family caregivers and the termination of home health care services for stroke patients. *Milbank Quarterly, 84*(2), 305–331.

Martin, K. S., & Norris, J. (1996). The Omaha System: A model for describing practice. *Holistic Nursing Practice, 11*(1), 75–83.

Martin, K. S., & Scheet, N. J. (1992). *The Omaha System: Applications for community health nursing.* Philadelphia: W. B. Saunders. Retrieved November 1, 2014, from http://www.omahasystem.org/interventionscheme.html

Meadows, P. (2009). Community health nursing. *American Journal of Nursing, 109,* 19. doi:10.1097/01.NAJ.0000343102.62178.80

Moorhead, S., Johnson, M., Maas, M., et al. (Eds.). (2013). *Nursing outcomes classification (NOC)* (5th ed.). St. Louis, MO: C. V. Mosby.

Nightingale, F. (1860/1969). *Notes on nursing: What it is, and what it is not.* New York: Dover.

Nurse researcher surveys infection prevention practices for home-care patients. (2012, June 25). *Infection Control Today.* Retrieved November 2, 2014, from http://www.infectioncontroltoday.com/news/2012/06/nurse-researcher-surveys-infection-prevention-practices-for-homecare-patients.aspx

The Omaha System. (2009, May 11; updated). *Solving clinical data-information: Problem rating scale for outcomes.* Retrieved from http://www.omahasystem.org/problemratingscaleforoutcomes.html

Pereira, J. A., Quach, S., Heidebrecht, C. L., et al. (2012). Barriers to the use of reminder/recall interventions for immunizations: A systematic review. *BMC Medical Informatics and Decision-Making, 12,* 145. doi:10.1186/1472-6947-12-145

Purnell, L. D. (2009). *Guide to culturally competent healthcare* (2nd ed.). Philadelphia: F. A. Davis.

Quad Council of Public Health Nursing Organizations. (2011). *Core competencies for public health nurses.* Washington, DC: Author.

Saba, V. (2007). *Clinical care classification (CCC) system manual: A guide to nursing documentation* (pp. 142–150). New York: Springer.

Saba, V. K. (2012.). Clinical care classification system (Version 2.5) (2nd ed.). New York: Springer. Retrieved September 13, 2013, from http://www.sabacare.com/Tables/Components.html

Selekman, J. (Ed.) (2012). *School nursing: A comprehensive text* (2nd ed.). Philadelphia: F. A. Davis.

Siegel, B. (1983). *Lillian Wald of Henry Street.* New York: Macmillan.

U.S. Department of Health and Human Services (USDHHS). (2008). *Healthy People 2020* objectives. Retrieved November 2, 2014, from http://www.healthypeople.gov/2020/topicsobjectives2020/default

Veenema, T. G. (Ed.). (2013). *Disaster nursing and emergency preparedness for chemical, biological, and radiological terrorism and other hazards* (3rd ed.). New York: Springer.

West Virginia Department of Military Affairs and Public Safety. (n.d.). *Ready WV: A family emergency guide.* West Virginia Office of Emergency Services. Retrieved November 5, 2014, from http://www.ready.wv.gov/SiteCollectionDocuments/GuideReaderSpreadRCPGP.pdf

CHAPTER 44

Allen, R., Judkins-Cohn, T., deVelasco, R., et al. (2013). Moral distress among healthcare professionals at a health system. *JONA's Healthcare Law, Ethics, and Regulation, 15*(3), 111–18.

American Association of Colleges of Nursing (AACN). (2008). *The essentials of baccalaureate education for professional nursing practice.* Washington, DC: Author. Retrieved September 29, 2013, from http://www.aacn.nche.edu/Education/pdf/BaccEssentials08.pdf

American Hospital Association. (2003). *Patient care partnership: Understanding expectations, rights and responsibilities.* Retrieved October 3, 2013, from http://www.aha.org/aha/issues/Communicating-With-Patients/pt-care-partnership.html

American Nurses Association (ANA). (1988). *Nursing and the human immunodeficiency virus: A guide for nursing's response to AIDS.* Kansas City, MO: Author.

American Nurses Association (ANA). (1991a). American Nurses Association: Position statement on HIV testing. Retrieved October 3, 2013, from http://www.nursingworld.org/MainMenuCategories/Policy-Advocacy/Position-Testing.htmls-and-Resolutions/ANAPositionStatements/Position-Statements-Alphabetically/HIV

American Nurses Association (ANA). (1991b). Equipment/safety procedures to prevent transmission of blood-borne diseases. Retrieved November 29, 2013, from http://nursingworld.org/MainMenuCategories/Policy-Advocacy/Positions-and-Resolutions/ANAPositionStatements/Position-Statements-Alphabetically/Equipment Safety-Procedures-to-Prevent-Transmission-of-Bloodborne-Diseases.html

American Nurses Association (ANA). (2001). *Code of ethics for nurses with interpretive statements.* Washington, DC: American Nurses Publishing. Retrieved October 3, 2013, from http://nursingworld.org/MainMenuCategories/EthicsStandards/CodeofEthicsforNurses/2110Provisions.aspx

American Nurses Association (ANA). (2010). *Nursing: Scope and standards of practice* (2nd ed.). Silver Spring, MD: Author.

American Nurses Association (ANA). (2011). Position statement on forgoing nutrition and hydration. Retrieved October 3, 2013, from http://www.nursingworld.org/MainMenuCategories/Policy-Advocacy/Positions-and-Resolutions/ANAPositionStatements/Position-Statements-Alphabetically/prtetnutr14451.pdf

American Nurses Association (ANA). (2012). Position statement on nursing care and do-not-resuscitate (DNR) and allow natural death (AND) decisions. Retrieved October 3, 2013, from http://www.nursingworld.org/dnrposition

American Nurses Association (ANA). (2013). Position statement on euthanasia, assisted suicide, and aid in dying. Retrieved October 3, 2013, from http://www.nursingworld.org/euthanasiaanddying

Attree, M. (2007). Factors influencing nurses' decisions to raise concerns about care quality. *Journal of Nursing Management, 15*(4), 392–402.

Balch, S. (2006). The dubious value of value neutrality. *Academic Questions, 19*(4), 44–48.

Bandman, E., & Bandman, B. (2002). *Nursing ethics through the life span* (4th ed.). Upper Saddle River, NJ: Prentice-Hall.

Bayles, M. (1984). *Reproductive ethics.* Englewood Cliffs, NJ: Prentice-Hall.

Beauchamp, T. L., & Childress, J. F. (2012). *Principles of biomedical ethics* (7th ed.). New York: Oxford University Press.

Buck, H. (2012). Refusing artificial nutrition and hydration in advanced illness. *Nursing2012, 42*(9), 12–13.

Burkhardt, M., & Nathaniel, A. (2014). *Ethics and issues in contemporary nursing* (4th ed.). Clifton Park, NY: Thomson Delmar Learning.

Burston, A., & Tuckett, A. (2012). Moral distress in nursing: Contributing factors, outcomes and interventions. *Nursing Ethics, 20*(3), 312–324.

Butts, J., & Rich, K. (2012). *Nursing ethics across the curriculum and into practice* (3rd ed.). Burlington, MA: Jones & Bartlett.

Cameron, B. (2004). Ethical moments in practice: The nursing "how are you" revisited. *Nursing Ethics, 11*(1), 53–62.

Catalano, J. T. (2012). *Nursing now!: Today's issues, tomorrow trends* (6th ed.). Philadelphia: F. A. Davis.

Clark, C. (2006). Moral character in social work. *The British Journal of Social Work, 36*(1), 75–89.

Cooper, R. (2012). Making the case for ethical decision-making models. *Nurse Prescribing, 10*(12), 607–622.

Curtin, L., & Flaherty, J. (1982). *Nursing ethics: Theories and pragmatics.* Bowie, MD: Robert J. Brady

Davis, S., Schrader, V., & Belcheir, M. (2012). Influencers of ethical beliefs and the impact on moral distress and conscientious objection. *Nursing Ethics, 19*(6), 738–749.

Dierckx de Casterlé, B., Izumi, S., Godfrey, N., et al. (2008). Nurses' responses to ethical dilemmas in nursing practice: Meta-analysis. *Journal of Advanced Nursing, 63*(6), 540–549.

Edwards, S. (2009). Three versions of ethics of care. *Nursing Philosophy, 19*(4), 231–240.

Edwards, S. (2011). Is there a distinctive care ethics? *Nursing Ethics, 18*(2), 184–191.

Epstein, E., & Delgado, S. (2010). Understanding and addressing moral distress. *The Online Journal of Issues in Nursing, 15*(3), Manuscript 1. Retrieved October 2, 2013, from http://www.nursingworld.org/MainMenuCategories/EthicsStandards/Courage-and-Distress/Understanding-Moral-Distress.html

Epstein, E., & Hamric, A. (2009). Moral distress, moral residue, and the crescendo effect. *Journal of Clinical Ethics, 20*(4), 330–342.

Gaudine, A., & Thorne, L. (2012). Nurses' ethical conflict with hospitals: A longitudinal study of outcomes. *Nursing Ethics, 19*(6), 727–737.

Gilligan, C. (1993). *In a different voice.* Cambridge, MA: Harvard University Press.

Gormley-Fleming, L., & Campbell, A. (2011). Factors involved in young people's decisions about their health care. *Nursing Children & Young People, 23*(9), 19–22.

Gruenewald, D. (2012). Can health care rationing ever be rational? *Journal of Law, Medicine & Ethics, 40*(1), 17–25.

ISNA Bulletin (2013). What do I do now? Ethical dilemmas in nursing and health care. *INSA Bulletin, 39*(2), 5–12.

International Council of Nurses (ICN). (revised 2012). *The ICN code of ethics for nurses.* Geneva, Switzerland: Author. Retrieved October 3, 2013, from http://www.icn.ch/images/stories/documents/about/icncode_english.pdf

Ivanov, L., & Oden, T. (2013). Public health nursing, ethics and human rights. *Public Health Nursing, 30*(3), 231–238.

Jameton, A. (1984). *Nursing practice: The ethical issues.* Englewood Cliffs, NJ: Prentice-Hall.

Jurchak, M., & Pennington, M. (2009). Fostering moral agency in new intensive care unit nurses. *Critical Care Nurse, 29*(6), 79–80.

Jones, A., Moss, A., & Harris-Kojetin, L. (2011). *Use of advance directives in long-term care* (NCHS Data Brief No. 54). Retrieved October 1, 2013, from http://www.cdc.gov/nchs/data/databriefs/db54.pdf

Husted, J., & Husted, G. (2008). *Ethical decision making in nursing and healthcare* (4th ed.). New York: Springer.

Kim, Y., Kang, S., & Ahn, J. (2013). Moral sensitivity relating to the application of the code of ethics. *Nursing Ethics, 20*(4), 470–478.

Kohlberg, L. (1968). Moral development. In *International encyclopedia of social science.* New York: Macmillan.

Kohlberg, L. (1981). *Essays on moral development* (Vols. 1–3). San Francisco: Harper & Row.

Kothari, S., & Kirschner, K. (2006). Abandoning the Golden Rule: The problem with "putting ourselves in the patient's place." *Topics in Stroke Rehabilitation, 13*(4), 68–73.

Lachman, V. (2012). Applying the ethics of care to your nursing practice. *MedSurg Nursing, 21*(2), 112–114, 116.

Landwehr, C. (2013). Procedural justice and democratic institutional design in health-care priority-setting. *Contemporary Political Theory*. Advance online publication. doi:10.1057/cpt.2012.28

Leininger, M. (2002). Culture care theory: A major contribution to advance transcultural nursing knowledge and practice. *Journal of Transcultural Nursing, 13*(3), 189–192.

Lekes, N., Joussemet, M., Koestner, R., et al. (2011). Transmitting intrinsic value from mother to adolescent: The moderating role of a supportive family environment. *Child Development Research, 2011*. Retrieved September 29, 2013, from http://www.hindawi.com/journals/cdr/2011/167146/cta/

Leuter, C., Petrucci, C., Mattei, A., et al. (2013). Ethical difficulties in nursing, educational needs and attitudes about using ethics resources. *Nursing Ethics, 20*(3), 348–358.

Milton, C., Peacock, S., Storch, J., et al. (2010). Moral distress among health care managers: Conditions, consequences and potential responses. *Healthcare Policy, 6*(2), 99–112.

Moore, L., & McAuliffe, E. (2012). To report or not to report? Why some nurses are reluctant to whistleblow. *Clinical Governance: An International Journal, 17*(4), 332–342.

National Conference of Commissioners on Uniform State Laws. (2006). Revised Uniform Anatomical Gift Act. Retrieved October 3, 2013, from http://www.uniformlaws.org/Act.aspx?title=Anatomical%20Gift%20Act%20(2006)

National Council of State Boards of Nursing. (2011). *A nurse's guide to professional boundaries*. Chicago, IL: Author. Retrieved October 4, 2013, from https://www.ncsbn.org/ProfessionalBoundaries_Complete.pdf

National League for Nursing. (2007). *Core values*. Retrieved October 4, 2013, from http://www.nln.org/aboutnln/corevalues.htm

Olsen, D. (2007). Ethical issues. Unwanted treatment: What are the ethical implications? *American Journal of Nursing, 107*(9), 51–53.

O'Mara, E., Jackson, L., Batson, C., et al. (2011). Will moral outrage stand up? Distinguishing among emotional reactions to a moral violation. *European Journal of Social Psychology, 41*(2), 173–179.

Paquin, S. (2011). Social justice advocacy in nursing: What is it? How do we get there? *Creative Nursing, 17*(2), 63–67.

Park, M. (2009). The legal basis of nursing ethics education. *Journal of Nursing Law, 13*(4), 106–113.

Peate, M., Watts, K., & Wakefield, C. (2013). The "value" of values clarification in cancer-related decision aids. *Patient Education & Counseling, 90*(2), 281–283.

Peters, K., Luck, L., Hutchinson, M., et al. (2011). The emotional sequelae of whistleblowing: Finding from a qualitative study. *Journal of Clinical Nursing, 20*(19/20), 2907–2914.

Pinquart, M., & Silbereisen, R. K. (2004). Transmission of values from adolescents to their parents: The role of value content and authoritative parenting. *Adolescence, 39*(153), 83–100.

Polzer Casarez, R., & Engebretson, J. (2012). Ethical issues of incorporating spiritual care into clinical practice. *Journal of Clinical Nursing, 21*(15/16), 2099–2107.

Potter, G., Clarke, C., Hackett, S., et al. (2013). Nursing students and geriatric care: The influence of specific knowledge on evolving values, attitudes, and actions. *Nurse Education in Practice, 13*(5), 449–453.

Purtilo, R. (2010). *Ethical dimensions in the health professions* (5th ed.). Philadelphia: W. B. Saunders.

Raths, L., Harmin, M., & Simon, S. (1978). *Values and teaching*. Columbus, OH: Merrill.

Ricker, F. (2013). Ethics and respect for each other. *Colorado Nurse, 113*(2), 1–5.

Roberts, D. (2012). For better or worse—values shape nursing practice. *MedSurg Nursing, 21*(1), 7.

Roe v. Wade, 410 U.S. 113 (1973). Retrieved November 30, 2013, from http://www.law.cornell.edu/supct/html/historics/USSC_CR_0410_0113_ZS.html

Schwarz, J. (2009). Stopping eating and drinking. *American Journal of Nursing, 10*(9), 53–62.

Scott, R. S. (1985). When it isn't life or death. *American Journal of Nursing, 85*(1), 19–20.

Steele, S. M., & Harmon, V. M. (1979). *Values clarification in nursing*. Norwalk, CT: Appleton-Century-Crofts.

Steele, S. M., & Harmon, V. M. (1983). *Values clarification in nursing* (2nd ed.). New York: Appleton-Lange.

Thiroux, J. (1977). *Ethics, theory and practice*. Philadelphia: MacMillan.

Tong, R., & Williams, N. (2009). Feminist Ethics. *The Stanford Encyclopedia of philosophy, 2011 edition*. Retrieved September 29, 2013, from http://plato.stanford.edu/entries/feminism-ethics/#FemAppEth

Tschundin, V. (2003). *Ethics in nursing: The caring relationship* (3rd ed.). Oxford: Butterworth & Heinemann.

Vanlaere, L., & Gastman, C. (2011). A personalistic approach to care ethics. *Nursing Ethics, 18*(2), 161–173.

Varcoe, C., Pauly, B., Storch, J., et al. (2012). Nurses' perceptions of and responses to morally distressing situations. *Nursing Ethics, 19*(4), 488–500.

Villers, M., & DeVon, H. (2012). Moral distress and avoidance behavior in nurses working in critical care and noncritical care units. *Nursing Ethics, 20*(5), 589–603.

Waugh, D. (1978). Moral development: Theory and process. In D. E. Reilly (Ed.), *Teaching and evaluating the affective domain in nursing programs* (pp. 17–30). New York: Charles B. Slack.

Webster, G. C., & Baylis, F. E. (2000). Moral residue. In S. B. Rubin & L. Zoloth (Eds.), *Margin of error: The ethics of mistakes in the practice of medicine* (pp. 217–230). Hagerstown, MD: University Publishing Group.

Whitehead, B., & Barker, D. (2010). Does the risk of reprisal prevent nurses blowing the whistle on bad practice. *Nursing Times, 106*(43), 12–15.

Wiegand, D., & Funk, M. (2012). Consequences of clinical situations that cause critical care nurses to experience moral distress. *Nursing Ethics, 19*(4), 479–487.

Wilkinson, J. M. (1987/1988). Moral distress in nursing practice: Experience and effect. *Nursing Forum, 23*, 16–29.

Wilkinson, J. M. (1997). *Toward a context-sensitive theory of nursing ethics: Classification and comparison of nurses' narratives from four time periods (1934, 1979, 1989 & 1995)* (Unpublished doctoral dissertation). University of Kansas, Kansas City.

Yoder-Wise, P. (2010). *Leading and managing in nursing* (5th ed.). St. Louis, MO: C. V. Mosby.

Zuzelo, P. R. (2007). Exploring the moral distress of registered nurses. *Nursing Ethics, 14*, 344–359.

CHAPTER 45

Admore v. Nurse Connection, Inc. WL 5874397 (Cir. Ct. Palm Beach Co., Fl. 2009). Retrieved October 20, 2013, from http://www.nursinglaw.com/whistleblowernurse.pdf

American Nurses Association (ANA). (n.d.a). Nurses' bill of rights. Retrieved October 19, 2013, from http://www.nursingworld.org/MainMenuCategories/WorkplaceSafety

/Healthy-Work-Environment/Work-Environment/Nurses BillofRights

American Nurses Association. (n.d.b). Scope and standards of practice. Retrieved October 19, 2013, from http://www.nursingworld.org/modelofpracticeregulation

American Nurses Association (n.d.c). Scope and Standards of Practice. Retrieved October 19, 2013, from http://www.nursingworld.org/scopeandstandardsofpractice

American Nurses Association (ANA). (2001). *Code of ethics for nurses with interpretive statements*. Washington, DC: American Nurses Publishing. Retrieved October 25, 2013, from http://www.nursingworld.org/MainMenuCategories/EthicsStandards/CodeofEthicsforNurses/Code-of-Ethics.pdf

American Nurses Association (ANA). (2007). *Registered nurse utilization of nursing assistive personnel* [Position statement]. Washington, DC: Author. Retrieved October 25, 2013, from http://gm6.nursingworld.org/MainMenuCategories/Policy-Advocacy/Positions-and-Resolutions/ANAPositionStatements/Position-Statements-Alphabetically/Registered-Nurses-Utilization-of-Nursing-Assistive-Personnel-in-All-Settings.html

American Nurses Association (ANA). (2010a). Position statement: Registered nurses roles and responsibilities in providing expert care and counseling at the end of life. Retrieved October 19, 2013, from http://www.nursingworld.org/MainMenuCategories/EthicsStandards/Ethics-Position-Statements/etpain14426.pdf

American Nurses Association (ANA). (2010b). *Nursing: Scope and standards of practice* (2nd ed.). Silver Spring, MD: Nursebooks.org.

American Nurse Association (ANA). (2012). Roles of state boards of nursing: Licensure, regulation and complaint investigation. Retrieved October 20, 2013, from http://www.nursingworld.org/MainMenuCategories/Tools/State-Boards-of-Nursing-FAQ.pdf

American Nurses Association (ANA). (2013). Position statements: Euthanasia, assisted suicide, and aid in dying. Retrieved October 24, 2013, from http://www.nursingworld.org/euthanasiaanddying

Americans With Disabilities Act (ADA) of 1990, Pub. L. No. 101–336, 104 Stat. 327, enacted July 26, 1990, codified at 42 U.S.C. § 12101 *et seq*. Retrieved October 19, 2013, from http://www.eeoc.gov/eeoc/history/35th/thelaw/ada.html

Americans With Disabilities Act (ADA) Amendments Act of 2008, 42 U.S.C.A § 12101. Retrieved October 19, 2013, from http://www.eeoc.gov/laws/statutes/adaaa.cfm

Anselmi, K. (2012). Nurses' personal liability vs. employer's vicarious liability. *MedSurg Nursing, 21*(1), 45–48.

Arnold, P. (2012). The importance of accurate documentation. *Australian Nursing Journal, 19*(10), 28.

Austin, S. (2008). 7 tips for safe nursing practice. *Nursing2008, 28*(3), 34–39.

Austin, S. (2011). Stay out of court with proper documentation. *Nursing2011, 41*(4), 24–29.

Balestra, M. (2012). The best defense for registered nurses and nurse practitioners: Understanding the disciplinary process. *Journal of Nursing Law, 15*(2), 39–44.

Banford, E., & Budake, A. (2012). Risk reduction for nursing—understanding your role in reducing liability exposure. *Bariatric Nursing & Surgical Patient Care, 7*(4), 183–185.

Barber v. Reinking, 411 P.2d 861 (Wash. 1966). *Legal Eagle.* Retrieved October 19, 2013, from http://www.leagle.com/xmlResult.aspx?xmldoc=196620768Wn2d139_1187.xml&docbase=CSLWAR1-1950-1985

Byrne v. Chester County Hospital, 519 Fed. Appx. 739 (2013).

Coulter v. Thomas, 33 S.W.3d 5229 (Ky. 2000). *Legal Eagle.* Retrieved October 19, 2013, from http://www.leagle.com/xmlResult.aspx?xmldoc=200055533SW3d522_1553.xml&docbase=CSLWAR2-1986-2006

Dollinger, M., & Dollinger, R. (2012). A new legal interpretation of duty for registered nurses. *Journal of Nursing Regulation, 3*(1), 21–25.

Equal Employment Opportunity Commission (EEOC). (n.d.). Facts about sexual harassment. Retrieved October 25, 2013, from http://www.eeoc.gov/eeoc/publications/fs-sex.cfm

Falls: Care plan not updated, jury finds negligence. (2010). *Legal Eagle Eye Newsletter for the Nursing Profession.* Retrieved October 23, 2013, from www.nursinglaw.com/fallcareplan4.pdf

Georgia Nurses Association. (n.d.). Nurse advocate program. The impaired nurse: Checklist for detecting potential chemical dependence in an employee. Retrieved October 24, 2013, from http://www.georgianurses.org/impaired_nurse.htm#pabi

Gonzales v. Carhart, 550 U.S. 124 (2007).

Griswold v. Connecticut, 381 U.S. 479 (1965).

Hanna, A., & Suplee, P. (2012). Don't cross the line, respecting professional boundaries. *Nursing2012, 42*(9), 40–47.

Health Insurance Portability and Accountability Act (HIPAA), 29 U.S.C.A § 167; 1181 *et seq*. Retrieved October 25, 2013, from http://www.hhs.gov/ocr/privacy/

Helm, A. (2003). *Nursing malpractice: Sidestepping legal minefields.* Philadelphia: Lippincott, Williams & Wilkins.

Hunsaker, A., & Mann, A. (2013). An analysis of the Patient Self-Determination Act of 1990. *Journal of Human Behavior in the Social Environment, 23*(7), 841–848.

Job Accommodation Network. (n.d.). Retrieved October 18, 2013, from http://AskJAN.org

Kansas State Board of Nursing. (1993; last amended 2007, April 20). Unprofessional conduct. Retrieved October 25, 2013, from http://www.ksbn.org/npa/pages/60-7-106.pdf

Legal Information Institute (LII). Maintained by Cornell University Law School. Retrieved October 24, 2013, from http://www.law.cornell.edu/

March, A. L., Cassandra, D. F., Adams, M. H., et al. (2011). The mock trial: A collaborative interdisciplinary approach to understanding legal and ethical issues. *Nurse Educator, 36*(2), 66–69.

Matt, S. (2012). Ethical and legal issues associated with bullying in the nursing profession. *Journal of Nursing Law, 15*(1), 9–13.

Mattox, E. (2012). Patient safety. Medical devices and patient safety. *Critical Care Nurse, 32*(4), 60–68.

Missouri Revised Statutes, Chapter 335, Section 335.016. (August 28, 2013). Retrieved October 24, 2013, from http://www.moga.mo.gov/statutes/C300-399/3350000016.HTM

National Council of State Boards of Nursing (NCSBN). (n.d.). Professional boundaries: A nurse's guide to the importance of appropriate professional boundaries. Retrieved October 24, 2013, from https://www.ncsbn.org/ProfessionalBoundariesbrochure.pdf

National Council of State Boards of Nursing (NCSBN). (2012). Nursing license verification. Retrieved December 10, 2013, from https://www.ncsbn.org/3942.htm

Nurse Connection, Inc. v. Admore, 48 So.3d 64 (Fla. Dist. Ct. App. 4th Dist. 2010).

Nurses Service Organization (NSO). (n.d.). Case study with risk management strategies. Retrieved December 10, 2013, from https://www.nso.com/pdfs/db/NP_SLCS_x-8610-0411_final_web.pdf?fileName=NP_SLCS_x-8610-0411_final_web.pdf&folder=pdfs/db&isLiveStr=Y

Nurses Service Organization (NSO). (2011). August 2011 Legal Case Study. Hatboro, PA: Author. Retrieved October 24, 2013, from http://www.nso.com/case-studies/article/293.jsp

Nurses Service Organization (NSO). (2012). Case study: Failure to adequately assess and monitor patient postoperatively resulting in patient's death. Retrieved October 24, 2013, from https://www.nso.com/pdfs/db/Nurse_SLCS_X-8540-0112_final_web.pdf?fileName=Nurse_SLCS_X-8540-0112_final_web.pdf&folder=pdfs/db&isLiveStr=Y

Nurses Service Organization (NSO). (2013a). Legal case study: Failure to properly control woman's post-cesarean section bleeding—death—$1.35 million settlement. Retrieved October 19, 2013, from http://www.nso.com/case-studies/casestudy-article/317.jsp

Nursing Service Organization (NSO). (2013b). Alleged failure to properly assess and monitor the impaired, restrained patient and failure to provide proper care in a safe environment. February 2013 Legal Case Study. Hatboro, PA: Author. Retrieved October 24, 2013, from https://www.nso.com/pdfs/db/RN_SLCSx-10116-0113_February2013.pdf?fileName=RN_SLCSx-10116-0113_February2013.pdf&folder=pdfs/db&isLiveStr=Y

Nurses Service Organization (NSO). (2013c). Woman falls while home health nurse is weighing her—fractured leg—surgery, rehab and need for continuing care—$791,573 verdict. January 2013 Legal Case Study. Hatboro, PA: Author. Retrieved October 24, 2013, from http://www.nso.com/case-studies/casestudy-article/315.jsp

O'Keefe, M. E. (Ed.). (2001). *Nursing practice and the law: Avoiding malpractice and other legal risks*. Philadelphia: F. A. Davis.

Pallacovitch v. Waterbury Hosp., 2012 Conn. Super. Lexis 1962 (Conn. Super. Ct., 2012).

Patient Self Determination Act of 1990, § 167; 4206 and 4751 of the Omnibus Reconciliation Act of 1990, Pub. L. No. 101-508.

Planned Parenthood v. Casey, 505 U.S. 833 (1992).

Reising, D. (2012). Make your nursing care malpractice-proof. *American Nurse Today, 7*(1), 24–29.

Rodas v. Seidlin, 656 F.3d 610 (7th Cir. 2011).

Roe v. Wade, 410 U.S. 113 (1973).

Shepard, L. (2009). *If that ever happen to me: Making life and death decisions after Terry Schaivo*. Chapel Hill: University of North Carolina Press.

Spoelstra, S. L., Given, B. A., & Given, C. W. (2012). *Fall prevention in hospitals: An integrative review. Clinical Nursing Research, 21*(1), 92–112.

Stenberg v. Carhart, 530 U.S. 914 (2000).

Sturgill v. Ashe Memorial Hosp., 652 S.E.2d 302 (N.C. App. 2007); reviewed denied, 658 S.E.2d 662 (N.C. 2008).

Thomas, C., & Siela, D. (2011). The impaired nurse: Would you know what to do if you suspected substance abuse. *American Nurse Today, 6*, 8. Retrieved October 24, 2013, from http://www.americannursetoday.com/article.aspx?id=8114&fid=8078

U.S. Department of Health and Human Services (USDHHS), Centers for Medicare & Medicaid Services. (updated 2012, March 26). Emergency Medical Treatment & Labor Act (EMTALA) resource. Retrieved October 24, 2013, from http://www.cms.hhs.gov/emtala/

Webster v. Reproductive Health Services, 492 U.S. 490 (1989).

Wellington, T. (2013, August 13). Police: School video "altered" in Danville principal, superintendent criminal case. *TheBurlingtonFreePress.Com*. Retrieved October 19, 2013, from http://www.burlingtonfreepress.com/apps/pbcs.dll/article?AID=2013308130019&gcheck=1&nclick_check=1

INDEX

Note: Page number followed by *f* refer to figures; page numbers followed by *t* refer to tables; page numbers followed by *b* refer to boxes; page numbers followed by *p* refer to procedures.

A

A-delta fibers, (V1) 793–794, (V1) 793*f*
Abbreviations
  for documentation, (V1) 378, (V2) 169–170
  drug name, error-prone, (V2) 480*t*
  error-prone, (V2) 478–479*t*
  medication-related, (V2) 477–478*t*
ABCDEE pain assessment, (V1) 799*b*
Abdellah, Faye G., nursing theory of, (V1) 146*t*
Abdomen
  assessment of, (V1) 504–505, (V1) 504*f*, (V1) 505*f*, (V1) 514*p*, (V2) 271–277*p*
  auscultation of, (V1) 505
  inspection of, (V1) 504–505, (V1) 505*f*
  movement of, in respiration, (V1) 445
  palpation of, (V1) 505
  percussion of, (V1) 505
  postoperative distention of, (V1) 1050*t*
Abdominal binder, (V1) 929, (V1) 930–931*p*, (V2) 697–699*p*
Abducens nerve (VI), testing, (V2) 288*p*
ABG analysis, (V1) 996, (V1) 997*t*, (V1) 998
Ablative surgery, (V1) 1027
ABO blood groups, (V1) 1019, (V1) 1019*t*
Abrasion, (V1) 581, (V1) 902*t*
Abscess, (V1) 902*t*. *See also* Infection(s)
Absorption, medication, (V1) 609–614. *See also* Medication(s), absorption of
Abstinence, (V1) 862, (V2) 654
Abstract, (V1) 1091
Abstract thinking, assessing, (V2) 286–287*p*
Abuse
  of adolescents, (V1) 191
  of alcohol, (V1) 1097
  assessing for, (V2) 63–66
    documentation of, (V2) 66–67
    evaluation in, (V2) 66
    focused health history in, (V2) 63–64
    focused physical assessment in, (V2) 64–65
    follow-up in, (V2) 65
    home care in, (V2) 66
    patient teaching in, (V2) 66
    for psychological abuse, (V2) 64
  of child, (V1) 183–184
    assessing for, (V2) 65–66
  history of, population vulnerability and, (V1) 1116
  identification of, (V2) 62
  of infant, (V1) 177
    assessing for, (V1) 178*b*
    detection and prevention of, (V1) 178*b*
  of older adult, (V1) 211
    assessing for, (V1) 214, (V2) 66
  of opioids, (V1) 806
  reporting regulations on, (V1) 1184
  sexual, (V1) 864–865
  substance. *See* Substance abuse
Abusive head trauma (AHT), to infant, (V1) 177
Acceptance
  in communication, (V1) 233
  as stage of dying, (V1) 353*b*
Accessory muscles, during inspiration, (V1) 946
Accessory nerve (XI), testing, (V2) 290*p*
Accidents, motor vehicle
  prevention of, (V1) 564–565
  risk factors for, (V1) 551
Accommodation
  in cognitive development, (V1) 167
  in culturally competent care, (V1) 323
  pupil, (V1) 494
    testing of, (V2) 243*p*
Accountability
  for decisions and actions, (V1) 107
  legal, (V1) 1162–1185, (V2) 905–911
Accreditation, (V1) 1171
Accreditation Commission on Education in Nursing (ACEN), (V1) 22
Accrediting bodies, for nursing education, (V1) 22
Acculturation, (V1) 305–306
Acetaminophen, (V1) 805
Achilles reflex, testing, (V2) 294*p*
Achondroplasia, (V1) 827
Acid, (V1) 989
Acid-base balance
  assessment of, (V1) 998–1001, (V2) 815–817
  critical thinking about, (V2) 818–819
  disorders of, (V1) 996, (V1) 997*t*
    nursing diagnosis for, (V1) 1001
    nursing interventions for, (V1) 1001–1015
    nursing outcomes for, (V1) 1001
  full-spectrum nursing and, (V2) 817–818
  knowledge map for, (V2) 821
  regulation of, (V1) 989, (V1) 991–992
Acidosis, (V1) 991, (V1) 996
  metabolic, (V1) 996, (V1) 997*t*, (V1) 999
  respiratory, (V1) 996, (V1) 997*t*
Acne, (V1) 581
Acoustic nerve (VIII) testing, (V2) 289*p*
Acrochordons, (V1) 491, (V2) 228
Acromegaly, head size and, (V1) 493
Actigraph, (V1) 891
Acting, in values clarification, (V1) 1156*t*
Active listening
  for enhancing therapeutic communication, (V1) 473–474, (V1) 474*f*
  for spirituality diagnoses, (V1) 340
Active range of motion (AROM), (V1) 820. *See also* Range of motion (ROM)
  for mobility, (V1) 843–844
Active transport, (V1) 985, (V1) 986, (V1) 987*f*, (V1) 987*t*
Activities of Daily Living (ADLs)
  for ambulation conditioning, (V1) 844, (V2) 638
  in older adult assessment, (V1) 213
Activity
  in infection prevention, (V1) 532–533
  level of
    bowel elimination and, (V1) 749
    energy expended by, (V1) 681*t*
    urinary function and, (V1) 719
Activity intolerance, (V1) 834
  exercise and, (V1) 834
  postoperative, (V2) 851
  sexuality and, (V1) 867
Activity theory, of psychosocial development of older adults, (V1) 207, (V1) 209, (V1) 209*f*
Actual nursing diagnosis, (V1) 66*t*
  goals for, (V1) 98, (V1) 99*t*
  intervention type related to, (V1) 110*t*
Acupressure, for pain, (V1) 802
Acupuncture
  for pain, (V1) 802
  in stress management, (V1) 259
Acute pain, (V1) 792, (V1) 797*b*
  postoperative, (V2) 851–852
Acute renal failure (ARF), definition of, (V1) 725*b*
Acute wound, (V1) 902
Adaptation(s)
  in cognitive development, (V1) 167
  definition of, (V1) 240
  hardiness and, (V1) 244
  health status and, (V1) 244
  in leadership, (V1) 1059
  as outcome of stress, (V1) 243
  perception of stressor and, (V1) 244
  personal factors influencing, (V1) 243–244
  stress and, (V1) 239–261, (V2) 92–101. *See also* Stress, adaptation to
  support system and, (V1) 244
Adapted physical activity (APA) programs, (V1) 206
Adaptive coping, (V1) 243
Addiction, (V1) 806. *See also* Substance abuse
Adhesive tape/strips, (V1) 905, (V1) 924, (V1) 929*p*
Adipose tissue, (V1) 898*f*, (V1) 899
Adjuvant analgesics, (V1) 805–806
Administrative law, (V1) 1163–1164
Admission, to nursing unit, (V1) 237*p*, (V2) 77–79*p*
Admission assessment, (V1) 47
Admission data form, (V1) 382–383, (V2) 171
Adolescent(s), (V1) 188–194
  abuse, neglect and violence involving, (V1) 191
  alcohol use by, (V1) 189–190
  anorexia nervosa in, (V1) 190
  assessment of, (V1) 191–193
  bulimia in, (V1) 190
  cardiovascular system in, (V1) 971–972
  cigarette smoking by, (V1) 971
  communication by, (V1) 465
  condom use by, (V1) 191
  depression in, (V1) 190
  development of
    cognitive, (V1) 168*t*, (V1) 189
    physical, (V1) 188–189, (V1) 188*b*

psychosexual, (V1) 167*t*
psychosocial, (V1) 168, (V1) 189, (V1) 189*f*
developmental tasks of, (V1) 166*t*
eating disorders in, (V1) 190
exercise guidelines for, (V1) 822*b*
grief in, (V1) 350
growth of, (V1) 189
health problems of, (V1) 189–191
health promotion for, (V1) 1101*t*
home poisoning risks for, (V1) 549
interventions for, (V1) 193–194
nutrition for, (V1) 684
oral sex among, (V1) 181
overweight/obesity in, (V1) 190–191
physical examination of, (V1) 487
pregnancy in, (V1) 191, (V1) 1097
pulmonary system in, (V1) 939–940
risky sexual behaviors by, (V1) 191
safety needs of, (V1) 548
sensory perception in, (V1) 774
sexuality of, (V1) 853–854
sexually transmitted infections in, (V1) 191
sleep for, (V1) 881, (V1) 881*t*, (V1) 885
stressors of, (V1) 242*b*
substance abuse by, (V1) 189
suicide by, (V1) 190
surgery and, (V1) 1028
tobacco use by, (V1) 190
web-based social networking among, (V1) 181
Adult(s)
bowel elimination in, (V1) 748
cohabiting, (V1) 288
exercise guidelines for, (V1) 822*b*
grief in, (V1) 350
middle, (V1) 196–200. *See also* Middle adult(s)
nutrition for, (V1) 684
obesity in, (V1) 826
older, (V1) 201–202, (V2) 72–75. *See also* Older adult(s)
safety needs of, (V1) 548
self-concept formation in, (V1) 264
sensory perception in, (V1) 774
skin of, (V1) 899
sleep for, (V1) 881, (V1) 881*t*, (V1) 885
young, (V1) 194–196. *See also* Young adult(s)
Advance directives, (V1) 355, (V1) 1165–1166
autonomy and, (V1) 1149
full-spectrum nursing model applied to, (V2) 89
informing patients about, (V1) 1161
Advanced practice nurses (APNs), expanded roles for, (V1) 28
Advice, offering, as barrier to therapeutic communication, (V1) 477
Advocacy, guidelines for, (V2) 899
Advocate, client
community nurse as, (V1) 1118
in ethical situations, (V1) 1160–1161
home health nurse as, (V1) 1127
Aerobic conditioning, (V1) 821
Aerobic exercise, (V1) 821
Aerosol foam, (V1) 611*t*
Aerosol spray, (V1) 611*t*
application of, (V2) 430*p*
Aerosol sprayers, (V1) 639
Aerosols, (V1) 612*t*
Aesthetic needs, (V1) 54
Afebrile, (V1) 425
Affective learning, (V1) 399*t*, (V1) 400
Affective responses. *See* Psychological responses
Affordable Care Act, (V1) 1065
African Americans
hair care for, (V1) 596–597
healers and practices of, (V1) 311*t*
pain perception and responses in, (V2) 127
values and health/illness beliefs of, (V1) 314*t*
Against medical advice, (V1) 1173
Age
in health-illness, (V1) 225
pharmacokinetics and, (V1) 617, (V1) 618*t*
population vulnerability and, (V1) 1116
surgery and, (V1) 1028
Age groups
distribution of, migration and, (V1) 202–203
as percentage of total population, (V1) 203, (V1) 203*f*
Ageism, (V1) 211–212
Agency for Health Care Policy and Research (AHCPR), pain-assessment approach by, (V1) 798–799, (V1) 799*b*
Agency for Healthcare Research and Quality (AHRQ), infection guidelines of, (V1) 518
Agglutination, in humoral immunity, (V1) 525
Aggregate(s)
of individuals, (V1) 115, (V1) 1115
of information, (V1) 1088
Aggressive communication, (V1) 468
Aging, (V1) 202–206
life expectancy and, (V1) 202
life-span perspective on, (V1) 203–204
perspectives on, (V1) 202–204
in place and alternatives, (V1) 204–205
sensory function changes with, (V1) 774*t*
theories of, (V1) 205–206
Agonist-antagonists, (V1) 806
Agonists, mu, (V1) 806
Air embolus, intravenous therapy and, (V1) 1015*t*
Air pollution, (V1) 940–941
reducing, (V1) 568
as safety hazard, (V1) 551
Air quality, (V1) 940–941
Airborne infection transmission, (V1) 521
Airborne precautions, (V2) 340–341
Airway, (V1) 935, (V1) 936*f*
artificial, (V1) 957–958, (V1) 966*p*. *See also* Mechanical ventilation
endotracheal, (V1) 957–958, (V1) 958*f*, (V2) 763
suctioning for, (V1) 960, (V1) 964–965*p*, (V2) 744–745*p*
ineffective clearance of, (V1) 951
chest physiotherapy for, (V1) 955, (V1) 955*f*, (V1) 963–964*p*, (V2) 728–730*p*
interventions and outcomes for, (V1) 2
preoperative, (V1) 1033
inflammation of, (V1) 944
lower, (V1) 935, (V1) 936*f*
suctioning of, (V1) 960, (V1) 964–965*p*
nasopharyngeal, (V1) 957, (V1) 957*f*, (V1) 966*p*, (V2) 760–761*p*
obstruction of, (V1) 944. *See also* Sleep apnea
in toddlers, (V1) 939
oropharyngeal, (V1) 957, (V1) 957*f*, (V1) 966*p*, (V2) 759–760*p*
postoperative, (V1) 1046
resistance of, (V1) 938
suctioning of, (V1) 959–960, (V1) 964–965*p*
upper, (V1) 935, (V1) 936*f*
suctioning of, (V1) 960, (V1) 965*p*, (V2) 749–751*p*
Alarm, infusion pump, (V1) 1011
Alarm stage, of general adaptation syndrome, (V1) 244–246
Albinism, (V1) 491
Albumin, serum levels of, nutritional levels and, (V1) 695
Alcohol
abuse of, (V1) 1097
cardiovascular effects of, (V1) 973
sexual function and, (V1) 858*t*
sleep and, (V1) 886
surgery and, (V1) 1029
teratogenic effects of, (V1) 171
use of
by adolescents, (V1) 190
health-illness and, (V1) 226
nutrition and, (V1) 686
treatment for, family support and, (V1) 297
Alcoholism, nutrition in, (V1) 689
Aldosterone, (V1) 988
in stress response, (V1) 245, (V1) 246*f*
Alert, description of, (V1) 507
Alginate dressing, (V1) 925*t*
Algor mortis, (V1) 367
Alkali, (V1) 989
Alkalosis, (V1) 991, (V1) 996
metabolic, (V1) 996, (V1) 997*t*
respiratory, (V1) 996, (V1) 997*t*
Allen's test, (V2) 271*p*
Allergic reactions, to medications, (V1) 620, (V1) 621*f*
Allergy/allergic reaction
cardiovascular effects of, (V1) 972
drug, in medication administration record, (V1) 387
food, bowel elimination and, (V1) 750–751
iodine, (V2) 787
latex, (V1) 1033, (V2) 849
pulmonary effects of, (V1) 940
in school-age child, assessment of, (V1) 186
shellfish, (V2) 787
surgery and, (V1) 1030
testing for, (V1) 948
transfusion, (V1) 1021*t*, (V2) 807*p*
Alopecia, (V1) 492, (V1) 596
Alopecia areata, (V1) 492, (V2) 313*f*
Alpha-linolenic acid, (V1) 673
Alpha waves, (V1) 882
Alternative care provider, on healthcare team, (V1) 20
Alternative healing, (V1) 313–315, (V1) 314*t*
definition of, (V1) 315
Alternatives
considering, in critical thinking, (V1) 35*t*, (V1) 36
exploring, in critical thinking, (V1) 35*t*, (V1) 36, (V2) 12
Altitude
cardiovascular effects of, (V1) 972
oxygen pressure and, (V1) 941
pulmonary effects of, (V1) 941
Altruism, as nursing value, (V1) 1146*t*
Aluets, healers and practices of, (V1) 311*t*

Alveolar-capillary gas exchange, (V1) 938, (V1) 938*f*
Alveolar-capillary membrane disorders, (V1) 944
Alveolar cells, (V1) 936, (V1) 937*f*
Alveoli, (V1) 936
Alzheimer's disease, (V1) 211. *See also* Dementia
Amblyopia, (V1) 495
Ambulation
  assisting with, (V1) 842*p*, (V1) 844–846, (V1) 845*f*, (V2) 632–634*p*
  mechanical aids for, (V1) 845–846, (V2) 639–640
Ambulatory care centers, (V1) 17, (V1) 17*f*
American Hospital Association (AHA)
  Patient Care Partnership of, (V1) 1153, (V1) 1154*b*, (V1) 1168–1169
  on teaching responsibilities, (V1) 398
American Nurses Association (ANA), (V1) 14
  Code of Ethics for Nurses of, (V1) 1152, (V1) 1153*b*, (V1) 1168
  on cultural competence, (V1) 315
  infection guidelines of, (V1) 518
  model of, for quality assurance, (V1) 25–26
  Nurses' Bill of Rights of, (V1) 1169
  nursing definition of, (V1) 7–8
  recommendations of, for healthcare reform, (V1) 24
  on safety, (V1) 546
  standards of care of, (V1) 12*t*, (V1) 1153, (V1) 1153*b*
  standards of clinical nursing practice of, (V1) 12, (V1) 13*t*
  standards of practice of, (V1) 1169
    for assessment, (V1) 45, (V1) 45*b*
    for diagnosis, (V1) 60*b*
    for evaluation, (V1) 130*b*
    for implementation, (V1) 121*b*
    for outcomes and planning, (V1) 86*b*
    for research utilization, (V1) 151
    for teaching responsibilities, (V1) 397
  standards of professional performance of, (V1) 13*t*
American Nurses Credentialing Centers (ANCC), Magnet Recognition Program of, (V1) 1059
Americans with Disabilities Act (ADA), (V1) 1166–1167
  Amendments Act of 2008, (V1) 294
Amino acids
  essential, (V1) 670, (V1) 670*t*
  nonessential, (V1) 670, (V1) 670*t*
Amphiarthroses, (V1) 818
Ampule(s), (V1) 643*f*
  drawing up medications from, (V1) 643, (V1) 657*p*, (V2) 435–436*p*
  mixing medication from vial and, (V2) 441*p*
ANA. *See* American Nurses Association (ANA)
Anabolism, definition of, (V1) 668
Anaerobic exercise, (V1) 821
Anal intercourse, (V1) 862
Anal sphincters, (V1) 747, (V1) 747*f*
  surgery on, bowel elimination and, (V1) 750
Analgesia
  intraspinal, (V1) 808–809, (V1) 809*f*
  patient-controlled, (V1) 809, (V1) 809*p*, (V2) 611–614*p*
  postoperative, (V1) 1047
  single-use anesthetic pump for, (V1) 1047, (V1) 1052
Analgesics, (V1) 804–809, (V1) 805*b*
  around-the-clock dosing for, (V1) 804–805
  endogenous, (V1) 794
  nonopioid, (V1) 805–806, (V1) 805*b*
  opioid, (V1) 806–807, (V1) 807*b*
    patient-controlled, (V1) 809, (V1) 809*p*, (V2) 611–614*p*
    preoperative, (V1) 1037*t*
  WHO three-step ladder for, (V1) 804, (V1) 804*f*
Analysis. *See* Diagnostic reasoning
Analytical reading, in evaluating quality of research, (V1) 157, (V1) 157*b*
Analyzing assumptions, in critical thinking, (V1) 35*t*, (V1) 36
Anaphylactic reactions, to medications, (V1) 620
Anaphylaxis, slow reacting substance of, (V1) 940
Androgyny, (V1) 851
Andropause, (V1) 197
Anemia, (V1) 976
Aneroid manometers, (V1) 449, (V1) 449*f*
Anesthesia
  bowel elimination and, (V1) 750
  complications of, nursing diagnosis for, (V1) 1042–1043
  epidural, (V1) 1041, (V1) 1042*f*
  general, (V1) 1040
  local, (V1) 1041
    for pain, (V1) 810
  malignant hyperthermia with, (V1) 1040
  peripheral nerve block for, (V1) 1041
  recovery from, (V1) 1045–1046, (V1) 1046*b*
  regional, (V1) 1041
  spinal, 1042*f*, (V1) 1041
  topical, (V1) 1041
    for pain, (V1) 810
  urinary function and, (V1) 720
Anesthesiologist, (V1) 1039
Angel of mercy image of nurse, (V1) 5
Anger
  management of, in stress management, (V1) 258
  in response to stress, (V1) 249
  as stage of dying, (V1) 353*b*
Angina pectoris, (V1) 975
Angiocaths, (V1) 1005
Angiogram, (V2) 767
Angiotensin II, (V1) 988
Angry clients, dealing with, (V2) 93–94*b*
Anhedonia, in depression, (V1) 279
Anilingus, (V1) 862
Animals, pathogens carried by, (V1) 551
  avoiding, (V1) 565
Anions, (V1) 984
Anisocoria, (V1) 494
Ankle, range of motion in, (V2) 646
Ankle-brachial index, (V2) 271*p*
Ankylosing spondylitis, (V1) 828
Ankylosis, (V1) 831
Anorexia nervosa, (V1) 704
  in adolescents, (V1) 190
Anosomia, (V1) 779
Antacids, bowel elimination and, (V1) 749
Antagonistic drug relationship, (V1) 621
Antalgic gait, (V1) 833
Anterior and posterior triangles, (V1) 497
Anterior chamber, inspection of, (V2) 243*p*
Anthropometric measurements, in body composition assessment, (V1) 692–693
Anti-incontinence devices, for urinary incontinence, (V1) 737
Anti-inflammatories, skin effects of, (V1) 900
Antianxiety agents
  preoperative, (V1) 1037*t*
  sexual function and, (V1) 858*t*
Antibiotics
  bowel elimination and, (V1) 749
  overuse of, for upper respiratory infections, (V1) 951–952
  preoperative, (V1) 1036–1037, (V1) 1037*t*
  prophylactic, (V1) 1036–1037
  skin effects of, (V1) 900
  surgery and, (V1) 1030*b*
Anticholesterol medications, (V1) 981
Anticholinergics
  for overactive bladder, (V1) 719
  preoperative, (V1) 1037*t*
  urinary retention from, (V1) 722*b*
Anticoagulants
  skin effects of, (V1) 900
  subcutaneous administration of, clinical insight on, (V2) 476*b*
  surgery and, (V1) 1030*b*
Anticonvulsants, sexual function and, (V1) 858*t*
Antidepressants
  sexual function and, (V1) 858*t*
  for sleep, (V1) 895
  tricyclic, urinary retention from, (V1) 722*b*
  for urinary incontinence, (V1) 719
Antidiuretic hormone (ADH), (V1) 988
  in stress response, (V1) 245, (V1) 246*f*
Antidysrhythmics, surgery and, (V1) 1030*b*
Antiembolism stockings, (V1) 980, (V1) 1054*p*, (V2) 829–832*p*
  postoperative use of, (V1) 1052–1053
  preoperative use of, (V1) 1037–1038, (V1) 1037*f*
Antihistamines
  preoperative, (V1) 1037*t*
  sexual function and, (V1) 858*t*
  urinary retention from, (V1) 722*b*
Antihypertensives
  sexual function and, (V1) 858*t*
  surgery and, (V1) 1030*b*
Antimicrobial dressing, (V1) 925*t*
Antimotility drugs, bowel elimination and, (V1) 749
Antipyretic medications, (V1) 426
Antiseptics, wound care and, (V1) 921
Antispasmodics
  for overactive bladder, (V1) 719
  urinary retention from, (V1) 722*b*
Anuria, definition of, (V1) 725*b*
Anus, (V1) 747, (V1) 747*f*
  assessment of, (V1) 511, (V1) 514–515*p*, (V2) 305–306*p*
Anxiety, (V1) 267–269
  abnormal, (V1) 267–268
  analysis/nursing diagnosis for, (V1) 277–278
  assessment for, (V1) 277
    guide for, (V2) 106
  chest pain and, (V1) 977, (V1) 979

complementary and alternative medicine for, (V1) 283*b*
coping with, (V1) 268–269
defense mechanisms for, (V1) 269
fear *vs.*, (V1) 267
interventions/implementation for, planning, (V1) 278–279
levels of, (V1) 267, (V1) 268*t*
minimizing, for sensory deprivation, (V1) 784
normal, (V1) 267
outcomes/evaluation for, planning, (V1) 278
pain and, (V1) 795
postoperative, (V2) 852
preoperative, (V1) 1032, (V2) 846
relieving
for confused client, (V1) 788
in stress management, (V1) 257–258
in response to stress, (V1) 249
sleep and, (V1) 880
standardized nursing languages for, (V2) 109–110
urinary function and, (V1) 718
urinary retention from, (V1) 722
Anxiolytics, preoperative, (V1) 1037*t*
AORN (Association of periOperative Registered Nurses), (V1) 1026–1027
Apex, of heart, (V1) 968
Apgar scoring system, (V1) 175, (V2) 67
Aphasia, assessing for, (V1) 472
Aphthous ulcers, (V1) 497
Apical pulse, (V1) 438
assessment of, (V2) 195–196*p*
when to take, (V1) 438–439, (V1) 439*f*
Apical-radial pulse
deficit in, assessing for, (V2) 197–198
when to take, (V1) 439
Apnea, (V1) 444, (V1) 444*t*, (V1) 946
mixed, (V1) 889
sleep, (V1) 888–889, (V1) 941
APNs. *See* Advanced practice nurses (APNs)
Apothecary system, of medication measurement, (V1) 622, (V2) 482
Appeal, in litigation, (V1) 1176
Appearance
personal, in nonverbal communication, (V1) 463–464
in physical examination, (V1) 488
Appendix, (V1) 746
Appetite
loss of, impaired nutrition from, interventions for, (V1) 698
patient's, stimulating, (V1) 705
Approval, expressing, as barrier to therapeutic communication, (V1) 476–477
Aquathermia pads, (V1) 932, (V1) 933*f*, (V2) 708
Aqueous solutions, (V1) 612*t*, (V1) 613*t*
Arab heritage, pain perception and responses in, (V2) 127
Arbitration, in resolution of litigation, (V1) 1176
Archetype, cultural, (V1) 308
Arm board, (V2) 787
Arm exercises, (V2) 638
Aromatherapy, (V1) 779, (V1) 779*b*
Arousal
level of, determining, (V2) 285*p*
sexual, disorders of, (V1) 865–866
Arousal mechanism, (V1) 772–773
Art activities, engaging in, in stress management, (V1) 259
Arterial blood gases (ABGs), (V1) 949, (V2) 767
acid-base balance and, (V1) 996, (V1) 997*t*, (V1) 998
sampling of, (V1) 445
Arterial blood oxygen saturation (SaO_2), (V1) 948, (V2) 726–728
Arterial oxygen saturation, (V1) 445
Arterial ulcers, (V1) 903*t*, (V1) 909
Arterioles, (V1) 969
Arteriosclerosis, (V1) 447
Artery(ies), (V1) 969. *See also* Cardiovascular system
autonomic nervous system effects on, (V1) 970–971
brachial, for blood pressure assessment, (V1) 451
carotid, (V1) 503
coronary, (V1) 970, (V1) 970*f*
disease of, (V1) 975
sleep and, (V1) 890
peripheral, (V1) 504
size and compliance of, in blood pressure regulation, (V1) 447
tone of, (V1) 970
Arthritis, (V1) 827–828
rheumatoid, (V2) 314*f*
Articular cartilage, (V1) 818
Articulation, (V1) 817
Artificial eyes, caring for, (V1) 598, (V1) 599*f*, (V1) 601*p*, (V2) 397–398*p*
Ascites, (V1) 984
Ascorbic acid. *See* Vitamin C
Asepsis. *See also* Gloving/gloves; Gown; Hygiene; Sterile technique
definition of, (V1) 533
intravenous catheter, (V2) 813–814
medical
definition of, (V1) 533
environmental cleanliness in, (V1) 534–535
hand hygiene in, (V1) 533–534, (V1) 533*f*
promoting, (V1) 516–544, (V2) 317–347
surgical, (V1) 538–542
tracheostomy care, (V1) 958, (V2) 736–741
wound, (V1) 928
Asian Americans
healers and practices of, (V1) 311*t*
pain perception and responses in, (V2) 127
values and health/illness beliefs of, (V1) 314*t*
Asian diet, (V1) 689
Asphyxia, birth, (V1) 175
Asphyxiation, in home, risk factors for, (V1) 350
Aspiration (needle), wound, (V1) 916
Aspiration (physiological)
prevention of, (V1) 959–960, (V2) 762
risk for, (V1) 951, (V1) 954
intraoperative, (V1) 1043, (V2) 848
Aspirin, (V1) 805
bowel elimination and, (V1) 749
cardiovascular disease prevention and, (V1) 973
surgery and, (V1) 1030*b*
Assault, (V1) 1173
and battery, (V1) 1173
Assertive communication, (V1) 468–469, (V1) 469*b*
techniques for, (V2) 212*b*
Assertiveness, for enhancing therapeutic communication, (V1) 474
Assessment(s), (V2) 15–25. *See also* Evaluation; *specific organ or body part*
acid-base balance, (V1) 2
of adolescent, (V1) 191–193
for anxiety, (V1) 277
bedside
brief, (V1) 515*p*, (V2) 306–307*p*
of sensory function, (V2) 606
of blood pressure, (V1) 449–453
of bowel elimination, (V1) 753–755
of breathing patterns, (V1) 945–946
of cardiovascular system, (V1) 976–978
in fluid and electrolyte assessment, (V1) 999
central venous access device in, (V1) 2
for chest pain, (V1) 976–977
circulation, (V2) 776
of client environment, (V1) 601
in collaborative care, (V1) 44–45
of communication, (V1) 472
community, (V1) 50–51, (V1) 1123
comprehensive (global), (V1) 47–48, (V1) 48*f*
for cough, (V1) 946–947
cultural, (V1) 50, (V1) 318–320
data sources in, (V1) 46, (V1) 47*t*
definition of, (V1) 44
delegation of, (V1) 45–46
for depression, (V1) 279–280, (V1) 281*b*
in discharge planning, (V1) 87
documentation of, (V1) 378
of dying patient, (V1) 357
for dyspnea, (V1) 946
electrolyte, (V1) 998–1001
for ethical decisions, (V1) 1154–1155
exercise, (V1) 832–834
of eyes, (V1) 597
failure to perform, malpractice claims for, (V1) 1177
for fall risk, (V1) 557–558
family, (V1) 50, (V1) 295–298
for fatigue, (V1) 977
of feet, (V1) 588
fluid, (V1) 998–1001
fluids and electrolytes, (V1) 999, (V2) 815–817
focused, (V1) 48–49
functional ability, (V1) 49–50, (V1) 50*b*
of grief and loss, (V1) 357, (V2) 153–154
guidelines and tools for
Discharge Planning Form as, (V2) 34
Instrumental Activities of Daily Living as, (V2) 18
Nursing Admission Data Form as, (V2) 19–22
of hair, (V1) 596
health, (V1) 479–515, (V2) 219–316. *See also* Health assessment
of health and illness, (V1) 233–234
health history in, (V1) 51–53, (V1) 52*t*
in health promotion, (V1) 233–234, (V1) 1102–1104
in home healthcare, (V1) 1131
implementation and, (V1) 120–121
of infant, (V1) 178

of infection and infection prevention, (V1) 529
initial (admission), (V1) 47
intake and output, (V1) 1000, (V2) 810–811
intraoperative, (V1) 1042
knowledge map for, (V2) 25
learning, (V1) 407–408
medication-related, (V1) 628
of middle adult, (V1) 198
mobility, (V2) 641–642
of mucous membranes, in fluid and electrolyte evaluation, (V1) 999
of nails, (V1) 589
of neonate, (V1) 175
of neurological system, in fluid and electrolyte assessment, (V1) 999
nursing, (V1) 481
in nursing process, (V1) 38, (V1) 38*f*, (V1) 43–58, (V2) 15–25
nutritional, (V1) 50, (V1) 691–695
of older adult, (V1) 212–215
ongoing, (V1) 47, (V1) 481
of oral cavity, (V1) 592
oxygenation, (V1) 945–947, (V2) 765–766
pain, (V2) 616–618
for pain, (V1) 50, (V1) 798–800
perioperative, (V1) 1032, (V2) 841–845
peripheral circulation, (V1) 977, (V2) 776
physical, (V1) 481–487. *See also* Physical examination
physical fitness/activity, (V1) 832–834
postoperative, (V1) 1046
preoperative, (V1) 1031–1032
of preschooler, (V1) 184
for pressure ulcer, (V1) 912–813, (V1) 917–918
professional standards for, (V1) 45, (V1) 45*b*
psychosocial, (V1) 50, (V1) 270–271
of pulmonary system, (V1) 945–949
of pulse, (V1) 437–440
purpose of, (V1) 44
reflecting critically about, (V1) 56–57
relation of, to other nursing process steps, (V1) 44, (V1) 44*f*
of respirations, (V1) 443–446, (V1) 946
in fluid and electrolyte evaluation, (V1) 999
safety
for fall prevention, (V2) 357*p*
S.A.S. Safety Assessment Scale as, (V2) 358
of school-age child, (V1) 186–187
of self-concept and self-esteem, (V1) 273–274
of sensory perception, (V1) 780–782
sexual health, (V1) 866–867, (V2) 656–657
of skin, (V1) 581, (V1) 913, (V2) 709–710
for fluid and electrolyte assessment, (V1) 999
for surgery, (V1) 1044
sleep, (V1) 891
special needs, (V1) 49–51
spiritual health, (V1) 50
of spirituality, (V1) 337–338
sputum, (V1) 946–947, (V2) 767
stress, (V1) 2
of stress and adaptation, (V1) 255–256
system-specific, (V1) 481
of temperature, (V1) 427–431. *See also* Temperature, assessment of
of toddler, (V1) 181
types of, (V1) 47–51
of urinary elimination, (V1) 723–726
wellness, (V1) 50
wound, (V1) 913, (V2) 709–710
of young adult, (V1) 196
Assignments, accepting, qualifications for, in minimizing malpractice risks, (V1) 1182
Assimilation
in cognitive development, (V1) 167
cultural, (V1) 306
Assistants, power of, (V1) 1066
Assisted living facilities (ALFs), (V1) 17, (V1) 205
Assisted suicide, (V1) 355–356
Associate degree, research and, (V1) 152
Associate degree nursing program, (V1) 10
Association of periOperative Registered Nurses (AORN), (V1) 1026–1027
Assumptions
analyzing, in critical thinking, (V1) 35*t*, (V1) 36
of nursing theory, (V1) 139
Asthma, (V1) 940
childhood, (V1) 186
teaching about, (V1) 187–188
peak flow monitoring and, (V1) 949, (V1) 950*f*
sleep and, (V1) 890
Astigmatism, definition of, (V1) 777*b*
Atelectasis, (V1) 939, (V1) 944, (V1) 1048*t*
Atheism, (V1) 335
Athletic performance, eating for, (V1) 687
Atomizers, (V1) 639
Atria, (V1) 968, (V1) 968*f*
Atrial natriuretic peptide (ANP), (V1) 988
Atrioventricular node, (V1) 969, (V1) 969*f*
Atrophy, (V1) 833*b*
Attitudes
critical thinking, (V1) 31–32
moral decisions and, (V1) 1144
Attuning, in communication, (V1) 233
Audio-recorded report, (V1) 390
Audiovisual media
reduced use of, for sensory overload, (V1) 785
for sensory deprivation, (V1) 784
Audit trail, (V1) 1089
Auscultation
of abdomen, (V1) 505, (V2) 273–274*p*
of blood pressure, (V1) 451–453
with palpation, (V1) 453
of blood vessels, (V2) 268*p*
of chest, (V2) 263–264*p*
of heart, (V1) 502–503
sites for, (V1) 502*f*, (V1) 502*t*
of lung, (V1) 976
performing, (V2) 309*p*
in physical examination, (V1) 485–486
of pulse, (V1) 437
Auscultatory gap, (V1) 453
Authoritarian leadership, (V1) 1058
Authority
in gaining knowledge, (V1) 152
power of, (V1) 1066
Authority gradient, (V1) 1068
Autocratic leadership, (V1) 1058
Autoimmune reaction theory of aging, (V1) 206
Autologous blood donation, (V1) 1020
Autolysis, (V1) 923
Automated Dispensing Cabinets (ADCs), in medication error prevention, (V1) 627
Automated dispensing system, for medications, (V1) 608
Automaticity, of heart, (V1) 969
Autonomic nervous system, (V1) 818
cardiovascular effects of, (V1) 970–971
Autonomous actions, (V1) 107
Autonomy
as ethical concept, (V1) 1149–1150
as nursing value, (V1) 1146*t*
in resolving dilemma, (V1) 1158
versus shame and doubt stage of psychosocial development, (V1) 168
Autonomy model, for discussing dilemma, (V1) 1160
Autopsy, (V1) 356
Avatars, (V1) 1082
Avoidance
change-related, (V1) 1070
of stressors, (V1) 250*t*
Awareness, contextual, in critical thinking, (V1) 34, (V1) 35*t*, (V2) 12
Axillae, assessment of, (V1) 498, (V1) 498*f*, (V2) 258*p*, (V2) 259*p*, (V2) 513*p*
Axillary temperature, assessment of, (V2) 186*p*
Ayurveda, (V1) 315
health described by, (V1) 223*b*
Ayurvedic medicine, (V1) 333

B

B cells, (V1) 525
Babinski reflex, (V1) 174
Baby-bottle tooth decay, (V1) 591
Baccalaureate degree in nursing, research and, (V1) 152
Baccalaureate degree nursing program, (V1) 10
Back injury
in healthcare workers, (V1) 556
prevention of, (V1) 825
in nurse, (V1) 836
Back massage, (V1) 893*p*, (V2) 664–665*p*
following bath, (V1) 582
Bacteria, urinary, (V2) 563
Bag bath, (V1) 583
Balance, (V1) 820
assessment of, (V1) 506, (V2) 280*p*
Bandages, (V1) 929, (V1) 931*p*, (V2) 699–703*p*. *See also* Dressing (wound)
circular turns for, (V2) 700
cloth, (V1) 929
elastic, (V1) 931
figure-8 turns for, (V2) 701
gauze, (V1) 929, (V1) 931
recurrent turns for, (V2) 701
rolled, (V1) 931
spiral turns for, (V2) 700–701
Barbiturates
preoperative, (V1) 1037*t*
for sleep, (V1) 895
Barcoding, for medications, (V1) 1084
Bargaining, as stage of dying, (V1) 353*b*

Bariatric surgery, nutrition and, (V1) 689–690
Barium enema, in GI tract studies, (V2) 595
Baroreceptors, (V1) 971
Barrel chest, (V1) 499, (V1) 500*f*
Bartholin's glands, palpation of, (V2) 302–303*p*
Basal metabolic rate (BMR), (V1) 424, (V1) 680
  calculating, (V1) 680*b*
  factors affecting, (V1) 680
Base, (V1) 989
  of support, (V1) 820, (V1) 820*f*
Basin and water bath, (V1) 583, (V2) 370–371*p*
Basin and water shampooing of hair, (V2) 385–387*p*
Bath/bathing, (V1) 600*p*
  for adult patient, guidelines for, (V1) 584*b*
  "assist," (V1) 582
  bag, (V1) 583
  basin and water, (V1) 583, (V2) 370–371*p*
  bed, (V1) 583
  complete, (V1) 582, (V2) 364–369*p*
  for dementia patients, (V1) 585
    clinical insights on, (V2) 402
  for morbidly obese patient, (V1) 585–586, (V1) 586*t*
  for older adults, (V1) 587
  partial, (V1) 582
  perineal care in, (V1) 584
  with prepackaged products, (V1) 583, (V2) 364–369*p*
  pressure ulcer prevention and, (V1) 918
  purposes of, (V1) 582
  sitz, (V1) 932, (V1) 932*f*
  therapeutic, (V1) 584, (V1) 932, (V1) 932*f*
  towel, (V1) 583, (V2) 369–370*p*
  tub, (V1) 584, (V1) 585*f*
    assisting with, clinical insights on, (V2) 401
  type of, (V1) 582–584
  water for, (V1) 583
  for wound, (V1) 918, (V2) 708, (V2) 709
Battery, (V1) 1173
Battle-ax image of nurse, (V1) 5
BE A.L.E.R.T. safety campaign, (V1) 705, (V1) 706*b*
Beard care, (V1) 597, (V1) 600*p*, (V2) 387–388*p*
Bed(s)
  adjustable, (V1) 836
  client moving in/from. *See* Position/positioning, bed for
  hospital, (V1) 602–603, (V1) 602*f*
    mattresses and linens for, (V1) 603
    monitoring devices for, use of, (V1) 573*p*, (V2) 350–351*p*
  leg exercises in, (V1) 1054*p*, (V2) 826–827*p*, (V2) 828–829*p*
  linens for, (V1) 918
  making, (V1) 603
    when occupied, (V1) 601*p*, (V2) 394–396*p*
    when unoccupied, (V1) 601*p*, (V2) 392–394*p*
  siderails for, (V1) 836
  support surfaces for, (V1) 919
Bed bath, (V1) 583
Bedpan
  placing and removing, (V1) 769*p*, (V2) 572–574*p*
  urine output measurement from, (V2) 532*p*
Bedrest, (V1) 830
  prevention of complications of, (V1) 832*b*
Bedside
  checking feeding tube placement at, (V1) 709
  urine testing at, (V2) 538–539*p*
Bedside assessment
  brief, (V1) 515*p*, (V2) 306–307*p*
  of sensory function, (V2) 606
Bedside report, (V1) 390
Bedsores. *See* Pressure ulcer(s)
Bedwetting, nocturnal, (V1) 890
Behavior(s)
  change in, for health promotion, (V1) 1099
  in depression, (V1) 279
  illness, stages of, (V1) 230–231
  inappropriate, (V1) 871
  moral, (V1) 1138
  nonverbal, in enhancing communication, (V2) 211*b*
  in physical examination, (V1) 488
  sick role, (V1) 230
  violent. *See* Violence
Behavioral interventions, for urinary incontinence, (V1) 736
Behavioral responses
  to stress, assessing, (V1) 255
  to stressors, (V1) 248*b*
Behavioral theory, of leadership, (V1) 1058
Behavioral therapy, for pain, (V1) 802–803
Being with, in caring, (V1) 39
Belief(s)
  health
    in health promotion assessment, (V1) 1103
    and illness, (V1) 310, (V1) 312*f*
  moral decisions and, (V1) 1144
  refutation of, for change, (V1) 1070
  spiritual. *See* Spirituality
Bell's palsy, face in, (V2) 237*f*
Belonging needs, (V1) 147, (V1) 147*f*
Beneficence
  as ethical concept, (V1) 1150–1151
  in resolving dilemma, (V1) 1158
Benner, Patricia, (V1) 139
  model of development of expertise of, (V1) 11–12
  nursing theory of, (V1) 145, (V1) 146*t*
Benner's "Novice to Expert," (V1) 139
Benzodiazepines, for sleep, (V1) 894–895
Bereavement. *See* Grief
Beta-adrenergic blocking agents, (V1) 974*t*, (V1) 981
Beta waves, (V1) 882
Beverages
  bedtime, (V1) 894
  sugary, (V1) 973
Bias
  as barrier to culturally competent care, (V1) 316
  in diagnostic reasoning, (V1) 72
Bicarbonate, (V1) 989, (V1) 991*t*
Biceps reflex, testing, (V2) 293*p*
Bicultural, (V1) 305
Bier (intravenous) block, (V1) 1041
Bile salts, in feces, (V1) 747
Bilirubin
  excess, in neonatal jaundice, (V1) 175
  urinary, (V2) 563
Bill of Rights, (V1) 1164
  Nurses', (V1) 1169
Binders, (V1) 928–929, (V1) 930–931*p*, (V2) 697–699*p*
Bioengineered skin, (V1) 920
Bioethics, definition of, (V1) 1139
Biofeedback
  in stress management, (V1) 259
  for urinary incontinence, (V1) 736
Biographical data, in nursing health history, (V1) 52*t*
Biological clocks, (V1) 881
Biological factors, in healing-illness, (V1) 224–225
Biological half-life, of drug, (V1) 617
Biological hazards, in healthcare facility, (V1) 555
Biological variations
  assessing for, (V2) 126
  culture and, (V1) 309
Biopsy, wound, (V1) 916
Biorhythms, (V1) 881
Bioterrorism, minimizing effects of, (V1) 543
Biotransformation, of drugs, (V1) 615
Biot's respirations, (V1) 444*t*, (V1) 946
Birth asphyxia, (V1) 175
Birth control pills. *See* Oral contraceptives (V1)
Birth defects, screening for, (V1) 172
Birth injuries, (V1) 175
Birthmarks, (V1) 491
Bisexuals, (V1) 852–853
Black heritage. *See* African Americans
Bladder
  irrigation of, (V1) 734*p*, (V1) 735, (V2) 553–556*p*
  neurogenic, (V1) 720
  overactive, (V1) 722
    medications for, (V1) 719
  in urine storage, (V1) 717
Bladder training, for urinary incontinence, (V1) 736, (V2) 558
Blastocyst, (V1) 170
Bleeding. *See also* Hemorrhage(s)
  external, (V1) 906
  internal, (V1) 906
  negative pressure wound therapy and, (V2) 685–690
  postoperative, (V1) 1049*t*
  stoma, (V1) 2
  venipuncture and, (V1) 2
  wound, (V1) 906
Blindness. *See also* Vision
  color, (V1) 494
Blisters, (V2) 312*f*
Blogging, (V1) 1081
Blood
  autologous, (V1) 1020
  donation of, (V1) 1015, (V1) 1019
  fecal occult, testing for, (V1) 755, (V1) 769*p*, (V2) 570–572*p*
  flow of
    to area, drug absorption and, (V1) 614
    local, in drug distribution, (V1) 615
  glucose in. *See* Blood glucose
  loss of. *See* Bleeding; Hemorrhage
    pulse and, (V2) 437
  pH of, (V1) 2
  transfusion of. *See* Blood transfusion
  typing and crossmatching of, (V1) 1019–1020, (V1) 1019*t*, (V2) 845
  viscosity of, in blood pressure regulation, (V1) 447
  volume of, in blood pressure regulation, (V1) 447
  whole, (V1) 1020

Blood clot. *See* Embolus; Thrombus
Blood gases, (V1) 949
  interpretation of, (V1) 2
Blood glucose, preoperative, (V1) 2
Blood glucose levels
  fingerstick, checking, (V1) 712*p*, (V2) 494–499*p*
  nutritional status and, (V1) 694–695
Blood groups, (V1) 1019, (V1) 1019*t*
Blood pressure (BP), (V1) 446–457
  adult, classification of, (V1) 447*t*
  assessment of, (V1) 449–453, (V2) 201–203*p*
    auscultation in, (V1) 451–453
    delegation of, (V2) 200
    direct, (V1) 449
    documentation of, (V2) 203
    ensuring accuracy of, (V1) 452*b*, (V2) 204
    equipment for, (V1) 449–451, (V1) 449*f*, (V1) 450*f*, (V2) 200
    in home care, (V2) 203
    indirect, (V1) 449
    palpation in, (V1) 453
      with auscultation, (V1) 453
    patient teaching of, (V2) 203
    site for, (V1) 451
  factors influencing, (V1) 448–449
  in fluid and electrolyte assessment, (V1) 999–1000
  lowering, alternative therapies for, (V1) 455*b*
  monitors of, electronic, (V1) 450
  normal, (V1) 422*t*, (V1) 446, (V1) 447*t*
  nursing diagnoses related to, (V1) 453–454
  orthostatic, (V1) 831, (V1) 993
  regulation of, (V1) 446–447
  self-monitoring of, teaching client, (V1) 450–451*b*
  spinal anesthesia effects on, (V1) 1041
Blood pressure cuff(s), (V1) 450*f*
  bladder sizes for, (V1) 452*t*
  size of, correct, determining, (V1) 450–451, (V1) 451*f*, (V2) 204
Blood pressure medications, skin effects of, (V1) 900
Blood studies, in renal function assessment, (V1) 726
Blood transfusion, (V1) 1015, (V1) 1018*p*, (V1) 1019–1020
  administration of, (V2) 804–808*p*
  autologous, (V1) 1020
  evidence-based studies on, (V1) 1022
  initiation of, (V1) 1020
  reaction to, (V1) 1018*p*, (V1) 1020, (V1) 1021*t*
  typing and crossmatching for, (V1) 1019–1020, (V1) 1019*t*, (V2) 845
  verifications for, (V1) 2
Blood urea nitrogen (BUN)
  in renal function assessment, (V1) 726
  in urinary elimination assessment, (V2) 563
Blood vessels. *See* Artery(ies); Capillaries; Vein(s)
  assessment of, (V1) 503–504, (V1) 514*p*, (V2) 265–271*p*
  central, (V1) 503–504, (V1) 503*f*
  networks of, (V1) 501
  peripheral, (V1) 504
Bloodborne pathogen exposure, instructions following, (V1) 54*b*, (V1) 542–543
BMI. *See* Body mass index (BMI)
Body
  mechanics of, (V2) 635
  shape and symmetry of, (V1) 506
Body alignment, (V1) 819
  assessment of, (V2) 641
Body composition
  analysis of, (V1) 682
  assessment of, (V1) 692–694
  basal metabolic rate and, (V1) 680
  evaluation of, measuring circumferences in, (V2) 515*p*
Body function, teaching about, (V1) 868–869
Body image
  actual, (V1) 265
  appearance and, (V1) 265
  disturbed, (V1) 274
    as etiology, (V1) 274–275
    as problem, (V1) 274
    sexuality and, (V1) 868
    wound and, (V1) 917
  function influencing, (V1) 265
  gradual changes in, (V1) 265
  ideal, (V1) 265
  influence of, on health, (V1) 266
  perceived, (V1) 265
  positive, promoting, (V1) 276
  in self-concept, (V1) 265–266
  sudden changes in, (V1) 265
Body language, interpreting, for enhancing therapeutic communication, (V1) 475
Body mass, pharmacokinetics and, (V1) 617
Body mass index (BMI)
  in body composition assessment, (V1) 693
  calculating, (V1) 693*b*
  in older adult assessment, (V1) 212
  in physical examination, (V1) 488–489
  of school-age child, assessment of, (V1) 186–187
Body mechanics, (V1) 819–820
  guidelines for, (V1) 820
  principles of, (V2) 635
Body piercings, (V1) 901
Body position, blood pressure and, (V1) 448
Body system framework, for assessment data, (V1) 54
Body systems
  functions of, differentiation of, (V1) 164–165
  growth rates for, (V1) 164
  review of, in nursing health history, (V1) 52*t*
Body temperature, (V1) 422–436. *See* Temperature
Body type, in physical examination, (V1) 488
Bone(s), (V1) 817, (V1) 817*f*
  disease of, (V1) 827
  fracture of, (V1) 828, (V1) 828*f*
  immobility effects on, (V1) 831
  osteoporosis in, (V1) 828
  tumors of, (V1) 828
Bone density scan, in older adult assessment, (V1) 213
Boots, (V1) 837
Borg Rate of Perceived Exertion Scale®, (V1) 822*b*
Borrowed servant doctrine, (V1) 1175
Botulinum toxin, for overactive bladder, (V1) 719
Boundaries, professional, in minimizing malpractice risks, (V1) 1182, (V1) 1182*b*
Bowel diversion, (V1) 751–752, (V1) 751*f*, (V1) 752*f*
  caring for patient with, (V1) 763–765
Bowel elimination, (V1) 744–770, (V2) 569–598
  activity level and, (V1) 749
  assessment of, (V1) 753–755
    guidelines for, (V2) 594
  developmental stage and, (V1) 748
  diverticulosis and, (V1) 751
  factors affecting, (V1) 748–751
  food allergies and, (V1) 750–751
  food intolerances and, (V1) 751
  hydration and, (V1) 749
  knowledge map on, (V2) 598
  medications and, (V1) 749, (V1) 749*b*
  nursing diagnoses related to, (V1) 756
  nursing interventions for, (V1) 756–763
  nursing outcomes for, (V1) 756
  nutrition and, (V1) 749
  pathological conditions and, (V1) 750–751
  personal factors affecting, (V1) 748–749
  pregnancy and, (V1) 750
  process of, (V1) 747–748
  sociocultural factors affecting, (V1) 748–749
  surgery/procedures and, (V1) 750
Bowel incontinence
  care map for, (V1) 768
  definition of, (V1) 756
  interventions for, (V1) 762–763
  nursing care plan for, (V1) 766–767
  skin integrity and, (V1) 918
Bowel preparation, (V1) 1036
Bowel sounds, auscultation of, (V1) 505, (V2) 274*p*
Bowel training, for bowel incontinence, (V1) 763
Bowlby, John, on grief, (V1) 347, (V1) 348*t*
Bowman's capsule, (V1) 715–716
Braces, (V1) 845–846
Brachial artery, for blood pressure assessment, (V1) 451
Brachial pulse, assessment of, (V2) 192*p*
Brachioradialis reflex, testing, (V2) 293*p*
Braden scale, (V1) 913, (V2) 711
Bradycardia, definition of, (V1) 440
Bradydysrhythmia, (V1) 978
Bradypnea, (V1) 444*t*, (V1) 946
Brain
  in breathing regulation, (V1) 938
  in pain modulation, (V1) 794, (V1) 795*f*
  sensory areas of, (V1) 773*f*
  in sleep regulation, (V1) 882–883
Brain natriuretic peptide (BNP), (V1) 988
Brain stem centers, in cardiovascular function, (V1) 971
Brain waves, (V1) 882–883, (V1) 883*f*
BRAT diet, for diarrhea, (V1) 759
Breach of duty, (V1) 1174
Breakthrough pain, (V1) 806
Breast(s)
  assessment of, (V1) 498, (V1) 498*f*, (V1) 513*p*, (V2) 257–259*p*
  cancer of
    prevention of, in young adults, interventions for, (V1) 196
    screening for, in health promotion assessment, (V1) 1104, (V2) 876

examination of, (V1) 869–970
clinical, (V1) 498
in older adult assessment, (V1) 213
self-examination of. *See* Breast self-examination (BSE)
Breast milk, in diarrhea management, (V1) 759
Breast self-examination (BSE), (V2) 67–68*p*
by adolescents, interventions for, (V1) 193–194
in older adult assessment, (V1) 213
patient teaching on, (V2) 259
teaching for, (V1) 869–870
Breath sounds, (V1) 445, (V1) 499–501, (V1) 501*f*, (V2) 264–265
absent, (V1) 946
adventitious, (V1) 500
diminished, (V1) 500, (V1) 946
misplaced, (V1) 500
Breathing. *See also* Respiration(s)
assessment of, (V1) 945–946
control of, (V1) 938–939
deep, (V1) 1054*p*, (V2) 826–827*p*, (V2) 829*p*
for secretion mobilization, (V1) 954
ineffective, (V1) 950
postoperative risk for, (V1) 1046
mechanics of, (V1) 442, (V1) 442*f*
periodic, in neonate, (V1) 173
sleep-related interruption in, (V1) 888–889
voluntary control of, (V1) 938
Brevity, in verbal communication, (V1) 462
Bricker's loop, (V1) 738
Bridge, (V1) 593
Bronchi, (V1) 935
Bronchial breath sounds, (V1) 499–500, (V1) 501*f*, (V2) 264
Bronchioles, (V1) 935
Bronchophony, (V1) 500, (V2) 264
Bronchoscopy, (V2) 767
Bronchospasm, (V1) 935
Bronchovesicular breath sounds, (V1) 500, (V1) 501*f*, (V2) 264
Bruits, in carotid arteries, (V1) 503
Bruxism, (V1) 890
BSE. *See* Breast self-examination (BSE)
Buccal administration of drugs, (V1) 611*t*
Buccal mucosa
assessment of, (V1) 497
medication administration by, (V1) 634–635
Buddhism, (V1) 333–334, (V1) 334*f*
Buffers, (V1) 989, (V1) 991
Bulimia nervosa, (V1) 704
in adolescents, (V1) 190
Bulking agents, (V1) 749*b*
Bunion, (V1) 587
Burnout, from failure of adaptive mechanisms, (V1) 254, (V1) 254*b*
Burns, (V1) 581
in home
causes of, (V1) 549
prevention of, (V1) 561–562
Bursae, (V1) 505, (V1) 506*f*
Business sense, in manager, (V1) 1061
Butterfly needle, (V1) 1005, (V1) 1005*f*
Butterfly (wing-tipped) catheter, (V1) 1005, (V1) 1005*f*, (V2) 785, (V2) 786

C

C fibers, (V1) 793*f*, (V1) 794
C-type natriuretic peptide (CNP), (V1) 988
Caffeine
nutrition and, (V1) 686
sleep and, (V1) 886
Calcium, (V1) 676, (V1) 677*t*, (V1) 827, (V1) 988–989, (V1) 990*t*
daily intake of, (V1) 992*t*
deficiency of, (V1) 988–989
imbalances in, (V1) 994–995*t*
in ovo-lacto vegetarian diet, (V1) 686
supplemental, (V1) 1002
Calcium channel blocking agents, (V1) 974*t*
Calculation skills, assessing, (V2) 286*p*
Calluses, (V1) 587
Calories, (V1) 679
for infants, (V1) 682
skin effects of, (V1) 899
Calyx(ces), (V1) 715, (V1) 715*f*
CAM. *See* Complementary and alternative medicine (CAM)
Cancer
breast
prevention of, in young adults, interventions for, (V1) 196
screening for, in health promotion assessment, (V1) 1104, (V2) 876
cervical, screening for, (V1) 511
in health promotion assessment, (V2) 876
in older adult assessment, (V1) 213
colon, screening for
in health promotion assessment, (V2) 876
in older adult assessment, (V1) 213
in middle adult, (V1) 198
prostate, screening for, in health promotion assessment, (V1) 1104, (V2) 876
sexuality and, (V1) 857
skin, screening for, in health promotion assessment, (V2) 876
testicular, screening for, in health promotion assessment, (V2) 876
Canes, (V1) 845, (V1) 845*f*, (V2) 639
Canker sores, (V1) 497
Cantor tube, (V2) 837
Capillaries, (V1) 969
Capillary blood glucose levels, checking, (V1) 712*p*, (V2) 494–499*p*
Capillary hemangioma, (V2) 312*f*
Capillary refill, assessing for, (V2) 236*p*, (V2) 271*p*
Capillary-tissue gas exchange, (V1) 938, (V1) 938*f*
Capitated costs, HMOs based on, (V1) 23
Capnography, (V1) 948
Capnometry test for feeding tube placement verification, (V1) 709, (V1) 710*f*
Capsule, (V1) 610*t*
timed-release, (V1) 610*t*
Captain of ship principle, (V1) 1175
Caput succedaneum, (V1) 175
Car safety seats, (V1) 566*t*
infant, interventions for, (V1) 179
Carbohydrates, (V1) 668, (V1) 669*t*, (V1) 670
sleep and, (V1) 886, (V1) 895
Carbon dioxide
excess of, (V1) 943*b*
low level of, (V1) 943
measurement of, (V1) 948, (V1) 949
partial pressure of, (V1) 949
transport of, (V1) 970
Carbon dioxide detector, (V1) 948
Carbon monoxide, (V1) 976
exposure to, in home, (V1) 549
interventions for, (V1) 560
Carbonic acid-sodium bicarbonate system, (V1) 989, (V1) 991
Cardiac arrest
exercise and, (V1) 823–824
in-hospital, (V1) 981
pain in, (V1) 798
resuscitation for, (V1) 981
Cardiac catheterization, (V2) 767
Cardiac cycle, (V1) 502, (V1) 968
Cardiac ischemia, (V1) 974–975
Cardiac monitoring, (V1) 977–978, (V1) 979*p*, (V2) 774–775*p*
Cardiac muscle, (V1) 818
Cardiac output
blood pressure and, (V1) 446–447
decrease in, (V1) 978
definition of, (V1) 436
Cardiac sphincter, (V1) 745
Cardioinhibitory center, (V1) 971
Cardiomyopathy, (V1) 974
Cardiopulmonary resuscitation, (V1) 981
"hands-only," (V1) 981–982
Cardiovascular system, (V1) 968–970. *See also* Artery(ies); Heart; Vein(s)
abnormalities of, (V1) 974–976
in adolescents, (V1) 971–972
age-related changes in, assessment for, (V1) 208*t*
in alarm stage, of stress response, (V1) 246, (V1) 246*f*
allergy effects on, (V1) 972
altitude effects on, (V1) 972
arteries of, (V1) 969, (V1) 970, (V1) 970*f*. *See also* Artery(ies)
arterioles of, (V1) 969
assessment of, (V1) 501–504, (V1) 976–978, (V2) 776
diagnostic testing in, (V1) 977–978, (V2) 777
dyspnea in, (V1) 977
fatigue in, (V1) 977
in fluid and electrolyte evaluation, (V1) 999
pain in, (V1) 976–977
peripheral circulation in, (V1) 977, (V2) 776
physical examination in, (V1) 976–977
risk factors in, (V1) 976
autonomic nervous system effects on, (V1) 970–971
blood vessels in, (V1) 503–504, (V1) 503*f*
brain stem center effects on, (V1) 971
capillaries of, (V1) 969
in children, (V1) 971
cigarette smoking effects on, (V1) 973
circulation promotion for, (V1) 979–980
clot prevention for, (V1) 980
cold effects on, (V1) 972
developmental stage and, (V1) 971–972
disease of, (V1) 974–976
sexuality and, (V1) 856
surgery and, (V1) 1029*b*
disorders of
from failure of adaptive mechanisms, (V1) 252*t*
in middle adult, (V1) 198
urinary function and, (V1) 720

effects of pain on, (V1) 798
environmental effects on, (V1) 972
exercise effects on, (V1) 823–824, (V1) 824*b*
full-spectrum nursing and, (V2) 777–778
heart in, (V1) 502–503, (V1) 502*f*, (V1) 502*t*
heat effects on, (V1) 972
immobility effects on, (V1) 831
lifestyle effects on, (V1) 972–973
medications for, (V1) 973, (V1) 974*t*, (V1) 981
in middle-aged adults, (V1) 972
of neonate, (V1) 173
nursing diagnosis for, (V1) 978–979
nursing interventions for, (V1) 979–982
nursing outcomes for, (V1) 979
nutrition effects on, (V1) 972–973
obesity effects on, (V1) 973
in older adults, (V1) 972
pain effects on, (V1) 798
postoperative complications of, (V1) 1049*t*
in pregnancy, (V1) 972
regulation of, (V1) 970–971
resuscitation for, (V1) 981–982
stress effects on, (V1) 972
structures of, (V1) 968–970
substance abuse effects on, (V1) 973
veins of, (V1) 969, (V1) 970*f*. *See also* Vein(s)
venous return promotion for, (V1) 980
venules of, (V1) 969
in young adults, (V1) 972
Care. *See* Healthcare; Nursing care
Care coordinator, home health nurse as, (V1) 1127
Care map, for ineffective sexuality patterns, (V1) 876
Care plan(s), (V1) 88–94
basic needs form in, (V1) 89, (V1) 89*f*
client profile form in, (V1) 89, (V1) 89*f*
comprehensive, information in, (V1) 88
computer, (V1) 94
using NOC with, (V1) 100
critical pathways in, (V1) 91, (V1) 93*f*
documents in, (V1) 89–94, (V1) 89*f*, (V1) 90*f*, (V1) 92–93*f*
electronic, Nursing Interventions Classification in, (V1) 115
evaluating and revising, (V1) 134–135
individualized, (V1) 89*f*, (V1) 91
writing process for, (V1) 94–95
for ineffective sexuality patterns, (V1) 872–875
integrated, (V1) 91
policies in, (V1) 89–90
procedures in, (V1) 89–90
protocols in, (V1) 90, (V1) 90*f*
special discharge, (V1) 89*f*, (V1) 91, (V1) 94
special teaching, (V1) 89*f*, (V1) 91, (V1) 94
outcomes for, (V1) 102
standardized, (V1) 91, (V1) 92
preprinted, (V1) 89, (V1) 89*f*
student, (V1) 94
mind-mapping, (V1) 94
unit standards of care in, (V1) 90
written, importance of, (V1) 88
Career roles, for nurses, expanded, (V1) 28–29
Caregiver
for older adult with dementia, support for, (V1) 219
role strain in, (V1) 1131–1132
assessing for, (V1) 298
interventions for, (V1) 300
standardized nursing languages for, (V2) 121
support for, in home care, (V1) 1135, (V1) 1135*b*
Carina tracheae, (V2) 743
Caring
definition of, (V1) 39
for family, (V1) 150
in full-spectrum nursing, (V1) 40–42, (V1) 40*f*, (V1) 40*t*
CaringBridge, (V1) 1081
Carminative enemas, (V1) 761, (V1) 761*t*
Carotid artery(ies), (V1) 503
auscultation of, (V2) 268*p*
palpation of, (V2) 267*p*
Carotid pulse, assessment of, (V2) 192*p*
Carotid stenosis, (V1) 503
Carriers, in chain of infection, (V1) 519
Cartilage, articular, (V1) 818
Cartridge, prefilled, and single-dose vial for IV administration, (V2) 442*p*
Case management, in work redesign, (V1) 24
Case manager
community nurse as, (V1) 1118–1119
role and function of, (V1) 6*t*
Case method of care, (V1) 15
Cast, in-home care of, (V1) 829
Casts, urinary, (V2) 563
Catabolism, definition of, (V1) 668
Cataplexy, (V1) 889
Cataracts, (V1) 494
congenital, (V1) 494
definition of, (V1) 777*b*
Catecholamines, (V1) 972
Catheter/catheterization
cardiac, (V2) 767
central. *See* Central venous access device
embolus with, (V1) 1015*t*
epidural, clinical insights on, (V2) 614–615
inside-the-needle, (V1) 1005, (V1) 1005*f*
midline peripheral, (V1) 1005
over-the-needle, (V1) 1005, (V1) 1005*f*, (V2) 785–786
peripherally inserted, (V1) 1007, (V1) 1007*f*
suction, (V1) 959, (V1) 959*f*
transtracheal, (V1) 957
urinary
condom
applying, (V1) 734*p*, (V2) 548–550
for urinary incontinence, (V1) 737
home care for, (V1) 1134
hydrogel coated, (V1) 730
indwelling, (V1) 730, (V1) 731*f*
care for patient with, (V1) 732, (V1) 735, (V2) 556–557
insertion of, (V2) 544–547*p*
measuring urine from, (V2) 532–533*p*
preoperative, (V1) 1036
removing, (V1) 734*p*, (V1) 735, (V2) 551–552*p*
for urinary incontinence, (V1) 737
urinary tract infections from, (V1) 721
insertion of, (V1) 732, (V2) 539–540*p*
irrigation of, (V1) 734*p*, (V2) 553–556*p*
polyvinyl chloride, (V1) 730
silicone (100%), (V1) 730
silicone elastomer-coated, (V1) 730
silver-alloy coated, (V1) 730
sizing of, (V1) 731
straight, (V1) 730
supplies for, (V1) 731–732
suprapubic, (V1) 730–731, (V1) 732*f*
Teflon-bonded, (V1) 730
types of, (V1) 730
for urinary retention, (V1) 730–732, (V1) 734*p*
valved, for urinary incontinence, (V1) 737
whistle-tipped, (V1) 959, (V1) 959*f*
wing-tipped (butterfly), (V1) 1005, (V1) 1005*f*, (V2) 785, (V2) 786
Yankauer, (V1) 959, (V1) 959*f*
Catholicism, Roman, (V1) 332
Cations, (V1) 984
Causation, (V1) 1174
CCC. *See* Clinical Care Classification (CCC)
Cecum, (V1) 746
Celibacy, (V1) 862, (V2) 654
Cell(s)
alveolar, (V1) 936, (V1) 937*f*
complete count of, (V1) 1000
Langerhans, (V1) 898
red, transfusion of, (V1) 1020. *See also* Blood transfusion
white, transfusion of, (V1) 1020. *See also* Blood transfusion
Cellular immunity, (V1) 526–527
Cellular malfunction theory of aging, (V1) 205–206
Cellular response, in inflammatory process, (V1) 247–248
Census tracts, (V1) 1115
Centenarians, (V1) 207
Center of gravity, (V1) 820, (V1) 820*f*
Centers for Disease Control and Prevention (CDC)
diseases reportable to, (V1) 863
guidelines of
infection, (V1) 518
for pathogen transmission prevention, (V1) 535, (V1) 536*p*
standard precautions of, clinical insight on, (V2) 337–338
transmission-based precautions of, (V1) 535
following, clinical insights on, (V2) 339–341
Centigrade-Fahrenheit conversion chart, (V2) 206
Centigrade temperature scale, (V1) 427, (V1) 427*f*
Central chemoreceptors, in regulation of respiration, (V1) 442
Central deafness, definition of, (V1) 778*f*
Central sleep apnea, (V1) 889
Central venous access devices (CVADs), (V1) 655, (V1) 655*f*, (V1) 659*p*, (V1) 1006–1007
assessment of, (V2) 813
care for, (V2) 813–814
dressing change for, (V2) 797–798*p*
extravasation and, (V2) 814
implantable, (V1) 1007–1008, (V1) 1008*f*
infiltration and, (V2) 814
maintenance interventions for, (V2) 813
medication administration through, (V2) 467–470*p*
nontunneled, (V1) 1007, (V1) 1007*f*
peripherally inserted, (V1) 1007, (V1) 1007*f*

placement of, (V2) 808–809*p*
tunneled, (V1) 1007, (V1) 1008*f*
Cerebellar function, assessment of, (V1) 509
Cerebral function, in neurological assessment, (V1) 507–508
Certification, (V1) 1171
Certified nurse midwife (CNM), advanced practice nurse as, (V1) 28
Certified registered nurse anesthetist (CRNA), advanced practice nurse as, (V1) 28
Cerumen, (V1) 495–496, (V1) 599
impacted, definition of, (V1) 778*f*
Cervical cancer screening, (V1) 511
in health promotion assessment, (V2) 876
in older adult assessment, (V1) 213
Cervical lymph nodes, assessment of, (V1) 498, (V2) 255*p*
Chair, transfer to, (V1) 841, (V1) 842*p*, (V1) 843, (V2) 628, (V2) 630–631*p*
Chancre, syphilitic, (V2) 315*f*
Change
implementation of, (V1) 1071
integration of, (V1) 1071
model of, (V1) 1069, (V1) 1069*f*
resistance to, (V1) 1070
reduction of, (V1) 1070, (V1) 1071*b*
transtheoretical model of, (V1) 1099
Change agent, role and function of, (V1) 6*t*
Changing subject, as barrier to therapeutic communication, (V1) 476
Channel, for message, (V1) 460–461
Chariker-Jeter (negative-pressure) dressing, (V1) 930*p*, (V2) 688*p*
Charitable organizations, as payor for healthcare, (V1) 21–22
Chart, (V1) 372. *See also* Documentation
Charting. *See also* Documentation
delegation of, (V1) 395
by exception (CBE), (V1) 374–375, (V1) 375*f*
in minimizing malpractice risks, (V1) 1179–1180
Checklist, surgical, (V2) 842–843
Cheilitis, (V2) 232
Cheilosis, (V1) 592
Chemical dependence, in workplace, signs of, (V1) 1183*b*
Chemical stimuli, (V1) 793
Chemical thermometers, disposable, (V1) 429–430, (V1) 430*t*
Chemoreceptors, (V1) 772, (V1) 938–939, (V1) 971
in regulation of respiration, (V1) 442
Chemotherapy
sexual function and, (V1) 858*t*
skin effects of, (V1) 900
Chest
assessment of, (V1) 499–501, (V1) 499*f*, (V1) 500*f*, (V1) 513*p*, (V2) 260–265*p*
barrel, (V1) 499, (V1) 500*f*
drainage of, (V1) 961–963, (V1) 963–964*p*, (V1) 965–966*p*, (V2) 755–759*p*
landmarks of, (V1) 499, (V1) 499*f*, (V1) 500*f*
movement of, in respiration, (V1) 445
percussion of, (V1) 955, (V1) 963–964*p*, (V2) 728–730*p*
retractions of, (V1) 946
shape and size of, (V1) 499
vibration of, (V1) 955, (V1) 963–964*p*, (V2) 728–730*p*
Chest pain, (V1) 798, (V1) 976–977
anxiety with, (V1) 977, (V1) 979
Chest physiotherapy, (V1) 955, (V1) 955*f*, (V1) 963–964*p*, (V2) 728–730*p*
Chest tube, (V1) 961–963, (V1) 965–966*p*, (V2) 755–759*p*
clinical insight on, (V2) 764–765
complications of, (V1) 963, (V2) 764–765
dry-seal, (V1) 962, (V1) 962*f*, (V2) 756, (V2) 765
monitoring of, (V2) 764–765
one-chamber, (V1) 962, (V1) 962*f*
portable, (V1) 962–963
safety for, (V2) 757–758
three-chamber, (V1) 962
two-chamber, (V1) 962
water-seal, (V1) 962, (V1) 962*f*, (V2) 756, (V2) 765
Chest vibration, (V1) 955, (V2) 728–730*p*
Chest x-ray, (V2) 767
preoperative, (V1) 1032, (V2) 845
Chewing, impaired, nutrition and, (V1) 689
Cheyne-Stokes respirations, (V1) 352, (V1) 444*t*, (V1) 946
Chief complaint, in nursing health history, (V1) 52*t*
Child(ren). *See also* Adolescent(s); Infant(s); Preschooler(s); School-age child(ren); Toddler(s)
abuse of, assessing for, (V2) 65–66
assessment of pain in, (V1) 799
bowel elimination in, (V1) 748
car safety seats for, (V1) 566*t*
cardiovascular system in, (V1) 971
cough in, (V1) 952
death of, as health disruption, (V1) 230
enuresis in, managing, (V1) 737, (V1) 737*b*
exercise guidelines for, (V1) 822*b*
firearm injuries to
prevention of, (V1) 562
risk factors for, (V1) 550
grief in, (V1) 350
honey for, (V1) 952
influenza in, (V1)
loss by, helping with, (V1) 367, (V1) 367*b*
medication dosage calculation for, (V2) 484
night terrors in, (V1) 890
nocturnal enuresis in, (V1) 890
obesity in, (V1) 826
oral medication administration for, (V1) 635, (V1) 636*b*
pain in, (V1) 796
pharmacokinetic processes in, (V1) 618*t*
poisoning risks for, in home, (V1) 548–549, (V1) 549*b*
interventions for, (V1) 560, (V1) 561*b*
promoting self-esteem in, (V1) 276*b*
pulmonary system of, (V1) 939
self-concept formation in, (V1) 264
sensory perception in, (V1) 774
sexual predator precautions for, (V1) 862
sexuality of, (V1) 853
skin of, (V1) 899
sleep for, (V1) 881, (V1) 881*t*, (V1) 885
stressors of, (V1) 242*b*
surgery for, (V1) 1028
teaching, (V1) 403
urinary elimination in, (V1) 718
young
families with, health risks for, (V1) 290–291
neurological exam in, (V1) 507
Childbearing couples, health risks for, (V1) 290, (V1) 290*f*
Childless couples, health risks for, (V1) 290
Children's Health Insurance Program (CHIP), as payor for healthcare, (V1) 21
Chinese heritage. *See also* Asian Americans
pain perception and responses in, (V2) 127
Chinese medicine, traditional, on health, (V1) 223*b*
Chiropractic adjustment, in stress management, (V1) 259
Chlamydia trachomatis infection, (V1) 863
Chloride, (V1) 989, (V1) 991*t*
Chloride channel activators, (V1) 749*b*
Choking, in infants/toddlers, (V1) 939
Choking rescue, (V1) 564, (V1) 564*f*
Cholesterol, (V1) 671, (V1) 977
functions of, (V1) 673
medications for, (V1) 981
skin and, (V1) 899
Choosing, in values clarification, (V1) 1156*t*
Christian Science, (V1) 332
Christianity, (V1) 331–332
Chronic disability, as family health risk, (V1) 293–294
Chronic illness
as family health risk, (V1) 293–294
host susceptibility and, (V1) 528
population vulnerability and, (V1) 1116
Chronic obstructive pulmonary disease (COPD), sleep and, (V1) 890
Chronic pain, (V1) 792, (V1) 797*b*
sexuality and, (V1) 867
Chronic wounds, (V1) 902. *See also* Pressure ulcer(s)
Chvostek's sign, (V2) 810
Cigarette smoking, (V1) 1097. *See also* Nicotine
by adolescents, (V1) 190, (V1) 971
cardiovascular effects of, (V1) 973
cessation of, (V1) 953
benefits of, (V1) 942*b*
5A's for, (V1) 953*b*
tips for, (V1) 954
health-illness and, (V1) 226
home fires from, (V1) 550
host susceptibility and, (V1) 528
nutrition and, (V1) 685–686
pulmonary effects of, (V1) 942
respiration and, (V1) 443
skin effects of, (V1) 901
sleep and, (V1) 886
surgery and, (V1) 1029
Cilia, (V1) 935
CINAHL (Cumulative Index for Nursing and Allied Health Literature), (V1) 1091, (V1) 1092*t*
Circadian rhythm(s), (V1) 881–882
body temperature and, (V1) 425
disorders of, (V1) 887
Circulating nurse, (V1) 1039, (V1) 1044
Circulation, skin and, (V1) 580
Circulatory system. *See also* Cardiovascular system
coronary, (V1) 501, (V1) 970. *See also* Heart
impaired, (V2) 776
critical thinking about, (V2) 778

disorders of, (V1) 830
exercise and, (V1) 824*b*, (V1) 973
full-spectrum nursing and, (V2) 777–778
impaired, skin and, (V1) 900
nursing interventions for, (V1) 979–980
peripheral, (V1) 977
pulmonary, (V1) 501. *See also* Pulmonary system
systemic, (V1) 501
transfusion-related overload of, (V1) 1021*t*
Circumcision, (V1) 176, (V1) 510
female, (V1) 855–856
Circumference
arm, in body composition evaluation, (V1) 692–693, (V2) 515*p*
hip, in body composition evaluation, (V1) 692–693, (V2) 515*p*
waist, in body composition evaluation, (V1) 692–693, (V2) 515*p*
Civil law, (V1) 1172–1176
claims under, litigation of, (V1) 1176–1177
Claims-made liability insurance, (V1) 1184
Clarifying, for enhancing therapeutic communication, (V1) 474
Clarity
for informed consent, (V1) 1034–1035, (V1) 1180
of urine, (V2) 562
in verbal communication, (V1) 462
CLAS standards, language-related, (V1) 322
Clavicle, fracture of, in neonate, (V1) 175
Clean-catch urine specimen collection, (V1) 733*p*, (V2) 535*p*
Clean-contaminated wounds, (V1) 902
Clean team, (V1) 1039
Clean wounds, (V1) 902
Cleansing enema, (V1) 760
administering, (V2) 575–577*p*
Client(s)
angry, dealing with, (V2) 93–94*b*
computer use by, (V1) 1084–1085
culture of, (V1) 33–34
dying. *See* Dying patient
environment of, (V1) 601–603. *See also* Environment, client
establishing trust with, in health promotion, (V1) 235–236
illness experience of
honoring, (V1) 234–236
unique, (V1) 230–232
individual differences in, (V1) 33
learning by. *See* Learning, client
as payor for healthcare, (V1) 20
perceptions of, in community assessment, (V1) 1123
placement of, CDC standard precautions on, (V2) 337
power of, (V1) 1066
praying with, (V2) 137–138
preparation of, for physical examination, (V1) 483
progress of, evaluation of, (V1) 131–134
roles of, (V1) 34
teaching. *See* Teaching, patient
transfer of. *See also* Bed(s), client moving in/from
operative suite, (V1) 1038–1039
postanesthesia care unit, (V1) 1045, (V1) 1045*f*
surgical nursing unit, (V1) 1046
uniqueness of, (V1) 33–34
values clarification for, assisting with, (V1) 1155
Client advocate
community nurse as, (V1) 1118
role and function of, (V1) 6*t*
Client educator
home health nurse as, (V1) 1127
role and function of, (V1) 6*t*
Clinical Care Classification (CCC), (V1) 74, (V1) 102, (V1) 115, (V1) 1132, (V1) 1133, (V2) 865, (V2) 891–892*b*
Clinical judgment, (V1) 5
Clinical nurse specialist (CNS), expanded roles for, (V1) 28
Clinical practice guidelines, (V1) 109–110, (V1) 109*b*
Clinical practice theory
application of, (V1) 143
definition of, (V1) 138
Clinical problem, identification of, in finding best evidence, (V1) 155–156
Clinical reasoning, (V1) 33*b*. *See also* Critical thinking; Diagnostic reasoning
Clinical support tools, (V1) 1088
Clitoris, (V1) 848, (V1) 849*f*
excision of, (V1) 855–856
inspection of, (V2) 302*p*
Clonus, (V1) 833*b*
Closed systems, in systems theory, (V1) 149
Closed wounds, (V1) 902
Clostridium difficile, resistant strains of, (V1) 523
Cloth bandages, (V1) 929
Clots. *See* Embolus; Thrombus
Clotting time, (V2) 715
Clubbing, of fingers, in hypoxia, (V1) 445, (V1) 492, (V1) 492*f*
Coaching, (V1) 1061
Coagulation disorders, surgery and, (V1) 1029*b*
Coagulation times, (V2) 715
Cocaine, teratogenic effects of, (V1) 171
Cochrane Library, (V1) 1092*t*
Code Blue, (V1) 981
Coercion, (V1) 1066
Cognition
changes in
age-related, assessment for, (V1) 209*t*
urinary function and, (V1) 720
in depression, (V1) 279
sleep and, (V1) 879–880
Cognitive ability, in self-care ability assessment, (V1) 577
Cognitive-behavioral therapy, for pain, (V1) 802–803
Cognitive development
of adolescent, (V1) 168*t*, (V1) 189
of infant, (V1) 168*t*, (V1) 176–177
of neonate, (V1) 174
of older adults, (V1) 207
of preschooler, (V1) 168*t*, (V1) 182
stages of, client teaching and, (V1) 403
of toddler, (V1) 168*t*, (V1) 180
of young adult, (V1) 195
Cognitive development theory, (V1) 165, (V1) 167, (V1) 168*t*
Cognitive function
impaired
clients with, enhancing communication with, (V1) 478, (V2) 213–214*b*
therapeutic communication and, (V1) 472
in neurological assessment, (V1) 508
nutrition and, (V1) 689
in older adults, promoting, (V1) 219
Cognitive impairment, self-care ability and, (V1) 576
Cognitive learning, (V1) 388*t*, (V1) 399
Cognitive level, hygiene and, (V1) 575
Cognitive needs, (V1) 54
Cognitive responses
to stress, assessing, (V1) 255
to stressors, (V1) 248*b*
Cognitive restructuring, in stress management, (V1) 260
Cognitive theory, of depression, (V1) 270
Cognitively impaired client
assessment of pain in, (V1) 799, (V1) 800
pain in, (V1) 796–797
skin breakdown in, (V1) 900
Coitus, (V1) 861
Coitus interruptus, (V2) 654
Cold. *See also* Hypothermia
cardiovascular effects of, (V1) 972
Cold (common), (V1) 952
Cold pack, (V2) 709
Cold therapy
clinical insights on, (V2) 709
for pain, (V1) 802
safety measures for, (V2) 709
for wounds, (V1) 931–933, (V2) 709
Colectomy, total, with ileoanal reservoir, (V1) 751–752, (V1) 751*f*
Colic, in infant, (V1) 177
interventions for, (V1) 179
Collaboration
in culturally competent care, (V1) 323
definition of, (V1) 28, (V1) 125
in discharge planning, (V1) 88
in implementation, (V1) 125
interprofessional, trend toward, (V1) 28
for sensory deprivation, (V1) 784
Collaborative care, assessment in, (V1) 44–45
Collaborative interventions, (V1) 107
Collaborative problems
diagnostic statement formats for, (V1) 78*f*, (V1) 79
evaluation of, (V1) 133–134
goals for, (V1) 98, (V1) 99*t*
intervention type related to, (V1) 110*t*
nursing and medical diagnoses and
comparison of, (V1) 63*t*
distinguishing between, (V1) 64*f*
perioperative, (V2) 848–849, (V2) 850
recognizing, (V1)64
Collaborative professional communication, (V1) 467–469, (V1) 467*b*
Collaborator, community nurse as, (V1) 1118
Collagen, (V1) 904
in older adults, (V1) 580*t*
Collagen dressing, (V1) 925*t*
Collective bargaining, influence of, on contemporary nursing practice, (V1) 26
Colloids, (V1) 985
Colon, (V1) 746–747. *See also* Bowel *entries*
Colon cancer screening
in health promotion assessment, (V2) 876
in older adult assessment, (V1) 213
Colonization, of wound, (V1) 901
Colonoscopy, fiberoptic, (V2) 595
Color blindness, (V1) 494

Color change test, (V2) 271*p*
Color vision, (V1) 494
testing of, (V2) 239*p*
Colorectal cancer screening, for middle adult, (V1) 198
Colostomy, (V1) 752, (V1) 752*f*, (V1) 857
caring for patient with, (V1) 763–765
dietary changes associated with, (V1) 765*b*
irrigation of, (V1) 765, (V1) 769–770*p*, (V2) 586–588*p*
Coma, (V1) 352
Glasgow coma scale for, (V2) 296
Comatose, description of, (V1) 507
Comfort, contexts of, (V1) 150
Comfort zone, change and, (V1) 1069, (V1) 1069*f*
Commands, for change, (V1) 1070
Commission on Collegiate Nursing Education (CCNE), (V1) 22
Commodity Supplemental Food Program, (V1) 697
Common cold, (V1) 952
Common law, (V1) 1164
Common sense, in gaining knowledge, (V1) 152
Communicable diseases
in preschooler, (V1) 183
reporting regulations on, (V1) 1184
Communication, (V1) 458–478, (V2) 210–218
across language barrier, (V2) 128
aggressive, (V1) 468
assertive, (V1) 468–469, (V1) 469*b*
techniques for, (V2) 212*b*
assessing, (V2) 287*p*
assessment guidelines and tools for, (V2) 215
with care, (V1) 474*b*
of care and concern in health promotion, (V1) 233
client-nurse
acceptance in, (V1) 233
attuning in, (V1) 233
enjoying in, (V1) 233
settling in, (V1) 233
for sexual counseling, (V1) 870–871
for sexual history, (V2) 653, (V2) 656–657
collaborative professional, (V1) 467–469, (V1) 467*b*
content of, (V1) 460
culture and, (V1) 308
definition of, (V1) 459, (V1) 459*b*
developmental variations in, (V1) 465
documentation in, (V1) 372
electronic, (V1) 1080–1082. *See also* Computer(s)
in end-of-life care
barriers to, (V1) 363*b*
therapeutic, (V1) 363
enhancing
with clients
from another culture, (V1) 478, (V2) 212–213*b*
with cognitive impairment, (V1) 478, (V2) 213–214*b*
with decreased level of consciousness, (V1) 478, (V2) 213–214*b*
with hearing or speech impairment, (V1) 478, (V2) 213*b*
through nonverbal behaviors, (V2) 211*b*
environment and, (V1) 465
as etiology of other nursing diagnoses, (V1) 473
factors affecting, (V1) 465–467
family patterns of, in family health assessment, (V1) 297
gender and, (V1) 465
group, (V1) 459
in group helping relationships, (V1) 471–472
with hearing impaired client, (V2) 604
impaired, urinary function and, (V1) 720
improving, (V1) 233–234
interpersonal, (V1) 459
intrapersonal, (V1) 459
knowledge map for, (V1) 219, (V2) 218
leadership and, (V1) 1067
levels of, (V1) 459–460
by manager, (V1) 1067
nonassertive, (V1) 468
nonverbal, (V1) 463–464
pain-related, (V2) 615
nurse-surgical team, (V1) 1038
nursing diagnoses related to, (V1) 472–473
with older adults, (V1) 217–219
with cognitive deficit, (V1) 218–219
passive, (V1) 467–468
patient rounds approach to, (V1) 469
personal space and, (V1) 465–466
as process, (V1) 460–461, (V1) 460*f*
public speaking as, (V1) 459–460
roles and relationships and, (V1) 467
SBAR model for, (V1) 469, (V2) 212*b*
patient safety and, (V1) 570
for sensory deprivation, (V1) 784
simplified, for confused client, (V1) 788
sociocultural factors and, (V1) 466
standardized tools for, (V1) 469
surgical team-nurse, (V1) 1038
in teaching/learning, (V1) 402
territoriality and, (V1) 466
therapeutic, definition of, (V1) 469
in therapeutic relationships, (V1) 469–478
verbal, (V1) 461–463
brevity in, (V1) 462
clarity in, (V1) 462
connotative meaning in, (V1) 461
credibility in, (V1) 462
definition of, (V1) 461
denotative meaning in, (V1) 461
humor in, (V1) 463
impaired, culture and, (V1) 320
intonation in, (V1) 462
pacing in, (V1) 461–462
relevance in, (V1) 462
timing in, (V1) 462
vocabulary in, (V1) 461
with visually impaired client, (V2) 604
Communicator, role and function of, (V1) 6*t*
Community(ies)
assessment of, (V1) 1123
components of, (V1) 1115
definition of, (V1) 1114
elder-friendly, (V1) 204
health of, indicators of, (V1) 1115–1116
retirement, (V1) 204–205
safety hazards in, (V1) 550–552
interventions for, (V1) 564–568
working within, (V1) 1118–1122
Community assessment, (V1) 50–51
Community-based care
definition of, (V1) 1116
home healthcare in, (V1) 1125–1135
nursing process applied to, (V1) 1124–1125
Community care, standardized nursing languages for, (V1) 115
Community health, patient-centered care in, promoting, (V1) 1119*b*
Community health centers, (V1) 17
Community health goals, (V1) 100–102
Community health nursing, (V1) 1116–1117, (V1) 1117*f*
Community nurses, roles of, (V1) 1118–1119
Community nursing, (V1) 1113–1136, (V2) 885–896
career opportunities in, (V1) 1121–1122, (V1) 1121*f*, (V1) 1123*f*
concept of, (V1) 1116–1118
interventions of, classification of, (V1) 1119–1120
knowledge map on, (V2) 896
Community-oriented nursing, (V1) 1117, (V1) 1117*f*
Comorbidities, (V1) 33
Compensation
in acid-balance imbalance, (V1) 992, (V1) 998
as defense mechanism, (V1) 250*t*
Compensatory justice, (V1) 1152
Competence, (V1) 1066, (V1) 1067
cultural, (V1) 150
for informed consent, (V1) 1180–1181
Complement activation, in humoral immunity, (V1) 526
Complement cascade, in defense against infection, (V1) 524
Complementary and alternative medicine/modalities (CAM), (V1) 315
for anxiety, (V1) 283*b*
aromatherapy in, (V1) 779*b*
for common cold, (V1) 952
for depression, (V1) 283*b*
in end-of-life care, (V1) 354*b*
evidence-based studies of, (V1) 975
guided imagery as, (V1) 803, (V1) 894
increased use of, (V1) 27
intercessory prayer as, (V1) 342*b*
for lowering blood pressure, (V1) 455*b*
in nursing health history, (V1) 52*t*
for pain, (V1) 801–804
for perimenopausal symptoms, (V1) 870
in preventing illness, (V1) 1117*b*
for spiritual care, (V1) 343*b*
in stress reduction, (V1) 258*b*
Complete blood count
in fluid and electrolyte assessment, (V1) 1000
preoperative, (V2) 845
Completeness, of informed consent, (V1) 1180
Compliance
arterial, in blood pressure regulation, (V1) 447
lung, (V1) 937
Comprehension, of informed consent, (V1) 1180
Comprehensive assessment, (V1) 47–48, (V1) 48*f*
Compress
cold, (V2) 709
heated, (V2) 708

Compression, pressure ulcers and, (V1) 908, (V1) 908*f*
Compression garments, (V1) 920
Compromise, in solving ethical problem, (V1) 1159
Computed tomography (CT)
  in body mass evaluation, (V1) 693
  in GI tract study, (V2) 595
  in urinary system assessment, (V2) 564–565
Computer(s), (V1) 1080
  in care management, (V1) 1083–1085
  client use of, (V1) 1084–1085
  definition of, (V1) 1080
  diagnosis assisted by, (V1) 71–72
  for documentation, (V1) 1084
  for e-mail, (V1) 1080–1081
  error reduction with, (V1) 1083–1084
  for evidence-based practice, (V1) 1089–1093
  evidence-based studies on, (V1) 1083
  for home care, (V1) 1082
  for interactive gaming, (V1) 1081–1082
  interventions generated by, (V1) 113, (V1) 114*f*
  for listserv mailing, (V1) 1081
  in long-distance communication, (V1) 1080–1082
  in nursing education, (V1) 1085
  for social networking, (V1) 1081
  for telehealth, (V1) 1082, (V1) 1082*f*
  for text messaging, (V1) 1080–1081
  for virtual learning, (V1) 1081–1082
  for web conferencing, (V1) 1081
Computer care plans, (V1) 94
  using NOC with, (V1) 100
Computerized physician order entry, (V1) 1084, (V1) 1088
Computerized physician/prescriber order entry (CPOE), (V1) 1078
Computerized Prescriber Order Entry (CPOE), (V1) 627
Conception, (V1) 170
Concepts, in nursing theory, (V1) 140
Conceptual framework, definition of, (V1) 141
Conceptual model, definition of, (V1) 141
Concrete operations stage, of cognitive development, (V1) 168*t*
Concreteness, in therapeutic communication, (V1) 471
Concussions, in school-age child, (V1) 186
Condom, (V2) 655
  adolescent use of, (V1) 191
  teaching about, (V2) 654
Condom catheters
  applying, (V1) 734*p*, (V2) 548–550*p*
  for urinary incontinence, (V1) 737
Conduction, in heat exchange with environment, (V1) 424, (V1) 424*f*
Conduction deafness, definition of, (V1) 778*b*
Confidentiality
  autonomy and, (V1) 1150
  of health records, (V1) 393–394
  maintaining, in minimizing malpractice risks, (V1) 1181
Conflict
  informal negotiation for, (V1) 1073
  levels of, (V1) 1071–1072
  resolution of, (V1) 1073
  win-win resolution of, (V1) 1072
Confrontation, in therapeutic communication, (V1) 471
Confused clients, interventions for, (V1) 787–788
Confusion
  minimizing, for sensory deprivation, (V1) 784
  pain and, (V1) 795
Congenital abnormalities, exercise and, (V1) 827
Congenital anomalies, (V1) 175
Congenital cataracts, (V1) 494
Conjunctiva
  disorders of, (V1) 493
  inspection of, (V2) 242*p*
Connecting phrase, in diagnostic statement, (V1) 77
Connotative meaning, in verbal communication, (V1) 461
Conscious sedation, (V1) 1040–1041
Consciousness
  level of
    assessing, (V1) 781
    decreased, clients with, enhancing communication with, (V1) 478, (V2) 213–214*b*
    in neurological assessment, (V1) 507
  postoperative, (V1) 1046
Consent
  informed, (V1) 1034–1035. *See* Informed consent
  for surgery, (V1) 1034–1035
Consequentialism, (V1) 1147–1148
Considering alternatives, in critical thinking, (V1) 35*t*, (V1) 36
Constant fever, (V1) 426
Constipation
  definition of, (V1) 756
  interventions for, (V1) 699, (V1) 759–762
  medications associated with, (V1) 753*b*
  opioid-related, (V) 807*b*
  postoperative, (V1) 1050*t*, (V2) 853–854
  in pregnancy, (V1) 750*b*
Constitution, definition of, (V1) 1163
Constitutional law, (V1) 1163
Consumers, healthcare, influence of, on contemporary nursing practice, (V1) 26
Contact lens care, (V1) 598, (V1) 598*b*, (V1) 601*p*, (V2) 390–391*p*
Contact precautions, (V2) 339
Contaminated wounds, (V1) 901, (V1) 902
Contextual awareness, in critical thinking, (V1) 34, (V1) 35*t*, (V2) 12
Continent ileostomy, (V1) 751, (V1) 751*f*
Continent urinary reservoir, (V1) 738, (V1) 739*f*
  interventions for patients with, (V1) 739
Continuing care retirement communities (CCRC), (V1) 204
Continuing education, (V1) 11
  participating in, in minimizing malpractice risks, (V1) 1182
Continuity of care, documentation in, (V1) 371
Continuous mechanical ventilation, (V2) 752
Continuous passive motion, (V1) 844
Continuous positive airway pressure (CPAP), (V2) 752
Continuous quality improvement (CQI) programs, (V1) 25
Contraception, (V2) 654–656
  teaching about, (V1) 870, (V2) 654
Contract law, (V1) 1172
Contractual agreements, definition of, (V1) 408
Contracture, immobility and, (V1) 831
Contralateral stimulation, for pain, (V1) 802
Controlled substances
  abuse of. *See* Substance abuse
  regulation of, (V1) 606–607, (V1) 607*f*
Controlling leadership, (V1) 1058
Contusion, (V1) 902*t*
Convalescence, in infection, (V1) 522
Convection, in heat exchange with environment, (V1) 424, (V1) 424*f*
Conversational dyspnea, (V1) 946
Conversion, as defense mechanism, (V1) 250*t*
Coordination, (V1) 820
  assessment of, (V1) 506, (V2) 280*p*
  definition of, (V1) 125
  in implementation, (V1) 125–126
Coping
  adaptive, (V1) 243
  with anxiety, (V1) 268–269
  approaches to, (V1) 243
  maladaptive, (V1) 243
Coping ability, developmental influences on, (V1) 225
Coping processes, family, in family health assessment, (V1) 297–298
Coping response(s)
  definition of, (V1) 240
  surgery and ineffective, (V1) 1033
Coping strategies, for stress, (V1) 242–243
Copper, (V1) 678*t*, (V1) 899
Cordotomy, for pain, (V1) 810
Corn, (V1) 587
Cornea
  inspection of, (V1) 494, (V2) 242*p*
  preventing damage to, with medication administration, (V1) 638
Corneal reflex, testing, (V2) 242*p*
Coronary arteries, (V1) 969, (V1) 969*f*. *See also* Heart
Coronary artery disease, (V1) 975
  sleep and, (V1) 890
Coronary circulation, (V1) 501
Correctional facility nursing, (V1) 1121
Corticosteroids, surgery and, (V1) 1030*b*
Cortisol, in stress response, (V1) 245, (V1) 245*f*
Cosmetic surgery, (V1) 1028
Cost containment, ethical issues for nurses and, (V1) 1142
Cough, (V1) 445
  assessment of, (V1) 946–947
  CDC standard precautions on, (V2) 337
  in children, (V1) 952
  honey for, (V1) 952
  over-the-counter medications for, (V1) 952
  for secretion mobilization, (V1) 954
  teaching for, (V1) 1054*p*, (V2) 826–827*p*, (V2) 829*p*
  tracheostomy care and, (V2) 740
Counseling
  in health promotion, (V1) 1107–1108
  nutritional, (V1) 696–697
  providing, in minimizing malpractice risks, (V1) 1181
  sexual health, (V1) 870–871
  for smoking cessation, (V1) 953
Counselor
  community nurse as, (V1) 1118
  role and function of, (V1) 6*t*

Countershock phase, of fight or flight reaction, (V1) 245
Courage, intellectual, (V1) 32
Crackles, (V1) 445, (V2) 265
Cradle boots, (V1) 837, (V2) 637
Cradle cap, (V1) 492
Cramping, menstrual, (V1) 869
Cranial nerve assessment, (V1) 508, (V1) 508*t*, (V1) 509*f*, (V2) 288–290*p*
Crawling reflex, (V1) 174, (V1) 174*f*
Cream(s), (V1) 611*t*, (V1) 612*t*
  application of, (V1) 636–637, (V2) 430*p*
Creatine, normal, (V2) 817
Creatine kinase-MB, (V2) 767
Creatinine
  levels of, in renal function assessment, (V1) 726
  serum levels of, protein metabolism and, (V1) 695
  in urinary elimination assessment, (V2) 563
Credentialing, (V1) 1171
Credé's maneuver, (V1) 729
Credibility, in verbal communication, (V1) 462
Credible sources, using, in critical thinking, (V1) 35*t*, (V1) 36
Crepitus, (V1) 506, (V1) 827, (V1) 914, (V2) 642
Crime, definition of, (V1) 1171
Crimean War, (V1) 3
Criminal law, (V1) 1171–1172
Crisis, from failure of adaptive mechanisms, (V1) 253–254
Crisis intervention
  guidelines for, (V2) 94*b*
  in stress management, (V1) 260–261
Criteria, in evaluation, (V1) 130
Critical pathways
  in patient care plans, (V1) 91, (V1) 93*f*
  in work redesign, (V1) 24
Critical thinking, (V1) 5
  about acid-base balance, (V2) 818–819
  in assessment, (V2) 23–24
  on bowel elimination, (V2) 596–597
  about circulation, (V2) 778
  on communication, (V1) 216–217
  on community and home nursing, (V2) 892–894
  on culturally competent nursing, (V2) 131–133
  definition of, (V1) 31–32, (V1) 32*b*
  in diagnosis, (V2) 29–30
  on documentation and reporting, (V2) 174
  about electrolytes, (V2) 818–819
  on ethical issues, (V2) 900–902
  in evaluation, (V2) 51
  in evidence-based practice, (V2) 55–57
  about exercise, (V2) 648–649
  on family issues, (V2) 122–123
  about fluids, (V2) 818–819
  in full-spectrum nursing, (V1) 40*t*, (V1) 41
  on grief and loss, (V2) 155–156
  on health promotion, (V2) 879–880
  on hygiene, (V2) 404–406
  in implementation, (V2) 51
  importance of, for nurses, (V1) 33–34
  on infection prevention, (V2) 345
  about informatics, (V2) 867–868
  knowledge map for, (V2) 14
  about leadership, (V2) 860–861
  on legal accountability, (V2) 908–910
  about management, (V2) 860–861
  on medication administration, (V2) 485–487
  model for, (V1) 34, (V1) 35–36*t*, (V1) 36, (V1) 37*f*
  about nursing, (V2) 8
  in nursing process, (V1) 31–32, (V1) 32*b*, (V1) 39, (V2) 10–14
  on nutrition, (V2) 526–527
  about oxygenation, (V2) 769
  about pain, (V2) 619–620
  on patient safety, (V1) 359–360
  about perioperative nursing, (V2) 856
  on personal view of health, (V2) 89
  about physical activity, (V2) 648–649
  in planning interventions, (V2) 41–43
  in planning outcomes, (V2) 37
  on self-concept disturbance, (V2) 113–114
  on sensory function, (V2) 607–608
  about sexual health, (V2) 658–659
  about sleep, (V2) 668–669
  on spiritual care, (V2) 143
  about stress/stressors, (V2) 99–100
  on teaching and learning, (V2) 180–182
  on urinary elimination, (V2) 566
  on vital sign measurement, (V2) 207–209
  about wounds, (V2) 718
Critical thinking attitudes, (V1) 32–33
Critical thinking skills, (V1) 32
Critically ill patient, oral care for, (V1) 593–594
Cross-dressing, (V1) 852
Crossmatching, for blood transfusion, (V1) 1019–1020, (V1) 1019*t*, (V2) 845
Crushing wound, (V1) 902*t*
Crust, (V2) 233
Crutches, (V1) 846, (V1) 846*f*
  sizing of, (V2) 639
  teaching for, (V2) 639–640
Crying, in infant, (V1) 177
Crystalloids, (V1) 985
Crystals, urinary, (V2) 563
CT colonographies, in older adult assessment, (V1) 213
Cues
  cluster, (V1) 67–68
  in diagnostic reasoning, (V1) 65–67, (V1) 67*b*
Cultural archetype, (V1) 308
Cultural assessment, (V1) 50, (V1) 318–320
  guidelines and tools for, (V2) 129–130
  health history in, (V1) 318
  models and tools for, (V1) 320
  physical assessment in, (V1) 319
  using transcultural assessment model, (V2) 130
Cultural assimilation, (V1) 306
Cultural awareness, definition of, (V1) 315
Cultural competence, (V1) 150, (V1) 302
  American Nurses Association on, (V1) 315
  definition of, (V1) 315
  for health assessment, (V1) 482*b*
  Leininger and, (V1) 316
  in nursing care, challenge to provide, (V1) 302–303
  pain assessment and, (V1) 799
  patient outcomes and, (V1) 316*b*
  Purnell model for, (V1) 315–316, (V1) 317*f*
  Quality and Safety Education for Nurses on, (V1) 315
  teaching and, (V1) 406*b*
Cultural influences
  on nutrition, (V1) 687, (V1) 689
  on urinary function, (V1) 719
Cultural sensitivity
  definition of, (V1) 315
  in end-of-life care, (V1) 366, (V1) 366*f*
Cultural stereotype, (V1) 308
Cultural stereotyping, as barrier to culturally competent care, (V1) 317
Culturally competent care, (V1) 315–316
  barriers to, (V1) 316–318
    language barriers as, (V1) 318
    racism as, (V1) 317
    sexism as, (V1) 317–318
  being considerate of cultural specifics in, (V1) 323*b*
  developing, (V1) 324
  providing, nursing strategies for, (V1) 321–323, (V1) 323*b*
Culturally sensitive care, standardized language for, (V1) 116
Culture, (V1) 302. *See also* Ethnicity; Race(s); Religion(s)
  biological variations and, (V1) 309
    assessing for, (V2) 126
  characteristics of, (V1) 303–304, (V1) 304*f*
  of clients, (V1) 33–34
  clients from another, enhancing communication with, (V1) 478, (V2) 212–213*b*
  communication and, (V1) 308
  concepts related to, (V1) 305–307
  definition of, (V1) 303
  dominant, (V1) 306
  economy and, (V1) 310
  education and, (V1) 309
  environmental control and, (V1) 309
  female genital mutilation and, (V1) 855–856
  health-illness practices and, (V1) 226–227
    possible effects of, (V1) 322*t*
    responding to, (V1) 321
  of healthcare, (V1) 310
  hygiene and, (V1) 575
  knowledge map for, (V2) 135
  law and, (V1) 310
  meaning of, (V1) 303–307
  of nursing, (V1) 312–313
  pain and, (V1) 796
  philosophy and, (V1) 309
  politics and, (V1) 310
  reasons to learn about, (V1) 302–303
  religion and, (V1) 309
  sensory function and, (V1) 775
  sexuality and, (V1) 855–856
  social organization and, (V1) 309
  space and, (V1) 308
  technology and, (V1) 309–310
  time orientation and, (V1) 308–309
Culture (laboratory)
  sputum, (V2) 767
  wound, (V1) 1 and (V1) 2 for sub-entries and this entry
    biopsy, (V1) 916, (V2) 673–675*p*, (V2) 715
    needle aspiration, (V1) 916
    swab, (V2) 673–675*p*
Culture specifics, (V1) 307, (V1) 308*f*
  affecting health, (V1) 308–310
  being considerate of, (V1) 323*b*
Culture universals, (V1) 307
Cumulative Index to Nursing and Allied Health Literature (CINAHL), (V1) 156, (V1) 1091, (V1) 1092*t*
Cunnilingus, (V1) 861

Cures, (V1) 329
CureTogether, (V1) 1081
Curiosity, intellectual, (V1) 32
Current Procedural Terminology (CPT), (V1) 74
Cushing's syndrome, face in, (V2) 237*f*
Custodial care facilities, (V1) 16
Cutaneous pain, (V1) 791
Cutaneous stimulation, (V1) 802
Cutaneous ureterostomy, (V1) 738
Cyanocobalamin, (V1) 675*t*
Cyanosis, (V1) 490*t*, (V2) 312*p*
definition of, (V1) 440
description of, (V1) 581
Cyst, (V2) 231
Cystitis, (V1) 720
Cystometry, (V2) 564
Cystoscopy, (V2) 564
Cytotoxic T cells, in cellular immunity, (V1) 526

D

Damages, (V1) 1174
Dance, in stress management, (V1) 259
Dandruff, (V1) 596
Dangling legs at bedside, (V1) 842, (V1) 842*p*, (V1) 844, (V2) 628*p*, (V2) 629–630*p*, (V2) 638
Data, (V1) 1079. *See also* Assessment(s)
analysis and interpretation of, in diagnostic reasoning, (V1) 65–68, (V1) 67*f*
for assessment
documentation of, (V1) 54, (V1) 56, (V1) 57*f*
organization of, (V1) 53–54, (V1) 55–56*t*
sources of, (V1) 46, (V1) 47*t*
validation of, (V1) 53
definition of, (V1) 1079
gaps in, identification of, in diagnostic reasoning, (V1) 68
inconsistencies in, identification of, in diagnostic reasoning, (V1) 68
knowledge map for, (V2) 870
objective, (V1) 46, (V1) 47*t*
primary, (V1) 46, (V1) 47*t*
reassessment, collection of, in evaluation, (V1) 132
secondary, (V1) 46, (V1) 47*t*
significant, in analyzing and interpreting data, (V1) 65–67
subjective, (V1) 46, (V1) 47*t*
Data security, for electronic health records, maintaining confidentiality of, (V1) 393–394
Database(s)
in community assessment, (V1) 1123
literature, (V1) 1091, (V1) 1092*b*, (V1) 1092*t*
nursing, (V1) 156
patient, assessment data in, (V1) 44
in problem-oriented record system, (V1) 374
Date rape, (V1) 865
Deafness. *See also* Hearing
central, definition of, (V1) 777*b*
conduction, definition of, (V1) 778*b*
nerve, definition of, (V1) 778*b*
Death, (V1) 345–368, (V2) 145–158. *See also* Dying; Grief; Loss
of child, as health disruption, (V1) 230
definition of, (V1) 351
in family, interventions for, (V1) 300
heart-lung, (V1) 351
higher-brain, (V1) 351
impending, as health disruption, (V1) 229
timeliness of, grief and, (V1) 349–350
whole-brain, (V1) 351
Deaths, unintentional, leading causes of, in U.S., (V1) 546*t*
Debridement, (V1) 922–923
autolytic, (V1) 923
enzymatic, (V1) 923
hydrotherapeutic, (V1) 923
maggot, (V1) 923
mechanical, (V1) 923
sharp, (V1) 923, (V1) 928
Decision making, (V1) 33*b*
in critical thinking, (V1) 35*t*, (V1) 36
ethical, (V1) 1154–1161. *See also* Ethical decision making
Decision-making, in management, (V1) 1061
Decongestants, (V1) 952
nasal, administration of, (V1) 638
Decubitus ulcers. *See* Pressure ulcer(s)
Deductive reasoning, (V1) 141, (V1) 142*f*
Deep breathing, (V1) 1054*p*, (V2) 826–827*p*, (V2) 829*p*
Deep somatic pain, (V1) 791, (V1) 797*b*
Deep tendon reflexes
assessment of, (V1) 508, (V1) 509*f*
testing, (V2) 292–294*p*
Deep vein thrombosis (DVT)
antiembolism stockings for prevention of, (V1) 980, (V1) 1037–1038, (V1) 1037*f*, (V1) 1054*p*, (V2) 829–832*p*
assessment for, (V1) 977
Defamation of character, (V1) 1172
Defecation
normal patterns of, (V1) 748
normal/regular, promoting, (V1) 757–758
process of, (V1) 747–748
Defendant, (V1) 1174
Defense mechanisms
for anxiety, (V1) 269
identification of, (V1) 165
against infection, (V1) 524–527
primary, (V1) 524
breaks in, host susceptibility and, (V1) 528
secondary, (V1) 524–525, (V1) 525*t*
supporting, (V1) 530, (V1) 532–533
tertiary, (V1) 525–527, (V1) 526*b*, (V1) 527*b*, (V1) 527*f*
psychological, (V1) 250–251*t*
Definition(s), in nursing theory, (V1) 140
Degenerative joint disease, (V2) 314*f*
Dehiscence, wound, (V1) 906–907, (V1) 907*f*
postoperative, (V1) 1051*t*
Dehydration, (V1) 823, (V1) 825, (V1) 993
skin and, (V1) 580
Delegation, (V1) 1067–1069
of adding medications to IV fluids, (V2) 457–458*p*
of administering feedings through gastric and enteric tubes, (V2) 502
ambulation assistance, (V2) 632
antiembolism stockings, (V2) 829
of apical pulse assessment, (V2) 195
of apical-radial pulse deficit assessment, (V2) 197–198
of artificial eye care, (V2) 397
of assessment, (V1) 45–46
of temperature, (V2) 185
of vital signs, (V1) 457
back massage, (V2) 664
bandaging, (V2) 699
of bathing
with basin and water, (V2) 370
with prepackaged bathing product, (V2) 364
towel, (V2) 369
of beard and mustache care, (V2) 387
of bed making, (V2) 392, (V2) 394
of bed monitoring device installation, (V2) 350
bed-to-chair transfer, (V2) 628
bed-to-stretcher transfer, (V2) 628
of bladder/catheter irrigation, (V2) 553
of blood pressure measurement, (V2) 200
blood transfusion, (V2) 804
of brushing and flossing of teeth, (V2) 377
cardiac monitoring, (V2) 774
central venous catheter placement, (V2) 808
of charting, (V1) 395
of checking fingerstick blood glucose levels, (V2) 494
chest tube, (V2) 755
of colostomy irrigation, (V2) 586
concerns about, (V1) 1068–1069
of condom catheter application, (V2) 549
of contact lens care, (V2) 390
coughing teaching, (V2) 826
dangling client's legs at bedside, (V2) 628
deep breathing teaching, (V2) 826
definition of, (V1) 126
of denture care, (V2) 380
of digital stool removal, (V2) 579
drain emptying, (V2) 706
drain shortening, (V2) 705
dry wound dressing, (V2) 680
endotracheal suctioning, (V2) 744
of enema administration, (V2) 575
of fecal drainage device placement, (V2) 589
of fecal occult blood testing, (V2) 570
five rights of, (V1) 126–127, (V2) 46*b*
of foot care, (V2) 374
gastric suctioning, (V2) 834
grid for, NCSBN, (V2) 47
guidelines for, in minimizing malpractice risks, (V1) 1181–1182
of hair shampooing, (V2) 384
of hearing aid care, (V2) 398
heparin lock, (V2) 800
hydrating dressing, (V2) 693
of hygiene care, (V1) 578
of incentive spirometry coaching, (V1) 954
of indwelling catheter removal, (V2) 551
of intradermal injection administration, (V2) 445
of intramuscular injection administration, (V2) 453
intravenous fluid/electrolyte change, (V2) 793
intravenous fluid/electrolyte discontinuation, (V2) 803
intravenous fluid/electrolyte regulation and maintenance, (V2) 788
intravenous fluid/electrolyte solution change, (V2) 793
leg exercise teaching, (V2) 826
logrolling, (V2) 623
lung percussion, (V2) 728

mechanical ventilation, (V2) 752
of medication administration, (V2) 410–411
oral, (V2) 414
of metered-dose inhaler administration, (V2) 423
moving up in bed, (V2) 623
of nasal medication administration, (V1) 424
nasopharyngeal suctioning, (V2) 749
nasopharyngeal tube, (V2) 760
nasotracheal suctioning, (V2) 746
needle aspiration culture, (V2) ch 35
negative pressure wound therapy, (V2) 685
of nutritional assessments, (V1) 695
of oral care for unconscious patient, (V2) 382
oropharyngeal airway, (V2) 759
orotracheal suctioning, (V2) 746
of ostomy appliance changing, (V2) 582
of otic medication administration, (V2) 422
oxygen therapy, (V2) 731
pain management, (V2) 611
patient-controlled analgesia, (V2) 611
of perineal care, (V2) 371
peripheral intravenous infusion, (V2) 783
of peripheral pulse assessment, (V2) 191
of placing and removing bedpan, (V2) 572
postural drainage, (V2) 728
pressure ulcer assessment, (V2) 709–710
pulse oximetry, (V2) 726–727
of rectal suppository insertion, (V2) 428
of respiration assessment, (V2) 198
of restraint application and removal, (V2) 352
of safety interventions, (V1) 572–573
saline lock, (V2) 800
sequential compression device, (V2) 832
of shaving patient, (V2) 389
skin closures, (V2) 695
sputum collection, (V2) 723–724
of subcutaneous injections, (V2) 448
suture/staple removal, (V2) 703
taping dressing, (V2) 678
tracheostomy care, (V2) 736–741
tracheostomy suctioning, (V2) 741, (V2) 744
transparent film dressing, (V2) 691
turning in bed, (V2) 623
upper airway suctioning, (V2) 749
of urinary catheter insertion, (V2) 540
of urine bedside testing, (V2) 538
of urine measuring, (V2) 531
of urine specimen collection, (V2) 534
of vaginal medication administration, (V2) 426
vibration therapy, (V2) 728
volume-control pump, (V2) 790
wet-to-damp dressing, (V2) 682
of wound assessment, (V1) 916–917
wound irrigation, (V2) 675–676
wound swab culture, (V2) 673
Delirium
assessing older adults for, (V1) 280
clients with, interventions for, (V1) 787–788
Delta waves, (V1) 883
Deltoid muscle injection site, (V1) 650–651, (V1) 650*f*, (V1) 659*p*, (V2) 451–452*p*
Dementia
bathing and, (V1) 585
clinical insights on, (V2) 402
clients with, interventions for, (V1) 787–788
depression differentiated from, (V2) 108
in older adults, (V1) 210–211
assessing for, (V1) 214, (V1) 280
interventions for, (V1) 218–219
normal aging changes distinguished from, (V1) 210*t*
oral care and, (V1) 595
pain assessment in, (V1) 799, (V1) 800
sexuality and, (V1) 864
validation theory and, (V1) 148
Democratic leadership, (V1) 1058
Demonstration, in patient teaching, (V1) 414, (V1) 417*t*
Denial
in coping with anxiety, (V1) 269
as defense mechanism, (V1) 250*t*
as stage of dying, (V1) 353*b*
Denotative meaning, in verbal communication, (V1) 461
Dental caries, (V1) 591–592
in infant, (V1) 177, (V1) 591
Dental health, in health promotion assessment, (V2) 876
Dental hygiene. *See also* Hygiene, oral
in preschooler, (V1) 184
in school-age child, assessment of, (V1) 186
Dentist, on healthcare team, (V1) 20
Dentition. *See also* Tooth (teeth)
of school-age child, (V1) 185
Denture care, (V1) 593, (V1) 600*p*, (V2) 380–381*p*
Denver Developmental Screening Test, (V1) 178
Deontology, (V1) 1148
Dependence
chemical, in workplace, signs of, (V1) 1183*b*
on drug, (V1) 622
level of, (V1) 833
opioid, (V1) 806
on others, in illness, (V1) 231
Dependent interventions, (V1) 107
Depersonalization, preventing, (V1) 273
Depilatory use, (V1) 597
Depo-Provera injection, (V2) 655
Depression, (V1) 269–270, (V1) 269*f*
in adolescents, (V1) 190
assessment continuum for, (V1) 280*f*
assessment for, (V1) 279–280
guide for, (V2) 107
causes of, (V1) 270
complementary and alternative medicine for, (V1) 293*b*
dementia differentiated from, (V2) 108
grief differentiated from, (V1) 357
interventions/implementation for, planning, (V1) 282
in middle adults, (V1) 270
nursing diagnosis for, (V1) 281
in older adults, (V1) 211, (V1) 270
assessing for, (V1) 214
nursing interventions for, (V1) 282–283
outcomes/evaluation for, planning, (V1) 281–282
pain and, (V1) 795, (V2) 616
referral for
evaluation for, (V2) 105
indications for, (V1) 280, (V1) 281*b*
in response to stress, (V1) 249
sleep and, (V1) 890
as stage of dying, (V1) 353*b*
standardized nursing languages for, (V2) 111–112
symptoms of, (V1) 279–280
treatment of, (V1) 270
truths and myths about, (V1) 269*t*
Dermatitis, (V1) 901
Dermis, (V1) 579, (V1) 898, (V1) 898*f*
of neonate, (V1) 173
in older adults, (V1) 580*t*
Desire, in sexual response cycle, (V1) 859
Desquamation, (V1) 579
Detrusor muscle, (V1) 717
Development. *See also under specific age group, e.g.*, Infant(s), development of
cardiovascular system and, (V1) 971–972
definition of, (V1) 164
delayed, sexuality and, (V1) 867
exercise and, (V1) 826
mobility and, (V1) 826
pain and, (V1) 796
patterns of, (V1) 164
principles of, (V1) 164–165
pulmonary function and, (V1) 939–940
sexuality and, (V1) 853–855
sleep and, (V1) 885
theories of, (V1) 148, (V1) 165–170, (V1) 166–167*t*
cognitive, (V1) 165, (V1) 167, (V1) 168*t*
developmental task theory as, (V1) 165, (V1) 166–167*t*
moral, (V1) 169–170
psychoanalytic, (V1) 165, (V1) 167*t*
through life span, knowledge map for, (V2) 71, (V2) 75
Developmental dysplasia of the hip (DDH), (V1) 827
Developmental stage
blood pressure and, (V1) 448
communication and, (V1) 465
in health-illness, (V1) 225
host susceptibility and, (V1) 528
hygiene and, (V1) 575
learning and, (V1) 403, (V1) 403*f*
of maturing female, (V2) 303–304*t*
moral decisions and, (V1) 1143
neurological exam and, (V1) 506–507
physical examination and, (V1) 486–487
pulse and, (V1) 437
respiration and, (V1) 442–443
safety and, (V1) 547–548
in self-concept, (V1) 264
sensory function and, (V1) 774–775, (V1) 774*t*
skin and, (V1) 580
temperature regulation and, (V1) 425
Developmental stressors, (V1) 240
Developmental task theory, (V1) 165, (V1) 166–167*t*
Developmental theories, (V1) 290
Diabetes mellitus
foot care and, (V1) 588
foot ulcers in, (V1) 909
gestational, monitoring for, (V1) 172
maternal, macrosomia and, (V1) 171
in older adults, race/ethnicity and, (V1) 210
physical findings in, (V1) 694*b*
preoperative medications in, (V1) 1029*b*
sexuality and, (V1) 856–857
sleep and, (V1) 890
surgery and, (V1) 1029*b*

type 2, childhood obesity and, (V1) 186
urinary tract infections and, (V1) 721
Diagnosis. *See also* Diagnostic statements, formats for
implementation and, (V1) 121
knowledge map on, (V2) 32
medical
nursing diagnosis and collaborative problems and
comparison of, (V1) 63*t*
distinguishing between, (V1) 64*f*
recognizing, (V1) 62–64
nursing, (V1) 59–83. *See also* Nursing diagnosis(es)
in nursing process, (V1) 38, (V1) 38*f*
Diagnostic and Statistical Manual (DSM-5), (V1) 74
Diagnostic (exploratory) surgery, (V1) 1027
Diagnostic reasoning, (V1) 65–73
computer-assisted diagnosing and, (V1) 71–72
critiquing, (V1) 73*b*
data analysis and interpretation in, (V1) 65–68, (V1) 67*f*
definition of, (V1) 65
drawing conclusions about health status in, (V1) 67*f*, (V1) 68–69
in health promotion, (V1) 234
reflecting critically on, (V1) 72–73
verifying problems with patient in, (V1) 67*f*, (V1) 69
Diagnostic related group, (V2) 865
Diagnostic related groups (DRGs), in reimbursement, (V1) 23
Diagnostic statements, (V1) 76–82
formats for, (V1) 77–80, (V1) 78*t*
for collaborative problems, (V1) 78*f*, (V1) 79
one-part, (V1) 77, (V1) 78*t*, (V1) 79
three-part, (V1) 77, (V1) 78*t*
two-part, (V1) 77, (V1) 78*t*
variations in, (V1) 78*f*, (V1) 79
quality of, judging guidelines for, (V1) 80–82
reflecting critically about, (V1) 80–82
writing, (V1) 76–80
Diagnostic testing
circulation-related, (V2) 777
of fluid, electrolyte, and acid-base balance, (V1) 1000–1001, (V2) 817
lung volumes and capacities, (V2) 766–767
oxygenation-related, (V2) 767
preoperative, (V2) 845
tuberculin skin, (V1) 947–948, (V2) 768
for wound assessment, (V2) 715
Diaphragm, (V1) 937, (V1) 937*f*
Diaphragm (contraceptive), (V2) 655–656
Diarrhea
definition of, (V1) 756
interventions for, (V1) 758–759
Diarthroses, (V1) 818
Diastole, (V1) 436, (V1) 502, (V1) 969
Diastolic pressure, (V1) 446
Diet
for fluid/electrolyte imbalance prevention, (V1) 1003
in pressure ulcer prevention, (V1) 915
sleep and, (V1) 886
Diet(s)
antigen-avoidance, (V1) 691
Asian, (V1) 689
calorie-protein push, (V1) 691
calorie-restricted, (V1) 690
changes in, associated with ostomy, (V1) 765*b*
diabetic, (V1) 690
in diarrhea management, (V1) 759
fat-restricted, (V1) 690
Hispanic, (V1) 689
Indian, (V1) 689
Mediterranean, (V1) 687
modified
by consistency, (V1) 690, (V1) 691*t*
by disease, (V1) 690–691
NPO, (V1) 690
protein controlled, (V1) 690
regular, (V1) 690
renal, (V1) 690
sodium-restricted, (V1) 690
special, (V1) 690–691
weight loss, (V1) 687
Dietary fiber, (V1) 668
Dietary history, (V1) 692
Dietary intake, impaired, interventions for, (V1) 698
Dietary Reference Intakes (DRIs), (V1) 646–665
for calcium, (V1) 992*t*
for minerals, (V1) 677–678*t*
for potassium, (V1) 677*t*
for Vitamin D, (V1) 992*t*
for vitamins, (V1) 674–676*t*
Dietary supplements, bowel elimination and, (V1) 749
Differentiated practice, (V1) 15
Diffusion, (V1) 986, (V1) 986*f*, (V1) 987*t*
Digital information sources, in patient teaching, (V1) 415–416, (V1) 418*t*
Digital rectal exam, in older adult assessment, (V1) 213
Dignity
human, as nursing value, (V1) 1146*t*
loss of, urinary function and, (V1) 719
respect for, do no harm and, (V1) 1150
Dilemma, ethical, (V1) 1156
Diploma nursing, research and, (V1) 152
Diploma nursing program, (V1) 10
Dipstick testing of urine, (V1) 725, (V1) 733*p*
Direct care agencies, (V1) 1126
Direct-care interventions, (V1) 106
Direct care provider
home health nurse as, (V1) 1127
role and function of, (V1) 6*t*
Directive leadership, (V1) 1058
Disability, chronic, as family health risk, (V1) 293–294
Disaccharides, (V1) 668
Disapproval, expressing, as barrier to therapeutic communication, (V1) 476–477
Disaster services nursing, (V1) 1122, (V1) 1122*b*
Discharge assessment/instructions form, (V2) 87
Discharge planning, (V1) 86–88, (V1) 237*p*, (V2) 83–85*p*
assessment in, (V1) 87
collaboration in, (V1) 88
definition of, (V1) 87
maintaining trust during, (V1) 236
for older adults, (V1) 88
written plans in, (V1) 87–88
Discharge Planning Form, (V2) 34
Discharge summary, (V1) 383, (V1) 383*f*
Disciplinary actions, for nurses, (V1) 1170–1171
Discipline, nursing as, (V1) 8
Discomfort zone, change and, (V1) 1069, (V1) 1069*f*
Discovery phase, in litigation, (V1) 1176
Discrimination, as barrier to culturally competent care, (V1) 317
Discriminatory sensations, testing, (V2) 292*p*
Disease. *See* Illness
Disease(s)
exercise and, (V1) 827–830
reportable, (V1) 863
Disengagement theory, of psychosocial development of older adults, (V1) 207
Disinfection, in medical asepsis, (V1) 534
Displacement
in coping with anxiety, (V1) 269
as defense mechanism, (V1) 250*t*
Dissociation, as defense mechanism, (V1) 250*t*
Distance
intimate, communication and, (V1) 466
personal, communication and, (V1) 466
public, communication and, (V1) 466
social, communication and, (V1) 466
Distraction, for pain, (V1) 803
Distress, (V1) 240. *See also* Stress; Stressor(s)
moral, (V1) 1140, (V1) 1141*f*
Distributive justice, (V1) 1151–1152
Disturbed body image, wounds and, (V1) 917
Disturbed sleep pattern, (V1) 891–892
Disuse syndrome, risk for, (V1) 834
Diuretics, (V1) 974*t*, (V1) 981
classes of, (V1) 719*b*
surgery and, (V1) 1030*b*
Diurnal variations, in blood pressure, (V1) 448
Diversions, urinary, caring for patients with, (V1) 738–739, (V2) 559
Diverticulosis, bowel elimination and, (V1) 751
DNAR order, (V1) 355, (V1) 356*b*, (V2) 152
Do Not Attempt Resuscitation (DNAR) order, (V1) 355, (V1) 356*b*, (V2) 152
Doctoral degree in nursing, research and, (V1) 152
Doctoral entry nursing program, (V1) 10
Documentation, (V1) 371–395, (V2) 161–176. *See also* Reporting
abbreviations for, (V1) 378, (V2) 169–170
of adding medications to IV fluids, (V2) 458
of administering feedings through gastric and enteric tubes, (V2) 506
of administering parenteral nutrition, (V2) 511
of admission of client to nursing unit, (V2) 79
antiembolism stockings, (V2) 831
of apical pulse assessment, (V2) 196
of apical-radial pulse deficit assessment, (V2) 198
of artificial eye care, (V2) 398
of assessment data, (V1) 54, (V1) 56, (V1) 57*f*
bandaging, (V2) 702
of bathing, (V2) 368
of beard and mustache care, (V2) 388

bed-chair transfer, (V2) 631
of bed monitoring device use, (V2) 351
bed-stretcher transfer, (V2) 631
binder, (V2) 699
of bladder/catheter irrigation, (V2) 555–556
of blood pressure measurement, (V2) 203
blood transfusion, (V2) 807
of breast examination findings, (V2) 259
of brief bedside assessment, (V2) 307
cardiac monitoring, (V2) 775
central venous access device, (V2) 809, (V2) 814
chest tube, (V2) 758
of colostomy irrigation, (V2) 588
of condom catheter application, (V2) 550
of contact lens care, (V2) 391
coughing, teaching of, (V2) 829
dangling legs at bedside, (V2) 631
deep breathing, teaching of, (V2) 829
delegation of, (V1) 395
of digital stool removal, (V2) 580–581
of discharge of client from healthcare facility, (V2) 85
drain emptying, (V2) 707
drain shortening, (V2) 706
dressing, taping of, (V2) 680
dry wound dressing, (V2) 682
electronic, (V1) 382
of enema administration, (V2) 578
of evaluative statement, (V1) 132–133, (V1) 134*f*
of fecal drainage device placement, (V2) 591
of fecal occult blood testing, (V2) 572
of fingerstick blood glucose levels, (V2) 497
of foot care, (V2) 376
forms for, (V1) 382–388, (V2) 171–173
admission data form as, (V1) 382–383, (V2) 171
checklists as, (V1) 384, (V1) 385*f*
discharge summary as, (V1) 383, (V1) 383*f*
flowsheets as, (V1) 383–384, (V2) 173
graphic records as, (V1) 383–384
input and output records as, (V1) 384, (V2) 172
integrated care plan as, (V1) 387–388
Kardex as, (V1) 387
medication administration records as, (V1) 384, (V1) 386–387, (V1) 386*f*
occurrence report as, (V1) 388, (V1) 388*f*
patient care summary as, (V1) 387, (V1) 388*f*
gastric suctioning, (V2) 838
of general survey, (V2) 226*p*
guidelines for, (V2) 164–168, (V2) 907
of hair assessment, (V2) 234
of hair shampooing, (V2) 387
of head and face assessment, (V2) 238
of hearing aid care, (V2) 400
heparin lock, (V2) 802
in home healthcare, (V1) 389
hydrating dressing, (V2) 694
of implementation, (V1) 128
of indwelling catheter insertion, (V2) 548
of indwelling catheter removal, (V2) 552
infusion pump, (V2) 792
of intradermal injection administration, (V2) 447
of intramuscular injection administration, (V2) 456
intraoperative nursing, (V1) 1044
intravenous fluid/electrolyte administration, (V2) 788, (V2) 790
intravenous fluid/electrolyte discontinuation, (V2) 804
intravenous fluid/electrolyte dressing change, (V2) 800
intravenous fluid/electrolyte solution/tubing change, (V2) 795
of IV push medication administration, (V2) 463
knowledge map for, (V2) 176
leg exercises, teaching of, (V2) 829
legal, (V1) 372
of lipid administration, (V2) 513
in long-term care, (V1) 389
mechanical ventilation, (V2) 754
of medication administration, (V2) 413–414
of medication administration through central venous access device, (V2) 470
of medication administration through enteral tube, (V2) 418
of medication administration to skin, (V2) 432
of metered-dose inhaler administration, (V2) 434
in minimizing malpractice risks, (V1) 1179–1180
moving and turning patient in bed, (V2) 627
moving in bed, teaching of, (V2) 829
of nail assessment, (V2) 236
of nasal medication administration, (V2) 425
of nasogastric and nasoenteric tubes, (V2) 502
nasopharyngeal suctioning, (V2) 751
nasopharyngeal tube, (V2) 761
nasotracheal suctioning, (V2) 748
negative pressure wound therapy, (V2) 690
nursing process and, (V1) 378
of ophthalmic medication administration, (V2) 421–422
of oral care, (V2) 379
of oral care for unconscious patient, (V1) 364
of oral medication administration, (V2) 418
oropharyngeal airway, (V2) 760
oropharyngeal suctioning, (V2) 751
orotracheal suctioning, (V2) 748
of ostomy appliance changing, (V2) 585
of otic irrigation, (V2) 602
of otic medication administration, (V2) 423
oxygen therapy, (V2) 733
pain management, (V1) 812
patient-controlled analgesia, (V2) 613–614
percussion therapy, (V2) 730
of perineal care, (V2) 374
of peripheral pulse assessment, (V2) 194
peripherally inserted central catheter, (V2) 814
of physical assessment findings, (V1) 511–512
of placing and removing bedpan, (V2) 574
position change, (V2) 627
postural drainage, (V2) 730
pulse oximetry, (V2) 728
of rectal suppository insertion, (V2) 429
of rectal tube insertion, (V2) 582
of removing nasogastric and nasoenteric tubes, (V2) 507
of respiration assessment, (V2) 199–200
of restraint use, (V2) 354
saline, (V2) 802
sequential compression device, (V2) 833
of shaving patient, (V2) 390
skin closures, (V2) 696
of skin lesions, (V2) 229, (V2) 229*f*
sputum collection, (V2) 726
standardized nursing languages in, importance of, (V1) 373
of subcutaneous injection administration, (V2) 450
suture/staple removal, (V2) 704
of teaching and learning, (V1) 419
of telephone orders, (V1) 391–392
of temperature assessment, (V2) 190
tracheostomy care, (V2) 740–741
tracheostomy suctioning, (V2) 744
of transfer of client to another unit, (V2) 81
of transfer of client to long-term care facility, (V2) 83
transfusion reaction, (V2) 807*p*
transparent film dressing, (V2) 692
of urine bedside testing, (V2) 539
of urine measurements, (V2) 534
of urine specimen collection, (V2) 537
use of, by healthcare providers, (V1) 372–373
of vaginal medication administration, (V2) 427
of verbal orders, (V1) 392
vibration therapy, (V2) 730
of vital signs, (V1) 422
wet-to-damp dressing, (V2) 685
wound irrigation, (V2) 678
wound swab culture, (V2) 675
Documents, in patient care plan, (V1) 89–94, (V1) 89*f*, (V1) 90*f*, (V1) 92–93*f*
Doing, in full-spectrum nursing, (V1) 40–41, (V1) 40*f*, (V1) 40*t*
Doing for, in caring, (V1) 39
Domestic abuse. *See also* Abuse
as family health risk, (V1) 294–295
of middle adult, (V1) 198
Domestic violence, (V1) 864–865
Dominant culture, (V1) 306
Dorsal recumbent position, (V1) 840
Dorsalis pedis pulse, assessment of, (V2) 192*p*
Dorsogluteal muscle injection site, (V1) 650
Dosage. *See* Medication(s), dosage of
Double-barreled colostomy, (V1) 752, (V1) 752*f*
Double locking, of controlled substances, (V1) 606
Douche, (V1) 638
Douching, teaching for, (V1) 869
Drain/drainage
chest, (V1) 961–963, (V1) 963–964*p*, (V1) 965–966*p*, (V2) 755–759*p*
complications of, (V1) 963, (V2) 764–765
Hemovac, (V1) 922, (V1) 922*f*
Jackson-Pratt, (V1) 922, (V1) 922*f*
Penrose, (V1) 922, (V1) 922*f*
postoperative, (V1) 1046
postural, (V1) 955, (V1) 963–964*p*, (V2) 728–730*p*
wound, (V1) 921–922, (V1) 922*f*
assessment of, (V1) 915
emptying of, (V1) 906, (V1) 931*p*, (V2) 706–707*p*

serosanguineous, (V1) 906
shortening of, (V1) 906, (V1) 931*p*, (V2) 705–706*p*
Dreams
erotic, (V1) 861
memory and, (V1) 879–880
Dress, in physical examination, (V1) 488
Dressing (wound)
absorbent, (V1) 925*t*
adhesive tape for, (V1) 905, (V1) 924, (V1) 929*p*
alginate, (V1) 925*t*
antimicrobial, (V1) 925*t*
asepsis for, (V1) 928
collagen, (V1) 925*t*
dry, (V1) 929*p*, (V2) 680–682*p*, (V2) 796–800*p*
foam, (V1) 926*t*
foam tape for, (V1) 924
gauze, (V1) 926*t*
antimicrobial, (V1) 925*t*
dry, (V2) 680–682*p*, (V2) 797*p*
peripheral IV, (V2) 787*p*, (V2) 797*p*
change of, (V1) 1012, (V1) 1017*p*, (V2) 796–800*p*
wet-to-damp, (V2) 682–685*p*
hydrating, (V1) 930*p*, (V2) 693–694*p*
hydrocolloid, (V2) 693–694*p*
hydrocolloids, (V1) 926–927*t*, (V1) 930*p*
hydrogel, (V1) 927*t*, (V1) 930*p*, (V2) 693–694*p*
moisture barriers, (V1) 927*t*
Montgomery straps for, (V1) 924, (V1) 928*f*
nonallergenic tape for, (V1) 924
paper tape for, (V1) 924
peripheral IV, change of, (V2) 787*p*, (V2) 796–800*p*
postoperative, (V1) 1046*b*
primary, (V1) 923
procedures for, gauze, (V1) 930*p*, (V2) 787*p*, (V2) 797*p*
secondary, (V1) 923
silver, (V1) 919
skin sealants, (V1) 927*t*
taping of, (V1) 929*p*, (V2) 678–680*p*
transparent film, (V1) 927*t*, (V1) 928*f*, (V1) 930*p*, (V2) 690–692*p*, (V2) 787*p*, (V2) 797*p*
types of, (V1) 925–927*t*
wet-to-damp, (V1) 930*p*, (V2) 682–685*p*
wet-to-dry, (V1) 923
Drip rate, for intravenous fluids and electrolytes, (V1) 1011, (V1) 1011*b*, (V1) 1016*p*, (V2) 788–790
Droplet infection transmission, (V1) 521
Droplet precautions, (V2) 340
Drowning
of children, (V1) 550
prevention of, (V1) 562, (V1) 564
toddler, (V1) 939
of toddlers, (V1) 181
Drowsiness, opioid-related, (V) 807*b*
Drug. *See* Medication(s)
Drug abuse, (V1) 1097
definition of, (V1) 622
Drug(s), over-the-counter, (V1) 895–896, (V1) 952
Dry dressing, application/removal of, (V2) 680–682*p*, (V2) 796–800*p*
Dry heat therapy, (V2) 708
Dry powder inhaler, (V1) 639
Dual-energy x-ray absorptiometry (DEXA), in body mass evaluation, (V1) 693
Dunn's health grid, (V1) 223–224, (V1) 224*f*
Duodenum, (V1) 746
Durable medical equipment (DME), (V1) 1126
Durable power of attorney (DPOA), (V1) 355
Durable power of attorney for healthcare (DPOA), (V1) 1165, (V1) 1166
Duty, (V1) 1174
breach of, (V1) 1174
Dwarfism, (V1) 827
Dying, (V1) 345–368, (V2) 145–158. *See also* End-of-life care
assessment during, (V1) 357
knowledge map for, (V2) 158
stages of, (V1) 352–353
physiological, (V1) 352–353
psychological, (V1) 353, (V1) 353*b*
Dying patient
caring for, (V1) 364–366
addressing cultural needs in, (V1) 366, (V1) 366*f*
meeting physiological needs in, (V1) 364, (V2) 148–149
meeting psychological needs in, (V1) 364–365, (V2) 149–150
meeting spiritual needs in, (V1) 365
families of, helping, (V1) 364, (V2) 147–148
Dysmenorrhea, (V1) 863
Dyspareunia, (V1) 865
Dyspnea, (V1) 444, (V1) 946
assessment of, (V1) 977
Dysrhythmia, definition of, (V1) 440
Dysrhythmias, (V1) 975, (V1) 978
airway suctioning and, (V2) 745
Dyssomnias, (V1) 886–887
Dysuria, definition of, (V1) 725*b*

E

E-cigarettes, (V1) 953
E-mail, (V1) 1080–1081
Ear(s). *See also* Hearing
assessment of, (V1) 495–496, (V2) 245–249*p*
external, examining, (V1) 495–496, (V1) 495*f*, (V2) 245–246*p*
hygiene care for, (V1) 599
inner, (V1) 495, (V1) 495*f*
irrigation of, (V1) 786*p*, (V2) 600–602*p*
medication administration into, (V1) 638, (V2) 422–423
middle, examining, (V1) 495–496, (V1) 495*f*
Eating disorders, (V1) 703–704, (V1) 704*b*
in adolescents, (V1) 190
Ecchymosis, (V1) 490*t*
Echinacea, for common cold, (V1) 952
Echocardiogram, (V2) 767
Economics
healthcare, (V1) 1065
hygiene and, (V1) 575
Economy
culture and, (V1) 310
national, influencing contemporary nursing practice, (V1) 26
Ectopy, (V1) 978
Ectropion, (V1) 493
Edema, (V1) 491, (V1) 993
assessing for, (V1) 491*t*, (V2) 228*p*
Edematous tissue, in inflammatory process, (V1) 247
Edentulism, in oldest-old, (V1) 206
medication(s)
allergic reactions to, (V1) 620, (V1) 621*f*
cumulative effect of, (V1) 621
idiosyncratic reactions to, (V1) 620–621
Education. *See also* Learning; Teaching
computers in, (V1) 1085
continuing, (V1) 11
participating in, in minimizing malpractice risks, (V1) 1182
culture and, (V1) 309
documentation in, (V1) 373
formal, (V1) 9–11
graduate nursing, (V1) 10
practical nursing, (V1) 10
registered nursing entry, (V1) 10
vocational nursing, (V1) 10
grief, providing, (V1) 367
health, in health promotion, (V1) 1108
in-service, (V1) 11
informal, (V1) 11
providing, in minimizing malpractice risks, (V1) 1181
Educator
community nurse as, (V1) 1118
home health nurse as, (V1) 1127
Effleurage, for pain, (V1) 802
Ego, in psychoanalytic theory of development, (V1) 165
Ego defense mechanisms, in response to stress, (V1) 249
Ego integrity, *versus* despair stage of psychosocial development, (V1) 169
Egophony, (V1) 500, (V2) 264
Ejaculation, (V1) 849, (V1) 860
Elastic bandages, (V1) 931
Elastic recoil, (V1) 937
Elastic stockings, (V1) 980
Elasticity, lung, (V1) 937
Elbow, range of motion in, (V2) 644
Elder-friendly communities, (V1) 204
Elder-friendly residences, (V1) 204
Elderberry, for common cold, (V1) 952
Elderly. *See* Adults, older
Elective surgery, (V1) 1028
teaching for, (V1) 1036
Electric heating pads, (V1) 932, (V2) 708
Electrical hazards
in healthcare facilities, (V1) 553–554
in healthcare facility, interventions for, (V1) 568
Electrical stimulation, for wound healing, (V1) 919–920
Electrical storms
as safety hazard, (V1) 552
safety measures for, (V1) 568
Electrocardiogram (ECG), 969*f*, (V1) 977–988, (V2) 767
electrode placement for, (V1) 977, (V1) 978*f*
preoperative, (V2) 845
Electroencephalogram, during sleep, (V1) 882–883
Electrolyte(s), (V1) 984–985, (V1) 990–991*t*. *See also* Fluid(s)
assessment of, (V1) 998–1001, (V2) 815–817
critical thinking about, (V2) 818–819
full-spectrum nursing and, (V2) 817–818
imbalance in, (V1) 993, (V1) 994–995*t*, (V1) 996
nursing diagnosis for, (V1) 1001
nursing interventions for, (V1) 1001–1015

nursing outcomes for, (V1) 1001
prevention of, (V1) 1002–1003
intravenous. *See* Intravenous fluids and electrolytes
knowledge map for, (V2) 821
normal levels of, (V1) 2
regulation of, (V1) 988–989
renal effects on, (V1) 992
respiratory effects on, (V1) 991–992
serum, (V1) 1000, (V2) 845
supplemental, (V1) 1002, (V1) 1003
Electrolytes, pathogen growth and, (V1) 520
Electronic blood pressure monitors, (V1) 450
Electronic care plans, Nursing Interventions Classification in, (V1) 115
Electronic cigarettes, (V1) 953
Electronic documentation, (V1) 382
for recording assessment data, (V1) 56, (V1) 58*f*
Electronic formularies, (V1) 606
Electronic health record, (V1) 1084, (V1) 1085–1089, (V1) 1086*f*
accessibility of, (V1) 1087, (V1) 1087*f*
adoption of, (V1) 1087
barriers to, (V1) 1088
audit trail for, (V1) 1089
benefits of, (V1) 1087–1088
error reduction with, (V1) 1088
ethical use of, (V1) 1088–1089
HIPAA regulations for, (V1) 1089
improved efficiency with, (V1) 1087
interoperability and, (V1) 1085
passwords for, (V1) 1088–1089, (V1) 1089*b*
privacy with, (V1) 1088
reduced redundancy and, (V1) 1087
research with, (V1) 1088
standardized languages for, (V1) 1085–1087
unintended consequences of, (V1) 1088
Electronic health record system, (V1) 375–377, (V1) 376*f*
Electronic health records, guidelines for, (V1) 393–394
Electronic thermometers, (V1) 428–429, (V1) 429*t*
infrared, (V1) 429, (V1) 430*t*
Elimination
bowel, (V1) 744–770, (V2) 569–598. *See also* Bowel elimination
by neonate, (V1) 173
urinary, (V1) 714–743, (V2) 530–568. *See also* Urinary elimination
Elixir, (V1) 610*t*
Embolus
air, (V1) 1015*t*
catheter, (V1) 1015*t*
postoperative, (V1) 1048*t*, (V1) 1049*t*
prevention of, (V1) 980
pulmonary, (V1) 944, (V1) 1048*t*
Embryo, (V1) 170
Embryonic phase, (V1) 170
Emergency care triage, telehealth for, (V1) 1082, (V1) 1082*f*
Emergency Medical Treatment and Active Labor Act (EMTALA), (V1) 1165
Emergency surgery, (V1) 1028
teaching for, (V1) 1036
Emotional disturbances, self-care ability and, (V1) 576
Emotional intelligence theory, of leadership, (V1) 1058
Emotional responses
to stress, assessing, (V1) 255
to stressors, (V1) 248*b*
Emotions
body temperature and, (V1) 425
learning and, (V1) 401
Emotion(s), pain and, (V1) 795–796
Empathy
intellectual, (V1) 32
in therapeutic communication, (V1) 470–471
Empowerment, sources of, (V1) 1066–1067
Enabling, in caring, (V1) 39
Encoding, of message, (V1) 460, (V1) 460*f*
Encopresis, in preschooler, (V1) 183
End-of-life care, (V1) 18, (V1) 353—354
assessment in, (V1) 357
communication in
barriers to, (V1) 363*b*
therapeutic, (V1) 363
complementary and alternative modalities in, (V1) 354*b*
hospice care in, (V1) 354
interventions in, planning for, (V1) 358
legal/ethical aspects of, (V1) 354–357
advance directives as, (V1) 355
assisted suicide as, (V1) 355–356
autopsy as, (V1) 356
DNAR order as, (V1) 355, (V1) 356*b*
euthanasia as, (V1) 356
organ donation as, (V1) 356–357
nursing care plan for, (V1) 359–361
nursing diagnoses in, (V1) 357–358
outcomes of, planning for, (V1) 358
palliative care in, (V1) 354
postmortem care in, providing, (V1) 366–367, (V2) 150–15
End-stage renal disease (ESRD), definition of, (V1) 725*b*
Endocrine system
age-related changes in, assessment for, (V1) 208*t*
disorders of, from failure of adaptive mechanisms, (V1) 252*t*
exercise effects on, (V1) 824*b*
pain effects on, (V1) 797–798
responses of, in fight or flight reaction, (V1) 245, (V1) 245*f*, (V1) 246*f*
Endogenous analgesia system, (V1) 794
Endogenous opioids, (V1) 794
Endorphins, in stress response, (V1) 245
Endotracheal airways, (V1) 957–958, (V1) 958*f*, (V2) 763
Endotracheal intubation, (V1) 957–958, (V1) 958*f*
clinical insight on, (V2) 763
dislodgement of, (V1) 958
suctioning for, (V1) 959–960, (V1) 959*f*, (V1) 964–965*p*, (V2) 744–745*p*
Endotracheal tubes, (V1) 958, (V1) 958*f*, (V2) 763
Enemas, (V1) 639, (V1) 769*p*
administering, (V2) 575–578*p*
barium, in GI tract studies, (V2) 595
for fecal impaction, (V1) 760–761
preoperative, (V1) 1036
Energy
needs for, calculating, (V1) 680, (V1) 681*t*
work-related use of, (V1) 1074
Energy balance, (V1) 679–682
Energy nutrients, (V1) 67–673. *See also* Nutrients, energy
Engel, George, on grief, (V1) 347, (V1) 348*t*
Enjoying, in communication, (V1) 233
Enteral administration of drugs, (V1) 610*t*
Enteral feedings. *See* Enteral nutrition
Enteral medication administration, (V1) 635
Enteral nutrition
administering feedings in, (V1) 710–711
aspiration prevention with, (V2) 762
Be A.L.E.R.T. safety campaign for, (V1) 705, (V1) 706*b*
closed system for, (V1) 711
continuous, (V1) 710
cyclic, (V1) 710–711
definition of, (V1) 705
gravity feedings for, (V1) 710
home care for, (V1) 1134
intermittent, (V1) 711, (V1) 712*p*
monitoring patient on, (V1) 711
open system for, (V1) 711
patients receiving, infection prevention in, (V2) 519*p*
providing, (V1) 705
pump-controlled infusions for, (V1) 710
risks associated with, (V1) 705
solutions for, types of, (V1) 710*b*
sputum collection and, (V2) 723–726
Enteral tube, medication administration through, (V2) 416–417*p*
Enteric tube(s)
administering feedings through, (V1) 712*p*, (V2) 502–506*p*
types of, (V1) 707
Enterococci, vancomycin-resistant, (V1) 523
Entropion, (V1) 493
Enuresis, (V1) 718, (V1) 723
definition of, (V1) 725*b*
managing, (V1) 737, (V1) 737*b*
nocturnal, (V1) 890
in preschooler, (V1) 183
Environment
body temperature and, (V1) 425
cardiovascular effects of, (V1) 972
client, (V1) 601–603
assessment of, (V1) 601
beds in. *See* Bed(s)
bedside equipment in, (V1) 602–603
clean
in medical asepsis, (V1) 534–535
providing, clinical insights on, (V2) 336
interventions for, (V1) 601–603
noise control for, (V1) 602
temperature control for, (V1) 602
ventilation for, (V1) 602
communication and, (V1) 465
exercise and, (V1) 827
for learning, (V1) 401–402, (V1) 402*f*
living, hygiene and, (V1) 575
in nursing theory, (V1) 142, (V1) 142*f*, (V1) 143
pharmacokinetics and, (V1) 617
preparation of, for physical examination, (V1) 483
protection of, in health promotion, (V1) 1099
protective, in special situations, (V1) 536
maintaining, (V2) 342–343
pulmonary system effects of, (V1) 940–941

sleep and, (V1) 886
stimuli in, assessing, (V1) 781–782
in systems theory, (V1) 148
Environmental control, culture and, (V1) 309
Environmental factors
in health-illness, (V1) 227
in host susceptibility, (V1) 528
Environmental influences, on urinary function, (V1) 718–719
Environmental theory, of depression, (V1) 270
Environmental tobacco smoke, (V1) 942
Enzymatic debridement, (V1) 923
Enzyme(s), digestive, secretion of, nutrition and, (V1) 689
Epiboly, (V1) 915
Epidemics, minimizing effects of, (V1) 543
Epidermis, (V1) 579, (V1) 898, (V1) 898*f*
of neonate, (V1) 173
in older adults, (V1) 580*t*
Epididymis, palpation of, (V2) 298–299*p*
Epidural administration of drugs, (V1) 613*t*
Epidural analgesia, (V1) 808–809, (V1) 809*f*
contraindications for, (V2) 614
Epidural anesthesia, 1042*f*, (V1) 1041
Epidural injection, (V1) 810
Epiglottis, (V1) 745, (V1) 935, (V1) 936*f*
Epilepsy, sleep and, (V1) 891
Epithelialization, (V1) 903, (V1) 904, (V1) 915*t*
Equianalgesia, (V1) 807–808
Equipment. *See also* Needle(s); Syringe(s)
accidents related to, (V1) 553
patient care, soiled, CDC standard precautions on, (V2) 337–338
personal protective, (V1) 535. *See also* Personal protective equipment (PPE)
potentially contaminated, control of, (V1) 536–538
safe use of, clinical insights on, (V2) 906
safety of, maintaining, (V1) 571
suppliers of, (V1) 22
surgical counts of, (V1) 1044
Erectile dysfunction (ED), (V1) 865–866
Erikson, Erik, psychosocial theory of, (V1) 263
Erogenous zones, (V1) 858
Erosion, (V2) 232
Erotic dreams, (V1) 861
Errors
in healthcare, as safety hazard, (V1) 552–553
medication, (V1) 625–628. *See also* Medication error(s)
treatment, avoiding, (V1) 1179
Error(s). *See also* Never events
of commission, (V1) 1083
electronic health record reduction of, (V1) 1088
in execution, (V1) 1083
handwriting and, (V1) 1088
of omission, (V1) 1083
in planning, (V1) 1083
Erythema, (V1) 490*t*
description of, (V1) 581
wound-related, (V1) 914
Eschar, (V1) 915, (V1) 915*t*
Eschatology, (V1) 328
Eskimos, healers and practices of, (V1) 311*t*
Esophageal reflux, interventions for, (V1) 699
Esophagogastroduodenoscopy (EGD), (V2) 595
Esophagus, (V1) 745
Essential hypertension, (V1) 454
Essential oils, for aromatherapy, (V1) 779*b*
Esteem and self-esteem needs, (V1) 54
Estrogen, for urinary incontinence, (V1) 719
Ethical agency, (V1) 1140–1142
Ethical concepts
autonomy as, (V1) 1149–1150
beneficence as, (V1) 1150–1151
fidelity as, (V1) 1151
justice as, (V1) 1151–1152
nonmaleficence as, (V1) 1150
veracity as, (V1) 1151
Ethical decision making, (V1) 1154–1161
assessment for, (V1) 1154–1155
Golden Rule and, (V2) 900
improving skills in, (V1) 1161
MORAL model for, (V1) 1157–1158. *See also* MORAL model for ethical decision making
obligations in, (V1) 1159–1161
problem *vs.* dilemma in, (V1) 1155–1157
recognizing ethical issues in, (V1) 1155
working through ethical problem in, (V1) 1157–1159
Ethical dilemma, (V1) 1156
Ethical issues, in healthcare, (V1) 1154
Ethical knowledge, (V1) 37
in full-spectrum nursing, (V1) 40*t*, (V1) 41
Ethical problem, working through, (V1) 1157
Ethics, (V1) 1137–1161, (V2) 897–904. *See also* Nursing ethics
code of, nursing, (V1) 1152, (V1) 1153*b*, (V1) 1168
definition of, (V1) 1138
feminist, (V1) 1148–1149
law and, (V1) 1138
placebo and, (V1) 812
study of, reasons for, (V1) 1139–1140
values and, (V1) 1144
Ethics committees, (V1) 1160
Ethics-of-care, (V1) 1149
Ethnic groups, (V1) 304
health disparities among, (V1) 302
Ethnicity, (V1) 304
knowledge map for, (V2) 135
nutrition and, (V1) 687, (V1) 689
Ethnocentrism, (V1) 306
as barrier to culturally competent care, (V1) 316–317
Etiology(ies)
in diagnostic statement, (V1) 76–77
interventions and, (V1) 80
problem, identification of, in drawing conclusions about health status, (V1) 69
Etiquette for patients, CDC standard precautions on, (V2) 337
Eupnea, (V1) 444*t*, (V1) 945
European Americans
healers and practices of, (V1) 311*t*
pain perception and responses in, (V2) 127
values and health/illness beliefs of, (V1) 314*t*
Eustress, (V1) 240
Euthanasia, (V1) 356
Evaluation, (V1) 129–136, (V2) 45–53. *See also* Assessment(s)
checklist for, (V2) 48–50
of collaborative problems, (V1) 133–134
criteria used in, (V1) 130
critical thinking and reasoning in, (V2) 51
in full-spectrum nursing, (V1) 129–130
in health promotion, (V1) 234
implementation and, (V1) 122
intermittent, (V1) 131
knowledge map for, (V2) 53
of learning, (V1) 416–417, (V1) 419
in nursing process, (V1) 38*f*, (V1) 39
ongoing, (V1) 131
outcomes, (V1) 131
of patient progress, (V1) 131–134
process, (V1) 131
of quality of care in healthcare setting, (V1) 135–136
reflecting critically about, (V1) 135
relation of, to other nursing process steps, (V1) 129
standards used in, 130*b*, (V1) 130
structure, (V1) 130–131
terminal, (V1) 131
tools for, (V2) 46, (V2) 48–50
types of, (V1) 130–131
Evaluative statement, recording of, (V1) 132–133, (V1) 134*f*
Evaporation, in heat exchange with environment, (V1) 424, (V1) 424*f*
Evidence, best, basing practice on, (V1) 155–159
Evidence-based practice (EBP)
anxiety and music therapy in, (V1) 284
being good nurse and doing right thing in, (V1) 42
on bowel diversions, (V1) 764
clinical practice guidelines in, (V1) 109–110, (V1) 109*b*
communication in, (V1) 464
community nursing interventions in, (V1) 1120
computers, (V1) 1089–1093
cultural competence in, (V1) 319
definition of, (V1) 108
delegation in, (V1) 128
depression in elderly in, (V1) 284
on documentation, (V1) 394–395
on end-of-life communication, (V1) 365
evidence reports in, (V1) 109
full-spectrum nursing model applied to, (V2) 55
grandparents raising grandchildren in, (V1) 299
on health promotion, (V1) 1107
hypertension, (V1) 975
on injection pain, (V1) 647
integrating research into, (V1) 158–159, (V1) 159*b*
key concepts in, (V1) 138, (V1) 138*f*
knowledge map for, (V2) 58
motivational nursing intervention efficacy, based on stages of change on self-care in heart failure patients in, (V1) 117
nursing assessment of risk of chemotherapy-induced febrile neutropenia in, (V1) 54
nursing diagnoses, interventions and outcomes in, (V1) 83
on nutrition and brain function, (V1) 667
on oral care, (V1) 595
outcomes related to dehydration in pediatric population in, (V1) 104
on patient teaching, (V1) 416

preventive sexual health promotion in, (V1) 129
resilience in, (V1) 232
on SBAR model for communication and patient safety, (V1) 570
sexuality, (V1) 860
siderail use in, (V1) 27
sleep disorders, (V1) 888
on spirituality at end of life, (V1) 330
steps in, (V1) 108–109, (V1) 109*f*
stress and adaptation in, (V1) 241
surgical safety checklist, (V2) 844
on surgical site infection prevention, (V1) 537
telehealth home monitoring for older adults in, (V1) 219
on temperature, (V1) 435–436
tension-type headache, (V1) 888
theory and research on, (V1) 137–159, (V2) 54–58
on time orientation for cognitive impairment, (V1) 788
unintentional torts in, (V1) 1175
on urinary retention, (V1) 731
whistleblowing in, (V1) 1141
wound cleansing, (V1) 921
Evisceration, (V1) 907, (V1) 907*f*
postoperative, (V1) 1051*t*
Evolution of nursing, knowledge map for, (V2) 9
Ewald tube, (V2) 837
Exacerbation, of chronic illness, (V1) 231
Excessive daytime sleepiness, (V1) 886–887
Excitement, in sexual response cycle, (V1) 859
Excoriation, (V1) 581, (V1) 901, (V2) 232
Excretion, of medications, (V1) 615–616
Exercise
blood pressure and, (V1) 448
body temperature and, (V1) 425
encouraging, for regular defecation, (V1) 757
for health promotion, (V1) 1106, (V1) 1106*f*
in infection prevention, (V1) 532–533
for middle adult, interventions for, (V1) 199
prolonged, basal metabolic rate and, (V1) 680
pulse and, (V1) 437
respiration and, (V1) 443
for school-age child, teaching about, (V1) 187
in stress management, (V1) 257, (V1) 258
for young adults, interventions for, (V1) 196
Exercise(s), (V1) 821. *See also* Mobility
activity tolerance and, (V1) 833
aerobic, (V1) 821
for ambulation conditioning, (V1) 844, (V2) 638
anaerobic, (V1) 821
assessment of, (V1) 832–834, (V2) 641–642
bedrest and, (V1) 830
benefits of, (V1) 822–823, (V1) 824*b*
bone disease effects on, (V1) 827–828
bone trauma effects on, (V1) 828–829
cardiac injury with, (V1) 823–824
cardiovascular benefits of, (V1) 824*b*, (V1) 973
circulatory disorders and, (V1) 830
definition of, (V1) 817
dehydration with, (V1) 823, (V1) 825
development and, (V1) 826
disease effects on, (V1) 827–830
duration of, (V1) 821
endocrine benefits of, (V1) 824*b*
environmental factors and, (V1) 827
fatigue and, (V1) 830
fitness program for, (V1) 821–822, (V1) 823
flexibility, (V1) 821
frequency of, (V1) 821
full-spectrum nursing and, (V2) 648
gastrointestinal system benefits of, (V1) 824*b*
guidelines for, (V1) 822*b*
for health promotion, (V1) 824*b*
heat exhaustion with, (V1) 825–826
hyperthermia with, (V1) 825
hypothermia with, (V1) 826
immune system benefits of, (V1) 824*b*
integumentary system effects of, (V1) 824*b*
intensity of, (V1) 822*b*
isokinetic, (V1) 821
isometric, (V1) 821
isotonic, (V1) 821
joint disease effects on, (V1) 827–828
knowledge map for, (V2) 650
leg, (V1) 1054*p*, (V2) 826–827*p*, (V2) 828–829*p*
lifestyle and, (V1) 826
mental health benefits of, (V1) 824*b*
modes of, (V1) 821
musculoskeletal benefits of, (V1) 824*b*
musculoskeletal disease effects on, (V1) 827–828
musculoskeletal injury with, (V1) 824–825
nervous system benefits of, (V1) 824*b*
nursing diagnosis for, (V1) 834
nutrition and, (V1) 826
obesity and, (V1) 826
objections to, (V1) 835*b*
for older adults, (V1) 821, (V1) 822*b*, (V1) 825
pelvic floor muscle, for urinary incontinence, (V1) 736, (V2) 558–559
promotion of, (V1) 834–835
pulmonary effects of, (V1) 824*b*, (V1) 941
for range of motion, (V1) 843–844
rate of perceived exertion scale in, (V1) 822*b*
resistance, (V1) 821
respiratory benefits of, (V1) 824*b*
respiratory disease and, (V1) 829–830
risks of, (V1) 823–826
safety for, (V1) 835
skin effects of, (V1) 824*b*, (V1) 901
sleep and, (V1) 886
stress and, (V1) 827
support system for, (V1) 827
talk test during, (V1) 822*b*
target heart rate in, (V1) 822*b*
tips for, (V1) 823
types of, (V1) 821
urinary system benefits of, (V1) 824*b*
Exhalation, (V1) 937, (V1) 937*f*
Exhaustion, heat, (V1) 426
Exhaustion stage, of general adaptation syndrome, (V1) 247
Exocrine glands, in drug excretion, (V1) 616
Expectorants, (V1) 952
Expectorated sputum, (V2) 724–725
Expert witness, (V1) 1174
Expertise
empowerment and, (V1) 1067
power of, (V1) 1066
sharing of, (V1) 1067
Expiration, mechanics of, (V1) 442, (V1) 442*f*
Expiratory reserve volume, (V2) 766
Exploratory (diagnostic) surgery, (V1) 1027
Exploring alternatives, in critical thinking, (V1) 35*t*, (V1) 36, (V2) 12
Expressive writing, for pain, (V1) 804
Extended care facilities, (V1) 16–17. *See also* Nursing homes
External respiration, (V1) 938, (V1) 938*f*
Extracellular fluid (ECF), (V1) 984, (V1) 985
Extracellullar fluid, (V1) 679
Extract, (V1) 610*t*
Extraocular movements, assessing, (V2) 240–241*p*
Extravasation, (V1) 1013*t*, (V2) 814. *See also* Infiltration
Exudate, (V1) 906
amount of, (V1) 914
color of, (V1) 914
drainage of. *See* Drain/drainage
odor of, (V1) 914
purosanguineous, (V1) 906
purulent, (V1) 906
sanguineous, (V1) 906
serosanguineous, (V1) 906
serous, (V1) 906
Exudate formation, in inflammatory response, (V1) 248
Eye(s). *See also* Vision
artificial, caring for, (V1) 598, (V1) 599*f*, (V1) 601*p*, (V2) 397–398*p*
assessment of, (V1) 493–495, (V2) 238–245*p*
for hygiene care, (V1) 597
defensive function of, (V1) 524
disorders of, (V2) 313*f*
external structures of, (V1) 493–494, (V1) 494*f*
hygiene care for, (V1) 597–599
internal structures of, (V1) 495
irrigation of, (V2) 421*p*
medication administration into, (V1) 638, (V2) 419–422*p*
Eye exam
for middle adult, (V1) 198
in older adult assessment, (V1) 213
Eye shields, (V1) 535*f*
assessing need for, (V2) 320
CDC standard precautions on, (V2) 337
donning, (V2) 321*p*
removing, (V2) 323*p*
Eyeglasses, caring for, (V1) 598
Eyelashes, inspection of, (V2) 241*p*
Eyelids
abnormal findings on, (V1) 493
drooping of, (V1) 493
inspection of, (V2) 241*p*

F

Face, assessment of, (V1) 493, (V2) 236–238*p*
Face mask, oxygen, (V1) 956, (V2) 733–734
Face masks, (V1) 535*f*
assessing need for, (V2) 320
donning, (V2) 321*p*
removing, (V2) 323*p*
Face tent, for oxygen therapy, (V2) 735

Face-to-face oral report, (V1) 390
Facebook, (V1) 1081
Facial expression, in nonverbal communication, (V1) 463, (V1) 463*f*
Facial nerve (VII), testing, (V2) 289*p*
FACT documentation system, (V1) 381
FACT format, for documenting care, (V2) 907
FACTUAL format, for charting, (V1) 1180
Fahrenheit-Centigrade conversion chart, (V2) 206
Fahrenheit temperature scale, (V1) 427, (V1) 427*f*
Failure to probe, as barrier to therapeutic communication, (V1) 476
Failure to thrive, of infant, (V1) 177
Fair-mindedness, (V1) 32–33
Faith, (V1) 328–329. *See also* Religion; Spirituality
Falls
  in healthcare facility, (V1) 553
    interventions for, (V1) 568, (V1) 569*b*
    risk assessment for, (V1) 557, (V1) 558*f*
  in home
    prevention of, (V1) 562, (V1) 563*b*
    risk factors for, (V1) 550
  prevention of
    Get Up and Go Test in, (V2) 357*p*
    nurse's legal responsibilities and, (V1) 1178*b*
    Timed Up & GO Test in, (V2) 357*p*
False imprisonment, (V1) 1173
False reassurance, as barrier to therapeutic communication, (V1) 477
Family(ies), (V1) 286–300, (V2) 118–124
  with adolescents, health risks for, (V1) 291, (V1) 291*f*
  blended, (V1) 288
  care of, theories useful for, (V1) 289–290
  caring for, (V1) 150
  as context for care, (V1) 288–289
  death in, interventions for, (V1) 300
  definition of, (V1) 287–289
  dual-earner, (V1) 287
  of dying patient, helping, (V1) 364, (V2) 147–148
  of dying patients, helping, (V1) 364
  extended, (V1) 288
  grandparent, (V1) 287
    evidence-based practice on, (V1) 299
  health assessment for, (V1) 295–298
    for caregiver role strain, (V1) 298
    conducting, (V2) 119–120
    family communication patterns in, (V1) 297
    family coping processes in, (V1) 297–298
    family health beliefs in, (V1) 296–297
    family health history in, (V1) 295–296, (V1) 296*f*, (V1) 297*b*
    guidelines and tools for, (V2) 120–121
  health risk factors for, (V1) 290–292, (V1) 292–295
    chronic illness and disability as, (V1) 293–294
    homelessness as, 294*f*, (V1) 294
    infectious diseases as, (V1) 293
    neglect in family as, (V1) 294–295
    poverty as, (V1) 292–293
    unemployment as, (V1) 292–293
    violence in family as, (V1) 294–295
  healthy, characteristics of, (V1) 298*b*
  illness within, interventions for, (V1) 300, (V1) 300*b*
  interventions/implementation for, planning, (V1) 298
  with middle-aged adults, health risks for, (V1) 291–292
  nursing diagnoses for, (V1) 298
  with older adults, health risks for, (V1) 292, (V1) 292*f*
  outcomes and evaluation for, planning, (V1) 298–299
  relationships with, in self-concept, (V1) 264–265
  sandwich, (V1) 288
  single-parent, (V1) 287–288
  step, (V1) 288
  structures of, changes in, (V1) 287–288
  subsystems of, (V1) 289
  as system, (V1) 289
  traditional, (V1) 287
  as unit of care, (V1) 289
  wellness of, promoting, (V1) 299
  with young adults, health risks for, (V1) 291
  with young children, health risks for, (V1) 290–291
Family assessment, (V1) 50
Family educator
  home health nurse as, (V1) 1127
  role and function of, (V1) 6
Family health, knowledge map for, (V2) 124
Family health history, in nursing health history, (V1) 52*t*
Family interactional theory, (V1) 289
Family nursing, approaches to, (V1) 288–289, (V1) 288*f*
Family support, for alcohol treatment, (V1) 297
Fantasy, sexual, (V1) 861
Fasciotomy, (V1) 1014*t*
Fasting blood sugar test, preoperative, (V2) 845
Fat(s)
  dietary, (V1) 672*t*
  monounsaturated, (V1) 672
  polyunsaturated, (V1) 672
  true, (V1) 671
Fat-soluble vitamins, (V1) 673, (V1) 676
  adult dietary reference intakes for, (V1) 674*t*
Fatigue, (V1) 830
  assessment of, (V1) 977
  exercise and, (V1) 830
  in healthcare workers, (V1) 882
  sexuality and, (V1) 867
Fatty acids
  essential, (V1) 673
  nonessential, (V1) 673
  saturated, (V1) 672
  trans-, (V1) 673
  unsaturated, (V1) 672
Fear(s)
  anxiety *vs.*, (V1) 267
  nursing interventions for, (V2) 846
  nursing outcomes for, (V2) 846
  pain and, (V1) 795
  postoperative, (V2) 846
  preoperative, (V1) 1032–1033, (V2) 846
  in response to stress, (V1) 249
  sexuality and, (V1) 867, (V1) 868
  about spirituality, (V1) 336–337
Febrile, (V1) 425
Fecal collection devices, external, for bowel incontinence, (V1) 762, (V1) 763*f*, (V1) 770*p*
Fecal drainage device
  external, (V2) 588
    applying, (V2) 589*p*
  indwelling
    care of patient with, (V2) 592
    inserting, (V1) 770*p*, (V2) 590–591*p*
Fecal drainage devices, indwelling, (V1) 763, (V1) 763*f*
Fecal impaction, (V1) 759–761
  digital removal of stool for, (V1) 761, (V1) 769*p*, (V2) 579–581*p*
  enemas for, (V1) 760–761, (V1) 769*p*
Fecal incontinence. *See* Bowel incontinence
Fecal occult blood, testing for, (V1) 755, (V1) 769*p*, (V2) 570–572*p*
Feces, (V1) 747
  fluid loss with, (V1) 987
  normal characteristics and variations in, (V1) 754*t*
Federal law, (V1) 1164–1167
Feedback
  in communication, (V1) 460*f*, (V1) 461
  evaluative, (V1) 1067
  in learning, (V1) 401
  in systems theory, (V1) 149
Feeding(s)
  enteral, (V1) 705–711. *See also* Enteral nutrition
  infant, (V1) 176, (V1) 682–683
Feeding tube(s)
  enteric
    administering feedings through, (V1) 712*p*, (V2) 502–506*p*
    types of, (V1) 707
  gastric, administering feedings through, (V1) 712*p*, (V2) 502–506*p*
  gastrostomy, (V1) 708
    percutaneous endoscopic, (V1) 708–709, (V1) 708*f*
  inserting, (V2) 498–502*p*
  jejunostomy, (V1) 708–709
  Levin, (V1) 707, (V1) 707*f*
  lumen of, (V1) 708
  medication administration through, (V2) 416–417*p*
  nasoenteric, (V1) 707, (V1) 708*f*, (V1) 712*p*. *See also* Nasoenteric feeding tube(s)
  nasogastric, (V1) 707, (V1) 712*p*. *See also* Nasogastric feeding tube(s)
  nasojejunal, (V1) 707
  placement of, checking, (V1) 709–710, (V2) 517–518*p*
  removing, (V1) 711, (V2) 506–507*p*
  Salem sump, (V1) 707, (V1) 707*f*
  selecting, (V1) 707–709
  sputum collection and, (V2) 723–726
Feelings, in depression, (V1) 279
Fellatio, (V1) 861
Felonies, definition of, (V1) 1171–1172
Female circumcision, (V1) 855–856
Female development, maturation status of, (V2) 303–304*t*
Female genitourinary system
  abnormalities of, (V2) 315*f*
  assessment of, (V1) 510–511, (V1) 510*f*, (V1) 514*p*
Feminist ethics, (V1) 1148–1149

Femoral hernias, palpation for, (V2) 299*p*, (V2) 303*p*
Femoral pulse, assessment of, (V2) 193*p*
Fencing reflex, (V1) 174
Fertilization, (V1) 170
Fetal alcohol syndrome, (V1) 175
Fetus
definition of, (V1) 170
development of, (V1) 170
Fever, (V1) 425–426
blood transfusion and, (V1) 1021*t*
constant, (V1) 426
in defense against infection, (V1) 524–525
intermittent, (V1) 426
phases of, (V1) 426
pulse and, (V1) 437
relapsing, (V1) 426
remittent, (V1) 426
respiration and, (V1) 443
skin breakdown and, (V1) 901
Fiber, dietary, (V1) 668
Fiberoptic colonoscopy, (V2) 595
Fibroblasts, (V1) 904
Fidelity
as ethical concept, (V1) 1151
in resolving dilemma, (V1) 1158
"Fight or flight" reaction, (V1) 244–246
Filipino heritage, pain perception and responses in, (V2) 127
Filtration, fluid, (V1) 986, (V1) 986*f*, (V1) 987*t*
Filtration pressure, (V1) 986
Finances, in health-illness, (V1) 227
Fingernails, hand hygiene and, (V2) 335
Fingers, range of motion in, (V2) 645
Fingerstick blood glucose levels, checking, (V1) 712*p*, (V2) 494–499*p*
Fire extinguishers, (V1) 570
Fire-hosing information, as barrier to therapeutic communication, (V1) 476
Firearm injuries, in home
prevention of, (V1) 562
risk factors for, (V1) 550
Fires
in healthcare facility, (V1) 553–554
preventing and responding to, (V1) 568, (V1) 570
home
causes of, (V1) 549–550
prevention of, (V1) 560–561
First-pass effect, (V1) 615
Fissure, (V2) 232
Fistula, wound-related, (V1) 907, (V1) 907*f*
Fitness, definition of, (V1) 817
5 A's for treating tobacco dependence, (V1) 953*b*
5 Cs of charting, (V2) 907
Flaccidity, muscle, (V1) 833*b*
Flap techniques, for wound healing, (V1) 920
Flatulence, managing, (V1) 758
Flatus, (V1) 747
Flexibility training, (V1) 821
Flora, in chain of infection, (V1) 519
Flow meter, oxygen, (V2) 731
Flow rate, intravenous fluid and electrolyte, (V1) 1011, (V1) 1011*b*, (V1) 1016*p*, (V2) 788–790
Flowsheets, (V1) 383–384, (V2) 173
Fluid(s)
in diarrhea management, (V1) 759
extracellullar, (V1) 679
for infants, (V1) 682
intake of
healthful, supporting, (V1) 757
promoting, (V1) 728, (V1) 728*b*
intracellular, (V1) 679
intravenous, adding medications to, (V2) 457–458*p*
pharmacokinetics and, (V1) 617
Fluid extract, (V1) 610*t*
Fluid(s), (V1) 984–988, (V2) 781–821. *See also* Electrolyte(s); Hydration
active transport of, (V1) 985, (V1) 986, (V1) 987*f*, (V1) 987*t*
assessment of, (V1) 998–1001, (V2) 815–817
balance of, (V1) 984
postoperative, (V1) 1046
for clot prevention, (V1) 980
critical thinking about, (V2) 818–819
deficient volume of, (V1) 992–993
risk for, (V1) 1046
weight and, (V1) 993, (V1) 1000
diffusion of, (V1) 986, (V1) 986*f*
distribution of, (V1) 984, (V1) 985*f*
excess volume of, (V1) 993
intravenous therapy and, (V1) 1015*t*
extracellular (ECF), (V1) 984, (V1) 985, (V1) 985*f*
filtration of, (V1) 986, (V1) 986*f*
full-spectrum nursing and, (V2) 817–818
hormonal regulation of, (V1) 987–988
hypertonic, (V1) 986
hypotonic, (V1) 986
imbalance in, (V1) 992–993
nursing diagnosis for, (V1) 1001
nursing interventions for, (V1) 1001–1015
nursing outcomes for, (V1) 1001
prevention of, (V1) 1002–1003
risk for, intraoperative, (V1) 1043, (V2) 849
insensible loss of, (V1) 987
intake of, (V1) 987, (V1) 1000. *See also* Intake and output (I&O)
facilitation of, (V1) 1003
modification of, (V1) 1003
interstitial, (V1) 984, (V1) 985*f*
intracellular, (V1) 984, (V1) 985*f*
intravascular, (V1) 984, (V1) 985*f*
intravenous. *See* Intravenous fluids and electrolytes
isotonic, (V1) 985–986
knowledge map for, (V2) 821
osmosis of, (V1) 985, (V1) 985*f*
output of, (V1) 987, (V1) 1000. *See also* Intake and output (I&O); Urine, collection of
passive transport of, (V1) 985–986
regulation of, (V1) 987–988
restriction of, facilitation of, (V1) 1003
sensible loss of, (V1) 987
third spacing of, (V1) 984
total, (V1) 984, (V1) 984*t*
transcellular, (V1) 984
Fluoride, (V1) 678*t*
Flushing, (V1) 490*t*
Foam
aerosol, (V1) 611*t*
open pore reticulated polyurethane, (V1) 930*p*
Foam dressing, (V1) 926*t*
Foam tape, (V1) 924
Focus charting, (V1) 380–381
Focused assessments, (V1) 48–49. *See also* Assessment(s)
Folacin, (V1) 675*t*
Folic acid deficiency, fetal risk from, (V1) 171
Folk healers and practices, (V1) 311*t*
Folk medicine, (V1) 313–315, (V1) 314*t*
Follower/followership, (V1) 1064–1065. *See also* Leadership
Fontanels, in neonatal skull, (V1) 173, (V1) 173*f*
Food(s)
allergies to, bowel elimination and, (V1) 750–751
causing diarrhea, (V1) 758
healthful intake of, supporting, (V1) 757
high-fiber, for constipation, (V1) 759
intolerances of, bowel elimination and, (V1) 751
Kosher, (V1) 331
nutritious
limited ability to purchase, interventions for, (V1) 699
on limited budget, (V1) 697, (V1) 698*b*
poor selection of, interventions for, (V1) 698
pulse and, (V1) 437
safety recommendations for, (V1) 565, (V1) 567*b*
Food frequency questionnaire, (V1) 692
Food guides, for older adults, (V1) 666
Food poisoning, (V1) 551
Food record, in nutritional screening, (V1) 692
Foodborne pathogens, (V1) 551
Foot cradles, (V1) 837, (V2) 637
Foot (feet)
care of
client teaching on, (V1) 589*b*
diabetic, (V1) 588
providing, (V2) 374–376*p*
deformities of, (V1) 827
developmental variations in, (V1) 587
hygiene for, (V1) 587–588
odor from, (V1) 587
problems of, (V1) 587
range of motion of, (V2) 646
Footboard, (V1) 837, (V1) 837*f*
Forearm support crutches, (V1) 846, (V1) 846*f*, (V2) 639–640
Forgiveness facilitation, for spirituality diagnoses, (V1) 341
Formal operations stage, of cognitive development, (V1) 168*t*
Formularies, (V1) 606
Formula(s), enteral, (V1) 710*b*
Fowler's positions, (V1) 837, (V1) 838*b*
Fraction of inspired oxygen, (V1) 949, (V2) 752
Fracture, (V1) 828, (V1) 828*f*
Fracture(s), of clavicle, in neonate, (V1) 175
Frail elderly, (V1) 207. *See also* Older adult(s), frail
Framework(s)
for assessment data organization, (V1) 53–54, (V1) 55–56*t*
conceptual, definition of, (V1) 141
ethical, (V1) 1145–1149
Framingham Heart Study, (V1) 138
Fraud, (V1) 1173
Freckles, (V1) 491

Fremitus, tactile, chest palpation for, (V2) 262–263*p*
French scale, for measuring feeding tube, (V1) 708
Frequency, definition of, (V1) 725*b*
Freud, Anna, (V1) 165
Freud, Sigmund, psychoanalytic theory of development of, (V1) 165, (V1) 167*t*
Friction, pressure ulcers and, (V1) 908, (V1) 908*f*
Friction-reducing devices, for position change, (V1) 840–841
Friction rub, (V2) 265
Frontal sinuses, transillumination of, (V2) 251*p*
Fruitarian diet, (V1) 686
Full Outline of UnResponsiveness (FOUR), (V2) 296
Full-spectrum nursing, (V1) 39–42, (V2) 11
  concepts used in, (V1) 39–40, (V1) 40*t*
  evaluation and, (V1) 129–130
  Golden Rule in, (V2) 900
  model for, (V1) 40*f*
    acid-base balance, (V2) 817–818
    advance directives, (V2) 89
    assessment, (V2) 22–23
    bowel elimination, (V2) 596
    care of older adults, (V2) 73–74
    circulation, (V2) 777–778
    communication, (V2) 216
    community nursing, (V2) 892
    culturally competent nursing, (V2) 131
    depressed single mother, (V2) 122
    depression, (V2) 113
    diagnosis, (V2) 28–29
    documentation and reporting, (V2) 174
    electrolytes, (V2) 817–818
    end-of-life care, (V2) 155
    evaluation, (V1) 129–130, (V2) 50
    evidence-based practice, (V2) 55
    exercise, (V2) 648
    health promotion, (V2) 879
    fluids, (V2) 817–818
    hearing deficit, (V2) 607
    hygiene, (V2) 404
    infection prevention, (V2) 345
    informatics, (V2) 866–867
    leadership, (V2) 860
    to legal accountability, (V2) 908
    management, (V2) 860
    medication administration, (V2) 484–485
    nutritional problems, (V2) 526
    oxygenation and, (V2) 768–769
    pain and, (V2) 619
    patient safety, (V2) 359
    perioperative nursing and, (V2) 855–856
    physical activity and, (V2) 648
    planning interventions, (V2) 41
    planning outcomes, (V2) 36
    sexual health and, (V2) 658
    sleep and, (V2) 667–668
    spiritual issues, (V2) 142
    stress, (V2) 98–99
    teaching and learning, (V2) 180
    urinary elimination, (V2) 565–566
    vital sign measurement, (V2) 206–207
    wounds and, (V2) 717–718
    young adult, (V2) 68–69
Full-thickness wounds, (V1) 902
Functional ability(ies)
  assessment of, (V1) 49–50, (V1) 50*b*
    for hygiene, (V2) 402
  in nursing health history, (V1) 52*t*
Functional dysrhythmia, (V1) 975, (V1) 978
Functional independence measure (FIM), (V1) 833
Functional limitations
  affecting nutrition, (V1) 689–690
  of oldest-old, (V1) 206–207
Functional nursing, (V1) 15
Functional residual capacity, (V2) 767
Functional status assessment, in older adult, (V1) 213
Fungal infection, of nails, (V2) 313*f*

G

Gag reflex, testing, (V2) 254*p*
Gait
  antalgic, (V1) 833
  assessment of, (V2) 642
  propulsive, (V1) 833
  scissors, (V1) 833
  spastic, (V1) 833
  steppage, (V1) 833
  waddling, (V1) 833
Gait(s)
  abnormal, (V2) 315*f*
  assessment of, (V2) 279*p*
  in nonverbal communication, (V1) 463
Gang rape, (V1) 865
Gas exchange, (V1) 938, (V1) 938*f*. *See* Respiration (gas exchange)
  alveolar cells in, (V1) 936, (V1) 937*f*
  external, (V1) 938, (V1) 938*f*
  impaired, (V1) 943, (V1) 943*b*, (V1) 951
  internal, (V1) 938, (V1) 938*f*
  problems with, (V1) 951
Gases, (V1) 612*t*
Gastric secretions, decreased, interventions for, (V1) 699
Gastric tubes, administering feedings through, (V1) 712*p*, (V2) 502–506*p*
Gastric ulcers, sleep and, (V1) 891
Gastrocolic reflex, (V1) 747
Gastroesophageal reflux, interventions for, (V1) 699
Gastroesophageal reflux disease, (V1) 940
Gastroesophageal sphincter, (V1) 745
Gastrointestinal motility, dysfunctional, definition of, (V1) 756
Gastrointestinal suction, (V1) 1053–1054, (V1) 1054–1055*p*, (V2) 834–839*p*
  tubes for, (V2) 837
Gastrointestinal system, postoperative complications of, (V1) 1050*t*
Gastrointestinal tract
  age-related changes in, assessment for, (V1) 208*t*
  in alarm stage, of stress response, (V1) 246, (V1) 246*f*
  anatomical structures of, (V1) 745–747, (V1) 745*f*
  defensive function of, (V1) 524
  disorders of, from failure of adaptive mechanisms, (V1) 252*t*
  in drug excretion, (V1) 615–616
  immobility effects on, (V1) 831
  pain effects on, (V1) 798
  physical activity effects on, (V1) 824*b*
  studies of
    direct visualization, (V2) 594–595
    indirect visualization, (V2) 595
  upper, (V1) 745
Gastrostomy button (G-button), (V1) 708–709, (V1) 709*f*
Gastrostomy tube (G-tube), (V1) 708
  medication administration by, (V1) 635
Gate-control theory, of pain, (V1) 794, (V1) 795*f*
Gauze bandages, (V1) 929, (V1) 931
Gauze dressing, (V1) 924*f*, (V1) 926*t*, (V1) 929, (V1) 930*p*, (V1) 931
  antimicrobial, (V1) 925*t*
  dry, (V2) 680–682*p*, (V2) 797*p*
  peripheral IV, (V2) 787*p*, (V2) 797*p*
  wet-to-damp, (V2) 682–685*p*
Gel, (V1) 611*t*
Gender, (V1) 851, (V1) 851*f*
  blood pressure and, (V1) 448
  body temperature and, (V1) 425
  communication and, (V1) 465
  disparities in life expectancy and, (V1) 202
  in health-illness, (V1) 224
  pharmacokinetics and, (V1) 617
  pulse and, (V1) 437
  in self-concept, (V1) 264
  as subculture, (V1) 307
Gender identity, (V1) 851–852
Gender roles, (V1) 851
General adaptation syndrome (GAS), 246*f*, (V1) 244–247, (V1) 245*f*
General system theory, in family care, (V1) 289
Generalizing results, in quantitative research, (V1) 153
Generativity, *versus* stagnation stage of psychosocial development, (V1) 169
Genetic factors, pharmacokinetics and, (V1) 617
Genetic theories of aging, (V1) 205
Genetics
  blood pressure and, (V1) 448
  in health-illness, (V1) 224
Genital human papillomavirus (HPV), (V1) 863
Genital warts, (V1) 863, (V2) 315*f*
Genitalia. *See also* Genitourinary system
  female, (V1) 510*f*, (V1) 848–849, (V1) 857
    inspection of, (V2) 301–302*p*
    mutilation of, (V1) 855–856
  male, (V1) 849, (V1) 850*f*
    inspection of, (V2) 297–298*p*
  self-stimulation of, (V1) 861
Genitourinary system
  age-related changes in, assessment for, (V1) 208*t*
  defensive function of, (V1) 524
  female
    abnormalities of, (V2) 315*f*
    assessment of, (V1) 509, (V1) 510–511, (V1) 510*f*, (V2) 301–304*p*
  immobility effects on, (V1) 831–832
  male
    abnormalities of, (V2) 31*f*
    assessment of, (V1) 509–510, (V1) 510*f*, (V1) 514*p*, (V2) 297–300*p*
  pain effects on, (V1) 798
  postoperative complications of, (V1) 1050*t*

Genogram, construction of, (V1) 206*f*, (V1) 296
Genomics, (V1) 295–296
Genuineness, in therapeutic communication, (V1) 471
Geranium, (V1) 952
Gestation, (V1) 170–172
  fetal development during, (V1) 170
  health problems during, (V1) 171
Gestational diabetes, monitoring for, (V1) 172
Gestures, in nonverbal communication, (V1) 464
Get Up and Go Test, (V2) 357*p*
Gilligan, Carol, moral development theory of, (V1) 169–170
Gingiva, (V1) 496, (V1) 590
  assessment of, (V1) 497, (V2) 252*p*
  hyperplasia of, from phenytoin, (V1) 591
Gingivitis, (V1) 497, (V1) 592
Ginkgo biloba, for depression, (V1) 283*b*
Ginseng, for depression, (V1) 283*b*
Gland(s)
  Bartholin's, palpation of, (V2) 302–303*p*
  exocrine, in drug excretion, (V1) 616
  prostate. *See* Prostate gland
  sebaceous, (V1) 579
    in older adults, (V1) 580*t*
  sweat, (V1) 579
    in older adults, (V1) 580*t*
  thyroid, assessment of, (V1) 498, (V2) 256*p*
  urethral, palpation of, (V2) 302–303*p*
Glasgow coma scale, (V2) 296
Glass thermometers, (V1) 428, (V1) 429*t*
Glaucoma, definition of, (V1) 777*b*
Global assessment, (V1)47
Global positioning systems, (V1) 1083
Glomerular filtration, (V1) 716
Glomerular filtration rate, (V1) 716
Glomerulus, (V1) 715–716
Glossitis, (V1) 497, (V1) 592
Glossopharyngeal nerve (IX), testing, (V2) 290*p*
Gloves
  CDC standard precautions on, (V2) 338
  sterile
    assessing need for, (V2) 320
    donning, (V1) 539*p*, (V1) 540–541, (V1) 541*f*, (V2) 322*p*
      closed method, (V2) 328–329*p*
      open method, (V2) 331–332*p*
    removing, (V2) 322–323*p*
    sizing of, (V2) 330
Gloving/gloves, for respiratory infection prevention, (V1) 953
Gluconeogenesis, (V1) 670
Glucose
  blood levels of. *See* Blood glucose levels
  preoperative, (V1) 2
  testing of, (V1) 977
  urinary, (V2) 563
Glucose intolerance, interventions for, (V2) 699
Glue, surgical, (V1) 906
Glycerides, (V1) 671
Glycogen, (V1) 668, (V1) 670
Glycogenolysis, (V1) 670
Goals
  achievement of, judging, in evaluation, (V1) 132
  for actual, risk, and possible nursing diagnoses, (V1) 98, (V1) 99*t*
  for cardiovascular problems, (V1) 979
  for collaborative problems, (V1) 98, (V1) 99*t*
  community (public) health, (V1) 100–102
  derivation of, from nursing diagnoses, (V1) 98I*t*
  essential *versus* nonessential, (V1) 98
  for fluid/electrolyte imbalances, (V1) 1001
  for groups, writing, (V1) 100–102
  health problems and, (V1) 80
  importance of, (V1) 95
  for intraoperative problems, (V1) 1043
  long-term, (V1) 96, (V1) 96*t*, (V1) 1074
  for mobility problems, (V1) 834
  nursing diagnoses and, (V1) 97–98, (V1) 97*t*
  nursing responsibility for, (V1) 95
  for pain management, (V1) 801
  patient, planning, (V1) 95–102
  reassessment for, (V1) 133*t*
  setting of, (V1) 1074
  for sexual problems, (V1) 868
  short-term, (V1) 96, (V1) 96*t*, (V1) 1074
  for sleep problems, (V1) 892
  statement of, components of, (V1) 96–97
  teaching, (V1) 409
  use of term, (V1) 95–96
  for wellness diagnosis, writing, (V1) 102
Goal(s), expected, reflecting critically about, (V1) 102–103
Goggles
  donning, (V2) 321*p*
  removing, (V2) 323*p*
Gonorrhea, (V1) 863
Good Samaritan laws, (V1) 1167–1168
Gordon's Functional Health Patterns, (V1) 55*t*
Gout, (V1) 828
Government financing, as payor for healthcare, (V1) 21
Government personnel, nurses as, licensure and, (V1) 1170
Gown, sterile
  assessing need for, (V2) 320
  donning, (V1) 539*p*, (V1) 540, (V2) 321*p*
    closed method, (V2) 328*p*, (V2) 329*p*
  removing, (V2) 323*p*
Gowns, CDC standard precautions on, (V2) 337
Graduate nursing education, (V1) 10
Gram, (V2) 481
Grand theory, (V1) 143
Grandparent families, (V1) 287
  evidence-based practice on, (V1) 299
Granulation tissue, (V1) 903, (V1) 904*f*, (V1) 915*t*
Graphic flow sheet, for recording assessment data, (V1) 56, (V1) 57*f*
Grasp reflex, (V1) 173, (V1) 174*f*
Gravity
  center of, (V1) 820, (V1) 820*f*
  for enteral feedings, (V1) 710
  line of, (V1) 820
Gravity drip
  for blood transfusion, (V2) 806*p*
  for intravenous infusion, (V2) 789
Grief, (V1) 347–351, (V2) 145–15. *See also* Death; Dying; Loss
  anticipatory, (V1) 351
    care map for, (V1) 362
    nursing care plan for, (V1) 359–361
  assessment guidelines for, (V2) 153–154
  bibliotherapy in, (V1) 364
  chronic, (V1) 351
  communication with people experiencing, (V2) 146–147
  complicated, (V1) 350–351
  delayed, (V1) 351
  depression differentiated from, (V1) 357
  developmental changes and, (V1) 350
  disenfranchised, (V1) 351
  as etiology, diagnosis of, (V1) 358
  expressing feelings in, (V1) 363*f*, (V1) 363
  facilitating work of, (V1) 363–364
  factors affecting, (V1) 349–350
  finding meaning in, (V1) 364
  knowledge map for, (V2) 158
  masked, (V1) 351
  as problem, diagnosis of, (V1) 357–358
  recalling memories in, (V1) 363
  as reconstructing meaning, (V1) 349
  stages of, (V1) 347, (V1) 348*t*
  types of, (V1) 350–351
  uncomplicated, (V1) 350
Grief education, providing, (V1) 367
Grooming, in physical examination, (V1) 488
Group acceptance, by adolescents, (V1) 189
Group B streptococcus, in pregnancy, screening for, (V1) 172
Group communication, (V1) 459
Group discussion, in patient teaching, (V1) 416, (V1) 417*t*
Group rape, (V1) 865
Group(s)
  communication in, (V1) 471–472
  successful, characteristics of, (V1) 472*b*
Groups, goals for, writing, (V1) 100–102
Growth
  of adolescent, (V1) 189
  definition of, (V1) 164
  of infant, (V1) 176
  of neonate, (V1) 172–173
  patterns of, (V1) 164
  periods of, basal metabolic rate and, (V1) 680
  of preschooler, (V1) 182
  principles of, (V1) 164–165
  of school-age child, (V1) 184–185
Growth factors, for wound healing, (V1) 920
Grunting, (V2) 265
  in respiration, (V1) 946
Guided imagery
  for pain, (V1) 803
  for sleep, (V1) 894

H

H_2 receptor antagonists, (V1) 1037*t*
Hair
  assessment of, (V1) 491–492, (V1) 512*p*, (V1) 596, (V2) 234*p*
  care of, (V1) 595–597
  color of, (V1) 491
  distribution of, (V1) 492
  loss of, (V1) 492, (V1) 596, (V2) 313*f*
  shampooing of, (V1) 596, (V1) 600*p*, (V2) 384–387*p*
  terminal, (V1) 595
  texture of, (V1) 491
  vellus, (V1) 595
Hair cells, as receptors, (V1) 772

Hair covers
assessing need for, (V2) 320–321
donning, (V2) 321*p*
removing, (V2) 323*p*
Hair follicles, in older adults, (V1) 580*t*
Half-and-half nails, (V1) 492, (V2) 313*f*
Halitosis, (V1) 591
Hallux valgus, (V1) 587
Hand hygiene, (V1) 538*p*
after PPE removal, (V2) 323*p*
with alcohol-based handrubs, (V1) 319–320*p*
CDC standard precautions on, (V2) 337
clinical insights on, (V2) 335
in home care, (V1) 1134, (V2) 888*b*
in medical asepsis, 533*f*, (V1) 533–534
soap and water for, (V2) 318–319*p*
surgical, (V1) 1026*b*
surgical scrub compared with, (V1) 540*t*
Hand rolls, (V1) 837, (V2) 637
Hand splint, (V1) 837
Handmaiden image of nurse, (V1) 5
Handoff report, giving, (V1) 389–390, (V1) 391*b*
Hand(s), range of motion in, (V2) 645
Hands-Only cardiopulmonary resuscitation, (V1) 981–982
Handwashing, surgical
brushless system for, (V1) 539*p*, (V2) 326–328*p*
traditional, (V1) 539*p*, (V2) 324–326*p*
Harassment, sexual, (V1) 871
Hard palate, assessment of, (V1) 497
Hardiness, (V1) 231–232, (V1) 232*f*
adaptation to stress and, (V1) 244
in health promotion assessment, (V1) 1103
Harris flush, (V1) 761
Haustra, (V1) 747
Haustral churning, (V1) 747
Havighurst, Robert, developmental task theory of, (V1) 165, (V1) 166–167*t*
Hay fever, (V1) 940
Hazardous waste, safe disposal of, (V1) 568
Hazards
environmental, in workplace, (V1) 941
oxygen, (V1) 956–957
Head, assessment of, (V1) 493–497, (V1) 513*p*, (V2) 236–238*p*
ears in, (V1) 495–496, (V1) 513*p*
eyes in, (V1) 493–495, (V1) 513*p*. *See also* Eye(s)
face in, (V1) 493, (V1) 513*p*
mouth in, (V1) 496–497, (V1) 496*f*, (V1) 513*p*
nose in, (V1) 496, (V1) 496*f*, (V1) 513*p*
oropharynx in, (V1) 496–497, (V1) 496*f*, (V1) 513*p*
skull in, (V1) 493
Head lice, (V1) 492, (V1) 596, (V2) 313*f*
Headache, tension-type, evidence-based study on, (V1) 888
Healing
in inflammatory response, (V1) 248
spiritual, (V1) 329
traditional/alternative, (V1) 313–315, (V1) 314*t*
Healing presence, in health promotion, (V1) 236
Healing touch, for pain, (V1) 803
Health
attainability of, (V1) 236, (V1) 238
beliefs about, (V1) 310, (V1) 312*f*
in family health assessment, (V1) 296–207
community, patient-centered care in, promoting, (V1) 1119*b*
concepts of, (V1) 222
conceptual models of, (V1) 223–224, (V1) 223*f*, (V1) 224*f*
culture specifics affecting, (V1) 308–310
disruptions of, (V1) 227–230
competing demands as, (V1) 229
imbalance as, (V1) 229–230
impending death as, (V1) 229
injury as, (V1) 227–228
isolation as, (V1) 230
loss as, (V1) 228–229
mental illness as, (V1) 228
pain as, (V1) 228
physical disease as, (V1) 227
unknown as, (V1) 229
eating for, (V1) 687
effects of mercury exposure on, (V1) 555*t*
experiencing, (V1) 221–238, (V2) 76–91
knowledge map for, (V2) 91
as individual experience, (V1) 222–223
influence of body image on, (V1) 266
influences on
biological, (V1) 224–225
cultural, (V1) 226–227, (V1) 308–310
environmental, (V1) 227
financial, (V1) 227
lifestyle choices as, (V1) 226
meaningful work as, (V1) 225
nutritional, (V1) 225
personal relationships as, (V1) 226, (V1) 226*t*
physical activity as, (V1) 225
religious, (V1) 227
sleep and rest as, (V1) 225
spiritual, (V1) 227
in nursing theory, (V1) 142, (V1) 142*f*, (V1) 143
promoting
communicating care and concern in, (V1) 233
nursing process in, (V1) 233–238
protection of. *See also* Illness prevention
health promotion *versus*, (V1) 1096
psychosocial, (V1) 263–267. *See also* Psychosocial health
spiritual beliefs and, (V1) 329–330
WHO definition of, (V1) 18
Health and Wellness Resource Center, (V1) 1092*t*
Health assessment, (V1) 479–515, (V2) 219–316
cultural adaptation for, (V1) 482*b*
definition of, (V1) 481
physical examination in, (V1) 481–487. *See also* Physical examination
Health behaviors, (V1) 1097
Health history
in cultural assessment, (V1) 318
family
in family health assessment, (V1) 295–296, (V1) 296*f*, (V1) 297*b*
in nursing health history, (V1) 52*t*
in health promotion assessment, (V1) 1102
past, in nursing health history, (V1) 52*t*
in pulmonary system assessment, (V2) 765
in self-care ability assessment, (V1) 576
sexual, (V2) 653, (V2) 656–657
sleep, (V2) 666
Health-illness continuum, (V1) 223, (V1) 223*f*
Health Insurance Portability and Accountability Act (HIPAA), (V1) 1164–1165
Health literacy, learning and, (V1) 405–406, (V1) 406*b*
Health maintenance organizations (HMOs), (V1) 23–24
Health policy, nurses' influence on, (V1) 29
Health practices, cultural, (V1) 310–312, (V1) 311*t*
Health problem(s)
definition of, (V1) 62
in diagnostic statement, (V1) 76
etiologies of, identification of, in drawing conclusions about health status, (V1) 69
goals and, (V1) 80
prioritizing, in diagnostic reasoning, (V1) 69–71
verification of, with patient, (V1) 69
Health promotion, (V1) 18, (V1) 1095–1109, (V2) 871–881
activities for, (V1) 257
analysis/nursing diagnosis in, (V1) 234
assessment for, (V1) 1102–1104
assessment in, (V1) 233–234
critical thinking on, (V1) 879–880
definition of, (V1) 1096
health protection *versus*, (V1) 1096
in infection prevention, (V1) 530, (V1) 532–533
interventions for, (V1) 1105–1108
NIC, selected, (V2) 877–878
knowledge map on, (V1) 881
models for, (V1) 1097–1099, (V1) 1098*f*, (V1) 1099*f*
nursing diagnoses related to, (V1) 1104
nursing outcomes for, (V1) 1104–1105, (V1) 1105*b*
planning interventions/implementation in, (V1) 234–238
planning/outcomes/evaluation in, (V1) 234
programs for, (V1) 1099–1100
throughout life span, (V1) 1100–1101*t*, (V1) 1100–1102
Health record(s), (V1) 372. *See also* Documentation
charting by exception in, (V1) 374–375, (V1) 375*b*
electronic, guidelines for, (V1) 393–394
electronic systems for, (V1) 375–377, (V1) 376*f*
paper
advantages and disadvantages of, (V1) 377, (V1) 377*b*
guidelines for, (V1) 392–393
problem-oriented systems for, (V1) 374
source-oriented systems for, (V1) 373–374
Health restoration, (V1) 18
Health risk, appraising, in health promotion, (V1) 1099–1100
Health risk appraisal (HRA), (V1) 1102
Health screening activities, in health promotion assessment, (V1) 1103–1104, (V2) 876

Health status
adaptation and, (V1) 244
client's perception of, in nursing health history, (V1) 52*t*
drawing conclusions about, in diagnostic reasoning, (V1) 67*f*, (V1) 68–69
racial/ethnic disparities in, (V1) 302
self-care ability and, (V1) 575–576
skin and, (V1) 580
Health teaching, for toddlers, (V1) 181
Healthcare
access to, racial/ethnic disparities in, (V1) 302
categories of, (V1) 17–18
culture of, (V1) 310
durable power of attorney for, (V1) 1165, (V1) 1166
economics of, (V1) 1065
ethical issues in, (V1) 1154
financing of, (V1) 20–22
high-tech *vs.* high-touch trends in, (V1) 29
holistic, (V1) 34
home, (V1) 1125–1135. *See also* Home healthcare
infections associated with, (V1) 517–518
locations for accessing, (V1) 15–17, (V1) 16*f*, (V1) 17*f*
ambulatory care centers as, (V1) 17, (V1) 17*f*
community health centers, (V1) 17
extended care facilities as, (V1) 16–17
home healthcare agencies as, (V1) 17
hospitals as, (V1) 15–16. *See also* Hospital(s)
independent living facilities as, (V1) 17
public health centers as, (V1) 17
primary, (V1) 18
quality of, racial/ethnic disparities in, (V1) 302
rationing of, (V1) 23
regulation of, (V1) 22
as right or privilege, (V1) 24–25
secondary, (V1) 18
settings for, expanded variety of, (V1) 27–28
socialized, (V1) 23
tertiary, (V1) 18
trends in, (V1) 27–29
Healthcare delivery system, (V1) 15–25
Healthcare facility. *See also* Hospital; Long-term care facility; Nursing homes
public safety room in, (V1) 571–572
safety hazards in, (V1) 552–557
biological, (V1) 55
equipment-related, (V1) 553
fires and electrical hazards as, (V1) 553–554
healthcare workers, (V1) 555–557
interventions for, (V1) 568–572
mercury exposure as, (V1) 555, (V1) 555*t*
never events and, (V1) 546, (V1) 553
restraint-related, (V1) 554
root cause analysis of, (V1) 553
violence in, coping with, (V1) 571–572
Healthcare jargon, (V1) 318
Healthcare policy, effects of, on care, (V1) 22–24
Healthcare proxy, (V1) 355
Healthcare reform
ANA recommendations for, (V1) 24
computers and. *See also* Electronic health record
effects of, on care, (V1) 22–24
issues related to, (V1) 24–25
Healthcare system
indigenous, (V1) 310, (V1) 311*t*
professional, (V1) 310, (V1) 312*t*
Healthcare team, members of, (V1) 18–20
Healthcare workers
hazards to, (V1) 555–557
infection control and prevention for, (V1) 542–543
Healthy meals, building, (V2) 513
Healthy People 2020, (V1) 826
Healthy People 2020 Goals, (V1) 1104, (V1) 1105*b*
Hearing. *See also* Ear(s)
assessing, (V1) 496, (V1) 513*p*, (V2) 247–248*p*
bedside assessment of, (V2) 606
changes in, with aging, (V1) 774*t*
deficits in, (V1) 777, (V1) 777*b*. *See also* Deafness
clients with, enhancing communication with, (V1) 478, (V2) 604
home care for, (V1) 787*b*
interventions for, (V1) 786
of neonate, (V1) 174
in oldest-old, (V1) 206
screening of, in older adults, (V2) 605
stimulation of, for sensory deprivation, (V1) 784
Hearing aids
care of, (V1) 599, (V1) 601*p*, (V2) 398–400*p*
types of, (V1) 599, (V1) 599*f*
Heart, (V1) 968–969, (V1) 968*f*
assessment of, (V1) 502–503, (V1) 514*p*, (V2) 265–271*p*
auscultation of, (V1) 502–503
sites for, (V1) 502*f*, (V1) 502*t*
autonomic nervous system effects on, (V1) 970
cycle of, (V1) 502, (V1) 968
electrical conduction of, (V1) 969, (V1) 969*f*
functions of, (V1) 501
blood pressure and, (V1) 446–447
immobility effects on, (V1) 831
inspection of, (V1) 502
monitoring of, (V1) 977–978, (V1) 979*p*, (V2) 774–776*p*
in older adults, (V1) 972
palpation of, (V1) 502
valvular abnormalities of, (V1) 975
Heart disease
sexuality and, (V1) 856
sleep and, (V1) 890
Heart failure, (V1) 974
Heart rate. *See also* Pulse
blood pressure and, (V1) 447
Heart sounds, (V1) 502–503
Heartbeat, (V1) 968, (V1) 969, (V1) 969*f*
irregular (dysrhythmias), (V1) 975, (V1) 978
Heat
cardiovascular effects of, (V1) 972
exchange of, between body and environment, (V1) 424, (V1) 424*f*
production of, in body, (V1) 424
Heat exhaustion, (V1) 426, (V1) 825–826
Heat stroke, (V1) 426
Heat therapy, (V1) 931–932
clinical insight on, (V2) 708
dry, (V1) 932, (V2) 708
for pain, (V1) 802
safety measures for, (V1) 932, (V2) 708
for wounds, (V1) 931–932
Heating pads, (V1) 932, (V2) 708
Heaves, precordial, (V1) 502
Heberden's nodes, (V2) 314*f*
Height
measurement of, in older adult assessment, (V1) 212
in physical examination, (V1) 488–489, (V1) 489*f*
Height–weight tables, (V1) 681
Heimlich maneuver, (V1) 564
Heimlich valve, (V2) 756
Helper T cells, in cellular immunity, (V1) 526
Helplessness, pain and, (V1) 795
Hemangioma, capillary, (V2) 312*f*
Hematocrit, normal, (V1) 993, (V1) 1000
Hematoma, (V1) 906
in IV therapy, (V1) 1013*t*
Hematuria, definition of, (V1) 725*b*
Hemiplegia, (V1) 833*b*
Hemodialysis, weighing with, (V1) 1000
Hemoglobin, (V1) 941, (V1) 948, (V1) 949
respiration and, (V1) 443
serum levels of, protein metabolism and, (V1) 695
test for, (V2) 767
urinary, (V2) 563
Hemorrhage(s). *See also* Bleeding
postoperative, (V1) 1049*t*, (V2) 852
splinter, (V1) 492
subconjunctival, (V1) 493, (V2) 313*f*
wound, (V1) 906
Hemorrhoids, (V1) 511
Hemostasis, wound, (V1) 903–904, (V1) 905*f*, (V1) 906
Hemothorax, (V1) 961
Hemovac drain, (V1) 922, (V1) 922*f*
Henderson, Virginia, nursing theory of, (V1) 144, (V1) 144*b*, (V1) 146*t*
Heparin, administering, (V1) 649
safe, (V1) 632
Heparin lock, (V1) 1017–1018*p*, (V2) 786*p*, (V2) 800–802*p*
Herbal preparations
for common cold, (V1) 952
skin effects of, (V1) 900
for sleep, (V1) 895–896
surgery and, (V1) 1028–1029
Hermaphrodite, (V1) 852
Hernia(s), (V1) 510
femoral, palpation for, (V2) 299*p*, (V2) 303*p*
inguinal, palpation for, (V1) 299*p*, (V2) 303*p*
locations of, (V2) 315*f*
umbilical, assessment for, (V2) 273*p*
Heroin, teratogenic effects of, (V1) 171
Herpes simplex lesions, (V2) 312*p*
Herpes vulvovaginitis, (V2) 315*f*
Heterosexuality, (V1) 852
High-Fowler's position, (V1) 837
High-top sneakers, (V1) 837
Hinduism, (V1) 333
Hip
developmental dysplasia of, (V1) 827
range of motion of, (V2) 645–646
Hip abduction pillows, (V1) 837, (V2) 637
HIPAA (Health Insurance Portability and Accountability Act), (V1) 1089

Hispanic Americans
diet of, (V1) 689
gender roles and, (V1) 855
healers and practices of, (V1) 311*t*
pain perception and responses in, (V2) 127
values and health/illness beliefs of, (V1) 314*t*
Histamine, (V1) 940
HITECH (Health Information Technology for Economic and Clinical Health) Act, (V1) 1087
Holistic care, standardized language and, (V1) 115–116
Holistic healthcare, (V1) 34
Holistic nursing, definition of, (V1) 138
Holistic nursing care, (V1) 149
Holmes-Rahe Readjustment Scale, (V2) 95
Holter monitoring, (V2) 767
Homan's sign, (V1) 977
Home. *See also* Home care; Home healthcare; Self-care
infection control in, (V1) 888*b*
oxygen administration in, (V1) 956*f*, (V2) 732–733
safety hazards in, (V1) 548–550
assessment of, (V1) 558
interventions for, (V1) 560–562, (V1) 563*b*
surgical discharge to, (V1) 1031
Home care
administering feedings through gastric and enteric tubes in, (V2) 505–506
administering lipids in, (V2) 513
administering parenteral nutrition in, (V2) 511
antiembolism stockings, (V2) 831
apical pulse assessment in, (V2) 196
apical-radial pulse deficit assessment in, (V2) 198
artificial eye care in, (V2) 398
bandaging, (V2) 702
bathing in, (V2) 368
binder, (V2) 699
bladder/catheter irrigation in, (V2) 555
blood pressure measurement in, (V2) 203
brushing and flossing of teeth in, (V2) 379
cardiac monitoring, (V2) 775
cast care, (V1) 829
checking fingerstick blood glucose levels in, (V2) 496–497
chest tube, (V2) 759
colostomy irrigation in, (V2) 588
condom catheter application in, (V2) 550
digital stool removal in, (V2) 580
discharge of patient to home, (V1) 1031
drain emptying, (V2) 707
dry wound dressing, (V2) 682
encouraging toddlers to eat in, (V1) 683*b*
endotracheal suctioning, (V2) 748
enema administration in, (V2) 578
fecal occult blood testing in, (V2) 572
foot care in, (V2) 376
gastric suctioning, (V2) 838
hair shampooing in, (V2) 387
hearing aid care in, (V2) 400
heparin lock, (V2) 802
hydrating dressing, (V2) 694
indwelling catheter insertion in, (V2) 548
indwelling catheter removal in, (V2) 552
infection control in, (V1) 1134, (V2) 888*b*
infection prevention in home and community in, (V1) 532*b*
informatics, (V1) 1082
infusion pump, (V2) 792
intramuscular injection administration in, (V2) 456
intravenous fluid/electrolyte administration, (V2) 788, (V2) 790
intravenous fluid/electrolyte dressing change, (V2) 799
intravenous fluid/electrolyte solution/tubing change, (V2) 795
IV push medication administration in, (V2) 462
lung care in, (V2) 264
mechanical ventilation, (V2) 754
medication administration in
through central venous access device in, (V2) 470
through enteral tube in, (V2) 418
metered-dose inhaler administration in, (V2) 434
mobility, (V1) 832
moving patient in bed, (V2) 627
moving patient out of bed, (V2) 631
nasogastric and nasoenteric tubes in, (V2) 501–502
nasopharyngeal suctioning, (V2) 751
nasotracheal suctioning, (V2) 748
negative pressure wound therapy, (V2) 690
nutritional support in, (V1) 707*b*
ophthalmic medication administration in, (V2) 421
oropharyngeal suctioning, (V2) 751
orotracheal suctioning, (V2) 748
ostomy appliance changing in, (V2) 585
otic irrigation in, (V2) 602
oxygen therapy, (V2) 732–733
peak flow meter, (V1) 950
percussion therapy, (V2) 730
perineal care in, (V2) 373–374
peripheral pulse assessment in, (V2) 194
postural drainage, (V2) 730
pulse oximetry, (V2) 728
removing nasogastric and nasoenteric tubes in, (V2) 507
respiration assessment in, (V2) 199
restraint use in, (V2) 354
reusing needles and syringes in, clinical insight on, (V2) 471*b*
safety interventions for, (V1) 560–564
saline lock, (V2) 802
self-administration of medications in, (V2) 413
for sensory deficits, (V1) 787*b*
shaving in, (V2) 390
skin assessment in, (V2) 229
sputum collection, (V2) 727
subcutaneous injection administration, (V2) 449–450
telehealth for, (V1) 1082, (V1) 1082*f*
temperature assessment in, (V2) 190
tracheostomy care, (V2) 740, (V2) 743–744
tracheostomy suctioning, (V2) 741–744
urine bedside testing in, (V2) 539
urine collection and measurement in, (V2) 533
vibration therapy, (V2) 730
wet-to-damp dressing, (V2) 684
wound irrigation, (V2) 678
Home health, standardized nursing languages for, (V1) 115
Home health nurses, (V1) 1127
Home health team, (V1) 1127
Home healthcare, (V1) 1125–1135
assessment in, (V1) 1131
caregiver support in, (V1) 1135, (V1) 1135*b*
client referral to, (V1) 1128–1129
concept of, (V1) 1125–1126
distinctive features of, (V1) 1125–1126, (V1) 1126*f*
documentation in, (V1) 389
funding sources for, (V1) 1128
future of, (V1) 1129
goals of, (V1) 1125
home health nurses in, (V1) 1127, (V1) 1128*t*
home safety promotion in, (V1) 1135
home visit in
conducting, (V1) 1130–1131, (V1) 1130*f*
preparation for, (V1) 1129–1130
responsibilities after, (V1) 1131
hospice nurses in, (V1) 1127–1128, (V1) 1128*t*
nursing diagnosis in, (V1) 1131–1132
nursing interventions in, (V1) 1133–1135
nursing outcomes in, (V1) 1132–1133
nursing process in, (V1) 1131–1135
providers of, (V1) 1126–1127
safety considerations in, (V2) 887*b*
Home healthcare agencies, (V1) 17
Home nursing, knowledge map on, (V2) 896
Homelessness, as family health risk, (V1) 294, (V1) 294*f*
Homemaker services, (V1) 1125
Homeostasis, (V1) 240
Homosexuality, (V1) 852
Honey, for common cold, (V1) 952
Honoring personhood, (V1) 149
Hope
inspiration of, for spirituality diagnoses, (V1) 341
in spirituality, (V1) 329
HOPE approach, to spiritual assessment, (V2) 140
Hopelessness
definition of, (V1) 341
in depression, (V1) 281
Hordeolum, (V2) 313*f*
Hormonal implant (contraception), (V2) 656
Hormone(s)
fluid and electrolyte balance regulation by, (V1) 987–988
immobility effects on, (V1) 831
in older adults, (V1) 580*t*
Hormone replacement therapy, (V1) 869
Hospice care, (V1) 354. *See also* End-of-life care
Hospice nurses, (V1) 1127–1128, (V1) 1128*t*
Hospice organizations, (V1) 1127
Hospital(s), (V1) 15–16
cardiac arrest in, (V1) 981
clot formation in, (V1) 980
design features of, evidence-based study on, (V1) 1072
environment of, sleep and, (V1) 886, (V1) 888
wait times and anxiety in, evidence-based study on, (V1) 1072
Hospital-based home health agencies, (V1) 1127
Hospital beds, (V1) 602–603, (V1) 602*f*

Hospital room, (V1) 601–603. *See also* Environment, client
hygiene for, (V1) 2
postoperative preparation of, (V1) 1039, (V2) 840
preparation of, for new client, (V2) 86*b*
Hospitalization
depersonalization during, preventing, (V1) 273
stress of, reducing, (V1) 260, (V1) 260*b*
Hospitalized child, helping, (V1) 188
Host susceptibility
in chain of infection, (V1) 519*f*, (V1) 521
factors increasing, (V1) 527–528
Hostility, in response to stress, (V1) 249
Hot packs, (V2) 708
Hot water bags/bottles, (V1) 932, (V2) 708
Household system, of medication measurement, (V1) 622, (V2) 482
Human dignity, as nursing value, (V1) 1146*t*
Human immunodeficiency (HIV) infection, as family health risk, (V1) 293
Human papillomavirus (HPV) infection, (V1) 863
Human patient simulator, (V1) 1085, (V1) 1085*f*
Human relations-based management, (V1) 1060
Human responses, in nursing diagnoses, (V1) 62
Humidifier, (V1) 955
Humidity, (V1) 941
evaporative water loss and, (V1) 424
Humility, intellectual, (V1) 32
Humor
for pain, (V1) 803
in stress management, (V1) 259, (V1) 259*f*
in verbal communication, (V1) 463
Humoral immunity, (V1) 525–526, (V1) 527*b*, (V1) 527*f*
Hydration
bowel elimination and, (V1) 749
for clot prevention, (V1) 980
for pressure ulcer prevention, (V1) 899–900
for pulmonary function, (V1) 955
for secretion mobilization, (V1) 955
skin effects of, (V1) 899–900, (V1) 918
urinary function and, (V1) 719
Hydrocephalus, (V1) 493
Hydrocolloid dressing, (V1) 926–927*t*, (V2) 693–694*p*
Hydrogel dressing, (V1) 927*t*, (V2) 693–694*p*
Hydrostatic pressure, (V1) 986
Hydrotherapy, (V1) 923
Hygiene, (V1) 574–603, (V2) 363–408
assessment guidelines for, (V2) 402–404
cognitive level and, (V1) 575
cultural influences on, (V1) 575
delegating care for, (V1) 578
dental
for preschooler, (V1) 184
of school-age child, assessment of, (V1) 186
developmental level and, (V1) 575
ear, (V1) 599
economic status and, (V1) 575
eye, (V1) 597–599
assessment guidelines for, (V2) 404
factors influencing, (V1) 575
foot, (V1) 587–588, (V1) 600*p*, (V2) 374–376*p*
assessment guidelines for, (V2) 403
hair, (V1) 595–597
assessment guidelines for, (V2) 403–404
hand, (V1) 538*p*. *See also* Hand hygiene
surgical, (V1) 1026*b*
in infection prevention, (V1) 530, (V1) 532
knowledge level and, (V1) 575
knowledge map for, (V2) 408
living environment and, (V1) 575
nail
assessment guidelines for, (V2) 403
care in, (V1) 588–590, (V1) 590*b*
nose, (V1) 599–500
oral, (V1) 590–595, (V1) 600*p*. *See also* Mouth; Tooth (teeth)
assessment in, (V1) 591, (V1) 592
guidelines for, (V2) 403
client teaching on, (V1) 593–594*b*
for critically ill patients, (V1) 593–594
for dementia patients, (V1) 595
denture care in, (V1) 593, (V2) 380–381*p*
evidence-based practice on, (V1) 595
nursing diagnoses for, (V1) 592
nursing interventions for, (V1) 593–595
nursing outcomes for, (V1) 593
for unconscious patients, (V1) 594, (V1) 600*p*, (V2) 382–384*p*
personal preferences on, (V1) 575
in physical examination, (V1) 488
pulmonary, (V1) 944
religious influences on, (V1) 575
scheduled care for, (V1) 578
self-care abilities for, assessing, (V2) 402
skin
assessment in, (V1) 581
guidelines for, (V2) 402–403
back message in, (V1) 582
bathing in, (V1) 582. *See also* Bath/bathing
breakdown and, (V1) 901
excessive/insufficient, (V1) 901
interventions for, (V1) 582
irrigation for, (V1) 921, (V1) 929*p*
nursing diagnoses for, (V1) 581–582
outcomes for, (V1) 582
perineal care in, (V1) 584
shower in, (V1) 583
for surgery, (V1) 1026, (V1) 1036
for wounds (irrigation), (V1) 921, (V1) 929*p*, (V2) 675–678
sleep, teaching of, (V1) 894, (V1) 895
spiritual influences on, (V1) 575
toileting, in promoting normal urination, (V1) 728–729
Hyperalgesia, (V1) 794
Hyperbaric oxygen therapy, for wound healing, (V1) 906, (V1) 920
Hypercalcemia, (V1) 995*t*
Hypercarbia, (V1) 943*b*, (V1) 949
Hyperemia
in inflammatory process, (V1) 247
reactive, (V1) 908
Hyperglycemia, nutritional status and, (V1) 694
Hyperhidrosis, (V1) 490
Hyperkalemia, (V1) 994*t*
Hypermagnesemia, (V1) 995*t*
Hypernatremia, (V1) 994*t*
Hyperopia, (V1) 494
definition of, (V1) 777*b*
Hyperperistalsis, (V1) 505, (V2) 274
Hyperphosphatemia, (V1) 995*t*
Hyperpyrexia, (V1) 425
Hypersomnia, (V1) 888
Hypertension, (V1) 454
alternative therapies for, (V1) 455*b*
evidence-based studies of, (V1) 975
interventions for, (V1) 455
in middle adult, (V1) 198
outcomes for, (V1) 454
pulmonary, (V1) 944
"white-coat," (V1) 448
Hyperthermia, (V1) 426
exercise and, (V1) 825–826
interventions for, (V1) 431, (V1) 433–434
malignant, (V1) 1040
nursing diagnoses for, (V1) 431
Hyperthyroidism, sleep and, (V1) 890
Hypertonic fluids, (V1) 1004
Hypertonic solutions, (V1) 986
for cleansing enemas, (V1) 760, (V1) 761*t*
Hypertrophy, muscle, (V1) 833
Hyperventilation, (V1) 446, (V1) 937
Hypervolemia, (V1) 993
Hypnosis, for pain, (V1) 803
Hypnotics, (V1) 894–895
preoperative, (V1) 1037*t*
Hypoactive sexual desire, (V1) 865
Hypocalcemia, (V1) 994–995*t*
Chvostek's sign for, (V2) 810
Trousseau's sign for, (V2) 810
Hypocarbia, (V1) 943*b*, (V1) 949
Hypochondriasis, from failure of adaptive mechanisms, (V1) 252
Hypoglossal nerve (XII) testing, (V2) 290*p*
Hypoglycemia, nutritional status and, (V1) 694
Hypokalemia, (V1) 994*t*
Hypomagnesemia, (V1) 995*t*
Hypomania, sexuality and, (V1) 857
Hyponatremia, (V1) 994*t*
Hypoperistalsis, (V1) 505, (V2) 274
Hypophosphatemia, (V1) 995*t*
Hypotension, (V1) 453–454
interventions for, (V1) 455
orthostatic (postural), (V1) 831, (V1) 993
outcomes for, (V1) 454
Hypothermia, (V1) 426–427
exercise and, (V1) 826
interventions for, (V1) 434–435
nursing diagnoses for, (V1) 431
Hypothyroidism, sleep and, (V1) 890
Hypotonic fluids, (V1) 1004
Hypotonic solutions
for cleansing enemas, (V1) 760, (V1) 761*t*
Hypotonic solutions, (V1) 986
Hypoventilation, (V1) 446, (V1) 937
Hypovolemia, (V1) 992–993
postoperative, (V1) 1049*t*
Hypovolemic shock, (V1) 993
Hypoxemia, (V1) 937, (V1) 943*b*
Hypoxia, (V1) 937, (V1) 943*b*
clinical signs of, (V1) 445
Hysterectomy, sexuality and, (V1) 857

I

Ice bag/collar, (V2) 709
ICN. *See* International Council of Nurses (ICN)
Icteric sclera, (V1) 493

Id, in psychoanalytic theory of development, (V1) 165
Identification, as defense mechanism, (V1) 250*t*
Identity
  gender, (V1) 851–852
  versus role confusion stage of psychosocial development, (V1) 168
  sexual, (V1) 851
Ileal conduit, (V1) 738, (V1) 738*f*
Ileal loop, (V1) 738
Ileal reservoir, (V1) 738
Ileoanal reservoir, total colectomy with, (V1) 751–752, (V1) 751*f*
Ileocecal valve, (V1) 746
Ileostomy, (V1) 751–752, (V1) 751*f*
  caring for patient with, (V1) 763–765
  dietary changes associated with, (V1) 765*b*
Ileum, (V1) 746
Ileus, paralytic, (V1) 1050*t*
  postoperative, (V1) 750
Illicit drugs, (V1) 622
Illness(es)
  affecting nutrition, (V1) 689–690
  basal metabolic rate and, (V1) 680
  beliefs about, (V1) 310, (V1) 312*f*
  blood pressure and, (V1) 448
  chronic, (V1) 231, (V1) 231*b*
    as family health risk, (V1) 293–294
    telehealth in self-management of, (V1) 228*b*
  communicable, reporting regulations on, (V1) 1184
  conceptual models of, (V1) 223–224, (V1) 223*f*, (V1) 224*f*
  diets modified by, (V1) 690–691
  emerging, awareness of, importance of, (V1) 522–523
  experience of, factors influencing, (V1) 230–23
  experiencing, (V1) 221–238, (V2) 76–91
    knowledge map for, (V2) 91
  in family member, interventions for, (V1) 300, (V1) 300*b*
  host susceptibility and, (V1) 528
  as lived experience, (V1) 222–223
  mental, as health disruption, (V1) 228
  nature of, experience of illness and, (V1) 231
  as outcome of stress, (V1) 243
  physical, as health disruption, (V1) 227
  present, in nursing health history, (V1) 52*t*
  prevention of, (V1) 18
    complementary and alternative medicine in, (V1) 1117*b*
    levels of, (V1) 1096–1097
  psychosocial, (V1) 267–270. *See also* Psychosocial illness
  pulse and, (V2) 437
  respiration and, (V1) 443
  sensory function and, (V1) 775
  sexuality and, (V1) 856–857
  sleep and, (V1) 880, (V1) 880*f*, (V1) 886
Illness behavior, stages of, (V1) 230–231
Illness practices, cultural, (V1) 310–312, (V1) 311*f*
Imagery, guided
  for pain, (V1) 803
  for sleep, (V1) 894
Imbalance, as health disruption, (V1) 229–230
Imbalanced nutrition, risk for, culture and, (V1) 320
Immediate postoperative phase, (V1) 1045
Immigrants, (V1) 305–306
Immobility/immobilization
  complications of, (V1) 830–832
  effects of, (V1) 831–832
  for pain, (V1) 802
  urinary function and, (V1) 720
Immune system
  disorders of, from failure of adaptive mechanisms, (V1) 252*t*
  exercise effects on, (V1) 824*b*
  sleep-related effects on, 880, (V1) 879
Immunity
  active, (V1) 525, (V1) 526*b*
  cellular, (V1) 526–527
  humoral, (V1) 525–526, (V1) 527*b*, (V1) 527*f*
  passive, (V1) 525, (V1) 526*b*
  specific, (V1) 525
Immunization(s)
  for adolescents, interventions for, (V1) 194
  for infants, interventions for, (V1) 179
  in infection prevention, (V1) 533
  influenza, (V1) 952
  for middle adults, interventions for, (V1) 199
  for older adults, (V1) 217, (V1) 218*f*
  for school-age children, assessment of, (V1) 187
  tetanus, (V1) 916
  for toddlers, (V1) 181
Immunocompromised patients, urinary tract infections in, (V1) 721
Immunoglobulins (Igs), classes of, (V1) 527*b*
Impacted cerumen, definition of, (V1) 778*f*
Impaction, fecal, (V1) 759–761
  digital removal of stool for, (V1) 761
  enemas for, (V1) 760–761
Impaired nurses, reporting regulations on, (V1) 1183
Impaired nursing practice, (V1) 1141
Implanted port, for fluid and electrolyte administration, (V1) 1007–1008, (V1) 1008*f*
Implementation, (V1) 120–128, (V1) 129*t*, (V2) 45–53
  assessment and, (V1) 120–121
  collaboration in, (V1) 125
  coordination in, (V1) 125–126
  critical thinking and reasoning in, (V2) 51
  delegation in, (V1) 126–127
  diagnosis and, (V1) 121
  documentation of, (V1) 128
  evaluation and, (V1) 122
  in health promotion, (V1) 234
  knowledge and skill needed for, (V1) 124–125
  knowledge map for, (V2) 53
  in nursing process, (V1) 38, (V1) 38*f*
  planning outcomes and, (V1) 121
  preparing for, (V1) 122–124, (V1) 123–124*t*
  reflecting critically about, (V1) 128, (V1) 129*t*
  relation of, to other nursing process steps, (V1) 120–122, (V1) 120*f*
  standards of practice for, (V1) 121*b*
  tools for, (V2) 46, (V2) 47
In-service education, (V1) 11
Inappropriate sexual behavior, (V1) 871
Incentive spirometry, (V1) 953–954, (V1) 1052, (V1) 1053
  postoperative, (V1) 1052
  teaching about, (V1) 1053
Incident reports, (V1) 388, (V1) 388*f*
  in minimizing malpractice risks, (V1) 1180
Incisional wound, (V1) 902*t*. *See also* Wound(s)
Incisors, (V1) 590
Incontinence
  bowel. *See* Bowel incontinence
  urinary, (V1) 722–723. *See also* Urinary incontinence
Incubation stage of infection, (V1) 522
Independent interventions, (V1) 107
Independent living facilities, (V1) 17
Independent thinking, (V1) 32
Indexes, nursing, (V1) 156
Indian diet, (V1) 689
Indiana pouch, (V1) 738
Indirect care agencies, (V1) 1126
Indirect-care interventions, (V1) 106
Inductive reasoning, (V1) 141, (V1) 142*f*
Industry, *versus* inferiority stage of psychosocial development, (V1) 168
Indwelling fecal drainage devices, for bowel incontinence, (V1) 763, (V1) 763*f*
Indwelling urinary catheter, (V1) 730, (V1) 731*f*
  care for patient with, (V1) 732, (V1) 735, (V2) 556–557
  insertion of, (V2) 544–547*p*
  measuring urine from, (V2) 532–533*p*
  removing, (V1) 734*p*, (V1) 735, (V2) 551–552*p*
Infant(s)
  abuse, neglect and violence involving, (V1) 177
  assessment of, (V1) 178, (V1) 178*b*
  bowel elimination in, (V1) 748
  car safety seats for, (V1) 566*t*
    interventions for, (V1) 179
  communication by, (V1) 465
  crying and colic in, (V1) 177
    interventions for, (V1) 179
  dental caries in, (V1) 177, (V1) 591
  development of
    cognitive, (V1) 168*t*, (V1) 176–177
    milestones of, (V1) 176*b*
    physical, (V1) 176
    psychosexual, (V1) 167*t*
    psychosocial, (V1) 168, (V1) 177
  developmental tasks of, (V1) 166*t*
  failure to thrive of, (V1) 177
  feeding of, (V1) 176
  gender and, (V1) 851, (V1) 851*f*
  growth of, (V1) 176
  health problems of, (V1) 177–178
  health promotion for, (V1) 1100*t*
  honey contraindication in, (V1) 952
  immunizations for, interventions for, (V1) 179
  interventions for, (V1) 178–179
  neurological exam in, (V1) 506
  newborn. *See* Neonate
  nutrition for, (V1) 682–683
  pain in, (V1) 796
  parent attachment to, (V1) 853, (V1) 853*f*
  physical examination of, (V1) 486
  pulmonary system of, (V1) 939, (V1) 971
  safety needs of, (V1) 547

self-concept formation in, (V1) 264
sensory perception in, (V1) 774
skin of, (V1) 899
sleep for, (V1) 881, (V1) 881*t*, (V1) 894
patterns of, (V1) 176
sudden infant death syndrome and, (V1) 178
interventions for, (V1) 179
surgical risks for, (V1) 1028
unintentional injury of, (V1) 177
interventions for, (V1) 179
urinary elimination in, (V1) 718
Infection(s). *See also* Pathogen(s)
acute, (V1) 522
blood transfusion and, (V1) 1021*t*
body defenses against, (V1) 524–527
primary, (V1) 524
secondary, (V1) 524–525, (V1) 525*t*
tertiary, (V1) 525–527, (V1) 526*b*, (V1) 527*b*, (V1) 527*f*
chain of, (V1) 518–521, (V1) 519*f*
chronic, (V1) 522
classification of, (V1) 521–522
control of, in home care, (V1) 1134, (V2) 888
convalescence stage of, (V1) 522
decline stage of, (V1) 522
endogenous, (V1) 522
exogenous, (V1) 521–522
fungal, of nails, (V2) 313*f*
healthcare-associated, (V1) 517–518
host susceptibility to, (V1) 519*f*, (V1) 522
factors increasing, (V1) 527–528
illness stage of, (V1) 522
incubation stage of, (V1) 522
intravenous therapy and, (V1) 1014*t*
knowledge about, importance of, (V1) 517–518
latent, (V1) 522
local, (V1) 521
nosocomial, (V1) 517
presence or risk of, tests for evaluating, (V2) 344
prevention of, (V1) 516–544, (V2) 317–347
asepsis in, (V1) 517, (V1) 533–542. *See also* Asepsis
assessment in, (V1) 529
client teaching in, (V1) 530, (V1) 531–532*b*
for healthcare workers, (V1) 542–543
in home and community, (V1) 532*b*
nursing diagnoses relevant to, (V1) 529
in patients receiving enteral feedings, (V2) 519*p*
professional standards and guidelines on, (V1) 518
wellness promotion in, (V1) 530, (V1) 532–533
primary, (V1) 521
prodromal stage of, (V1) 522
respiratory tract, (V1) 939, (V1) 943–944
obesity and, (V1) 941
prevention of, (V1) 951–953
secondary, (V1) 521
sexually transmitted, (V1) 863
in adolescents, (V1) 863
teaching about, (V1) 870
stages of, (V1) 522
systemic, (V1) 521
in toddler, (V1) 181
upper respiratory, prevention of, (V1) 1108*b*
urinary tract, (V1) 720–721. *See also* Urinary tract infection (UTI)
wound, (V1) 901, (V1) 906
risk for, (V1) 917
surgical risk for, (V1) 1028, (V1) 1029*t*, (V1) 1046
Infection preventionist nurse, role of, (V1) 542
Infectious agent, in chain of infection, (V1) 519, (V1) 519*f*
Infectious disease(s)
emerging, definitions of, (V1) 522
as family health risk, (V1) 293
Infectious microorganisms, in neonate, (V1) 175
Inferences, in drawing conclusions about health status, (V1) 68–69
Infibulation, (V1) 855
Infiltration, intravenous therapy and, (V1) 1013*t*
Inflammation, (V1) 904
in defense against infection, (V1) 524
in humoral immunity, (V1) 526
urinary retention from, (V1) 721
Inflammatory response, (V1) 247–248, (V1) 247*b*
Influenza, (V1) 943–944
as family health risk, (V1) 293
vaccine against, (V1) 952
Informatics, (V1) 1077–1094, (V2) 864–870. *See also* Computer(s); Electronic health record
critical thinking about, (V2) 867–868
data and, (V1) 1079
definition of, (V1) 1079
evidence-based studies on, (V1) 1083
full-spectrum nursing and, (V2) 866–867
in home care, (V1) 1082
information and, (V1) 1079
knowledge and, (V1) 1079–1080
knowledge map for, (V2) 870
research with, (V1) 1089–1093
wisdom and, (V1) 1080
wound care and, (V1) 914
Information. *See also* Data; Informatics; Nursing research
aggregated, (V1) 1088
definition of, (V1) 1079
fire-hosing, as barrier to therapeutic communication, (V1) 476
Information literacy, (V1) 1089, (V1) 1090*b*. *See also* Informatics; Literature; Nursing research
Information processing, (V1) 1080
Informed consent
autonomy underlying, (V1) 1149
elements of, (V1) 1180–1181
nurse's role in, (V1) 1181
for nursing research, (V1) 154–155
obtaining, in minimizing malpractice risks, (V1) 1180–1181
surgical, (V1) 1034–1035
Infrared electronic thermometers, (V1) 429, (V1) 430*t*
Infusion pump
home care for, (V2) 792
for intravenous fluids and electrolytes, (V1) 1011, (V2) 790–792
Ingrown toenail, (V1) 587
Inguinal hernias, palpation for, (V2) 299*p*, (V2) 303*p*
Inhalation, (V1) 936–937, (V1) 937*f*
Inhalations, respiratory, (V1) 639–640, (V1) 639*f*
Inhaler
dry powder, (V1) 639
metered-dose, (V1) 639–640, (V1) 639*f*, (V1) 640*f*, (V1) 657*p*
administering, (V2) 432–434*p*
Initial assessment, (V1) 47
Initiative, *versus* guilt stage of psychosocial development, (V1) 168
Injection(s)
accounting for needle "dead space" in, (V1) 644
comfort and safety considerations for, (V1) 645–646
developmental stage and, (V1) 646
discomfort minimization for, (V1) 645–646
drawing up medication for, (V1) 643, (V1) 643*f*
equipment for, (V1) 640–643
needles as, (V1) 640–641, (V1) 641*f*. *See also* Needle(s)
syringes as, (V1) 641–643, (V1) 641*f*, (V1) 642*f*. *See also* Syringe(s)
intradermal, (V1) 613*t*, (V1) 646–647, (V1) 658*p*
administration of, (V2) 445–447*p*
sites for, (V1) 646*f*
intramuscular, (V1) 649–652. *See also* Intramuscular injection(s)
mixing medications for, (V1) 643–644
needlestick injury prevention in, (V1) 644–645, (V1) 645*f*, (V2) 355*p*
reconstituting medications for, (V1) 643
subcutaneous, (V1) 647–649, (V1) 658*p*. *See also* Subcutaneous injections
Injury(ies)
back
in healthcare workers, (V1) 556
prevention of, (V1) 825
in nurse, (V1) 836
firearm, in home
prevention of, (V1) 562
risk factors for, (V1) 550
as health disruption, (V1) 227–228
history of, population vulnerability and, (V1) 1116
host susceptibility and, (V1) 528
needlestick
in healthcare workers, (V1) 556
prevention of, (V1) 644–645, (V1) 645*f*, (V2) 355*p*
radiation, in healthcare workers, (V1) 556
risk factors for, individual, (V1) 548*t*
unintentional
of infant, (V1) 177
interventions for, (V1) 179
in school-age child, (V1) 186
of toddler, (V1) 181
Inpatient, definition of, (V1) 15
Input, in systems theory, (V1) 148
Input and output record, (V1) 384, (V2) 172
Inquiry, in critical thinking, (V1) 35*t*, (V1) 36
Insects, pathogens carried by, (V1) 551
Insensible fluid loss, (V1) 987
Insensible water loss, (V1) 424
Inside-the-needle catheters, (V1) 1005, (V1) 1005*f*
Insomnia, (V1) 887, (V1) 891. *See also* Sleep

Inspection
of abdomen, (V1) 504–505, (V1) 505*f*, (V2) 272–273*p*
of heart, (V1) 502
in physical examination, (V1) 485
for pressure ulcers, (V1) 918
of skin, (V1) 918
Inspiration
in gaining knowledge, (V1) 152
mechanics of, (V1) 442, (V1) 442*f*
Inspiratory capacity, (V2) 767
Inspiratory reserve volume, (V2) 766
Instillations, performing, (V1) 637–638, (V1) 637*f*
Institute for Healthcare Improvement (IHI), (V1) 1027
Institute of Medicine (IOM), report of, on patient safety, (V1) 546
Institutional review boards, overseeing nursing research, (V1) 155
Instrumental Activities of Daily Living (IADLs), (V2) 18
in older adult assessment, (V1) 213
Insulin
administration of, home care for, (V1) 1134
appearance of, (V1) 648–649
basal, (V1) 648
categories of, (V1) 648
correction, (V1) 648
functions of, (V1) 670
injection of, (V1) 648–649
equipment for, (V1) 649
prandial, (V1) 648
preprandial, (V1) 648
storing, (V1) 649
two kinds of, mixing, in one syringe, clinical insight on, (V2) 475–476*b*
Insulin syringe, (V1) 642, (V1) 642*f*
Insurance
liability, professional, (V1) 1184
private
employment-based, as payor for healthcare, (V1) 21
individual, as payor for healthcare, (V1) 20–21, (V1) 20*f*
reimbursement for home care by, (V1) 1128
Intake and output (I&O)
in fluid and electrolyte assessment, (V1) 1000
guidelines for, (V2) 810–811
intraoperative, (V1) 1044
postoperative, (V1) 1046
Intake and output (I&O) sheet, (V1) 56
Integrated care plan, (V1) 387–388
Integrated delivery networks (IDNs), (V1) 24
Integrity, as nursing value, (V1) 1146*t*
Integumentary system. *See* Hair; Nail(s); Skin
Intellectual courage, (V1) 32
Intellectual curiosity, (V1) 32
Intellectual empathy, (V1) 32
Intellectual humility, (V1) 32
Intellectual perseverance, (V1) 32
Intellectualization, as defense mechanism, (V1) 250*t*
Intensive care unit (ICU), sensory overload in, (V1) 776*b*
Intensivist, (V1) 1082
Intentional torts, (V1) 1172–1173
Intercostal muscles, (V1) 937, (V1) 937*f*
Intercostal retraction, in respiration, (V1) 445
Interdependent interventions, (V1) 107
Interleukin secretion, in cellular immunity, (V1) 526
Intermittent bladder/catheter irrigation, (V2) 553–554*p*
Intermittent claudication, (V1) 980
Intermittent evaluation, (V1) 131
Intermittent fever, (V1) 426
Intermittent mandatory ventilation, (V2) 752
Intermittent urinary catheterization, (V2) 540–543*p*
Internal bleeding, (V1) 906
Internal respiration, (V1) 938, (V1) 938*f*
International Classification for Nursing Practice (ICNP), (V1) 74, (V2) 866
International Council of Nurses (ICN), (V1) 14
Code of Ethics of, (V1) 1152
nursing definition of, (V1) 7
International nursing, (V1) 1122, (V1) 1123*f*
Internet, for nursing research, (V1) 1091–1092, (V1) 1092*t*, (V1) 1093*t*
Internet-based formularies, (V1) 606
Interpersonal communication, (V1) 459
Interpreters, (V1) 322, (V2) 616
communicating through, (V2) 128
Interprofessional collaboration, trend toward, (V1) 28
Intersexuality, (V1) 852
Interstitial fluid, (V1) 984, (V1) 985*f*
Interventions. *See* Nursing interventions
Interview(s)
closed questions in, (V1) 51, (V1) 53*t*
closing, (V2) 18*b*
conducting, (V2) 17*b*
directive, (V1) 51
nondirective, (V1) 51
nursing, in comprehensive assessment, (V1) 48, (V1) 49*f*
to obtain nursing health history, (V1) 51–53, (V1) 52*t*
open-ended questions in, (V1) 51, (V1) 53*t*
preparing for, (V1) 51–53, (V2) 16*b*
for sexual history, (V2) 653, (V2) 656–657
Intestine
large, (V1) 746–747, (V1) 746*f*. *See also* Bowel *entries*
small, (V1) 746, (V1) 746*f*
surface area of, nutrition and, (V1) 689
Intimacy, *versus* isolation stage of psychosocial development, (V1) 168–169
Intimate distance, communication and, (V1) 466
Intimate partner abuse. *See also* Abuse; Domestic abuse
in young adults, (V1) 195–196
Intimate partner violence, (V1) 864–865
Intonation, in verbal communication, (V1) 462
Intracellular fluid (ICF), (V1) 679, (V1) 984, (V1) 985*f*
Intractable pain, (V1) 792
Intradermal injections, (V1) 613*t*, (V1) 646–647, (V1) 658*p*
administration of, (V2) 445–447*p*
sites for, (V1) 646*f*
Intramuscular injection(s), (V1) 613*t*, (V1) 649–652, (V1) 659*p*
administration of, (V2) 453–456*p*
Z-track technique for, (V1) 651, (V2) 455–456*p*
aspiration before, (V1) 649
deltoid site for, (V1) 650–651, (V1) 650*f*, (V1) 659*p*, (V2) 451–452*p*
dorsogluteal site for, (V1) 650
needle selection for, (V1) 651, (V1) 652*t*
rectus femoris site for, (V1) 651, (V1) 659*p*, (V2) 453*p*
site selection for, (V1) 650–651, (V1) 650*f*, (V1) 651*f*, (V1) 658*p*, (V2) 451–453*p*
vastus lateralis site for, (V1) 651, (V1) 651*f*, (V1) 659*p*, (V2) 452*p*
ventrogluteal site for, (V1) 650, (V1) 650*f*, (V1) 658*p*, (V2) 451*p*
Intraoperative nursing, (V1) 1039–1045
anesthesia in, (V1) 1040–1042, (V1) 1042*f*
assessment for, (V1) 1042
clean team in, (V1) 1039
client positioning in, (V1) 1044
documentation in, (V1) 1044
intake and output monitoring in, (V1) 1044
nursing diagnosis for, (V1) 1042–1043
nursing interventions for, (V1) 1043–1045
nursing outcomes for, (V1) 1043
personnel in, (V1) 1039
questionnaire for, (V2) 844
safety measures in, (V1) 1044
skin preparation in, (V1) 1043–1044
specimen handling in, (V1) 1044
sterile field maintenance in, (V1) 1044, (V2) 840
sterile team in, (V1) 1039
supplies in, (V1) 1044
Intraosseous devices, for fluid and electrolyte administration, (V1) 1008
Intrapersonal communication, (V1) 459
Intraspinal administration of drugs, (V1) 613*t*
Intrathecal administration of drugs, (V1) 613*t*
Intrauterine device, (V2) 655
Intravaginal support device, for urinary incontinence, (V1) 737
Intravascular fluid, (V1) 984, (V1) 985*f*
Intravenous fluids
adding medications to, (V2) 457–458*p*
and electrolytes, (V1) 1003–1022. *See also* Blood transfusion
administration set for, (V1) 1009, (V1) 1009*f*
change of, (V1) 1012, (V1) 1017*p*
air embolus with, (V1) 1015t
asepsis technique for, (V1) 1004, (V2) 813
butterfly (wing-tipped) catheter for, (V1) 1005, (V1) 1005*f*, (V2) 785, (V2) 786
catheter diameter for, (V1) 1008
catheter embolus with, (V1) 1015*t*
central venous access device for, (V1) 1006–1007, (V1) 1007*f*, (V1) 1018*p*. *See also* Central venous access device
dressing change for, (V1) 1012, (V1) 1017*p*, (V2) 797–800*p*
complications of, (V1) 1011–1012, (V1) 1013–1015*t*
discontinuation of, (V1) 1012, (V1) 1015, (V1) 1018*p*, (V2) 803–804*p*
therapy duration for, (V1) 1009
thrombophlebitis with, (V1) 1014*t*
tunneled central venous catheters for, (V1) 1007, (V1) 1008*f*
venipuncture for, (V1) 1009–1010
volume-control set for, (V1) 1010–1011, (V1) 1016*p*, (V2) 790–792*p*

dressing for, (V2) 787*p*
change of, (V1) 1012, (V1) 1017*p*, (V2) 796–800*p*
drip chamber for, (V1) 1009, (V1) 1009*f*
drip rate for, (V1) 1011, (V1) 1011*b*, (V1) 1016*p*, (V2) 788–790
extension tubing for, (V1) 1009, (V2) 784–785
extravasation with, (V1) 1013*t*, (V2) 814
filters for, (V1) 1009
flow rates for, (V1) 1011, (V1) 1011*b*
regulation of, (V1) 1016*p*, (V2) 788–790
fluid overload with, (V1) 1015*t*
glass bottle for, (V1) 1009, (V2) 784
gravity flow for, (V1) 1010, (V2) 789
hematoma with, (V1) 1013*t*
implanted ports for, (V1) 1007–1008, (V1) 1008*f*
infection with, (V1) 1014*t*
prevention of, (V1) 1006–1007
infiltration with, (V1) 1013*t*, (V2) 814
infusion pump for, (V1) 1011
infusion speed for, (V1) 1009, (V1) 1010, (V1) 1011*b*
initiation of, (V1) 1008–1011, (V1) 1016*p*
injection port for, (V1) 1009
inside-the-needle catheter for, (V1) 1005, (V1) 1005*f*
intraosseous devices for, (V1) 1008
macrodrip chamber for, (V1) 1009
microdrip chamber for, (V1) 1009
midline peripheral catheter for, (V1) 1005
monitoring of, (V1) 1010–1011
multiple lines for, (V1) 1011
nerve injury with, (V1) 1014*t*
nontunneled central venous catheters for, (V1) 1007, (V1) 1007*f*
over-the-needle catheter for, (V1) 1005, (V1) 1005f, (V2) 785–786
peripheral intravenous lock for, (V1) 1006, (V1) 1006*f*, (V1) 1012, (V1) 1017–1018*p*, (V2) 786*p*, (V2) 800–802*p*
peripheral site for, (V1) 1009
peripheral vascular access devices for, (V1) 1005, (V1) 1005*f*, (V2) 785–786
peripherally inserted central catheters for, (V1) 1007, (V1) 1007*f*
phlebitis with, (V1) 1013–1014*t*
regulation and maintenance for, (V1) 1010–1011, (V1) 1016*p*
septicemia with, (V1) 1014*t*
solution for, (V1) 1009, (V2) 784
change of, (V1) 1012, (V1) 1016–1017*p*, (V2) 793–795*p*
Intravenous (IV) infusion pumps
piggyback setup with, intermittent infusion using, (V2) 466–467*p*
smart, in medication error prevention, (V1) 627
Intravenous (IV) medication administration, (V1) 612–613*t*, (V1) 652–655
adding medications to large-volume infusions in, (V1) 652–653, (V2) 457–458*p*
central venous access devices for, (V1) 655, (V1) 655*f*, (V1) 659*p*
complications of, preventing, (V1) 652
home care for, (V1) 1134
intermittent infusion in, (V1) 653–654, (V1) 654*f*, (V1) 659*p*, (V2) 463–467*p*
IV push medications in, (V1) 653, (V1) 659*p*, (V2) 459–463*p*
using prefilled cartridge and single-dose vial, (V2) 442*p*
volume-control infusion sets for, (V1) 654, (V1) 655*f*
Intravenous (IV) medications
extravasation of, (V1) 1013*t*, (V2) 814
infiltration with, (V1) 2
Intravenous (IV) therapy, (V1) 1004
Intravenous pyelogram (IVP), (V2) 564
Intuition
in gaining knowledge, (V1) 152
listening and, (V1) 150
Invasion of privacy, (V1) 1173
Invasive procedures, host susceptibility and, (V1) 528
Iodine, (V1) 678*t*
Ionization, drug absorption and, (V1) 614
Iris, inspection of, (V2) 243*p*
Irish heritage, pain perception and responses in, (V2) 127
Iron, (V1) 678, (V1) 678*t*
bowel elimination and, (V1) 749
in ovo-lacto vegetarian diet, (V1) 686
Irrigation(s)
bladder, (V1) 734*p*, (V1) 735, (V2) 553–556*p*
catheter, (V1) 734*p*, (V2) 553–556*p*
colostomy, (V1) 765, (V1) 769–770*p*, (V2) 586–588*p*
nasogastric tube, (V1) 1055*p*, (V2) 836*p*
ophthalmic, (V2) 421*p*
otic, (V1) 786*p*, (V2) 600–602*p*
performing, (V1) 637–638, (V1) 637*f*
wound, (V1) 921, (V1) 929*p*, (V2) 675–678*p*
Ischemia, cardiac, (V1) 974–975
Ishihara cards, (V1) 494, (V2) 239
Islam, (V1) 333
Isokinetic exercise, (V1) 821
Isolation
as health disruption, (V1) 230
patient in, supporting psychological needs of, (V1) 538
protective, (V1) 536–537
supplies used in, disposing of, (V1) 537–538
transmission-based, (V1) 537
Isometric exercise, (V1) 821
Isotonic exercise, (V1) 821
Isotonic fluids, (V1) 1004
Isotonic solution, (V1) 985–986
Issues, exploring, in enhancing therapeutic communication, (V1) 475
Italian heritage, pain perception and responses in, (V2) 127
IV. *See* Intravenous *entries*
IV piggyback setup, for intermittent infusions, (V1) 654

J

Jackson-Pratt drains, (V1) 922, (V1) 922*f*
Japanese heritage. *See also* Asian Americans
pain perception and responses in, (V2) 127
Jargon, (V1) 318
Jaundice, (V1) 490*t*, (V2) 312*p*
description of, (V1) 581
neonatal, (V1) 175
skin in, (V1) 580
Jehovah's Witnesses, (V1) 332
Jejunostomy tube (J-tube, PEJ), (V1) 708–709
Jejunum, (V1) 746
Jelly, (V1) 611*t*, (V1) 612*t*
Jewelry, hand hygiene and, (V2) 335
Jewish heritage, pain perception and responses in, (V2) 127
Johnson, Dorothy, nursing theory of, (V1) 146*t*
Joint(s)
ankylosis of, (V1) 831
classification of, (V1) 817–818
degenerative disease of, (V2) 314*f*
disease of, (V1) 827–828
function assessment of, (V2) 642
mobility of, (V1) 506, (V1) 827–828
range of motion testing for, (V2) 643–647
synovial, (V1) 818, (V1) 818*t*
Joint Commission, the, (V1) 22
accreditation standards of, (V1) 1154
on assessment, (V1) 45
infection guidelines of, (V1) 518
patient safety goals of, (V1) 552*b*
on safety, (V1) 546, (V1) 559*b*, (V1) 1027
on surgical safety, (V1) 1027
on teaching responsibilities, (V1) 398
Joint mobility. *See* Mobility
Journal writing
for pain, (V1) 804
in stress management, (V1) 259
Journals, nursing, (V1) 157
refereed, (V1) 157
Judaism, (V1) 331
Judgment
assessing, (V2) 287*p*
clinical, (V1) 5
Judicial law, (V1) 1164
Jugular veins, (V1) 504
auscultation of, (V2) 268*p*
Jugular venous pressure, measuring, (V2) 266–267*p*
Justice
compensatory, (V1) 1152
distributive, (V1) 1151–1152
as ethical concept, (V1) 1151–1152
procedural, (V1) 1152
social, as nursing value, (V1) 1146*t*

K

K-complexes, (V1) 883
Kardex, (V1) 387
Karnofsky Performance scale, in functional ability assessment, (V1) 50
Katz Index of ADL scale, in functional ability assessment, (V1) 49, (V1) 50*b*
Kava, for depression, (V1) 283*b*
Kegel exercises, for urinary incontinence, (V1) 736
Keloid, (V2) 233
Keofeed tube, (V2) 837
Keratinocytes, (V1) 898
Ketones, urinary, (V2) 563
Ketosis, blood glucose levels and, (V1) 694
Kidney(s)
disease of
end-stage, (V1) 725*b*
surgery and, (V1) 1029*b*
in drug excretion, (V1) 615
in electrolyte regulation, (V1) 992

failure of
acute, definition of, (V1) 725*b*
postoperative, (V1) 1050*t*
functions of, (V1) 715, (V1) 715*f*
Kidney stones, (V1) 831
urinary tract infections and, (V1) 721
Kilocalories, (V1) 679
Kinesthesia
bedside assessment of, (V2) 606
changes in, with aging, (V1) 774*t*
Kinesthetic sense
deficits in, home care for, (V1) 787*b*
impaired, (V1) 790
testing of, (V2) 291*p*
King, Imogene, nursing theory of, (V1) 146*t*
Kinsey, Alfred C., (V1) 852
Kith, (V1) 288
Knee, range of motion in, (V2) 646
Knowing, in caring, (V1) 39
Knowledge
client's
deficient, preoperative, (V1) 1033, (V2) 847
sexual, (V1) 856
deficient
as etiology, (V1) 408
in home care, (V1) 1132
incorrect uses of, (V1) 408
NOC outcomes for, (V1) 409
as primary problem, (V1) 408
definition of, (V1) 1079
ethical, (V1) 37
in full-spectrum nursing, (V1) 40*t*, (V1) 41
gaining, methods of, (V1) 152–153
general, assessing, (V2) 286*p*
nursing, kinds of, (V1) 36–37
practical, (V1) 37
in full-spectrum nursing, (V1) 40*f*, (V1) 41
self-, (V1) 37
in diagnostic reasoning, (V1) 72
in full-spectrum nursing, (V1) 40*t*, (V1) 41
theoretical, (V1) 37
in diagnostic reasoning, (V1) 72
in full-spectrum nursing, (V1) 40*t*, (V1) 41
transformation of data into, (V1) 1079–1080, (V1) 1080*f*
Knowledge level, hygiene and, (V1) 575
Knowledge map
on acid-base balance, (V2) 821
activity, (V2) 650
assessment, (V2) 25
bowel elimination, (V2) 598
circulation, (V2) 780
communication, (V2) 218
community and home nursing, (V2) 896
critical thinking, (V2) 14
culture and ethnicity, (V2) 135
development through life span, (V2) 71
older adults, (V2) 75
diagnosing, (V2) 32
documentation and reporting, (V2) 176
electrolytes, (V2) 821
evaluation, (V2) 53
evidence-based practice, (V2) 58
evolution of nursing, (V2) 9
exercise, (V2) 650
experiencing health and illness, (V2) 91
family health, (V2) 124
fluids, (V2) 821
health promotion, (V1) 881
homeostasis, (V2) 821
hygiene, (V2) 408
implementation, (V2) 53
infection prevention, (V2) 347
informatics, (V2) 870
interventions, (V2) 44
laws and regulations, (V2) 911
leadership, (V2) 863
loss, grief, and dying, (V2) 158
management, (V2) 863
medication administration, (V2) 489
mobility, (V2) 650
nursing ethics, (V2) 904
nutrition, (V2) 529
oxygenation, (V2) 771, (V2) 780
pain, (V2) 621
perioperative nursing, (V2) 858
physical examination, (V2) 316
planning, (V2) 39
on pressure ulcer, (V2) 721
psychosocial health and illness, (V2) 117
safety, (V2) 362
on sensory perception, (V2) 609
sexuality, (V2) 661
skin and wounds, (V2) 721
sleep and rest, (V2) 670
spirituality, (V2) 144
stress and adaptation, (V2) 101
teaching and learning, (V2) 183
urination, (V2) 568
vital signs, (V2) 209
Kock pouch, (V1) 751, (V1) 751*f*
Kohlberg, Lawrence, moral development theory of, (V1) 169
Korotkoff sounds, (V1) 452, (V1) 453*f*
Kosher foods, (V1) 331
Kussmaul's respirations, (V1) 444*t*, (V1) 946
Kwashiorkor, (V1) 703
Kyphosis, (V2) 314*f*
description of, (V1) 506, (V2) 261
thoracic cage and, (V1) 499

L

Labia majora, (V1) 848, (V1) 849*f*
excision of, (V1) 855–856
Labia minora, (V1) 848, (V1) 849*f*
excision of, (V1) 855–856
Labor market, nursing, (V1) 1065
Laboratory specimens. *See* Specimen(s)
Laboratory studies. *See* Diagnostic testing
Laceration, (V1) 902*t*
Lacrimal ducts, inspection of, (V2) 242*p*
Lactation, nutrition in, (V1) 684
Lacto-vegetarians, (V1) 686
Lactose intolerance, bowel elimination and, (V1) 751
Laissez-faire leadership, (V1) 1058
Langerhans cells, (V1) 898
Language(s)
nursing. *See* Standardized nursing languages
patronizing, as barrier to therapeutic communication, (V1) 477
Language barrier(s)
communicating across, (V2) 128
to culturally competent care, (V1) 319
interpreters/translators and, (V1) 322
to therapeutic communication, (V1) 472
Large intestine, (V1) 746–747, (V1) 746*f*. *See also* Bowel *entries*
Larynx, (V1) 935
Lateral positions, (V1) 837, (V1) 838*b*, (V1) 839
Lateral recumbent position, (V1) 837, (V1) 839
Latex allergy, (V1) 1033, (V1) 1043, (V2) 849
Latinos. *See* Hispanic Americans
Laughter, in pain management, (V1) 803
Lavage. *See* Irrigation(s)
Law(s). *See also* Legal issues
administrative, (V1) 1163–1164
civil, (V1) 1172–1176
common, (V1) 1164
constitutional, (V1) 1163
contract, (V1) 1172
criminal, (V1) 1171–1172
culture and, (V1) 310
ethics and, (V1) 1138
federal, (V1) 1164–1167
Good Samaritan, (V1) 1167–1168
guiding nursing practice, (V1) 1164–1171
judicial, (V1) 1164
knowledge map for, (V2) 911
mandatory reporting, (V1) 1167
sources of, (V1) 1163–1164, (V1) 1164*t*
state, (V1) 1167–1168
statutory, (V1) 1163
tort, (V1) 1172–1176
types of, (V1) 1163–1164
Law concept of, (V1) 1163
Lawton Instrumental Activities of Daily Living (IADL), (V2) 18
Lawton Instrumental Activities of Daily Living (IADL) scale, in functional ability assessment, (V1) 49–50
Laxatives
bowel elimination and, (V1) 749
for constipation, (V1) 759
patient teaching on, (V1) 760*b*
types of, (V1) 749*b*
Leader, role and function of, (V1) 6
Leadership, (V1) 1057–1059, (V2) 859–863. *See also* Management
authoritarian, (V1) 1058
communication and, (V1) 1067
critical thinking about, (V2) 860–861
democratic, (V1) 1058
full-spectrum nursing and, (V2) 860
knowledge map for, (V2) 863
in manager, (V1) 1060
participative, (V1) 1058
preparation for, (V1) 1061–1064
theories of, (V1) 1057–1058
behavioral, (V1) 1058
emotional intelligence, (V1) 1058
laissez-faire, (V1) 1058
situational, (V1) 1058–1059
task *vs.* relationship, (V1) 1058
trait, (V1) 1057–1058
transactional, (V1) 1059, (V1) 1059*t*
transformational, (V1) 1059, (V1) 1059*t*
Learning, (V1) 396–419, (V2) 177–183. *See also* Education
affective, (V1) 399*t*, (V1) 400
assessment guidelines for, (V2) 179
basic concepts and principles of, (V1) 398–407
client
active involvement in, (V1) 401
assessment for, (V1) 407–408

barriers to, (V1) 406–407, (V1) 407*b*
communication for, (V1) 402
content amount and complexity for, (V1) 402
cultural factors in, (V1) 403, (V1) 405, (V1) 406*b*
developmental stage and, (V1) 403
emotions and, (V1) 401
environment for, (V1) 401–402, (V1) 402*f*
factors affecting, (V1) 400–406
feedback in, (V1) 401
health literacy and, 406*b*, (V1) 405–406
motivation for, (V1) 400
readiness for, (V1) 400–401
repetition in, (V1) 401
scheduling session for, (V1) 402, (V1) 402*b*
by special populations, (V1) 402–403
timing and, (V1) 401
cognitive, (V1) 399, (V1) 399*t*
in culturally competent care, (V1) 323
definition of, (V1) 398
documentation of, (V1) 419
domains of, (V1) 398–400, (V1) 399*t*
active verbs for, (V1) 409It
evaluation of, (V1) 416–419
knowledge map for, (V2) 183
objectives of, (V1) 409
psychomotor, (V1) 399–400, (V1) 399*t*
sleep and, (V1) 879–880
Lecture, in patient teaching, (V1) 416, (V1) 417*t*
Leg(s)
dangling from bedside, (V1) 842*p*, (V2) 628*p*, (V2) 629–630*p*, (V2) 638
exercises for, (V1) 1054*p*, (V2) 826–827*p*, (V2) 828–829*p*
Legal considerations, on medications, (V1) 607–608
Legal documentation, (V1) 372
Legal issues, (V1) 1162–1185, (V2) 905–911. *See also* Law; Malpractice
Legislation
drug, U.S., (V1) 606
influence of, on contemporary nursing practice, (V1) 26
Legislators, in healthcare regulation, (V1) 22
Leininger, Madeleine, nursing theory of, (V1) 145, (V1) 146*t*
Leisure activities, in stress management, (V1) 257
Lens
inspection of, (V1) 494, (V2) 242*p*
opacities of, (V1) 494
Lethargic, description of, (V1) 507
Leukocyte esterase, urinary, (V2) 563
Leukocytes, in inflammatory process, (V1) 247
Leukopenia, (V1) 695
Leukoplakia, (V1) 497
Levin tube, (V1) 707, (V1) 707*f*, (V2) 837
Levine Myra, nursing theory of, (V1) 146*t*
Levine technique, (V2) 674
Liability
definition of, (V1) 1163
vicarious, (V1) 1175–1176
Liability insurance, professional, (V1) 1184
Libel, (V1) 1172
Libido, (V1) 859
low, (V1) 865
Lice, head, (V1) 492, (V1) 596, (V2) 313*f*
Licensing bodies, for nursing, (V1) 22
Licensure, requirements for, (V1) 1169–1170
Life expectancy, (V1) 202
Life span, (V1) 163–220, (V2) 61–75. *See also* Development; Growth
adolescence in, (V1) 188–194. *See also* Adolescent(s)
development through, knowledge map on, (V2) 71
gestational period in, (V1) 170–172
health promotion throughout, (V1) 1100–1101*t*, (V1) 1100–1102
infancy in, (V1) 176–179
middle adulthood in, (V1) 196–200. *See also* Middle adult(s)
neonatal period in, (V1) 172–176. *See also* Neonate
older adulthood in, (V1) 201–222, (V2) 72–75. *See also* Older adult(s)
preschoolers in, (V1) 182–184. *See also* Preschooler(s)
school-age children in, (V1) 184–188. *See also* School-age child(ren)
stressors throughout, (V1) 242*b*
toddlerhood in, (V1) 179–182. *See also* Toddler(s)
young adulthood in, (V1) 194—196. *See also* Young adult(s)
Life-span perspective, on aging, (V1) 203–204
Life stress review, in health promotion assessment, (V1) 1103
Lifestyle
blood pressure and, (V1) 448
cardiovascular effects of, (V1) 972–973
changes in, for health promotion, (V1) 1099, (V1) 1106
support for, (V1) 1108
effects of depression on, (V1) 279
exercise and, (V1) 826
in health promotion assessment, (V1) 1102
guidelines and tools for, (V2) 873–875
mobility and, (V1) 826
nutrition and, (V1) 685–687
pulmonary system effects of, (V1) 941–942
sedentary, (V1) 834
health status and, (V1) 1097
sensory function and, (V1) 775
sexuality and, (V1) 856
skin and, (V1) 580
skin effects of, (V1) 901
sleep and, (V1) 885–886
Lifestyle choices, in health-illness, (V1) 226
Lifestyle modifications, for urinary incontinence, (V1) 736, (V2) 558
Lifting, technique for, (V1) 825
Lifts, precordial, (V1) 502
Ligaments, (V1) 818
trauma to, (V1) 829
Light
pathogen growth and, (V1) 520
in sleep therapy, (V1) 886
Line of gravity, (V1) 820
Linens
hospital bed, (V1) 603
in pressure ulcer prevention, (V1) 918
Liniment, (V1) 611*t*
Linoleic acid, (V1) 673
Lipid(s), (V1) 669*t*, (V1) 671–673
administering, (V1) 713*p*, (V2) 511–513*p*
functions of, (V1) 673
sources of, (V1) 671–673
types of, (V1) 671–673, (V1) 671*b*
Lipid panel screening
in health promotion assessment, (V2) 876
for middle adult, (V1) 198
in older adult assessment, (V1) 213
Lipoproteins, (V1) 671
high-density, (V1) 672
low-density, (V1) 671–672
Lips, assessment of, (V1) 497
Liquid oxygen units, (V1) 956*f*
List. *See also* Checklist
work-related use of, (V1) 1074
Listening
active
for enhancing therapeutic communication, (V1) 473–474, (V1) 474*f*
for spirituality diagnoses, (V1) 340
intuition and, (V1) 150
Listserv, (V1) 1081
Liter, (V2) 481
Literacy, information, (V1) 1089, (V1) 1090*b*
Literature, nursing
databases for, (V1) 1091, (V1) 1092*t*
search of, (V1) 156–157
Litigation in civil claims, (V1) 1176–1177
Lived experience, illness as, (V1) 222–223
Liver
in drug excretion, (V1) 615
palpation of, (V2) 276*p*
surgery and, (V1) 1029*b*
Living will, (V1) 355, (V1) 1166, (V1) 1166*b*
Livor mortis, (V1) 367
Local adaptation syndrome (LAS), (V1) 247–248
Local anesthesia, (V1) 810
Locus of control, in self-concept, (V1) 265
Logical reasoning, (V1) 141
in gaining knowledge, (V1) 152
Logrolling, (V1) 840, (V1) 842, (V2) 626–627*p*
Long-term care, documentation in, (V1) 389
Long-term care facility, (V1) 16
transferring patient to, (V1) 237*p*, (V2) 81–82*p*
Long-term goals, (V1) 1074
Loop-acting diuretics, (V1) 719*b*
Loop colostomy, (V1) 752, (V1) 752*f*
Lordosis, (V2) 314*f*
description of, (V1) 506
Loss, (V1) 346–347, (V2) 145–158. *See also* Death; Dying; Grief
actual, (V1) 346
of aspects of self, (V1) 347
assessment guidelines for, (V2) 153–154
environmental, (V1) 347
as etiology, diagnosis of, (V1) 358
external, (V1) 346–347
as health disruption, (V1) 228–229
helping children deal with, (V1) 367, (V1) 367*b*
internal, (V1) 347
knowledge map for, (V2) 158
perceived, (V1) 346
physical, (V1) 346
as problem, diagnosis of, (V1) 357–358
psychological, (V1) 346
of significant relationships, (V1) 347

Lotion(s), (V1) 611*t*
application of, (V1) 636–637, (V2) 430*p*
in pressure ulcer prevention, (V1) 918
Love, in spirituality, (V1) 329
Love and belonging needs, (V1) 54
Love needs, (V1) 147, (V1) 147*f*
Lower respiratory tract infections, (V1) 944
Lozenge, lipid-soluble, (V1) 611*t*
Lubricant laxatives, (V1) 749*b*
Luer-lock syringe tip, (V1) 641, (V1) 642*f*
Lumen, of feeding tube, (V1) 708
Lung(s), (V1) 935–936, (V1) 936*f*. *See also* Pulmonary system; Respiration(s)
assessment of, (V1) 499–501, (V1) 501*f*, (V1) 513*p*, (V2) 260–265*p*
cancer of, (v1) 942
compliance of, (V1) 937
in drug excretion, (V1) 616
elasticity of, (V1) 937
in electrolyte regulation, (V1) 991–992
fluid loss from, (V1) 987
immobility effects on, (V1) 831
percussion of, (V1) 955, (V1) 963–964*p*, (V2) 728–730*p*
receptors of, (V1) 939
recollapse of, (V2) 764
reexpansion of, (V2) 764
vibratory therapy for, (V1) 955, (V1) 963–964*p*, (V2) 728–730*p*
Lung sounds, (V1) 445, (V1) 449–501, (V1) 501*f*, (V2) 264–265
normal, (V2) 264–265
Lung volumes, (V2) 766–767
Lymph nodes, cervical, assessment of, (V1) 498, (V2) 255*p*
Lymphocytes, (V1) 671
B, (V1) 525
serum levels of, protein metabolism and, (V1) 695
in specific immunity, (V1) 525
T, (V1) 525
in cellular immunity, (V1) 526–527, (V1) 527*f*

M

Maceration, (V1) 581, (V1) 900, (V1) 914
Macrosomia, maternal diabetes and, (V1) 171
Macular degeneration, definition of, (V1) 777*b*
Macule, (V2) 230
Maggot debridement, (V1) 923
Magnesium, (V1) 677*t*, (V1) 678, (V1) 989, (V1) 990–991*t*
imbalances in, (V1) 989, (V1) 995*t*
Magnetic resonance imaging (MRI)
in body mass evaluation, (V1) 693
in GI tract study, (V2) 595
Mainstream smoke, (V1) 942
Maintaining belief, in caring, (V1) 39
Major depressive disorder, criteria for, (V1) 269
Major surgery, (V1) 1028
Maladaptive coping, (V1) 243
Male chauvinism, as barrier to culturally competent care, (V1) 317–318
Male genitourinary system
abnormalities of, (V2) 315*f*
assessment of, (V1) 510, (V1) 510*f*, (V1) 514*p*
Malignancy(ies), oral, (V1) 592
Malignant hyperthermia, (V1) 1040
Malingering, from failure of adaptive mechanisms, (V1) 252–253
Malnutrition
definition of, (V1) 703
protein-calorie, chronic diseases and, (V1) 689
severe, signs of, (V1) 703
Malpractice, (V1) 1174
avoiding, (V1) 1179–1185, (V2) 907
common causes of, (V1) 1177–1178, (V1) 1177*b*
definition of, (V1) 1163
failure to assess and diagnose and, (V1) 1177
failure to evaluate and, (V1) 1178
failure to implement plan of care and, (V1) 1178
failure to plan and, (V1) 1178
risks for, minimizing, (V1) 1179–1185
Mammary glands, (V1) 848
Mammogram
for middle adult, (V1) 198
in older adult assessment, (V1) 213
Mammography, (V1) 498
Managed care, (V1) 23–24
Management, (V1) 1059–1060, (V2) 859–863. *See also* Leadership; Manager
challenges in, (V1) 1065
of change, (V1) 1069–1071
communication and, (V1) 1067
of conflict, (V1) 1071–1073
critical thinking about, (V2) 860–861
delegation in, (V1) 1067–1069. *See also* Delegation
empowerment and, (V1) 1066–1067
full-spectrum nursing and, (V2) 860
healthcare economics and, (V1) 1065
human relations-based, (V1) 1059
knowledge map for, (V2) 863
labor market and, (V1) 1065
power sources and, (V1) 1066
scientific, (V1) 1059
servant leadership theory of, (V1) 1059
theories of, (V1) 1059
theory X of, (V1) 1059
theory Y of, (V1) 1059
of time, (V1) 1073–1075
Manager. *See also* Management
activities of, (V1) 1061
business sense of, (V1) 1061
clinical expertise of, (V1) 1061
decisional activities of, (V1) 1061
definition of, (V1) 1059–1060
effective, (V1) 1059–1061
informational responsibilities of, (V1) 1061
interpersonal activities of, (V1) 1061
leadership by, (V1) 1060. *See also* Leadership
preparation of, (V1) 1061–1064
role and function of, (V1) 6*t*
Mandatory reporting laws, (V1) 1167
Mandatory reporting regulations, in minimizing malpractice risks, (V1) 1183–1184
Mania, sexuality and, (V1) 857
Mannequins, for teaching, (V1) 1085, (V1) 1085*f*
Manual of the International Classification of Disease and Related Health Problems (ICD-10), (V1) 74
Marasmus, definition of, (V1) 703
Marriage, (V1) 854, (V1) 855
Marriage and family therapist, on healthcare team, (V1) 19
Mask(s)
CDC standard precautions on, (V2) 337
face, (V1) 535*f*
oxygen, (V2) 731–735*p*
Maslow, Abraham, self-actualization and self-transcendence theory of, (V1) 263–264
Maslow's Hierarchy of Human Needs, (V1) 147–148, (V1) 1070
as assessment data framework, (V1) 54
nurses' use of, (V1) 147–148, (V1) 147*f*
in prioritizing problems, (V1) 70, (V1) 70*f*, (V1) 71*t*
Mass peristalsis, (V1) 747
Massage
back, (V1) 802, (V2) 664–665
following bath, (V1) 582
for pain, (V1) 802
for postoperative pain, (V1) 1047
in pressure ulcer prevention, (V1) 918
for sleep promotion, (V1) 893*p*
in stress management, (V1) 259
Mastectomy, (V1) 857
Master's degree in nursing, research and, (V1) 152
Master's entry nursing program, (V1) 10
Mastication, (V1) 745
Masturbation, (V1) 861
Maternal age, fetal health and, (V1) 171
Maternal changes, during pregnancy, (V1) 170–171
Maternal health, fetal health and, (V1) 171
Maternal nutrition, fetal health and, (V1) 171, (V1) 172
Mathematical skills, assessing, (V2) 286*p*
Mattress, (V1) 836
hospital bed, (V1) 603
Maxillary sinuses, transillumination of, (V2) 251*p*
McCaffery, Margo, (V1) 791
MDROs. *See* Multidrug-resistant organisms (MDROs)
Mead, Margaret, on self-concept, (V1) 264
Meals
assisting patient with, (V2) 516–517*p*
assisting patients with, (V1) 699
healthy, building, (V2) 513
Meaning
exploring, for spirituality diagnoses, (V1) 340
of work, (V1) 1066
Mechanical aids
for ambulation, (V2) 639–640
for transfer, (V1) 841, (V1) 841*f*, (V1) 843*f*
Mechanical debridement, (V1) 923
Mechanical stimuli, (V1) 793
Mechanical ventilation, (V1) 960–961, (V1) 960*f*, (V1) 965*p*, (V2) 752–754*p*
dysfunctional weaning from, (V1) 951
evidence-based studies of, (V1) 961
modes of, (V2) 752
negative pressure, (V1) 960
pneumonia associated with, (V1) 961
positive pressure, (V1) 960
suctioning and, (V2) 741–748
terminology for, (V2) 752
Mechanistic nursing, definition of, (V1) 138

Mechanoreceptors, (V1) 772
Meconium, (V1) 173, (V1) 748
Mediastinum, (V1) 935
Mediation, in resolution of litigation, (V1) 1176
Medicaid
  as payor for healthcare, (V1) 21
  reimbursement for home care by, (V1) 1128
Medical diagnosis
  nursing diagnosis and collaborative problems and comparison of, (V1) 63*t*
    distinguishing between, (V1) 64*f*
  recognizing, (V1) 62–64
Medical malpractice statutes, (V1) 1168
Medical record, (V1) 372. *See also* Documentation
Medicare
  "never events" and, (V1) 546, (V1) 553, (V1) 1027
  as payor for healthcare, (V1) 21
  public policy and, (V1) 23
  reimbursement for home care by, (V1) 1128
Medicated enemas, (V1) 761
Medication(s). *See also* Drug *entries*
  abbreviations related to, (V2) 478*t*
  absorption of, (V1) 609–614
    blood flow to area and, (V1) 614
    ionization and, (V1) 614
    pH and, (V1) 614
    route of administration and, (V1) 609, (V1) 610–613*t*, (V1) 614
    solubility of drug and, (V1) 614
  addition of, to intravenous fluids, (V2) 457–458*p*
  administration of, (V1) 604–660, (V2) 409–490. *See also* Medication administration
  adverse reactions to, (V1) 619, (V1) 619*b*
  allergies to, in medication administration record, (V1) 387
  antidiarrheal, (V1) 758–759
  associated with constipation, (V1) 753*b*
  barcoding of, (V1) 627, (V1) 1084
  biological half-life of, (V1) 617
  blood pressure and, (V1) 448
  bowel elimination and, (V1) 749
  cardiovascular, (V1) 973, (V1) 974*t*, (V1) 981
  cardiovascular effects of abused, (V1) 973
  causing taste disturbance, (V1) 778*b*
  chemotherapeutic effects of, (V1) 619
  classification of, (V1) 606
  controlled substances as, regulation of, (V1) 606–607, (V1) 607*f*
  dependence on, (V1) 622
  distribution of, (V1) 614–615
  dosage of
    calculation of, (V1) 622, (V2) 482–484
      for child, (V2) 484
    designations of, error-prone, (V2) 479*t*
    measurement systems for, (V1) 622, (V2) 481–482
    measurements for, (V1) 622
    measuring, when changing needles, clinical insight on, (V2) 474–475*b*
  drawing up, (V1) 643, (V1) 657*p*, (V2) 435–439*p*
  duration of action of, (V1) 616, (V1) 616*f*
  effectiveness of, concepts relevant to, (V1) 616–617, (V1) 616*f*
  enteric-coated, (V1) 614
  excretion of, (V1) 615–616
  extravasation of, (V1) 1013*t*, (V2) 814
  host susceptibility and, (V1) 528
  for hypertension, administering, (V1) 455
  illicit, (V1) 622
    abuse of, (V1) 1097
  incompatibilities of, (V1) 621
  injury risk from, (V1) 629
  IV push, administering, (V1) 653, (V1) 659*p*, (V2) 459–463*p*
  legal considerations on, (V1) 607–608
  liquid, pouring, (V1) 634, (V1) 634*f*
  listings and directories of, (V1) 606–607
  local effects of, (V1) 609
  management of, in home care, assisting with, (V1) 1133–1134
  metabolism of, (V1) 615
  minimum effective concentration of, (V1) 616, (V1) 616*f*
  misuse of, (V1) 629
  mixing, in same syringe, (V1) 643–644, (V1) 657–658*p*, (V2) 439–441*p*
  names of, (V1) 605–606
    brand, (V1) 605
    chemical, (V1) 605
    generic, (V1) 605
    official, (V1) 606
    proprietary, (V1) 605
  nonprescription, (V1) 606
  nutrition and, (V1) 690
  for older adults with depression, (V1) 282
  onset of action of, (V1) 616, (V1) 616*f*
  oral problems from, (V1) 591
  over-the-counter, (V1) 606
    for cough and cold, (V1) 952
    for sleep, (V1) 895–896
  overuse of, (V1) 629
  palliative effects of, (V1) 618
  pathogens resistant to, (V1) 522–523
  peak action of, (V1) 616, (V1) 616*f*
  peak level of, (V1) 616, (V1) 616*f*, (V1) 617
  pharmacodynamics of, (V1) 618–622. *See also* Pharmacodynamics
  pharmacokinetics of, (V1) 609–618. *See also* Pharmacokinetics
  as poisoning risk in home, (V1) 549
    interventions for, (V1) 560, (V1) 560*f*
  preoperative, (V1) 1036–1037, (V1) 1037*t*
  prescription, (V1) 606
  prescriptions for, (V1) 623–625. *See also* Prescription(s)
  prn, (V1) 608
  protein-binding capacity of, distribution and, (V1) 615
  pulmonary system, (V1) 973, (V1) 974*t*
  pulmonary system effects of, (V1) 942–943
  pulse and, (V1) 437
  quality of, mechanisms promoting, (V1) 606–609
  reconstituting, (V1) 643
    clinical insight on, (V2) 473*b*
  respiration and, (V1) 443
  respiratory, (V1) 951
  restorative effects of, (V1) 619
  rights of, (V1) 631–634
  safety of, mechanisms promoting, (V1) 606–609
  self-administration of, teaching patients about, (V1) 630
  sensory function and, (V1) 775
  sexual function and, (V1) 857, (V1) 858*t*
  side effects of, (V1) 619
  with similar-sounding names, (V1) 625*b*
  skin effects of, (V1) 900, (V1) 901*f*
  sleep and, (V1) 886
  solubility of, (V1) 614
  stock supply of, (V1) 608
  storage of, safe, (V1) 630
  storing and distributing systems for, (V1) 608–609, (V1) 608*f*
  substitutive effects of, (V1) 618–619
  suppliers of, (V1) 22
  supportive effects of, (V1) 618
  surgical risk and, (V1) 1028–1029, (V1) 1030*b*
  systemic effects of, (V1) 609
  teratogenic, (V1) 171
  therapeutic level of, (V1) 616
  therapeutic range of, (V1) 616–617
  timed-release, (V1) 614
  tolerance to, (V1) 621
  toxic reactions to, (V1) 620
  transdermal, (V1) 637, (V1) 637*f*
  trough level of, (V1) 616–617
  underuse of, (V1) 629
  unit-dose system for, (V1) 608, (V1) 608*f*
    prefilled, clinical insight on, (V2) 472*b*
  urinary function and, (V1) 719
  for urinary incontinence, (V1) 738
  urinary retention from, (V1) 721, (V1) 722*b*
Medication administration, (V1) 604–660, (V2) 409–490
  assessment for, (V1) 628
  central venous access device for, (V2) 467–470*p*
  inhalation for, (V1) 639–640, (V1) 639*f*, (V1) 640*f*
  instillations for
    ophthalmic, (V1) 638, (V1) 656*p*, (V2) 419–422*p*
    otic, (V1) 638, (V1) 656*p*, (V2) 422–423*p*
    rectal, (V1) 639
    vaginal, (V1) 638–639
  by intermittent infusion, (V2) 463–467*p*
  interventions for, (V1) 629
  intravenous, (V1) 652–655. *See also* Intravenous (IV) medication administration
  knowledge map for, (V2) 489
  noncompliance with, (V1) 629
  nursing diagnosis for, (V1) 628–629
  oral, 634*f*, (V1) 634–636, (V1) 656*p*, (V2) 414–419*p*
    buccal, (V1) 634–635
    for children, (V1) 635, (V1) 636*b*
    contraindications to, (V1) 635
    enteral, (V1) 635
    with objectionable taste, (V1) 635
    for older adults, (V1) 636
    pouring liquid medications for, (V1) 634, (V1) 634*f*
    sublingual, (V1) 634–635
    with swallowing difficulty, (V1) 635
    through enteral tube, (V2) 416–417*p*
  outcomes for, (V1) 629

parenteral, (V1) 612–613*t*, (V1) 640–655. *See also* Injection(s)
intradermal, (V1) 613*t*, (V1) 646–647, (V1) 658*p*
intramuscular, (V1) 613*t*. *See also* Intramuscular injection(s)
intravenous, (V1) 612–613*t*. *See also* Intravenous (IV) medication administration
subcutaneous, (V1) 613*t*. *See also* Subcutaneous injection(s)
safe, for inpatients, ensuring, (V1) 631–634
right documentation in, (V1) 633–634, (V1) 633*f*
right dose in, (V1) 632
right drug in, (V1) 631–632
right patient in, (V1) 633
right route in, (V1) 632–633
right time in, (V1) 632
three checks in, (V1) 631
steps to follow for, (V2) 410–414*p*
topical, (V1) 636–639
irrigations/instillations as, (V1) 637–638, (V1) 637*f*
nasal, (V1) 638, (V1) 656*p*, (V2) 424–425*p*
ophthalmic, (V1) 638, (V2) 419–422*p*
otic, (V1) 638, (V2) 422–423*p*
rectal, (V1) 639, (V1) 657*p*
transdermal, (V1) 637, (V1) 637*f*, (V1) 657*p*
vaginal, (V1) 638–639, (V1) 656–657*p*, (V2) 426–427*p*
Medication administration record (MAR), (V1) 384, (V1) 386–387, (V1) 386*f*
documenting drug administration in, (V1) 633–634, (V1) 633*f*
Medication error(s), (V1) 625–628
abbreviations, symbols, and dose designations contributing to, (V2) 478–481*t*
avoidance of, (V1) 625–628, (V1) 1179
automated systems and, (V1) 1084
error-prevention technology in, (V1) 625, (V1) 627
causes of, (V1) 626*b*
for older adults, reducing risk for, (V1) 637*b*
pediatric considerations on, (V1) 627–628
taking action after, (V1) 628, (V2) 477*b*
Medication history, in nursing health history, (V1) 52*t*
Meditation
evidence-based studies of, (V1) 975
in stress management, (V1) 258–259
Mediterranean diet, (V1) 687
MEDLINE, (V1) 1091, (V1) 1092*t*
Medulla, renal, (V1) 715, (V1) 715*f*
Mees' lines, (V1) 492
Melanocytes, (V1) 898
in older adults, (V1) 580*t*
Melatonin, for sleep, (V1) 895
Membrane permeability, in drug distribution, (V1) 616
Memory, assessing, (V2) 285–286*p*
Memory T cells, in cellular immunity, (V1) 527
Menarche, (V1) 189, (V1) 853
Menopause, (V1) 197, (V1) 854
teaching about, (V1) 869
Menstrual cycle, (V1) 849, (V1) 850
dysfunction of, (V1) 863–864
Menstruation
onset of (menarche), (V1) 853
painful, (V1) 863–864
teaching about, (V1) 869
Mental health disorders
self-care ability and, (V1) 576
sexuality and, (V1) 857
Mental health specialist, referral to, indications for, (V1) 280, (V1) 281*b*
Mental illness, as health disruption, (V1) 228
Mental state
exercise effects on, (V1) 824*b*
in physical examination, (V1) 488
Mental status
assessing, (V1) 781
in neurological assessment, (V1) 508
surgery and, (V1) 1028
Mentee, (V1) 1064*b*
Mentor, (V1) 1062–1063, (V1) 1064*b*
Mentoring, in patient teaching, (V1) 414, (V1) 418*t*
Mercury exposure
health effects of, (V1) 555*t*
in healthcare facility, (V1) 555
from spills, reducing, (V1) 572*b*
reducing, (V1) 571
Mercury manometers, (V1) 449–450, (V1) 449*f*
Message, in communication, (V1) 460, (V1) 460*f*
Meta-analysis, definition of, (V1) 151
Metabolic acidosis, (V1) 996, (V1) 997*t*, (V1) 999
Metabolic alkalosis, (V1) 996, (V1) 997*t*
Metabolic disorders, urinary function and, (V1) 720
Metabolic panel, preoperative, (V2) 845
Metabolism
in alarm stage, of stress response, (V1) 246, (V1) 246*f*
definition of, (V1) 668
in heat production, (V1) 424
immobility effects on, (V1) 831
of medications, (V1) 615
sleep and, (V1) 879
Meter, (V2) 481
Metered-dose inhalers (MDIs), (V1) 639–640, (V1) 639*f*, (V1) 640*f*, (V1) 657*p*
administering, (V2) 423–434*p*
Methadone, teratogenic effects of, (V1) 171
Methamphetamines, teratogenic effects of, (V1) 171
Methicillin-resistant *Staphylococcus aureus* (MRSA), (V1) 523
community-acquired, preventing, patient teaching on, (V1) 531–532*b*
in toddlers, (V1) 182
Metric system, of medication measurement, (V1) 622, (V2) 481
Mexican heritage. *See also* Hispanic Americans
pain perception and responses in, (V2) 127
Microcephaly, (V1) 493
Micronutrients, (V1) 673–679
minerals as, (V1) 676–679
vitamins as, (V1) 673–676
Microorganisms
in chain of infection, (V1) 519
infectious, in neonate, (V1) 175
Micturition, (V1) 717
definition of, (V1) 725*b*
Middle adult(s), (V1) 196–200
analysis/diagnosis for, (V1) 199
assessment of, (V1) 198
cancer in, (V1) 198
cardiovascular disease in, (V1) 198
cardiovascular system in, (V1) 972
depression in, (V1) 270
development of
physical, (V1) 196–197
psychosocial, (V1) 169, (V1) 197, (V1) 197*f*
developmental tasks of, (V1) 166–167*t*
domestic abuse of, (V1) 198
health problems of, (V1) 197–198
health promotion for, (V1) 1101*t*
hypertension in, (V1) 198
interventions for, (V1) 198–199
planning, (V1) 200
neglect of, (V1) 198
obesity in, (V1) 198
physical examination of, (V1) 487
planning outcomes/evaluation for, (V1) 199–200
pulmonary system of, (V1) 940
sexuality in, (V1) 854
sleep for, (V1) 881, (V1) 881*t*, (V1) 885
stressors of, (V1) 242*b*
violence against, (V1) 198
Midlife crisis, (V1) 197
Midline peripheral catheter, (V1) 1005
Migration, age group distribution and, (V1) 202–203
Milia, (V1) 491
in neonate, (V1) 173, (V2) 228
Military image of nurse, (V1) 5
Military personnel, nurses as, licensure and, (V1) 1170
Milk, breast, in diarrhea management, (V1) 759
Miller–Abbott tube, (V2) 837*t*
Milliequivalent, (V1) 984
Milliequivalent system for medication measurement, (V1) 622, (V2) 482
Milligram, (V1) 984
Mind-mapping student care plans, (V1) 94
Mineral(s), (V1) 676–679
for infants, (V1) 682
major, (V1) 676, (V1) 677*t*
supplemental, (V1) 696–697
trace, (V1) 676, (V1) 678*t*
Minimization, as defense mechanism, (V1) 250*t*
Minor surgery, (V1) 1028
Minority groups, (V1) 306
Minute ventilation, (V1) 941
Miosis, (V1) 494
Miracles, (V1) 329
Misdemeanor, definition of, (V1) 1172
Mixed apnea, (V1) 889
Mobility, (V1) 820, (V1) 826. *See also* Exercise(s); Immobility
assessment of, (V1) 832–834, (V1) 913, (V2) 641
decreased, postoperative, bowel elimination and, (V1) 750
development and, (V1) 826
disease and abnormalities and, (V1) 827–830
environmental factors and, (V1) 827
impaired, (V1) 834
sexuality and, (V1) 867
skin breakdown and, (V1) 899

in-home assessment for, (V1) 832
joint, (V1) 827–828. *See also* Range of motion
knowledge map for, (V2) 650
lifestyle and, (V1) 826
limited, self-care ability and, (V1) 575–576
nursing diagnosis for, (V1) 834
nursing interventions for, (V1) 834–846. *See also* Ambulation; Exercise(s); Position/positioning; Range of motion (ROM)
nursing outcomes for, (V1) 834
nutrition and, (V1) 826
postoperative, (V1) 1046
in self-care ability assessment, (V1) 577
stress and, (V1) 827
teamwork on outcomes for, (V1) 830
Model(s)
conceptual, definition of, (V1) 141
definition of, (V1) 141
full-spectrum nursing, (V1) 40*f*. *See also* Full-spectrum nursing, models for
health promotion, (V1) 1097–1099, (V1) 1098*f*, (V1) 1099*f*
Moist heat therapy, (V1) 932, (V1) 932*f*, (V2) 708
Moisture
excess skin, (V1) 900–901
management of, (V1) 918
pressure ulcers and, (V1) 908, (V1) 908*f*
pathogen growth and, (V1) 520
skin and, (V1) 580
Moisture-associated skin damage (MASD), (V1) 901
Moisture barriers, (V1) 927*t*
Molars, (V1) 590
Moles, (V1) 491
Mongolian spots, in neonate, (V1) 173
Monogamy, serial, (V1) 854
Monosaccharides, (V1) 668
Mons pubis, (V1) 848
Montgomery straps, (V1) 924, (V1) 928*f*
Mood, immobility effects on, (V1) 832
Moral agency, (V1) 1140–1142
Moral behavior, (V1) 1138
Moral decisions
attitudes and, (V1) 1144
beliefs and, (V1) 1144
developmental stage and, (V1) 1143
factors affecting, (V1) 1143–1154
values and, (V1) 1143–1144
Moral development theory
Gilligan's, (V1) 169–170
Kohlberg's, (V1) 169
Moral distress, (V1) 1140, (V1) 1141*f*
Moral frameworks, (V1) 1145–1149
MORAL model for ethical decision making
action in, (V1) 1158
clinical insights on, (V2) 899
dilemma in, (V1) 1157
evaluation in, (V1) 1158
information gaps in, (V1) 1157
options in, (V1) 1157–1158
resolution in, (V1) 1158
Moral outrage, (V1) 1140–1141
Morals, definition of, (V1) 1138
Morbid obesity, bathing and, (V1) 585–586, (V1) 586*t*
Mormonism, (V1) 332
Moro reflex, (V1) 174
Morphine, teratogenic effects of, (V1) 171
Morse Fall Scale, (V1) 557
Morula, (V1) 170
Mosquitoes, pathogens carried by, (V1) 551
avoiding, (V1) 565
Motivation, for learning, (V1) 400
Motor cortex, in breathing, (V1) 938
Motor development, of infants, (V1) 176, (V1) 176*b*
Motor function, assessment of, (V1) 509
Motor vehicle accidents
prevention of, (V1) 564–565
risk factors for, (V1) 551
Mottling, (V1) 490*t*
Mourning. *See* Grief
Mouth
assessment of, (V1) 496–497, (V1) 496*f*, (V2) 251–254*p*
defensive function of, (V1) 524
in digestion, (V1) 745
dry, interventions for, (V1) 699
hygiene for, (V1) 590–595. *See also* Hygiene, oral
malignancies of, (V1) 592
problems of, (V1) 591–592
Movement. *See also* Gait; Immobility/immobilization; Mobility/ Range of motion (ROM); Walking
assessment of, (V1) 506
physiology of, (V1) 817–818
MRSA. *See* Methicillin-resistant *Staphylococcus aureus* (MRSA)
Mu agonists, (V1) 806
Mucous membranes, assessment of, (V1) 999
Multicultural, (V1) 305
Multicultural population, ethical issues for nurses and, (V1) 1142
Multidrug-resistant organisms (MDROs), (V1) 523
preventing, (V1) 535–536
transmission of, preventing, clinical insight on, (V2) 341–342
Multitasking, (V1) 1075
Murmur(s), heart, (V1) 502, (V1) 503
assessing, (V2) 269*p*
Muscarinic receptor antagonists, for bladder disorders, (V1) 719
Muscle(s), (V1) 818. *See also* Musculoskeletal system
atrophy of, (V1) 831, (V1) 833*b*
cardiac, (V1) 818. *See also* Heart
clonus of, (V1) 833*b*
extension and flexion of, (V1) 819*f*
flaccidity of, (V1) 833*b*
function of, (V1) 506
hypertrophy of, (V1) 833*b*
immobility effects on, (V1) 831
injection of. *See* Injection(s), intramuscular
skeletal, (V1) 818
movement of, in heat production, (V1) 424
smooth, (V1) 818
spasms of. *See* Clonus
strength assessment of, (V2) 642
strength of, testing, (V2) 283–284*p*
Musculoskeletal system
age-related changes in, assessment for, (V1) 208*t*
in alarm stage, of stress response, (V1) 246, (V1) 246*f*
assessment of, (V1) 505–506, (V1) 514*p*, (V2) 277–284*p*
congenital abnormalities of, (V1) 827
disorders of
atlas of, (V2) 314*f*
from failure of adaptive mechanisms, (V1) 252*t*
exercise effects on, (V1) 824–825, (V1) 824*b*
immobility effects on, (V1) 831
pain effects on, (V1) 798
trauma to, (V1) 828–829
Music listening, in stress management, (V1) 259
Music therapy
for pain, (V1) 803
for sleep, (V1) 894
Mustache care, (V1) 597, (V1) 600*p*, (V2) 387–388*p*
Mutual Recognition Model (MRM) Nurse Licensure Compact, (V1) 1170
Mydriasis, (V1) 494
Myopia, (V1) 494
definition of, (V1) 777*b*
Myotonia, (V1) 859
MyPlate, (V1) 665–666, (V1) 666*f*
vegan, (V1) 688*f*

N

Nail(s)
assessment of, (V1) 492–493, (V1) 512–513*p*, (V1) 589, (V2) 235–236*p*
black, (V1) 492
care of, (V1) 588–590, (V1) 590*b*
color of, (V1) 492
disorders of, (V1) 588, (V2) 313f
in older adults, (V1) 580*t*
pulse oximetry and, (V2) 727
shape of, (V1) 492, (V1) 492*f*
texture of, (V1) 492–493, (V2) 235
Nail polish, pulse oximetry and, (V2) 727
NANDA-I nursing diagnosis(es), (V1) 2
for activity and exercise problems, (V1) 2
associated with stress, (V2) 97–98
for community health problems, (V1) 1123–1124
components of, (V1) 74–75
descriptors for, (V2) 27–28*b*
for fluid and electrolyte imbalances, (V1) 2
for impaired skin integrity, (V1) 2
infection-related, (V1) 529
interventions linked to, (V1) 114, (V1) 115*t*
outcomes linked to, (V1) 100*b*
for pain, (V1) 800
for pulmonary system problems, (V1) 951
for sexual problems, (V1) 867
NANDA-I spirituality diagnoses, (V1) 338, (V1) 339*b*
NANDA-I system, critiquing, (V1) 82
NANDA-I Taxonomy of Nursing Diagnosis, (V1) 74
NANDA-I Taxonomy of Nursing Diagnosis II, (V1) 55*t*
NANDA International, (V1) 74
NAP. *See* Nursing assistive personnel (NAP)
Narcolepsy, (V1) 889
Narcotics, teratogenic effects of, (V1) 171
Narrative format, for documentation, (V1) 379
Nasal cannula, for oxygen therapy, (V1) 956, (V2) 731–732

Nasal flaring, (V1) 946
Nasal medications, (V1) 638
Nasoenteric feeding tube(s), (V1) 707, (V1) 708*f*
  inserting, (V1) 712*p*, (V2) 498–502*p*
  removing, (V1) 712*p*, (V2) 506–507*p*
Nasogastric feeding tube(s), (V1) 707
  inserting, (V1) 712*p*, (V2) 498–502*p*
  irrigation of, (V1) 1055*p*, (V2) 836*p*
  medication administration by, (V1) 635
  removing, (V1) 712*p*, (V2) 506–507*p*
  suctioning of, (V1) 1053–1054, (V1) 1054–1055*p*, (V2) 834–839*p*
Nasojejunal feeding tube, (V1) 707
Nasopharyngeal airway, (V1) 957, (V1) 957*f*, (V1) 966*p*, (V2) 760–761*p*
  suctioning of, (V2) 749–751*p*
Nasotracheal suctioning, (V1) 960, (V2) 746–748*p*
National Council Licensure Exam (NCLEX), (V1) 12
National economy, influencing contemporary nursing practice, (V1) 26
National Formulary (NF), (V1) 606
National League of Nursing (NLN), (V1) 14
National Priorities Partnership, (V1) 1027
National School Lunch and Breakfast Programs, (V1) 697
National Student Nurses Association (NSNA), (V1) 14
Native Americans
  healers and practices of, (V1) 311*t*
  pain perception and responses in, (V2) 127
  religions of, (V1) 334
  values and health/illness beliefs of, (V1) 314*t*
Natriuresis, (V1) 988
Natural family planning, (V2) 654
Naturally occurring retirement communities (NORCs), (V1) 204
Nature, *versus* nurture in growth and development, (V1) 164
Naughty nurse image, (V1) 5
Nausea
  impaired nutrition from, interventions for, (V1) 698
  opioid-related, (V) 807*b*
  patients with, interventions for, (V2) 516*p*
  postoperative, (V1) 1050*t*, (V2) 853
Navajo Indian heritage. *See also* Native Americans
  pain perception and responses in, (V2) 128
NCLEX. *See* National Council Licensure Exam (NCLEX)
Nebulization, (V1) 639
Nebulizer(s)
  for secretion mobilization, (V1) 955
  types of, (V1) 639, (V1) 639*f*
Neck
  assessment of, (V1) 497–498, (V1) 513*p*, (V2) 255–256*p*
  range of motion in, (V2) 643
Needle(s), (V1) 640–641
  bevel of, (V1) 641, (V1) 641*f*
  CDC standard precautions on, (V2) 337
  changing, measuring dosage when, clinical insight on, (V2) 474–475*b*
  dead space in, accounting for, (V1) 644
  filter, (V1) 641
  gauge of, (V1) 640, (V1) 641*f*
  length of, (V1) 641
  recapping
    for contaminated needle, (V1) 644–645, (V1) 658*p*
    for sterile needle, (V1) 645, (V1) 658*p*, (V2) 444–445*p*
    using one-handed technique, (V2) 443–444*p*
  reusing, in home care, clinical insight on, (V2) 471*b*
  safety, (V1) 641, (V1) 641*f*, (V1) 1005, (V1) 1005*f*
  selection of
    for intramuscular injections, (V1) 651, (V1) 652*t*
    for subcutaneous injections, (V1) 648
  transfer, (V1) 653, (V1) 653*f*
Needle aspiration culture, (V1) 916
Needleless connection, for intermittent infusions, (V1) 654
Needlestick injuries
  in healthcare workers, (V1) 555
  prevention of, (V1) 644–645, (V1) 645*f*, (V2) 355*p*
Needs, human, Maslow's Hierarchy of, (V1) 147–148, (V1) 1070. *See also* Maslow's Hierarchy of Human Needs
Negative pressure ventilation, (V1) 960
Negative pressure wound therapy, (V1) 919, (V1) 930*p*, (V2) 685–690*p*
Neglect
  of adolescent, (V1) 191
  in family, as family health risk, (V1) 294–295
  of infant, (V1) 177
  of middle adult, (V1) 198
  of preschooler, (V1) 183–184
  of young adult, (V1) 195–196
Negligence, (V1) 1174, (V1) 1175
Negotiation
  in culturally competent care, (V1) 321, (V1) 323
  for problem-solving, (V1) 1073
  in resolution of litigation, (V1) 1176
Neobladder, (V1) 738
  interventions for patients with, (V1) 739, (V2) 559
Neonate. *See also* Infant(s)
  assessment of, (V1) 175
  cardiovascular system of, (V1) 173
  dermis of, (V1) 173
  development of
    cognitive, (V1) 174
    physical, (V1) 172–174, (V1) 174*f*
    psychosocial, (V1) 174–175
  elimination by, (V1) 173
  epidermis of, (V1) 173
  growth of, (V1) 172–173
  health problems of, (V1) 175
  hearing of, (V1) 174
  interventions for, (V1) 175–176
  jaundice in, (V1) 175
  neuromuscular system of, (V1) 173–174, (V1) 174*f*
  pain in, (V1) 796
  premature, pulmonary system of, (V1) 939
  respirations in, (V1) 173
  sensory perception in, (V1) 774
  sleep for, (V1) 881, (V1) 881*t*
  smell sense in, (V1) 174
  thermoregulation in, (V1) 173
  touch in, (V1) 174
  vision of, (V1) 174
Nephrons, in urine formation, (V1) 715–716, (V1) 716*f*
Nephropathy, definition of, (V1) 725*b*
Nephrotoxic, definition of, (V1) 725*b*
Nerve(s)
  cranial, assessment of, (V1) 508, (V1) 508*t*, (V1) 509*f*, (V2) 288–290*p*
  injury to, in IV therapy, (V1) 1014*t*
  peripheral, in pain transmission, (V1) 793–794, (V1) 795*f*
Nerve block, (V1) 1041
  for pain, (V1) 810
Nerve deafness, definition of, (V1) 778*f*
Nervous system, (V1) 818. *See* Neurological system; Sensation; Sensory perception
  in breathing regulation, (V1) 938–939
  in cardiovascular regulation, (V1) 970–971
  conditions of, urinary function and, (V1) 720
  disorders of, (V1) 829
  exercise effects on, (V1) 824*b*
  in movement, (V1) 818
  in pain transmission, (V1) 793–794
  in pulmonary disease, (V1) 944
  in sleep regulation, (V1) 883, (V1) 884
Networking, (V1) 1061
Neuman, Betty
  on health, (V1) 1096
  nursing theory of, (V1) 146*t*
Neuman's continuum, (V1) 224, (V1) 224*f*
Neurectomy, for pain, (V1) 810
Neurocognitive disorders, (V1) 280
Neurogenic bladder, (V1) 720
Neuroleptics
  preoperative, (V1) 1037*t*
  for restless leg syndrome, (V1) 887
Neurological system
  age-related changes in, assessment for, (V1) 208*t*
  assessment of, (V1) 506–509, (V1) 514, (V2) 284–296*p*
    cerebral function and, (V1) 507–508
    cranial nerve function and, (V1) 508, (V1) 508*t*, (V1) 509*f*
    developmental considerations for, (V1) 506–507
    in fluid and electrolyte assessment, (V1) 999
    motor and cerebellar function and, (V1) 509
    reflex function and, (V1) 508, (V1) 509*f*
    sensory function and, (V1) 509
  disorders of
    pulmonary effects of, (V1) 944
    surgery and, (V1) 1029*b*
    urinary retention from, (V1) 721
Neuromuscular system, of neonate, (V1) 173–174, (V1) 174*f*
Neuropathic pain, (V1) 792
Neuropathy, peripheral, blood glucose levels and, (V1) 694
Neutralization, in humoral immunity, (V1) 525
"Never events," (V1) 546, (V1) 553, (V1) 1027
Nevi, (V1) 491
Nevus flammeus, (V2) 312*f*
Newborn. *See* Neonate

Newman, Margaret, nursing theory of, (V1) 146*t*
Niacin, (V1) 675*t*
Nicotine. *See also* Cigarette smoking
  sleep and, (V1) 886
  teratogenic effects of, (V1) 171
Nicotine replacement therapy, (V1) 953
Night terrors, (V1) 890
Nightingale, Florence, (V1) 3–4, (V1) 5*f*, (V1) 1066
  health defined by, (V1) 223*b*
  in history of nursing research, (V1) 151
  nursing theory of, (V1) 144
Nightmares, (V1) 890
Nirvana, (V1) 333
Nitrite, urinary, (V2) 563
Nitrogen balance, (V1) 671
Nits, (V1) 492
NLN. *See* National League of Nursing (NLN)
"No," (V1) 1075
Nociceptive pain, (V1) 792
Nociceptors, (V1) 792
Nocturnal frequency, in older adults, (V1) 718
Nocturia, definition of, (V1) 725*b*
Nocturnal enuresis, (V1) 723, (V1) 890
  in children, (V1) 718
  definition of, (V1) 725*b*
Nodule, (V2) 231
Noise control
  for client environment, (V1) 602
  for sensory overload, (V1) 785
Noise pollution
  reducing, (V1) 568
  as safety hazard, (V1) 552
Non-luer-lock syringe tip, (V1) 641, (V1) 642*f*
Non-rapid eye movement (NREM) sleep, (V1) 883, (V1) 884*t*
Nonadherence, (V1) 629
Nonallergenic tape, (V1) 924
Nonassertive communication style, (V1) 468
Nonbenzodiazepines, for sleep, (V1) 894
Noncompliance, (V1) 629
  culture and, (V1) 320
Nonelectrolytes, (V1) 984
Nonmaleficence
  as ethical concept, (V1) 1150
  in resolving dilemma, (V1) 1158
Nonnursing models, for assessment data organization, (V1) 54
Nonopioid, (V1) 805–806, (V1) 805*b*
Nonselective debridement, (V1) 923
Nonshivering thermogenesis, (V1) 424
Nonsteroidal anti-inflammatory drugs (NSAIDs), (V1) 805, (V1) 805*b*
  bowel elimination and, (V1) 749
  skin effects of, (V1) 900
  surgery and, (V1) 1030*b*
Nontunneled central venous catheters, (V1) 1007, (V1) 1007*f*
Nonverbal behaviors, in enhancing communication, (V2) 211*b*
Nonverbal communication, (V1) 463–464
  pain-related, (V2) 615
Normothermia, for surgical client, (V1) 1036
Norton scale, (V1) 913, (V2) 712
Nose
  assessment of, (V1) 496, (V1) 496*f*, (V2) 249–251*p*
  hygiene care for, (V1) 599–600
  medication administration into, (V1) 638, (V2) 424–425*p*
Nosocomial infections, (V1) 517
Notifiable diseases, (V1) 863
NPO, (V1) 690
NREM (non-rapid eye movement) sleep, (V1) 883, (V1) 884*t*
NSNA. *See* National Student Nurses Association (NSNA)
Numerical Rating Scale, for pain, (V2) 617
Nurse(s)
  circulating, (V1) 1039, (V1) 1044
  disciplinary actions for, (V1) 1170–1171
  education for, (V1) 9–12. *See also* Education
  employment of, (V1) 1065
  empowerment of, (V1) 1066–1067
  impaired, reporting regulations on, (V1) 1183
  inappropriate sexual behavior toward, (V1) 871
  licensure of, requirements for, (V1) 1169–1170
  moral problems of, (V1) 1142
  position in healthcare organization, ethical problems and, (V1) 1142
  power of, (V1) 1066
  as professional, (V1) 5
  qualities of, (V1) 9*b*
  role of, (V1) 30–31*b*
  roles and functions of, (V1) 6*t*
  scope of practice of, (V1) 1170
  study of ethics by, reasons for, (V1) 1139–1140
Nurse administrator, advanced practice nurse as, (V1) 28
Nurse anesthetist (CRNA), (V1) 1039
Nurse assistive personnel (NAP), delegation to. *See* Delegation
Nurse educator, advanced practice nurse as, (V1) 28
Nurse entrepreneur, advanced practice nurse as, (V1) 28
Nurse informaticist, advanced practice nurse as, (V1) 28
Nurse informatics specialist, (V1) 1079
Nurse practice acts, (V1) 12, (V1) 607, (V1) 1168, (V1) 1169–1171
  assessment in, (V1) 45
Nurse practitioner (NP), advanced practice nurse as, (V1) 28
Nurse researcher, advanced practice nurse as, (V1) 28
Nurse sexual assault examiner, (V1) 865
Nurses' Bill of Rights, (V1) 1169
Nursing
  community, (V1) 1113–1136, (V2) 885–896. *See also* Community nursing
  contemporary, (V1) 6–15
  culture of, (V1) 312–313
  definition of, (V1) 6–9, (V1) 8*b*
    of American Nurses Association, (V1) 7–8
    importance of, (V1) 8
    of International Council of Nurses, (V1) 7
  as discipline, (V1) 8
  evolution of, (V2) 7–9
    knowledge map on, (V2) 9
  family, (V1) 288–289
  full-spectrum, (V1) 5, (V1) 6*t*, (V1) 39–42. *See also* Full-spectrum nursing
  functional, (V1) 15
  historical context of, (V1) 4–5
  images of, (V1) 4–5
  as occupation, (V1) 8
  primary, (V1) 15
  as profession, (V1) 8, (V1) 9*t*
  spirituality in, (V1) 326
  team, (V1) 15
  trends in, (V1) 27–29
Nursing activities
  for cardiovascular problems, (V1) old p. 909–912
  for drain maintenance, (V1) old p. 854
  for fear, (V2) 846
  for mobility problems, (V1) 834
  for pain, (V1) 801
  for pressure ulcer prevention, (V1) 917–919
  for sexual problems, (V1) 868
  for sleep problems, (V1) 893
  for wound problems, (V1) 919–920
Nursing admission assessment, (V1) 56
Nursing Admission Data Form, (V2) 19–22
Nursing assessment. *See also* Assessment(s)
  definition of, (V1) 481
Nursing assistive personnel (NAP)
  appropriate use of, (V1) 126
  delegation to. *See* Delegation
  on healthcare team, (V1) 19
  increased use of, (V1) 29
  power of, (V1) 1066
Nursing care
  continuity of, documentation in, (V1) 371
  cultural competence in, challenge to provide, (V1) 302–303
  documenting, guidelines for, (V1) 392–395
  end-of-life, (V1) 353–354. *See also* End-of-life care
  holistic, (V1) 149
  models of, (V1) 15
  postmortem, (V1) 366–367
  purposes of, (V1) 15
  recipients of, (V1) 14–15
Nursing care facilities, (V1) 205
Nursing code of ethics, (V1) 1152
Nursing diagnosis(es), (V1) 59–83, (V2) 26–32. *See also* Diagnostic statements, formats for
  actual, (V1) 66*t*
  for anxiety, (V1) 277–278
  assessment and, (V1) 44
  for blood pressure disorders, (V1) 453–454
  for bowel elimination problems, (V1) 756
  for cardiovascular problems, (V1) 978–979
  for communication problems, (V1) 472–473
  for community health problems, (V1) 1123–1124
  computer-assisted, (V1) 71–72
  culturally sensitive, (V1) 320
  definition of, (V1) 61
  for depression, (V1) 281
  deriving goals and interventions from, (V1) 98*t*
  documentation of, (V1) 378
  for eyes, (V1) 597
  failure to make, malpractice claims for, (V1) 1177
  for fall risk, (V1) 558–559
  for family, (V1) 298
  for feet, (V1) 588
  for fluid/electrolyte imbalances, (V1) 1001
  goals and, (V1) 97–98, (V1) 97t, (V1) 99*t*
  for growth and development, (V1) 199
  for hair, (V1) 596

for health and illness, (V1) 234
in health promotion, (V1) 234, (V1) 1104
in home healthcare, (V1) 1131–1132
for infection, (V1) 529
for intraoperative problems, (V1) 1042–1043
knowledge map for, (V2) 32
of loss and grief
as etiology, (V1) 358
as problem, (V1) 357–358
medical diagnosis and collaborative problems and
comparison of, (V1) 63*t*
distinguishing between, (V1) 64*f*
medication-related, (V1) 628–629
for mobility problems, (V1) 834
for nails, (V1) 589
NANDA-I. *See* NANDA-I nursing diagnosis(es)
nutritional, (V1) 695–696
for older adult, (V1) 215
for oral cavity, (V1) 592
origins of, (V1) 61–62
for overweight/obesity, (V1) 700
for pain, (V1) 800–801
for postoperative problems, (V1) 1046–1047, (V2) 846–855
potential, (V1) 66*t*
for preoperative problems, (V1) 1032–1033, (V2) 846–855
professional standards for, (V1) 60*b*
psychosocial, (V1) 271
for pulmonary system problems, (V1) 978–979
for pulse abnormalities, (V1) 440
recognizing, (V1) 62
relation of, to outcomes and interventions, (V1) 80
for respiratory alterations, (V1) 446
review of, in intervention selection, (V1) 111, (V1) 111*f*
risk, (V1) 66*t*
for self-concept and self-esteem issues, (V1) 274–275
for sensory-perceptual problems, (V1) 782
for sexuality, (V1) 867–868
for skin problems, (V1) 581–582, (V1) 917, (V2) 716–717
for sleep problems, (V1) 891–892
for spirituality, (V1) 338–340
standardized language for, (V2) 27–28*b*
for stress and adaptation, (V1) 256
stress-related, standardized outcomes and interventions for, (V2) 98
syndrome, (V1) 66*t*
for teaching, (V1) 408
for temperature regulation alterations, (V1) 431
terminology of, (V1) 61, (V1) 62*t*
types of, (V1) 64–65, (V1) 65*f*, (V1) 66*t*
for underweight/undernutrition, (V1) 703–704
for urinary elimination problems, (V1) 727
wellness, (V1) 66*t*
Nursing discharge summary, (V1) 56
Nursing education, nursing theories in, 143
Nursing ethics, (V2) 897–904
consequentialism and, (V1) 1147–1148
cost containment and, (V1) 1142
definition of, (V1) 1139
deontology and, (V1) 1148
ethics-of-care and, (V1) 1149
feminist ethics and, (V1) 1148–1149
frameworks for, (V1) 1145–1149
increased consumer awareness and, (V1) 1142
knowledge map on, (V2) 904
multicultural population and, (V1) 1142
nature of profession and, (V1) 1143
professional guidelines for, (V1) 1152–1154
societal factors and, (V1) 1142
technology and, (V1) 1142
Nursing health history
components of, (V1) 52*t*
interviewing to obtain, (V1) 51–53, (V1) 52*t*
Nursing history
in chronic wound assessment, (V1) 912–913, (V2) 709
in fluid and electrolyte assessment, (V1) 999
in mobility assessment, (V1) 832–833
preoperative, (V1) 1031
in skin assessment, (V1) 912–913, (V2) 709
Nursing home, (V1) 16
transferring patient to, (V1) 237*p*, (V2) 81–82*p*
Nursing informatics specialist, (V1) 1079. *See also* Informatics
Nursing interventions
for adolescent, (V1) 193–194
for anxiety, (V1) 278–279
for blood pressure disorders, (V1) 454–456
for bowel elimination problems, (V1) 756–767
for client environment, (V1) 601–603
collaborative, (V1) 107
for communication problems, (V1) 473–478
for community health problems, (V1) 1124
computer-generated, (V1) 113, (V1) 114*f*
culturally appropriate, (V1) 321–323
definition of, (V1) 106
dependent, (V1) 107
for depression, (V1) 282–284
derivation of, from nursing diagnoses, (V1) 98*t*
direct-care, (V1) 106
documentation of, (V1) 378
etiologies and, (V1) 80
for eyes, (V1) 597–599
for family, (V1) 299–300
for feet, (V1) 588
for fluid/electrolyte imbalances, (V1) 1001–1012, (V1) 1015, (V1) 1019–1020
for growth and development, (V1) 200
for hair care, (V1) 596–597
for health and illness, (V1) 234–238
for health promotion, (V1) 1105–1108
in home healthcare, (V1) 1133–1135
independent, (V1) 107
indirect-care, (V1) 106
individualized and standardized, (V1) 113, (V1) 113*t*
for infant, (V1) 178–179
for infection and infection prevention, (V1) 530–533
interdependent, (V1) 107
intraoperative, (V1) 1043–1045
knowledge map on, (V2) 44
for loss and grief, (V1) 358–368
for medical asepsis, (V1) 535–538
for medication administration, (V1) 629
for middle adult, (V1) 198–199
for mobility problems, (V1) 834–846
for nails, (V1) 590
for neonate, (V1) 175–176
nursing diagnosis and, (V1) 80
for nutrition problems, (V1) 696–699
for older adult, (V1) 215–219
for oral cavity, (V1) 593–595
for overweight/obesity, (V1) 701–703
for pain, (V1) 801–810
planning of, (V1) 105–118, (V2) 40–44
applying full-spectrum nursing model to, (V2) 41
critical thinking in, (V2) 41–43
in health promotion, (V1) 234
standardized language use in, (V1) 113–116
for postoperative problems, (V1) 1047, (V1) 1052–1054, (V2) 846–855
for preoperative problems, (V2) 846–855
for preschooler, (V1) 184
problem status influencing, (V1) 110, (V1) 110*t*
psychosocial, (V1) 273
for pulmonary system problems, (V1) 979–982
for pulse abnormalities, (V1) 441
for safety, (V1) 559–573
for school-age child, (V1) 187–188
selection of, (V1) 107–113
nursing research influencing, (V1) 108
process for, (V1) 110–113, (V1) 111*f*, (V1) 112*t*, (V1) 113*t*
theories influencing, (V1) 107–108
for self-concept and self-esteem issues, (V1) 275–277
for sensory-perceptual problems, (V1) 782–489
for sexual problems, (V1) 868–871
for skin hygiene, (V1) 582–587
for sleep problems, (V1) 892–896
for spiritual care, (V1) 340–343
standardized language and, (V1) 116
for stress and adaptation, (V1) 256–261
to support spirituality, (V2) 140–142
for teaching, (V1) 409–416
for temperature regulation alterations, (V1) 431, (V1) 433–435
for toddler, (V1) 181–182
for underweight/undernutrition, (V1) 704–713
for urinary elimination problems, (V1) 727–742
wellness, standardized language and, (V1) 116
for young adult, (V1) 196
Nursing Interventions Classification (NIC), (V1) 113–115, (V2) 865
in electronic care plans, (V1) 115
interventions in
appropriate, locating, (V1) 114–115, (V1) 115*t*
example of, (V1) 114*b*
Omaha system and, (V2) 890–891
Nursing interview
in comprehensive assessment, (V1) 48, (V1) 49*f*
for sexual history, (V2) 653, (V2) 656–657
Nursing journals, (V1) 1091
Nursing Management Minimum Data Set (NMMDS), (V2) 865

Nursing Minimum Data Sets (NMDS), (V2) 866
Nursing models, for assessment data organization, (V1) 54, (V1) 55–56*t*
Nursing orders, (V1) 116–118
  components of, (V1) 116–117
  reflecting critically about, (V1) 117–118
Nursing outcomes
  for anxiety, (V1) 278
  for blood pressure disorders, (V1) 454
  for bowel elimination problems, (V1) 756
  for cardiovascular problems, (V1) 979
  for communication problems, (V1) 473
  for community health, (V1) 1124
  culturally sensitive, (V1) 321
  for depression, (V1) 281–282
  desired, review of, in intervention selection, (V1) 111, (V1) 112*t*
  documentation of, (V1) 378
  expected, reflecting critically about, (V1) 102–103
  for eyes, (V1) 597
  for fall risk, (V1) 559
  for family, (V1) 298–299
  for feet, (V1) 588
  for fluid/electrolyte imbalance, (V1) 1001
  for growth and development, (V1) 199–200
  for hair care, (V1) 596
  for health and illness, (V1) 234
  for health promotion, (V1) 1104–1105
  in home healthcare, (V1) 1132–1133
  for infection, (V1) 530
  intraoperative, (V1) 1043
  for loss and grief, (V1) 358
  for medication administration, (V1) 629
  for mobility problems, (V1) 834
  for nails, (V1) 590
  NOC definition of, (V1) 99
  nursing diagnosis and, (V1) 80
  for nutrition, (V1) 696
  for older adult, (V1) 215
  for oral problems, (V1) 593
  for overweight/obesity, (V1) 700–701
  for pain management, (V1) 801
  planning and evaluation of, documentation in, (V1) 371
  planning of, (V1) 84–104, (V2) 33–39
    applying full-spectrum nursing model to, (V2) 36
    critical thinking in, (V2) 37
    in health promotion, (V1) 234
    implementation and, (V1)121
    patient care plans in, (V1) 88–94
    for psychosocial issues, (V1) 271–273
    relation of, to nursing process steps, (V1) 85, (V1) 87*f*
  postoperative, (V1) 1047, (V2) 846–855
  preoperative, (V1) 1034, (V2) 846–855
  for pulmonary system problems, (V1) 951
  for pulse abnormalities, (V1) 440–441
  for self-concept and self-esteem issues, (V1) 275
  for sensory-perceptual problems, (V1) 782
  for sexual problems, (V1) 868
  for skin problems, (V1) 582
  for sleep problems, (V1) 892
  for spirituality, (V1) 340
  standardized terminology for, (V1) 99–100, (V1) 100*t*, (V2) 35
  for stress and adaptation, (V1) 256
  for teaching, (V1) 408–409
  for temperature regulation alterations, (V1) 431
  for underweight/undernutrition, (V1) 704
  for urinary elimination problems, (V1) 727
  use of term, (V1) 95–96
  for wounds, (V1) 917
Nursing Outcomes Classification (NOC), (V1) 99, (V2) 865
  with computer care plans, (V1) 100
  measurement scales of, (V2) 35
  Omaha system and, (V2) 889
  outcomes in
    community health, (V1) 101, (V2) 889
    components of, (V1) 99–100
Nursing practice
  contemporary, factors influencing, (V1) 26–29
  laws and regulations guiding, (V1) 1164–1171
  nursing care in, (V1) 14–15
  nursing theories in, (V1) 143
  regulation of, (V1) 12
  scope of, (V1) 1170
  unauthorized, reporting regulations on, (V1) 1184
Nursing process
  application of, to community-based care, (V1) 1124–1125
  assessment in, (V1) 38, (V1) 38*f*, (V1) 43–58, (V2) 15–25. *See also* Assessment
  critical thinking in, (V1) 31–32, (V1) 32*b*, (V1) 39, (V2) 10–14
  definition of, (V1) 37–38
  diagnosis in, (V1) 38, (V1) 38*f*, (V1) 59–83. *See also* Nursing diagnosis
  evaluation in, (V1) 38*f*, (V1)39, (V1) 129–136. *See also* Evaluation
  in full-spectrum nursing, (V1) 40*t*, (V1) 41
  in home care, (V1) 1131–1135
  implementation in, (V1) 38, (V1) 38*f*, (V1) 119–128, (V1) 120–128, (V1) 129*t*. *See also* Implementation
  phases of, (V1) 38, (V1) 39*f*
    overlapping, (V1) 60–61, (V1) 61*f*
  planning in, (V1) 38, (V1)38*f*
  planning interventions in, (V1) 105–118. *See also* Nursing interventions, planning of
  planning outcomes in, (V1) 84–104. *See also* Nursing outcomes, planning of
  in promoting health, (V1) 233–238
Nursing research, (V1) 150–159
  appraisal of, (V1) 157–158
  approaches to, (V1) 153—154, (V1) 153*t*
  barriers to using, (V1) 159*b*
  best evidence from, basing practice on, (V1) 155–159
  definition of, (V1) 151
  educational competencies for, (V1) 151
  educational preparation for, (V1) 152
  gaining knowledge for, (V1) 152–153
  history of, (V1) 151–152
  importance of, (V1) 138–139
  influencing intervention selection, (V1) 108
  integration of, into practice, (V1) 158–159, (V1) 159*b*
  nursing theories in, (V1) 143
  online sources of, (V1) 1091, (V1) 1092*t*
  participants in, rights of, (V1) 154–155
  phases of process of, (V1) 154
  priorities for, development of, (V1) 152
  qualitative approach to, (V1) 153*t*, (V1) 154
  quality of, evaluating, (V1) 157–158, (V1) 157*b*
  quantitative approach to, (V1) 153–154, (V1) 153*t*
  utilization of, ANA standards for, (V1) 151
  World Wide Web sites for, (V1) 1091–1092, (V1) 1093*t*
Nursing theory(ies)
  assumptions of, (V1) 139
  of Betty Neuman, (V1) 146*t*
  caring, originators of, (V1) 145
  clinical practice
    application of, (V1) 143
    definition of, (V1) 138
  components of, (V1) 139–140
  concepts in, (V1) 140
    essential, (V1) 142–143
  definitions of, (V1) 140
  developing, (V1) 138
  development of, (V1) 141–142, (V1) 142*f*
  of Dorothea Orem, (V1) 146*t*
  of Dorothy Johnson, (V1) 146*t*
  environment in, (V1) 142, (V1) 142*f*, (V1) 143
  of Ernestine Wiedenbach, (V1) 146*t*
  of Faye Abdellah, (V1) 146*t*
  of Florence Nightingale, (V1) 144
  grand, (V1) 143
  health in, (V1) 142, (V1) 142*f*, (V1) 143
  of Hildegard Peplau, (V1) 144–145, (V1) 146*t*
  of Ida Jean Orlando, (V1) 146*t*
  of Imogene King, (V1) 146*t*
  importance of, (V1) 138–139
  interventions/implementation based on, planning, (V1) 149–150
  of J. Wrubel, (V1) 146*t*
  of Jean Watson, (V1) 146*t*
  of Madeleine Leninger, (V1) 145, (V1) 146*t*
  of Margaret Newman, (V1) 146*t*
  of Martha Rogers, (V1) 146*t*
  of Myra Levine, (V1) 146*t*
  in nursing education, (V1) 143
  in nursing practice, (V1) 143
  in nursing research, (V1) 143
  originators of, (V1) 143–146, (V1) 146*t*
  of Patricia Benner, (V1) 145, (V1) 146*t*
  phenomena in, (V1) 139–140
  of Rosemarie Rizzo Parse, (V1) 146*t*
  of Sr. Callista Roy, (V1) 146*t*
  statements in, (V1) 140
  use of, (V1) 143
  of Virginia Henderson, (V1) 144, (V1) 144*b*, (V1) 146*t*
Nurture, *versus* nature in growth and development, (V1) 164
Nutrient(s)
  energy, (V1) 667–673
    carbohydrates as, (V1) 668, (V1) 669*t*, (V1) 670
  essential, water as, (V1) 670
  imbalance of, physical examination findings in, (V1) 694
  for infectious organisms, (V1) 519–520
Nutrition, (V1) 661–713, (V2) 491–529
  for adolescents, (V1) 684
  for adults, (V1) 684
  assessment of, (V1) 691–695
    focused, (V1) 692–695, (V2) 522–525*p*
  for athletic performance, (V1) 687
  bowel elimination and, (V1) 749

cardiovascular effects of, (V1) 972–973
counseling on, (V1) 696–697
cultural practices and, (V1) 687, (V1) 689
definition of, (V1) 664
disease processes affecting, (V1) 689–690
enteral, (V1) 705–711. *See also* Enteral nutrition
ethnic practices and, (V1) 687, (V1) 689
exercise and, (V1) 826
factors affecting, (V1) 682–691
functional limitations affecting, (V1) 689–690
for health, (V1) 687
for health promotion, (V1) 1105–1106
for infants, (V1) 682–683
interventions for, (V1) 178–179
in infection prevention, (V1) 530
information sources for, (V1) 664–667
interventions for, (V1) 696
knowledge map on, (V2) 529
for lactating women, (V1) 684
lifestyle and, (V1) 685–687
maternal, fetal health and, (V1) 171, (V1) 172
for middle adult, interventions for, (V1) 199
mobility and, (V1) 826
nursing diagnoses related to, (V1) 695–696
nursing outcomes for, (V1) 696
for older adults, (V1) 684–685, (V1) 685*t*
for oldest-old, (V1) 206
parenteral, (V1) 711, (V1) 713. *See also* Parenteral nutrition (PN)
for pregnant women, (V1) 684
for preschoolers, (V1) 683
in pressure ulcer prevention, (V1) 918–919
problems with, screening for, (V2) 521–522*p*
pulmonary effects of, (V1) 941
religious practices and, (V1) 687, (V1) 689
for school-age child, (V1) 683–684
assessment of, (V1) 186
teaching about, (V1) 187
skin effects of, (V1) 899, (V1) 918–919
in stress management, (V1) 257
for toddlers, (V1) 683
urinary function and, (V1) 719
vegetarian, (V1) 686–687, (V1) 688*f*
for weight loss, (V1) 687
Nutrition Fact Label, (V1) 666–667, (V1) 668*f*
Nutritional assessment, (V1) 50
in health promotion assessment, (V1) 1103
Nutritional disorders, surgery and, (V1) 1029*b*
Nutritional factors, in healing-illness, (V1) 225
Nutritional needs, special, supporting, (V1) 698–699
Nutritional problems, screening for, (V1) 691
Nutritional status
laboratory values indicating, (V1) 694–695
preoperative, (V1) 1036
skin and, (V1) 580
tests reflecting, norms for, (V2) 525*p*
wound assessment and, (V1) 915
Nutritionist, on healthcare team, (V1) 20
Nutritive enemas, (V1) 761

O

OASIS (Outcome and Assessment Information Set), (V1) 389
Obesity, (V1) 699–700
in adolescents, (V1) 190–191
preventing and treating, interventions for, (V1) 193
bathing and, (V1) 585–586, (V1) 586*t*
binder application and, (V2) 698
blood pressure and, (V1) 448
cardiovascular effects of, (V1) 973
in children, (V1) 186
teaching about, (V1) 187
definition of, (V1) 699
as etiology of other problems, (V1) 700
exercise and, (V1) 826
health risks from, (V1) 1097
interventions for, (V1) 701–703
in middle adult, (V1) 198
in older adults, (V1) 700
population vulnerability and, (V1) 1116
pulmonary system effects of, (V1) 941
respiratory tract infection and, (V1) 941
sleep apnea and, (V1) 941
in young adults, (V1) 196
Objective data, (V1) 46, (V1) 47*t*
Oblique position, (V1) 839, (V1) 839*f*
Observation(s)
in comprehensive assessment, (V1) 47, (V1) 48*b*, (V1) 48*f*
sharing, in enhancing therapeutic communication, (V1) 475
Observation skills
in improving communication, (V1) 234
in promoting health, (V1) 234
Obstructive sleep apnea, (V1) 889
Occupation
hazards of, (V1) 941
nursing as, (V1) 8
Occupation health nursing, (V1) 1121
Occupational therapist, on healthcare team, (V1) 19
Occurrence report, 388*f*, (V1) 388
Occurrence-type liability insurance, (V1) 1184
Oculomotor nerve (III) testing, (V2) 288*p*
Odor(s)
control of, for sensory overload, (V1) 785
exudate, (V1) 915
foot, (V1) 587
menstrual, (V1) 869
urinary, (V2) 562
wound, (V2) 689, (V2) 710
Oil-retention enemas, (V1) 761, (V1) 761*t*
administering, (V2) 577*p*
Oils, essential, for aromatherapy, (V1) 779*b*
Ointment(s), (V1) 611*t*
application of, (V1) 636–637, (V2) 430*p*
ophthalmic, (V1) 638
Old age, as subculture, (V1) 307
Older adulthood, stages of, (V1) 206–207
Older adult(s), (V1) 201–222, (V2) 72–75
abuse of, (V1) 211
assessing for, (V1) 214, (V2) 66
ageism and, (V1) 211–212
aging and, (V1) 202–206. *See also* Aging
analysis/diagnosis for, (V1) 215
applying full-spectrum nursing model to, (V2) 73–74
assessment of, (V1) 212–215
for depression, dementia, or delirium, (V1) 280
in frail elderly, (V1) 215
in middle-old, (V1) 214–215, (V1) 214*f*
in oldest-old, (V1) 215
in young-old, (V1) 214
balance exercises for, (V1) 821
bathing for, (V1) 587
calcium deficiency in, (V1) 989
cardiac efficiency in, (V1) 972
cardiovascular system in, (V1) 972
communicating with, (V1) 217–219
communication by, (V1) 465
constipation in, (V1) 759
dementia in, (V1) 210–211, (V1) 210*t*
assessing for, (V1) 214
interventions for, (V1) 218–219
depression in, (V1) 211, (V1) 270
assessing for, (V1) 214
nursing interventions for, (V1) 282–283
development of
cognitive, (V1) 207
physical, (V1) 207, (V1) 208–209*t*
psychosocial, (V1) 207, (V1) 209
developmental changes of, (V1) 207–219
discharge planning for, (V1) 88
empowerment of, (V1) 217
exercise guidelines for, (V1) 822*b*
falls by. *See* Falls
female, urinary tract infections in, (V1) 720
food guides for, (V1) 666
foot problems of, (V1) 587
frail, (V1) 207
assessment for, (V1) 215
interventions for, (V1) 216–217
functional abilities preservation for, (V1) 217
grief in, (V1) 350
growing proportion of, in U.S., influencing contemporary nursing practice, (V1) 26
health problems of, (V1) 209–212
health promotion for, (V1) 1101*t*
hearing screening in, (V2) 605
in high-conflict scenarios, (V1) 1072
illness prevention for, (V1) 217
immunizations for, (V1) 217, (V1) 218*f*
impaired nutritional status in, screening for, (V2) 521–522*p*
interventions/implementation for, (V1) 215–219
light therapy for, (V1) 886
medication errors for, reducing risk for, (V1) 637*b*
middle-old, (V1) 206
assessment for, (V1) 214–215, (V1) 214*f*
interventions for, (V1) 216
motor vehicle safety recommendations for, (V1) 565
neurological exam in, (V1) 507
nutrition for, (V1) 684–685, (V1) 685*t*
obesity in, (V1) 700
oldest-old, (V1) 206–207
assessment for, (V1) 215
interventions for, (V1) 216
oral medication administration for, (V1) 636
outcomes/evaluation for, (V1) 215
pain in, (V1) 796, (V1) 810–811
pharmacokinetic processes in, (V1) 618*t*
physical examination of, (V1) 487
polypharmacy in, (V1) 211
with pressure ulcers, (V1) 900
psychosocial development in, (V1)169
pulmonary system of, (V1) 940
residential alternatives for, (V1) 204–205
restless leg syndrome in, (V1) 887
safety needs of, (V1) 548
sensory perception in, (V1) 774

sexuality of, (V1) 854–855
skin of, (V1) 899
changes in, (V1) 580, (V1) 580*t*
sleep for, (V1) 880, (V1) 881, (V1) 885
stressors of, (V1) 242*b*
surgery for, (V1) 1028, (V1) 1030, (V1) 1032, (V1) 1033, (V1) 1033*t*
antiembolism stockings and, (V1) 1038. *See also* Antiembolism stockings
evidence-based studies of, (V1) 1040
postoperative pain management and, (V1) 1047
teaching about, (V1) 1036
teaching, (V1) 403, (V1) 404–405*t*
urinary elimination in, (V1) 718
urinary incontinence and, (V1) 722
ventilation in, (V1) 940
walking assistance for, (V1) 844–845
young-old, (V1) 206
assessment for, (V1) 214
interventions for, (V1) 215–216
Olfaction, in physical examination, (V1) 486
Olfactory nerve (I), testing, (V2) 288*p*
Oliguria, definition of, (V1) 725*b*
Omaha System, (V1) 74, (V1) 102, (V1) 115, (V2) 865
for community health problems, (V1) 1124, (V2) 888–891, (V2) 889*b*, (V2) 891*b*
Omega-3, (V1) 673
Omega-6, (V1) 673
One-to-one instruction, in patient teaching, (V1) 414, (V1) 418*t*
Ongoing assessment, (V1) 47
Ongoing evaluation, (V1) 131
Ongoing groups, communication in, (V1) 471
Onychomycosis, (V1) 492
Open-pore reticulated polyurethane foam therapy, (V1) 930*p*, (V2) 687*p*
Open systems, in systems theory, (V1) 149
Open wounds, (V1) 902
Ophthalmic medications, (V1) 638
administration of, (V2) 419–422*p*
Ophthalmoscopy, assessing internal structures of eye via, (V2) 244*p*
Opioid Risk Tool, (V1) 806
Opioids (narcotics), (V1) 806–807
abuse of, (V1) 806
agonist-antagonist, (V1) 806
constipation with, (V) 807*b*
drowsiness with, (V) 807*b*
effectiveness of, (V1) 806
endogenous, (V1) 794
epidural, (V1) 808–809, (V1) 809*f*
equianalgesia for, (V1) 807–808
intra-articular, (V1) 808
intramuscular, (V1) 808
intraspinal, (V1) 808–809, (V1) 809*f*
intravenous, (V1) 808
misconceptions about, (V1) 806
mu agonist, (V1) 806
nasal, (V1) 808
nausea with, (V) 807*b*
oral, (V1) 808
paradoxical reaction to, (V1) 807
patient-controlled, (V1) 809, (V1) 809*p*, (V2) 611–614*p*
physical dependence on, (V1) 806
pruritus with, (V) 807*b*
psychological dependence on, (V1) 806
rectal, (V1) 808
respiratory depression with, (V) 807*b*
route of administration for, (V1) 808
sedation with, (V1) 806
sexual function and, (V1) 858*t*
side effects of, (V1) 807, (V1) 807*b*
subcutaneous, (V1) 808
surgery and, (V1) 1030*b*
tolerance to, (V1) 806
transdermal, (V1) 808
vomiting with, (V) 807*b*
Optic nerve (II) testing, (V2) 288*p*
Oral administration of drugs, (V1) 610*t*
Oral care. *See* Hygiene, oral
Oral cavity. *See* Mouth
Oral contraceptives, (V2) 655
nutrition and, (V1) 685
teaching about, (V1) 870
Oral-genital stimulation, (V1) 861
Oral medication administration, (V1) 634*f*, (V1) 634–636. *See also* Medication administration, oral
Oral mucosa, inspection of, (V2) 252*p*
Oral reporting, (V1) 389–392
Oral reports, giving, (V2) 163
Oral sex, adolescent, (V1) 191
Oral temperature, (V2) 186–187*p*
Orchiectomy, (V1) 857
Order(s)
questioning, (V1) 392
standing, (V1) 624
telephone
documentation of, (V1) 391–392
taking, (V2) 164
verbal
documentation of, (V1) 392
taking, (V2) 164
Orem, Dorothea, nursing theory of, (V1) 146*t*
Orem's Self-Care Model, (V1) 56*t*
Organ donation, (V1) 356–357
Organisms, pathogenic, in chain of infection, (V1) 519
Organizations, nursing, (V1) 12, (V1) 14
Orgasm, (V1) 860
disorders of, (V1) 866
Orientation
level of, determining, (V2) 285*p*
in neurological assessment, (V1) 507
promoting, for confused client, (V1) 788
Orientation phase, of therapeutic relationship, communication in, (V1) 469
Orlando, Ida Jean, nursing theory of, (V1) 146*t*
Oropharyngeal airway, (V1) 957, (V1) 957*f*, (V1) 966*p*, (V2) 759–760*p*
Oropharynx
assessment of, (V1) 496*f*, (V1) 497, (V2) 251*p*, (V2) 254*p*
suctioning of, (V2) 749–751*p*
Orotracheal tube, (V1) 958, (V1) 958*f*
suctioning of, (V1) 960, (V1) 965*p*, (V2) 745–748*p*
Orthopnea, (V1) 444, (V1) 946
Orthopneic position, (V1) 839*f*
Orthostatic (postural) hypotension, (V1) 453, (V1) 831, (V1) 993
Osmolality, (V1) 985
serum, (V1) 1000–1001
urine, (V1) 1001
Osmols, (V1) 985
Osmosis, (V1) 985–986, (V1) 985*f*, (V1) 987*t*
Osmotic laxatives, (V1) 749*b*
Osmotic pressure, (V1) 986
Ossicles, (V1) 495
Osteoarthritis, (V1) 827
Osteoblasts, (V1) 817
Osteoclasts, (V1) 817
Osteogenesis imperfecta, (V1) 827
Osteomyelitis, (V1) 828, (V1) 923
Osteoporosis, (V1) 828
chest size and, (V1) 499
in older adults, gender and, (V1) 210
screening for, for middle adult, (V1) 198
Ostomy. *See also* Colostomy; Ileostomy
Ostomy appliance, changing, (V1) 769*p*, (V2) 582–585*p*
Ostomy care, guidelines for, (V2) 593
Otic medications, (V1) 638
Otitis externa, (V1) 495
Otitis media, (V1) 495
definition of, (V1) 778*f*
Otosclerosis, definition of, (V1) 778*f*
Otoscopic examination, (V1) 495–496, (V2) 246–247*p*
Outcome, NOC definition of, (V1) 99
Outcome and Assessment Information Set (OASIS), (V1) 389
Outcomes. *See* Nursing outcomes
Outcomes evaluation, (V1) 131
Outpatient, definition of, (V1) 15
Output, in systems theory, (V1) 149
Outrage, moral, (V1) 1140–1141
Ova (eggs), (V1) 848
Ovary, (V1) 849*f*
Over-the-counter medications
for cough and cold, (V1) 952
for sleep, (V1) 895–896
Over-the-needle catheter, (V1) 1005, (V1) 1005*f*, (V2) 785–786
Overweight, (V1) 699–700. *See also* Obesity
in adolescents, (V1) 190–191
definition of, (V1) 699
interventions for, (V1) 701–703
Ovo-lacto vegetarians, (V1) 686
Ovulation, (V1) 849
Oximetry, pulse, (V1) 445
Oxygen. *See also* Oxygen therapy
altitude and, (V1) 941, (V1) 972
hyperbaric, for wound, (V1) 906, (V1) 920
inspired fraction of, (V1) 949
liquid, (V1) 956*f*
partial pressure of, (V1) 949
pathogen growth and, (V1) 520
saturation of, (V1) 949
pulse oximetry for. *See* Pulse oximetry
toxicity of, (V1) 957
transport of, (V1) 970
abnormalities of, (V1) 976
Oxygen concentrator, (V1) 956
Oxygen saturation, measurement of, (V1) 445
Oxygen therapy, (V1) 955–957, (V1) 964*p*, (V2) 731–735*p*
face masks for, (V1) 956, (V2) 733–734
face tent for, (V2) 735
fires and, (V1) 957
hazards of, (V1) 956–957
home, (V1) 956*f*, (V2) 732–733
nasal cannula for, (V1) 956, (V2) 731–732
safety precautions for, (V2) 763
T-piece for, (V2) 735

tank for, (V1) 956*f*, (V2) 731
rupture with, (V1) 957
tracheostomy collar for, (V2) 735
transtracheal, (V1) 957
Oxygenation, (V1) 934–966, (V2) 722–771. *See also* Cardiovascular system; Gas exchange; Oxygen therapy; Pulmonary system; Respiration(s)
critical thinking about, (V2) 769
definition of, (V1) 935
diagnostic testing for, (V1) 977, (V2) 766–768
focused assessment of, (V2) 765–766
full-spectrum nursing and, (V2) 768–769
inadequate, (V1) 943
knowledge map for, (V2) 771
tests of, (V1) 948

P

P wave, (V1) 978
Pacific Islanders
healers and practices of, (V1) 311*t*
values and health/illness beliefs of, (V1) 314*t*
Pacing, in verbal communication, (V1) 461–462
Paget's disease, (V1) 827
Pain, (V1) 790–815, (V2) 610–621
acupressure for, (V1) 802
acupuncture for, (V1) 802
acute, (V1) 792, (V1) 797*b*
postoperative, (V1) 1047
analgesics for, (V1) 804–809, (V1) 805*b*
acetaminophen, (V1) 805
adjuvant, (V1) 805–806
around-the-clock dosing for, (V1) 804–805
nonopioid, (V1) 805–806, (V1) 805*b*
NSAID, (V1) 805, (V1) 805*b*
opioid, (V1) 806–807
abuse of, (V1) 806
effectiveness of, (V1) 806
equianalgesia for, (V1) 807–808
misconceptions about, (V1) 806
patient-controlled, (V1) 809, (V1) 809*p*, (V2) 611–614*p*
route of administration for, (V1) 808–809
side effects of, (V1) 807, (V1) 807*b*
WHO three-step ladder and, (V1) 804, (V1) 804*f*
anesthesia for, (V1) 810
assessment of, (V1) 50, (V1) 798–800
in children, (V1) 799
in difficult-to-assess patient, (V1) 799
guidelines for, (V1) 799, (V2) 615–616
history in, (V2) 616
nonverbal signs in, (V1) 799, (V2) 615, (V2) 616–617
scales for, (V1) 800, (V2) 616, (V2) 617
verbal expressions in, (V2) 615–616
blood pressure and, (V1) 448
bodily response to, (V1) 797–798, (V1) 797*b*
breakthrough, (V1) 806
cardiovascular response to, (V1) 798
care map for, (V1) 815
cause of, (V1) 792
chemical measures for, (V1) 810
chest, (V1) 798, (V1) 976–977
in children, (V1) 796, (V1) 799
chronic, (V1) 792, (V1) 797*b*
sexuality and
cognitive-behavioral interventions for, (V1) 802–803
cognitive impairment and, (V1) 796–797
cold therapy for, (V1) 802
complementary and alternative modalities for, (V1) 801–804
contralateral stimulation for, (V1) 802
critical thinking about, (V2) 619–620
culture and, (V1) 796
cutaneous, (V1) 791
cutaneous stimulation for, (V1) 802
definition of, (V1) 791
development and, (V1) 796
diaphragmatic breathing for, (V1) 803
diary for, (V2) 618
distraction for, (V1) 803
duration of, (V1) 792
effleurage for, (V1) 802
emotional response to, (V1) 795–796
endocrine response to, (V1) 797–798
endogenous analgesia system in, (V1) 794
expressive writing for, (V1) 804
factors that influence, (V1) 795–797
fear and, (V1) 795
full-spectrum nursing model and, (V2) 619
gastrointestinal system response to, (V1) 798
gate-control theory of, (V1) 794, (V1) 795
genitourinary system response to, (V1) 798
guided imagery for, (V1) 803
as health disruption, (V1) 228
heat therapy for, (V1) 802, (V2) 708
humor for, (V1) 803
hypnosis for, (V1) 803
immobilization for, (V1) 802
incidence of, (V1) 791
intractable, (V1) 792
knowledge map for, (V2) 621
massage for, (V1) 802
medications for, bowel elimination and, (V1) 749
misconceptions about, (V1) 810, (V1) 811*t*
misjudgment of, (V2) 615
modulation of, (V1) 794, (V1) 795*f*
musculoskeletal response to, (V1) 798
nerve block for, (V1) 810
neuropathic, (V1) 792
nociceptive, (V1) 792
nonverbal cues in, (V1) 2, (V1) 799
nursing diagnosis for, (V1) 800–801
nursing interventions for, (V1) 801–812
delegation of, (V1) 801*b*, (V2) 611
documentation for, (V1) 812
evaluation of, (V1) 812–813
example of, (V1) 813, (V1) 815
nonpharmacological, (V1) 801–804
pharmacological, (V1) 804–809
nursing outcomes for, (V1) 801
in older adults, (V1) 810–811
origin of, (V1) 791–792
PENS for, (V1) 802
perception of, (V1) 794
phantom, (V1) 792
physiology of, (V1) 793–794
placebo for, (V1) 812
postoperative management of, (V1) 1047, (V1) 1052, (V1) 1052*f*
previous experience of, (V1) 795–796
psychogenic, (V1) 792
pump for, (V1) 1052*f*
quality of, (V1) 792
radiating, (V1) 791–792
radiofrequency ablation therapy for, (V1) 810
referred, (V1) 792, (V1) 792*f*
relaxation techniques for, (V1) 803
respiration and, (V1) 443, (V1) 798
responses to, cultural influences on, (V1) 319
self-care ability and, (V1) 575
in self-care ability assessment, (V1) 577
self-report of, (V1) 798
with sexual intercourse, (V1) 868
sleep and, (V1) 880, (V1) 890
sociocultural factors and, (V1) 796
somatic, (V1) 791, (V1) 797*b*
spinal cord stimulator for, (V1) 802
spiritual, components of, (V1) 338, (V1) 339*f*
subjective nature of, (V1) 791
in substance-abusing clients, (V1) 811–812
superficial, (V1) 791
surgery for, (V1) 810
teaching about, (V1) 812
TENS for, (V1) 802
therapeutic touch for, (V1) 803
threshold for, (V1) 794
tolerance to, (V1) 794
transduction of, (V1) 793
transmission of, (V1) 793–794, (V1) 793*f*
unrelieved, (V1) 797–798
visceral, (V1) 791
as vital sign, (V1) 798–799
wound, (V1) 915, (V1) 917
Pain disorder, from failure of adaptive mechanisms, (V1) 252
Pain history, (V2) 616
Pain scales, (V1) 800, (V2) 617
Pain threshold, (V1) 794
Pain tolerance, (V1) 794
PAINAD (Pain Assessment in Advanced Dementia), (V1) 799
Painkillers, prescription, deaths from, (V1) 549
Palate, hard and soft, assessment of, (V1) 497
Palliative care, (V1) 354. *See also* End-of-life care
surgery in, (V1) 1027
Pallor, (V1) 490*t*
definition of, (V1) 440
description of, (V1) 581
Palmar grasp reflex, (V1) 173, (V1) 174*f*, (V2) 294
Palpation
of abdomen, (V1) 505, (V2) 275–277*p*
of anus, (V2) 305*p*
of axillae and clavicular lymph nodes, (V2) 259*p*
of blood pressure, (V1) 453
of breasts, (V2) 258–259*p*
of chest, (V2) 262–263*p*
of ear external structures, (V2) 246*p*
of eye external structures, (V2) 244*p*
of face, (V2) 238*p*
of hair, (V2) 234*p*
of head, (V2) 237*p*
of heart, (V1) 502
of liver, (V2) 276*p*
in male genitourinary system assessment, (V2) 298–299*p*
of peripheral pulses, (V2) 270*p*

of precordium, (V2) 267–268*p*
of pulse, (V1) 437
of rectum, (V2) 305*p*
respiratory assessment, (V1) 945
of scalp, (V2) 234*p*
of skin, (V2) 227–238*p*
of spleen, (V2) 276*p*
Pandemic
definition of, (V1) 522
preparing clients for, (V1) 543, (V1) 544*b*
Pantothenic acid, (V1) 675*t*
Papanicolaou (Pap) smear, (V1) 511
in health promotion assessment, (V2) 876
in older adult assessment, (V1) 213
Paper tape, (V1) 924
Papule, (V2) 230
Paradigm, definition of, (V1) 140
Paradoxical reaction, to opioids, (V1) 807
Paralysis, (V1) 833*b*
Paralytic ileus, (V1) 831
postoperative, (V1) 750
Paraphilias, (V1) 862
Paraplegia, (V1) 833*b*
Parasites, urinary, (V2) 563
Parasomnias, (V1) 887, (V1) 890
Parasympathetic fibers, (V1) 970
Parenteral medication administration, (V1) 640–655. *See also* Medication administration, parenteral
Parenteral nutrition (PN)
administering, (V1) 712–713*p*, (V2) 508–511*p*
patients receiving, interventions for, (V2) 520*p*
providing, (V1) 711, (V1) 713
safe use of, (V1) 706*b*
solutions for, (V1) 711
Parenteral therapy, (V1) 1003–1004. *See also* Intravenous fluids, and electrolytes
Parenting
cough and cold medication self-care for, (V1) 952
impaired, culture and, (V1) 320
infant attachment in, (V1) 853, (V1) 853*f*
Paresis, (V1) 833*b*
Paresthesias, (V1) 833*b*
Parish nursing, (V1) 1121, (V1) 1121*f*
Parkinson's disease, (V1) 829, (V1) 845
Paronychia, (V2) 313*f*
Parotitis, (V1) 497
Paroxysmal nocturnal dyspnea, (V1) 946
Parse, Rosemarie Rizzo, nursing theory of, (V1) 146*t*
Partial pressure
of carbon dioxide, (V1) 949
of oxygen, (V1) 949
Partial-thickness wounds, (V1) 902
Partial thromboplastin time, (V2) 715
Passive communication style, (V1) 467–468
Passive range of motion, (V1) 844
for mobility, (V1) 844, (V2) 638
Passive relaxation, in stress management, (V1) 258
Passive transport, (V1) 985
Password, for electronic health record, (V1) 1088–1089, (V1) 1089*b*
Paste, (V1) 611*t*
Patch(es)
for drug administration, (V1) 637, (V1) 637*f*
transdermal, (V1) 611*t*
Patellar reflex, testing, (V2) 293*p*
Paternalism, beneficence and, (V1) 1151
Pathogen(s). *See also* Infection(s)
aerobic, (V1) 520
anaerobic, (V1) 520
bloodborne, exposure to, instructions following, (V1) 542–543, (V1) 543*b*
in chain of infection, (V1) 519
definition of, (V1) 551
drug-resistant, (V1) 522–523
emerging, awareness of, importance of, (V1) 522–523
foodborne, (V1) 551
transmission of, preventing, CDC guidelines for, (V1) 535, (V1) 536*p*
vectorborne, (V1) 551
fighting, (V1) 565
waterborne, (V1) 551
Pathological states, pharmacokinetics and, (V1) 617
Patient. *See* Client(s)
Patient benefit model, for discussing dilemma, (V1) 1160
Patient Care Partnership, (V1) 1153, (V1) 1154*b*, (V1) 1168–1169
Patient care plans, (V1) 88–94. *See also* Care plan(s)
Patient care summary, (V1) 387, (V1) 388*f*
Patient-controlled analgesia, (V1) 809, (V1) 809*p*, (V2) 611–614*p*
oral, (V1) 808
Patient database, assessment data in, (V1) 44
Patient education form, (V2) 88
Patient rounds approach to communication, (V1) 469
Patient Self-Determination Act (PSDA), (V1) 355, (V1) 1165–1166, (V1) 1165*b*
PatientsLikeMe, (V1) 1081
Patronizing language, as barrier to therapeutic communication, (V1) 477
Peak expiratory flow rate, (V1) 949
Peak flow meter, (V1) 949, (V1) 950*f*
home use of, (V1) 950
Pectoriloguy, whispered, (V1) 500, (V2) 264
Pediculosis, (V1) 492, (V1) 596, (V2) 313*f*
Peer relationships, in self-concept, (V1) 264–265
Pelargonium sidoides, (V1) 952
Pelvic examination, in older adult assessment, (V1) 213
Pelvic floor muscle exercises, for urinary incontinence, (V1) 736, (V2) 558–559
Pelvic inflammatory disease, (V1) 863
Pen devices, insulin, (V1) 649
Pender's Health Promotion Model, (V1) 1098, (V1) 1098*f*
Penetrating wound, (V1) 902, (V1) 902*t*
Penis, (V1) 849, (V1) 950*f*
erectile dysfunction of, (V1) 865–866
medications for
inflammation of, (V1) 865
palpation of, (V2) 298*p*
phimosis of, (V1) 865
Penrose drain, (V1) 922, (V1) 922*f*
PENS (percutaneous electrical stimulation), for pain, (V1) 802
Peplau, Hildegard E., nursing theory of, (V1) 144–145, (V1) 146*t*
Perception(s), (V1) 771–789, (V2) 599–609
client, in community assessment, (V1) 1123
definition of, (V1) 772
developmental influences on, (V1) 225
pain, (V1) 794
sensory. *See* Sensory perception
tactile, impaired, (V1) 779
Percussion
of abdomen, (V1) 505, (V2) 274–275*p*
of chest, (V2) 263*p*, (V2) 728–730*p*
of lung, (V2) 728–730*p*
performing, (V2) 308*p*
in physical examination, (V1) 485
Percutaneous electrical stimulation (PENS), for pain, (V1) 802
Percutaneous endoscopic gastrostomy (PEG) tube, (V1) 708–709, (V1) 708*f*
Perfusion
blood pressure and, (V1) 446
definition of, (V1) 436
pulse and, (V1) 436
Pericardial effusion, (V1) 984
Pericardium, (V1) 968
Perineal care, (V1) 584, (V1) 600*p*, (V2) 371–374*p*
in urinary incontinence, (V1) 736
Perineum, surgery on, bowel elimination and, (V1) 750
Periodic breathing, in neonate, (V1) 173
Periodicals, (V1) 1091
Periodontal disease, (V1) 592
Perioperative nursing, (V1) 1025, (V2) 825–858
critical thinking about, (V2) 856
definition of, (V1) 1026
full-spectrum nursing and, (V2) 855–856
intraoperative, (V1) 1039–1045. *See also* Intraoperative nursing
knowledge map for, (V2) 858
"never events" and, (V1) 1027
Perioperative Nursing Data Set for, (V1) 1030–1031, (V2) 866
postoperative, (V1) 1045–1054. *See also* Postoperative nursing
preoperative, (V1) 1027–1039. *See also* Preoperative nursing
safety for, (V1) 1026–1027, (V1) 1026*b*, (V1) 1031
Perioperative Nursing Data Set (PNDS), (V1) 74, (V1) 1030–1031, (V2) 866
Perioperative Patient-Focused Model, (V1) 1031
Peripheral arterial insufficiency, (V1) 980
Peripheral artery disease, (V1) 980
Peripheral chemoreceptors, in regulation of respiration, (V1) 442
Peripheral intravenous lock, (V1) 1006, (V1) 1006*f*, (V1) 1017–1018*p*, (V2) 786*p*
Peripheral nerve catheter pain management therapy, (V1) 809
Peripheral nerve(s), in pain transmission, (V1) 795*f*, (VI) 793–794
Peripheral neuropathy, blood glucose levels and, (V1) 694
Peripheral pulses
assessment of, (V2) 191–194*p*, (V2) 270*p*
brachial, (V2) 192*p*
carotid, (V2) 192*p*
delegation of, (V2) 191
documentation of, (V2) 194*p*
dorsalis pedis, (V2) 192*p*
femoral, (V2) 193*p*
in home care, (V2) 194*p*
patient teaching on, (V2) 194*p*

popliteal, (V2) 193*p*
posterior tibial, (V2) 193*p*
radial, (V2) 191*p*
temporal, (V2) 194*p*
sites for, (V1) 438, (V1) 439*f*
Peripheral resistance, in blood pressure regulation, (V1) 447
Peripheral vascular access devices, (V1) 1005, (V1) 1005*f*
Peripheral vascular system, disorders of, (V1) 975
Peripheral vision, (V1) 495
testing of, (V2) 240*p*
Peripherally inserted central catheter (PICC)
care for, (V2) 813–814
fluids/electrolyte administration by, (V1) 1007, (V1) 1007*f*
dressing changes for, (V2) 798–799*p*
evidence-based study on, (V1) 1022
infiltration and extravasation and, (V2) 814
Peristalsis
in colon, (V1) 747
in esophagus, (V1) 745
nutrition and, (V1) 689
Peroxide, for wound irrigation, (V2) 677
PERRLA, (V1) 494
Perseverance, intellectual, (V1) 32
Persistent vegetative state (PVS), (V1) 352
Personal appearance, in nonverbal communication, (V1) 463–464
Personal distance, communication and, (V1) 466
Personal factors
affecting bowel elimination, (V1) 748–749
in urinary function, (V1) 718–719
Personal identity
disturbed, (V1) 274
in self-concept, (V1) 266
Personal preferences, hygiene and, (V1) 575
Personal presence, (V1) 150
Personal protective equipment (PPE), (V1) 535
donning, (V1) 538*p*, (V1) 539*p*, (V2) 320–322*p*
removing, (V1) 538*p*, (V2) 322–324*p*
Personal relationships, in health-illness, (V1) 226, (V1) 226*f*
Personal space, communication and, (V1) 465–466, (V1) 466*f*
Personality
age-related changes in, assessment for, (V1) 209*t*
sensory function and, (V1) 775
Personhood, honoring, (V1) 149
Perspiration, (V1) 987
PES format, (V1) 77
Pessary
definition of, (V1) 725*b*
for urinary incontinence, (V1) 737
Pet therapy, for sensory deprivation, (V1) 784
Petechiae, (V1) 490*t*, (V2) 313*f*
pH, (V1) 989
blood, (V2) 817
buffer effects on, (V1) 989, (V1) 991
of local environment, drug absorption and, (V1) 614
pathogen growth and, (V1) 520
renal effects on, (V1) 992
respiratory effects on, (V1) 991–992
scale for, (V1) 996*f*
urinary, (V2) 562, (V2) 817
Phagocytes, in fever, (V1) 426
Phagocytosis
in defense against infection, (V1) 524, (V1) 525*t*
in humoral immunity, (V1) 525, (V1) 527*f*
Phantom pain, (V1) 792
Pharmacist
for drug information, (V1) 606
on healthcare team, (V1) 20
Pharmacodynamics, (V1) 618–622
definition of, (V1) 618
drug abuse or misuse and, (V1) 621–622
medication interactions in, (V1) 621
primary therapeutic effects in, (V1) 618–619
chemotherapeutic, (V1) 619
palliative, (V1) 618
restorative, (V1) 619
substitutive, (V1) 618–619
supportive, (V1) 618
secondary therapeutic effects in, (V1) 619–621
adverse reactions as, (V1) 619, (V1) 619*b*
allergic reactions as, (V1) 620
cumulative effect as, (V1) 621
idiosyncratic reactions as, (V1) 620–621
side effects as, (V1) 619
toxic reactions as, (V1) 620
Pharmacokinetics, (V1) 609–618
absorption in, (V1) 609–614. *See also* Medication(s), absorption of
definition of, (V1) 609, (V1) 609*f*
distribution in, (V1) 614–615
excretion in, (V1) 615–616
factors affecting, (V1) 617–618
metabolism in, (V1) 615
Pharmacology texts, for drug information, (V1) 606
Pharmacopoeia, (V1) 606
Pharyngeal airways, (V1) 957, (V1) 957*f*
Pharynx, (V1) 745, (V1) 935
suctioning of, (V2) 749–751*p*
Phenomena, in nursing theory, (V1) 139–140
Phenytoin (Dilantin), gingival hyperplasia from, (V1) 591
Philosophy, culture and, (V1) 309
Phlebitis, intravenous therapy and, (V1) 1013–1014*t*
Phonation, (V1) 497
Phosphate, (V1) 989, (V1) 991*t*
Phosphate buffer system, (V1) 991
Phosphorus, (V1) 677*t*
Photoreceptors, (V1) 772
Physiatrist, on healthcare team, (V1) 19
Physical activity. *See also* Exercise(s)
assessment of, (V1) 832–834, (V2) 641–642
baseline, (V1) 821
critical thinking about, (V2) 648–649
definition of, (V1) 817, (V1) 821
factors affecting, (V1) 826–830
full-spectrum nursing and, (V2) 648
guidelines for, (V1) 822*b*
health-enhancing, (V1) 821
in health-illness, (V1) 225
knowledge map for, (V2) 650
nursing diagnosis for, (V1) 834
tolerance for, (V1) 833, (V2) 642
Physical assessment. *See also* Physical examination
definition of, (V1) 481
Physical disease, as health disruption, (V1) 227
Physical examination, (V1) 481–487, (V2) 219–316
abdomen in, (V1) 504–505, (V1) 504*f*, (V1) 505*f*, (V1) 514*p*
of adolescents, (V1) 487
appearance in, (V1) 488
auscultation in, (V1) 485–486
axillae in, (V1) 498, (V1) 498*f*, (V1) 513*p*
bedside, brief, (V1) 515*p*
behavior in, (V1) 488
body type in, (V1) 488
breasts in, (V1) 498, (V1) 498*f*, (V1) 513*p*
cardiovascular system in, (V1) 501–504, (V1) 514*p*, (V1) 976–977, (V2) 776
chest in, (V1) 499–501, (V1) 499*f*, (V1) 500*f*, (V1) 513*p*
client positioning for, (V1) 483–485*t*
comprehensive, (V1) 481
in comprehensive assessment, (V1) 47–48, (V1) 48*f*
cultural adaptation for, (V1) 482*b*
definition of, (V1) 481
developmental stage and, (V1) 486–487
documentation of findings of, (V1) 511–512
dress in, (V1) 488
equipment needed for, (V2) 221–222
in fluid and electrolyte assessment, (V1) 999–1000
focused, (V1) 481
general survey in, (V1) 487–489, (V1) 512*p*, (V2) 221–226*p*
genitourinary system in, (V1) 509–511, (V1) 510*f*, (V1) 514*p*
grooming in, (V1) 488
hair in, (V1) 491–492, (V1) 512*p*
head in, (V1) 493–497, (V1) 513*p*
in health promotion assessment, (V1) 1102
guidelines and tools for, (V2) 872–873*t*
height in, (V1) 488–489, (V1) 489*f*
hygiene in, (V1) 488
of infants, (V1) 486, (V2) 223
in infection prevention, (V1) 529
inspection in, (V1) 485
integumentary system in, (V1) 489–493
knowledge map for, (V2) 316
lungs in, (V1) 499–501, (V1) 501*f*, (V1) 513*p*
mental state in, (V1) 488
of middle adults, (V1) 487
in mobility assessment, (V1) 832–833
musculoskeletal system in, (V1) 505–506, (V1) 514*p*
nails in, (V1) 492–493, (V1) 512–513*p*
neck in, (V1) 497–498, (V1) 513*p*
neurological system in, (V1) 506–509, (V1) 514*p*
of older adults, (V1) 487, (V2) 223
olfaction in, (V1) 486
percussion in, (V1) 485
posture in, (V1) 488
preparing for, (V1) 481–483
of preschoolers, (V1) 486, (V2) 223
purposes of, (V1) 481
in respiratory function assessment, (V1) 945
of school-age children, (V1) 486–487, (V2) 223
in sexual health assessment, (V1) 866–867
skin in, (V1) 489–491, (V1) 512*p*
speech in, (V1) 488

system-specific, (V1) 481
techniques for, (V1) 485–486
of toddlers, (V1) 486, (V2) 223
types of, (V1) 481
vital signs in, (V1) 488
weight in, (V1) 488–489
wound, (V2) 710
of young adults, (V1)487
Physical fitness assessment, in health promotion assessment, (V1) 1102
Physical functioning, in self-care ability assessment, (V1) 577
Physical therapist, on healthcare team, (V1) 19
Physician, on healthcare team, (V1) 19
Physician's assistants (PAs), on healthcare team, (V1) 19
Physician's Desk Reference (PDR), (V1) 606
Physiological barriers, to therapeutic communication, (V1) 472
Physiological effects, of depression, (V1) 280
Physiological needs, (V1) 54, (V1) 147, (V1) 147*f*
of dying patient, meeting, (V1) 364, (V2) 148–149
Physiological responses, to stress, assessing, (V1) 255
Physiological stressors, (V1) 240
Physiological theories, of depression, (V1) 270
Physiotherapy, chest, (V1) 955, (V1) 955*f*, (V1) 963–964*p*, (V2) 728–730*p*
Piaget, Jean, cognitive development theory of, (V1) 165, (V1) 167, (V1) 168*t*
PICOT questions
acupuncture for neuropathic pain, (V1) 880
formulating, (V1) 156, (V1) 156*b*
metabolic acidosis, (V1) 999
pressure ulcers and malnourished older adult, (V1) 900
risk for surgical infection in older adults, (V1) 1030
Piercings
adolescents and, (V1) 189
body, (V1) 901
Piggyback setup for IV medication administration, (V1) 654, (V1) 654*f*
intermittent infusion using, (V2) 465–467*p*
Pill, (V1) 610*t*
Pillows, (V1) 836
hip abduction, (V1) 837, (V2) 637
in pressure ulcer prevention, (V1) 926*t*
Piloerection, in increasing temperature, (V1) 423
Pinworms, assessing for, (V1) 755
Placebo, pain relief with, (V1) 812
Plaintiff, (V1) 1174
Plan of care, in problem-oriented record system, (V1) 374
Planning
definition of, (V1) 85
discharge, (V1) 86–88. *See also* Discharge planning
formal, (V1) 85
if outcomes, (V1) 84–104, (V2) 33–39. *See also* Nursing outcomes, planning of
informal, (V1) 85
initial, (V1) 85–86
of interventions, (V1) 105–118, (V2) 40–44. *See also* Nursing interventions, planning of
knowledge map for, (V2) 39
in nursing process, (V1) 38, (V1) 38*f*
nursing process steps related to, (V1) 85
ongoing, (V1) 86
Plantar warts, (V1) 587
Plaque, dental caries and, (V1) 591–592
Plasma derivatives, (V1) 1020
Plasma transfusion, (V1) 1020
Plateau phase, in sexual response cycle, (V1) 859–860
Platelet-derived growth factor, (V1) 906
Platelet transfusion, (V1) 1020. *See also* Blood transfusion
Play, infant, interventions for, (V1) 179
Pleading, in litigation, (V1) 1176
PLISSIT (permission, limited information, specific suggestions, intensive therapy) model, for sexual counseling, (V1) 870–871
Pneumatic compression devices, (V1) 980
Pneumonia, (V1) 944
healthcare-associated, (V1) 953
postoperative, (V1) 1048*t*
prevention of, (V1) 952–953
ventilator-associated, (V1) 961
rate of, improving, (V1) 531*b*
Pneumothorax, (V1) 961
Point of maximal impulse (PMI), (V1) 502
Point of service (POS), (V1) 24
Poisoning
food, (V1) 551
home hazards for, (V1) 548–549, (V1) 549*b*
interventions for, (V1) 560, (V1) 561*b*
of preschooler, (V1) 183
Politics, culture and, (V1) 310
Pollution
air, (V1) 940–941
noise
reducing, (V1) 568
as safety hazard, (V1) 552
reducing, (V1) 565, (V1) 567
as safety hazard, (V1) 551–552
Polydipsia, blood glucose levels and, (V1) 694
Polygamy, (V1) 855
Polyphagia, blood glucose levels and, (V1) 694
Polypharmacy, injury risk from, (V1) 629
Polysomnography, (V1) 891
Polyuria, definition of, (V1) 725*b*
Popliteal pulse, assessment of, (V2) 193*p*
Population(s)
age groups as percentage of, (V1) 203, (V1) 203*f*
definition of, (V1) 1114–1115
diversity of, 303*b*, (V1) 302
multicultural, ethical issues for nurses and, (V1) 1142
special, learning by, (V1) 402–403
vulnerable
characteristics of, (V1) 1116
as subcultures, (V1) 306–307, (V1) 306*f*
Port, implantable, for fluid and electrolyte administration, (V1) 1007, (V1) 1008*f*
Port-wine stain, (V2) 312*f*
Portal of entry, in chain of infection, (V1) 519*f*, (V1) 521
Portal of exit, in chain of infection, (V1) 519*f*, (V1) 520–521
Position/positioning, (V1) 835–836
bed for
client moving in/from, (V1) 840–841, (V1) 843
to chair, (V1) 841, (V1) 842*p*, (V1) 843, (V2) 628, (V2) 630–631*p*
dangling legs at bedside, (V1) 842*p*, (V2) 628*p*, (V2) 629–630*p*, (V2) 638
delegation of, (V2) 623, (V2) 628
exercise for, (V1) 1054*p*
friction-reducing devices for, (V1) 840–841
knowledge map for, (V2) 650
logrolling, (V1) 840, (V1) 842*p*, (V2) 626–627*p*
mechanical lift for, (V1) 841, (V1) 841*f*, (V1) 843*f*
moving up, (V1) 840, (V1) 842*p*, (V2) 624–625*p*
for pressure ulcer prevention, (V1) 919
rule of 30 for, (V1) 919
to stretcher, (V1) 842*p*, (V2) 628–629*p*
transfer board for, (V1) 841
turning in, (V1) 840, (V1) 842*p*, (V2) 625–626*p*
teaching client to move in, (V1) 1054*p*, (V2) 826–827*p*, (V2) 827–828*p*, (V2) 829*p*
transferring patients out of, (V1) 841–843, (V1) 842*p*
belt for, (V1) 843, (V1) 843*f*
board for, (V1) 841, (V1) 841*f*
change in, pulse and, (V1) 437
devices for, (V1) 836–837, (V2) 636–637
dorsal recumbent, (V1) 484*t*
foot cradles for, (V1) 837, (V2) 637
footboard for, (V1) 837, (V1) 837*f*
Fowler's, (V1) 837, (V1) 838*b*
hand rolls for, (V1) 837, (V2) 637
hand/wrist splints for, (V1) 837
high-top sneakers for, (V1) 837
hip abduction pillows for, (V1) 837, (V2) 637
intraoperative, (V1) 1044, (V2) 850
for intravenous infusion, (V1) 1010
knee-chest, (V1) 485*t*
lateral, (V1) 837, (V1) 837*t*
lateral recumbent, (V1) 485*t*, (V1) 837, (V1) 839
lithotomy, (V1) 484*t*
for maximum ventilation, (V1) 953
mechanical lift for, (V1) 841, (V1) 841*f*, (V1) 843*f*
for normal defecation, assisting with, (V1) 757
for normal urination, assisting with, (V1) 727
oblique, (V1) 839, (V1) 839*f*
orthopneic, (V1) 839*f*
for physical examination, (V1) 483–485*t*
pillows for, (V1) 836, (V1) 837
pressure-ulcer prevention and, (V1) 919
prone, (V1) 484*t*, (V1) 838*b*, (V1) 839–840
respiration and, (V1) 443
for respiration assessment, (V1) 946
Rule of 30 and, (V1) 919
sandbags for, (V1) 837
scoot sheet in, (V1) 840, (V1) 841*f*
semi-Fowler's, (V1) 837
Sims', (V1) 484*t*, (V1) 839*b*, (V1) 840
sitting, (V1) 483*t*

standing, (V1) 483*t*
standing assist device for, (V1) 843, (V1) 843*f*
supine, (V1) 483*t*, (V1) 839*b*, (V1) 840
surgical, (V1) 1044
risk for injury with, (V1) 1043
techniques for, (V1) 837, (V1) 838–839*t*, (V1) 839–840
bed-bound patient, (V1) 838*b*
trapeze bar for, (V1) 836–837
trochanter rolls for, (V1) 837, (V2) 636
of unconscious client, (V1) 1046
for ventilation, (V1) 946
Positive end-expiratory pressure (PEEP), (V2) 752
Positive inotropes, (V1) 974*t*, (V1) 981
Positive pressure ventilation, (V1) 960, (V1) 960*f*
Positive self-talk, in stress management, (V1) 260
Possible nursing diagnosis
goals for, (V1) 98, (V1) 99*t*
intervention type related to, (V1) 110*t*
Post-traumatic stress disorder (PTSD), from failure of adaptive mechanisms, (V1) 253
Postanesthesia care unit, (V1) 1045, (V1) 1045*f*, (V1) 1046
Postanesthesia phase, (V1) 1045
Posterior tibial pulse, assessment of, (V2) 193*p*
Postmortem care, providing, (V1) 366–367, (V2) 150–151
Postoperative nursing, (V1) 1045–1054
anesthesia assessment in, (V2) 845
anesthesia recovery in, (V1) 1045–1046, (V1) 1046*b*
antiembolism stockings in, (V1) 1052–1053, (V1) 1054*p*, (V2) 829–832*p*
assessment in, (V1) 1046
collaborative problems in, (V1) 1048–1051*t*
gastrointestinal suction in, (V1) 1053–1054, (V1) 1054–1055*p*
incentive spirometry in, (V1) 1052
nursing diagnosis for, (V1) 1046–1047
nursing interventions for, (V1) 1047, (V1) 1052–1054
nursing outcomes for, (V1) 1047
pain management in, (V1) 1047, (V1) 1052
recovery room, (V1) 1039, (V2) 840
report for, (V1) 1045*b*
sequential compression devices in. *See* Sequential compression devices
surgical unit for, (V1) 1046
teaching in, (V1) 1052
Postoperative transsexuals, (V1) 852
Postural drainage, (V1) 955, (V1) 963–964*p*, (V2) 728–730*p*
Postural hypotension, (V1) 453
Posture, (V1) 819
assessment of, (V2) 277–278*p*
in nonverbal communication, (V1) 463
in physical examination, (V1) 488
self-care for, (V1) 819
Postvoid residual urine (PVR), (V1) 729
measuring, (V1) 733*p*
Potassium, (V1) 677*t*, (V1) 988, (V1) 990*t*
imbalances in, (V1) 994*t*
normal, (V2) 817
supplemental, (V1) 1002
Potassium-sparing diuretics, (V1) 719*b*
Potential nursing diagnosis, (V1) 66*t*
intervention type related to, (V1) 110*t*
Poverty, as family health risk, (V1) 292–293
Powder, (V1) 610*t*
prescribed, application of, (V2) 430
Power, (V1) 1065–1066. *See also* Leadership; Management
expertise and, (V1) 1066
sources of, (V1) 1066–1067
Powerlessness
culture and, (V1) 320
in depression, (V1) 281
PPE. *See* Personal protective equipment (PPE)
Practical knowledge, (V1) 37
in full-spectrum nursing, (V1) 40*t*, (V1) 41
Practical nursing education, (V1) 10
Pratt's sign, (V1) 977
Prayer
intercessory, (V1) 342*b*
for spirituality diagnoses, (V1) 341–342, (V1) 342*b*, (V1) 342*f*
Praying, with patients, (V2) 137–138
Pre-interaction phase, of therapeutic relationship, communication in, (V1) 469
Prealbumin, (V2) 715
serum levels of, nutritional levels and, (V1) 695
Precautions, latex, (V1) 2
Preceptor, (V1) 1062–1063
Precordium, (V1) 502. *See* Heart
Preexisting conditions, surgery and, (V1) 1028, (V1) 1029*t*
Preferred provider organizations (PPOs), (V1) 24
Pregnancy
adolescent, (V1) 191, (V1) 1097
preventing, interventions for, (V1) 193
bowel elimination and, (V1) 750
cardiovascular system in, (V1) 972
constipation in, (V1) 750*b*
exercise guidelines for, (V1) 822*b*
health promotion during, (V1) 1100*t*
maternal changes during, (V1) 170–171
nutrition in, (V1) 684
pharmacokinetics and, (V1) 617
pulmonary system in, (V1) 941
teen, (V1) 191, (V1) 1097
urinary tract infections in, (V1) 720
Prehypertension, (V1) 454
Prejudices, as barrier to culturally competent care, (V1) 317
Premature ejaculation, (V1) 866
Premature infant. *See also* Infant(s)
pulmonary system of, (V1) 939
Premenstrual dysphoric disorder, (V1) 864
Premenstrual syndrome, (V1) 863–864
teaching about, (V1) 869
Preoperational stage, of cognitive development, (V1) 168*t*
Preoperative nursing, (V1) 1031–1039
antiembolism stockings in, (V1) 1037–1038, (V1) 1037*f*, (V1) 1054*p*, (V2) 829–832*p*
assessment in, (V1) 1031–1032, (V2) 841
for discharge to home, (V1) 1031
bowel preparation in, (V1) 1036
checklist in, (V1) 1042, (V2) 842–843
client transfer in, (V1) 1038–1039
consent form in, (V1) 1034–1035
coordination in, (V1) 1034
diagnostic testing in, (V2) 845
identity check in, (V1) 1038
medication administration in, (V1) 1036–1037, (V1) 1037*t*
normothermia maintenance in, (V1) 1036
nurse-surgical team communication in, (V1) 1038
nursing diagnosis for, (V1) 1032–1033
nursing history for, (V1) 1031
nursing interventions for, (V1) 1034–1039
nursing outcomes for, (V1) 1034
nutritional status monitoring in, (V1) 1036
for older adults, (V1) 1032, (V1) 1033, (V1) 1033*t*
patient preparation in, (V1) 1034, (V1) 1036–1038
Perioperative Nursing Data Set for, (V1) 1030–1031, (V2) 866
physical assessment in, (V1) 1032
postoperative room preparation in, (V1) 1039, (V2) 840
prosthesis removal in, (V1) 1037
screening tests in, (V1) 1032
site marking in, (V1) 1038
skin preparation in, (V1) 1036
teaching in, (V1) 1034, (V1) 1035–1036, (V2) 839
urinary elimination in, (V1) 1036
Preoperative transsexuals, (V1) 852
Presbycusis, definition of, (V1) 778*f*
Presbyopia, (V1) 494
definition of, (V1) 777*b*
Preschooler(s)
abuse, neglect and violence involving, (V1) 183–184
assessment of, (V1) 184
car safety seats for, (V1) 566*t*
cardiovascular system in, (V1) 971
communicable diseases in, (V1) 183
communication by, (V1) 465
development of
cognitive, (V1) 168*t*, (V1) 182
physical, (V1) 182, (V1) 182*b*
psychosexual, (V1) 167*t*
psychosocial, (V1) 168, (V1) 183, (V1) 183*f*
sensorimotor, (V1) 182
developmental tasks of, (V1) 166*t*
enuresis in, (V1) 183
growth of, (V1) 182
health problems of, (V1) 183–184
health promotion for, (V1) 1101*f*
interventions for, (V1) 184
nutrition for, (V1) 683
physical examination of, (V1) 486
poisoning in, (V1) 183
pulmonary system of, (V1) 939
safety needs of, (V1) 547
sleep for, (V1) 881, (V1) 881*t*, (V1) 885
surgery and, (V1) 1028
Prescription, electronic, (V1) 1084
Prescription painkillers, deaths from, (V1) 549
Prescription(s), (V1) 623–625
abbreviations used in, (V1) 623–624
automatic stop dates for, (V1) 624
communication of, (V1) 624
elements of, (V1) 623
example of, (V1) 623*f*
incorrect, handling, (V1) 624–625
prn, (V1) 624
single, (V1) 624

STAT, (V1) 624
telephone, (V1) 624
types of, (V1) 624
verbal, (V1) 624
verification of, (V1) 623
written, (V1) 624
standard, (V1) 624
Presence, for spirituality diagnoses, (V1) 340
Pressure
atmospheric, (V1) 941
filtration, (V1) 986
hydrostatic, (V1) 986
osmotic, (V1) 986
Pressure-redistributing devices, in pressure ulcer prevention, (V1) 919
Pressure support ventilation, (V2) 752
Pressure ulcer(s), (V1) 581, (V1) 903*t*
assessment of, (V1) 912–813, (V1) 916–918
at admission, (V1) 913
Braden scale in, (V1) 913, (V2) 711
healing chart for, (V2) 714
history in, (V1) 912–913, (V2) 709
laboratory data in, (V2) 715
Norton scale in, (V1) 913, (V2) 712
physical examination in, (V1) 913–916, (V2) 710
PUSH tool in, (V2) 713
scales for, (V1) 913, (V1) 917–918, (V2) 711, (V2) 712
care competencies for, (V1) 920–925, (V1) 928–929, (V1) 931–933
contributing factors of, (V1) 908*f*
development of, (V1) 908, (V1) 908*f*
on feet, (V1) 587
friction and, (V1) 908, (V1) 908*f*
knowledge map for, (V2) 721
malnourished older adult with, (V1) 900
moisture and, (V1) 908, (V1) 908*f*
nursing diagnosis for, (V1) 917
nursing interventions for, (V1) 917–919
nursing outcomes for, (V1) 917
patient teaching for, (V1) 920
pressure points and, (V1) 909*f*
preventive measures for, (V1) 917–919
shearing and, (V1) 908, (V1) 908*f*
skin inspection for, (V1) 918
staging of, (V1) 909, (V1) 910–912*t*
surgery and, (V1) 1044
teaching about, (V1) 920
unstageable (eschar), (V1) 915, (V1) 915*t*
Pretrial motions, in litigation, (V1) 1176
Prevention
aspiration, (V1) 954, (V2) 762
back injury, (V1) 825, (V1) 836
clot, (V1) 980
electrolyte imbalance, (V1) 1002–1003
embolus, (V1) 980
immobility complications, (V1) 832*b*
pneumonia, (V1) 952–953
pressure ulcer, (V1) 917–919
pulmonary system infection, (V1) 952–953
sexually transmitted infections, (V1) 870
thrombus, (V1) 980
Primary data, (V1) 46, (V1) 47*t*
Primary intention healing, (V1) 903, (V1) 904*f*
Primary nursing, (V1) 15
Printed materials, in patient teaching, (V1) 414, (V1) 418*t*
Prioritizing problems, in diagnostic reasoning, (V1) 69–71
Privacy
autonomy and, (V1) 1150
for electronic health record, (V1) 1088
invasion of, (V1) 1173
lack of, urinary function and, (V1) 718
maintaining, in minimizing malpractice risks, (V1) 1181
providing
for normal defecation, (V1) 757
for normal urination, (V1) 727
violation of, (V1) 1165
Prizing, in values clarification, (V1) 1156*t*
prn medications, (V1) 608
Problem-Intervention-Evaluation (PIE) system for documentation, (V1) 379
Problem list, in problem-oriented record system, (V1) 374
Problem-oriented record systems, (V1) 374
Problem-solving, (V1) 5, (V1) 33*b*
Problems. *See* Collaborative problems; Health problem(s)
Procedural justice, (V1) 1152
Process, communication as, (V1) 460–461, (V1) 460*f*
Process evaluation, (V1) 131
Process recordings, in enhancing therapeutic communication, (V1) 475
Procurement surgery, (V1) 1028
Prodromal stage of infection, (V1) 522
Profession, nursing as, (V1) 8, (V1) 9*t*
Professional, nurse as, (V1) 5
Professional boundaries, in minimizing malpractice risks, (V1) 1182, (V1) 1182*b*
Professional communication, collaborative, (V1) 467–469, (V1) 467*b*
Professional liability insurance, (V1) 1184
Professional standards. *See* Standards of practice
Professional values, (V1) 1145
Progress notes
formats for, (V1) 378–382
in problem-oriented record system, (V1) 374
Progressive relaxation, in stress management, (V1) 258
Progressive (sequential) relaxation
for pain, (V1) 803
for sleep, (V1) 894
Projection, as defense mechanism, (V1) 250*t*
Prone position, (V1) 838*b*, (V1) 839–840
Propositions, in nursing theory, (V1) 140
Proprietary home health organizations, (V1) 1127
Proprioceptors, (V1) 772
Propulsive gait, (V1) 833, (V2) 315*f*
Prospective reimbursement system, (V1) 23
Prostaglandins, in fever, (V1) 426
Prostate gland
assessment of, (V1) 511
cancer of, screening for, in health promotion assessment, (V1) 1104, (V2) 876
exam of, for middle adult, (V1) 198
hypertrophy of
urinary function and, (V1) 720
urinary retention from, (V1) 721
urinary tract infections and, (V1) 720
removal of, sexuality and, (V1) 857
Prostatectomy, (V1) 857
Prostatic specific antigen (PSA), serum level of, in older adult assessment, (V1) 213
Prostheses, preoperative removal of, (V1) 1037
Prosthetic eyes, caring for, (V1) 598, (V1) 599*f*, (V1) 601*p*, (V2) 397–398*p*
Protective isolation, (V1) 536–537. *See also* Isolation
Protein(s), (V1) 669*t*, (V1) 670–671
complete, (V1) 670
functions of, (V1) 671
incomplete, (V1) 670
for infants, (V1) 682
metabolism of, (V1) 670–671
serum markers of, (V1) 695
in ovo-lacto vegetarian diet, (V1) 686
plasma, (V1) 1020
drugs binding to, (V1) 615
serum levels of, nutritional levels and, (V1) 695
skin effects of, (V1) 899
storage of, (V1) 670–671
urinary, (V2) 562
Protein system, (V1) 991
Proteinuria, definition of, (V1) 725*b*
Pruritus, (V1) 581
opioid-related, (V) 807*b*
Pseudo-narcolepsy, (V1) 889
Psoriasis, (V2) 233
Psychoanalytic theory, of development, (V1) 165, (V1) 167*t*
Psychodynamic theories, of depression, (V1) 270
Psychogenic pain, (V1) 792
Psychological dependence, on opioids, (V1) 806
Psychological factors/functioning
immobility effects on, (V1) 831
pain and, (V1) 797*b*
pharmacokinetics and, (V1) 617–618
Psychological needs
of dying patient, meeting, (V1) 364–365, (V2) 149–150
of patient in isolation, supporting, (V1) 538
Psychological responses, to stress, (V1) 248–249, (V1) 248*b*, (V1) 250–251*t*
Psychological safety, (V1) 1071*b*, (V1) 1070
Psychomotor learning, (V1) 399–400, (V1) 399*t*
Psychosexual development, of infant, (V1) 167*t*
Psychosis
anxiety contributing to, (V1) 269
sexuality and, (V1) 857
Psychosocial assessment, (V1) 50
Psychosocial development
of adolescent, (V1) 168, (V1) 189, (V1) 189*f*
of infant, (V1) 168, (V1) 177
of middle adult, (V1) 169, (V1) 197, (V1) 197*f*
of neonate, (V1) 174–175
of older adults, (V1) 207, (V1) 209
of preschooler, (V1) 168, (V1) 183, (V1) 183*f*
of school-age child, (V1) 168, (V1) 185, (V1) 185*f*
of toddler, (V1) 168, (V1) 180–181
of young adult, (V1) 168–169, (V1) 195
Psychosocial development theory, (V1) 209
Psychosocial health
assessment of, (V1) 270–271
definition of, (V1) 263, (V1) 263*f*
and illness, (V1) 262–285, (V2) 102–117
knowledge map for, (V2) 117
nursing care promoting, (V1) 270–285

Psychosocial illness, (V1) 267–270
anxiety as, 268*t*, (V1) 267–269. *See also* Anxiety
depression as, (V1) 269–270. *See also* Depression
interventions/implementation for, (V1) 273
knowledge map for, (V2) 117
nursing diagnosis of, (V1) 271
implications of, (V1) 272*t*
nursing outcomes for, (V1) 271–273
sexuality and, (V1) 857
Psychosocial stressors, (V1) 240
Psychosocial theory, (V1) 263–264
PsycINFO 1887, (V1) 1092*t*
Pterygium, (V1) 493, (V2) 313*f*
Ptosis, (V1) 493
Puberty, (V1) 853
onset of, (V1) 189
skin at, (V1) 899
Public distance, communication and, (V1) 466
Public financing, as payor for healthcare, (V1) 21
Public health centers, (V1) 17
Public health clinic nursing, (V1) 1121–1122
Public health goals, (V1) 100–102
Public health nursing, (V1) 1117, (V1) 1117*f*
Public home health agencies, (V1) 1126
Public records, in community assessment, (V1) 1123
Public relations, (V1) 1061
Public speaking, (V1) 459–460
Puerto Rican heritage. *See also* Hispanic Americans
pain perception and responses in, (V2) 127
Pulmonary circulation, (V1) 501
Pulmonary embolism, (V1) 980
Pulmonary function studies, (V2) 767
Pulmonary hypertension, (V1) 944
Pulmonary system, (V1) 935–936. *See also* Airway; Lung(s); Respiration(s)
abnormalities of, (V1) 944
in adolescents, (V1) 939–940
in adults, (V1) 940
air pollution effects on, (V1) 940–941
allergy effects on, (V1) 940
altitude effects on, (V1) 941
alveolar-capillary membrane abnormalities of, (V1) 944
assessment of, (V1) 945–949
arterial blood gases in, (V1) 949
breathing patterns in, (V1) 945–946
capnography in, (V1) 948
cough in, (V1) 946–947
in oxygenation assessment, (V2) 766
peak flow monitoring in, (V1) 949
physical examination in, (V1) 945–947
pulse oximetry in, (V1) 948, (V1) 948*f*, (V1) 963*p*, (V2) 726–728, (V2) 762
respiratory effort in, (V1) 946
risk factors in, (V1) 945
skin testing in, (V1) 947–948
spirometry in, (V1) 948
sputum in, (V1) 947, (V1) 947*b*, (V2) 767
atelectasis of, (V1) 939, (V1) 944
central nervous system abnormality effects on, (V1) 944
cigarette smoking effects on, (V1) 942
circulation abnormalities of, (V1) 944
developmental stage and, (V1) 939–940
disease effects on, (V1) 943–944
embolus of, (V1) 944
environmental effects on, (V1) 940–941
exercise effects on, (V1) 941
functions of, (V1) 936–938
promotion of, (V1) 979–980
tests of, (V2) 767
hypertension of, (V1) 944
in infant, (V1) 939
infection of, (V1) 943–944
prevention of, (V1) 952–953
lifestyle effects on, (V1) 941–942
medication effects on, (V1) 942–943
in middle-aged adults, (V1) 940
neuromuscular abnormality effects on, (V1) 944
nursing diagnosis for, (V1) 949–951
nursing interventions for, (V1) 951–963
airway suctioning in, (V1) 959–960, (V1) 965*p*, (V2) 749–751
artificial airways in, (V1) 957–958
chest tubes in, (V1) 961–963, (V2) 755–759, (V2) 764–765
mechanical ventilation in, (V1) 965*p*
oxygen therapy in, (V1) 955–957
respiratory function in, (V1) 951–954
secretions mobilization in, (V1) 954–955
nursing outcomes for, (V1) 951
nutrition effects on, (V1) 941
obesity effects on, (V1) 941
obstructive abnormalities of, (V1) 944
occupational hazard effects on, (V1) 941
in older adults, (V1) 940
pregnancy effects on, (V1) 941
in preschool children, (V1) 939
in school-age children, (V1) 939
stress effect on, (V1) 940
structural abnormalities of, (V1) 944
substance abuse effects on, (V1) 941–942
in toddlers, (V1) 939
in young adults, (V1) 940
Pulse, (V1) 436–441, (V1) 833
apical, (V1) 438
assessment of, (V2) 195–196*p*
when to take, (V1) 438–439, (V1) 439*f*
apical-radial
deficit in, assessing for, (V2) 197–198
when to take, (V1) 439
assessment of, (V1) 437–440
data collected during, (V1) 439–440
equipment for, (V1) 437–438, (V1) 438*f*
sites for, (V1) 438–439
bilateral equality of, (V1) 440
definition of, (V1) 436
in fluid and electrolyte assessment, (V1) 999
nursing diagnoses related to, (V1) 440
nursing interventions for, (V1) 441
peripheral
assessment of, (V2) 191–194*p*, (V2) 270*p*
sites for, (V1) 438, (V1) 439*f*
production and regulation of, (V1) 436
quality of, (V1) 440
rate of, (V1) 440
factors influencing, (V1) 436–437
normal, (V1) 422*t*, (V1) 436
rhythm of, (V1) 440
volume of, (V1) 440
Pulse oximetry, (V1) 445, (V1) 948, (V1) 948*f*, (V1) 963*p*, (V2) 726–728*p*
clinical insight on, (V2) 762
Pulse pressure, (V1) 446
Pump(s)
anesthetic, (V1) 1047, (V1) 1052
infusion
for fluids and electrolytes, (V1) 1011, (V2) 790–792
home care for, (V2) 792
insulin, (V1) 649
sequential compression. *See* Sequential compression devices
Puncture, (V1) 902*t*
Pupil(s)
accommodation of, testing of, (V2) 243*p*
inspection of, (V1) 494, (V2) 243*p*
Pupillary reaction to light, testing, (V2) 243*p*
Purnell model, for cultural competence, (V1) 315–316, (V1) 317*f*
Purosanguineous exudate, (V1) 906
Purulent exudate, (V1) 906
PUSH tool, (V1) 916, (V2) 713
Pustule, (V2) 231
Pyelogram, (V2) 564
Pyelonephritis, (V1) 720
Pyorrhea, (V1) 592
Pyrexia, (V1) 425–426. *See also* Fever
Pyridoxine, (V1) 675*t*
Pyrogens, (V1) 426
Pyuria, definition of, (V1) 725*b*

Q

QRS complex, (V1) 978
QSEN competency(ies), (V1) 7*b*
quality improvement as, (V1) 136
Quadriceps drills, for ambulation conditioning, (V1) 844, (V2) 638
Quadriplegia, (V1) 833*b*
Qualitative approach, to nursing research, (V1) 153*t*, (V1) 154
Quality and Safety Education for Nurses (QSEN)
on cultural competence, (V1) 315
infection guidelines of, (V1) 518
quality improvement competency of, (V1) 25*b*
on safety competence, (V1) 546
Quality assurance, ANA model for, (V1) 25–26
Quality assurance (QA) programs, (V1) 136
Quality improvement, documentation in, (V1) 371
Quality improvement programs, continuous, (V1) 25
Quality of care, in healthcare setting, evaluating, (V1) 135–136, (V1) 136*b*
Quantitative approach, to nursing research, (V1) 153–154, (V1) 153*t*
Quasi-intentional torts, (V1) 1172
Question, searchable, formulating, (V1) 156, (V1) 156*b*
Questions, excessive, as barrier to therapeutic communication, (V1) 475
Question(s), "no" response to, (V1) 1075

R

Race(s), (V1) 304–305
blood pressure and, (V1) 448
definition of, (V1) 304
disparities in life expectancy and, (V1) 202
health disparities among, (V1) 302

Racism, as barrier to culturally competent care, (V1) 317
Radial pulse, assessment of, (V2) 191*p*
Radiating pain, (V1) 791–792
Radiation, in heat exchange with environment, (V1) 424, (V1) 424*f*
Radiation injury, in healthcare workers, (V1) 556
Radio Frequency Identification Detectors, (V1) 1083
Radiofrequency ablation therapy, for pain, (V1) 810
Radiography, chest, (V2) 767
  preoperative, (V2) 1032
Rales, (V2) 265
Rando, Theresa, on grief, (V1) 347, (V1) 348*t*
Range of motion (ROM), (V1) 820
  active, (V1) 820
    and passive, testing, (V1) 506, (V2) 282–283*p*
  ankle, (V2) 646
  elbow, (V2) 644
  exercises for, (V1) 843–844
  fingers, (V2) 645
  foot, (V2) 646
  hand, (V2) 645
  hip, (V2) 645–646
  knee, (V2) 646
  for mobility, (V1) 820, (V1) 844
  neck, (V2) 643
  passive, (V1) 844
  shoulder, (V2) 643–644
  testing of, (V2) 643–647
  thumb, (V2) 645
  toes, (V2) 647
  trunk, (V2) 647
  wrist, (V2) 644
Rape, (V1) 865
Rape-trauma syndrome, (V1) 868
Rapid eye movement (REM) sleep, (V1) 883, (V1) 884*t*
  disorders of, (V1) 890
Rastafarianism, (V1) 334–335
Rate
  drip, for intravenous fluids/electrolytes, (V1) 1011, (V1) 1011*b*, (V1) 1016*p*, (V2) 788–790
  flow, for intravenous fluids/electrolytes, (V1) 1011, (V1) 1011*b*
  of perceived exertion (RPE) scale, (V1) 822*b*
  respiratory, (V1) 937
Rationalization, as defense mechanism, (V1) 251*t*
Rationing, of healthcare, (V1) 23
Reaction formation, as defense mechanism, (V1) 251*t*
Reactive hyperemia, (V1) 908
Readiness, for learning, (V1) 400–401
Reading, analytical, in evaluating quality of research, (V1) 157, (V1) 157*b*
Real Time Location Systems, (V1) 1083
Reanastomosis, for bowel diversion, (V1) 751
Reasoning
  deductive, (V1) 141, (V1) 142*f*
  definition of, (V1) 141
  diagnostic, (V1) 65–73. *See also* Diagnostic reasoning
  inductive, (V1) 141, (V1) 142*f*
  logical, (V1) 141
    in gaining knowledge, (V1) 152
Reasons, seeking, as barrier to therapeutic communication, (V1) 475
Reassessment, in evaluation, (V1) 132
Rebound effect, from nasal decongestants, (V1) 638
Rebound phenomenon, (V1) 932
Receiver, of message, (V1) 460*f*, (V1) 461
Reception, (V1) 772
Receptors
  baroreceptor, (V1) 971
  lung, (V1) 939
  pain, (V1) 794
Reconstructive surgery, (V1) 1027
Recording. *See* Documentation
  of assessment data
    guidelines for, (V1) 54, (V1) 56
    tools for, (V1) 56, (V1) 57*f*
  process, in enhancing therapeutic communication, (V1) 475
Records, public, in community assessment, (V1) 1123
Recovery, from illness, (V1) 231
Recovery stage, of general adaptation syndrome, (V1) 247
Recreational therapist, on healthcare team, (V1) 19
Rectal suppository, (V1) 639
  inserting, (V1) 657*p*, (V2) 428–429*p*
Rectal temperature, (V2) 187–188*p*
Rectal tube, inserting, (V1) 769*p*, (V2) 581–582*p*
Rectum, (V1) 747, (V1) 747*f*
  assessment of, (V1) 511, (V1) 514–515*p*, (V2) 305–306*p*
  medication administration into, (V1) 639
  surgery on, urinary function and, (V1) 720
Rectus femoris muscle injection site, (V1) 651, (V1) 659*p*, (V2) 453*p*
Red blood cells, transfusion of, (V1) 1020. *See also* Blood transfusion
Refereed journals, (V1) 157
Referrals
  for depression
    evaluation for, (V2) 105
    indications for, (V1) 280, (V1) 281*b*
  to home healthcare, (V1) 1128–1129
  for spiritual care, (V1) 342–343
  for stress management, (V1) 261
Referred pain, (V1) 792, (V1) 792*f*
Reflecting critically, in critical thinking, (V1) 35*t*, (V1) 36
Reflective skepticism, in critical thinking, (V1) 36, (V1) 36*t*, (V2) 12
Reflex(es)
  Babinski, (V1) 174
  corneal, testing, (V2) 242*p*
  crawling, (V1) 174, (V1) 174*f*
  deep tendon
    assessment of, (V1) 508, (V1) 509*f*
    testing, (V2) 292–294*p*
  fencing, (V1) 174
  gag, testing, (V2) 254*p*
  gastrocolic, (V1) 747
  grasp, (V1) 173, (V1) 174*f*, (V2) 294
  Moro, (V1) 174
  neonatal, (V1) 173–174, (V1) 174*f*
  rooting, (V1) 173, (V2) 294
  startle, (V1) 174
  stepping, (V1) 174, (V1) 174*f*
  sucking, (V1) 173
  superficial, assessment of, (V1) 508, (V2) 294*p*
  swallowing, (V1) 173
  tonic neck, (V1) 174, (V1) 174*f*, (V2) 294
Reflex incontinence, (V1) 723
Reflex pain response, (V1) 247
Reflexology, in stress management, (V1) 259
Refractometer, (V1) 726, (V1) 726*f*
Refractory period, in sexual response cycle, (V1) 860
Regeneration, in healing, (V1) 248
Regenerative/epithelial healing, (V1) 903, (V1) 904, (V1) 915*t*
Regional anesthesia, (V1) 1041
Registered nurse, expertise power of, (V1) 1066
Registered nurse first assistant, (V1) 1039
Regression, as defense mechanism, (V1) 251*t*
Regulations, knowledge map on, (V2) 911
Rehabilitation centers, (V1) 16–17
Reimbursement, documentation in, (V1) 373
Relapsing fever, (V1) 426
Relationship(s)
  communication and, (V1) 467
  focus on, in leadership, (V1) 1058
  group helping, communication in, (V1) 471–472
  intimate, (V1) 861. *See also* Sexual health; Sexuality
    abuse in, (V1) 864
    negative, (V1) 864
  therapeutic, (V1) 469. *See also* Therapeutic relationships
Relaxation
  definition of, (V1) 258
  sequential. *See* Progressive (sequential) relaxation
  techniques for, in stress management, (V1) 258
Relaxation therapy
  for pain, (V1) 803
  for sleep, (V1) 894
Relevance, in verbal communication, (V1) 462
Reliability
  of evaluation criterion, (V1) 130
  of research study, (V1) 158
Religion(s), (V1) 305, (V1) 305*f*
  culture and, (V1) 309
  definition of, (V1) 326–328
  in health-illness, (V1) 227
  major, (V1) 331–335
    Atheism as, (V1) 335
    Buddhism as, (V1) 333–334, (V1) 334*f*
    Christian Science as, (V1) 332
    Christianity, (V1) 331–332
    Hinduism as, (V1) 333
    Islam as, (V1) 333
    Jehovah's Witnesses as, (V1) 332
    Judaism as, (V1) 331
    Mormonism as, (V1) 332
    Native American, (V1) 334
    Rastafarianism as, (V1) 334–335
    Roman Catholicism as, (V1) 332
    Seventh Day Adventism as, (V1) 332
  personal biases regarding, (V1) 335
  sexuality and, (V1) 856
  spirituality vs, (V1) 327*t*
Religious beliefs
  hygiene and, (V1) 575
  nutrition and, (V1) 687, (V1) 689

REM (rapid eye movement) sleep, (V1) 883, (V1) 884*t*
disorders of, (V1) 890
Reminiscence, for older adults, (V1) 282
Reminiscence therapy, for spirituality diagnoses, (V1) 340
Remission, of chronic illness, (V1) 231
Remittent fever, (V1) 426
Renal calculi, (V1) 831
urinary function and, (V1) 720
Renal cells, urinary, (V2) 563
Renal disease
end-stage, (V1) 725*b*
surgery and, (V1) 1029*b*
Renal failure
acute, definition of, (V1) 725*b*
postoperative, (V1) 1050*t*
Renal pelvis, (V1) 715, (V1) 715*f*
Renin, (V1) 988
Renin-angiotensin system, (V1) 988
Repair, in healing, (V1) 248
Repetition, for learning, (V1) 401
Report(s)
audio-recorded, (V1) 390
bedside, (V1) 390
handoff, giving, (V1) 389–390, (V1) 391*b*
incident, (V1) 388, (V1) 388*f*
in minimizing malpractice risks, (V1) 1180
oral
face-to-face, (V1) 390
giving, (V2) 163
transfer, (V1) 390–391
Reportable diseases, (V1) 863
Reporting. *See also* Documentation
knowledge map for, (V2) 176
mandatory, regulations on, in minimizing malpractice risks, (V1) 1183–1184
in minimizing malpractice risks, (V1) 1179
oral, (V1) 389–392
Repression, as defense mechanism, (V1) 251*t*
Reproductive system. *See also* Genitourinary system
female, (V1) 848–849, (V1) 849*f*
male, (V1) 849, (V1) 850*f*
teaching about, (V1) 868–869
Research
documentation in, (V1) 373
nursing, (V1) 150–159. *See also* Nursing research
Research consumer, (V1) 6*t*
Reservoir, in chain of infection, (V1) 519–520, (V1) 519*f*
Residence(s), elder-friendly, (V1) 204
Residual volume (pulmonary), (V2) 766
Resistance (physiological), airway, (V1) 938
Resistance stage, of general adaptation syndrome, (V1) 246–247
Resistance training, (V1) 821
Resolution phase, in sexual response cycle, (V1) 860
Resources, limited, population vulnerability and, (V1) 1116
Respect
in culturally competent care, (V1) 323
for dignity, do no harm and, (V1) 1150
in therapeutic communication, (V1) 471
Respiration(s), (V1) 441–446. *See also* Breathing; Pulmonary system
arterial oxygen saturation and, (V1) 445
assessment of, (V1) 443–446, (V1) 946, (V2) 198–200
data collected during, (V1) 443–446
equipment for, (V1) 443
in fluid and electrolyte assessment, (V1) 999
Biot's, (V1) 444*t*, (V1) 946
chemical aspects of, (V1) 441
chest and abdomen movement in, (V1) 445
Cheyne-Stokes, (V1) 352, (V1) 444*t*, (V1) 946
definition of, (V1) 936, (V1) 938
depth of, (V1) 937
exercise and, (V1) 824*b*
factors influencing, (V1) 442–443
Kussmaul's, (V1) 444*t*, (V1) 946
mechanical aspects of, (V1) 441
medications and, (V1) 942–943
in neonate, (V1) 173
opioid-related depression of, (V) 807*b*
pain and, (V1) 798
pH and, (V1) 991–992
position and, (V1) 946, (V1) 953
rate of, (V1) 937
normal, (V1) 422*t*, (V1) 442
regulation of, (V1) 442
stress and, (V1) 940
Respiration (gas exchange), (V1) 938, (V1) 938*f*
alveolar cells in, (V1) 936, (V1) 937*f*
external, (V1) 938, (V1) 938*f*
impaired, (V1) 943, (V1) 943*b*, (V1) 951
internal, (V1) 938, (V1) 938*f*
problems with, (V1) 951
Respirator, N-95
assessing need for, (V2) 320
donning, (V2) 321*p*
Respiratory acidosis, (V1) 996, (V1) 997*t*
Respiratory alkalosis, (V1) 996, (V1) 997*t*
Respiratory care, home care for, (V1) 1134
Respiratory depth, (V1) 444
Respiratory distress, in neonate, (V1) 175
Respiratory distress syndrome, (V1) 939
Respiratory effort, (V1) 444
Respiratory hygiene, CDC standard precautions on, (V2) 337
Respiratory (pulmonary) arrest, (V1) 981
Respiratory rate, (V1) 443–444, (V1) 444*t*
Respiratory rhythm, (V1) 444
Respiratory system. *See also* Pulmonary system; Respiration(s)
age-related changes in, assessment for, (V1) 208*t*
in alarm stage, of stress response, (V1) 246, (V1) 246*f*
defensive function of, (V1) 524
disease of, (V1) 829–830
exercise and, (V1) 829–830
sexuality and, (V1) 856
surgery and, (V1) 1029*b*
disorders of, from failure of adaptive mechanisms, (V1) 252*t*
exercise effects on, (V1) 824*b*
inhalation in drug administration to, (V1) 639–640, (V1) 639*f*
pain effects on, (V1) 798
upper, infections of, prevention of, (V1) 1108*b*
Respiratory therapist, on healthcare team, (V1) 19
Respiratory tract infection, (V1) 939, (V1) 943–944
obesity and, (V1) 941
prevention of, (V1) 951–953
Respite care, (V1) 1126
Respondeat superior, (V1) 1176
Rest, (V1) 879
adequate, promoting, for sensory overload, (V1) 785
in health-illness, (V1) 225
in infection prevention, (V1) 532
in stress management, (V1) 257
Restating, for enhancing therapeutic communication, (V1) 474
Restitution, as defense mechanism, (V1) 251*t*
Restless leg syndrome (RLS), (V1) 887
Restraints
preventing need for, (V1) 570–571
safety hazards related to, (V1) 554
use of, (V1) 573*p*, (V2) 352–354*p*
clinical insight on, (V2) 356
Resuscitation
cardiopulmonary, (V1) 981
patient, CDC standard precautions on, (V2) 337
Retention enemas, (V1) 760–761
Reticular activating system, (V1) 882, (V1) 882*f*
Reticular activating system (RAS), (V1) 772–773
Reticular formation, (V1) 882
Retirement communities, (V1) 204–205
Retractions, chest, (V1) 946
Retrograde ejaculation, (V1) 866
Retroperitoneum, (V1) 715
Retrospective audit programs, (V1) 25
Retrospective reimbursement system, (V1) 23
Return-flow enemas, (V1) 761
administering, (V2) 578*p*
Rewards, power of, (V1) 1066
Rheumatoid arthritis, (V1) 827–828, (V2) 314*f*
Rhizotomy, for pain, (V1) 810
Rhonchi, (V1) 445, (V2) 265
Rhythm
cardiac, irregular, (V1) 978
respiratory, (V1) 444
Riboflavin, (V1) 674*t*
Richmond Agitation-Sedation Rating Scale, (V2) 618
Rights
of delegation, (V1) 126–127, (V2) 46*b*
of medication, (V1) 631–634
Rigor mortis, (V1) 366
Ringworm, (V2) 313*f*
Rinne test, (V1) 496, (V2) 248–249*p*
Risk, health, appraising, in health promotion, (V1) 1099–1100, (V1) 1102
guidelines and tools for, (V2) 873–875
Risk nursing diagnosis, (V1) 66*t*
goals for, (V1) 98, (V1) 99*t*
intervention type related to, (V1) 110*f*
Ritual, bedtime, (V1) 893–894
Rodents, pathogens carried by, (V1) 551
avoiding, (V1) 565
Rogers, Martha, nursing theory of, (V1) 146*t*
Role(s)
communication and, (V1) 467
gender, (V1) 851
Role enhancement, facilitating, (V1) 277

Role modeling
in health promotion, (V1) 1106–1107
in patient teaching, (V1) 415, (V1) 418*t*
Role performance
ineffective, (V1) 274
in self-concept, (V1) 266
Role strain, caregiver
assessing for, (V1) 298
interventions for, (V1) 300
Rolled bandages, (V1) 931
ROM. *See* Range of motion (ROM)
Roman Catholicism, (V1) 332
Romberg test, (V1) 496, (V2) 249*p*
Room. *See* Environment, client; Hospital room
Root cause analysis (RCA), of healthcare errors, (V1) 553
Rooting reflex, (V1) 173
Roy, Sr. Callista, nursing theory of, (V1) 146*t*
Roy Adaptation Model, (V1) 55*t*
Rule of 30, (V1) 919
Rural healthcare, telehealth for, (V1) 1082, (V1) 1082*f*

S

S-Adenosyl Methionine (SAMe), for depression, (V1) 283*b*
Sacral nerve stimulator, for urinary incontinence, (V1) 737, (V1) 738
Safe harbor laws, (V1) 1184
Safety
assessment for, (V1) 557–558
chest tube, (V2) 757–758
for cold therapy, (V1) 1, (V2) 709
culture of, creating, (V1) 547*b*
for electric heating pads, (V2) 708
for enteral feedings, (V1) 705, (V1) 706*b*
environmental hazards and
in community, (V1) 550–552
interventions for, (V1) 564–568
in healthcare facility, (V1) 552–557
interventions for, (V1) 568–572
in home, (V1) 548–550
assessment of, (V1) 558
interventions for, (V1) 560–564
of equipment, maintaining, (V1) 571
in equipment use, clinical insights on, (V2) 902
for exercising, (V1) 835
factors affecting, (V1) 546–548
for heat therapy, (V1) 1, (V2) 708
home, promoting, in home care, (V1) 1135
in home care, considerations for, (V2) 886*b*
importance of, (V1) 546
interventions for, (V1) 559–573
knowledge map for, (V2) 362
medication
mechanisms promoting, (V1) 606–609
medication errors and, (V1) 626*b*
technologies for, (V1) 625, (V1) 627
limitations of, (V1) 627*b*
nursing diagnoses related to, (V1) 558–559
outcomes for, (V1) 559
oxygen therapy, (V1) 2
patient
goals of The Joint Commission for, (V1) 552*b*
maintaining, in minimizing malpractice risks, (V1) 1181
promoting, (V1) 545–573, (V2) 348–362
for school-age child
assessment of, (V1) 186
teaching, (V1) 187
for sleep, (V1) 884
SPEAK UP on, (V1) 559*b*
Safety and security needs, (V1) 54
Safety assessment scale (SAS), (V1) 558
Safety needs, (V1) 147, (V1) 147*f*
Safety syringes, (V1) 642–643, (V1) 642*f*
St. John's wort, for depression, (V1) 283*b*
Salem sump tubes, (V1) 707, (V1) 707*f*, (V2) 837
Saline lock, (V1) 1017–1018*p*, (V2) 786*p*, (V2) 800–802*p*
for wound care, (V1) 921
evidence-based studies of, (V1) 921
Sambucus nigra, for common cold, (V1) 952
Sandbags, (V1) 837
Sanguineous exudate, (V1) 906
Sanitation, (V1) 351
S.A.S. Safety Assessment Scale, (V2) 358
Saturation of oxygen, (V1) 949
SBAR model, for team communication, (V1) 469, (V2) 212*b*
patient safety and, (V1) 570
Scalds, in home
causes of, (V1) 549
prevention of, (V1) 561–562
Scales, (V2) 233
Scalp, assessment of, (V1) 492
Scar, (V2) 233
Scheduling, work-related use of, (V1) 1073, (V1) 1074
Scholarly journals, (V1) 1091
School-age child(ren), (V1) 184–188
assessment of, (V1) 184, (V1) 186–187
asthma in, (V1) 186
car safety seats for, (V1) 566*t*
cardiovascular system in, (V1) 971
cognitive development of, (V1) 168*t*
communication by, (V1) 465
dentition of, (V1) 185
development of
physical, (V1) 184–185
psychosexual, (V1) 167*t*
psychosocial, (V1) 168, (V1) 185, (V1) 185*f*
developmental tasks of, (V1) 166*t*
growth of, (V1) 184–185
health problems of, (V1) 185–186
health promotion for, (V1) 1101*t*
hospitalized, helping, (V1) 188
interventions for, (V1) 184, (V1) 187–188
nutrition for, (V1) 683–684
obesity in, (V1) 186
physical examination of, (V1) 486–487
pulmonary system in, (V1) 939
safety needs of, (V1) 547
sexuality of, (V1) 853
sleep for, (V1) 881, (V1) 881*t*, (V1) 885
unintentional injuries in, (V1) 186
visual acuity of, (V1) 185
School nursing, (V1) 1121
School readiness, assessment for, (V1) 184
Scientific inquiry, definition of, (V1) 152–153
Scientific management, (V1) 1060
Scientific method
characteristics of, (V1) 153*b*
in gaining knowledge, (V1) 152–153
Scissors gait, (V1) 833, (V2) 315*f*
Sclera
disorders of, (V1) 493
inspection of, (V2) 242*p*
Scoliosis, (V1) 827, (V2) 314*f*
description of, (V1) 506, (V2) 261
screening of school-age child for, (V1) 187
thoracic cage and, (V1) 499
Scoot sheet, (V1) 840, (V1) 841*f*
Screener and Opioid Assessment for Patients with Pain (SOAPP), (V1) 806
Screening
preoperative, (V1) 1012
substance abuse, (V1) 806
Scrotum, palpation of, (V2) 298–299*p*
Scrub nurse, (V1) 1039, (V1) 1044
Sebaceous glands, (V1) 579, (V1) 898*f*
in older adults, (V1) 580*t*
Second-hand smoke, (V1) 942
Secondary data, (V1) 46, (V1) 47*t*
Secondary intention healing, (V1) 903, (V1) 904*f*
Secretions, mobilization of, (V1) 954–955
Security needs, (V1) 147, (V1) 147*f*
Sedation
conscious, (V1) 1040–1041
opioid-related, (V1) 806
rating scale for, (V2) 618
Sedatives, for sleep, (V1) 894–895
Sedentary lifestyle, (V1) 834
Seizures, (V1) 780
patient at risk for, interventions for, (V1) 789
precautions for, clinical insights on, (V2) 602–603
Self
changing perception of, in stress management, (V1) 260
"dynamic," (V1) 264
preparation of, for performing physical examination, (V1) 481–482
sense of, loss of, as health disruption, (V1) 228–229
transcendence of, (V1) 148
values clarification for, (V1) 1155
when dealing with dying patient, taking care of, (V1) 367–368
Self-actualization needs, (V1) 54, (V1) 147–148, (V1) 147*f*
Self-administration, of medications, (V1) 609
Self-awareness, nurse, spiritual care and, (V1) 327*b*
Self-care
back injury prevention, (V1) 825
cardiopulmonary resuscitation, (V1) 982
cigarette smoking cessation, (V1) 954
contact lens care in, (V1) 598*b*
cough and cold medications, (V1) 952
electrolyte supplements, (V1) 1002
fitness program, (V1) 823
fluid and electrolyte imbalance prevention, (V1) 1002
food safety in, (V1) 567*b*
foot care in, client teaching on, (V1) 589*b*
healthcare worker fatigue, (V1) 882
hygiene
assessment for, (V1) 576–577
nursing diagnoses for, (V1) 577
nursing interventions for, (V1) 577–578
nursing outcomes for, (V2) 577
oral, client teaching on, (V1) 593–594*b*
incentive spirometry, (V1) 1053

informatics in, 1085*f*, (V1) 1084–1085
nail care in, client teaching on, (V1) 590*b*
nutritious food on limited budget in, (V1) 698*b*
older adult exercise, (V1) 825
postoperative teaching topics, (V1) 1052
posture, (V1) 819
promoting health and safety through, (V1) 579
sexual predator precautions, (V1) 862
sleep hygiene, (V1) 895
surgical site infection prevention, (V1) 1035
upper respiratory infection prevention in, (V1) 1108*b*
weight loss tips in, (V1) 701–702*b*
Self-care ability, health status and, (V1) 575–576
Self-catheterization
intermittent
teaching clients about, (V2) 560
for urinary incontinence, (V1) 737
for urinary retention, (V1) 730
Self-concept, (V1) 264–265
components of, (V1) 265–267, (V1) 267*f*
definition of, (V1) 264
disturbed
assessing for, (V2) 103
as etiology, (V1) 274–275
as problem, (V1) 274
factors affecting, (V1) 264–265
formation of, (V1) 264
personal identity and, (V1) 266
promoting, (V1) 275–276
role performance and, (V1) 266
self-esteem and, (V1) 266–267, (V1) 273–276
sexual identity and, (V1) 851
Self-esteem
inventory for, (V2) 104
low
chronic or situational, (V1) 274
sexuality and, (V1) 867
promoting, (V1) 275–276
in children, (V1) 276*b*
self-concept and, (V1) 266–267, (V1) 273–276
Self-esteem needs, (V1) 147, (V1) 147*f*
Self-examination
breast, (V1) 869–870
teaching about, (V1) 869–870
testis, (V1) 870
Self-help groups, communication in, (V1) 471–472
Self-knowledge, (V1) 37
in diagnostic reasoning, (V1) 72
in full-spectrum nursing, (V1) 40*t*, (V1) 41
about sexuality, (V1) 856
Self-report
about pain, (V1) 798
about sleep, (V1) 891
Self-stimulation, for sensory deprivation, (V1) 784
Selye, Hans, (V1) 148
Semen, ejaculation of, (V1) 849, (V1) 860
Semi-Fowler's position, (V1) 837
Semi-vegetarians, (V1) 686
Sender, of message, (V1) 460, (V1) 460*f*
Sengsten–Blakemore tube, (V2) 837*t*
Seniors. *See* Older adult(s)
Sensation(s), (V1) 771–789, (V2) 599–609
deep, testing, (V2) 291*p*
discriminatory, testing, (V2) 292*p*
kinesthetic, testing, (V2) 291*p*
postoperative, (V1) 1046
responding to, (V1) 773
of skin, diminished, (V1) 900
superficial, testing, (V2) 290–291*p*
Sensible fluid loss, (V1) 987
Sensorimotor development, of preschooler, (V1) 182
Sensorimotor stage, of cognitive development, (V1) 168*t*
Sensoristasis, definition of, (V1) 775
Sensory aids, use of, assessing, (V1) 781
Sensory alterations
communication by older adults and, (V1) 465
therapeutic communication and, (V1) 472
Sensory areas, of brain, (V1) 773*f*
Sensory deficit(s), (V1) 777–780
auditory, (V1) 777, (V1) 778*b*
gustatory, (V1) 777–779, (V1) 778*b*
interventions for, (V1) 785–787
kinesthetic, (V1) 780
olfactory, (V1) 779
self-care ability and, (V1) 576
in self-care ability assessment, (V1) 577
tactile, (V1) 779
visual, (V1) 777, (V1) 777*b*
Sensory deprivation, (V1) 775–776
interventions for, (V1) 783–784
signs of, (V1) 776*b*
Sensory experience, components of, (V1) 772–773
Sensory function
alterations in, (V1) 775–780
assessment of, (V1) 509, (V1) 514*p*
bedside assessment of, (V2) 606
changes in
with aging, (V1) 774*t*
assessment of, (V1) 781
culture and, (V1) 775
developmental variations in, (V1) 774–775, (V1) 774*t*
factors affecting, (V1) 773–775
illness and, (V1) 775
impaired, risk factors for, assessing for, (V1) 605–606
lifestyle and, (V1) 775
medications and, (V1) 775
optimal, promoting, (V1) 783
personality and, (V1) 775
stress and, (V1) 775
Sensory functions, assessment tools for, (V2) 605–606
Sensory overload, (V1) 776–777
in ICU, (V1) 776*b*
interventions for, (V1) 784–785
signs of, (V1) 776*b*
Sensory perception
assessment of, (V1) 780–782
impaired, risk factors for, assessing, (V1) 781
knowledge map for, (V2) 609
nursing diagnoses related to, (V1) 782
nursing interventions for, (V1) 782–789
nursing outcomes for, (V1) 782
Sensory receptors, (V1) 772
Sensory system
age-related changes in, assessment for, (V1) 208*t*
assessment of, (V2) 284–292*p*
Septicemia, (V1) 1014–1015*t*
Sequential compression devices, (V1) 980, (V1) 1054*p*, (V2) 832–833*p*
postoperative use of, (V1) 1052–1053, (V1) 1053*f*
Sequential relaxation. *See* Progressive (sequential) relaxation
Serial monogamy, (V1) 854
Serosanguineous exudate, (V1) 906
Serous exudate, (V1) 906
Serum electrolytes, (V1) 1000, (V2) 845
Serum osmolality, (V1) 1000–1001
Servant leadership, (V1) 1060
Set point, temperature, (V1) 426
Settling, in communication, (V1) 233
Seventh Day Adventism, (V1) 332
Sex chromosomes, (V1) 851
Sexism, as barrier to culturally competent care, (V1) 317–318
Sexual abuse, (V1) 864–865
Sexual assault, (V1) 864
clinical insights on, (V2) 652–653
Sexual assault nurse examiner, (V1) 865
Sexual behaviors, risky, in adolescents, (V1) 191
Sexual dysfunction, (V1) 867
Sexual harassment, (V1) 864, (V1) 1182
Sexual health, (V1) 847–877, (V2) 651–661. *See also* Sexuality
anal stimulation and, (V1) 862
assessment of, (V1) 866–867
celibacy and, (V1) 862
counseling for, (V1) 870–871
critical thinking about, (V2) 658–659
definition of, (V1) 858
erotic dreams and, (V1) 861
fantasies and, (V1) 861
full-spectrum nursing and, (V2) 658
intercourse and, (V1) 861
intimacy and, (V1) 861
knowledge map for, (V2) 661
masturbation and, (V1) 861
oral-genital stimulation and, (V1) 861
paraphilias and, (V1) 862
sexual response cycle in, (V1) 858–861, (V1) 858*f*
shared touching and, (V1) 861
teaching about, (V1) 868–870
body function, (V1) 868–869
contraception, (V1) 870
douching, (V1) 869
infection prevention, (V1) 870
menopause, (V1) 869
menstruation, (V1) 869
premenstrual syndrome, (V1) 869
reproduction, (V1) 868–869
self-examination, (V1) 869–870
Sexual history, (V1) 866, (V2) 653
guidelines and questions for, (V2) 656–657
Sexual identity, (V1) 851
Sexual intercourse, (V1) 861. *See also* Sexual health; Sexuality
arousal disorders and, (V1) 865–866
erectile dysfunction and, (V1) 865–866
orgasmic disorders and, (V1) 866
painful, (V1) 868
Sexual orientation, (V1) 852–853
emerging, in adolescents, (V1) 189
Sexual partners, multiple, host susceptibility and, (V1) 528

Sexual response cycle, (V1) 858–861
in older adults, (V1) 859
Sexuality, (V1) 849, (V1) 851
activity intolerance and, (V1) 867
adolescent, (V1) 853–854
adult, (V1) 854–855
arousal disorders and, (V1) 865–866
birth through preschool, (V1) 853
care map for, (V1) 876
chronic low self-esteem and, (V1) 867
chronic pain and, (V1) 867
culture and, (V1) 855–856
delayed development and, (V1) 867
dementia and, (V1) 864
development of, (V1) 853–855
dysmenorrhea and, (V1) 863
evidence-based studies of, (V1) 860
expression of, (V1) 861–862
fatigue and, (V1) 867
fear and, (V1) 867, (V1) 868
gender and, (V1) 851–852
illness and, (V1) 856–857
impaired physical mobility and, (V1) 867
inappropriate, (V1) 871
ineffective patterns of, (V1) 867
infection and, (V1) 863
knowledge about, (V1) 856
lifestyle and, (V1) 856
low libido and, (V1) 865
medical effects on, (V1) 863–864
misconceptions about, (V1) 869
negative relationships and, (V1) 864
nursing care plan for, (V1) 872–875
nursing diagnosis for, (V1) 867–868
nursing interventions for, (V1) 868–871
nursing outcomes for, (V1) 868
older adult, (V1) 854–855, (V1) 859*b*, (V1) 860
orgasmic disorders and, (V1) 866
premenstrual syndrome and, (V1) 863–864
psychiatric disorders and, (V1) 857
rape and, (V1) 865
religion and, (V1) 856
school age through puberty, (V1) 853–854
self-care deficits and, (V1) 867
self-knowledge about, (V1) 856
sexual harassment and, (V1) 864
sexual orientation and, (V1) 852–853
sexual response cycle disorders and, (V1) 865–866
sexually transmitted infection and, (V1) 863
Sexually transmitted infections (STIs), (V1) 863
in adolescents, (V1) 191
preventing, interventions for, (V1) 193
prevention of, teaching for, (V1) 870
in young adults, (V1) 195
Selye, Hans, response-based model of stress of, (V1) 242
Shaken baby syndrome, (V1) 177
Shampooing of hair, (V1) 596, (V1) 600*p*, (V2) 384–387*p*
Shared touching, (V1) 861
Sharp debridement, (V1) 923, (V1) 928
Sharps
CDC standard precautions on, (V2) 337
disposal of, (V1) 538
surgical count of, (V1) 1044
Shaving, (V1) 597, (V1) 601*p*, (V2) 389–390*p*
preoperative, 1035
Shearing forces, pressure ulcers and, (V1) 908, (V1) 908*f*
Shivering, (V1) 933
Shock
hypovolemic, (V1) 993
risk for, (V1) 979
Shock phase, of fight or flight reaction, (V1) 245
Shoe, high-top, (V1) 837
Shoe covers
assessing need for, (V2) 321
donning, (V2) 321*p*
removing, (V2) 323*p*
Short-term goals, (V1) 1074
Shoulder, range of motion in, (V2) 643–644
Shower
assisting with, clinical insights on, (V2) 401
in skin hygiene, (V1) 583
Side-stream smoke, (V1) 942
Siderails, (V1) 836
as restraints, (V1) 554
use of, evidence-based practice on, (V1) 27
SIDS. *See* Sudden infant death syndrome (SIDS)
Sigma Theta Tau International (STTI), (V1) 14
Sigmoidoscopy, (V2) 595
Significant data, in analyzing and interpreting data, (V1) 65–67
Silence, in enhancing therapeutic communication, (V1) 475
Silver dressing, (V1) 919
Simple Descriptor Scale, for pain, (V2) 617
Sims' position, (V1) 839*b*, (V1) 840
Single-use anesthetic pump, (V1) 1047, (V1) 1052
Sinoatrial node, (V1) 969, (V1) 969*f*
Sinuses, assessment of, (V2) 249–251*p*
Situational stressors, (V1) 240
Situational theory, of leadership, (V1) 1058–1059
Sitz bath, (V1) 932, (V1) 932*f*, (V2) 708
Skeletal muscle movement, in heat production, (V1) 424
Skeleton, (V1) 817–818
Skene's ducts, palpation of, (V2) 302–303*p*
Skepticism, reflective, in critical thinking, (V1) 36, (V1) 36*t*, (V2) 12
Skilled care facilities, (V1) 16
Skilled nursing services, (V1) 1125, (V1) 1126*b*
Skills, critical thinking, (V1) 32
Skin
adult, (V1) 899
age-related changes in, assessment for, (V1) 208*t*
age-related variations in, (V1) 899
anatomy and physiology of, (V1) 579
ascorbic acid effects on, (V1) 899
assessment of, (V1) 489–491, (V1) 581, (V2) 226–229*p*
biocultural variations in, (V1) 319
in fluid and electrolyte assessment, (V1) 999
history in, (V2) 709
surgical, (V1) 1044
bioengineered, (V1) 920
breakdown of. *See also* Pressure ulcer(s); Wound(s)
circulatory impairment and, (V1) 900
cognitive impairments and, (V1) 900
fever and, (V1) 901
impaired mobility and, (V1) 899
infection and, (V1) 901
lifestyle and, (V1) 901
medications and, (V1) 900
moisture and, (V1) 900–901
nutritional status and, (V1) 899–900
sensory impairments and, (V1) 900
café-au-lait spots on, (V1) 489
calorie intake and, (V1) 899
capillary hemangiomas on, (V1) 489
care of, (V1) 579–587
changes in, in older adults, (V1) 580, (V1) 580*t*
of children, (V1) 899
cholesterol effects on, (V1) 899
cigarette smoking effects on, (V1) 901
color of, (V1) 489, (V1) 490*t*
changes in, atlas of, (V2) 312*f*
cyanosis of, (V1) 490*t*, (V2) 312*f*
daily inspection of, (V1) 918
defensive function of, (V1) 524
developmental stage effects on, (V1) 899
diminished sensation of, (V1) 900
diseases of, (V1) 580
disorders of, nursing diagnosis of, (V1) 581
dry, (V1) 581
ecchymosis of, (V1) 490*t*
edema and, (V1) 491
erythema of, (V1) 490*t*
exercise effects on, (V1) 824*b*, (V1) 901
factors affecting, (V1) 580
fever and, (V1) 901
fluid loss through, (V1) 987
flushing of, (V1) 490*t*
functions of, (V1) 579
growths on, in older adults, (V1) 580*t*
hair removal from, preoperative, (V1) 1035
hydration effects on, (V1) 899–900
hygiene for, (V1) 581–587. *See also* Hygiene, skin
immobility effects on, (V1) 899
impaired circulation and, (V1) 900
infant, (V1) 899
infection of, (V1) 901
risk for, (V1) 917
integrity of, (V1) 898
impaired, (V1) 917
risk of impaired, (V1) 917
integrity of, impaired, (V1) 917
as etiology, (V1) 582
as problem, (V1) 581
risk for, (V1) 917
intraoperative preparation of, (V1) 1043–1044
itching of, (V1) 899
jaundice of, (V1) 490*t*, (V2) 312*f*
lesions of, (V1) 491, (V2) 312–313*f*
describing, (V2) 229*b*, (V2) 230–233*p*
identification of, (V2) 228*p*
maceration of, (V1) 900
medication administration to, (V1) 611*t*, (V1) 657*p*, (V2) 430–432*p*
medication effects on, (V1) 900, (V1) 901*f*
moistness of, (V1) 900–901, (V1) 908, (V1) 918
moisture of, (V1) 490
mongolian spots on, (V1) 489
mottling of, (V1) 490*t*
nutrition effects on, (V1) 899
of obese patient, care of, (V1) 586*t*

older adult, (V1) 899
pain in, (V1) 791
pallor of, (V1) 490*t*
petechiae of, (V1) 490*t*
piercings of, (V1) 901
preoperative preparation of, (V1) 1036
protein effects on, (V1) 899
at puberty, (V1) 899
regeneration of, (V1) 903, (V1) 904, (V1) 915*t*
screening of, in health promotion assessment, (V2) 876
striae of, (V1) 491
structure of, (V1) 898–899, (V1) 898*f*
surgical preparation of
tanning effects on, (V1) 901
tattoos of, (V1) 901
temperature of, (V1) 489
tenting of, (V1) 491
texture of, (V1) 490–491, (V2) 227*p*
tuberculin testing of, (V1) 947–948, (V2) 768
turgor of, (V1) 491, (V2) 227*p*
Skin closures, (V1) 905, (V2) 695–696*p*
placement of, (V1) 930*p*
Skin sealants, (V1) 927*t*
Skin tags, (V1) 491, (V2) 228
Skin temperature, using chemical strip thermometer, (V2) 189*p*
Skin testing, tuberculin, (V1) 947–948, (V2) 768
Skinfold thickness, measurement of, (V2) 514*p*
in body composition assessment, (V1) 692
Skull, assessment of, (V1) 493
Slander, (V1) 1172
Slang, (V1) 318
Sleep, (V1) 878–896, (V2) 662–670
adequate, promoting, for sensory overload, (V1) 785
for adolescents, (V1) 885
for adults, (V1) 885
age and, (V1) 885
alcohol and, (V1) 886
assessment of, (V1) 891, (V2) 666
asthma and, (V1) 890
back massage for, (V1) 893*p*, (V2) 664–665
bedtime rituals and routines for, (V1) 893–894
beverages before, (V1) 894
caffeine and, (V1) 886
care scheduling for, (V1) 893
for children, (V1) 885
circadian rhythms and, (V1) 881–882
comfort promotion for, (V1) 893
COPD and, (V1) 890
coronary artery disease and, (V1) 890
critical thinking about, (V2) 668–669
definition of, (V1) 879
depression and, (V1) 890
development and, (V1) 881, (V1) 885
diabetes mellitus and, (V1) 890
diet and, (V1) 886
disorders of, (V1) 886–890
secondary, (V1) 890
disorders provoked by, (V1) 890–891
dreaming during, (V1) 880, (V1) 884, (V1) 890
electroencephalogram during, (V1) 882–883
energy output during, (V1) 879
enhanced, readiness for, (V1) 891
environmental factors and, (V1) 886
epilepsy and, (V1) 891
evidence-based studies of, (V1) 888
exercise and, (V1) 886
full-spectrum nursing and, (V2) 667–668
functions of, (V1) 879–880
gastric ulcers and, (V1) 891
in health-illness, (V1) 225
for health promotion, (V1) 1106
hospitalization and, (V1) 886, (V1) 888
hygiene teaching for, (V1) 894, (V1) 895
illness and, (V1) 880, (V1) 880*f*
importance of, (V1) 879–880
for infants, (V1) 881, (V1) 881*t*, (V1) 894
in infection prevention, (V1) 532
intestinal ulcers and, (V1) 891
knowledge map for, (V2) 670
lifestyle factors and, (V1) 885–886
medications and, (V1) 886
medications for, (V1) 894–896
for newborns, (V1) 894
nicotine and, (V1) 886
NREM (non-rapid eye movement), (V1) 883, (V1) 884*t*
nursing diagnosis for, (V1) 891–892
nursing interventions for, (V1) 892–896
nursing outcomes for, (V1) 892
for older adults, (V1) 880, (V1) 885
pain and, (V1) 880, (V1) 890
physiology of, (V1) 881–883
quality of, (V1) 885–886
regulation of, (V1) 882–883
relaxation strategies for, (V1) 894
REM (rapid eye movement), (V1) 883, (V1) 884*t*
requirements for, (V1) 880–881, (V1) 881*t*
restful environment for, (V1) 893
snacks before, (V1) 894
stages of, (V1) 883, (V1) 883*f*, (V1) 884*t*
for stress, (V1) 880
in stress management, (V1) 257
thyroid disease and, (V1) 890
for young adults, (V1) 885
Sleep apnea, (V1) 888–889
Sleep deprivation, (V1) 882, (V1) 887–888, (V1) 891
Sleep diary, (V1) 891, (V2) 667
Sleep history, (V1) 891, (V2) 666
Sleep patterns
disturbed, (V1) 891–892
preoperative, (V1) 1033, (V2) 847
in infants, (V1) 176
of school-age child, assessment of, (V1) 186
Sleep-provoked disorders, (V1) 890–891
Sleep study, (V1) 891
Sleep-wake schedule disorders, (V1) 887
Sleeptalking, (V1) 890
Sleepwalking, (V1) 890
safety for, (V1) 894
Slings, for wounds, (V1) 928
Slough, (V1) 915, (V1) 915*t*
Slow-reacting substance of anaphylaxis, (V1) 940
Slow-wave sleep, (V1) 890
Small intestine, (V1) 746, (V1) 746*f*
Smell
bedside assessment of, (V2) 606
changes in, with aging, (V1) 774*t*
deficits in
home care for, (V1) 787*b*
interventions for, (V1) 786
diminished sense of, impaired nutrition from, interventions for, (V1) 698
in neonate, (V1) 174
stimulation of, for sensory deprivation, (V1) 784
structures concerned with, (V1) 778*f*
Smoking. *See* Cigarette smoking
Smooth muscle, (V1) 818
Snacks, bedtime, (V1) 894
Sneakers, high-top, (V1) 837
Snellen chart, (V1) 494
Snoring, (V1) 889
SOAP/SOAPIE/SOAPIER format, for documentation, (V1) 379–380
SOAR (strengths, opportunities, aspirations, results) planning, (V1) 1062, (V1) 1063*t*
Social distance, communication and, (V1) 466
Social history, in nursing health history, (V1) 52*t*
Social interaction, for sensory deprivation, (V1) 784
Social justice, as nursing value, (V1) 1146*t*
Social justice model, for discussing dilemma, (V1) 1160
Social networking, (V1) 1081
web-based, among adolescents, (V1) 191
Social organization, culture and, (V1) 309
Social theory, of depression, (V1) 270
Social worker, on healthcare team, (V1) 20
Socialization, (V1) 305
professional, (V1) 11
Socialized healthcare, (V1) 23
Society, trends in, influencing contemporary nursing practice, (V1) 26–27
Sociocultural factors. *See also* Culture
affecting bowel elimination, (V1) 748–749
communication and, (V1) 466
pain and, (V1) 796
Sociocultural influences, on urinary function, (V1) 718–719
Sodium, (V1) 677*t*, (V1) 678, (V1) 988, (V1) 990*t*, (V1) 1002
imbalances in, (V1) 994*t*
normal, (V2) 817
Sodomy, (V1) 862
Soft palate, assessment of, (V1) 497
Soil pollution, as safety hazard, (V1) 552
Solubility, of medications, (V1) 614
Solutes, (V1) 984
Solution(s), (V1) 610*t*, (V1) 612*t*, (V1) 613*t*
hypertonic, (V1) 986
hypotonic, (V1) 986
isotonic, (V1) 985–986
ophthalmic, (V1) 638
parenteral fluid/electrolyte. *See* Intravenous fluids, and electrolytes, solution for
parenteral nutrition, (V1) 711
Somatic nervous system, (V1) 818
Somatization, from failure of adaptive mechanisms, (V1) 252
Somatoform disorders, from failure of adaptation to stress, (V1) 252–253
Somnambulism, (V1) 890
Source-oriented record systems, (V1) 373–374
Space
culture and, (V1) 308
personal, communication and, (V1) 465–466, (V1) 466*f*

Spastic gait, (V1) 833, (V2) 315*f*
Spasticity, (V1) 833*b*
Special needs assessments, (V1) 49–51
Special populations, learning by, (V1) 402–403
Special-purpose forms, (V1) 56
Special teaching, care plans for, (V1) 89*f*, (V1) 91, (V1) 94
  outcomes for, (V1) 102
Specialty and categorical programs, as payor for healthcare, (V1) 21
Specific gravity, of urine, (V1) 717, (V1) 726, (V1) 993, (V2) 562, (V2) 817
  measuring, (V1) 733–734*p*
Specimen(s)
  safe handling of, (V1) 538
  stool, handling of, (V1) 755
  urine
    clean-catch, (V1) 724
      collecting, (V1) 733*p*, (V2) 535*p*
    freshly voided, (V1) 724
    sterile, (V1) 725
      obtaining, (V1) 733*p*, (V2) 536*p*
    24-hour, (V1) 724
      collecting, (V1) 733*p*, (V2) 536–537*p*
Speculum exam, (V1) 511
  assisting with, (V2) 309–310*p*
Speech, in physical examination, (V1) 488
Speech and language therapist, on healthcare team, (V1) 19
Speech impairment, clients with, enhancing communication with, (V1) 478, (V2) 213*b*
Sphincter(s)
  anal, (V1) 747, (V1) 747*f*
    surgery on, bowel elimination and, (V1) 750
  cardiac, (V1) 745
  gastroesophageal, (V1) 745
  urethral, (V1) 717
Sphygmomanometer, (V1) 449–450, (V1) 449*f*
SPICES assessment, (V1) 487
Spinal anesthesia, (V1) 1041, (V1) 1042*f*
Spinal cord injury, sexuality and, (V1) 857
Spinal cord stimulator, for pain, (V1) 802
Spindles, (V1) 883
Spine, curvatures of, (V1) 819*f*
Spirits, (V1) 610*t*
S-P-I-R-I-T assessment, (V2) 139
Spiritual beliefs, health and, (V1) 329–330
Spiritual care, (V1) 150
  barriers to, (V1) 335–337
  complementary and alternative modalities for, (V1) 343*b*
  interventions for, standardized language for, (V1) 116
  nurse self-awareness and, (V1) 327*b*
  personal biases and, (V1) 335
  provider of, on healthcare team, (V1) 20
Spiritual healing, (V1) 329
Spiritual health assessment, (V1) 50
Spiritual needs, of dying patient, meeting, (V1) 365
Spiritual pain, components of, (V1) 338, (V1) 339*f*
Spiritual responses, to stress, (V1) 249, (V1) 251
Spiritual support, for spirituality diagnoses, (V1) 341
Spirituality, (V1) 325–344, (V2) 136–144
  assessment of, (V1) 337–338
    data sources for, (V1) 337–338
    HOPE approach to, (V2) 140
    S-P-I-R-I-T assessment in, (V2) 139
    tools for, (V1) 338
  core issues of, (V1) 328–329
  definition of, (V1) 328
  as etiology, (V1) 338
  faith in, (V1) 328–329
  fears about, (V1) 336–337
  in health-illness, (V1) 227
  hope in, (V1) 329
  hygiene and, (V1) 575
  interventions for, standardized, (V1) 340–342
  knowledge map for, (V2) 144
  love in, (V1) 329
  in nursing, history of, (V1) 326
  nursing diagnoses for, (V1) 338–340
  standardized nursing language for, (V2) 140
  vs. religion, (V1) 327*t*
Spirometry, (V1) 948, (V1) 1053
  incentive, (V1) 953–954, (V1) 1052, (V1) 1053
    postoperative, (V1) 1052
    teaching about, (V1) 1053
Spleen, palpation of, (V2) 276*p*
Splint, hand/wrist, (V1) 837
Splinter hemorrhages, (V1) 492
Splinting (breathing), (V1) 798
Spokesperson, (V1) 1061
Spondylitis, ankylosing, (V1) 828
Sponge (contraceptive), (V2) 655
Sports, in stress management, (V1) 259
Sprain, (V1) 829
Spray, (V1) 611*t*
  aerosol, (V1) 611*t*
    application of, (V2) 430*p*
Spray injectors, for insulin, (V1) 649
Sputum
  assessment of, (V1) 947, (V2) 767
  collection of, (V1) 947, (V1) 963*p*, (V2) 723–726*p*
  color of, (V1) 947*b*
  expectoration of, (V2) 724–725
  postural drainage for, (V1) 955, (V1) 963–964*p*, (V2) 728–730*p*
Squamous cells, urinary, (V2) 563
Stairs, crutch walking on, (V2) 639–640
Standard precautions, clinical insight on, (V2) 337–338
Standardized language, definition of, (V1) 73
Standardized nursing languages, (V1) 1085–1087, (V2) 865–866
  for anxiety, (V2) 109–110
  for caregiver role strain, (V2) 121
  for depression, (V2) 111–112
  for diagnosis, (V1) 73–76. *See also* NANDA-I nursing diagnosis
  for health promotion diagnoses, (V2) 877
  holistic care and, (V1) 115–116
  for home health and community care, (V1) 115, (V1) 1132, (V2) 888–892
  importance of, (V1) 373
  for outcomes, (V1) 99–100, (V1) 100*f*
  for spirituality, (V2) 140
  for stress, (V2) 97–98
Standards, in evaluation, (V1) 130
Standards of practice, (V1) 12
  ANA, (V1) 1169. *See also* American Nurses Association (ANA), standards of practice of
  documentation in, (V1) 372–373
  following, in minimizing malpractice risks, (V1) 1179
Standing assist devices, (V1) 843, (V1) 843*f*
Standing orders, (V1) 624
Staples
  removal of, (V2) 703–704*p*
  stuck, (V2) 704
Startle reflex, (V1) 174
Stasis ulcer, (V2) 232
State boards of nursing, (V1) 22
State laws, (V1) 1167–1168
Statements, in nursing theory, (V1)140
Statins, (V1) 981
Statistical Nomenclature of Medicine Clinical Terminology (SNOMED CT), (V2) 866
Statute(s)
  definition of, (V1) 1163
  medical malpractice, (V1) 1168
Statutory law, (V1) 1163
Statutory rape, (V1) 865
Steppage gait, (V1) 833, (V2) 315*f*
Stepping reflex, (V1) 174, (V1) 174*f*
Stereotype(s)
  cultural, (V1) 308
  in diagnostic reasoning, (V1) 72
Stereotyping
  as barrier to therapeutic communication, (V1) 477
  cultural, as barrier to culturally competent care, (V1) 317
Sterile, definition of, (V1) 538
Sterile fields
  adding sterile solutions to, (V1) 542, (V2) 334*p*
  adding supplies to, (V1) 541–542, (V2) 333*p*
  preparing and maintaining, (V1) 539*p*, (V1) 541, (V2) 332–333*p*
    clinical insight on, (V2) 343–344
Sterile gown and gloves, donning, (V1) 539*p*, (V1) 540–541, (V1) 541*f*
Sterile team, (V1) 1039
Sterile technique, (V1) 539
  in nursing care, (V1) 541–542
  tracheostomy care, (V2) 736–741
  wound culture, (V2) 673–675
  wound irrigation, (V2) 675–678
Sterility, common breaks in, (V1) 542*b*
Sterilization, in medical asepsis, (V1) 535
Sterilization (biological), (V2) 656
Sterols, (V1) 671
Stertor, (V1) 445
Stethoscope, in pulse assessment, (V1) 437–438, (V1) 438*f*
Stimulant laxatives, (V1) 749*b*
Stimulants, sexual function and, (V1) 858*t*
Stimulus(i)
  adaptation to, (V1) 773
  contrast in, (V1) 773
  control of, for sensory overload, (V1) 784–785
  environmental, assessing, (V1) 781–782
  intensity of, (V1) 773
  pain-related, (V1) 793
  prior experience with, (V1) 773
  sexual, (V1) 859
Stockings, antiembolism, (V1) 980, (V1) 1054*p*, (V2) 829–832*p*
  postoperative use of, (V1) 1052–1053
  preoperative use of, (V1) 1037–1038, (V1) 1037*f*

Stoma, in bowel diversion, assessing, (V1) 764, (V1) 764*f*
Stomach, (V1) 745
function of, nutrition and, (V1) 689
Stomatitis, (V1) 592
Stool
digital removal of, for fecal impaction, (V1) 761, (V1) 769*p*, (V2) 579–581*p*
laboratory studies of, (V1) 755
occult blood in, testing for, (V1) 755, (V1) 769*p*, (V2) 570–572*p*
Stool softeners, (V1) 749*b*
Storms, electrical
as safety hazard, (V1) 552
safety measures for, (V1) 568
Strabismus, (V1) 495
definition of, (V1) 777*b*
Strain, (V1) 829
Stratum corneum, (V1) 898, (V1) 898*f*
Stratum germinativum, (V1) 898, (V1) 898*f*
Streamlining, work-related, (V1) 1075
Street talk, (V1) 318
Streptococcus, group B, in pregnancy, screening for, (V1) 172
Stress
adaptation to, (V1) 239–261, (V2) 92–101
analysis/nursing diagnosis of, (V1) 256
failure of, (V1) 251–254
knowledge map for, (V2) 101
planning interventions/implementation for, (V1) 256–257
planning outcomes/evaluation of, (V1) 256
assessment for, guidelines and tools for, (V2) 95–97
blood pressure and, (V1) 448
body temperature and, (V1) 425
bowel elimination and, (V1) 750
cardiovascular effects of, (V1) 972
change and, (V1) 1071
coping strategies for, (V1) 242–243
definition of, (V1) 240
exercise for, (V1) 827
in health promotion assessment, (V1) 1103, (V2) 875
of hospitalization, reducing, (V1) 260, (V1) 260*b*
knowledge map for, (V2) 101
management of
techniques for, (V1) 258–259
in workplace, (V1) 261
minimizing, for sensory overload, (V1) 785
models of, (V1) 240, (V1) 242
multiple responsibilities and, (V1) 241
NANDA-I nursing diagnoses associated with, (V2) 97–98
nursing diagnoses related to, standardized outcomes and interventions for, (V2) 98
outcomes of, (V1) 243
pulmonary system effects of, (V1) 940
pulse and, (V1) 437
reduction of
complementary and alternative medicine modalities in, (V1) 258*b*
food in, nutrition and, (V1) 685
in infection prevention, (V1) 533
respiration and, (V1) 443
respiratory, (V1) 939
response-based model of, (V1) 242
responses to
assessing, (V1) 255
organic, (V1) 252, (V1) 252*t*
psychological, (V1) 248–249, (V1) 248*b*, (V1) 250–251*t*, (V1) 253–254
spiritual, (V1) 249, (V1) 251
sensory function and, (V1) 775
sleep for, (V1) 880
Stress and adaptation theory, (V1) 148
Stressor(s)
adapting to, (V1) 243
altering, (V1) 243
avoiding, (V1) 243
changing perception of, in stress management, (V1) 260
definition of, (V1) 240
developmental, (V1) 240
external, (V1) 240
internal, (V1) 240
perception of, adaptation and, (V1) 244
physiological, (V1) 240
psychosocial, (V1) 240
responses to, (V1) 244–251
general adaptation syndrome as, (V1) 244–247, (V1) 245*f*
local adaptation syndrome as, (V1) 247–248
physiological, (V1) 255*b*
situational, (V1) 240
throughout life span, (V1) 242*b*
types of, (V1) 240
Stretcher, transfer to, (V2) 628–629
Stretching injury, (V1) 829
Striae, (V1) 491
Stridor, (V1) 445, (V1) 946, (V2) 265
Stroke, (V1) 829
ambulation assistance and, (V2) 634
heat, (V1) 426
Stroke volume
blood pressure and, (V1) 447
definition of, (V1) 436
Structural-functional family theories, (V1) 289
Structure evaluation, (V1) 130–131
STTI (Sigma Theta Tau International), (V1) 14
Student responsibilities, (V1) 1184–1185
Stuporous, description of, (V1) 507
Stye, (V2) 313*f*
Subconjunctival hemorrhage, (V1) 493, (V2) 313*f*
Subculture(s), (V1) 306
gender as, (V1) 307
nursing, (V1) 312–313
old age as, (V1) 307
vulnerable populations as, (V1) 306–307, (V1) 306*f*
Subcutaneous injection(s), (V1) 613*t*, (V1) 647–649
administration of, (V2) 448–451*p*
of anticoagulants, clinical insight on, (V2) 476*b*
for insulin administration, (V1) 648–649
needle selection for, (V1) 648
site selection for, (V1) 647, (V1) 648*f*
Subcutaneous layer, (V1) 898*f*, (V1) 899
Subcutaneous tissues, in older adults, (V1) 580*t*
Subjective data, (V1) 46, (V1) 47*t*
Subjects, in quantitative research, (V1) 153
Sublimation, as defense mechanism, (V1) 251*t*
Sublingual administration of drugs, (V1) 611*t*
Sublingual mucosa, medication administration by, (V1) 634–635
Substance abuse, (V1) 1097
by adolescents, (V1) 190
interventions for, (V1) 193
cardiovascular effects of, (V1) 973
health-illness and, (V1) 226
host susceptibility and, (V1) 528
pain management and, (V1) 806
pulmonary effects of, (V1) 941–942
surgery and, (V1) 1029
by young adult, (V1) 195
Substance addiction, maternal, neonatal problems from, (V1) 175
Substernal retraction, in respiration, (V1) 445
Substituted liability, (V1) 1175–1176
Subsystems
definition of, (V1) 148
of family, (V1) 289
Sucking reflex, (V1) 173
Suctioning
airway, (V1) 959–960, (V1) 959*f*, (V1) 965*p*, (V2) 749–751*p*
endotracheal, (V1) 960, (V1) 964–965*p*, (V2) 744–745*p*
gastrointestinal, (V1) 1053–1054, (V1) 1054–1055*p*, (V2) 834–839*p*
nasogastric, (V1) 1053–1054, (V1) 1054–1055*p*, (V2) 834–839*p*
nasopharyngeal, (V2) 749–751*p*
nasotracheal, (V1) 960, (V1) 965*p*, (V2) 746–748*p*
oropharyngeal, (V2) 749–751*p*
orotracheal, (V1) 960, (V1) 965*p*, (V2) 745–748*p*
sputum collection, (V1) 963*p*, (V2) 725–726
tracheostomy, (V1) 960, (V1) 964–965*p*, (V2) 741–744*p*
Sudden infant death syndrome (SIDS), (V1) 178
interventions for, (V1) 179
maternal cocaine abuse and, (V1) 171
Suffocation, in home
prevention of, (V1) 562
risk factors for, (V1) 350
Suicide
by adolescents, (V1) 190
assisted, (V1) 355–356
prevention of, interventions for, (V1) 283–284
risk for
cues indicating, (V1) 281*b*
in older adults with depression, (V1) 282
Summarizing conversation, in enhancing therapeutic communication, (V1) 475
Superego, in psychoanalytic theory of development, (V1) 165
Superficial reflexes, assessment of, (V1) 508
Superficial wounds, (V1) 902
Superinfections, (V1) 524
definition of, (V1) 528
Supine position, (V1) 839*b*, (V1) 840
Supplemental Nutrition Assistance Program (SNAP), (V1) 697
Supplement(s)
calcium, (V1) 1002
electrolyte, (V1) 1002, (V1) 1003
garlic
potassium, (V1) 1002
Suppliers, medical equipment, (V1) 22

Supplies. *See also* Equipment; Needle(s); Syringe(s)
potentially contaminated, control of, (V1) 536–538
providing healthcare industry with, (V1) 22
Support surfaces, in pressure ulcer prevention, (V1) 919
Support system(s)
adaptation and, (V1) 244
assessing, (V1) 255
for exercise, (V1) 827
identifying and using, in stress management, (V1) 260
Suppository(ies), (V1) 612*t*
rectal, (V1) 639
inserting, (V1) 657*p*, (V2) 428–429*p*
vaginal, (V1) 638
Suppressor T cells, in cellular immunity, (V1) 527, (V1) 527*f*
Suprapubic catheter, (V1) 730–731, (V1) 732*f*
Suprasternal retraction, in respiration, (V1) 445
Suprasystems, (V1) 289
Supraventricular dysrhythmia, (V1) 978
Surfactant, (V1) 936
Surgery
ablative, (V1) 1027
age and, (V1) 1028
alcohol use and, (V1) 1029
allergies and, (V1) 1029
body system classification of, (V1) 1027
bowel elimination and, (V1) 750
cardiovascular disease and, (V1) 1029*b*
checklists for, (V2) 842–843, (V2) 844
for children, (V1) 1028
cigarette smoking and, (V1) 1028
classification of, (V1) 1027–1028
coagulation disorders and, (V1) 1029*b*
complications of
nursing diagnosis for, (V1) 1042
postoperative, (V1) 1048–1051*t*
consent form for, (V1) 1034–1035
cosmetic, (V1) 1028
delayed recovery from, (V1) 1047, (V2) 854–855
diabetes mellitus and, (V1) 1029*b*
diagnostic (exploratory), (V1) 1027
elective, (V1) 1028
teaching for, (V1) 1036
emergency, (V1) 1028
teaching for, (V1) 1036
equipment counts in, (V1) 1044
fear and, (V1) 1032–1033, (V2) 846
hand hygiene for, (V1) 1026*b*
herbal preparations and, (V1) 1028–1029
infectious disorders and, (V1) 1029*b*
liver disease and, (V1) 1029*b*
major, (V1) 1028
medications and, (V1) 1028–1029, (V1) 1030*b*
mental status and, (V1) 1028
minor, (V1) 1028
neurological disorders and, (V1) 1029*b*
nursing before. *See* Preoperative nursing
nursing care after. *See* Postoperative nursing
nursing during. *See* Intraoperative nursing
nutritional disorders and, (V1) 1029*b*
for older adults, (V1) 1028, (V1) 1030, (V1) 1032, (V1) 1033, (V1) 1033*t*
antiembolism stockings and, (V1) 1038. *See also* Antiembolism stockings
evidence-based studies of, (V1) 1040
teaching about, (V1) 1036
palliative, (V1) 1027
personal habits and, (V1) 1029
preexisting conditions and, (V1) 1028
procurement, (V1) 1028
purpose classification of, (V1) 1027–1028
reconstructive, (V1) 1027
renal disease and, (V1) 1029*b*
respiratory disorders and, (V1) 1029*b*
risk classification of, (V1) 1028
risk factors and, (V1) 1028–1030
safety measures for, (V1) 1026–1027, (V1) 1038
sexuality and, (V1) 857
substance abuse and, (V1) 1029
teaching for
postoperative, (V1) 1052
preoperative, (V1) 1034, (V1) 1035–1036
transplant, (V1) 1028
two-minute briefings for, (V1) 1038
urgency classification of, (V1) 1028
urgent, (V1) 1028
urinary function and, (V1) 720
for wound healing, (V1) 920
wound infection with, (V1) 1028, (V1) 1029*t*
wrong patient, wrong site, wrong surgery check for, (V1) 1038
Surgical attire, donning, (V1) 540–541, (V1) 541*f*
Surgical glue, (V1) 906
Surgical handwashing, (V1) 539*p*
Surgical nursing unit, client transfer to, (V1) 1046. *See also* Postoperative nursing
Surgical scrub
hand hygiene compared with, (V1) 540*t*
performing, (V1) 540
Surgical staples, (V1) 905–906, (V1) 905*f*
removal of, (V1) 931*p*, (V2) 703–704*p*
Suspension, (V1) 610*t*
Sustained-release medications, (V1) 614
Suture(s), (V1) 905
removal of, (V1) 931*p*, (V2) 703–704*p*
Swab culture, (V1) 916, (V1) 929*p*, (V2) 673–675*p*
Swallowing, impaired
interventions for, (V1) 699
interventions for patients with, (V2) 515*p*
nutrition and, (V1) 689
Swallowing reflex, (V1) 173
Sweat glands, (V1) 579
in older adults, (V1) 580*t*
Swelling, wound-related, (V1) 914
SWOT (strengths, weaknesses, opportunities, threats) analysis, (V1) 1062, (V1) 1062*t*
Symbols, error-prone, (V2) 481*t*
Sympathectomy, for pain, (V1) 810
Sympathetic fibers, (V1) 970
Sympathetic nervous system, in stress response, (V1) 246
Symptoms, experiencing, (V1) 230
Synarthroses, (V1) 817
Synchronized intermittent mandatory ventilation, (V2) 752
Synchrony, (V1) 881
Syndactylism, (V1) 827
Syndrome nursing diagnosis, (V1) 66*t*
diagnostic statement for, (V1) 77
Synergistic drug relationship, (V1) 621
Synovial fluid, (V1) 818
Synovial joints, (V1) 818, (V1) 818*t*
range of motion testing for, (V2) 643–647
Syphilis, (V1) 863
Syphilitic chancre, (V2) 315*f*
Syringe(s), (V1) 641–643, (V1) 641*f*, (V1) 642*f*
for administering feedings through gastric and enteric tubes, (V2) 504–505*p*
disposable
prefilled, self-contained system, (V1) 642, (V1) 642*f*
for subcutaneous injection, (V1) 649
insulin, (V1) 642, (V1) 642*f*
mixing two kinds of insulin in, clinical insight on, (V2) 475–476*b*
parts of, (V1) 641*f*
prefilled unit-dose, (V1) 642, (V1) 642*f*
reusing, in home care, clinical insight on, (V2) 471*b*
safety, (V1) 642–643, (V1) 642*f*
standard, (V1) 642, (V1) 642*f*
tuberculin, (V1) 642, (V1) 642*f*
types of, (V1) 642–643, (V1) 642*f*, (V1) 643*f*
for wound irrigation, (V2) 675, (V2) 677
Syrup, (V1) 610*t*
System, definition of, (V1) 148
System theory, (V1) 148–149
Systemic circulation, (V1) 501
Systole, (V1) 436, (V1) 502, (V1) 969
Systolic pressure, (V1) 446

T

T binder, (V1) 929, (V1) 930–931*p*, (V2) 697*p*, (V2) 698–699*p*
T cells, (V1) 525
in cellular immunity, (V1) 526–527, (V1) 527*f*
T-piece, for oxygen therapy, (V2) 735
T wave, (V1) 978
Tablet, (V1) 610*t*
lipid-soluble, (V1) 611*t*
timed-release, (V1) 610*t*
Tachycardia, definition of, (V1) 440
Tachydysrhythmia, (V1) 975, (V1) 978
Tachypnea, (V1) 444*t*, (V1) 946
Tactile fremitus, chest palpation for, (V2) 262–263*p*
Taenia coli, (V1) 747
Talk test, (V1) 822*b*
Tandem setup, for intermittent infusions, (V1) 654
Tanner staging, (V2) 300
Tanning, (V1) 901
Taping
chest tube, (V2) 757
dressing, (V2) 678–680*p*
Target area, local blood flow in, drug distribution and, (V1) 615
Target heart rate, in exercise, (V1) 822*b*
Tartar, dental caries and, (V1) 592
Task focus, in leadership, (V1) 1058
Task groups, communication in, (V1) 471–472
Task *versus* relationship theories of leadership, (V1) 1058

Taste
bedside assessment of, (V2) 606
changes in, with aging, (V1) 774*t*
deficits in, (V1) 777–779, (V1) 778*b*
home care for, (V1) 787*b*
interventions for, (V1) 786
diminished sense of, impaired nutrition from, interventions for, (V1) 698
Tattoos, (V1) 901
adolescents and, (V1) 189
Taxonomy, definition of, (V1) 74
Taxonomy of Nursing Practice (NANDA-I/NOC/NIC), (V1) 55*t*
Taylor, Frederick, (V1) 1060
Teaching, (V1) 396–49, (V1) 396–419, (V2) 177–183. *See also* Education
adding medications to IV fluids, (V2) 458
administering feedings through gastric and enteric tubes, (V2) 505
administering lipids, (V2) 513
administering parenteral nutrition, (V2) 511
ambulation assistance, (V2) 634
apical pulse assessment, (V2) 196
apical-radial pulse deficit assessment, (V2) 198
artificial eye care, (V2) 397
bandaging, (V2) 702
barriers to, (V1) 406–407, (V1) 407*b*
bathing procedure, (V2) 368
bed monitoring device, (V2) 351
blood pressure measurement, (V2) 203
blood transfusion, (V2) 807
body function, (V1) 868–869
breast self-examination, (V1) 869–870, (V2) 259
brushing and flossing of teeth, (V2) 379
canes, (V2) 639
cardiac monitoring, (V2) 775
cardiopulmonary resuscitation, (V1) 981–982
checking fingerstick blood glucose levels, (V2) 496
chest tube, (V2) 759
collaborative patient partnership, (V1) 415*b*
colorectal cancer, (V2) 276
colostomy irrigation, (V2) 588
contact lens care, (V1) 598*b*, (V2) 391
contraception, (V1) 870, (V2) 654
coughing, (V1) 1054*p*, (V2) 826–827*p*, (V2) 829*p*
crutches, (V2) 639–640
deep breathing and coughing, (V1) 1054*p*, (V2) 826–827*p*, (V2) 829*p*
definition of, (V1) 398
digital stool removal, (V2) 580
documentation of, (V1) 419
douching, (V1) 869
drain shortening, (V2) 706
dry wound dressing, (V2) 682
effective, tips for, (V1) 410*b*
endotracheal suctioning, (V1) 748
enema administration, (V2) 578
fecal occult blood testing, (V2) 572
five rights of, (V1) 398*b*
fluid and electrolyte imbalance prevention, (V1) 1002
foot care, (V1) 589*b*
gastric suctioning, (V2) 838
goals of, (V1) 409
hair assessment, (V2) 234
hair shampooing, (V2) 387
Hands-Only CPR, (V1) 981–982
health promotion, (V1) 1108
hearing aid care, (V2) 400
hearing assessments, (V2) 249
heart disease, (V2) 270
heparin lock, (V2) 802
hydrating dressing, (V2) 694
incentive spirometry, (V1) 1053
indwelling catheter removal, (V2) 552
infection prevention, (V1) 530, (V1) 531–532*b*
infusion pump, (V2) 792
intermittent self-catheterization, (V2) 560
intradermal injection administration, (V2) 447
intravenous fluid/electrolyte administration, (V2) 788, (V2) 790
intravenous fluid/electrolyte discontinuation, (V2) 804
intravenous fluid/electrolyte dressing change, (V2) 799
intravenous fluid/electrolyte solution/tubing change, (V2) 795
IV push medications, (V2) 462
knowledge map for, (V2) 183
laxative use, (V1) 760*b*
leg exercises, (V1) 1054*p*, (V2) 826–827*p*, (V2) 828–829*p*
lung cancer prevention, (V2) 264
mechanical ventilation, (V2) 754
medication administration, (V2) 413
cutaneous, (V2) 430–432
nasal, (V2) 425
ophthalmic, (V2) 421
to self, (V1) 630
vaginal, (V2) 427
medication administration through central venous access device, (V2) 470
menopause, (V1) 869
menstruation, (V1) 869
metered-dose inhaler administration, (V2) 434
moving in bed, (V2) 627*p*
by client, (V2) 826–827*p*, (V2) 827–828*p*, (V2) 829*p*
moving out of bed, (V2) 631
nail care, (V1) 590*b*
nasogastric and nasoenteric tubes, (V2) 501
nasopharyngeal suctioning, (V2) 751
nasotracheal suctioning, (V2) 748
neck assessment, (V2) 256
nutritious food on limited budget, (V1) 698*b*
oral care for unconscious patient, (V2) 384
oral hygiene, (V1) 593–594*b*
oral medication administration, (V2) 417
oropharyngeal suctioning, (V2) 751
orotracheal suctioning, (V2) 748
ostomy appliance changing, (V2) 585
otic irrigation, (V2) 602
oxygen therapy, (V2) 732
pain management, (V1) 812
passive range of motion, (V2) 638
patient-controlled analgesia, (V2) 613
percussion therapy, (V2) 730
perineal care, (V2) 373
peripheral pulse assessment, (V2) 194
planning outcomes for, (V1) 408–409
plans for
content in, (V1) 410
creating, (V1) 410–416
example of, (V1) 411–413
instructional materials in, (V1) 410
scheduling and sequencing in, (V1) 410
strategies in, (V1) 410
selecting, (V1) 414–416
position change, (V2) 627
postural drainage, (V2) 730
premenstrual syndrome, (V1) 869
preoperative, (V1) 1034, (V1) 1035–1036, (V2) 839
preparing for pandemic disease outbreak, 544*b*, (V1) 543
pressure ulcer prevention, (V1) 920
pulse oximetry, (V2) 728
rectal suppository insertion, (V2) 429
rectal tube insertion, (V2) 582
removing nasogastric and nasoenteric tubes, (V2) 507
reproduction, (V1) 868–869
respiration assessment, (V2) 199
responsibilities for, (V1) 397–398
restraint use, (V2) 354
saline lock, (V2) 802
of self-care for hypertension, (V1) 455, (V1) 456*b*
self-monitoring of blood pressure, (V1) 450–451*b*
sensory perceptual health, (V1) 783*b*
sequential compression device, (V2) 833
sexual health, (V1) 868–870
sexual predator precautions, (V1) 862
shaving techniques, (V2) 390
skin assessment, (V2) 229
skin closures, (V2) 696
sleep hygiene, (V1) 894, (V1) 895
special. *See* Special teaching
sputum collection, (V2) 726
sterile gown and glove procedure, (V2) 330
subcutaneous injection administration, (V2) 449
suture/staple removal, (V2) 704
taping dressing, (V2) 678–680
temperature assessment, (V2) 190
testicular self-examination, (V1) 870
tracheostomy care, (V2) 740
tracheostomy suctioning, (V2) 745
transparent film dressing, (V2) 692
upper respiratory infection prevention, (V1) 1108*b*
upper respiratory tract infection prevention, (V1) 951–953
urinary tract infection prevention, (V1) 729*b*
urine bedside testing, (V2) 539
urine output recording, (V2) 533
urine specimen collection, (V2) 537
vibration therapy, (V2) 730
walker, (V2) 639
wet-to-damp dressing, (V2) 685
wound healing, (V1) 920
wound irrigation, (V2) 678
Team nursing, (V1) 15
Technetium scan, (V2) 767
Technicians, power of, (V1) 1066
Technologist, on healthcare team, (V1) 19
Technology
culture and, (V1) 309–310
ethical issues for nurses and, (V1) 1142

TED hose. *See* Antiembolism stockings
Teens. *See* Adolescent(s)
Telehealth, (V1) 1082, (V1) 1082*f*
in self-management of chronic illness, (V1) 228*b*
Telemetry, for cardiac monitoring, (V2) 775
Telephone counseling, in health promotion, (V1) 1107–1108
Telephone orders
documentation of, (V1) 391–392
taking, (V2) 164
Telephone prescriptions, (V1) 624
Temperature, (V1) 422–436
assessment of, (V1) 427–431, (V1) 428*p*, (V2) 185–190*p*
axillary, (V2) 186*p*
delegation of, (V2) 185
documentation of, (V2) 190
equipment for, (V1) 428–430, (V2) 185*f*. *See also* Thermometer(s)
home care for, (V2) 190
oral, (V2) 186–187*p*
patient teaching on, (V2) 190
rectal, (V2) 187–188*p*
sites for, (V1) 430–431, (V1) 432–433*t*
skin, using chemical strip thermometer, (V2) 189*p*
temporal artery, (V2) 188*p*
tympanic membrane, (V2) 188–189*p*
basal metabolic rate and, (V1) 680
behavioral control of, (V1) 423–424
Centigrade-Fahrenheit conversion chart for, (V2) 206
for client environment, (V1) 602
core, (V1) 423
decreasing, (V1) 423
definition of, (V1) 422
developmental level and, (V1) 425
elevated. *See* Fever
evidence-based practice on, (V1) 435–436
factors influencing, (V1) 425–427
in fluid and electrolyte assessment, (V1) 999
imbalanced, risk for
intraoperative, (V1) 1043, (V2) 848
nursing diagnoses for, (V1) 431
increasing, (V1) 423
interventions for, (V1) 431, (V1) 433–435
measurement scales for, (V1) 427
normal, (V1) 423, (V1) 423*f*
nursing diagnoses related to, (V1) 431
outcomes for, (V1) 431
pathogen growth and, (V1) 520
preoperative maintenance of, (V1) 1036
regulation of, (V1) 423–424
Temperature (ambient)
cardiovascular effects of, (V1) 972
pulmonary effects of, (V1) 941
Temporal artery temperature, (V2) 188*p*
Temporal pulse, assessment of, (V2) 194*p*
Temporomandibular joint (TMJ) syndrome, (V1) 493
Tendons, (V1) 818
TENS (transcutaneous electrical nerve stimulation), (V1) 802
Teratogens, (V1) 171
Terminal evaluation, (V1) 131
Terminal hair, (V1) 595
Termination phase, of therapeutic relationship, communication in, (V1) 470
Terminology, standardized. *See* Standardized nursing languages
Territoriality
communication and, (V1) 466
culture and, (V1) 308
Tertiary healing, (V1) 903, (V1) 904*f*
Testes, palpation of, (V2) 298–299*p*
Testicular cancer screening, in health promotion assessment, (V2) 876
Testicular self-examination (TSE), (V1) 870, (V2) 68*p*
by adolescents, interventions for, (V1) 194
Testis (testes), (V1) 849, (V1) 950*f*
Tetanus immunization, wound assessment and, (V1) 916
Text messaging, (V1) 1080–1081
Textbooks, (V1) 1090
Theology, (V1) 327
Theoretical knowledge, (V1) 37
in diagnostic reasoning, (V1) 72
in full-spectrum nursing, (V1) 40*t*, (V1) 41
Theory(ies). *See also* Nursing theory(ies)
developmental, (V1) 148, (V1) 165–170, (V1) 166–167*t*. *See also* Development, theories of
influencing intervention selection, (V1) 107–108
leadership, (V1) 1057–1059
management, (V1) 1059–1060
non-nursing, use of, (V1) 146–149
practical knowledge about, (V1) 149–150
stress and adaptation, (V1) 148
system, (V1) 148–149
Theory X, (V1) 1060
Theory Y, (V1) 1060
validation, (V1) 148
Theory X managers, (V1) 1060
Theory Y managers, (V1) 1060
Therapeutic bath, (V1) 584, (V1) 932, (V1) 932*f*, (V2) 708, (V2) 709
Therapeutic communication
assessment of, (V1) 472
barriers to, (V1) 475–478
characteristics of, (V1) 470–471
definition of, (V1) 469
in end-of-life care, (V1) 363
enhancing, interventions for, (V1) 473–475
interventions for, planning, (V1) 473–475
nursing diagnoses related to, (V1) 472–473
Therapeutic relationships, (V1) 469–478
limits and boundaries of, (V1) 470*b*
skills needed in, (V1) 471*b*
Therapeutic touch, for pain, (V1) 803
Therapists, on healthcare team, (V1) 19
Therapy groups, communication in, (V1) 472
Thermal stimuli, (V1) 793
Thermogenesis, nonshivering, (V1) 424
Thermography, breast, (V1) 498
in older adult assessment, (V1) 213
Thermometer(s)
chemical strip, (V1) 429–430, (V1) 430*t*
skin temperature using, (V2) 189*p*
electronic, (V1) 428–429, (V1) 429*t*
infrared, (V1) 429, (V1) 430*t*
glass, (V1) 428, (V1) 429*t*
Thermoreceptors, (V1) 772
Thermoregulation, (V1) 423–424
ineffective, nursing diagnoses for, (V1) 431
in neonate, (V1) 173
Theta waves, (V1) 883
Thiamin, (V1) 674*t*
Thiazide diuretics, (V1) 719*b*
Thinking
critical, (V1) 5. *See* Critical thinking
in diagnostic reasoning, (V1) 73
in full-spectrum nursing, (V1) 40–41, (V1) 40*f*, (V1) 40*t*
independent, (V1) 32
Thinking processes, complex, (V1) 3*b*
Third spacing, (V1) 984
Thirst, (V1) 987
Thoracentesis. *See also* Chest tube
Thought processes, assessing, (V2) 286*p*
Thrills, (V1) 502
Throat, (V1) 935
Throat culture, (V2) 767
Thrombophlebitis
intravenous therapy and, (V1) 1014*t*
postoperative, (V1) 1049*t*
sequential compress device prevention of, (V1) 1054*p*, (V2) 832–833*p*
Thrombus prevention, (V1) 980
Throughput, in systems theory, (V1) 148
Thrush, (V1) 497
Thumb, range of motion of, (V2) 645
Thyroid gland, assessment of, (V1) 498, (V2) 256*p*
Thyroid hormone, (V1) 988
Thyroid-stimulating hormone (TSH), in stress response, (V1) 245
Thyroxine, basal metabolic rate and, (V1) 424
Ticks, avoiding, (V1) 565
Tidal volume, (V1) 444, (V2) 752, (V2) 766
Time
lack of, urinary function and, (V1) 718
management of, (V1) 1073–1075, (V1) 1075*b*, (V1) 1075*t*
Time inventory, (V1) 1074
Time management, in stress management, (V1) 257
Time orientation
culture and, (V1) 308–309
in neurological assessment, (V1) 507
Timed-release medications, (V1) 614
Timed Up & Go Test, (V2) 357*p*
Timing
for learning, (V1) 401
in verbal communication, (V1) 462
Tincture, (V1) 610*t*
Tinea pedis, (V1) 587
Tinnitus, definition of, (V1) 778*f*
Tissue(s)
impaired integrity of, (V1) 917
risk for, (V1) 917
ineffective perfusion of, (V1) 979, (V1) 1046
risk for, (V1) 979
in wounds, (V1) 915, (V1) 915*t*
Tissue biopsy, (V1) 916
Tissue growth factors, for wound healing, (V1) 920
TMJ (temporomandibular joint) syndrome, (V1) 493
Tobacco use. *See* Cigarette smoking
Toddler(s), (V1) 179–182
airway obstruction in, (V1) 939
assessment of, (V1) 181
car safety seats for, (V1) 566*t*
communication by, (V1) 465

development of
cognitive, (V1) 168*t*, (V1) 180
physical, (V1) 179–180, (V1) 180*b*, (V1) 180*f*
psychosexual, (V1) 167*t*
psychosocial, (V1) 168, (V1) 180–181
developmental tasks of, (V1) 166*t*
drowning in, (V1) 939
health problems of, 181
health promotion for, (V1) 1101*t*
immunizations for, (V1) 181
infections in, (V1) 181
interventions for, (V1) 181–182
nutrition for, (V1) 683
physical examination of, (V1) 486
pulmonary system of, (V1) 939
safety needs of, (V1) 547
sexuality of, (V1) 853
sleep for, (V1) 881, (V1) 881*t*, (V1) 885
surgical risks for, (V1) 1028
toilet training delays in, (V1) 181
unintentional injury to, (V1) 181
Toenail, ingrown, (V1) 587
Toes, range of motion in, (V2) 647
Toilet training, delayed, in toddler, (V1) 181
Tolerance
to drugs, (V1) 621
exercise, (V1) 833, (V2) 642
opioids, (V1) 806
pain, 794
Tone, vascular, (V1) 970
Tongue, assessment of, (V1) 497, (V2) 253–254*p*
Tonic neck reflex, (V1) 174, (V1) 174*f*
Tonicity, (V1) 985
Tooth (teeth)
assessment of, (V1) 497, (V2) 253*p*
brushing and flossing, (V1) 600*p*, (V2) 377–380*p*
decay of
baby-bottle, (V1) 591
in infant, (V1) 177
deciduous, (V1) 590, (V1) 590*f*
developmental variations in, (V1) 590–591, (V1) 590*f*, (V1) 591*f*
grinding of, (V1) 890
primary, eruption of, (V1) 176
problems of, (V1) 591
nutrition and, (V1) 689
wisdom, (V1) 590
Topical anesthesia, (V1) 810
Topical anesthetic, (V1) 1041
Topical medication administration, (V1) 636–639
inhalation in, (V1) 612*t*
instillations for, (V1) 612*t*
skin, (V1) 611*t*, (V1) 657*p*, (V2) 430–432*p*
Tort(s)
intentional, (V1) 1172–1173
quasi-intentional, (V1) 1172
unintentional, (V1) 1174–1176
Tort law, (V1) 1172–1176
Total body water, (V1) 984, (V1) 984*t*
Touch
bedside assessment of, (V2) 606
changes in, with aging, (V1) 774*t*
deficits in
home care for, (V1) 787*b*
interventions for, (V2) 786–787
impaired sense of, (V1) 779
in nonverbal communication, (V1) 464, (V1) 464f
sense of, in neonate, (V1) 174
shared, (V1) 861
for spirituality diagnoses, (V1) 340
stimulation of, for sensory deprivation, (V1) 784
Touch therapies, in stress management, (V1) 259
Towel bath, (V1) 583, (V2) 369–370*p*
Toxic fumes, (V1) 941
Toxic reactions, to medications, (V1) 620
Toxins
take-home, (V1) 550
prevention of, (V1) 564
workplace, (V1) 941
Trachea, (V1) 935, (V1) 936*f*
suctioning of, (V1) 964–965*p*, (V2) 741–745*p*
Tracheostomy, (V1) 957, (V2) 736–741*p*
clinical insight on, (V2) 763
dislodgement of, (V2) 740
patient and family involvement in care of, (V1) 959
stabilizer removal from, (V2) 739
suctioning of, (V1) 960, (V1) 964–965*p*, (V2) 741–745*p*
Tracheostomy collar, (V2) 735
Tracheostomy stabilizers, removal of, (V2) 739
Tracheostomy tubes, (V1) 958, (V2) 736, (V2) 740
Tradition, in gaining knowledge, (V1) 152
Traditional healing, 314*t*, (V1) 313–315
Trait theory, of leadership, (V1) 1057–1058
Tranquilizers, surgery and, (V1) 1030*b*
Trans-fatty acids, (V1) 673
Transactional theory of leadership, (V1) 1059, (V1) 1059*t*
Transcellular fluid, (V1) 984
Transcendence of self, (V1) 148
Transcultural assessment model, for cultural assessment, (V2) 130
Transcutaneous electrical nerve stimulation (TENS), (V1) 802
Transdermal medication/patch, (V1) 611*t*, (V1) 637, (V1) 637*f*
application of, (V2) 431–432*p*
Transduction, of pain, (V1) 793
Transfer, client
to another unit, (V1) 237*p*, (V2) 80–81*p*
to long-term care facility, (V1) 237*p*, (V2) 81–82*p*
maintaining trust during, (V1) 236
operative suite, (V1) 1038–1039
postanesthesia care unit, (V1) 1045, (V1) 1045*f*, (V1) 1046
surgical nursing unit, (V1) 1046
Transfer belt, (V1) 843, (V1) 843*f*
Transfer board, (V1) 841, (V1) 841*f*
Transfer needles, (V1) 653, (V1) 653*f*
Transfer report, (V1) 390–391
Transfer roller sheet, (V1) 840, (V1) 840*f*
Transferrin, serum levels of, nutritional levels and, (V1) 695
Transformational theory, of leadership, (V1) 1059, (V1) 1059*t*
Transfusion reaction, (V1) 1021*t*, (V2) 807*p*
Transgendered identity, (V1) 851
Transillumination, of sinuses, (V2) 251*p*
Transitional cells, urinary, (V2) 563
Translators, (V1) 433, (V2) 128
Transmission
mode of, in chain of infection, (V1) 519*f*, (V1) 521
of pain, (V1) 793–794, (V1) 793*f*
Transmission-based precautions, (V1) 535
following, clinical insight on, (V2) 339–341
Transmucosal administration of drugs, (V1) 611*t*
Transparent film dressing, (V1) 927*t*, (V1) 928*f*, (V1) 930*p*, (V2) 690–692*p*, (V2) 787*p*, (V2) 797*p*
Transpersonal caring moments, (V1) 149–150
Transplant surgery, (V1) 1028
Transsexuality, (V1) 851–852
Transtheoretical model of change, (V1) 1099
Transtracheal catheter, (V1) 957
Transvestite, (V1) 852
Trapeze bar, (V1) 836–837
Trauma. *See* Injury(ies)
exercise and bone, (V1) 828–829
Treadmill test, (V2) 767
Treatment failure, as health disruption, (V1) 230
Tremor, (V1) 833*b*
Triage, telehealth for, (V1) 1082, (V1) 1082*f*
Trial and error, in gaining knowledge, (V1) 152
Trial process, in litigation, (V1) 1176
Triangles, anterior and posterior, (V1) 497
Triangular arm binder/sling, (V1) 928, (V1) 930–931*p*, (V2) 697*p*, (V2) 698*p*, (V2) 699*p*
Triceps reflex, testing, (V2) 293*p*
Tricyclic antidepressants
for sleep, (V1) 895
urinary retention from, (V1) 722*b*
Trigeminal nerve (V), testing, (V2) 289*p*
Trimesters, fetal development by, (V1) 170
Trochanter rolls, (V1) 837, (V2) 636
Troche, (V1) 611*t*
Trochlear nerve (IV) testing, (V2) 288*p*
Troponin, (V2) 767
Trousseau's sign, (V2) 810
Trunk, range of motion of, (V2) 647
Trust
establishing
for enhancing therapeutic communication, (V1) 474
in health promotion, (V1) 235–236
maintaining during transitions, in health promotion, (V1) 236
versus mistrust stage of psychosocial development, (V1) 168
TSE. *See* Testicular self-examination (TSE)
Tub bath, (V1) 584, (V1) 585*f*
assisting with, clinical insights on, (V2) 401
Tubal ligation, (V2) 656
Tube(s)
feeding. *See* Feeding tube(s)
rectal, inserting, (V1) 769*p*, (V2) 581–582*p*
Tuberculin skin testing, (V1) 947–948, (V2) 768
Tuberculin syringe, (V1) 642, (V1) 642*f*
Tubular reabsorption, (V1) 716
Tubular secretion, (V2) 716
Tunnel wound, (V1) 902*t*, (V1) 914
Tunneled central venous catheters, (V1) 1007, (V1) 1008*f*
24-hour recall, in nutritional assessment, (V1) 692
24-hour urine specimen, (V1) 734
collection of, (V1) 733*p*, (V2) 536–537*p*

Twitter, (V1) 1081
Two-minute briefings, (V1) 1038
Two-point discrimination, in testing tactile perception, (V1) 779
Tympanic membrane, (V1) 496, (V1) 599
Tympanic membrane temperature, (V2) 188–189*p*
Tympanites, (V1) 1050*t*

U

U wave, (V1) 978
Ulcer(s), (V2) 232
  aphthous, (V1) 497
  arterial, (V1) 903*t*, (V1) 909
  diabetic foot, (V1) 909
  duodenal, sleep and, (V1) 891
  foot, diabetic, (V1) 909
  gastric, sleep and, (V1) 891
  intestinal, sleep and, (V1) 891
  pressure, (V1) 581. *See* Pressure ulcer(s)
  venous stasis, (V1) 903*t*, (V1) 909
Ultrasonic nebulizer, (V1) 639
Ultrasonography
  in GI tract study, (V2) 595
  in urinary system assessment, (V2) 564
Ultrasound therapy, for wound healing, (V1) 920
Umbilical hernia, (V1) 510
  assessment for, (V2) 273*p*
Unauthorized practice, reporting regulations on, (V1) 1184
Unconscious client
  eye care for, (V1) 598
  interventions for, (V1) 789
  oral care for, (V1) 594, (V1) 600*p*, (V2) 382–384*p*
  positioning of, (V1) 1046
Unconscious mind, in psychoanalytic theory of development, (V1) 165
Undermining, of wound, (V1) 914
Underwater weighing, in body composition assessment, (V1) 694
Underweight/undernutrition, (V1) 703–713. *See also* Malnutrition
  interventions for, (V1) 704–713
    enteral nutrition as, (V1) 705–711. *See also* Enteral nutrition
    parenteral nutrition as, 713, (V1) 711. *See also* Parenteral nutrition (PN)
  nursing outcomes for, (V1) 704
Undifferentiated sexual state, (V1) 852
Unemployment, as family health risk, (V1) 292–293
Uniform Determination of Death Act, (V1) 351, (V1) 352*b*
Unintentional torts, (V1) 1174–1176
Unit-dose system, for medication storage and distribution, (V1) 608, (V1) 608*f*
Unit-dose systems for medications, (V1) 608, (V2) 608*f*
  prefilled, clinical insight on, (V2) 472*b*
Unit system for medication measurement, (V1) 622, (V2) 482
United States Department of Agriculture (USDA), dietary guidelines of, (V1) 665, (V1) 665*b*
United States Pharmacopoeia (USP), (V1) 606
United States Public Health Service (USPHS), goals of, (V1) 100–101
Unknown, as health disruption, (V1) 229
Unresponsiveness, full outline of, (V2) 296
Upper respiratory infections (URIs), (V1) 939, (V1) 943–944, (V1) 951–952
  obesity and, (V1) 941
  prevention of, (V1) 951–953
Urea, serum levels of, protein metabolism and, (V1) 695
Ureterostomy, cutaneous, (V1) 738
Ureters, in urine transport, (V1) 716–717
Urethra, in urine transport, (V1) 717
Urethral glands, palpation of, (V2) 302–303*p*
Urethral meatus, inspection of, (V2) 302*p*
Urethral meatus plug, for urinary incontinence, (V1) 737
Urethral sphincter
  external, (V1) 717
  internal, (V1) 717
Urethritis, (V1) 720
Urgency, definition of, (V1) 725*b*
Urgent surgery, (V1) 1028
Urinal, urine output measurement from, (V2) 532*p*
Urinalysis
  findings in, (V2) 562–563
  in fluid/electrolyte assessment, (V1) 1001
  preoperative, (V2) 845
Urinary bladder, in urine storage, (V1) 717
Urinary catheter. *See* Catheter(s), urinary
Urinary catheterization
  intermittent, (V2) 540–543*p*
  for urinary retention, (V1) 730–732, (V1) 734*p*
Urinary diversion(s)
  caring for patents with, (V1) 738–739, (V2) 559
  interventions for patients with, (V1) 739
  types of, (V1) 738, (V1) 738*f*, (V1) 739*f*
Urinary elimination, (V1) 714–743, (V2) 530–568
  assessment of, (V1) 723–726
    blood studies in, (V1) 726, (V2) 563
    diagnostic procedures in, (V1) 726
    nursing history in, (V1) 723, (V2) 561
    physical assessment in, (V1) 723, (V2) 561–562*p*
    urine assessment in, (V1) 723–726, (V2) 562–563
  factors affecting, (V1) 718–723
    activity level as, (V1) 719
    anesthesia as, (V1) 720
    developmental, (V1) 718
    environmental, (V1) 718–719
    hydration as, (V1) 719
    medications as, (V1) 719, (V1) 719*b*
    nutritional, (V1) 719
    pathological, (V1) 720
    personal, (V1) 718–719
    sociocultural, (V1) 718–719
    surgery as, (V1) 720
  interventions for, (V1) 727–732
  nursing diagnoses related to, (V1) 727
  outcomes for, (V1) 727
Urinary incontinence, (V1) 722–723
  behavioral interventions for, (V1) 736
  biofeedback for, (V1) 736
  bladder training for, (V1) 736
  caring for patients with, (V2) 558–559
  cognitive changes and, (V1) 720
  complementary alternative methods for, (V1) 737
  devices for, (V1) 738
  established, (V1) 722
  functional, (V1) 723
  lifestyle modification for, (V1) 736
  managing, (V1) 728*b*
  medications for, (V1) 719, (V1) 738
  mixed, (V1) 722
  nursing interventions for, (V1) 736–739
  overflow, (V1) 722
  pelvic floor muscle rehabilitation for, (V1) 736
  perineal skin care in, (V1) 736
  pressure ulcer prevention and, (V1) 918
  reflex, (V1) 723
  sacral nerve stimulation for, (V1) 737, (V1) 738
  scheduled voiding for, (V1) 736
  stress, (V1) 722
    care map for, (V1) 743
    nursing care plan for, (V1) 740–742
  supportive interventions for, (V1) 736
  surgical treatment for, (V1) 738
  transient, (V1) 722
  treatments for, (V1) 737–738
  types of, (V1) 722–723
  urge, (V1) 722
  vaginal weight training for, (V1) 736
Urinary meatus, (V1) 717
Urinary retention, (V1) 721–722
  interventions for, (V1) 729–732, (V1) 735
  medications associated with, (V1) 722*b*
Urinary system
  in alarm stage, of stress response, (V1) 246
  direct visualization studies of, (V2) 564
  exercise effects on, (V1) 824*b*
  functions of, (V1) 715–717
  indirect visualization studies of, (V2) 564–565
  organs of, (V1) 715
Urinary tract infections (UTIs), (V1) 720–721
  with indwelling catheters, prevention of, (V1) 732, (V1) 735
  postoperative, (V1) 1050*t*
  preventing, client teaching on, (V1) 729*b*
  recognizing and treating, (V1) 721
  risk factors for, (V1) 720–721
  urinary function and, (V1) 720
Urination, (V1) 717
  assessment of, intake/output measurement in, (V2) 810–811
  fluid loss with, (V1) 987
  knowledge map on, (V2) 568
  normal, promoting, (V1) 727–729
  normal patterns of, (V1) 717
  postoperative retention of, (V1) 1050*t*, (V2) 854
  terms associated with, (V1) 725*b*
Urine
  assessment of, (V1) 723–726
    dipstick testing in, (V1) 725, (V1) 733*p*, (V2) 538*p*
    intake and output measurement in, (V1) 723–724, (V1) 733*p*
    obtaining samples for urine studies in, (V1) 724–725, (V1) 733*p*, (V2) 534–538*p*
    routine urinalysis in, (V1) 725–726
    specific gravity in, (V1) 726, (V1) 733–734*p*, (V2) 538–539*p*, (V2) 562

formation of, nephrons in, (V1) 715–716, (V1) 716*f*
normal, characteristics of, (V1) 717–718
osmolality of, (V1) 1001
output of, (V1) 987
measuring, from bedpan or urinal, (V2) 532*p*
specific gravity of, normal, imbalances in, 995*t*
specimens of. *See* Specimen(s), urine
storage of, bladder in, (V1) 717
transport of, (V1) 716–717
Urobilinogen, urinary, (V2) 563
Urostomy, caring for patients with, (V1) 738–739
U.S. drug legislation, (V1) 606
Uterus, (V1) 849*f*
removal of, sexuality and, (V1) 857
Utilitarianism, (V1) 1147–1148
Utilization review, documentation in, (V1) 373

V

Vaccines, for influenza, (V1) 952
Vacuum-assisted wound closure, (V1) 919, (V2) 687*p*
Vagina, (V1) 848, (V1) 849*f*
introitus of, inspection of, (V2) 302*p*
involuntary closure of, (V1) 855–856
medication administration into, (V1) 638–639, (V2) 426–427*p*
muscle tone of, assessment of, (V2) 303*p*
surgery on, urinary function and, (V1) 720
Vaginal douche, teaching for, (V1) 869
Vaginal ring, (V2) 655
Vaginal weight training, for urinary incontinence, (V1) 736
Vaginismus, (V1) 865
Vagus nerve (X) testing, (V2) 290*p*
Validating message, for enhancing therapeutic communication, (V1) 474
Validation, of data for assessment, (V1) 53
Validation theory, (V1) 148
Validity
of evaluation criterion, (V1) 130
of research study, (V1) 158
Value(s), (V2) 897–904
clarification of, (V1) 1155, (V1) 1156*t*
definition of, (V1) 1143–1144
ethics and, (V1) 1144
moral decisions and, (V1) 1143–1144
nursing, behaviors and, (V1) 1146–1147*t*
professional *versus* personal, (V1) 1144–1145
transmission of, (V1) 1145, (V1) 1147*t*
Value neutrality, (V1) 1145
Value set, (V1) 1144
Value system, (V1) 1144
personal, (V1) 1144–1145
Valves, heart
abnormalities of, (V1) 975
Vancomycin-resistant *Enterococci*, (V1) 523
Vascular response, in inflammatory process, (V1) 247
Vascular system. *See also* Artery(ies); Vein(s)
assessment of, (V1) 503–504, (V1) 514*p*, (V2) 265–271*p*
central vessels of, (V1) 503–504, (V1) 503*f*
peripheral vessels of, (V1) 504
autonomic nervous system effects on, (V1) 970–971
peripheral, abnormalities of, (V1) 975
Vasectomy, (V2) 656
Vasocongestion, (V1) 859
Vasoconstriction, in increasing temperature, (V1) 423
Vasodilation, in decreasing temperature, (V1) 423
Vasodilators, (V1) 974*t*, (V1) 981
Vasomoter center, (V1) 971
Vastus lateralis muscle injection site, (V1) 651, (V1) 651*f*, (V1) 659*p*, (V2) 452*p*
Vector in infection transmission, (V1) 521
Vectorborne pathogens, (V1) 551
avoiding, (V1) 565
Vegans, (V1) 686
Vegetarianism, nutrition and, (V1) 686–687, (V1) 688*f*
Vegetative state, persistent, (V1) 352
Vein(s), (V1) 969
access to. *See* Central venous access device; Intravenous *entries;* Venipuncture
jugular, (V1) 504
auscultation of, (V2) 268*p*
peripheral, (V1) 504
Vellus hair, (V1) 595
Venipuncture, for intravenous fluid and electrolyte administration, (V2) 785, (V2) 812
Venous return, promotion of, (V1) 980
Venous star, (V2) 313*f*
Venous stasis
immobility with, (V1) 831
ulcers with, (V1) 903*t*, (V1) 909
Ventilation. *See also* Lung(s); Mechanical ventilation; Pulmonary system; Respiration(s)
for client environment, (V1) 602
impaired, (V1) 951
problems with, (V1) 951
pulmonary, (V1) 936–938
adequacy of, (V1) 937
in older adults, (V1) 940
position for, (V1) 946
Ventilator-associated pneumonia, (V1) 961
evidence-based studies of, (V1) 961
rate of, improving, (V1) 531*b*
Ventilator-perfusion scan, (V2) 767
Ventilators, (V1) 960, (V1) 960*f*
Ventricles, (V1) 968, (V1) 968*f*
Ventricular dysrhythmia, (V1) 978
Ventrogluteal muscle injection site, (V1) 650, (V1) 650*f*, (V1) 658*p*, (V2) 451*p*
Venturi mask, for oxygen therapy, (V2) 734
Venules, (V1) 969
Veracity
as ethical concept, (V1) 1151
in resolving dilemma, (V1) 1158
Verbal communication, (V1) 461–463. *See* Communication, verbal
Verbal orders
documentation of, (V1) 392
taking, (V2) 164
Verbal prescriptions, (V1) 624
Vernix caseosa, (V1) 899
in neonate, (V1) 173
Vesicles, (V2) 230, (V2) 312*f*
Vesicular breath sounds, (V1) 500, (V1) 501*f*, (V2) 264
Vestigial organ, appendix as, (V1) 746
Vial(s), (V1) 643*f*
drawing up medications from, (V1) 643, (V1) 657*p*, (V2) 437–439*p*
mixing medication from ampule and, (V2) 441*p*
single-dose, and prefilled cartridge for IV administration, (V2) 442*p*
two, mixing medication from, (V2) 439–440*p*
Vibration, chest, (V1) 955, (V2) 728–730*p*
Vicarious liability, (V1) 1175–1176
Villi, in small intestine, (V1) 746
Violence
domestic, (V1) 864–865. *See also* Abuse; Domestic abuse
in healthcare facility, coping with, (V1) 571–572
risk factors for, assessing, (V1) 558
sexual, (V1) 864
toward adolescent, (V1) 191
toward healthcare workers, (V1) 556–557
toward infant, (V1) 177
toward middle adult, (V1) 198
toward preschooler, (V1) 183–184
toward school-age child, intervention for, (V1) 188
toward young adult, (V1) 195
Virchow's triad, (V1) 831
Virtual learning, (V1) 1081–1082
Virulence of organisms, (V1) 519
Visceral pain, (V1) 791
Viscosity, blood, in blood pressure regulation, (V1) 447
Vision. *See also* Eye(s)
bedside assessment of, (V2) 606
changes in, with aging, (V1) 774*t*
color, (V1) 494
testing of, (V2) 239*p*
deficits in
home care for, (V1) 787*b*
interventions for, (V1) 785
distance, testing of, (V1) 494, (V2) 238*p*
impaired, (V1) 777, (V1) 777*b*
communicating with clients with, (V2) 604
near, testing of, (V1) 494, (V2) 239*p*
of neonate, (V1) 174
in oldest-old, (V1) 206
peripheral, (V1) 495
testing of, (V2) 240*p*
stimulation of, for sensory deprivation, (V1) 784
Vision screening
for preschooler, (V1) 184
for school-age child, (V1) 187
Visual acuity, (V1) 494
of school-age child, (V1) 185
Visual Analog Scale, for pain, (V2) 617
Visual fields, testing of, (V1) 494–495
Visual stimuli, control of, for sensory overload, (V1) 784
Visualization, in stress management, (V1) 259
Vital capacity, (V2) 767
Vital signs, (V1) 420–457, (V2) 184–209. *See also* Blood pressure; Pulse; Respiration(s); Temperature
assessment of, (V1) 422
average, for adults, (V1) 422*t*
definition of, (V1) 421–422
delegating, (V1) 457

documentation of, (V1) 422
evaluating, (V1) 457
in fluid/electrolyte balance assessment, (V1) 999–1000
graphic flowsheet for, (V2) 205
knowledge map for, (V2) 209
knowledge map on, (V2) 209
in older adult assessment, (V1) 212
pain as, (V1) 798–799
in physical examination, (V1) 488
postoperative, (V1) 1046
Vitamin(s), (V1) 673–676
fat-soluble, (V1) 673, (V1) 676
adult dietary reference intakes for, (V1) 674*t*
for infants, (V1) 682
supplemental, (V1) 696–697
water-soluble, (V1) 676
adult dietary reference intakes for, (V1) 674–676*t*
Vitamin A, (V1) 674*t*
Vitamin B_6, (V1) 675*t*
Vitamin B_{12}, (V1) 675*t*
in ovo-lacto vegetarian diet, (V1) 686
Vitamin C, (V1) 676*t*, (V1) 952
for common cold, (V1) 952
skin and, (V1) 899
Vitamin D, (V1) 674*t*, (V1) 827
deficiency of, (V1) 827
formation of, skin in, (V1) 579
in ovo-lacto vegetarian diet, (V1) 686
recommended daily intake of, (V1) 992*t*
Vitamin E, (V1) 674*t*
Vitamin K, (V1) 674*t*
Vitiligo, (V2) 312*f*
Vocabulary, in verbal communication, (V1) 461
Vocational nursing education, (V1) 10
Voiding, (V1) 717
scheduled, for urinary incontinence, (V1) 736, (V2) 558
Voiding reflex center, (V1) 717
Volume-control infusion sets, (V1) 654, (V1) 655*f*
administering medication by intermittent infusion using, (V2) 464*p*
for fluid and electrolytes, (V2) 790–792*p*
Voluntariness, in informed consent, (V1) 1180
Voluntary home health agencies, (V1) 1126–1127
Vomiting
opioid-related, (V) 807*b*
postoperative, (V1) 1050*t*
Von Bertalanffy, Ludwig, (V1) 148
Voodoo, (V1) 310, (V1) 312*f*
Vulnerable populations
characteristics of, (V1) 1116
as subcultures, (V1) 306–307, (V1) 306*f*
Vulva, (V1) 848
Vulvovaginitis, herpes, (V2) 315*f*

W

Waddling gait, (V1) 833, (V2) 315*f*
Wakefulness, (V1) 884*t*
brain activity during, (V1) 883
Walkers, (V1) 845, (V1) 846*f*
sizing of, (V2) 639
teaching for, (V2) 639
Walking, assistance for
conditioning exercises in, (V2) 638
critical aspects of, (V1) 842*p*, (V2) 632–634*p*
mechanical aids for, (V1) 845–846, (V2) 639–640
for older adults, (V1) 844–845
standing assist devices in, (V1) 843, (V1) 843*f*
transfer belt in, (V1) 843, (V1) 843*f*
Warts
genital, (V1) 863, (V2) 315*f*
plantar, (V1) 587
Waste
hazardous, safe disposal of, (V1) 568
solid, safe disposal of, (V1) 568
Water
bath, (V1) 583
as essential nutrient, (V1) 679
total body, (V1) 984, (V1) 984*t*
for wound care, (V1) 921
evidence-based studies of, (V1) 921
Water contamination, as safety hazard, (V1) 551–552
Water-soluble vitamins, (V1) 676
adult dietary reference intakes for, (V1) 674–676*t*
Waterborne pathogens, (V1) 551
Watson, Jean, (V1) 139, (V1) 139*f*
on health, (V1) 223*b*, (V1) 1096
nursing theory of, (V1) 146*t*
ten caring processes of, (V1) 140*b*
Watson's Science of Human Caring, (V1) 139
Wear-and-tear theory of aging, (V1) 205
Web conferencing, (V1) 1081
Web site, evaluation of, (V1) 1093*t*
Webcast, (V1) 1081
Weber test, (V1) 496, (V2) 248*p*
Webinar, (V1) 1081
Weighing, underwater, in body composition assessment, (V1) 694
Weight
assessment of, for fluid and electrolyte status, (V1) 1000
body water and, (V1) 984, (V1) 984*t*
fluid loss and, (V1) 993
loss of
dieting for, (V1) 687
tips for, (V1) 701–702*b*
pharmacokinetics and, (V1) 617
in physical examination, (V1) 488–489
standards for, (V1) 681–682
Wellness. *See also* Health; Health promotion
assessment of, in health promotion, (V1) 1099–1100
envisioning, in health promotion, (V1) 235
Wheel of, (V1) 1098–1099, (V1) 1099*f*
Wellness assessment, (V1) 50
Wellness diagnosis
intervention type related to, (V1) 110*t*
teaching for, (V1) 408
Wellness intervention, standardized language for, (V1) 116
Wellness nursing diagnosis, (V1) 66*t*
diagnostic statements for, (V1) 77
expected outcomes for, (V1) 99*t*
goals for, writing, (V1) 102
Wet-to-damp dressing, (V2) 682–685*p*
Wet-to-dry dressings, (V1) 923
Wheal, (V2) 231
Wheel of Wellness, (V1) 1098–1099, (V1) 1099*f*
Wheelchair, impaired mobility with, (V2) 834
Wheezes, (V1) 445, (V2) 265
Wheezing, (V1) 946
Whirlpool therapy, (V1) 923
Whispered pectoriloguy, (V1) 500, (V2) 264
Whistle-tipped suction catheter, (V1) 959, (V1) 959*f*
Whistleblowing, (V1) 1140–1141
White blood cells (WBCs)
count of, (V2) 767
transfusion of, (V1) 1020. *See also* Blood transfusion
types and function of, (V1) 525*t*
WHO three-step analgesic ladder, (V1) 804, (V1) 804*f*
Whole blood, (V1) 1020
Wiedenback, Ernestine, nursing theory of, (V1) 146*t*
Wikis, (V1) 1081
Will, living, (V1) 355, (V1) 1166, (V1) 1166*b*
Win-win resolution, (V1) 1072
Windshield survey, in community assessment, (V1) 1123
Wing-tipped catheter, (V1) 1005, (V1) 1005*f*, (V2) 785, (V2) 786
Wisdom, definition of, (V1) 1080
Withdrawal method, for family planning, (V2) 654
Witness, expert, (V1) 1174
Women, Infants, and Children (WIC), (V1) 697
Women's movement, influence of, on contemporary nursing practice, (V1) 26
Wong-Baker FACE Pain Rating Scale, (V2) 617
Worden, William, on grief, (V1) 347, (V1) 348*t*
Work
meaningful, (V1) 1066
in health-illness, (V1) 225
organization of, (V1) 1074–1075
streamlining of, (V1) 1075
Work environment
nutrition and, (V1) 685
stress management in, (V1) 261
Work redesign, in healthcare reform, (V1) 24
Work-related social groups, communication in, (V1) 472
Working phase, of therapeutic relationship, communication in, (V1) 470
Workplace
chemical dependence in, signs of, (V1) 1183*b*
hazardous substances of, (V1) 941
World Health Organization (WHO)
analgesia three-step ladder of, (V1) 804, (V1) 804*f*
health defined by, (V1) 18, (V1) 223*b*
on health promotion, (V1) 1096
surgical checklist of, (V1) 1042
World Wide Web, for nursing research, (V1) 1091–1092, (V1) 1093*t*
Wound(s), (V1) 901–933
acute, (V1) 902
appearance of, (V2) 710
asepsis for, (V1) 928
assessment of
diagnostic testing, (V2) 715
physical examination, (V2) 710
treated wounds, (V1) 913–915
untreated wounds, (V1) 916, (V2) 710
care of, in home care, (V1) 1134

chronic, (V1) 902, (V1) 903*t*, (V1) 907. *See also* Pressure ulcer(s)
clean, (V1) 902, (V1) 915*t*
clean-contaminated, (V1) 902
cleansing of
evidence-based studies of, (V1) 921
irrigation for, (V1) 921, (V2) 675–678
closed, (V1) 902
closures for, (V1) 905–906, (V2) 695–696*p*
contaminated, (V1) 901, (V1) 902
crepitus with, (V1) 914
critical thinking about, (V2) 718
crushing, (V1) 902*t*
culture of, (V1) 916
biopsy, (V1) 916, (V2) 715
needle aspiration, (V1) 916
swab, (V1) 916, (V1) 929*p*, (V2) 673–675*p*
depth of, (V1) 902
discoloration with, (V1) 910, (V1) 914
drain for
emptying of, (V1) 906, (V1) 931*p*, (V2) 706–707*p*
shortening of, (V1) 906, (V1) 931*p*, (V2) 705–706*p*
dressings for, (V1) 925–927. *See also* Dressing (wound)
epiboly of, (V1) 915
erythema with, (V1) 914
eschar of, (V1) 915, (V1) 915*t*
full-spectrum nursing and, (V2) 717–718
full-thickness, (V1) 902
granulation with, (V1) 903, (V1) 904*f*, (V1) 915*t*
healing of, (V1) 903–904
closures for, (V1) 905–906, (V2) 695–696*p*
complications of, (V1) 906–907
dehiscence and, (V1) 906–907, (V1) 907*f*
drainage for, (V1) 906
evisceration and, (V1) 907, (V1) 907*f*
fistula and, (V1) 907, (V1) 907*f*
granulation tissue in, (V1) 903, (V1) 904*f*, (V1) 915*t*
hemorrhage with, (V1) 906
infection and, (V1) 906
inflammatory phase of, (V1) 903–904, (V1) 905*f*
maturation phase, (V1) 904, (V1) 905*f*
phases of, (V1) 903–904, (V1) 905*f*
primary, (V1) 903, (V1) 904*f*
proliferative phase of, (V1) 904, (V1) 905*f*
regenerative/epithelial, (V1) 903, (V1) 904, (V1) 915*t*
secondary, (V1) 903, (V1) 904*f*
tertiary, (V1) 903, (V1) 904*f*
hemorrhage with, (V1) 906
hemostasis in, (V1) 903–904, (V1) 905*f*, (V1) 906
hyperbaric oxygen therapy for, (V1) 906, (V1) 920
incisional, (V1) 902*t*
infection of, (V1) 901, (V1) 902, (V1) 906
postoperative, (V1) 1051*t*
irrigation of, (V2) 675–678*p*
knowledge map for, (V2) 721
maceration of, (V1) 914
negative pressure therapy for, (V1) 930*p*, (V2) 685–690*p*
nonhealing of, (V1) 920
nursing diagnosis for, (V1) 917, (V2) 716–717
nursing interventions for, (V1) 917–933, (V2) 716–717
absorption dressings in, (V1) 925*t*
adjunctive therapies in, (V1) 919–920
alginate dressings in, (V1) 925*t*
antimicrobial dressings in, (V1) 925*t*
autolysis in, (V1) 923
bandages in, (V1) 928, (V1) 929, (V1) 931*p*, (V2) 699–703
barrier ointments in, (V1) 927*t*
binders in, (V1) 928–929, (V2) 697–699*p*
biotherapeutic debridement in, (V1) 923
cleansing in, (V1) 920–921
cold therapy in, (V1) 931–933, (V2) 709
collagen dressings in, (V1) 925*t*
debridement in, (V1) 922–923
drainage devices and, (V1) 921–922, (V2) 706–707*p*
dressing in, (V1) 923, (V1) 925–927*t*, (V1) 928. *See also* Dressing (wound)
enzymatic debridement in, (V1) 923
foam dressings in, (V1) 925*t*
gauze dressings in, (V1) 925*t*
heat therapy in, (V1) 931–932, (V2) 708
hydrocolloid dressings in, (V1) 925–926*t*, (V2) 693–694*p*
hydrogel dressings in, (V1) 927*t*, (V2) 693–694*p*
hydrotherapeutic debridement in, (V1) 923
infection control in, (V1) 924, (V1) 925
irrigation in, (V1) 921, (V1) 929*p*, (V2) 675–678*p*
maggot debridement in, (V1) 923
mechanical debridement in, (V1) 923
moisture provision in, (V1) 923–924, (V2) 708
sealant dressings in, (V1) 927*t*
sharp debridement in, (V1) 923, (V1) 928
tips for, (V1) 920
transparent film dressings in, (V1) 927*t*, (V1) 928*f*, (V1) 930*p*, (V2) 690–692*p*
nursing outcomes for, (V1) 917, (V2) 716–717
nutritional status and, (V1) 915
open, (V1) 902
pain with, (V1) 915
partial-thickness, (V1) 902
penetrating, (V1) 902, (V1) 902*t*
physical examination of, (V1) 710
platelet-derived growth factor for, (V1) 906
puncture, (V1) 902*t*
regenerative/epithelial healing of, (V1) 903, (V1) 904, (V1) 915*t*
size of, (V1) 914
slough with, (V1) 915, (V1) 915*t*
soak for, (V2) 708, (V2) 709
superficial, (V1) 902
surgical, (V1) 1028
dehiscence of, (V1) 1051*t*
evisceration of, (V1) 1051*t*
infection of, (V1) 1028, (V1) 1029*t*, (V1) 1046
surgical closure of, (V1) 905–906
surgical risk and, (V1) 1028, (V1) 1029*t*
swelling with, (V1) 914
tissues of, (V1) 915, (V1) 915*t*
tunnel, (V1) 902*t*, (V1) 914
types of, (V1) 902, (V1) 902*t*, (V1) 914
undermining in, (V1) 914
Wrist
range of motion in, (V2) 644
splint for, (V1) 837
Writing, journal, for pain, (V1) 804
Written prescriptions, (V1) 624
Wrong patient, wrong site, wrong surgery check, (V1) 1038
Wruble, J., nursing theory of, (V1) 146*t*

X

X-ray, abdominal flat plate, (V2) 595
Xerosis, (V1) 899
Xerostomia, impaired taste from, (V1) 778

Y

Yankauer suction tube, (V1) 959, (V1) 959*f*
Yeast, urinary, (V2) 563

Yoga, evidence-based studies of, (V1) 975
Young adult(s), (V1) 194–196
applying full-spectrum nursing model to, (V2) 68–69
assessment of, (V1) 196
cardiovascular system in, (V1) 972
development of
cognitive, (V1) 195
physical, (V1) 194–195
psychosexual, (V1) 167*t*
psychosocial, (V1) 168–169, (V1) 195
developmental tasks of, (V1) 166*t*
health problems of, (V1) 195–196
health promotion for, (V1) 1101*t*
interventions for, (V1) 196
intimate partner abuse, neglect, and violence among, (V1) 195–196
obesity in, (V1) 196
physical examination of, (V1) 487
sexuality of, (V1) 854
sexually transmitted infections in, (V1) 195
sleep for, (V1) 881, (V1) 881*t*, (V1) 885
stressors of, (V1) 242*b*
substance abuse and violence among, (V1) 195
surgery and, (V1) 1028
YouTube, (V1) 1081

Z

Z-stroke technique, (V2) 674
Z-track technique, for intramuscular injection, (V1) 651, (V2) 455–456*p*
Zinc, (V1) 678*t*
in ovo-lacto vegetarian diet, (V1) 686
skin and, (V1) 899

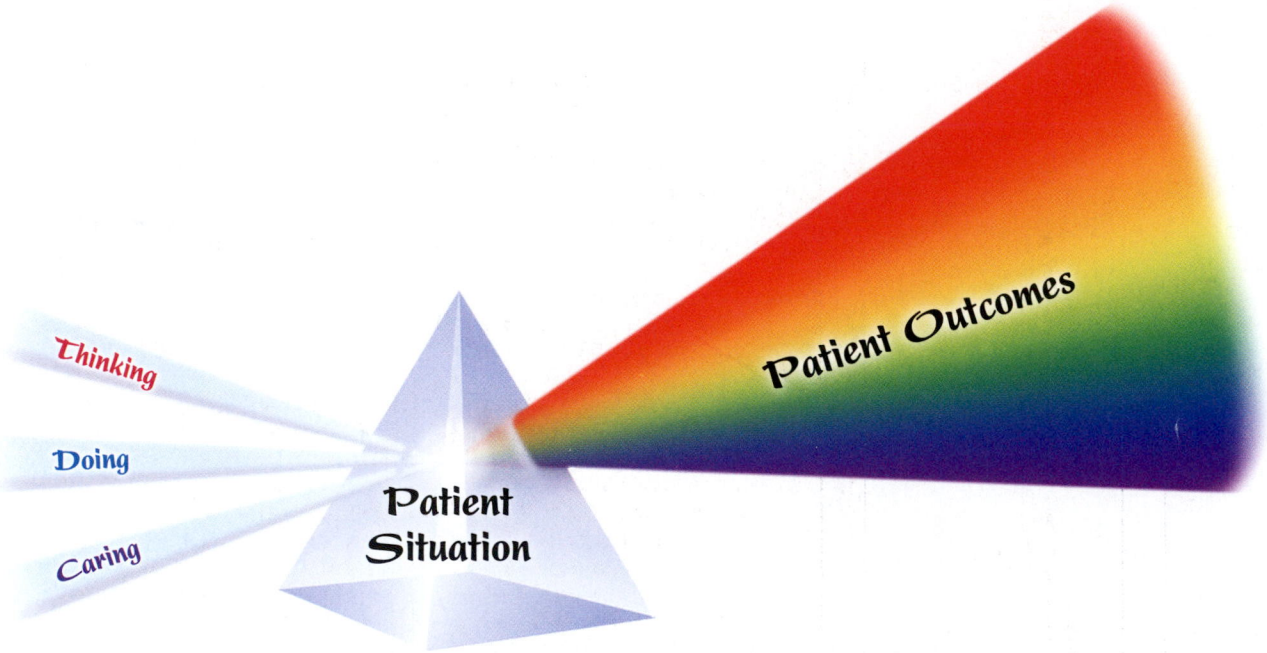

This illustration depicts the full-spectrum model of nursing used throughout this learning package. A full-spectrum nurse uses critical thinking and the nursing process to apply various types of knowledge (theoretical, practical, ethical, and self-knowledge) to the patient situation to bring about desired health outcomes. Truly, thinking and doing.